The Clinical Chemistry of Laboratory Animals

Third Edition

The Clinical Chemistry of Laboratory Animals

Third Edition

Edited by:

David M. Kurtz and Gregory S. Travlos

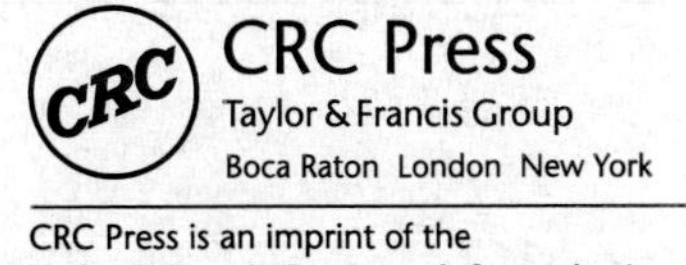

CRC Press is an imprint of the
Taylor & Francis Group, an **informa** business

Book Cover by:

David A. Sabio
Experimental Pathology Laboratories, Inc.
Research Triangle Park, NC

CRC Press
Taylor & Francis Group
6000 Broken Sound Parkway NW, Suite 300
Boca Raton, FL 33487-2742

First issued in paperback 2020

ISBN 13: 978-0-367-57035-4 (pbk)
ISBN 13: 978-1-4200-9113-7 (hbk)

Library of Congress Cataloging-in-Publication Data

Names: Kurtz, David M., editor. | Travlos, Gregory S., editor.
Title: Clinical chemistry of laboratory animals / [edited by] David M. Kurtz and Gregory S. Travlos.
Description: Third edition. | Boca Raton : Taylor & Francis, 2017. | Includes
bibliographical references and index.
Identifiers: LCCN 2016055474 | ISBN 9781420091137 (hardback : alk. paper)
Subjects: | MESH: Animals, Laboratory--metabolism | Clinical Chemistry
Tests--methods
Classification: LCC SF996.5 | NLM QY 50 | DDC 636.088/5--dc23
LC record available at https://lccn.loc.gov/2016055474

Visit the Taylor & Francis Web site at
http://www.taylorandfrancis.com

and the CRC Press Web site at
http://www.crcpress.com

Dedication

To Cat

To Kim, Hannah and Kyle

To Judith S. Prescott

To Our Authors

Contents

List of Contributors

Kirstin F. Barnhart, DVM, PhD, DACVP
MD Anderson Cancer Center
University of Texas
Houston, Texas

Susan J. Borghoff, PhD, DABT
ToxStrategies, Inc.
Cary, North Carolina

Guy F. Bouchard, DVM, MS, DACT
Sinclair Research Center, LLC
Auxvasse, Missouri

Denise Bounous, DVM, PhD, DACVP
Bristol-Myers Squibb Co.
Princeton, New Jersey

Larry D. Brown, DVM, PhD, DACVPM
Sinclair Research Center, LLC
Auxvasse, Missouri

Stan W. Casteel, DVM, PhD, Dipl. ABVT
University of Missouri
Columbia, Missouri

Charles B. Clifford, DVM, PhD, DACVP
Charles River Laboratories, Inc. (Retired)
Willmington, Massachusetts

Lesley A. Colby, DVM, MS, DACLAM
University of Washington
Seattle, Washington

Ralph L. Cooper, PhD
U.S. Environmental Protection Agency (Retired)
Research Triangle Park, North Carolina

Tara Cotroneo, DVM, DACLAM
Wayne State University
Detroit, Michigan

Lori K. Davis, PhD
Impact Pharmaceutical Services
Research Triangle Park, North Carolina

Carolina Escobar, DVM
ESA Diagnóstico
HQ Diagnostc, Santiago, Chile

Nancy E. Everds DVM, DACVP
Seattle Genetics, Inc.
Seattle, Washington

Andrea J. Fascetti, VMD, PhD, DACVIM
College of Veterinary Medicine
University of California
Davis, California

Craig A. Fletcher, DVM, PhD, DACLAM
University of North Carolina
Chapel Hill, North Carolina

James G. Fox, DVM, MS, DACLAM
Massachusetts Institute of Technology
Cambridge, Massachusetts

Jerome M. Goldman, PhD
U.S. Environmental Protection Agency (Retired)
Research Triangle Park, North Carolina

Carol B. Grindem, DVM, PhD, DACVP
College of Veterinary Medicine
North Carolina State University
Raleigh, North Carolina

Anna Hampton, DVM, DACLAM, DACAW, CPIA
Duke University
Durham, North Carolina

Claudia Harper, DVM, DACLAM
Cambridge, MA

Ernie Harpur, BSc, PhD, FATS, FBTS, FRSB
Newcastle University
Newcastle upon Tyne NE2 4HH, UK

Holly L. Jordan DVM, PhD, DACVP
Covance Laboratories, Inc.
Madison, Wisconsin

Grace E. Kissling, PhD
National Institute for Environmental Health Science
Research Triangle Park, North Carolina

Jennifer A. Larson, MS, DVM, PhD
College of Veterinary Medicine
University of California
Davis, California

Isabel A. Lea, PhD
Integrated Laboratory Systems, Inc.
Durham, North Carolina

Bruce E. LeRoy, DVM, PhD, DACVP
AbbVie, Inc.
Abbott Park, Illinois

Dana N. LeVine, DVM, PhD, DACVIM
College of Veterinary Medicine
Iowa State University
Ames, Iowa

Richard H. Luong, BVSc, DACVP
Stanford University
Stanford, California
and IDEXX Laboratories, Inc.
Westbrook, Maine

Owen P. McGuiness, PhD
Vanderbilt University School of Medicine
Nashville, Tennessee

Jennifer A. Neel, DVM, DACVP
College of Veterinary Medicine
North Carolina State University
Raleigh, North Carolina

Peter O'Brien, DVM, PhD, DVSC, DACVP, DECVP, FRCPath
School of Veterinary Medicine
University College Dublin
Belfield 4, Dublin, Ireland

Claire Louise Parry PhD, MSc, BSc. (Hons), CBiol MSB, FIBMS
AstraZeneca, Inc.
Cheshire, UK

Mary M. Patterson, MS, DVM, DACLAM
Massachusetts Institute of Technology
Cambridge, Massachusetts

Lila Ramaiah, DVM, PhD, DACVP
Bristol-Myers Squibb Co.
New Brunswick, New Jersey

Allison R. Rogala, DVM, DACLAM
University of North Carolina
Chapel Hill, North Carolina

Robert B. Rucker, MS, PhD
University of California
Davis, California

Patrick Sharp, DVM, DACLAM
National University of Singapore
Republic of Singapore

Masakasu Shiota, PhD, DVM
Vanderbilt University School of Medicine
Nashville, Tennessee

Joe H. Simmons, MS, DVM, PhD, DACLAM
MD Anderson Cancer Center
University of Texas
Houston, Texas

Alain Stricker-Krongrad, PhD, MSc
Sinclair Research Center, LLC
Auxvasse, Missouri

M. Michael Swindle, DVM, DACLAM
Medical University of South Carolina
Charleston, South Carolina

Lindsay Tomlinson, DVM, DVSc, DACVP, DABT
Pfizer, Inc.
Cambridge, Massachusetts

Gregory S. Travlos, DVM, DACVP
National Institute of Environmental Health Science (NIEHS)
Research Triangle Park, North Carolina

Barbara von Beust, Dr. Med. Vet., PhD, DACVP, DECVCP
Independent Consultant Winterthur, Zurich

Dana Walker, DVM, MS, PhD, DACVP
Novartis Institute of Biomedial Research (NIBR)
Cambridge, Massachusetts

Julia Whitaker, MS, DVM, DACLAM
University of North Carolina
Chapel Hill, North Carolina

Charles E. Wiedmeyer, DVM, PhD, DACVP
College of Veterinary Medicine
University of Missouri
Columbia, Missouri

List of Reviewers

Glen Almond, DVM, Msc, PhD
College of Veterinary Medicine
North Carolina State University
Raleigh, North Carolina

Jill Ascher, MA, DVM, MPH, DACLAM
Marshall BioResources
North Rose, New York

Adam Aulbach, DVM, DACVP
MPI Research
Mattawan, Michigan

Beth A. Bauer, DVM, DACLAM
IDEXX BioResearch, Inc.
Columbia, MO

J. David Becherer, PhD
Viamet Pharmaceuticals, Inc.
Durham, NC

Cory Brayton, DVM, DACLAM, DACVP
School of Medicine
Johns Hopkins University
Baltimore, MD

Kathleen K. Brown, DVM, PhD, DACVIM
GlaxoSmithKline
Research Triangle Park, NC

Roger D. Cox, PhD
MRC Harwell
Oxford, UK

Daniela Ennulat, DVM, PhD, DACVP
GlaxoSmithKline
King of Prussia, PA

Ellen W. Evans, DVM, PhD, DACVP
Pfizer, Inc.
Groton, CT

James R. Fahey, MS, PhD, DVM
The Jackson Laboratory
Bar Harbor, ME

Richard E. Fish, DVM, PhD, DACLAM
College of Veterinary Medicine
North Carolina State University
Raleigh, NC

Kendall Frazier, DVM, PhD, DACVP, DABT, FIATP
GlaxoSmithKline
King of Prussia, PA

Robert L. Hall, DVM, PhD, DAVCP
Covance Laboratories, Inc.
Madison, WI

Claire Hankenson, DVM, DACLAM
Michigan State University
East Lansing, MI

K.C. Hayes, DVM, PhD
Brandeis University
Waltham, MA

Kristin Henson, DVM, MS, DACVP
Novartis Pharmaceuticals Corporation
East Hanover, NJ

Armando R. Irizarry Rovira, DVM, PhD, DACVP
Eli Lilly and Company
Cumberland, IN

Christopher Jerome, BVetMed, PhD
Wake Forest Innovations
Center for Industry Research Collaborations
Winston Salem, NC

Michael L. Kent, MS, PhD
Oregon State University
Corvallis, OR

Urmila P. Kodavanti, PhD, DABT
U.S. Environmental Protection Agency
Research Triangle Park, NC

Kenneth S. Latimer, DVM, PhD, DACVP
College of Veterinary Medicine
University of Georgia
Athens, GA

Casey J. LeBlanc, DVM, PhD, DACVP
College of Veterinary Medicine
University of Tennessee
Knoxville, TN

Michelle Leland, DVM, DACLAM
University of Texas Health Sciences Center
San Antonio, TX

Kristie Mozzachio, DVM, DACVP
Mozzachio Mobile Veterinary Services
Hillsborough, NC

Doug Neptun, PhD, Bsc
Antech Diagnostics GLP (Retired)
Durham, NC

Jack Oliver, BS, MS, DVM, PhD
College of Veterinary Medicine
University of Tennessee
Knoxville, TN

Glen Otto, DVM, DACLAM
University of Texas
Austin, TX

Vincent Poitout, DVM, PhD
University of Montréal
Montréal, QC

Kathleen Pritchett-Corning, DVM, DACLAM, MRCVS
Harvard University
Cambridge, MA

George E. Sanders, DVM, MS
University of Washington School of Medicine
Seattle, WA

Eric Schultze, DVM, PhD, DACVP
Eli Lilly and Company
Cumberland, IN

Elizabeth Skuba, DVM, MVSc,
Novartis Institutes for Biomedial Research (NIBR)
East Hanover, NJ

Steven A. Smith, MS, DVM, PhD
Virginia Polytechnic Institute and State University
Blacksburg, VA

Philip F. Solter, DVM, PhD, DACVP DACVIM
College of Veterinary Medicine
University of Illinois
Urbana, IL

Dinesh Stanislaus, PhD
GlaxoSmithKline
King of Prussia, PA

Stephen A. Stimpson, PhD
GlaxoSmithKline

Mark A. Suckow, BS, DVM, DACLAM
University of Minnesota
Minneapolis, MN

Mike Talcott, DVM, DACLAM
Washington University School of Medicine
St. Louis, MO

Douglas K. Taylor, DVM, DACLAM
Emory University
Atlanta, GA

Patricia V. Turner, BSc, MS, DVM, DVSc, DACLAM, DABT
Ontario Veterinary College
University of Guelph
Guelph, ON

Dana Walker, DVM, MS, PhD, DACVP
Novartis Institute of Biomedial Research (NIBR)
Cambridge, MA

Ida Washington, DVM, DACLAM
Magee-Women's Research Institute
Pittsburgh, PA

Janet Welter, DVM, MPH, PHD, DACLAM
University of Wisconsin
Madison, Wisconsin

Philip A. Wood, DVM, PhD
Sanford|Burnham Medical Research Institute
Orlando, FL

1 The Laboratory Mouse

Richard H. Luong

CONTENTS

1.1 INTRODUCTION

The origin of the laboratory mouse lies in pet mice bred by mouse fanciers in Europe throughout the 1800s. These "fancy mice" in turn, were derived from several wild Asian mice species that were selected and mated for desirable traits in Asia before the seventeenth century. Although not appreciated initially, several desirable traits of these so-called "fancy-mice" were genetic in origin. In the early 1900s, biologists conducted Mendelian genetic experiments with fancy-mice (Rader, 2004; Paigen, 2003a). By 1909, the first inbred strain, the *dba* (DBA/2) mouse, was created by selecting for homozygosity of three recessive coat color alleles: *d* dilute, *b* brown, *a* nonagouti (Paigen, 2003a). By the 1970s, more than 250 strains of inbred mice had been created and used extensively in various fields of biomedical research, including cancer, biology, immunology, and genetics. Their use has expanded further with the advent of transgenic technologies in the 1980s (Paigen, 2003a). Outbred mice, especially the "Swiss" stocks, also have been extensively used for diverse research applications.

Practical and scientific advantages of mice in research include small size, ease of handling, low housing costs, short generation time, fecundity, short time to maturation, genetically homogenous populations (inbred strains) with well-defined traits, 95% genetic homology with humans, and genetic and phenotypic disease homologies between mice and humans (Paigen, 2003b).

Currently, more than 450 major inbred mouse strains and 13,000 unique strains of genetically engineered mice are available for research (National Center for Research Resources, 2004), and mouse gene knockout initiatives ongoing in several countries can be anticipated to increase the numbers further. However, common strains and stocks will be emphasized in this chapter. Further, online resources and information on inbred and genetically engineered mice (and their use as models for disease) not mentioned in this chapter are available to the biomedical researcher, including (but not limited to) the following:

- Mouse Phenome Database (The Jackson Laboratory, Bar Harbor, ME; http://phenome.jax.org/)
- Mouse Genome Informatics (The Jackson Laboratory, Bar Harbor, ME; http://www.informatics.jax.org/
- Knockout Mouse Project (http://www.knockoutmouse.org/)
- Mutant Mouse Regional Resource Centers (MMRRC Informatics, Coordination and Service Center, Bar Harbor, ME; http://www.mmrrc.org/)
- National Toxicology Program (http://ntp.niehs.nih.gov/)
- Europhenome Mouse Phenotyping Resource (http://www.europhenome.org/databrowser/viewer.jsp)
- Charles River Laboratories (http://www.criver.com/find-a-model)

There are many indications for performing clinical chemistry (along with other clinical and anatomic pathology testing) in laboratory mice. First, clinical chemistry may help with the characterization or validation of a disease and/or disease model in mice. Second, clinical chemistry is a critical component during phenotypic assessment of genetically engineered mice and new strains of inbred mice. Finally, clinical chemistry is strongly recommended for nonclinical toxicity and safety studies, and in fact, may be mandated by Federal Drug Administration (FDA) or other regulatory bodies (Weingand et al., 1992).

Clinical chemistry capabilities applicable to laboratory mice have expanded recently from about 20 tests on serum, plasma, and urine, to hundreds of biomarkers that can be quantified in increasingly smaller specimen sample sizes. Certainly, these assays will increase in significance and utility in the foreseeable future. However, the aim of this chapter is to provide information and resources regarding the more traditional bioanalytes assessed in the laboratory mouse.

1.2 UNIQUE PHYSIOLOGICAL CHARACTERISTICS OF THE LABORATORY MOUSE

The main physiological characteristic of laboratory mice relevant to clinical chemistry is their size, which in turn affects the sample volume, sampling frequency, and sample collection of both blood and urine, and potentially limits the number of bioanalytes that can be analyzed per sample and over time.

The metabolism of mice is also relatively high (961 kJ/kg bodyweight), compared to other larger mammalian research species (Terpstra, 2001). Their high metabolism and nocturnal feeding makes *ad libitum* access to food and water, the preferred method for mice. Most mouse activity (e.g., eating, drinking, and locomotion) occurs during darkness, even among blind mice that completely lack photoreceptors (Foster et al., 1991; Foster and Hankins, 2002). Circadian and ultradian variations in some blood and urine bioanalytes (e.g., glucose, lactate, lipids, and proteins) have been identified (discussed further in the following section). Thus, time of day should be considered when scheduling blood collections. In general, nonfasting levels of bioanalytes are routinely used for the assessment of blood and urine of laboratory mice. Depending on study requirements, withholding food for 4–18 hours has been recommended for the examination of fasting levels of certain bioanalytes (e.g., glucose, triglycerides, nonesterified fatty acids, total cholesterol, and insulin; Clapham et al., 2000). Regarding animal health and welfare, it must be stressed, however, that withholding food or water from mice for more than 18 hours is not advisable. Indeed, approval from Institutional Animal Care and Use Committee (IACUC) or Ethics Committees is usually required to pursue studies involving food and water deprivation or restriction.

Corticosterone is the predominant circulating glucocorticoid in laboratory mice (Spackman and Riley, 1978). It is their primary glucocorticoid regulator of carbohydrate, protein, and fat metabolism and modifies the host response to stress and immune response. In contrast, the main role of corticosterone in humans is as an intermediate metabolite in aldosterone biosynthesis, with corticosterone having only weak glucocorticoid and mineralocorticoid activity.

Lipid metabolism in laboratory mice has some significant differences compared to that of humans. In contrast to humans, laboratory mice carry most of their cholesterol as high-density lipoproteins (HDL), and lack cholesteryl ester transfer protein (CETP), which in other species (e.g., humans), is responsible for exchange of triglycerides for cholesteryl esters from very-low-density lipoproteins (VLDL) and low-density lipoproteins (LDL) to HDL, and vice versa (Lusis, 2000; Fernandez and Volek, 2006). Similar to humans, mice synthesize B apolipoproteins (apoB-100 and apoB-48) in the liver and small intestine; they are essential components for the transport of lipids in plasma. Both apoB-100 and apoB-48 are derived from a common structural gene, and apoB-48 results from an enzymatic editing of a single codon of the apoB mRNA. In mammals, due to the abundance of apolipoprotein B mRNA editing enzyme gene expression in the small intestine, effectively all B apolipoproteins produced at this location is apoB-48 (essential for production of chylomicrons). In humans, the liver is missing apolipoprotein B mRNA editing enzyme, and only apoB-100 is produced (needed for hepatic production of VLDL). In murine liver, however, there is a significant editing of apoB mRNA transcripts; thus, hepatic secretion of both apoB-100 and apoB-48 occurs. The reader is referred to the review of Kim and Young (1998) for more detail regarding mouse B apolipoproteins.

Bile acid metabolism in laboratory mice and humans also differ. Bile acids consist of a heterogeneous group of structurally different, hepatic-derived molecules that are the metabolic breakdown products of cholesterol. In humans, the primary bile acids are cholic acid (CA), chenodeoxycholic acid (CDCA), deoxycholic acid (DCA), and lithocholic acid (LCA), along with their glycine and taurine conjugates (Argmann et al., 2006b). However, in mice, the primary bile acids are CA and CDCA-derived muricholic acid (MCA), along with their taurine conjugates but a virtual absence of glycine bile acid conjugates.

1.3 METHODOLOGY FOR SAMPLE COLLECTION

1.3.1 Blood Collection

1.3.1.1 Collection Volume Limits and Frequency of Collection

Blood collection is the most common experimental procedure performed in the laboratory mouse, and often an essential component of most biomedical research. However, the major limiting factor in blood collection in the laboratory mouse is their size, which limits the total amount of blood that can be collected, as well as the frequency at which the blood is collected. Diehl et al. (2001) and Donovan and Brown (2005) provide good reviews of the amount of blood and the frequency of collection that can be obtained from live, healthy adult mice.

The circulating blood volume in a healthy, adult mouse is approximately 63–80 mL/kg (average 72 mL/kg). For single sampling purposes, not more than 15% of circulating blood volume can be sampled at any one time (allowing for a 4-week postcollection rest period) without any long-term adverse effects on health and physiology (such as hypovolemic shock and anemia) and allowing for adequate tissue repair at the site of collection (Diehl et al., 2001; Donovan and Brown, 2005). Additionally, not more than 20% of circulating blood volume can be removed over 24-hour period without any lasting adverse health and pathophysiologic effects, as well as effects on the concentration of bioanalytes and/or half-life other biomarkers being examined (allowing for a 3-week postcollection rest period) (Diehl et al., 2001; Donovan and Brown, 2005). Table 1.1 provides a summary of the circulating blood volume of healthy adult laboratory mice of different weights. Table 1.2 outlines the recommended maximum blood sample volume limits (as a percentage of circulating blood volume) and postcollection recovery periods in healthy adult laboratory mice, based on sampling frequency over a 24-hour period. Table 1.3 details the recommended maximum blood sample volumes from healthy adult mice of different weights, based on the blood sample volume limits presented in Table 1.2. Repeated blood sampling, especially over a short period of time (e.g., 24 hours) can result in alterations in the concentration of certain bioanalytes. While the volumes described above and in Table 1.2 list the maximum acceptable volumes published in the literature, individuals should check with their IACUC or Ethics Committee on limits to survival blood collection.

The limits that the size of laboratory mice has on blood volume collection can be somewhat overcome by collecting terminal blood samples (Donovan and Brown, 2005). At least half (50%) of the circulating blood volume can be obtained terminally via cardiocentesis (often termed cardiac puncture) by a trained individual (technique discussed in the following section), which is summarized in Table 1.3.

There are several factors, however, that must be considered when deciding how much blood should be collected for clinical chemistry from a live laboratory mouse, given the overall low blood volume collection limits. First, most bioanalytes and biomarkers are performed on serum or plasma samples. Given that the normal hematocrit of the laboratory mouse has a conservative reference range of 35%–50%, the serum or plasma collection limit may be a little as 50% and at the most 65% of the total blood volume collected in the healthy adult mouse. Second, blood is often collected from a single mouse for competing purposes beyond clinical chemistry, such as hematology, serology, immunology, and pharmacotoxicology. For example, Table 1.4 summarizes the volume of serum or plasma that is required to run certain clinical chemistry bioanalytes using a Siemens (Dade Behring) Xpand Integrated Chemistry System (Deerfield, Illinois) at the Diagnostic Laboratory of the Veterinary Services Center at Stanford University, Stanford, California (please note that these values are specific for this analyzing system and therefore may differ from other analyzing systems

TABLE 1.1
Summary of the Circulating Blood Volume of Healthy Adult Laboratory Mice of Different Weights

	Circulating Blood Volume (mL)		
Weight (g)	**Minimum**	**Mean**	**Maximum**
10	0.63	0.72	0.80
11	0.69	0.79	0.88
12	0.76	0.86	0.96
13	0.82	0.94	1.04
14	0.88	1.01	1.12
15	0.95	1.08	1.20
16	1.01	1.15	1.28
17	1.07	1.22	1.36
18	1.13	1.30	1.44
19	1.20	1.37	1.52
20	1.26	1.44	1.60
21	1.32	1.51	1.68
22	1.39	1.58	1.76
23	1.45	1.66	1.84
24	1.51	1.73	1.92
25	1.58	1.80	2.00
26	1.64	1.87	2.08
27	1.70	1.94	2.16
28	1.76	2.02	2.24
29	1.83	2.09	2.32
30	1.89	2.16	2.40
31	1.95	2.23	2.48
32	2.02	2.30	2.56
33	2.08	2.38	2.64
34	2.14	2.45	2.72
35	2.21	2.52	2.80
36	2.27	2.59	2.88
37	2.33	2.66	2.96
38	2.39	2.74	3.04
39	2.46	2.81	3.12
40	2.52	2.88	3.20

Source: Diehl, K.H. et al.: A good practice guide to the administration of substances and removal of blood, including routes and volumes. *J Appl Toxicol.* 2001. 21. 20. Copyright Wiley-VCH Verlag GmbH & Co. KGaA. Reprinted with permission.

in other reference laboratories; please check with the reference laboratory that will be used to obtain more specific information regarding the exact amounts of serum or plasma amounts required for their analyzing systems). A quick perusal of this reveals that a significant amount of serum (and therefore the amount of whole blood) that is required just for clinical chemistry purposes only. Third, the amount of actual serum required is greatly influenced by laboratory equipment and procedural methodology. For example, smaller amounts of serum are required for clinical chemistry analyzers that are based on microfluorescent immunoassays (MFIAs) technologies. Conversely, all chemistry analyzers require slightly more serum than required for proper bioanalyte analysis due to the issue of dead volume, which is the amount of serum that is not recoverable due to handling and processing

TABLE 1.2
Recommended Maximum Blood Sample Volume Limits (As a Percentage of Circulating Blood Volume) and Post-Collection Recovery Periods in Healthy Adult Laboratory Mice, Based on Sampling Frequency within a 24-h Period

Sampling Frequency within 24 Hours	Blood Sample Volume Limits (% of Circulating Blood Volume)	Approximate Recovery Period
Single (e.g., toxicity study)	7.5%	1 week
	10%	2 weeks
	15%	4 weeks
Multiple (e.g., toxicokinetic study)	7.5%	1 week
	10%–15%	2 weeks
	20%	3 weeks

Source: Diehl, K.H. et al.: A good practice guide to the administration of substances and removal of blood, including routes and volumes. *J Appl Toxicol.* 2001. 21. 20. Copyright Wiley-VCH Verlag GmbH & Co. KGaA. Reprinted with permission.

(in container reservoirs such as pipettes, serum tubes, and wells). Additionally, the amount of serum required might be increased if repeated testing or re-validation is required for any particular sample. Fourth, blood is often collected from mice with disease, and the disease state in turn may decrease the total circulating blood volume (e.g., via dehydration). Finally, the site of blood collection may influence the amount of blood that can be collected (discussed in the following section). All of these factors may therefore decrease blood volume available (or conversely, increase the blood volume that must be collected) for clinical chemistry. Therefore, the biomedical researcher wishing to perform clinical chemistry on laboratory mice must plan ahead to optimize the blood collection volume required, based on the factors just discussed. For example, the researcher might have to limit the number of bioanalytes that are assessed when dealing with smaller mice or diseased mice, or with mice that require simultaneous analysis of certain bioanalytes and other tests (such as serology).

1.3.1.2 Primary Sites for Collection and Restraint

There are four primary sites for routine blood collection in the adult laboratory mouse: the retro-orbital sinus, the tail vein, the superficial temporal vein (often called the submandibular or facial vein), and cardiocentesis (Argmann and Auwerx, 2006a; Diehl et al., 2001; Donovan and Brown, 2005). The choice of which blood collection site to be used will depend on the quantity of blood required, the frequency of blood collection, animal welfare and/or protocol restrictions, and (in this author's experience) the skill of collector. Most sites require some sort of physical and/or anesthetic restraint. Table 1.5 provides a summary of these four sites, whereas Tables 1.6 and 1.7 provide an outline of recommended injectable and inhalational anesthetic agents, respectively, that can be used for blood collection. Investigations into other blood collections sites (such as saphenous vein, tail clip, tail vein cut) have been recently described (Abaton et al., 2008; Argmann and Auwerx, 2006a), but these have not been reviewed here.

Regardless of the bleeding site and general anesthetic used, the author strongly recommends that individuals seek training in collection techniques and proper anesthesia from experienced laboratory animal care and technical staff, as to minimize any adverse effects on the welfare and health of the mice used for bleeding. Indeed, at some institutions, mandatory training for bleeding and anesthesia of laboratory mice might be a regulatory requirement, so consultation with animal care and technical staff is advised in any case. Additionally, regardless of site used, aseptic technique should be used. For survival procedures, the animal should also be assessed for adequate hemostasis, 30–60 minutes after blood collection (Donovan and Brown, 2005). Finally, the use of anticoagulants should be considered when plasma is required, with the choice of anticoagulant based on the clinical chemistry bioanalytes being performed (see the following section).

TABLE 1.3
Recommended Maximum Blood Sample Volumes from Healthy Adult Mice of Different Weights, Based on the Blood Sample Volume Limits Presented in Table 1.2

	Maximum Blood Sample Volumes (mL), Based on Percentage Blood Collection Volume Limits				
	Live Mouse				Euthanized Mouse
Weight (g)	7.5%	10.0%	15.0%	20.0%	50.0%
10	0.05	0.07	0.11	0.14	0.36
11	0.06	0.08	0.12	0.16	0.40
12	0.06	0.09	0.13	0.17	0.43
13	0.07	0.09	0.14	0.19	0.47
14	0.08	0.10	0.15	0.20	0.50
15	0.08	0.11	0.16	0.22	0.54
16	0.09	0.12	0.17	0.23	0.58
17	0.09	0.12	0.18	0.24	0.61
18	0.10	0.13	0.19	0.26	0.65
19	0.10	0.14	0.21	0.27	0.68
20	0.11	0.14	0.22	0.29	0.72
21	0.11	0.15	0.23	0.30	0.76
22	0.12	0.16	0.24	0.32	0.79
23	0.12	0.17	0.25	0.33	0.83
24	0.13	0.17	0.26	0.35	0.86
25	0.14	0.18	0.27	0.36	0.90
26	0.14	0.19	0.28	0.37	0.94
27	0.15	0.19	0.29	0.39	0.97
28	0.15	0.20	0.30	0.40	1.01
29	0.16	0.21	0.31	0.42	1.04
30	0.16	0.22	0.32	0.43	1.08
31	0.17	0.22	0.33	0.45	1.12
32	0.17	0.23	0.35	0.46	1.15
33	0.18	0.24	0.36	0.48	1.19
34	0.18	0.24	0.37	0.49	1.22
35	0.19	0.25	0.38	0.50	1.26
36	0.19	0.26	0.39	0.52	1.30
37	0.20	0.27	0.40	0.53	1.33
38	0.21	0.27	0.41	0.55	1.37
39	0.21	0.28	0.42	0.56	1.40
40	0.22	0.29	0.43	0.58	1.44

Source: Diehl, K.H. et al.: A good practice guide to the administration of substances and removal of blood, including routes and volumes. *J Appl Toxicol.* 2001. 21. 19. Copyright Wiley-VCH Verlag GmbH & Co. KGaA. Reprinted with permission.

Total serum or plasma yield is expected to be not more than 50%-65% of these values.

Blood collection from a newborn mouse is much more challenging, but can be accomplished by administrating two units of heparin subcutaneously before decapitation (Loeb, 1998). Subsequently, up 40 μL of blood (approximately 20 μL of plasma) can then be collected from the decapitation site. However, blood collected by decapitation is subject to contamination (e.g., with particulate matter, cerebrospinal fluid (CSF) fluid, ingesta, and infectious agents), which may interfere with or invalidate any bioanalyte results acquired.

TABLE 1.4
Minimum Volume of Serum or Plasma Required for Individual Clinical Chemistry Bioanalytes Using a Siemens (Dade Behring) Xpand Integrated Chemistry System (Deerfield, Illinois) at the Diagnostic Laboratory of the Veterinary Services Center at Stanford University, Stanford, CA

Bioanalyte	Sample Volume (μL)—Plasma or Serum
Dead volume	30
Albumin	5
Alkaline phosphatase	7
Amylase	14
Alanine aminotransferase	35
Aspartate aminotransferase	40
Blood urea nitrogen	3
Calcium	5
Cholesterol	3
Creatine kinase (total)	14
Creatine kinase—MB	14
Creatinine	20
Bilirubin (total)	28
Bilirubin (direct)	31
CO_2 (enzymatic)	5
Electrolytes (sodium, potassium, chloride)	10
Glucose	3
Gamma-glutamyl transpeptidase	32
High-density lipoprotein	3
Hemoglobin (A1C)	3
Immunoglobulin (indirect)	Calculation (total protein – albumin)
Iron (total)	50
Iron (binding capacity)	25
Lactate	4
Lactate dehydrogenase	14
Low-density lipoprotein	3
Lipase	4
Phosphorus	3
Total protein	15
Triglycerides	5
Troponin I	50
Uric acid	5

These values are in addition to the dead volume of the system (30 μL). *These values are specific for this instrument* and should be expected to differ from requirements for other reference laboratories. Always check with the reference laboratory regarding volume requirements and submission recommendations for their analyzing systems.

1.3.1.3 Handling and Storage

Proper handling and storage of the blood sample is imperative, not only for producing suitable and reliable data, but also for maximizing the amount of suitable blood that can be used for clinical chemistry and other purposes. Regardless of whether serum or plasma is to be used, it is best to process any blood for clinical chemistry within the first 2 hours after collection. The following

TABLE 1.5
Primary Sites for Routine Blood Collection in Adult Laboratory Mouse

	Retro-Orbital Plexus	Tail Vein	Superficial Temporal Vein	Cardiocentesis
Survival procedure	Yes	Yes	Yes	No
Tissue damage	Moderate to high	Moderate	Moderate	n/a
Repeat sampling	Yes, use contralateral plexus for each subsequent bleed	Yes	Yes, use contralateral vein for each subsequent bleed	n/a
Type of restraint	General anesthesia	Physical restraint; general anesthesia	Physical restraint; general anesthesia	Immediately after carbon dioxide euthanasia
Blood collection equipment required	• Blood capillary tube • Sterile saline or phosphate-buffered solution (PBS) • Sterile gauze swab or sponge	• 25–27 G needle • Blood capillary tube • Sterile gauze sponge	• GoldenRod animal lancet (MEDIpoint, Mineola, NY; http://www.medipoint.com) or 18–22G needle • Blood capillary tube or 1.0 mL centrifuge tube • Sterile gauze sponge	• 100% alcohol solution • 22–27G needle attached to 1.0–3.0 mL syringe
Amount of blood collected	<0.4 mL	<0.3 mL	<0.4 mL	0.5–1.0 mL
Procedure	• Anesthetize animal • Introduce the end of the blood capillary tube at the medial canthus of the orbit • Slowly, with axial rotation, advance the tip of the capillary tube gently toward the rear of the socket until blood flows into the tube • Remove the capillary tube and dab excess blood from the site with a gauze sponge or swab moistened with saline or PBS	• Physically restrain or anesthetize animal • Visualize a sampling site of the lateral tail vein at approximately the midpoint on the length of the tail • Extend the tail with one hand, and with the other handle, insert the needle 3–4 mm into the lateral tail vein • Collect blood from the hub of the needle with the blood capillary tube • Remove needle from tail vein and apply gauze sponge with gentle pressure on the bleeding site to ensure hemostasis	• Physically restrain or anesthetize animal • Scruff the neck and base of tail • Visualize the sampling site on the jaw, slightly in front of the angle on the mandible • Puncture the skin at a 90° angle until the tip of the lancet or needle is just through the skin • Collect the droplets of blood directly into centrifuge tube • Loosen the grip on the neck and apply pressure with a gauze sponge to ensure hemostasis	• Euthanize the mouse humanely via carbon dioxide asphyxiation • Place the animal in dorsal recumbency and saturate the ventral cranial abdomen with 100% alcohol • Insert needle just below and slightly to the left of the xiphoid cartilage at the base of the sternum at a 15–20° angle • Advance the needle slowly, applying slight negative pressure on the barrel of the syringe (blood will flow into the hub when the tip has entered one of the chambers of the heart). Aspirate gently until blood flow ceases
Disadvantages	• Mixing of venous and arterial blood • Stimulation of sympathetic nervous system • ↑ glucose	–	–	• ↑ glucose • ↑ creatine kinase • ↑ troponin

Sources: Diehl, K.H. et al.: A good practice guide to the administration of substances and removal of blood, including routes and volumes. *J Appl Toxicol*. 2001. 21. 20. Copyright Wiley-VCH Verlag GmbH & Co. KGaA. Reprinted with permission; Davis, K.H.: Mouse and rat anesthesia and analgesia. *Curr Protoc Neurosci*. 2005.Supplement 33. A.4G.1–A.4G.9. Copyright Wiley-VCH Verlag GmbH & Co. KGaA. Reprinted with permission.

TABLE 1.6
Injectable Anesthetic Agents Recommended for Bleeding Mice

Agent	Dosage (mg/kg); Route of administration	Duration of surgical anesthesia (min)
Pentobarbital	40–70; Intraperitoneal (IP)	20–40
Ketamine + xylazine	60–100 + 5–20; IP	20–25
Ketamine + xylazine + acepromazine	60–100 + 5–10 + 5–10; IP	20–30
Tribromoethanol[a]	125–160; IP	15–30
Propofol	12–26; Intravenous (IV)	5–10

[a] Tribromoethanol (TBE) is not available as a pharmaceutical grade compound, and TBE solutions exposed to heat or light can break down to potentially irritating and toxic byproducts. *In-vivo* use has been associated with post-procedural, clinical problems. Individuals should check with their Institutional Animal Care and Use (IACUC) or Ethics Committee prior to use.

Sources: Davis, J.A.: Mouse and rat anesthesia and analgesia. *Curr Protoc Neurosc i.* 2008. Supplement 42.A.4B.1–A.4B.21. Copyright Wiley-VCH Verlag GmbH & Co. KGaA. Reprinted with permission; Buitrago, S. et al.: Safety and efficacy of various combinations of injectable anesthetics in BALB/c mice. *J Am Assoc Lab Anim Sci.* 2008. 47. 11–17. Copyright Wiley-VCH Verlag GmbH & Co. KGaA.

TABLE 1.7
Inhalational Anesthetic Agents Recommended for Bleeding Mice

Agent	Induction (%)	Maintenance (%)
Isoflurane	5.0	1.0–1.5

Source: Davis J.A.: Mouse and rat anesthesia and analgesia. *Curr Protoc Neurosci.* 2008. Supplement 42. A.4B.1–A.4B.21. Copyright Wiley-VCH Verlag GmbH & Co. KGaA. Reprinted with permission.

If used with nitrous oxide (N_2O), reduction of the induction and maintenance percentage of the inhalational agent is required. Any inhalational agent should be used with a precision vaporizer and an adequate gaseous scavenging system

recommendations are adapted from the Diagnostic Laboratory of the Veterinary Services Center at Stanford University, Stanford, CA. For the interested biomedical researcher, Henry et al. (2001) provides more comprehensive discussions and guidelines for blood handling and storage.

1.3.1.4 Serum

Immediately after blood collection, place the blood in a 1 mL blood centrifuge tube (without any anticoagulants or preservatives). Allow the blood to clot for 30–60 minutes at ambient room temperature. Centrifuge the clotted blood sample for 10–15 minutes at a relative centrifugal force (RCF) of 14,000 *g*. Pipette the separated serum and transfer to a clean blood centrifuge tube. Recentrifuge the serum sample for another 2–3 minutes at 14,000 *g* to separate any remaining red blood cells. Pipette the clean serum and transfer to a clean blood centrifuge tube, and cap the tube tightly to prevent evaporation.

1.3.1.5 Plasma

Blood must be thoroughly mixed with an anticoagulant at the time of blood collection or immediately after blood collection. For the former, the sterile 1 mL syringe used for blood collection may be "primed" with the anticoagulant prior to blood collection by sterilely drawing 1 mL of the anticoagulant from the vial into the syringe, and then reinstilling the entire amount of the anticoagulant back into the vial. For the latter, add not more than 150 µL of anticoagulant to the 1 mL blood centrifuge tube used for blood collection. In either case, ensure that the blood is thoroughly mixed with the anticoagulant after the blood has been collected and introduced to the anticoagulant. Centrifuge the blood sample for 10–15 minutes at a RCF of 14,000 *g*. Pipette the separated plasma and transfer to a clean blood centrifuge tube. Recentrifuge the plasma sample for another 2–3 minutes at 14,000 *g* to separate out any remaining red blood cells. Pipette the clean plasma and transfer to a clean blood centrifuge tube, and cap the tube tightly to prevent evaporation.

1.3.1.6 Choice of Anticoagulant

The choice of anticoagulant will depend on the bioanalyte being analyzed and/or the preferences of the laboratory in which the clinical chemistry is run. Additionally, the choice of anticoagulant may be influenced if other concurrent tests beyond clinical chemistry are required (such hematology and serology). Therefore, the biomedical researcher is strongly encouraged to contact the laboratory used prior to blood collection to ensure that the blood collected is introduced with the correct anticoagulant (if required). A common anticoagulant used for clinical chemistry is lithium heparin, which in general, has little effect on the values of most bioanalytes (Wiedmeyer et al., 2007). However, a main disadvantage of using lithium heparin is that it does not contain cell preservatives, which precludes analysis for hematology (if concurrently required) unless blood smears are performed immediately after blood collection (Wiedmeyer et al., 2007). Another common anticoagulant used in the laboratory setting is ethylenediaminetetraacetic acid (EDTA). Although it is used extensively for hematology, it is not generally a suitable anticoagulant for clinical chemistry because its strong chelation properties interfere with calcium-dependent enzyme reactions of several bioanalytes (e.g., alkaline phosphatase) and the values of certain electrolytes (such as sodium or potassium). Similarly, the anticoagulant sodium citrate also strongly chelates with calcium, which makes it useful for analyzing clotting factor levels but not for general clinical chemistry.

1.3.1.7 Storage

Most bioanalytes are best analyzed at ambient room temperatures within the first 2 hours of collection. If the serum or plasma sample cannot be processed for clinical chemistry within this 2-hour time period, then place the sample (in its capped tube) into a refrigerator at 4°C for short-term storage (<1 week) or into a non-frost-free freezer at –20°C or colder for long-term storage (1 week to 6 months). There are some exceptions to these storage recommendations. For example, unless ammonia, lactate, and the bioanalytes of blood gas are analyzed immediately after collection, the serum or plasma samples should be stored in ice baths or –4°C to maintain accurate levels of these bioanalytes. Additionally, bilirubin will degrade upon exposure to direct light. Therefore, blood destined for bilirubin analysis should be stored via a lightproof method (e.g., wrapping the blood sample container with aluminum foil). Furthermore, if lactate dehydrogenase is the bioanalyte of interest, storage at room temperature is recommended.

1.3.2 Urine Collection and Storage

The body size and physiology of the laboratory mouse limits the total amount of urine that can be collected, as well as the frequency at which the urine is collected. The total urinary bladder volume of an adult mouse is normally less than 0.5 mL, and the total urinary output per day is less than 1.5–2 mL (Jung et al., 2003). The laboratory mouse also urinates frequently in small amounts, usually 0.1–0.3 mL per urination. All of these factors limit the amount of urine that can be collected at any one time, and therefore the number of bioanalytes that can be assessed from any one urine sample.

Table 1.8 outlines the different methods of collecting urine from the laboratory mouse (Cohen et al., 2007). The mouse should not be fasted prior to urine collection, in order to minimize any

TABLE 1.8
Methods for Collecting Fresh Voided Urine in Laboratory Mouse. The Mouse Should Not Be Fasted Prior to Collection

Method	Procedure	Advantages	Disadvantages
Routine collection of fresh voided urine	• Secure a large piece of clean parafilm to a solid surface with a raised edge • Pick the mouse up by gently squeezing the skin behind the ears to secure the head • Place the mouse on the parafilm allowing the mouse to grab the raised edge with the front feet • With the free hand, gently massage the lateral abdomen of the mouse just cranial to the pelvis to induce the mouse to void • Pipette up the voided urine and place in a small centrifuge tube	• Survival procedure • Relatively stress-free for mouse • Relatively easy procedure • Relatively clean urine sample collected	• Small volume of urine collected (0.1-0.3 mL)
Collection in metabolism cage	• Acclimatize mouse to the metabolism cages for at least 48 hours (ensure provision of food and water) • Collect urine after desired time period (2-24 hours) • For collections greater than 4 hours, ice and/or antimicrobial agents may be required in the collection point	• Relatively large volume of urine collected (1.0-2.0 mL)	• Ice used for preserving urine may dilute out urine bioanalytes and change solubility characteristics of sediments and other constituents • Urine contamination high • Requires use of antimicrobials to minimize urine contamination
Collection after euthanasia	• Humanely euthanize mouse via carbon dioxide asphyxiation • Using aseptic techniques, expose the urinary bladder by incising through the abdominal skin and body wall along the ventral midline • Aspirate urine directly from the urinary bladder via a 25 g needle attached to a 1.0 mL syringe	• Sterile urine collected	• Non-survival procedure • Mouse may involuntarily void urine at time of euthanasia • Small volume of urine collected (0.1–0.5 mL)

Source: Reprinted from Cohen, A.M. et al., *Toxicol Pathol.*, 35, 339–340, 2007. Copyright © 2007 SAGE Publications. With permission of SAGE Publications.

changes to urine bioanalyte and sediment content. Furthermore, the urine is best collected at night or in the first 2 hours of the light cycle if possible. Ideally, urinalysis should be performed immediately after urine collection. If immediate urinalysis is not possible, storing urine samples in an airtight container (e.g., an Eppendorf tube) to prevent evaporation, and in a refrigerator at 4°C (to limit bacterial growth) is recommended.

To mitigate the small urine volume limitations associated with mouse urinalysis, the dilution of urine samples can be performed to effectively increase the volume size. However, this may (and often does) introduce errors in the accuracy of any results generated for urinalysis. Pooling urine samples from multiple mice from single research group can also increase the total amount of urine collected. The main disadvantage of this technique is that it does not allow specific results to be related back to specific individuals from that group.

1.4 PREANALYTICAL SOURCES OF VARIATION

1.4.1 Sex

While variations in the levels of sex hormones are expected in most mammalian species, other less obvious yet significant variances in bioanalytes in the laboratory mouse have been attributed to sex. Corticosterone levels are reported to be higher in female mice than in male mice (Ottenweller et al., 1979; Scheving et al., 1983). Male mice have a well-defined diurnal concentration pattern, with a maximum concentration of 9 µg/dL at the start of the dark cycle and a minimum concentration of 5 µg/dL shortly before the end of the dark cycle (Ottenweller et al., 1979). In contrast, female mice have a minimum concentration of 13.5 µg/dL at the beginning of the dark cycle and a maximum of 40 µg/dL well into the dark period (Scheving et al., 1983). More recently, Laviola et al. (2002) confirmed this trend of sex differences in corticosterone levels in laboratory mice, with female adult mice having higher overall levels of corticosterone than males, although the significant sex differences were not noted between younger mice, 30–45 day old male and female mice.

Pickering and Pickering (1984) demonstrated that serum alkaline phosphatase activity is lower in males than in females, whereas serum alanine aminotransferase and aspartate aminotransferase activity is higher in males. Lactate dehydrogenase levels have been shown to be higher in males compared to females of the BALB/c strain (Frith et al., 1980). Male C57BL/6 mice exhibited higher glomerular filtration rate than female mice, as determined by a greater fluorescein isothiocyanate (FITC)-labeled inulin clearance rate (Qi et al., 2004).

Additional reviews and resources that document sex-related differences in bioanalytes include Loeb et al. (1996); Serfilippi et al. (2003), the Mouse Phenome Database (The Jackson Laboratory, Bar Harbor, ME; http://phenome.jax.org/), the National Toxicology Program (http://ntp.niehs.nih.gov/), the Europhenome Mouse Phenotyping Resource (http://www.europhenome.org/databrowser/viewer.jsp); and Charles River (http://www.criver.com/find-a-model).

1.4.2 Age

Loeb et al. (1996) reviews effects of age on clinical chemistry values in five inbred strains and two F1 hybrids. Glucose levels demonstrated the most dramatic changes, decreasing throughout life at an approximate rate of 2 mg/dL per month in both sexes of DBA, B6C3F1, C57BL/6J, and CBA/J mice, and in male BALB/cByJ and DBA/2J mice. Scrofano et al. (1998) found similar decreases in glucose as a function of age in a cohort of Emory mice. Other bioanalytes that decreased with age included: alkaline phosphatase activity in both sexes of BALB/c and C57BL/6, triglycerides in male and female C57BL/6, DBA, B6C3F1, B6D2F1 mice. Bioanalytes that increased with age included phosphorus in both sexes of BALB/c and C57BL/6; aspartate aminotransferase and alanine aminotransferase activities in both sexes of BALB/c and C57BL/6, and in female DBA and male B6D2F1 mice; total protein and gamma-globulins levels in both sexes of BALB/c and C57BL/6 (Loeb et al., 1996). More recently, Laviola et al. (2002) showed that younger 30–45-day-old mice have higher levels of corticosterone compared to older adult mice.

Additional reviews and resources that document sex-related differences in bioanalytes include the Mouse Phenome Database (The Jackson Laboratory, Bar Harbor, ME; http://phenome.jax.org/), the

National Toxicology Program (http://ntp .niehs.nih.gov/), and the Europhenome Mouse Phenotyping Resource (http://www.europhenome.org/databrowser/viewer.jsp).

1.4.3 Genetics

Genetic-associated variations (including those related to strain) have been noted for diverse clinical pathology bioanalytes and continue to be identified as mouse genome and phenome projects progress, and as genetically engineered mice and their background "control" strains are analyzed further. At least 14 inbred strains (including AKR/J, DBA/2J, FVB/N, some A strains, non-obese diabetic (NOD) strains and many BXD recombinant inbred strains) lack the fifth complement component, C5 (hemolytic complement) (Goldman and Goldman, 1976; Lake, 2009). Strain-associated variations in serum cholesterol (Dunnington et al., 1981; Maier et al., 2007; Meade and Gore, 1982); serum testosterone (Ivanyi et al., 1972); serum cortisol-binding protein (Goldman et al., 1977); serum protein (Borovkov and Svirdov, 1975; Loeb, 1997); and urine albumin excretion (Maier et al., 2007) are documented. Male Swiss-Webster mice possess a higher glomerular filtration rate than male C57BL/6 mice, as determined by a greater FITC-labeled inulin clearance rate (Qi et al., 2004).

Additional reviews and resources that document genetic- and strain-related differences in bioanalytes include Loeb et al. (1996); Serfilippi et al. (2003), the Mouse Phenome Database (The Jackson Laboratory, Bar Harbor, ME; http://phenome.jax.org/), the National Toxicology Program (http://ntp .niehs.nih.gov/), the Europhenome Mouse Phenotyping Resource (http://www.europhenome.org/databrowser/viewer.jsp); and Charles River (http://www.criver.com/find-a-model).

1.4.4 Health Status

It is beyond the scope of this material to discuss bioanalyte variability related to specific pathologic conditions that affect the health status of laboratory mice. In general, however, many diseases may induce similar nonspecific clinical signs of ill-health (e.g., dehydration, infection, and inanition due to illness, inability to access food, experimental protocol, or other causes) that may in turn alter bioanalytes. Furthermore, specific treatment for diseases conditions (such as antimicrobials, anti-inflammatory drugs, and immunomodulatory drugs) may furthermore introduce variability in bioanalyte levels.

Dehydration will in general cause concentration of proteins in the blood, resulting in hyperproteinemia in an otherwise healthy laboratory mouse. Generalized acute systemic inflammation (such as with acute, recent infection by a micro-organism or elements of micro-organisms, such as endotoxin/lipopolysaccharide; or with acute, recent administration of biologics or small molecules that may modulate the immune system) manifest with transient or sustained elevations in acute-phase proteins (mainly increases in serum amyloid A, with moderate or minor increased in α1-acid glycoprotein, haptoglobin, fibrinogen, and α2-macroglobulin) (Watterson et al., 2009). The effects of nutrition on the health status of laboratory mice are discussed in the following section.

Of particular note to laboratory mice is infection by lactate dehydrogenase-elevating virus (LDEV). This is a murine-specific arterivirus that may rarely cause clinical disease in susceptible mouse strains (immunosuppressed C58 and AKR) under specific conditions (Percy and Barthold, 2007). Regardless of strain and the manifestation of clinical disease, however, LDEV infection in laboratory mice is associated with a persistent elevation in lactate dehydrogenase (LDH) activity (and to a lesser degree, other enzyme-based bioanalytes such as isocitrate dehydrogenase, malate dehydrogenase, phoshphoglucose isomerase, glutathione reductase, aspartate transaminase, glutamate oxaloacetate transaminase, and alanine transaminase) in plasma or serum. This persistent elevation of enzymes is caused by viral infection and destruction of a nonessential population of murine macrophages that normally clear these enzymes (Riley et al., 1978; Plagemann et al., 1995).

Therefore, infections by LDEV in a mouse colony with subclinical infections may introduce variability into clinical chemistry results that are obtained.

1.4.5 Nutritional Status

1.4.5.1 Diet

Diet is known to influence the blood levels of many bioanalytes. Perhaps the best studied of these is the effect of atherogenic diets on serum cholesterol (Morrisett et al., 1982). Similarly, significant differences in both serum cholesterol and blood urea nitrogen are seen in mice maintained on a semipurified (AIN-76) diet (Greenman et al., 1982). Also, Cederroth et al. (2008) recently demonstrated that soy-fed mice showed reduced serum insulin levels (related to reduce pancreatic insulin content).

Immunocompromised mice are often administered antimicrobial-supplemented feed or water as a prophylactic treatment for *Pneumocystis murina* pneumonia. Recently, Altholtz et al. (2006) demonstrated that certain trimethoprim-sulfamethoxazole-medicated feeds may cause dose-dependent hypothyroidism in C57BL/6 mice, with significant decreases in plasma thyroxine (T_4) levels and increases in thyroid-stimulating hormone (TSH) levels. The mouse is unique among mammals because its muscles do not contain carnosine or anserine (Brewer, 1986). Carnosine serves as a source of histidine when its dietary intake is low, and mice on histidine-free diets show signs of histidine deficiency (Parker et al., 1985).

1.4.5.2 Fasting

Mice and rats are generally nocturnal. Overnight fasting impacts their period of greatest activity and may constitute a different or greater stressor compared to overnight fasting of diurnal species. Overnight fasting in BALB/c mice has been reported to decrease plasma glucose and plasma lactate levels (Young, 2005). Muglia et al. (2001) demonstrated that stressing healthy mice via fasting resulted in robust corticosterone production. Lipid metabolism is also altered by fasting of mice with longer periods of fasting (8–16 hours) resulting in higher circulating levels of free fatty acids and triglycerides than short periods of fasting (2 hours) (Argmann et al., 2006b). Similarly, bile acids are lower in fasted mice (Argmann et al., 2006b).

1.4.5.3 Caloric Restriction

Energy (or caloric) restricted diets can significantly change the clinical chemistry profile of laboratory mice. In one large study of 100 mice (Williams et al., 2007), a 30% energy restriction in C57BL/6 mice resulted in significant decreases in glucose, triglycerides, and cholesterol. Scrofano et al. (1998) found similar result in a cohort of Emory mice on long term, 50% caloric restriction, with decreases in glucose and cholesterol as well.

1.4.6 Environment

Environmental factors have been recognized as early as the 1940s to affect the results of scientific studies using laboratory mice. In one early study by Chance (1947), the degree of hydration, exposure to noise, degree of confinement, and environmental temperatures was shown to affect the metabolism and toxicity of drugs in mice. Subsequently, these same housing environmental factors have also been shown to influence bioanalyte values (Besch, 1985; Boyd, 1983; Jensen and Rasmussen, 1963; Laber et al., 2008; Lindsey et al., 1978; Serrano, 1971). For example, in one recent study, Laber et al. (2008) demonstrated that housing density influences stress and immune parameters in BALB/c and C57BL/6. Specifically, BALB/c and C57BL/6 mice housed at 10 animals per cage (compared to 2 or 5 animals per cage) demonstrated significant negative effects on stress (increased corticosterone levels) and immune parameters (decreased helper T-cell levels). Lower testosterone levels were noted in male mice in overcrowded (9 mice per cage) cages when compared to noncrowded (3 mice per cage) cages (Laviola et al., 2001).

1.4.7 Circadian Rhythm

Cyclic biorhythms, whether circadian or ultradian, influence blood levels of various bioanalytes in laboratory mice, with the most extensively researched being the hormone of hypothalamic-pituitary-adrenal gland axis. Blood levels of corticotrophin-releasing hormone (CRH), adrenocorticotropic hormone (ACTH), corticosterone, growth hormone (GH), and luteinizing hormone (LH) may peak one or more times daily (Loeb, 1997; Muglia et al., 2001). ACTH release is episodic (not at fixed intervals) and does not involve steroid feedback, and to visualize episodic cycling; samples must be collected at 5–30-minute intervals (Edwardson and Hough, 1975; Woodman, 1997). ACTH concentration peaks in the early evening in mice and can be reversed by reversing the light cycle (Halberg et al., 1965; Krieger, 1979). In terms of corticosterone, female mice have a minimum concentration of 13.5 μg/dL at the beginning of the dark cycle and a maximum of 40 μg/dL well into the dark period (Scheving et al., 1983). In contrast, male mice have a maximum concentration of 9 μg/dL at the start of the dark cycle and a minimum concentration of 5 μg/dL shortly before the end of the dark cycle (Ottenweller et al., 1979). These findings illustrate the importance that must be given to the timing of sample collection in laboratory mice.

1.4.8 Pregnancy

Holinka et al. (1979) found that estradiol levels significantly increased after day 17 of gestation in younger pregnant mice (3–7 months of age) when compared to older pregnant mice (11–12 months of age), attributing this difference to longer gestation time in the older mice.

1.4.9 Stress

Stress may result in alterations in clinicopathologic parameters can be attributed to stress in mice. Landi et al. (1982, 1985) found that plasma corticosterone concentrations in mice tested on arrival, or 24 or 48 hours after arrival (by plane or truck transport) were significantly higher than those of control mice. Muglia et al. (2001) reinforce these findings by demonstrating that stressing healthy mice via physical restraint for 20 minutes or acute, overnight fasting resulting in robust corticosterone production. Even handling prior to blood collection can profoundly alter serum corticosterone levels (MacLeod and Shapiro, 1988).

1.4.10 Anesthesia

Variations associated with the anesthesia have been described by Chuang and Luo (1997). In these studies, higher glucose levels were reported with tail vein blood collection in laboratory mice anesthetized with pentobarbital or methoxyflurane (compared with conscious mice); and after collection from the orbital plexus after pentobarbital or proparacaine hydrochloride administration. However, methoxyflurane had no glucose-elevating effect on samples collected from the orbital plexus. Ether inhalation has also been demonstrated to cause increased corticosterone production in healthy mice (Muglia et al., 2001).

1.4.11 Specimen Collection and Handling

1.4.11.1 Interfering Constituents

The effect of sample storage at various temperatures and for varying periods has been described. Falk et al. (1981) evaluated the effect of storage time (after freezing) on 20 serum bioanalytes in 6 laboratory species, and found that in the mouse, only creatine kinase activity changed significantly with storage up to 28 days.

Hemolysis is a common problem during blood collection in mice. Hemolyzed samples are associated with changes in various enzymes, such as increased total protein, alanine aminotransferase, aspartate aminotransferase, lactate dehydrogenase, potassium, and creatine kinase levels, and decreased phosphorus and lipase levels (Latimer et al., 2003). The effect of lipemia on clinical chemistry values has been reviewed for domestic animals (Latimer et al., 2003), which include increased glucose, calcium, phosphorus, and total bilirubin values, and decreased total protein, albumin, sodium, and potassium values.

1.4.11.2 Site of Sampling

Patrick et al. (1983) found that terminal cardiac puncture was associated with higher glucose and lower creatine kinase levels. O'Brien et al. (1997) demonstrated higher cardiac troponin levels in mice after terminal cardiocentesis as well. Increased alanine aminotransferase and aspartate aminotransferase levels are observed with terminal cardiac puncture in mice as well (Luong, 2009).

1.5 BASIC METHODOLOGY FOR COMMON PROCEDURES

1.5.1 Adrenocorticotropin Hormone Stimulation Test

Purpose of test: To assess adrenal gland corticosteroid-production function by measuring the corticosteroid response to exogenous adrenocorticotropin hormone administration.
Procedure:

1. Obtain 50 µL of plasma. Label sample as "baseline plasma."
2. Inject adrenocorticotropin (10 µg/kg body weight) intraperitoneally.
3. Obtain 50 µL of plasma 1 hour after adrenocorticotropin injection. Label sample with the appropriate time point.
4. Submit plasma samples for corticosterone and/or aldosterone analysis.

Source: Muglia et al. (2000).

1.5.2 Water Deprivation

Purpose of test: To differentiate between the causes of polydipsia, including: primary polydipsia, neurogenic diabetes insipidus, and nephrogenic diabetes insipidus.
Procedure:
Note: Obtain approval from institutional animal care and use committee/welfare and ethics committee BEFORE carrying out any water deprivation studies on mice.

1. Maintain mouse with normal access to food and water for a predetermined time (e.g., 1 week).
2. Obtain 10 µL of plasma. Ensure proper labeling of sample as "baseline plasma."
3. Immediately deprive mouse of water for a predetermined length of time (e.g., 6, 12, 24, 36, or 48 hours). Allow normal access to food during this period.

4. Obtain 10 μL of plasma at the end of the water deprivation period. Ensure proper labeling of sample with the appropriate time point.
5. Submit plasma samples for plasma osmolality and/or antidiuretic hormone (arginine vasopressin) analysis.

Sources: Kessler et al. (2007) and Tsunematsu et al. (2008).

1.5.3 Ammonia Tolerance Test

Purpose of test: To assess liver function, specifically hepatic functional mass and integrity of the enterohepatic circulation.
Procedure:

1. Fast mouse for 8–12 hours.
2. Administer a 5% ammonium chloride solution (100 mg/kg body weight) orally via oral gavage.
3. Obtain 20 μL of blood at predetermined time points after ammonium chloride administration (e.g., 5, 10, 15, 20, and 30 minutes). Immediately separate blood for plasma separation (place blood sample on ice if there is even the slightest delay between collection and plasma separation). Ensure proper labeling of samples with appropriate time points.
4. Submit plasma samples for ammonia level analysis.

Source: Hiroyama et al. (2007).

1.5.4 Indocyanine Green Elimination Test

Purpose of test: To assess liver function, specifically hepatic functional mass and integrity of the enterohepatic circulation.
Procedure:

1. Dissolve indocyanine green (ICG) dye in a minimum volume of water, and then dilute the dissolved ICG dye with Phosphate Buffered Saline (PBS) at 0.1 mg/mL.
2. Fast mouse for 8-12 hours.
3. Inject the ICG solution (0.5 mg/kg body weight) intravenously into the tail vein.
4. Obtain 20 μL of plasma at predetermined time points after ICG solution injection (e.g., 5, 10, and 15 minutes). Ensure proper labeling of samples with appropriate time points.
5. Submit plasma samples for ICG elimination rate analysis.

Source: Hiroyama et al. (2007).

1.5.5 Bile Acids—Pre- and Postprandial

Purpose of test: To assess liver function, specifically biliary system function, hepatic functional mass and integrity of the enterohepatic circulation.
Procedure:

1. Fast mouse for 8–12 hours.
2. Obtain 20 μL of plasma. Ensure proper labeling of sample as "preprandial plasma."
3. Feed mouse.
4. Obtain 20 μL of plasma at predetermined time points after feeding (e.g., 15 and 30 minutes). Ensure proper labeling of sample as "postprandial plasma."
5. Submit plasma samples for bile acid analysis.

Source: Argmann et al. (2006b).

1.5.6 Bromosulphthalein Clearance

Purpose of test: To assess liver function, specifically hepatic functional mass and integrity of the enterohepatic circulation.
Procedure:

1. Inject bromosulphthalein (BSP) (125 mg/kg body weight) intravenously into the tail vein.
2. Obtain 20 μL of plasma at predetermined time points after BSP injection (e.g., 10, 20, and 30 minutes). Ensure proper labeling of samples with appropriate time points.
3. Submit plasma samples for BSP clearance analysis.

Source: Hurwitz et al. (1985).

1.5.7 Low-Dose Dexamethasone Suppression Test

Purpose of test: In conjunction with other tests (such as the high-dose dexamethasone suppression test), to differentiate between the causes of hyperadrenocorticism, including primary hyperadrenocorticism (Cushing's syndrome), and secondary hyperadrenocorticism (Cushing's disease, ectopic adrenocorticotropin hormone syndrome).
Procedure:

1. Obtain 50 μL of plasma. Ensure proper labeling of sample as "baseline plasma."
2. Inject dexamethasone (0.03 μg/kg body weight) intraperitoneally.
3. Obtain 50 μL of plasma 6 hours after dexamethasone injection. Ensure proper labeling of sample with the appropriate time point.
4. Submit plasma samples for corticosterone analysis.

Source: Ridder et al. (2005).

1.5.8 High-Dose Dexamethasone Suppression Test

Purpose of test: In conjunction with other tests (such as the low-dose dexamethasone suppression test), to differentiate between the causes of hyperadrenocorticism, including primary hyperadrenocorticism (Cushing's syndrome), and secondary hyperadrenocorticism (Cushing's disease, ectopic adrenocorticotropin hormone syndrome).
Procedure:

1. Obtain 50 μL of plasma. Ensure proper labeling of sample as "baseline plasma."
2. Inject dexamethasone (1 mg/kg body weight) intraperitoneally.
3. Obtain 50 μL of plasma 6 hours after dexamethasone injection. Ensure proper labeling of sample with the appropriate time point.
4. Submit plasma samples for corticosterone analysis.

Source: McGill et al. (2005).

1.5.9 Intraperitoneal Glucose Tolerance Test

Purpose of test: To differentiate between the causes of hyperglycemia, including impaired fasting glycemia, impaired glucose tolerance, and diabetes mellitus.
Procedure:

1. Fast mouse for 8–12 hours.
2. Inject a 20% glucose solution (1.5–2.0 g/kg body weight) intraperitoneally.

3. Obtain 5–20 μL of plasma at predetermined time points after glucose solution administration (e.g., 0, 15, 30, 60, 90, and 120 minutes). Ensure proper labeling of samples with appropriate time points.
4. Submit plasma samples for glucose level analysis.

Sources: Heikkinen et al. (2007) and Yamada et al. (1997).

1.5.10 Oral Glucose Tolerance Test

Purpose of test: To differentiate between the causes of hyperglycemia, including impaired fasting glycemia, impaired glucose tolerance, and diabetes mellitus.
Procedure:

1. Fast mouse for 8–12 hours.
2. Administer a 20% glucose solution (1.5–2.0 g/kg body weight) via oral gavage.
3. Obtain 5–20 μL of plasma at predetermined time points after glucose solution administration (e.g., 0, 15, 30, 60, 90, and 120 minutes). Ensure proper labeling of samples with appropriate time points.
4. Submit plasma samples for glucose level analysis.

Source: Heikkinen et al. (2007).

1.5.11 Inulin Clearance—Single Bolus Injection Method

Purpose of test: To assess renal function by determining glomerular filtration rate.
Procedure:

1. Dissolve 5% FITC-labeled inulin in 0.9% NaCl by heating the solution in boiling water.
2. Dialyze the solution in 1000 mL of 0.9% NaCl at room temperature for 24 hours using a 1000-Da cutoff dialysis membrane to remove residual FITC not bound to inulin. Wrap the dialysis bottle with aluminum foil during the procedure. The resulting FITC-labeled inulin concentration is 3%.
3. Sterilize the dialyzed 3% FITC-labeled inulin solution by filtration through a 0.22 μm filter.
4. Inject the dialyzed 3% FITC-labeled inulin solution (3.74 μL/g body weight) intravenously, or retro-orbitally (under light anesthesia of approximately 20 seconds induced using isoflurane).
5. Obtain 10 μL of plasma at predetermined time points after dialyzed 3% FITC-labeled inulin solution administration (e.g., 3, 7, 10, 15, 35, 55, and 75 minutes). Ensure proper labeling of samples with appropriate time points.
6. Obtain as much urine as possible at the mid- and end time-points. Ensure proper labeling of samples with appropriate time points.
7. Submit plasma and urine samples for determination of FITC-labeled inulin clearance analysis.

Source: Qi et al. (2004).

1.5.12 TSH (Thyrotropin) Stimulation Test

Purpose of test: In conjunction with other tests (such as the thyrotropin-releasing hormone stimulation test), to differentiate between the causes of hypothyroidism, including primary hypothyroidism and secondary hypothyroidism.

Procedure:

1. Obtain 50 μL of serum. Ensure proper labeling of sample as "baseline serum."
2. Inject bovine TSH /thyrotropin (2.5 units/kg body weight) intraperitoneally.
3. Obtain 50 μL of serum 120 minutes after TSH /thyrotropin injection. Ensure proper labeling of sample with the appropriate time point.
4. Submit serum samples for triiodothyronine (T_3) analysis.

Source: Yamada et al. (1997).

1.5.13 Thyrotropin-Releasing Hormone Stimulation Test

Purpose of test: In conjunction with other tests (such as the TSH stimulation test), to differentiate between the causes of hypothyroidism, including primary hypothyroidism and secondary hypothyroidism.
Procedure:

1. Obtain 50 μL of serum. Ensure proper labeling of sample as "baseline serum."
2. Inject thyrotropin-releasing hormone (5 μg/kg body weight) intraperitoneally.
3. Obtain 50 μL of serum 30 and 120 minutes after thyrotropin-releasing hormone injection. Ensure proper labeling of sample with appropriate time point.
4. Submit baseline and 30-minute serum samples for thyroid-stimulating hormone analysis, and baseline and 120-minute serum samples for triiodothyronine (T_3) analysis.

Source: Yamada et al. (1997).

1.6 REFERENCE RANGES

Reference ranges refer to the range of a bioanalyte or biomarker in a population that has not been selected for the presence of disease or abnormality, and are used as a comparison to determine the presence or absence of disease or abnormality in a particular individual or group of individuals of diagnostic or research interest. Reference ranges and historical control data can be useful in designing experiments, but should be used with extreme caution in analysis and interpretation of experimental results. Sufficient sample size of concurrent relevant control animals should be included in the experimental design (i.e., baseline reference ranges should be compiled a sufficient sample size of individuals from the population of wild-type mice from which transgenic and knock-out (KO) mice were derived).

Protocol details regarding procurement of reference range or historical control data may have more value than the data itself in terms of obtaining useful or comparable data. As discussed throughout this chapter, collection methods and equipment (e.g., type or volume of anticoagulant, instrumentation, analysis method, or reagents), signalment (including genetic background), diets, housing, handling, and health status, are some of the factors that can influence results. Therefore, it is imperative that when publishing clinical chemistry data, sufficient details should be provided in the materials and methods sections that allow for replication the protocols used.

Tables 1.9 and 1.10 summarize clinical chemistry data in three strains of laboratory mice, whereas Table 1.11 summarizes the clinical urine data in laboratory mice. Moreover, the following resources may provide information on other outbred strains of mice, inbred strains of mice, and genetically modified mice: Loeb et al. (1996); Serfilippi et al. (2003), the Mouse Phenome Database (The Jackson Laboratory, Bar Harbor, ME; http://phenome.jax.org/), the National Toxicology Program (http://ntp.niehs.nih.gov/), the Europhenome Mouse Phenotyping Resource (http://www.europhenome.org/databrowser/viewer.jsp); and Charles River (http://www.criver.com/find-a-model).

TABLE 1.9

Clinical Chemistry Reference Ranges for CD-1 Outbred Laboratory Mice

	Male			Female		
Bioanalyte	**Mean**	**2 SD**	***n***	**Mean**	**2 SD**	***n***
Glucose (mg/dL)						
6–8 weeks	230	185–270	20	265	207–320	20
19–21 weeks	270	210–319	20	255	175–335	20
32–34 weeks	239	195–283	20	238	156–320	20
Blood urea nitrogen (mg/dL)						
6–8 weeks	33	23–43	20	28	21–35	20
19–21 weeks	22	17–29	20	23	17–29	20
32–34 weeks	20	17–23	20	23	14–32	20
Creatinine (mg/dL)						
6–8 weeks	0.5	0.2–0.8	20	0.6	0.4–0.8	20
19–21 weeks	0.7	0.4–1.0	20	0.5	0.3–0.7	20
32–34 weeks	0.5	0.3–0.7	20	0.5	0.3–0.7	20
Calcium (mg/dL)						
6–8 weeks	12.2	12.0–12.4	20	9.3	8.4–10.2	20
19–21 weeks	11.6	11.3–11.9	20	11.6	11.1–12.1	20
32–34 weeks	11.3	10.6–12.0	20	10.7	10.1–11.3	20
Phosphorus (mg/dL)						
6–8 weeks	13.2	7.8–18.6	20	11.2	7.4–15.0	20
19–21 weeks	9.0	8.3–9.7	20	10.1	9.0–11.2	20
32–34 weeks	11.5	9.6–13.4	20	10.1	8.8–11.4	20
Total bilirubin (mg/dL)						
6–8 weeks	0.2	0.1–0.3	20	0.3	0–0.5	20
19–21 weeks	0.2	0–0.4	20	0.3	0.2–0.4	20
32–34 weeks	0.2	0–0.4	20	0.3	0.1–0.5	20
Cholesterol (mg/dL)						
6–8 weeks	61	31–91	20	59	41–77	20
19–21 weeks	81	66–96	20	65	49–81	20
32–34 weeks	85	67–103	20	72	46–98	20
Iron (mg/dL)						
6–8 weeks	299	187–411	20	322	210–434	20
19–21 weeks	214	168–260	20	332	270–394	20
32–34 weeks	331	219–443	20	325	173–477	20
Alkaline phosphatase (IU/L)						
6–8 weeks	166	86–246	20	162	118–206	20
19–21 weeks	80	66–94	20	54	28–80	20
32–34 weeks	85	72–118	20	55	35–75	20
Aspartate aminotransferase (IU/L)						
6–8 weeks	248	24–472	20	137	87–187	20
19–21 weeks	124	68–180	20	153	55–251	20
32–34 weeks	127	65–189	20	208	132–284	20

(*Continued*)

TABLE 1.9 (*Continued*)

Clinical Chemistry Reference Ranges for CD-1 Outbred Laboratory Mice

	Male			Female		
Bioanalyte	**Mean**	**2 SD**	***n***	**Mean**	**2 SD**	***n***
Alanine aminotransferase (IU/L)						
6–8 weeks	109	28–190	20	103	56–159	20
19–21 weeks	84	22–146	20	106	28–184	20
32–34 weeks	118	66–170	20	101	59–143	20
Sodium (mEq/L)						
6–8 weeks	147	144–150	20	152	147–157	20
19–21 weeks	148	143–153	20	147	145–149	20
32–34 weeks	148	146–151	20	147	145–149	20
Potassium (mEq/L)						
6–8 weeks	5.5	4.7–6.3	20	5.2	4.2–6.2	20
19–21 weeks	5.1	3.8–6.4	20	7.4	4.8–10.0	20
32–34 weeks	8.8	7.3–10.3	20	8.2	6.5–9.9	20
Chloride (mEq/L)						
6–8 weeks	112	104–120	20	114	109–119	20
19–21 weeks	107	103–111	20	102	96–108	20
32–34 weeks	110	101–119	20	105	102–108	20
Total protein (g/dL)						
6–8 weeks	4.3	3.0–5.6	20	4.7	4.2–5.2	20
19–21 weeks	4.5	4.2–4.8	20	5.6	5.2–6.0	20
32–34 weeks	5.2	4.6–5.8	20	5.5	5.0–6.0	20
Albumin (g/dL)						
6–8 weeks	2.6	1.8–3.4	20	3.3	2.9–3.7	20
19–21 weeks	2.4	2.1–2.7	20	3.2	3.0–3.4	20
32–34 weeks	2.8	2.4–3.2	20	3.0	2.7–3.3	20
Globulin (g/dL)						
6–8 weeks	1.7	1.2–2.2	20	1.4	1.2–1.6	20
19–21 weeks	2.1	1.8–2.4	20	2.4	2.0–2.8	20
32–34 weeks	2.4	2.0–2.8	20	2.4	2.0–2.8	20
A/G ratio						
6–8 weeks	1.60	1.30–1.90	20	1.30	1.03–157	20
19–21 weeks	1.12	0.90–1.34	20	1.33	1.57–1.90	20
32–34 weeks	1.16	0.96–1.36	20	1.25	1.01–1.49	20

Source: Reprinted from Charles River Laboratories Research Models and Services, *Charles River- CD-1 and CF-1 Mice: Baseline Hematology and Clinical Chemistry Values as a Function of Sex and Age*, Wilmington, MA, Charles River, Epub 2005 Nov 11, available at: http://www.criver.com/SiteCollectionDocuments/rm_rm_r_hematology_sex_age_outbred_mice.pdf. May 15, 2010. With permission.

All values are performed on nonfasting animals and on serum, unless otherwise noted. Blood obtained via terminal cardiocentesis.

TABLE 1.10
Clinical Chemistry Reference Ranges for C57BL/6 Inbred and BALB/c Inbred Laboratory Mice

	C57BL/6						BALB/c					
	Male			Female			Male			Female		
Bioanalyte	**Mean**	**2 SD**	***n***	**Mean**	**2 SD**	***n***	**Mean**	**2 SD**	***n***	**Mean**	**2 SD**	***n***
Glucose (plasma, 4-hour fast) (mg/dL)												
8 weeks	156	97–215	54	176	113–239	30	114	65–163	22	112	79–145	20
16 weeks	159	109–209	30	152	94–210	30	97	62–132	20	115	152–83	20
52 weeks	–	–	–	–	–	–	–	–	–	–	–	–
Blood urea nitrogen (plasma) (mg/dL)												
8 weeks	24.2	18–27	54	27.1	19–35	30	20.0	13.7–26.3	22	17.0	13.6–20.4	20
16 weeks	26.7	18–22	30	22.3	16–29	30	24.2	19.3–29.1	20	20.9	16.0–25.8	20
26 weeks	–	–	–	27.8	23–33	4	22.1	14.4–29.8	8	24.6	17.2–32.0	8
52 weeks	26.2	21–31	8	26.8	21–32	6	21.0	14.9–27.1	7	–	–	–
Creatinine (mg/dL)												
8 weeks	–	–	–	–	–	–	–	–	–	–	–	–
16 weeks	–	–	–	–	–	–	–	–	–	–	–	–
26 weeks	–	–	–	–	–	–	–	–	–	–	–	–
52 weeks	–	–	–	–	–	–	–	–	–	–	–	–
Calcium (mg/dL)												
8 weeks	10.4	8.8–12.1	54	10.6	9.9–12.2	30	9.49	10.3–10.6	22	10.2	9.5–10.9	20
16 weeks	10.9	9.9–11.9	30	10.4	9.7–11.1	30	9.81	9.4–10.2	20	9.77	9.3–10.2	20
26 weeks	9.70	8.8–10.6	4	9.39	8.9–9.9	8	9.45	9.2–9.7	8	9.49	9.0–10.0	8
52 weeks	10.6	10.1–11.1	8	10.2	9.6–10.8	8	9.62	8.0–11.3	8	9.24	8.8–9.7	7
Phosphorus (mg/dL)												
8 weeks	10.3	5.7–14.9	54	10.3	6.5–14.1	30	8.99	6.3–11.7	22	9.46	7.5–11.4	20
16 weeks	9.26	6.7–11.8	30	10.0	7.0–13.0	30	7.92	4.8–11.1	20	7.11	5.1–9.2	20
26 weeks	7.02	6.2–7.0	4	7.24	5.2–9.3	8	5.41	4.4–6.4	8	5.91	4.6–7.2	8
52 weeks	6.86	5.6–8.1	8	6.77	5.4–8.1	8	5.53	1.4–9.7	8	5.31	4.0–6.6	7

(Continued)

TABLE 1.10 (*Continued*)
Clinical Chemistry Reference Ranges for C57BL/6 Inbred and BALB/c Inbred Laboratory Mice

	C57BL/6						BALB/c					
	Male			Female			Male			Female		
Bioanalyte	**Mean**	**2 SD**	***n***	**Mean**	**2 SD**	***n***	**Mean**	**2 SD**	***n***	**Mean**	**2 SD**	***n***
Total bilirubin (mg/dL)												
8 weeks	0.486	0.35–0.62	7	0.500	0.17–0.83	4	–	–	–	–	–	–
26 weeks	0.370	0.34–0.40	3	0.379	0.21–0.55	7	0.360	0.2–0.5	8	0.383	0.1–0.6	8
52 weeks	0.577	0.58–0.75	6	0.474	0.19–0.76	8	0.426	0.1–0.7	8	0.289	0.1–0.4	7
Cholesterol (mg/dL)												
8 weeks	100	76.2–123.8	54	79.2	61.5–96.9	30	78.0	63.5–92.5	22	80.0	64.3–95.7	20
16 weeks	93.3	72.9–113.7	30	69.8	57.7–81.9	30	113	91.2–134.8	20	68.9	54.7–83.1	20
52 weeks	–	–	–	–	–	–	–	–	–	–	–	–
Iron (mg/dL)												
8 weeks	–	–	–	–	–	–	–	–	–	–	–	–
26 weeks	124	110–138	4	156	59.6–252.4	8	241	200–282	8	253	200–306	8
52 weeks	171	108–234	7	178	104–252	8	197	82–312	8	205	172–238	7
Alkaline phosphatase (IU/L)												
8 weeks	–	–	–	–	–	–	–	–	–	–	–	–
26 weeks	68.2	60.3–76.1	4	95.1	48.7–141.5	8	78.1	71.2–85.0	8	88.5	69.6–107.4	8
52 weeks	83.5	63.1–103.9	8	129	45.4–212.6	8	80.1	30.9–129.3	8	77.1	43.5–110.7	8
Aspartate aminotransferase (IU/L)												
8 weeks	85.7	35.7–135.7	7	90.4	37.6–143.2	7	–	–	–	–	–	–
16 weeks	–	–	–	–	–	–	–	–	–	–	–	–
52 weeks	–	–	–	–	–	–	–	–	–	–	–	–

(*Continued*)

TABLE 1.10 (*Continued*)
Clinical Chemistry Reference Ranges for C57BL/6 Inbred and BALB/c Inbred Laboratory Mice

	C57BL/6						BALB/c					
	Male			Female			Male			Female		
Bioanalyte	**Mean**	**2 SD**	***n***	**Mean**	**2 SD**	***n***	**Mean**	**2 SD**	***n***	**Mean**	**2 SD**	***n***
Alanine aminotransferase (plasma) (IU/L)												
8 weeks	57.3	0–137.1	54	43.1	13.9–72.3	30	58.8	0–135.8	22	68.0	15.8–120.2	20
16 weeks	79.0	0–228.2	30	39.9	0–101.5	30	81.7	0–236.5	20	57.5	0–138.1	20
26 weeks	–	–	–	31.0	24.7–37.3	4	57.1	16.9–97.3	8	44.8	15.2–74.4	8
52 weeks	34.8	16.4–53.2	8	43.4	36.7–50.1	5	46.4	25.6–67.2	8	–	–	–
Creatine kinase (IU/L)												
8 weeks	799	0–2021	52	720	0–1810	30	428	0–1002	22	768	0–1752	20
16 weeks	601	61–1141	30	358	0–986	30	443	0–903	20	609	0–1441	20
52 weeks	–	–	–	–	–	–	–	–	–	–	–	–
Lipase (IU/L)												
8 weeks	–	–	–	–	–	–	–	–	–	–	–	–
26 weeks (plasma)	92.0	52.6–131.4	4	98.8	58.2–139.4	4	71.4	58.3–84.5	8	81.8	61.2–102.4	8
52 weeks (plasma)	57.4	39.4–75.4	8	74.3	50.3–98.3	7	51.4	40.7–62.1	8	–	–	–
Sodium (mEq/L)												
8 weeks	–	–	–	–	–	–	–	–	–	–	–	–
26 weeks	150	135–165	4	150	143–157	8	155	151–159	8	159	153–165	6
52 weeks	154	149–159	8	148	144–152	8	151	143–159	8	154	148–160	8
Potassium (mEq/L)												
8 weeks	–	–	–	–	–	–	–	–	–	–	–	–
26 weeks	5.17	4.9–5.4	4	6.33	5.5–7.1	8	6.85	5.7–8.0	8	7.11	5.5–8.8	8
52 weeks	5.62	4.4–6.8	8	5.51	4.7–6.3	8	6.79	4.9–8.7	8	6.20	5.2–7.2	8

(*Continued*)

TABLE 1.10 (*Continued*)
Clinical Chemistry Reference Ranges for C57BL/6 Inbred and BALB/c Inbred Laboratory Mice

	C57BL/6						BALB/c					
	Male			Female			Male			Female		
Bioanalyte	**Mean**	**2 SD**	***n***	**Mean**	**2 SD**	***n***	**Mean**	**2 SD**	***n***	**Mean**	**2 SD**	***n***
Chloride (mEq/L)												
8 weeks	–	–	–	–	–	–	–	–	–	–	–	–
26 weeks	111	99–123	4	121	114–128	8	119	117–121	8	123	112–134	8
52 weeks	112	107–117	8	114	109–119	8	114	107–121	8	116	112–120	8
Total protein (plasma) (g/dL)												
8 weeks	6.04	4.9–7.1	54	6.09	5.2–7.0	30	5.38	4.9–5.8	22	5.70	5.1–6.3	20
16 weeks	6.41	5.8–7.0	30	6.39	5.5–7.3	30	5.91	5.5–6.3	20	5.60	5.2–6.0	20
26 weeks	–	–	–	5.82	5.4–6.2	4	5.74	5.4–6.1	8	5.77	5.4–6.1	8
52 weeks	5.91	5.4–6.5	8	6.14	5.6–6.7	8	5.50	5.2–5.8	8	–	–	–
Albumin (g/dL)												
8 weeks	3.69	2.9–4.5	54	3.89	3.4–4.4	30	3.21	2.9–3.5	22	3.78	3.4–4.1	20
16 weeks	3.94	3.5–4.4	30	4.22	3.7–4.7	30	2.70	2.5–2.9	20	2.77	2.5–3.0	20
26 weeks	–	–	–	2.98	2.9–3.1	4	2.73	2.5–2.9	8	2.81	2.6–3.0	8
52 weeks	3.80	3.4–4.2	8	3.97	3.6–4.4	6	3.38	3.1–3.6	8	–	–	–
Globulin (g/dL)												
8 weeks	–	–	–	–	–	–	–	–	–	–	–	–
16 weeks	–	–	–	–	–	–	–	–	–	–	–	–
52 weeks	–	–	–	–	–	–	–	–	–	–	–	–
A/G ratio												
8 weeks	–	–	–	–	–	–	–	–	–	–	–	–
16 weeks	–	–	–	–	–	–	–	–	–	–	–	–
52 weeks	–	–	–	–	–	–	–	–	–	–	–	–

Source: Various Investigators, May 15, 2010, *Blood Chemistry Data*. Mouse Phenome Database website, Bar Harbor, Maine, The Jackson Laboratory,. http://phenome.jax.org/db/q?rtn=meas/catlister&req=Cblood+chemistry.

All values are performed on nonfasting animals and on serum, unless otherwise noted. Site and method of collection unspecified.

TABLE 1.11
Urine Chemistry Data for Several Strains of Laboratory Mice

Bioanalyte	Value	Units
Urine output (Jung et al., 2003; Takahasi et al., 2007; Yang and Bankir et al., 2005)	1.3-2.0	mL/day
pH (Kovacikova et al., 2006)	5.0–6.6	~
Specific gravity (Luong, 2009)	1.022–1.048	~
Osmolality (Takahasi et al., 2007)	1919–2650	mOsm/kgH_2O
Creatinine (Qi et al., 2004)	372–462	µg/day
Glucose (Luong, 2007)	0.5–3.2	mg/day
Protein (Luong, 2007)	0.5–2.7	mg/day
Urea (Yang and Bankir, 2005)	130	mmol/day/kg body weight
Sodium (Jung et al., 2003; Yang and Bankir, 2005)	0.15–0.29	mmol/day
Potassium (Jung et al., 2003)	0.34–0.37	mmol/day
Chloride (Jung et al., 2003)	0.28–0.34	mmol/day
Glomerular filtration rate	~	~
Creatinine clearance (Takahasi et al., 2007)	302–346	µL/min
FITC-labeled inulin clearance (Qi et al., 2004)	283–351	µL/min

Sources: Jung, J.Y. et al., *Am J Physiol Renal Physiol.*, 285, 1210–24, 2003; Kovacikova, J. et al., *Kidney Intl.*, 70, 1706–1716, 2003; Luong, R. 2009. Unpublished data; Qi, Z. et al., *Am J Physiol Renal Physiol.*, 286, F590–F596, 2004; Takahasi, N. et al. *Kidney Intl.*, 71, 266–271, 2007; Yang, B. and Bankir, L. *Am J Physiol Renal Physiol.*, 288, F881–F896, 2005.

REFERENCES

Abaton, O.I., Welch, K.B., and Nemzek, J.A. 2008. Evaluation of saphenous venipuncture and modified tail-clip blood collection in mice. *J Am Assoc Lab Anim Sci.* 47:8–15.

Altholtz, L.Y., La Perle, K.M.D., and Quimby, F.W. 2006. Dose-dependent hypothyroidism in mice induced by commercial trimethoprim-sulfamethoxazole rodent feed. *Comp Med.* 56:395–401.

Argmann, C.A. and Auwerx, J. 2006a. Collection of blood and plasma from the mouse. *Curr Protoc Mol Biol.* S75:29A.3.1–29A.3.4.

Argmann, C.A., Houten, S.M., Champy, M.F., et al. 2006b. Lipid and bile acid analysis. *Curr Protoc Mol Biol.* S75:29B.2.1–29B.2.24.

Besch, E.L. 1985. Definition of laboratory animal environmental conditions. In *Animal Stress*. Ed. G.P. Moberg, pp. 297–315. Bethesda, MD: American Physiological Society.

Borovkov, A. and Svirdov, S. 1975. Albumin content in blood of inbred mice strains. *Genetika.* 17:1690–1692.

Boyd, J.W. 1983. The mechanisms relating to increases in plasma enzymes and isoenzymes in diseases of animals. *Vet Clin Pathol.* 12:9–24.

Brewer, N.R. 1986. A note about histidine. *Synapse.* 19:12.

Buitrago, S., Martin, T.E., Tetens-Woodring, J., et al. 2008. Safety and efficacy of various combinations of injectable anesthetics in BALB/c mice. *J Am Assoc Lab Anim Sci.* 47:11–17.

Cederroth, C.R., Vinciguerra, M., Gjinovci, A. 2008. Dietary phytoestrogens activate AMP-activated protein kinase with improvement in lipid and glucose metabolism. *Diabetes.* 57:1176–1185.

Chance, M.R.A. 1947. Factors influencing the toxicity of sympathomimetic amines to solitary mice. *J Pharmacol Exp Ther.* 89:289–296.

Charles River Laboratories Research Models and Services. 2005. *Charles River—CD-1 and CF-1 Mice: Baseline Hematology and Clinical Chemistry Values as a Function of Sex and Age*. Wilmington, MA: Charles River, Epub 2005 Nov 11. Available at: http://www.criver.com/SiteCollectionDocuments/rm_rm_r_hematology_sex_age_outbred_mice.pdf. May 15, 2010.

Chuang, T. and Luo, J. 1997. Influence of blood collection sites and use of anesthesia on plasma glucose concentration in mice. *Contemp Top Lab Anim Sci.* 36:64–65.

Clapham, J.C., Arch, J.R.S., Chapman, H., et al. 2000. Mice overexpressing human uncoupling protein-3 in skeletal muscle are hyperphagic and lean. *Nature.* 406:415–418.

Cohen, A.M., Ohnishi, T., Clark, N.M., et al. 2007. Investigations of rodent urinary bladder carcinogens: collection, processing, and evaluation of urine and bladders. *Toxicol Pathol.* 35:337–47.

Davis, J.A. 2008. Mouse and rat anesthesia and analgesia. *Curr Protoc Neurosci.* (Suppl 42):A.4B.1–A.4B.21.

Diehl, K.H., Hull, R., Morton, D., et al. 2001. A good practice guide to the administration of substances and removal of blood, including routes and volumes. *J Appl Toxicol.* 21:15–23.

Donovan, J. and Brown, B. 2005. Blood collection. *Currt Protoc Neurosci.* S33:A.4G.1–A.4G.9.

Dunnington, E.A., White, J.M., and Vinson, W.E. 1981. Selection for serum cholesterol, voluntary physical activity, 56-day body weight, and feed intake in random bred mice. II. Correlated response. *Can J Genet Cytol.* 23:545–555.

Edwardson, J.A. and Hough, C.A.M. 1975. The pituitary-adrenal system of the genetically obese mouse. *J Endocrinol.* 65:99–107.

Falk, H.B., Schroer, R.A., Novak, J.J., et al. 1981. The effect of freezing on various serum chemistry parameters of common laboratory animals. *Clin Chem.* 27:1039–1041.

Fernandez, M.L. and Volek, J.S. 2006. Guinea pigs: A suitable animal model to study lipoprotein metabolism, atherosclerosis and inflammation. *Nutr Metab.* 3:17.

Foster, R.G. and Hankins, M.W. 2002. Non-rod, non-cone photoreception in the vertebrates. *Prog Retin Eye Res.* 21:507–527.

Foster, R.G., Provencio, I., Hudson, D., et al. 1991. Circadian photoreception in the retinally degenerate mouse (rd/rd). *J Comp Physiol A Neuroethol Sens Neural Behav Physiol.* 169:39–50.

Frith, C.H., Suber, R.L., and Umholtz, R. 1980. Hematologic and clinical chemistry findings in control BALB/c and C57BL/6 mice. *Lab Anim Sci.* 30:835–840.

Goldman, A.S., Katsumata, M., Yaffe S.J., et al. 1977. Palatal cytosol cortisol-binding protein associated with cleft palate susceptibility and H-2 genotype. *Nature.* 265:643–645.

Goldman, M.B. and Goldman J.N. 1976. Relationship in the functional levels of early components of complement to the H-2 complex of mice. *J Immunol.* 117:1584–1588.

Greenman, D.L., Fullerton, F., Gough, B., et al. 1982. Clinical chemistry and hematology of mice: A comparison of cereal-based and semipurified diets. *Lab Anim Sci.* 32:414.

Halberg, F., Galichich, J.H., and Ungar, F. 1965. Circadian rhythmic pituitary adrenocorticotropic activity, rectal temperature, and pinnal mitosis of starving, dehydrated c mice. *P Soc Exp Biol Med.* 118:414–419.

Heikkinen, S., Argmann, C.A., Champy, M.F., et al. 2007. Evaluation of glucose homeostasis. *Curr Protoc Mol Biol.* S77:29B.3.1–29B.3.22.

Henry, J.B., Davey, F.R., Herman, C.J., et al. 2001. *Clinical Diagnosis and Management by Laboratory Methods*, 20th edition. Philadelphia, PA: Saunders.

Hiroyama, M., Aoyagi, T., Fujiwara, Y., et al. 2007. Hyperammonaemia in V1a vasopressin receptor knockout mice caused by the promoted proteolysis and reduced intrahepatic blood volume. *J Physiol.* 581:1183–1192.

Holinka, C.F., Tseng, Y.C., and Finch, C.E. 1979. Impaired preparturitional rise of plasma estradiol in aging C57BL/6J mice. *Biol Reprod.* 21:1009–1013.

Hurwitz, A, Fischer, H.R., Innis, J.D., et al. 1985. Opioid effects on hepatic disposition of dyes in mice. *J Pharmacol Exp Ther.* 232:617–623.

Ivanyi, P., Hampl, R., Starka, L., et al. 1972. Genetic association between H-2 gene and testosterone metabolism in mice. *Nature (New Biology).* 238:280–282.

Jensen, M.M. and Rasmussen, A F. 1963. Stress and susceptibility to viral infection. *J Immunol.* 90:17–20.

Jung, J.Y., Madsen, K.M., Han, K.H., et al. 2003. Expression of urea transporters in potassium-depleted mouse kidney. *Am J Physiol Renal Physiol.* 285:1210–1224.

Kessler, M.S., Murgatroyd, C., Bunck, M., et al. 2007. Diabetes insipidus and, partially, low anxiety-related behaviour are linked to a SNP-associated vasopressin deficit in LAB mice. *Eur J Neurosci.* 26:2857–2864.

Kim, E. and Young, S.G. 1998. Genetically modified mice for the study of apolipoprotein B. *J Lipid Res.* 39:703–723.

Kovacikova, J., Winter, C., Loffing-Cueni, D., et al. 2006. The connecting tubule is the main site of the furosemide-induced urinary acidification by the vacuolar H+-ATPase. *Kidney Int.* 70:1706–1716.

Krieger, D.T. 1979. Rhythms in CRF, ACTH, and corticosteroids. In *Endocrine Rhythms.* Ed. D.T. Krieger, pp. 123–142. New York, NY: Raven Press.

Laber, K., Veatch, L.M., Lopez, M.F., et al. 2008. Effects of housing density on weight gain, immune function, behavior, and plasma corticosterone concentrations in BALB/c and C57BL/6 mice. *J Am Assoc Lab Anim Sci.* 47:16–23.

Lake, J. 2009. Complement C5 deficiency in inbred mouse strains. *J Immunol.* 182:134.61.

Landi, M., Kreider, J.W., Lang, C.M., et al. 1982. Effect of shipping on the immune function of mice. *Am J Vet Res.* 43:1654–1657.

Landi, M., Kreider, J.W., Lang, C.M., et al. 1985. Effect of shipping on the immune functions of mice. In *The Contribution of Laboratory Animal Science to the Welfare of Man and Animals*, Eds. J. Archibald, J. Ditchfield, and H.C. Rowsell, pp. 11–18. Stuttgart: Gustav Fischer Verlag.

Latimer, K.S., Mahaffey, E.A., and Prasse, K.W. 2003. *Duncan and Prasse's Veterinary Laboratory Medicine Clinical Pathology*, 4th edition. Ames, IA: Iowa Stress Press.

Laviola, G., Adriani, W., Morley-Fletcher, S., et al. 2002. Peculiar response of adolescent mice to acute and chronic stress and to amphetamine: Evidence of sex differences. *Behav Brain Res.* 130:117–125.

Lindsey, J.R., Conner, M.W., and Baker, H.J. 1978. Physical, chemical, and microbial factors affecting biologic response. In *Laboratory Animal Housing*. Eds. E.L. Besch, H.L. Foster, S.J. Goldstein, et al., pp. 31–43. Washington, DC: National Academy of Sciences.

Loeb, W.F. 1997. Clinical biochemistry of laboratory rodents and rabbits. In *Clinical Biochemistry of Domestic Animals*. Eds. J.J. Kaneko, J.W. Harvey, and M.L. Brass, pp. 845–899. San Diego, CA: Academic Press.

Loeb, W.F. 1998. Personal correspondence.

Loeb, W.F., Das, S.R., Harbour, L.S, et al. 1996. Clinical biochemistry. In *Pathobiology of the Aging Mouse*. Eds. U. Mohr, D.L. Dungworth, C.C. Capan, W.W. Carlton, J.P. Sundberg, and J.M. Ward, pp. 3–19. Washington, DC: ILSI Press.

Lusis, A.J. 2000. Atherosclerosis. *Nature.* 407:233–241.

MacLeod, J.N. and Shapiro, B.H. 1988. Repetitive blood sampling in unrestrained and unstressed mice using a chronic indwelling right atrial catheterization apparatus. *Lab Anim Sci.* 38:603–608.

Maier, S.M., Gross, J.K., Hamlin, K.L, et al. 2007. Proteinuria of nonautoimmune origin in wild-type FVB/NJ mice. *Comp Med.* 57:255–266.

Meade, C.J. and Gore, V.A. 1982. An H-2-associated difference in murine serum cholesterol levels. *Experientia.* 38:1106–1107.

McGill, B.E., Bundle, S.F., Yaylaoglu, M.B., et al. 2006. Enhanced anxiety and stress-induced corticosterone release are associated with increased *Crh* expression in a mouse model of Rett syndrome. *Proc Natl Acad Sci USA.* 103:18267–18272.

Morrisett, J.D., Kim, H.S., Patsch, J.R., et al. 1982. Genetic susceptibility and resistance to diet-induced atherosclerosis and hyperlipoproteinemia. *Arteriosclerosis.* 2:312–324.

Muglia, L.J., Jacobson, L., Luedke, C., et al. 2000. The physiology of corticotrophin-releasing hormone deficiency in mice. *J Clin Invest.* 105:1269–1277.

Muglia, L.J., Jacobson, L., Weninger, S.C., et al. 2001. Corticotropin-releasing hormone links pituitary adrenocorticotropin gene expression and release during adrenal insufficiency. *Peptides.* 22:725–731.

National Center for Research Resources. 2004. *Accelerating and Enhancing Research from Basic Discovery to Improved Patient Care*. Available at: http://www.ncrr.nih.gov/publications/about_ncrr/brochure.pdf

O'Brien, P.J., Dameron, G.W., Beck, M.L., et al. 1997. Cardiac troponin T is a sensitive, specific biomarker of cardiac injury in laboratory animals. *Lab Anim Sci.* 47:486–495.

Ottenweller, J.E., Meier, A.H., Russo, A.C., et al. 1979. Circadian rhythms of plasma corticosterone binding activity in the rat and mouse. *Acta Endocrinol.* 91:150–157.

Paigen, K. 2003a. One hundred years of mouse genetics: An intellectual history: I. The classical period (1902–1980). *Genetics.* 163:1–7.

Paigen, K. 2003b. One hundred years of mouse genetics: An intellectual history: II. The molecular revolution (1981–2002). *Genetics.* 163:1227–1235.

Parker, C.J., Riess, G.T., and Sardesai, V.M. 1985. Essentiality of histidine in adult mice. *J Nutr.* 115:824–826.

Patrick, D.H., Werner, R.M., and Lewis, L.L. 1983. Clinical chemistry values of the N: NIH(S) mice and parameter variations due to sampling techniques. *Lab Anim Sci.* 33:504.

Percy, D.H. and Barthold, S.W. 2007. Mouse. In *Pathology of Laboratory Rodents and Rabbits*, pp. 3–125. Iowa: Blackwell Publishing.

Pickering C.E. and Pickering R.G. 1984. Alkaline phosphatase activity of the mouse. *Comp Biochem Physiol C.* 79:417–424.

Plagemann, P.G., Rowland, R.R., Even, C., et al. 1995. Lactate dehydrogenase-elevating virus: An ideal persistent virus? *Springer Semin Immun.* 17:167–186.

Qi, Z., Whitt, I., Mehta, A., et al. 2004. Serial determination of glomerular filtration rate in conscious mice using FITC-inulin clearance. *Am J Physiol Renal Physiol.* 286:F590–F596.

Rader, K. 2004. *Making Mice: Standardizing Animals for American Biomedical Research, 1900–1955.* Princeton, NJ: Princeton University Press.

Ridder, A., Chourbaji, S., Hellweg, R., et al. 2005. Mice with genetically altered glucocorticoid receptor expression show altered sensitivity for stress-induced depressive reactions. *J Neurosci.* 25:6243–6250.

Riley, V., Spackman, D.H., Santisteban, G.A., et al. 1978. The LDH virus: an interfering biological contaminant. *Science.* 200:124–126.

Scheving, L.E., Tsai, T.H., Powell, E.W., et al. 1983. Bilateral lesions in the suprachiasmatic nuclei affect circadian rhythms and H-thymidine incorporation into deoxyribonucleic acid in mouse intestinal tract, mitotic index of corneal epithelium, and serum corticosterone. *Anat Rec.* 205:239–249.

Serrano, L.J. 1971. Carbon dioxide and ammonia in mouse cages: Effects of cage covers, population, and activity. *Lab Anim Sci.* 21:75–85.

Scrofano, M.M., Jahngen-Hodge, J., Nowell Jr., T.R., et al. 1998. The effects of aging and calorie restriction on plasma nutrient levels in male and female Emory mice. *Mech Ageing Dev.* 105:31–44.

Serfilippi, L.M., Pallman, D.R., and Russell, B. 2003. Serum clinical chemistry and hematology reference values in outbred stocks of albino mice from three commonly used vendors and two inbred strains of albino mice. *Contemp Top Lab Anim Sci.* 42:46–52.

Spackman, D.H. and Riley, V. 1978. Corticosterone concentrations in the mouse. *Science.* 200:87.

Takahasi, N., Boysen, G., Li, F., et al. 2007. Tandem mass spectrometry measurements of creatinine in mouse plasma and urine for determining glomerular filtration rate. *Kidney Int.* 71:266–271.

Terpstra, A.H. 2001. Differences between humans and mice in efficacy of the body fat lowering effect of conjugated linoleic acid: Role of metabolic rate. *J Nutr.* 131:2067–2068.

Tsunematsu, T., Fu, L.Y., Yamanaka, A., et al. 2008. Vasopressin increases locomotion through a V1a receptor in orexin/hypocretin neurons: Implications for water homeostasis. *J Neurosci.* 28:228–238.

Various Investigators. May 15, 2010. *Blood Chemistry Data.* Mouse Phenome Database website. Bar Harbor, ME: The Jackson Laboratory. Available at: http://phenome.jax.org/db/q?rtn=meas/catlister&req=Cblood+chemistry.

Watterson, C., Lanevschi, A., Horner, J., et al. 2009. A comparative analysis of acute-phase proteins as inflammatory biomarkers in preclinical toxicology studies: Implications for preclinical to clinical translation. *Toxicolo Pathol.* 37:28–33.

Weingand, K., Bloom, J., Carakostas, M., et al. 1992. Clnical pathology testing recommendations for nonclinical toxicity and safety studies. AACC-DACC/ASVCP Joint Task Force. *Toxicol Pathol.* 20:539–543.

Wiedmeyer, C.E., Ruben, D., and Franklin, C. 2007. Complete blood count, clinical chemistry, and serology profile by using a single tube of whole blood from mice. *J Am Assoc Lab Anim Sci.* 47:16–23.

Williams, E.A., Perkins, S.N., Smith, N.C.P., et al. 2007. Carbohydrates versus energy restriction: Effects on weight loss, body composition and metabolism. *Ann Nutr Metab.* 51:232–243.

Woodman, D.D. 1997. *Laboratory Animal Endocrinology.* West Sussex: John Wiley and Sons, Ltd.

Yamada, M., Saga, Y., Shibusawa, N., et al. 1997. Tertiary hypothyroidism and hyperglycemia in mice with targeted disruption of the thyrotropin-releasing hormone gene. *P Natl Acad Sci USA.* 94:10862–10867.

Yang, B. and Bankir, L. 2005. Urea and urine collecting ability: New insights from studies of mice. *Am J Physiol Renal Physiol.* 288:F881–F896.

Young, A. 2005. Effects on plasma glucose and lactate. *Adv Pharmacol.* 52:193–208.

2 The Laboratory Rat

Nancy E. Everds and Lila Ramaiah

CONTENTS

2.1 INTRODUCTION

The laboratory rat is one of the most extensively used animal models in biomedical research. A recent PubMed search of the National Library of Medicine indicated that more than 36,000 articles concerning rats were published in a single year. Rats are second only to mice in terms of numbers of animals used in biomedical research. Nevertheless, more than 50% scientific articles are published about rats than mice (Hendrich, 2006). Much of the research conducted on rats uses clinical chemistry parameters as important endpoints because they enable correlation of clinical signs and histopathology and are highly translatable to studies conducted in humans. Clinical chemistry endpoints constitute widely accepted and accessible first-tier biomarkers. A selection of important research areas and examples of rat models are listed in Table 2.1. Several recent reviews that include information concerning clinical chemistry of laboratory rats are available (Car et al., 2006; Evans, 2009; Peterino et al., 2006; Gosselin et al., 2009).

Rats have a number of attributes that make them particularly useful as animal models for biomedical research. They are generally healthy and robust research animals, have tolerance to manipulations (e.g., telemetry, implantation, catheterization, cannulation), and are easily trained for use in behavioral, cognitive, and neurological research. Rats are less expensive to maintain than other larger species such as rabbits, dogs, sheep, or pigs, and are more suitable for chronic or aging studies

TABLE 2.1
Important Rat Research Areas Using Clinical Chemistry as Key Endpoints

System	Models or Diseases	Rat Model
Gastrointestinal	Protein losing enteropathy, digestion	Many
Stress	Restraint stress, repeated variable stress, conditional stress	Many
Nutritional	Zucker obese rat, caloric restriction	Zucker Diabetic Fatty (ZDF)
Protein biochemistry	Analbuminemic rats	Nagase analbuminemic rats
Hepatology	Toxicity, regeneration	Many
Endocrinology	Type II diabetes	Zucker Diabetic Fatty (ZDF), Cohen diabetic rat, Toto-Kakizaki (GK)
	Type I diabetes	Biomedical Research Models BBDP, BBDP/Wor
	Hypercholesterolemia	EXHC
	Hyperlipemia	FCH
Neurologic	Epilepsy, experimental autoimmune encephalitis	Genetically Epilepsy-Prone Rats (GEPR/3, GEPR-9), WAG/Rij; EAE rats (Lewis, Dark Agouti)
Pulmonary	Asthma	Brown Norway
Renal	Polycystic kidney disease, compensatory renal hyperplasia	CyCy strain of Han:SPRD; CRJ:CD (SD) BR (Japan)
Acid/base	Acid loading, base loading	Many
Inflammation	Interleukin, acute phase, cytokine research	Many
Cardiovascular	Hypertension	Spontaneous hypertension (SHR) Obese spontaneously hypertensive (SHROB) Spontaneous hypertensive heart failure (SHHF) Fawn hooded hypertensive (FHH) Dahl/salt-sensitive (DSS)
	Stroke	SHR/stroke-prone (SHR/SP)
Toxicology	Acute, screening, and long-term toxicity and carcinogenicity	Wistar, Sprague-Dawley (SD) Fischer 344
Oncology	Prostate cancer	Noble (NBL)
	Pituitary tumors	Wistar Furth Rat (WF)
	Leukemia	AKR
Bone biology	Ovariectomized rat for osteoporosis	Many
Aging/gerontology		F344, BN, F344BNF1 hybrid
Immunodeficient	Nude athymic	Nude (NIH-Foxn1)
Ophthalmology	Cornea, lens, and retinal disorders	Many, RCS rat

Source: Reprinted from *The Laboratory Rat, 2nd edition,* Owens, D.R, Spontaneous, surgically, and chemically induced models of disease, pp. 711–732, Copyright (2006), with permission from **Elsevier**.

owing to their shorter lifespan. Compared to mice, the larger size of rats makes them easy to handle, and amenable to surgical procedures and functional studies. In addition, larger volumes of rat blood can be collected on multiple occasions, such that several parameters can be evaluated over time on a single animal. Disadvantages of rats compared to mice include higher expense of husbandry, longer generation time, greater quantities of test article required to achieve an equivalent mg/kg body weight dose, and very limited availability of rats with targeted mutations (e.g., transgenic, knock-in, and knock-out strains).

Rats are classified as outbred stocks and inbred strains. Commonly used outbred stocks include Sprague-Dawley and Wistar rats. Outbred stocks are closed colonies of more or less genetically heterogenous animals bred to maintain maximum heterozygosity by minimizing inbreeding. Because each animal is genetically unique, outbred stocks more accurately mimic the genetic variability in the human population than inbred strains. In addition, outbred stocks are considered to be more robust than inbred strains, since they tend not to suffer from inbreeding depression that results from increased homozygosity. Examples include differences in life spans, disease resistance, reproductive capacity, growth rate, and size. However, these stocks are also genetically undefined and experimental designs necessitate larger sample sizes than inbred strains due to interindividual genetic variability of outbred stocks.

Rat strains and stocks exhibit drift in physical and physiologic characteristics over time, affecting attributes including weight, growth rate, fertility, and lifespan. This drift occurs in both inbred and outbred rats but is more pronounced in outbred stocks particularly if small populations are maintained as the stock becomes partially inbred with resultant loss of heterozygosity. Effects can be minimized by regularly migrating breed stocks within a given outbred colony. Unless breed stock is regularly migrated among extant colonies of a given stock, drift will occur among various breeding facilities of a given supplier. For example, differences in incidence of chronic progressive nephrosis in Sprague-Dawley rats from different breeders may affect the interpretation of nephrotoxicity (Palm, 1998). Genetic drift, as well as changes in reagent systems and instrumentation, may affect the clinical pathology parameters. Because of the effects of drift in physiologic characteristics and changes in analytic procedures, relevant reference intervals for clinical chemistry parameters should include data collected from animals from a single supplier over a time span within a few years of the data being evaluated.

Inbred strains are genetically uniform strains originating from at least 20 consecutive brother-to-sister matings and maintained by continued brother-to-sister mating. In contrast to outbred stocks, properly maintained inbred strains are genetically uniform. Their defined and uniform genetic background minimizes interindividual variability in results. In addition, the inherent susceptibility or resistance of an inbred strain to a particular disease may make them ideal animal models for a wide variety of diseases. However, inbred strains are more prone to strain-specific phenotypes and lesions due to fixation of homozygous traits. Commonly used inbred strains include Brown Norway, Fischer 344, and Lewis rats. Lines of inbred strains separated for more than 10 generations of brother-to-sister inbreeding will show evidence of drift and are considered to be substrains.

Congenic strains are a type of inbred strain in which the genetic locus or phenotype from one inbred strain is introduced into the genome of another inbred strain by a series of selective backcrosses followed by 20 consecutive brother-to-sister matings. Consomic strains are similar to congenic strains, but an entire chromosome (rather than a fraction of a chromosome) is replaced in the inbred strain's genome. In addition, a few recombinant inbred rat strains have been developed. Related sets of recombinant inbred rat strains are studied in conjunction for identifying the location and linkage of polygenic traits (Hedrich, 2006).

Nomenclature for rat genes, strains, and stocks follows a standardized system, which allows quick recognition of the type of rat under consideration. This system is organized by the Rat Genome and Nomenclature Committee (RGNC) and curated by the Rat Genome Database. For outbred rat stocks, the first part of the name indicates the registered laboratory (e.g., Han, Crl, Hsd, Tac). The laboratory code is followed by a colon and then the specific stock name in uppercase letters. Thus, Crl:SD is the Charles River Sprague-Dawley. For inbred strains, the rules for rats are similar to those for mice. These detailed rules can be found at the website http://rgd.mcw.edu/nomen/nomen.shtml#StrainNomenclature (accessed on 9 August 2009). Further explanation about inbred strain nomenclature and extensive lists of rat strains can be found in Suckow et al. (2006), as well as vendor websites and publicly available databases (http://www.informatics.jax.org/external/festing/rat/STRAINS.shtml). Selected examples of some common spontaneous mutant or

TABLE 2.2
Examples of Strains and Stocks of Laboratory Rats

Inbred Rats	Outbred Rats	Hybrid Rats	Mutant Rats	Congenic Rats
Brown Norway	Sprague-Dawley	FBNF1/Hsd	Athymic Nude	PVG.DA-RT1^av1
Fischer 344	Wistar	LBNF1/Hsd	DPPIV Deficient	PVG.AO-RT1^u
Lewis	Long-Evans	DALF1/OlaHsd	HIV-1 Zucker	PVG.R8/OlaHsd
SHR		WAGBNF1/RijHsd	Dwarf-4	
Dahl Salt-Sensitive/ Resistant		WAGBUFF1		
Wistar Furth				
Wistar Kyoto				

genetically modified strains are provided in Table 2.1, and examples of common stocks and strains used in laboratory research are provided in Table 2.2.

2.2 HISTORY OF LABORATORY RATS

The modern laboratory rat is considered to be derived from naturally occurring albino mutants of the wild Norway rat (*Rattus norvegicus*), which originated in China but is now found on all continents except Antarctica. Albino Norway rats were bred in the nineteenth century as show animals and eventually became utilized in research laboratories. Brief histories of four commonly used stocks and strains are presented below:

- Wistar rats are outbred rats that originated from albino Norway rats transported from the University of Chicago to the Wistar Institute in Pennsylvania. Currently, Wistar rats contribute to more strains and stocks of rats than other type of rat.
- Sprague-Dawley rats are outbred rats originating from a white Wistar female and a hooded male that is half-white. The male was subsequently bred to females of successive generations of offspring. The colony was the basis on which Sprague-Dawley Inc. was established. The Crl:CD rat was developed in the 1950s from cesarean-derived SD rats.
- Lewis rats are inbred rats that were originated by Dr. Margaret Lewis in her laboratory at the Wistar Institute in the 1920s.
- Fischer 344 or F344 rats are albino inbred rats that originated in the lab of Curtiss and Dunning at the Columbia University Institute for Cancer Research in 1920. The colony eventually was migrated to the National Institutes of Health (NIH) in 1951 (Lindsay and Baker, 2006).

2.3 ANATOMIC AND PHYSIOLOGIC CHARACTERISTICS OF LABORATORY RATS

Laboratory rats, like several rodent species, are nocturnal. Laboratory rats breed throughout the year with a gestation period of approximately 21–23 days. Puberty is highly variable among strains with reports ranging from 40 to 70 days of age. While rats reach full sexual maturity at a young age (approximately 7–10 weeks of age), growth continues past sexual maturity for both males and females (Creasy, 2003; Mitchell and Creasy, 2007). The lifespan of a laboratory rat ranges from 2.5 to 3 years. Rats are social animals and will sleep together with cage mates.

Although wild rats are omnivores, laboratory diets for rats usually contain vegetable protein and no animal protein. Dietary protein exceeding 12%–15% has been associated with chronic nephropathy in rats (Keenan et al., 2000). The use of fish protein in rat chow has declined in Europe but may still occur in Japan.

Anatomic and physiologic features unique to rats must be considered when interpreting clinical chemistry endpoints. While thorough descriptions of these can be observed in textbooks such as The Laboratory Rat (Suckow et al., 2006), a short list of some rat peculiarities that influence clinical chemistry results is presented below:

- **Growth/maturation**: Rats have slow bone maturation compared to other mammals, with ossification occurring after 1 year of age. Peak growth rates occur at 7 weeks of age. Androgens, which help to maintain skeletal integrity, decline in aged nongrowing rats, resulting in accelerated bone turnover and osteopenia.
- **External ophthalmic veins:** In contrast to the mouse, which has an orbital venous *sinus* in the retro-orbital space, the rat has an orbital venous *plexus* formed by numerous anastomoses between the dorsal and ventral external ophthalmic veins (Timm, 1979).
- **Stomach:** Rats are unable to vomit owing to a limiting ridge that separates the forestomach from the glandular stomach. Gastric secretions in the rat are limited to pepsinogen C and Cathepsin D and E, in contrast to other species that also secrete pepsinogen A (Senoo, 2000).
- **Alkaline phosphatase (ALP)**: In rats, serum ALP activity is composed of activities from liver/bone isoenzymes and intestinal isoenzymes (Hoffmann et al., 1994). The liver and bone isoforms of ALP are products of the same gene (tissue nonspecific ALP isoenzyme) differing by posttranslational modifications. The intestinal and bone isoforms predominate in serum of rats, in contrast to other species, in which the liver isoform of ALP predominates. This results in more prominent effects on ALP due to feeding (intestinal) and body mass or growth (bone).
- **Amylase**: The rat has four salivary and liver amylase isozymes and two pancreatic amylase isozymes (Robinovitch and Sreebny, 1972). Amylase is present at higher concentrations in the salivary gland in rats and mice than that in other laboratory animals. Considerations for an increase in amylase include increases in food consumption and sialadenosis (Arglebe et al., 1978; Nagy et al., 2001; Proctor et al., 1990).
- **Insulin**: The rat has two nonallelic genes coding for insulin, and two proinsulins, whereas other species studied have one (Evans, 2009).
- **Acute phase proteins:** α-2 macroglobulin (A2MG), α-1 acid glycoprotein (AGP or A1AG), and thiostatin (α_1-major acute protein) are the major acute phase proteins in the rat (Gentry, 1999; Watterson, 2009).
- **Liver**: Gamma-glutamyltransferase (GGT) and total bilirubin concentrations are low to undetectable (depending on methodology) in the rat. Microsomal induction has been associated with decreased and increased serum liver enzymes in rats (Smith et al., 2002). The rat has no gall bladder. Biliary ducts from each hepatic lobe join to form the common bile duct and empty directly into the descending duodenum. Unlike species with gall bladders, the bile of rats is not concentrated and stored during periods of fasting.
- **Lipid profile:** In contrast to humans and nonhuman primates, high-density lipoproteins (HDL) cholesterol predominates over low-density lipoproteins (LDL) cholesterol in rats (Kieft et al., 1991). This may be due to the absence of cholesteryl ester transfer protein (CETP) in the rat (Guyard-Dangremont et al., 1998; Turk and Laughlin, 2004).
- **Corticosteroid:** Corticosterone, as opposed to cortisol, is the predominant form of corticosteroid in the rat and mouse (Rosol et al., 2001).

- **Thyroid hormone:** In the rat (and mouse), thyroxine and triiodothyronine have short half-lives (12–24 hours) because they are not transported bound to globulins (Capen et al., 2002).
- **Urine protein:** Male rats produce alpha 2-microglobulin (~20 kDa), a testosterone-dependent sex-associated protein produced by the liver that is hypothesized to act as the carrier for volatile substances important for pheromonal communication (Dinh et al., 1965; Mancini et al., 1989). Alpha 2-microglobulin is the major urinary protein in male rats in contrast to other laboratory animals and female rats, in which albumin predominates.

2.4 GENETIC CHARACTERISTICS AND BACKGROUND LESIONS

Phenotypic differences between rats of different genetic backgrounds can be quite useful when modeling particular diseases. However, these differences also have a considerable impact on many research endpoints. Genetic background may influence baseline clinical pathology tests in healthy animals (see Table 2.3, Sprague-Dawley vs. Wistar). In addition, there are many genetic differences with respect to organ function (e.g., kidney, liver, immune), xenobiotic metabolism, susceptibility to toxicity, carcinogenesis and spontaneous diseases, and aging diseases (Kacew et al., 1995; Firriolo et al., 1995; Hackbarth et al., 1981; Suckow et al., 2006; Evans, 2009). Therefore, choice of genetic background is an important consideration in experimental design and maintenance of historical control data.

2.5 METHODOLOGY FOR SAMPLE COLLECTION

2.5.1 Blood Collection (for Serum or Plasma)

Blood collection volume is an important consideration in rats, owing to their relatively small size. This is particularly true when multiple sampling intervals are required. Volume limits for collection of blood from rats vary from institution to institution on the basis of the local Institutional Animal Care and Use Committee (IACUC) or Ethics Committee guidelines. IACUCs or Ethics Committees usually limit blood collection to 10% of total blood volume, with additional collections permitted on a rolling accrual basis. As a general guideline, for a single collection (every 2–3 weeks), 10%–15% of total blood volume may be collected without adverse effects to the animal such as anemia, hypoxia, and hypotension. For repeated collections, 1% of the total blood volume may be collected daily, or no more than a total of 20% over a period of 3 weeks. Rat circulating blood volume is estimated to be 6.4% of body weight, or 57–69 mL/kg (McGuill and Rowan, 1989; Suckow et al., 2006). The maximum volume that can be collected from an adult rat in a terminal procedure depends on the site of collection, anesthetic used, skill of the phlebotomist, size of the animal, and hydration status but can range from 5 to 10 mL. The volume of blood that can be safely withdrawn as a survival procedure is dependent on these same characteristics, as well as IACUC or Ethics Committee requirements.

The preferred site for blood collection from rats depends on the volume and type of blood required (serum, plasma, or whole blood), sampling frequency (single vs. multiple collections), state of consciousness (anesthetized or unanesthetized), timing during experiment (interim or terminal time point), skill of phlebotomist, and IACUC or Ethics Committee requirements. For survival procedures, the chief blood collection sites are retro-orbital, tail vein (using a hypodermic needle or a nick), lateral saphenous vein, and jugular vein, while the sublingual and metatarsal veins are used less commonly. Historically, blood collection from the retro-orbital plexus was used commonly as a survival procedure. Today, its use as a survival procedure is discouraged because collection of blood from this site is associated with greater tissue injury and thus may affect animal welfare. Multiple survival collections are facilitated by pre-placement of a catheter in any one of several vessels (Thrivikraman et al, 2002). The chief sites used for terminal blood collection under anesthesia are retro-orbital plexus, abdominal aorta, abdominal vena cava, and heart. Specialized studies sometimes require decapitation; this is mostly performed for very young rats or for some hormonal research. When performing multiple collections, it is preferable to consistently collect from the same site owing to the differences between collection sites for a number of clinical pathology parameters (Van Herck et al., 2001; Dameron et al., 1992; Suber et al., 1985; Neptun et al., 1985).

The best method of blood collection is one that is the least stressful and most humane, yet provides a sufficient quantity of a quality blood sample. Major stressors for rats are listed in Table 2.4; several of these stressors are unavoidable during blood collection. While all blood collection methods require training, some methods (most notably jugular collections) must be performed regularly in order to maintain proficiency. Ongoing training for all methods of collection of blood should be conducted to ensure collection of a quality sample with minimal stress to the rat. Table 2.5 provides a list of the major sites of collection and their attributes.

2.5.2 Urine Collection

In rats, urine may be collected by free catch, timed collection into metabolic cages (e.g., Nalgene cages or wire-bottom cages), and cystocentesis, catheterization, or cystotomy at necropsy (Kurien et al., 2004; Cohen et al., 2007). Each method has advantages and disadvantages as detailed below.

Free catch collections are quick and yield clean samples (i.e., without contamination by water, food or feces). However, collected volumes are small (usually <0.5 mL) and may be insufficient for analysis in many animals on a given day. Success in collection of urine samples by free catch may be dependent on genetic background characteristics (Sprague-Dawley rats are easier than Wistar), sex (females are easier than males), time of day (first in the morning is usually most successful), and technique of the collector. In general, free catch is more successful with gentle, slow, and quiet handling of rats (Cohen et al., 2007). Light stimulation around the region of the bladder facilitates collections by promoting micturition. However, this method must not be used repeatedly because it has been shown to lead to necrosis and regenerative hyperplasia of the urothelium when performed several times weekly (Cohen et al., 1996).

In large rat studies, the most common method of urine collection is the timed (e.g., 16–24 hours of overnight collection, daytime collection, or other interval) collection. Urine is freely voided into trays placed beneath cages or into metabolic cages designed to minimize contamination from water, food, and feces. The main advantage of timed collections over other urine collection methods is that volumes are generally sufficient for analysis (approximately 0.5–20 mL depending on elapsed time) from most or all animals. In addition, timed sampling can be coordinated with experimental manipulations or pharmacodynamics of a test article (e.g., 0–4 and 4–24 hours post-dose). To improve accuracy of timed collections, bladders may be completely emptied prior to the start of collection by light stimulation of the region around the bladder to promote micturition. Timed collections minimize effects of diurnal fluctuations on urine constituents, although short timed collections can still show wide variability and analytes must be corrected for volume or creatinine concentrations (Haas et al., 1997). The disadvantages of metabolic cages are requirements for specialized caging and cage changing, delay between sample collection and analysis, and potential contamination of urine with hair, feces, test articles, water, food, and bacterial growth. There is a large variety of specially designed cages for rat urine collections, and each design has advantages and disadvantages. Optimally designed caging serves food and water outside the main collection area. The flooring optimally has pore sizes small enough to catch feces but large enough that urine droplets are not caught in the mesh flooring by capillary action. Placement of rats into wire-bottomed metabolic caging has been shown to be relatively nonstressful for rats (Eriksson et al., 2004).

Urine collected in metabolic cages can be collected at room temperature or cooled depending on the duration of collection (e.g., 5 hours vs. overnight) and stability of parameters to be

TABLE 2.3
Serum Clinical Chemistry Normative Data for Rat Stocks (Mean ± SD [Ref Interval])

Analyte	Abbreviation	Units	Stock: Sprague-Dawley M	Sprague-Dawley F	Wistar M	Wistar F
Acetylcholinesterase	**AchE**					
<6 months (Aleman et al., 1998)		U	0.27 ± 0.07	0.34 ± 0.07	–	–
6–18 months (Aleman et al., 1998)		U	0.29 ± 0.08	0.37 ± 0.09	–	–
18–32 months (Aleman et al., 1998)		U	0.29 ± 0.06	0.36 ± 0.06	–	–
Acid Phosphatase	**AP**					
<6 months (Aleman et al., 1998)		IU	37.9 ± 9.8	30.5 ± 9.0	–	–
6–18 months (Aleman et al., 1998)		IU	33.9 ± 13.5	25.0 ± 9.9	–	–
18–32 months (Aleman et al., 1998)		IU	30.3 ± 10.7	26.7 ± 6.9	–	–
Adrenaline						
Unknown (BW = 160–200 g) (Budohoski et al., 1987)		pg/mL	–	–	13 ± 4 $n = 5$	–
Adrenocorticotropic Hormone	**ACTH**					
Unstressed (Márquez et al., 2004)		pg/mL	~70–150	–	–	–
Stressed (Márquez et al., 2004)		pg/mL	1000–3000	–	–	–
10–12 weeks (Atkinson and Waddell, 1997)		pg/mL	–	–	24.4 (14.8–38.3)	
10–12 weeks—estrus (Atkinson and Waddell, 1997)		pg/mL	–	–	–	30.2 (16.5–43.9)
10–12 weeks—diestrus (Atkinson and Waddell, 1997)		pg/mL	–	–	–	33.4 (17.5–49.3)
10–12 weeks—proestrus (Atkinson and Waddell, 1997)		pg/mL	–	–	–	28.0 (17.5–38.4)
Alanine Aminotransferase	**ALT**					
3–7 weeks (Giknis and Clifford, 2006)		U/L	30 (27–35) $n = 146$	25 (23–28) $n = 146$	–	–

(*Continued*)

TABLE 2.3 (*Continued*)
Serum Clinical Chemistry Normative Data for Rat Stocks (Mean ± SD [Ref Interval])

			Stock			
			Sprague-Dawley		Wistar	
Analyte	Abbreviation	Units	M	F	M	F
Alanine Aminotransferase	ALT					
8–12 weeks (Giknis and Clifford, 2006)		U/L	34 (28–40) $n = 725$	29 (25–36) $n = 724$	–	–
8–16 weeks (Giknis and Clifford, 2008)		U/L	–	–	28 ± 7 (18–45) $n = 164$	25 ± 9 (16–48) $n = 157$
13–22 weeks (Giknis and Clifford, 2006)		U/L	35 (27–46) $n = 666$	32 (25–45) $n = 678$	–	–
≥17 weeks (Giknis and Clifford, 2008)		U/L	–	–	30 ± 8 (19–48) $n = 87$	30 ± 15 (14–64) $n = 87$
23–47 weeks (Giknis and Clifford, 2006)		U/L	47 (26–97) $n = 375$	51 (24–172) $n = 381$	–	–
48–65 weeks (Giknis and Clifford, 2006)		U/L	46 (24–81) $n = 55$	38 (23–117) $n = 55$	–	–
88–150 weeks (Giknis and Clifford, 2006)		U/L	52 (29–96) $n = 70$	60 (28–186) $n = 70$	–	–
Albumin						
3–7 weeks (Giknis and Clifford, 2006)		g/dL	3.6 (3.2–4.7) $n = 146$	–	–	–
8–12 weeks (Giknis and Clifford, 2006)		g/dL	3.6 (3.3–4.6) $n = 724$	3.9 (3.5–5.1) $n = 724$	–	–
8–16 weeks (Giknis and Clifford, 2008)		g/dL			4 ± 0.4 (3.4–4.8) $n = 164$	4.4 ± 0.5 (3.6–5.5) $n = 159$
13–22 weeks (Giknis and Clifford, 2006)		g/dL	3.7 (3.3–4.6) $n = 661$	4.2 (3.5–5.3) $n = 673$	–	–
≥17 weeks (Giknis and Clifford, 2008)		g/dL	–	–	4.1 ± 0.3 (3.6–4.7) $n = 10$	4.6 ± 0.5 (3.7–5.8) $n = 77$

(*Continued*)

TABLE 2.3 (*Continued*)
Serum Clinical Chemistry Normative Data for Rat Stocks (Mean ± SD [Ref Interval])

			Stock			
			Sprague-Dawley		Wistar	
Analyte	**Abbreviation**	**Units**	**M**	**F**	**M**	**F**
Albumin						
23–47 weeks (Giknis and Clifford, 2006)		g/dL	4.5 (3.7–5.0) $n = 356$	5.4 (4.5–6.6) $n = 363$	–	–
48–65 weeks (Giknis and Clifford, 2006)		g/dL	4.6 (4.1–5.2) $n = 55$	5.6 (4.6–6.7) $n = 55$	–	–
88–150 weeks (Giknis and Clifford, 2006)		g/dL	4.4 (2.0–5.0) $n = 48$	4.7 (2.1–6.7) $n = 50$	–	–
Albumin: Globulin Ratio	**A/G**					
3–7 weeks (Giknis and Clifford, 2006)		Ratio	1.6 (1.3–2.9) $n = 146$	1.8 (1.3–3.8) $n = 146$	–	–
8–12 weeks (Giknis and Clifford, 2006)		Ratio	1.4 (1.1–2.7) $n = 693$	1.6 (1.3–2.9) $n = 724$	–	–
8–16 weeks (Giknis and Clifford, 2008)		Ratio	–	–	2 ± 0.2 (1.58–2.67) $n = 144$	2.2 ± 0.34 (1.71–3) $n = 139$
13–22 weeks (Giknis and Clifford, 2006)		Ratio	1.3 (1.1–1.9) $n = 661$	1.4 (1.1–2.0) $n = 673$	–	–
≥17 weeks (Giknis and Clifford, 2006)		Ratio	–	–	1.91 ± 0.24 (1.5–2.33) $n = 66$	2.31 ± 0.34 (1.64–3.07) $n = 65$
23–47 weeks (Giknis and Clifford, 2006)		Ratio	1.4 (1.1–1.9) $n = 345$	1.7 (1.0–1.7) $n = 138$	–	–
48–65 weeks (Giknis and Clifford, 2006)		Ratio	2.1 (0.9–2.3) $n = 55$	1.8 (1.4–2.3) $n = 55$	–	–
88–150 weeks (Giknis and Clifford, 2006)		Ratio	1.9 (1.6–2.4) $n = 59$	1.7 (1.2–2.4) $n = 60$	–	–

(*Continued*)

TABLE 2.3 (*Continued*)
Serum Clinical Chemistry Normative Data for Rat Stocks (Mean ± SD [Ref Interval])

Analyte	Abbreviation	Units	Stock			
			Sprague-Dawley		Wistar	
			M	F	M	F
Alkaline phosphatase	**ALP**					
3–7 weeks (Giknis and Clifford, 2006)		U/L	233 (201–268) $n = 146$	162 (133–219) $n = 146$	–	–
8–12 weeks (Giknis and Clifford, 2006)		U/L	160 (136–188) $n = 719$	113 (90–147) $n = 695$	–	–
8–16 weeks (Giknis and Clifford, 2008)		U/L	–	–	113 ± 44 (62–230) $n = 163$	59 ± 28 (26–147) $n = 159$
13–22 weeks (Giknis and Clifford, 2006)		U/L	125 (104–160) $n = 646$	83 (65–117) $n = 658$	–	–
≥17 weeks (Giknis and Clifford, 2008)		U/L	–	–	66 ± 21 (36–131) $n = 88$	30 ± 11 (18–62) $n = 87$
23–47 weeks (Giknis and Clifford, 2006)		U/L	105 (53–226) $n = 330$	130 (19–205) $n = 357$	–	–
48–65 weeks (Giknis and Clifford, 2006)		U/L	96 (68–148) $n = 52$	55 (13–89) $n = 55$	–	–
88–150 weeks (Giknis and Clifford, 2006)		U/L	3.7 (2.1–4.9) $n = 60$	44 (10–219) $n = 60$	–	–
Ammonia	**NH_3**					
6–7 weeks (Kawai et al., 2009)		μg/dL	–	–	53 (46–58)	–
Amylase						
>17 weeks (Giknis and Clifford, 2006)		U/L	–	–	1557 ± 316 (1223–2109) $n = 10$	1211 ± 215 (866–1642) $n = 11$

(*Continued*)

TABLE 2.3 (*Continued*)
Serum Clinical Chemistry Normative Data for Rat Stocks (Mean ± SD [Ref Interval])

			Stock			
			Sprague-Dawley		Wistar	
Analyte	Abbreviation	Units	M	F	M	F
Aspartate Aminotransferase	**AST**					
3–7 weeks (Giknis and Clifford, 2006)		U/L	106 (94–116) *n* = 146	94 (78–109) *n* = 146	–	–
8–12 weeks (Giknis and Clifford, 2006)		U/L	101 (87–114) *n* = 725	96 (85–123) *n* = 724	–	–
8–16 weeks (Giknis and Clifford, 2008)		U/L	–	–	105 ± 20 (74–143) *n* = 164	102 ± 31 (65–203) *n* = 158
13–22 weeks (Giknis and Clifford, 2006)		U/L	91 (77–110) *n* = 666	93 (72–116) *n* = 678	–	–
≥17 weeks (Giknis and Clifford, 2008)		U/L	–	–	96 ± 24 (63–175) *n* = 88	101 ± 36 (64–222) *n* = 87
23–47 weeks (Giknis and Clifford, 2006)		U/L	90 (57–114) *n* = 375	97 (62–226) *n* = 381	–	–
48–65 weeks (Giknis and Clifford, 2006)		U/L	103 (48–159) *n* = 55	90 (50–128) *n* = 55	–	–
88–150 weeks (Giknis and Clifford, 2006)		U/L	105 (61–246) *n* = 70	150 (54–586) *n* = 70	–	–
Bicarbonate (Arterial)	**HCO_3**					
Adult (Ziomber et al., 2008)		mmol/L	27.7 ± 0.7 *n* = 10	–	–	–
Bicarbonate (Venous)	**TCO_2**					
Adult – Fed (Levine et al., 1988)		mEq/L	30.2 ± 0.5 *n* = 23	–	–	–

(*Continued*)

TABLE 2.3 (*Continued*)
Serum Clinical Chemistry Normative Data for Rat Stocks (Mean ± SD [Ref Interval])

			Stock			
			Sprague-Dawley		Wistar	
Analyte	**Abbreviation**	**Units**	**M**	**F**	**M**	**F**
Bicarbonate (Venous)	**TCO_2**					
Adult – Fasted (Levine et al., 1988)		mEq/L	24.9 ± 0.6 *n* = 22	–	–	–
Bilirubin—Direct	**cBili**					
8–16 weeks (Giknis and Clifford, 2008)		mg/dL	–	–	0.04 ± 0.01 (0.03–0.05) *n* = 109	0.04 ± 0.01 (0.2–0.6) *n* = 95
≥17 weeks (Giknis and Clifford, 2008)		mg/dL	–	–	–	0.04 ± 0.01 (0.03–0.07) *n* = 50
Bilirubin—Indirect	**uBili**					
8–16 weeks (Giknis and Clifford, 2008)		mg/dL	–	–	0.06 ± 0.03 (0.01–0.12) *n* = 139	0.08 ± 0.03 (0.03–0.15) *n* = 133
≥17 weeks (Giknis and Clifford, 2008)		mg/dL	–	–	0.06 ± 0.03 (0–0.1) *n* = 66	0.08 ± 0.03 (0.02–0.13) *n* = 65
Bilirubin—Total	**tBili**					
3–7 weeks (Giknis and Clifford, 2006)		mg/dL	0.6 (0.1–1.0) *n* = 146	0.6 (0.1–1.0) *n* = 146	–	–
8–12 weeks (Giknis and Clifford, 2006)		mg/dL	0.6 (0.1–1.0) *n* = 723	0.6 (0.2–1.0) *n* = 724	–	–
8–16 weeks (Giknis and Clifford, 2008)		mg/dL	–	–	0.09 ± 0.03 (0.05–0.15) *n* = 165	0.11 ± 0.03 (0.05–0.18) *n* = 157
13–22 weeks (Giknis and Clifford, 2006)		mg/dL	0.6 (0.2–1.0) *n* = 666	1.1 (0.2–2.0) *n* = 678	–	–
≥17 weeks (Giknis and Clifford, 2008)		mg/dL	–	–	0.1 ± 0.04 (0.04–0.2) *n* = 78	0.13 ± 0.04 (0.07–0.21) *n* = 77

(*Continued*)

TABLE 2.3 (*Continued*)
Serum Clinical Chemistry Normative Data for Rat Stocks (Mean ± SD [Ref Interval])

			Stock			
			Sprague-Dawley		Wistar	
Analyte	**Abbreviation**	**Units**	**M**	**F**	**M**	**F**
Bilirubin—Total	**tBili**					
23–47 weeks (Giknis and Clifford, 2006)ß		mg/dL	0.1 (0.1–0.2) $n = 365$	0.1 (0.1–0.2) $n = 372$	–	–
48–65 weeks (Giknis and Clifford, 2006)		mg/dL	0.1 (0.0–0.2) $n = 55$	0.2 (0.1–0.3) $n = 55$	–	–
88–150 weeks (Giknis and Clifford, 2006)		mg/dL	0.1 (0.0–0.4) $n = 60$	0.1 (0.1–0.2) $n = 60$	–	–
Blood Urea Nitrogen	**BUN/UN**					
3–7 weeks (Giknis and Clifford, 2006)		mg/dL	12 (10–13) $n = 146$	12 (10–13) $n = 146$	–	–
8–12 weeks (Giknis and Clifford, 2006)		mg/dL	14 (13–16) $n = 724$	13 (11–16) 724	–	–
8–16 weeks (Giknis and Clifford, 2008)		mg/dL	–	–	17 ± 2.9 (12–25) $n = 164$	19 ± 3.7 (13–27) $n = 158$
13–22 weeks (Giknis and Clifford, 2006)		mg/dL	13 (10–16) $n = 661$	13 (11–17) $n = 673$	–	–
≥17 weeks (Giknis and Clifford, 2008)		mg/dL	–	–	16 ± 2.3 (11–20) $n = 87$	17 ± 3.9 (12–25) $n = 88$
23–47 weeks (Giknis and Clifford, 2006)		mg/dL	15 (10–22) $n = 350$	16 (11–25) $n = 337$	–	–
48–65 weeks (Giknis and Clifford, 2006)		mg/dL	13 (8–16) $n = 55$	13 (8–17) $n = 55$	–	–
88–150 weeks (Giknis and Clifford, 2006)		mg/dL	17 (8–24) $n = 51$	17 (9–39) $n = 55$	–	–

(*Continued*)

TABLE 2.3 (*Continued*)
Serum Clinical Chemistry Normative Data for Rat Stocks (Mean ± SD [Ref Interval])

Analyte	Abbreviation	Units	Stock: Sprague-Dawley M	Sprague-Dawley F	Wistar M	Wistar F
Calcium (Ionized)	**iCa**					
Adult (Fryer et al., 2007)		mg/dL	1.24 ± 0.03 $n = 6$	–	–	–
Calcium (Total)	**tCa**					
3–7 weeks (Giknis and Clifford, 2006)		mg/dL	10.0 (9.4–11.4) $n = 146$	10.1 (9.4–11.3) $n = 146$	–	–
8–12 weeks (Giknis and Clifford, 2006)		mg/dL	10.0 (9.4–11.0) $n = 718$	10.1 (9.5–11.0) $n = 724$		
8–16 weeks (Giknis and Clifford, 2008)		mg/dL	–	–	10.4 ± 0.5 (9.5–11.5) $n = 165$	10.5 ± 0.4 (9.7–11.2) $n = 159$
13–22 weeks (Giknis and Clifford, 2006)		mg/dL	10.2 (9.6–10.9) $n = 661$	10.3 (9.6–11.2) $n = 673$	–	–
≥17 weeks (Giknis and Clifford, 2008)		mg/dL	–	–	10.3 ± 0.7 (9.1–11.9) $n = 78$	10.6 ± 0.7 (9.5–12.1) $n = 77$
23–47 weeks (Giknis and Clifford, 2006)		mg/dL	10.9 (9.9–11.9) $n = 350$	11.7 (10.2–12.6) $n = 356$	–	–
48–65 weeks (Giknis and Clifford, 2006)		mg/dL	10.9 (9.6–12.4) $n = 55$	11.1 (10.1–12.6) $n = 55$	–	–
88–150 weeks (Giknis and Clifford, 2006)		mg/dL	11.7 (9.6–13.1) $n = 70$	10.9 (9.0–13.4) $n = 60$	–	–
Chloride	**Cl**					
3–7 weeks (Giknis and Clifford, 2006)		mmol/L	102 (100–105) $n = 146$	105 (100–108) $n = 146$	–	–

(*Continued*)

TABLE 2.3 (*Continued*)
Serum Clinical Chemistry Normative Data for Rat Stocks (Mean ± SD [Ref Interval])

			Stock			
			Sprague-Dawley		Wistar	
Analyte	**Abbreviation**	**Units**	**M**	**F**	**M**	**F**
Chloride	**Cl**					
8–12 weeks (Giknis and Clifford, 2006)		mmol/L	104 (102–105) $n = 720$	105 (103–107) $n = 723$	–	–
8–16 weeks (Giknis and Clifford, 2008)		mmol/L	–	–	130 ± 1 (100–106) $n = 165$	103 ± 2 (100–107) $n = 159$
13–22 weeks (Giknis and Clifford, 2006)		mmol/L	104 (101–107) $n = 658$	105 (101–108) $n = 667$	–	–
≥17 weeks (Giknis and Clifford, 2008)		mmol/L	–	–	103 ± 2 (98–106) $n = 78$	102 ± 3 (97–106) $n = 77$
23–47 weeks (Giknis and Clifford, 2006)		mmol/L	106 (97–110) $n = 350$	103 (95–111) $n = 356$	–	–
48–65 weeks (Giknis and Clifford, 2006)		mmol/L	103 (97–110) $n = 55$	104 (96–107) $n = 55$	–	–
88–150 weeks (Giknis and Clifford, 2006)		mmol/L	103 (90–132) $n = 71$	105 (90–110) $n = 71$	–	–
Cholesterol (Total)	**Chol**					
3–7 weeks (Giknis and Clifford, 2006)		mg/dL	67 (56–92) $n = 146$	80 (69–92) $n = 146$	–	–
8–12 weeks (Giknis and Clifford, 2006)		mg/dL	62 (54–74) $n = 709$	75 (67–87) $n = 708$	–	–
8–16 weeks (Giknis and Clifford, 2008)		mg/dL	–	–	58 ± 13 (37–85) $n = 165$	48 ± 13 (24–73) $n = 158$
13–22 weeks (Giknis and Clifford, 2006)		mg/dL	65 (55–89) $n = 666$	78 (66–97) $n = 673$	–	–

(*Continued*)

TABLE 2.3 (*Continued*)
Serum Clinical Chemistry Normative Data for Rat Stocks (Mean ± SD [Ref Interval])

			Stock			
			Sprague-Dawley		Wistar	
Analyte	Abbreviation	Units	M	F	M	F
Cholesterol (Total)	**Chol**					
≥17 weeks (Giknis and Clifford, 2008)		mg/dL	–	–	59 ± 15 (37–95) $n = 68$	50 ± 19 (23–97) $n = 67$
23–47 weeks (Giknis and Clifford, 2006)		mg/dL	92 (62–234) $n = 375$	97 (47–182) $n = 357$	–	–
48–65 weeks (Giknis and Clifford, 2006)		mg/dL	82 (58–164) $n = 55$	93 (56–148) $n = 55$	–	–
88–150 weeks (Giknis and Clifford, 2006)		mg/dL	116 (50–204) $n = 60$	99 (36–161) $n = 60$	–	–
Corticosterone	**Cort**					
8 weeks—unstressed (Márquez et al., 2004)		µg/dL	<10	–	–	–
8 weeks—stressed (Márquez et al., 2004)		µg/dL	(10–50)			
10–12 weeks (Atkinson and Waddell, 1997)		ng/mL			102 (0–206)	–
10–12 weeks—estrus (Atkinson and Waddell, 1997)		ng/mL	–	–	–	129 (0–293)
10–12 weeks—diestrus (Atkinson and Waddell, 1997)		ng/mL	–	–	–	208 (43–373)
10–12 weeks—proestrus (Atkinson and Waddell, 1997)		ng/mL	–	–	–	246 (20–472)
Creatine Kinase	**CK**					
3–7 weeks (Giknis and Clifford, 2006)		U/L	657 (515–710) $n = 135$	499 (401–531) $n = 135$	–	–
8–12 weeks (Giknis and Clifford, 2006)		U/L	362 (344–380) $n = 724$	443 (420–466) 364	–	–
8–16 weeks (Giknis and Clifford, 2008)		U/L	–	–	658 ± 343 (162–1184) $n = 45$	575 ± 260 (163–1085) $n = 46$

(Continued)

TABLE 2.3 (*Continued*)
Serum Clinical Chemistry Normative Data for Rat Stocks (Mean ± SD [Ref Interval])

			Stock			
			Sprague-Dawley		Wistar	
Analyte	**Abbreviation**	**Units**	**M**	**F**	**M**	**F**
Creatine Kinase	**CK**					
13–22 weeks (Giknis and Clifford, 2006)		U/L	320 (203–437) $n = 471$	280 (180–381) $n = 449$	–	–
≥17 weeks (Giknis and Clifford, 2008)		U/L	–	–	846 ± 246 (460–1230) $n = 46$	702 ± 261 (218–1320) $n = 45$
23–47 weeks (Giknis and Clifford, 2006)		U/L	240 (56–477) $n = 118$	237 (117–633) $n = 119$	–	–
48–65 weeks (Giknis and Clifford, 2006)		U/L	234 (68–1218) $n = 50$	171 (58–740) $n = 41$	–	–
88–150 weeks (Giknis and Clifford, 2006)		U/L	229 (59–396) $n = 70$	81 (20–241) $n = 70$	–	–
Creatinine	**Creat**					
3–7 weeks (Giknis and Clifford, 2006)		mg/dL	0.5 (0.5–0.6) $n = 146$	0.6 (0.5–0.6) $n = 146$	–	–
8–12 weeks (Giknis and Clifford, 2006)		mg/dL	0.5 (0.5–0.6) $n = 724$	0.6 (0.5–0.6) $n = 724$	–	–
8–16 weeks (Giknis and Clifford, 2008)		mg/dL	–	–	0.3 ± 0.1 (0.2–0.5) $n = 163$	0.4 ± 0.1 (0.2–0.6) $n = 159$
13–22 weeks (Giknis and Clifford, 2006)		mg/dL	0.6 (0.4–0.6) $n = 661$	0.6 (0.4–0.7) $n = 673$	–	–
≥17 weeks (Giknis and Clifford, 2008)		mg/dL	–	–	0.4 ± 0.1 (0.3–0.5) $n = 88$	0.4 ± 0.1 (0.3–0.6) $n = 88$
23–47 weeks (Giknis and Clifford, 2006)		mg/dL	0.7 (0.5–0.8) $n = 350$	0.8 (0.5–0.9) $n = 357$	–	–

(*Continued*)

TABLE 2.3 (*Continued*)
Serum Clinical Chemistry Normative Data for Rat Stocks (Mean ± SD [Ref Interval])

			Stock			
			Sprague-Dawley		Wistar	
Analyte	**Abbreviation**	**Units**	**M**	**F**	**M**	**F**
Creatinine	**Creat**					
48–65 weeks (Giknis and Clifford, 2006)		mg/dL	0.7(0.6–0.8) 55	0.7 (0.6–0.9)n = 55	–	–
88–150 weeks (Giknis and Clifford, 2006)		mg/dL	0.6 (0.4–0.9) n = 60	0.5 (0.3–0.9) n = 60	–	–
Estradiol						
4.7 weeks (Shin et al., 2009)		pg/mL	28.7 ± 8.89n = 10	–	–	–
Adult—Diestrus 1 (Flores et al., 2008)	Strain: CIIZ-V	pg/mL	–	57.3 ± 6.0 n = 29	–	–
Adult—Diestrus 2 (Flores et al., 2008)		pg/mL	–	49.1 ± 5.0 n = 30	–	–
Adult—Proestrus (Flores et al., 2008)		pg/mL	–	144.0 ± 11.8 n = 25	–	–
Adult—Estrus (Flores et al., 2008)		pg/mL	–	22.5 ± 2.9 n = 18	–	–
Free Fatty Acid						
Adult (BW = 150–180 g) (Kannappan and Anuradha, 2009)		mg/dL	–	–	25.68 ± 2.42 n = 12	–
Follicle Stimulating Hormone (for adult female—list specific stage of estrous)	**FSH**					
12–16 weeks (Ansari-Lari and Taniceh, 2009)		IU/L	14.04 ± 3.27n = 22	–	–	–
>8.5 weeks intact (Woodruff et al., 1996)		ng/mL	11.6		–	–
>8.5 weeks castrated (Woodruff et al., 1996)		ng/mL	63	–	–	–
>8.5 weeks metestrus (Woodruff et al., 1996)		ng/mL	–	5.5	–	–
>8.5 weeks proestrus (Woodruff et al., 1996)		ng/mL	–	4.8	–	–

(*Continued*)

TABLE 2.3 (*Continued*)
Serum Clinical Chemistry Normative Data for Rat Stocks (Mean ± SD [Ref Interval])

			Stock			
			Sprague-Dawley		Wistar	
Analyte	**Abbreviation**	**Units**	**M**	**F**	**M**	**F**
Follicle Stimulating Hormone (for adult female—list specific stage of estrous)	**FSH**					
>8.5 weeks ovariectomized (Woodruff et al., 1996)		ng/mL	–	44.9	–	–
Adult estrus (BW = 180–220g) (Sánchez-Criado et al., 1997)		µg/L	–	3.5 ± 0.4 $n = 7$	–	–
Adult metestrus (BW = 180–220 g) (Sánchez-Criado et al., 1997)		µg/L	–	4.0 ± 0.5 $n = 7$	–	–
Globulin	**Glob**					
8–16 weeks (Giknis and Clifford, 2008)		g/dL	–	–	2 ± 0.2 (1.5–2.5) $n = 144$	2 ± 0.2 (1.5–2.4) $n = 139$
≥17 weeks (Giknis and Clifford, 2008)		g/dL	–	–	2.1 ± 0.2 (1.8–2.5) $n = 66$	1.9 ± 0.2 (1.6–2.3) $n = 65$
Glucose						
3–7 weeks (Giknis and Clifford, 2006)		mg/dL	136 (85–167) $n = 146$	145 (100–179) $n = 146$	–	–
8–12 weeks (Giknis and Clifford, 2006)		mg/dL	146 (112–176) $n = 724$	160 (113–185) $n = 724$	–	–
8–16 weeks (Giknis and Clifford, 2008)		mg/dL	–	–	165 ± 123 (70–208) $n = 165$	117 ± 25 (76–175) $n = 159$
13–22 weeks (Giknis and Clifford, 2006)		mg/dL	157 (121–197) $n = 661$	159 (120–186) $n = 673$	–	–
≥17 weeks (Giknis and Clifford, 2008)		mg/dL	–	–	141 ± 19 (106–184) $n = 78$	119 ± 16 (89–163) $n = 77$

(*Continued*)

TABLE 2.3 (*Continued*)
Serum Clinical Chemistry Normative Data for Rat Stocks (Mean ± SD [Ref Interval])

Analyte	Abbreviation	Units	Stock			
			Sprague-Dawley		Wistar	
			M	F	M	F
Glucose						
23–47 weeks (Giknis and Clifford, 2006)		mg/dL	115 (92–138) *n* = 350	115 (95–152) *n* = 337	–	–
48–65 weeks (Giknis and Clifford, 2006)		mg/dL	109 (89–165) *n* = 55	105 (81–146) *n* = 55	–	–
88–150 weeks (Giknis and Clifford, 2006)		mg/dL	120 (49–167) *n* = 51	112 (54–15) *n* = 55	–	–
Gamma-Glutamyltransferase	**GGT**					
3–7 weeks (Giknis and Clifford, 2006)		U/L	0.05 (0–3.00) *n* = 136	0.0 (0.0–1.0) *n* = 141	–	–
8–12 weeks (Giknis and Clifford, 2006)		U/L	0.5 (0.0–1.0) *n* = 579	0.2 (0.0–0.4) *n* = 579	–	–
13–22 weeks (Giknis and Clifford, 2006)		U/L	0.5 (0.0–1.0) *n* = 565	0.5 (0.0–1.0) *n* = 557	–	–
23–47 weeks (Giknis and Clifford, 2006)		U/L	0.5 (0.0–3.0) *n* = 278	0.5 (0.0–1.0) *n* = 286	–	–
48–65 weeks (Giknis and Clifford, 2006)		U/L	1.0 (0.0–2.0) *n* = 55	1.0 (0.0–2.0) *n* = 55	–	–
88–150 weeks (Giknis and Clifford, 2006)		U/L	2.4 (0.0–4.1) *n* = 50	1.0 (0.0–3.6) *n* = 50	–	–
Glutamate Dehydrogenase	**GDH/GLDH**					
10 weeks (O'Brien et al., 2002)		IU/L	7.6 ± 0.4 *n* = 16	–	–	–

(*Continued*)

TABLE 2.3 (*Continued*)
Serum Clinical Chemistry Normative Data for Rat Stocks (Mean ± SD [Ref Interval])

			Stock			
			Sprague-Dawley		Wistar	
Analyte	**Abbreviation**	**Units**	**M**	**F**	**M**	**F**
Glutamate Dehydrogenase	**GDH/GLDH**					
unknown (BW = 250–280 g) (Conybeare et al., 1988)		IU/L	–	–		13.8 ± 2.0 $n = 9$
Insulin						
unknown (BW = 160–200 g) (Budohoski et al., 1987)		µU/mL	–	–	37 ± 3 $n = 9$	–
Insulin						
Adult (BW = 150–180g) (Kannappan and Anuradha, 2009)		µU/mL	–	–	46.58 ± 3.87	–
Lactate Dehydrogenase	**LDH**					
3–7 weeks (Giknis and Clifford, 2006)		U/L	744 (569–890) $n = 130$	423 (317–476) $n = 130$	–	–
8–12 weeks (Giknis and Clifford, 2006)		U/L	389 (360–418) $n = 724$	411 (401–422) $n = 354$	–	–
13–22 weeks (Giknis and Clifford, 2006)		U/L	479 (431–526) $n = 448$	386 (246–525) $n = 444$	–	–
≥17 weeks (Giknis and Clifford, 2008)		U/L	–	–	1305 ± 510 (272–1965) $n = 10$	971 ± 438 (256–1552) $n = 10$
23–47 weeks (Giknis and Clifford, 2006)		U/L	256 (105–652) $n = 46$	210 (76–953) $n = 33$	–	–
48–65 weeks (Giknis and Clifford, 2006)		U/L	194 (61–241) $n = 50$	209 (71–268) $n = 42$	–	–

(*Continued*)

TABLE 2.3 (*Continued*)
Serum Clinical Chemistry Normative Data for Rat Stocks (Mean ± SD [Ref Interval])

			Stock			
			Sprague-Dawley		Wistar	
Analyte	**Abbreviation**	**Units**	**M**	**F**	**M**	**F**
Lipase						
≥17 weeks (Giknis and Clifford, 2008)		U/L	–	–	9 ± 2 (7–14) $n = 10$	7 ± 0 (7–8) $n = 11$
Luteinizing Hormone	**LH**					
4.7 weeks (Shin et al., 2009)		pg/mL	23.3 ± 8.520 $n = 10$	–	–	–
12–16 weeks (Ansari-Lari and Taniceh, 2009)		IU/L	0.29 ± 0.09 $n = 22$	–	–	–
Adult estrus (BW = 180–220 g) (Sánchez-Criado et al., 1997)		μg/L	–	0.3 ± 0.1 $n = 7$	–	–
Adult metestrus (BW = 180–220 g) (Sánchez-Criado et al., 1997)		μg/L	–	0.2 ± 0.1 $n = 7$	–	–
Magnesium	**Mg**					
≥17 weeks (Giknis and Clifford, 2008)		mg/dL	–	–	2.1 ± 0.1 (1.9–2.2) $n = 15$	2.2 ± 0.1 (1.9–2.4) $n = 15$
Noradrelanine						
Unknown (BW = 160–200 g) (Budohoski et al., 1987)		pg/mL	–	–	14 ± 5 $n = 5$	–
Parathyroid Hormone	**PTH**					
Adult (Fryer et al., 2007)		pg/mL	72 ± 16 $n = 6$	–	–	–

(*Continued*)

TABLE 2.3 (*Continued*)
Serum Clinical Chemistry Normative Data for Rat Stocks (Mean ± SD [Ref Interval])

			Stock			
			Sprague-Dawley		Wistar	
Analyte	**Abbreviation**	**Units**	**M**	**F**	**M**	**F**
Phosphorus	**P**					
3–7 weeks (Giknis and Clifford, 2006)		mg/dL	9.2 (8.5–10.3) *n* = 146	8.0 (6.7–9.6) *n* = 146	–	–
8–12 weeks (Giknis and Clifford, 2006)		mg/dL	8.1 (7.3–10.0) *n* = 672	7.0 (6.2–9.1) *n* = 674	–	–
8–16 weeks (Giknis and Clifford, 2008)		mg/dL	–	–	8.04 ± 1.22 (5.58–10.41) *n* = 164	7.92 ± 1.51 (5.02–10.7) *n* = 158
13–22 weeks (Giknis and Clifford, 2006)		mg/dL	7.7 (7.0–9.5) *n* = 636	6.6 (5.6–8.6) *n* = 649	–	–
≥17 weeks (Giknis and Clifford, 2008)		mg/dL	–	–	6.23 ± 1.24 (3.64–8.4) *n* = 78	6.66 ± 1.15 (4.53–9.51) *n* = 77
23–47 weeks (Giknis and Clifford, 2006)		mg/dL	7.7 (5.5–9.2) *n* = 350	6.7 (3.3–8.4) *n* = 356	–	–
48–65 weeks (Giknis and Clifford, 2006)		mg/dL	8.0 (5.9–10.5) *n* = 55	7.2 (5.0–13.4) *n* = 55	–	–
88–150 weeks (Giknis and Clifford, 2006)		mg/dL	6.6 (4.1–8.7) *n* = 50	6.2 (4.0–8.7) *n* = 60	–	–
Potassium	**K**					
3–7 weeks (Giknis and Clifford, 2006)		mmol/L	5.2 (4.7–6.1) *n* = 146	4.9 (4.3–6.0) *n* = 146	–	–
8–12 weeks (Giknis and Clifford, 2006)		mmol/L	5.2 (4.7–6.2)725	4.8 (4.2–6.1) *n* = 723	–	–
8–16 weeks (Giknis and Clifford, 2008)		mmol/L	–	–	4.48 ± 0.44 (3.82–5.55) *n* = 165	4.07 ± 0.37 (3.31–4.9) *n* = 158
13–22 weeks (Giknis and Clifford, 2006)		mmol/L	5.3 (4.6–6.1) *n* = 658	4.9 (4.3–5.9) *n* = 667	–	–

(*Continued*)

TABLE 2.3 (*Continued*)
Serum Clinical Chemistry Normative Data for Rat Stocks (Mean ± SD [Ref Interval])

Analyte	Abbreviation	Units	Stock: Sprague-Dawley M	Stock: Sprague-Dawley F	Stock: Wistar M	Stock: Wistar F
Potassium	**K**					
≥17 weeks (Giknis and Clifford, 2008)		mmol/L	–	–	4.55 ± 0.53 (3.88–6.11) $n = 78$	4.07 ± 0.42 (3.37–5.11) $n = 77$
23–47 weeks (Giknis and Clifford, 2006)		mmol/L	6.3 (5.0–7.3) $n = 350$	5.7 (4.2–6.7) $n = 356$	–	–
48–65 weeks (Giknis and Clifford, 2006)		mmol/L	6.0 (9.6–12.2) $n = 55$	5.6 (4.1–6.9) $n = 55$	–	–
88–150 weeks (Giknis and Clifford, 2006)		mmol/L	6.2 (4.0–6.7) $n = 71$	5.7 (4.1–6.3) $n = 71$	–	–
Prolactin						
Adult (BW = 180–200 g) (Hattori et al., 2007)		μg/L	–	–	15.8 ± 4.4 $n = 9$	–
Progesterone (for adult female—list specific stage of estrous)	**Prog**					
Adult—Diestrus 1 (Flores et al., 2008)	Strain: CIIZ-V	ng/mL	–	22.9 ± 1.9 $n = 29$	–	–
Adult—Diestrus 2 (Flores et al., 2008)		ng/mL	–	8.0 ± 1.1 $n = 30$	–	–
Adult—proestrus (Flores et al., 2008)		ng/mL	–	11.1 ± 1.9 $n = 25$	–	–
Adult—estrus (Flores et al., 2008)		ng/mL	–	17.3 ± 2.4 $n = 18$	–	–
Sodium	**Na**					
3–7 weeks (Giknis and Clifford, 2006)		mmol/L	143 (141–148) $n = 146$	143 (140–147) $n = 146$	–	–

(*Continued*)

TABLE 2.3 (*Continued*)
Serum Clinical Chemistry Normative Data for Rat Stocks (Mean ± SD [Ref Interval])

			Stock			
			Sprague-Dawley		Wistar	
Analyte	**Abbreviation**	**Units**	**M**	**F**	**M**	**F**
Sodium	**Na**					
8–12 weeks (Giknis and Clifford, 2006)		mmol/L	144 (141–150) *n* = 725	–	–	–
8–16 weeks (Giknis and Clifford, 2006)		mmol/L	–	–	146 ± 2 (142–151) *n* = 164	144 ± 2 (140–150) *n* = 159
13–22 weeks (Giknis and Clifford, 2008)		mmol/L	144 (141–149) *n* = 658	143 (141–148) *n* = 667	–	–
≥17 weeks (Giknis and Clifford, 2008)		mmol/L	–	–	143 ± 2 (137–147) *n* = 78	141 ± 3 (135–146) *n* = 77
23–47 weeks (Giknis and Clifford, 2006)		mmol/L	149 (143–157) *n* = 350	148 (147–156) *n* = 356	–	–
48–65 weeks (Giknis and Clifford, 2006)		mmol/L	147 (141–156) *n* = 55	146 (141–151) *n* = 55	–	–
88–150 weeks (Giknis and Clifford, 2006)		mmol/L	142 (141–156) *n* = 60	145 (139–151) *n* = 71	–	–
Sorbitol Dehydrogenase	**SDH**					
10 weeks (O'Brien et al., 2002)		IU/L	19 ± 6.8 *n* = 9	–	–	–
Testosterone						
4.7 weeks (Shin et al., 2009)		ng/mL	2.1 ± 0.31 *n* = 10	–	–	–
12–16 weeks (Ansari-Lari and Taniceh, 2009)		ng/mL	2.94 ± 1.08 *n* = 22	–	–	–
Adult (BW = 180–200g) (Hattori et al., 2007)		μg/L	–	–	3.46 ± 0.47 *n* = 21	

(*Continued*)

TABLE 2.3 (*Continued*)
Serum Clinical Chemistry Normative Data for Rat Stocks (Mean ± SD [Ref Interval])

			Stock			
			Sprague-Dawley		Wistar	
Analyte	**Abbreviation**	**Units**	**M**	**F**	**M**	**F**
Testosterone						
Adult—Diestrus 1 (Flores et al., 2008)	Strain: CIIZ-V	ng/mL	–	8.5 ± 2.3 $n = 29$	–	–
Adult—Diestrus 2 (Flores et al., 2008)		ng/mL	–	54.5 ± 8.4 $n = 30$	–	–
Adult—Proestrus (Flores et al., 2008)		ng/mL	–	99 ± 14.1 $n = 25$	–	–
Adult—Estrus (Flores et al., 2008)		ng/mL	–	<2 $n = 18$	–	–
Total Protein	**TP**					
3–7 weeks (Giknis and Clifford, 2006)		g/dL	5.9 (5.6–6.4) $n = 146$	6.0 (5.7–6.4) $n = 146$	–	–
8–12 weeks (Giknis and Clifford, 2006)		g/dL	6.2 (5.9–6.6) $n = 723$	6.4 (6.1–7.0) $n = 724$	–	–
13–22 weeks (Giknis and Clifford, 2006)		g/dL	6.4 (6.0–7.1) $n = 661$	6.7 (6.4–7.5) $n = 673$	–	–
8–16 weeks (Giknis and Clifford, 2008)		g/dL	–	–	6 ± 0.5 (5.2–7.1) $n = 164$	6.3 ± 0.5 (5.5–7.7) $n = 159$
≥17 weeks (Giknis and Clifford, 2008)		g/dL	–	–	6.3 ± 0.5 (5.6–7.6) $n = 77$	6.6 ± 0.7 (5.7–8.3) $n = 77$
23–47 weeks (Giknis and Clifford, 2006)		g/dL	6.9 (6.3–8.1) $n = 359$	7.2 (6.7–9.1) $n = 366$	–	–
48–65 weeks (Giknis and Clifford, 2006)		g/dL	6.4 (6.2–7.2) $n = 55$	7.2 (6.7–8.9) $n = 55$	–	–
88–150 weeks (Giknis and Clifford, 2006)		g/dL	6.0 (4.6–7.9) $n = 70$	5.7 (6.2–8.6) $n = 70$	–	–

(*Continued*)

TABLE 2.3 (*Continued*)
Serum Clinical Chemistry Normative Data for Rat Stocks (Mean ± SD [Ref Interval])

			Stock			
			Sprague-Dawley		Wistar	
Analyte	Abbreviation	Units	M	F	M	F
Triglycerides	**Trig**					
3–7 weeks		mg/dL	60 (53–73) *n* = 146	54 (41 + 66) *n* = 146	–	–
8–12 weeks (Giknis and Clifford, 2006)		mg/dL	73 (61–99) *n* = 653	60 (42–74)642	–	–
8–16 weeks (Giknis and Clifford, 2008)		mg/dL	–	–	44 ± 21 (20–114) *n* = 163	28 ± 8 (14–46) *n* = 159
13–22 weeks (Giknis and Clifford, 2006)		mg/dL	76 (62–92) *n* = 661	61 (51–75) *n* = 673	–	–
≥17 weeks (Giknis and Clifford, 2008)		mg/dL	–	–	62 ± 32 (27–160) *n* = 77	42 ± 35 (16–175) *n* = 76
23–47 weeks (Giknis and Clifford, 2006)		mg/dL	94 (46–208) *n* = 319	67 (30–205) *n* = 357	–	–
48–65 weeks (Giknis and Clifford, 2006)		mg/dL	110 (78–274) *n* = 55	84 (61–259) *n* = 55	–	–
88–150 weeks (Giknis and Clifford, 2006)		mg/dL	187 (81–329) *n* = 50	138 (31–289) *n* = 60	–	–
Cardiac Troponin I	**cTnI**					
Adult (Erenna – Singulex) (Schultze et al., 2009)		pg/mL	4.94 (1–15)		–	–
Tri-iodothyronin (total)	**tT3**					
6 months (Silvestri et al., 2008)		ng/dL	–	–	96.4 ± 11.8 *n* = 5	–
12 months (Silvestri et al., 2008)		ng/dL	–	–	95.6 ± 10.4 *n* = 5	–

(*Continued*)

TABLE 2.3 (*Continued*)
Serum Clinical Chemistry Normative Data for Rat Stocks (Mean ± SD [Ref Interval])

Analyte	Abbreviation	Units	Stock: Sprague-Dawley M	Stock: Sprague-Dawley F	Stock: Wistar M	Stock: Wistar F
Tri-iodothyronin (total)	**tT3**					
24 months (Silvestri et al., 2008)		ng/dL	–	–	28.2 ± 10.7 $n = 5$	–
Tri-iodothyronin (free)	**fT3**					
6 months (Silvestri et al., 2008)		ng/dL	–	–	2.60 ± 0.21 $n = 5$	–
12 months (Silvestri et al., 2008)		ng/dL	–	–	2.40 ± 0.19 $n = 5$	–
24 months (Silvestri et al., 2008)		ng/dL	–	–	1.30 ± 0.11 $n = 5$	–
Thyroid Stimulating Hormone	**TSH**					
6 months (Silvestri et al., 2008)		ng/dL	–	–	0.63 ± 0.03 $n = 5$	–
12 months (Silvestri et al., 2008)		ng/dL	–	–	0.62 ± 0.02 $n = 5$	–
24 months (Silvestri et al., 2008)		ng/dL	–	–	0.60 ± 0.02 $n = 5$	–
Thyroxine (total)	**tT4**					
6 months (Silvestri et al., 2008)		μg/dL	–	–	6.03 ± 0.59 $n = 5$	–
12 months (Silvestri et al., 2008)		μg/dL	–	–	4.20 ± 0.75 $n = 5$	–
24 months (Silvestri et al., 2008)		μg/dL	–	–	2.85 ± 0.80 $n = 5$	–

(*Continued*)

TABLE 2.3 (*Continued*)
Serum Clinical Chemistry Normative Data for Rat Stocks (Mean ± SD [Ref Interval])

			Stock			
			Sprague-Dawley		Wistar	
Analyte	**Abbreviation**	**Units**	**M**	**F**	**M**	**F**
Thyroxine (free)	**fT4**					
6 months (Silvestri et al., 2008)		µg/dL	–	–	1.30 ± 0.11 n = 5	–
12 months (Silvestri et al., 2008)		µg/dL	–	–	0.68 ± 0.13 n = 5	–
24 months (Silvestri et al., 2008)		µg/dL	–	–	0.28 ± 0.13 n = 5	–
Urea			–	–	–	–
<4 weeks (Petterino and Argentino-Storino, 2006)		mmol/L	14.7 ± 3.7 (6.6–31.4) n = 162	16.9 ± 3.6 (6.9–30.5) n = 162	–	–
13 weeks (Petterino and Argentino-Storino, 2006)		mmol/L	16.2 ± 4.4 (10.8–34.4) n = 160	17.9 ± 3.7 (11.1–31.7) n = 158	–	–
<6 months (Aleman CL et al., 1998)		mmol/L	7.21 ± 2.04	7.76 ± 2.26	–	–
6–18 months (Aleman CL et al., 1998)		mmol/L	6.09 ± 1.54	6.49 ± 1.09	–	–
18–32 months (Aleman CL et al., 1998)		mmol/L	6.31 ± 0.63	4.67 ± 0.75	–	–
Uric Acid						
Young (Hilltop Lab Animals, 2010)		mg/dL	(0.8–1.9)	(0.7–1.3)	(1.2–2.0)	(0.9–1.9)
Mature (Hilltop Lab Animals, 2010)		mg/dL	(0.5–1.6)	(0.4–2.5)	(0.7–1.5)	(0.9–1.2)

TABLE 2.4
Stressors for Laboratory Rats

Emotional Stress	Physical Stress
Restraint	Cold
Immobilization	Heat
Aggression	Fasting
Single housing	Blood collection
Change in housing	Immobilization
Transport	Illness
Chronic variable stress	Anesthesia
	Noise
	Dosing

analyzed. Water evaporation, solute decomposition, and bacterial growth can be minimized by collecting samples into cooled containers. If urine is collected in a cooled container, care must be taken so that the cooling system does not decrease the ambient temperature, cause stress to the animals housed in the metabolic cages, or cause water condensation within the underlying cage or on the inner surface of the collection container. In addition, collection of urine over ice changes the solubility characteristics of urine and may result in *ex vivo* crystallization or precipitation of solutes. The use of preservatives such as boric acid, thymol, toluene, and Stabilur® is not required and may even interfere with some analyses. For example, sodium azide and thimerosal at concentrations higher than 0.1% inhibit the enzymatic reaction for the detection of microalbumin. Conversely, preservatives and/or stabilizers may be required when control of bacterial contamination is a prerequisite or for detection of urinary enzymes (e.g., urine metabonomics, nuclear magnetic resonance [NMR]) (Evans, 2009).

The main advantage to collecting urine at necropsy is that sample deterioration and contamination are minimized and specialized caging is not required. Disadvantages of this technique are that they yield small volumes (usually <0.5 mL), urine will likely not be collected from all animals, and they may be technically challenging or time-consuming. The ability to collect urine samples at necropsy is dependent on having minimal pre-necropsy procedures and manipulations to minimize voiding prior to necropsy.

There are no specific storage requirements for rat urine compared to other species. Best practices minimize growth of bacterial contaminants. The containers and cleaning products used for urine collection and storage must be nonreactive with urine constituents. Samples should be stored at 2°C–6°C and are generally stable for less than 72 hours. Freezing samples at –20°C may falsely decrease the concentrations or activities of proteins including albumin, beta 2-microglobulin, GGT, and glutathione-*S*-transferase (GST) (Elving et al., 1989; Brinkman et al., 2005; Evans, 2009).

2.6 SOURCES OF VARIATION

The major preanalytical and analytical sources of variation in clinical chemistry parameters for laboratory rats are listed in Table 2.6. The sources of variability can be divided into those concerning inherent animal properties (e.g., age) and husbandry (e.g., caging), those concerning procedures conducted in conjunction with blood collection (e.g., collection site), and those occurring post-collection in the clinical chemistry laboratory (e.g., storage duration). There is a multitude of variables that can affect laboratory result outcomes including, but not limited to, considerations such as age, sex, strain, route of exposure, diet, caging, overnight fasting, handling, restraint, anesthetic, type of tube (anticoagulant or serum type), the use of anticoagulants, the site of collection,

TABLE 2.5
Sites for Blood Collection for Laboratory Rats

Site	Restraint	Survival or Terminal	Quantity	Potential for Contamination of Blood by Other Substances	Phlebotomist Skill	Collection Equipment	Comments	Selected References
Retro-orbital plexus	Anesthesia required	Terminal or survival in some geographic areas	~1–2 mL[a]	Moderate	Moderate	Capillary tube	Not approved by some Institutional Animal Care and Use Committees (IACUCs)	van Herck et al. (1998)
Dorsal and lateral tail veins	Tube-type restrainer or manual	Survival	0.1–0.2 mL	Low	Moderate	21 g needle		Conybeare (1988)
Ventral tail artery	Anesthesia optional	Survival	0.2–3 mL	Low	Moderate	19–27 g needle		Joslin (2009)
Tail incision	Tube-type restrainer or manual	Survival	0.1–0.3 mL	High	Moderate	Incision in vein		Fluttert (2000)
Jugular vein	Manual restraint or rodent bleed board without anesthesia, or anesthesia	Survival	~1–2 mL[a]	Low	High	Syringe and 23–25 g needle		Koch (2006)
Sublingual vein	Anesthesia required	Survival	~0.1–0.2mL	Moderate	Moderate	23g needle and syringe		Zeller et al. (1998)
Saphenous vein	Manual restraint or anesthesia	Survival	~1–2 mL[a]	High	High	23 g needle		Beeton et al. (2007) and Hem et al. (1998)
Indwelling catheter	Yes or No, depending on apparatus	Survival	~1–2 mL[a]	Low	Low	Preplaced catheter	Requires surgery; catheter maintenance	Thrivikraman KV(2002)
Decapitation	Anesthesia optional	Terminal	Entire blood volume	High	High	Guillotine	Used for neonates and stress studies	Koch (2006)
Abdominal aorta or vena cava	Anesthesia required	Terminal	Entire blood volume	Low	Low	Syringe and needle or vacutainer system		Koch (2006)
Cardiac	Anesthesia required	Terminal	Entire blood volume	High	Moderate	Syringe and needle	Generally abdominal vena cava or aorta preferable	Koch (2006)

[a] Volume collected generally limited by IACUC or Ethics Committee requirements.

TABLE 2.6
Sources of Variation in Rat Clinical Chemistry Parameters

Intrinsic	Blood Collection Procedures	Laboratory Procedures
Genetic background	Handling	Order of processing/analysis
Sex	Restraint	Laboratory instruments/ methodology
Supplier	Anesthesia	Sample handling and processing
Age	Skill of phlebotomist	
Housing/bedding	Site of collection	
Diet/nutrition	Volume collected	
Fasting status	Anticoagulant	
	Sample matrix	
	Order of collection	

and sample storage conditions. The following is a description of some of the more prominent concerns when clinical chemistry assessments are to be evaluated.

2.6.1 Sex and Age

Clinical chemistry parameters that are consistently higher in males compared to female rats are serum ALP and triglycerides, and urine protein and ketones (Zhang et al., 2004; Charles River, Inc., 1993; Harlan Research Models and Services, 2009).

Male rats between 8 and 60 weeks old show higher serum ALP activity compared to female rats primarily due to the predominance of the bone isoenzyme, with a lesser contribution from the liver isoenzyme (Hoffmann et al., 1994). Male rats have higher triglycerides compared to female rats due to the testosterone-mediated reduction of postheparin-lipoprotein lipase activity in males (Reaven, 1978, Shearer et al., 2000).

Sexually mature male rats show slightly more urine protein compared to female rats. Prior to 100 days of age, this is due to high urinary concentrations of the androgen-dependent rat prostatic protein alpha 2μ-globulin (Alt et al., 1980; Goldstein et al., 1988). Some nephrotoxicants cause accumulation of this male rat major urinary protein in secondary lysozomes of renal tubules, resulting in a male rat-specific nephrotoxicity (Hard et al., 1993). In addition, male rats are susceptible to the development of age-related nephropathy (Doi et al., 2007). Because of this condition, the primary urinary protein in aging male rats older than 200 days is albumin and is associated with chronic renal disease (Goldstein et al., 1988; Loeb, 1999). Urine from fasted male rats often has trace urine ketones, whereas urine from female rats is negative by the dipstick method.

Clinical chemistry values that decrease with age in rats include phosphorus and ALP (Lillie et al., 1996; Hoffmann et al., 1994; Wolford et al., 1987). Clinical chemistry values that increase and become more variable with age in rats include aspartate aminotransferase (AST), alanine aminotransferase (ALT), glutamate dehydrogenase (GLDH), cholesterol, and triglycerides (Lindena et al., 1980; O'Brien et al., 2000; Waner et al., 1991; Wolford et al., 1987; Charles River Laboratories, Inc., 1993). In general, clinical chemistry values of younger rats (less than 6 months old) exhibit less interindividual variability (lower coefficient of variation (CV)%) compared to older animals (Charles River, Inc., 1993). In older animals, the high degree of heterogeneity due to age-related changes and spontaneous disease may obscure compound effects, making clinical pathology testing less informative.

Young rats tend to have higher ALP owing to higher bone, as well as intestinal and liver ALP isoenzymes; the activity of these isoenzymes decreases during aging, with the biggest decrease in bone ALP. Adult activities are reached by 34 weeks of age in both sexes (Hoffmann et al., 1994).

Urinary protein, especially albumin, increases from about 8 to 14 months of age in both sexes (Robinson and Evans, 1996).

2.6.2 Genetic Influence

Undoubtedly, several strain- and stock-related differences occur for clinical chemistry parameters of rats. Unfortunately, there are no published studies comparing full chemistry panels of commonly used rat strains and stocks on a side-to-side basis (within the same lab and at the same time). Some documented strain differences are listed below:

- Multilaboratory genetic background differences have been reported for AST (F344 > SD), ALP (F344 > SD > Wistar), creatinine (F344 > SD or Wistar), and creatine kinase (SD > Wistar or F344) (Matsuzawa et al., 1993).
- Sprague-Dawley rats excrete approximately twice as much urinary protein when compared to Han Wistar rats (Ramaiah et al., 2009). This may relate to Sprague-Dawley's susceptibility to chronic progressive nephropathy. Susceptibility to urolithiasis is also greater in SD rats than that in Wistar, likely due to higher protein and magnesium excretion in SD rats (Brdicka, 1984).
- Bilirubin is higher in mutant strains (e.g., Gunn rat) which cannot convert bilirubin to glucuronide because they lack uridine diphosphate (UDP)-glucuronate glucuronyltransferase activity (Wolf et al., 1979; Robinson, 1971).
- Wistar rats may be more sensitive to anesthesia (ketamine/xylazine followed by 5 hours of isoflurane) than Sprague-Dawley rats. Wistar rats anesthetized with this regimen have decreased blood pH and increased lactate, creatinine, ALT, AST, and lactate dehydrogenase (LDH) compared to similarly treated Sprague-Dawley rats (Siller-Matula and Jilma, 2008).
- Rats from different genetic backgrounds may vary in their stress response to restraint. After a given stressor, Fischer rats tend to exhibit greater changes in stress-related parameters, while SD and Wistar rats are intermediate, and Long-Evans rats exhibit very low stress responses (Dhabhar et al., 1997).

2.6.3 Nutritional Status

Rats are extensively utilized in nutrition research. A thorough review of the effects of dietary manipulation on clinical chemistry parameters is beyond the scope of this chapter. However, a brief discussion of the effects of diet restriction on clinical chemistry is presented below. Effects of fasting are discussed as a part of preanalytical variables impacting clinical chemistry parameters.

In rats, short-term dietary restriction of ≤ 2 weeks can result in decreased globulins and cholesterol, increased bilirubin, and electrolyte disturbances related to the severity of the restriction (Levin et al., 1993). Long-term restriction decreased total protein, albumin, globulin, triglycerides, phosphorus, potassium, and increased ALP, ALT, AST, urea nitrogen, and sodium, and either decreased or increased glucose (Schwartz et al., 1973; Oishi et al., 1979; Boiziau et al., 1996). Urine protein excretion is decreased in diet-restricted rats compared to ad libitum-fed rats (Gumprecht et al., 1993).

2.6.4 Caging

Housing type (wire-bottom vs. solid-bottom caging) has been shown to exhibit little or only transient effects on clinical chemistry parameters in rats (Sauer et al., 2006). A change in caging causes a transient, 8–10-fold increase in corticosterone. Corticosterone concentrations peak approximately 40 minutes after a rat is placed in a new cage and return to baseline after 2 hours (Fluttert et al., 2000).

2.6.5 Circadian Rhythm

Most diurnal variations in clinical chemistry parameters can be attributed to light/dark cycles, hypothalamic–pituitary axis rhythms (circadian and ultradian), and feeding cycles. The nocturnal feeding habits of rats are likely responsible for the circadian rhythms of serum ALP and urine volume, urinary protein excretion, and fractional excretion of phosphorus, sodium, chloride, potassium, and calcium (Ramaiah et al., 2009). Circadian variations in urinary analytes that are independent of feeding habits exist for glomerular filtration rate and renal excretion of potassium, calcium, and phosphorus (Rabinowitz et al., 1987; Ramaiah et al., 2009). In addition, diurnal variations have been reported for tacrolimus-induced nephrotoxicity in rats (Yamauchi et al., 2004). A circadian rhythm of urinary immunoglobulin excretion in rats has been reported following the subcutaneous implantation of a lymphoid tumor that produced immunoglobulin light chains (Nelson et al., 1974).

Diurnal differences in hormone concentrations in rats are well documented. Diurnal rhythms are observed for a wide variety of hormones, including but not limited to melatonin, adrenocorticotropic hormone (ACTH), corticosterone, aldosterone, thyroxine, intermedin, calcitonin (and calcium), follicle stimulating hormone, thyrotropin, and prolactin (Levinson, 1940; Nathanielsz, 1969; Milhaud et al., 1972; McLean et al., 1977; Kimura and Kawakami, 1980; Szafarczyk et al., 1985; Kant et al., 1986; Laakset al., 1990; Atkinson and Waddell, 1997; Lightman et al., 2000; Evans, 2009). Minor diurnal variations have also been reported for glucose, triglycerides, cholesterol, and amino acids (Kaminsky and Kosenko, 1986; Marrino et al., 1987; Eriksson et al., 1989).

A circadian rhythm has been demonstrated for markers of bone metabolism. Studies using dietary calcium restriction found a circadian rhythm in total calcium concentration (Hirsch and Hagaman, 1982; Lausson et al., 1985). The bone metabolic markers reported to exhibit a circadian rhythm include ALP, procollagen type I C-terminal peptide (PICP), type I C-terminal telopeptide (ICTP), hydroxyproline (HYP), and Ca. These variations appear to be regulated by melatonin and light/dark cycles. In addition, ICTP and Ca concentrations correlate positively with daily fluctuation of insulin-like growth factor-1 (IGF-1) (Ostrowska et al., 2003).

2.6.6 Effects of Estrous Cycle, Pregnancy, or Lactation

The effect of the rat estrus cycle on routine clinical chemistry parameters has not been described. Effects of the estrus cycle on plasma corticosterone have been documented, with lowest concentrations at estrus and highest concentrations at proestrus. The differences are most pronounced at the peak of the circadian rhythm (Atkinson and Waddell, 1997). Effects of pregnancy on clinical chemistry parameters have been evaluated in several studies with generally concordant results (LaBorde et al., 1999; Papworth and Clubb, 1995a, 1995b; Liberati et al., 2004; de Rijk et al., 2002; Horne and Fergusen, 1972). Most of the changes in the dams occur near term. ALP, glucose, bilirubin, total protein, albumin, sodium, and chloride are fairly consistently reported to be decreased near termination of pregnancy. The mechanism underlying the decreases in the latter four parameters may be the characteristic plasma volume expansion that occurs in pregnancy in many species. The largest magnitude of change occurs for triglycerides (a three- to fourfold increase). Postnatally, most values return to baseline within a short period of time. During lactation, calcium and parathyroid hormone (PTH) concentrations are increased compared to non-lactating controls (Gonen et al., 2005).

2.6.7 Fasting

Fasting of rats prior to measurement of clinical chemistry parameters is a practice with advantages and disadvantages, and the decision to fast or not should be made on a case-by-case basis (Matsuzawa and Sakazume, 1994). The advantages of fasting are that it yields data that is less variable and minimizes changes related to test article effects on food consumption. In contrast, allowing access to food prior to blood collection maintains the normal feeding schedule of rats (e.g., prevents a nonphysiologic catabolic state that may obfuscate effects). In addition, fasting status can affect the rate of test article absorption and clearance from the stomach. Regardless of fasting status, consistency must be maintained among the treatment of all animals.

In general, fasting of rats for up to 24 hours results in decreased serum ALP, bilirubin, cholesterol, triglycerides, glucose, and total protein. Most parameters recover within 6 hours of refeeding (Maejima and Nagase, 1991; Mitev et al., 1993; Thompson et al., 1989; Matsuzawa and Sakazume, 1994; Waner and Nyska, 1994).

Serum ALP of rats is more influenced by status of food intake than that of other species (Evans, 2009). Fasting decreases serum ALP activities in the rat. Feeding, especially with a high fat meal, results in increased ALP within approximately 7 hours (Eliakim et al., 1991; Hoffmann et al., 1994). The influence of feeding status on ALP in the rat is at least partially due to its longer half-life (54.1–68.3 minutes for the second elimination phase; Young et al., 1984). Intestinal ALP (IAP) of the rat is the product of two separate genes that share only 79% sequence homology (Engle and Alpers, 1992), unlike other species that have different isoforms of intestinal ALP due to posttranslational modifications. The intestinal alkaline phosphatase (IAP)-II isoenzyme is most responsive to feeding of a fat meal (Eliakim et al., 1990).

Fasting of rats also results in an initial fall in water intake coupled with an increase in urine output (Thompson et al., 1987; Apostolou et al., 1976; Pickering and Pickering, 1984). After 24 hours of fasting, rats begin to conserve sodium, unlike other species that exhibit natriuresis (Van Liew et al., 1978).

2.6.8 Handling

Entry of a caretaker into an animal room and movement of cages causes increases in plasma protein, glucose, pyruvate, and lactate, along with other indicators of excitement/stress (heart rate, hematocrit, hemoglobin, plasma protein) (Gärtner et al., 1980). Routine cage changing alters behavior and cardiovascular parameters in rats, but clinical chemistry parameters were not investigated (Duke et al., 2001). Anesthetizing rats in their home cages has been shown to be less stressful than removing animals and placing them in an induction chamber, although the effect on standard clinical chemistry parameters was not determined (Fomby et al., 2004). Limited data exists on the effects on clinical chemistry parameters of picking up rats from their home cage. Picking up rats behind the front legs results in twofold higher serum creatine kinase activities compared to picking rats up by the tail, even if rats are handled for 30 seconds or less (Yerroum et al., 1999).

2.6.9 Restraint

Light restraint of rats for 6 hours, allowing movement of limbs but restriction of relocation (vertical 23°C water immersion to the level of the xyphoid process while confined within a firmly fitted stainless mesh cage), results in increases in creatine kinase (CK), AST, ALT, LDH, amylase, lipase, urea nitrogen, creatinine, and glucose; some of the increases are quite dramatic (Arakawa et al., 1997). Recovery for most parameters is partial or complete by 24 hours. These increases in serum enzymes are blocked by pretreatment with β-adrenergic agonists, suggesting that stress associated with restraint, rather than the physical restraint itself, is responsible for these effects. When exposed to repeated consistent handling or mild restraint, rats may become habituated. Habituation results in attenuation of the increase in ACTH, corticosterone, and glucose in some stress models (Márquez et al., 2004).

2.6.10 Anesthesia

Some anesthetics have significant effects on clinical chemistry parameters in rats. Inhalation anesthetics have the least effects, and are generally the method of choice for rat anesthesia, provided that proper protection is afforded the experimenter (e.g., backdraft tables, scavenging systems). Generally speaking, all inhalation anesthetics have some effects on clinical chemistry when compared with unanesthetized rats (Deckardt et al., 2007). Historical publications addressing effects of anesthesia commonly include experiments using ether, an anesthetic that is infrequently used at the present time. Many of these studies also include collection of blood from the retro-orbital plexus as a survival procedure. As noted previously, collection from this site is now limited in some geographical areas to terminal procedures under anesthesia.

Inhalation anesthetics such as isoflurane provide sufficient depth and length of anesthesia for most blood collection procedures. Isoflurane anesthesia for less than 10 minutes has little to no impact on routine clinical chemistry parameters for rats (unpublished observation; Saha et al., 2005). Blood collected from the jugular vein of isoflurane anesthetized non-cannulated rats had similar but slightly higher serum corticosterone and glucose concentrations compared to blood collected from non-anesthetized rats with cannulated jugular veins, suggesting that the anesthetic procedure is slightly stressful (Vachon and Moreau, 2001). Rats rapidly recover from short-term isoflurane without deleterious effects. Ether or halothane/O_2/N_2O anesthesia increase glucose; ether also increases pyruvate and lactate (de Haan et al., 2002; Gärtner et al., 1980). CO_2 or CO_2/O_2 combinations have been used for immobilization of rats for blood collection but are more stressful than isoflurane (Altholtz et al., 2006). Compared to animals exposed only to room air, animals immobilized with CO_2 or CO_2/O_2 mixtures prior to retro-orbital plexus blood collection have higher serum glucose concentrations and lower calcium concentrations and CK and ALT activities (Walter, 1999). CO_2 anesthesia is inappropriate for studies in which blood gas parameters are measured (e.g., Gaspari et al., 2007).

Injectable anesthetics (generally given intramuscularly or intraperitoneally) are also used for rat anesthesia. Intramuscular injection of anesthetics causes alterations in serum activities of muscle enzymes, increasing AST, ALT, CK, and LDH. Other muscle-specific parameters such as skeletal troponin and aldolase would likely also be affected. Xylazine alone or in combination with ketamine increases glucose (Saha et al., 2005; Rodrigues et al., 2006). Intraperitoneal injections of saline cause markedly increased corticosterone, indicating stress; these changes likely occur with intraperitoneal injections of pentobarbital as well (personal observation). Intraperitoneal pentobarbital may also result in hemolysis, with resultant effect on clinical chemistry parameters.

2.6.11 Site of Blood Collection

Because methods vary widely among the numerous studies examining effects of site of collection on clinical chemistry parameters, consistency among the results is limited (Van Herck et al., 2001; Dameron et al., 1992; Suber et al., 1985; Neptun et al., 1985). In addition, such studies are invariably complicated by differences in anesthesia, collection device, and volume collected among the different sites of blood collection, making interpretation of data even more difficult. These publications, like those evaluating effects of anesthetics (e.g., ether), include data from procedures that, at the current time, are less frequently used or only used in limited geographic areas. The following studies illustrate the differences observed depending on the experimental conditions used.

Comparing heart (H), retro-orbital plexus (O), and tail collection (T), Suber found the following effects for various clinical chemistry parameters: ALP (O>H=T), LDH (H=T>O), AST, ALT, GGT, creatinine (H>O=T), urea nitrogen (H=O=T). Comparing retro-orbital plexus to posterior vena cava, Dameron observed mostly minor effects except for magnesium and phosphorus, which were both higher in the posterior vena cava. Neptun et al. (1985) examined five sites of collection and found that, for most parameters, tail and retro-orbital plexus samples of blood deviated most from the grand mean of all methods, and that exsanguination and small volume collection from the identical site resulted in significantly different results (Neptun et al., 1985). Blood collected from the retro-orbital plexus of rats under ether anesthesia had lower glucose and total bile acid concentrations and higher cholesterol and triglyceride concentrations and sorbitol dehydrogenase (SDH) activity (Khan et al., 1996). Finally, samples collected from two periorbital sites (retro-orbital plexus and dorsal anastomotic orbital vein), sublingual vein, and abdominal aorta, all under ether anesthesia showed significant increases for creatine kinase, LDH, and AST activities in the peripheral sites, compared to that in the abdominal aorta (Bernardi et al., 1996).

Decapitation has been considered to be essential for stress studies in which ACTH and catecholamine concentrations are measured. However, recent literature in mice and rats suggests that retro-orbital or arterial cannulation (mice) or tail vein collection (rats) are equal or superior to decapitation (Vahl et al., 2005; Grouzmann et al., 2003).

Some sites for blood collection have been reported to be inappropriate for certain parameters. Compared to the blood collected from a tail vein, the blood collected from the retro-orbital plexus or from the heart results in increased creatine kinase activity. Creatine kinase and AST activities are highly increased when blood is repeatedly collected from the retro-orbital plexus compared to that collected from the sublingual vein (Mahl et al., 2000). Blood collection by puncture of heart has been shown to alter cardiac troponin concentrations as well as creatine kinase activities (Bachmaier et al., 1995).

2.6.12 Volume of Blood Collected

Although IACUC guidelines allow blood collection volumes that are acceptable in terms of animal welfare, these volumes are considerably sufficient to affect the clinical pathology parameters in subsequent blood draws. In addition, blood collection may potentiate or obfuscate test article effects on hematologic and clinical chemistry parameters (Furuhama et al., 1987). Published data on the effect of repeated blood sampling on clinical chemistry parameters in rats is limited; however, single or repeated phlebotomies may increase serum glucose, regardless of site (Mahl et al., 2000). In addition, clinical chemistry parameters measured when limited blood is collected may differ from those measured in blood collected from the same site during exsanguination (Neptun et al., 1985).

2.6.13 Post-Collection Processing Artifacts

Interferences: As with other species, hemolysis, lipemia, and icterus can influence results of clinical chemistry parameters. The level at which these interferents affect results is dependent on instrumentation and methodology used in the laboratory. Each laboratory should establish its own levels of acceptable hemolysis, lipemia, and icterus; and develop criteria for unacceptable levels of interference. Species-specific interferences that affect rats are effects of hemolysis and platelet counts on potassium concentrations. Hemolysis as an interferent is similar for rats, humans, and other species with similar biochemical RBC composition. Rat red blood cells contain high concentrations of potassium relative to serum such that hemolysis in rats increases serum potassium concentrations (Harvey, 1997). Because rats, like mice, have high numbers of platelets (approximately 900–1500 × $10^3/\mu L$), formation of a clot releases sufficient amounts of potassium to result in substantial differences between plasma (non-clotted) and serum (clotted) potassium concentrations (Sevastos et al., 2008). This effect is exaggerated in rats with increased platelets.

Evaporation during processing and analysis can affect clinical chemistry results due to the small volume of serum/plasma available from rats. Evaporative concentration of analytes usually is most noticeable for sodium and chloride, since these parameters have such a narrow range of values in health. To minimize the effect of evaporation, it is important to keep samples covered, to run samples in a timely fashion, and to randomize or stratify collection and analysis across groups in order to minimize the consequence of evaporation.

Refrigerated and frozen stability for clinical chemistry parameters of the rat has been reported in the literature and is generally similar to the stability for human parameters (Cray et al., 2009). Freezing and storing serum samples at –70°C is preferable to freezing and storing at –20°C. Of the common clinical chemistry parameters measured, CK, CO_2, and ALT have the lowest stability when rat serum samples are frozen at –70°C. Because stability is dependent on methodology, it is important for each laboratory to establish stability under the conditions in which it operates. For example, recently, it has been shown that the CK activity of rats can be almost doubled by maintaining the serum sample at room temperature rather than at 4°C prior to analysis (Goicoechea et al., 2008).

2.7 REFERENCE INTERVALS FOR LABORATORY RATS

Reference intervals for clinical chemistry parameters of laboratory rats are available from numerous sources, including this book (Table 2.3), for rats of various ages, strains, and sexes. As mentioned in the previous sections, several preanalytical factors influence the result generated for a given clinical chemistry parameter. In addition to the preanalytical factors described earlier in this chapter, other procedures within a laboratory also affect results, including sample handling, instrumentation, assay methodology, and laboratory data review procedures (Matsuzawa et al., 1997). For these reasons, the most useful clinical chemistry reference intervals are those generated within each laboratory based on routine conditions (Hall, 1997). Reference intervals are useful tools to gauge the magnitude of changes and to determine whether they are adverse or not (Table 2.7). However, they should not be relied upon to determine the relatedness of a change to an experimental treatment. To interpret changes in clinical pathology endpoints, test values must be compared to that from concurrent controls, using reference intervals as supportive data if necessary. A robust change from controls may be within the reference interval but may still be consistent with a treatment-related effect. This is particularly true for stocks/strains of rats (vs. large animals), where the inter-individual homogeneity and more animals per group enables detection of subtle changes.

TABLE 2.7
Quantitative Urinalysis Normative Data for Male Han Wistar—Crl:WI(Han)—Rats Age 11–15 Weeks

Analyte	Units	Mean ± SD	Ref Interval	*n*
Water intake	mL/hour	1.24 ± 0.75	(0.08–2.45)	192
Volume (20 hours)	mL/hour	1.04 ± 0.61	(0.23–2.23)	192
Osmolality	mOsm/kg H_2O	664 ± 593	(205–2118)	191
Free water clearance		–0.33 ± 0.49	(–1.03–0.60)	174
pH		6.6 ± 0.5	(5.8–7.0)	192
Sodium (Na)				
Concentration	mmol/L	43 ± 42	(10–19)	192
Rate of excretion	µmol/hour	30 ± 12	(12–52)	192
Fractional excretion	%	0.12 ± 0.06	(0.05–0.21)	174
Chloride (Cl)				
Concentration	mmol/L	48 ± 60	(20–211)	192
Rate of excretion	µmol/hour	32 ± 18	(14–72)	192
Fractional excretion	%	0.15 ± 0.06	(0.07–0.25)	174
Potassium (K)				
Concentration	mmol/L	90.3 ± 95.9	(23.6–351.2)	192
Rate of excretion	µmol/hour	59 ± 28	(31–130)	192
Fractional excretion	%	8.3 ± 3.2	(3.9–14)	174
Calcium				
Concentration	mmol/L	0.87 ± 0.86	(0.05–2.71)	192
Rate of excretion	µmol/hour	0.6 ± 0.5	(0.1–1.4)	192
Fractional excretion	%	0.12 ± 0.10	(0.02–0.29)	192
Phosphorus				
Concentration	mmol/L	38.6 ± 29.1	(12.0–103.7)	192
Rate of excretion	µmol/hour	27.2 ± 7.2	(16.1–39.0)	192
Fractional excretion	%	7.5 ± 2.8	(3.5–12.4)	174

(Continued)

TABLE 2.7 (*Continued*)
Quantitative Urinalysis Normative Data for Male Han Wistar—Crl:WI(Han)—Rats Age 11–15 Weeks

Analyte	Units	Mean ± SD	Ref Interval	*n*
Creatinine				
Concentration	mmol/L	5.0 ± 3.3	(1.6–10.6)	192
Rate of excretion	μmol/hour	3.6 ± 0.9	(2.2–5.2)	192
Renal clearance	μL/minutes	3102 ± 1170	(1598–5104)	174
Urea nitrogen				
Concentration	mmol/L	397 ± 378	(113–1366)	160
Rate of excretion	μmol/hour	250 ± 102	(150–498)	160
Renal clearance	μL/minutes	706 ± 193	(382–1015)	142
Albumin	mg/L	<6.3	<6.3	159
Protein concentration				
Concentration	g/L	0.47 ± 0.50	(0.09–1.57)	192
Rate of excretion	μg/hour	285 ± 182	(142–567)	192
Ratio to creatinine (UPC)	ratio	0.79 ± 0.62	(0.32–1.66)	200
Glucose				
Concentration	mmol/L	0.57 ± 0.93	(0.11–2.72)	192
Rate of excretion	μmol/hour	0.34 ± 0.32	(0.12–1.01)	192
Fractional excretion	%	0.027 ± 0.013	(0.011–0.043)	174

Note: Huntingdon Life Sciences Historical Control Database for Renal Safety Pharmacology. February 2010 (unpublished). Vehicle-treated control Han Wistar males aged 11–15 weeks; 20-hour overnight urine collection in metabolic cage into cooled container.

REFERENCES

Alemán, C.L., Más, R.M., Rodeiro, I., et al. 1998. Reference database of the main physiological parameters in Sprague-Dawley rats from 6 to 32 months. *Lab Anim.* 32:457–466.

Alt, J.M, Hackbarth, H., Deerberg, F., and Stolte, H. 1980. Proteinuria in rats in relation to age-dependent renal changes. *Lab Anim.* 14:95–101.

Altholtz, L.Y., Fowler, K.A., Badura, L.L., and Kovacs, M.S. 2006. Comparison of the stress response in rats to repeated isoflurane or CO2:O2 anesthesia used for restraint during serial blood collection via the jugular vein. *J Am Assoc Lab Anim Sci.* 45:17–22.

Ansari-Lari, M., and Taniceh, N. 2009. Changes in sex hormones and offspring sex ratio following gasoline exposure in male rats. *Comp Clin Pathol.* 18:43–45

Apostolou, A., Saidt, L., and Brown, W.R. 1976. Effect of overnight fasting of young rats on water consumption, body weight, blood sampling, and blood composition. *Lab Anim Sci.* 26(6 Pt 1):959–960.

Arakawa, H., Kodama. H., Matsuoka, N., and Yamaguchi, I. 1997. Stress increases plasma enzyme activity in rats: Differential effects of adrenergic and cholinergic blockades. *J Pharmacol Exp Ther.* 280:1296–1303.

Arglebe, C., Bremer, K., and Chilla, R. 1978. Hyperamylasaemia in isoprenaline-induced experimental sialadenosis in the rat. *Arch Oral Biol.* 23:997–999.

Atkinson, H.C., and Waddell, B.J. 1997. Circadian variation in basal plasma corticosterone and adrenocorticotropin in the rat: Sexual dimorphism and changes across the estrous cycle. *Endocrinology.* 138:3842–3848.

Bachmaier, K., Mair, J., Offner, F., Pummerer, C., and Neu, N. 1995. Serum cardiac troponin T and creatine kinase–MB elevations in murine autoimmune myocarditis. *Circulation.* 92:1927–1932.

Beeton, C., Garcia, A., and Chandy, K.G. 2007. Drawing blood from rats through the saphenous vein and by cardiac puncture. *J Vis Exp.* 7:266.

Bernardi, C., Moneta, D., Brughera, M., et al. 1996. Hematology and clinical chemistry in rats: Comparison of different blood collection sites. *Comp Haematol Int.* 6:160–166.

Boiziau, JL., Jabes, F., and Deshayes, C. 1996. The effect of food restriction on body weights and clinical chemistry in Sprague Dawley rats. *Toxicol Lett.* 88(Suppl 1): 107.

Brdicka, R. 1984. Urinary proteins: Interstrain differences in the laboratory rat. *Anim Blood Groups Biochem Genet.* 15:79–83.

Brinkman, J.W., de Zeeuw, D., Duker JJ., et al. 2005. Falsely low urinary albumin concentrations after prolonged frozen storage of urine samples. *Clin Chem.* 51:2181–2183.

Budohoski, L., Challiss, R.A.J., Dubaniewicz, A., et al. 1987. Effects of prolonged elevation of plasma adrelanine concentration in vivo on insulin-sensitivity in soleus muscle of the rat. *Biochem J.* 244:655–660.

Capen, C.C., DeLellis, R.A., Yarrington, J.T. 2002. Chapter 41: Endocrine system. In *Handbook of Toxicologic Pathology*, 2nd edition, Vol. 2. W.B. Hashek, C.G. Rousseaux, and M.A. Wallig. San Diego, CA: Academic Press.

Car, B.D. 2006. Chapter 6: Clinical pathology of the rat. In *The Laboratory Rat*, 2nd edition. Eds. M. Suckow, S.H. Weisbroth, C.L. Franklin. Worcester, MA: Elsevier Academic Press.

Charles River, Inc. 1993. Serum Chemistry Parameters for the Crl:CD®BR Rat. Charles River Research Models and Services (general page with links to specific strains). Available at: http://www.criver.com/files/pdfs/rms/cd/rm_rm_d_cd_rat.aspx (Accesssed 21 April 2017).

Cohen, S.M., Cano, M., Anderson, T., and Garland, E.M. 1996. Extensive handling of rats leads to mild urinary bladder hyperplasia. *Toxicol Pathol.* 24:251–257.

Cohen, S.M., Ohnishi, T., Clark, N.M., He, J., and Arnold, L.L. 2007. Investigations of rodent urinary bladder carcinogens: Collection, processing, and evaluation of urine and bladders. *Toxicol Pathol.* 35:337–347.

Conybeare, G., Leslie, G.B., Angles, K., Barrett, R.J., Luke, J.S., and Gask, D.R. 1988. An improved simple technique for the collection of blood samples from rats and mice. *Lab Anim.* 22:177–182.

Cray, C., Rodriguez, M., Zaias, J., and Altman, N.H. 2009. Effects of storage temperature and time on clinical biochemical parameters from rat serum. *J Am Assoc Lab Anim Sci.* 48:202–204.

Creasy, D.M. 2003. Evaluation of testicular toxicity: A synopsis and discussion of the recommendation proposed by the Society of Toxicologic Pathology. *Birth Defects Res, B Dev Reprod Toxicol.* 68:408–415.

Dameron, G.W., Weingand, K.W., Duderstadt, J.M., et al. 1992. Effect of bleeding site on clinical laboratory testing of rats: Orbital venous plexus vs. posterior vena cava. *Lab Anim Sci.* 42(3):299–301.

de Haan, M., van Herck, H., Tolboom, J.B., Beynen, A.C., and Remie, R. 2002. Endocrine stress response in jugular-vein cannulated rats upon multiple exposure to either diethyl-ether, halothane/O2/N2O or sham anaesthesia. *Lab Anim.* 36:105–114.

de Rijk, E.P., van Esch, E., and Flik, G. 2002. Pregnancy dating in the rat: Placental morphology and maternal blood parameters. *Toxicol Pathol.* 30:271–282.

Deckardt, K., Weber, I., Kaspers, U., Hellwig, J., Tennekes, H., and van Ravenzwaay, B. 2007. The effects of inhalation anaesthetics on common clinical pathology parameters in laboratory rats. *Food Chem Toxicol.* 45(9):1709–1718.

Dhabhar, F.S., McEwen, B.S., and Spencer, R.L. 1997. Adaptation to prolonged or repeated stress–comparison between rat strains showing intrinsic differences in reactivity to acute stress. *Neuroendocrinology.* 65:360–368.

Dinh, B.L., Tremblay, A., and Dufour, D. 1965. Immunochemical study on rat urinary proteins: Their relation to serum and kidney proteins (chromatographic separation of the major urinary protein). *J Immunol.* 95:574–582.

Doi, A.M., Hill, G., Seely, J., Hailey, J.R., Kissling, G., and Bucher, J.R. 2007. Alpha 2u-globulin nephropathy and renal tumors in national toxicology program studies. *Toxicol Pathol.* 35:533–540.

Duke, J.L., Zammit, T.G., and Lawson, D.M. 2001. The effects of routine cage-changing on cardiovascular and behavioral parameters in male Sprague-Dawley rats. *Contemp Top Lab Anim Sci.* 40:17–20.

Eliakim, R., Mahmood, A., and Alpers, D.H. 1991. Rat intestinal alkaline phosphatase secretion into lumen and serum is coordinately regulated. *Biochim Biophys Acta.* 1091:1–8.

Eliakim, R., Seetharam, S., Tietze, C.C., and Alpers, D.H. 1990. Differential regulation of mRNAs encoding for rat intestinal alkaline phosphatase. *Am J Physiol Gastrointest Liver Physiol.* 259:G93–G98.

Elving, L.D., Bakkeren, J.A., Jansen, M.J., de Kat Angelino, C.M., de Nobel, E., and van Munster, P.J. 1989. Screening for microalbuminuria in patients with diabetes mellitus: Frozen storage of urine samples decreases their albumin content. *Clin Chem.* 35:308–310.

Engle, M.J., and Alpers, D.H. 1992. The two mRNAs encoding rat intestinal alkaline phosphatase represent two unique nucleotide sequences. *Clin Chem.* 38:2506–2509.

Eriksson, E., Royo, F., Lyberg, K., Carlsson, H.E., and Hau, J. 2004. Effect of metabolic cage housing on immunoglobulin A and corticosterone excretion in faeces and urine of young male rats. *Exp Physiol.* 89:427–433.

Eriksson, T., Wiesel, K., Voog, L., and Hagman, M. 1989. Diurnal rhythms in rat plasma amino acids. *Life Sci.* 45:979–986.

Evans, G. 2009. *Animal Clinical Chemistry*. London: Taylor & Francis.

Firriolo, J.M., Morris, C.F., Trimmer, G.W., Twitty, L.D., Smith, J.H., and Freeman, J.J. 1995. Comparative 90-day feeding study with low-viscosity white mineral oil in Fischer-344 and Sprague-Dawley-derived CRL: CD rats. *Toxicol Pathol.* 23:26–33.

Flores, A., Gallegos, A.I., Velasco, J., et al. 2008. The acute effects of bilateral ovariectomy or adrenalectomy on progesterone, testosterone and estradiol serum levels depend on the surgical approach and the day of the estrous cycle when they are performed. *Reprod Biol Endocrinol.* 6:48.

Fluttert, M., Dalm, S., and Oitzl, M.S. 2000. A refined method for sequential blood sampling by tail incision in rats. *Lab Anim.* 34:372–378.

Fomby, L.M., Wheat, T.M., Hatter, D.E., Tuttle, R.L., and Black, C.A. 2004. Use of CO2/O2 anesthesia in the collection of samples for serum corticosterone analysis from Fischer 344 rats. *Contemp Top Lab Anim Sci.* 43:8–12.

Fryer, R.M., Segreti, J.A., Widomski, D.L., et al. 2007. Systemic activation of the calcium sensing receptor produces acute effects on vascular tone and circulatory function in uremic and normal rats: Focus on central versus peripheral control of vascular tone and blood pressure by cinacalcet. *J Pharmacol Exp Ther.* 323(1):217–226.

Furuhama, K., Kato, M., Suzuki, N., Igarashi, K., and Onodera, T. 1987. The influence of single or repeated phlebotomy on the physiological condition of normal and diseased rats. *J Toxicol Sci.* 12:1–9.

Gärtner, K., Büttner, D., Döhler, K., Friedel, R., Lindena, J., and Trautschold, I. 1980. Stress response of rats to handling and experimental procedures. *Lab Anim.* 14: 267–274.

Gaspari, R.J., and Paydarfar, D. 2007. Pathophysiology of respiratory failure following acute dichlorvos poisoning in a rodent model. *Neurotoxicology.* 28:664–671.

Gentry, P. 1999 Acute phase proteins. In *The Clinical Chemistry of Laboratory Animals*. Eds. W.F. Loeb and F.W. Quimby, 2nd edition, pp. 336–398. Philadelphia, PA: Taylor & Francis.

Giknis, M.L.A. and Clifford, C.B. 2006. *Clinical Laboratory Parameters for Crl:CD(SD) Rats*. Charles River Laboratories. Available at: http://www.criver.com/files/pdfs/rms/cd/rm_rm_r_clinical_parameters_cd_rat_06.aspx (Accessed 21 April 2017).

Giknis, M.L.A., and Clifford, C.B. 2008. Clinical Laboratory Parameters for Crl:WI(Han). Available at http://www.criver.com/files/pdfs/rms/wistarhan/rm_rm_r_wistar_han_clin_lab_parameters_08.aspx (Accessed 21 April 2017).

Goicoechea, M., Cía, F., San José, C., et al. 2008. Minimizing creatine kinase variability in rats for neuromuscular research purposes. *Lab Anim.* 42:19–25.

Goldstein, R.S., Tarloff, J.B., and Hook, J.B. 1988. Age-related nephropathy in rats. *FASEB J.* 2:2241–2251.

Gonen, E., Sahin, I., Ozbek, M., Kovalak, E., Yologlu, S., and Ates, Y. 2005. Effects of pregnancy and lactation on bone mineral density, and their relation to the serum calcium, phosphorus, calcitonin and parathyroid hormone levels in rats. *J Endocrinol Invest.* 28: 322–326.

Gosselin, S., Ramaiah, L., and Earl, L. 2009. Clinical chemistry in toxicity testing: Scope and methods. In *General and Applied Toxicology*, 3rd edition, Vol. 3. Eds. B. Ballantyne, T.C. Marrs, T. Syversen, pp. 707–742. Chichester: Wiley & Sons.

Grouzmann, E., Cavadas, C., Grand, D., et al. 2003. Blood sampling methodology is crucial for precise measurement of plasma catecholamines concentrations in mice. *Pflugers Arch.* 447:254–258.

Gumprecht, L.A., Long, C.R., Soper, K.A., Smith, P.F., Haschek-Hock, W.M., and Keenan, K.P. 1993. The early effects of dietary restriction on the pathogenesis of chronic renal disease in Sprague-Dawley rats at 12 months. *Toxicol Pathol.* 21:528–537.

Guyard-Dangremont, V., Desrumaux, C., Gambert, P., Lallemant, C., and Lagrost, L. 1998. Phospholipid and cholesteryl ester transfer activities in plasma from 14 vertebrate species. Relation to atherogenesis susceptibility. *Comp Biochem Physiol B Biochem Mol Biol.* 120:517–525.

Haas, M., Kluppel, A.C., Moolenaar, F., Meijer, D.K., de Jong, P.E., and de Zeeuw, D. 1997. Urine collection in the freely moving rat: Reliability for measurement of short-term renal effects. *J Pharmacol Toxicol Methods.* 38:47–51.

Hackbarth, H., Baunack, E., and Winn, M. 1981. Strain differences in kidney function of inbred rats: 1. Glomerular filtration rate and renal plasma flow. *Lab Anim.* 15:125–128.

Hall, R.L. 1997. Lies, damn lies, and reference intervals (or hysterical control values for clinical pathology data). *Toxicol Pathol.* 25:647–649; discussion 650–651.

Hard, G.C., Rodgers, I.S., Baetcke, K.P., Richards, W.L., McGaughy, R.E., and Valcovic, L.R. 1993. Hazard evaluation of chemicals that cause accumulation of α 2u-globulin, hyaline droplet nephropathy, and tubule neoplasia in the kidneys of male rats. *Environ Health Perspect.* 99:313–349.

Harlan Research Models and Services. 2009. (General page with links to specific strains.) Available at http://www.envigo.com/products-services/research-models-services/ (Accessed 21 April 2017).

Harvey, J.W. 1997. Chapter 7: The erythrocyte. In *Clinical Biochemistry of Domestic Animals,* 5th edition. Eds. J.J. Kaneko, J.W. Harvey, M.L. Bruss., pp. 157–203. San Diego, CA: Academic Press.

Hattori, N., Nakayama, Y., Kitagawa, K., Li, T., and Inagaki, C. 2007. Development of anti-PRL (prolactin) autoantibodies by homologous PRL in rats: A model for macroprolactinemia. *Endocrinology.* 148(5):2465–2470.

Hedrich, H.J. 2006. Chapter 3: Taxonomy and stocks and strains In *The Laboratory Rat,* 2nd edition. Eds. M. Suckow, S.H. Weisbroth, and C.L. Franklin, pp. 128–143. Worcester, MA: Elsevier Academic Press.

Hem, A., Smith, A.J., and Solberg, P. 1998. Saphenous vein puncture for blood sampling of the mouse, rat, hamster, gerbil, guinea pig, ferret and mink. *Lab Anim.* 32:364–368.

Hilltop Lab Animals. 2010. Available at: http://hilltoplabs.com/public/sdblood.html and http://hilltoplabs.com/public/wiblood.html (Accessed 21 April 2017). Scottdale, PA.

Hirsch, P.F. and Hagaman, J.R. 1982. Feeding regimen, dietary calcium, and the diurnal rhythms of serum calcium and calcitonin in the rat. *Endocrinology.* 110:961–968.

Hoffmann, W.E., Everds, N., Pignatello, M., Solter, P.F. 1994. Automated and semiautomated analysis of rat alkaline phosphatase isoenzymes. *Toxicol Pathol.* 22:633–638.

Horne, C.H. and Ferguson, J. 1972. The effect of age, sex, pregnancy, oestrogen and progestogen on rat serum proteins. *J Endocrinol.* 54:47–53.

Joslin, J.O. 2009. Blood collection techniques in exotic small mammals. *J Exot Pet Med.* 18(2): 117–139.

Kacew, S., Ruben, Z., and McConnell, R.F. 1995. Strain as a determinant factor in the differential responsiveness of rats to chemicals. *Toxicol Pathol.* 23:701–714; discussion 714–715.

Kaminsky, Y.G. and Kosenko, E.A. 1986. Blood glucose and liver glycogen in the rat. Effects of chronic ethanol consumption and its withdrawal on the diurnal rhythms. *FEBS Lett.* 200:217–220.

Kannappan, S. and Anuradha, C.V. 2009. Insulin sensitizing actions od fenugreek seed polyphenols, quercetin & metformin in a rat model. *Indian J Med Res.* 129(4):401–408.

Kant, G.J., Mougey, E.H., and Meyerhoff, J.L. 1986. Diurnal variation in neuroendocrine response to stress in rats: Plasma ACTH, beta-endorphin, beta-LPH, corticosterone, prolactin and pituitary cyclic AMP responses. *Neuroendocrinology.* 43:383–390.

Kawai, H., Kudo, N., Kawashima, Y., and Mitsumoto, A. 2009. Efficacy of urine bile acid as a non-invasive indicator of liver damage in rats. *J Toxicol Sci.* 34(1):27–38.

Keenan, K.P., Coleman, J.B., McCoy, C.L., Hoe, C-M., Soper, K.A., and Laroque, P. 2000. Chronic nephropathy in ad libitum overfed Sprague Dawley rats and its early attenuation by increasing degrees of dietary (caloric) restriction to control growth. *Toxicol Pathol.* 28:788–798.

Khan, K.N., Komoscar, W.J., Das, I., et al. 1996. Effect of bleeding site on clinical pathologic parameters in Sprague-Dawley rats: Retro-orbital venous plexus versus abdominal aorta. *Contemp Top Lab Anim Sci.* 35:63–66.

Kieft, K.A., Bocan, T.M., and Krause, B.R. 1991. Rapid on-line determination of cholesterol distribution among plasma lipoproteins after high-performance gel filtration chromatography. *J Lipid Res.* 32:859–866.

Kimura, F. and Kawakami, M. 1980. Two daily surges of prolactin secretion in the immature female rat. *Endocrinology.* 107:172–175.

Koch, M.A. 2006. Chapter 18: Experimental modeling and Research methodology. In *The Laboratory Rat,* 2nd edition. Eds. M. Suckow, S.H. Weisbroth, and C.L. Franklin. pp. 587–626. Worcester, MA: Elsevier Academic Press.

Krinke, G.J. 2000. History, strains and models. In *The Laboratory Rat (Handbook of Experimental Animals).* Eds. G.R. Bullock and T Bunton, pp. 3–16. London: Academic Press.

Kurien, B.T., Everds, N.E., and Scofield, R.H. 2004. Experimental animal urine collection: a review. *Lab Anim.* 38:333–361.

Laakso, M.L., Porkka-Heiskanen, T., Stenberg, D., Johansson, G., and Männistö, P.T. 1990. Lighting conditions affect serum and pituitary TSH in male rats. *Am J Physiol.* 259(2 Pt 1):E162–169.

LaBorde, J.B., Wall, K.S., Bolon, B., et al. 1999. Haematology and serum chemistry parameters of the pregnant rat. *Lab Anim.* 33:275–287.

Lausson, S., Staub, J.F., Milhaud, G., and Perault-Staub, A.M. 1985. Circadian variations in plasma calcium and calcitonin: Effect of calcium deficiency and fasting. *J Endocrinol.* 107:389–395.

Levin, S., Semler, D., and Ruben, Z. 1993. Effects of two weeks of feed restriction on some common toxicologic parameters in Sprague-Dawley rats. *Toxicol Pathol.* 21:1–14.

Levine, D.Z., Iacovitti, M., Nash, L., and Vandorpe, D. 1988. Secretion of bicarbonate by rat distal tubules in vivo. Modulation by overnight fasting. *J Clin Invest.* 81(6):1873–1878.

Levinson, L. 1940. Diurnal variation of intermedin in the blood of the albino rat. *Proc Natl Acad Sci U S A.* 26:257–258.

Liberati, T.A., Sansone, S.R., and Feuston, M.H. 2004. Hematology and clinical chemistry values in pregnant Wistar Hannover rats compared with nonmated controls. *Vet Clin Pathol.* 33:68–73.

Lightman, S.L., Windle, R.J., Julian, M.D., et al. 2000. Significance of pulsatility in the HPA axis. *Novartis Found Symp*, 227:244–257; discussion 257–260.

Lillie, L.E., Temple, N.J., and Florence, L.Z. 1996. Reference values for young normal Sprague-Dawley rats: Weight gain, haematology and clinical chemistry. *Hum Exp Toxicol.* 15:612–616.

Lindena, J., Friedel, R., Rapp, K., Sommerfeld, U., Trautschold, I., and Deerberg, F. 1980. Long-term observation of plasma and tissue enzyme activities in the rat. *Mech Ageing Dev.* 14:379–407.

Lindsay, J.R. and Baker, H.J. 2006. Chapter 1: Historical foundations. In *The Laboratory Rat*, 2nd Edition. Eds. M. Suckow, S.H. Weisbroth, C.L. Franklin, pp. 1–52. Worcester, MA: Elsevier Academic Press.

Loeb, W.F. 1999. Chapter 2: The rat. In *The Clinical Chemistry of Laboratory Animals*, 2nd edition. Eds. W.F. Loeb and F.W. Quimby, pp. 33–48. Philadelphia, PA: Taylor & Francis.

Maejima, K. and Nagase, S. 1991. Effect of starvation and refeeding on the circadian rhythms of hematological and clinico-biochemical values, and water intake of rats. *Jikken Dobutsu.* 40:389–393.

Mahl, A., Heining, P., Ulrich, P., et al. 2000. Comparison of clinical pathology parameters with two different blood sampling techniques in rats: Retrobulbar plexus versus sublingual vein. *Lab Anim.* 34:351–361.

Mancini, M.A., Majumdar, D., Chatterjee, B., and Roy, A.K. 1989. Alpha 2u-globulin in modified sebaceous glands with pheromonal functions: Localization of the protein and its mRNA in preputial, meibomian, and perianal glands. *J Histochem Cytochem.* 37:149–157.

Márquez, C., Nadal, R., and Armario, A. 2004. The hypothalamic–pituitary–adrenal and glucose responses to daily repeated immobilisation stress in rats: Individual differences. *Neuroscience.* 123:601–612.

Marrino, P., Gavish, D., Shafrir, E., and Eisenberg, S. 1987. Diurnal variations of plasma lipids, tissue and plasma lipoprotein lipase, and VLDL secretion rates in the rat. A model for studies of VLDL metabolism. *Biochim Biophys Acta.* 920:277–284.

Matsuzawa, T., Hayashi, Y., and Nomura, M. 1997. A survey of the values of clinical chemistry parameters obtained for a common rat blood sample in ninety-eight Japanese laboratories. *J Toxicol Sci.* 22:25–44.

Matsuzawa, T., Nomura, M., and Unno, T. 1993. Clinical pathology reference ranges of laboratory animals. Working Group II, Nonclinical Safety Evaluation Subcommittee of the Japan Pharmaceutical Manufacturers Association. *J Vet Med Sci.* 55:351–362.

Matsuzawa, T. and Sakazume, M. 1994. Effects of fasting on haematology and clinical chemistry values in the rat and dog. *Comp Haematol Int.* 4:152–156.

McGuill, M.W. and Rowan, A.N. 1989. Biological effects of blood loss: Implications for sampling volumes and techniques. *ILAR News.* 31:5–20.

McLean, B.K., Rubel, A., and Nikitovitch-Winer, M.B. 1977. Diurnal variation of follicle stimulating hormone (FSH) in the male rat. *Neuroendocrinology.* 23: 23–30.

Milhaud, G., Perault-Staub, A.M., and Staub, J.F. 1972. Diurnal variation of plasma calcium and calcitonin function in the rat. *J Physiol.* 222:559–567.

Mitchell, D.J. and Creasy, D.M. 2007. Sexual maturity and age of animals in preclinical studies to support 'first in man' studies. *Toxicol Sci.* 96:58.

Mitev, Y., Almeida, O.F., and Patchev, V. 1993. Pituitary-adrenal function and hypothalamic beta-endorphin release in vitro following food deprivation. *Brain Res Bull.* 30(1–2):7–10.

Nagy, A., Barta, A., Varga, G., and Zelles, T. 2001. Changes of salivary amylase in serum and parotid gland during pharmacological and physiological stimulation. *J Physiol Paris.* 95(1–6):141–145.

Nathanielsz, P. W. 1969. A circadian rhythm in the disappearance of thyroxine from the blood in the calf and the thyroidectomized rat. *J Physiol.* 204:79–90.

Nelson, W., Zinneman, H., Selden, J., Schaper, K., Halberg, F., and Bazin, H. 1974. Circadian rhythm in Bence-Jones protein excretion by Lou rats bearing a transplantable immunocytoma responsive to adriamycin treatment. *Int J Chronobiol.* 2:359–365.

Neptun, D.A., Smith, C.N., and Irons, R.D. 1985. Effect of sampling site and collection method on variations in baseline clinical pathology parameters in Fischer-344 rats. 1. Clinical chemistry. *Fundam Appl Toxicol.* 5(6 Pt 1):1180–1185.

O'Brien, P.J., Slaughter, M.R., Polley, S.R., and Kramer, K. 2000. Advantages of glutamate dehydrogenase as a blood biomarker of acute hepatic injury in rats. *Lab Anim.* 36:313–321.

Oishi, S., Oishi, H., and Hiraga, K. 1979. The effect of food restriction for 4 weeks on common toxicity parameters in male rats. *Toxicol Appl Pharmacol.* 47:15–22.

Ostrowska, Z., Kos-Kudla, B., Marek, B., and Kajdaniuk, D. 2003. Influence of lighting conditions on daily rhythm of bone metabolism in rats and possible involvement of melatonin and other hormones in this process. *Endocr Regul.* 37:163–174.

Owens, D.R. 2006. Chapter 23: Spontaneous, surgically, and chemically induced models of disease. In *The Laboratory Rat.* Eds. M. Suckow, S.H. Weisbroth, and C.L. Franklin, pp. 711–732. Worcester, MA: Elsevier Academic Press.

Palm, M. 1998. The incidence of chronic progressive nephrosis in young Sprague-Dawley rats from two different breeders. *Lab Anim.* 32:477–482.

Papworth, T.A. and Clubb, S.K. 1995a. Clinical pathology in the female rat during the pre- and postnatal period. *Comp Haematol Int.* 5:13–24.

Papworth, TA. and Clubb, S.K. 1995b. Clinical pathology of the neonatal rat. *Comp Haematol Int.* 5:237–250.

Petterino, C. and Argentino-Storino, A. 2006. Clinical chemistry and haematology historical data in control Sprague-Dawley rats from pre-clinical toxicity studies. *Exp Toxicol Pathol.* 57:213–219.

Pickering, R.G. and Pickering, C.E. 1984. The effects of reduced dietary intake upon the body and organ weights, and some clinical chemistry and haematological variates of the young Wistar rat. *Toxicol Lett.* 21:271–277.

Proctor, G.B., Asking, B., and Garrett, J.R. 1990. Factors influencing the movement of parotid amylase into the serum of rats on feeding. *Exp Physiol.* 75:709–712.

Rabinowitz, L., Berlin, R., and Yamauchi, H. 1987. Plasma potassium and diurnal cyclic potassium excretion in the rat. *Am J Physiol.* 253(6 Pt 2): F1178–1181.

Ramaiah, L., Miyamoto, M., Spatzier, B.N., and Kelly, C.M. 2009. Optimizing interpretive value of quantitative urinalysis in renal safety pharmacology. In Poster at *American College of Veterinary Pathology Annual Meeting*. Monterey, CA, 2009.

Reaven, G.M. 1978. Effect of age and sex on triglyceride metabolism in the rat. *J Gerontol.* 33:368–371.

Robinovitch, M.R., and Sreebny, L.M. 1972. On the nature of the molecular heterogeneity of rat parotid amylase. *Arch Oral Biol.* 17:595–600.

Robinson, J. and Evans, G.O. 1996. Preanalytical and analytical variables. In: *Animal Clinical Chemistry*. Ed. G.O. Evans, pp. 21–31. London: Taylor & Francis.

Robinson, S.H., Yannoni, C., and Nagasawa, S. 1971. Bilirubin excretion in rats with normal and impaired bilirubin conjugation: Effect of phenobarbital. *J Clin Invest.* 50:2606–2613.

Rodrigues, S.F., de Oliveira, M.A., Martins, J.O., et al. 2006. Differential effects of chloral hydrate- and ketamine/xylazine-induced anesthesia by the s.c. route. *Life Sci.* 79:1630–1637.

Rosol, T.J., Yarrington, J.T., Latendresse, J., and Capen, C.C. 2001. Adrenal gland: Structure, function, and mechanisms of toxicity. *Toxicol Pathol.* 29:41–48

Saha, J.K., Xia, J., Grondin, J.M., Engle, S.K., and Jakubowski, J.A. 2005. Acute hyperglycemia induced by ketamine/xylazine anesthesia in rats: Mechanisms and implications for preclinical models. *Exp Biol Med (Maywood).* 230:777–784.

Sánchez-Criado, J.E., Tébar, M., Ruiz, A., and Padrón, L. 1997. The steroid antagonist RU486 given at prooestrus induces hypersecretion of follicle-stimulating hormone from oestrus afternoon to early metoestrus in the rat. *Eur J Endocrinol.* 137(3):281–286.

Sauer, M.B., Dulac, H., Clark, S., et al. 2006. Clinical pathology laboratory values of rats housed in wire-bottom cages compared with those of rats housed in solid-bottom cages. *J Am Assoc Lab Anim Sci.* 45:30–35.

Schultze, E.A., Carpenter, K.H., Wians, F.H., et al. 2009. Longitudinal studies of cardiac troponin-I concentrations in serum from male Sprague Dawley rats: Baseline reference ranges and effects of handling and placebo dosing on biological variability. *Toxicol Path.* 37(6):754–760.

Schwartz, E., Tornaben, J.A., and Boxill, G.C. 1973. The effects of food restriction on hematology, clinical chemistry and pathology in the albino rat. *Toxicol Appl Pharmacol.* 25:515–524.

Senoo, H. 2000. Digestion, metabolism. In *The Laboratory Rat.* Ed. G.J. Krinke, pp. 359–383. London: Academic Press.

Sevastos, N., Theodossiades, G., and Archimandritis, A.J. 2008. Pseudohyperkalemia in serum: A new insight into an old phenomenon. *Clin Med Res.* 6:30–32.

Shearer, G.C., Joles, J.A., Jones, H., Walzem, R.L., and Kaysen, G.A. 2000. Estrogen effects of triglyceride metabolism in analbuminemic rats. *Kidney Int.* 57:2268–2274.

Shin, J.H., Kim, T.S., Kang, I.H., Kang, T.S., Moon, H.J., and Han, S.Y. 2009. Effects of postnatal administration of diethylstilbestrol on puberty and thyroid function in male rats. *J Reprod Dev.* 55(5):461–466.

Siller-Matula, J.M. and Jilma, B. 2008. Strain differences in toxic effects of long-lasting isoflurane anaesthesia between Wistar rats and Sprague Dawley rats. *Food Chem Toxicol.* 46:3550–3552.

Silvestri, E., Lombardi, A., de Lange, P., et al. 2008. Age-related changes in renal and hepatic cellular mechanisms associated with variations in rat serum thyroid hormone levels. *Am J Physiol Endocrinol Metab.* 294(6):E1160–E1168.

Smith, G.S., Hall, R.L., and Walker, R.M. 2002. Chapter 6: Applied clinical pathology in preclinical testing. In *Handbook of Toxicologic Pathology*, 2nd edition, Vol. 1. Eds. W.B. Hashek, C.G. Rousseaux, and M.A. Wallig. San Diego, CA: Academic Press.

Suber, R.L. and Kodell, R.L. 1985. The effect of three phlebotomy techniques on hematological and clinical chemical evaluation in Sprague-Dawley rats. *Vet Clin Pathol.* 14:23–30.

Suckow, M., Weisbroth, S.H., and Franklin, C.L. 2006. *The Laboratory Rat*, 2nd edition. Worcester, MA: Elsevier Academic Press.

Szafarczyk, A., Alonso, G., Ixart, G., Malaval, F., and Assenmacher, I. 1985. Diurnal-stimulated and stress-induced ACTH release in rats is mediated by ventral noradrenergic bundle. *Am J Physiol.* 249(2 Pt 1): E219–E226.

Thompson, C.S., Mikhailidis, D.P., Gill, D.S., Jeremy, J.Y., Bell, J.L., and Dandona, P. 1989. Effect of starvation and sampling time on plasma alkaline phosphatase activity and calcium homeostasis in the rat. *Lab Anim.* 23:53–58.

Thompson, C.S., Mikhailidis, D.P., Jeremy, J.Y., Bell, J.L., and Dandona, P. 1987. Effect of starvation on biochemical indices of renal function in the rat. *Br J Exp Pathol.* 68:767–775.

Thrivikraman, K.V., Huot, R.L., and Plotsky, P.M. 2002. Jugular vein catheterization for repeated blood sampling in the unrestrained conscious rat. *Brain Res Brain Res Protoc.* 10:84–94.

Timm, K.I. 1979. Orbital venous anatomy of the rat. *Lab Anim Sci.* 29:636–638.

Turk, J.R. and Laughlin, M.H. 2004. Physical activity and atherosclerosis: Which animal model? *Can J Appl Physiol.* 29:657–683.

Vachon, P. and Moreau, J.P. 2001. Serum corticosterone and blood glucose in rats after two jugular vein blood sampling methods: Comparison of the stress response. *Contemp Top Lab Anim Sci.* 40:22–24.

Vahl, T.P., Ulrich-Lai, Y.M., Ostrander, M.M., et al. 2005. Comparative analysis of ACTH and corticosterone sampling methods in rats. *Am J Physiol Endocrinol Metab.* 289: E823–828.

Van Herck, H., Baumans, V., Brandt, C.J., et al. 2001. Blood sampling from the retro-orbital plexus, the saphenous vein and the tail vein in rats: Comparative effects on selected behavioral and blood variables. *Lab Anim.* 35:131–139.

Van Liew, J.B., Eisenbach, G.M., Dlouha, H., and Boylan, J.W. 1978. Renal sodium conservation during starvation in the rat. *J Lab Clin Med.* 91:650–659.

Walter, GL. 1999. Effects of carbon dioxide inhalation on hematology, coagulation, and serum clinical chemistry values in rats. *Toxicol Pathol.* 27:217–225.

Waner, T. and Nyska, A. 1994. The influence of fasting on blood glucose, triglycerides, cholesterol, and alkaline phosphatase in rats. *Vet Clin Pathol.* 23:78–80.

Waner, T., Nyska, A., and Chen, R. 1991. Population distribution profiles of the activities of blood alanine and aspartate aminotransferase in the normal F344 inbred rat by age and sex. *Lab Anim.* 25:263–271.

Watterson, C. 2009. Chapter 8: Proteins. In *Animal Clinical Chemistry*. Ed. G. Evans, pp. 159–181. London: Taylor & Francis.

Wolf, C.F., Gans, H., Subramanian, V.A., and McCoy, C.H. 1979. A rat model for study of bilirubin conjugation by a cultured cell/ artificial capillary liver assist device. *Int J Artif Organs.* 2:97–103.

Wolford, S.T., Schroer, R.A., Gallo, P.P., et al. 1987. Age-related changes in serum chemistry and hematology values in normal Sprague-Dawley rats. *Fundam Appl Toxicol.* 8:80–88.

Woodruff, T.K., Besecke, L.M., Groome, N., Draper, L.B., Schwartz, N.B., Weiss, J. 1996. Inhibin A and inhibin B are inversely correlated to follicle-stimulating hormone, yet are discordant during the follicular phase of the rat estrous cycle, and inhibin A is expressed in a sexually dimorphic manner. *Endocrinology.* 137(12):5463–547.

Yamauchi, A., Oishi, R., and Kataoka, Y. 2004. Tacrolimus-induced neurotoxicity and nephrotoxicity is ameliorated by administration in the dark phase in rats. *Cell Mol Neurobiol.* 24:695–704.

Yerroum, M., Braconnier, F., and Chariot, P. 1999. Influence of handling procedures on rat plasma creatine kinase activity. *Muscle Nerve.* 22:1119–1121.

Young, G.P., Rose, I.S., Cropper, S., Seetharam, S., and Alpers, D.H. 1984. Hepatic clearance of rat plasma intestinal alkaline phosphatase. *Am J Physiol.* 247(4 Pt1):G419–G426.

Zeller, W., Weber, H., Panoussis, B., Bürge, T., and Bergmann, R. 1998. Refinement of blood sampling from the sublingual vein of rats. *Lab Anim.* 32:369–376.

Zhang, Z-P., Tianm Y-H., Li, R., et al. 2004. The comparison of the normal blood biochemical values of Wistar rats with different age and sex. *Asian J Drug Metab Pharmacokinet.* 4:215–218.

Ziomber, A., Machnik, A., Dahlmann, A., et al. 2008. Sodium-, potassium-, chloride-, and bicarbonate-related effects on blood pressure and electrolyte homeostasis in deoxycorticosterone acetate-treated rats. *Am J Physiol Renal Physiol.* 295(6):F1752–1763.

3 The Laboratory Rabbit

Anna Hampton, Tara Cotroneo, and Lesley A. Colby

CONTENTS

3.1 USE OF RABBITS IN BIOMEDICAL RESEARCH

Rabbits (*Oryctolagus cuniculus*) have long been used as research animal models. Many of their anatomic and physiologic features make them uniquely suited for use in research. Following centuries of domestication, rabbits thrive in captivity. In addition, their ability to produce large numbers of offspring at short and predictable intervals not only supports their ready availability but also facilitates their study over multiple generations. The body size of a rabbit is small enough to permit animals to be acquired and housed economically and at high densities. However, they are sufficiently large, especially when compared to mice and rats, for facilitating instrumentation and visualization of anatomic regions as well as collection of sizable tissue samples. Currently, with recent expansions in transgenic technology, numerous strains of rabbits are being developed to more closely model diseases and conditions of interest. Therefore, rabbits are considered valuable experimental animal models.

3.1.1 Examples of Existing Rabbit Models

While many breeds of rabbits have been used in research including the Flemish Giant and the Polish rabbit (Kraus et al., 1984), the two breeds used most commonly are the New Zealand White (NZW) and the smaller Dutch Belted with mature body weights of approximately 5–6 kg and 1.5–2 kg, respectively (Brewer, 2006). Rabbits have been used in the study of a diverse array of scientific areas including cancer, cardiovascular disease, aging, ophthalmology, reproductive physiology, and infectious and parasitic diseases. They are also commonly employed in the production of antibodies and in pharmaceutical and environmental safety testing. Although samples for clinical chemistry analytes may be collected from any experimental model, discussion of rabbit models in this chapter will focus on those most applicable to veterinary clinical chemistry.

Within the field of cancer research, many of the frequently published rabbit models involve tumors known to spontaneously develop in the rabbit *in situ* (e.g., spontaneous endometrial adenocarcinoma [Baba and von Haam, 1972; Elsinghorst et al.,1984]) or as a sequela of a viral infection (e.g., myxomatosis and rabbit papillomavirus) (Suckow et al., 2002). Many models involve the purposeful inoculation of transplantable tumors including the VX-2 carcinoma (Gu et al., 2007; Kreuter et al., 2008), Brown-Pearce carcinoma, and Greene melanoma (Shikishima, 2004). More recently, transgenic rabbits such as the HLA-A2.1 rabbit and rabbits genetically modified to express oncogenes have been produced to closely model human cancer conditions (Hu et al., 2007; Fan and Watanabe, 2003).

Perhaps, the most well-recognized rabbit models are those used in cardiovascular research. Rabbits were the first and are currently one of the most common animal species used to model human atherosclerosis. Initially, rabbits were selected as they were found to quickly develop hypercholesterolemia when fed a high-cholesterol diet and then progress to develop arterial mineralization (Yanni, 2004).

The Watanabe Heritable Hyperlipidemic (WHHL) rabbit is the predominant rabbit strain used as a model of atherosclerosis and is a well-accepted model of human familial hypercholesterolemia. An inbred strain derived from a male mutant Japanese rabbit, the WHHL rabbit possesses a single mutation in the low-density lipoprotein (LDL) receptor gene resulting in reduced LDL catabolism and lipoprotein accumulation in the plasma. As a sequela to their hypercholesterolemia and hypertriglyceridemia, WHHL rabbits consistently develop aortic and coronary atherosclerosis at 4–5 months of age as well as skin xanthomas (Aliev and Burnstock, 1998; Norido et al., 1993). The WHHL rabbit has been used to study characteristics and development of atherosclerosis as well as to assess experimental therapies (Aliev and Burnstock, 1998). The general health characteristics, development of lesions, and biochemical profile of the WHHL rabbit have been described (Aliev and Burnstock, 1998; Norido et al., 1993).

Another well-known, but less frequently used rabbit model of atherosclerosis is the St. Thomas' Mixed Hyperlipidaemic (SMHL) rabbit (previously known as the St. Thomas Hospital rabbit). The SMHL rabbit is used as a model of human familial combined hyperlipidemia (FCHL), a genetic disorder of unknown etiology (de Roos et al., 2005). Similar to the WHHL rabbit, the SMHL rabbit developed as a result of a spontaneous mutation and maintains a combined hyperlipidemia with significantly elevated levels of plasma cholesterol and triglycerides. However, hyperlipidemia in the SMHL rabbit is attributed not to an LDL receptor defect as in the WHHL rabbit but to an increased production rate of apolipoprotein B (apoB)-containing lipoproteins (de Roos et al., 2005). One disadvantage of many rabbit models, both those induced by high-cholesterol diets and those developed through a spontaneous mutation (e.g., WHHL), is that lesions do not develop in the same locations as in humans. Transgenic strains derived both from NZW and WHHL strains as well as additional experimental techniques are being developed to address this issue and to examine unique aspects of the disease (Moghadasian et al., 2001; Brousseau and Hoeg, 1999; Yanni, 2004).

Rabbits are also commonly used in a wide range of other cardiovascular diseases including myocardial infarction and cardiomyopathy. For instance, the Watanabe Heritable Hyperlipidemic Myocardial Infarct (WHHLMI) strain of rabbit has been developed through selective breeding of WHHL rabbits to spontaneously develop myocardial infarction that is uniquely similar to the human condition (Shiomi et al., 2003). The β-MyHC-Q transgenic rabbit is a valuable model of human familial hypertrophic cardiomyopathy (Marian et al., 1999).

Recently, the rabbit has been increasingly studied as a model of Alzheimer's disease following the observation that cholesterol-fed rabbits develop many of the neuropathologic features of the condition including central accumulation of amyloid-beta in the nervous tissue and development of cognitive deficits (Woodruff-Pak, 2008; Sparks, 2008).

The rabbit has been used as an animal model of several ophthalmologic conditions. It has the advantage over many smaller species (e.g., mice and rats) of a large globe (eye) for which diagnostic and therapeutic interventions developed for use in humans can easily be applied (Shikishima, 2004). The spectrum of ophthalmologic studies utilizing rabbits include contact lens-associated corneal hypoxia (McCanna et al., 2008), dry eye (Schrader et al., 2008), and most notably glaucoma and uveal melanoma. Buphthalmia, or enlargement of the eye (also termed congenital or infantile glaucoma) is one of the most common inherited diseases in domestic rabbits (Brock, 2012). The buphthalmic (*bu/bu*) NZW rabbit had been commonly used as an animal model of glaucoma as the disease frequently occurs spontaneously in this breed (Hanna et al., 1962; Tesluk et al., 1982). Treatments for uveal melanoma have been extensively evaluated (Brock, 2012) following the implantation of a melanoma cell line in the immuno-privileged anterior chamber of a rabbit's eye. The most frequently utilized tumor line in the rabbit model is the Greene melanoma, a tumor line originally derived from a hamster amelanotic melanoma (Shikishima, 2004).

The reproductive physiology of the rabbit has been well studied. Rabbits and humans share many similar hematological and biochemical trends during pregnancy (Wells et al., 1999). The tightly controlled timing of rabbit ovulation and subsequent egg maturation and development have made them useful in studies of egg maturation, fertilization, cleavage, and implantation. The anatomy of a female rabbit's uterus and two cervices (opening separately into the vagina) prevents the migration of embryos between uterine horns as in most other species allowing separate fetal populations in the same animal (Kozma et al., 1974). Rabbits have also been used extensively to study fetal development and to evaluate the potential teratogenic effects of substances proposed for human administration (Hartman, 1974; Wells et al., 1999). Smaller breeds are often preferred for studies to test novel compounds as a smaller quantity of drug is required when administered on a per body weight basis (Spence, 2003).

Rabbit models continue to fill an important role in the study of infectious and parasitic diseases. Although consistent or expanding in some areas (e.g., tuberculosis and microsporidiosis), the use of rabbits is being largely surpassed by that of transgenic rodent models (Basaraba, 2008; Wasson and Peper, 2000).

Many treatment, diagnostic, and testing modalities incorporate use of purposefully produced monoclonal or polyclonal antibodies. Rabbits have been consistently used for decades in the production of polyclonal antibodies (Suckow et al., 2002). Detailed descriptions of the procedure have been published (Hendriksen and Hau, 2003; Cooper and Patterson, 2008). Rabbits are an almost ideal species for this purpose as they have readily accessible blood vessels for blood collection, are of significant body size (especially when compared to rodents) to permit frequent collection of large volumes of blood, and often have strong immunologic responses to administered immunogens (Stills, 1994).

Rabbits are regularly utilized in the safety testing of pharmaceuticals, biologic materials, and medical devices. In the past, rabbits were commonly used for evaluating the degree of ocular or dermal irritation induced by substances prior to their approval for human use. Common tests included the Draize rabbit eye and skin irritancy tests. Numerous alternative tests have been developed resulting in a substantial reduction in the number of rabbits used for these types of tests. These include the red blood cell, hemoglobin denaturation, bovine corneal opacity and permeability, isolated chicken eye, isolated rabbit eye, and the chorioallantoic membrane test methods to evaluate eye irritation (NICEATM, 2006). Cell culture systems, transcutaneous electrical resistance assays, and commercially produced *in vitro* tests are among the alternatives used to evaluate skin irritation (Vinardell and Mitjans, 2008). Rabbits were also historically used in an *in vivo* test to evaluate the presence of bacterial endotoxins or other pyrogens in substances produced for human administration. The rabbit pyrogen test has been largely replaced with alternative tests such as the limulus amoebocyte lysate assay (Hartung, 2002). The suitability of these and other alternative tests for safety testing of pharmaceuticals, biologic materials, and medical devices are periodically reviewed for acceptance by the United States, Europe, and other region's regulatory agencies. In some instances, no one test is accepted as a total replacement for an animal-based test. Rather, conduct of a series of alternative tests may be accepted in full or partial replacement of the relevant animal-based test.

3.1.2 Mutant and Genetically Modified Strains

Inbred strains of rabbits have been developed to decrease the biologic variability present in outbred stocks. However, while inbred animals are genetically uniform, significant experimental variability can be induced through minor environmental alterations (Napier, 1963). On average, the reproductive efficiency of inbred rabbit strains may be lower than that of outbred stocks partially owing to decreased litter size and increased mortality rates (Fox, 1974). As a result of this and an increased susceptibility to disease, it is not uncommon for lines of inbred strains to be lost within the first few generations of inbreeding (Napier, 1963). Although many inbred strains of rabbits (e.g., WHHL, WHHLMI, SMHL) have been developed, few are commercially available. Many stocks and strains have been preserved through cryopreservation (Joly et al., 2012).

Many of the transgenic technologies initially developed in the mouse have been adapted for use in the rabbit. Numerous transgenic rabbit strains have been developed for a wide variety of uses including as specially designed models of disease (e.g., cardiovascular disease and acquired immunodeficiency syndrome [AIDS]) and as live bioreactors for the large-scale production of biologically active recombinant proteins (e.g., human interleukin-2, erythropoietin, and growth hormone) (Fan and Watanabe, 2003). Compared to other species, the rabbit is highly suited to use as a bioreactor owing to its size and reproductive and physiologic characteristics. Colonies of transgenic rabbits expressing human genes can be maintained free of selected diseases and intensively reared within strictly controlled environmental conditions. As a consequence of their highly efficient reproductive physiology, rabbits produce large volumes of protein-rich milk that can be collected and processed to yield recombinant proteins for therapeutic, diagnostic, and research applications at relatively low cost compared to that from larger agricultural species (Fan and Watanabe, 2003).

Numerous spontaneous mutations have been identified and are frequently selected for study in rabbit colonies (Fox, 1974; Lindsey and Fox, 1994). These include buphthalmia (Fox et al., 1969) and mandibular prognathism (Fox and Crary, 1971) in the NZW used as models for human glaucoma and prognathism, respectively, and the Pelger-Huet anomaly (Lindsey and Fox, 1994).

3.2 UNIQUE PHYSIOLOGICAL CHARACTERISTICS OF RABBIT

The rabbit possesses many unusual or unique anatomical and physiological characteristics on which researchers can capitalize when designing scientific studies. Rabbit breeds vary greatly in size and include the large Flemish giant with an adult weight of approximately 9 kg and the Polish rabbit with an adult weight frequently less than 1 kg (Yanni, 2004). In addition, rabbits possess a very light and fragile skeletal system, accounting for only 7%–8% of the total body weight (Suckow and Douglas, 1997; Brewer, 2006). In contrast, they are heavily muscled (approximately 50% body weight) with much of their muscle mass associated with the rear legs (Donnelly, 2003). As a result, rabbits are prone to lumbar back fractures if they are not handled and restrained appropriately (Bergdall and Dysko, 1994). The fasting metabolic rate of the rabbit is high when compared to that of other animals of their size. For instance, the fasting metabolic rate of a 2 kg rabbit is approximately 120 kcal/day or 750 kcal/m^2 (Brewer, 2006). Lacking sweat glands over the majority of their body, rabbits are most comfortable in cool environmental temperatures. Their pinnae (external ears) represent a large portion of their total body surface, approximately 12% in NZW (Donnelly, 2003). Their ears are utilized in thermoregulation, providing a means to help cool the body, and are vascularized with proportionately large blood vessels facilitating arterial and venous access (Brewer, 2006). Furthermore, the thymus persists into adulthood (Donnelly, 2003). Cortisol is the major plasma glucocorticoid (Lassen, 2004).

Compared to other common laboratory animals, the rabbit has a high number of basophils in its peripheral circulation (Kozma et al., 1974). The rabbit polymorphonuclear leukocyte is referred to as a heterophil not a neutrophil due to the presence of large granules that can be easily visualized on routine bloodstains. The Pelger-Huet anomaly is inherited as a partial dominant trait and is observed in varying frequencies across rabbit strains. In this anomaly, the heterophil is hyposegmented due to the incomplete differentiation of granulocytes (McLaughlin and Fish, 1994). Similar to the mouse and rat, the rabbit is a steroid sensitive species in which lymphopenia is induced through lympholysis following exposure to stressors or exogenous glucocorticoids (Toth and January, 1990).

All rabbit teeth are open-rooted (hypsodontic) and grow continuously throughout life. A normal anatomic feature that distinguishes all lagomorphs is the "peg" teeth, a second set of upper incisors located immediately behind the more visible front upper incisors. Three layers of striated muscle extend the full length of the esophagus and include the cardiac portion of the stomach (Kraus et al., 1984). The gastrointestinal tract and its contents can account for 10%–20% of an animal's body weight. The stomach of a rabbit is rarely empty even after prolonged fasts and may contain 15% of the intestinal contents. Furthermore, rabbits are not able to vomit due to the anatomic position of their well-developed cardia relative to the other portions of the stomach (Brewer, 2006; Donnelly, 2003).

Compared to other segments of the gastrointestinal tract, the cecum is disproportionately large, accounting for approximately 40% of the total digestive tract (Brewer, 2006) and with a capacity approximately 10 times that of the stomach (Suckow et al., 2002). This large structure plays a vital role in supporting the nutritional health of the animal. It is within the cecum that a high concentration of microorganisms converts substances within the ingesta to highly nutritive components of the cecotrophs.

Coprophagy, the eating of feces, is a normal behavior of rabbits. Produced in the evening, cecotrophs are soft fecal pellets that are high in B-complex vitamins, electrolytes, water, and protein and are low in fiber. In contrast, the firmer fecal pellets produced during the day are composed predominantly of undigested fiber (Suckow and Douglas, 1997; Kraus et al., 1984). Rabbits will consume the cecotrophs as they are passed from the anus. Thus, housing rabbits on raised surfaces, through which fecal pellets can fall, will not prohibit their coprophagic behavior. It is interesting to note that germ-free rabbits do not consume their cecotrophs (Kozma et al., 1974), presumably due to the lack of additional nutrients.

Two distinctive structures composed of gut-associated lymphoid tissue, the sacculus rotundus and the cecal appendix, are present in the rabbit gastrointestinal tract. The sacculus rotundus (also known as the cecal tonsil) is a distinctive structure at the terminal ileum. The cecal appendix is a long, thin structure at the distal end of the cecum (Suckow and Douglas, 1997).

The water consumption rate of rabbits spans a wide range (50–150 mL/kg of body weight/day) and, at its upper end, is higher than that of most other mammals (Cizek, 1961). However, they have a remarkable ability to withstand significant levels of dehydration, up to 48% of their body weight (Brewer, 2006). Rabbits tend to drink copious quantities of water when food is withheld, which is enough to alter their serum electrolyte balance (Cizek, 1961). If water is withheld, food consumption decreases (Cizek, 1961).

As indicated in Table 3.1, many of the enzymes traditionally assessed to evaluate liver function are produced by multiple tissues in the rabbit, as is true in many mammal species. Therefore, it is important to recognize all sources of an enzyme when interpreting clinical chemistry data (Benson and Paul-Murphy, 1999; McLaughlin and Fish, 1994).

Additional factors that must be considered when interpreting enzyme levels in the rabbit and other species include the means by which the enzyme is released into the blood (e.g., leakage from the extracellular space following cell injury or following increased production); the duration of enzyme activity once in the blood; tissue specificity of the enzyme; and the methods used to collect, store, and analyze the blood sample (Lassen, 2004). It is also important to consider the degree of muscle trauma induced during blood collection through such procedures as restraint, administration of injections, decapitation, or surgical incisions as they may result in significant elevation of enzymes present in both the liver and the muscle, thereby making evaluation of liver function difficult.

On a per weight basis, rabbits produce a relatively high volume of bile. The components of bile acid differ significantly in the rabbit when compared to other mammals. For instance, over 80% of rabbit bile acid is composed of deoxycholic acid while it is composed of limited chenodeoxycholic acid, the primary bile acid in several mammals (Taylor et al., 1981). Rabbits possess a gallbladder

TABLE 3.1
Tissue Origin of Enzymes Commonly Measured in Blood

Enzyme	Tissue Source of Enzyme
Alanine aminotransferase (ALT)	Liver, cardiac muscle
Aspartate aminotransferase (AST)	Liver, cardiac and skeletal muscle, kidney, pancreas
Creatine kinase (CK)	Cardiac, skeletal, and smooth muscle; brain
Gamma glutamyltransferase (GGT)	Liver including bile duct epithelial cells (the major source of the enzyme), renal epithelium
Alkaline phosphatase (ALP)	Several tissues including osteoblasts, renal tubular epithelium, intestinal epithelium, liver, and placenta. Rabbits are unique in having three ALP isoenzymes (one intestinal and two liver/kidney forms) as opposed to the two isoenzymes (intestinal and liver/kidney/bone forms) of most other mammals.
Glutamate dehydrogenase (GD)	Liver, cardiac and skeletal muscle, kidney, brain, leukocytes
Lactate dehydrogenase (LDH)	Cytoplasm of almost all cells of the body. The rabbit has multiple isoenzymes of LDH that correspond with isoenzymes 1–5 of humans.
Alpha-amylase	Pancreas, salivary glands, liver

Sources: Benson, K.G. and Paul-Murphy, J., *Vet Clin North Am Exot Anim Pract*, 2, 539–551, 1999; McLaughlin, R.M. and Fish, R.E., *The Biology of the Laboratory Rabbit*, Academic Press, San Diego, 1994; Lindena, J. et al., *J Clin Chem Clin Biochem*, 24, 35–47, 1986; Lassen, E.D., *Veterinary Hematology and Clinical Chemistry*, Lippincott Williams & Wilkins, Philadelphia, 2004; Campbell, T.W., *Veterinary Hematology and Clinical Chemistry*, Lippincott Williams & Wilkins, Philadelphia, 2004.

and the common bile duct enters the duodenum separately from the pancreatic duct thereby making it relatively easy to cannulate (Brewer, 2006). Unlike most other mammals where bilirubin is the only heme end product excreted in bile, rabbits excrete both biliverdin (70%) and bilirubin (30%) in the bile. Bilirubin found in the bile and in plasma is most frequently in its conjugated form (McLaughlin and Fish, 1994). Biliverdin is not normally present in the plasma (Lassen, 2004). Some rabbits produce a liver enzyme, atropinesterase, which allows them to quickly and efficiently metabolize the antimuscarinic agent atropine (Sawin and Glick, 1943; van Zutphen, 1974) that may be administered to control respiratory tract secretions and heart rate. The gene responsible for production of the enzyme is inherited with incomplete dominance.

There are many unique characteristics of the rabbit kidney that make it a useful model for a variety of research focuses (Brewer, 2006). The anatomic structure of the rabbit kidney is simple with a single papilla and calyx. The rabbit is unique in that its renal tubules can be dissected without disrupting the basement membrane, making it useful for studies in renal tubule physiology (Brewer, 2006). The number of glomeruli in the kidneys is not static at birth but rather varies over time. Furthermore, ectopic glomeruli may be present in the kidney of adult rabbits (Brewer, 2006). Plasma urea nitrogen and creatinine can be used as markers for estimating rabbit renal function (Lassen, 2004; Campbell, 2004).

The volume of urine produced by a rabbit can vary widely (20–350 mL/kg/day) although a range of 20–75 mL/kg/day is typical (Kozma et al., 1974; Washington and Van Hoosier, 2012). Daily urine volume is influenced by many variables including an animal's food and water consumption, level of physical activity, and environmental temperature (Kozma et al., 1974). Crystalluria is a normal finding in rabbits with calcium carbonate, ammonium magnesium phosphate (triple phosphate), and anhydrous calcium carbonate crystals frequently produced (Benson and Paul-Murphy, 1999; McLaughlin and Fish, 1994). Urine is usually basic (pH 7.6–8.8) and with a specific gravity between 1.003 and 1.036. However, urine pH may become acidic (pH 6–7) during a fast (Kojima and Tanaka, 1974). Casts should not been seen although trace protein or glucose and an occasional WBC may normally be detected in urine (Kozma et al., 1974, 1967; McLaughlin and Fish, 1994). Red urine may be observed and should not automatically be assumed to be hematuria as dietary porphyrins may be excreted in the urine causing a red discoloration.

Rabbits are unlike most other mammals with regard to calcium metabolism and excretion. While most mammals maintain serum calcium levels within a tightly controlled range, the serum calcium level of rabbits is directly influenced by dietary calcium. Rabbit plasma calcium levels are frequently higher (13–15 mg/dL) than that observed in other species (Buss and Bourdeau, 1984; Brewer, 2006). Moreover, while most mammals' primary route of calcium excretion is through bile, the rabbit excretes calcium predominately through urine (Donnelly, 2003; Suckow and Douglas, 1997). Their fractional urinary excretion of calcium ranges from 45% to 60% as compared to less than 2% in most other mammals (Buss and Bourdeau, 1984).

Rabbits fed a high calcium diet can have secondary changes to their urine such as a very thick, cloudy, white, pasty consistency or calcium carbonate crystalluria. This is especially true in obese and sedentary rabbits. When coupled with an increased urinary pH, these rabbits are predisposed for development of urolithiasis (Hoefer, 2000; Pare and Paul-Murphy, 2004). Prolonged intake of elevated dietary levels of calcium can lead to calcification of the aorta and kidney (Donnelly, 2003). This effect is exaggerated if vitamin D is coadministered (Buss and Bourdeau, 1984). Rabbits may also absorb excess calcium from a calcium-rich water source. Diets low in calcium elicit a parathyroid hormone-mediated, tubular reabsorption of calcium with resultant hypocalcuria. A diet low in phosphorus causes a rapid increase in calcium excretion and phosphorus reabsorption by the kidneys (McLaughlin and Fish, 1994). Therefore, due to the noted influence of calcium, phosphorus, and vitamin D on rabbit kidney function, researchers should consider the level of these nutrients in the diet when using rabbit tissues in isolated renal tubule perfusion studies (Buss and Bourdeau, 1984).

The timing of sexual maturity is influenced not only by the age of an individual but also by the mature body weight of the breed or strain. In general, smaller breeds tend to reach sexual maturity at an earlier age than larger breeds (Kozma et al., 1974; Donnelly, 2003). For instance, the age at sexual maturity for the smaller Dutch Belted rabbit is approximately 4 months as opposed to 5–7 months for the larger NZW and 9–12 months for the Flemish Giant (Suckow et al., 2002; Morrell, 1995).

Female rabbits do not exhibit an estrous cycle although they do have predictable periods of sexual receptivity. They are induced ovulators. The timing of ovulation is very predictable, 10–13 hours post-copulation or following injection of luteinizing hormone, human chorionic gonadotropin, or gonadotropic releasing hormone (Foote and Simkin, 1993; Kozma et al., 1974; Suckow and Douglas, 1997; Morrell, 1995). Their ova are large and develop rapidly (Brewer, 2006). They have a duplex uterus, consisting of two uterine horns each communicating with the vaginal chamber through separate cervixes (Brewer, 2006).

An approximately 16-day pseudopregnancy can result from sterile matings with a male, mounting by another female, or the presence of another buck nearby (Kozma et al., 1974; Suckow et al., 2002; Napier, 1963). Pseudopregnancy can also be reliably induced with administration of luteinizing hormone (Brewer, 2006). During this time, females may display many of the behavioral and physiological characteristics of pregnancy including nest building and milk production (Kozma et al., 1974; Napier, 1963). Matings will not be successful during pseudopregnancy as ovulation is suppressed during this time (Napier, 1963). Progesterone assays can be used to diagnose pregnancy (Morrell, 1995).

Gestation is approximately 31–32 days in duration with an average litter size of eight. Longer gestations may occur if the litter size is small. The rabbit has a hemochorial type of placentation, similar to that in the human. Maternal and fetal circulations are in very close contact allowing a high degree of placental transfer of substances from the dam to the offspring. Most passive transfer of immunity (globulins) occurs in utero with very little passive transfer through consumption of colostrum (Kozma et al., 1974; Suckow and Douglas, 1997). Dams produce approximately 160–220 g of milk per day and may allow kits to nurse for up to 10 weeks although weaning usually occurs by 5–8 weeks of age (Suckow et al., 2002).

Kits are altricial at birth and are ectotherms until day 7. They nurse only once daily for approximately 3–5 minutes at consistent times each day, often in the morning (Brewer, 2006). While nursing, a kit may consume milk equivalent to 20% of its body weight (Alus and Edwards, 1977). When raised with their dams, kits will consume milk exclusively up to 10 days of age. By 20 days of age, they will convert to a diet primarily of solid food and start to display coprophagy, consuming only a small amount of milk by approximately 30 days. During this time, the size of the cecum and the amount of cecal fermentation increases to accommodate the transitioning diet (Alus and Edwards, 1977).

Artificial insemination of females has been developed and is useful for controlled and efficient management of reproduction and to exclude transmission of pathogens either between breeders or from dam to offspring. Fresh or cryopreserved sperm can be used (Morrell, 1995). Embryo transfer was first developed in the rabbit and it has since been utilized to develop specific pathogen-free (SPF) and transgenic colonies of rabbits (Forcada and Lopez, 2000; Watanabe et al., 2005).

3.3 METHODOLOGY FOR SAMPLE COLLECTION

3.3.1 Blood Collection

As detailed in Table 3.2, the common sites for phlebotomy in a rabbit include jugular vein, ear vasculature, cephalic vein, lateral saphenous vein, and the heart. Removal of the fur over the venipuncture site will often improve visualization of peripheral vessels. The recommended restraint technique and amount of blood that can be collected varies with each site. In general, potential venipuncture complications include hemorrhage, bruising, thrombosis, and stress secondary to improper restraint. Procedures such as proper restraint technique, proper preparation of the venipuncture site, and application of adequate pressure to the venipuncture site after blood collection should reduce the rate of complications (Joint Working Group on Refinement, 1993).

TABLE 3.2
Comparison of Blood Collection Sites

Blood Collection Site or Method	Relative Collection Volume (+ to +++)	General Anesthesia Required	Multiple Collections Recommended from Site
Marginal ear vein/ central ear artery	++	No (use of local anesthetic recommended)	Yes
Jugular vein	+++	No	Yes
Cephalic vein	+	No	Yes
Saphenous vein	+	No	Yes
Cardiac puncture	+++	Yes	No

Source: Adapted from Joint Working Group on Refinement, *Lab Anim*, 27, 1–22, 1993.

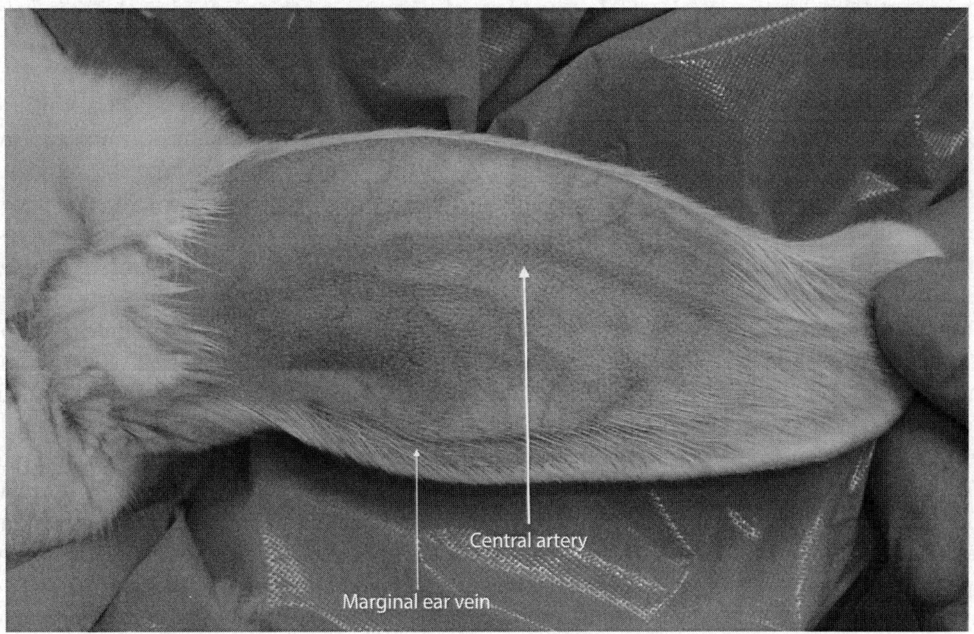

FIGURE 3.1 **(See color insert.)** Marginal ear vein and central ear artery.

3.3.1.1 Primary Sites for Collection

3.3.1.1.1 Ear Vessels

The marginal ear vein and central ear artery (Figure 3.1) are vessels commonly utilized for blood collection. The amount of blood that can be obtained from these vessels varies with the technique. A small amount of blood can be obtained through cannulation of the marginal ear vein with a 25–27 gauge (G) needle. With this technique, blood is allowed to passively enter the blood collection equipment. It is important to note that vessels collapse easily if a syringe or vacuum tubes are used (Mader, 2004). Vasodilation is recommended to facilitate obtaining a larger blood sample. The optimal method to induce vasodilation is heavily influenced by the animal handler's experience and comfort with a method and the potential influence of the method on experimental requirements and results. Dilation of the local vasculature can be achieved by warming the ear with a low wattage heat bulb or topical application of 40% D-limonene, 2% nitroglycerin ointment, or citrus oil (Adams, 2002; Hrapkiewicz et al., 2007; Smith et al., 1988). For example, the application of 2 mL of 25%–40% D-limonene to the ear surface will result in vasodilation in 2–5 minutes lasting for at least 10 minutes (Bivin, 1994; Lacy et al., 1987). If a topical vasodilator agent is used it must be cleaned from the ear such as with 70%–95% ethanol following blood collection (Lacy et al., 1987) to minimize skin irritation.

Systemic administration of pharmacologic agents can be used to facilitate blood collection by inducing dilation of peripheral vasculature and reducing stress (Ludders et al., 1987). However, it must be noted that administration of any pharmacologic agent has the potential to affect blood parameters (Bivin, 1994). Therefore, the possible effects induced by a substance on parameters of interest in each experimental study must be considered prior to substance administration. Acepromazine maleate is one pharmacologic agent commonly used to induce a light sedation and vasodilation (Hrapkiewicz et al., 2007). Recommended dose ranges of acepromazine for this procedure most frequently vary between 0.5 and 5.0 mg/kg and differ largely on the level of animal sedation intended. Local anesthetics such as topical lignocaine-prilocaine (EMLA) cream applied to the collection site 1 hour prior to blood collection can be utilized to decrease induced pain or discomfort (Hrapkiewicz et al., 2007). A variety of techniques are described in the literature to help facilitate collection of a larger blood sample from the ear vasculature. Selected techniques are described here.

One method involves the placement of a hub-less 18 G needle into a dilated central ear artery (Bivin, 1994). This technique allows for the collection of 35–85 mL of blood in 1–3 minutes (Bivin, 1994). If more blood is required, an additional 10–15 mL can be collected from the vasculature of the other ear using the same technique (Bivin, 1994). In another method, a 22 G double-head needle or a standard 22 G needle and extension set assembly is inserted into the dilated ear vessel and then coupled with a vacuum blood collection tube. With this method, up to 20 mL of blood can be collected from a 4 kg rabbit (Barrera and Young, 1997). Although not often currently utilized, a miniperistaltic pump can be used with catheterization of the central ear artery to reliably obtain up to 40 mL of blood (Bivin, 1994; Ludders et al., 1987; Stickrod et al., 1981). Alternatively, if frequent and repeated blood collection is required, an indwelling catheter can be placed and maintained in the ear vasculature (Smith et al., 1988).

A negative sequela that can occur with ear venipuncture regardless of the technique used is thrombosis with subsequent epithelial sloughing. This complication occurs more often in rabbits with small ears and vasculature (Mader, 2004). Discomfort may also occur with venous and arterial blood collection involving a larger gauge needle. To help alleviate this potential discomfort, a topical anesthetic such as EMLA cream can be utilized. The hair overlying the marginal ear vein should be removed and 1 mL of EMLA cream applied topically 1 hour prior to the venipuncture procedure (Flecknell et al., 1990). In addition, it is essential that direct pressure be maintained on the vessel puncture site after blood collection to promote hemostasis. Prolonged pressure may be required with puncture of the central ear artery.

3.3.1.1.2 Jugular Vein

Jugular venipuncture can be performed in an awake rabbit with manual restraint provided by two technicians. This technique is useful when blood volumes greater than 0.5 mL are required (Benson and Paul-Murphy, 1999). The rabbit is placed on its stomach with its front legs held down off the edge of a table and its head extended up toward the ceiling (Figure 3.2) (Mader, 2004). When extending the head upward, it is important to be cautious not to overextend the neck and interfere with respiration. Alternatively, the rabbit can be placed on its back with its neck extended parallel to the table by the phlebotomist (Figure 3.3). The needle is inserted into the jugular vein near the base of the neck, the needle tip directed toward the head (Benson and Paul-Murphy, 1999). Chemical restraint may be required in rabbits that are not conditioned to human handling or are fractious with restraint.

The jugular vein is the preferred site for long-term venous catheterization. Catheterization is recommended when multiple blood samples are needed as this can help reduce the stress associated

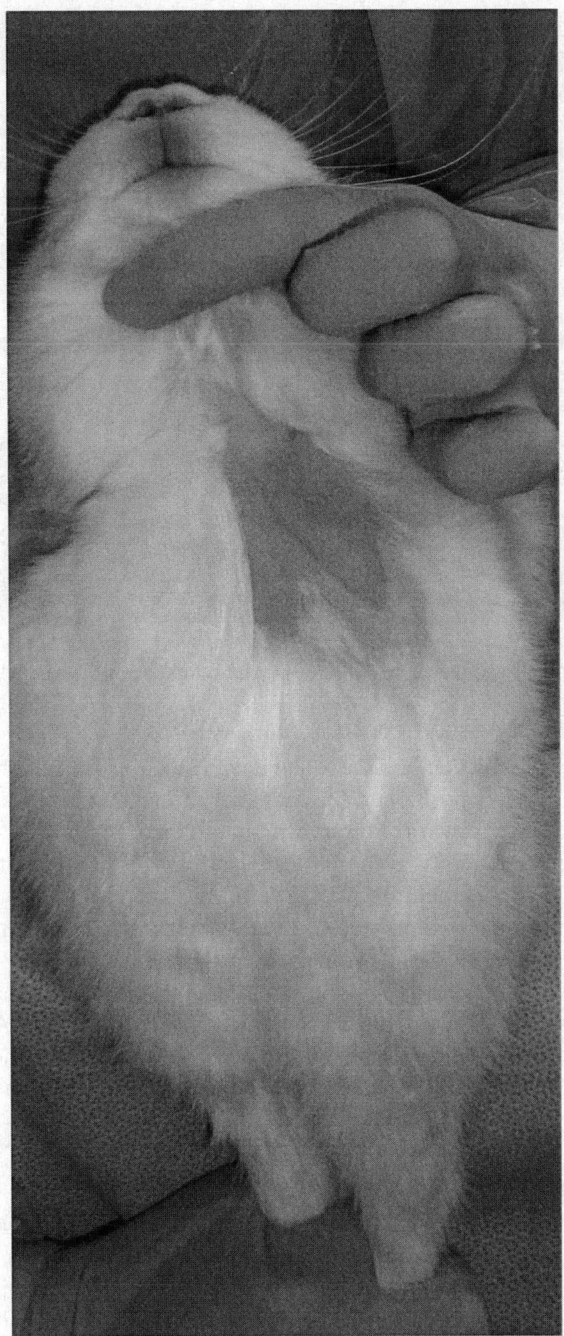

FIGURE 3.2 Manual restraint for jugular venipuncture.

with repeated venipunctures. A plastic over-the-needle catheter can be placed in the jugular vein and maintained for approximately 1–2 days. An anticoagulant such as heparin should be left in the catheter between sample collections. Long-term catheter placement often requires surgery to expose the vessel and experienced personnel with surgical skills to perform the procedure is essential (Joint Working Group on Refinement, 1993).

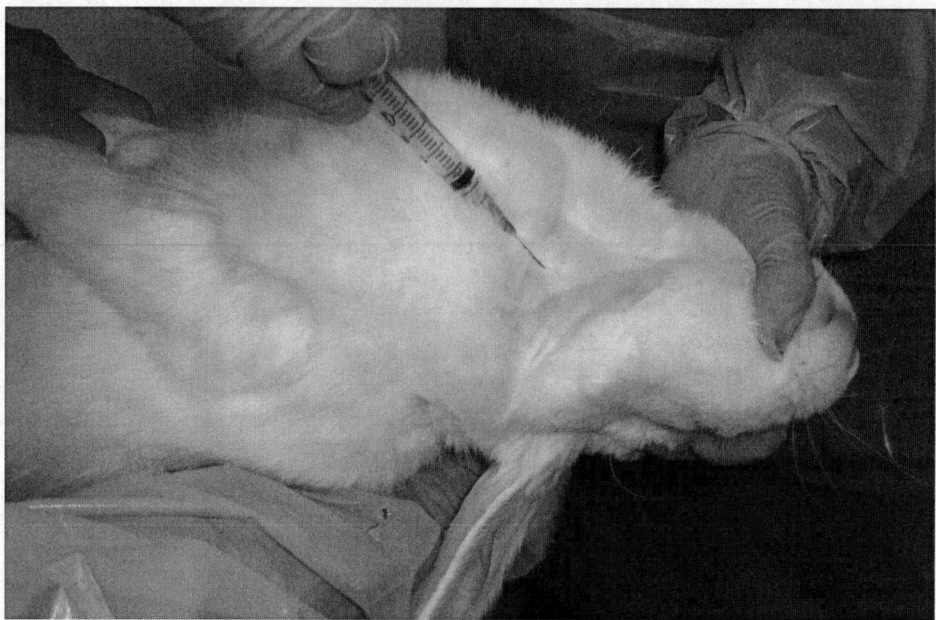

FIGURE 3.3 (See color insert.) Manual restraint for jugular venipuncture with rabbit in dorsal recumbency.

3.3.1.1.3 Lateral Saphenous and Cephalic Veins

The cephalic vein of the rabbit can be used when only a small blood sample is needed (Stein and Walshaw, 1996). The rabbit is positioned for cephalic venipuncture by placing it on its stomach and extending the forelimb forward. Pressure is maintained around the upper forelimb by an assistant. Since the cephalic vein is a common site for catheter placement in rabbits, the vessel should not be utilized for venipuncture if future catheter placement is indicated (Graham, 2006). The lateral saphenous vein courses medial-to-lateral across the lateral aspect of the distal tibia (Mader, 2004). In the rabbit, this vein is flat and easily collapsible (Benson and Paul-Murphy, 1999). To access the vein, it is best to restrain the animal on its side with an assistant compressing the vein just above the caudal portion of the hock (Mader, 2004). A small gauge needle (>25 G) and 1 mL syringe should be utilized for venipuncture of both the cephalic and lateral saphenous veins (Benson and Paul-Murphy, 1999). In addition, shaving the region may improve visualization.

3.3.1.1.4 Cardiocentesis

Cardiocentesis (often termed as cardiac puncture) can be utilized to obtain a large amount of blood from live animals and for terminal exsanguinations (Bivin, 1994). However, artificially high levels of enzymes produced by striated and cardiac muscles (e.g., lactate dehydrogenase, aspartate aminotransferase, creatine kinase, and troponin) may contaminate the sample secondary to the inherent invasiveness of cardiac puncture (McLaughlin and Fish, 1994. Owing to the need for full animal restraint and the invasiveness of the procedure, this procedure must only be performed on fully anesthetized animals and at most institutions may only be performed as a terminal procedure. Sterile technique must be employed if the animal is allowed to recover from the anesthetic episode. Both ventral and lateral approaches can be utilized to access the heart. For the ventral approach, the anesthetized rabbit is placed on its back and may be stabilized in a restraining board to facilitate proper positioning (Bivin, 1994). A 18 G, 1.5 inch needle is inserted in a cranio-dorsal direction at a 30° angle to the plane of the sternum and immediately caudal to the xyphoid process (Bivin, 1994). Alternatively, the lateral technique is performed by inserting the needle through the lateral chest wall at the site of maximum pulse intensity (Adams, 2002). The needlepoint can lacerate tissues if it is moved inappropriately while in the chest. Therefore, the needle must always be introduced along a straight line and not be repositioned while in the chest cavity. If the needle is not in the proper location, it should be completely removed from the chest cavity and then redirected prior to reinsertion (Bivin, 1994). Although not often currently utilized, a miniperistaltic pump can be used to facilitate blood collection during a terminal cardiac puncture. Blood volumes up to 190 mL can be obtained (Adams, 2002; Stickrod et al., 1981).

Several animal health complications can occur following cardiocentesis. Improper needle placement or repositioning may cause lacerations of the lung, the cardiac muscle, or blood vessels. Lung lacerations may cause a lung to collapse or the chest to inappropriately fill with air. Laceration of the cardiac muscle may cause accumulation of blood within the pericardial sac, potentially resulting in cardiac tamponade and subsequent shock and death. Laceration of blood vessels will result in uncontrolled internal bleeding. Given the severe potential complications, the authors very highly recommend that cardiocentesis be performed only as a terminal procedure. If performed as a recovery procedure, it is essential that personnel be highly trained and proficient prior to attempting the procedure and the animal be closely monitored during and after the procedure (Bivin, 1994).

3.3.1.2 Methods of Restraint

The most appropriate restraint mechanism to be employed will vary based on the selected blood collection technique as well as the temperament of the rabbit. Generally, samples can be obtained from the ear vessels with manual restraint of the animal or use of a restraint box. Commonly, rabbits can be calmed by covering their eyes or placing them on their backs (Graham, 2006). In addition, rabbits can often be calmed and easily restrained by wrapping them firmly in a towel (Benson and Paul-Murphy, 1999). Restraint boxes (Figures 3.4 and 3.5) are useful for blood collection because they provide secure restraint and easy access to the animal's head. Regardless of the restraint technique implemented, it is vital that the rabbit's hindquarters be appropriately supported in order to prevent spinal fractures. Chemical restraint may be indicated to reduce stress and the chance of injury with fractious rabbits or rabbits not acclimated to frequent handling and restraint.

3.3.1.3 Collection Volume and Frequency

The circulating blood volume of a mature rabbit is estimated to be 44–70 mL/kg of lean body weight. Many factors must be considered when determining the maximum volume of blood that can be safely collected from an individual. For instance, the total blood volume per kg body weight is

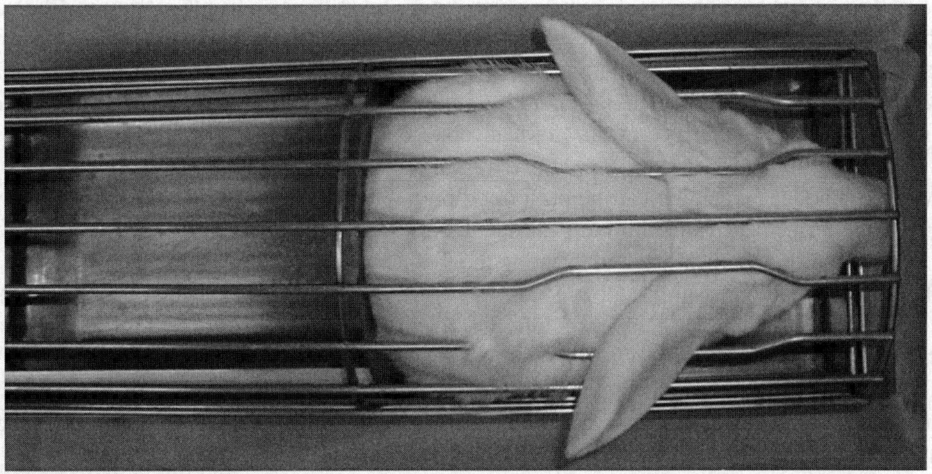

FIGURE 3.4 Top view of rabbit restrainer.

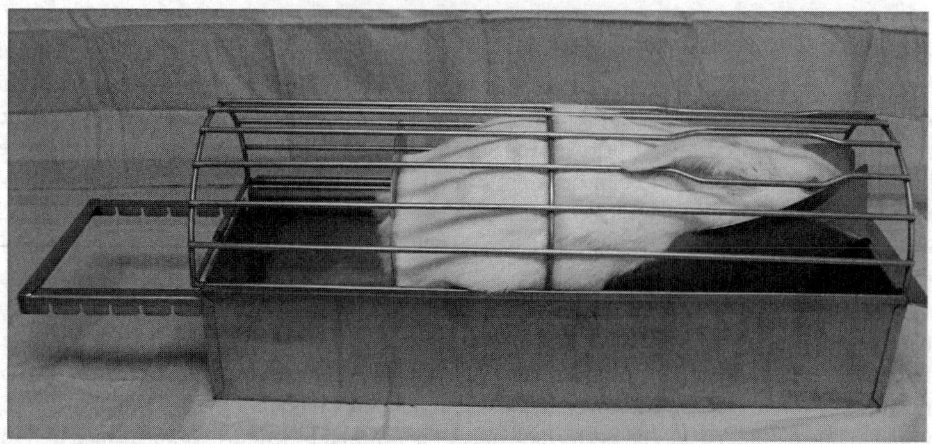

FIGURE 3.5 Side view of rabbit restrainer.

directly impacted by an animal's body composition and age with lower total blood volume for obese and older animals. The frequency and volume of prior blood collections must also be considered. In general, up to 10% of the circulating blood volume of a healthy adult rabbit can be withdrawn at one time point every 2–4 weeks without inducing clinical signs (Joint Working Group on Refinement, 1993; Diehl et al., 2001). Alternatively, up to 1.0% of the circulating blood volume can be collected every 24 hours if multiple, successive samples are required. Since animals may not respond uniformly to repeated blood collection, it is ideal to monitor an individual's complete blood count over time (Joint Working Group on Refinement, 1993; Benson and Paul-Murphy, 1999).

3.3.2 Urine Collection

Standard techniques for rabbit urine collection include free catch, cystocentesis, and urinary catheter placement. If it is necessary to collect urine over an extended period of time, use of a commercially produced metabolism cage is recommended (Bivin, 1994). Use of metabolic cages is considered to be one of the least stressful methods of urine collection and allows for accurate quantification of urine production (Kurien et al., 2004). However, this technique does not eliminate urine contamination, which may adversely affect urinalysis parameters. Urine can be easily obtained in rabbits less than 10 days of age by manually stimulating urination. This is done by firmly restraining the young rabbit on its back with its head toward the wrist of the handler (Kurien et al., 2004). The other hand is used to stroke the abdomen beginning in the region of the stomach and ending in the region of the bladder (Kurien et al., 2004). Stroking should continue until urine is expelled. Excessive pressure or restraint should be avoided as they may have adverse consequences for the rabbit including internal injury or suffocation (Kurien et al., 2004).

Manual bladder expression can be performed on an awake animal; however, the procedure is more easily performed if the animal is anesthetized. Manual bladder expression is performed by palpating the abdomen, locating and isolating the bladder in the caudal ventral abdomen, and then applying firm steady pressure to the bladder. Urine is collected as it is expelled from the urethra. Excessive pressure can cause bladder rupture. The technique should be avoided if there is a possibility of urinary blockage (Bivin, 1994).

Cystocentesis is a reliable method to collect urine directly from the bladder and avoid contamination from the lower genito-urinary tract and environment (Kurien et al., 2004). Unless a rabbit is highly accustomed to restraint and manual manipulations, it is strongly recommended that the rabbit be anesthetized or sedated to facilitate the cystocentesis procedure. The rabbit is placed in dorsal recumbency and the bladder is palpated in the caudal ventral abdomen. The bladder is stabilized between the thumb and forefinger and raised to the abdominal wall. The overlying skin is cleaned with an antiseptic solution and a 23–25 G needle (attached to a sterile syringe) is inserted through the skin directly into the bladder (Mader, 2004; Bivin, 1994).

An additional method of urine collection is the placement of a urinary catheter, which due to anatomical structure, is easier to accomplish in male rabbits (Bivin, 1994). It is recommended that the rabbit be sedated or anesthetized for this procedure (Graham, 2006). Sterile technique must be followed when performing all urinary catheterizations to avoid inducing a urinary tract infection. To catheterize a male, the rabbit is placed in a sitting position, the penis extruded by applying pressure to the surrounding tissues, and a well-lubricated, sterile 9 French catheter introduced into the urethra (Bivin, 1994). Females are placed on their stomach and the urethral opening is located on the floor of the vagina (Graham, 2006). The distance from the urethra to the neck of the bladder should be approximated and the catheter should not be inserted beyond this distance. The bladder can be evacuated by attaching a syringe to the catheter and gently aspirating urine. Care must be taken not to apply excessive suction through the catheter as this can cause damage to the urethra or bladder wall and contaminate the specimen with blood.

Ideally, urine should be examined and processed within 30 minutes of collection (Latimer et al., 2003). However, urine can be refrigerated up to 12 hours post-collection for culture and up to 48 hours for sediment evaluation (Loeb and Quimby, 1989).

3.4 PREANALYTICAL SOURCES OF VARIATION

When interpreting results obtained from blood chemistry and urinalysis, it is important to consider the wide source of potential variations resulting from the experimental procedures; environmental conditions; as well as the strain, breed, and/or individual animal. Sources of variation to be considered include the genetic variability within and between animal colonies, an animal's reproductive status, stress-induced metabolic changes from animal handling and transportation (both during and immediately prior to sample collection), administration of xenobiotics to the animals (e.g., anesthetics and experimental compounds), the vessel and anatomic location accessed for sample collection, the quality and source of testing reagents, and the equipment and analytic methods used to process and evaluate samples (McLaughlin and Fish, 1994; Lindena and Trautschold, 1986). Catheterization of vessels should be considered if multiple blood samples must be collected because it may decrease stress experienced by the animal and minimize tissue trauma. Meaningful and reliable results can only be obtained by recognizing and controlling these and other sources of variability.

3.4.1 Sex

Variations between sexes may be noted in selected biochemical parameters; however, these variations are typically slight and most frequently fall within normal reference ranges established for rabbits as a species. In the adult rabbit, sex variations are noted in cholesterol, typically with higher values in female rabbits (Mortensen and Frandsen, 1996; Kozma et al., 1974; Fox, 1989). Variation in cholesterol levels is typically not seen prior to adulthood (McLaughlin and Fish, 1994). Higher plasma albumin levels and lower alpha band protein levels may be seen in female than in male NZW rabbits (Kozma et al., 1967). When evaluating renal values, serum creatinine levels may be significantly higher in male than in female NZW rabbits (Aleman et al., 2000). Conversely, females tend to have a significantly higher serum blood urea nitrogen (BUN) level compared to that of males although strain variations may exist (Fox et al., 1970). In addition, total protein and phosphorous levels may be influenced by the sex of the rabbit (McLaughlin and Fish, 1994; Fox et al., 1970). Overall, it is important to consider the influence of sex on the variability of blood parameters when evaluating clinical pathologic findings. This is especially true when comparing values obtained from both sexes either within or between studies.

3.4.2 Age

A rabbit's age and stage of growth can significantly affect clinical pathologic parameters. For some parameters, values may fluctuate over time in young animals until reaching more consistent values in adulthood. Hormonal influence, bone growth, diet, and general physiologic changes in a growing rabbit can influence biochemistry values. In general, alkaline phosphatase (ALP) is two to four times higher in young animals compared to that in adults (McLaughlin and Fish, 1994). At birth, serum cholesterol levels are similar to adult levels; however, as the rabbit matures, cholesterol levels rapidly rise then gradually decline back to adult levels. Additionally, cholesterol levels may increase with advancing age in adult rabbits (Fox, 1989). Typically, total serum protein levels increase with age in young rabbits. This may be attributed to the rise in globulin levels as the immune system is exposed to a greater number of antigens (McLaughlin and Fish, 1994; Fox, 1989; Laird and Fox, 1970). In NZW rabbits, it has been shown that triglyceride levels tend to decrease with age (Mortensen and Frandsen, 1996). Variations in glucose levels are observed between age groups. In young rabbits, glucose values can vary in relation to the timing of nursing (McLaughlin and Fish, 1994). In addition, young rabbits tend to have a lower fibrinogen level compared to that of older rabbits (Benson and Paul-Murphy, 1999). Because of these potential variations, it is important to consider the influence of age when analyzing blood chemistry values in rabbits.

Variations in hormone levels can also be seen in growing rabbits. One parameter to note is protein-bound iodine (PBI), which is an indicator of thyroid function and reflects blood levels of tri-iodothyronine (T_3) and tetraiodothyronine (T_4). PBI levels increase rapidly in growing rabbits for the first few days of life and then decrease until adult levels are reached (McLaughlin and Fish, 1994; Campbell, 2004; Laird and Fox, 1970).

Animal age may also influence the urinalysis. For instance, young healthy rabbits can have a small amount of albumin in their urine and trace proteinuria may be detectable in normal adults (Hoefer, 2000). Suckling rabbits should have clear urine in contrast to the yellow-, orange-, or red-tinged urine observed in adults (Harkness and Wagner, 1995).

3.4.3 Strain/Breed

Numerous breeds and strains of domestic rabbits have been developed, many with unique physical or physiological features. Parameters that may be affected by breed or strain include total protein, γ-globulins, blood glucose, BUN, inorganic phosphorus, cholesterol, ALP, and electrolyte concentrations (McLaughlin and Fish, 1994; Fox and Laird, 1970; Fox, 1989; Campbell, 2004).

Variations in hormone parameters can also be seen. Serum PBI (reflecting serum thyroid hormone levels), serum iron, total iron binding capacity, and growth hormone levels vary between inbred strains of rabbits. In general, the closer the genetic relationship of these strains, the less variation is seen. Furthermore, genetics can influence the plasma aldosterone concentration in rabbits. This makes it important to define the source, strain, age, and sex of rabbits in studies that relate to these endocrine functions (Schindler et al., 1974; Fox, 1974, 1989; Campbell, 2004).

Although there are several different rabbit breeds, the NZW and Dutch Belted rabbits are the most common breeds used in a research setting. Variations in biochemical parameters have been noted between these breeds. For instance, Dutch Belted rabbits have higher total protein and lower blood glucose levels than NZWs. In addition, Dutch Belted rabbits had a slightly higher sodium and chloride level compared to that of NZW rabbits (Kozma et al., 1974). Although these variations are subtle, they can play an important role when these parameters are specifically evaluated in a research setting.

3.4.3.1 WHHL Rabbits

As stated earlier in this chapter, WHHL rabbits have been developed as a model of human familial hypercholesterolemia. The single-gene mutation of the WHHL results in the absence of LDL membrane receptors. This missing receptor characterizes the strain and leads to a significant increase of serum lipid levels. Because of these changes, WHHL rabbits are used as an animal model for the study of familial hypercholesterolemia, lipid metabolism, and cardiovascular atherosclerosis (Norido et al., 1993).

Because of the unique genetic makeup of this inbred strain, selected biochemical parameters of the WHHL can vary from outbred rabbits. WHHL rabbits have been purposely bred for hypercholesterolemia, thus homozygous WHHL rabbits have an elevated cholesterol and serum triglyceride level compared to that of other domesticated rabbit breeds (Norido et al., 1993). In contrast, heterozygous WHHL rabbits tend to have blood lipid levels similar to outbred, normolipidemic rabbits (Mortensen and Frandsen, 1996). Hyperlipidemia develops rapidly with age. For example, a 45-day-old WHHL rabbit has a greater than 10-fold higher lipid level than that of NZW rabbit controls. This elevation will gradually decrease as the rabbit ages, but still remains significantly elevated (Norido et al., 1993). Plasma cholesterol and triglyceride levels fluctuate as a WHHL rabbit ages and are influenced by the animal's sex. Females tend to have a higher cholesterol level than that of WHHL males, with the variation occurring earlier in heterozygous than homozygous rabbits. Furthermore, lipid levels can vary during the reproductive phases of the female. During gestation, heterozygous WHHL females typically show a decrease in the total cholesterol and LDL levels, reaching their lowest values during lactation, when values may be significantly lower than at mating. However, during gestation and lactation an increase in very low-density lipoprotein (VLDL) levels and a decrease in high-density lipoprotein (HDL) levels have been noted, which tend to reach their extremes during gestation (Mortensen and Frandsen, 1996). WHHL rabbits have been specifically bred for the changes that are seen physiologically, clinically, and in their biochemistry. When looking at specific changes in these selected parameters, knowing the normal changes to expect in WHHL rabbits is of paramount importance.

3.4.4 Nutritional Status

3.4.4.1 Diet Composition

A rabbits' cholesterol level can be easily manipulated by diet composition. Because of this, rabbit models are frequently used to study cholesterol metabolism. A rabbit fed a diet high in cholesterol will quickly develop a dose-dependent increase in serum cholesterol with a more pronounced effect noted in female rabbits. This rise in serum cholesterol can take several weeks to return to normal after discontinuing the high cholesterol diet (Borgman and Wardlaw, 1975; McLaughlin and Fish, 1994). Similarly, an increase in VLDL and LDL can be seen when feeding a diet high in cholesterol (Campbell, 2004). Serum cholesterol levels can also be influenced by dietary sucrose levels, the presence of fishmeal, the lysine-to-arginine ratio, the type of dietary protein, and the protein–fat interaction (McLaughlin and Fish, 1994; Sebesteny et al., 1985). Interestingly, it has been shown that a semi-synthetic diet high in casein and dextrose can elevate serum cholesterol, lipase, creatine kinase (CK), aspartate aminotransferase (AST), and alanine aminotransferase (ALT) in NZW rabbits. These values typically return to normal after discontinuing the diet (Hausner et al., 1995). Furthermore, female NZW rabbits may show an increase in plasma triglycerides if maintained completely on a liquid diet (Latour et al., 1998). It is important to note that serum cholesterol levels can be influenced by breed when a special cholesterol diet is fed (Adams et al., 1972).

Rabbits are unique in their metabolism and excretion of calcium. Serum calcium levels are not homeostatically regulated but vary directly with the dietary levels of calcium. Serum calcium can reach levels as high as 15 mg/dL due to dietary influences alone (Brewer, 2006; Hrapkiewicz et al., 2007; Suckow and Douglas, 1997). In contrast, due to rapid changes in parathyroid hormone and calcitonin levels, a four-time increase in dietary vitamin D has no effect on serum calcium levels. However, in some rabbits, a vitamin D deficiency can lead to a severe hypophosphatemia. Phosphorus levels can also be affected by the diet with a high phosphorous diet inducing elevated serum phosphorus levels (McLaughlin and Fish, 1994). Although rare, nutritional secondary hyperparathyroidism can occur in the rabbit (Hoefer, 2000). Other factors that can be influenced by diet composition include protein and BUN levels. A high protein diet can cause an elevation in BUN values (Hoefer, 2000; Donnelly, 2003). Likewise, a decrease in dietary protein or protein restriction results in decreased BUN levels (McLaughlin and Fish, 1994).

As noted previously in this chapter, the concentrations of calcium present in the blood and urine is strongly influenced by dietary calcium levels. Diets high in calcium will directly influence select clinical chemistry values and may induce significant physiologic abnormalities. In addition, diets high in porphyrins, tannins, and other phenolic compounds often result in highly pigmented urine, ranging from a dark red to orange. This can be a normal variation; however, further diagnostics are required to differentiate pigment from blood (Hrapkiewicz et al., 2007; McLaughlin and Fish, 1994).

Small variations in diet composition can influence a variety of clinical pathology parameters. Therefore, the composition of all food sources (both routinely provided feed and food treats) must be determined and then evaluated for their potential influence on research outcomes.

3.4.4.2 Acute Fasting

There are numerous circumstances that may require a short period of fasting in a rabbit, the most common being preparation for sedation or anesthesia prior to a surgical procedure or sample collection. The necessity of fasting rabbits prior to anesthesia has been debated. Although rabbits cannot vomit, fasting prior to anesthesia or an oral procedure may be beneficial as it can reduce the amount of food remnants in the oral cavity and oropharynx. In addition, acute fasting can reduce the amount of digesta in the gastrointestinal tract. This decreases pressure on the diaphragm during anesthesia and may aid in visualization during a laparotomy or gastrointestinal surgery (Lipman et al., 2008). Plasma glucose levels are directly affected by the food consumption of an animal with the postprandial blood glucose concentration typically peaking 3 hours after a meal. These fluctuations in blood glucose levels in response to food consumption tend to decrease with age (Fox, 1989; Campbell, 2004). Administration of glucose to fasted rabbits may cause an increase in bilirubin excretion, thereby causing a decrease in plasma bilirubin and unconjugated liver bilirubin (McLaughlin and Fish, 1994). Furthermore, acute fasting can cause a decrease in urinary pH due to an induced catabolic state (Hoefer, 2000). Overall, a healthy adult rabbit can tolerate a short period of dietary restriction while still maintaining normal blood glucose levels. The effects of fasting may be more pronounced in geriatric, debilitated, or young rabbits or in all rabbits during prolonged periods of fasting.

3.4.4.3 Long-Term Dietary Restriction

Longer periods of caloric restriction can cause a greater variation in clinical pathology parameters and have a more detrimental effect on a rabbit's health. In the neonate, glycogen stores are depleted and blood glucose levels drop following 6 hours of food restriction. As the rabbit ages, the glycogen stores become sufficient to maintain blood glucose levels for longer periods of time (McLaughlin and Fish, 1994). Adult rabbits can maintain their serum glucose levels after 4 days of fasting. Continued maintenance of blood glucose values may be due to coprophagy or a residual bolus of food being continually digested in the intestinal tract during the fasting period (Fox, 1989; Kozma et al., 1974). Prolonged fasting or anorexia can be associated with abnormalities in gluconeogenesis and biliary metabolism and may result in a dramatic increase in plasma triglyceride levels (Harkness and Wagner, 1995). Bilirubinuria may develop secondary to starvation in the form of conjugated bilirubin (Hoefer, 2000; DiBartola, 1995). Rabbits often become polydipsic during periods of food deprivation. This can lead to loss of sodium due to urine excretion and a secondary hyponatremia (McLaughlin and Fish, 1994). Long-term caloric restriction can lead to progressive deterioration in the rabbit's general health and can be life threatening.

3.4.5 Housing Environment

Rabbits typically can adapt to gradual environmental changes and can be housed in a wide array of environmental climates and caging. Domesticated rabbits prefer a cool climate, with the recommended dry-bulb housing temperature ranging between 61 and 72 °F (16°C–22°C). When changing a rabbit's primary and secondary enclosure temperature, a gradual change is always recommended to allow the rabbit to adapt physiologically, behaviorally, and morphologically (Institute of Laboratory Animal Resources, 2011). Exposure to extreme cold can cause an increase in total protein levels and fibrinogen while causing a decrease in serum albumin levels (Harkness and Wagner, 1995; Fox, 1989; Sutherland et al., 1958).

Heat stress has been shown to increase AST, BUN, and creatinine levels. The associated hyperthermia can increase blood glucose levels, further increase BUN levels, and cause hyperproteinemia (McLaughlin and Fish, 1994; Campbell, 2004). In addition, heat stress can lead to a significant elevation in plasma corticosterone levels (Besch and Brigmon, 1991). Thus, it is important to avoid environmental temperature extremes in rabbits as it can not only affect blood parameters but also may affect their overall health status.

In addition to temperature changes, bedding, caging, and housing density may affect blood parameters. Chronic exposure to softwood bedding material (e.g., cedar wood) may increase liver enzymes (Johnston and Nevalainen, 2003). It has been shown that germ-free rabbits have a lower γ-globulin level compared to that of conventionally housed rabbits (Kozma et al., 1974). Maternal, prenatal γ-globulin levels in colostrum-deprived, newborn rabbits disappear rapidly. As the kit is exposed to environmental microflora the γ-globulin levels begin to increase. This process typically takes 4–5 weeks. Moreover, in the absence of environmental microflora, only a low γ-globulin level is reached (Wostmann, 1961). In addition to their caging and bedding, animal housing density has been shown to affect blood parameters in the rabbit. Specifically, group housed animals tend to have elevated plasma cortisol levels when compared to individually housed animals, with significant differences seen at day 8 (Fuentes and Newgren, 2008). Furthermore, a significant decrease in ALP levels has been noted in pair-housed compared to individually housed NZW rabbits (Nevalainen et al., 2007).

3.4.6 Circadian Rhythm

The biology of the rabbit's circadian rhythm is complicated by many external factors. Rabbits in the wild are primarily nocturnal and demonstrate a pattern of leaving their burrows at dusk and returning in the early morning (Jilge and Hudson, 2001). Laboratory rabbits in well-controlled conditions also demonstrate a clear pattern of increased motor activity, food and water intake, urination, and hard feces excretion during the dark hours (Jilge and Hudson, 2001). Rabbits are sensitive to environmental influences and may demonstrate a diurnal rhythm when housed in captivity (Jilge and Hudson, 2001; Jilge, 1991). The rabbit's circadian rhythm has been shown to cause fluctuation in clinical chemistry and blood hormone parameters (Piccione et al., 2007; Lesault et al., 1991a, 1991b). Owing to the circadian variation associated with some parameters, it is important that the time samples collected for accurate comparison between time points are consistent. Serum cholesterol and BUN concentrations demonstrated circadian rhythm variation in rabbits kept on a 12-hour light/dark cycle and *ad libitum* feeding (Piccione et al., 2007). Furthermore, serum iron and PBI levels vary with the time of day (McLaughlin and Fish, 1994).

In addition to changes in blood chemistry parameters levels of blood hormones such as glucocorticoids, adrenocorticotropic hormone (ACTH), follicle stimulating hormone (FSH), luteinizing hormone (LH), prolactin, and insulin vary with the time of day (Lassen, 2004; Lesault et al., 1991a, 1991b; Szeto et al., 2004; Cano et al., 2005). The glucocorticoid hormones, corticosterone, and cortisol peak during the afternoon and are lowest in the morning (Szeto et al., 2004). Although plasma glucose levels remain stable in fed and fasted rabbits during a 24-hour period, blood insulin levels show diurnal variation (Lesault et al., 1991a, 1991b). Rabbit kits have a diurnal variation of FSH, LH, and prolactin. Prolactin has a similar circadian pattern in adult male and female rabbits with peak values in the afternoon and early morning (Cano et al., 2005).

3.4.7 Estrous Cycle, Pregnancy, or Lactation

It is important to consider an animal's reproductive state as it can have a direct effect on biochemical blood parameters. Ovulation is induced in rabbits, occurring on average 10–13 hours after natural mating. Several hormonal fluctuations occur near ovulation. Luteinizing hormone increases rapidly, peaks approximately 90 minutes postcoitus, and returns to basal levels within 6 hours. Follicle stimulating hormone levels spike at both 3.5 and 24 hours postcoitus. Plasma progesterone levels rise after coitus and ovulation (Orstead et al., 1988).

Information has been published on the hematologic and biochemical values of young, pregnant NZW (Tables 3.3 and 3.4), and DB rabbits (Table 3.4) as well as the expected rate of spontaneous fetal abnormalities in these breeds (Spence, 2003).

Several clinical chemistry parameters are significantly influenced over the approximately 31–32-day gestation period. Alkaline phosphatase, BUN, cholesterol, creatinine, and total protein decrease throughout gestation (Wells et al., 1999). Conversely, ALT and AST may progressively increase (Wells et al., 1999). Glucose is more variable and may begin a steady decrease around mid-gestation until parturition (Wells et al., 1999). In addition, an insulin-resistant state develops around day 24–30 of gestation (Hauguel et al., 1987). This condition is secondary to a decrease in insulin responsiveness in both glucose producing and utilizing tissues (Hauguel et al., 1987). Triglycerides may demonstrate a rise followed by a precipitous fall at the end of gestation (Wells et al., 1999). Total cholesterol is lower during gestation compared to values at mating (Mortensen and Frandsen, 1996). Calcium and phosphorus values also exhibit an overall decrease during pregnancy (Wells et al., 1999). Sodium, potassium, and chloride levels demonstrate a slight decrease, which is likely secondary to water retention (Hauguel et al., 1987).

Hormone levels are strongly influenced by the stage of gestation and the period of lactation. Estradiol 17β and progesterone levels increase during pregnancy (Kriesten and Murawski, 1988). Serum cortisol elevates during the final days of pregnancy (Kriesten and Murawski, 1988).

During the period of lactation, total cholesterol and triglycerides are decreased compared to their levels at mating (Mortensen and Frandsen, 1996). Oxytocin and prolactin levels vary in the dam concurrent with the once daily nursing of her kits. Estradiol is present throughout the lactation period but at lower concentrations than during pregnancy (González-Mariscal et al., 2007). Progesterone is absent during the lactation period (González-Mariscal et al., 2007).

3.4.8 Stress

Stress has been demonstrated to cause significant variations in physiologic parameters. A variety of environmental conditions may induce stress in rabbits including animal transport, handling, and restraint. Stress will generally result in an increased circulating level of glucocorticoid hormones (Toth and January, 1990). Increased levels of noise such as that produced by machinery (e.g., facility cage wash equipment) may produce physiologic changes in the rabbit such as elevations in blood glucose and corticosteroid levels (Hrapkiewicz et al., 2007; Fletcher, 1976). Social pairings can also stimulate an increase in glucocorticoid hormones that correlates with exhibition of defensive behaviors (Szeto et al., 2004). Conditioning animals to handling and new procedures prior to beginning a study can minimize stress and the associated physiologic consequences. Furthermore, allowing at least 48 hours for rabbits to acclimate to a new environment after shipping may decrease stress-related variables (Fowler, 1995). However, the appropriate length of the acclimation period must be determined for each anticipated stressor and evaluated parameter.

TABLE 3.3
Changes in Biochemical Parameter during Gestation in the New Zealand White Rabbit

Day of gestation		AST (IU/L)	ALT (IU/L)	ALP (IU/L)	BilT (mg/L)	Chol (g/L)	Tg (g/L)	Glu (g/L)	Urea (g/L)	Creat (mg/L)	TP (g/L)	Ca (mg/L)	P (mg/L)	Na (mEq/L)	K (mEq/L)	Cl (mEq/L)
−1	Mean	12	46	247	2	0.69	0.53	1.23	0.55	12	61	163	51	142	4.6	107
	SD	5.3	17.4	57.6	0.5	0.2	0.2	0.2	0.1	1.8	2.9	12.5	6.1	2.0	0.9	2.5
	n	90	90	90	89	90	90	90	90	90	90	90	90	89	89	89
7	Mean	20*	49	193*	2	0.60*	0.78*	1.40*	0.37*	12	63*	159	55*	144*	4.3*	104*
	SD	6.6	16.0	33.7	0.9	0.2	0.3	0.2	0.0	1.7	3.0	21.7	6.5	1.9	0.4	2.1
	n	29	29	29	27	28	29	29	29	29	28	28	28	29	29	29
10	Mean	20*	47	204*	2	0.58*	0.68*	1.31	0.41*	12	61	161*	51	144	4.0*	104*
	SD	3.7	15.9	37.3	0.7	0.2	0.2	0.1	0.1	1.1	2.8	6.0	5.4	2.9	0.4	2.3
	n	25	25	25	21	25	25	25	25	25	25	25	25	24	24	24
13	Mean	20*	51*	189*	2	0.54*	0.90*	1.35*	0.38*	12*	60	160	53	137*	4.1*	104*
	SD	9.1	21.7	35.6	0.8	0.2	0.4	0.1	0.0	1.6	2.6	5.1	4.8	1.3	0.3	1.8
	n	29	29	29	29	29	29	29	29	29	29	29	29	29	29	29
16	Mean	21*	59	190*	2	0.27*	1.02*	1.34	0.35*	11*	57*	156*	48*	138*	4.0*	105*
	SD	14.2	37.6	71.6	15.3	16.0	15.9	15.8	16.0	13.9	19.5	54.9	16.7	49.6	15.1	36.3
	n	25	25	25	25	25	25	25	25	25	25	25	25	25	25	25
19	Mean	28*	64*	159*	2	0.15*	1.33*	1.33*	0.35*	12	57*	154	47*	137*	4.1*	103*
	SD	13.5	27.0	36.8	0.7	0.1	0.6	0.1	0.0	1.1	1.7	5.1	3.9	1.9	0.4	1.7
	n	29	29	29	29	29	29	29	29	29	29	29	29	29	29	29
22	Mean	30*	56	153*	2	0.08*	0.86*	1.28	0.31*	10*	56*	151*	43*	136*	3.9*	100*
	SD	16.0	21.4	40.2	0.6	0.0	0.2	0.1	0.0	1.0	2.3	4.8	4.3	3.1	0.3	3.4
	n	25	25	25	22	25	25	25	25	25	25	25	25	25	25	25
25	Mean	40*	67*	113*	2	0.06*	0.39*	1.15*	0.32*	10*	48*	141*	41*	139*	4.1*	108*
	SD	28.4	35.7	35.7	0.9	0.0	0.2	0.1	0.0	0.9	2.6	5.2	3.1	1.8	0.5	2.2
	n	29	29	29	27	29	29	29	29	29	29	29	29	28	28	28
28	Mean	23*	44	85*	2	0.06*	0.28*	1.13*	0.30*	10*	47*	138*	39*	141*	4.2*	108
	SD	8.5	14.7	25.9	0.5	0.0	0.1	0.1	0.0	1.1	3.9	6.6	3.5	1.4	0.4	1.7
	N	25	25	25	11	25	25	25	25	25	25	25	25	25	25	25

Source: Reprinted from Wells, M.Y. et al., *Toxicol Pathol*, 27, 370–379, 1999. With permission.
BilT, total bilirubin; Chol, cholesterol; Tg, tryglycerides; Glu, glucose; Creat, creatinine; TP, total protein.
* $p < .05$ (paired t-tests, comparison with pretest values, day 1).

TABLE 3.4
Serum Biochemistry Values of Dutch Belted and New Zealand White Rabbits at Gestational Day 21

Parameter	Units	*n*	Min	Max	Mean	SD	95% CI
Dutch Belted							
A/G ratio	na	125	2.1	6.3	3.238	0.9724	3.065–3.41
Albumin	g/dL	125	3.3	5.1	4.13	0.3665	4.065–4.194
ALK phosphatase	U/L	125	27	108	48.69	16.25	45.81–51.56
ALT	U/L	125	15	81	31.27	9.589	29.57–32.97
AST	U/L	125	8	386	25.81	33.54	19.87–31.74
Calcium	mg/dL	125	11.9	15.1	13.42	0.6038	13.31–13.52
Chloride	mEq/L	125	93	109	100.1	2.69	99.67–100.6
Cholesterol	mg/dL	125	7	28	12.98	3.568	12.34–13.61
Creatinine	mg/dL	125	0.8	1.5	1.094	0.118	1.074–1.115
Glucose	mg/dL	125	77	202	122.5	17.77	119.3–125.6
Phosphorus	mg/dL	125	2.6	6.3	4.617	0.6726	4.498–4.736
Potassium	mEq/L	125	3	6	3.852	0.386	3.784–3.92
Sodium	mEq/L	125	134	153	139	2.718	138.5–139.5
Total protein	g/dL	125	4.1	6.4	5.486	0.3706	5.42–5.551
Triglycerides	mg/dL	125	35	264	122	41.91	114.6–129.5
Urea nitrogen	mg/dL	125	10	26	15.66	2.902	15.14–16.17
New Zealand White	–	–	–	–	–	–	–
A/G ratio	na	247	1.5	4.9	2.655	0.7131	2.566–2.745
Albumin	g/dL	247	3.2	4.8	3.926	0.2621	3.893–3.959
ALK phosphatase	U/L	247	19	200	59.27	21.31	56.6–61.94
ALT	U/L	247	16	285	44.31	25.27	41.14–47.47
AST	U/L	247	9	203	27.58	18.4	25.27–29.88
Calcium	mg/dL	247	9.7	14.9	12.8	0.6086	12.73–12.88
Chloride	mEq/L	247	92	110	101.1	2.857	100.8–101.5
Cholesterol	mg/dL	247	6	122	17.35	9.16	16.2–18.5
Creatinine	mg/dL	247	0.9	8	1.216	0.4599	1.158–1.273
Glucose	mg/dL	247	104	176	128.3	11.2	126.9–129.7
Phosphorus	mg/dL	247	2.8	18.5	4.577	1.064	4.444–4.711
Potassium	mEq/L	247	3.1	6.5	3.957	0.4129	3.906–4.009
Sodium	mEq/L	247	129	151	138.7	2.888	138.3–139
Total protein	g/dL	247	4.6	6.4	5.485	0.3116	5.446–5.524
Triglycerides	mg/dL	247	47	1146	144.4	87.99	133.4–155.4
Urea nitrogen	mg/dL	247	8	220	14.11	13.52	12.41–15.8

Source: Reprinted from Spence, S., *Birth Defects Res B Dev Reprod Toxicol*, 68, 439–48, 2003. With permission.

3.4.9 Anesthesia

Anesthetic agents can directly affect blood parameters. It is therefore important to choose an appropriate anesthetic regimen based on the parameters of interest. As illustrated in Table 3.5, studies have demonstrated fluctuations in biochemistry parameters throughout anesthetic episodes and up to 24 hours postanesthesia in NZW rabbits. However, the values remained within the normal reference range for rabbits in most cases. The degree of fluctuation varies with the anesthetic agent.

TABLE 3.5
Influence of Commonly Utilized Anesthetic Agents on the Clinical Chemistry Values of NZW Rabbits

	Ketamine-Xylazine[a,b,c,d,e]	Ketamine-Diazepam[a,b,c,d,e]	Fentanyl-Droperidol[a,c,e]	Thiopentone[a,e,f]	Pentobarbitone[a,e,f]	Halothane[g,h]	Isoflurane[g,h]
ALT	↑↑	↑↑	NC	↑↑	NC	↑	NC
AST	↑↑↑	↑↑↑	NC	↑↑	↓↓	↑↑↑	↑
ALP	↓↓	↓↓	NC	↓	↑	NC	NC
GGT	NC	NC	NC	↑↑	↑↑	–	–
Glucose	↑↑↑	↑↑	NC	NC	NC	↑↑↑	↑↑
BUN	↑↑	↑↑	NC	↑↑	NC	↑	↑
Creatinine	↑↑	↑↑↑	NC	NC	NC	↑	↑
LDH	↑	↑↑↑	–	NC	↓↓	–	–
Triglycerides	↑↑↑	↑↑↑	–	NC	NC	–	–
Cholesterol	NC	↑	–	NC	↑	–	–
Sodium	↑	↑↑	–	↑	NC	–	–
Calcium	↑	NC	–	NC	NC	–	–
Phosphorus	NC	↑↑	NC	NC	NC	–	–
Chloride	NC	↑	–	NC	NC	–	–
Potassium	↑	NC	–	NC	↓	–	–

NC, no change; –, indicates value was not evaluated; ↑, 25%–50% change at one or more time points; ↑↑, 50%–100% change at one or more time points; ↑↑↑, >100% change at one or more time points (% variation based on the maximum variation observed during the anesthetic episode).

[a] Compared with control animals.
[b] Gil et al. (2004).
[c] Gonzalez Gil et al. (2003).
[d] Gonzalez Gil et al. (2002).
[e] Illera et al. (2000).
[f] Gonzalez Gil et al. (2005).
[g] Compared with baseline values.
[h] Gil et al. (2007).

Based on this, to limit study variation, it is important that a consistent regimen of anesthesia be utilized for all animals on a study. In addition, the time at which samples are collected for a study should be standardized for a predetermined duration of anesthesia.

Similarly, blood hormone values can be influenced by anesthetic administration. For instance, serum ACTH, cortisol, corticosterone, and serotonin levels all vary with the administration of a variety of anesthetic agents (Gil et al., 2007; Illera et al., 2000).

3.4.10 Specimen Collection and Handling Artifacts

Proper collection and handling of blood samples is important to ensure accurate results. Prolonged exposure to erythrocytes can cause a spurious decrease in glucose (due to consumption by the red blood cell [RBC]) and an elevation of AST, lactate dehydrogenase (LDH), and inorganic phosphorus (Loeb, 1997). Erythrocytes should be promptly separated from serum or plasma to help minimize these effects. In addition, poor venipuncture technique or inappropriate equipment may result in hemolysis, which can cause artificial changes to blood parameters such as an increase in LDH, AST, creatine kinase, total protein, and potassium (Melillo, 2007). Moreover, lipemic samples can induce change in blood parameters and should be avoided.

While either serum or plasma can be used for the analysis of most blood chemistry parameters, variations may be observed in some chemistry values such as globulin and total protein (Loeb, 1997). For routine serum collection, the blood sample is typically allowed to clot for 30–45 minutes followed by centrifugation (Fox, 1989). Rabbit blood clots quickly at room temperature. When plasma collection is required, whole blood should be mixed with an anticoagulant during or immediately after collection in order to reduce clotting (Melillo, 2007) and then centrifuged immediately. The appropriate size collection tube must be chosen based on the anticipated sample volume in order to prevent significant dilution of the sample with the anticoagulant (Murray, 2000). However, the relative volume of anticoagulant required for the rabbit may vary due to their variable serum calcium levels (Bjoraker and Ketcham, 1981). Anticoagulants can interfere with some blood parameters. Heparin is often preferred over other anticoagulants, as it has a minimal effect on many biochemical parameters (Melillo, 2007).

3.5 COMMON PROCEDURES

Very few clinical pathology diagnostic procedures have been described in the rabbit. Some of these procedures may be invasive and only have experimental value. The value of these tests in a clinical setting is debatable. Even though the test can be performed, the results may be difficult to interpret in the context of disease.

3.5.1 Liver Function Evaluation

3.5.1.1 Sulfobromophthalein Clearance

Sulfobromophthalein (BSP) is a cholephilic dye that is cleared almost exclusively by the liver though bile; 75% of this is in the conjugated form (McLaughlin and Fish, 1994). Because of this, evaluation of BSP clearance can be utilized to measure liver function in the rabbit. Acquiring the BSP clearance rate requires injecting BSP intravenously and then measuring the plasma concentration at a given time point. At an intravenous dose of 60 mg/kg, the plasma clearance rate in the rabbit is approximately 1.8 mg/min and the BSP excretory capacity is 0.85 mg/min/kg, which is four times faster than in the dog (Klaassen and Plaa, 1967). BSP retention or a reduction in the normal clearance rate indicates a loss in liver function. It is important to note that biliary excretion is crucial to BSP clearance; thus if a biliary or posthepatic obstruction is present, the test is considered invalid.

Furthermore, BSP clearance rates can be falsely elevated if shock, dehydration, or competitive drugs are present (Jenkins, 2000).

3.5.1.2 Indocyanine Green Clearance

Measured clearance of the dye indocyanine green (ICG) from the blood can also be used to assess liver function (Plaa and Charbonneau, 2008; Klaassen and Plaa, 1969). Although similar in principle to BSP clearance testing, ICG clearance testing has some noted advantages (Plaa and Charbonneau, 2008; Cherrick et al., 1960). ICG is rapidly and completely bound to plasma protein and is excreted in bile in an unconjugated form. The dye does not undergo biotransformation prior to excretion. In addition, no extrahepatic methods of elimination have been identified. The ICG clearance assay is technically easy to perform. A known quantity of ICG is administered intravenously to the animal. At predetermined times plasma is collected from the animal and the concentration of ICG determined through spectrophotometric analysis. ICG is not irritating to subcutaneous tissues therefore tissues should not be damaged following inadvertent extravascular administration. Furthermore, as ICG administration does not stimulate a notable immune response, ICG can be administered multiple times to the same animal without apparent adverse effects.

In the rabbit as in other species (e.g., dog and rat), plasma clearance of ICG is exponential over at least a 32-minute period. Bile flow may be decreased with high ICG doses. The optimal dose of ICG for testing in the rabbit is 25–30 mg/kg. The half-life maximum clearance rates have been estimated over multiple doses (Klaassen and Plaa, 1969).

3.5.2 Renal Function

3.5.2.1 Inulin Clearance

Rabbit renal function can be estimated by measuring the excretion pattern of exogenously administered inulin or endogenously produced creatinine. Inulin is an exogenous compound that is cleared from plasma freely and exclusively by glomerular filtration and is not secreted or metabolically altered by the renal tubules. Because of this, inulin clearance from plasma is considered the gold standard in determining the glomerular filtration rate (GFR) in the rabbit (Hoefer, 2000).

The rabbit must be anesthetized for this procedure, thus the effect of the anesthetic agent on the GFR must be considered. Intravenous access is obtained and a method for collecting urine throughout the procedure is initiated. These can be achieved through use of an intravenous catheter and a urethral or ureter catheter, respectively. During this procedure, it is recommended that additional intravenous fluids be given to maintain hydration. Following anesthesia, inulin is administered intravenously first at an induction dose of 150 mg and then at a constant rate infusion of 3% inulin at 0.1 mL/min. A steady-state plasma inulin level is achieved after an hour of infusion. At this time, urine is collected for an hour and blood samples are collected at 0, 30, and 60 minutes. Inulin concentrations are determined in the urine and blood samples, and the rate of inulin clearance is calculated by the following equation (Homayoon et al., 1997; Wong et al., 1986):

$$\text{plasma clearance (mL/min)} =$$
$$[\text{urine flow (mL/min)} \times \text{inulin concentration in urine}] / \text{inulin concentration in plasma}$$

The normal renal clearance rate of inulin in the rabbit is 7.0 (5.0–8.4) mL/min/kg (Kozma et al., 1974). With this information, information on the GFR can be extrapolated.

In the rabbit, glomerular clearance of endogenous creatinine is identical to glomerular clearance of inulin; thus, measuring the rate of plasma creatinine clearance by the kidney provides an accurate estimate of the GFR (Buss and Bourdeau, 1984). Measuring creatinine clearance is less time consuming and invasive than measuring inulin clearance. Both endogenous and exogenous creatinine can be used. However, this test requires the quantitative collection of urine for 24 hours. The reported creatinine clearance rate in the rabbit is 3.2 (2.2–4.2) mL/min/kg (Hoefer, 2000). Although it is a technically easier procedure and is less invasive, it is not considered the gold standard for measuring GFR, thus inulin clearance is used more frequently in a research setting.

3.5.3 Adrenal Function

3.5.3.1 ACTH Stimulation Assay

Although not frequently performed, the adrenocorticotropic hormone (ACTH) stimulation assay evaluates the adrenal gland–pituitary gland axis. In this test, ACTH is administered IM at a dose of 6 μg/kg and plasma coricosterone levels measured at time 0 and 30 minutes. In a rabbit with normal adrenal gland function, the baseline (T0) corticosterone level is 1.52 ± 0.52 μg/dL and raises to 19.9 ± 7.9 μg/dL 30 minutes after ACTH administration (Rosenthal, 2000). Although adrenal dysfunction is rare in the rabbit, this can be a valuable test experimentally and diagnostically if an adrenal-pituitary dysfunction is suspected.

3.6 CONCLUSION

The rabbit is a valuable and frequently utilized laboratory animal species. It has many characteristics that make it especially suited for use in research such as its ease of handling and sample collection, physical size, fecundity, and unique physiologic and biochemical characteristics. In addition, distinct breeds and strains of rabbits can be produced through natural breeding and genetic modification. However, with the rabbit, as with all species, both internal and external factors exist that can adversely affect test findings. Recognizing and controlling for these factors is of utmost importance in the conduct of research utilizing the rabbit.

TABLE 3.6
Clinical Chemistry Data for Rabbits

Analyte	Typical Value	Reference
Adrenocorticotropin hormone (ACTH)	25 pg/dL	Campbell (2004)
Alanine aminotransferase (ALT)	25–65 IU/L	Suckow et al. (2002)
Albumin	2.7–5.0 g/dL	Suckow et al. (2002)
Alkaline phosphatase (ALP)	10–86 IU/L	Suckow et al. (2002)
Amylase	200–500 IU/L	Suckow et al. (2002)
Aspartate aminotransferase (AST)	20–120 IU/L	Suckow et al. (2002)
Bicarbonate (Total CO_2)	19–27 mEq/L	Mitruka and Rawnsley (1981)
Bilirubin (total)	0.2–0.5 mg/dL	Suckow et al. (2002)
Blood urea nitrogen (BUN)	5–25 mg/dL	Suckow et al. (2002)
Calcium	5.60–12.1 mg/dL	Suckow et al. (2002)
Chloride	92–120 mEq/L	Suckow et al. (2002)
Cholesterol	10–100 mg/dL	Suckow et al. (2002)
Corticosterone	1.54 μg/dL	Suckow et al. (2002)
Cortisol	2.6–3.8 μg/dL	Campbell (2004)
Creatine kinase (CK)	25–120 IU/L	Suckow et al. (2002)
Creatinine	0.5–2.6 mg/dL	Suckow et al. (2002)

(Continued)

TABLE 3.6 (*Continued*)
Clinical Chemistry Data for Rabbits

Analyte	Typical Value	Reference
Estradiol (basal level of preovulatory females)	3 pg/mL	DePaolo and Masoro (1989)
Follicle stimulating hormone (FSH)—estrus	1.6–2.2 ng/mL	Orstead et al. (1988)
Follicle stimulating hormone (FSH)—pseudopregnancy	1.1–2.3 ng/mL	Orstead et al. (1988)
Gamma glutamyl transpeptidase (GGT)	10–98 IU/L	Suckow et al. (2002)
Globulin	1.5–2.7 gm/dL	Suckow et al. (2002)
Glucose	74–148 mg/dL	Suckow et al. (2002)
Glutamate dehydrogenase (GDH)	16 U/L	Kaneko (1989)
Insulin	24–36 μU/mL	Lesault et al. (1991a)
Iron	190–210 mg/dL	Fox et al. (1974)
Lactate dehydrogenase (LHD)	33.5–129 IU/L	Suckow et al. (2002)
Luteinizing hormone (LH)—estrus	0.28 ng/mL	Orstead et al. (1988)
LH—pseudopregnancy	0.43–0.68 ng/mL	Orstead et al. (1988)
Magnesium	2.0–5.4 mg/dL	Suckow et al. (2002)
Phosphorous	4.0–6.0 mg/dL	Suckow et al. (2002)
Potassium	305–7.0 mEq/L	Suckow et al. (2002)
Progesterone (female, basal)	<1 ng/mL	DePaolo and Masoro (1989)
Progesterone (female, 6 hours postcoitus)	8 ng/mL	DePaolo and Masoro (1989)
Progesterone (female, 10 days postcoitus)	15–20 ng/mL	DePaolo and Masoro (1989)
Sodium	125–150 mEq/L	Suckow et al. (2002)
Sorbitol dehydrogenase (SDH)	170–177 U	Suckow et al. (2002)
Testosterone (male, peak of 4–5 hours cycle)	3–5 ng/mL	DePaolo and Masoro (1989)
Total protein	5.0–7.5 gm/dL	Suckow et al. (2002)
Triglycerides	50–200 mg/dL	Suckow et al. (2002)
Tri-iodothyronin (T3)	130–143 ng/dL	Campbell (2004)
Thyroid stimulating hormone (TSH)	40–100 μU/mL	Campbell (2004)
Thyroxine (T4)	1.7–2.4 μg/dL	Campbell (2004)
Uric acid	1.0–4.3 mg/dL	Suckow et al. (2002)

TABLE 3.7
Urine Chemistry Data for Adult Rabbits

Analyte	Typical Value	Reference
Volume	20–350 mL/kg/day; average 130 mL/kg	Kozma et al. (1974), and Mitruka and Rawnsley (1981)
pH	7.6–8.8 ± 8.2	McLaughlin and Fish (1994), and Kozma et al. (1974)
Specific Gravity	1.003–1.036	Kozma et al. (1974), and Mitruka and Rawnsley (1981)
Creatinine	20.0–80.0 mg/kg/day	Mitruka and Rawnsley (1981)
Glucose	Occasional traces	Kozma et al. (1974)
Protein	0.74–1.86 mg/kg/day	Mitruka and Rawnsley (1981)
Electrolytes		
Sodium	50.0–70.0 mg/kg/day	Mitruka and Rawnsley (1981)
Potassium	40.0–55.0	Mitruka and Rawnsley (1981)
Chloride	190.0–300.0 mg/kg/day	Mitruka and Rawnsley (1981)
Calcium	12.1–19.0 mg/kg/day	Mitruka and Rawnsley (1981)

(*Continued*)

TABLE 3.7 (*Continued*)
Urine Chemistry Data for Adult Rabbits

Analyte	Typical Value	Reference
Phosporous	10.0–60.0 mg/kg/day	Mitruka and Rawnsley (1981)
Magnesium	0.65–4.20 mg/kg/day	Mitruka and Rawnsley (1981)
Glomerulare Filtration Rate	7 mL/min/kg as measured by inulin clearance	Kaplan and Timmons (1979)
	1.8 mg/min/kg as measured by BSP clearance	Kozma et al. (1974)
Sediment		
RBCs/hp	Rare	Kozma et al. (1974)
WBC/hpf	Rare	Kozma et al. (1974)
Casts	Absent to rare	Mader (2004)
Epithelial cells	Absent to rare	Mader (2004)
Bacteria	Absent to rare	Mader (2004)
Crystals	Ammonium magnesium phosphate, calcium carbonate monohydrate, anhydrous calcium carbonate	Mader (2004)

3.7 REFERENCE RANGES

Clinical chemistry data for rabbits and urine chemistry data for adult rabbits are given, respectively, in Tables 3.6 and 3.7.

REFERENCES

Adams, R.J. 2002. Techniques of experimentation. In *Laboratory Animal Medicine*. Ed. J.G. Fox. New York, NY: Academic Press.

Adams, W.C., Gaman, E.M., and Feigenbaum, A.S. 1972. Breed differences in the responses of rabbits to atherogenic diets. *Atherosclerosis.* 16(3):405–411.

Aleman, C.L., Noa, M., Mas, R., et al. 2000. Reference data for the principal physiological indicators in three species of laboratory animals. *Lab Anim.* 34(4):379–85.

Aliev, G. and Burnstock, G. 1998. Watanabe rabbits with heritable hypercholesterolaemia: A model of atherosclerosis. *Histol Histopathol.* 13(3):797–817.

Alus, G. and Edwards, N.A. 1977. Development of the digestive tract of the rabbit from birth to weaning. *Proc Nutr Soc.* 36(1):3A.

Baba, N. and von Haam, E. 1972. Animal model: Spontaneous adenocarcinoma in aged rabbits. *Am J Pathol.* 68(3):653–656.

Barrera, J. and Young, J.D. 1997. A simple technique for collection of large amounts of blood from tranquilized or anesthetized rabbits. *Contemp Top Lab Anim Sci.* 36(3):81–82.

Basaraba, R.J. 2008. Experimental tuberculosis: The role of comparative pathology in the discovery of improved tuberculosis treatment strategies. *Tuberculosis (Edinb).* 88(1 Suppl):S35–S47.

Benson, K.G. and Paul-Murphy, J. 1999. Clinical pathology of the domestic rabbit. Acquisition and interpretation of samples. *Vet Clin North Am Exot Anim Pract.* 2(3):539–551, v.

Bergdall, V.K. and Dysko, R.C. 1994. Metabolic, traumatic, mycotic, and miscellaneous diseases. In *The Biology of the Laboratory Rabbit*. Ed. P.J. Manning, D.H. Ringler, and C.E. Newcomer. San Diego, CA: Academic Press.

Besch, E.L. and Brigmon, R.L. 1991. Adrenal and body temperature changes in rabbits exposed to varying effective temperatures. *Lab Anim Sci.* 41(1):31–34.

Bivin, W.S. 1994. Basic biomethodology. In *The Biology of the Laboratory Rabbit*. Eds. P.J. Manning, D.H. Ringler, C.E. Newcomer, and S.H. Weisbroth. San Diego, CA: Academic Press.

Bjoraker, D.G. and Ketcham, T.R. 1981. 3.8% sodium citrate (1:9) is an inadequate anticoagulant for rabbit blood with high calcium. *Thromb Res.* 24(5–6):505–508.

Borgman, R.F. and Wardlaw, F.B. 1975. Serum cholesterol concentrations and cholelithiasis in rabbits as influenced by the form of dietary fat. *Am J Vet Res.* 36(1):93–95.

Brewer, N.R. 2006. Biology of the rabbit. *J Am Assoc Lab Anim Sci.* 45(1):8–24.

Brock, K., Gallaugher, L., Bergdall, V.K., and Dysko, R.C. 2012. Mycoses and non-infectious diseases. In *The Laboratory Rabbit, Guinea Pig, Hamster, and Other Rodents.* Ed. M.A. Suckow, K.A. Stevens, and R.P. Wilson, pp. 503–528. San Diego, CA: Academic Press.

Brousseau, M.E. and Hoeg, J.M. 1999. Transgenic rabbits as models for atherosclerosis research. *J Lipid Res.* 40(3):365–375.

Buss, S.L. and Bourdeau, J.E. 1984. Calcium balance in laboratory rabbits. *Miner Electrolyte Metab.* 10(2):127–132.

Campbell, T.W. 2004. Clinical chemistry of mammals: Laboratory animals and miscellaneous species. In *Veterinary hematology and clinical chemistry.* Ed. M. Thrall. Philadelphia, PA: Lippincott Williams & Wilkins.

Cano, P., Jimenez-Ortega, V., Alvarez, M.P., Alvarino, M., Cardinali, D.P., and Esquifino, A.I. 2005. Effect of rabbit doe-litter separation on 24-hour changes of luteinizing hormone, follicle stimulating hormone and prolactin release in female and male suckling pups. *Reprod Biol Endocrinol.* 3:50.

Cherrick, G.R., Stein, S.W., Leevy, C.M., and Davidson, C.S. 1960. Indocyanine green: Observations on its physical properties, plasma decay, and hepatic extraction. *J Clin Invest.* 39:592–600.

Cizek, L.J. 1961. Relationship between food and water ingestion in the rabbit. *Am J Physiol.* 201:557–566.

Cooper, H.M. and Patterson, Y. 2008. Production of polyclonal antisera. *Curr Protoc Immunol.* Chapter 2:Unit 2.4.1–2.4.10.

de Roos, B., Caslake, M.J, Milliner, K., Benson, G.M., Suckling, K.E., and Packard, C.J. 2005. Characterisation of the lipoprotein structure in the St. Thomas' Mixed Hyperlipidaemic (SMHL) rabbit. *Atherosclerosis.* 181(1):63–68.

DePaolo, LV. and Masoro, E.J. 1989. Endocrine hormones in laboratory animals. In *The Clinical Chemistry of Laboratory Animals.* Eds. W.F. Loeb, and F.W. Quimby. New York, NY: Pergamon Press.

DiBartola, S.P. 1995. Clinical approach and laboratory evaluation of renal disease. In *Textbook of Veterinary Internal Medicine: Diseases of the Dog and Cat.* Eds. S.J. Ettinger, and E.C. Feldman. Philadelphia, PA: W.B. Saunders.

Diehl, K.H., Hull, R., Morton, D., et al. 2001. A good practice guide to the administration of substances and removal of blood, including routes and volumes. *J Appl Toxicol.* 21(1):15–23.

Donnelly, T.M. 2003. Basic anatomy, physiology, and husbandry. In *Ferrets, Rabbits, and Rodents Clinical Medicine and Surgery.* Eds. K.E. Quesenberry, and J.W. Carpenter. St. Louis, MO: Saunders.

Elsinghorst, T.A., Timmermans, H.J., and Hendriks, H.G. 1984. Comparative pathology of endometrial carcinoma. *Vet Q.* 6(4):200–208.

Fan, J. and Watanabe, T. 2003. Transgenic rabbits as therapeutic protein bioreactors and human disease models. *Pharmacol Ther.* 99(3):261–282.

Flecknell, P.A., Liles, J.H., and Williamson, H.A. 1990. The use of lignocaine-prilocaine local anaesthetic cream for pain-free venepuncture in laboratory animals. *Lab Anim.* 24(2):142–146.

Fletcher, J.L. 1976. Influence of noise on animals. In *Laboratory Animal Handbooks 7: Control of the Animal House Environment.* Ed. T. McSheehy. London: Laboratory Animals.

Foote, R.H. and Simkin, M.E. 1993. Use of gonadotropic releasing hormone for ovulating the rabbit model. *Lab Anim Sci.* 43(4):383–355.

Forcada, F. and Lopez, M. 2000. Repeated surgical embryo recovery and embryo production in rabbits. *Anim Reprod Sci.* 64(1–2):121–126.

Fowler, M.E. 1995. *Restraint and Handling of Wild and Domestic Animals*, 2nd edition. Ames, IA: Iowa State University Press.

Fox, J.G. 1989. The clinical chemistry of laboratory animals. In The Clinical Chemistry of Laboratory Animals. Eds. W.F. Loeb, and F. Quimby. New York, NY: Pergamon Press.

Fox, R.R. 1974. Taxonomy and genetics. In *The Biology of the Laboratory Rabbit.* Eds. S.H. Weisbroth, R.E. Flatt, and A.L. Kraus. New York, NY: Academic Press.

Fox, R.R. 1989b. The rabbit. In *The Clinical Chemistry of Laboratory Animals.* Eds. W.F. Loeb, and F.W. Quimby. New York, NY: Pergamon Press.

Fox, R.R. and Crary, D.D. 1971. Mandibular prognathism in the rabbit. Genetic studies. *J Hered.* 62(1):23–27.

Fox, R.R., Crary, D.D., Babino, E.J, Jr., and Sheppard, L.B. 1969. Buphthalmia in the rabbit. Pleiotropic effects of the (bu) gene and a possible explanation of mode of gene action. *J Hered.* 60(4):206–212.

Fox, R.R. and Laird, C.W. 1970. Biochemical parameters of clinical significance in rabbits. II. Diurnal variations. *J Hered.* 61(6):265–268.

Fox, R.R., Laird, C.W., Blau, E.M., Schultz, H.S., and Mitchell, B.P. 1970. Biochemical parameters of clinical significance in rabbits. I. Strain variations. *J Hered.* 61(6):261–265.

Fox, R.R., Laird, C.W., Kirshenbaum, J., and Meier, H. 1974. Effect of strain, sex, and circadian rhythm on rabbit serum bilirubin and iron levels. *Proc Soc Exp Biol Med.* 145(2):421–427.

Fuentes, G.C. and Newgren, J. 2008. Physiology and clinical pathology of laboratory new zealand white rabbits housed individually and in groups. *J Am Assoc Lab Anim Sci.* 47(2):35–38.

Gil, A.G., Silvan, G., and Illera, J.C. 2007. Pituitary-adrenocortical axis, serum serotonin and biochemical response after halothane or isoflurane anaesthesia in rabbits. *Lab Anim.* 41(4):411–419.

Gil, A.G., Silvan, G., Illera, M., and Illera, J.C. 2004. The effects of anesthesia on the clinical chemistry of New Zealand White rabbits. *Contemp Top Lab Anim Sci.* 43(3):25–29.

Gonzalez Gil, A., Illera, J.C., Silvan, G., and Illera, M. 2003. Effects of the anaesthetic/tranquillizer treatments on selected plasma biochemical parameters in NZW rabbits. *Lab Anim.* 37(2):155–161.

Gonzalez Gil, A., Illera, J.C., Silvan, G., Lorenzo, P.L., and Illera, M. 2002. Changes in hepatic and renal enzyme concentrations and heart and respiratory rates in new zealand white rabbits after anesthetic treatments. *Contemp Top Lab Anim Sci.* 41(6):30–32.

Gonzalez Gil, A., Silvan, G., and Illera, J.C. 2005. Effects of barbiturate administration on hepatic and renal biochemical parameters in new zealand white rabbits. *Contemp Top Lab Anim Sci.* 44(6):43–45.

González-Mariscal, G., McNitt J.I., and Lukefahr, S.D. 2007. Maternal care of rabbits in the lab and on the farm: Endocrine regulation of behavior and productivity. *Hormones and Behavior.* 52(1):86–91.

Graham, J. 2006. Common procedures in rabbits. *Vet Clin North Am Exot Anim Pract.* 9(2):367–388, vii.

Gu, T., Li, C.X., Feng, Y., Wang, Q., Li, C.H., and Li, C.F. 2007. Trans-arterial gene therapy for hepatocellular carcinoma in a rabbit model. *World J Gastroenterol.* 13(14):2113–2117.

Hanna, B.L., Sawin, P.B., and Sheppard, L.B. 1962. Recessive buphthalmos in the rabbit. *Genetics.* 47:519–529.

Harkness, J.E. and Wagner, J.E. 1995. *The Biology and Medicine of Rabbits and Rodents*, 4th edition. Baltimore, MD: Williams & Wilkins.

Hartman, H.A. 1974. The fetus in experimental teratology. In *The Biology of the Laboratory Rabbit.* Eds. S.H. Weisbroth, R.E. Flatt, and A.L. Kraus. New York, NY: Academic Press.

Hartung, T. 2002. Comparison and validation of novel pyrogen tests based on the human fever reaction. *Altern Lab Anim.* 30(2 Suppl):49–51.

Hauguel, S., Gilbert M., and Girard, J. 1987. Pregnancy-induced insulin resistance in liver and skeletal muscles of the conscious rabbit. *Am J Physiol.* 252(2 Pt 1):E165–E169.

Hausner, E.A., Schlingmann, K.L., Chen, H.W., et al. 1995. Hepatic and adrenal changes in rabbits associated with hyperlipidemia caused by a semi-synthetic diet. *Lab Anim Sci.* 45(6):663–670.

Hendriksen, C. and Hau, J. 2003. Production of polyclonal and monoclonal antibodies. In *Handbook of Laboratory Animal Science*. Eds. J. Hau, and G.L. Van Hoosier. Boca Raton, FL: CRC Press.

Hoefer, H.L. 2000. Rabbit and ferret renal disease diagnosis In *Laboratory Medicine: Avian and Exotic Pets.* Ed. A.M. Fudge. Philadelphia, PA: Saunders.

Homayoon, K.A., Salle, J.L., McLorie, G.A., Bagli, D.J., Agarwal, S.K., and Khoury, A.E. 1997. Correlation of inulin with creatinine clearance in partial unilateral ureteral obstruction for determination of differential glomerular filtration rate in rabbits. *Contemp Top Lab Anim Sci.* 36(6):44–46.

Hrapkiewicz, K., Medina, L., and Holmes, D.D. 2007. *Clinical Laboratory Animal Medicine: An Introduction*, 3rd edition. Ames, IA: Blackwell Publishing.

Hu, J., Peng, X., Budgeon, L.R., Cladel, N.M., Balogh, K.K., and Christensen, N.D. 2007. Establishment of a cottontail rabbit papillomavirus/HLA-A2.1 transgenic rabbit model. *J Virol.* 81(13):7171–7177.

Illera, J.C., Gonzalez Gil, A., Silvan, G., and Illera, M. 2000. The effects of different anaesthetic treatments on the adreno-cortical functions and glucose levels in NZW rabbits. *J Physiol Biochem.* 56(4):329–336.

Institute of Laboratory Animal Resources (U.S.). 2011. *Guide for the Care and Use of Laboratory Animals*, 8th edition. Washington, D.C: National Academy Press.

Jenkins, J.R. 2000. Rabbit and ferret liver and gastrointestinal testing. In *Laboratory Medicine: Avian and Exotic Pets*. Ed. A.M. Fudge. Philadelphia, PA: Saunders.

Jilge, B. 1991. The rabbit: A diurnal or a nocturnal animal? *J Exp Anim Sci.* 34(5–6):170–183.

Jilge, B. and Hudson, R. 2001. Diversity and development of circadian rhythms in the European rabbit. *Chronobiol Int.* 18(1):1–26.

Johnston, N.A. and Nevalainen, T. 2003. Impact of the biotic and abiotic enviroment on animal experiments. In *Handbook of Laboratory Animal Science*. Eds. J. Hau, and G. Van Hoosier, 2nd edition, Boca Raton, FL: CRC Press.

Joint Working Group on Refinement. 1993. Removal of blood from laboratory mammals and birds. First report of the BVA/FRAME/RSPCA/UFAW Joint Working Group on Refinement. 1993. *Lab Anim.* 27(1):1–22.

Joly, T., Neto, V., and Salvetti, P. 2012. Cryopreservation of genetic diversity in Rabbit Species (*Oryctolagus cuniculus*). In *Current Frontiers in Cryopreservation*. Ed. I. Katkov, pp. 179–186. Rijeka: InTech Europe.

Kaneko, J.J. 1989. Appendixes. In *Clinical Biochemistry of Domestic Animals*. Ed. J.J. Kaneko. San Diego, CA: Academic Press.

Kaplan, H.M. and Timmons, E.H. 1979. *The Rabbit: A Model for the Principles of Mammalian Physiology and Surgery*. New York, NY: Academic Press.

Klaassen, C.D. and Plaa, G.L. 1967. Species variation in metabolism, storage, and excretion of sulfobromophthalein. *Am J Physiol.* 213(5):1322–1326.

Klaassen, C.D. and Plaa, G.L. 1969. Plasma disappearance and biliary excretion of indocyanine green in rats, rabbits, and dogs. *Toxicol Appl Pharmacol.* 15(2):374–384.

Kojima, S. and Tanaka, R. 1974. Factors influencing absorption and excretion of drugs. III. Effect of fasting on absorption and excretion of sodium salicylate and aspirin in rabbits. *Chem Pharm Bull (Tokyo).* 22(10):2270–2275.

Kozma, C.K., Macklin, L., Cummins, L., and Mauer, R. 1974. Anatomy, physiology, and biochemistry of the rabbit. In *The Biology of the Laboratory Rabbit*. Eds. S.H. Weisbroth, R. Flatt, and A. Kraus. New York, NY: Academic Press.

Kozma, C.K., Pelas, A., and Salvador, R.A. 1967. Electrophoretic determination of serum proteins of laboratory animals. *J Am Vet Med Assoc.* 151(7):865–869.

Kraus, A.L., Weisbroth, S.H., Flatt, R.E., and Brewer, N. 1984. Biology and diseases of rabbits. In *Laboratory Animal Medicine*. Eds. J.G. Fox, B.J. Cohen, and F.M. Loew. Orlando, FL: Academic Press.

Kreuter, K.A., El-Abbadi, N., Shbeeb, A., et al. 2008. Development of a rabbit pleural cancer model by using VX2 tumors. *Comp Med.* 58(3):287–293.

Kriesten, K. and Murawski, U. 1988. Concentrations of serum cortisol, progesterone, estradiol-17 beta, cholesterol and cholesterol ester in the doe during the reproductive stadium, in the fetal serum, in the amniotic fluid and in the milk of rabbits, as well as correlations between these parameters. *Comp Biochem Physiol A Comp Physiol.* 90(3):413–420.

Kurien, B.T., Everds, N.E., and Scofield, R.H. 2004. Experimental animal urine collection: A review. *Lab Anim.* 38(4):333–361.

Lacy, M.J., Kent, C.R., and Voss, E.W, Jr. 1987. D-Limonene: An effective vasodilator for use in collecting rabbit blood. *Lab Anim Sci.* 37(4):485–487.

Laird, C.W. and Fox, R.R. 1970. The effect of age on cholesterol and PBI levels in the 3–3c hybrid rabbit. *Life Sci II.* 9(21):1243–1253.

Lassen, E.D. 2004. Laboratory evaluation of the liver. In *Veterinary Hematology and Clinical Chemistry*. Ed. M.A. Thrall. Philadelphia, PA: Lippincott Williams & Wilkins.

Latimer, K.S., Mahaffey, E.A., Prasse, K.W., and Duncan, J.R. 2003. *Duncan & Prasse's Veterinary Laboratory Medicine: Clinical Pathology*, 4th edition. Ames, IA: Iowa State Press.

Latour, M. A., Hopkins, D., Kitchens, T., Chen, Z., and Schonfeld, G. 1998. Effects of feeding a liquid diet for one year to New Zealand White rabbits. *Lab Anim Sci.* 48(1):81–84.

Lesault, A., Elchinger, B., and Desbals, B. 1991a. Circadian rhythms of food intake, plasma glucose and insulin levels in fed and fasted rabbits. *Horm Metab* Res. 23(11):515–516.

Lesault, A., Elchinger, B., and Desbals, B. 1991b. Circadian variations and extraadrenal effect of ACTH on insulinemia in rabbit. *Horm Metab* Res. 23(10):461–464.

Lindena, J. and Trautschold, I. 1986. Catalytic enzyme activity concentration in plasma of man, sheep, dog, cat, rabbit, guinea pig, rat and mouse. Approach to a quantitative diagnostic enzymology, I. Communication. *J Clin Chem Clin Biochem.* 24(1):11–18.

Lindena, J., Sommerfeld, U., Hopfel, C., and Trautschold, I. 1986. Catalytic enzyme activity concentration in tissues of man, dog, rabbit, guinea pig, rat and mouse. Approach to a quantitative diagnostic enzymology, III. Communication. *J Clin Chem Clin Biochem.* 24(1):35–47.

Lindsey, J.R. and Fox, R.R. 1994. Inherited diseases and variations. In *The Biology of the Laboratory Rabbit*. Eds. P.J. Manning, D.H. Ringler, and C.E. Newcomer. San Diego, CA: Academic Press.

Lipman, N.S., Marini, R.P., and Flecknell, P.A. 2008. Anesthesia and analgesia in rabbits. In *Anesthesia and Analgesia in Laboratory Animals*. Eds. R.F. Fish, M.J. Brown, P.J. Danneman, and A.Z. Karas. San Diego, CA: Academic Press.

Loeb, W.F. 1997. Clinical biochemistry of laboratory rodents and rabbits. In *Clinical Biochemistry of Domestic Animals*. Eds. J.J. Kaneko, J.W. Harvey, and M. Bruss. San Diego, CA: Academic Press.

Loeb, W.F. and Quimby, F.W. 1989. *The Clinical Chemistry of Laboratory Animals*. New York, NY: Pergamon Press.

Ludders, J.W., Thomas, C.B., Sharp, P., and Sedgwick, C.J. 1987. An anesthetic technique for repeated collection of blood from New Zealand white rabbits. *Lab Anim Sci.* 37(6):803–805.

Mader, D.R. 2004. Rabbits basic approach to veterinary care. In *Ferrets, Rabbits, and Rodents: Clinical Medicine and Surgery.* Eds. K.E. Quesenberry, and J.W. Carpenter. St. Louis, MO: Saunders.

Marian, A.J., Wu, Y., Lim, D.S., et al. 1999. A transgenic rabbit model for human hypertrophic cardiomyopathy. *J Clin Invest.* 104(12):1683–1692.

McCanna, D.J., Driot, J.Y., Hartsook, R., and Ward, K.W. 2008. Rabbit models of contact lens-associated corneal hypoxia: A review of the literature. *Eye Contact Lens.* 34(3):160–165.

McLaughlin, R.M. and Fish, R.E. 1994. Clinical biochemistry and hematology. In *The Biology of the Laboratory Rabbit.* Eds. P.J. Manning, D.H. Ringler, and C.E. Newcomer. San Diego, CA: Academic Press.

Melillo, A. 2007. Rabbit clinical pathology. *Journal of Exotic Pet Medicine.* 16(3):135–145.

Mitruka, B.M. and Rawnsley, H.M. 1981. *Clinical Biochemical and Hematological Reference Values in Normal Experimental Animals and Normal Humans*, 2nd edition. New York, NY: Masson Pub. USA.

Moghadasian, M.H., Frohlich, J.J., and McManus, B.M. 2001. Advances in experimental dyslipidemia and atherosclerosis. *Lab Invest.* 81(9):1173–1183.

Morrell, J. M. 1995. Artificial insemination in rabbits. *Br Vet J.* 151(5):477–488.

Mortensen, A. and Frandsen, H. 1996. Reproductive performance and changes in blood lipids in breeding females and in growing Watanabe heritable hyperlipidaemic and New Zealand White rabbits. *Lab Anim.* 30(3):252–259.

Murray, M. 2000. Rabbit and ferret laboratory medicine. In *Laboratory Medicine: Avian and Exotic Pets.* Ed. A.M. Fudge. Philadelphia, PA: Saunders.

Napier, R.A.N. 1963. Rabbits. In *Animals for Research.* Ed. W. Lane-Petter. New York, NY: Academic Press.

Nevalainen, T.O., Nevalainen, J.I., Guhad, F.A., and Lang, C.M. 2007. Pair housing of rabbits reduces variances in growth rates and serum alkaline phosphatase levels. *Lab Anim.* 41(4):432–440.

NICEATM, Interagency Coordinating Committee on the Validation of Alternative Methods (ICCVAM) and National Toxicology Program (NTP) Interagency Center for the Evaluation of Alternative Toxicological Methods. 2006. ICCVAM Test Method Evaluation Report In Vitro Ocular Toxicity Test Methods for Identifying Severe Irritants and Corrosives.

Norido, F., Zatta, A., Fiorito, C., Prosdocimi, M., and Weber, G. 1993. Hematologic and biochemical profiles of selectively bred WHHL rabbits. *Lab Anim Sci.* 43(4):319–323.

Okubo, N., Hombrouck, C., Fornes, P., et al. 2000. Cardiac troponin I and myocardial contusion in the rabbit. *Anesthesiology.* 93(3): 811–817.

Orstead, K.M., Hess, D.L., and Spies, H.G. 1988. Pulsatile patterns of gonadotropins and ovarian steroids during estrus and pseudopregnancy in the rabbit. *Biol Reprod.* 38(4):733–743.

Pare, J.A. and Paul-Murphy, J. 2004. Disorders of the reproductive and urinary systems. In *Ferrets, Rabbits and Rodents Clincal Medicine and Surgery.* Eds. K.E. Quesenberry, and J.W. Carpenter. St. Louis, MO: Saunders.

Piccione, G., Caola, G., and Refinetti, R. 2007. Daily rhythms of liver-function indicators in rabbits. *J Physiol Sci.* 57(2):101–105.

Plaa, G.L. and Charbonneau, M. 2008. Detection and evaluation of chemically induced liver injury. In *Principles and Methods of Toxicology.* Ed. A.W. Hayes. Boca Raton, FL: CRC Press/Taylor & Francis Group.

Rosenthal, K.L. 2000. Ferret and rabbit endocrine disease diagnosis In *Laboratory Medicine: Avian and Exotic Pets.* Ed. A.M. Fudge. Philadelphia, PA: Saunders.

Sawin, P.B. and Glick, D. 1943. Atropinesterase, a genetically determined enzyme in the rabbit. *Proc Natl Acad Sci U S A.* 29(2):55–59.

Schindler, W.J., Hutchins, M.O., Laird, C.W., Fox, R.R., and Meier, H. 1974. Effect of strain and sex variation on growth hormone in rabbit serum. *Proc Soc Exp Biol Med.* 147(3):820–822.

Schrader, S., Mircheff, A K., and Geerling, G. 2008. Animal models of dry eye. *Dev Ophthalmol.* 41:298–312.

Sebesteny, A., Sheraidah, G.A., Trevan, D.J., Alexander, R.A., and Ahmed, A.I. 1985. Lipid keratopathy and atheromatosis in an SPF laboratory rabbit colony attributable to diet. *Lab Anim.* 19(3):180–188.

Shikishima, K. 2004. Methods for subchoroidal implantation of Greene melanoma in rabbits. *Int J Clin Oncol.* 9(2):79–84.

Shiomi, M., Ito, T., Yamada, S., Kawashima, S., and Fan, J. 2003. Development of an animal model for spontaneous myocardial infarction (WHHLMI rabbit). *Arterioscler Thromb Vasc Biol.* 23(7):1239–1244.

Smith, P.A., Prieskorn, D.M., Knutsen, C.A., and Ensminger, W.D. 1988. A method for frequent blood sampling in rabbits. *Lab Anim Sci.* 38(5):623–625.

Sparks, D.L. 2008. The early and ongoing experience with the cholesterol-fed rabbit as a model of Alzheimer's disease: The old, the new and the pilot. *J Alzheimers Dis.* 15(4):641–656.

Spence, S. 2003. The Dutch-Belted rabbit: An alternative breed for developmental toxicity testing. *Birth Defects Res B Dev Reprod Toxicol.* 68(5):439–448.

Stein, S. and Walshaw, S. 1996. Rabbits. In *Handbook of Rodent and Rabbit Medicine*. Eds. K. Laber-Laird, M.M. Swindle, and P.A. Flecknell. Tarrytown, NY: Pergamon.

Stickrod, G., Ebaugh, T., and Garnett, C. 1981. Use of a mini-peristaltic pump for collection of blood from rabbits. *Lab Anim Sci.* 31(1):87–88.

Stills, H.F. 1994. Polyclonal antibody production. In *The Biology of the Laboratory Rabbit*. Eds. P.J. Manning, D.H. Ringler, and C.E. Newcomer. San Diego, CA: Academic Press.

Suckow, M. A. and Douglas, F.A. 1997. *The Laboratory Rabbit, The Laboratory Animal Pocket Reference Series*. Boca Raton, FL: CRC Press.

Suckow, M.A., Brammer, D.W., Rush, H.G., and Chrisp, C.C. 2002. Biology and diseases of rabbits. In *Laboratory Animal Medicine*. Eds. J.G. Fox, L.C. Anderson, F.M. Loew, and F.W. Quimby. New York, NY: Academic Press.

Sutherland, G.B., Trapani, I.L., and Campbell, D.H. 1958. Cold adapted animals. II. Changes in the circulating plasma proteins and formed elements of rabbit blood under various degrees of cold stress. *J Appl Physiol.* 12(3):367–372.

Szeto, A., Gonzales, J.A., Spitzer, S.B., et al. 2004. Circulating levels of glucocorticoid hormones in WHHL and NZW rabbits: Circadian cycle and response to repeated social encounter. *Psychoneuroendocrinology.* 29(7):861–866.

Taylor, W., Ellis, W.R., and Bell, G.D. 1981. The effect of cholesterol feeding on gallbladder bile acids of the rabbit. Evidence that lithocholic acid is a primary bile acid in the rabbit. *Biochem J.* 198(3):639–643.

Tesluk, G.C., Peiffer, R.L., and Brown, D. 1982. A clinical and pathological study of inherited glaucoma in New Zealand white rabbits. *Lab Anim.* 16(3):234–239.

Toth, L.A. and January, B. 1990. Physiological stabilization of rabbits after shipping. *Lab Anim Sci.* 40(4):384–387.

van Zutphen, L.F. 1974. Serum esterase genetics in rabbits. I. Phenotypic variation of the prealbumin esterases and classification of atropinesterase and cocainesterase. *Biochem Genet.* 12(4):309–326.

Vinardell, M.P. and Mitjans, M. 2008. Alternative methods for eye and skin irritation tests: An overview. *J Pharm Sci.* 97(1):46–59.

Washington, I.M. and Van Hoosier, G. 2012. Clinical biochemistry and hematology. In *The Laboratory Rabbit, Guinea Pig, Hamster, and Other Rodents*. Eds. M.A. Suckow, K.A. Stevens, and R.P. Wilson, pp. 57–116. San Diego, CA: Academic Press.

Wasson, K. and Peper, R.L. 2000. Mammalian microsporidiosis. *Vet Pathol.* 37(2):113–128.

Watanabe, N., Nakagawa, H., Kitajima, S., et al., 2005. Establishment of a SPF colony of human apo(a) transgenic rabbits by frozen-thawed embryo transfer. *Exp Anim.* 54(4):353–357.

Wells, M.Y., Decobecq, C.P., Decouvelaere, D.M., Justice, C., and Guittin, P. 1999. Changes in clinical pathology parameters during gestation in the New Zealand white rabbit. *Toxicol Pathol.* 27(3):370–379.

Wong, N.L., Whiting, S.J., Mizgala, C.L., and Quamme, G.A. 1986. Electrolyte handling by the superficial nephron of the rabbit. *Am J Physiol.* 250(4 Pt 2):F590–F595.

Woodruff-Pak, D.S. 2008. Animal models of Alzheimer's disease: Therapeutic implications. *J Alzheimers Dis.* 15(4):507–521.

Wostmann, B.S. 1961. Recent studies on the serum proteins of germfree animals. *Ann NY Acad Sci.* 94:272–283.

Yanni, A.E. 2004. The laboratory rabbit: An animal model of atherosclerosis research. *Lab Anim.* 38(3):246–256.

4 The Laboratory Dog

Julia Whitaker, Allison R. Rogala,
Dana N. LeVine, and Craig A. Fletcher

CONTENTS

4.1 USE OF DOGS IN BIOMEDICAL RESEARCH

Dogs have been used in research since the seventeenth century (Gay, 1984; Kohn, 1995). As dogs are popular companion animals, there is a wealth of information on congenital or acquired diseases in dogs (or particular breeds of dogs) from clinical practice, as well as information from research studies. The dog is a common animal model for several reasons, including its relatively large body size, tractable behavior, and an organ system that is comparable to humans (Loeb, 1999; Tsai et al., 2007). Surgical models were developed in dogs for cardiopulmonary bypass, coronary artery bypass, aortic aneurysm repair, congenital heart defect correction, and heart valve replacement (Kohn, 1995). Canines are used for research in transplantation (kidney, lung, and heart), joint prostheses, gastrointestinal (GI) surgery, chronic pancreatitis, hemorrhagic pancreatitis, endocarditis (Kohn, 1995), aging, amyloidosis, radiation treatment, treatment of cardiogenic shock, and intervertebral disk disease (Gay, 1984). In pulmonary research, dogs have been used to study pulmonary inflammation, airway hyperresponsiveness (Chapman, 2008), chronic bronchitis, asthma, emphysema, and obstructive airway disease (Gay, 1984). In order to cover all the diseases for which dogs can serve as animal models, an entire book would be needed. In fact, a book of animal models, including the canine models, has already been written: *Spontaneous animal models of human disease* (Andrews et al., 1979).

In this chapter, we have limited our coverage to only some of the diseases for which the dog is an animal model. While Beagles are the standard research dog (Loeb, 1999), spontaneous diseases that arise in other breeds provide many models for similar, or even identical, diseases in humans. There are many cardiovascular diseases and conditions for which dogs serve as models. Recent interest in human familial dilated cardiomyopathy (DCM) has prompted a number of researchers to investigate the genetic basis of canine DCM (Moïse, 1999). It is clear that dogs, similar to humans, have a prolonged presymptomatic phase of the disease extending over years. Dog breeds affected by DCM include the large and giant breeds (Boxers, Great Dane, Weimaraners, Doberman Pinscher, German Shepherd, Irish Wolfhound, Newfoundland, Standard Poodle, and St. Bernard), and spaniels (Cockers and Springers) (Andrews et al., 1979; Moïse, 1999). Within these breeds, the disease is prevalent in certain family lines and therefore the disease has long been suspected to have a genetic basis. An autosomal dominant transmission has been reported in Irish Wolfhounds, Newfoundlands and Dobermans (Andrews et al., 1979; Dukes-McEwan et al., 2003; Moïse, 1999). Patent Ductus Arteriosus (PDA) with features either similar or identical to human disease occurs in Poodles (Kohn, 1995). Subvalvular aortic stenosis (SAS), defined as a congenital ridge or ring of fibrous tissue located below the aortic valve, is the second most common cardiovascular malformation in the dog. It is observed frequently in the Newfoundland, Golden Retriever, Rottweiler, German Shepherd, and other breeds (Buchanan, 1999). In dogs with SAS, the S-T segment, the flat, isoelectric section of the electrocardiogram (ECG) between the end of the S wave and the beginning of the T wave, appears to be depressed below the ECG baseline, presumably as a result of injury to the myocardium. The S-T segment depression (STD) is believed to be a clinically useful indicator of myocardial ischemia in both human patients with aortic stenosis and dogs with SAS. However, it is possible that the degree of myocardial ischemia that develops with SAS in the dog is less than that in the human patient because of the substantial cardiac collateral circulation observed in the dog (Davainis et al., 2004). Pulmonic stenosis (PS) in Beagles is phenotypically most similar to valvular PS in people (Andrews et al., 1979; Kohn, 1995). The pulmonary valve lesions of dogs affected with PS vary in severity and in various combinations. Lesions in some dogs are similar to what has been called pulmonary valve dysplasia in humans. Valvular PS, pulmonary valve dysplasia, and intermediate forms of these lesions can occur in members of the same litter of Beagles, indicating that these two types of pulmonary valve deformity are not separate etiologic or developmental entities in the Beagle (Patterson et al., 1981). A Tetralogy of Fallot model was developed in Keeshond dogs, and it closely resembles tetralogy of Fallot in man (Andrews et al., 1979; Kohn, 1995). Cardiac sudden death models exist within the German Shepherd, which mimics abnormal ventricular repolarization, and in the Boxer, which is similar to arrhythmogenic right ventricular dysplasia. Additional cardiac disease models include Sick Sinus Syndrome in Miniature Schnauzers, atrial standstill in English Springer Spaniels, and tricuspid valve dysplasia in Labrador Retrievers (Moïse, 1999).

Dogs also serve as models for hematologic disorders. Cyclic hematopoiesis (an intracellular protein trafficking defect) in the gray collie is a simple autosomal recessive trait with episodes of neutropenia that mimics the human disease and has been employed for the development of novel therapeutics with translational implications (Dysko et al., 2002; Yanay et al., 2006). There is a canine leukocyte adhesion deficiency (CLAD) (Parker et al., 2010) similar to leukocyte adhesion deficiency in humans in which dogs and children develop life-threatening bacterial infections due to mutations in the leukocyte integrin CD18 (Hunter et al., 2011). Dogs with CLAD are used as gene therapy models for this disorder (Hunter et al., 2011). Three spontaneously occurring coagulation factor deficiencies that occur in dogs—Hemophilia A (Factor VIII deficiency), Hemophilia B (Factor IX deficiency), and FVII deficiency—are similar to their human counterparts both phenotypically and in their response to therapeutic intervention (Knudsen et al., 2010). Thus, these canine bleeding disorders provide excellent models of some of the most prevalent inherited human coagulopathies and are good predictors of efficacy of treatment in human hemophilia (Knudsen et al., 2010; Nichols et al., 2009). Dogs affected with Hemophilia A and Hemophilia B are now used in gene therapy trials for the treatment of these disorders (Tsai et al., 2007; Nichols et al., 2009). Hemophiliac dogs are useful for studying recombinant FVIIa (rFVIIa) treatment of hemophilia (in patients with factor inhibitors) because the interaction of human rVIIa with canine tissue factor (TF) recapitulates that of the human proteins (Knudsen et al., 2010). Factor VII deficiency is described in the Alaskan Klee Kai, Alaskan Malamute, Beagle (research colony and companion dogs), among others (Kaae et al., 2007; Macpherson et al., 1999). The disease in Beagles is autosomal recessive, and although heterozygotes are asymptomatic carriers, dogs may have reduced clotting activity as demonstrated by thromboelastography (Fleischer et al., 2008; Callan et al., 2006). Canine Factor VII deficiency can be mild in presentation, or even asymptomatic, but can significantly impact research, as reduced FVII activity can alter hemostatic or cardiovascular endpoints (Callan et al., 2006). Thus, researchers using Beagles for studies that could be influenced by FVII deficiency should be aware of this defect and screen for both homo- and heterozygotes as needed. Von Willebrand's Disease (VWD) is the most prevalent inherited bleeding disorder in both dogs and humans, and dogs with VWD provide an excellent model for novel VWD therapeutics (Nichols et al., 2009; Kohn, 1995).

In musculoskeletal research, one of the well-developed canine models is that of Duchenne Muscular Dystrophy. Although this devastating muscle wasting disorder currently has no treatment, canine models are indispensable for studying disease pathogenesis and the development of therapies (Nakamura and Takeda, 2011). While numerous dog breeds with naturally occurring dystrophin-deficient muscular dystrophy have been characterized clinically, Golden retriever muscular dystrophy (GRMD) has been the most extensively examined and studied at the molecular level (Baltzer et al., 2007; Nakamura and Takeda, 2011). Duchenne Muscular Dystrophy in Golden Retrievers is caused by a mutation in the dystrophin gene resulting in the deficiency of dystrophin, a cytoskeletal protein that connects the muscle contractile machinery to the cell membrane (Dysko et al., 2002; Tsai et al., 2007; Sharp et al., 1992; Allen and Whitehead, 2011). The phenotype of GRMD closely mirrors that of human DMD with its severe skeletal and cardiac defects (Nakamura and Takeda, 2011). Gene therapy, exon-skipping therapy, and mesoangioblast stem cell treatments for DMD are being studied in GRMD with some preliminary success (Nakamura and Takeda, 2011; Sampaolesi et al., 2006).

Similar storage diseases affect dogs and humans. The autosomal recessive copper storage disease of Bedlington Terriers is presently the best characterized copper storage disease. The Bedlington defect in biliary copper excretion leads to hepatic copper accumulation and chronic progressive hepatitis and cirrhosis (Vonk et al., 2008). The clinical phenotype of copper storage disease in Bedlingtons is similar to Wilson disease in people, although neurologic defects observed in people are absent in the dogs (Vonk et al., 2008). The genetic mutation is different in people and dogs, with a deletion in the *COMMD1* gene affecting Bedlingtons and mutations in the *ATP7B* gene causing Wilson disease (Vonk et al., 2008). Both mutations, however, result in impaired intracellular copper transport (Vonk et al., 2008). Dogs have several lysosomal storage diseases, including Mucopolysaccharidosis (MPS) I & VII, glycogen storage Ia (glucose-6-phosphatase), globoid cell leukodystrophy (galactocerebrosidase), and G_{M1} gangliosidosis (β-D-galactosidase) (Ellinwood et al., 2004). Glycogen storage disease Ia in the Maltese dog due to defective glucose-6-phosphatase activity is similar clinically, biochemically, and pathologically to the human disease. The canine model of lysosomal storage diseases is routinely used in retroviral and adenoviral vector gene therapy experiments. Dogs are also a model of cognitive aging (the role of mitochondria in oxidative stress and dementia) and Alzheimer's disease and are used to investigate novel cognitive-enhancing therapeutics for both age-associated memory disorder and dementia (Ikeda-Douglas et al., 2005; Studzinski et al., 2005).

Canine atopic dermatitis (AD) is remarkably similar to human AD and provides a tool for unraveling the pathogenesis of the human disease and investigating therapeutics (Marsella and Girolomoni, 2009). The dog is also an important animal model for periodontal disease because canine gingiva reacts similarly to human gingiva in response to dental plaque accumulation. The Beagle is the primary breed used in periodontal studies (Andrews et al., 1979).

There are several canine ophthalmic disease models, such as progressive retinal atrophy and collie eye anomaly (Parker et al., 2010). Glaucoma is inherited as a simple autosomal recessive trait in the Beagle (Andrews et al., 1979). Dogs are a model for cataracts, in part because the lens/globe ratio is closest to that in humans among the common lab animals, other than nonhuman primates (Andrews et al., 1979). Retinitis pigmentosa (RP, or progressive retinal degeneration) in humans is phenotypically and molecularly similar to progressive retinal atrophy (PRA) in dogs (Tsai et al., 2007). Identification of the causative genetic mutation of progressive rod-cone degeneration (PRCD), a late-onset, autosomal recessive form of PRA in dogs (a mutation in the *PRCD* gene) led to the discovery of the same mutation in a woman with RP whose genetic defect had been previously unknown (Tsai et al., 2007; Zangerl et al., 2006). Another canine hereditary retinal degeneration, the RPE65-/- dog, suffers from early severe visual impairment that models the childhood blindness of Leber congenital amaurosis (LCA) (Acland et al., 2001). Gene therapy with adeno-associated virus carrying wild-type RPE65 restored vision to an affected dog and paved the way for successful gene therapy in humans with LCA (Tsai et al., 2007; Acland et al., 2001; Ashtari et al., 2011). The renal diseases for which the dog serves as an animal model include ectopic ureter urolithiasis, nephrogenic diabetes insipidus (NDI), and hereditary renal diseases including hereditary nephritis in various breeds, renal dysplasia in Lhaso Apsos and Shih Tzus, and Fanconi Syndrome in Basenjis (Andrews et al., 1979). Hereditary nephritis (HN) affects several dog breeds including Samoyeds (X-linked dominant), English Cocker Spaniel (autosomal recessive), mixed breed dogs (X-linked dominant), Bull Terriers, and Dalmatians (autosomal dominant) (Vaden, 2010). Canine HN, a defect in the basement membrane collagen type IV, serves as a model for human Alport syndrome (Vaden, 2010). HN in people and dogs is similar, except that the auditory and ophthalmologic abnormalities described in humans are uncommon in affected dogs (Tsai et al., 2007; Vaden, 2010). Currently, the only treatment for Alport syndrome is dialysis or renal transplant. However, the results of the preliminary studies of gene therapy that replaces the defective collagen gene in Samoyeds with HN are promising (Tsai et al., 2007; Harvey et al., 2003).

Many naturally occurring cancers in dogs share features with human cancers including histological appearance, tumor genetics, and biological behavior (Paoloni and Khana, 2008). Studying canine cancer can both identify genetic defects and environmental risk factors (in pet dogs) for similar human neoplasias (Paoloni and Khana, 2008). Furthermore, dogs provide a mechanism for evaluating novel cancer therapeutics, especially because survival studies in dogs can be much shorter in dogs than in people (Paoloni and Khana, 2008; Rowell et al., 2011). Some of the canine models for cancer include melanoma, gastric carcinoma, hemangiosarcoma, lymphoma, malignant histiocytosis (Shearin and Ostrander, 2010), and osteosarcoma (OSA; Rowell et al., 2011). Cytogenic aberrations are similar in dogs and people with non-Hodgkin lymphoma, and both have similar response profiles to different chemotherapeutic agents (Breen and Modiano, 2008; Paoloni and Khana, 2008). OSA in dogs recapitulates the human form of the cancer in terms of biologic behavior—such as propensity for pulmonary metastasis—and genetics, including frequent genome alterations affecting the oncogenes MYC and KIT in both species (Rowell et al., 2011). OSA, which is 20 times more prevalent in dogs than humans, makes canine OSA an incredibly useful tool for studying cellular pathways of disease and investigating therapeutics (Rowell et al., 2011). The Scottish terrier has a 20-fold increased risk of developing transitional cell carcinoma, which makes this breed a good genetic and therapeutic model for human invasive urinary bladder cancer (Shearin and Ostrander, 2010; Mohammed et al., 2003).

Genetics is an area in which there is growing interest in using dogs as animal models. There are about 450 known hereditary diseases in dogs, with over half being clinically similar to corresponding human diseases (Tsai et al., 2007). The complete canine genome sequence is now available. The genetic analysis tools now available in canine research include dense linkage and radiation hybrid maps, oligo-based microarrays, and single nucleotide polymorphism (SNP) arrays (Tsai et al., 2007). Many cancer loci have been identified in dogs and, in general, humans are genetically more homologous with dogs than with mice (Shearin and Ostrander, 2010). Hematopoietic Stem Cell (HSC) gene therapy is expanding in dogs because they offer a few advantages over nonhuman primate models: larger litters, easier to handle, and easier collection of bone marrow biopsies (Trobridge and Kiem, 2010). In addition, unlike in the mouse, canine $CD34^+$ bone marrow cells are similar to human *in vitro* and *in vivo* canine models of hematopoietic diseases, and leukocyte antigen-matched transplants are available (Trobridge and Kiem, 2010). As so many diseases are associated with particular breeds, the advances in genetic testing for breed genetic contribution is important. There is an SNP database searchable by chromosome and breed available online for dogs through the Broad Institute at MIT and the Inherited Diseases in Dogs (IDID) web site lists diseases of dog breeds that are likely either completely or partially transmitted genetically (Fleischer et al., 2008). In addition, the Canine Inherited Disorders Database (CIDD) is searchable by organ system and by breed (Fleischer et al., 2008). Genetic testing is commercially available that can identify the breed of origin with 99% certainty (Fleischer et al., 2008).

4.2 UNIQUE PHYSIOLOGICAL CHARACTERISTICS OF DOG

The physiology of the dog is similar in most aspects to other animals used in research. Some physiologic features that are unique to the dog or unlike other research animals are highlighted in this section. Dogs are often used in pharmacologic studies. The overall dimensions of the canine gastrointestinal tract (GIT) are sufficiently similar to the human GIT to allow the dog to be used as a preclinical model for oral drugs that are intended for subsequent testing in humans (Dressman, 1986). The stomach of the dog has three types of glandular mucosa: cardiac mucosa (narrow zone around cardia), fundic glands (about 2/3 of mucosa of stomach), and pyloric mucosa (lining aboral portion). The size of each region is proportional to that of the human stomach in contrast to the pig (in which cardiac portion is large) or the rat (in which stratified nonglandular portion is large) (Kohn, 1995). However, several features of canine GI anatomy affect drug absorption and metabolism in dogs, and it must be considered when extrapolating canine bioavailability studies to humans. The pylorus of the stomach serves as a sieve, restricting the passage of materials on the basis of size so that only digestible-sized material enters the small intestine, the major site of absorption (Martinez and Papich, 2009). The canine stomach has a smaller pyloric sieve (>2–3 mm) than the human stomach (>7 mm), meaning that larger nondisintegrating dosage forms will stay in the canine stomach longer than the human stomach (Sagawa and Sutton 2006; Martinez and Papich, 2009). In dogs, the impact of food effects on oral drug bioavailability is dramatic, in that meals may result in delayed gastric emptying (Martinez and Papich, 2009). This effect is much more pronounced than that observed in humans (Martinez and Papich, 2009). In several drug studies, administering drugs to fed dogs compared to fasted dogs caused a delay in tablet emptying from the stomach, leading to delayed drug absorption and altered pharmacokinetics (Martinez and Papich, 2009). A much smaller food effect was observed in parallel studies in humans (Martinez and Papich, 2009). The small intestine of the dog is shorter than the human, which may result in lower absorptive capacity, although the fact that intestinal permeability is greater in the dog than the human helps compensate for the shorter small intestine (Sagawa and Sutton 2006). The body size variation among breeds results in differences in pyloric sieving (larger dogs have larger sieves) and potentially intestinal permeability, which in turn result in breed variability in pharmacokinetic studies (Fleischer et al., 2008; Martinez and Papich, 2009; Randell et al., 2001). Sighthounds have lower volume of distribution of lipophilic compounds (like propofol), a result of their lower percentage body fat as compared with other breeds (Fleischer et al., 2008). The canine heart has extramural coronary blood vessels that differ from humans by having an increased frequency of interarterial anastomoses (Kohn, 1995). The main blood supply to the sinus node is from the right coronary artery, with a large supply of anastomoses, making experimental-induced ischemia via ligation difficult (Kohn, 1995).

There are over 12 canine blood groups, and dogs can currently be classified as positive or negative for the following blood types: dog erythrocyte antigen (DEA) 1.1, 1.2, 3, 4, 5, 7, 8, and Dal (Kohn, 1995; Hohenhaus, 2004; Blais et al., 2007; Kessler et al., 2010). Although dogs that have never been transfused do have naturally occurring alloantibodies against some blood group antigens, unlike in other species these antibodies appear to have limited clinical significance (Hohenhaus, 2004). Furthermore, unlike humans, pregnancy has not been shown to induce alloantibodies in bitches (Blais et al., 2009).The most immunogenic of the DEA is 1.1 and transfusion of DEA 1.1 positive erythrocytes into a previously sensitized DEA 1.1 negative recipient can result in a severe hemolytic transfusion reaction (Hohenhaus, 2004). A canine universal donor is often defined as a dog negative for DEA 1.1, 1.2, 3, 5, and 7, and positive for DEA 4. Given that this definition is somewhat restrictive, ideally a donor dog should at least be DEA 1.1 negative (Hohenhaus, 2004).

In contrast to human, rat, or nonhuman primate erythrocytes, canine erythrocytes have high sodium to potassium ratio, meaning that hemolysis does not affect potassium levels as much as in other species (Evans, 2009). The major anaphylactic shock organ in the dog is the liver, instead of the lung, which is the shock organ in other animals and humans. The first signs of anaphylaxis in the dog are GI such as diarrhea and vomiting, due to hepatic vein congestion and portal hypertension (Waddell, 2010). GI signs may then progress to respiratory distress, and collapse secondary to hypovolemic shock (Waddell, 2010). Dogs with anaphylaxis may also demonstrate generalized wheals, angioedema, and pruritis. In severe cases, angioedema of the larynx and pharynx can result in respiratory distress secondary to upper airway obstruction (Waddell, 2010). Dogs have some unique features that can affect their response in toxicity studies. Dogs lack N-acetyltransferase, which detoxifies sulfonamides and predisposes them to sulfonamide hypersensitivity (Fleischer et al., 2008). Different breeds have different levels of thiopurine S-methyltransferase (TMPT) activity, an enzyme that plays an important role in metabolism of thiopurine drugs. Dogs with lower TMPT activity are predisposed to azothioprine toxicity. There are breed differences in inhibition of platelet aggregation in response to arachidonic acid, which must be considered when using the dog for coagulation or cardiovascular studies (Fleischer et al., 2008). Different cytochrome P450 (CYP) oxidative enzyme variations exist among breeds of dogs, so breed variation should be considered when studying pharmacokinetics of drugs that are metabolized by P450 (Fleischer et al., 2008). The Collie MDR-1 mutation results in increased toxicity after administration of compounds with *p*-glycoprotein substrates (for example, ivermectin) (Fleischer et al., 2008). The predisposition to sulfonamide polyarthopathy in large breeds may be the result of a limited capacity to detoxify hydroxylamine metabolites of sulfonamides (Fleischer et al., 2008).

The dog has some unique reproductive features. Unlike many other species, the dog is nonseasonal and monoestrous, ovulating only once or twice a year at a 5–12 month interval (Songsasen and Wildt, 2007). Estrous cycle intervals increase with age from 7.5 months to 12–15 months near the end of life (Cunningham, 1997). Canine proestrus does not begin within 48 hours of the end of luteal phase, the proestrual bitch is under the influence of estrogen and this is the dominant hormone during this stage of the cycle. Estrogen is responsible for most of the clinical signs observed in bitches during proestrus, because this hormone stimulates growth and activity of the glandular epithelium of the uterus and promotes swelling and increased vascularity of the lining of the uterus (mucosa). Serum progesterone concentrations during proestrus are at basal levels (<0.5 ng/mL) and then start a gradual rise at the end of proestrus. Preovulatory follicular luteinization (transformation of the estrogen secreting follicle to a progesterone secreting structure), unique to the canine, is responsible for this increase in progesterone concentration (Wildt et al., 1979). The long lifespan of semen means fertilization can occur in the oviduct as late as eight days after coitus, but oocytes are usually viable only 12–24 hours once ovulated (Dysko et al., 2002).

Dogs also have some endocrine idiosyncracies. In dogs, only approximately 15% of the triiodothyronine (T_3) and thyroxine (T_4) is reabsorbed from the intestinal tract (vs. 79%–100% in primates) so dogs have a higher thyroxine production rate and replacement requirement (Engelking, 2002). Thyroxine (T_4) values in several animals, including the dog, are lower than in humans (Evans, 2009) because their thyroid transport proteins have a comparatively lower affinity for T_4 (Loeb, 1999). Dogs with diabetes mellitus in the majority of cases are hypoinsulinemic with mild to severe ketosis and are similar to humans with type 1 diabetes (Engelking, 2002). In a minority of cases, diabetic dogs are hyperinsulinemic, have elevated growth hormone, and are similar to humans with type 2 diabetes (Engelking, 2002).

Isoenzymes of alkaline phosphatase (ALP) from intestine and kidney have a short half-life and do not contribute substantially to total ALP in serum (Loeb, 1999). Serum ALP is increased in the dog by biliary stasis, elevated glucocorticoids (GCs; exogenous or endogenous), or osteoblastic hyperactivity, each of which induces a specific isoenzyme (Loeb, 1999). The ability of glucocorticoids to induce ALP activity, termed "steroid-induced ALP," is a unique canine feature (Evans, 2009). Via the biliary or GC mechanism, serum activity of ALP may be increased by 10–60 times that of the upper reference value, in contrast to less-pronounced increases due to osteoblastic hyperactivity (Loeb, 1999).

In dogs, stress will only cause a mild increase in glucose, compared to the dramatic increases it can induce in cats and nonhuman primates (Loeb, 1999). The estrus cycle in the bitch does not cause a change in baseline blood glucose or insulin values, but the cycle does impair glucose tolerance during estrus (Loeb, 1999). Cortisol is the major glucocorticoid in dogs, as in humans and nonhuman primates (vs. corticosterone in rodents) (Evans, 2009). C-reactive protein is the primary acute phase protein in the dog (also in nonhuman primates and humans) (Evans, 2009).

Canines can excrete bilirubin easily via the kidney (Loeb, 1999). Accordingly, conjugated bilirubin may be found in the urine before bilirubinemia is detected (Evans, 2009). Increases of serum urea nitrogen occur rather readily in canines. Decreased urine osmolality and specific gravity are more highly sensitive determinants of renal capacity than blood urea nitrogen (BUN) or creatinine (Loeb, 1999). Other (nonrenal) factors can increase BUN or creatinine. There can be increases in plasma urea and creatinine postprandially, which vary with diet (Evans, 2009). Plasma creatinine measurement can be falsely elevated by up to 45% by endogenous noncreatinine chromogens (such as bilirubin and ketones) (Evans, 2009). There are four isoenzymes of amylase identified in the dog. Isoenzyme 3 is of pancreatic origin (>50%), whereas isoenzyme 4 is found in all tissues. Pancreatic serum amylase is removed by a mechanism other than a renal one, or it is inactivated by the kidney, such that the high serum amylase is not followed by the high amylase levels in urine, in contrast to what occurs in humans (Loeb, 1999). Dexamethasone can have greater effect in the altering levels of serum lipase than that of serum amylase (Evans, 2009). There are sex differences in the values of *N*-acetyl-β-glucosaminidase, in that males have higher values (which are also true in rats) (Evans, 2009).

Total cholesterol and triglycerides do not vary across breeds, but high-density lipoprotein (HDL) and low-density lipoprotein (LDL) levels are breed-dependent (Fleischer et al., 2008) and primary hyperlipoproteinemias have been reported in several breeds of dogs including the Beagle (Elliott and Schenck, 2010). Serum cholesterol in the dog is primarily HDL cholesterol, in contrast to humans (Evans, 2009). Intact female dogs have higher HDL cholesterol than do intact male dogs (Johnson, 2005; Loeb, 1999). Cholesterol ester transfer protein (CETP) activity is low in the dog (Evans, 2009). This means that dogs are unable to perform cholesterol shuttling and therefore do not form cholesterol ester-rich LDL. In humans, cholesterol-ester rich LDL can be removed from circulation by macrophages lining arteries. Ingestion of oxidized LDL and the foam cell formation of macrophages are the hallmark of atherosclerosis development. As dogs lack CETP activity, they are resistant to the development of atherosclerosis, and are therefore a poor model for human cholesterol disorders (Johnson, 2005). Furthermore, the canine lack of CEPT leads to the formation of a unique HDL molecule that is cholesterol-ester rich called HDL_1. This HDL isoform is absent in humans (Johnson, 2005). The cholesterol-ester rich HDL can be removed from the circulation by endocytosis in the liver (Johnson, 2005).

4.3 METHODOLOGY FOR SAMPLE COLLECTION

4.3.1 Blood Collection (for Serum or Plasma)

Inconsistent data can result from factors such as variability in sample collection and handling methods (McGuill and Rowan, 1989), the stress levels of the dogs, or the signalment of the dogs used. To minimize these variables, it is important that dogs should be properly acclimated to their environment and to restraint during routine procedures. Environmental enrichment programs should be in place and a reward-based training program can be used to encourage dogs to readily accept common procedures such as blood draws; therefore, anesthesia or sedation is rarely necessary for minor procedures. For the safety of both the animals and the handlers, it is important that dogs with good dispositions be selected. Handlers must also demonstrate patience and should be skilled at both handling and sample collection techniques.

The preferred collection sites in the dog are the jugular, cephalic, and lateral saphenous veins (Morton et al., 1993). Large volume samples are best drawn from the jugular vein, as its thicker wall is less likely to collapse under the pressure asserted by a large syringe. Smaller samples (<5 cc) can be easily drawn from the cephalic or saphenous veins, but care must be taken to use a small amount of pressure. This can be accomplished by asserting a slow, steady pull on the syringe plunger and by utilizing only small 1, 3, or 5 cc syringes. Blood withdrawn from the saphenous vein provides the benefit of allowing the collector to be positioned away from the dog's mouth and face; however, this vein will typically "roll" more than the cephalic. It is important to prepare all necessary sample collection items and have them readily accessible prior to bringing the dog to the procedure area. Select a needle and syringe size appropriate for the size of the dog and the quantity of blood to be collected. An 18–20-G, 1 inch needle will yield the best results and can be used in larger dogs; however, a 22-G needle may be necessary for smaller dogs but can result in hemolysis (Weiser, 2004). The area surrounding the venipuncture site can be clipped to better visualize the vessel and allow for more thorough cleaning of the region.

It is very important to the safety of both the dogs and staff that dogs be firmly yet gently restrained during the procedures. When dogs are placed on an elevated structure such as a table, a handler should have a hand on the dog at all times. To obtain blood from the right jugular vein, with the dog either sitting or in sternal recumbency, the holder stands on the left side of the dog and cradles his or her right arm over and around the thorax of the dog with his or her fingertips at the point of the right shoulder. The left hand of the holder cradles the chin of the dog while gently directing the nose up and slightly to the left. The phlebotomist occludes the vessel with the nondominant thumb by applying gentle pressure to the ventral region of the jugular furrow to the right of the trachea (Taylor, 2010). This will cause the vessel to become distended with blood and stand out from the surrounding tissues. The holder can be asked to redirect the head of the dog to allow better visualization and distention of the vein. However, in some heavier dogs, the vein may not become visually apparent and hence must be palpated. Once the vein is identified, 70% alcohol is applied to the area. The needle is directed through the skin and then into the vessel with the needle bevel facing the phlebotomist and the syringe held at approximately 20–30° from the neck of the dog. Care must be taken to neither puncture through the other side of the vessel nor pierce surrounding structures such as the recurrent laryngeal nerve or the trachea. Once blood is visualized in the hub of the needle, a gentle force can be applied to fill the syringe. Too much pressure may result in the collapse of the vein and hemolysis of the sample. Once the syringe has been filled, the pressure is released, both by releasing the syringe plunger and by removing the finger from occluding the vessel. The needle is removed and digital pressure is maintained over the venipuncture site for approximately 60 seconds to minimize the hematoma formation.

The reverse can be done to collect from the left jugular vein. Vacutainer-type needles, which seat directly into the vacutainer tubes, can also be used as an alternative to a syringe.

Collection from the cephalic vein can be accomplished similarly with the holder restraining the head of the dog from behind with the upper arm and the trunk region against the back of the dog for preventing backward movement. The other hand holds off the vessel by placing the proximal medial portion of the thumb over the vessel, and rolling the vessel laterally and proximally to straighten the vessel. Downward pressure is then applied to occlude the vessel. The phlebotomist holds the carpus and/or metacarpus in the palm of the nondominant hand with the thumb placed lateral to the vein to stabilize while blood is collected as previously described.

To restrain a dog for phlebotomy of the lateral saphenous vein, the dog is placed in lateral recumbency. The forearm of the arm nearest the head gently keeps the head of the dog from rising and the hands are used to secure the forelimbs. The other arm applies gentle pressure on the upside of the lateral hip while the hand rolls the vessel while stabilizing the upside leg from which the blood will be drawn.

When drawing blood from peripheral veins such as the cephalic and saphenous, the needle may mistakenly be placed completely through the vessel resulting in what is termed a "blown" vein. For this reason, the attempts for collection should begin distally with further attempts being moved proximally. Repeat attempts should be very limited. If damage has occurred to the vessel, a small pressure bandage is placed on the site for a short period of time to minimize hematoma formation.

If multiple blood draws will be necessary over a short period of time, cannulation can be considered. Indwelling long catheters provide the advantage of providing a repeated sampling port without necessitating repeated venipuncture. However, their initial placement requires sedation or anesthesia, depending on the temperament of the dog. A long catheter (18–20 gauge) can be placed in a central vein (jugular or lateral saphenous fed to the femoral vein). The area where the catheter is to be placed is shaved and sterilely prepared. The authors often use a local subcutaneous lidocaine injection to numb the area of catheter placement. A stab incision is made with a blade, and the catheter is then placed in the vein. This catheter is sutured in place and wrapped, with wooden splints (popsicle sticks) on either side of the leg to help stabilize the bandage. Dogs usually tolerate these catheters well, although placing an Elizabethan collar is recommended as a precaution. When sampling blood, it is recommended that a "dump" sample the volume of the catheter (usually 3–6 mL) be taken in a syringe prior to obtaining your sample. The "dump" sample can be collected in a heparinized syringe so that it can be returned to the dog after the sample is taken. The catheter should be flushed with saline after each sample is taken, and flushed every 6 hours to retain patency. An indwelling long catheter can be kept in place for up to 3 days.

Sample volume limitations are typically set by each research institution's animal care and use committee. Many such standards are based upon the 1993 recommendation of the Joint Working Group on Refinement that a single collection is limited to a quantity equal or less than 10% of the animal's circulating blood volume, which can then be repeated in 3–4 weeks (Morton et al., 1993). The circulating blood volume of a mature, healthy dog ranges from 79 to 90 mL/kg (Morton et al., 1993) but can be lower in obese dogs and may vary according to the breed. Other institutions have set the recommendation of 1% of total body weight every 3 weeks (McGuill and Rowan, 1989). The physiologic responses to the blood loss can be offset by the administration of intravenous (IV) fluids to compensate for the volume lost. Advances in technology have led to the ability to analyze smaller quantities than were previously necessary. Whittemore and Flatland compared the chemistry and CBC blood values obtained from healthy dogs using both standard and microsample blood collection tubes and found no statistically significant difference between the two (Whittemore and Flatland, 2010).

An arterial sample can be collected from either the femoral or the dorsal pedal arteries. The sample can be collected with a 22- or 25-gauge needle attached to a heparinized 3 cc syringe or an arterial blood gas syringe containing a lyophilized heparin tablet (Taylor, 2010). Firm pressure should be placed over the collection site for at least three minutes to mitigate hematoma formation (Taylor, 2010).

4.3.2 Urine Collection

Urine samples are also commonly collected to evaluate parameters such as renal clearance of a compound, glomerular filtration rate (GFR), or the health status of the urinary tract. This can be accomplished via free-catch, catheterization, or cystocentesis. Although a free catch sample is not suitable for culture, it should be obtained mid-stream as the initial void may contain a higher number of contaminants from the vulvar and preputial skin, which can interfere with protein values and sediment analysis (Reine and Langston, 2005). Free-catch samples are relatively easy to obtain in housebroken dogs, but timing can be more challenging in a kennel setting.

Urinary catheterization of the dog is achieved by threading an appropriately sized sterile red rubber catheter along the urethra. While some male dogs may allow the procedure without sedation, some males and most females will require sedation. The male dog is positioned in lateral recumbency and the penis extruded from the prepuce, and the tip gently wiped with dilute chlorhexidine solution (Reine and Langston, 2005). The catheter tip is dipped in a sterile lubricant, carefully and gently inserted into the external urethral orifice, and then advanced just into the bladder. The wrapped catheter can be held against the dog prior to unwrapping for estimating the point on the catheter that will be visible once the tip has entered the bladder. The first 5–6 mL should be discarded for analyzing the remaining sample (Taylor, 2010).

The female dog is typically sedated and placed sternally with the hindlimbs hanging off the back end of the procedure table with the pelvis elevated by sandbags placed under the inguinal region. The external genitalia is cleansed with dilute chlorhexidine scrub and a sterilized speculum is placed to allow visualization of the tubercle residing on the ventral floor of the vaginal vault. The urethral orifice lies centrally on the dorsal aspect of this tubercle. The catheter tip is lubricated with a sterile lubricant and gently directed under the index finger of a sterile gloved hand into the orifice into the bladder lumen. Once the bladder has been reached, urine should stream from the free end of the catheter. As with the male, the first few milliliters of urine should be discarded (Reine and Langston, 2005). In both cases, the free end of the catheter should be clamped off with a hemostat prior to withdrawal from the urethra. With experience and knowledge of the structures, catheters may be placed using a blind digital approach.

Should there be a need for continuous sampling or quantitation of output, an indwelling catheter can be secured in place. The strong disadvantage to the use of this method, however, is the high risk for ascending infection. Two recent studies have reported that the respective overall rates of nosocomial bacteriuria in a small animal hospital setting are 10.3% and 9.8% (Smarick et al., 2004; Sullivan et al., 2010). The risk of infection can best be mitigated by establishing protocols to ensure strict sterile technique at the point of insertion, proper care of the catheter system while in use, and the selection of a catheter made of a material resistant to the growth of a biofilm layer. A foley catheter impregnated with antimicrobials is a good selection, as the balloon anchors the catheter into the bladder and the material may decrease the risk of ascending infection. The foley catheter is inserted as described previously such that the balloon is inside the bladder. The location of the catheter can be checked via an abdominal radiograph if necessary. The balloon is then filled with the amount of sterile water or saline indicated on the package insert, and the catheter is gently pulled caudally to settle the balloon into the trigone of the bladder. The sterile attachment of a collection bag to the catheter constitutes a "closed collection system."

Standardized collection bags offer the advantage of an antireflux chamber and ports to allow removal of urine from the system without opening the system (Bard Medical, Gainesville, VA). Alternatively, some small animal hospitals adapt used fluid bags (which have never contained dextrose) as reservoirs. The disadvantage of using this system is the need to open the system for urine drainage and the lack of the antireflux chamber; yet in one study, no difference was observed in the rate of nosocomial infections among dogs in which either system was used (Sullivan et al., 2010).

With either system, the bag should be placed at a level lower than the bladder to ensure outward flow. To facilitate this, an optional IV drip set can be added to extend the length of the system. The catheter can be secured to the prepuce or the perivaginal skin by the placement of two sutures through a tape "butterfly," created by sticking an approximately 6–8 cm section of tape across the catheter near the skin region to be sutured. Then, pressing the sticky sides of the tape together such that the catheter is secured in the middle with a "wing" on either side. The proximal tubing can also be taped to the hindlimb for added security.

Indwelling catheters should remain in the dog for the shortest amount of time necessary to complete the study as the incidence of infection increases with time. Proper catheter maintenance entails frequently checking patency of lines and security of connection points as well as cleansing of the lines and vaginal or preputial orifices with a dilute chlorhexidine solution. Sterile technique, including the use of sterile gloves, should always be followed any time the catheter is handled.

Urinary samples can be collected via cystocentesis when a sterile sample is necessary for culture. However, the use of this collection method introduces the risk of damaging the bladder wall or worse yet, puncturing an abdominal structure other than the bladder itself. The use of an ultrasound to guide collection may decrease the risk of damage and facilitate recognition of the bladder. Regardless, it is absolutely imperative that the dog is still while the needle is within the abdomen. With the dog in lateral recumbency, the bladder is palpated and held in the nondominant hand. Excessive pressure on the bladder either during or immediately following collection can cause urine leakage into the abdomen, and therefore it should be avoided. Alcohol is applied to the skin overlying the bladder and a 22-g 1½ inch needle attached to a 6 cc syringe placed through the lateral abdominal wall and into the bladder. The needle is directed slightly caudally so the needle is maintained in the lumen of the bladder as the bladder wall retracts (Reine and Langston, 2005). Care is taken to avoid piercing the finger of the nondominant hand. The syringe plunger is only pulled back once the needle tip is in the bladder lumen to avoid aspirating tissue into the sample. If the bladder is not hit, redirection of the needle intra-abdominally is contraindicated as this can cause damage to surrounding structures. Instead, a second attempt should be made using a clean needle. Keep in mind that if the bladder is relatively empty, a cystocentesis may not be possible until the bladder fills sufficiently. Pressure against the plunger should also be released prior to removal of the needle from the bladder once the sample has been collected.

Alternatively, a ventral approach to the bladder may be easier in overweight dogs or others in which the bladder is difficult to palpate. As in the lateral approach, the dog is held very still, but in dorsal recumbency. The bladder is not palpated, but rather a blind stick is utilized in this approach, subsequently increasing the potential risk of damage to other organs. On the female, the needle is inserted along the midline of the caudal abdomen about midway between the umbilicus and the brim of the pelvis. This site typically corresponds to the lowest point of the abdomen in dorsal recumbency; thus, the optimal site (on the female, but not the male) can often be identified by dousing the caudal abdomen with a 70% alcohol solution and identifying the area the solution settles into as the lowest point. The needle is inserted perpendicular to the skin at the point where the liquid pools. On male dogs, the collection site is accessed by gently retracting the prepuce and penis or by approaching lateral to the penis.

4.4 PREANALYTICAL SOURCES OF VARIATION

4.4.1 Animal Source and Selection

The number of dogs used in research has been on a downward trend over the last 20 years. The United States and Japan are the main world users of dogs in research and testing (ILAR, 1994). The United States Department of Agriculture (USDA) collects annual statistics on the use of some laboratory animals (Prescott et al., 2004). Dogs used in research are generally segregated into two classes: purpose-bred (Class A) and random source (Class B). Facilities can purchase dogs through USDA designated Class A or B licensed dealers, respectively. Class A dealers breed and raise dogs on their own premises in closed or stable colonies and are the major source of dogs used in biomedical research in the United States. Class B dealers are involved in the purchase of dogs from other individuals (including animals from municipal pounds) and subsequent resale of animals to research facilities (USDA, 1985).

Dogs from Class A dealers have known genetic backgrounds and medical histories (e.g., vaccination status, exposure to infectious diseases) and usually have received veterinary care throughout their stay at the facility. Random-source dogs are obtained from any source that did not breed and raise the animals on their premises. These dogs will have unknown or incomplete medical histories. Once random-source dogs have been quarantined, vaccinated, and determined free of parasites and any other medical or biological anomaly, they are considered "conditioned."

To minimize animal variability, animal resource programs should provide normal, healthy, well-adapted animals that represent a physiological model characterized by a narrow range of physical, behavioral, and clinical parameters. Dogs that are purpose-bred should arrive at the facility adequately vaccinated and from disease-free colonies compatible with the current animal program health status or be segregated upon arrival. It is helpful to obtain the animals from the same dealer to take advantage of group immunities (Meunier, 2006). In general, closed colonies are easier to manage and help ensure a disease-free population. Newly introduced dogs and staff with dogs at home pose a potential risk to the animal colony. The use of dedicated work clothing and segregating animal groups from the same vendor source together maintains a disease-free health status. In some cases, the diseases can be subclinical but this can still affect research results in terms of blood values, immune suppression, healing times, and so on (NRC, 1994).

Most dogs used in research and testing are Beagles, although other breeds (e.g., canine familial disorders, mongrel foxhounds) are purpose-bred for use in research (Meunier, 2006). The Beagle was originally chosen for use in the laboratory owing to its placid temperament, and it can easily be housed in kennels. In addition, its relatively small size and ease of access to the cephalic vein for blood sampling allows for dosing and measuring body responses with relative ease (ILAR, 1994).

4.4.2 Sex

The importance of classifying clinical chemistry data groups by sex is generally accepted and has been justified for certain parameters by statistical testing (Maxwell and Delaney, 1985). Significant differences between males and females exist in many chemistry values depending on the breed size and hormone levels but lack clinical relevance in most cases (Kley et al., 2003). The differences between males and females become less obvious with age (Kaspar and Norris, 1977). For example, with increasing age in the Beagle, serum cholesterol levels are initially higher in females, but increase faster in males over time, so that after a 10-year span the values are at similar levels.

4.4.3 Age

In neonates and geriatric animals, the ranges for many tests tend to show greater variation compared to late juveniles and mature adults (Evans, 2009). Plasma alkaline phosphatase (ALP) is probably the best-known example of an age-dependent parameter. The presence of higher calcium and phosphorus concentrations in young dogs attributed to skeletal growth and increased osseous activity is attributed to high skeletal ALP isoenzyme in young growing animals (Sanecki et al., 1993). Creatine kinase activity is higher in young dogs and decreases when the animals reach adulthood (Kaspar and Norris, 1977; Kraft et al., 1995; Keller and Wall, 1982). Plasma total protein, albumin (Alb), total bilirubin, creatinine, urea, alanine aminotransferase (ALT), gamma-glutamyl transferase (GGT), and iron all tend to increase with age, reflecting changes in muscle mass and immune maturity and possibly a decrease in the GFR. The age-associated increase for total bilirubin is also considered to be due to increasing hemoglobin concentrations (Kraft et al., 1995). Furthermore, increased immune stimulation results in an elevated globulin fraction, but also to an increasing albumin production, as a result of better liver function and intestinal absorption (Hall, 2006).

4.4.4 Breed

Bred and raised for laboratory use, the Beagle is the standard research dog in toxicology studies (Dysko et al., 2002). The breed is fairly uniform and tends to be free of breed-related diseases except for coagulation factor VII deficiency, which is often asymptomatic and can be detected by the one-stage prothrombin time test (PTT). Random source or pound dogs are generally unacceptable due to nonuniformity. However, breeds other than Beagles and purpose-bred mongrels are occasionally used for special purposes, such as when a larger body size than that of the Beagle is required. Significant breed effects have been found among many clinical chemistry parameters. Reference ranges for total protein, creatine, total bilirubin, potassium, calcium, amylase, ALP, GGT, and lipase varies among breeds. However, lower total protein concentrations for retrievers, lower total bilirubin concentrations for terriers, higher total bilirubin for mastiff-type dogs, and lower lipase activity for sled-type dog are the only clinical chemistries found to be significantly statistically different among breeds (Kley et al., 2003). Prestudy clinical pathology testing is useful for general health screening of dogs before studies commence.

4.4.5 Nutritional Status

Feeding regimens at facilities vary and should be dependent on study requirements. There are basically three methods of feeding dogs: free choice (ad libitum), time limited, or food limited (Meunier, 2006). Upon arrival to a new facility, a dog may not adapt readily to dietary and environmental changes. Therefore, close attention should be paid to be certain that an animal is eating adequately and maintaining its weight. Ideally, the facility should provide a diet that is the same as that of the kennel of origin. The diet can then be changed over several days to a new food if a diet change is necessary. Adult dogs can adapt to one meal per day feeding (Morris et al., 2005). In contrast to ad libitum feeding used for some other laboratory animal species, dogs should be meal fed an optimal amount of food to prevent obesity (Fillman-Holliday et al., 2002). Adult dogs that are consuming food voluntarily should be fed relative to their body condition and not necessarily by a formula (Morris and Rogers, 2000). Eating habits vary among dogs. For example, if provided free choice feeding, some dogs may demonstrate an eating pattern more like cats (e.g., eating several times between the light and the dark period) (Meunier, 2006). This may result in over-feeding or under-feeding dogs that are pair housed.

The diet composition can impact the clinical chemistry values of the dog. Dietary protein intake, urea production rates, and the renal and extrarenal urea excretion will impact blood urea nitrogen (BUN) levels. For example, over-feeding, feeding high protein diets, upper gastrointestinal bleeding, and disorders that increase endogenous protein catabolism can alter the amino acids absorbed in the gastrointestinal tract and contribute to an increase in BUN caused by increased hepatic ureagenesis. Animal manipulations prior to sequential blood sampling in toxicological studies should be similar with respect to food and water intake to minimize within-animal variations of plasma and urinary chemistry values. Fasting is characterized by low glucose concentrations, and accordingly, low levels of insulin and high glucagon. Daily level variations of serum lipids (nonesterified fatty acids (NEFA), triglycerides, phospholipids, total cholesterol, and total lipids) occur in healthy dogs, particularly in temporal relationship to lighting and fasting cycles. Bertolucci et al. found levels of serum NEFA patterns were significantly higher during fasting due to mobilization of adipose tissue NEFA mediated by the decrease in insulin with its lipolytic effects (Bertolucci et al., 2008). Blood glucose will increase, while triglycerides, urea nitrogen, calcium, inorganic phorshorus, and ALP have all been shown to decrease with fasting (Matsuzawa et al., 1993). In addition, Lawler et al. (2007) studied the effects of 25% diet restriction in dogs. The study showed that lifetime food restriction resulted in erythrocyte levels slightly higher among dogs fed ad libitum—a possible reflection of the need to support both higher body fat mass and lean mass that uses energy less efficiently. Among serum biochemistry variables, glucose and triglycerides were lower, while creatinine was slightly higher (in the absence of renal disease or failure) over the life spans of diet-restricted dogs (Lawler et al., 2007).

4.4.6 Housing Environment and Stress

Extreme and continuous stress can significantly affect experimental outcomes due to neuroendocrine effects (Clark et al., 1997). Stressed animals may divert energy into adaption, generally at the expense of other biological processes such as behavior, immune function, growth, and reproduction. It is important to anticipate the stressful events that dogs may experience to prevent physiological changes during data collection.

Dog pens are usually constructed of concrete, stainless steel, galvanized metal, and wood. Stainless steel is preferable to galvanized metal, which may damage the feet or flake away if the quality of the galvanization is poor. Flaking galvanized metal may have toxic effects due to the zinc being absorbed during licking (Dysko et al., 2002; Prescott et al., 2004). Dogs should be housed in pairs or groups whenever possible. Boredom in dogs may have as much effect as any stressor on the overall well-being of an animal. As demonstrated in previous studies, animals will subject themselves to aversive conditions or engage in stereotypic behavior, including self-mutilation, to attain some stimulation (Wemelsfelder, 1990). An enriched environment is very important, whether or not a dog is bored. Primary sources of enrichment include interaction with people and/or a conspecific companion and the provision of manipulanda. Enrichment allows the dog to work off extra energy and occupy its mind, which will aid the animal to behave more naturally in a restricted environment. Enriched animals learn to cope better with stressful situations (Loveridge, 1998). It is important to establish that the introduction of environmental enrichment does not interfere with experimental data being measured, for example, foreign body ingestion. It is essential to select dogs that are well socialized to people and with other dogs. Most Class A research dogs are raised in a research facility, and habituated to people during their sensitive socialization periods and become adapted to these specific surroundings. These animals tend to be less fearful or reactive to procedures (Hirsjarvi and Junnila, 1986). Social isolation or restriction is regarded as a major stressor for a social species like the dog (Wolfle, 1990). Furthermore, dogs housed singly are usually less active or exhibit more repetitive nonsocial repetitive behaviors (Hubrecht et al., 1992; Hughes et al., 1989). The withdrawal of a conspecific contact can be detrimental, particularly, to dogs used to such contact. It is important for facility personnel to handle dogs from the time they arrive and throughout their lives to provide and develop environmental diversification and trusting relationships.

4.4.7 Transportation

Transportation is an especially powerful stressor for dogs (Kuhn et al., 1991). Transporting animals can produce a number of effects ranging from weight loss, altered immune function and behavior, and changes in blood characteristics linked with stress and shock reactions (Tuli et al., 1994). Even moving within a facility can cause an animal stress (Swallow et al., 2005). With this in mind, a period of acclimation is useful following transportation, prior to the beginning an experimental study. This allows animals a period of time for physiological, psychological, and nutritional stabilization before their use. The length of time for stabilization will depend on the type and duration of animal transportation, the dogs involved, and the intended use of the animals (Obernier and Baldwin, 2006; NRC, 1996). If dogs are to be paired or group housed, it is advisable to pair- or group-house dogs upon arrival. Ideally, animals should be purchased from a sole vendor. Preexisting stable groups will enhance the acclimation period within the new facility by minimizing dog-to-dog aggression and utilizing group immunity to prevent the spread of disease (Prescott et al., 2004). When forming a new pair or group, potential for conflict may be reduced by housing together individuals of different ages and/or body weights. Quarantine periods vary between institutions and depend on the animal source, health history, and current health status on the animal colony at the receiving institution. Most institutions recommend 7–14 days for newly purchased dogs and allow at least 3 days for animals to acclimate when they have been moved in individual containers between buildings on-site and/or entering an acute terminal study (Prescott et al., 2004). At least 24 hours should be permitted for acclimatization when there is a permanent change of pen location, assuming similar husbandry and care procedures are (Prescott et al., 2004).

4.4.8 Circadian Rhythm—Time of Collection

It is well known that there is diurnal variation in plasma corticosteroids in the dog (Reilly, 1998). Plasma levels of hormones and metabolites (including insulin, testosterone, and growth hormones) have shown diurnal variations (Fukuda, 1990), which may cause variation in clinical chemistry parameters. In particular, it should be taken into account that total lipids, total cholesterol, phospholipids, and triglycerides show daily rhythmicity in dogs maintained under 12:12-hour light:dark cycles (Bertolucci et al., 2008). Samples should be collected and synchronized, if needed, in a manner harmonious with the natural circadian cycle of the study cohort. Seasonal effects alter analyte values in most species. Among clinical chemistry, the parameters found to show seasonal effects with highest values in the summer were creatinine, phosphorus, uric acid, total protein, globulin, lactate dehydrogenase, γ-glutamyl transpeptidase, and total and direct bilirubin (Sothern et al., 1993). Significant circannual variation with highest values in winter was found in urea nitrogen, amylase, glucose, chloride, albumin, ALP, alanine aminotransferase, calcium, and sodium (Sothern et al., 1993).

4.4.9 Pregnancy, Parturition, and Lactation

Pregnancy, parturition, and lactation can influence plasma protein concentrations. For example, serum albumin may decrease due to dilutional effects secondary to water retention and globulin levels may increase in preparation of pregnancy to facilitate passive transfer to offspring, respectively.

4.4.10 Anesthesia

Anesthetic agents induce two types of artifact into data values: physiological and biochemical. Physiological effects are produced by alterations in blood pressure and cardiac output, respiration, and excitement, whereas biochemical effects are the result of enzyme induction, tissue hypoxia, and direct toxic damage. Xylazine and medetomidine are sedative analgesic/muscle relaxants routinely used in dogs and are reported to interfere with growth hormone, glucagon, insulin, glucose, follicle-stimulating hormone, and possibly antidiuretic hormone (Greene and Thurmon, 1988). Horber et al. (1990) found that isoflurane induces a mild hypoinsulinemia in dogs. Thiopental sodium has been the major anesthetic agent used to induce dogs for major surgery; however, at the time of publication, its future availability is questionable. Researchers have found that thiopental sodium promotes insulin responsiveness to glucose plasma levels (Ishihara et al., 1981). IV glucose tolerance tests during infusion of thiopentone indicated an increased insulinogenic index compared to halothane. The anesthetic used should minimize struggling and muscle activity. Muscle activity above resting levels may produce significant effects on many analytes. Potassium is released from the liver, and serum creatine kinase, plasma lactate, and circulating leukocytes and erythrocytes may be increased as animals struggle or become excited (Garber and Carey, 1984).

4.4.11 Specimen Collection/Handling Artifact

The deleterious effects of storage are the result of multiple factors operating on the sample. Storage conditions for one analyte (serum creatine kinase) are not necessarily ideal for others (isoenzymes of lactate dehydrogenase) (Reilly, 1998). Factors affecting storage include: evaporation, interaction of the sample with the container (for example, platelet clumping), temperature, light, and humidity. Erythrocyte lysis or hemolysis in serum and plasma is a common collection artifact best avoided. Hemolysis is the breakdown of erythrocytes (*in vivo*-circulating blood *after* blood collection). Poor venipuncture technique, prolonged blood storage, temperature extremes (hot or cold enough to freeze the cells), and certain anticoagulants (fluoride-oxalate) will cause artifactual hemolysis. Hemolysis after blood collection or due to a difficult venipuncture is an artifact, whereas *in vivo* hemolysis signifies a disease process. However, erythrocytes are also more fragile in lipemic samples and tend to lyse more readily in these samples even if the blood is stored or handled correctly. Artifactual hemolysis can mimic intravascular hemolysis and it can be very difficult to tell them apart (particularly in the laboratory setting where clinical correlation is unavailable). Upon blood collection, it is important to determine if the sample has hemolyzed and either redrawn the sample or document the hemolysis appropriately in the record. With this in mind, if the animal is anemic and has hemoglobinuria, true intravascular hemolysis (or a pathological hemolytic anemia) is likely. The canine erythrocyte is high in sodium and low in potassium, in contrast to that of rat, the nonhuman primates, or man whose erythrocytes are low in sodium and high in potassium (Harris and Kellermeyer 1970). Hemolysis can artifactually increase or decrease normal substances in the serum or interfere with results from spectrophotometer assays. Specimens must be handled in a timely manner and stored appropriately. Lipemia, the presence of visibly detectable lipid in serum or plasma, is much more common in the dog than in other laboratory animals. Lipemia will invalidate or interfere with analytic methodologies by falsely decreasing the concentrations of analytes within the serum. With some analyzers and reagents, hemolysis and lipemia will cause artifactually high bilirubin values.

Samples collected from different sites in the animal do not necessarily have comparable analyte values (Garber and Carey, 1984). Leukocyte, platelet, and erythrocyte numbers vary dependent on sampling site and may lead to sample contamination. In addition to variations in leukocyte and differential counts, variations are commonly found in red blood cell (RBC), hemoglobin (HGB), and hematocrit (HCT) values when comparing sampling sites (Reilly, 1998). The method of sample collection and processing can also influence analyte concentration. For example, hemolysis results in a significant reduction or elevation depending on measurable analyte. Mechanical injury to and subsequent damage to tissue may release an analyte into circulation (e.g., cardiac stick not appropriate site for creatine kinase (CK) or tropinin) resulting in high plasma values. The canine cephalic vein is smaller than the jugular vein and, consequently, is more susceptible to trauma during blood sample collection. The jugular vein is ideal for repeat serial sampling, compared to samples collected from the cephalic vein. In order to minimize the influences of variables it is important that the blood should be collected in the same manner (e.g., ideally same handler and/or phlebotomist) at each sampling time and that the volume of blood be limited to the minimum required to perform the desired analysis. When collecting urine for clinical chemistry evaluation every effort must be made to avoid contamination with food, drinking water, and feces.

Appropriate blood tubes (various anticoagulant, nonanticoagulant, or serum separator) can be selected based on experimental design, but consistency is essential. Switching between tube types may cause analyte measurements to vary, especially if switching between plasma (e.g., green or lavender tops) and serum (e.g., red tops). If utilizing the services of a clinical pathology reference lab or core-lab, be certain to check their tube preferences and volume requirements prior to commencing your study. Gel separator tubes may confer an advantage in obtaining "clean" (cell-free) serum or plasma from small specimens; however, caution should be used if the serum is also utilized for pharmacologic studies or therapeutic drug monitoring as the gel substance may bind the drug metabolite to be measured, causing falsely decreased measurements. Lithium heparin anticoagulant tubes are useful when hematology [complete blood count (CBC)] evaluations are to be performed on the same specimen. The fluid phase of blood should be removed from cellular elements as soon as separation has occurred because the cells left in contact will metabolize certain chemical components in the serum. Glucose will be metabolized by cells, thus decreasing measured values at the rate of approximately 10% per hour if left in contact with red blood cells. Harvested serum should be analyzed quickly; otherwise, it can be stored in a refrigerator for 24–48 hours or frozen afterward at −70°F. All samples should be handled in the same manner. Serum enzymes, as a general rule, should be analyzed within 24 hours of collection. ALT, aspartate aminotransferase (AST), ALP, CK, and amylase are satisfactorily stable (>70% activity) when stored at 4°C (Loeb, 1999). Samples stored in frost-free and nonfrost-free −20°C freezers should not differ significantly through day 90, but repeated freeze/thaw cycles may result in statistically significant difference in some parameters. Factors such as storage time and temperature should be considered when designing any retrospective study (Cray, 2009). In addition to sources of variation that occur before sample analysis, the analytical procedure (e.g., analyzer, quantitative methodology) itself is a source of variation. It is important to caution that one must use reference ranges specific to a machine or reference lab and to use other reference ranges (including those in this chapter) only as guides. Analytic variation is minimized by robust quality control systems and appropriate study design (Hall and Everds, 2007).

4.5 BRIEF DESCRIPTION OF COMMON PROCEDURES

4.5.1 Adrenal Function Testing

4.5.1.1 Hyperadrenocorticism Diagnosis

Given the high incidence of hyperadrenocorticism (HAC; Cushing's syndrome) in dogs, dogs demonstrating cardinal features of the disease (such as polyuria and polyphagia, a pendulous abdomen, and hair loss) should be evaluated for HAC (Willeberg and Priester, 1982; Kooistra and Galac, 2010).

The ideal screening test in a calm dog is a urine cortisol:creatinine ratio (UCCR) measured on a *voided* urine specimen. Because urine is stored in the bladder for several hours, urinary cortisol measurement integrates the impact of pulsatile ACTH secretion and variable plasma cortisol concentrations over time (Kooistra and Galac, 2010). Basal UCCR in healthy dogs varies from 0.3 to 8.3 × 10^{-6} (Kooistra and Galac, 2010). Given the high predictive value of a negative test result (0.98) (Rijnberk et al., 1988), a UCCR in this normal range accurately rules out HAC. However, since stress can generate false positives (the test is sensitive but not specific), the positive predictive value of the UCCR is only 0.88 (Rijnberk et al., 1988). An elevated UCCR requires further diagnostics to confirm the HAC diagnosis: a low-dose dexamethasone suppression test (LDDST) or an adrenocorticotropic stimulation test.

HAC can be diagnosed by testing the integrity of the glucocorticoid feedback system on the hypothalamic–pituitary–adrenal axis via the LDDST (Kooistra and Galac, 2010). The LDDST is the most sensitive (95%) test for HAC in dogs and is considered by many to be the test of choice for HAC diagnosis in dogs (Feldman, 2009; Behrend and Kennis, 2010). The specificity of the LDDST can be low (40%–50%), especially when measured in a population of sick dogs (Kaplan et al., 1995). In the LDDST, 0.01 mg dexamethasone sodium phosphate per kg of body weight is administered IV. Cortisol measurements are performed using plasma or serum (ethylenediaminetetraacetic acid or EDTA) collected before, and at 4 and 8 hours after dexamethasone administration. Cooling of plasma is not necessary, but serum should be stored and shipped frozen (−20°C) (Behrend et al., 1998). An 8-hour plasma cortisol >1.4 µg/dL is consistent with the diagnosis of HAC (Feldman, 2009). Only the 8 hour sample is necessary for HAC diagnosis, but the 4-hour sample may be useful in determining if the hypercortisolism is adrenal or pituitary-dependent (Kooistra and Galac,

2010). If the 8 hour sample is consistent with HAC and the plasma cortisol concentration at 4 or 8 hours is ≥50% lower than the baseline value, the hypercortisolism is pituitary-dependent (Kooistra and Galac, 2010). The high-dose dexamethasone suppression test (HDDST) is a discriminatory test used in dogs already diagnosed with HAC in order to determine if the dog has PDH or ADH. It is performed just as the LDDST except that a higher dose of dexamethasone (0.1 mg/kg) is administered (Feldman, 2009).

An alternative diagnostic test for HAC is the adrenocorticotropic hormone stimulation (ACTH) test. Because of its low sensitivity, (80%, meaning 20% of dogs with HAC will have test results within the reference range) some clinicians no longer recommend this diagnostic approach for dogs with hypercortisolism (Feldman, 2009; Behrend and Kennis, 2010). Furthermore, due to the cost of ACTH (see below), the ACTH test is markedly more expensive than the LDDST and may be cost-prohibitive in the research setting. However, since the ACTH test is used to monitor therapy of HAC, others still employ it as a diagnostic test in order to obtain baseline therapeutic parameters. The ACTH stimulation is the test of choice for initial testing in dogs with history of exogenous steroids (suspected iatrogenic HAC) (Scott-Montcrieff, 2010). The ACTH stimulation test is also the only test that is capable of diagnosing atypical HAC, as discussed below. The specificity of the ACTH stimulation test is higher than that of the LDDST (85%–90%) (Melian et al., 2010). Finally, the ACTH stimulation test remains the gold standard for diagnosis of hypoadrenocorticism.

Caution must be taken in interpreting an ACTH stimulation test result in dogs with nonadrenal illness. It is possible for stressed and sick dogs without HAC to have exaggerated ACTH test responses (Behrend and Kennis, 2010). Fourteen to 36% of dogs with nonadrenal illness but without HAC have ACTH stimulation results consistent with HAC (Chastain et al., 1986; Kaplan et al., 1995). However, both the UCC and the LDDST generate even more false positive results (76% and 56%, respectively) than the ACTH stimulation test in dogs with nonadrenal illness (Kaplan et al., 1995). The ACTH test is the best choice for HAC diagnosis in dogs with concurrent disease, but ideally testing a sick dog for HAC should be avoided altogether (Chastain et al., 1986; Kaplan et al., 1995).

The ACTH stimulation test assesses the adrenal gland's cortisol producing capacity in response to a maximal stimulus (Klein and Peterson, 2010). It is conducted as follows:

1. Draw a baseline blood sample for plasma (EDTA tube) or serum (plain tube) preparation (serum or plasma depends on your laboratory's requirements). Centrifuge the samples (allow non-anticoagulated samples to clot first) and collect serum or plasma. Ensure serum is kept cold (–20°C); plasma does not need to be cooled (Behrend et al., 1998).
2. Inject ACTH gel (2.2 mg/kg intramuscularly (IM) or cosyntropin (5 μg/kg IV; maximum dose 250 μg/dog; see Table 4.1).
3. Collect a blood sample 1 and 2 hours after ACTH gel administration or just 1 hour after cosyntropin administration. We recommend collecting a second plain tube for serum preparation and storing frozen serum in case testing for atypical HAC becomes necessary (Cook, 2011).
4. Centrifuge the samples (allow non-anticoagulated samples to clot first) and collect serum or plasma. Ensure serum is kept cold.
5. Measure cortisol levels in baseline and poststimulation samples.

Available formulations of ACTH include synthetic ACTH and gel preparations (Klein and Peterson, 2010). These products are costly and sometimes plagued by poor availability (Kemppainen et al., 2005). Gel preparations are administered at a dose of 2.2 mg/kg IM, and blood samples must be collected at both 1 and 2 hours post-ACTH stimulation because of variability in the time to peak response among different compounded products (Kemppainen et al., 2005).

Standardly, ACTH stimulation involves 250 μg synthetic ACTH (cosyntropin, Cortrosyn; Amphastar Pharmaceuticals, Rancho Cucamonga, CA) given IV or IM followed by blood

TABLE 4.1
Cortrosyn Dosing Regimen Used for the ACTH Stimulation test to Diagnose HAC or Hypoadrenocorticism in Dogs

Weight (kg)	Dose (mcg)
<5	25
5–10	50
10–15	75
15–20	100
20–25	125
25–30	150
30–40	200
40–50	225
>50	250 (1 vial)

Source: Papich, M.G. *Saunders Handbook of Veterinary Drugs*, Saunders Elsevier, St. Louis, MO, 2007.

sampling one hour later (Klein and Peterson, 2010). Alternatively, a more cost effective approach employs a lower (5 µg/kg) IV cosyntropin dose (Klein and Peterson, 2010). This low-dose ACTH stimulation test (5 µg/kg) when compared with the standard dose (250 µg/dog) resulted in maximal stimulation of the adrenal cortex in normal dogs and dogs with HAC (Kerl et al., 1999), and produced equivalent results to the standard dose of 250 µg/dog in dogs with suspected hypoadrenocorticism (Lathan et al., 2008). The cosyntropin dose regimen based on the low-dose ACTH protocol currently used for diagnosis of both hyper- and hypo-adrenocorticism at the NCSU College of Veterinary Medicine is detailed in Table 4.1. To maximize the financial benefit of the low-dose ACTH protocol, cosyntropin can be stored stably in frozen aliquots (-20°C) in plastic syringes for up to 6 months (Frank and Oliver, 1998). Care should be taken when aliquoting the drug since the reconstituted cosyntropin does not contain preservatives (Klein and Peterson, 2010).

The ACTH stimulation test is useful in diagnosing the syndrome of atypical HAC, a syndrome that has been rarely documented in dogs (Benitah et al., 2005; Behrend and Kennis, 2010). In this syndrome, increased circulating concentrations of adrenal hormones other than cortisol (such as progesterone or 17-hydroxyprogesterone) are proposed to cause clinical signs that are indistinguishable from those due to excess glucocorticoids (Scott-Moncrieff, 2010). These dogs have clinical signs and/or laboratory abnormalities consistent with HAC, but have LDDST or ACTH stimulation tests (Behrend and Kennis, 2010). An extended panel of adrenal corticosteroids should be measured before and after ACTH stimulation in dogs with clinical and laboratory evidence of HAC, but normal cortisol testing. The protocol is the same as that of the ACTH stimulation test, but pre- and poststimulation serum is submitted for an extended panel of adrenal steroid measurement (currently being performed at the Clinical Endocrinology Service at the University of Tennessee) (Scott-Moncrieff, 2010). Serum can be stored at −20°C to −70°C for at least 1 month before measuring these hormone concentrations and can be measured on the same sample collected for serum cortisol measurement (Benitah et al., 2005). Increases (1.5–2 times greater than the upper end of the reference range) in 2–3 adrenal steroid hormone concentrations are supportive of atypical HAC (Scott-Moncrieff, 2010). Levels of adrenal sex steroid hormones must be considered in the context of sex and neuter status (Benitah et al., 2005). The reader is referred to Betinah et al. for reference intervals for serum 17-hydroxyprogesterone concentrations in healthy dogs of different sex and neuter status following ACTH stimulation (Benitah et al., 2005). The specificity of the adrenal sex hormone testing, however, has not been evaluated, and some debate whether sex hormone elevation is truly a form of HAC or simply a nonspecific reflection of nonadrenal illness (Behrend and Kennis, 2010). Sex hormone concentrations of normal dogs, HAC dogs, and dogs with nonadrenal illness can overlap (Scott-Moncrieff, 2010). Interpretation of the extended adrenal steroid panel must be performed with the understanding that there is limited published information relating elevations in these cortisol precursors to clinical signs and that some authors are not convinced that an atypical HAC syndrome truly exists in dogs (Behrend and Kennis, 2010; Cook, 2011).

4.5.1.2 Hypoadrenocorticism Diagnosis

The gold standard for diagnosing hypoadrenocorticism in dogs is an ACTH stimulation test, which demonstrates an inability of the zona fasciculata and reticularis to produce cortisol response to a maximal stimulus (Klein and Peterson, 2010). However, the measurement of a normal, resting cortisol concentration can exclude a diagnosis of hypoadrenocorticism, avoiding the cost of the ACTH stimulation test (Lennon et al., 2007). Dogs with basal cortisol levels ≥2 μg/dL are very unlikely to have hypoadrenocorticism (Lennon et al., 2007). A baseline cortisol <2 μg/dL is nondiagnostic, and requires further evaluation with an ACTH stimulation test. For dogs with basal cortisol levels ≥ 2 μg/dl in which a strong suspicion for hypoadrenocorticism remains, a full ACTH stimulation test should be performed (Lennon et al., 2007).

The protocol for the ACTH stimulation to diagnosis hypoadrenocorticism is the same as that to diagnose HAC. To confirm the diagnosis, pre and post-ACTH cortisol concentrations should be less than 2 μg/dL (Scott-Moncrieff, 2010a). While in normal dogs, synthetic ACTH can be administered IV or IM to ensure adequate absorption, IV cosyntropin is recommended in dehydrated dogs like those in Addisonian crisis (Hansen et al., 1994; Peterson et al., 1996).

4.5.2 Thyroid Function Testing

Although hypothyroidism is one of the most common canine endocrinopathies, diagnosis can be challenging. Usually, a combination of low plasma total thyroxine (TT_4) concentration and elevated thyroid stimulating hormone (TSH) is diagnostic for hypothyroidism (Diaz Espineira et al., 2007). Unfortunately, TSH concentrations are normal in up to one third of dogs with primary hypothyroidism (Ramsey et al., 1997; Scott-Moncrieff et al., 1998b; Diaz Espineira et al., 2007). This, coupled with the fact that plasma TT4 concentrations are frequently decreased in dogs with nonthyroidal illness (euthyroid sick), makes it challenging to differentiate between dogs with hypothyroidism and those that are euthyroid sick (Diaz Espineira et al, 2007). Further tests of thyroid function become necessary.

4.5.2.1 Thyrotropin (TSH) Response Test

The TSH response test is considered by some authors as the most accurate test for thyroid gland function (Feldman and Nelson, 1996). It tests the thyroid gland's reserve by evaluating the thyroid gland's responsiveness to exogenous TSH administration. Most importantly, the TSH response test is the best biochemical thyroid function test for differentiating between true hypothyroidism and the euthyroid sick syndrome in dogs (Feldman and Nelson, 2004; Diaz Espineira et al., 2007). However, the "gold standard" status of the TSH response test for hypothyroidism diagnosis has recently been questioned because it can still falsely classify euthyroid sick dogs as hypothyroid (Diaz Espineira et al., 2007; Daminet et al., 2007). Thyroid pertechnetate uptake may be the only reliable way to distinguish between dogs with nonthyroidal illness and those with primary hypothyroidism (Diaz Espineira et al., 2007).

Recombinant human TSH (rhTSH) (Thyrogen, Genzyme Corporation, Cambridge, MA) is the recommended pharmaceutic for the TSH response test. Reconstituted rhTSH can be stored in plastic syringes for up to 8 weeks at −20°C or 4 weeks at 4°C, making use of this expensive product more cost-effective (De Roover et al., 2006; Daminet et al., 2007). The traditionally used bovine TSH is no longer available as a pharmaceutical preparation (Boretti et al., 2006). We do not recommend use of chemical grade bovine TSH as life-threatening reactions can occur in dogs following its administration (Scott-Moncrieff, 2010b).

The protocol using rhTSH is as follows:

1. Collect a blood sample in a plain tube. Following clot retraction at room temperature, harvest serum via low-speed centrifugation. Transfer to *plastic* tubes for storage at −20°C until subsequent hormone assay (Boretti et al., 2006). Samples can be shipped without cooling if assayed within 5 days (Behrend et al., 1998).
2. Administer 150 μg rhTSH IV per dog. Use of a lower dose (75 μg), especially in a diseased dog or a dog taking medications known to affect thyroid function, may lead to an inappropriate diagnosis of hypothyroidism (Boretti et al., 2009).
3. Collect a blood sample 6 hours later and harvest serum as above. Serum must be stored in plastic tubes (Behrend et al., 1998).
4. Measure pre- and post-TSH serum TT_4 concentrations.

The expectation is that there will be minimal change in post-TSH TT_4 concentration compared with basal concentration in dogs with hypothyroidism (Boretti et al., 2006). If both pre and post-TSH serum TT_4 concentrations are below the reference range for basal TT_4, a diagnosis of hypothyroidism is likely; if post-TSH TT_4 is >2.5 μg/dL and increased to at least 1.5 times basal TT_4 concentration, dogs are classified as being euthyroid (Scott-Moncrieff, 2010b). Post-TSH serum TT_4 values between 1.6 and 2.5 μg/dL are nondiagnostic (Boretti et al., 2009).

Because thyroxine causes thyroid atrophy, dogs being treated with thyroxine cannot be tested with the TSH response test until they have been off supplementation for 6-8 weeks (Scott-Moncrieff, 2010b).

4.5.2.2 Thyrotropin-Releasing Hormone (TRH) Response Test

The TRH response test can be used to evaluate thyroid function in dogs in place of the TSH response test (Feldman and Nelson, 2004). An expected normal response to the TRH test would be the endogenous production of TSH by the pituitary gland with subsequent increase in serum TT_4 concentration due to stimulation of the thyroid gland (Lothrop et al., 1984). However, the TRH response test is less reliable than the TSH response test for the diagnosis of canine hypothyroidism because normal dogs have a small, inconsistent increase in serum TT_4 and some sick euthyroid dogs fail to respond to TRH (Frank, 1996; Kemppainen and Behrend, 2001); thus, this test cannot be used to differentiate primary hypothyroidism from euthyroid illness (Frank, 1996; Diaz Espineira et al., 2007). Furthermore, dogs with primary hypothyroidism have an unusual blunted response to TRH administration: they produce minimal or no TSH in response to TRH (Diaz Espineira et al., 2007; Diaz-Espineira et al., 2008). We would expect primary hypothyroid dogs to produce exaggerated TSH in response to TRH because of the reduced negative feedback of thyroxine on the pituitary. In people, TRH stimulation does indeed lead to this expected exaggerated release of TSH in patients with primary hypothyroidism; people with condary hypothyroidism have a blunted TSH response to TRH (Diaz-Espineira et al., 2008). Therefore, in people the TRH response test can differentiate primary from secondary hypothyroidism. However, in dogs the TRH response test cannot be used to differentiate primary from secondary hypothyroidism since all hypothyroid dogs have a blunted TSH response in the TRH test (Scott-Moncrieff and Nelson, 1998a; Diaz-Espineira et al., 2008). In sum, clinical utility of the TRH response test in dogs is limited.

The protocol for the TRH response test is as follows (Feldman and Nelson, 2004):

1. Collect baseline blood samples, centrifuge, and harvest serum, transfer to a plastic tube.
2. Give 200 µg TRH per dog IV.
3. Collect blood 30 minutes and 4 hours after TRH administration. Centrifuge and harvest serum, transfer to *plastic* tubes (Behrend et al., 1998).
4. Store at −20°C until measurement can be performed. Samples can be shipped at ambient temperature as long as they are assayed within 5 days (Behrend et al., 1998). Measure serum TT_4 concentration at 0 and 4 hours; measure serum TSH at 0 and 30 minutes.

Although higher doses of TRH have been evaluated (>0.1 mg/kg TRH), increasing the dosage of TRH does not increase the magnitude of TT_4 stimulation, but does increase the occurrence of adverse effects due to the central cholinergic properties of TRH such as salivation, miosis, vomiting, urination, defecation, tachycardia, and tachypnea (Lothrop et al., 1984; Feldman and Nelson, 2004).

One schematic for interpreting results of the TRH response test is as follows:

- Euthyroidism likely: post-TRH TT_4 concentration >2 µg/dL and relative increase in TSH >100% at 30 minutes post-TRH (Scott-Moncrieff, 2010b).
- Possible hypothyroid diagnosis: Post-TRH TT_4 is <1.5 µg/dL (Scott-Moncrieff, 2010b).
- Post-TRH serum TT_4 concentrations between 1.5 and 2 µg/dL are nondiagnostic (Feldman and Nelson, 2004).

4.5.3 Liver Function Testing

4.5.3.1 Pre- and Postprandial Bile Acids

Measurement of serum bile acids provides a simple, highly specific test of liver function and perfusion that evaluates the enterohepatic circulation of bile acids (Center et al., 1991; Webster, 2010). After meal ingestion, cholecystokinin (CCK) release stimulates gallbladder contraction and subsequent release of bile acids to intestine. From the ileum, bile acids are transported back to portal circulation, where they are removed by hepatocytes and recycled back into the biliary system (Ruland et al., 2010; Webster, 2010). Postprandial entry of bile into the small intestine leads to an increase in bile acids in portal circulation that exceeds the hepatic clearing capacity, leading to a small transient postprandial increase in serum bile acids in dogs with normal hepatic function (Center, 1993; Ruaux et al., 2002). If enterohepatic circulation is disrupted, serum bile acids increase above normal concentrations. This can occur due to loss of functional hepatic mass, due to portosystemic shunting of blood, or due to cholestasis (Bain, 2003; Ruland et al., 2010).

Although fasting serum bile acids can be measured and interpreted alone, the best application of the serum bile acid test involves a paired pre- and postprandial bile acids measurement to optimize the chance of detecting elevated values (Balkman et al., 2003). In detecting shunting associated with portosystemic vascular anomalies (PSVA) and cirrhosis, the postprandial serum bile acid concentration is more sensitive than the fasting bile acid concentration (Center et al., 1991).

To obtain the preprandial sample, the dog is fasted for 12 hours and blood is drawn into a plain tube for serum preparation. A meal is then fed. The meal must have adequate fat or amino acid content to lead to CCK release and gallbladder contraction. Ideally, the dog should be fed a typical sized meal (Center, 1993). Minimally, at least two teaspoons of food for dogs less than 5 kg and two tablespoons of food for dogs greater than 5 kg should be consumed (Webster, 2010). If the dog will not eat voluntarily, the food can be ground in a blender and syringe-fed (Center, 1993). To ensure test accuracy, the dog must be observed to eat the meal (Webster, 2010). Blood is then sampled for postprandial serum bile acids measurement 2 hours after feeding. Although serum bile acids are stable at room temperature, hemolysis and lipemia must be avoided as they interfere with the spectrophotometric endpoints of most commonly used assays for bile acids (Webster, 2010). Hemolyzed samples cannot be analyzed accurately, but lipemia can be cleared by high-speed centrifugation of the sera (Center, 1993).

About 20% of dogs have higher fasting than 2-hour postprandial bile acids due to differences in the rates of gastric emptying, gallbladder contraction, and enteric motility (Center, 1993; Balkman et al., 2003). The accuracy of the postprandial bile acids measurement depends on the meal adequately stimulating CCK release and subsequent gall bladder contraction. Variables such as the rate of gastric emptying, anorexia, and vomiting can influence postprandial bile acid concentrations (Bridger et al., 2008). To ensure adequate gall bladder contraction, injection of a CCK analog (ceruletide) has been proposed as an alternative testing procedure (Bridger et al., 2008). Ceruletide serum bile acid stimulation has been shown to perform equally well as postprandial bile acids stimulation in dogs with portosystemic shunts (Bridger et al., 2008). The test needs to be evaluated more extensively for accuracy in the context of other liver diseases and for potential side effects such as pancreatitis induction (Webster, 2010).

Maltese dogs can have elevated postprandial bile acids in the absence of hepatobiliary disease (Tisdall et al., 1995). The reason for this breed-anomaly is unknown but necessitates the use of the ammonia tolerance test (ATT) to evaluate liver function in Maltese.

When interpreting serum bile acid levels, we need to remember that the test is only capable of discriminating normal from abnormal hepatic function (Webster, 2010). Bile acids values do not indicate the type of hepatobiliary disease (Center, 1993). Furthermore, the histologic severity of the disease or the degree of portovascular shunting is not well correlated with the degree of bile acid elevation (Center, 1993; Webster, 2010).

4.5.3.2 Ammonia Tolerance Test (ATT)

The liver detoxifies ammonia that is generated in the GIT by degradation of amines, amino acids, purines, bacterial hydrolysis of urea, and intestinal deamination of glutamine (Walker et al., 2001; Webster, 2010). Ammonia that is released from the gut into portal circulation is converted by hepatocytes to urea and is used in glutamine synthesis in the liver and other tissues (Walker et al., 2001; Webster, 2010). In hepatic synthetic failure, or when blood is shunted away from the liver, ammonia escapes hepatic metabolism, leading to hyperammonemia (Webster, 2010). Since the hepatic urea cycle normally operates at only 60% capacity, hepatic synthetic failure must be advanced to cause hyperammonemia (Webster, 2010). Unlike serum bile acids, plasma ammonia is not influenced by cholestasis (Gerritzen-Bruning et al., 2006). Like bile acid testing, ammonia levels only assess the hepatic function and not the underlying reason for the dysfunction (e.g., portosystemic shunting vs. hepatocellular disease).

In dogs, fasting blood ammonia elevation has a sensitivity of 100% for congenital PSVA and 86% for acquired shunts; the specificity of fasting hyperammonemia for portosystemic shunting is 89% (Gerritzen-Bruning et al., 2006). Elevated fasting ammonia in dogs is more specific for the detection of portosystemic shunting than are elevated fasting serum bile acids (Gerritzen-Bruning et al., 2006; Ruland et al., 2010). The sensitivity of blood ammonia levels for detection of portosystemic shunting is increased by sampling 6 hours after feeding (Walker et al., 2001). Elevated blood ammonia levels are less common in dogs with parenchymal liver disease in the absence of acquired shunting, making blood ammonia an insensitive test for detecting hepatocellular disease regardless of feeding status (Walker et al., 2001; Webster, 2010).

Hyperammonemia has also been reported in dogs without liver disease. Increased plasma ammonia can occur with urea-cycle enzyme deficiencies or conditions resulting in decreased availability of urea-cycle substrates (Webster, 2010). Hyperammonemia was reported in a dog with selective cobalamin deficiency that led to urea cycle dysfunction and in two dogs with a deficiency of the urea cycle enzyme arginosuccinate synthetase (Strombeck et al., 1975a; Battersby et al., 2005). Transient hyperammonemia occurs in Irish Wolfhound puppies under 4 months of age due to an incompletely characterized urea cycle enzyme deficiency (Zandvliet and Rothuizen,

2007). These nonhepatic causes of hyperammonemia should be considered when interpreting plasma ammonia levels or ATT results. False negative baseline ammonia levels have also been documented (Webster, 2010).

Improper sample handling can lead to artificially increased plasma ammonia and reduced specificity of the test (Gerritzen-Bruning et al., 2006). Samples should be drawn directly into cold, closed ammonia-free lithium heparin or EDTA tubes (anticoagulant depends on the method of measurement). The sample should be put on melting ice, spun in a refrigerated centrifuge, and ammonia measured within 30 minutes to avoid *in vitro* generation of ammonia (Hitt and Jones, 1986). Hemolysis or failure to immediately separate erythrocytes from plasma (within 20 minutes) can also lead to spurious ammonia increases because erythrocytes contain three times more ammonia than plasma (Prytz et al., 1970; Webster, 2010). A baseline sample from a normal dog should always be submitted as a quality control of sample management and the assay (Center, 2003). Samples cannot be frozen and stored (Hitt and Jones, 1986; Webster, 2010).

The diagnostic accuracy of blood ammonia concentrations, especially in identifying dogs with PSVA, is increased significantly by the ATT (Meyer et al., 1978). Before performing an ATT, a baseline ammonia level should always be measured. An ATT should be avoided in dogs in which the baseline ammonia is already increased, as this could cause severe neurologic decompensation (Bain, 2003). Since ammonia is one of the factors responsible for hepatic encephalopathy (HE), an ATT could exacerbate HE and is thereby contraindicated dogs with suspected HE (Strombeck et al., 1975b; Berent and Weisse, 2010).

The ATT can be performed by administration of ammonium chloride orally or rectally. The rectal route is better tolerated, easy to perform, and avoids the aspiration potential of PO ammonia administration or vomiting subsequent to PO administration (Walker et al., 2001; Berent and Tobias, 2009). Blood is drawn for ammonia measurement before and 30 minutes after ammonium chloride administration. To administer ammonium chloride per rectum, a cleansing enema is first performed. Thirty minutes later, ammonium chloride (2mL/kg of a 5 % ammonium chloride solution in water, not to exceed 3 g) is administered via a lubricated urinary catheter inserted at least 20 cm beyond the anal spinchter (Rothuizen and van den Ingh, 1982). Ammonia should be retained in the rectum for 5 minutes by digital pressure on the anus (Tisdall et al., 1995).

4.5.4 Renal Function Testing

4.5.4.1 Glomerular Filtration Rate

GFR is the best and most sensitive indicator of overall renal function (Heiene and Lefebvre, 2007). Increases in plasma urea and creatinine levels only occur once 75% or more of the renal functional mass has been lost. Early renal dysfunction is better identified by measuring GFR because GFR is directly related to functional renal mass (Heiene and Lefebvre, 2007; DiBartola, 2010).

GFR can be estimated by the renal clearance of a filtration marker by measuring marker levels in the plasma and urine, or by plasma clearance by measuring only plasma marker levels (Heiene and Moe, 1998). Although urinary inulin clearance is considered the gold standard for GFR measurement, the lack of general availability of inulin and laboratories that measure inulin preclude its common use (Bexfield et al., 2008). Iohexol and creatinine can be used in place of inulin as both substances meet the characteristics of ideal GFR markers: they are freely filtered, not reabsorbed, secreted, or extrarenally excreted, and are not metabolized (Heiene and Lefebvre, 2007).

Urinary clearance methods in general are cumbersome. Complete bladder emptying is required so that GFR is not underestimated. However, when bladder catheterization is used to ensure complete bladder emptying and urine collection, there is a risk of introducing infection (Heiene and Moe, 1998). For this reason, only plasma clearance methods are described here.

Single injection plasma clearance methods have been developed using inulin, iohexol, or creatinine to estimate GFR. Plasma clearance of these substances is calculated as quotient of administered dose divided by area under plasma concentration versus time curve (AUC) (DiBartola, 2010). The accuracy of plasma clearance methods depends on the pharmacokinetic model used to calculate AUC and the timing and number of samples used to make calculations (DiBartola, 2010). Extensive comparison of different methods of plasma clearance estimation of GFR in dogs has been reviewed elsewhere (Heiene and Moe, 1998). Plasma inulin clearance is significantly higher than urinary clearance, suggesting that there are other nonrenal routes of removal of inulin from plasma, thus making the plasma inulin clearance an inferior method for GFR measurement (Watson et al., 2002).

In contrast to what is observed in human medicine, GFR in dogs does not necessarily decrease with age (Bexfield et al., 2008). One study found that only in the smallest weight quartile of dogs was there an age-related decrease in GFR (Bexfield et al., 2008). GFR is, however, much higher in puppies than in mature dogs (Laroute et al., 2005). A significant negative linear relationship has been described in dogs between body weight and GFR (Bexfield et al., 2008). Thus, in interpreting GFR values, body size and age (for small dogs and puppies) of the patient should be considered (Bexfield et al., 2008).

Fasting prior to and during GFR studies is important because protein intake can influence GFR in individual dogs, with increases in GFR occurring 1.5–8 hours after protein ingestion (Brown and Finco, 1992). Free access to water is equally important during these studies because dehydration decreases GFR in dogs (Tabaru et al., 1993).

4.5.4.2 Iohexol Plasma Clearance

Iohexol is an iodinated, water-soluble nonionic low osmolar contrast agent used to estimate GFR (DiBartola, 2010). Unlike inulin, iohexol is stable in plasma so blood samples can be sent for lab analysis without special handling, making the iohexol plasma measurement more practical (Heiene and Lefebvre, 2007). Iohexol measurement is performed in many laboratories, and iohexol itself is widely available. Accurate GFR results using plasma iohexol measurements have been described in dogs (Goy-Thollot et al. 2006; Heiene et al., 2010). Some experts believe that iohexol could replace inulin as a reference marker (Brown and O'Reilly, 1991).

Although the ideal GFR marker is nontoxic, rare toxic reactions to iohexol are possible (allergy, skin reactions, and reversible nephropathy) (Cochran, 2005; Heiene and Lefebvre, 2007; Heiene et al., 2010). Iohexol has been shown to affect GFR in dogs potentially through effects on adenosine receptors (Arakawa et al., 1996). In dogs with normal renal function, renal plasma flow, and GFR increased after iohexol injection. In dogs with experimentally induced renal insufficiency, a low dose of iohexol did not change GFR, but a high dose of iohexol first increased and then reduced renal plasma flow and GFR (Arakawa et al., 1996). Despite these caveats, the iohexol plasma clearance in dogs appears comparable to other methods of GFR estimation (Heiene et al., 2010).

Iohexol clearance can be determined via protocols that minimize the number of blood samples that are required. These limited sampling strategies yield similar results to the 9- and 10-sample reference methods, and are probably acceptable for most clinical and research situations (Goy-Thollot et al., 2006; Heiene and Lefebvre, 2007). If necessary for the application, accuracy can be increased by increasing the sampling frequency (Heiene et al., 2010). A 3-sample method described by Heiene and colleagues for determining the iohexol clearance that appears to optimize accuracy and practicality is detailed below (Heiene and Lefebvre, 2007; Heiene et al., 2010):

1. Withhold food for 12 hours prior to procedure.
2. Provide free access to water during the study; withhold food.
3. Weigh the dog.

4. Take a baseline blood sample in heparinized tubes for plasma preparation. Volume of blood drawn depends on the requirements of the laboratory being used for iohexol measurement. At the time of writing, the Diagnostic Center for Population and Animal Health at Michigan State University was measuring iohexol via HPLC with a minimum sample volume of 1.2 mL. Contact the laboratory prior to performing the test. Some laboratories require serum rather than plasma.
5. Administer iohexol (300 mg iodine/mL) solution as an IV bolus via a peripheral IV catheter. Give 1 mL/kg to dogs without azotemia and 0.5 mL/kg to azotemic dogs.
6. Flush the catheter with 2 mL saline after injection and begin timing. Remove the catheter after flushing.
7. Sample blood at 2, 3, and 4 hours after administration from a different site from where iohexol was given. Indwelling sampling catheters (separate from the catheter through which iohexol was infused) may be used for blood collection, but the first milliliter of blood collected from the sampling catheter at each time-point must be discarded and the catheter flushed with saline following each sample collection (Heiene et al., 2010). Record the exact time of sampling.
8. Prepare plasma from blood samples via centrifugation and send to a laboratory.
9. Clearance is then calculated using a 1-compartmental model (CL_{1comp}), using the formula CL_{1comp} = dose/AUC, where AUC = C_0/k, C_0 is concentration at time 0, and k is the elimination rate constant corresponding to the terminal monoexponential phase of the concentration-time curve (Heiene and Moe, 1999; Bexfield et al., 2008). This value is then corrected to account for having neglected the first part of the concentration–time curve with the dog-specific equation generated by Heiene and colleagues:

$$\text{Clearance} = 0.03 + \left(1.06 \times \text{CL}_{1\text{comp}}\right) - (0.07012 \times \left[\text{CL}_{1\text{comp}}\right]^2) \text{ (Heiene et al., 2010)}$$

In an extended-sample protocol, samples are collected at the following times after iohexol administration: 5, 15, 30, and 60 minutes and 2, 3, 4, 5, and 6 hours (Heiene et al., 2010). Clearance is then calculated as the quotient of dose divided by the AUC, where AUC calculated using a noncompartmental (trapezoidal) method (Heiene et al., 2010). No correction is needed, as the distribution phase of the concentration–time curve is not being neglected. Such extended and more frequent sampling times are recommended in cases of severely decreased renal function, or when extreme accuracy in GFR calculation is necessary (Bexfield et al., 2008). However, the optimal time points for sample collection in dogs with poor kidney function have not yet been determined (Heiene et al., 2010).

4.5.4.3 Creatinine Clearance

Plasma exogenous creatinine clearance is another method that is practical, cost-effective, and comparable to urine inulin clearance (Watson et al., 2002). Laboratory analysis of creatinine is widely available. While the accuracy of endogenous creatinine clearance is impeded by measurement of noncreatinine chromagens by many creatinine assays, exogenous administration of creatinine increases plasma concentrations of creatinine, thereby minimizing the effect of these substances. One drawback to exogenous creatinine clearance measurement is that creatinine has a volume of distribution and half-life that are three times greater than the corresponding parameters for other markers, thus requiring longer sampling times (Heiene and Lefebvre, 2007). Male dogs do have minimal renal tubular creatinine secretion, but this does not appear to impact exogenous creatinine clearance measurements (O'Connell et al., 1962; Watson et al., 2002).

The following protocol for exogenous creatinine clearance is adapted from Heiene and Lefebrve (Heiene and Lefebvre, 2007):

1. Fast the dog overnight. This is essential because plasma creatinine may change postprandially (Watson et al., 2002).
2. Provide water during the test; withhold food.
3. Weigh the patient.
4. Take a baseline blood sample for basal creatinine value measurement. Plasma or serum can be collected depending on what your laboratory is equipped to measure.
5. Prepare an 80 mg/mL creatinine solution by dissolving anhydrous creatinine (Sigma–Aldrich) in distilled water or 0.9% saline. Filter sterilize with a 0.2 µm filter.
6. Administer 1 mL/kg creatinine as a bolus via a peripheral IV catheter. Flush with 2 mL saline. Begin timing. Remove the catheter.
7. Sample blood (1 mL) at 10 minutes, 1, 2, 6, and 10 hours after creatinine administration.
8. Measure creatinine of all samples on the analyzer within the same batch for consistency.
9. Determine plasma clearance by dividing the dose by the area under the curve from the plasma creatinine versus time profile with AUC calculated from a noncompartmental approach (Watson et al., 2002). AUC is calculated by the trapezoidal rule (Watson et al., 2002). The reader is referred to the appendix of the article by Watson et al. for an example of this calculation (Watson et al., 2002). In creating the plasma versus time curve, basal values should be subtracted from the measured values of creatinine after administration.

Dogs with severe renal dysfunction may require sampling between 10 and 24 hours for more accurate GFR estimation, but the exact schedule necessary is unknown (Watson et al., 2002). As with determination of iohexol clearance, the accuracy of GFR measurement by exogenous creatinine clearance will be increased by increasing the number of blood samples taken to 10 over a 24-hour period (Watson et al., 2002).

4.5.4.4 Modified Water Deprivation Test (WDT)/ADH Response Test

In dogs with confirmed polyuria and polydipsia, the WDT can be performed as a provocative test of urine-concentrating ability. Administering just oral desmopressin in the absence of the rest of the WDT has been advocated as an alternative test (Syme, 2007). These tests should *only* be performed to distinguish between primary NDI, psychogenic (primary) polydipsia, and central diabetes insipidus (CDI) (Heiene and Lefebvre, 2007). All other causes of polyuria/polydipsia must be ruled out before considering these tests (Syme, 2007). The WDT should not be performed in patients who are azotemic, dehydrated, or have known renal disease or causes of secondary NDI (Heiene and Lefebvre, 2007). Dogs with secondary NDI such as pyelonephritis, hyercalcemia, renal insufficiency, pyometra, and HAC and dogs with partial CDI have similar WDT results (Syme, 2007). If all secondary NDI causes are not ruled out prior to the WDT, it may be impossible to distinguish dogs with secondary NDI from those with partial CDI and the test may cause significant patient morbidity (Nichols, 2001; Syme, 2007). The WDT is difficult to perform, unpleasant for the dog, and potentially dangerous if the dog is not appropriately monitored for signs of dehydration or neurologic signs secondary to hypernatremia (Heiene and Lefebvre 2007; Syme, 2007). Results of the test can also be confusing and inconclusive, especially with partial deficiency syndromes (Feldman and Nelson, 2004).

The WDT works on the principal that if the dog loses 5% body weight due to water deprivation, plasma osmolality will thereby increase sufficiently to stimulate maximal ADH secretion (Syme, 2007). If the kidneys can respond to this ADH stimulus, urine concentration will similarly increase (Feldman and Nelson, 2004). If the dog has normal ADH production, the exogenous ADH administration should not further increase the urine concentration, as the kidney should have been fully stimulated by endogenous ADH (Syme, 2007).

TABLE 4.2

Protocol for the Modified Water Deprivation Test [Adapted from Feldman and Nelson (2004) and Syme (2007)]

Phase I. Preparation for the test

1. Gradually withhold water over 3-5 days. Restrict water to 120 mL/kg/day 72 hours before, to 90 mL/kg/day 48 hours before, and to 60 mL/kg/day 24 hours before the WDT.[a] These volumes of water should be given in 6–8 aliquots through the day.
2. Fast the dog for 12 hours, allow access to water.

Phase II. Water deprivation

1. Withhold food and all water.
2. Place an indwelling urinary catheter (ideally) and empty the urinary bladder.
3. Weigh the patient (exactly).
4. Measure urine specific gravity and osmolality.
5. Take a plasma/serum sample to measure creatinine/BUN and sodium concentration and osmolality.
6. Document the dog's baseline hydration and CNS status.
7. Completely empty the bladder every 1–2 hours.
8. Measure urine osmolality and specific gravity at each interval.
9. Weigh the dog after each urine collection.
10. Recheck serum/ plasma sodium and creatinine/BUN every 2–4 hours.
11. Check the hydration and CNS status each hour.
12. Stop Phase II if:
    a. The dog loses 5% of its body weight
    b. The dog is clinically dehydrated or ill
    c. Urine specific gravity >1.030
    d. Neurologic signs occur
    e. Hypernatremia or azotemia are identified
    f. After 3% body weight loss has occurred, when changes in urine concentration plateau so that there is <5% (or <30 mOsm/kg) increase in urine osmolality between three consecutive determinations, 1 hour apart.[a]
    NOTE. False plateaus can be detected with urine specific gravity; urine osmolality is more reliable.
13. On completion of phase II:
    a. Empty bladder
    b. Measure urine osmolality and specific gravity
    c. Measure plasma/ serum osmolality
    d. Measure plasma/serum creatinine/BUN and sodium

Phase III. Response to exogenous ADH

1. Administer aqueous vasopressin (Pitressin) IM (0.55 U/kg, maximum total dose 5 U).
2. Continue withholding food and water.
3. Empty the bladder every 30 minutes for 2 hours.
4. Measure urine osmolality and specific gravity at each interval.
5. With each urine collection, take serum/plasma for osmolality measurement.
6. Check serum/plasma creatinine/BUN and sodium.
7. Check hydration and CNS status.

Phase IV. Test End

1. Introduce small amounts of water (10–20 mL/kg) every 30 minutes for 2 hours.
2. Monitor for vomiting, check hydration and CNS status. (Acute water overload and cerebral edema can result if water is not reintroduced gradually.)[b]
3. If dog has tolerated water reintroduction, return to ad lib water 2 hours after ending test.

[a] Adapted from DiBartola (2006).

[b] Adapted from Nichols (2001).

TABLE 4.3
Expected Results of the Water Deprivation and ADH Administration Phases of the Modified Water Deprivation Test

Diagnosis	Response to Water Deprivation to 5% Loss Body Weight	Response to ADH Administration Following Water Deprivation
Normal	Urine concentrates to mean peak osmolality of 2,289 mOsm/kg (range 1,768–2,738 mOsm/kg); mean urine SG 1.062 (range 1.050–1.076)[a]	<10% increase in urine osmolality[b]
Psychogenic (primary) polydipsia	Urine concentrates to osmolality > plasma osmolality; urine SG up to 1.030	<10% increase in urine osmolality
Central diabetes insipidus	*Complete CDI*: Urine osmolality does not increase above that of plasma (290–310 mOsm/kg); urine SG < 1.012 *Partial CDI*: Urine osmolality may increase > plasma osmolality; urine SG 1.012–1.020	*Complete CDI*: Urine osmolality increases by 50%–800% of pre-ADH value; urine SG > 1.025 *Partial CDI*: Urine osmolality increases by 10%–50% of pre-ADH value; urine SG > 1.025
Primary nephrogenic diabetes insipidus	Urine osmolality ≤ plasma	No change in urine osmolality/ urine SG

Source: Syme, H.M., In J. Elliott and G.F. Grauer [Eds.], *BSAVA Manual Series*, Quedgeley, British Small Animal Veterinary Association, pp. 8-25, 2007.

Secondary NDI should be excluded before performing the test (see text); results of secondary NDI may overlap with those of partial CDI.SG, specific gravity.

[a] Hardy and Osborne (1979).

[b] Mulnix et al. (1976).

Because dogs with primary polydipsia likely have renal medullary washout, they will not be able to concentrate their urine effectively in the face of water deprivation (Syme, 2007). For this reason, the gradual (modified) WDT is considered superior to the WDT because the associated gradual water deprivation allows time for correction of the medullary washout prior to the WDT (Syme, 2007). In the traditional WDT, dogs with primary polydipsia can be mistakenly identified as having (NDI) due to their medullary washout.

The modified WDT is described in Table 4.2, a protocol adapted from Syme and Feldman and Nelson (Feldman and Nelson, 2004; Syme, 2007). In normal dogs, sufficient dehydration to induce maximal urine concentration usually occurs after a mean of 42 hours, but may not occur until after 96 hours (Hardy and Osborne, 1979). In dogs with polyuria and polydipsia, time until reaching 5% dehydration, that is, the completion of the first phase of the test, may range from a few hours to 12 hours (DiBartola, 2006).

If a dog does not concentrate urine during water deprivation, either the kidneys cannot respond to ADH (NDI) or an ADH deficiency exists (CDI) (Hardy and Osborne, 1979). In dogs with complete CDI, urine osmolality will increase by 50% or more following administration of vasopressin. In the partial forms of central CDI, urine osmolality after vasopressin will increase, though less dramatically (≥10%), and in NDI there will be very little or no rise in urine osmolality (Kooistra and Galac, 2010). Table 4.3 summarizes the expected modified WDT results for each syndrome. Some authors have advocated incorporating plasma vasopressin measurements into phase II of the WDT to improve its accuracy in discriminating between the different disorders affecting urine concentration (Feldman and Nelson, 2004). However, the erratic vasopressin responses to osmolality that have been documented in some dogs make the utility of vasopressin measurement questionable (van Vonderen et al., 2004). One complicating factor in interpreting the WDT in dogs is that psychogenic polydipsia may not be a uniform syndrome in dogs (van Vonderen et al., 1999). Some dogs with psychogenic polydipsia have abnormalities in their vasopressin release and thus have WDT results consistent with partial CDI (van Vonderen et al., 1999; Rijnberk, 2010). Dogs with HAC may also have similar WDT results to those of dogs with psychogenic polydipsia and partial CDI. HAC must be considered in a dog with equivocal WDT results, especially given the greater frequency of HAC compared to the relatively rare CDI, NDI, and psychogenic polydipsia (Feldman and Nelson, 2004).

An alternative to the modified WDT is a response to oral desmopressin, in which dogs receive oral desmopressin (0.05–0.2 mg/dog every 8 hours) for 5–7 days (Syme, 2007). The dog is monitored for resolution of polyuria/polydipsia. Urine specific gravity is evaluated before and after desmopressin treatment. Only dogs with CDI will respond to desmopressin by concentrating their urine to >1.025 SG. Dogs with NDI or primary polydipsia will not respond or respond minimally and cannot be differentiated from each other by this test (Feldman and Nelson, 2004; Syme, 2007). Water intoxication is a potential complication of this test if dogs continue to be polydipsic during the antidiuretic effects of vasopressin (Hardy and Osborne, 1982).

4.6 REFERENCE RANGES IN THE DOG

Analyte		Concentration	Units	Reference
Ammonia	–	45–120	µg/dL	Silverstein and Hopper (2009)
Bile acids	Fasting	<10	µM	Silverstein and Hopper (2009)
	Radioimmunoassay	0.2–4.3	µmol/L	Counsell and Lumsden (1988)
	Enzymatic	0–8.6	µmol/L	
Cardiac troponin I	–	0.00–0.11	ng/mL	Payne et al. (2011)
Cardiac troponin T	–	<0.05	ng/mL	Tarducci et al. (2004)
Gamma-glutamyl transferase(GGT)		1.2–6.4	U/L	Kaneko et al. (2008)
Ornithine carbamyl transferase (OTC)		2.7 (±) 0.7	U/L	Kaneko et al. (2008)
Sorbitol dehydrogenase (SDH)	–	2.9–8.2	U/L	Kaneko et al. (2008)
Thyroid function				
Triiodothyronine (T3)	–	48–154	ng/dL	Silverstein and Hopper (2009)
Thyroxine (T4) serum	–	20–55	nmol/L	Kemppainen and Behrend (2001)
	–	1.5–4.3	µg/dL	Kemppainen and Behrend (2001)
Free T4	Dialysis	10.0–45.0	pmol/L	Kemppainen and Behrend (2001)

(continued)

Analyte		Concentration	Units	Reference
Thyroid stimulating hormone (TSH)	–	<0.5	ng/mL	Kemppainen and Behrend (2001)
	–	0–0.41	ng/mL	Ramsey et al. (1997)
Adrenal function				
Plasma ACTH	–	10–70	pg/mL	Feldman and Nelson (2004)
Resting cortisol	–	13.8–137.9	nmol/L	Klein and Peterson (2010)
		0.5–6.0	µg/dL	Feldman and Nelson (2004)
17-hydroxyprogesterone	–	<0.33–0.63	ng/ml	Ristic (2002)
Pancreatic/Diabetic regulation				
Insulin	–	5–20	U/mL	Feldman and Nelson (2004)
Glucose	–	70–110	mg/dL	Feldman and Nelson (2004)
Fructosamine	–	192.6–357.4	µmol/L	Coppo and Coppo (1997)
	–			
	–			
Parathyroid function				
Total calcium	–	9.0–11.7	mg/dL	Feldman and Nelson (2004)
	–	2.2–3.9	mmol/L	
	–			
Ionized calcium	–	4.6–5.6	mg/dL	Feldman and Nelson (2004)
	–	1.12–1.42	mmol/L	
	–			
Parathyroid hormone (PTH)	–	2–13	pmol/L	Feldman and Nelson (2004)
Parathyroid hormone-related protein (PTH-P)	–	<2	pmol/L	Feldman and Nelson (2004)
	–			
1,25-Dihydroxyvitamin D (Calcitriol)	Adults	20–50	pg/mL	Rosol et al. (2000)
	10–12 week old	60–120	pg/mL	
Reproductive hormones				
Estradiol	–	44.6–120.3	pg/mL	Frank et al. (2010)
	Peak 24 hours prior to LH peak	68.9 (±) 11.0	ng/mL	Nett et al. (1975)
	Basal levels	17.8 (±) 6.3	ng/mL	

(*continued*)

Analyte		Concentration	Units	Reference
Luteinizing hormone (LH)	Proestrus	2.8 (±) 0.1	ng/mL	Nett et al. (1975)
	Early estrus	35.5 (±) 10.0	ng/mL	
	Early diestrus	2.2 (±) 0.1	ng/mL	
	Intact male	0.2–12.0	ng/mL	DePalatis et al. (1978)
	Castrated male	9.8 (±) 2.7	ng/mL	
	Male Beagles	4.6 (±) 2.7	ng/mL	Urhausen et al. (2009)
Progesterone	Proestrus	1.7 (±) 0.3	ng/mL	Nett et al. (1975)
	Early estrus	3.5 (±) 0.3	ng/mL	
	Day 5 after LH peak	23.3 (±) 2.8	ng/mL	
	One day prior to whelping	3.3 (±) 1.2	ng/mL	
	Day of whelping	1.1 (±) 0.2	ng/mL	
Prolactin	Male	<6.0	ng/mL	Corrada et al. (2006)
	Male beagles	3.8 (±) 0.9	ng/mL	Urhausen et al. (2009)
Testosterone	Intact male	0.4 - 6.0	ng/mL	DePalatis et al. (1978)
	Castrated male	Undetectable		
Gastrointestinal absorption and digestion				
Cobalamin	–	284–836	ng/L	Silverstein and Hopper (2009)
Folate	–	7.5–17.5	µg/dL	Silverstein and Hopper (2009)
Iron	–	94–122	µg/dL	Silverstein and Hopper (2009)
	–			
Pepsin-like immunoreactivity (PLI)	–	4.4–276.1	µg/L	Silverstein and Hopper (2009)
Trypsin-like immunoreactivity (TLI)	–	5–35	µg/L	Silverstein and Hopper (2009)
Serum gastrin	–	<100	pg/mL	Altschul et al. (1997)
		10–40	pg/mL	Green and Gartrell (1997)

(continued)

Because methodologies and analyzers may vary, it is best to use the reference ranges of the reference laboratory generating the results.

REFERENCES

Acland, G.M., Aguirre, G.D., Ray, J. et al. 2001. Gene therapy restores vision in a canine model of childhood blindness. *Nat Genet.* 28(1): 92–95.

Allen, D.G. and Whitehead, N.P. 2011. Duchenne muscular dystrophy—What causes the increased membrane permeability in skeletal muscle? *Int J Biochem Cell Biol.* 43(3): 290–294.

Altschul, M., Simpson, K.W., Dykes, N.L., Mauldin, E.A., Reubi, J.C., and Cummings, J.F. 1997. Evaluation of somatostatin analogues for the detection and treatment of gastrinoma in a dog. *J Sm Anim Pract.* 38:286.

Andrews, E.J., Ward, B.C., and Altman, N.H. Eds. 1979. *Spontaneous Animal Models of Human Disease*, Vol. 1 and 2. New York, NY: Academic Press.

Arakawa, K., Suzuki, H., Naitoh, M., et al. 1996. Role of adenosine in the renal responses to contrast medium. *Kidney Int.* 49(5):1199–206.

Ashtari, M., Cyckowski, L.L., Monroe, J.F., et al. 2011. The human visual cortex responds to gene therapy-mediated recovery of retinal function. *J Clin Invest.* 121(6):2160–2168.

Bain, P.J. 2003. Liver. In *Duncan & Prasse's Veterinary Laboratory Medicine: Clinical Pathology*. Eds. K.S. Latimer, E.A. Mahaffey, K.W. Prasse, and J.R. Duncan, pp. 193–213. Ames, IA: Iowa State Press.

Balkman, C.E., Center, S.A., Randolph, J.F., et al. 2003. Evaluation of urine sulfated and nonsulfated bile acids as a diagnostic test for liver disease in dogs. *J Am Vet Med Assoc.* 222(10):1368–1375.

Baltzer, W.I., Calise, D.V., Levine, J.M., et al. 2007. Dystrophin-deficient muscular dystrophy in a Weimaraner. *J Am Anim Hosp Assoc.* 43:227–232.

Battersby, I.A., Giger, U., and Hall, E.J. 2005. Hyperammonaemic encephalopathy secondary to selective cobalamin deficiency in a juvenile Border collie. *J Small Anim Pract.* 46(7):339–344.

Behrend, E.N., Kemppainen, R.J., and Young, D.W. 1998. Effect of storage conditions on cortisol, total thyroxine, and free thyroxine concentrations in serum and plasma of dogs. *J Am Vet Med Assoc.* 212(10):1564–1568.

Behrend, E.N. and Kennis, R. 2010. Atypical Cushing's syndrome in dogs: Arguments for and against. *Vet Clin North Am Small Anim Pract.* 40(2):285–296.

Benitah, N., Feldman, E.C., Kass, P.H., and Nelson, R.W. 2005. Evaluation of serum 17-hydroxyprogesterone concentration after administration of ACTH in dogs with hyperadrenocorticism. *J Am Vet Med Assoc.* 227(7):1095–1101.

Berent, A.C. and Tobias, K.M. 2009. Portosystemic vascular anomalies. *Vet Clin North Am Small Anim Pract.* 39(3):513–541.

Berent, A.C. and Weisse, C. 2010. Hepatic vascular anomalies. In *Textbook of Veterinary Internal Medicine: Diseases of the Dog and the Cat.* Eds. S.J. Ettinger and E.C. Feldman, pp. 1649–1672. St. Louis, MO: Elsevier Saunders.

Bertolucci, C., Fazio, F., and Piccione, G. 2008. Daily rhythms of serum lipids in dogs: Influences of lighting and fasting cycles. *Comp Med.* 58(5):485–489.

Bexfield, N.H., Heiene, R., Gerritsen, J., et al. 2008. Glomerular filtration rate estimated by 3-sample plasma clearance of iohexol in 118 healthy dogs. *J Vet Intern Med.* 22(1):66–73.

Blais, M.C., Berman, L., Oakley, D.A., and Giger, U. 2007. Canine Dal blood type: A red cell antigen lacking in some Dalmatians. *J Vet Int Med.* 21(2):281–286.

Blais, M.C., Rozanski, E.A., Hale, A.S., Shaw, S.P., and Cotter, S.M. 2009. Lack of evidence of pregnancy-induced alloantibodies in dogs. *J Vet Int Med.* 23(3):462–465.

Boretti, F.S, Sieber-Ruckstuhl, N.S., Favrot, C., et al. 2006. Evaluation of recombinant human thyroid-stimulating hormone to test thyroid function in dogs suspected of having hypothyroidism. *Am J Vet Res.* 67(12):2012–2016.

Boretti, F.S, Sieber-Ruckstuhl, N.S., Wenger-Riggenbach, B., et al. 2009. Comparison of 2 doses of recombinant human thyrotropin for thyroid function testing in healthy and suspected hypothyroid dogs. *J Vet Int Med.* 23(4):856–861.

Breen, M. and Modiano, J.F. 2008. Evolutionarily conserved cytogenetic changes in hematological malignancies of dogs and humans—Man and his best friend share more than companionship. *Chromosome Res.* 16(1):145–154.

Bridger, N., Glanemann, B., and Neiger, R. 2008. Comparison of postprandial and ceruletide serum bile acid stimulation in dogs. *J Vet Int Med.* 22(4):873–878.

Brown, S.A. and Finco, D.R. 1992. Characterization of the renal response to protein ingestion in dogs with experimentally induced renal failure. *Am J Vet Res.* 53(4):569–573.

Brown, S.C. and O'Reilly, P.H. 1991. Iohexol clearance for the determination of glomerular filtration rate in clinical practice: Evidence for a new gold standard. *J Urol.* 146(3):675–679.

Buchanan, J.W. 1999. Prevalence of cardiovascular disorders. In *Textbook of Canine and Feline Cardiology. Principles and Clinical Practice*. Ed. P.R. Fox, D. Sisson, and N.S. Moise, pp. 457–470. Philadelphia, PA: WB Saunders.

Callan, M.B., Aljamali, M.N., Margaritis, P. et al. 2006. A novel missense mutation responsible for factor VII deficiency in research Beagle colonies. *J Thromb Hemost.* 4(12):2616–2622.

Center, S.A. 1993. Serum bile acids in companion animal medicine. *Vet Clin North Am Small Anim Pract.* 23(3):625–657.

Center, S.A. 2003. *Portosystemic Shunts in the Dog and Cat., Block V Class Notes.* Cornell University College of Veterinary Medicine, Ithaca, NY.

Center, S.A., ManWarren, T., Slater, M.R., and Wilentz, E. 1991. Evaluation of twelve-hour preprandial and two-hour postprandial serum bile acids concentrations for diagnosis of hepatobiliary disease in dogs. *J Am Vet Med Assoc.* 199(2):217–226.

Chapman, R.W. 2008. Canine models of asthma and COPD. *Pul Pharmacol Ther.* 21(5):731–742.

Chastain, C.B., Franklin, R.T., Ganjam, V.K., and Madsen, R.W. 1986. Evaluation of the hypothalamic pituitary-adrenal axis in clinically stressed dogs. *J Am Anim Hosp Assoc.* 22:435–442.

Clark, J.D., Rager, D.R., and Calpin, J.P. 1997. Animal well-being II. Stress and distress. *Lab Anim Sci.* 47:571–579.

Cochran, S.T. 2005. Anaphylactoid reactions to radiocontrast media. *Curr Allergy Asthma Rep.* 5(1):28–31.

Cook, A.K. 2011. *Atypical Cushing's. Proceedings of the AAHA/OVMA Conference*, Toronto, Ontario. CD ROM.

Coppo, J.A. and Coppo, N.B. 1997. Serum fructosamine: A reference interval for a heterogeneous canine population. *Vet Res Commun.* 21(7):471–476.

Corrada, Y., Rimoldi, I., Arreseigor, S., et al. 2006. Prolactin reference range and pulsatility in male dogs. *Theriogenology.* 66:1599–1602.

Counsell, L.J. and Lumdsen, J.H. 1988. Serum bile acids: Reference values in healthy dogs and comparison of two kit methods. *Vet Clin Pathol.* 17:71–74.

Cunningham, J.G. Ed. 1997. *Textbook of Veterinary Physiology*. Philadelphia, PA: WB Saunders.

Daminet, S., Fifle, L., Paradis, M., Duchateau, L., and Moreau, M. 2007. Use of recombinant human thyroid-stimulating hormone for thyrotropin stimulation test in healthy, hypothyroid and euthyroid sick dogs. *Can Vet J.* 48(12):1273–1279.

Davainis, G., Meurs, K., and Wright, N. 2004. The relationship of resting S-T segment depression to the severity of subvalvular aortic stenosis and the presence of ventricular premature complexes in the dog. *J Am Anim Hosp Assoc.* 40:20–23.

DePalatis, L., Moore, J., and Falvo, R.E. 1978. Plasma concentrations of testosterone and LH in the male dog. *J Reprod Fert.* 52:201–207.

De Roover, K., Duchateau, L., Carmichael, N., van Geffen, C., and Daminet, S. 2006. Effect of storage of reconstituted recombinant human thyroid-stimulating hormone (rhTSH) on thyroid-stimulating hormone (TSH) response testing in euthyroid dogs. *J Vet Int Med.* 20(4):812–817.

Diaz-Espineira, M.M., Galac, S., Mol, J.A., Rijnberk, A., and Kooistra, H.S. 2008. Thyrotropin-releasing hormone-induced growth hormone secretion in dogs with primary hypothyroidism. *Domest Anim Endocrinol.* 34(2):176–181.

Diaz Espineira, M.M., Mol, J.A., Peeters, M.E., et al. 2007. Assessment of thyroid function in dogs with low plasma thyroxine concentration. *J Vet Int Med.* 21(1):25–32.

DiBartola, S.P. 2006. Disorders of sodium and water: Hypernatremia and hyponatremia. In *Fluid, Electrolyte, and Acid-Base Disorders in Small Animal Practice.* Ed. S.P. DiBartola, pp. 47–79. St. Louis, MO: Saunders Elsevier.

DiBartola, S.P. 2010. Clinical approach and laboratory evaluation of renal disease. In *Textbook of Veterinary Internal Medicine: Diseases of the Dog and the Cat.* Eds. S.J. Ettinger and E.C. Feldman, pp. 1955–1969. St. Louis, MO: Elsevier Saunders.

Dressman, J.B. 1986. Comparison of canine and human gastrointestinal physiology. *Pharm Res.* 3(3):123–131.

Dukes-McEwan, J., Borgarelli, M., Tidholm, A., et al. 2003. Proposed guidelines for the diagnosis of canine idiopathic dilated cardiomyopathy. *J Vet Cardiol.* 5(2):7–19.

Dysko, R.C., Nemzek, J.A., Levin, S.I., et al. 2002. Biology and diseases of dogs. In *Laboratory Animal Medicine.* Eds. J.G. Fox, L.C. Anderson, F.M. Loew, and F.W. Quimby, pp. 395–458. San Diego, CA: Academic Press.

Ellinwood, N.M., Vite, C.H., and Haskins, M.E. 2004. Gene therapy for lysosomal storage diseases: The lessons and promise of animal models. *J Gene Med.* 6:481–506.

Elliott, D. and Schenck, P.A. 2010. Dietary and medical considerations in hyperlipidemia. In *Textbook of Veterinary Internal Medicine: Diseases of the Dog and the Cat.* Eds. S.J. Ettinger and E.C. Feldman, Vol. 1, pp. 710–715. St. Louis, MO: Elsevier Saunders.

Engelking, L.R. 2002. *Review of Veterinary Physiology.* Chap. 140 and 141, pp. 585–599. Jackson, MI: Teton New Media.

Evans, G.O. Ed. 2009. *Animal Clinical Chemistry: A Practical Handbook for Toxicologists and Biomedical Researchers.* Boca Raton, FL: CRC Press, Taylor & Francis Group.

Feldman, E. 2009. *Diagnosis & Treatment of Canine Cushing's I: Diagnosis of Hyperadrenocorticism (Cushing's Syndrome) in Dogs—Which Tests are Best? Proceedings of the Western Veterinary Conference*, Las Vegas, NV. Available at: http://www.vin.com/Members/Proceedings/Proceedings.plx?CID=wvc2009&PID=pr50766&O=VIN (Accessed 4 July, 2011).

Feldman, E.C. and Nelson, R.W. 1996. *Canine and Feline Endocrinology and Reproduction*. Philadelphia, PA: Saunders.

Feldman, E.C. and Nelson, R.W. 2004. *Canine and Feline Endocrinology and Reproduction*. St. Louis, MO: WB Saunders.

Fillman-Holliday, D. and Landi, M.S. 2002. Animal care best practices for regulatory testing. *ILAR J.* 43(Suppl_1):S49–S58.

Fleischer, S., Sharkey, M., Mealey, K., et al. 2008. Pharmacogenetic and metabolic differences between dog breeds: Their impact on canine medicine and use of the dog as a preclinical model. *Am Assoc Pharm Sci J.* 10(1):110–119.

Frank, L.A. 1996. Comparison of thyrotropin-releasing hormone (TRH) to thyrotropin (TSH) stimulation for evaluating thyroid function in dogs. *J Am Vet Med Assoc.* 32(6):481–487.

Frank, L.A., Mullins, R., and Rohrbach, B.W. 2010. Variability of estradiol concentration in normal dogs. *Vet Dermatol.* 21:490–493.

Frank, L.A. and Oliver, J.W. 1998. Comparison of serum cortisol concentrations in clinically normal dogs after administration of freshly reconstituted versus reconstituted and stored frozen cosyntropin. *J Am Vet Med Assoc.* 212(10):1569–1571.

Fukuda, S. 1990. Circadian rhythm of serum testosterone levels in male beagle dogs—Effects of lightning time zone. *Exp Anim.* 39(1):65–68

Garber, C.C. and Carey, R.N. 1984. Evaluation methods. In *Clinical Chemistry—Theory, Analysis and Correlation*. Eds. L.A. Kaplan and A.J. Pesce, pp. 338–359. St. Louis, MO: CV Mosby.

Gay, W.I. 1984. Health benefits of animal research. *Physiologist.* 27(3):133–141.

Gerritzen-Bruning, M.J., van den Ingh, T.S., and Rothuizen, J. 2006. Diagnostic value of fasting plasma ammonia and bile acid concentrations in the identification of portosystemic shunting in dogs. *J Vet Int Med.* 20(1):13–19.

Goy-Thollot, I., Besse, S., Garnier, F., Marignan, M., and Barthez, P.Y. 2006. Simplified methods for estimation of plasma clearance of iohexol in dogs and cats. *J Vet Int Med.* 20(1):52–56.

Green, R.A. and Gartrell, C.L. 1997. Gastrinoma: A retrospective study of four cases (1985–1995). *J Am Anim Hosp Assoc.* 33:524.

Hall, R.L. 2006. Animal models in toxicology. In *Clinical Pathology of Laboratory Animals*. Ed. S.C. Gad, 2nd edition, Chap. 12, pp. 787–830. Boca Raton, FL: CRC Press.

Hall, R.L. and Everds, N.E. 2007. Priniciples of clinical pathology for toxicology studies. In *Principles and Methods of Toxicology.* Ed. A.W. Hayes, 5th edition. Philadelphia, PA: CRC Press.

Hansen, B.L., Kemppainen, R.J., and MacDonald, J.M. 1994. Synthetic ACTH (cosyntropin) stimulation tests in normal dogs: Comparison of intravenous and intramuscular administration. *J Am Vet Med Assoc.* 30:38–41.

Hardy, R.M. and Osborne, C.A. 1979. Water deprivation test in the dog: Maximal normal values. *J Am Vet Med Assoc.* 174(5):479–483.

Hardy, R.M. and Osborne, C.A. 1982. Reposital vasopressin response test in clinically normal dogs undergoing water diuresis: Technique and results. *Am J Vet Res.* 43(11):1991–1993.

Harvey, S.J., Zheng, K., Jefferson, B., et al. 2003. Transfer of the alpha 5(IV) collagen chain gene to smooth muscle restores in vivo expression of the alpha 6(IV) collagen chain in a canine model of Alport syndrome. *Am J Pathol.* 162(3):873–885.

Heiene, R., Eliassen, K.A., Risoen, U., Neal, L.A., and Cowgill, L.D. 2010. Glomerular filtration rate in dogs as estimated via plasma clearance of inulin and iohexol and use of limited-sample methods. *Am J Vet Res.* 71(9):1100–1107.

Heiene, R. and Lefebvre, H.P. 2007. Assessment of renal function. *BSAVA Manual of Canine and Feline Nephrology and Urology*. Eds. J. Elliott and G.F. Grauer, pp. 117–125. Quedgeley: British Small Animal Veterinary Association.

Heiene, R. and Moe, L. 1998. Pharmacokinetic aspects of measurement of glomerular filtration rate in the dog: A review. *J Vet Int Med.* 12(6):401–414.

Heiene, R. and Moe, L. 1999. The relationship between some plasma clearance methods for estimation of glomerular filtration rate in dogs with pyometra. *J Vet Int Med.* 13(6):587–596.

Hirsjarvi, P. and Junnila, M. 1986. Happy rats-reliable results. *Acta Physiol Scand.* 128(Suppl 554):32.

Hitt, M.E. and Jones, B.D. 1986. Effects of storage temperature and time on canine plasma ammonia concentrations. *Am J Vet Res.* 47(2):363–364.

Hohenhaus, A.E. 2004. Importance of blood groups and blood group antibodies in companion animals. *Transfus Med Rev.* 18(2):117–126.

Horber, F.F., Krayer, S., Rehder, K., and Haymond, M.W. 1988. Anesthesia with halothane and nitrous oxide alters protein and amino acid metabolism in dogs. *Anesthesiology.* 69:319–326.

Hubrecht, R.C., Serpell, J.A., and Poole, T.B. 1992. Correlates of pen size and housing conditions on the behaviour of kennelled dogs. *Appl Anim Behav Sci.* 34(4):365–383.

Hughes, H.C., Campbell, S., and Kenney, C. 1989. The effects of cage size and pair housing on exercise of beagle dogs. *Lab Anim Sci.* 39(4):302–305.

Hunter, M.J., Zhao, H., Tuschong, L.M., et al. Gene therapy for canine leukocyte adhesion deficiency with lentiviral vectors using the murine stem cell virus and human phosphoglycerate kinase promoters. *Hum Gene Ther.* 22(6):689–696.

Ikeda-Douglas, C.J., de Rivera, C., and Milgram, N.W. 2005. Pharmaceutical and other commercial uses of the dog model. *Prog Neuro-Psychopharmacol Biol Psychiatry.* 29:355–360.

Institute of Laboratory Animal Resources. 1994. *Laboratory Animal Management: Dogs.* Washington, DC: National Academies Press.

Ishihara, H., Kallus, F.T., Giesecke, A.H., Jr. 1981. Intravenous glucose tolerance test during anaesthesia in dogs: Insulin response and glucose clearance. *Can Anaesth Soc J.* 28:381–386.

Johnson, M.C. 2005. Hyperlipidemia disorders in dogs. *Comp Cont Educ Pract.* 27:361–371.

Kaae, J.A., Callanand, M.B., and Brooks, M.B. 2007. Hereditary factor VII deficiency in the Alaskan Klee Kai dog. *J Vet Int Med.* 21(5):976–981.

Kaplan, A.J., Peterson, M.E., and Kemppainen, R.J. 1995. Effects of disease on the results of diagnostic tests for use in detecting hyperadrenocorticism in dogs. *J Am Vet Med Assoc.* 207(4):445–451.

Kaneko, J.J., Harvey, J.W., and Bruss, M. 2008. *Clinical Biochemistry of Domestic Animals.* Amsterdam: Academic Press/Elsevier.

Kaspar, L.V. and Norris, W.P. 1977. Serum chemistry values of normal dogs (beagles): Associations with age, sex, and family line. *Lab Anim Sci.* 27:980–985.

Keller, P. and Wall, M. 1982. Plasma enzyme activity in the dog. Effects of age and sex. *Schweiz Arch Tierheilkd.* 124:83–95.

Kemppainen, R.J. and Behrend, E.N. 2001. Diagnosis of canine hypothyroidism. Perspectives from a testing laboratory. *Vet Clin North Am Small Anim Pract.* 31(5):951–962, vii.

Kemppainen, R.J., Behrend, E.N., and Busch, K.A. 2005. Use of compounded adrenocorticotropic hormone (ACTH) for adrenal function testing in dogs. *J Am Anim Hosp Assoc.* 41(6):368–372.

Kerl, M.E., Peterson, M.E., Wallace, M.S., Melian, C., and Kemppainen, R.J. 1999. Evaluation of a low-dose synthetic adrenocorticotropic hormone stimulation test in clinically normal dogs and dogs with naturally developing hyperadrenocorticism. *J Am Vet Med Assoc.* 214(10):1497–1501.

Kessler, R.J., Reese, J., Chang, D., et al. 2010. Dog erythrocyte antigens 1.1, 1.2, 3, 4, 7, and Dal blood typing and cross-matching by gel column technique. *Vet Clin Pathol.* 39(3):306–316.

Klein, S.C. and Peterson, M.E. 2010. Canine hypoadrenocorticism: Part II. *Can Vet J.* 51(2):179–184.

Kley S., Tschudi, P., Busato, A., and Gaschen, F. 2003. Establishing canine clinical chemistry reference values for the Hitachi ® 912 using the International Federation of Clinical Chemistry (IFCC) recommendations. *Comp Clin Pathol.* 12(2):106–112.

Knudsen, T., Kristensen, A.T., Sorensen, B.B., et al. 2010. Characterization of canine coagulation factor VII and its complex formation with tissue factor: Canine-human cross-species compatibility. *J Thromb Haemost.* 8(8):1763–1772.

Kohn, D.F. 1995. Dogs. In *The Experimental Animal in Biomedical Research.* Ed. B.E. Rollin, vol. 2, pp. 435–455. Boca Raton, FL: CRC Press.

Kooistra, H.S. and Galac, S. 2010. Recent advances in the diagnosis of Cushing's syndrome in dogs. *Vet Clin North Am Small Anim Pract.* 40(2):259–267.

Kraft, W., Hartmann, K., and Dereser, R. 1995. Dependency on age of laboratory values in dogs and cats. 1. Enzyme activities in blood serum. *Tierärztl Prax.* 23:502–508.

Kuhn, G., Lichtwald, K., Hardegg, W., and Abel, H.H. 1991. The effect of transportation stress on circulating corticsteroids, enzyme activities and hematological values in laboratory dogs. *J Exp Anim Sci.* 34:99–104.

Laroute, V., Chetboul, V., Roche, L., et al. 2005. Quantitative evaluation of renal function in healthy Beagle puppies and mature dogs. *Res Vet Sci.* 79(2):161–167.

Lathan, P., Moore, G.E., Zambon, S., and Scott-Moncrieff, J.C. 2008. Use of a low-dose ACTH stimulation test for diagnosis of hypoadrenocorticism in dogs. *J Vet Int Med.* 22(4):1070–1073.

Lawler, D.F., Larson, B.T., Ballam, J.M. et al., 2008. Diet restriction and ageing in the dog: Major observations over two decades. *Br J Nutr.* 99(4):793–805.

Lennon, E.M., Boyle, T.E., Hutchins, R.G., et al. 2007. Use of basal serum or plasma cortisol concentrations to rule out a diagnosis of hypoadrenocorticism in dogs: 123 cases (2000–2005). *J Am Vet Med Assoc.* 231(3):413–416.

Loeb, W.F. 1999. The dog. In *Clinical Chemistry of Laboratory Animals.* Eds. W.F. Loeb and F.W. Quimby, pp. 85–102. Philadelphia, PA: Taylor & Francis.

Lothrop, C.D., Jr., Tamas, P.M., and Fadok, V.A. 1984. Canine and feline thyroid function assessment with the thyrotropin-releasing hormone response test. *Am J Vet Res.* 45(11):2310–2313.

Loveridge, G.G, 1998. Environmentally enriched dog housing. *Appl Anim Behav Sci.* 59:101–113.

Macpherson, R., Scherer, J., Ross, M.L., et al. 1999. Factor VII deficiency in a mixed breed dog. *J Can Vet.* 40:503–505.

Marsella, R. and Girolomoni, G. 2009. Canine models of atopic dermatitis: A useful tool with untapped potential. *J Invest Dermatol.* 129:2351–2357.

Martinez, M.N. and Papich, M.G. 2009. Factors influencing the gastric residence of dosage forms in dogs. *J Pharm Sci.* 98(3):844–860.

Matsuzawa, T., Nomura, M., and Uno, T. 1993. Clinical pathology reference ranges of laboratory animals. Working Group II, Nonclinical Safety Evaluation Subcommittee of the Japan Pharmaceutical Manufacturers Association. *J Vet Med Sci.* 55(3):351–362.

Maxwell, S.E. and Delaney, H.D. 1985. Measurement and statistics: An examination of construct validity. *Psychol Bull.* 97:85–93.

McGuill, W.M. and Rowan, A.N. 1989. Biological effects of blood loss: Implications for sampling volumes and techniques. *Inst Lab Anim Res News.* 31(4):5–20.

Melian, C., Perez-Alenza, M.D., and Peterson, M.E. 2010. Hyperadrenocorticism in dogs. In *Textbook of Veterinary Internal Medicine: Diseases of the Dog and the Cat.* Eds. S.J. Ettinger and E.C. Feldman, Vol. 2, pp. 1816–1840. St. Louis, MO: Elsevier Saunders.

Meunier, L.D. 2006. Selection, acclimation, training, and preparation of dogs for the research setting. *J Inst Lab Anim Res.* 47:326–347.

Meyer, D.J., Strombeck, D.R., Stone, E.A., Zenoble, R.D., and Buss, D.D. 1978. Ammonia tolerance test in clinically normal dogs and in dogs with portosystemic shunts. *J Am Vet Med Assoc.* 173(4):377–379.

Mohammed, S.I., Craig, B.A., Mutsaers, A.J., et al. 2003. Effects of the cyclooxygenase inhibitor, piroxicam, in combination with chemotherapy on tumor response, apoptosis, and angiogenesis in a canine model of human invasive urinary bladder cancer. *Mol Cancer Ther.* 2(2):183–188.

Moïse, N.S. 1999. Inherited arrhythmias in the dog: Potential experimental models of cardiac disease. *Cardiovasc Res.* 44:37–46.

Morris, J.G. and Rogers, Q.R. 2000. Nutrition of healthy dogs and cats in various stages of adult life. In *Textbook of Veterinary Internal Medicine: Diseases of the Dog and Cat.* Eds. S.J. Ettinger and E.C. Feldman, Vol. 1, pp. 236–240. Philadelphia, PA: WB Saunders.

Morris, J.G., Rogers, Q.R., and Fascetti, A.J. 2005. Nutrition of healthy dogs and cats in various stages of adult life. In *Textbook of Veterinary Internal Medicine: Diseases of the Dog and Cat.* Eds. S.J. Ettinger and E.C. Feldman, Vol. 1, pp. 555–560. Philadelphia: WB Saunders.

Morton, D.B., Abbot, D., Barclay, R., et al. 1993. Removal of blood from laboratory animals and birds. First report of the BVA/FRAME/RSPCA/UFAW Joint Working Group on Refinement. *Lab Anim.* 27:1–22.

Mulnix, J.A., Rijnberk, A., and Hendriks, H.J. 1976. Evaluation of a modified water-deprivation test for diagnosis of polyuric disorders in dogs. *J Am Vet Med Assoc.* 169(12):1327–1330.

Nakamura, A. and Takeda, S. 2011. Mammalian models of Duchenne Muscular Dystrophy: Pathological characteristics and therapeutic applications. *J Biomed Biotechnol.* 2011:184393.

Nett, T.M., Akbar, A.M., Phemister, R.D., et al. 1975. Levels of luteinizing hormone, estradiol and progesterone in serum during the estrous cycle and pregnancy in the beagle bitch. *Proc Soc Exp Biol Med.* 148:134–139.

Nichols, R. 2001. Polyuria and polydipsia. Diagnostic approach and problems associated with patient evaluation. *Vet Clin North Am Small Anim Pract.* 31(5):833–844, v.

Nichols, T.C., Dillow, A.M., Franck, H.W., et al. 2009. Protein replacement therapy and gene transfer in canine models of hemophilia A, hemophilia B, von willebrand disease, and factor VII deficiency. *J Inst Lab Anim Res.* 50(2):144–167.

NRC (National Research Council).. 1994. *Laboratory Animal Management Dogs.* Washington, DC: National Academy Press.

NRC (National Research Council).. 1996. *Guide for the Care and Use of Laboratory Animals.* 7th edition. Washington, DC: National Academy Press.

Obernier, J.A. and Baldwin, R.L. 2006. Establishing an appropriate period of acclimation following transportation of laboratory animals. National Research Council. *ILAR J.* 47(4):364–369.

O'Connell, J.B., Romeo, J.A., and Mudge, G.H. 1962. Renal tubular secretion of creatinine in the dog. *Am J Physiol.* 203(6):985–990.

Paoloni, M. and Khanna, C. 2008. Translation of new cancer treatments from pet dogs to humans. *Nat Rev Cancer.* 8(2):147–156.

Papich, M.G. 2007. *Saunders Handbook of Veterinary Drugs.* St. Louis, MO: Saunders Elsevier.

Parker, H.G., Shearin, A.L., and Ostrander, E.A. 2010. Man's best friend becomes best in show:Genomeanalyses in the domestic dog. *Annu Rev Genet.* 44:309–336.

Patterson, D.F., Haskins, M.E., and Ma Schnarr, W.R. 1981. Hereditary dysplasia of the pulmonary valve in beagle dogs: Pathologic and genetic studies. *Am J Cardiol.* 47(3):631–641.

Payne, E.E., Roberts, B.K., Schroeder, N., Burk, R.L., and Schermerhorn, T. 2011. Assessment of a point-of-care cardiac troponin I test to differentiate cardiac from noncardiac causes of respiratory distress in dogs. *J Vet Emerg Crit Care.* 21(3):217–225.

Peterson, M.E., Kintzer, P.P., and Kass, P.H. 1996. Pretreatment clinical and laboratory findings in dogs with hypoadrenocorticism: 225 cases (1979–1993). *J Am Vet Med Assoc.* 208(1):85–91.

Prescott, M.J., Morton, D.B., Anderson, D., et al. 2004. Refining dog husbandry and care. *Lab Anim.* 38(Suppl 1):1–96.

Prytz, B., Grossi, C.E., and Rousselot, L.M. 1970. In vitro formation of ammonia in blood of dog and man. *Clin Chem.* 16(4):277–279.

Randell, S.C., Hill, R.C., Scott, K.C., Omori, M., and Burrows, C.F. 2001. Intestinal permeability testing using lactulose and rhamnose: a comparison between clinically normal cats and dogs and between dogs of different breeds. *Res Vet Sci.* 71(1):45–49.

Ramsey, I.K., Evans, H., and Herrtage, M.E. 1997. Thyroid-stimulating hormone and total thyroxine concentrations in euthyroid, sick euthyroid and hypothyroid dogs. *J Small Anim Pract.* 38(12):540–545.

Reilly, J. 1998. Variables in animal based research: Part 2. Variability associated with experimental conditions and techniques. Australian and New Zealand Council for the Care of Animals in Research and Teaching (ANZCCART) News 11, Insert 1–12. Available at: http://www.adelaide.edu.au/ANZCCART/

Reine, N.J. and Langston, C.E. 2005. Urinalysis interpretation: How to squeeze out the maximum information from a small sample. *Clin Tech Small Anim Prac.* 20(1):2–10.

Rijnberk, A. 2010. Diabetes insipidus. In *Textbook of Veterinary Internal Medicine: Diseases of the Dog and the Cat.* Eds. S.J. Ettinger and E.C. Feldman, Vol. 2, pp. 1716–1722. St. Louis, MO: Elsevier Saunders.

Rijnberk, A., van Wees, A., and Mol, J.A. 1988. Assessment of two tests for the diagnosis of canine hyperadrenocorticism. *Vet Rec.* 122(8):178–180.

Ristic, J.M., Ramsey, I.K., Heath, E.M., Evans, H.J., and Herrtage, M.E. 2002. The use of 17-hydroxyprogesterone in the diagnosis of canine hyperadrenocorticism. *J Vet Intern Med.* 16:433.

Rosol, T.J., Chew, D.J., Nagode, L.A., et al. 2000. Disorders of calcium. In *Fluid Therapy in Small Animal Practice.* Ed. S.P. DiBartola, 2nd edition, pp 108–162. Philadelphia, PA: WB Saunders.

Rothuizen, J. and van den Ingh, T.S. 1982. Rectal ammonia tolerance test in the evaluation of portal circulation in dogs with liver disease. *Res Vet Sci.* 33(1):22–25.

Rowell, J.L., McCarthy, D.O., and Alvarez, C.E. 2011. Dog models of naturally occurring cancer. *Trends Mol Med.* 17(7):380–388.

Ruaux, C.G., Steiner, J.M., and Williams, D.A. 2002. Postprandial changes in serum unconjugated bile acid concentrations in healthy beagles. *Am J Vet Res.* 63(6):789–793.

Ruland, K., Fischer, A., and Hartmann, K. 2010. Sensitivity and specificity of fasting ammonia and serum bile acids in the diagnosis of portosystemic shunts in dogs and cats. *Vet Clin Pathol.* 39(1):57–64.

Sagawa, K. and Sutton, S. 2006. GI physiology: Species comparison. In Abstract from *American Association of Pharmaceutical Scientists Annual Meeting*. San Antonio, TX.

Sampaolesi, M., Blot, S., D'Antona, G., et al. 2006. Mesoangioblast stem cells ameliorate muscle function in dystrophic dogs. *Nature.* 444(7119):574–579.

Sanecki, R.K., Hoffmann, W.E., Hansen, R., et al. 1993. Quantification of bone alkaline phosphatase in canine serum. *Vet Clin Pathol.* 22:17–23.

Scott-Moncrieff, J.C. 2010a. Hypoadrenocorticism. In *Textbook of Veterinary Internal Medicine : Diseases of the Dog and the Cat.* Eds. S.J. Ettinger and E.C. Feldman, Vol. 2, pp. 1847–1857. St. Louis, MO: Elsevier Saunders.

Scott-Moncrieff, J.C. 2010b. Hypothyroidism. In *Textbook of Veterinary Internal Medicine: Diseases of the Dog and the Cat.* Eds. S.J. Ettinger and E.C. Feldman, Vol. 2, pp. 1751–1761. St. Louis, MO: Elsevier Saunders.

Scott-Moncrieff, J.C. and Nelson, R.W. 1998a. Change in serum thyroid-stimulating hormone concentration in response to administration of thyrotropin-releasing hormone to healthy dogs, hypothyroid dogs, and euthyroid dogs with concurrent disease. *J Am Vet Med Assoc.* 213(10):1435–1438.

Scott-Moncrieff, J.C., Nelson, R.W., Bruner, J.M., and Williams, D.A. 1998b. Comparison of serum concentrations of thyroid-stimulating hormone in healthy dogs, hypothyroid dogs, and euthyroid dogs with concurrent disease. *J Am Vet Med Assoc.* 212(3):387–391.

Scott-Montcrieff, J. 2010. *Hyperadrenocorticism in the Dog & Cat: Clinical Presentation & Diagnosis. Proceedings of the ACVIM Forum*, Anaheim, CA. Available at: http://www.vin.com/Members/Proceedings/Proceedings.plx?CID=acvim2010&PID=pr55859&O=VIN (Accessed 4 July, 2011).

Sharp, N.J., Kornegay, J.N., Van Camp, S.D., et al. 1992. An error in dystrophin mRNA processing in golden retriever muscular dystrophy, an animal homologue of Duchenne muscular dystrophy. *Genomics.* 13(1):115–121.

Shearin, A.L. and Ostrander, E.A. 2010. Leading the way: Canine models of genomics and disease. *Dis Model Mech.* 3:27–34.

Silverstein, D.C. and Hopper, K. 2009. *Small Animal Critical Care Medicine*. St. Louis, Mo: Saunders/Elsevier.

Smarick, S.D., Haskins, S.C., Aldrich, J., et al. 2004. Incidence of catheter-associated urinary tract infection among dogs in a small animal intensive care unit. *J Am Vet Med Assoc.* 224(12):1936–1940.

Songsasen, N. and Wildt, D.E. 2007. Oocyte biology and challenges in developing in vitro maturation systems in the domestic dog. *Anim Reprod Sci.* 98(1–2):2–22.

Sothern, R.B., Farber, M.S., and Gruber, S.A. 1993. Circannual variations in baseline values in dogs. *Chronobiol Int.* 10:364–382.

Strombeck, D.R., Meyer, D.J., and Freedland, R.A. 1975a. Hyperammonemia due to a urea cycle enzyme deficiency in two dogs. *J Am Vet Med Assoc.* 166(11):1109–1111.

Strombeck, K.R., Weiser, M.G., and Kaneko, J.J. 1975b. Hyperammonemia and hepatic encephalopathy in the dog. *J Am Vet Med Acssoc.* 166(11):1105–1108.

Studzinski, C.M., Araujo, J.A., and Milgram, N.W. 2005. The canine model of human cognitive aging and dementia: Pharmacological validity of the model for assessment of human cognitive-enhancing drugs. *Prog Neuropsychopharmacol Bio Psychiatry.* 29(3):489–498.

Sullivan, L.A., Campbell, V.L., and Onuma, S.C. 2010. Evaluation of open versus closed urine collection systems and development of nosocomial bacteriuria in dogs. *J Am Vet Med Assoc.* 237(2):187–190.

Swallow, J., Anderson, D., Buckwell, A.C., et al. 2005. Guidance on the transport of laboratory animals: Report of the Transport Working Group established by the Laboratory Animal Science Association (LASA). *Lab Anim.* 39:1–39.

Syme, H.M. 2007. Polyuria and polydypsia. *BSAVA Manual Series*. Eds. J. Elliott and G.F. Grauer, pp. 8–25. Quedgeley: British Small Animal Veterinary Association.

Taylor, S.M. 2010. *Small Animal Clinical Techniques*, pp. 1–19, 147–158. St. Louis, MO: Saunders/Elsevier.

Tabaru, H., Finco, D.R., Brown, S.A., and Cooper, T. 1993. Influence of hydration state on renal functions of dogs. *Am J Vet Res.* 54(10):1758–1764.

Tarducci, A., Abate, O., Borgarelli, M., Borrelli, A., Zanatta, R., and Cagnasso, A. 2004. Serum values of cardiac troponin-T in normal and cardiomyopathic dogs. *Vet Res Commu.* 28(Suppl 1):385–388.

Tisdall, P.L., Hunt, G.B., Tsoukalas, G., and Malik, R. 1995. Post-prandial serum bile acid concentrations and ammonia tolerance in Maltese dogs with and without hepatic vascular anomalies. *Aust Vet J.* 72(4):121–126.

Trobridge, G.D. and Kiem, H-P. 2010. Large animal models of hematopoietic stem cell gene therapy. *Gene Ther.* 17:939–948.

Tsai, K.L., Clark, L.A., and Murphy, K.E. 2007. Understanding hereditary diseases using the dog and human as companion model systems. *Mamm Genome.* 18:444–451.

Tuli, J.S., Smith, J.A., and Morton, D.B. 1994. Stress measurements in mice after transportation. *Lab Anim.* 29:132–138.

Urhausen, C., Seefeldt, A., Eschricht, F.M., et al. 2009. Concentrations of prolactin, LH, testosterone, TSH, and thyroxine in normospermic dogs of different breeds. *Reprod. Dom. Anim.* 44(Suppl 2):279–282.

Vaden, S.L. 2010. Glomerular diseases. In *Textbook of Veterinary Internal Medicine: Diseases of the Dog and the Cat.* Eds. S.J. Ettinger and E.C. Feldman, Vol. 2, pp. 2021–2047. St. Louis, MO: Elsevier Saunders.

van Vonderen, I.K., Kooistra, H.S., Sprang, E.P., and Rijnberk, A. 1999. Disturbed vasopressin release in 4 dogs with so-called primary polydipsia. *J Vet Int Med.* 13(5):419–425.

van Vonderen, I.K., Kooistra, H.S., Timmermans-Sprang, E.P., et al. 2004. Vasopressin response to osmotic stimulation in 18 young dogs with polyuria and polydipsia. *J Vet Int Med.* 18(6):800–806.

Vonk, W.I., Wijmenga, C., and van de Sluis, B. 2008. Relevance of animal models for understanding mammalian copper homeostasis. *Am J Clin Nutr.* 88(3):840S–845S.

Waddell, L. 2010. Systemic anaphylaxis. In *Textbook of Veterinary Internal Medicine: Diseases of the Dog and the Cat*. Eds. S.J. Ettinger and E.C. Feldman, pp. 531–547. St. Louis, MO: Elsevier Saunders.

Walker, M.C., Hill, R.C., Guilford, W.G., et al. 2001. Postprandial venous ammonia concentrations in the diagnosis of hepatobiliary disease in dogs. *J Vet Int Med.* 15(5):463–466.

Watson, A.D., Lefebvre, H.P., Concordet, D., et al. 2002. Plasma exogenous creatinine clearance test in dogs: Comparison with other methods and proposed limited sampling strategy. *J Vet Int Med.* 16(1):22–33.

Webster, C.R.L. 2010. History, clinical signs, and physical findings in hepatobiliary disease. In *Textbook of Veterinary Internal Medicine: Diseases of the Dog and the Cat*, Eds. S.J. Ettinger and E.C. Feldman, Vol. 2, pp. 1612–1625. St. Louis, MO: Elsevier Saunders.

Weiser, G. 2004. Sample collection, processing, and analysis of laboratory service options. In *Veterinary Hematology and Clinical Chemistry*. Ed. M. Thrall, pp. 39–53. Philadelphia, PA: Lippincott Williams & Wilkins.

Wemelsfelder, F. 1990. Boredom and laboratory animal welfare. In: *The Experimental Animal in Biomedical Research, A Survey of Scientific and Ethical Issues for Investigators*. Ed. B.E. Rollin, Vol. 1, pp. 243–272. Boca Raton, FL: CRC Press.

Whittemore, J.C. and Flatland, B. 2010. Comparison of biochemical variables in plasma samples obtained from healthy dogs and cats by use of standard and microsample blood collection tubes. *J Am Vet Med Assoc.* 327(3):288–292.

Wildt, D.E., Panko, W.B., Chakraborty, P.K., et al. 1979. Relationship of serum estrone, estradiol-17 beta and progesterone to LH, sexual behavior and time of ovulation in the bitch. *Biol Reprod.* 20:648–658.

Willeberg, P. and Priester, W.A. 1982. Epidemiological aspects of clinical hyperadrenocorticism in dogs (canine Cushing's syndrome). *J Am Anim Hosp Assoc.* 18:717–724.

Wolfle, T.L. 1990. Policy, program and people: The three P's to wellbeing. In: *Canine Research Environment*. Eds. J.A. Mench and L. Krulisch, pp. 41–47. Greenbelt, MD: Scientists Center for Animal Welfare.

Wolford, S.T., Schroer, R.A., Gohs, F.X., et al. 1986. Reference range data base for serum chemistry and hematology values in laboratory animals. *J Toxicol Environ Health.* 18(2):161–188.

Yanay, O., Brzezinski, M., Christensen, J., et al. 2006. An adult dog with cyclic neutropenia treated by lentivirus—Mediated delivery of granulocyte colony-stimulating factor. *Hum Gene Ther.* 17(4):464–469.

Zandvliet, M.M. and Rothuizen, J. 2007. Transient hyperammonemia due to urea cycle enzyme deficiency in Irish wolfhounds. *J Vet Int Med.* 21(2):215–218.

Zangerl, B., Goldstein, O., Philp, A.R., et al. 2006. Identical mutation in a novel retinal gene causes progressive rod-cone degeneration in dogs and retinitis pigmentosa in humans. *Genomics.* 88(5):551–563.

5 The Laboratory Pig

Alain Stricker-Krongrad, Larry D. Brown, Guy F. Bouchard, M. Michael Swindle, and Stan W. Casteel

CONTENTS

5.1 INTRODUCTION

The pig has become an important tool as a laboratory animal for biomedical research. The increasing importance of swine as an animal model for human diseases and testing is related to the highly correlated anatomical and physiological similarities between the two species, and to a lesser justification, the lowered animal rights group interest in swine use as compared to primate [nonhuman primate (NHP)] or dog use. For example, because swine demonstrate similarities to man in cardiovascular anatomy and physiology (e.g., comparable heart-to-body size ratio, coronary vasculature anatomy, lipoprotein structure/profile, development of hypercholesterolemia and atherosclerosis, tendency toward obesity, insulin resistance, and susceptibility to a variety of stress factors), they have become a valuable animal model for cardiovascular research. Concordance between swine and human dermal wound healing studies was 78% while a significantly lower concordance was reported for rodents (Sullivan et al., 2001). Pigs are monogastric omnivores and exhibit a resemblance to man in dietary habits and digestive physiology. Numerous references describe similarities between pigs and humans, thus laying the foundation for the extrapolation of experimental pig data to humans (Horstman et al., 1960; Bustad and McClellan, 1966; McClellan, 1968; Douglas, 1972; Mitruka et al., 1976; Tumbleson, 1986; Swindle and Adams, 1988; Swindle et al., 1992; Tumbleson and Schook, 1996; Brown and Terris, 1996; Reeds and Odle, 1996; Mortensen et al., 1998; Swindle and Smith, 1998, 2000; Schook et al., 2005; Vodicka et al., 2005; Svendsen, 2006; Nunoya et al., 2007).

Besides the obvious functional and anatomical similarities, swine provide other advantages for the biomedical investigator. As intelligent, sociable, and trainable animals, they are adaptable to a wide variety of experimental conditions. They are readily available at a relatively lower cost as compared to primates and are capable of producing large litters in a reasonably short period of time. Though considered large laboratory animals along with dogs, ruminants, and primates, miniature and young domestic pigs are of manageable size and can accommodate performance of complicated surgical techniques, dosing of test article by all routes, serial blood collections, and many other research manipulations. "Micropigs" or microswine offer even greater advantages regarding size, handling ease, and food and caging requirements. Examples of microswine include the Micro-Yucatan, currently marketed by Sinclair BioResources, LLC, and the Göttingen Minipig® (Ellegaard Göttingen Minipigs A/S), which is marketed by Marshall BioResources. Pigs can be downsized as evidenced by these Micros but along with the smaller size from inbreeding comes higher rates of birth defects. Swine models are acceptable surrogates for the canine and primate models in most regulatory safety studies (Jacobs, 2006). In summary, there are good scientific, economic, and sociological reasons why domestic swine and miniswine are appropriate research models.

5.2 USE OF PIGS IN BIOMEDICAL RESEARCH

The anatomy of the pig was documented in the twelfth century by Copho, a professor teaching anatomy at Salernum, Italy, in his treatise entitled *Anatomica Porci*. Earlier Greek works on porcine anatomy also existed. In 1543, Andreas Vesalius, a Flemish anatomist from Brussels, taught anatomy at the University of Padua, Italy, where he performed vivisection on pigs for teaching medical students (Ball, 1910). Since early times, the truffle-loving pig with the exquisite olfactory sense has found refined use as a teaching tool and an animal model, especially in agricultural, biomedical, and nutrition research.

The laboratory swine (*Sus scrofa*) has been utilized as a mammalian model for human nutrition and biology research, gnotobiology, toxicology testing, and experimental surgical modeling for many decades and is well established (Phillips and Tumbleson, 1986; Miller and Ullrey, 1987; Lunney, 2007; Swindle and Smith, 2008; Swindle, 2007; Gad et al., 2008). The United States Department of Agriculture (USDA)–National Agriculture Library (NAL) Information Resources on Swine in Biomedical Research (Swindle and Smith, 2000) addresses comparative anatomy and physiology of research swine in some detail. Most miniature swine organs and systems are physiologically mature by sexual maturity (4–6 months) (Swindle and Smith, 2008). The similarity in size, physiology, and in organ development and disease progression make the swine an ideal model for studies during almost all developmental periods (fetal, perinatal, juvenile, adolescence, adulthood, geriatric). The United States Food and Drug Administration (FDA, 2000), Buelke-Sam (2002), Beck et al. (2006), and Padgett (2009) have addressed approximate ages of miniswine, which are comparable to human developmental periods for central nervous system (CNS) and reproductive development up through adolescence. Since biological systems may develop, advance, or mature at differing timeframes, the age equivalent period for CNS and brain may not necessarily apply for skeletal, immunological, reproductive, or other systems.

Similarities to human organ size and human leukocyte antigen (HLA) haplotyping (compared to swine leukocyte antigen [SLA]) have made the swine the primary choice for organ, tissue, and cell xenograft transplantation procedures. Genetically altered (knock-out or gene insertion) porcine models show promise for xenotransplantation research (Prather et al., 2003). The ability to use matched littermates facilitates comparison of genetically homogeneous treatment and control animals. The U.S. National Swine Resource and Research Center (NSRRC), established in 2003 at the University of Missouri in Columbia, Missouri, facilitates specialized genetic studies as a resource for frozen embryos, germplasm, cells, tissues, and organs.

Because of the considerable skin surface area in young adult swine, control and treatment dermal application or wound sites can be placed side by side for ready comparison. Swine skin is fixed or tightly adherent to the hypodermis and heals primarily by re-epithelialization like that of humans rather than primarily by contraction as in loose-skinned rodents or rabbits.

The ease of deliberately timing studies— imaging internal vessels, organs, and bone using standard technologies (fluoroscopy, dual Energy x-ray [DEXA], computed axial tomography [CT], magnetic resonance imaging [MRI], intravascular ultrasound [IVUS]); and collecting necropsy specimens, repeated peripheral blood, urine, synovial fluid, and cerebrospinal fluid (CSF) samples of generous quantity—has provided evidence that the pig is a workable biomedical model.

Over the past 50 years, application of the pig as a research model has expanded to include models for many experimental biomedical designs, including paradigms for the study of a wide variety of human disease conditions, biological processes/mechanisms, and for preclinical testing (Table 5.1). Animal models, such as swine, are necessary for study of human disease biology, processes, pathology, treatment modalities, surgical methods, and for testing of potential pharmaceutical drugs, biologics, and implantable biomedical devices. Miniature swine models are extensively used in preclinical safety and efficacy studies, and applications listed in Table 5.1.

Porter (1993) and Pond and Mersmann (2001) have identified current domestic pig breeds of the world. As adapted from Porter (1993), Pond and Mersmann (2001) listed 172 breeds of domestic pigs and, as adapted from Panepinto (1996), 24 breeds of miniature swine. Panepinto (1996) has reviewed the history and background of miniature swine breeds used in worldwide research. Swindle and Smith (2008) suggest there are over 50 miniature swine breeds worldwide but only a few are important in biomedical research. Common miniature swine used in research include the Yucatan, Hanford, Sinclair S-1, Ossabaw, Göttingen, Banna, Vietnamese Potbellied, and Meishan (Swindle and Smith, 2008). Table 5.2 lists almost all historical and contemporary miniature and microswine lineages. The Vita Vet or Pitman Moore, Chicago Medical School, Labco, and Nebraska are historical miniature swine strain names. Reference data, including clinical pathology, are usually available either from the literature or from companies or institutes producing or using each contemporary breed, strain, or lineage of miniature swine.

Domestic swine breeds commonly used in biomedical, nutritional, agricultural, and environmental research in North America include the Yorkshire, Yorkshire-cross, and Duroc, while in European research settings the Landrace or Landrace-cross and British Large White are most popular. Other domestic breeds such as the Pig Improvement Company (PIC), United States, genetic lines from Franklin, Kentucky, are in use for environmental Superfund soil oral bioavailability studies (Casteel et al., 1997). Select miniature swine lineages have found

TABLE 5.1
Applications of Swine Models in Biomedical Research and Preclinical Testing

Alcoholism	Metabolism
Anesthesiology	Melanoma or cancer research
Atherosclerosis and heart disease	Myocardial infarction
Behavior	Neonatology
Biomaterials testing	Neuroscience and stroke
Cardiopulmonary surgery	Nutrition
Cardiovascular pharmacology	Ophthalmology
Congenital heart disease	Organ, tissue, or cell xenotransplantation
Cosmetic and cutaneous biology/testing	Osteochondrosis
Dental and gingivitis research	Osteoporosis
Dermatotoxicology	Gastric ulcers
Developmental immunology	Pharmaceutical toxicity/safety
Device safety	Photobiology and photoaging
Diabetes	Radiation therapy, radiology, imaging
Digestion and gastroenterology	Renal function/disease, nephrology/urology
Dialysis	Septic shock
Endotoxic shock	Skeletal research
Endoscopic and laparoscopic training	Surgical modeling
Environmental bioavailability	Stress
Exercise physiology/energetics	Tissue engineering
Ex vivo testing of skin, organs, cells, tissues	Thrombosis
Genetics	Trauma or traumatology
Hemorrhagic shock and hemostasis	Vaccine safety and infectious disease models
Hypotension/hypertension	Whole body composition
Immunology	Wound healing

Intended to present examples but not an exhaustive list of uses.

application in specific research categories but almost all lineages function equally well for most applications. Popular North American miniature swine lineages and example uses include the Micro- or Mini-Yucatan for ventricular septum defect (VSD), diabetes, and wound healing; the Sinclair S-1 for osteoporosis, malignant melanoma, and dental models; and the Hanford for atherosclerosis and dermal toxicology testing. The thrifty feral island Ossabaw miniature pig has recently been applied to diabetes and cardiometabolic syndrome model research (Sturek et al., 2007). The Standard or Mini Yucatan is commonly used in the research and contract research organization (CRO) settings in the United States. Domestic swine are applied widely for many models such as familial hypercholesterolemia (FHC) and atherosclerosis, hypertrophic dermal scarring (Duroc), wound healing and thermal burns (Yorkshire), neonatal or pediatric nutrition, trauma, surgical training, metabolism, stent and other cardiovascular studies.

5.3 UNIQUE PHYSIOLOGICAL CHARACTERISTICS OF THE LABORATORY PIG

Swine models show important anatomical, physiological, and biochemical concordance with higher-order mammals, especially humans. This is the main reason why they are valuable for biomedical research. Only a few dissimilar unique aspects exist such as the neurogenic instead of myogenic heart conduction, a paucity of eccrine glands in the skin, the lack or low activity of CYP2B, CYP2C, and CYP22D and low drug sulfation activity. Ornithine carbamoyltransferase (OCT) is an enzyme that is liver-specific in the pig and could be useful for the detection of hepatocellular injury

TABLE 5.2
Miniature and Micro Swine Lineages

Mini	Mini (*Continued*)
Standard Yucatan (Mexican Hairless)[a,b]	Guanxi bama (China)[e]
Hanford[a,b]	Meishan (China)[e]
Hormel-Hanford (FDA)[b]	Kunekune (New Zealand)[f]
Sinclair S-1 (Hormel or Minnesota)[a,b]	Collared Peccaries (Javelina, not a true pig, *Tayassu pecari*) (Mexico, Southwest United States)[f]
Ossabaw[a,b]	Westran (Australia)[f]
Chicago Medical School (CMS)[g]	Kangaroo Island (South Australia)[f]
Pitman-Moore[g] (Distributed by Vita-Vet Labs)	Labco[g] (Yucatan in early 1960s)
NIH Minipig	Nebraska Minipig[g]
Munchener Troll (Munich, West Germany, Eastern Europe)[c]	Juliani (Painted Miniature)
MeLiM (Libechov)(Czechoslovakia)[c]	African Pigmy (Guinea Hogs)[f]
Mini-Lewe (Czechoslovakia, Eastern Europe)	Vita Vet Lab Minipig[g] (Florida Swamp Pig)
Minisib (Siberia, Russia)[e]	Kakhetian (Georgia, Russia)
Svetlogorsk (Russia)	Nepal Bl. Minipig
Mangalica (Hungary)	Sevanetian Minipig
Am. Esseks	Taiwan Minipig
Beltsville (Maryland, USA)	Vietnamese Potbellied
Corsican (Corsica)	Lan Yu (Taiwan)
Hurrah (Nepal)	
Clawn (Japan)[d]	**Micro**
Ohmini (Japan)[d]	Göettingen Minipig (Denmark/Germany/Europe)[a–c]
NIBS Minipig (Japan)[d]	Micro Yucatan (Sinclair)[a, b]
Lee Sung (Taiwan)[e]	PWG T-Type Micro-pig® (PWG Genetics Korea, Ltd., Kyoungki-Do, Korea)[a,e]
Wu-zhishan (China)[e]	Mexican Cuino[f]
Chinese Experimental Miniature (Guizhou) (China)[e]	West African Dwarf (Nigerian Black or Ashanti)[f]
Banna (China)[e]	Chinese Dwarf[f]
Xiang (China)[e]	Criollo (Latin America)[f]
Diannan Small-Ear (China)[e]	Black Hairless[f]
Tibetan Minipig (China)[e]	Nilo (Brazil)[f]

[a] Commercially available
[b] Popular in North America for biomedical research
[c] Popular in Europe for biomedical research
[d] Popular in Japan for biomedical research
[e] Popular in Asia for biomedical research
[f] Potentially Useful for biomedical research
[g] Historical breeds/lineages

(Cornelius, 1989); it has been recommended as a useful serum marker of liver damage in the pig (Wilson et al., 1972). Arginase and sorbital dehydrogenase (SDH, also called iditol dehydrogenase or IDH) are other liver-specific enzymes in swine (Kahn, 2008a, 2008b). The $T_{1/2}$ of SDH in swine is reported to be only 1.6 hours (Hoffmann and Solter, 2008; Boyd, 1983), which limits its usefulness in most long-term toxicology studies but it may have utility in acute hepatocellular testing.

Gad et al. (2008) has reported that swine have a liver cytochrome P-450 system that is comparable to humans, although there are a few exceptions for certain cytochromes P450 (CYP) isoenzymes and the amounts and activities of specific enzyme isoforms occasionally vary between minipigs and humans. In swine, there is a low level of CYP2C, and CYP2D is absent (Swindle, 2007).

Swine are useful models for atherosclerosis, coronary heart disease, and obesity, because pigs and humans have similar lipoprotein patterns (Mahley and Weisgraber, 1974); the majority of the plasma cholesterol is carried as low-density lipoprotein (LDL) in pigs and humans (Attie et al., 1992); vascular plaques readily forms in swine on high-fat high-cholesterol (HFHC) diets, especially after intimal or vascular wall damage by balloon; and both have a similar propensity for obesity. In the progression of these lesions, vascular streaks precede complex vascular lesions containing cholesterol clefts and macrophages. There are multiple techniques for acceleration of the natural tendency for formation of arteriosclerotic or atherosclerotic plaque lesions in swine, as follows:

1. Dietary HFHC (2%–4% cholesterol, 40% dietary fat; generalized lesions in 6 months) (Swindle and Smith, 2008)
2. Balloon catheter denuding of specific intimal sites (coronaries, iliacs) with HFHC diet (lesions by 3 months) (Swindle and Smith, 2008; Gal and Isner, 1992) (for laser angioplasty denuding, see White et al., 1988; also White and Ramee, 1989)
3. Overstretching of arterial wall by catheter balloon (Gerdes et al., 1996; Saitoh et al., 1998; Eto et al., 2000)
4. Diabetes plus HFHC diet (Gerrity et al., 2001; Dixon et al., 2002)
5. Blood flow stenosis by aneroid or ligation restriction (carotids) (Ishii et al., 2006; Shi et al., 2009)

Attie et al. (1992) described a mutant, spontaneously hypercholesterolemic pig resembling FHC in humans (Type Ha), which is the most common type of hypercholesterolemia involving an increase in LDL. The mutant pigs had increased LDL and normal LDL receptor activity (Rapacz et al., 1986). Two variants of the familial hypercholesterolemic pigs, Lpb5.1 and Lpb5.2, were described, and both had alterations of the predominant apoprotein, apo-B, which serves as the ligand for the receptor. The altered protein caused a decreased affinity of LDL for the receptor, resulting in a decreased clearance rate of LDL from the blood. The Lpb5.1 pigs displayed an approximately threefold increase of serum cholesterol concentration, while the Lpb5.2 pigs had only a moderate 20%–25% increase. Besides the cholesterol concentration difference, the cholesterol increase in the Lpb5.1 pigs was characterized by a marked elevation in the concentration of a more buoyant form of LDL; there was a greater cholesterol ester/protein ratio than that found for the denser form of LDL. The Lpb5.2 pigs did not demonstrate an increase of this buoyant LDL variant. Additionally, the more buoyant form of LDL was catabolized more slowly than the denser LDL (Checovich et al., 1988). Small dense LDL (sdLDL) is less buoyant and more atherogenic in humans so buoyancy or flotation rate of LDL is a logical interest factor for atherosclerosis researchers (Norata et al., 2009). Hasler-Rapacz et al. (1995) reported that the University of Wisconsin domestic herd of complex familial hypercholesterolemia (c-FHC) phenotype pigs were characterized by elevated levels of total plasma cholesterol (TC) and apoB and reduced levels of high-density lipoprotein cholesterol (HDL-C) and apoA-l is associated with the spontaneous atherosclerotic lesions in the swine. Certain apo B genotypes (Lpb2/3, 3/3, 3/5, 5/5, 3/8) of these animals developed stenotic coronary lesions containing necrotic cores, fibrous caps, calcification, neovascularization, hemorrhage, and fissuring, which resembled advanced coronary artery disease (CAD) in humans (Prescott et al., 1995). The familial dyslipidemia appeared to be polygenic.

Aminophenylboronic acid affinity chromatography methods have been used to demonstrate that pigs have lower glycosylated hemoglobin (A1c) values than other commonly used laboratory animal species (e.g., the dog, rat, mouse, gerbil, and rabbit) and man (Rendell et al., 1985).

Spontaneous, genetically manipulated (e.g., transgenic or knockout), and conventionally induced models are available. Most organs and systems in pigs are physiologically mature by sexual maturity (Swindle and Smith, 2008), which occurs at a relatively young age (4–6 months) in minipigs. As the knowledge base expands, further unique aspects of swine models may be uncovered.

5.4 METHODOLOGY FOR SAMPLE COLLECTION

5.4.1 Blood Collection

Blood collection from swine can be a labor-intensive procedure that, in most instances, requires special restraint methods and/or equipment. For example, Carle and Dewhirst (1942) described a method for blood collection from the anterior vena cava during which a hog snare was used to immobilize the animal for venipuncture. A number of restraining devices have been described (Bustad and McClellan, 1966; Earl, 1968; Huhn et al., 1969; Mackellar, 1970; Terris et al., 1986; Tumbleson et al., 1968), and methods of physical and chemical restraint have been reviewed (Panepinto, 1986; Riebold and Thurmon, 1986). More established techniques of restraint, including the snare and V-trough, were designed for livestock handling and, as a forceful means of restraint, can cause stress to the animal. There are less stressful methods, including a hoisting rack, a portable confinement unit, farrowing crates, tethering, the Panepinto sling, and socialization to facilitate little or no restraint.

In young and adult pigs, blood collection has been accomplished from several sites; the site for collection depends on the frequency of sampling and the volume of blood required. For single blood samples, methods have been described for collection from the orbital sinus (Huhn et al., 1969; Muirhead, 1981) and by cardiac puncture (Calvert et al., 1977). Venous sites include the auricular veins (Muirhead, 1981), cranial vena cava (Brown, 1979; Carle and Dewhirst, 1942), cephalic vein (Tumbleson et al., 1968), and lateral saphenous vein (Bobbie and Swindle, 1986). The auricular and lateral saphenous veins can be visualized for venipuncture while the cephalic vein and cranial vena cava are usually blindly approached for percutaneous venipuncture. The cranial vena cava is the venous site of choice for procedures requiring a large volume of blood. Swindle (2007), Popesko (1984), and Ghoshal (1975) have previously addressed anatomical considerations for swine vascular access.

For serial blood sampling, indwelling catheters have been implanted in one of several vessels such as the external jugular (Bailie et al., 1986; Brown et al., 1973; Rodriguez and Kunavongkrit, 1983; Takahashi, 1986; Terris et al., 1986; Wingfield et al., 1974), ear vein (Bustad, 1966), femoral vein (Brown et al., 1978), vena cava via the external jugular (Ford and Maurer, 1978), midsacral artery or subcutaneous (SC) abdominal vein (Witzel et al., 1973), abdominal aorta via the superficial femoral artery (Weiskopf et al., 1986), medial saphenous vein (Bobbie and Swindle, 1986), pulmonary artery via the innominate vein (Weiskopf et al., 1986), and carotid artery (Bossone and Hannon, 1985; Hannon et al., 1981a, 1981b; Terris et al., 1986). Fleming and Arce (1986) described a method of portal vein and carotid artery catheterization which, with appropriate familiarization of the animals regarding handling procedures and personnel, allowed the collection of timed serial samples with minimal stress to the animals. Techniques for the chronic implantation of catheters in fetal pigs have also been reviewed (Hill, 1986; Randall, 1986; Spencer et al., 1986).

5.4.1.1 Restraint for Venipuncture

Agricultural methods of restraint such as snout tying or snaring and squeeze chutes should be avoided where possible in research swine. These methodologies are stressful to the pig and make it more difficult for personnel to interact with the animals when they are on a chronic study. Vocalization during this type of restraint is stressful to personnel who are working with the animals, and the pig stress response also causes variability in many blood values. Swine may be restrained in humane restraint slings or with the use of minimal manual restraint in smaller animals.

If animals need to be chemically restrained, several methods may be utilized. Administration of diazepam 0.5–5 mg/kg *per os* (PO) in a food treat or by SC injection will provide relaxation for most swine within approximately 15 minutes postadministration. Diazepam sedation will last for 4–6 hours. Swine may also be induced under gas anesthesia with isoflurane or sevoflurane delivered via a face mask for blood sampling. In large and/or fractious animals, intranasal (IN) administration of 0.2–0.4 mg/kg midazolam is very effective in providing short-term sedation in <5 minutes after administration. The sedation lasts approximately 20 minutes. For IN administration, the injectable agent is pulled into a syringe, the needle is removed, and the solution is rapidly injected into a nostril while the pig is being distracted with a hand-held food treat or toy. The object for distraction is held above the level of the pig's head causing the snout to be elevated.

5.4.1.2 Venipuncture Sites and Techniques

Bleeding sites may be rotated between the vessels discussed in this section. Lidocaine patches can be used to desensitize the skin to repeated needle sticks (Swindle, 2007; Hawk et al., 2005). For chronic projects involving frequent blood samples, the implantation of catheters or vascular access ports may be indicated. Short-term catheterization with intravenous catheters (Intracath™ with through the needle introducer, Becton Dickinson) may also be performed for up to 3 days (Swindle, 2007; Swindle et al., 2005). Yen (2001) has reviewed blood sampling and surgical techniques in research swine.

Retro-orbital bleeding has been described in the agricultural literature but it should be avoided because it is both distressing to the pig and may cause ocular complications. Vacutainers can be used for the larger vessels but they will not function well for the cephalic, coccygeal, and auricular veins. Alcohol applied to the skin over the superficial veins will facilitate the identification and dilation of the vessels.

5.4.1.2.1 Cranial Vena Cava

The cranial vena cava (precava) is the largest vessel that is commonly accessed for blood samples (Figure 5.1). The sample size from this vessel is only limited by the amount of blood which can be safely removed without causing harm to the animal (generally not to exceed 1% of the total blood volume for nonterminal procedures). Examples of clinical signs resulting from excess blood removal include death, collapse, pale mucous membranes, lethargy, anemia, bruising, hematoma, and avoidance behavior. This occurs very infrequently with large animal miniature swine models. Animals may be positioned in a restraint sling or placed in dorsal recumbency to access this vessel. The vessel is always accessed from the right side of the thoracic inlet to avoid the vagus and recurrent laryngeal nerves which are more prominent on the left side. The needle is advanced at

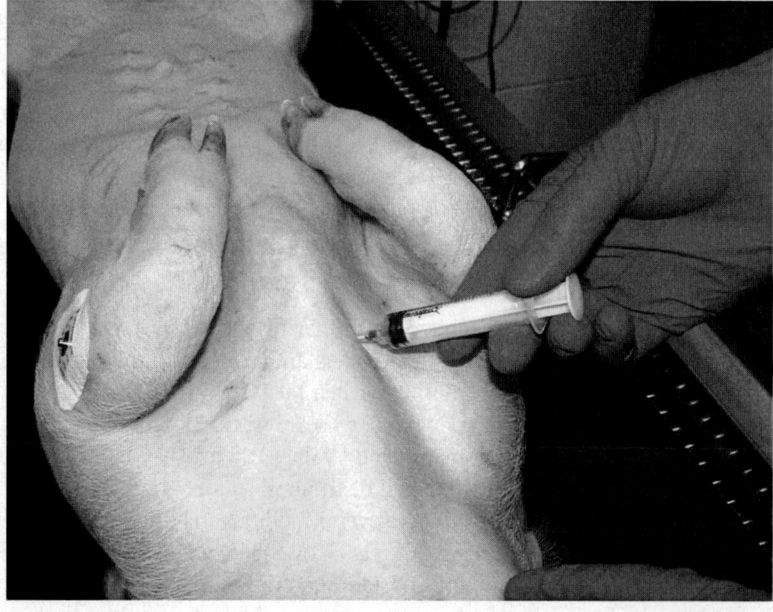

FIGURE 5.1 **(See color insert.)** Cranial vena cava venipuncture.

a 45° angle toward the left shoulder of the pig. Repeated blood sampling from this area will result in hematoma or blood clot formation in the thoracic inlet, because it is not possible to stop leakage from the venipuncture with digital pressure. In swine <50 kg the vessel can be accessed using a 20 gauge (G), 1.5″ needle. For animals >50 kg, needles as large as 18 G, 2.5″ may have to be used (Swindle, 2007; Hawk et al., 2005).

5.4.1.2.2 External Jugular Vein

The external jugular vein can be accessed in the jugular furrow which is visualized after extending the neck and retracting the forelegs caudally (Figure 5.2). The vein runs along a line drawn from the caudal aspect of the mandible to the thoracic inlet on the same side. The amount of blood that can be withdrawn from this vessel is also unlimited, but generally it is used for samples <20 mL because of the manipulations of the pig that are required. This is a large blood vessel which can be accessed with a 20 G, 1.0–1.5″ needle in most swine (Swindle, 2007; Hawk et al., 2005).

5.4.1.2.3 Internal Jugular Vein and Carotid Artery

The internal jugular vein, carotid artery, and vagus nerve are all located in a sheath on either side of the trachea on the ventral surface of the cervical vertebrae (Figure 5.3). Positioning of the head and neck are the same as for the external jugular vein. The carotid pulse can be used to locate these vessels. The vein will be slightly lateral to the artery and the nerve. The carotid artery is frequently used as the vascular access site for terminal bleeding under general anesthesia. These vessels can be accessed with a 20 G, 1.0–1.5″ needle. Bradycardia or arrhythmias may occur if the vagus nerve is accidentally stimulated with the needle (Swindle, 2007; Hawk et al., 2005).

5.4.1.2.4 Cephalic Vein

The cephalic vein can be accessed along the cranial surface of the radius on the foreleg and also as it crosses the ventral surface of the neck to enter the external jugular vein at the thoracic inlet (Figures 5.4 and 5.5). A tourniquet is placed around the foreleg at the level of the proximal radius and the elbow (ulnar head) is pressed to extend the leg. In order to access the vessel on the ventral surface of the neck the animal is placed in dorsal recumbency and digital pressure is applied to the thoracic

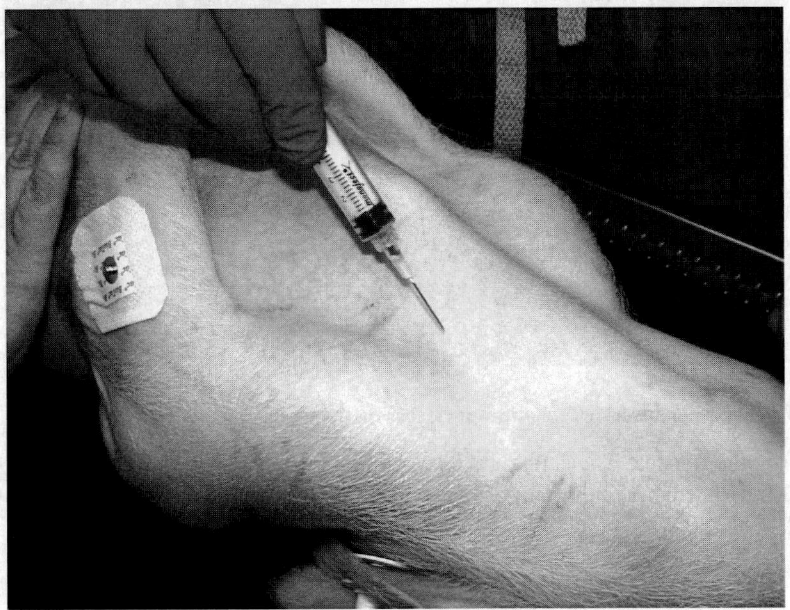

FIGURE 5.2 **(See color insert.)** External jugular vein accesses.

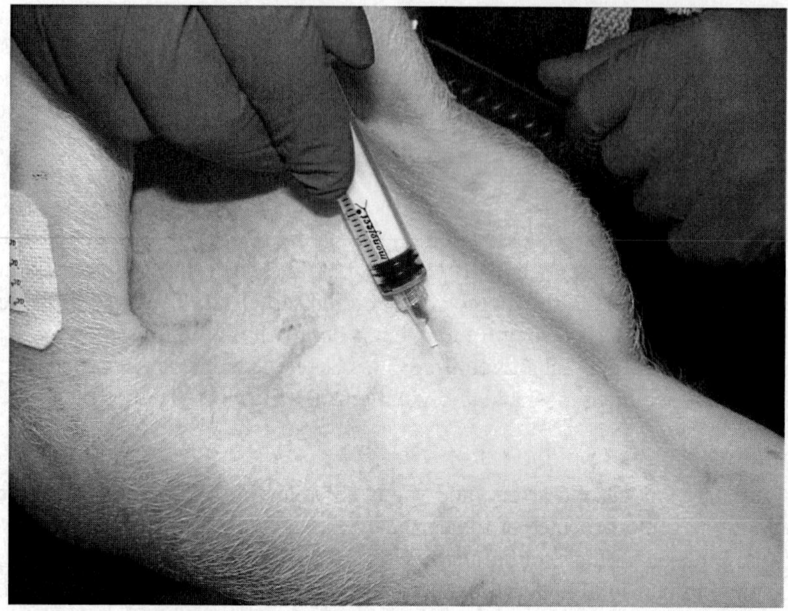

FIGURE 5.3 **(See color insert.)** Internal jugular vein and carotid artery access.

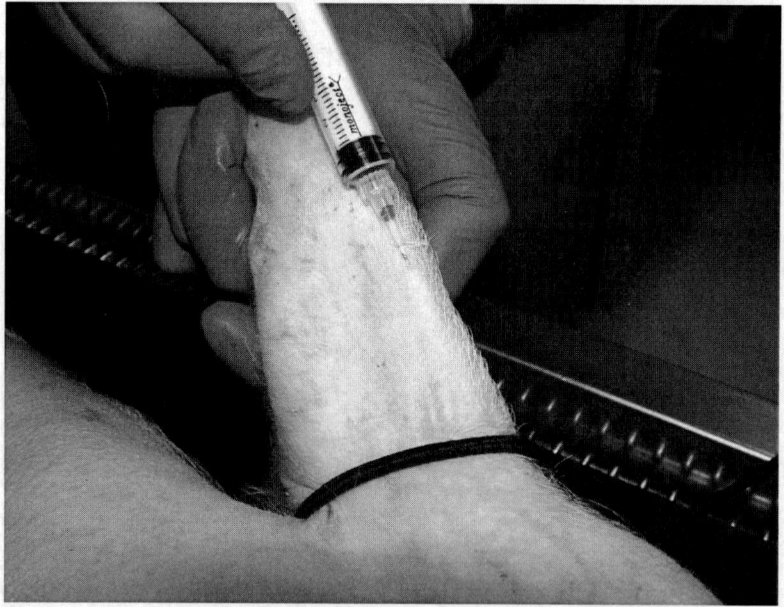

FIGURE 5.4 **(See color insert.)** Cephalic vein access on the foreleg.

inlet alongside the trachea. The cephalic vein can then be visualized. This vessel can be accessed with a 20 G, 1.0″ needle. The amount of blood that can be withdrawn is usually < 5 mL (Swindle, 2007; Hawk et al., 2005).

5.4.1.2.5 Femoral Vein and Artery

The femoral artery and vein are located in the femoral groove formed by the borders of the sartorius and gracilis muscles (Figure 5.6). They may be located by palpation of the femoral pulse or

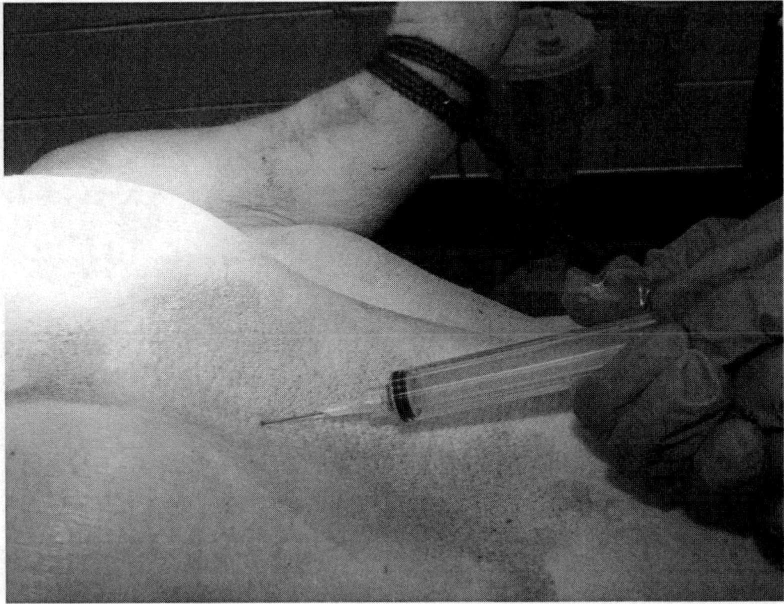

FIGURE 5.5 **(See color insert.)** Cephalic vein access on the neck.

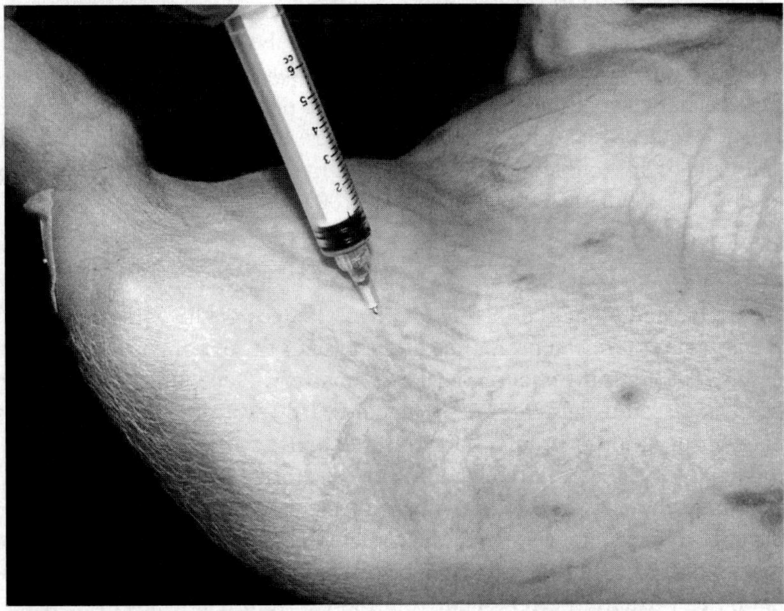

FIGURE 5.6 **(See color insert.)** Femoral artery and vein access.

by following the pulse of the medial saphenous artery, which disappears as this superficial vessel disappears into the femoral groove (Figure 5.7). The vessels are located under the medial edge of the gracilis muscle rather than directly in the groove. The pig is placed in dorsal recumbency and the rear leg is gently extended to access this site. Sedation is required for this procedure. The femoral vessels can be accessed with 20 G, 1.0–1.5″ needles. The amount of blood that can be withdrawn is usually 5–10 mL (Swindle, 2007; Hawk et al., 2005).

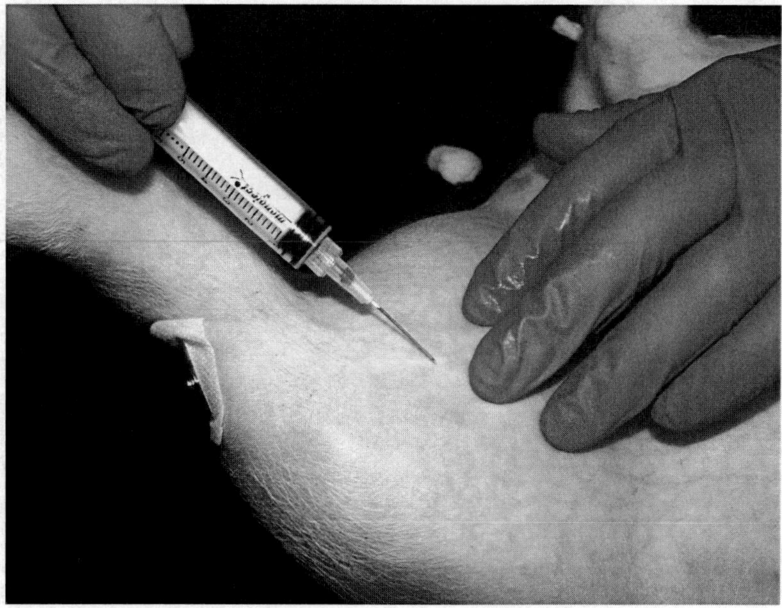

FIGURE 5.7 **(See color insert.)** Medial saphenous artery access.

5.4.1.2.6 Cranial Abdominal (External Mammary) Vein

The cranial abdominal vein is located along the deep lateral edge of the most cranial three mammary glands (Figure 5.8). This vessel greatly enlarges in sows that have had litters. Digital pressure is applied at the caudal edge of the last rib along the line of mammary glands to distend this vessel. This vessel can be accessed using 20 G, 1.0″ needles. In animals that have not reached sexual maturity, usually only 5 mL of blood can be obtained. In sows that have had litters, volumes up to 20 mL can be obtained (Swindle, 2007; Hawk et al., 2005).

5.4.1.2.7 Ear (Auricular) Vein

The ear veins are located along the medial and lateral edges of the dorsal aspect of the pinnae (Figure 5.9). Digital pressure can be applied at the base of the ear or a tourniquet can be used to dilate the vessels. The central vessel on the ear is an artery. Depending upon the size of the pig the veins can be accessed using 20–22 G, 1″ needles. However, it is better to access them with a butterfly catheter or an intravascular catheter. Use of 18″ intravenous catheters (Intracath™) will allow you to pass a catheter into the maxillary or external jugular vein in most animals. For this technique, the catheter is passed to the base of the ear and then the ear is pulled cranially and a finger is used to facilitate passage of the catheter beyond the base of the ear into the larger vessels. Catheters placed in the ear veins can be maintained successfully for up to 3 days. Only 1–2 mL of blood can usually be obtained from the ear vein itself; however, if the method of passing a catheter is used then the amount of blood that can be obtained is unlimited (Swindle, 2007; Hawk et al., 2005).

5.4.1.2.8 Tail (Coccygeal) Vein

The coccygeal veins accompany the artery on the ventral surface of the tail. These vessels may be accessed by raising the tail and performing venipuncture at the base of the tail (Figure 5.10). These vessels can be accessed using 20 G, 1.0″ needles. Only 1–2 mL of blood can be obtained from these vessels (Swindle, 2007; Hawk et al., 2005).

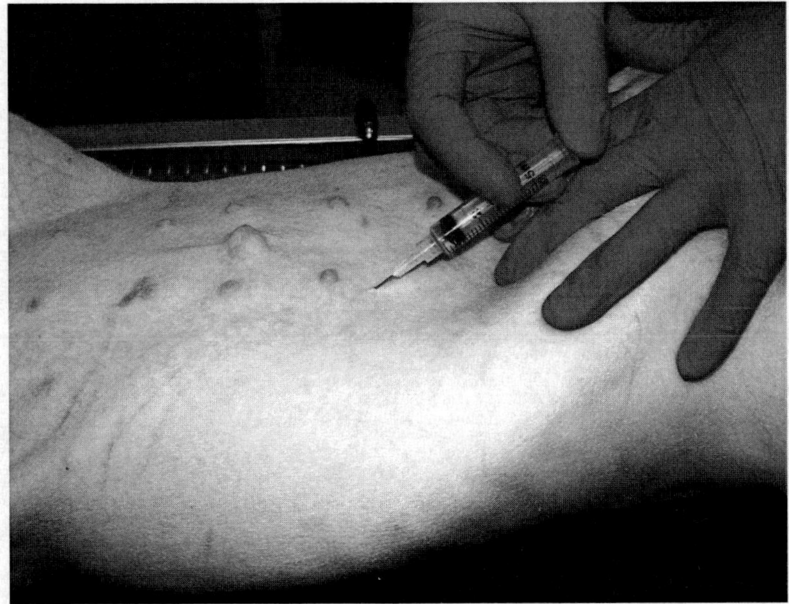

FIGURE 5.8 **(See color insert.)** Cranial abdominal vein access.

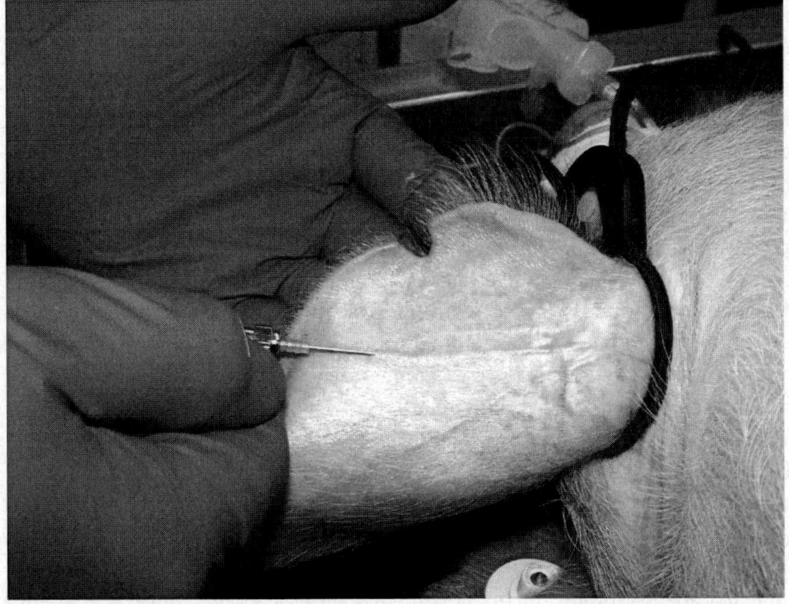

FIGURE 5.9 **(See color insert.)** Ear vein access with a catheter.

5.4.2 Urine Collection

Timed urine collections can be performed for swine with the use of metabolism cages. Equipment and methods for timed urine collection from male and female pigs of various sizes have been reviewed (Terris et al., 1986). Since these authors suggested that most of the methods and equipment available did not allow adequate freedom of movement for the experimental animals, they described a portable metal unit that did allow more motion. They indicated, however, that the urine

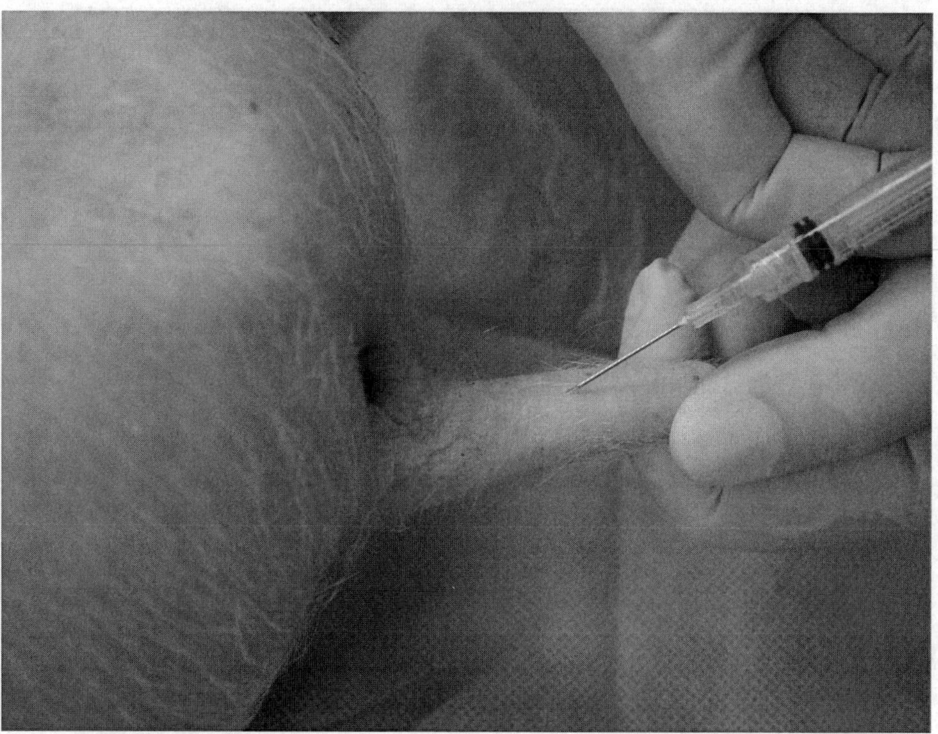

FIGURE 5.10 Coccygeal vein access.

was obtained from an unrefrigerated collecting pan, and there were no provisions for the quantitative separation of urine and feces, which can significantly impact results of urinalysis.

Metabolism cages for swine are commercially available and can be used for collection of total urine volume over time. Invariably these urine samples will become mixed with feces, food, and water, and potential contamination has to be taken into consideration when using this methodology. Assimos et al. (1986) described the use of a metabolism cage for the collection of a timed urine sample that allowed the animals to eat, drink, and sleep; urine was transported through a central floor port via a hose to a refrigerated container. Assimos et al. indicated that there was little fecal contamination of the collected urine. Urine samples were, however, filtered through a #1 Whatman filter paper prior to analysis.

Other methods of urine collection have involved catheterization and surgical techniques. For example, renal clearance studies have been performed on catheterized gilts using a 16 Fr Foley retention catheter (Zatzman et al., 1986). Also, surgical cannulation of ureters (O'Hagan and Zambraski, 1986) and an *in situ* isolated kidney preparation (Loveday et al., 1989) have been used for urine collection in pigs.

It is possible to collect samples during normal urination of a caged animal by manually catching the urine in a suitable container. However, collection of an adequate and clean sample from a pig by using this method would be haphazard at best. Cystocentesis has been used to collect urine but the bladder of the pig is thin walled and can easily be sucked onto the needle tip during cystocentesis if excess positive suction with the syringe is applied while collecting urine (Wills et al., 1997).

The most reliable method for the collection of an uncontaminated urine sample in the pig involves acute or chronic catheterization of the urinary bladder. Females are more easily catheterized and can be done so in either dorsal or ventral recumbency. Animals should be anesthetized or sedated when performing this procedure. Catheters used in females should either have some degree of stiffness or have a stylette inserted into them prior to attempting the catheterization (Figure 5.11).

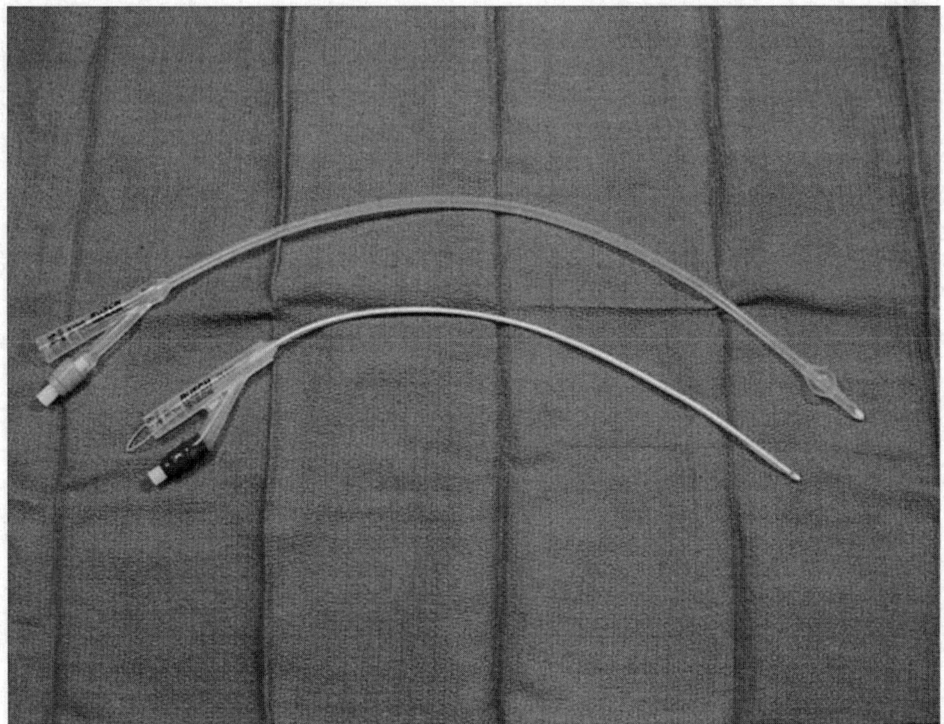

FIGURE 5.11 Foley urinary catheters composed of 100% silicone with retention balloons.

Flexible rubber catheters tend to bend and not advance retrograde into the bladder. The urethral opening is on the floor of the vagina a short distance beyond the caudal edge of the pubis. The urinary papilla can be visualized and catheterized directly if a vaginal speculum is utilized to spread the vaginal opening laterally and a laryngoscope or endoscope with a light is then inserted to press the dorsal surface of the vagina. With the female in sternal position, the papilla becomes evident and the catheter can be inserted directly. The urethra can also be catheterized directly if the animal is in dorsal recumbency and a catheter is slid along the ventral floor of the vagina into the urethra. Catheterization is facilitated if a sterile lubricant is applied to the tip of the catheter. Catheters with balloons can be inflated to be chronically maintained in the bladder or the catheter may be sewn to the vagina. The catheter can be plugged and periodically opened and a sample collected with the animal either sedated or restrained in a sling (Figure 5.12). Catheter sizes from 5 to 14 Fr will fit pigs between 10 and 70 kg (Swindle, 2007).

Male pigs are more difficult to catheterize due to the anatomy of the penis. Obstacles include the preputial diverticulum, the corkscrew-shaped tip of the penis, and the sigmoid flexure on the ventral surface of the pubis. While catheterization of males is not routinely performed, a recent abstract (Hite, 2009) presented a technique for catheterization of male pigs by using a guide wire. In larger pigs, the urethra can be palpated as it crosses the caudal aspect of the pubic bone to enter the pelvic cavity, and this portion of the urethra can be percutaneously or surgically approached and an indwelling catheter inserted into the bladder. Retention of a chronic catheter is performed in the same manner as for the female (Swindle, 2007).

Alternatively an indwelling catheter can be surgically implanted into the bladder of either gender with a midline or paramedian surgical approach in the caudal abdomen cranial to the pubis. The bladder catheter can be sutured into place and exteriorized for collection with sedation or restraint in a sling when a sample is required. Human pediatric collection bags have an adhesive edge and can be placed over the vulva of a female for short-term collection (Swindle, 2007).

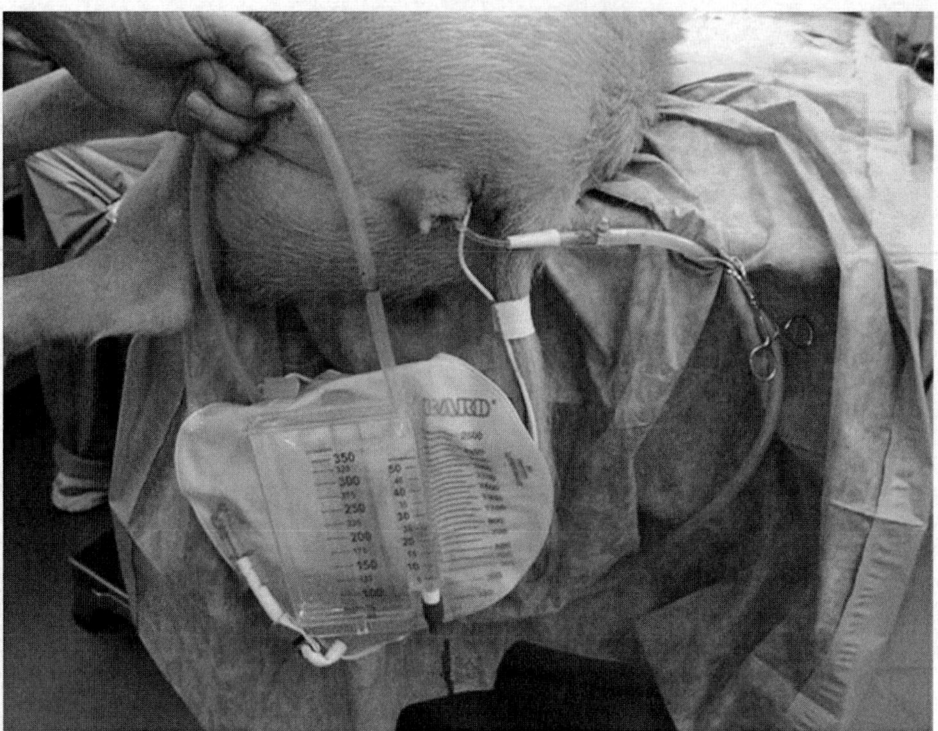

FIGURE 5.12 Urinary catheterization of a female with a urinary collection bag attached.

5.5 PREANALYTICAL SOURCES OF VARIATION

Besides choosing appropriate endpoints for analysis, the research investigator must consider several preanalytical sources of variation prior to the inclusion of clinical chemistry evaluations in any study design involving swine (Tumbleson and Schmidt, 1986).

5.5.1 Gender

As observed in many other species, gender differences for clinical chemistry values have been documented in swine. For example, for Sinclair (S-1) miniature swine evaluated in a 36-month study, serum urea nitrogen decreased for female pigs after 13 months and up to 24 months of age when urea nitrogen concentration stabilized for the remainder of the study (Hutcheson et al., 1979). In males, serum urea nitrogen increased from 7 to 24 months of age and then remained stable. Additionally, 5- to 36-month-old female Sinclair miniature pigs had higher cholesterol and triglyceride concentrations than males (Tumbleson et al., 1976a). There were no gender differences for serum total protein, creatinine, inorganic phosphorus, calcium, sodium, potassium, and chloride concentrations between male and female Sinclair (S-1) miniature pigs (Hutcheson et al., 1979; Tumbleson et al., 1976b). Tumbleson et al. (1976b) reported that, at 14 months of age, albumin concentration was 3.7 and 3.9 g/dL for male and female minipigs, respectively. By 36 months of age, albumin concentrations declined to 3.0 g/dL for male and 3.1 g/dL for female minipigs. It has been reported that serum cholesterol in swine decreases with age (Tumbleson et al., 1976a).

In Yucatan miniature swine, no gender differences were observed for clinical chemistry reference values of animals ranging in age between 8 and 54 months (Radin et al., 1986). In another study, however, Yucatan miniature swine with an average age of approximately 35 weeks demonstrated gender differences for several clinical chemistry reference values (Parsons and Wells, 1986). The authors demonstrated higher serum creatinine (123.8 vs. 106.1 μmol/L), triglyceride (341 vs. 192 mg/L) concentrations, and lactate dehydrogenase (LDH) activity (557 vs. 451 U/L) and a lower albumin concentration (46 vs. 53 g/L) for female and male minipigs, respectively. Additionally, female Yucatan swine have been observed to have greater concentrations of cholesterol along with higher HDL and LDL fractions when compared to male Yucatan swine (Thomas et al., 2002). These authors also noted a more pronounced increase in cholesterol, HDL, and LDL in female Yucatan swine placed on a high-fat diet when compared to male swine.

In a study evaluating age, gender, and line differences for hematological and biochemical variables in Göttingen miniature pigs, Oldigs (1986) indicated that in general gender differences were small and not important; a gender effect, however, was demonstrated for creatine kinase (CK) activity. The general lack of a gender effect was related to the fact that castrated male pigs were evaluated. A more recent study of Göttingen pigs, using data at both 8-week and 8-month ages, indicates that female pigs, while having similar blood glucose levels to intact males of similar age, have higher insulin levels along with higher levels of total cholesterol, triglyceride, HDL-C, and lower free fatty acids (Christoffersen et al., 2007).

A study evaluating lipid parameters in Meishan pigs comparing castrated and intact males to female animals at 5 months of age found that total cholesterol, triglycerides, LDL, and phospholipids were higher in female animals than intact males. These parameters were reportedly not significantly different between females and males that had been castrated at 1 month of age (Kojima et al., 2008).

5.5.2 Age

In swine, age-dependent changes occur for a variety of clinical chemistry variables, and many of these changes occur within the first days, even hours, of life. For example, Tumbleson et al. (1972) described the changes in concentrations, or activities, of 20 biochemical variables for crossbred pigs during late fetal (gestational days 85, 92, 99, and 106) and neonatal (birth, 12 hours, 1, 2, 3, 4, 5, 6, and 7 days) life. Calcium concentration was higher (approximately 14.1 mg/dL) at gestational days 85 and 92, declined to a low of 10.7 mg/dL at birth, and increased to approximately 12.2 mg/dL after 1 day of age. Inorganic phosphorus and potassium concentrations demonstrated a pattern similar to that reported for calcium. Inorganic phosphorus concentration was approximately 8.3 mg/dL at gestational days 85, 92, and 99, declined to a low of 4.5 mg/dL at birth, and increased to approximately 9.1 mg/dL after 2 days of age. Potassium concentration was approximately 8.2 mg/dL at gestational days 85 and 92, declined to a low of 5.1 mg/dL at birth, and increased to approximately 6.2 mg/dL after 12 hours of age. Chloride concentration was lower (approximately 108.5 mg/dL) during late fetal life but after birth increased to approximately 118 mg/dL after 4 days. Creatinine concentration was higher (approximately 3.8 mg/dL) during late fetal life, declined to 1.65 mg/dL at birth, but then increased to approximately 2.2 mg/dL after birth. In general, urea nitrogen concentration was similar during fetal (approximately 17 mg/dL) and neonatal life (approximately 18 mg/dL); however, 12 hours after birth, urea nitrogen was increased (27.9 mg/dL). Glucose was higher during fetal life (approximately 143 mg/dL), declined to 54 mg/dL at birth, but then increased to approximately 123 mg/dL after day 5. Cholesterol was low during fetal life and at birth (approximately 61 mg/dL), increased to a peak of 197 mg/dL at day 4, and then decreased 140 mg/dL at day 7. In general, neonatal serum activities of LDH, alkaline phosphatase (ALP), and aspartate aminotransferase (AST) were higher than during late fetal life; marked increases of activity occurred either at birth (ALP) or 12 hours after birth (LDH and AST). Total protein, albumin, and globulin concentrations were markedly lower during fetal life and at birth than after birth. For example, total protein concentration was approximately 2.75 mg/dL for piglets prior to or at parturition; after birth, the concentration increased to approximately 7.5 mg/dL. While albumin also was higher 12 hours after birth, the concentration continued to increase during the first week, α-globulin increased from fetal concentrations of approximately 0.82–1.17 mg/dL at birth, increased again to 2.07 mg/dL at day 3, and then decreased to 1.48 mg/dL at day 7. Additionally, γ-globulin increased from fetal concentrations (approximately 0.65 mg/dL) to 3.67 mg/dL at 12 hours, and then declined thereafter to 1.79 mg/dL at day 7.

In neonates, albumin was lower in weak or underweight piglets, and α-fetoprotein, α2-macroglobulin, α2-antitrypsin inhibitor, and α1-protease inhibitor levels were lower in those that were weak, underweight, stillborn, or traumatized (Svendsen et al., 1986).

Glucose concentrations were higher in stillborn and weakborn piglets compared to unaffected piglets (Svendsen et al., 1986). In a 28-day study by Khan et al. (1986), neonatal, colostrum-free, Hormel:Hanford piglets demonstrated an increase in serum glucose and total protein concentrations at 6–8 hours of age (post-colostrum ingestion); these values continued to rise until stabilization by day 7 postpartum. Total and direct bilirubin also increased markedly at 6–8 hours postpartum and remained stable to the end of the study. Globulin concentrations dramatically increased by 6–8 hours postpartum and remained high at day 3; concentrations then declined, almost returning to precolostral concentrations by day 28. Cholesterol and albumin concentrations also increased from birth; these values, however, continued to increase to the end of the study at day 28 postpartum. Creatinine concentrations decreased 50% from birth to day 3 but stabilized. Slight increases of calcium and phosphorus concentrations occurred by day 3 postpartum. There was an increase in the activities of alanine aminotransferase (ALT), AST, LDH, ALP, and γ-glutamyl transpeptidase (GGT) by 6–8 hours postpartum. By day 3, however, AST, ALP, and GGT activities declined to or below the activity levels at birth. There was a progressive increase of LDH activity; similar findings for LDH were reported for miniature and crossbred domestic pigs (Earl et al., 1971; Tumbleson and Kalish, 1972). Weaned Pitman-Moore miniature pigs showed age-related decreases of ALP and increases of urea nitrogen, albumin, and calcium from 14 to 28 days of age (Filer et al., 1986).

In the Ossabaw obese pig, plasma insulin concentrations were greater than those for conventional breeds at 10 weeks of age (Wangsness et al., 1981); they were not hyperglycemic at 10 weeks or 5 months of age (Wangsness et al., 1981; Martin et al., 1972).

In one 8-week study, crossbred domestic swine, from birth (pre-colostrum) to 8 hours of age (postcolostrum), demonstrated increases of total protein, urea nitrogen, total bilirubin, and activities of LDH, AST, and ALP (Tumbleson and Kalish, 1972). Concentrations of sodium, chloride, and potassium decreased. There was no change in cholesterol concentration during the first 24 hours postpartum, but cholesterol increased from 1 to 3 days postpartum and then declined to 6 weeks of age.

Alterations in clinical chemistry analyses have been observed once piglets are weaned from the sow. For example, McClellan et al. (1966) evaluated the clinical chemistry variables for miniature swine from weaning to 6 years. They reported that serum cholesterol was highest at weaning, declining to a stable concentration (80–100 mg/dL) by 3 months of age. Urea nitrogen and creatinine concentrations increased from weaning, stabilizing at approximately 19 mg/dL at 3 months of age for the former and 1.6 mg/dL at 3 years for the latter. Protein increased and inorganic phosphorus decreased from weaning, but they stabilized at 6 months and 4 years, respectively. ALP activity decreased markedly from weaning to 1 year, then slowly decreased to a stable level at 3 years. In another study, ALP activity declined for conventional and miniature pigs up to 20 weeks of age (Pond et al., 1968). In crossbred swine, after weaning at 5 weeks of age, potassium concentrations increased while sodium and chloride concentrations decreased (Tumbleson and Kalish, 1972).

In Sinclair miniature swine, age variances in several analytes have been reported. Serum cholesterol has been shown to decrease with age, from 5 to 36 months (Tumbleson et al., 1976a). In a separate study, Tumbleson et al. (1976b) demonstrated increases of serum total protein concentration, from 6.4 g/dL at 1 month to 8.2 g/dL at 10 months; afterward, protein values remained stable to 36 months of age. Globulin concentrations increased, from 2.8 g/dL at 1 month to 4.9 g/dL at 36 months. Albumin concentrations dropped from 3.6 g/dL at 1 month to 3.0 g/dL at 3 months, increased to approximately 3.8 g/dL at 14 months, and decreased to approximately 3.0 g/dL at 36 months. Similar findings for proteins were reported for conventional swine (Miller et al., 1961).

For Sinclair miniature swine at 1–36 months of age, serum urea nitrogen increased after 1–2 months (Hutcheson et al., 1979). After 13 months, the serum urea nitrogen decreased for the female pigs, becoming stable after 24 months. In males, however, serum urea nitrogen began to increase after 7 months, stabilizing after 24 months. Serum creatinine was similar for male and female pigs, decreasing from 1 to 20 months; after 20 months, creatinine concentration increased to the end of the study at 36 months. The decrease in inorganic phosphorus concentration throughout the first 3 years of life was similar for males and females (Hutcheson et al., 1979); comparable findings were reported for gilts, ranging in age from 4 to 10 months (Hlousek, 1978). In male and female Sinclair swine up to 3 years old, calcium was highest in young animals, decreasing from 1 to 28 months (Hutcheson et al., 1979). In contrast, serum calcium and magnesium were lowest in the youngest gilts, ranging in age from 4 to 10 months (Hlousek, 1978). During the first 3 years of life, male and female Sinclair swine demonstrated decreases in serum sodium from 20 to 36 months, potassium during the first 12 months, and chloride during the first 30 months (Hutcheson et al., 1979).

In Göttingen miniature pigs between the ages of 60 and 276 days, Oldigs (1986) demonstrated a decrease of ALP, leucine aminopeptidase (LAP), and LDH activity with advancing age. Age effects were also found for sodium, phosphorus, phospholipid, and iron concentrations. A study examining parameters related to metabolic syndrome in Göttingen pigs at 8 weeks and 8 months of age (before and after sexual maturity) found that triglyceride decreased significantly with age in male pigs while cholesterol decreased in both sexes with increased age, though the decrement was greater in males. HDL-C was noted to decrease with age in both sexes as well (Christoffersen et al., 2007).

Amoss and Beattie (1986) demonstrated that during the first year of life, Sinclair boars had low (<200 pg/mL) serum testosterone concentrations until 20 weeks of age, when testosterone began increasing, reaching maximum concentration (approximately 1300 pg/mL) at 32 weeks. In the boars, changes of serum estradiol coincided with changes in testosterone and were <20 pg/mL until 20 weeks of age, reaching maximum concentration of approximately 250 pg/mL at 32 weeks. Estradiol concentrations for Sinclair gilts less than 30-weeks-old were approximately 16.5 pg/mL; these increased to approximately 23.7 pg/mL for gilts 30 weeks or older. No pre-luteinizing hormone (LH) estradiol surges were observed in this study; however, pre-LH estradiol surges of up to 85 pg/mL have been documented (Shearer et al., 1972). The development of the LH surge mechanism is an age-dependent process (Elsaesser et al., 1992). Immature gilts have shown a delayed, low-amplitude LH surge in response to administration of estradiol benzoate. Further, the maturation of the LH surge mechanism is estrogen dependent and ovarian secretions of estrogens appear to be required for the final peripubertal maturation maintenance of this mechanism in the sexually mature gilt. Testosterone concentrations were consistently low (<25 pg/mL) for gilts. Orchidectomy or ovariectomy at 6 weeks of age caused serum testosterone to decrease to <20 pg/mL and remain at these concentrations for the first year. Estradiol concentrations of both orchidectomized and ovariectomized animals were similar to those for gilts; that the estradiol originated from the adrenal cortex or peripheral conversion of an adrenal cortical metabolite was suggested.

Ford and Christenson (1986) reported that serum testosterone exhibits three periods of elevated concentrations for developing male pigs. Baseline testosterone for developing and neonatal males was <1 ng/mL. Testosterone concentrations were increased in fetuses at gestational days 35–40 (approximately 5 ng/mL), and postnatally during the first month (approximately 1.5 ng/mL) and after 4 months of age (ranging between 3 and 6 ng/mL). Concentrations of follicle-stimulating hormone (FSH), LH, and testosterone were greater for Meishan boars than Duroc or white composite breeds (Borg et al., 1993; Wise et al., 1994, 1996; Zanella et al., 1996). Mean FSH concentrations were approximately 550 ng/mL for Meishan boars versus approximately 100 ng/mL for composite animals. Additionally, Meishan boars have been divided into high- and low-FSH secreters (>750 and <500 ng/mL, respectively). Baseline testosterone concentrations were approximately 14 and 2 ng/mL for Meishan and composite boars, respectively, while LH concentrations were approximately 1.5 and 0.2 ng/mL, respectively. Orchidectomy caused a significant increase of serum gonadotropin concentrations compared to levels in intact boars (Minton and Wettemann, 1988).

In another study, castration caused a greater increase of FSH concentration in the white composite breed (190% increase) versus the Meishan breed (28% and 82% increase for high- and low-FSH secreters, respectively) (Zanella et al., 1996).

Basal concentrations and clearance rates of adrenocorticotropic hormone (ACTH), growth hormone, thyroxine, and prolactin have been determined for the fetal pig (Spencer et al., 1986). McCauley and Hartmann (1984) demonstrated that newborn pigs had 12 times higher cortisol concentrations than adults. The cortisol levels decreased rapidly after birth, slightly increased at weaning, then decreased to adult concentrations by 21 days postweaning.

5.5.3 Stage of Reproductive Cycle/Estrus/Pregnancy/Gestation/Lactation

A study examining lipoproteins in conjunction with 17β-estradiol in the estrous cycle of Yucatan swine revealed that total cholesterol, total HDL, and LDL were all elevated at the point of higher 17β-estradiol levels in the cycle (Liu et al., 2004). In an evaluation of the effects of the estrous cycle on biochemical variables in sows, Tewes et al. (1977) reported that cyclical changes occurred for blood pH, bicarbonate, total CO_2, base excess, and protein and glucose concentrations. The pH, bicarbonate, total CO_2, and base excess levels were lowest during proestrus. Glucose concentrations were low during the luteal phase, increased after luteolysis, and then decreased again during the follicular phase. Protein concentrations were greatest at ovulation and lowest at the end of the luteal phase of the estrous cycle.

Reports looking at the effects of gestation, parturition, and lactation on clinical chemistry endpoints have demonstrated a variety of findings. For example, gestation caused a decrease in serum concentrations of cholesterol, urea nitrogen, and α-globulin and an increase of β-globulin for Sinclair miniature swine (Tumbleson et al., 1970). Gotze et al. (1984), however, reported that sodium, total protein, calcium, inorganic phosphorus, blood urea nitrogen (BUN), cholesterol, and ALP were similar for pregnant and nonpregnant gilts. In a study on 1-year-old domestic crossbred swine, gilts, and sows, serum concentrations of total protein, globulin, cholesterol, and calcium were decreased in lactating swine, compared to gestating swine (Reese et al., 1984). Additionally, CK activity and concentrations of creatinine and triglycerides were increased in these gestating swine, compared to lactating swine (Reese et al., 1984).

In a hyperphagic obesity study, pregnant and nonpregnant sows were allowed to overeat or were intake-restricted (Hausman et al., 1986). The pregnant sows had an approximately 30% decrease in the glucose clearance rate, which was most pronounced in the overfed pregnant sows, showing an approximate 60% decrease.

In their evaluations of the effects of pregnancy on biochemical variables in sows, Tewes et al. (1979a) reported that plasma proteins increased during gestation and demonstrated peak concentrations at 6 and 12 weeks postbreeding. Plasma protein concentrations then declined to prebreeding levels at parturition. These investigators also demonstrated that glucose, inorganic phosphorus, and LDH levels were lower, but stable, for pregnant versus nonpregnant sows. A decrease of plasma LDH activity during gestation has been reported for the pig (Nachreiner and Ginther, 1972).

In sows, blood glucose decreased during lactation (Tewes et al., 1979b; Tumbleson et al., 1970); decreases in serum total protein, albumin, and β-globulin were also observed. Tumbleson et al. (1970) also reported decreases for calcium and sodium in lactating sows while no changes in inorganic phosphorus occurred.

For the sow, serum activities of AST and CK increased immediately after parturition to 24 hours postpartum (Bostedt, 1978). After parturition, GGT decreased until the second day and remained decreased at 3 weeks postpartum. By 3 weeks postpartum, activities of AST, ALT, LDH, and glutamate dehydrogenase (GDH) were the same as prepartum levels; the activities of GGT, creatine phosphokinase (CPK), and SDH were decreased. In another study, glucose, inorganic phosphorus, and LDH activity were decreased for 2 weeks postpartum, and plasma protein decreased during lactation (Tewes et al., 1979b). Serum proteins (total, albumin, β-globulin), glucose, calcium, and sodium were decreased, and cholesterol and ALP activity were increased during lactation in Sinclair miniature swine (Tumbleson et al., 1970).

5.5.4 Breed/Lineage/Genetics

Breed and line differences in preanalytical clinical biochemistry determinations and reference ranges have been described. The Ossabaw obese pig had lower growth hormone and higher insulin values than conventional swine (Kasser et al., 1981; Wangsness et al., 1981). Pigs genetically selected for obesity generally had lower growth hormone concentrations (Althen and Gerrits 1976; Lund-Larsen and Bakke, 1975). Pond et al. (1968) compared conventional and miniature pigs up to 20 weeks of age. Serum cholesterol was lower in suckling miniature pigs, and urea nitrogen was lower in miniature pigs from 10 to 12 weeks of age. ALP activity declined more rapidly for miniature pigs during the first 6 weeks of the study; they also had higher serum protein concentrations throughout the study. In another study, plasma sodium, potassium, and glucose concentrations were higher, and bicarbonate, urea nitrogen, and creatinine concentrations were lower in the Kangaroo Island strain of pig compared to an equivalent population of domesticated Large White breed pigs from Australia (McIntosh and Pointon, 1981). It also has been reported that the Hormel:Hanford strain of miniature pig has approximately a 50% lower serum creatinine concentration than the Sinclair strain (Hutcheson et al., 1979).

Oldigs (1986) examined line differences for hematological and biochemical variables in 204 (120 white and 84 colored) Göttingen miniature pigs and demonstrated that the white line had higher values for ALP, CK, and GGT activity; no differences were observed for aldolase (ALD), ALT, AST, LAP, and LDH. Additionally, the white line had higher total protein, albumin, and β-globulin concentrations and lower concentrations of α-globulin, iron, creatinine, urea nitrogen, and triglyceride. Another study also reported the breeding family of Göttingen pig can affect triglyceride and cholesterol levels (Christoffersen et al., 2007).

The Ossabaw pig, a feral strain of obese pig living on Ossabaw Island off the Georgia coast, has lower growth hormone and higher T3, insulin, triglyceride, and cholesterol concentrations than conventional breeds (Etherton and Kris-Etherton, 1980; Martin et al., 1972; Wangsness et al., 1981). During fasting, Ossabaw pigs had lower concentrations of growth hormone and T4 and higher glucagon and free fatty acid concentrations than Yorkshire pigs (Wangsness et al., 1981).

High-ovulating Meishan sows have had greater baseline estradiol and higher and longer estradiol peaks than large-white hybrid sows (Hunter et al., 1996). Mean baseline estradiol concentrations were approximately 70 pmol/L for Meishan sows versus approximately 43 pmol/L for hybrid animals; estradiol peaks were approximately 105 and 78 pmol/L for Meishan and hybrid sows, respectively. Mean inhibin concentration was higher for the Meishan sows (approximately 1.0 μg/L) than for large-white hybrid sows (approximately 0.75 μg/L). LH and FSH secretion did not differ between the breeds; however, the time from the onset of the LH surge to the increase in plasma progesterone was shorter for the Meishan sows.

5.5.5 Health Status

Changes in swine lymphoid cell numbers are commonly associated with viral (lymphopenia or lymphocytosis), bacterial (neutrophilia), and parasitic disease (monocytic or eosinophilic responses). Shifts in clinical chemistry parameters are also reported for inflammatory processes (Odink et al., 1990) and common swine diseases (Friendship and Henry, 1992). Many of these changes occur in plasma proteins, especially the acute phase plasma proteins (haptoglobin, C-reactive protein, and serum amyloid A [SAA]) (Petersen et al., 2004). Researchers have shown that respiratory infections caused by different serotypes of *Actinobacillus pleuropneumoniae* (Agersø et al., 1998; Hall et al., 1992; Heegaard et al., 1998), *Mycoplasma hyorhinis* (Magnusson et al., 1999), or porcine reproductive and respiratory syndrome virus (Asai et al., 1999) are reflected by increased haptoglobin concentration.

In an *Escherichia coli* sepsis model, septic animals had increases of ALP, AST, and ALT activities, suggesting hepatic injury, and increases of urea nitrogen and creatinine, indicating impairment of renal function (Hoban et al., 1992). Microscopically, lesions of thrombosis and vasculitis were observed in several organs, including the liver and kidney, and there were cortical infarcts in the kidneys. In a total parenteral nutrition model, sepsis related to catheter implantation was preceded by glucosuria, and as the sepsis resolved, so did the glucosuria; no other changes of urine or serum chemistries were observed (Buckley et al., 1986). Straw et al. (2006) discuss many porcine disease and intoxication conditions that affect serum biochemical parameters.

5.5.6 Nutritional Status/Diet

Fasting in pigs can alter a variety of blood constituents. Fasting for 27 hours caused an increase in serum cholesterol and total protein concentrations of 3-month-old pigs (Kornegay et al., 1964). Prolongation of the fast to 167 hours caused decreases of glucose, calcium, sodium, urea nitrogen, and ammonia concentrations. In another study, fasting for 115 hours caused increases of bilirubin, CPK, total protein, albumin, globulin, cholesterol, phospholipids, free fatty acids, and urea nitrogen, and decreases of ALP, chloride, calcium, magnesium, and triglycerides (Baetz and Mengeling, 1971).

The effects of short-term starvation (up to 5 days) on hepatic ketone body production were investigated in the conscious unrestrained miniature pig (Muller et al., 1982). During starvation, arterial free fatty acid and glucagon concentrations increased (in addition to ketones), and arterial insulin levels decreased. Cortisol levels remained unchanged.

Fasting pigs for various durations has resulted in increased total protein, albumin, and globulin concentrations (Kornegay et al., 1964; Baetz and Mengeling, 1971), but chronic diet restriction caused no effects in serum total protein or its electrophoretic patterns (Wilson et al., 1972). Protein-restricted diets fed to swine, however, have led to decreased concentrations of total protein and albumin (Pond and Houpt, 1978; Rippel et al., 1965; Tumbleson, 1973; Wilson et al., 1972; Yen et al., 1982), and pigs fed a diet containing cornstarch as the source of carbohydrate demonstrated a slight decrease of serum total protein compared to those fed a glucose-containing diet (Mateo and Veum, 1980). Lowered diet consumption for cornstarch was recorded. The globulin fractions are also susceptible to alterations in nutrition. Increases in absolute and relative concentrations of α-globulin have been reported for pregnant (Rippel et al., 1965) and growing (Tumbleson, 1973) swine during periods of protein restriction. Absolute and relative β-globulin concentrations were decreased and absolute and relative γ-globulin concentrations were increased in malnourished swine (Baetz and Mengeling, 1971; Tumbleson, 1973). In contrast, α-globulin decreased with increased duration of food-intake restriction for male collard peccaries (Lochmiller et al., 1985). Yen et al. (1982) have shown that serum transferrin (a major β1-globulin) concentration is a good indicator of protein status in swine. Total β-globulin decreased with increased duration of intake restriction for male collard peccaries and was reflected by decreases of both β1- and β2-globulin (Lochmiller et al., 1985). β-Globulin also decreased in protein-restricted malnourished swine (Tumbleson, 1973). γ-Globulin concentrations were increased in malnourished swine (Baetz and Mengeling, 1971; Tumbleson, 1973) and intake-restricted male collard peccaries (Lochmiller et al., 1985). Total serum protein and albumin concentrations were not affected for intake-restricted male and female collard peccaries (Lochmiller et al., 1985).

Serum urea nitrogen and creatinine concentrations can be influenced by extrarenal factors such as nutritional status. For example, prolonged fasting has caused decreased (Kornegay et al., 1964) and increased urea nitrogen concentrations (Baetz and Mengeling, 1971; Wilson et al., 1972). The effects of long-term severe undernutrition of the wild boar resulted in increased creatinine and, initially, slightly decreased then increased urea nitrogen concentrations (Wolkers et al., 1994). In intake-restricted male collard peccaries, serum urea nitrogen was increased after 9 weeks of feed restriction, though creatinine concentrations were not affected (Lochmiller et al., 1985). Protein source and concentration of the diet are important factors determining serum urea nitrogen concentrations. For example, groups of pigs maintained on diets of different protein concentrations demonstrated that the higher the protein content of the diet, the higher the blood urea nitrogen concentration (Wilson et al., 1972). In neonatal pigs, serum urea nitrogen increased with greater concentrations of soy proteins in the diet, as compared to milk proteins (Veum et al., 1986). In another neonatal pig study, urea nitrogen levels were markedly lower for diets containing casein as a protein source in lieu of dried egg albumen (Watkins and Veum, 1986). Additionally, the type of carbohydrate in the diet can affect urea nitrogen levels. For example, Mateo and Veum (1980) fed pigs a diet containing glucose, sucrose, or cornstarch as sources of carbohydrate. The cornstarch diet caused a decrease in serum urea nitrogen concentration, compared to the glucose- and sucrose-containing diets.

Fasting of pigs caused decrease of calcium, chloride, magnesium, and sodium concentrations (Baetz and Mengeling, 1971; Kornegay et al., 1964). In Yucatan swine, it has been shown that feeding low-phosphorus or low-calcium diets increased production of 1,25-dihydroxycholecalciferol, approximately 2.5-fold and fourfold, respectively. Metabolic clearance of the vitamin decreased with the low-calcium diet but not the low-phosphorus diet (Fox and Ross, 1985). Inorganic phosphorus was decreased in pregnant and lactating sows (Tewes et al., 1979a, 1979b).

In swine, there are reports indicating that during fasting or low-protein diets glucose concentrations are maintained (Atinmo et al., 1974; Baetz and Mengeling, 1971; Doornenbal et al., 1983; Grandhi and Strain, 1982; Tumbleson et al., 1972); however, in 3-month-old pigs, prolongation of a fast to 167 hours caused decreases in glucose concentrations (Kornegay et al., 1964). Also in an experimental fast of prepubertal (130 days old) mixed breed gilts, blood glucose was reported to be decreased throughout the fast; however, insulin levels were not noted to decrease until the 28-hour period of the fast (Barb et al., 2001). Serum glucose concentrations were consistently lower in intake-restricted male and female collard peccaries (Lochmiller et at., 1985). Fifteen-days-old baby pigs reared artificially and fed diets containing glucose, sucrose, or cornstarch as carbohydrate sources plus isolated soybean protein were evaluated for alterations of serum glucose, total protein, and urea nitrogen (Mateo and Veum, 1980). The diet containing sucrose caused a slight decrease in serum glucose compared to the glucose-fed group, but values were considered within the reference range. When cornstarch instead of glucose was utilized as the source of carbohydrates decreases in serum glucose, total protein, and urea nitrogen occurred. Sows allowed *ad lib* access to feed from 60 days of gestation were evaluated for altered glucose tolerance (Weldon et al., 1994). Compared to sows fed a standard level of feed, the *ad lib* sows were less tolerant of glucose infusion in the form of an intravenous glucose tolerance testing (IVGTT) on day 1 of lactation. Nonesterified fatty acids were greater in the *ad lib* sows than in sows fed at a standard level, and release of nonesterified fatty acids in response to an epinephrine challenge also was greater in the *ad lib* sows. Insulin concentrations were not affected by feeding status.

Fasting of pigs has increased serum concentrations of cholesterol, phospholipids, and free fatty acids, and decreased triglycerides (Baetz, 1973; Baetz and Mengeling, 1971; Kornegay et al., 1964). A study of Göttingen swine fasted for a period of 48 hours reported that bilirubin level increased and magnesium decreased in males (Tsutsumi et al., 1999). Long-term and severe undernutrition causing increased nonesterified fatty acid concentrations in the wild boar has also been reported (Wolkers et al., 1994). Serum triglyceride concentrations decreased and nonesterified fatty acids increased in intake-restricted (25% of *ad lib*) male collard peccaries, though cholesterol concentrations were not altered (Lochmiller et al., 1985). Female collard peccaries, restricted to 55% of *ad lib* intake, exhibited increased nonesterified fatty acid concentrations but no changes in the triglyceride concentrations.

Besides diet restriction or undernutrition, altering diet composition or components can also affect lipid profiles. For example, feeding a semisynthetic diet containing 0.25% cholesterol to Pitman-Moore miniature pigs for 28 days resulted in approximately a fourfold increase in serum cholesterol (Filer et al., 1986). Addition of 15% cellulose to the diet dampened the response, as the serum cholesterol increased only twofold. In another study, feeding a HFHC diet to crossbred domestic pigs for 6 months induced an approximately sixfold increase in cholesterol concentration with concomitant increases in very-low-density lipoprotein (VLDL), LDL, and HDL-C of approximately eightfold, sevenfold, and twofold, respectively; triglyceride concentrations were not affected (Fuster et al., 1986). A study using young Bama miniswine fed a high-fat, high-sucrose, high-cholesterol diet produced a linear increase in serum glucose over a 5-month period resulting in a level 2.15-fold higher than control at 5 months. Insulin levels began to increase at 2 months, peaked at 4 months, and declined from that point. Total cholesterol and triglyceride significantly increased over control from the first month onward (Liu et al., 2007). A high-fat diet in Yucatan swine also produced increases in cholesterol, LDL, and HDL over normal fed in a 20- and 24-week study (Thomas et al., 2002; Otis et al., 2003). Additionally, sows fed a high cholesterol and fat diet during lactation showed increased serum and milk cholesterol concentrations, resulting in higher serum cholesterol concentrations in the nursing offspring (Heald and Naseem, 1986). In protein-restricted malnourished swine, cholesterol and triglyceride concentrations were higher than for *ad lib* controls (Tumbleson, 1973).

Serum enzyme activities also can be affected by nutritional status. It has been demonstrated that fasting increases the serum activity of CK and decreases the activity of ALP (Baetz and Mengeling, 1971). Long-term and severe undernutrition caused decreased serum ALP activity in the wild boar (Wolkers et al., 1994). In male collard peccaries restricted to 25% of *ad lib* intake, serum ALP activity doubled after 3 weeks of restriction; thereafter, ALP activity decreased to control levels by 9 weeks of restriction (Lochmiller et al., 1985). The activities of LDH, GGT, AST, and ALT were unaffected; although total LDH activity was not altered, there was an increase in the percentage of LDH1 and LDH2 in the LDH isoenzyme profiles of the intake-restricted animals. In female collard peccaries restricted to 55% of *ad lib* intake, serum activity of AST increased.

Fasting pigs for up to 167 hours caused decreases in calcium, chloride, magnesium, and sodium concentrations (Baetz and Mengeling, 1971; Kornegay et al., 1964). In diet-restricted male collard peccaries, serum concentrations of copper, calcium, magnesium, sodium, and chloride were decreased, compared to the *ad lib* control animals; there also were relationships between intake and phosphorus, potassium, zinc, and iron concentrations (Lochmiller et al., 1985). In protein-restricted malnourished swine, inorganic phosphorus and calcium concentrations decreased, while potassium concentration increased (Tumbleson, 1973).

Endocrine function can also be affected by nutritional status. Male collard peccaries restricted to 25% of *ad lib* intake had approximately one-half the triiodothyronine (T3) but not thyroxine (T4) concentration, compared to controls; testosterone concentration also was approximately 50% lower (Lochmiller et al., 1985). Female collard peccaries restricted to 55% of *ad lib* intake, however, demonstrated a consistent decrease in serum T4 but not T3 concentrations.

Cholesterol concentration increased in neonatal pigs 2 days postpartum and remained elevated during the nursing period (Mersmann et al., 1979; Tumbleson and Kalish, 1972); triglyceride concentrations in the piglets also increased during nursing and decreased after weaning. Serum total lipid, cholesterol, HDL, and LDL were low in neonates compared to adult pigs but increased to an elevated concentration after colostrum/milk ingestion (Johansson and Karlsson, 1982). By 8 weeks, total lipid, cholesterol, and LDL decreased to adult concentrations; HDL remained elevated. In the sow, serum cholesterol was increased during lactation (Tumbleson et al., 1970).

There are breed and line differences affecting preanalytical clinical biochemistry determinations and reference ranges. Ossabaw obese pigs had higher triglyceride and cholesterol concentrations at 10–12 months of age than conventional breeds (Etherton and Kris-Etherton, 1980). For genetically selected obese lines, lower growth hormone and higher fasting free fatty acids were the most common findings. Lower growth hormone concentrations in weanling pigs, or pigs of 90–95 kg, have also been observed for conventional breeds selected for obesity (Althen and Gerrits, 1976; Lund-Larsen and Bakke, 1975). From birth to 5–6 months of age, these pigs were not hyperglycemic, hyperinsulinemic, hypertriglyceridemic, or hypercholesterolemic, and they all exhibited a normal glucose tolerance (Mersmann et al., 1973). In the fed state, obese pigs had higher free fatty acid concentrations than lean pigs (Mersmann and MacNeil, 1985); the reverse was true for the fasted state (Bakke, 1975; Mersmann and MacNeil, 1985). A line of domestic pigs selected for leanness had higher fasting free fatty acid concentrations than control pigs (Gregory et al., 1980). In contrast, Ossabaw pigs did not have lower fasting free fatty acid concentrations, as had been observed for the genetically selected lines (Wangsness et al., 1981). One line of obese pig had higher plasma cortisol concentrations (Lunstrom et al., 1983) and a higher fasting glucose (Bakke, 1975).

Increasing lipid or cholesterol content in the diet caused increases of serum cholesterol concentration, with a large increase of cholesterol content occurring in the LDL fraction and a modest increase in the HDL fraction (Beynen et al., 1983; Kim et al., 1984); however, the magnitude of serum cholesterol increase can be altered by the type of lipid added to the diet. For example, the addition of corn oil to the diet resulted in lower serum cholesterol concentrations than the addition of butter (Kim et al., 1984). Including propionic acid or calcium propionate in the diet caused decreases of serum cholesterol, HDL-C, LDL cholesterol, and triglycerides (Thacker and Bowland, 1986). Dietary whey lessened the increases of serum cholesterol in pigs fed a hypercholesterolemic (high-cholesterol) diet. Serum cholesterol concentrations in these animals were similar to pigs fed non-cholesterol supplemented diets, with or without whey (Beames et al., 1986).

Foudin et al. (1986) demonstrated that, in boars, voluntary consumption of alcohol for a period of 17 weeks caused serum triglyceride concentrations to increase, peaking at 4 weeks and remaining increased to the end of the 17-week test period. Triglyceride concentrations increased twofold within 3 days post-alcohol removal, after which they began to decline. During alcohol consumption, the triglyceride concentration elevation was attributed to increases of 16:0, 18:0, and 18:1 fatty acids; 18:2 fatty acids decreased. The increase that occurred during withdrawal was attributed to triglycerides containing 18:1, 18:2, and 16:0 fatty acids.

The source and concentration of protein in the diet are important determining factors for serum urea nitrogen concentrations. Groups of pigs maintained on diets of different protein concentrations demonstrated that the higher the protein content of the diet, the higher the blood urea nitrogen concentrations (Wilson et al., 1972). In neonatal pigs, serum urea nitrogen increased with greater concentrations of soy proteins in the diet, compared to milk proteins (Veum et al., 1986). Piglets fed diets containing a 50:50 ratio of casein:whey protein had lower plasma urea nitrogen concentrations than those fed diets containing casein:whey at ratios of 80:20 or 0:100 (Newport and Henschel, 1986). The authors suggested that the equal proportions of protein types caused an improvement in protein utilization. It was indicated that casein is the predominant protein of cow milk, whey predominates in human milk, and sow milk contains approximately equal proportions of both. In another neonatal pig study, urea nitrogen levels were markedly lower for diets containing casein as a protein source as compared to those containing dried egg albumen (Watkins and Veum, 1986). That the type of carbohydrate in the diet can affect urea nitrogen levels was exemplified by the work of Mateo and Veum (1980), who fed pigs diets containing glucose, sucrose, or cornstarch as sources of carbohydrate. The use of cornstarch in the diet caused a decrease in serum urea nitrogen concentration, compared to diets containing glucose and sucrose.

Gestation caused a decrease in urea nitrogen concentration (Tumbleson et al., 1970); this phenomenon was not observed by Gotze et al. (1984). Oldigs (1986) demonstrated that a white line of Göttingen miniature pig had creatinine and urea nitrogen concentrations that were lower than for a colored line.

The fact that urea nitrogen and creatinine concentrations are affected by age differences has been documented. Urea nitrogen increased (Tumbleson and Kalish, 1972) and creatinine decreased (Khan et al., 1986) in neonatal pigs from birth to 72 hours of age. After weaning, urea nitrogen and creatinine concentrations increased, stabilizing at 3 months for urea nitrogen and at 3 years for creatinine (McClellan et al., 1966). Similar findings occurred for urea nitrogen in Sinclair miniature swine (Hutcheson et al., 1979). In Yucatan miniature swine, a gender difference was observed for creatinine, 123.8 for female versus 106.1 μmol/L for male (Parsons and Wells, 1986); no gender difference was observed for Sinclair miniature pigs (Hutcheson et al., 1979).

5.5.7 Housing Environment/Enrichment

Researchers examining salivary cortisol levels in pigs housed in an enriched or barren pen environment noted a blunted circadian rhythm of cortisol in pigs in the barren environment during light but not dark periods (de Groot et al., 2001).

5.5.8 Circadian Rhythm

Circadian rhythms also exist for certain biochemical constituents. In a study to evaluate the role of the photoperiod on the secretion of cortisol and melatonin in boars, Minton et al. (1989) demonstrated a circadian rhythm for cortisol and that the rhythm shifted in conjunction with a 6-hour phase shift advance. In general, higher cortisol concentrations were observed during the late subjective evening and darkphase, while lower concentrations occurred about 6–10 hours after onset of the lightphase. Circadian rhythms of ACTH, prolactin, and melatonin have also been investigated (Griffith and Minton, 1991, 1992).

A study of diurnal variation in Göttingen swine found that glutamic oxaloacetic transaminase (aspartate transaminase) increased from morning through afternoon then decreased from midnight to early morning in both male and female animals. Urea nitrogen was described as decreasing in morning in both sexes and increasing through the afternoon and into the night for males but increasing in females only in afternoon. Calcium levels in female swine decreased in the morning and increased through the afternoon into night. Inorganic phosphorus was reported to decrease in the afternoon and increase from midnight to morning in both males and females. All of these variations were reportedly eliminated by fasting the animals (Tsutsumi et al., 1999).

Yorkshire gilts (110-day-old), maintained under 14-hour light/10-hour dark lighting conditions, were placed into two groups that were 180° out of phase. When estradiol (15 mg/kg) was administered intramuscular (IM) during the subjective light phase, the LH surges demonstrated a biphasic pattern with lower peaks (between 4 and 8 ng/mL). When estradiol was administered during the subjective dark phase, the LH surges demonstrated a single higher peak (between 8 and 12 ng/mL). This pattern reversed when the light regime was reversed, suggesting an interaction between light–dark cycle and estrogen affecting the release of LH in the pig. For all gilts, baseline LH concentrations were <2 ng/mL, and LH peaks were >5 ng/mL (Evans et al., 1994).

5.5.9 Stress

In studies requiring clinical chemistry analyses, the effect of experimental procedures upon the analytes considered for evaluation is often a concern. Acute responses to stress-inducing factors such as introduction to a new environment, introduction of a gilt to a boar, unfamiliar or rough handling procedures, restraint, transportation, and mixing of unfamiliar swine have been reported (Barnett et al., 1982, 1984; Spencer and Hallet, 1986; Wade et al., 1986). For example, sling restraint of untrained pigs caused immediate increases in epinephrine and norepinephrine concentrations and slower increases of ACTH, cortisol, aldosterone, and renin concentrations (Wade et al., 1986). The use of a maxillary sling restraint resulted in increased concentrations of cortisol, ACTH, lactate, and glucose (Brenner et al., 1979).

Spencer and Hallet (1986) demonstrated that the stress of loading for transport resulted in rapid increases of plasma glucose, insulin, lactate, and thyroxine, reaching peak values within 10 minutes. Triiodothyronine and cortisol also increased but did not reach peak concentrations until 15–20 minutes poststress. The values for all analytes returned to baseline by 1 hour postloading. In the same study, free fatty acid concentrations were immediately decreased, remained decreased for an hour, and then increased to above baseline at approximately 110 minutes poststress, remaining elevated at 210 minutes. Detectable somatomedin activity by bioassay was rapidly depressed and remained decreased for > 2 hours. In other studies on the response to the stress of transport and slaughter, increased activities of CK, LDH, AST, malic dehydrogenase (MDH), ALP, and isocitric dehydrogenase (ICDH) occurred, as well as increases in concentrations of urea nitrogen and potassium (Lengerken and Pfeiffer, 1978; Moss and McMurray, 1979; Yu et al., 2007). One study also found serum proteins such as major acute phase protein (Pig-MAP), haptoglobin, SAA, C-reactive protein were increased over control in two boars after 24 hours of transport (Piñeiro et al., 2007).

Thermal stress has been shown to cause changes in acid–base balance, demonstrated as respiratory alkalosis and characterized by increased blood pH and decreased PCO_2 (Bartko et al., 1984). In their studies of halothane-induced physiological changes, Henning et al. (1986) indicated that it had been reported that exogenously induced hyperthermia in stress-susceptible pigs led to an increase of lactic acid concentration and activities of ALT, AST, LDH, and CK and a decrease in plasma base excess. They also pointed out that stress-susceptible pigs have been identified by increased CK activity 24 hours after treadmill exercise; pH decreases and increases of lactic acid and LDH have also been observed after exercise in stress-susceptible pigs.

Parsons et al. (1986) demonstrated that with endurance training, pigs developed clinical chemistry changes similar to those in marathon runners (Wood and Haskell, 1979): total cholesterol decreased while HDL-C increased. Also, iron concentration decreased while the hemoglobin content remained the same. Like humans, pigs become acidotic with exercise.

In a study determining the effects of floor temperature, supplemental heat, and drying on piglet survival, McGinnis et al. (1981) demonstrated that T4 concentrations at 5 days of age were lower for male pigs, pigs on the warmer floor, and pigs given supplemental heat. No treatment effects were noted for T3 concentrations.

Short-term overcrowding caused mild increases of glucose concentration and ALD activity (Kolataj et al., 1988). Barnett et al. (1983) reported that chronic stress was associated with higher concentrations of total protein and glucose and lower uric acid. In their review of handling and housing practices and chronic stress, Barnett and Hemsworth (1986) reported that unpleasant rough handling, administered either on a regular or irregular basis, resulted in increased free corticosteroid concentrations.

Housing methods, resulting in a high level of confinement (tether stalls), have caused higher corticosteroid concentrations when compared to those in group-housed animals (Barnett and Hemsworth, 1986). The pigs in tether stalls displayed aggressive behavior compared to group-housed animals in which a social order was established and little aggression observed. Baldi et al. (1989) also demonstrated that cortisol, proteins, and CK levels were negatively correlated with social hierarchy.

Pigs housed with adequate space had higher CK values than those housed under restricted (50%) space (Meldrum et al., 1986). The increases were related to greater space for movement and fighting among the pigs with adequate space versus those in cramped conditions.

Chronic increases of cortisol have been reported in space-restricted pigs but providing straw reduced cortisol concentrations (Warnier and Zayan, 1985). In contrast, crowding crossbred male pigs did not alter cortisol concentrations when compared to uncrowded animals (Meunier-Salaun et al., 1987; Pearce and Paterson, 1993). Tethered pigs (Von Borell and Ladewig, 1989) and crowded pigs (Meunier-Salaun et al., 1987) have demonstrated higher cortisol responses to an ACTH challenge than non-tethered, group-housed pigs or those housed in lower densities.

In an evaluation of intensive housing for prepartum, crossbred gilts and sows, Becker et al. (1986) described the changes in cortisol concentrations related to tethering versus individual housing (gestation stalls and pens). The authors indicated that chronic restrictive housing is not a chronic stress based on the circadian rhythm of cortisol and its responses to ACTH and dexamethasone administration. They showed that, depending on the animals' previous housing experience, placement of prepartum gilts and sows in tether or gestation stalls did not necessarily result in increased cortisol concentrations. The cortisol circadian rhythm of gilts placed in tether stalls became altered for a period of 3–8 days, after which the animals adapted.

Acute responses to stress factors can alter some hormone concentrations such as epinephrine, norepinephrine, ACTH, cortisol, aldosterone, and renin (Barnett et al., 1982, 1984; Spencer and

Hallet, 1986; Wade et al., 1986). For example, sling restraint of untrained pigs caused increases in epinephrine, norepinephrine, ACTH, cortisol, and aldosterone concentrations and renin activity (Wade et al., 1986). The stress of physical restraint for blood collection of swine resulted in increased concentrations of cortisol and ACTH (Brenner et al., 1979). The stress of loading for transport resulted in rapid increases of insulin, T4, T3, and cortisol concentrations (Spencer and Hallet, 1986); the values for analytes peaked within 10–20 minutes and returned to baseline by 1 hour postloading. Bioassayable somatomedin activity was also rapidly depressed and remained decreased for >2 hours. Housing methods may likewise alter cortisol concentrations (Barnett and Hemsworth, 1986) or cortisol response to ACTH challenge (Meunier-Salaun et al., 1987; Pearce and Paterson, 1993; Von Borell and Ladewig, 1989).

5.5.10 Effects of Anesthesia

Malignant hyperthermia (MH) is a slight risk when anesthetizing pigs. It may occur in any breed but is commonly encountered in Hampshire, Landrace, Pietrain, Poland China, and Yorkshire breeds (McGrath et al., 1981). Halothane triggers MH in susceptible pigs, resulting in a marked decrease of arterial pH and an increase of arterial blood lactate that occurs almost immediately after administering the anesthetic (Nelson, 1986). Succinylcholine can initiate an episode and increase the incidence in swine anesthetized with halothane (Nelson, 1986). Isoflurane, enflurane (Nelson, 1986), sevoflurane (Shulman et al., 1981), and chloroform (Hall et al., 1972) can also trigger an episode, while barbiturates (Gronert, 1980), narcotics, and nitrous oxide (Nelson, 1986) do not. In some highly susceptible animals, restraint-associated stress can initiate the syndrome (Riebold and Thurmon, 1986).

In a study of halothane-induced MH, Landrace piglets were exposed to the anesthetic for 5 minutes, and several biochemical variables were serially evaluated (Henning et al., 1986). Stress-susceptible animals showed a more pronounced decrease in blood pH during inhalation and slower recovery than resistant animals; the positive pigs also showed a more pronounced increase of pCO_2 during inhalation. Lactate increased more during inhalation and demonstrated a slower recovery in the reactors: lactate concentrations increased from approximately 9 mg/dL at baseline to 75 mg/dL at the onset of halothane inhalation, increasing again to 95 mg/dL at the end of the 5-minute exposure. Peak concentrations of 106 mg/dL occurred at 15 minutes postinhalation. LDH activity progressively increased in the reactors, starting 60 minutes postinhalation, and at 120 and 180 minutes, LDH activity was approximately 2170 and 2680 mU/mL. Preinhalation LDH activity for the reactors was approximately 700 mU/mL. In their discussion, these authors indicated that a similar response had been reported for CK activity. Henning et al. (1986) also demonstrated that AST activity progressively increased, starting 60 minutes postinhalation, peaking at approximately 75 mU/mL at 180 minutes, and not returning to basal activity (approximately 16 mU/mL) until 96 hours postinhalation. ALT activity progressively increased, starting 180 minutes postinhalation, peaking at approximately 41 mU/mL between 24 and 48 hours, and not returning to basal activity (approximately 30 mU/mL) until 96 hours postinhalation.

A study using Yucatan swine reported that isoflurane anesthesia caused decreased glucose tolerance and decreased insulin levels (Laber-Laird et al., 1992). This decreased glucose-induced insulin secretion is also reported with sevoflurane anesthesia (Saho et al., 1997). Another study reported that ketamine–xylazine combination anesthesia resulted in decreased insulin levels in female Yucatan swine (Heim et al., 2002). Use of a telazol–ketamine–xylazine mixture in mixed breed swine resulted in decreased LH levels in barrows and increased cortisol levels in barrows and gilts (Clapper, 2008). ALT has been used to evaluate potential hepatic damage caused by anesthetics (Weiskopf et al., 1992) and sepsis (Hoban et al., 1992). Epinephrine, norepinephrine, and vasopressin concentrations and renin activity have been used to evaluate responses to alterations of blood pressure by anesthetic agents (Weiskopf et al., 1992). Increasing the depth of anesthesia caused increases in vasopressin concentrations and renin activity. In a model of hemorrhagic shock, rapid blood loss resulted in changes in vasoactive hormones characterized by increases in plasma renin activity and concentrations of epinepherine, norepinepherine, vasopressin, aldosterone, ACTH, and cortisol (Hannon, 1992).

5.5.11 Blood Collection Site and Handling

The use of physical restraint for blood collection in swine can be stressful; for example, the use of maxillary sling restraint resulted in increased concentrations of cortisol, ACTH, lactate, and glucose (Brenner et al., 1979). There also appears to be significant intra-animal variability in stress response when this type of restraint is used.

The effect of the site of blood collection has been investigated and differences, such as those in concentrations of plasma amino acids, have been described (Stockland et al., 1971). CPK activity was higher for samples collected from the anterior vena cava than those from the auricular vein (Bruss and Becker, 1981). Flushing the needle in the anterior vena cava with saline after insertion ameliorated this effect. A study examining the feasibility of using tibial intraosseous blood sampling as compared to auricular venous sampling found that, though many blood chemistry parameters were comparable to the venous sample, potassium and AST were higher in intraosseous samples (Greco et al., 2001). Researchers examining LH and progesterone levels in the jugular vein and caudal vena cava of Landrace and Hungarian Mangalica swine reported that the caudal vena cava had a higher mean level of progesterone (Brussow et al., 2008). Baldi et al. (1989) showed that the different techniques of blood sampling influenced LDH and CK activities. Researchers examined blood obtained by jugular venipuncture as compared to blood drawn from a cannula placed in the anterior vena cava. They noted jugular CK, AST, total bilirubin, GGT, albumin, and total protein were increased while Na, CO_2, and P were decreased as compared to cannula samples. They also report statistical differences in chemistry values when comparing results of experienced versus inexperienced samplers (Dubreuil et al., 1990). The effect of repeated blood sampling in weanling pigs has been described as well (Kornegay, 1967). In a comparison between the use of an indwelling catheter and an external jugular venipuncture, total protein, albumin, and creatinine concentrations were increased for catheter-collected blood (Tumbleson, 1986). No changes were observed for cholesterol, lipoproteins, triglycerides, urea nitrogen, or protein electrophoresis. As mentioned in Section 5.5.10, certain anesthetics and, in some highly susceptible individuals, restraint-associated stress can initiate a MH response.

Serum testosterone and estradiol concentrations can vary depending on the sampling site. Testosterone concentrations for blood collected from the testicular vein of white composite breed boars were approximately 40 times higher than the values (approximate mean value of 80 ng/mL) obtained for blood collected from the jugular vein (approximate mean value of 2 ng/mL) (Wise et al., 1996).

Unilateral ovariectomy caused FSH, but not LH, to increase 24 hours postsurgery; bilateral ovaricetomy induced both FSH and LH to increase (Redmer et al., 1984). Unilateral ovariectomy also caused ovarian venous blood estradiol concentrations to be increased at 2 and 4 days postsurgery; 8 days postsurgery, estradiol concentrations were similar to sham control values (Redmer et al., 1984). The estradiol concentration for peripheral blood collected from the jugular vein, however, did not demonstrate these changes. In another study, plasma estrone concentration in blood collected from the jugular vein was unchanged for unilaterally ovariohysterectomized white composite breed gilts at days 30, 31, 38, and 45 of pregnancy (Vallet and Christenson, 1994).

Hemolysis interfered with several biochemical analyses, and hemoglobin added as blood hemolysate, caused increases of creatinine, total protein, albumin, inorganic phosphorus, calcium, potassium, total bilirubin, ALT, AST, and LDH (Dorner et al., 1983). Bilirubin was affected starting at a hemoglobin concentration of 54 mg/dL, and ALT and AST activity increases started at 133 and 215 mg/dL, respectively. The other affected variables demonstrated increases at 400 mg/dL. The authors concluded that if serum contained hemoglobin at 400 mg/dL (cherry red), the sample should not be tested. If serum contained <100 mg/dL hemoglobin, the effect was insignificant and the sample was acceptable for biochemical analyses. In another study, free hemoglobin of <500 mg/dL had no effect on the analyses of creatinine, urea, inorganic phosphorus, sodium, calcium, copper, and CK (Naumann et al., 1983). Hemoglobin concentrations of at least 180 mg/dL caused interference with total protein, albumin, potassium, zinc, and ALP; hemoglobin >500 mg/dL caused interference with urea, inorganic phosphorus, γ-globulin, ceruloplasmin, and AST analyses. Hemolysis was not influenced by relative centrifugal force during the separation of serum from cells, and there were no differences in the concentrations or activities of 14 serum variables in pig blood centrifuged at various forces between 2.5 and 45,000×*g* for 10 minutes (Mulder and Tumbleson, 1972).

5.5.12 Experimental Manipulation

In immature domestic pigs, loss of 50% (but not 30%) of the estimated blood volume over a 1-hour period resulted in increased serum concentrations of glucose, lactate, arterial PO_2, urea nitrogen, creatinine, sodium, magnesium, and inorganic phosphorus; there were decreases in arterial pH, arterial PCO_2, bicarbonate, base excess, potassium, total protein, albumin, and globulin (Hannon and Bossone, 1986). For the most part, these changes were partially resolving 5 hours posthemorrhage.

Hannon (1992) reviewed the physiological responses to hemorrhagic hypotension in pigs. Significant rapid blood loss resulted in increased concentrations of creatinine and urea nitrogen due to decreased renal clearance. There were decreases in urine volume and in sodium, potassium, and osmolal excretion related to decreased renal blood flow. Decreases in arterial pH, arterial PCO_2, and bicarbonate were related to increased lactic acid concentrations. Protein decreases were related to a shift of water from the extravascular to intravascular space. It was suggested that potassium decreases were related to increased cellular glucose utilization. It was noted, however, that pigs subjected to prolonged hemorrhagic hypotension using the Wiggers method demonstrated increases of plasma potassium and phosphorus concentrations; these changes were rarely observed for fixed-volume hemorrhage paradigms. Vasoactive hormones demonstrated increases in plasma renin activity, epinephrine, norepinephrine, vasopressin, aldosterone, ACTH, and cortisol; fixed-volume and Wiggers models of hemorrhage gave qualitatively similar hormone responses. Increases in the activities of hepatic transaminases may also occur during prolonged fixed-pressure hemorrhage, though function tests were not compromised.

Surgical manipulations can also alter chemistry values. For example, a 95%–98% small intestinal bypass caused decreases of albumin, total protein, calcium, and cholesterol concentrations; urine protein excretion decreased, and there was an increase in the urine activity of β-galactosidase (Assimos et al., 1986). The authors also observed that similar postoperative decreases of albumin, total protein, calcium, and cholesterol have been reported for humans. Splenectomy resulted in alterations of the resting arterial PO_2, pH, arterial PCO_2, and bicarbonate values (Hannon et al., 1990). Hepatotoxic effects resulting in cholestasis and characterized by marked increases of total and direct bilirubin (>11 and >5 mg/dL, respectively) occurred after chronic intravenous hyperalimentation (Cohen et al., 1986). Additionally, activities of ALP, LDH, and AST were increased.

5.6 BRIEF DESCRIPTION OF COMMON AND SPECIALIZED PROCEDURES

Common clinical chemistry procedures in swine biomedical research models include serum biochemistry panels, clotting factors, urinalysis, serum protein and immunoglobulin profiles, plasma lipoprotein and triglyceride profiles, blood gases and electrolytes, cardiac, liver, and kidney function analytes, and hormone bioassays. Nutritionists are also targeting minerals, vitamins, sugars, proteins, metabolites, and other nutritional factors in blood. Categorized typical and special biochemistry parameters for swine models are listed in Table 5.3.

TABLE 5.3
Swine Peripheral Venous Blood Serum Biochemistry Parameters

Category	Parameter [a]	Units
Electrolytes/Ions		
Cations	Sodium	mmol/L or mEq/L
	Calcium	mg/dL
	Potassium	mmol/L
	Iron	μg/dL or μmol/L
	Magnesium	mg/dL
Anions	Chloride	mmol/L or mEq/L
	Bicarbonate (TCO^2)	mmol/L or mEq/L
	Phosphorus/phosphate	mg/dL
	Anion gap	mmol/L
	Osmolality	mOsm/kg
Carbohydrates	Glucose	mg/dL
	Fructosamine	mmol/L
Metabolic Products	Urea or blood urea nitrogen (BUN)	mg/dL
	Creatinine	mg/dL
	BUN/creatinine ratio	ratio
	Total bilirubin	mg/dL
	Direct bilirubin	mg/dL
	Indirect bilirubin	mg/dL
	Lactate	nmol/L or mg/dL
	Uric acid	mg/dL
Proteins	Total protein	g/dL
	Albumin	g/dL
	Globulin (α,ß,γ)	g/dL
	A/G ratio	ratio
	Fibrinogen [b]	mg/dL or μmol/L
	Immunoglobulins	mg/dL or μmol/L
Lipids	Cholesterol	mg/dL
	High-density lipoprotein (HDL)	mmol/L
	LDL	mmol/L
	Very-low-density lipoprotein (VLDL), IDL	mmol/L
	Triglycerides	mg/dL
	Free fatty acids	mg/dL
Enzymes	Alkaline phosphatase (ALP)	IU/L or μkat/L
	Aspartate aminotransferase (AST)	IU/L or μkat/L
	Alanine aminotransferase (ALT)	IU/L or μkat/L
	Gamma-glutamyl transferase (GGT)	IU/L or μkat/L
	Lactate dehydrogenase (LDH)	IU/L or μkat/L
	Creatine phosphokinase (CPK)	IU/L or μkat/L
	Sorbital dehydrogenase (SDH) or iditol dehydrogenase (IDH)	IU/L
	Ornithine carbamoyltransferase (OCT)	IU/L
	Isocitric dehydrogenase (ICDH)	IU/L

(Continued)

TABLE 5.3 (*Continued*)
Swine Peripheral Venous Blood Serum Biochemistry Parameters

Category	Parameter[a]	Units
	Malic dehydrogenase *(MDH)*	IU/L
	Lipase	IU/L
	Amylase	IU/L
	Arginase	IU/L
Hormones	*Total T3*	ng/mL
	Total T4	μg/mL
	Free T4	ng/mL
	ACTH	pg/mL
	Cortisol	μg/dL or mg/mL
	Insulin	μIU/mL
	Corticotropin-releasing factor (CRF) or corticotropin-releasing hormone (CRH)	
	Glucagon	
	Insulin-like growth factor 1 (ILGF-1/ IGF-1)	ng/mL
	C-peptide	
	Follicle-stimulating hormone (FSH)	ng/mL or μIU/mL
	Leutinizing hormone (LH)	ng/mL or μIU/mL
	Somatostatin	pmol/L
	GH (somatrophin)	ng/mL
	Somatomedin (Substance P)	U/mL
	Estrogen	nmol/L or ng/mL
	Testosterone	nmol/L or ng/mL
	ß-Endorphin	pg/mL
	Epinephrine	pg/mL
	Renin	ng A1/mL/h
Vitamins	*Cobalamin (Vit B_{12})*	ng/L
	Folate	μg/L
Other	*Pig-MAP (major acute phase protein-)*	
	Haptoglobin (HPT)	ng/mL or g/L
	Heat shock protein (HSP-)	
	C-reactive protein (CRP)	mg/dL
	Serum amyloid A (SAA)	
	Leptin, resistin, ghrelin	ng/mL
	B_2 microglobin	
	Neopterin	nmol/L

[a] Typical analytes are in regular font (non italics); special (non-routine) analytes are in italics.

[b] Plasma fibrinogen. Enzymes units are occasionally reported as μkat/L, an SI unit; for conversion of μkat/L to IU/L, multiply μkat/L by 60.

Additionally, sophisticated toxicogenomics technologies (proteomic, genomic, or metabolomic) procedures for assaying unique biochemical entities can include molecular biology (polymerase chain reaction [PCR]), immunology, or classical chemistry (tandem mass spectrometry [MS/MS], nuclear magnetic resonance [NMR]) methods (NRC, 2007). Established biochemical markers are now reported in the swine literature, such as troponin for cardiac and skeletal muscle function (O'Brien et al., 1997). Other potential biomarkers or biosignatures include sialic acid, acute phase proteins (B_2 microglobulin, C-reactive protein [CRP], haptoglobin, SAA), leptin, and metallothionein for environmental metal exposures.

Specialized biochemical tests in swine include ACTH response testing, sulfobromophthalein (BSP) clearance, glucose tolerance testing, dexamethasone suppression test (DST), inulin and creatinine clearance, and thyrotropin-releasing hormone (TRH) stimulation test. Of these tests, the glucose tolerance testing is the most commonly practiced at Sinclair Research Center.

5.6.1 ACTH Stimulation Testing

The ACTH stimulation test is used to assess the functional state of the adrenal gland. Following ACTH administration, the adrenal should respond by releasing glucocorticosteroid hormone (cortisol). If no increase in cortisol is noted, the adrenal may be fatigued. A chronically stressed animal will normally have higher levels of cortisol post-ACTH challenge than will unstressed animals. Becker et al. (1986) described an ACTH stimulation test in the pig using 10 International Units (IU) of ACTH IV and collecting samples at 0, 15, and 30 minutes, and 1, 2, 4, 6, and 8 hours postinjection. In a different study, response to an exogenous ACTH challenge was performed by collecting blood via an indwelling jugular catheter every 15 minutes from 12.00 to 16.30 hours. During the collection period, 25 IU ACTH/pig was administered by IM injection at 13.55 hours (Pearce and Paterson, 1993).

5.6.2 BSP Clearance

BSP is a cholephilic dye that is used for testing hepatic function (portal circulation, function of hepatocytes, patency of biliary tract) (Cornelius, 1989). In their reviews, Wilson et al. (1972) and Cornelius (1989) cited reports investigating the use of BSP clearance as a test for hepatic function in the pig. BSP retention for 100 kg pigs (administered 6 mg BSP/kg) was 3%–4% at 15 minutes postadministration. In another study, after intravenous (IV) administration of 5 mg BSP/kg, 30 kg pigs had a 5-minute retention of 5.3% ± 2.0%; the retention at 10 minutes was 1.4% ± 0.9% and at 15 minutes 0.6% ± 0.6%. In that study, after a protein-deficient diet for approximately 5 months, the BSP retentions were between 10.5% and 16.7%, 1.7% and 6.0%, and 0.6% and 2.6% for 5, 10, and 15 minutes postadministration, respectively. Chloroform toxicosis increased the BSP retention in the protein-deficient pigs by three- to fourfold. In another investigation, 6 hours after intragastric administration of aflatoxin to pigs, BSP half-time increased from baseline (approximately 2 minutes) to approximately 19 minutes. Another report suggested that BSP retained at >0.3 mg dye/100 mL at 30 minutes postinjection of 5 mg/kg was indicative of hepatic dysfunction. In their review, Wilson et al. (1972) concluded that the BSP function test, while difficult to perform, was a useful test for hepatic function in the pig.

5.6.3 Glucose Tolerance Testing

Oral or intravenous glucose tolerance testing is frequently used to evaluate swine models of the metabolic syndrome (Larsen et al., 2002; Shoumin et al., 2004). Diabetes research (Bellinger et al., 2006; Larsen and Rolin, 2004) has made significant strides using these swine models. Renner et al. (2010) have created RIP II-GIPR^{dn} transgenic swine with glucagon-like peptide 1 receptor (GLP-1) and glucose-dependent insulinotropic polypeptide (GIP) receptor deficiency, disturbed incretin function, and glucose intolerance for Type 2 diabetes modeling. Researchers have also studied the use of insulin sensitivity testing in swine as a potential alternative to the longer time course of the glucose tolerance testing (Otis et al., 2003; Christoffersen et al., 2009). Swine oral and intravenous glucose tolerance tests (OGTT and IVGTT, respectively) are well established. Stimulation tests were performed in swine after an overnight fast and insulin therapy had been stopped for 30 hours (Mullen et al., 1992). The IVGTT was performed by IV injection of 0.5 g/kg glucose of a 50% solution and collection of blood samples at 0, 5, and 10 minutes, and every 10 minutes thereafter up to 60 minutes (Mullen et al., 1992). Additionally, blood samples collected at –15 and 2.5 minutes were used to calculate *K* values. In another study, the IVGTT was performed using an injection of 0.5 g glucose/kg given intravenously over 2 minutes, with blood samples collected at 0, 3, 5, 7, 10, 20, 30, 45, 60, and 90 minutes post glucose administration; *K* values were determined from the IVGTT data (DaFoe et al., 1989). An OGTT can be performed by giving 1.75 g glucose/kg in solution PO or 2 g glucose/kg mixed with a small amount of feed. Blood can be collected every 15 minutes up to 90 minutes (Wilson et al., 1986) or every 30 minutes up to 120 minutes (Mullen et al., 1992). Intravenous arginine tests have been performed by giving 0.5 g arginine/kg as a 0.6 g/mL solution during a 1-minute period. Blood was collected at 15 minute intervals, and concentrations of glucose, insulin, glucagon, somatostatin, and/or C-peptide were measured (Mullen et al., 1992). A tolbutamide response has also been used in the pig (Romsos et al., 1971). OGTT, IVGTT, isoglycemic and euglycemic clamps, hyperinsulinemia, and modified insulin tolerance tests are a few of the many diabetic protocols performed in swine models (Christoffersen et al., 2009).

5.6.4 Dexamethasone Suppression Test (DST)

The DST is classically used to assess pituitary–adrenal disturbances induced by chronic stress (Hay et al., 2000). Determination of blood cortisol levels before and after administration of dexamethasone also assists in diagnosing Cushing's syndrome and identifying the cause (i.e., primary disease due to adrenocortical tumors versus secondary hyperadrenocorticism from pituitary adenoma), depending on the protocol and dose used. Dexamethasone suppresses pituitary secretion of ACTH in normal animals and therefore the blood level of cortisol is decreased postadministration; low doses do not suppress cortisol levels in dogs and putatively in pigs with pituitary-dependent Cushing's syndrome, while high doses do cause suppression. High-dose dexamethasone administration differentiates between pituitary tumor and tumor elsewhere, such as the adrenal or another location. Cortisol production by functional adrenal tumors is not affected by dexamethasone. Urinary measurements of swine cortisol were as useful as blood cortisol determinations (Hay et al., 2000). The stress application for the DST has more utility than for Cushing's disease confirmation in research swine but the test will function for both purposes.

5.6.5 Inulin and Creatinine Clearance

This test is a procedure by which the filtering capacity of the glomeruli (the main filtering structures of the kidney) is determined by measuring the rate at which inulin, the test substance, is cleared from blood plasma. Inulin is the most accurate substance to measure this capacity because it is a small inert polysaccharide molecule that readily passes through the glomeruli into the urine without being reabsorbed by the renal tubules. The steps involved in this measurement, however, are quite involved; consequently, inulin is seldom used in clinical testing, although it is used in the research setting. Creatinine clearance is the more practical procedure used to assess renal function (Wendt et al., 1990; Bauer et al., 2000).

5.7 SUMMARY AND CONCLUSIONS

Swine have become increasingly important research models for the study of human disease and preclinical testing. Clinical biochemistry analysis is an important component of these studies to qualify animals for study and evaluate the post-dosing effect of the candidate drug, device, or procedure. Understanding and appreciating preanalytical sources of variation which can impact changes in biochemical parameter levels in biological fluids (blood, serum, plasma, urine, CSF, synovial fluid, peritoneal fluid, pleural fluid, ocular fluid) is important when conceiving experimental designs and during data interpretation. These potential preanalytical chemistry-impacting factors include age, sex, breed/genetics, fasting/feeding regimen/diet, health status, anesthesia, collection site, handling of animals or samples, housing/environment/enrichment, season, time of day/circadian rhythm, estrus/pregnancy/parturition/lactation, experimental manipulation, and stress. Availability of lineage- and age-specific reference ranges for biochemical parameters are useful during analyte data analysis and interpretation of shifts from baseline or control animal ranges. Multiple sources for domestic swine and miniature swine reference ranges have been cited. Reference ranges are provided in tabular form for selected representative breeds (Appendices A and B). While published reference ranges are helpful, use of pretest, concurrent or parallel control group and historical laboratory ranges are recommended, when available.

Evaluation of clinical chemistry variables has been an important part of investigations using swine research models. This review has provided general information concerning biochemical assays and factors affecting their variability and application for swine in a biomedical research setting.

5.8 REFERENCE VALUES

The concept of reference values and intervals are discussed in detail by Stockham and Scott (2008). Reference values for a wide variety of blood chemistry variables have been established and reported for several breeds and ages of pigs (Eisenhauer et al., 1994; Hannon et al., 1990; Horstman et al., 1960; Khan et al., 1986; McIntosh and Pointon, 1981; Parsons and Wells, 1986; Pond and Houpt, 1978; Radin et al., 1986; Tumbleson and Schmidt, 1986; Rispat et al., 1993; Oldigs, 1986; Hutcheson et al., 1979; McClellan et al., 1966; Miller et al., 1961; Burks et al., 1977; Drougas et al., 1996; Dungan et al., 1995), including fetal pigs (Spencer et al., 1986). Multiple veterinary biochemistry, clinical pathology, toxicology, and other laboratory reference textbooks offer reference biochemistry ranges for swine (Duncan and Prasse, 1986; Meyer et al., 1992; Kaneko et al., 1997; Plumb, 2005; Swindle, 2007; Gad, 2008; Evans, 2009). The Merck Manual (Kahn, 2008a, 2008b) and Oregon State Veterinary Diagnostic Laboratory (2009) offer online domestic swine reference ranges. Reference domesticated swine chemistry data (biochemical values [2–4 months age], blood gas and acid base status, plasma electrolytes and metabolites, plasma hormone concentrations, porcine serum constituents, serum constituents in pregnant and lactating females) are presented in Appendix A (Tables A.1 through A.6). Reference chemistry and urinalysis data for representative ages of Yucatan miniature swine are also presented in Appendix B. Appendix C presents key references on clinical chemistry of laboratory swine. Sinclair BioResources, LLC, offers clients a "Miniature Swine Book of Normals 2011" CD which covers serum chemistry for the Yucatan and other lineages (Sinclair S-1, Micro-Yucatan, Hanford), plus normals for hematology, EKG, organ weights, histopathology and gross necropsy findings, and many other categories of data. Marshall BioResources has published "Reference Data Guide 2008," which offers serum chemistry and other data on the Göttingen Minipig®. Because numerous factors can affect biochemical profiles of swine, these values should be used as general guidelines and should not preclude the use of individual animal pretest evaluations, concurrent control animal data for individual studies, and historical control data established by the laboratory controlling the study or individual animal samples. However, sometimes published reference ranges are the only data available for comparison.

Potential treatment group serum chemistry comparisons include the use of the historical control data ranges, pretest data for individual animals (these data serve as internal control data for each animal), and the concurrent control group data range. Wells and Gosselin (1996) have outlined methods for clinical pathology data interpretation. Predose baseline biochemical data are of value for qualification of an animal's health for study assignment. Comparison to historical institute normal/control data or reference ranges from the clinical pathology laboratory is commonly practiced. Study control animal group data collected at the same time point (concurrent) is most useful for comparison to study treatment group changes. Published reference ranges from the literature become very important when these values are the sole source for comparison.

DNA or protein microarray screening and biomarker research may also change the regulatory framework and the way in which traditional xenobiotic, drug, and new chemical entity (NCE) safety and efficacy studies are conducted, including the selection of biochemical profile parameters. However, adoption of novel markers by regulatory arms has been slow because of rigorous validation requirements, so the standard safety testing biochemistry profile will not be likely to change in the near future.

With large-scale studies involving hundreds or even thousands of samples in multiple treatment groups, it is difficult to interpret the resulting complex, high-density clinical chemistry data. Using a heat map to visualize large-scale chemistry data in a graphic facilitates the identification of previously unrecognized trends (Auman et al., 2007). This technique is simple to implement and maintains the biological integrity of the data. The value of this clinical chemistry data transformation and visualization will manifest itself through integration with other high-density data, such as genomics data, to study biology and toxicology at the systems level.

Values obtained for a particular analyte may vary among laboratories depending on prevailing conditions, experimental protocol, instrumentation, reagents, and method of analysis. Thus, individual laboratories should establish in-house reference values appropriate for the animals and laboratory conditions in which their studies are conducted.

Preanalytical sources of variation are common for clinical biochemistry determinations and reference ranges. For example, factors including gender, age, breed, and diet can affect variables such as serum protein, urea nitrogen, cholesterol concentrations and activities of ALT, ALP, AST, GDH, LDH, and SDH(Wilson et al., 1972). Understanding potential preanalytical sources of variation for different parameters are important for successful research or preclinical testing with porcine models.

ACKNOWLEDGMENT

We wish to thank Gregory S. Travlos, the author of this chapter in the second edition of this book, for his vision and contributions to this chapter.

REFERENCES

Agersø, H., Friis, C., and Nielsen J.P. 1998. Penetration of amoxycillin to the respiratory tract tissues and secretions in *Actinobacillus pleuropneumoniae* infected pigs. *Res Vet Sci.* 64:251–257.

Althen, T.G. and Gerrits, R.J. 1976. Pituitary and serum growth hormone levels in Duroc and Yorkshire swine genetically selected for high and low backfat. *J Anim Sci.* 42:1490–1497.

Amoss, M.S. and Beattie, C.W. 1986. Influence of gonadal steroid hormones upon the growth of melanoma in Sinclair swine. In *Swine in Biomedical Research.* Ed. M.E. Tumbleson, pp. 689–698. New York, NY: Plenum Press.

Asai, T., Mori, M., Okada, M., Uruno, K., Yazava, S., and Shibata, I. 1999. Elevated serum haptoglobin in pigs infected with porcine reproductive and respiratory syndrome virus. *Vet Immunol Immunopathol.* 70:143–148.

Assimos, D.G., Boyce, W.H., Lively, M., et al., 1986. Porcine urologic models including jejunoileal bypass. In *Swine in Biomedical Research.* Ed. M.E. Tumbleson, pp. 399–424. New York, NY: Plenum Press.

Atinmo, T., Pond, W.G., and Barnes, R.H. 1974. Effect of dietary energy vs. protein restriction on blood constituents and reproductive performance in swine. *J Nutr.* 104:1033–1040.

Attie, A.D., Aiello, R.J., and Checovich, W.J. 1992. The spontaneously hypercholesterolemic pig as an animal model of human hypercholesterolemia. In *Swine as Models in Biomedical Research.* Ed. M.M. Swindle, pp. 141–155. Ames, IA: Iowa State University Press.

Auman, J.T., Boorman, G.A., Wilson, R.E., Travlos, G.S., and Paules, R.S. October 22, 2007. Heat map visualization of high-density clinical chemistry data. *Physiol Genomics.* 31(2):352–6.

Baetz, A.L. 1973. The effect of fasting on the serum lipid components in swine and ponies. In *Advances in Automated Analysis. 1972 Technicon International Congress*, Vol. 7, pp. 73–75. Tarrytown, NY: Mediad Incorporated.

Baetz, A.L. and Mengeling, W.L. 1971. Blood constituent changes in fasted swine. *Am J Vet Res.* 32:1491–1499.

Bailie, M.B., Wixson, S.K., and Landi, M.S. 1986. Vascular-access-port implantation for serial sampling in conscious swine. *Lab Anim Sci.* 36(4):431–433.

Bakke, H. 1975. Serum levels of non-esterifled fatty acids and glucose in lines of pigs selected for gain and thickness of backfat. *Acta Agr Scand.* 25:113–116.

Baldi, A., Verga, M., Maffii, M., Canali, E., Chiaraviglio, D., and Ferrari, C. 1989. Effects of blood sampling procedures, grouping, and adrenal stimulation on stress responses in the growing pig. *Reprod Nutr Dev.* 29:95–103.

Ball, J.M. 1910. *Andreas Vesalius, The Reformer of Anatomy.* St Louis, MO: Medical Science Press. Stanford University Libraries. Available at: http://www.archive.org/stream/andreasvesalius00ballgoog/andreasvesalius00ballgoog_djvu.txt.

Barb, C.R., Barrett, J.B., Kraeling, R.R., and Rampacek, G.B. 2001. Serum leptin concentrations, luteinizing hormone and growth hormone secretion during feed and metabolic fuel restriction in the prepuberal gilt. *Domest Anim Endocrinol.* 20(1):47–63.

Barnett, J.L., Cronin, G.M., Hemsworth, P.H., and Wingfield, C.G. 1984. The welfare of confined sows: Physiological, behavioural and production responses to contrasting housing systems and handler attitudes. *Annales De Recherches Veterinares.* 15:217–226.

Barnett, J.L. and Hemsworth, P.H. 1986. The impact of handling and environmental factors on the stress response and its consequences in swine. *Lab Anim Sci.* 36:366–369.

Barnett, J.L., Hemsworth, P.H., and Cronin, G.M. 1982. The effect of mating on plasma corticosteroids in the female pig and the influences of individual and group penning on this response. *Gen Comp Endocrinol.* 47:516–521.

Barnett, J.L., Hemsworth, P.H., and Hand, A.M. 1983. Effects of chronic stress on some blood parameters in the pig. *Appl Anim Ethol.* 9:273–277.

Bartko, P., Vrzgula, L., Paulikova, I., and Reichel, P. 1984. Vplyv Tepelneho Stresu na Acidobazicku Homeostazu Osipanych. *Veterinarni Medicina (Praha).* 29:337–344.

Bauer, R., Walter, B., and Zweiner, U. 2000. Comparison between inulin clearance and endogenous creatinine clearance in newborn normal weight and growth restricted newborn piglets. *Exp Toxicol Pathol.* 52(4):367–372.

Beames, C.G., Jr., Maxwell, C.V., Norton, S.A., and Bond, G.A. 1986. Whey and cholesterol in swine. In *Swine in Biomedical Research.* Ed. M.E. Tumbleson, pp. 1041–1046. New York, NY: Plenum Press.

Beck, M.J., Padgett, E.L., Bowman, C.J., et al. 2006. Non juvenile toxicology testing. In *Developmental and Reproductive Toxicology: A Practical Approach.* Ed. R.D. Hood, 2nd edition, pp. 263–328. New York, NY: Informa Healthcare.

Becker, B.A., Ford, J.J., Nienaber, J.A., Hahn, G.L., and Christenson, R.K. 1986. Endocrine and behavior changes associated with intensive housing systems for swine. In *Swine in Biomedical Research.* Ed. M.E. Tumbleson, pp. 173–189. New York, NY: Plenum Press.

Bellinger, D.W., Merricks, E.P., and Nichols, T.C. 2006. Swine models of type 2 diabetes mellitus: Insulin resistance, glucose tolerance, and cardiovascular complications. *ILAR J.* 47(3):243–258.

Beynen, A.C., Schouten, J.A., Terpstra, A.H.M., and Visser, J. 1983. Density profile and cholesterol concentration of serum lipoproteins in pigs (*Sus scrofa domestica*) fed a hypercholesterolemic diet. *Zeitschrift Fur Versuchstierkunde.* 25:333–337.

Bobbie, D.L. and Swindle, M.M. 1986. Porcine urologic models including jejunoileal bypass. In *Swine in Biomedical Research.* Ed. M.E. Tumbleson, pp. 273–277. New York, NY: Plenum Press.

Borg, K.E., Lundstra, D. D., and Christenson, R.K. 1993. Semen characteristics, testicular size, and reproductive hormone concentrations in mature Duroc, Meishan, Fengjing, and Minzhu boars. *Biol Reprod.* 49:515–521.

Bossone, C.A. and Hannon, J.P. 1985. A multi-isotope procedure for simultaneously estimating the volume of body fluid compartments of swine. Technical Report 201. Presidio of San Francisco, CA: Letterman Army Institute of Research.

Bostedt, H. 1978. Das Schwein in der Ante- und Postpartalen Periode. II Mitteilung: Aktivitatsmessungen der Enzyme GOT, GPT, LDH, CPK, SDH, GLDH Sowie g-GT im Blutserum. *Berliner Und Munchener Tierarztliche Wochenschrift.* 91:51–53.

Boyd, J.W. 1983. The mechanism relating to increases in plasma enzymes and isoenzymes in diseases of animals. *Vet Clin Pathol.* 12:9–24.

Brenner, K.-V., Gurtler, H., and Ziebarth, S. 1979. Reaktion von Schweinen auf Eine Fixation Mittels Oberkieferschlinge Anhand von Klinisch-Chemischen Parametern im Blut. *Montaschefte Fur Veterinaermedizin.* 34:28–31.

Brown, C.M. 1979. A method for collecting blood from hogs using the thoracic inlet. *VM SAC.* 74:361–363.

Brown, D. and Terris, J. 1996. Swine in physiological and pathophysiological research. In: *Advances in Swine in Biomedical Research.* Eds. M.E. Tumbleson, and L.B. Schook, pp. 5–6. New York, NY: Plenum Press.

Brown, D.E., King, G.J., and Hacker, R.R. 1973. Polyurethane indwelling catheters for piglets. *J Anim Sci.* 37:303–304.

Brown, J.R., Tyeryar, E.A., Harrington, D.A., and Hilmas, D.E. 1978. Femoral venipuncture for repeated blood sampling in miniature swine. *Lab Anim Sci.* 28:339–342.

Bruss, M.L. and Becker, H.N. 1981. Effect of method of blood sampling on serum creatine kinase concentrations in swine. *Am J Vet Res.* 42:528–531.

Brussow, K.P., Schneider, F., Tuchscherer, A., Egerszegi, L., and Ratky, J. Comparison of luteinizing hormone, leptin, and progesterone levels in the systemic circulation (Vena jugularis) and near the ovarian circulation (Vena cava caudalis) during the oestrous cycle in Mangalica and Landrace gilts. *J Reprod Dev.* 2008, 54(6) 431–438.

Buckley, D.C., Mirtallo, J.M., and Kudsk, K.A. 1986. Total parenteral nutrition in swine. In *Swine in Biomedical Research.* Ed. M.E. Tumbleson, pp. 1147–1151. New York, NY: Plenum Press.

Buelke-Sam, J. 2002. *Postnatal Evaluation in Developmental and Juvenile Toxicity Studies, presented at the Henry Stewart Conference; Meeting FDA, EPA, OECD, and ICH Regulatory Requirements for Reproductive Toxicology Data Submissions.* Washington, DC: Georgetown University Conference Center, 2002.

Burks, M.F., Tumbleson, M.E., Hicklin, K.W., Hutcheson, D.P., and Middleton, C.C. 1977. Age and sex related changes of hematologic parameters in Sinclair (S-1) miniature swine. *Growth.* 41(1):51–62.

Bustad, L.K. 1966. Pigs in the laboratory. *Sci Am.* 214:94–100.

Bustad, L.K. and McClellan, R.O., Eds. 1966. *Swine in Biomedical Research.* Seattle, WA: Frayn Printing Co.

Calvert, G.D., Scott, P.J., and Sharpe, D.N. 1977. Percutaneous cardiac puncture in domestic pigs. *Aust Vet J.* 53:337–339.

Carle, B.N. and Dewhirst, W.H., Jr. 1942. A method for bleeding swine. *J Am Vet Med Assoc.* 101:495–496.

Casteel, S.W., Cowart, R.P., Weis, C.P., et al. 1997. Bioavailability of lead to juvenile swine dosed with soil from the smuggler mountain NPL site of Aspen, Colorado. *Toxicol Sci.* 36(2):177–187.

Checovich, W.J., Fitch, W.L., Krauss, R.M., et al. 1988. Defective catabolism and abnormal composition of low-density lipoproteins from mutant pigs with hypercholesterolemia. *Biochem.* 27:1934–1941.

Christoffersen, B., Ribel, U., Raun, K., Golozoubova, V., and Pacini, G. 2009. Evaluation of different methods for assessment of insulin sensitivity in Goettingen minipigs: Introduction to a new, simpler method. *Am J Physiol Regul Integr Comp Physiol.* 297(4):R1195–R1201.

Christoffersen, B.O., Grand, N., Golozoubova, V., Svendsen, O., and Raun, K. 2007. Gender-associated differences in metabolic syndrome-related parameters in Göttingen minipigs. *Comp Med.* 57: 493–504.

Clapper, J.A. 2008. Effects of two different anaesthetics on serum concentrations of cortisol and luteinizing hormone in barrows and gilts. *Lab Anim.* 42(1):83–91.

Cohen, I.T., Meunier, K.M., Lipman, R.D., and Ellis, N.G. 1986. Chronic intravenous hyperalimentation in the neonatal piglet. In *Swine in Biomedical Research.* Ed. M.E. Tumbleson, pp. 1265–1275. New York, NY: Plenum Press.

Cornelius, C.E. 1989. Liver function. In *Clinical Biochemistry of Domestic Animals.* Ed. J.J. Kaneko, pp. 364–397. New York, NY: Academic Press.

DaFoe, D.C., Campbell, D.A. Jr., Rosenberg, L., et al. 1989. No improvement of pancreas transplant endocrine function by exogenous insulin infusion (Islet Rest) in the postoperative period. *Transplantation.* 48:22–26.

de Groot, J., de Jong, I.C., Prelle, I.T., and Koolhaas, J.M. 2001. Immunity in barren and enriched housed pigs differing in baseline cortisol concentration. *Physiol Behav.* 71(3–4):217–223.

Dixon, J.L., Shen, S., Vuchetich, J.P., Wysocka, E., Sun, G.Y., and Sturek M. 2002. Increased atherosclerosis in diabetic dyslipidemic swine: Protection by atorvastatin involves decreased VLDL triglycerides but minimal effects on the lipoprotein profile. *J Lipid Res.* 43:1618–1629.

Doornenbal, H., Tong, A.K.W., Martin, A.H., and Sather, A.P. 1983. Studies on the performance, development, and carcass composition of the growing pig: Effects of sex, feeding regime, and age on blood serum parameters. *J Anim Sci.* 63:977–984.

Dorner, J.L., Hoffman, W.E., and Filipov, M.M. 1983. Effect of in vitro hemolysis on values for certain porcine serum constituents. *Vet Clin Pathol.* 12:15–19.

Douglas, W.R. 1972. Of pigs and men and research: A review of applications and analogies of the pig, Sus scrofa, in human medical research. *Space Life Sci.* 3:226–234.

Drougas, J.G., Barnard, S.G., Wright, J.K., et al. 1996. A model for the extended studies of hepatic hemodynamics and metabolism in swine. *Lab Anim Sci.* 46(6):648–655.

Dubreuil, P., Couture, Y., Tremblay, A., and Martineau, G.P. 1990. Effects of experimenters and different blood sampling procedures on blood metabolite values in growing pigs. *Can J Vet Res (Revue canadienne de recherche veterinaire).* 54(3):379–382.

Duncan, J.R. and Prasse, K.W. 1986. Appendix 1 Reference Values. In: *Veterinary Laboratory Medicine: Clinical Pathology*, pp. 232–234. Ames, IO: Iowa State University Press.

Dungan, L.J., Wiest, D.B., Fyfe, D.A., Smith, A.C., and Swindle, M.M. 1995. Normal hematology, serology, and serum protein electrophoresis values in fetal Yucatan miniature swine. *Lab Anim Sci.* 45(3):285–289.

Earl, F.L. 1968. Housing and handling of miniature swine. *Lab Anim Care.* 18:110–115.

Earl, F.L., Melveger, B.E., Reinwall, J.E., and Wilson, R.L. 1971. Clinical laboratory values of neonatal and weanling miniature pigs. *Lab Anim Sci.* 21:754–759.

Eisenhauer, C.L., Matsuda, L.S., and Uyehara, C.F. 1994. Normal physiologic values of neonatal pigs and the effects of isoflurane and pentobarbital anesthesia. *Lab Anim Sci.* 44:245–252.

Elsaesser, F., Parvizi, N., and Foxcroft, GR. 1992. Control of the LH surge mechanism in the female pig. *J Physiol Pharmacol.* 43(4 Suppl 1):69–78.

Etherton, T.D. and Kris-Etherton, P.M. 1980. Characterization of plasma lipoproteins in swine with different propensities for obesity. *Lipids.* 15:823–289.

Eto, Y., Shimokawa, H., Hiroki, J., et al. 2000. Gene transfer of dominant negative Rho kinase suppresses neointimal formation after balloon injury in pigs. *Am J Physiol Heart Circ Physiol.* 278: H1744–H1750.

Evans, G.O. Ed. 2009. *Animal Clinical Chemistry: A Practical Handbook for Toxicologists and Biomedical Researchers*, 2nd edition, 368pp. Boca Raton, FL: CRC Press.

Evans, N.M., Evans, F.D., Maher, A., Friendship, R., and Hacker, R.R. 1994. Influence of light-dark cycles on estradiol-17b induced luteinizing hormone patterns of the prepuberal gilt. *J Anim Sci.* 72:1995–2000.

Filer, L.J., Andersen, D.W., and Cotton, R.H. 1986. Effect of fiber on growing pigs. In *Swine in Biomedical Research.* Ed. M.E. Tumbleson, pp. 701–708. New York, NY: Plenum Press.

Fleming, S.E. and Arce, D. 1986. Using the pig to study digestion and fermentation in the gut. In *Swine in Biomedical Research.* Ed. M.E. Tumbleson, pp. 123–134. New York, NY: Plenum Press.

Food and Drug Administration (FDA). 2000. Guidance for Industry: E11 Clinical Investigation of Medicinal Products in the Pediatric Population. ICH December 2000. 14pp. Available at: http://www.fda.gov/downloads/RegulatoryInformation/Guidances/ucm129477.pdf

Ford, J.J. and Christenson, R.K. 1986. Differentiation of sexual behavior. In *Swine in Biomedical Research.* Ed. M.E. Tumbleson, pp. 191–200. New York, NY: Plenum Press.

Ford, J.J. and Maurer, R.R. 1978. Simple technique for chronic venous catheterization of swine. *Lab Anim Sci.* 28:615–618.

Foudin, L., Sun, G.Y., and Tumbleson, M.E. 1986. Ethanol effects on serum lipids of Sinclair (S-1) miniature swine. In *Swine in Biomedical Research.* Ed. M.E. Tumbleson, pp. 611–622. New York, NY: Plenum Press.

Fox, T. and Ross, R. 1985. Effects of low phosphorus and low calcium diets on the production and metabolic clearance rates of 1,25-Dihydroxycholecalciferol in pigs. *J Endocrinol.* 105:169–173.

Friendship, R.M., Henry, S.C. 1992. Cardiovascular system, hematology, and clinical chemistry. In *Diseases of Swine.* Eds. A.D. Leman, B.E. Straw, W.L. Mengeling, S. D'Allaire, and D.J. Taylor, 7th edition, pp. 3–11. Ames, IA: Iowa State University Press.

Friendship, R.M, Lumsden, J.H., McMillan, I., and Wilson, M.R. 1984. Hematology and biochemistry reference values for Ontario swine. *Can J Comp Med.* 48:390–393.

Fuster, V., Badimon, L., Badimon, J.J., Turitto, V., Lie, J.T., and Bowie, E.J.W. 1986. Experimental approach to vascular disease in swine with Von Willebrand's disease. In *Swine in Biomedical Research.* Ed. M.E. Tumbleson, Vol. 3, pp. 1527–1541. New York, NY: Plenum Press.

Gad, S.C., Dincer, Z., Svendsen, O., and Skaanild, M.T. 2008. The minipig. In *Animal Models in Toxicology.* Ed. S.C. Gad, Chap. 10, pp. 731–771. New York, NY: Informa Healthcare.

Gal, D. and Isner, J.M. 1992. Atherosclerotic Yucatan microswine as a model for novel cardiovascular interventions and imaging. In: *Swine as Models in Biomedical Research.* Ed. M.M. Swindle, pp. 118–140. Ames, IA: Iowa State University Press.

Gerdes, C., Faber-Steinfeld, V., Yalkinoglu, O., and Wohlfeil, S. October, 1996. Comparison of the effects of the thrombin inhibitor r-hirudin in four animal models of neointima formation after arterial injury. *Arterioscler Thromb Vasc Biol.* 16(10):1306–1311.

Gerrity, R.G., Natarajan, R., Nadler, J.L., and Kimsey, T. 2001. Diabetes-induced accelerated atherosclerosis in swine. *Diabetes.* 50:1654–1665.

Ghoshal, N.G. 1975. Heart and arteries. In *Sisson and Grossman's the Anatomy of the Domestic Animals.* Ed. R. Getty, Chap. 44, Vol. 2, pp. 1306–1342. Philadelphia, PA: W.B. Saunders.

Gotze, M., Bergfeld, J., Wollenhaupt, K., and Brussow, K.P. 1984. Stoffwechseluntersuchungen Bei Graviden und Nichtgraviden Jungsauen. *Archiv Fur Experimentelle Veterinarmedizin.* 38:120–128.

Grandhi, R.R. and Strain, J.H. 1982. Blood metabolic levels in feed-restricted hogs. *Can J Anim Sci.* 62:315–319.

Greco, S.C., Talcott, M.R., LaRegina, M.C., and Eisenbeis, P.E. 2001. Use of intraosseous blood for repeated hematologic and biochemical analyses in healthy pigs. *Am J Vet Res.* 62(1):43–47.

Gregory, N.G., Wood, J.D., Enser, M., Smith, W.C., and Ellis, M. 1980. Fat mobilisation in large white pigs selected for low backfat thickness. *J Sci Food Agric.* 31:567–572.

Griffith, M.K. and Minton, J.E. 1991. Free-running rhythms of adrenocorticotropic hormone (ACTH), cortisol, and melatonin in pigs. *Domest Anim Endocrinol.* 8:201–208.

Griffith, M.K. and Minton, J.E. 1992. Effect of light intensity on circadian profiles of melatonin, prolactin, ACTH, and cortisol in pigs. *J Anim Sci.* 70:492–498.

Gronert, G.A. 1980. Malignant hyperthermia. *Anesthesiol.* 53:395–423.

Hall, L.W., Trim, C.M., and Woolf, N. 1972. Further studies of porcine malignant hyperthermia. *Br Med J.* 2:145–148.

Hall, W.F., Eurell, T.E., Hansen, T.E., and Herr, W.F. 1992. Serum haptoglobin concentration in swine naturally or experimentally infected with *Actinobacillus pleuropneumoniae. J Am Vet Med Assoc.* 201:1730–1733.

Hannon, J.P. 1992. Hemorrhage and hemorrhagic shock in swine: A review. In *Swine as Models in Biomedical Research.* Ed. M.M. Swindle, pp. 197–245. Ames, IA: Iowa State University Press.

Hannon, J.P. and Bossone, C.A. 1986. The conscious pig as a large animal model for studies of hemorrhagic hypotension. In *Swine in Biomedical Research.* Ed. M.E. Tumbleson, pp. 1413–1428. New York, NY: Plenum Press.

Hannon, J.P., Bossone, C.A., and Wade, C.E. 1990. Normal physiological values for conscious pigs used in biomedical research. *Lab Anim Sci.* 40:293–298.

Hannon, J.P., Jennings Jr., P.B., and Dixon, R.S. 1981a. Physiologic Aspects of Porcine Hemorrhage. II. Alterations in Heart Rate and Arterial Pressure During Fifty Percent Blood Loss in the Conscious Animal. Technical Report 94. Presidio of San Francisco, CA: Letterman Army Institute of Research.

Hannon, J.P., Jennings Jr., P.B., and Dixon, R.S. 1981b. Physiologic Aspects of Porcine Hemorrhage. III. Heart Rate and Arterial Blood Pressure Changes During Spontaneous Recovery from 30 and 50 Percent Blood Volume Loss in the Conscious Animal. Technical Report 95. Presidio of San Francisco, CA: Letterman Army Institute of Research.,

Hasler-Rapacz, J., Prescott, M.F., Von-Linden-Reed, J., Repacz, J.M. Jr, Hu, Z., and Rapacz, J. 1995. Elevated concentrations of plasma lipids and apolipoproteins B, C-III, and E are associated with the progression of coronary artery disease in familial hypercholesterolemic swine. *Arterioscler Thromb Vasc Biol.* 15(5):583–592.

Hausman, D.B., Kasser, T.R., Seerley, R.W., and Martin, R.J. 1986. Studies of gestational diabetes using the pig as a model. In *Swine in Biomedical Research.* Ed. M.E. Tumbleson, pp. 561–572. New York, NY: Plenum Press.

Hawk, C.T., Leary, S.L., and Morris, T.H. 2005. *Formulary for Laboratory Animals*, 3rd edition. Ames, IA: Blackwell Publishing.

Hay, M., Meunier-Salaun, M.C., Brulaud, F., Monnier, M., and Mormede, P. 2000. Assessment of hypothalamic-pituitary-adrenal axis and sympathetic nervous system activity in pregnant sows through the measurement of glucocorticoids and catecholamines in urine. *J Anim Sci.* 78:420–428.

Heald, F.P. and Naseem, S.M. 1986. Effect of high cholesterol diet during lactation on cholesterol metabolism in offspring of Yorkshire swine. In *Swine in Biomedical Research.* Ed. M.E. Tumbleson, pp. 1573–1582. New York, NY: Plenum Press.

Heegaard, P.M.H., Klausen, J., Nielsen, J.P., et al. 1998. The porcine acute phase response to infection with *Actinobacillus pleuropneumoniae*. Haptoglobin, C-reactive protein, major acute phase protein and serum amyloid A protein are sensitive indicators of infection. *Comp Biochem Physiol B Biochem Mol Biol.* 119:365–373.

Heim, K.E., Morrell, J.S., Ronan, A.M., and Tagliaferro, A.R. 2002. Effects of ketamine-xylazine and isoflurane on insulin sensitivity in dehydroepiandrosterone sulfate-treated minipigs (Sus scrofa domestica). *Comp Med.* 52(3):233–237.

Henning, M., Kallweit, E., and Smidt, D. 1986. Halothane-induced physiologic changes in the venous blood of pigs. In *Swine in Biomedical Research.* Ed. M.E. Tumbleson, pp. 1451–1458. New York, NY: Plenum Press.

Hill, D.E. 1986. Swine in perinatal research: An overview. In *Swine in Biomedical Research.* Ed. M.E. Tumbleson, pp. 1155–1159. New York, NY: Plenum Press.

Hite, C.M. 2009. Urinary catheterization of male swine. Denver, CO: American Association of Laboratory Animal Science—National Meeting.

Hlousek, A. 1978. Age-dependent changes in biochemical composition of blood in gilts from large-scale piggeries. *Acta Veterinaria Brno.* 47:15–21.

Hoban, L.D., Paschall, J.A., Eckstein, J., et al. 1992. Awake porcine model of intraperitoneal sepsis. In *Swine as Models in Biomedical Research.* Ed. M.M. Swindle, pp. 246–264. Ames, IA: Iowa State University Press.

Hoffmann, W.E. and Solter, P.F. 2008 Ch 12. Diagnostic enzymology of domestic animals. In *Clinical Biochemistry of Domestic Animals.* Eds. Kaneko JJ., et al., 6th edition, p. 357. Academic Press.

Horstman, V.G., Clarke, W.J., Hackett, P.L., Kerr, M.E., Pershing, R.L., and Bustad, L.K. 1960. Anatomical and physiological data in miniature swine. In *Hanford Biology Research Annual Report for 1959*, pp. 59–67. Hanford Atomic Products Operation USAEC Report HW 65500. Richland, Washington DC: Hanford Laboratories.

Huhn, G.G., Osweiler, G.D., and Switzer, W.P. 1969. Application of the orbital sinus bleeding technique to swine. *Lab Anim Care.* 19:403–405.

Hunter, M.G., Picton, H.M., Biggs, C., Mann, G.E., McNeilly, A.S., and Foxcroft, G.R. 1996. Periovulatory endocrinology in high ovulating Meishan sows. *J Endocrinol.* 150:141–147.

Hutcheson, D.P., Tumbleson, M.E., and Middleton C.C. 1979. Serum electrolyte concentrations in Sinclair (S-1) miniature swine from 1 through 36 months of age. *Growth.* 43:62–70.

Ishii, A., Viñuela, F., Murayama, Y., et al. 2006. Swine model of carotid artery atherosclerosis: Experimental induction by surgical partial ligation and dietary hypercholesterolemia. *AJNR Am J Neuroradiol.* 27(9):1893–1899.

Jacobs, A. 2006. Use of nontraditional animals for evaluation of pharmaceutical products. *Summ Expert Opin Drug Metab Toxicol.* 2(3):345–349.

Johansson, M.B.N. and Karlsson, B.W. 1982. Lipoprotein and lipid profiles in the blood serum of the fetal, neonatal, and adult pig. *Biol Neonate.* 42:127–137.

Kahn, C.M. Ed. 2008a. Merck Veterinary Manual Online. Reference Guides. Serum Biochemistry Reference Ranges. Merial. Available at: http://www.merckvetmanual.com/mvm/htm/bc/tref7.htm.

Kahn, C.M. Ed. 2008b. Merck veterinary manual online. Serum enzyme concentrations. In: *Hepatic Disease in Large Animals: Introduction.* Whitehouse Station, NJ: Merial/Merck & Co. Available at: http://www.merckvetmanual.com/mvm/index.jsp?cfile=htm/bc/22800.htm.

Kaneko, J.J. Harvey, J.W., and Bruss. M.L. 1997. Appendix VIII. Blood analyte reference values in large animals. In: *Clinical Biochemistry of Domestic Animals*, 5th edition, p. 890. San Diego, CA: Academic Press.

Kasser, T.R., Martin, R.J., Gahagan, J.H., and Wangsness, P.J. 1981. Fasting plasma hormones and metabolites in feral and domestic newborn pigs. *J Anim Sci.* 53:420–426.

Khan, M.A., Sager, A.O., Khattak, Z.R., Braunberg, R.C., Sobotka, T.J., and Travlos, G.S. 1986. Baseline biochemical and hematological parameters of neonatal miniature piglets: model for perinatal toxicology. In *Proceedings of the 13th International Congress of Nutrition* (held under the auspices of the International Union of Nutritional Science). Eds. T.G. Taylor and N.K. Jenkins, pp. 656–658. Brighton, UK, 18–23 August.

Kim, D.N., Schmee, J., Lee, K.T., and Thomas, W.A. 1984. Hypo-atherogenic effect of dietary corn oil exceeds hypo-cholesterolemic effect in swine. *Atherosclerosis.* 52:101–113.

Kojima, M., Sekimoto, M., and Degawa, M. 2008. Gender-related differences in the level of serum lipids in Meishan pigs. *J Health Sci.* 54(1):97–100.

Kolataj, A., Dziewiecki, C., Piekarzewska, A., et al. 1988. Effect of fasting and crowding on some physiological indicators in pigs. *Pig News Inf.* 9:265–268.

Kornegay, E.T. 1967. Daily and twice daily repeated blood sampling in weanling pigs. *Am J Vet Res.* 28:839–844.

Kornegay, E.T., Miller, E.R., Brent, B.E., Long, C.H., Ullrey, D.E., and Hoefer, J.A. 1964. Effect of fasting and refeeding on body weight, rectal temperature, blood volume, and various blood constituents in growing swine. *J Nutr.* 84:295–304.

Laber-Laird, K., Smith, A., Swindle, M.M., and Colwell, J. 1992. Effects of isoflurane anesthesia on glucose tolerance and insulin secretion in Yucatan minipigs. *Lab Anim Sci.* 42(6):579–581.

Larsen, M.O., and Rolin, B. 2004. Use of the Göttingen minipig as a model of diabetes with special focus on type 1 diabetes research. *ILAR J.* 45(3):303–313.

Larsen, M.O., Rolin, B., Wilkin, M., Carr, R.D., and Svendsen, O. 2002. High-fat high-energy feeding impairs fasting glucose and increases fasting insulin levels in the Göttingen minipig. *Ann New York Acad Sci.* 967:414–423.

Lengerken, G., and Pfeiffer, H. 1978. Einfluss von Transport und Schlachtung auf die Variabilitat Biochemischer Kennwerte im Blutplasma von Hybridschweinen. *Montaschefte Fur Veterinaermedizin.* 32:620–624.

Liu, Y., Rector, R.S., Thomas, T.R., et al. 2004. Lipoproteins during the estrous cycle in swine. *Metabolism.* 53(2):140–141.

Liu, Y., Wang, Z., Yin, W., et al. 2007. Severe insulin resistance and moderate glomerulosclerosis in a minipig model induced by high-fat/ high-sucrose/ high-cholesterol diet. *Exp Anim.* 56(1):11–20.

Lochmiller, R.L., Hellgren, E.C., Varner, L.W., et al. 1985. Physiological responses of the adult male collard peccary, Tayassu tajacu (Tayassuidae), to severe dietary restriction. *Comp Biochem Physiol.* 82:49–58.

Loveday, J.A., Gonzaludo, G.A., Sondeen, J.L., et al. 1989. Renal hemodynamics and function in conscious swine: Surgical preparation of a single kidney model. *FASEB.* 3:A1018.

Lund-Larsen, T.R. and Bakke, H. 1975. Growth hormone and somatomedin activities in lines of pigs selected for rate of gain and thickness of backfat. *Acta Agriculturae Scandinavica.* 25:231–234.

Lunney, J.K. 2007. Advances in swine biomedical model genomics. *Int J Biol Sci.* 3(3):179–184.

Lunstrom, K., Dahlberg, E., Nyberg, L., Snochowski, M., Standal, N., and Edqvist, L-E. 1983. Glucocorticoid and androgen characteristics in two lines of pigs selected for gain and thickness of backfat. *J Anim Sci.* 56:401–409.

Mackellar, J.C. 1970. Collection of blood samples and smears for diagnosis. *Vet Rec.* 86:302–306.

Magnusson, U., Wilkie, B., Artursson, K., and Mallard, B. 1999. Interferon-alpha and haptoglobin in pigs selectively bred for high and low immune response and infected with Mycoplasma hyorhinitis. *Vet Immunol Immunopathol.* 68:131–137.

Mahley, R.W. and Weisgraber, K.H. 1974. An electrophoretic method for the quantitative isolation of human and swine plasma lipoproteins. *Biochem.* 13:1964–1969.

Martin, R.J., Gobble, J.L., Hartsock, T.H., Graves, H.B., and Ziegler, J.H. 1972. Characterization of an obese syndrome in the pig. *Proceed Soc Exp Biol Med.* 143:198–203.

Mateo, J.P. and Veum, T.L. 1980. Utilization of glucose, sucrose, and corn starch with isolated soybean protein by 15-day-old baby pigs reared artificially. *Nutr Rep Int.* 22:419–430.

McCauley, I. and Hartmann, P.E. 1984. Changes in piglet leucocytes, B lymphocytes, and plasma cortisol from birth to three weeks after weaning. *Res Vet Sci.* 37:234–241.

McClellan, R.O. 1968. Applications of swine in biomedical research. *Lab Anim Care.* 18:120–126.

McClellan, R.O., Vogt, C.S., and Ragan, H.A. 1966. Age-related changes in hematological and serum biochemical parameters in miniature swine. In *Swine in Biomedical Research.* Eds. L.K. Bustad, and R.O. McClellan, pp. 597–610. Seattle, WA: Frayn Printing Co.

McGinnis, R.M., Marple, D.N., Ganjam, V.K., Prince, T.J., and Pritchett, J.F. 1981. The effects of floor temperature, supplemental heat and drying at birth on neonatal swine. *J Anim Sci.* 53:1424–1432.

McGrath, C.J., Rempel, W.E., Addis, P.B., and Crimi, A.J. 1981. Acepromazine and droperidol inhibition of halothane-induced malignant hyperthermia. *Am J Vet Res.* 42:195–198.

McIntosh, G.H., Pointon, A. 1981. The Kangaroo Island strain of pig in biomedical research. *Aust Vet J.* 57:182–185.

Meldrum, J.B., Troutt, H.F., Kornegay, E.T., Ehrich, M.F., and Chickering, W.R. 1986. Influence of selenium, zinc, and restricted floor space on glutathione peroxidase and creatinine phosphokinase activities and on production performance in weanling pigs. In *Swine in Biomedical Research.* Ed. M.E. Tumbleson, pp. 1069–1076. New York, NY: Plenum Press.

Mersmann, H.J., Arakelian, M.C., and Brown, L.J. 1979. Plasma lipids in neonatal and growing swine. *J Anim Sci.* 48:554–558.

Mersmann, H.J. and MacNeil, M.D. 1985. Relationship of plasma lipid concentrations to fat deposition in pigs. *J Anim Sci.* 61:122–128.

Mersmann, H.J., Pond, W.G., and Yen, J.T. 1973. Plasma glucose, insulin, and lipids during growth of genetically lean and obese swine. *Growth.* 46:189–198.

Meunier-Salaun, M.C., Vantrimponte, M.N., Raab, A., and Dantzer, R. 1987. Effect of floor area restriction upon performance, behavior, and physiology of growing-finishing pigs. *J Anim Sci.* 64:1371–1377.

Meyer, D.J., Coles, E.H., and Rich, L.J. 1992. Table 2. Normal serum chemistry values for adult animals and Table 5. Normal ranges of serum chemistry values for adult animals expressed in international units. In: *Veterinary Laboratory Medicine: Interpretation and Diagnosis*, pp. 329–331. Philadelphia, PA: W.B. Saunders Company.

Miller, E.R. and Ullrey, D.E. 1987. The pig as a model for human nutrition. *Annu Rev Nutr.* 7:361–382.

Miller, E.R., Ullrey, D.E., Ackerman, I., Schmidt, D.A., Hoefer, J.A., and Luecke, R.W. 1961. Swine hematology from birth to maturity. I. Serum Proteins. *J Anim Sci.* 20:31–35.

Minton, J.E., Davis, D.L., and Stevenson, J.S. 1989. Contribution of the photoperiod to circadian variations in serum cortisol and melatonin in boars. *Domes Anim Endocrinol.* 6:177–181.

Minton, J.E. and Wettemann, R.P. 1988. The influence of photoperiod and hemicastration on growth and testicular and endocrine functions of boars. *Dome Anim Endocrinol.* 5:71–80.

Mitruka, B.M., Rawnsley, H.M., and Vadehra, D.V. 1976. *Animals for Medical Research: Models for the Study of Human Disease*, 591pp. New York, NY: John Wiley & Sons.

Mortensen, J.T., Brinck, P., and Lichtenberg, J. 1998. The minipig in dermal toxicology. In: Svendsen O. *The Minipig in Toxicology, Scand J Lab Anim Sci.* 25(Suppl 1):77–83.

Moss, B.W. and McMurray, C.H. 1979. The effect of the duration and type of stress on some serum enzyme levels in pigs. *Res Vet Sci.* 26:1–6.

Muirhead, M.R. 1981. Blood sampling in pigs. *In Practice.* 3(5):16–20.

Mulder, J.B. and Tumbleson, M.E. 1972. Effect of relative centrifugal force, during separation of serum from cells, on serum biochemic values. In *Advances in Automated Analysis. 1970 Technicon International Congress*, Vol. 2, pp. 169–173. Mt. Kisco, NY: Futura Publishing Company.

Mullen, Y., Taura, Y., Nagata, M., Miyazawa, K., and Stein, E. 1992. Swine as a model for pancreatic beta-cell transplantation. In *Swine as Models in Biomedical Research.* Ed. M.M. Swindle, pp. 16–34. Ames, IA: Iowa State University Press.

Muller, M.J., Paschen, U., and Seitz, H.J. 1982. Starvation-induced ketone body production in the conscious unrestrained miniature pig. *J Nutr.* 112:1379–1386.

Nachreiner, R.F. and Ginther, O.J. 1972. Porcine agalactia: Hematologic, serum chemical, and clinical changes during the preceding gestation. *Am J Vet Res.* 33:799–809.

Naumann, J., Neumann, G., and Schmoranzer, A. 1983. Der Einfluss Einer Unterschiedlich Starken Hamolyse auf Chemisch-Klinische Parameter des Schweines. *Monatsch Veterinaermed.* 38:131–133.

Nelson, T.E. 1986. Malignant hyperthermia: A pharmacogenetic disease of man and pigs. In *Swine in Biomedical Research.* Ed. M.E. Tumbleson, pp. 261–272. New York, NY: Plenum Press.

Newport, M.J. and Henschel, M.J. 1986. Influence of casein and whey protein content of milk on protein digestion and growth in the piglet. In *Swine in Biomedical Research.* Ed. M.E. Tumbleson, pp. 755–758. New York, NY: Plenum Press.

Norata, G.D., Raselli, S., Grigore, L., et al. October, 2009. Small dense LDL and VLDL predict common carotid artery IMT and elicit an inflammatory response in peripheral blood mononuclear and endothelial cells. *Atherosclerosis.* 206(2):556–62.

NRC. 2007. *Applications of Toxicogenomic Technologies to Predictive Toxicology and Risk Assessment.* National Academy of Sciences Board on Environmental Studies and Toxicology, Board on Life Sciences. National Research Council of the National Academies. Washington, DC: National Academies Press, 22–44.

Nunoya, T., Shibuya, K., Saitoh, T., et al. 2007. Use of miniature pig for biomedical research, with reference to toxicological studies. *J Toxicol Pathol.* 20(3):125–132.

O'Brien, P.J., Landt, Y., and Ladenson, J.H. 1997. Differential reactivity of cardiac and skeletal muscle from various species in a cardiac troponin I immunoassay. *Clin Chem.* 43:2333–2338.

O'Hagan, K.P. and Zambraski, E.J. 1986. Kidney function in deoxycorticosterone acetate (DOCA) treated hypertensive Yucatan miniature swine. In *Swine in Biomedical Research.* Ed. M.E. Tumbleson, pp. 1779–1787. New York, NY: Plenum Press.

Odink, J., Smeets, J.F., Visser, I.J., Sandman, H., and Snijders, J.M. 1990. Hematologic and clinicochemical profiles of healthy swine and swine with inflammatory processes. *J Anim Sci.* 68:163–170.

Oldigs, B. 1986. Effects of internal factors upon hematological and clinical chemical parameters in the Göttingen miniature pig. In *Swine in Biomedical Research.* Ed. M.E. Tumbleson, pp. 809–813ssss. New York, NY: Plenum Press.

Oregon State Veterinary Diagnostic Laboratory University. 2009. Biochemistry Reference Ranges. Available at: http://oregonstate.edu/vetmed/sites/default/files/CP_Biochemistry_Reference_Ranges_04_09.pdf.

Otis, C.R., Wamhoff, B.R., and Sturek, M. 2003. Hyperglycemia-induced insulin resistance in diabetic dyslipidemic Yucatan swine. *Comp Med.* 53(1):53–64.

Padgett, E.L. The minipig as a model for juvenile toxicity testing, nonclinical juvenile toxicology. In Abstract from *Powerpoint Presentation at 3rd Minipig Research Forum*, Nov 2009, The National Conference Center, Lansdowne, Virginia, Slides 22–23, October 15–16, 2009.

Panepinto, L.M. 1986. Laboratory methodology and management of swine in biomedical research. In *Swine in Biomedical Research.* Ed. M.E. Tumbleson, pp. 97–109. New York, NY: Plenum Press.

Panepinto, L.M. 1996. Miniature swine breeds used worldwide in research. In *Advances in Swine in Biomedical Research—Vol 2.* Eds. M.E. Tumbleson and L.B. Schook, pp. 681–691. New York, NY: Plenum Press.

Parsons, A.H., Smith, S.C., Kertzer, R., and Salkovitz, I.R. 1986. Endurance exercising miniature pigs—A review of methodology. In *Swine in Biomedical Research.* Ed. M.E. Tumbleson, pp. 143–151. New York, NY: Plenum Press.

Parsons, A.H. and Wells, R.E. 1986. Serum biochemistry of healthy Yucatan miniature pigs. *Lab Anim Sci.* 36:428–430.

Pearce, G.P. and Paterson, A.M. 1993. The effect of space restriction and provision of toys during rearing on the behavior, productivity, and physiology of male pigs. *Appl Anim Behav Sci.* 36:11–28.

Petersen, H.H., Nielsen, J.P., and Heegaard, P.M.H. 2004. Application of acute phase protein measurements in veterinary clinical chemistry. *Vet Res.* 35:163–187.

Phillips, R.W. and Tumbleson, M.E. 1986. Models. In *Swine in Biomedical Research.* Ed. M.E. Tumbleson, Vol. 1, pp. 437–440. New York, NY: Plenum Press.

Piñeiro, M., Piñeiro, C., Carpintero, R., et al. 2007. Characterisation of the pig acute phase protein response to road transport. *Vet J.* 173(3):669–674.

Plumb, D.C. 2005. Reference laboratory values: sheep, goats and swine. In: *Plumb's Veterinary Drug Handbook*, 5th edition, p. 881. Ames, IA: Blackwell Publishing.

Pond, W.G., Banis, R.J., Van Vleck, L.D., Walker, E.F., Jr., and Chapman, P. 1968. Age changes in body weight and in several blood components of conventional versus miniature pigs. *Proceed Soc Exp Biol Med.* 127:895–900.

Pond, W.G. and Houpt, K.A. 1978. *The Biology of the Pig.* Ithaca, NY: Cornell University Press, Comstock Publishing Associates.

Pond, W.G. and Mersmann H.J. 2001. *The Biology of the Pig.* Ithaca, NY: Cornell University Press.

Popesko, P. 1984. *Atlas of Topographic Anatomy of the Domestic Animals*, Vol. 1, pp. 98–110. Philadelphia, PA: W.B. Saunders.

Porter V. 1983. *Pigs: A Handbook to the Breeds of the World.* Ithaca, NY: Cornell University Press.

Prather, R.S., Hawley, R.J., Carter, D.B., et al. 2003. Transgenic swine for biomedicine and agriculture. *Theriogenol.* 59:115–123.

Prescott, M.F., Hasler-Repacz, J., von-Linden-Reed, J., and Rapacz, J. 17 January, 1995. Familial hypercholesterolemia associated with coronary atherosclerosis in swine bearing different alleles for apolipoprotein B. *Ann NY Acad Sci.* 748:283–292.

Radin, M.J., Weiser, M.G., and Fettman, M.J. 1986. Hematologic and serum biochemical values for Yucatan miniature swine. *Lab Anim Sci.* 36:425–427.

Randall, G.C.B. 1986. Chronic implantation of catheters and other surgical techniques in fetal pigs. In *Swine in Biomedical Research.* Ed. M.E. Tumbleson, pp. 1179–1185. New York, NY: Plenum Press.

Rapacz, J., Hasler-Rapacz, J., Taylor, K.M., Checovich, W.J., and Attie, A.D. 1986. Lipoprotein mutations in pigs are associated with elevated plasma cholesterol and atherosclerosis. *Science.* 234:1573–1577.

Redmer, D.A., Christenson, R.K., Ford, J.J., and Day, B.N. 1984. Effect of unilateral ovariectomy on compensatory ovarian hypertrophy, peripheral concentrations of follicle-stimulating hormone and luteinizing hormone, and ovarian venous concentrations of estradiol-17b in prepuberal gilts. *Biol Reprod.* 31:59–66.

Reeds, P. and Odle, J. 1996. Pigs as models for nutrient functional interaction. In *Advances in Swine in Biomedical Research*. Eds. M.E. Tumbleson, and L.B. Schook, pp. 709–711. New York, NY: Plenum Press.

Reese, D.E., Peo, Jr. E.R., Lewis, A.J., and Hogg, A. 1984. Serum chemical values of gestating and lactating swine: Reference values. *Am J Vet Res.* 45:978–980.

Rendell, M., Stephen, P.M., Paulsen, R., et al. 1985. An interspecies comparison of normal levels of glycosylated hemoglobin and glycosylated albumin. *Comp BiochemPhysiol B.* 81:819–822.

Renner, S., Fehlings, C., Herbach, N., et al. 2010. Glucose intolerance and reduced proliferation of pancreatic β-cells in transgenic pigs with impaired glucose-dependent insulinotropic polypeptide function. *Diabetes.* 59(5):1228–1238.

Riebold, T.W. and Thurmon, J.C. 1986. Anesthesia in swine. In *Swine in Biomedical Research.* Ed. M.E. Tumbleson, pp. 243–254. New York, NY: Plenum Press.

Rippel, R.H., Harmon, B.G., Jensen, A.H., Norton, H.W., and Becker, D.E. 1965. Response of the gravid gilt to levels of protein as determined by nitrogen balance. *J Anim Sci.* 24:209–215.

Rispat, G., Slaoui, M., Weber, D., Salemink, P., Berthoux, C., and Shrivastava, R. 1993. Haematological and plasma biochemical values for healthy Yucatan micropigs. *Lab Anim.* 27:368–373.

Rodriguez, H. and Kunavongkrit, A. 1983. Chronical venous catheterization for frequent blood sampling in unrestrained pigs. *Acta Vet Scand.* 24:318–320.

Romsos, D.R., Leveille, G.A., and Allee, G.L. 1971. Alloxan diabetes in the pig (Sus domesticus). Response to glucose, tolbutamide, and insulin administration. *Comp Biochem Physiol A Comp Physiol.* 40:557–568.

Saho, S., Kadota, Y., Sameshima, T., Miyao, J., Tsurumaru, T., and Yoshimura, N. 1997. The effects of sevoflurane anesthesia on insulin secretion and glucose metabolism in pigs. *Anesth Analg.* 84(6):1359–1365.

Saitoh, S., Saito, T., Ohwada, T., et al. 1998. Morphological and functional changes in coronary vessel evoked by repeated endothelial injury in pigs. *Cardiovasc Res.* 38:772–781.

Schook, L.B., Beattie, C., Beever, J., et al. 2005. Swine in biomedical research: Creating the building blocks of animal models. *Anim Biotechnol.* 16:183–190.

Shearer, H., Purvis, K., Jenkin, G., and Haynes, N.B. 1972. Peripheral plasma progesterone and oestradiol-17b levels before and after puberty in gilts. *J Reprod Fertil.* 30:347–360.

Shi, Z.-S., Feng, L., He, X., et al. 2009. Vulnerable plaque in a swine model of carotid atherosclerosis. *AJNR Am J Neuroradiol.* 30:469–472.

Shoumin, X., Weidong, Y., Zongbao, W., et al. 2004. A minipig model of high-fat/high-sucrose diet-induced diabetes and atherosclerosis. *Int J Exp Pathol.* 85(4):223–231.

Shulman, M., Baverman, B., Ivankovick, A. D., and Gronert, G. 1981. Sevoflurane triggers malignant hyperthermia in swine. *Anesthesiol.* 54:259–260.

Spencer, G.S.G. and Hallett, K.G. 1986. Hormone and metabolite changes with stress in pigs. In *Swine in Biomedical Research.* Ed. M.E. Tumbleson, pp. 159–165. New York, NY: Plenum Press.

Spencer, G.S.G., Garssen, G.J., Macdonald, A.A., Colenbrander, B., Hallett, K.G., and Bevers, M.M. 1986. Clearance rates of some hormones in the fetal pig. In *Swine in Biomedical Research.* Ed. M.E. Tumbleson, pp. 1239–1243. New York, NY: Plenum Press.

Stockham, S.L. and Scott, M.A. 2008. *Fundamentals of Veterinary Clinical Pathology*, 2nd edition, p. 16. Ames, IA: Wiley-Blackwell Publishing.

Stockland, W.L., Meade, R.J., Tumbleson, M.E., and Palm, B.W. 1971. Influence of site of sampling and stage of fast on concentrations of all free amino acids in the plasma and liver in the young pig. *J Anim Sci.* 32:1143–1152.

Straw, B.E., Zimmerman, J.J., D'Allaire, S., and Taylor, D.J. 2006. *Diseases of Swine*, 9th edition, 1153 pp. Hoboken, NJ: Blackwell Publishing.

Sturek, M., Alloosh, M., Wenzel, J.P., et al. 2007. Ossabaw island miniature swine: Cardiometabolic syndrome assessment. In *Swine in the Laboratory: Surgery, Anesthesia, Imaging and Experimental Techniques*. Ed. M.M. Swindle, 2nd edition, pp. 397–402. Boca Raton, FL: CRC Press.

Sullivan, T.P., Eaglstein, W.H., Davis, S.C., and Mertz, P. 2001. The pig as a model for human wound healing. *Wound Repair Regen.* 9:66–76.

Svendsen, J., Westrom, B.R., Svendsen, L.S., Bengtsson, A.-C., Ohlsson, B., and Karlsson, B.W. 1986. Some blood serum characteristics of newborn, unaffected pigs and of pigs dying within the perinatal period: Stillborn intrapartum pigs, weakborn pigs, underweight pigs, and traumatized pigs. In *Swine in Biomedical Research.* Ed. M.E. Tumbleson, pp. 1277–1288. New York, NY: Plenum Press.

Svendsen, O. 2006. The minipig in toxicology. *Exp Toxicol Pathol.* 57(5–6):335–339.

Swindle, M.M. Ed. 2007. *Swine in the Laboratory: Surgery, Anesthesia, Imaging, and Experimental Techniques*, 2nd edition, p. 471. Boca Raton, FL: CRC Press, Taylor & Francis Group.

Swindle, M.M. and Adams R.J. Eds. 1988. *Experimental Surgery and Physiology: Induced Animal Models of Human Disease.* Baltimore, MD: Williams and Wilkins.

Swindle, M.M., Moody, D.C., and Phillips, L.D. Eds. 1992. *Swine as Models in Biomedical Research.* Ames, IA: Iowa State University Press.

Swindle, M.M., Nolan, T., Jacobson, A., Wolf, P., Dalton, M.J., and Smith, A.C. 2005. Vascular access port (VAP) usage in large animal species. *Contemp Topic Lab Anim Sci.* 44(3):7–17.

Swindle, M.M. and Smith, A.C. 1998. Comparative anatomy and physiology of the pig. *Scand J Lab Anim Sci.* 25:11–21.

Swindle, M.M. and Smith, A.C. 2000. Information Resources on Swine in Biomedical Research 1990–2000. Available at: https://pubs.nal.usda.gov/sites/pubs.nal.usda.gov/files/swine.pdf.

Swindle, M.M. and Smith, A.C. 2008. Swine in biomedical research. In *Sourcebook of Models for Biomedical Research.* Ed. P.M. Conn, Chap. 26, pp. 233–239. Totowa, NJ: Humana Press.

Takahashi, H. 1986. Long-term blood-sampling technique in piglets. *Lab Anim.* 20:206–209.

Terris, J.M., Martin, T.V., and Simmonds, R.C. 1986. Metabolism unit, confinement unit, and placement of indwelling catheters for use with swine. In *Swine in Biomedical Research.* Ed. M.E. Tumbleson, pp. 111–121. New York, NY: Plenum Press.

Tewes, H., Steinbach, J., and Smidt, D. 1977. Investigations on the blood composition of sows during the reproductive cycle. I. Blood changes during the oestrus cycle. *Zuchthygiene.* 12:117–124.

Tewes, H., Steinbach, J., and Smidt, D. 1979a. Investigations on the blood composition of sows during the reproductive cycle. II. Blood changes during pregnancy. *Zuchthygiene.* 14:111–116.

Tewes, H., Steinbach, J., and Smidt, D. 1979b. Investigations on the blood composition of sows during the reproductive cycle. III. Blood changes during lactation. *Zuchthygiene.* 14:159–164.

Thacker, P.A. and Bowland, J.P. 1986. Effects of propionate on serum lipids and lipoproteins in the pig. In *Swine in Biomedical Research.* Ed. M.E. Tumbleson, pp. 745–754. New York, NY: Plenum Press.

Thomas, T.R., Pellechia, J., Rector, R.S., Sun, G.Y., Sturek, M.S., and Laughlin, M.H. 2002. Exercise training does not reduce hyperlipidemia in pigs fed a high-fat diet. *Metabolism.* 51(12):1587–1595.

Tsutsumi, H., Monnai, Y., Ishii, H., Tanioka, Y., and Tanigawa, M. 1999. Diurnal variations and effects of fasting on blood constituents in minipigs. *Exp Anim.* 48(4):247–254.

Tumbleson, M.E. 1973. Protein-calorie undernutrition in young Sinclair (S-1) miniature swine: Serum biochemic and hematologic values. In *Advances in Automated Analysis. 1972 Technicon International Congress*, Vol. 7, pp. 51–71. Tarrytown, NY: Mediad Incorporated.

Tumbleson, M.E. Ed. 1986. *Swine in Biomedical Research*, Vol. 1–3. New York, NY: Plenum Press.

Tumbleson, M.E., Burks, M.F., Spate, M.P., Hutcheson, D.P., and Middleton, C.C. 1970. Serum biochemical and hematological parameters of Sinclair (S-1) miniature sows during gestation and lactation. *Can J Comp Med.* 34:312–319.

Tumbleson, M.E., Donemert, A.R., and Middleton, C.C. 1968. Techniques for handling miniature swine for laboratory procedures. *Lab Anim Care.* 18:584–587.

Tumbleson, M.E., Hicklin, K.W., and Burks, M.F. 1976a. Serum cholesterol, triglyceride, glucose, and total bilirubin concentrations, as functions of age and sex, in Sinclair (S-1) miniature swine. *Growth.* 40:293–300.

Tumbleson, M.E., Hutcheson, D.P., and Fogg, T.J. 1972. Serum biochemic values of fetal and neonatal crossbred swine. In *Advances in Automated Analysis. 1970 Technicon International Congress*, Vol. 2, pp. 149–156. Mt. Kisco, NY: Futura Publishing Company.

Tumbleson, M.E., Hutcheson, D.P., and Middleton, C.C. 1976b. Serum protein concentrations and enzyme activities, as a function of age and sex, in Sinclair (S-1) miniature swine. *Growth.* 40:53–68.

Tumbleson, M.E. and Kalish, P.R. 1972. Serum biochemical and hematological parameters in crossbred swine from birth through eight weeks of age. *Can J Comp Med.* 36:202–209.

Tumbleson, M.E. and Schook, L.B. Eds. 1996. *Advances in Swine in Biomedical Research. Proceedings of an International Symposium on Advances in Swine in Biomedical Research held at the University of Maryland*, University College Park, MD, October 22–25, 1995, 2 Vols, Plenum Press.

Tumbleson, M.E. and Schmidt, D.A. 1986. Swine clinical chemistry. In *Swine in Biomedical Research*. Ed. M.E. Tumbleson, pp. 783–807. New York, NY: Plenum Press.

Vallet, J.L. and Christenson, R.K. 1994. Effect of esterone treatment from day 30 to day 45 of pregnancy on endometrial protein secretion and uterine capacity. *J Anim Sci.* 72:3188–3195.

Veum, T.L., Zamora, R.G., and Sherry, M.P. 1986. Utilization of soybean and milk proteins by neonatal pigs reared artificially. In *Swine in Biomedical Research*. Ed. M.E. Tumbleson, pp. 1113–1124. New York, NY: Plenum Press.

Vodicka, P., Smetana, K., Jr, Dvorankova, B., et al. 2005. The miniature pig as an animal model in biomedical research. *Ann N Y Acad Sci.* 1049:161–71.

Von Borell, E. and Ladewig, J. 1989. Altered adrenocortical response to acute stressors or ACTH (1–24) in intensively housed pigs. *Domes Anim Endocrinol.* 6:299–309.

Wade, C.E., Hannon, J.P., Bossone, C.A., Hunt, M.M., and Rodkey, W.G. 1986. Cardiovascular and hormonal responses of conscious pigs during physical restraint. In *Swine in Biomedical Research*. Ed. M.E. Tumbleson, pp. 1395–1404. New York, NY: Plenum Press.

Wangsness, P.J., Acker, W.A., Burdete, J.H., Krabill, L.F., and Vasilatos, R. 1981. Effect of fasting on hormones and metabolites in plasma of fast-growing, lean, and slow-growing obese pigs. *J Anim Sci.* 52:69–74.

Warnier, A. and Zayan, R. 1985. Effects of confinement upon behavioral and hormonal responses and production indices in fattening pigs. In *Social Space for Domestic Animals*. Ed. R. Zayan, pp. 128–150. Dordrecht: Martinus-Nijhoff.

Watkins, K.L. and Veum, T.L. 1986. Utilization of soybean and milk proteins by neonatal pigs reared artificially. In *Swine in Biomedical Research*. Ed. M.E. Tumbleson, pp. 1125–1135. New York, NY: Plenum Press.

Weiskopf, R.B., Bogetz, M.S., Reid, I.A., Roizen, M.F., and Keil, L.C. 1986. Cardiovascular, endocrine, and metabolic responses of conscious swine to hemorrhage. In *Swine in Biomedical Research*. Ed. M.E. Tumbleson, pp. 1405–1411. New York, NY: Plenum Press.

Weiskopf, R.B., Holmes, M.A., Eger II, E.I., et al. 1992. Use of swine in the study of anesthetics. In *Swine as Models in Biomedical Research*. Ed. M.M. Swindle, pp. 96–117. Ames, IA: Iowa State University Press.

Weldon, W.C., Lewis, A.J., Louis, G.F., Kovar, J.L., and Miller, P.S. 1994. Postpartum hypophagia in primiparous sows: II. Effects of feeding level during gestation and exogenous insulin on lactation feed intake, glucose tolerance, and epinephrine-stimulated release of nonesterified fatty acids and glucose. *J Anim Sci.* 72:395–403.

Wells, M.Y. and Gosselin, S. 1996. Reporting clinical pathology results. In: *Presenting Toxicology Results: How to Evaluate Data and Write Reports*. Ed. G.J. Nohynek, Chap. 7, pp. 63–74. London: Taylor & Francis.

Wendt, M., Waldmann, K.H., and Bickhardt, K. 1990. Comparative studies of the clearance of inulin and creatinine in swine. *Zentralbl Veterinarmed A.* 37(10):752–759.

White C.J. and Ramee S.R. 1989. Swine models of atherosclerosis. In *Atherosclerosis and Arteriosclerosis: Human Pathology and Experimental Methods and Models*. Ed. R.A. White, Chap. 9, pp. 207–234. Boca Raton, FL: CRC Press.

White, C.J., Ramee, S.R., Card, H.G., et al. 1988. Laser angioplasty: An atherosclerotic swine model. *Lasers Surg Med.* 8(3):318–321.

Wills, R.W., Zimmerman, J.J., Yoon, K.J., et al. 1997. Porcine reproductive and respiratory syndrome virus: Routes of excretion. *Vet Microbiol.* 57:69–81.

Wilson, J.D., Dhall, D.P., Simeonovic, C.J., and Lafferty, K.J. 1986. Induction and management of diabetes mellitus in the pig. *Aust J Expl Biol Med Sci.* 64:489–500.

Wilson, G.D.A., Harvey, D.G., and Snook, C.R. 1972. A review of factors affecting blood biochemistry in the pig. *Br Vet J.* 128:596–610.

Wingfield, W.E., Tumbleson, M.E., Hicklin, K.W., and Mather, E.C. 1974. An exteriorized cranial vena caval catheter for serial blood sample collection from miniature swine. *Lab Anim Sci.* 24:359–361.

Wise, T., Lundstra, D.D., and Ford, J.J. 1994. Changes in serum testosterone and FSH in Cross-Breed (CX) and Meishan (MS) boars after castration and in response to steroidal challenge. *Biol Reprod.* 50(Suppl 1):50.

Wise, T., Lundstra, D.D., and Ford, J.J. 1996. Differential pituitary and gonadal function of Chinese Meishan and European white composite boars: Effects of gonadotropin-releasing hormone stimulation, castration, and steroidal feedback. *Biol Reprod.* 54:146–153.

Witzel, D.A., Littledike, E.T., and Cook, H.M. 1973. Implanted catheters for blood sampling in swine. *Cornell Vet.* 63:432–435.

Wolkers, J., Wensing, T., Groot Bruinderink, G.W.T.A., and Schonewille, J.T. 1994. The effect of undernutrition on haematological and serum biochemical variables in wild boar (Sus scrofa). *Comp Biochem Physiol.* 108:431–437.

Wood, P.D. and Haskell, W.L. 1979. The effect of exercise on plasma high density lipoproteins. *Lipids.* 14:417–427.

Yen, J.T. 2001. Blood sampling and surgical techniques. In *Swine Nutrition.* Eds. A.J. Lewis, and L. Lee Southern, Chap. 42, pp. 961–983. Boca Raton, FL: CRC Press.

Yen, J.T., Pond, W.G., and Stone, R.T. 1982. Serum transferrin and albumin in protein-deficient young pigs. *Nutr Rep Int.* 25:561–566.

Yu, H., Bao, E.D., Zhao, R.Q., and Lv, Q.X. 2007. Effect of transportation stress on heat shock protein 70 concentration and mRNA expression in heart and kidney tissues and serum enzyme activities and hormone concentrations of pigs. *Am J Vet Res.* 68(11):1145–1150.

Zanella, E.L., Ford, J.J., Wise, T., and Hamernik, D.L. 1996. Pituitary relationship of gonadotropins and messenger ribonucleic acid for gonadotropin subunits in white composite and Meishan boars. *Biol Reprod.* 54:154–159.

Zatzman, M.L., Swartz, H.A., Hicklin, K.W., and Tumbleson, M.E. 1986. Renal function of limit fed and ad libitum fed miniature swine. In *Swine in Biomedical Research.* Ed. M.E. Tumbleson, pp. 1767–1777. New York, NY: Plenum Press.

APPENDIX A

Reference Ranges for Domestic Swine

TABLE A.1
Biochemical Values—Domestic Farm Swine (2–4 Months of Age)

Parameter	Units	Presurgery Baseline Values (Mean ± SEM)
Sodium (Na)	mEq/L	142 ± 1
Potassium (K)	mEq/L	4.8 ± 0.2
Chloride (Cl)	mEq/L	101 ± 1
Calcium (Ca)	mg/dL	10 ± 0.1
Phosphorous (P)	mg/dL	9.5 ± 0.4
Iron (Fe)	µg/dL	137 ± 20
Total protein	g/dL	5.6 ± 0.1
Albumin	g/dL	3.1 ± 0.1
Globulin	g/dL	2.5 ± 0.1
Urea	mg/dL	10 ± 1
Creatinine	mg/dL	1.2 ± 0.1
Bicarbonate	mEq/L	26 ± 1
Hemoglobin	g/dL	11.2 ± 0.3
Bilirubin	mg/dL	0.15 ± 0.04
Alkaline phosphatase	IU/L	164 ± 12
Alanine aminotransferase (ALT)	IU/L	38 ± 3
Aspartate aminotransferase (AST)	IU/L	39 ± 3
Lactate dehydrogenase (LDH)	IU/L	622 ± 51
Prothrombin time	sec	11.2 ± 0.3

Source: Drougas, J.G. et al., *Lab Anim Sci.*, 46, 648–655, 1996. With permission.

Animals were 8–16-weeks-old, crossbred (Yorkshire × Hampshire × Duroc), domestic swine. Gender included female (*n* = 18), castrate male (*n* = 5), and intact male (*n* = 4). Body weight range was 20.6–70.7 kg (mean 30.6 ± 9.8kg).

TABLE A.2
Blood Gas and Acid–Base Status—Domestic Swine

Measurement	*N*	Mean	SD	Range
Blood Oxygenation				
Arterial PO_2 (mmHg)	36	82	4.2	73–92
Arterial HbO_2 (%)	18	94	0.7	92–95
Arterial O_2 capacity (mL/dL)	21	13.1	1.04	10.1–14.2
Arterial O_2 content (mL/dL)	21	12.4	1.62	8.7–15.1
Arterial carboxyhemoglobin (%)	18	4	0.4	4–5
Arterial methemoglobin (%)	18	1	0.3	0.6–1.8
Mixed venous PO_2 (mmHg)	22	41	3.3	32–45
Mixed venous HbO_2 (%)	22	60	5.7	48–71
Mixed venous O_2 Content (mL/dL)	20	8.0	1.27	5.3–10.8
Art.-ven. O_2 cont. diff. (mL/dL)	26	4.3	0.43	3.4–5.7
Acid–Base Status				
Arterial pH	36	7.48	0.033	7.40–7.53
Arterial PCO_2 (mmHg)	36	40	2.3	35–44
Arterial plasma HCO_3 (mEq/L)	36	29	2.2	22–33
Arterial buffer base (mEq/L)	40	45	3.3	40–52
Mixed venous pH	23	7.42	0.024	7.38–7.48
Mixed venous PCO_2 (mmHg)	22	49	3.2	44–55
Mixed venous plasma HCO_3 (mEq/L)	14	31	2.1	28–35

Source: Hannon, J.P. et al., *Lab Anim Sci.*, 40, 293–298, 1990. With permission.
The values are normal for 20–25 kg Yorkshire/Duroc cross farm pigs.

TABLE A.3
Plasma Electrolytes and Metabolites—Domestic Swine

Measurement	*N*	Mean	SD	Range
Cations				
Sodium (mEq/L)	35	138	3.49	129–143
Potassium (mEq/L)	35	4.4	0.37	3.9–4.1
Magnesium (mEq/L)	17	1.4	0.18	1.2–1.9
Calcium (mEq/L)	15	4.8	0.29	4.5–5.6
Anions				
Chloride (mEq/L)	17	106	7.8	93–126
Bicarbonate (mEq/L)	36	29	2.2	22–33
Phosphate (mEq/L)	17	4.0	0.58	3.1–5.1
Plasma albumin (mEq/L)	40	7.6	0.80	6.2–9.2
Plasma globulin (mEq/L)	40	6.1	0.90	4.8–7.8
Metabolites				
Glucose (mM/L)	33	4.6	0.66	2.6–6.5
Lactate (mM/L)	33	1.0	0.26	0.5–1.5

(*Continued*)

TABLE A.3 (*Continued*)
Plasma Electrolytes and Metabolites—Domestic Swine

Measurement	*N*	Mean	SD	Range
Urea (mM/L)	17	3.2	1.15	2.0–5.4
Creatinine (μM/L)	17	89	19.5	62–131
Free Fatty Acids				
Lauric (μM/L)	18	6	0.59	5–7
Myristic (μM/L)	18	11	2.67	7–16
Palmitic (μM/L)	18	147	66.0	147–249
Palmitoleic (μM/L)	18	30	8.9	9–43
Steric (μM/L)	18	121	38.2	58–188
Oleic (μM/L)	18	244	100.6	89–394
Linoleic (μM/L)	18	115	32.2	46–169
Linolinic (μM/L)	18	8	4.7	1–16
Arachadonic (μM/L)	18	42	3.3	14–62
Total free fatty acids (μM/L)	18	0.8	0.07	0.1–1.1

Source: Hannon, J.P. et al., Lab Anim Sci., *40, 293–298, 1990. With permission.*
Note: The values are normal for 20–25 kg Yorkshire/Duroc cross farm pigs.

TABLE A.4
Plasma Hormone Concentrations—Domestic Swine

Measurement	*N*	Mean	SD	Range
Adrenocorticotropic hormone (ACTH) (pg/mL)	17	34	23.5	11–96
β-Endorphin (pg/mL)	8	56	20.2	33–90
Cortisol (μg/dL)	18	4.3	1.43	1.8–7.9
Aldosterone (ng/dL)	17	3.4	2.89	1.6–6.1
Total T3 (ng/dL)	14	28	5.2	22–40
Total T4 (μg/dL)	14	2.6	0.50	1.8–3.5
Free T4 (ng/dL)	14	0.32	0.055	0.20–0.39
Insulin (μg/dL)	18	4.2	2.98	1.0–11.0
Glucagon (pg/mL)	18	237	73.9	156–407
Glucagon/insulin ratio ($\times 10^{-6}$)	18	56	76.9	24–333
Vasopressin (pg/mL)	17	1.0	0.33	0.5–1.9
Renin activity (ngA1/mL/hr)	18	1.24	1.450	0.12–6.24
Epinephrine (pg/mL)	15	69	45.8	20–132
Norepinephrine (pg/mL)	17	179	90.0	53–332

Source: Hannon, J.P. et al., *Lab Anim Sci.*, 40, 293–298, 1990. With permission.
The values are normals for 20–25 kg Yorkshire/Duroc cross farm pigs.

TABLE A.5
Porcine Serum Constituents—Domestic Swine

	Unit of Measure	Weaner		Feeder		Gilts		Sows	
		X	SD	*X*	SD	*X*	SD	*X*	SD
Ions									
Calcium	mmol/L	2.61	0.27	2.54	0.18	2.57	0.15	2.55	0.20
Phosphorus	mmol/L	2.75	0.45	2.75	0.27	2.33	0.21	1.97	0.28
Iron	mmol/L	21	8	22	9	23	6	22	6
Metabolites									
Glucose	mmol/L	5.4	0.9	5.5	1.0	4.6	0.7	4.4	0.7
Urea nitrogen	mmol/L	5.30	1.30	5.30	1.40	5.60	1.80	5.30	1.50
Creatinine	mmol/L	102	22	126	19	166	27	160	32
Cholesterol	mmol/L	2.19	0.52	2.27	0.41	2.03	0.31	1.99	0.35
Bilirubin	mmol/L	2.0	0.7	1.7	0.9	1.7	0.5	1.7	0.9
Proteins									
Total protein	g/L	56	7	68	7	72	4	77	6
Albumin	g/L	27	5	31	6	38	3	37	3
Albumin/globulin	g/g	1	0.4	0.9	0.2	1.1	0.2	0.9	0.2
Enzymes									
Alanine aminotransferase	U/L	27	9	29	7	32	9	33	11
Aspartate aminotransferase	U/L	37	12	35	12	28	13	24	9
Alkaline phosphatase	U/L	517	172	406	141	234	73	110	54

Source: Friendship, R.M. et al., *Can J Comp Med*., 48, 390–393, 1984. With permission.

Data represent mean (*X*) and standard deviation (SD) for 85–109 domestic pigs in each class. Pigs on 11 different farms were sampled with approximately 10 pigs/class/farm. Breed nonspecified commercial pigs in various age groups (weanling, feeder, adult breeder) were housed on farms in Ontario, Canada.

TABLE A.6
Serum Constituents in Pregnant and Lactating Females—Domestic Swine

		Late Gestation Gilts (*n* = 33)		Lactation Day 14 Sows (*n* = 13)	
Variable	**Unit of Measure**	*X*	SD	*X*	SD
Ions					
Calcium	mmol/L	2.52	0.30	2.70	0.25
Phosphorus	mmol/L	1.65	0.19	1.58	0.17
Iron	µmol/L	25.3	6.2	25.9	6.2
Sodium	mmol/L	141.2	9.1	139.4	7.5
Potassium	mmol/L	6.5	0.8	6.9	0.9
Metabolites					
Glucose	mmol/L	4.86	0.73	5.28	0.69
Urea nitrogen	mmol/L	3.14	0.57	4.93	0.89
Creatinine	µmol/L	212	27	177	25
Cholesterol	mmol/L	1.93	0.42	3.46	0.76

(Continued)

TABLE A.6 (*Continued*)
Serum Constituents in Pregnant and Lactating Females—Domestic Swine

Variable	Unit of Measure	Late Gestation Gilts (n = 33)		Lactation Day 14 Sows (n = 13)	
		X	SD	*X*	SD
Proteins					
Total protein	g/L	62	9	66	7
Albumin	g/L	39	5	38	4
Globulin	g/L	23	5	28	5
Enzymes					
Aspartate aminotransferase	µkat/L	0.213	0.173	0.202	0.060
Alkaline phosphatase	µkat/L	1.35	0.34	1.09	0.40

Source: Reese, D.E. et al., *Am J Vet Res.*, 45, 978–980, 1984. With permission.
Data represent mean (*X*) and standard deviation (SD); adult 1-year-old domestic crossbred swine, gilts, and sows.

APPENDIX B

Reference Ranges for Miniature Swine (Yucatan)

TABLE B.1
Clinical Chemistry Data for Yucatan Miniature Swine

Serum Analyte	Yucatan[a]		Range[b]	
	Male	Female	Male	Female
Alanine aminotransferase (ALT) (IU/L)				
Weanling (32–35 days)	26 ± 8	28 ± 7	17–44	18–43
Juvenile (3–6 months)	34 ± 8	36 ± 5	22–50	24–44
Adult (6–12 months)	43 ± 11	33 ± 8	20–59	21–46
Aspartate aminotransferase (AST) (IU/L)				
Weanling (32–35 days)	40 ± 43	52 ± 70	14–215	17–351
Juvenile (3–6 months)	42 ± 16	39 ± 8	26–81	28–61
Adult (6–12 months)	32 ± 9	28 ± 11	21–52	17–65
Lactate dehydrogenase (LDH) (IU/L)				
Weanling (32–35 days)	719 ± 585	587± 53	382–1753	508–641
Juvenile (3–6 months)[c]	760 ± 180	788 ± 179	462–1290	588–1710
Adult (6–12 months)	435 ± 61	444 ± 65	309–564	363–615
Gamma-glutamyl transferase (GGT) (IU/L)				
Weanling (32–35 days)	44 ± 10	38 ± 10	27–66	24–65
Juvenile (3–6 months)	56 ± 9	53 ± 12	40–75	38–98
Adult (6–12 months)	35 ± 13	35 ± 7	17–65	23–49
Creatine phosphokinase (CPK) (IU/L)				
Weanling (32–35 days)	Not performed	Not performed	Not performed	Not performed
Juvenile (3–6 months)[c]	717 ± 995	704.4 ± 1159	105–5160	132–5999
Adult (6–12 months)	488 ± 332	613 ± 438	142–1410	219–1778

(*Continued*)

TABLE B.1 (*Continued*)
Clinical Chemistry Data for Yucatan Miniature Swine

Serum Analyte	Yucatan[a]		Range[b]	
	Male	Female	Male	Female
Alkaline phosphatase (ALP) (IU/L)				
Weanling (32–35 days)	172 ± 41	176 ± 43	72–239	68–259
Juvenile (3–6 months)	92 ± 17	101 ± 19	67–120	64–130
Adult (6–12 months)	106 ± 26	105 ± 28	73–167	66–163
Blood urea nitrogen (BUN) (mg/dL)				
Weanling (32–35 days)	15 ± 3	14 ± 4	9–23	8–24
Juvenile (3–6 months)	8 ± 2	10 ± 5	3–13	6–25
Adult (6–12 month)	21 ± 5	17 ± 3	12–32	12–25
Creatinine (CREAT) (mg/dL)				
Weanling (32–35 days)	0.7 ± 0.1	0.7 ± 0.1	0.5–0.9	0.4–0.9
Juvenile (3–6 months)	0.8 ± 0.2	0.9 ± 0.2	0.5–1.2	0.6–1.2
Adult (6–12 months)	1.2 ± 0.2	1.2 ± 0.2	1.0–1.6	0.9–1.5
Glucose (GLU) (mg/dL)				
Weanling (32–35 days)	92 ± 13	91 ± 20	63–110	36–115
Juvenile (3–6 months)	72 ± 11	80 ± 6	56–102	71–90
Adult (6–12 months)	110 ± 34	91 ± 22	66–174	57–139
Sodium (Na) (mmol/L)				
Weanling (32–35 days)	139 ± 4	139 ± 2	130–154	134–144
Juvenile (3–6 months)	139 ± 4	138 ± 5	133–145	126–147
Adult (6–12 months)	143 ± 4	139 ± 2	136–150	136–143
Potassium (K) (mmol/L)				
Weanling (32–35 days)	5.2 ± 0.8	5.3 ± 0.8	4.1–6.7	4.0–7.5
Juvenile (3–6 months)	4.6 ± 1.2	4.2 ±1.0	3.6–8.9	3.5–7.8
Adult (6–12 months)	4.6 ± 1.0	4.4 ± 0.5	1.5–6.3	3.4–5.3
Chloride (CL) (mmol/L)				
Weanling (32–35 days)	105 ± 5	104 ± 2	99–123	99–108
Juvenile (3–6 months)	98 ± 3	98 ± 5	91–101	88–103
Adult (6–12 months)	101 ± 4	102 ± 3	95–110	101–107
Bicarbonate (CO_2) (mmol/L)				
Weanling (32–35 days)	22 ± 4	21 ± 3	14–28	16–28
Juvenile (3–6 months)	22 ± 2	22 ± 2	17–26	17–26
Adult (6–12 months)	30 ± 5	30 ± 5	21–42	25–41
Total bilirubin (TBIL) (mg/dL)				
Weanling (32–35 days)	0.3 ± 0.1	0.2 ± 0.2	0.1–0.6	0.1–0.6
Juvenile (3–6 months)	0.2 ± 0.1	0.2 ± 0.1	0.1–0.5	0.1–0.5
Adult (6–12 months)	0.1 ± 0.1	0.1 ± 0.1	0.0–0.2	0.1–0.2
Total protein (TPRO) (g/dL)				
Weanling (32–35 days)	5.3 ± 0.4	5.4 ± 0.4	4.6–5.9	4.2–6.0
Juvenile (3–6 months)	6.3 ± 0.4	6.0 ± 0.3	5.7–7.0	5.5–6.6
Adult (6–12 months)	8.3 ± 0.5	8.3 ± 0.7	7.4–9.4	6.5–9.6

(*Continued*)

TABLE B.1 (*Continued*)
Clinical Chemistry Data for Yucatan Miniature Swine

Serum Analyte	Yucatan[a] Male	Yucatan[a] Female	Range[b] Male	Range[b] Female
Albumin (ALB) (g/dL)				
Weanling (32–35 days)	3.5 ± 0.3	3.4 ± 0.4	2.9–3.9	2.4–3.9
Juvenile (3–6 months)	4.0 ± 0.3	3.7 ± 0.2	3.6–4.6	3.4–4.0
Adult (6–12 months)	4.3 ± 0.5	4.1 ± 0.4	3.6–5.5	3.0–4.6
Globulin (GLOB) (g/dL)				
Weanling (32–35 days)	1.9 ± 0.2	2.0 ± 0.2	1.5–2.3	1.4–2.4
Juvenile (3–6 months)	2.3 ± 0.2	2.3 ± 0.3	2.0–2.7	1.8–2.9
Adult (6–12 months)	4.1 ± 0.6	4.2 ± 0.4	2.8–5.0	3.5–5.0
A/G ratio (A/G) (Ratio)				
Weanling (32–35 days)	1.93 ± 0.30	1.86 ± 0.43	1.39–2.89	1.04–2.95
Juvenile (3–6 months)	1.79 ± 0.22	1.64 ± 0.27	1.41–2.10	1.17–2.22
Adult (6–12 months)	1.09 ± 0.28	0.98 ± 0.10	0.80–1.82	0.85–1.22
Calcium (CA) (mg/dL)				
Weanling (32–35 days)	10.0 ± 0.4	9.9 ± 0.6	9.1–11.2	8.4–10.5
Juvenile (3–6 months)	9.5 ± 1.4	9.5 ± 0.8	3.6–10.3	6.3–10.4
Adult (6–12 months)	11.3 ± 0.6	10.9 ± 0.7	10.3–12.2	9.1–11.8
Phosphorus (PHOS) (mg/dL)				
Weanling (32–35 days)	8.6 ± 0.7	8.3 ± 0.8	7.0–9.4	6.3–10.3
Juvenile (3–6 months)	7.7 ± 0.6	7.2 ± 0.6	6.5–9.1	6.3–8.4
Adult (6–12 months)	8.4 ± 0.8	7.9 ± 0.6	6.8–10.0	7.0–9.2
Cholesterol (CHOL) (mg/dL)				
Weanling (32–35 days)	66 ± 12	73 ± 18	35–85	47–113
Juvenile (3–6 months)	73 ± 14	83 ± 12	58–98	61–109
Adult (6–12 months)	80 ± 24	83 ± 18	37–116	56–142
Triglyceride (TRIG) (mg/dL)				
Weanling (32–35 days)	53 ± 42	48 ± 12	23–233	29–81
Juvenile (3–6 months)	31 ± 13	41 ± 32	16–62	19–170
Adult (6–12 months)	35 ± 14	54 ± 23	16–64	24–111
Lipase (LIP) (IU/L)				
Weanling (32–35 days)	Not performed	Not performed	Not performed	Not performed
Juvenile (3–6 months)	Not performed	Not performed	Not performed	Not performed
Adult (6–12 months)	7 ± 3	9 ± 3	2–13	3–15
Amylase (AMY) (IU/L)				
Weanling (32–35 days)	Not performed	Not performed	Not performed	Not performed
Juvenile (3–6 months)	Not performed	Not performed	Not performed	Not performed
Adult (6–12 months)	1507 ± 584	1657 ± 331	17–2898	1176–2188
Direct bilirubin (DBILI) (mg/dL)				
Weanling (32–35 days)	Not performed	Not performed	Not performed	Not performed
Juvenile (3–6 months)[d]	0.0 ± 0.0	0.0 ± 0.0	0.03–0.06	0.03–0.05
Adult (6–12 months)	0.05 ± 0.05	0.07± 0.05	0.0–0.10	0.00–0.10

(*Continued*)

TABLE B.1 (*Continued*)
Clinical Chemistry Data for Yucatan Miniature Swine

	Yucatan[a]		Range[b]	
Serum Analyte	**Male**	**Female**	**Male**	**Female**
Indirect bilirubin (IBILI) (mg/dL)				
Weanling (32–35 days)	Not performed	Not performed	Not performed	Not performed
Juvenile (3–6 months)[d]	0.1 ± 0.0	0.1 ± 0.0	0.07–0.12	0.02–0.09
Adult (6–12 months)	0.07± 0.06	0.04 ± 0.06	0.00–0.20	0.00–0.20
Uric acid (UA) (mg/dL)				
Weanling (32–35 days)	Not performed	Not performed	Not performed	Not performed
Juvenile (3–6 months)	Not performed	Not performed	Not performed	Not performed
Adult (6–12 months)[c]	3.6 ± 7.1	7.1 ± 7.1	0.0–29.7	0.0–29.7

Source: Rispat, G. et al., *Lab Anim.*, 27, 368–373, 1993.

[a] Values are given as mean ± standard deviation.

[b] Values are smallest and largest observed values.

[c] 20–80 weeks Yucatan, $n = 36$ males and 35 females.

Original Rispat et al. values in μkat/L were multiplied by 60 to yield IU/L. All other data from Sinclair Research Center, LLC, unless otherwise stated: 32–35 days: $n = 24$ males, 25 females; 3–6 months: $n = 20$ males, 20 females; 6–12 months: $n = 19$ males, 19 females. Analysis by ANTECH Diagnostics or ANTECH GLP.

TABLE B.2
Urine Chemistry Data for Young Adult Yucatan Miniature Swine (6 months)

	Yucatan[a]		Range[b]	
	Male	**Female**	**Male**	**Female**
Urine Analyte				
pH[a]	7.8 ± 1.3	8.0 ± 1.6	6–9	5.5–9
Specific gravity[a]	1.010 ± 0.004	1.020 ± 0.005	1.005–1.016	1.009–1.025
Osmolality[a] (mOSMO)	365 ± 107.9	635 ± 160.0	220–530	279–801
Creatinine (mg/dL)[a]	45 ± 16.4	63 ± 11.6	23–70	43–82
Glucose (mg/dL)[a]	1.4 ± 1.3	2.1 ± 0.8	0.0–3	1–3
Total protein (mg/dL)[a]	9.1 ± 6.8	12.6 ± 4.4	2–24	6–20
Urine Enzymes				
Alkaline phosphatase (ALP) (IU/L)[a]	5.9 ± 5.5	1.0 ± 0.00	1–15	1–1
Aspartate aminotransferase (AST) (IU/L)[a]	3.9 ± 2.4	2.4 ± 1.2	0.5–7	1–4
Alanine aminotransferase (ALT) (IU/L)[a]	4.1 ± 4.0	0.5 ± 0.0	0.5–9.0	0.5–0.5
Creatine phosphokinase (CPK) (IU/L)[a]	1.0 ± 0.0	1.8 ± 1.8	1–1	1–6
Gamma-glutamyl transferase (GGT) (IU/L)[a]	15.3 ± 4.1	2.0 ± 0.9	9–23	1–3
Lactate dehydrogenase (LDH)[a]	9.3 ± 2.6	12.4 ± 2.5	6–14	7–15
N-acetyl-(beta)-D-glucosaminidase (NAG)[a]	18.9 ± 14.3	19.3 ± 8.8	0.5–36	9.8–33.8
Urine Electrolytes				
Sodium (mEq/L)[a]	62.6 ± 24.8	19.2 ± 6.0	20.2–90.7	9.4–24.3
Potassium (mEq/L)[a]	77.8 ± 27.8	238.3 ± 157.5	38.8–119.3	69.6–600
Chloride (mEq/L)[a]	70.5 ± 26.9	54.1 ± 20.7	24.0–100.6	29.0–89.1
Calcium (mg/dL)[a]	5.7 ± 3.1	2.6 ±1.7	1.3–9.5	0.5–4.3

(*Continued*)

TABLE B.2 (*Continued*)
Urine Chemistry Data for Young Adult Yucatan Miniature Swine (6 months)

	Yucatan[a]		Range[b]	
	Male	**Female**	**Male**	**Female**
Phosphorus (mg/dL)[a]	17.5 ± 11	19.3 ± 7.1	5.0–30.9	5.0–28.7
Magnesium (mg/dL)[a]	10.7 ± 6.8	21.3 ±15.8	1.2–20.6	8.9–58.0

[a] An *n* of 10 animals of each gender is represented. All samples were collected by cystocentesis of approx. 6-month-old animals; samples were spun, aliquoted off, frozen, then shipped to laboratory; ½ the limit of detection was used for samples reported out as < value and ≥ value reported as the value. Analytical methods are outlined below. Analysis was performed by Antech GLP, Morrisville, NC. Values are given as mean ± standard deviation.

[b] Values are smallest and largest observed values. All data from Sinclair Research Center, LLC, unless otherwise stated.

TABLE B.3
Miniswine Urinalysis Analytical Methods[a]

Test	Method	Instrument	Reagent	Units
pH	Dipstick	Bayer Clinitek 200+	Siemens	None
Specific gravity	Visual	Refractometer	NA	None
OSMO	Freezing point depression	Osmometer	NA	mOSMO
Creatinine	Modified jaffe, kinetic	Olympus 640e	Olympus	mg/dL
Glucose	Hexokinase, UV/NAD	Olympus 640e	Olympus	mg/dL
Total protein	Pyrogallol Red Dye	Olympus 640e	Olympus	mg/dL
ALP	*p*-Nitrophenyl phosphate, IFCC	Olympus 640e	Olympus	U/L
ALT	UV/NADH, IFCC	Olympus 640e	Olympus	U/L
AST	UV/NADH, IFCC	Olympus 640e	Olympus	U/L
Creatine kinase	ADP/ATP, IFCC	Olympus 640e	Olympus	U/L
GGT	Szasz	Olympus 640e	Olympus	U/L
LDH	Lactate-pyruvate, IFCC	Olympus 640e	Olympus	U/L
NAG	Enzymatic hydrolysis of 2-methyoxy-4-(2'-nitrovinyl)-phenyl 2 acetaminido-2-deoxy-β-D-glucopyranoside (MNP-GIcNAc)	Olympus 640e	Olympus	U/L
Calcium	Arsenazo	Olympus 640e	Olympus	mg/dL
I. Phosphorus	Phosphohmolybdate complex	Olympus 640e	Olympus	mg/dL
Magnesium	Xylidyl blue	Olympus 640e	Olympus	mg/dL
Sodium	ISE	Olympus 640e	Olympus	mEq/L
Potassium	ISE	Olympus 640e	Olympus	mEq/L
Chloride	ISE	Olympus 640e	Olympus	mEq/L

[a] Performed by ANTECH GLP, Morrisville, NC (Aug 2009).

APPENDIX C

Selected References: Clinical Chemistry Reference Data Sources for Laboratory Swine

Baetz, A.L. 1970. Phosphatase, phosphokinase, and transferase levels in blood and tissues of domestic animals. In *Advances in Automated Analysis*. 1969 Technicon International Congress, Vol. 3, pp. 163–167. Tarrytown, NY: Mediad Incorporated.

Brechbuler, T., Kaeslin, M., and Wyler, F. 1984. Reference values of various blood constituents in young minipigs. *J Clin Chem Clin Biochem.* 22:301–304.

Burks, M., Tumbleson, M.E., Hicklin, K.W., Hutcheson, D.P., and Middleton, C.C. 1977. Age and sex related changes of hematologic parameters in Sinclair (S-1) miniature swine. *Growth.* 41:51–62.

Chen, Y., Qin, S., Ding, Y., et al. 2011. Reference values of biochemical and hematological parameters for Guizhou minipigs. *Exp Biol Med.* 236(4):477–482.

Copland, J.W. 1975. Some normal biochemical parameters of pigs in Papua New Guinea. *Trop Anim Health Prod.* 8(1):71–81.

Drougas. J.G., Barnard S.G., Wright J.K., et al. 1996. A model for the extended studies of hepatic hemodynamics and metabolism in swine. *Lab Anim Sci.* 46(6):648–655.

Dungan, L.J., Wiest, D.B., Fyfe, D.A., Smith, A.C., and Swindle, M.M. 1995. Hematology, serology and serum protein electrophoresis in fetal miniature Yucatan swine: normal data. *Lab Anim Sci.* 45(3):285–289.

Dupont, J., Oh, S.Y., O'Deen, L., et al. 1986. Synthesis and disappearance of cholesterol and bile acids in miniature swine. In *Swine in Biomedical Research.* Ed. M.E. Tumbleson, pp. 821–838. New York, NY: Plenum Press.

Earl, F.L., Melveger, B.E., Reinwall, J.E., and Wilson, R.L. 1971. Clinical laboratory values of neonatal and weanling miniature pigs. *Lab Anim Sci.* 21:754–759.

Eisenhauer, C.L., Matsuda, L.S., and Uyehara, C.F. 1994. Normal physiologic values of neonatal pigs and the effects of isoflurane and pentobarbital anesthesia. *Lab Anim Sci.* 44:245–252.

Ellegaard, L.S., Jørgensen, K.D., Klastrup, S., Hansen, A.K., and Svendsen. O. 1995. Hematological and clinical chemistry values in 3- and 6-month-old Göttingen minipigs. *Scand J Lab Anim Sci.* 22:239–248.

Friendship, R.M., Lumsden, J.H., McMillan, I., Wilson, M.R. 1984. Hematology and biochemistry reference values for Ontario swine. *Can J Comp Med.* 48:390–393.

Gad, S.C., Dincer, Z., Skaanild, A.T. 2008. The minipig. In *Animal Models in Toxicology.* Ed. S.C. Gad, pp. 732–767. Zug: Informa Healthcare.

Hannon, J.P., Bossone, C.A., and Wade, C.E. 1990. Normal physiological values for conscious pigs used in biomedical research. *Lab Anim Sci.* 40:293–298.

Heath, M.F., Evans, R.J., Gresham, A.C. 1991. Blood biochemical reference ranges for sows under modern management conditions. *Br Vet J.* 147(4):331–339.

Horstman, V.G., Clarke, W.J., Hackett, P.L., Kerr, M.E., Pershing, R. L., and Bustad, L.K. 1960. Anatomical and physiological data in miniature swine. In *Hanford Biology Research Annual Report for 1959*, pp. 59–67. Hanford Atomic Products Operation USAEC Report HW 65500. Richland, Washington DC: Hanford Laboratories.

Hutcheson, D.P., Tumbleson, M.E., and Middleton C.C. 1979. Serum electrolyte concentrations in Sinclair (S-1) miniature swine from 1 through 36 months of age. *Growth.* 43:62–70.

Khan, M.A., Sager, A.O., Khattak, Z.R., Braunberg, R.C., Sobotka, T.J., and Travlos, G.S. 1986. Baseline biochemical and hematological parameters of neonatal miniature piglets: model for perinatal toxicology. In *Proceedings of the 13th International Congress of Nutrition* (held under the auspices of the International Union of Nutritional Science). Eds. T.G. Taylor and N.K. Jenkins, pp. 656–658. Brighton, UK, 18–23 August.

Kojima, M., Sekimoto, M., and Degawa, M. 2008. Gender-related differences in the level of serum lipids in Meishan pigs. *J Health Sci.* 54(1):97–100.

Kramer, J.W. 1989. Clinical enzymology. In *Clinical Biochemistry of Domestic Animals.* Ed. J.J. Kaneko, pp. 338–363. New York, NY: Academic Press.

Lochmiller, R.L. and Grant, W.E. 1984. Serum chemistry of the collared peccary (Tayassu tajacu). *J Wildl Dis.* 20(2):134–140.

McClellan, R.O., Vogt, C.S., and Ragan, H.A. 1966. Age-related changes in hematological and serum biochemical parameters in miniature swine. In *Swine in Biomedical Research.* Eds. L.K. Bustad, and R.O. McClellan, pp. 597–610. Seattle, WA: Frayn Printing Co.

McIntosh, G.H., and Pointon, A. 1981. The Kangaroo island strain of pig in biomedical research. *Aust Vet J.* 57:182–185.

Miller, E.R., Ullrey, D.E., Ackerman, I., Schmidt, D.A., Hoefer, J.A., and Luecke, R.W. 1961. Swine hematology from birth to maturity. I. Serum proteins. *J Anim Sci.* 20:31–35.

Odink, J., Smeets, J.F., Visser, I.J., Sandman, H., and Snijders, J.M. 1990. Hematologic and clinicochemical profiles of healthy swine and swine with inflammatory processes. *J Anim Sci.* 68:163–170.

Oldigs, B. 1986. Effects of internal factors upon hematologic and clinical chemical parameters in the Gottinger miniature pig. In *Swine in Biomedical Research.* Ed. M.E. Tumbleson, Vol. 2, pp. 809–813. New York, NY: Plenum Press.

Parsons, A.H. and Wells, R.E. 1986. Serum biochemistry of healthy Yucatan miniature pigs. *Lab Anim Sci.* 36(4):428–430.

Radin, M.J., Weiser, M.G., and Fettman. M.J. 1986. Hematologic and serum biochemical values for Yucatan miniature swine. *Lab Anim Sci.* 36:425–427.

Reese, D.E., Peo, Jr. E.R., Lewis, A.J., and Hogg, A. 1984. Serum chemical values of gestating and lactating swine: Reference values. *Am J Vet Res.* 45:978–980.

Rispat, G.M., Slaoui, M., Weber, D., Salemink, P., Berthoux, C., and Shrivastava, R. 1993. Hematological and plasma biochemical values for healthy Yucatan micropigs. *Lab Anim.* 27:368–373.

Swindle, M.M., Smith, A.C., Laber, K., Goodrich, J.A., and Bingel S.A. 2003. Biology and medicine of swine. In *Laboratory Animal Medicine and Management.* Eds. J.D. Reuter, and M.A. Suckow. Ithaca, NY: International Veterinary Information Service (www.ivis.org).

Tanaka, H., Igarashi, T., Lefor, A.T., and Kobayashi, E. 2009. The effects of fasting and general anesthesia on serum chemistries in KCG miniature pigs. *J Am Assoc Lab Anim Sci.* 48(1): 33–38.

Travlos, G.S. 1999. The laboratory pig. In *The Clinical Chemistry of Laboratory Animals.* Eds. F.W. Quimby, and W.F. Loeb, 2nd edition, Chap. 7, pp. 103–135. Philadelphia, PA: Taylor & Francis. (Appendices, p. 643).

Tumbleson, M.E., Burks, M.F., Spate, M.P., Hutcheson, D.P., and Middleton, C.C. 1970. Serum biochemical and hematological parameters of Sinclair (S-1) miniature sows during gestation and lactation. *Can J Comp Med.* 34:312–319.

Tumbleson, M.E., Donemert, A.R., and Middleton, C.C. 1968. Techniques for handling miniature swine for laboratory procedures. *Lab Anim Care.* 18:584–587.

Tumbleson, M. E., Hicklin, K.W., and Burks, M.F. 1976. Serum cholesterol, triglyceride, glucose, and total bilirubin concentrations, as functions of age and sex, in Sinclair (S-1) miniature swine. *Growth.* 40:293–300.

Tumbleson, M.E., Hutcheson, D.P., and Fogg, T.J. 1972. Serum biochemical values of fetal and neonatal crossbred swine. In *Advances in Automated Analysis. 1970 Technicon International Congress*, Volume 2, 149–156. Mt. Kisco, NY: Futura Publishing Company.

Tumbleson, M.E., Hutcheson, D.P., and Middleton, C.C. 1976. Serum protein concentrations and enzyme activities, as a function of age and sex, in Sinclair (S-1) miniature swine. *Growth.* 40:53–68.

Tumbleson, M. E. and Kalish, P. R. 1972. Serum biochemical and hematological parameters in crossbred swine from birth through eight weeks of age. *Can J Comp Med.* 36:202–209.

Tumbleson, M.E., Middleton, C.C., Tinsley, O.W., and Hutcheson, D.P. 1969. Serum biochemical and hematologic parameters of Hormel miniature swine from four to nine months of age. *Lab Animal Care.* 19:345–351.

Tumbleson, M.E. and Schmidt, D.A. 1986. Swine clinical chemistry. In *Swine in Biomedical Research.* Ed. M.E. Tumbleson, pp. 783–807. New York, NY: Plenum Press.

Verheyen, A.J.M., Maes, D.G., Mateusen, B.,et al. 2007. Serum biochemical reference values for gestating and lactating sows. *Vet J.* 174(1):92–98.

Weissinger, J., Wolf, P., and Bloor, C. 1980. Serum enzyme abnormalities in swine associated with systemic infection and fever. *Enzyme.* 25(5):342–345.

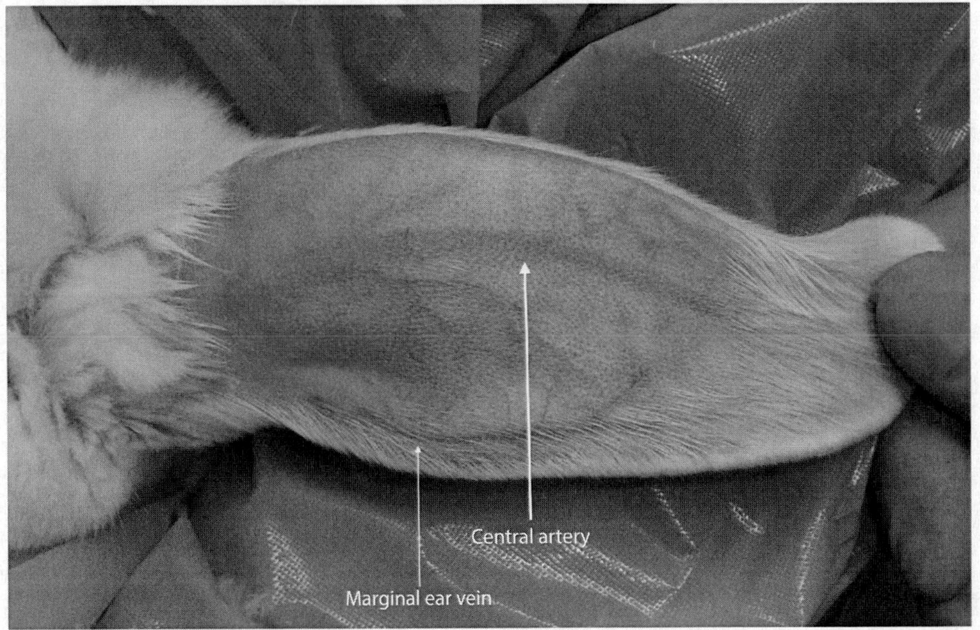

FIGURE 3.1 Marginal ear vein and central ear artery.

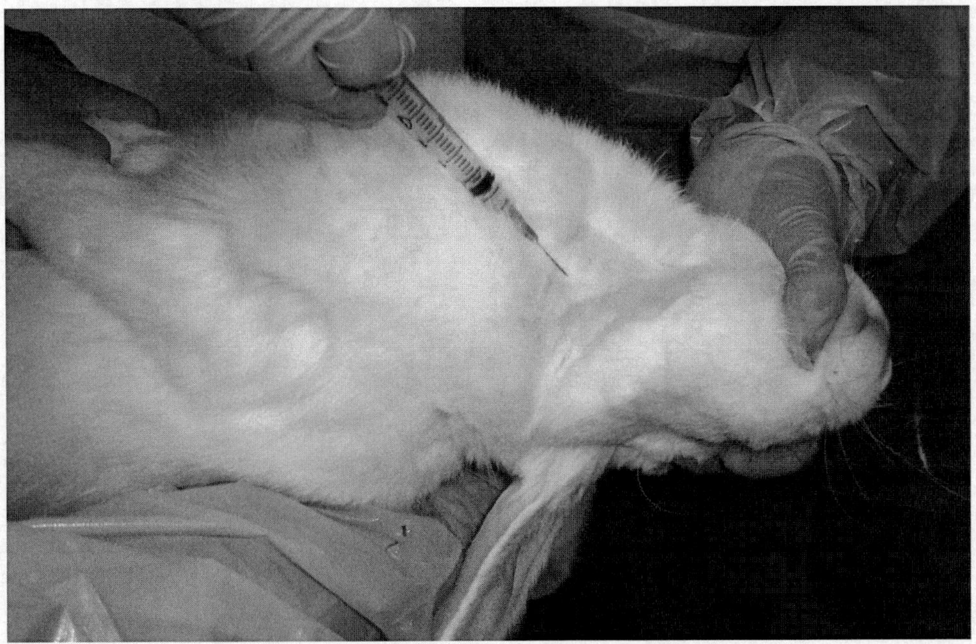

FIGURE 3.3 Manual restraint for jugular venipuncture with rabbit in dorsal recumbency.

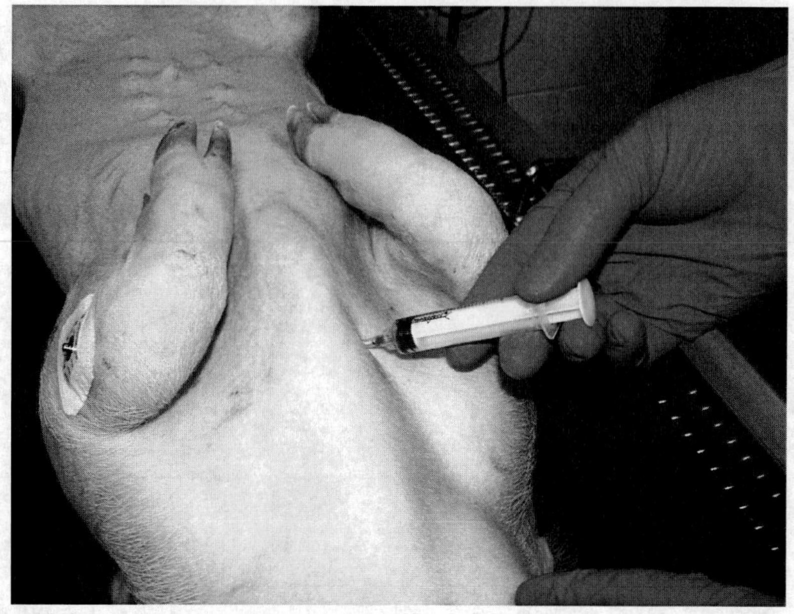

FIGURE 5.1 Cranial vena cava venipuncture.

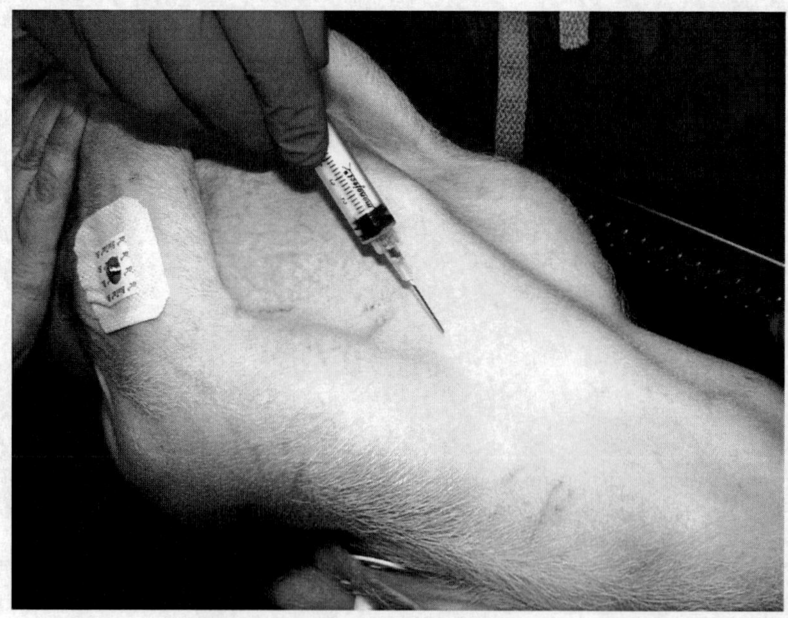

FIGURE 5.2 External jugular vein accesses.

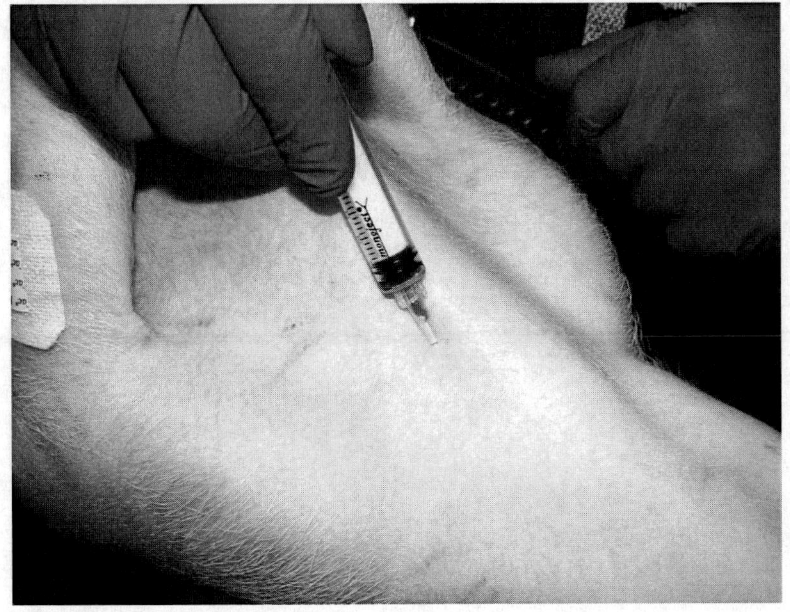

FIGURE 5.3 Internal jugular vein and carotid artery access.

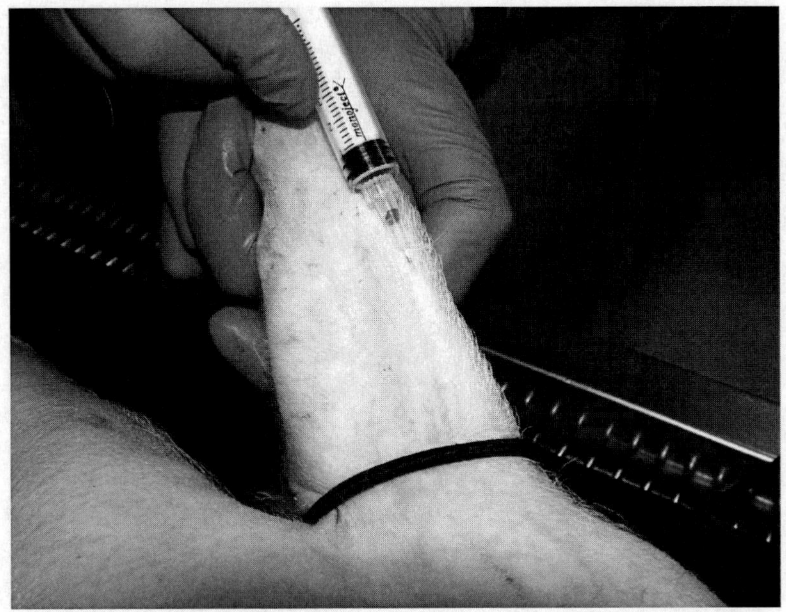

FIGURE 5.4 Cephalic vein access on the foreleg.

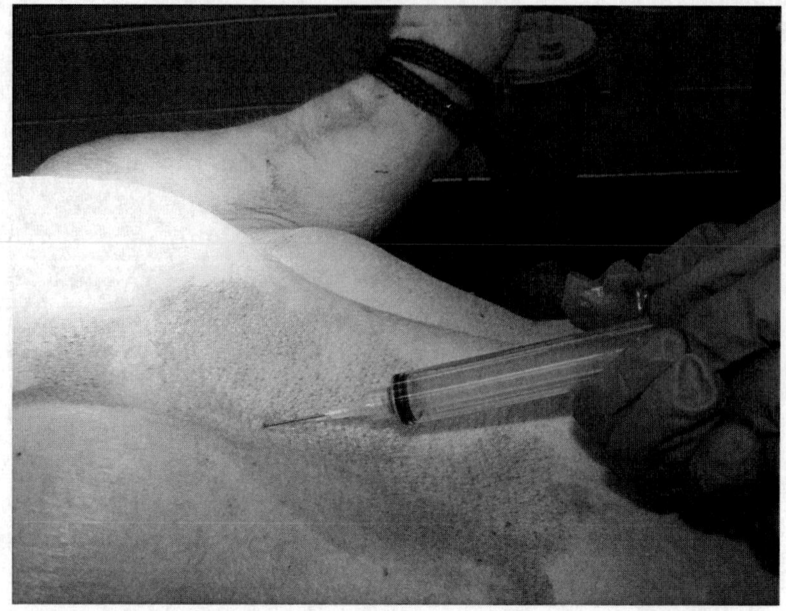

FIGURE 5.5 Cephalic vein access on the neck.

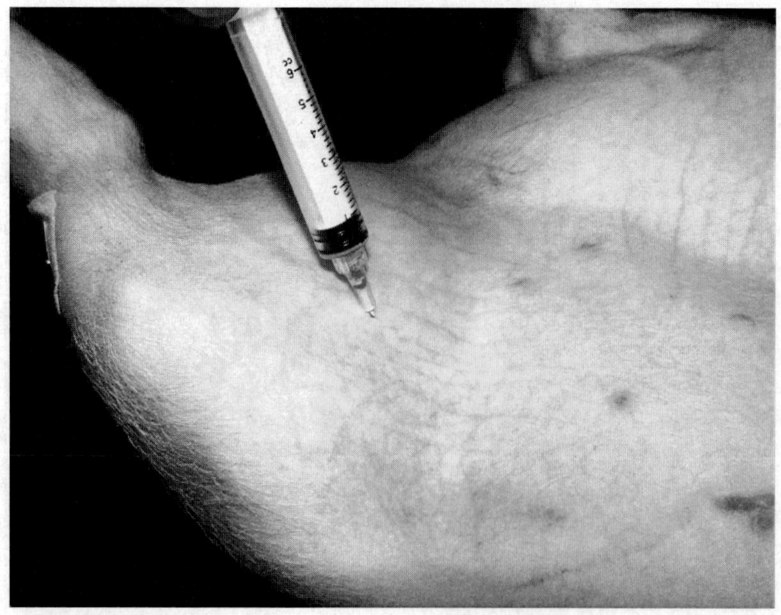

FIGURE 5.6 Femoral artery and vein access.

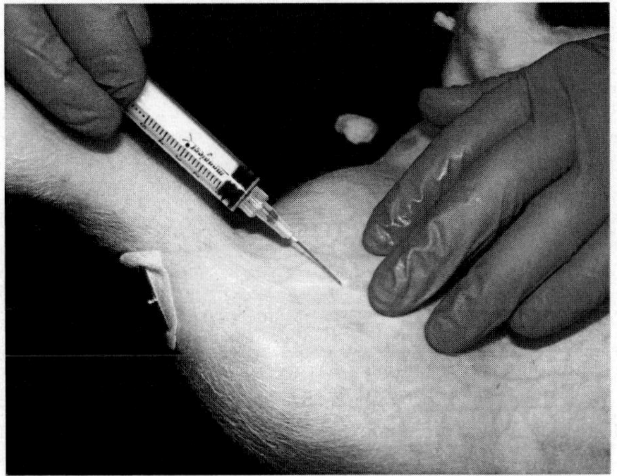

FIGURE 5.7 Medial saphenous artery access.

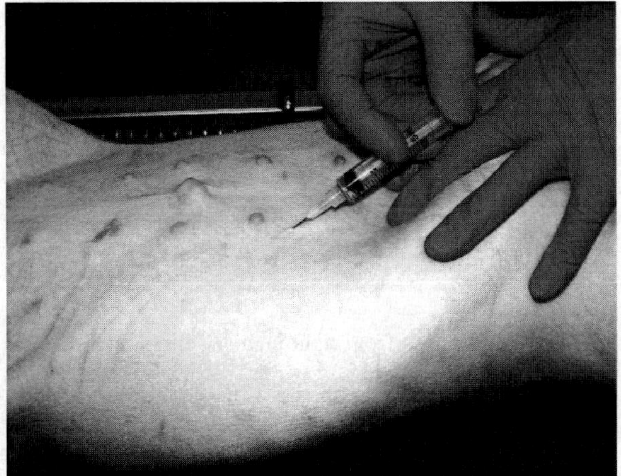

FIGURE 5.8 Cranial abdominal vein access.

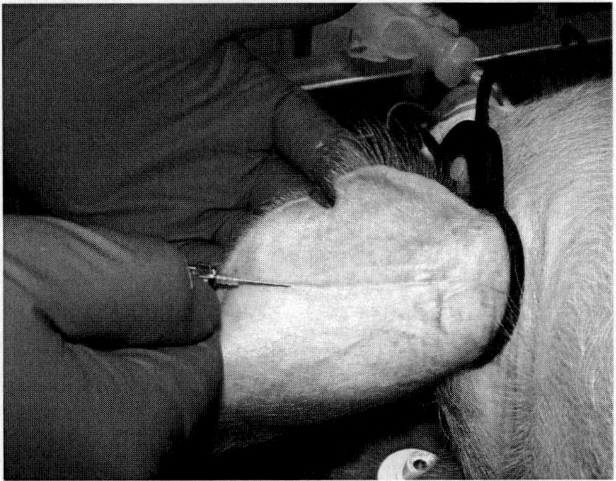

FIGURE 5.9 Ear vein access with a catheter.

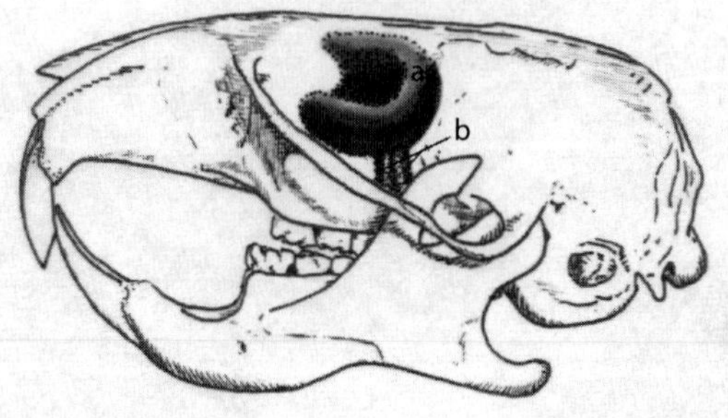

FIGURE 7.1 Hamster skull—showing location of the orbital venous sinus. Since the orbital venous sinus resides in the caudal one-half to two-thirds of the orbit, the microhematocrit tube should be inserted into the lateral canthus of the eye in a posterior and medial direction. (a) Orbital venous sinus. (b) External ophthalmic veins.

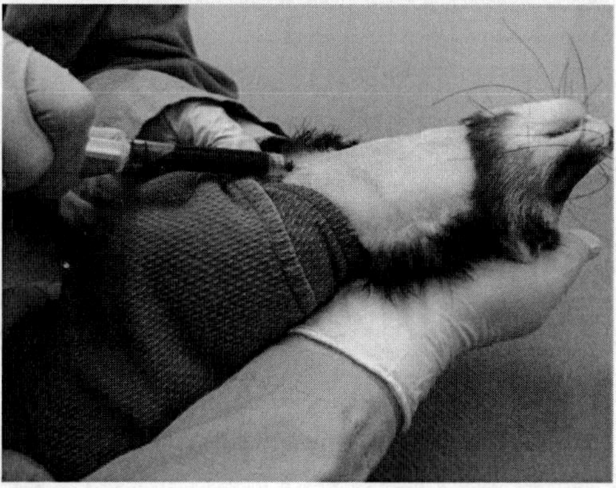

FIGURE 9.1 Restraint for blood collection from right jugular vein in an awake ferret. Clipping the hair at the venipuncture site is recommended.

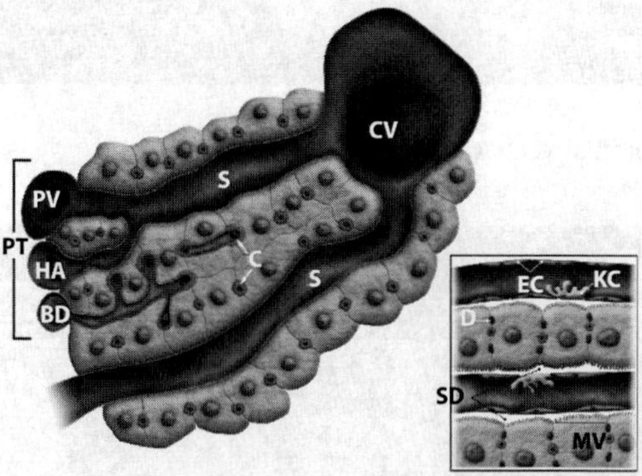

FIGURE 11.1 Schematic presentation of the liver microanatomy. Hepatic sinusoids (S) are surrounded by one to two layers of cords of hepatocytes. The portal veins (PV), hepatic arterioles (HA), and bile ductules (BD) comprise the portal triad (PT). Blood flows from the portal triad (PV and HA) through the sinusoids to the central vein (CV). Bile flows from the bile canaliculi (C) to the BD of the PT. The inset depicts a close up of the sinusoids lined by fenestrated epithelia (EC) and Kupffer cells (KC). A perisinusoidal space (aka, space of Disse [SD]) is located between the hepatocytes and sinusoids. The basolateral hepatocyte surface has microvilli (MV) that extend into the SD that allows plasma components from the sinusoids to be absorbed by the hepatocytes. Bile canaliculi are formed on the lateral surface of adjacent hepatocytes and the hepatocytes attach to their neighbors with specialized junctions (desmosome; D). Original concept by Chuck Wiedemeyer and Greg Travlos; drawing by David Sabio.

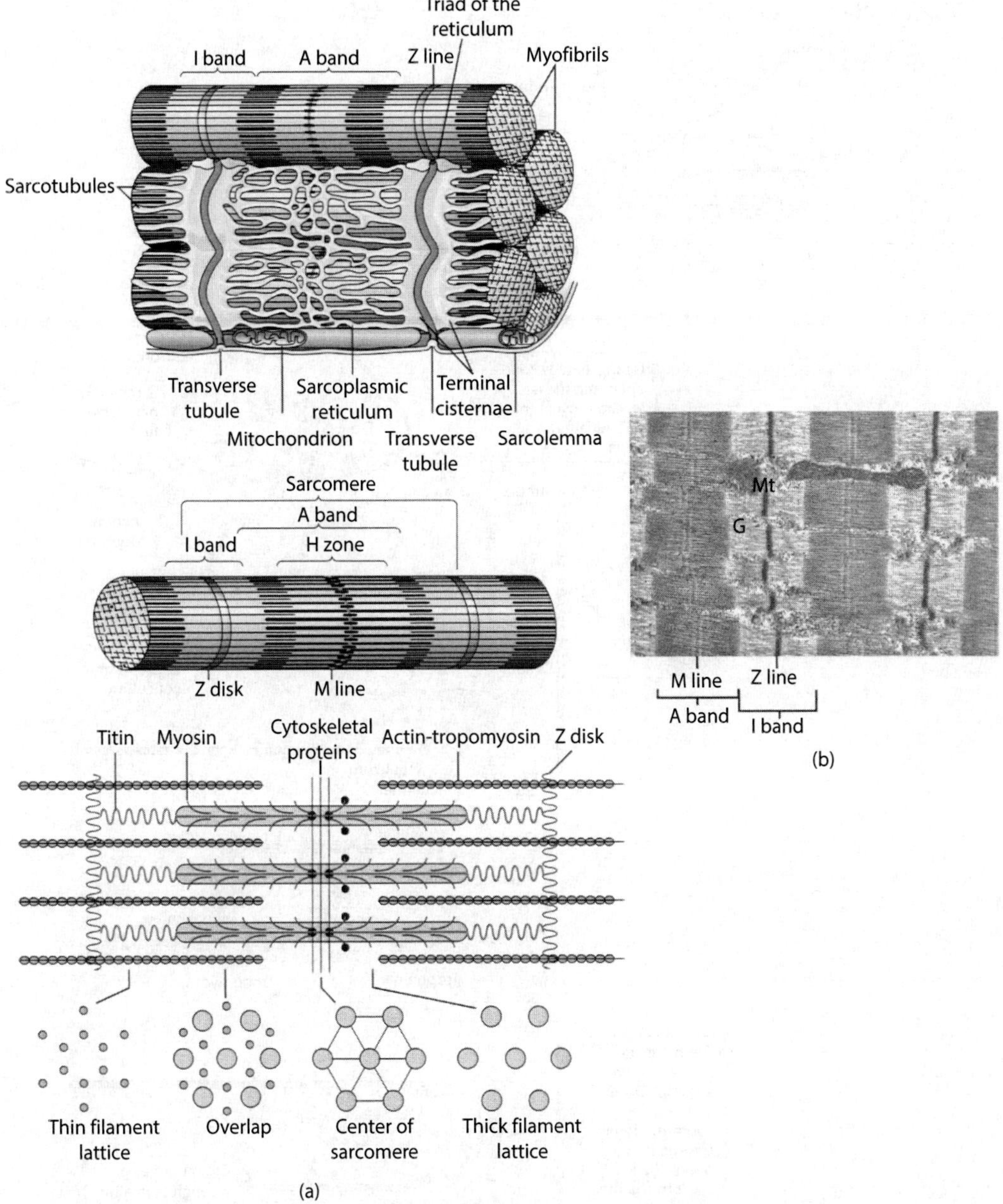

FIGURE 14.2 Myofiber structure. (a) Schematic representation of myofiber orientation, secondary organelles, and ultrastructural arrangement of cytoskeletal proteins within sarcomeres. (From Copstead-Kirhorn, L.E. and Banasik, J.L., *Pathophysiology Biological and Behavioral Perspective*, Saunders, St. Louis, 2005.) (b) Skeletal muscle, longitudinal section, normal mammalian skeletal muscle. Sarcomeres are defined by Z lines, A bands composed of thick myosin filaments, and I bands composed of thin actin filaments. Dense M lines with adjacent clear H zones occur in the center of the A band. Mitochondria (Mt) and glycogen (G) are interspersed between the myofibrils. Transmission electron microscopy (TEM). Uranyl acetate and lead citrate stain. (Courtesy of Dr. BA Valentine, College of Veterinary Medicine, Oregon State University). (Reprinted from *Pathologic Basis of Veterinary Disease*, 4th edition, McGavin, M.D. and Zachary, J.F, 976, Copyright (2007), with permission from Mosby Elsevier.)

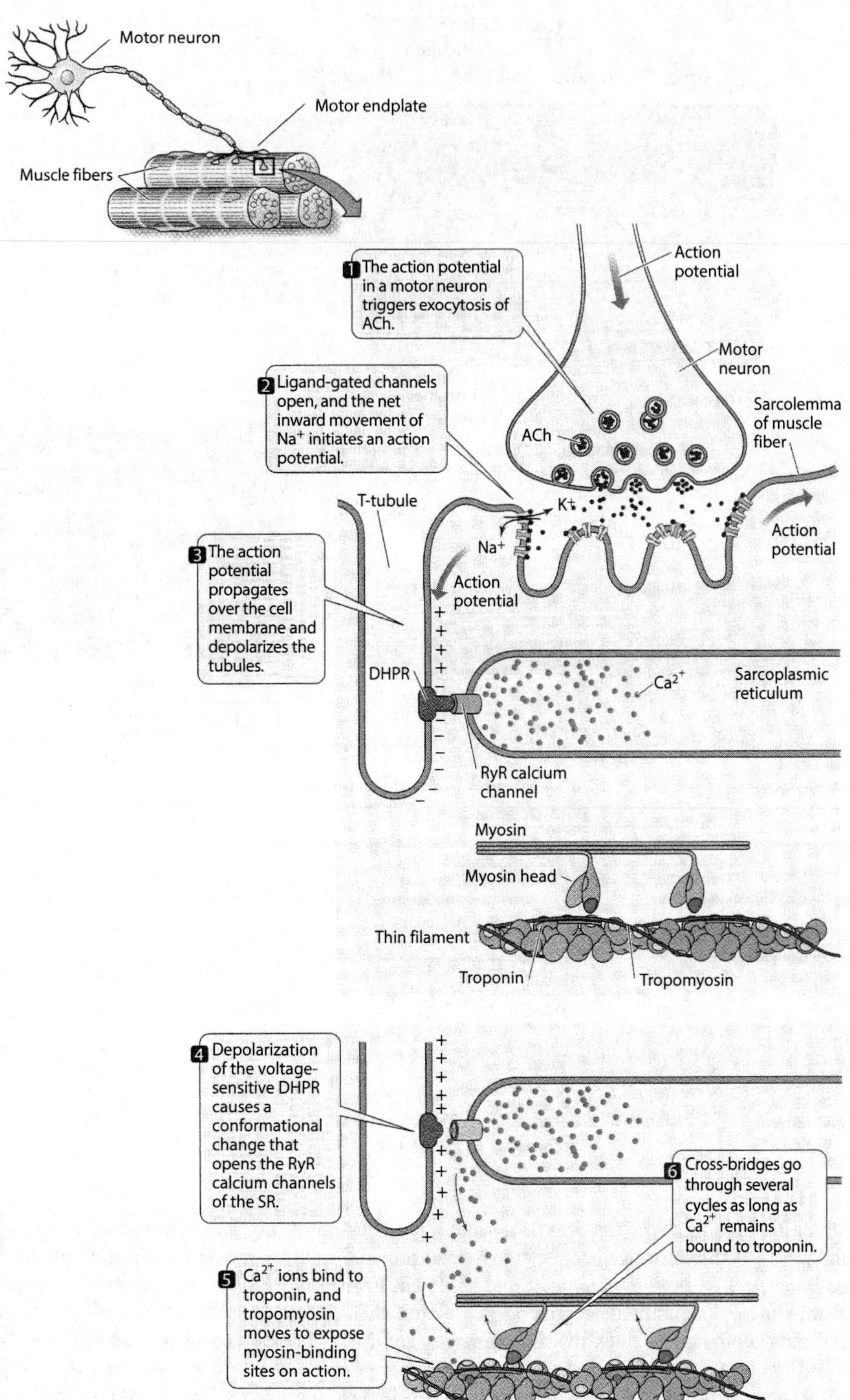

FIGURE 14.4 Excitation–contraction coupling is accomplished by the interactions of components in two intimately associated membrane systems: the transverse tubular system and the sarcoplasmic reticulum. (After Silverthorn, D.U., *Human Physiology: An Integrated Approach*, Pearson/Benjamin Cummings, San Francisco, 2004; Reprinted from Hill, R.W. et al., *Animal Physiology* Sinauer Associates, Sunderland, 2004, 471. With permission.)

6 The Nonhuman Primate

Kirstin F. Barnhart

CONTENTS

6.1 TAXONOMY

Nonhuman primates (NHPs) belong to the order Primata, which is composed of three suborders: (1) Prosimii, considered as pre-primates, is rarely used in research; (2) Anthropoidea, which contains the true primates, is divided into two infraorders: the Platyrrhine or New World (NW) monkeys and the Catarrhine, consisting of Old World (OW) monkeys, apes, and humans; and (3) Tarsioidea, a newly recognized order, represents the bridge between pre-primates and true primates. NW monkeys are found in Central and South America and consist of two families: (1) Callitrichidae, which include marmosets and tamarins, and (2) Cebidae, which include owl and squirrel monkeys (Fortman et al., 2002). Although many Prosimian NHPs are nocturnal, owl monkeys are the only nocturnal species of simian NHPs and the only nocturnal NHP that is commonly used in research. OW monkeys and apes originate from Africa and Asia. Of all the apes, only the chimpanzee has played a prominent role in biomedical research; however, in recent years, the use of the chimpanzee has decreased substantially due to the high costs associated with housing and ethical considerations.

6.2 UNIQUE PHYSIOLOGICAL CHARACTERISTICS AND USE IN BIOMEDICAL RESEARCH

The most widely used NHP species in biomedical research are the OW monkeys that belong to the Cercopithecinae subfamily: the cynomolgus monkey (*Macaca fascicularis*), the rhesus monkey (*Macaca mulatta*), and the baboon (*Papio* spp.). Macaques are robust, sexually dimorphic animals with a large geographic distribution. Rhesus monkeys are the larger of the two macaque species with adult females typically weighing from 4 to 9 kg and adult males from 6 to 11 kg. Cynomolgus monkeys are smaller; adult males and females typically weigh 4–8 kg and 2–6 kg, respectively (Fortman et al., 2002).

Both the rhesus monkey and the cynomolgus monkey play important roles in biomedical research, vaccine studies, and pharmaceutical development. The majority of preclinical safety studies that require NHPs are conducted in one of these two species. Cynomolgus monkeys are the most widely used macaque in pharmaceutical studies due to several important advantages over rhesus monkeys; they are less aggressive, cheaper, and smaller so they can be housed more efficiently and require less test article for preclinical safety assessment. Both the rhesus and cynomolgus monkeys have factored heavily in neuroscience studies, particularly those involving aging and behavior.

Rhesus monkeys are a highly relevant and well-characterized model for studying human obesity and associated comorbidities, particularly type II diabetes mellitus (Hansen and Bodkin, 1986; Bodkin et al., 1989, 1993a; Hotta et al., 2001). Numerous reports have documented the importance of this model to human medicine (Bodkin et al., 1993b, 2000). More recently, the cynomolgus monkey (Wagner et al., 2001) and baboons (Chavez et al., 2008, 2009) have also been developed as models for obesity and type II diabetes. Similar to humans, the incidence of type II diabetes in each of these three species is associated with increasing age and body weight (Hotta et al., 2001; Hansen and Bodkin, 1993; Wagner et al., 1996; Chavez et al., 2009). The pathogenesis of type II diabetes in NHPs parallels that of the human disease. The initial phase, which includes normal glucose tolerance and insulin resistance with compensatory hyperinsulinemia, is followed by continued alterations in carbohydrate metabolism (Wagner et al., 2001; Bodkin, 2000).

For over 20 years, the rhesus monkey has served as an important model for human immunodeficiency virus (HIV) research. Although chimpanzees are susceptible to infection with HIV-1, they have functioned primarily as an apathogenic model (Juompan et al., 2008). Following exposure to human-adapted variants, the vast majority of chimpanzees control infection and are relatively resistant to developing acquired immunodeficiency syndrome (AIDS) because they avoid the immunopathologic events that affect the function of lymphoid tissues (Rutjens et al., 2010; Henney et al., 2006). In contrast, rhesus macaques infected with certain strains of SIV (e.g., SIVmac) or the chimeric SIV/HIV virus termed simian hybrid immunodeficiency virus (SHIV) recapitulate many of the pathologic events that occur in human AIDS (Baroncelli et al., 2008).

Baboons are a sexually dimorphic and relatively large NHP. Adult males and females weigh approximately 22–30 kg and 11–15 kg, respectively. *Papio anubis* (olive baboon) and *Papio cynocephalus* (yellow baboon) are the most common species used in biomedical research (Fortman et al., 2002). Given their size and robust nature, these Cercopithecine primates are amenable to multiple blood collections and a relatively large amount of blood product can be obtained for diagnostic and experimental purposes.

The baboon has also served as an important model for researching human disease, particularly in the areas of obesity, reproduction, surgery, and vascular research. Reproductively, the baboon shares many anatomic and physiologic features with humans (Nyachieo et al., 2007). They have similar placentation, particularly in the initial stages and can serve as a model for studying transplacental transport (Carter, 2007; Van Calsteren et al., 2009). Endometrial function, including uterine receptivity and embryo implantation, is also similar, and studies have shown that fetal loss and maternal risk factors associated with stillbirths in baboons were similar to those in women.

Baboons have also served as effective large animal models for certain areas of cardiac and vascular research. Baboons develop atherosclerosis both naturally and experimentally and are the most relevant model for investigating the effect of circulating risk factors on endothelial dysfunction and arterial wall susceptibility to vascular disease (Wang et al., 2004). In cardiac xenotransplantation, the orthotopic pig-to-baboon model is the accepted preclinical model (Brandl et al., 2005). Following lipopolysaccharide administration, the kinetics of cytokine release, hemodynamic changes, and hematologic alterations are similar to humans; consequently, the baboon can function as a model for trauma, shock, and sepsis studies (Redl and Bahrami, 2005).

The African green monkey (*Cercopithecus aethiops*) is another member of the Cercopithecinae subfamily that has also been referred to as a vervet monkey or a grivet. Recently, the African green monkey is being explored in pharmaceutical research as an alternative to macaques, which have practical limitations that include relatively high cost and short supply. (Ward et al., 2008). Recent reports by Ward et al. (2008, 2009) concluded that the African green monkey may be an appropriate NHP for modeling both oral and intravenous pharmacokinetics and drug–drug interactions. African green monkeys have fulfilled other important roles in vaccine development biomedical research. They are frequently used as a model for presymptomatic Parkinson's disease and have been utilized in developing vaccines for plague and respiratory syncytial virus (Sato, 2008; Patterson and Carrion, 2005; Pessiglione et al., 2003).

Chimpanzees (*Pan troglodytes*) are the only Great Apes that have played an important role in biomedical research. They have had limited but very important roles in vaccine and small molecule development for hepatitis C virus (HCV), behavioral and evolutionary studies, and certain safety and efficacy studies of therapeutics such as monoclonal antibodies that require a high degree of homology with humans. To date, the chimpanzee is the only established model of HCV infection that is susceptible to viral infection (Brass et al., 2007). Historically, chimpanzees were crucial to the successful development of a vaccine for Hepatitis B virus (HBV) in humans, and critical work with chimpanzees is ongoing to develop a vaccine against antiviral drug-resistant HBV mutants (Prince and Brotman, 2001; Kamili et al., 2009).

The most commonly used NW monkeys in biomedical research include three members of the family Callitrichidae: common marmoset (*Callithrix jacchus*), cotton-top tamarin (*Sanguinus oedipus*), and the moustached tamarin (*Sanguinus mystax*); and two members of the family Cebidae: the owl monkey (*Aotus trivirgatus*) and the squirrel monkey (*Saimiri* spp.) (Fortman et al., 2002). In general, NW monkeys provide practical, economic primate models for institutions lacking the space and/or resources to house larger primates.

Although not widely used, marmosets have been used in pharmaceutical research due to several beneficial qualities that include decreased test article dosages, smaller housing requirements due to its small size, reduced biohazardous risks as compared to macaques, and the ease of reproduction in captivity. Despite these benefits, the inability to obtain large blood volumes and the lack of assays validated specifically for marmosets can pose substantial disadvantages (Zuhlke and Weinbauer, 2003). Additionally, captive-bred marmosets develop a frequently fatal disease termed Wasting Marmoset Syndrome (WMS) that has limited their usefulness in toxicology studies. WMS is generally considered a type of inflammatory bowel disease with many potential causes including viral diseases, nutritional imbalances, and nematodes. To date, the exact cause of WMS remains unknown (Sousa et al., 2008; Gore et al., 2001).

The common marmoset has been used extensively in infectious disease research and is probably the most widely used NW monkey in drug development and preclinical studies. Marmosets are highly susceptible to herpes simplex virus-1 encephalitis and have been used to model hepatitis A virus, malaria and measles (Blagbrough and Zara, 2009; Mansfield, 2003). Marmosets can be infected with GB virus B (GBV-B) and thus, serve as a surrogate model for studying HCV infection. GBV-B is a flavivirus similar to HCV that shares similar mechanisms for processing viral gene products. Both viruses result in persistent infections in their respective host, and infected marmosets develop similar hepatic pathology to humans infected with HCV (Jacob et al., 2004; Weatherford et al., 2009; Mansfield, 2003).

Marmosets have also been used widely in neurologic research, particularly in the areas of Parkinson's disease and multiple sclerosis. Several mechanisms for recapitulating the pathogenesis and clinical outcome of Parkinson's disease have been established in the marmoset in part because of the diversity of behavioral assessments available for this species as well as its suitability for stereotaxic surgery (Eslamboli, 2005). Infectious allergic encephalitis in marmosets following immunization with myelin or myelin proteins creates an inflammatory demyelinating disease similar to multiple sclerosis. Another unique characteristic of marmosets is that they give birth to twin or triplet siblings that are full bone marrow chimeras. This feature allows for transfer of functional T-cell populations ('t Hart et al., 2000; Massacesi et al., 1995).

Although the natural host is still unknown, the GB viruses (GBV-A and GBV-B) were originally identified and cloned from pooled tamarin sera that were obtained from experimentally inoculated animals (Simons et al., 1995). Like the marmoset, GBV-B-infected tamarins have served as a surrogate model for HCV research. Cotton-top tamarins routinely live for greater than 20 years in captivity and naturally deposit AB amyloid into plaques and blood vessels in the brain; consequently, they may represent a model for the pathogenesis of early Alzheimer's disease (Lemere et al., 2008).

Additionally, cotton-top tamarins spontaneously develop colitis in captivity and the wild. In chronic cases, the colitis may progress to colorectal cancer. These findings have allowed the tamarin to become a resource for investigating therapeutics directed at key mediators of colonic inflammation (Tobi et al., 2000; Watkins et al., 1997).

The owl monkey is an unusual NW monkey in that it is nocturnal and displays no sexual dimorphism. The most important characteristic of the owl monkey that has led to its establishment as a laboratory primate is its susceptibility to *Plasmodium falciparum* and *Plasmodium vivax*. The World Health Organization has recommended this species as a model for evaluating malaria vaccines (Nino-Vasquez et al., 2000). Similar to the marmoset, the owl monkey is highly susceptible to herpes simplex virus-1 encephalitis and has served as one of the standard NHP models for this infection (Blagbrough and Zara, 2009). In addition, it is a useful model for studying hepatitis A (Purcell and Emerson, 2001).

Similar to the owl monkey, several malarial strains have been adapted to squirrel monkeys, and this species has become an alternative malarial model that accurately recapitulates most of the clinical pathologic changes of human malaria (Contamin et al., 2000). Until recently, an animal model demonstrating BK virus had not been described. BK virus is a polyomavirus that causes several clinical syndromes including interstitial nephritis and cystitis in immunosuppressed humans, particularly transplant patients. Zaragoza et al. (2005) demonstrated that squirrel monkeys could be successfully infected with BK virus and potentially used as a model for testing antiviral agents intended for human use. Squirrel monkeys also contribute to studies on Alzheimer's disease. Aging squirrel monkeys naturally develop senile plaques and cerebral amyloid angiopathy, which may exacerbate the dementia associated with this disease (Elfenbein et al., 2007).

6.3 METHODOLOGY FOR SAMPLE COLLECTION

6.3.1 Blood Collection

Blood from NHPs can be collected from a number of venipuncture sites depending on the size of the animal, the method of restraint, and the sample volume required. Depending on the species, animals are restrained manually, chemically, or physically with squeeze cages or chairs. Some animals, particularly chimpanzees and macaques, may be trained to extend an arm from the cage for venipuncture (Coleman, 2008). The most common site for the collection of large blood volumes is the femoral vein. The cephalic vein of the forearm, the saphenous vein on the caudal aspect of the hind limb, the coccygeal vein of the tail, and the jugular vein can also be used. For small samples, a sterile lancet may be used to puncture the marginal ear vein, a finger or a heel. The preferred methods for blood collection from commonly used NHPs are provided in Table 6.1. The average circulating blood volume of rhesus macaques, cynomolgus macaques, and marmosets has been estimated as 56, 65, and 70 mL/kg, respectively. Guidelines for the maximum amount of blood that can be taken in a single sample or multiple samplings have been established. Up to 15% of the animal's blood volume typically can be removed in a single collection without causing significant disturbance to the animal's normal physiology. The recovery period for single samplings ranging from 7.5% to 15% of total blood volume is 1 and 4 weeks, respectively. A higher blood volume (20%) can be collected in a 24-hour period through multiple samplings for toxico- or pharmacokinetic studies (Diehl et al., 2001). Individuals are recommended to check with their Institutional Animal Care and Use Committee (IACUC) or Ethics Committee for specific guidelines or limits on blood volume collection.

6.3.2 Urine Collection

Urine collection in the NHP can be performed using methods similar to other species. NHPs can be trained to urinate into pans or other collection devices. Sterile collection via catheterization or cyctocentesis should be performed in sedated or anesthetized animals (Wolf and White, 2012).

TABLE 6.1
Blood Collection Sites

Species	Site	Needle Gauge	Reference
Marmoset	Femoral vein	25–26, 23–27	Hearn (1987) Fortman et al. (2002)
Squirrel monkey	Femoral vein	21–23	Bernacky et al. (2002)
	Femoral vein (large samples > 0.25 mL) Lateral tail veins (large samples > 0.25 mL) Saphenous veins (small samples)	23–27	Brady (2000)
Owl monkey	Femoral vein[a]	23–27	Baer (1994)
Macaques	Femoral vein[a]	20–23 (if greater than 3 kg)	Fortman et al. (2002) Dysko and Hoskins (1995)
Baboons	Femoral vein[a]	20–23 (if greater than 3 kg)	Fortman et al. (2002)
Chimpanzees	Femoral vein Antecubital vein Saphenous veins	18–22	Hanley (2009)

[a] Alternative sites include cephalic, saphenous, tail, and jugular veins.

6.4 PREANALYTICAL SOURCES OF VARIATION

Given the complex taxonomy and longevity of NHPs, many sources of preanalytical variability exist that can have a significant impact on the results of biochemical analyses. These include sex, age, breed/strain/geographical origin, nutritional status, time in captivity, husbandry practices, stress, anesthesia, menstruation, and pregnancy. Consideration should be given to the potential effects of these variables when interpreting bioanalytical data.

6.4.1 Sex

Sex has a wide range of effects on biochemical analytes in all NHP species used in biomedical research. Ideally, sex-specific reference intervals should be utilized when interpreting biochemical data. For example, in a study of 80 male and 60 female African green monkeys, males had significantly higher levels of total bilirubin, direct bilirubin, creatinine, glucose, phosphorus, calcium total CO_2, and potassium (Sato et al., 2005). A second study by Liddie et al. (2010) that determined chemistry values for 331 African green monkeys also showed significant elevations for total bilirubin and creatinine in male monkeys; while females had significantly higher alkaline phosphatase (ALP), aspartate aminotransferase (AST), cholesterol, blood urea nitrogen (BUN), triglycerides, and creatine kinase (CK). Although some of the same sex-based trends identified for African green monkeys were also seen in cynomolgus monkeys, for certain analytes, the opposite trend was reported. Creatinine, albumin, gamma glutamyl transferase (GGT), CK, amylase calcium, phosphorus, and sodium were significantly higher in males, while globulin total bilirubin, triglycerides, and chloride were significantly higher in females (Schuurman and Smith, 2005). Sodium, uric acid, AST, and CK are reportedly higher in male chimpanzees than females (Howell et al., 2003). Male baboons greater than 5 years of age had increased creatinine levels as compared to females of similar age due to their larger muscle mass (Harewood et al., 1999). Additionally, male rhesus monkeys demonstrated that serum ALP activity is approximately 1/3 times higher than females. Beland et al. (1979) reported higher serum ALP values in female squirrel monkeys (*Saimiri sciureus*) than in males.

The effect of sex on bone markers was studied in Mauritian cynomolgus monkeys. Important markers of bone formation, osteocalcin (OC), bone-specific alkaline phosphatase (BALP), and carboxy-terminal propeptide of type I procollagen (PICP) were statistically higher in young males than young females. Several markers of bone resorption including free deoxypyridinoline (DPD), urinary carboxyterminal pyridinoline cross-linked telopeptide of type I collagen (CTX-1), and serum CTX-1 were also statistically higher in young males as compared to females. No significant differences were noted between males and females for urinary pyridiniums, urinary N-telopeptide (NTX-1), and pyridinoline cross-linked carboxyterminal telopeptide of type I collagen (ICTP) (Chen et al., 2000).

6.4.2 Age

Significant changes in the level of many biochemical analytes occur throughout neonatal development. Hseih et al. (2008) reported significant changes in 11/23 analytes in neonatal baboons from 6 to 12 weeks postpartum. Serum cortisol levels are reportedly lower in infant and juvenile squirrel monkeys than in adults (Kaack et al., 1979a). Neonatal physiological hyperbilirubinemia, comparable to that in human infants, has been described in newborn rhesus monkeys.

BUN and/or creatinine increased in aged cynomolgus and rhesus monkeys (Kapeghian et al., 1984; Smucny et al., 2001). Decreased albumin, calcium, and total protein, and increased globulin and triglycerides have also been described as an effect of aging in rhesus monkeys (Smucny et al., 2001, 2004; Nakamura et al., 1998). Biologically significant changes in clinical chemistry parameters occurred in both male and female chimpanzees from middle to old age. BUN, creatinine, sodium, potassium, and globulin increased while phosphorus, chloride, and albumin decreased (Videan et al., 2008).

C-reactive protein (CRP) is an acute phase reactant that has been used extensively in human medicine as a marker of acute inflammation. Male and female chimpanzees younger than 3 years of age had mean CRP levels of 0.65 and 0.60, respectively. Males and females 7 years or older had mean CRP levels of 0.86 and 1.08, respectively (Lamperez et al., 2005).

Young growing animals have high serum BALP activity, proportional to their growth rates, and total serum ALP has been shown to decline throughout life in male rhesus monkeys (Perretta et al., 1991; Lane et al., 1999). In baboons, a drop in ALP gives clear indication of the completion of skeletal maturation in both males and females (Harewood, 1999). This trend has been reported in many other NHP species (Sato, 2005; Kapeghian et al., 1984; Beland et al., 1979). Lane et al. (1999) attributed the decrease in total ALP in rhesus monkeys to a lower percentage of BALP. Juvenile animals had approximately 91% BALP and 9% liver-specific ALP; whereas, adult animals dropped to 88% and 12% and old animals dropped to 85% and 15% of bone-specific and liver-specific ALP, respectively.

Bone turnover is elevated during growth and development as evidenced by increased levels of serum OC and ICTP in female rhesus monkeys (Colman et al., 1999). The osteopenic, ovariectomized, aged cynomolgus monkey has been established as a model for human osteoporosis. Legrand et al. (2003) demonstrated that three major markers of bone formation (ALP, OC, and PICP) and a single marker of bone resorption, NTX-1, were statistically higher in young female cynomolgus monkeys as compared to mature females. An additional study in female cynomolgus monkeys showed that procollagen type 1 *N*-terminal propeptide decreases with age while PICP does not change and tartrate resistant acid phosphatase (TrACP) fluxuates throughout the entire lifespan (Chen et al., 2000).

Sato et al. (2005) reported that yearling and juvenile African green monkeys have elevated calcium levels that generally normalize at the time of skeletal maturity and phosphorus values that steadily decline through the yearling and juvenile stages. In chimpanzees and baboons as well as African green monkeys, serum creatinine levels have been positively correlated with body weight, and creatinine fluxuations that can occur during the growth phase are generally absent once growth is stabilized (Eder 1996; Sato 2005; Harewood et al., 1999). Phosphorus values decreased from yearlings to juveniles in African green monkeys (Sato, 2005). Although these age-related trends in calcium phosphorus and creatinine were described for three NHP species, similar trends are commonly noted in other NHPs.

Age can have a significant effect on blood gas values. In aged squirrel monkeys, PaO_2, pH, TCO_2, base excess, and HCO_3 were significantly decreased as compared to young monkeys (Brizzee et al., 1988).

Although it is often assumed that glucose regulation becomes progressively impaired with age, a study in nondiabetic rhesus monkeys showed that fasting plasma glucose, the mean level of fasting insulin, glucose and insulin levels 2 hours following an oral glucose tolerance test (OGTT), and the area under the curve for insulin do not change significantly with age. This trend is not seen for diabetic animals, which show significant decreases in glucose tolerance by middle age (Tigno et al., 2004).

Age-related decreases in the basal levels of several steroid hormones, dehydroepiandrosterone, dehydroepiandrosterone sulfate, pregnenolone, and 17-hydroxy-pregnenolone were identified in male baboons. These decreases occur similarly in man and may be caused by decreased adrenal cortical cell capacity (Goncharova and Lapin, 2000). Consistent with observations in man and rat, serum cholesterol and triglycerides levels increase with age in adult rhesus monkeys (Szymanski and Kritchevsky, 1980).

6.4.3 Strain/Breed

Biologically relevant differences in blood and urine analyte between various strains and species of monkeys highlight the importance of interpreting reference ranges from animals of different origin with caution. The geographical origin or strain of a particular NHP species can have significant effects on serum biochemistry. Notable differences exist in cynomolgus monkeys that originate from Mauritius as compared to those from Southeast Asia (China, Vietnam, and Philippines). These differences are likely related to the isolated geography and lower degree of genetic variability in monkeys of Mauritian origin (Leuchte et al., 2004). As compared to monkeys of Southeast Asian origin, Mauritian monkeys have approximately 20%–40% higher serum enzyme activity of glutamate dehydrogenase (GDH), alanine aminotransferase (ALT), ALP, and GGT, approximately 25% higher total bilirubin, lower serum high-density lipoprotein (HDL) cholesterol and higher free fatty acid levels, and approximately 40% lower CRP (Zuehlke et al., 2006). Minor differences include slightly lower creatinine levels and slightly higher phosphorus levels in Chinese, Vietnamese, and Philippine monkeys (Zuehlke et al., 2006; Drevon-Gaillot et al., 2006).

Several genetic markers have shown that rhesus monkeys originating from India are divergent from those from Mainland China. A study by Champoux et al. (1996) showed that total protein was higher in Chinese–Indian hybrid rhesus monkey infants from age 14 to 150 days of age as compared to Indian derived. In addition, GGT activity was notably higher in the Chinese–Indian hybrid monkeys from days 90 to 150.

Weller et al. (1996) measured many of the same urine and serum analytes from one squirrel monkey species, *Saimiri peruviensis*, and one owl monkey species, *Aotus nancymae*. Despite the fact that squirrel and owl monkeys share similar characteristics in geographical origin, distribution, and body weight, a majority of the analytes demonstrated significant differences between the two species. Only serum calcium, creatinine, and phosphorus, and urine sodium, potassium clearance, glucose clearance, and the fractional excretion of sodium were comparable. Additionally, blood and urine analytes were compared between two species of owl monkeys, *A. nancymae and Aotus vociferans*. While the majority of the parameters were similar between the two owl monkey species, significant differences still existed. Serum calcium, phosphorus, sodium, potassium, and BUN were significantly higher in *A. nancymae* while urine calcium, calcium clearance, and fractional excretion of calcium were higher in *A. vociferans* (Weller et al., 1993a).

Amylase activity in the tissues and serum of several species of NHPs has been described by McGeachin and Akin (1982). Rhesus monkeys, squirrel monkeys, and Great Apes all demonstrated high levels of amylase activity in the pancreas, whereas only rhesus monkeys and Great Apes had high amylase activity in the parotid salivary gland. Both the parotid and salivary glands from squirrel monkeys reportedly contain very low levels of salivary amylase. In general, OW monkeys including rhesus, cynomolgus, and African green monkeys have notably high serum amylase levels (typically 600–1200 IU/L) as compared to humans and other NHP species (Gatesman, 1992; Altshuler and Stowell, 1972). Serum amylase values from Great Apes are similar to humans. In a study that determined reference ranges for six species of apparently healthy marmosets, serum amylase values were shown to be elevated as compared to humans and Great Apes but significantly lower than macaques and African green monkeys. Normal serum amylase values for several species of baboons were similar to marmosets (Gatesman, 1992). Increased adrenalin has been associated with elevated amylase, and the effects of stress due to handling and restraint may contribute to some degree to the elevated amylase in NHPs as compared to humans.

Bahr et al. (2000) compared the metabolism and excretion of cortisol among the common marmoset, cynomolgus monkeys, and chimpanzees through quantitation of urinary and fecal cortisol. In all three species, cortisol metabolites (>80%) were excreted predominantly in the urine; however, native cortisol was the major urinary excretory product only in the marmoset. Relatively small amounts of cortisol were found in the urine from chimpanzees and cynomolgus monkeys. A small amount of native cortisol was detected in marmoset feces, but cortisol was virtually absent from the other two species.

Phenotype was shown to have an effect on blood gas parameters in normal Colombian and Bolivian squirrel monkeys. The $PaCO_2$, CO_2, HCO_3, and base excess were all significantly lower in Colombian monkeys as compared to Bolivian (Brizzee et al., 1988).

Creatine kinase activity in owl monkeys was similar to cynomolgus monkeys, lower than red-bellied tamarin and the common marmoset but substantially higher than humans and most other animal species (Weller et al., 1991a).

6.4.4 Nutritional Status

6.4.4.1 Dietary Protein

The amount and type of protein in the diet may affect biochemical parameters. In African green monkeys, Johnson et al. (2001) showed that ALT was elevated on a high protein diet consisting of maize and legumes. Total protein, albumin, bilirubin, and glucose were significantly elevated on a high protein diet consisting of milk solids. Neither diet had a significant effect on AST or GGT. The effect of a high and low-protein diet on the renal function of baboons with experimentally impaired renal function was studied by Bourgoignie et al. (1994). Animals had unilateral nephrectomy and partial infarction of the contralateral kidney, and they were fed diets containing 8% or 25% casein. Animals that fed the high protein diet had lower serum creatinine and higher serum and urine urea nitrogen. Glomerular filtration rate, as determined by inulin clearance, and creatinine clearance were substantially higher in the animals fed the high protein diet.

6.4.4.2 Bilirubin

In general, normal bilirubin metabolism in NHPs strongly resembles that of humans. In addition, the genetic syndrome of fasting hyperbilirubinemia, which occurs in Bolivian and Peruvian squirrel monkeys but not in Brazilian or Guyanese squirrel monkeys, in many aspects resembles Gilbert's syndrome of benign, chronic nonhemolytic unconjugated hyperbilirubinemia in man (Cornelius and Freedland, 1992; Portman et al., 1984). The mechanism of fasting hyperbilirubinemia in affected squirrel monkey species may be attributed to two different components of bile metabolism. In Bolivian squirrel monkeys, increased bilirubin turnover/production with a twofold increase in endogenous bilirubin excretion into bile occurred following a 24-hour fast (Myers et al., 1991).

Second, a decreased hepatic conjugation potential for bilirubin developed secondary to reduced uridine diphosphate glucuronyltransferase activity (Cornelius and Freedland, 1992; Portman et al., 1984). Postprandially or following the administration of glucose, affected monkeys have concentrations of serum bilirubin comparable to those of unaffected squirrel monkeys.

Gartner et al. (1997) characterized the hepatic transport and metabolism of bilirubin in normal rhesus monkey neonates. In this study, physiologic unconjugated hyperbilirubinemia was shown to have a biphasic pattern. Phase I was characterized by a rapid increase in serum bilirubin concentration by 19 hours and an equally rapid decline by 48 hours following parturition. Phase II was characterized by a stable elevation that was approximately four times greater than normal adult levels from 48 to 96 hours after birth followed by a decline to normal adult concentrations.

6.4.4.3 Dietary Lipids

Similar to humans, the amount of dietary cholesterol can significantly alter certain serum biochemistry parameters. A study in cynomolgus monkeys showed that increased dietary cholesterol caused a marked increase in cholesterol and serum triglycerides and a marked decrease in HDL cholesterol. In addition, slight elevations in BUN, uric acid, and AST were observed (Bush, 1985). Neonatal baboon infants frequently receive formulas supplemented with dietary long-chain polyunsaturated fatty acids (LCPUFA). Although most parameters were unaffected by these supplements, triglycerides were significantly decreased at all levels of LCPUFA and calcium was significantly decreased at high levels of LCPUFA (Hseih et al., 2008).

6.4.4.4 Caloric Restriction

Rhesus monkeys that received a calorie-restricted diet had reduced blood glucose and insulin levels, improved insulin sensitivity, and decreased triglycerides and cholesterol levels (Mattison et al., 2017; Higami et al., 2005). In fasting rhesus monkeys and baboons, Goodner et al. (1977) observed periodic oscillations of insulin, glucose, and glucagon. Glucose and insulin oscillated in phase with each other and out of phase with glucagon. No similar effect has been observed in man. In rhesus monkeys, these oscillations had a periodicity of 9 minutes, and c-peptide oscillated in phase with insulin. The release of insulin and c-peptide was equimolar (Koerker et al., 1978).

Food restriction also induces a significant delay in skeletal development. Rhesus monkeys that received 30% less food per body weight had a reduced but otherwise normal skeleton, lower level of total serum ALP activity, and normal levels of parathyroid hormone (PTH), calcium, phosphorus, and OC (Lane et al., 1999).

6.4.4.5 Obesity

Female cynomolgus monkeys show similar obesity characteristics to humans. In a study of eight females, aged 6–34 years, serum insulin, leptin, glucose, and triglyceride positively correlated with body weight (Chen et al., 2002). In geriatric cynomolgus monkeys, obesity was associated with higher fasted blood sugar, acetylated hemoglobin, and triglycerides but comparable levels of cholesterol, low-density lipoprotein (LDL)/HDL, and insulin (Zuehlke et al., 2006).

Obese male rhesus monkeys had markedly elevated serum insulin values and slightly elevated fasting serum glucose values when compared with nonobese controls (Jen et al., 1985). Anticipation of feeding did not affect serum insulin levels in rhesus monkeys (Natelson et al., 1982).

In African green monkeys, Meis and Rose (1983) determined that feeding resulted in rapid elevation of cortisol, with a subsequent decrease to minimal values 5 hours after feeding. Feeding, rather than exposure to light, synchronized the circadian rhythm of cortisol.

6.4.5 Housing Environment and Social Status

Transferring a NHP to a new facility shortly before initiation of an experimental study may confound the assessment of biochemical parameters as the monkeys begin to adapt to new surroundings.

A study by Hassimoto et al. (2004) showed that ALP, glucose, and sodium significantly decreased following a 6-month acclimation period. Yoshida (1981) found that the average value from over 200 cynomolgus monkeys for BUN, glucose, and albumin gradually increased during a 6-month interval following importation. It was postulated that these changes might have resulted in part from nutritional changes. In the same study, ALT and AST also increased 6 months following importation. The reason for the increased enzyme levels was not determined.

A monkey's social status within a colony can affect cortisol levels and glucocorticoid regulation. In a colony of common marmosets, morning plasma cortisol and ACTH levels were determined before, and 1, 2, and 3 days following dexamethasone administration. Subordinate animals had low baseline cortisol levels as compared to dominant animals; however, no differences were noted at any time point for ACTH suggesting that adrenocorticotropic hormone (ACTH) secretion may be restrained by a steroid-independent mechanism (Saltzman, 2004). Similarly, dominant male cynomolgus monkeys showed higher baseline cortisol levels than subordinate, but the adrenal response differed in that subordinate monkeys showed enhanced responsiveness (Czoty et al., 2008).

The relationship between dominance in the troop and resting cortisol was studied in male African green monkeys. In stable groups, dominant and subordinate males had similar cortisol values. However, in unstable groups, males becoming dominant had higher serum cortisol values than did subordinate males (McGuire et al., 1986).

6.4.6 Circadian Rhythm

Circadian periodicities have been demonstrated in many species. For example, in the rhesus monkey, cortisol levels decrease throughout the day with the lowest levels in the evening, whereas in the squirrel monkey, values are highest at the start of the light period and lowest 4 hours after the onset of darkness (Garg et al., 1978; Leshner et al., 1978; Quabbe et al., 1982; Rose et al., 1978; Wilson et al., 1978). Although light cycles are frequently related to circadian rhythms, one study in rhesus monkeys demonstrated that the marked differences occurring between day and night for testosterone, cortisol, prolactin, and luteinizing hormone were not principally determined by photoperiodicity (Dubey et al., 1983).

A study in cynomolgus macaques provided evidence of circadian rhythms in calcium metabolism. These rhythms showed partial similarity to humans, but the authors stated that endogenous corticosteroid release associated with stress in the monkeys might have affected some findings. Serum total calcium (reflection of albumin) increased at night while a distinct rhythm for ionized calcium was not identified. Serum phosphorus also displayed a circadian rhythm that was higher at night. In contrast to humans, however, parathyroid hormone and ALP failed to show a rhythmic change (Hotchkiss and Jerome, 1998b).

In owl monkeys, total serum protein displays clear diurnal rhythmicity with peak levels at the beginning of the light cycle and a total fluctuation of approximately 10%. In addition, serum iron showed a marked bimodal rhythmicity with fluctuations of approximately 60% (Klein et al., 1985).

6.4.7 Effects of Estrous Cycle, Pregnancy, Lactation, and Menopause

Baboons and macaques are an important model for physiological changes associated with menopause due to reproductive similarities with humans that include a menstrual cycle, natural menopause, and bone-remodeling processes in both cancellous and cortical bone (Colman et al., 1999). Many studies have examined the effect of natural menopause or surgically induced menopause through ovariectomy on serum biomarkers. In rhesus monkeys, OC was elevated after natural menopause. ICTP and ALP were not elevated, which likely reflects the lack of specificity for these markers (Colman et al., 1999).

Lees et al. (1998) studied changes in bone biomarkers in cynomolgus monkeys during pregnancy and lactation. They concluded that urinary pyridinium did not change while BALP and bone Gla protein (BGP) were below baseline throughout pregnancy with the lowest levels occurring in the third trimester. In contrast, BALP, BGP, and urinary pyridiniums were increased during lactation. Both urinary CTX-1 and OC have a significant circatrigintan (menstrual) rhythm in cynomolgus monkeys, and urinary CTX-1 was markedly decreased when estrogen levels were maximal (Hotchkiss et al., 2000).

Baboons and chimpanzees display marked turgescence and detumescence of the sex skin in association with the follicular and luteal phases of the menstrual cycle, respectively. In baboons, plasma volume contracts during turgescence and up to 2 L of extracellular fluid (ECF) can accumulate in the perineum. During detumescence, the ECF is rapidly "auto-infused" back into the circulation (Harewood et al., 2000). These fluid shifts can affect biochemical indices and the renin–angiotensin–aldosterone (RAA) system (Table 6.2). Plasma renin activity is significantly increased in the follicular phase and suppressed in the luteal phase. The activity of the RAA system is considerably greater during the menstrual cycle of baboons as compared to normal adult males. In a study of baboons (Harewood et al., 2000), alterations in red blood cell indices were consistent with a contracted plasma volume in the follicular phase and an expanded plasma volume in the luteal phase. However, increased total protein and albumin in the luteal phase as compared to the follicular phase did not correlate with plasma volume, and the reason for this finding was not determined (Harewood et al., 1996, 2000).

Pregnancy alters numerous biochemical parameters in many NHP species and humans. Harewood et al. (2000) described in detail the changes identified at various stages of gestation in the baboon. Decreased sodium, potassium, BUN, creatinine, cholesterol, and osmolality developed in early gestation and persisted throughout pregnancy. Total protein, albumin, and ALP were reduced from mid-gestation. Additionally, calcium decreased throughout pregnancy and iron concentration was elevated.

Meis et al. (1982) reported that during gestation, cynomolgus monkeys had a decrease in fasting glucose and an increase in the peak plasma insulin response to glucose challenge. Peak plasma insulin response remained elevated during lactation, but glucose clearance rates were unaffected. Serum cholesterol is decreased in pregnant rhesus macaques, pigtail macaques (*Macaca nemestrina*), and baboons. In pigtail macaques, this is associated with a decrease in HDL cholesterol (Rudel et al., 1981a).

Pregnant female squirrel monkeys have lower total protein, albumin, and total cholesterol levels. ALP activity increases in late pregnancy and throughout nursing (Suzuki et al., 1996). In pregnant marmosets, biochemical parameters were reported to be generally within the reference range with the exception of lower glucose, AST, and BUN (Casetti et al., 1995).

TABLE 6.2
Plasma Analytes to Assess the Renin–Angiotensin–Aldosterone System in Baboons (Mean ± SEM)

	Female Follicular Phase (*N* = 10)	Female Luteal Phase (*N* = 10)	Female Lactating (*N* = 16–19)	Adult Males (*N* = 6–10)
Plasma renin activity (fmol/L/second)	2081 ± 927	1051 ± 966	1654 ± 693	841 ± 331
Angiotensin I (pg/mL)	96 ± 6	101 ± 10	–	–
Angiotensin II (pg/mL)	32 ± 6	21 ± 4	30 ± 10	6.5 ± 3
Aldosterone (pg/mL)	1938 ± 400	1059 ± 400	1880 ± 1370	287 ± 45

Source: Harewood, W.J. et al., *J Med Primatol*, 25, 267–271, 1996.

Fecal cortisol concentrations are significantly affected by reproductive status. Wild, cycling, female chacma baboons displayed relatively high levels of cortisol during pregnancy while the lowest cortisol levels occurred during the menstrual cycle (Weingrill et al., 2004). Elevated fecal cortisol levels have also been found in late gestation in black tufted-ear marmosets (Smith et al., 1997) and cotton-top tamarins (Ziegler et al., 1995).

6.4.8 Stress

As in many other mammals, NHP species commonly display elevated glucose levels in association with stress. Glucose levels greater than 200 mg/dL are common in squirrel and owl monkeys. Lambeth et al. (2006) demonstrated that chimpanzees that trained to voluntarily present for an injection had much less stress and lower glucose levels as compared to chimpanzees that had to be involuntarily restrained.

Glucocorticoid release is an important biomarker for stress in NHP that is frequently used by primatologists and clinicians to evaluate the level of stress caused by husbandry practices, experimental procedures, and other manipulations. Basal cortisol levels in primates vary according to psychosocial factors such as rank in dominance heirarchy, individual personality, and social group composition (Bentson et al., 2003). Cortisol levels from normal animals may also vary as a result of immobilization, psychological stress associated with blood collection, and anesthetic reagents used for chemical restraint. One study showed that the stress of capture caused an elevation in plasma cortisol for 60 minutes in rhesus monkeys (Blank et al., 1983). An additional study in rhesus monkeys showed that blood sampling does not affect cortisol levels in animals trained to extend an arm; conversely, cortisol levels increase in untrained monkeys. In physically restrained rhesus monkeys, plasma ACTH and cortisol were elevated within 15 minutes after the start of restraint (Norman and Smith, 1992).

Juvenile rhesus monkey offspring of stressed mothers also showed higher ACTH and cortisol levels as compared to control offspring (Clarke et al., 1994). The excitement of restraint induces hyperglycemia more readily and to a greater degree in small, NW monkeys than in macaques, baboons, or chimpanzees (Dubey et al., 1983).

Testosterone levels declined progressively in serial samples obtained from cage-restrained male rhesus monkeys; however, this decrease was not detected when serial blood samples were collected following ketamine injections (Puri, 1981).

6.4.9 Anesthesia

Blood collection from NHP frequently requires chemical restraint. The most commonly used anesthetic agent is ketamine hydrochloride, but other agents such as tiletamine-zolazepam (Telazol®), pentobarbital, propofol, isoflurane, and sevoflurane are frequently used. Hom et al. (1999) reported no significant differences in biochemical parameters from rhesus monkeys anesthetized with ketamine, pentobarbital, isoflurane, and propofol with the exception of triglycerides, which are elevated with propofol administration due to the presence of soybean oil. Woodward and Weld (1997) also reported minimal significant differences in rhesus monkeys anesthetized with ketamine, ketamine/acepromazine, or Telazol®. Potassium was significantly elevated in animals administered Telazol®; however, the difference was not considered biologically relevant.

Although the choice of inhalant anesthetic regimen has little effect on chemistry parameters, many changes have been described in rhesus monkeys prior to and 15 minutes after an intramuscular injection of ketamine. Sodium, potassium, chloride, calcium, glucose, total protein, albumin, total cholesterol, lactate dehydrogenase (LDH), GGT, ALP, and ALT were significantly decreased and BUN and CK were significantly increased following the ketamine injection (Bennett et al., 1992). Conversely, few alterations were detected in marmosets before and shortly after ketamine administration. AST and CK were significantly increased and GGT was decreased (Taglioni et al., 1996). Administration of ketamine and diazepam for 150 minutes in baboons also resulted in minimal changes in blood parameters (du Plooy et al., 1998). Soma et al. (1995) showed that increases in AST, ALT, LDH, and CK occurred following an initial three weekly injections of sevoflurane; however, with continued dosing three times per week for 7 weeks, these elevations were resolved. These findings suggested that tolerance develops following multiple periods of anesthesia. Although ketamine injections caused a sustained elevation in cortisol in baboons, this pharmacologic effect was absent in rhesus monkeys given ketamine (Bentson et al., 2003).

A number of anesthetic regimens have been shown to decrease ionized calcium and PTH in humans and animals. Following isoflurane anesthesia in cynomolgus monkeys, ionized calcium was significantly decreased and both PTH and OC were significantly increased. Serum fluoride levels were elevated following isoflurane anesthesia and fluoride has been shown to decrease ionized calcium. Although increased fluoride may have contributed to the decrease in calcium, other factors likely contributed. The elevation in PTH and OC was presumed to be secondary to the decrease in ionized calcium (Hotchkiss et al., 1998a).

6.4.10 Sample Collection

The method selected for sample collection can have significant effects on laboratory values. A recent study compared values from samples obtained by venipuncture with samples obtained by an indwelling venous catheter connected to a subcutaneous vascular access port. Serum obtained by venipuncture had higher levels of potassium, phosphorus, and LDH that may have been caused by erythrocyte hemolysis. Serum obtained from the indwelling catheter had an elevated glucose level that may have resulted from the 50% dextrose and heparin used to maintain patency (Iliff et al., 2003).

6.4.11 Sample Hemolysis

Hemolysis in marmosets affects both AST and ALT with a greater effect on ALT (Cowie and Evans, 1985). LDH increases even with low levels of hemolysis. Higher levels of hemolysis correlate with increased levels of ALT, isocitrate dehydrogenase, glutathione reductase, bilirubin, AST, and sorbitol dehydrogenase (SDH) (Davy et al., 1984a). In tamarins, moderate hemolysis caused significant elevations in albumin, total protein, potassium, AST, and total bilirubin. Severe hemolysis additionally caused an elevation in phosphorus and a decrease in ALT and carbon dioxide (Ramer et al., 1995).

6.4.12 Sample Storage

Few reports that specifically address the affects of storage on primate sera or plasma exist in the literature. In cotton-top tamarins, biologically relevant differences in clinical chemistry analytes were not detected between fresh sera and sera stored frozen at –70°C for 4 weeks (Ramer, 1995). Kuo et al. (2008) found that in sera from cynomolgus monkeys AST, ALT, and SDH were stable for up to 24 hours at both room and refrigerated temperatures, and up to 3 months at –80°C. In addition, AST and SDH were stable for up to 3 months at –20°C, but ALT became unstable by 7 days at –20°C. Short-term stability (24 and 48 hours) of multiple enzymes in sera from common marmosets has been described. Refrigerated conditions (4°C) were considered optimal for AST, LDH, and GGT while freezing at –20°C was considered optimal for ALP. Both SDH and GGT were stable at 4°C or –20°C for 48 hours, but 4°C was considered optimal for SDH. The stability of SDH in marmoset sera differs from human sera in which SDH has been reported to be extremely unstable at both room and refrigerated temperatures (Davy et al., 1984b).

6.5 SPECIFIC SERUM CHEMISTRY ANALYTES IN NHPs

6.5.1 Blood Gas

Reported values for arterial and/or venous blood gas analysis in rhesus monkeys, squirrel monkeys, and baboons are detailed in Tables 6.3 and 6.4.

6.5.2 Bone Biomarkers

NHP are frequently used in bone research owing to the similarities in reproductive physiology and skeletal structure as compared with humans. Bone metabolism studies commonly use biomarkers in blood and urine to assess bone formation and resorption. Reference ranges for markers of formation and resorption were established for young (2–3 years) and mature (>10 years) Mauritian cynomolgus monkeys (Table 6.5).

6.5.3 Calcium and Phosphorus

Serum parathyroid hormone and calcitonin in the rhesus monkey are known to have some degree of cross-reactivity with the human hormones, and human assays have been successfully validated and adapted for use in the rhesus monkey (Arnaud et al., 2002). A calcitonin radioimmunoassay was validated for rhesus monkeys by Hargis et al. (1978). The assay used a ^{131}I-labeled synthetic human tracer and showed that the mean basal concentration of calcitonin in plasma from normal rhesus monkeys was not significantly different from normal human plasma and that rhesus monkey calcitonin responds to changes in serum calcium concentration similarly to human calcitonin.

A study by Fincham et al. (1993) demonstrated sufficient cross-reactivity between humans and African green monkeys for intact parathyroid hormone using a commercially available immunoradiometric diagnostic kit. A second radioimmunoassay that was validated for parathyroid hormone in healthy rhesus monkeys showed very similar hormone levels as compared to humans. In addition,

TABLE 6.3
Arterial Blood Gas Analysis in Rhesus Macaques, Colombian, and Bolivian Squirrel Monkeys (Mean ± SD)

		Rhesus[a,b]	Colombian[c]		Bolivian[c]	
		Male	Young	Old	Young	Old
Parameter	Units	N = 33	N = 4	N = 3	N = 4	N =
Age	Years	3–5	5.67 ± 0.00	17.69 ± 0.05	10.48 ± 1.85	15.48 ± 0.93
PaO_2	mmHg	88.06 ± 7.49	114.05 ± 2.93	102.03 ± 9.65	104.8 ± 8.59	98.00 ± 4.27
$PaCO_2$	mmHg	38.19 ± 3.77	23.45 ± 1.59	24.70 ± 2.43	29.35 ± 2.05	26.60 ± 0.75
O_2 saturation	%	96.53 ± 1.00	95.77 ± 0.66	93.67 ± 1.44	95.88 ± 0.79	93.12 ± 0.85
pH		7.39 ± 0.03	7.20 ± 0.02	7.11 ± 0.03	7.22 ± 0.04	7.12 ± 0.01
TCO_2	mEq/L	24.71 ± 2.75	9.58 ± 0.42	8.53 ± 1.27	12.70 ± 0.47	9.38 ± 0.32
HCO_3	mEq/L	23.53 ± 2.65	8.85 ± 0.44	7.77 ± 1.21	11.78 ± 0.5	8.48 ± 0.32
Base excess	mEq/L	NA	−17.5 ± 0.53	−20.13 ± 1.72	−14.18 ± 1.56	−19.40 ± 0.55

Source: Hom, G.J. et al., *Contemp Top Lab Anim Sci,* 38, 60–64, 1999; Brizzee, K.R. et al., *Lab Anim Sci,* 38, 200–202, 1988.

[a] Sedation with ketamine.

[b] Hom et al. (1999).

[c] Brizzee et al. (1988).

TABLE 6.4
Arterial and Venous Blood Gas References in Pregnant Female Baboons ($N = 13$; Mean ± SD)

Parameter	Units	Mean ± SD	Range
Arterial			
pH	–	7.39 ± 0.03	7.31–7.43
PaO_2	torr	82.23 ± 8.42	70.0–96.0
$PaCO_2$	torr	39.69 ± 3.86	35.0–48.0
HCO_3	mEq/L	23.29 ± 2.79	21.1–32.0
Base excess		–0.70 ± 2.32	–3.0–5.8
O_2 saturation	%	96.11 ± 0.75	94.0–97.5
Mixed Venous			
pH	–	7.38 ± 0.03	7.31–7.44
PvO_2	torr	50.15 ± 4.24	45.0–57.0
$PvCO_2$	torr	40.92 ± 4.13	36.0–50.0
HCO_3	mEq/L	23.19 ± 2.24	20.4–29.3
Base excess	–	–0.80 ± 2.41	–3.9–5.8
O_2 saturation	%	74.32 ± 3.52	69.0–82.0

Source: Cissik, J.H. et al., *Am J Primatol*, 11, 277–284, 1986.

TABLE 6.5
Bone Biomarkers in Mauritian Cynomolgus Monkeys (Mean ± SEM)

Measurement	Units	Sample	Young Male (2–3 years)	Young Female (2–3 years)	Mature Female (>10 years)
Bone Formation					
Bone alkaline phosphatase (BALP)	IU/L	Serum	462 ± 19	340 ± 14	111 ± 6
Osteocalcin (OC)	ng/mL	Serum	49 ± 2	38 ± 1	23 ± 1
Procollagen type I C propeptide (PICP)	ng/mL	Serum	373 ± 26	285 ± 38	115 ± 4
Bone Resorption					
Pyridinoline	nmol/L	Serum	2.55 ± 0.01	–	–
C-terminal cross-linking telopeptide of type I collagen (ICTP)	mg/L	Serum	23.0 ± 5.0	24.1 ± 1.0	–
C-telopeptide (CTX-1)	nmol/L	Serum	13.1 ± 0.8	9.8 ± 0.6	–
C-telopeptide (CTX-1)	nmol/L	Urine	2045 ± 998	1381 ± 153	–
Deoxypyridinoline (DPD)	nM/mM	Urine	17.2 ± 0.6	12.9 ± 0.3	–
N-telopeptide (NTX-1)	nMmM	Urine	571 ± 54	622 ± 3	116 ± 7

Source: Legrand, J-J. et al., *Biomarkers,* 8, 63–77, 2003.

a study of rhesus parathyroid hormone and calcium levels following experimentally induced hypocalcemia and hypercalcemia demonstrated a very similar physiologic response between monkeys and humans (Hargis et al., 1977).

An extensive study of calcium kinetics in African green monkeys as a model for man has been reported (Fincham et al., 1993). Parathyroid hormone responded to chelation-induced hypocalcemia by a fourfold increase within 10 minutes, followed by an increase in calcium and a decrease in parathyroid hormone. Published normal values for analytes associated with calcium metabolism in several NHP species are provided in Table 6.6.

TABLE 6.6
Markers of Calcium Metabolism

	Rhesus Macaque[a,b]			Rhesus[c,d]	African Green[c,e,f]					Baboon[g,h]
Age (years)	6.8 ± 0.5	16.7 ± 0.7	25.5 ± 0.5	Juvenile (3–4)	Subadult	Subadult	5–10	5–10	5–10	Adult
Sex	F	F	F	M	M	F	M	F	Both	F
Number	12	30	16	7	10	14	5	3	8	8
Parathyroid hormone (pg/mL)	21.8 ± 2.7	28.9 ± 2.9	32.6 ± 4.7	32 ± 30	–	–	–	–	–	–
Parathyroid hormone (pmol/L)	–	–	–	–	–	–	–	–	9.93 ± 6.08 (6.5–24.3)	2.91–4.57
25-hydroxyvitamin D (ng/mL)	138.7 ± 9.2	128.7 ± 9.1	137.5 ± 6.3	–	–	–	–	–	–	–
1,25-dihydroxyvitamin D (pg/mL)	–	–	–	195 ± 48	–	–	–	–	–	–
Ionized calcium (mmol/L)	–	–	–	–	1.05 ± 0.03	1.10 ± 0.03	1.09 ± 0.02	1.11 ± 0.02	1.1 ± 0.02	1.31–1.37
Calcitonin (pg/mL)	–	–	–	40 ± 14	–	–	–	–	–	–

Source: Colman, R.J. et al., *J Clin Endocrinol Metab.*, 84, 4144–4148, 1999; Arnaud, S.B. et al., *Am J Physiol Endocrinol Metab.*, 282, E514–E521, 2002; Fincham, J.E. et al., *J Med Primatol.*, 22, 246–252, 1993; Leszczyzynski, J.K. et al., *Comp Med.*, 52, 563–567, 2002.

[a] Mean ± SEM.
[b] Colman et al. (1999).
[c] Mean ± SD.
[d] Arnaud et al. (2002).
[e] Range.
[f] Fincham et al. (1993).
[g] Mean ± 2SD.
[h] Leszcyzynski et al. (2002).

6.5.4 Skeletal and Cardiac Biomarkers

6.5.4.1 Lactate Dehydrogenase

As in most animal species, cynomolgus monkeys have five LDH isoenzymes. Isoenzymes 1–3 are the most prevalent and similar quantities of each are found in serum (on average 22%–28%). Isoenzyme 5 is the least prevalent. In many species, including cynomolgus monkeys, the activity of isoenzymes 1 and 2 is high in the myocardium, kidneys, and brain; however, monkeys also have a high percentage of these isoenzymes in red blood cells (Preus et al., 1989). In rhesus monkeys, substantial day-to-day variability and diurnal variation for LDH were documented. In addition to these normal physiologic fluxuations, the stress of both physical and chemical restraint procedures can cause significant LDH elevations (Scott et al., 1976).

6.5.4.2 Creatine Kinase

CK is a cytoplasmic enzyme that originates primarily from brain, skeletal muscle, cardiac muscle, and smooth muscle. Although brain contains a high level of CK activity locally, it is not known to cause an increase in serum CK activity (Stockham and Scott, 2008). The primary cause of CK elevation in NHP is skeletal muscle injury. Vahle (1998) studied the distribution of total CK in cynomolgus monkeys. He found the highest activities (6,000–12,000 IU/g of wet weight) in pectoral and gastrocnemius muscles, slightly less in the diaphragm, approximately 2000 IU/g in the esophagus, heart freewall, and heart septum, and minute activities in the stomach, cerebrum, colon, jejunum, and urinary bladder.

The activity of CK and its isoenzymes have been used to evaluate myocardial damage in NHP; however, this testing strategy lacks a high degree of specificity and sensitivity for myocardial injury and has been replaced largely by highly specific markers such as cardiac troponin I (CTnI) or T (CTnT) and the brain natriuretic peptides. At least three isoenzymes have been identified in all evaluated mammalian species: BB (or CK-1), MB (or CK-2), and MM (or CK-3). A fourth isoenzyme, mitochondrial CK (or CK-Mt) has been detected in some species but is currently of limited diagnostic utility for preclinical studies (Walker, 2006). In humans, the activity of CK-BB is almost entirely in the brain while CK-MM activity is found in both skeletal and cardiac muscle, and CK-Mt activity occurs in the mitochondria of many tissues. Although the majority of CK-MB activity occurs in cardiac muscle, skeletal muscle also contributes to elevations in this isoenzyme.

Although specific studies have not been published for many NHP species regarding the specific distribution of CK isoenzyme activity, it is likely that the trends are similar to humans. In a study of CK isoenzyme distribution in cynomolgus monkeys, MM was the only isoenzyme found in skeletal muscles; from heart muscle, it was predominantly MM with about 10% MB. In the cerebrum, stomach, jejunum, colon, and bladder, it was predominantly BB. In the diaphragm and esophagus, it was predominantly MM with traces of MB and BB (Vahle, 1998). A second study performed in cynomolgus monkeys showed that total CK content was higher in skeletal muscle than that in heart muscle and the CK-MB/total CK ratio was lower in skeletal muscle than that in heart muscle. As a reference, the mean activity of total CK and CK isoenzymes in skeletal and cardiac muscle from cynomolgus monkeys is provided in Table 6.7 (Fredericks et al., 2001). Although CK determination alone is not specific or sensitive enough to reliably indicate cardiac disease, a study by Gozalo et al. (2008) suggested that CK, AST, CK/AST ratio, LDH, and proteinuria together may provide a reliable way to diagnose clinical and/or subclinical cardiomyopathy.

6.5.4.3 Cardiac Troponin I and T

Cardiac troponin I (CTnI) and T (CTnT) possess high sensitivity and specificity for myocardial injury and have been used effectively in NHP to identify cardiac disease and assess drug-induced myocardial injury in preclinical studies (Minomo et al., 2009). Quantitative assessment of these markers in cynomolgus monkeys showed that the mean content of both CTnI and CTnT in skeletal muscle was less than 0.6% of that found in cardiac muscle (Fredericks et al., 2001). Numerous

TABLE 6.7
Mean Activity (SD) of Total Creatine Kinase (CK) and CK Isoenzymes per mg of Protein in Cynomolgus Monkeys

		Total CK	CK-MM (CK-3)	CK-MB (CK-2)	CK-BB (CK-1)
Cardiac	U per mg/protein	24.90 (28.90)	23.40 (29.81)	1.2 (0.93)	0.30 (0.28)
	% of total CK	NA	94.07	4.62	1.31
Skeletal	U per mg/protein	56.10 (33.04)	53.00 (32.03)	1.5 (1.46)	1.70 (2.05)
	% of total CK	NA	94.43	2.72	2.94

Source: Fredericks, S. et al., *Clin Chim Acta,* 304, 65–74, 2001.

commercial assays are available for monitoring CTnI. Different analytical characteristics associated with each assay have made harmonization difficult and values obtained from different assays should be evaluated with caution. A recent study by Apple et al. (2008) showed good CTnI immunoreactivity for rhesus and cynomolgus monkeys by using nine different commercially available assays. CTnT assays are produced by a single vendor and therefore pose less of a heterogeneity problem. Rhesus and cynomolgus monkeys show good and weak responses to this assay, respectively.

6.5.4.4 Atrial and Brain Natriuretic Peptides

Atrial and brain natriuretic peptides (ANP and BNP, respectively) are structurally related hormones secreted from the heart following increased tension of the atrial or ventricular wall, respectively. In humans, BNP has been correlated well with the severity of left ventricular dysfunction, and several recent publications have suggested that this association is also present in NHP (Ely et al., 2011; Izumi et al., 2009). A study by Wondergem et al. (1999) concluded that the plasma concentration of ANP was an important parameter for subclinical cardiac damage; however, the literature contains little recent information regarding the utility of ANP as a cardiac biomarker in NHP. Although few comprehensive studies have been published to date regarding the utility of these cardiac biomarkers in evaluating cardiac disease and myocardial injury in preclinical studies, the early evidence indicates that these hormones have conserved function across species and will likely be important cardiac biomarkers for NHP in the future (Walker, 2006). Currently, commercial assays with known cross-reactivity to ANP and BNP in some NHP species are readily available.

6.5.5 Cortisol

Cortisol (the primary glucocorticoid of NHPs) and corticosterone are heavily metabolized by the liver and intestinal bacteria prior to fecal elimination; consequently, the most reliable assays for most NHP species use group-specific antibodies for glucocorticoid metabolites (Heistermann et al., 2006). Bahr et al. (2000) recommended measurement of fecal 11,17-dioxoandrostanes rather than native cortisol as a more effective noninvasive way to measure adrenal function. Quantitation of urinary cortisol is an alternative noninvasive method frequently used to assess the level of stress associated with procedures and husbandry practices in captive NHPs (Paramastri et al., 2007).

A method of detecting cortisol in salivary specimens was also developed for squirrel monkeys to avoid the stress associated with venipuncture. Specimens were collected on cotton-tipped applicators and analyzed by immunoassay with time-resolved fluorescence detection (Fuchs et al., 1997).

The corticosteroid binding proteins of NHPs have been studied and are quite similar to human with several notable exceptions. Squirrel monkeys, marmosets, and tamarins are unique among NHPs in that they maintain a high circulating level of free plasma cortisol and a low corticosteroid-binding globulin (CBG) binding capacity. The magnitude of the increase in free plasma cortisol in squirrel monkeys is approximately 10-fold higher than that of the humans (Klosterman et al.,

1986). Despite this marked elevation, squirrel monkeys maintain normal electrolytes and blood pressures (Scammell, 2006). A recent study identified several alterations in cortisol metabolism that likely contribute to the adaptive mechanisms that minimize the effects of high cortisol in squirrel monkeys. These included increased peripheral 11β-hydroxysteroid dehydrogenase-2 activity and increased 6β-hydroxycortisol in the urine (Scammell, 2006).

6.5.6 C-Reactive Protein

CRP is an acute-phase reactant produced by the liver that is very sensitive to inflammation and correlates well with the other indicators of inflammation. In recent years, the interest in CRP as a marker for inflammation in toxicology, virology, and microbiology studies has grown. CRP is measured by a variety of immunoassay methods, the majority of which are human-specific. It is important to validate these assays in each NHP, as significant differences in cross-reactivity may exist. A monkey-specific enzyme-linked immunosorbent assay (ELISA) for CRP was developed using sera from several macaque species that displayed greater sensitivity than that of the human-specific assay (Jinbo et al., 1998).

6.5.7 Hepatic Enzymes

6.5.7.1 Alanine Aminotransferase and Aspartate Aminotransferase

In marmosets, Mohr et al. (1971) showed the highest activity of ALT to occur in the liver, though cardiac muscle and kidney also had substantial quantities of the enzyme. The highest level of AST activity occurred in cardiac muscle. Although other tissues had activities of only one-third or one-fourth of that in cardiac muscle (by wet weight), tissues having relatively high activity included the liver, skeletal muscle, kidney, and brain.

The differences in ALT values among healthy chimpanzees, as well as the responses of ALT to inoculation with HCV, have been shown to be genetic in origin (Williams-Blangero et al., 1994). This underscores the importance of pre-study testing in primates, in which, typically, few animals per treatment group are used and animals are not inbred. In NHPs, ALT is not as specific for liver cell injury as it is in the dog, rat, or mouse.

Both hepatic injury and muscle injury can cause equally high elevations in ALT and AST. Mild to moderate elevations in ALT and AST of skeletal muscle origin are commonly seen in NHP species following normal chemical restraint, administration of intravenous substances, and blood collection procedures. Consequently, caution must be taken in attributing elevations of ALT and AST to hepatic injury when concurrent elevations in creatine kinase and/or lactate dehydrogenase are present.

6.5.7.2 Alkaline Phosphatase

In NHPs, the biliary and osteoblastic isoenzymes are the principal components of serum activity; however, the sensitivity of ALP as an indicator of cholestasis and biliary disease is much poorer than in many other laboratory animals such as the dog. This is particularly true in macaques, where the normal range of enzyme activity can be as high as 1500 IU/L, and the activity level in individual animals can vary considerably over time (Hall and Everds, 2003).

6.5.7.3 Gamma Glutamyltransferase

The tissue distribution of GGT was studied in baboons and macaques. In both species, GGT was found primarily in liver, pancreas, and kidney (Braun et al., 1980). In macaques, GGT has been described as a more sensitive and specific marker for biliary disease than ALP (Hall and Everds, 2003). In rhesus and cynomolgus monkeys, GGT levels are markedly higher in young animals of both sexes and decrease with age (Perretta et al., 1991). This trend is similar to humans in which the neonatal GGT activity is five to seven times higher than the upper limit of the adult reference range with adult levels being reached by approximately 7 months of age (Cabrera-Abreu and Green, 2002). In chimpanzees, GGT levels have less daily intraindividual variation than AST or ALT, and smaller changes are considered more significant than comparable changes in AST or ALT. The initial increase in GGT may follow ALT or occur simultaneous. In most cases, it is the last enzyme to return to normal (Valenza and Muchmore, 1985).

6.5.8 Iron Metabolism

The amount of iron in commercially available primate diets can have a substantial impact on analytes used to determine iron status. This is particularly true for NW monkeys such as lemur, squirrel monkeys, and owl monkeys, which frequently develop hemosiderosis in captivity owing to excessive dietary supplementation (Barnhart, 2008; Wood et al., 2003; Glenn et al., 2006; Miller et al., 1997; Smith et al., 2008). The reasons for this iron sensitivity are not completely understood, but they may be related to increased iron absorption as a physiologic adaptation to an arboreal habitat. In a recent report, the incidence of elevated serum iron (>160 µg/dL) was 34.3% in owl monkeys and 35.6% in squirrel monkeys with serum iron ranging from162 to 351 µg/dL. Total iron binding capacity (TIBC) was frequently markedly elevated, ranging from 243 to 950 µg/dL, and percent iron saturation ranged from 35.5% to 97.6% (Barnhart, 2008). Monkeys that chronically receive high levels of dietary iron are at risk for hepatic hemosiderosis. Removing iron from the diet and adding iron-chelators such as tannins and phytates has been shown to effectively prevent this syndrome (Wood et al., 2003). A recent study in marmosets suggested that ferritin, serum iron, and percent transferrin saturation could be used to assess the severity of hemosiderosis (Smith et al., 2008).

Iron accumulation has not been reported for OW monkeys. Reference values for parameters to assess iron metabolism in normal cynomolgus monkeys are provided in Table 6.8.

6.5.9 Lipids and Lipoproteins

Cholesterol, triglycerides, and lipoproteins have been studied very extensively in NHPs, particularly with respect to models of dyslipoproteinemia and atherosclerosis. Many of these studies were performed in animals fed experimental diets (Portman et al., 1985; Spray et al., 1994; Rudel et al., 1981b; Srinivasan et al., 1974). Determination of serum cholesterol before and after a high-cholesterol diet allows for the classification of *M. mulatta* and other primate species into high- and low-cholesterol responder categories that are believed to be genetically controlled (Bhattacharyya and Eggen,

TABLE 6.8
Iron Metabolism in Cynomolgus Monkeys

	Males (N = 35) (2 months to 15 years)		Females (N = 31)[a] (1.5 months to 8 years)	
Measurement	**Mean ± SD**	**Range**	**Mean ± SD**	**Range**
Ferritin (ng/mL)	11 ± 0.03	1–42	13 ± .03	1–62
Iron (µg/dL)	99 ± 37	30–154	110 ± 39	34–184
Total transferrin (mg/dL)	452 ± 40	368–553	465 ± 74	340–658
Total iron binding capacity (TIBC; µg/dL)	317 ± 28	258–387	326 ± 52	238–461
Unsaturated iron binding capacity (UIBC; µg/dL)	217 ± 45	116–293	216 ± 50	125–328
Saturated iron-transferrin (%)	31 ± 12	9–61	34 ± 11	11–56

Source: Giulietti, M. et al., *Comp Biochem Physiol,* 114, 181–184, 1996.

[a] Nonpregnant.

1983). In addition, variation in plasma lipid and lipoprotein response to a high-cholesterol diet in cynomolgus monkeys (*M. fascicularis*) was attributed to additive genetic effects (Spray et al., 1994).

The lipoprotein profile of cynomolgus monkeys is very similar to that of humans with approximately equal amounts of HDL- and LDL-cholesterol and little very low-density lipoprotein (VLDL) cholesterol. Both density-gradient centrifugation and fast protein liquid chromatography have been used to quantitate lipoproteins in NHP (Lehmann et al., 1993). Reference ranges for lipoproteins and lipids in healthy, young adult cynomolgus monkeys are provided in Table 6.9.

Brazilian squirrel monkeys on a lithogenic diet were highly susceptible to cholelithiasis, whereas Bolivian males were resistant. This was associated with HDL-2, which is high in the Brazilian subspecies and low in the Bolivian subspecies. The transport of cholesterol to bile is attributed to HDL-2 (Portman et al., 1985).

Serum lipid profiles were compared in lean and obese chimpanzees (Steinetz et al., 1996). The obese animals had higher total cholesterol, LDL-cholesterol, and triglycerides, though the differences were not statistically significant (Table 6.10).

Sera from many NHP including chimpanzees, rhesus, cynomolgus, squirrel, and owl monkeys frequently have high serum triglyceride levels with no visible evidence of lipemia. The most likely reason for this finding is an increase in free glycerol in the serum. A study in baboons showed that free glycerol concentrations are highly variable and may account for 32% of the serum triglyceride levels (Mott and Rogers, 1978). Most standard assays for serum triglyceride actually measure total triglyceride, which includes free glycerol. Triglyceride blanking to correct for endogenous glycerol may be performed by quantitating the glycerol prior to adding lipase, which is the necessary enzyme for calculating total triglycerides (Rifai and Warnick, 2006). Possible causes of the increased glycerol include stressful situations such as restraint and disease that increase epinephrine, which activates hormone-sensitive lipase, resulting in glycerol release into the circulation (Mott and Rogers, 1978).

TABLE 6.9
Lipoprotein and Lipids in Rhesus and Cynomolgus Monkeys (Mean ± SD)

	Cynomolgus[a]	**Rhesus**[b]
	***N* = 19** **2–7 years**	***N* = 11** **10–30 years** **Obese, Nondiabetic**
Total cholesterol (mmol/L)	4.41 ± 1.06	Mean = 145 Range = 128–245
Free cholesterol (mmol/L)	0.83 ± 0.17	–
Triglycerides (mmol/L)	0.45 ± 0.11	Mean = 55 Range = 19–96
Phospholipids (mmol/L)	2.67 ± 0.47	–
HDL total cholesterol (mmol/L)	1.93 ± 0.60	–
HDL free cholesterol (mmol/L)	0.38 ± 0.13	–
HDL triacylglycerols (mmol/L)	0.26 ± 0.09	–
HDL phospholipids (mmol/L)	1.87 ± 0.42	–
Low-density lipoprotein (mg/dL)	–	72 ± 15
High-density lipoprotein (mg/dL)	–	81 ± 22
Very low-density lipoprotein (mg/dL)	–	12 ± 13

Source: Aouidet, A. et al., *J Clin Chem Clin Biochem,* 28, 251–252, 1990; Najafian, B. et al., *Diabetes Metab Res Rev,* 27, 341–347, 2010.

Note: Mean and range are measured in mg/dL.

[a] Aouidet et al. (1990).

[b] Najafian et al. (2010).

TABLE 6.10
Lipoprotein Cholesterol Levels for Lean and Obese Chimpanzees (Mean ± SD)

Analyte	Lean Males	Lean Females	Obese Males	Obese Females
Number	12	5	1	13
Average age, years (mean ± SD)	27 ± 5[a]	23 ± 1	21	28 ± 4[a]
Average weight, kg (mean ± SD)	53.9 ± 6.0	54.2 ± 6.8	55	60.9 ± 8.3
Total cholesterol	207 ± 63	248 ± 64	210	232 ± 55
High-density lipoprotein (HDL) cholesterol	44 ± 12	61 ± 15	39	46 ± 15
Low-density lipoprotein cholesterol	148 ± 61	160 ± 61	156	166 ± 49
Ratio of total cholesterol to HDL cholesterol	5.0 ± 2.3	4.1 ± 0.5	5.4	5.3 ± 1.4

Source: Steinetz, BG. et al., *J Med Primatol,* 25, 17–25, 1996.

[a] Age not known for all animals, average based on $n = 10$.

6.5.10 Pepsinogen I

Pepsinogen I is the inactive precursor to pepsin that is produced and secreted by the gastric chief cells. The majority of pepsinogen I is secreted into the gastric lumen and converted into pepsin in the presence of hydrochloric acid. A small amount of pepsinogen I is also present in blood. Lynch et al. (2004) evaluated a human ELISA for measuring pepsinogen I in cynomolgus monkeys and concluded that serum pepsinogen I provides a sensitive and specific biomarker for gastric toxicity for preclinical studies.

6.5.11 Protein

In owl monkeys, a positive linear relationship between serum total calcium and both albumin and protein have been identified. The findings were similar to dogs, and the adjusted formula for calcium based on albumin concentration for dogs correlated with monkeys and could be potentially used to provide an accurate estimate of total calcium in monkeys (Weller et al., 1990).

Changes in serum proteins of *M. fascicularis* during lactation have been studied (D'Ovidio and Turillazzi, 1994). During the 48 weeks of lactation, the absolute values of α1 and γ globulins decreased while α2 and β globulins increased. Several positive acute-phase proteins including α1 acid glycoprotein, haptoglobin, and ceruloplasmin, as well as the negative acute-phase protein transferrin were decreased. It was considered likely that these trends were caused by estrogen and progesterone variations after delivery.

6.5.12 Uric Acid

Serum uric acid is an insensitive indicator of renal function in certain NHP species that has limited diagnostic applications. Despite its lack of practical application, uric acid production has important evolutionary implications. Uric acid is a product of purine metabolism that is converted to the more soluble and readily excreted allantoin by the copper-binding enzyme urate oxidase (uricase). During primate evolution, uricase activity was lost and eventually silenced due to genetic mutations; consequently, NHP species that underwent mutation developed elevated levels of uric acid (Oda et al., 2002; Johnson et al., 2009). Johnson et al. (2005) theorized that these mutations occurred as a way of increasing blood pressure in response to a low-sodium and low-purine diet. OW monkeys, including baboons and rhesus monkeys, have a moderate degree of urate oxidase activity and a low serum uric acid level (Christen et al., 1970). Similar to humans, urate oxidase activity is not detectable in liver homogenates from chimpanzees, which have serum uric acid levels of approximately 3 mg/dL (Johnson et al., 2009; Friedman et al., 1985). With some exceptions, most NW monkeys have high urate oxidase activity in the liver and consequently low serum uric acid levels. In a study by Christen et al. (1970), one tamarin (*S. oedipus*), one wooley monkey, and two Cebus monkey species showed moderate serum uric acid levels.

6.5.13 Serum Amyloid A

Serum amyloid A (SAA) is an apoprotein of monkey HDL and lymph chylomicrons that is released as part of the acute-phase response (Parks and Rudel, 1985). Commercially available ELISA kits for human diagnostics have been used successfully to detect SAA in primate sera; however, validation of the assay must be performed for the specific species of interest. Hukkanen et al. (2006) recently reported that an immunoassay developed by different companies performed with varying results in NHPs.

6.5.14 Sex Hormones and Gonadotropins

NHPs have been extensively utilized in investigations of pituitary and sex hormone responses due to their similarities to humans in these respects. Table 6.11 provides reference values for some analytes used to assess endocrine function in NHP.

6.5.14.1 Testosterone

In male cynomolgus monkeys, normal androgen levels can be segregated into four phases: neonatal, infancy, prepubertal, and pubertal. The neonatal period is associated with elevated testosterone and dihydrotestosterone (DHT) levels that have been attributed to testicular steroidogenic activity. Levels of these hormones subsequently decreased throughout the infancy and prepubertal phases before sharply increasing with the onset of puberty (Meusy-Dessolle and Dang, 1985). The average levels for testosterone at each phase are provided in Table 6.12. Unlike testosterone and DHT, D4-androstenedione remained relatively constant from birth to 3 years of age with a decrease from 3 to 4.5 years (Meusy-Dessolle and Dang, 1985). High serum testosterone levels of testicular origin are also present in neonatal male rhesus monkeys and pigtail macaques, whereas neonatal females have testosterone levels

TABLE 6.11
Measurements of Endocrine Function in Nonhuman Primates (NHPs)

	Baboons (*Papio ursinus*) (Mean Value)[a]		Rhesus (Mean ± SEM)[b]	
	Wild Caught (*N* = 6)	Captive Bred (*N* = 9)	Young Female (*N* = 9)	Aged Female (*N* = 10)
Cortisol (nmol/L)	1206.00	1273.56	–	–
Corticotrophin (pg/mL)	26.33	44.3	–	–
Prolactin (μM/mL)	110.00	130.56	–	–
Testosterone (nmol/L)	0.7	0.7	–	–
β-Endorphin (fmol/mL)	12.83	12.11	–	–
Melatonin (pg/mL)	15.83	14.44	–	–
Luteinizing hormone (ng/mL)	–	–	15.1 ± 1.6	43.3 ± 11.8
Estradiol (pg/mL)	–	–	84.1 ± 16.0	39.6 ± 13.3
Progesterone (ng/mL)	–	–	0.46 ± 0.08	0.40 ± 0.07
Insulin-like growth factor-1 (ng/mL)	–	–	281 ± 32	134 ± 23

Source: De Wet, E.H. et al., *SAMS,* 84, 302–303, 1994; Woller, M.J. et al., *J Clin Endocrinol Metab,* 87, 5160–5167, 2002.

[a] De Wet et al. (1994).

[b] Woller et al. (2002).

TABLE 6.12
Testosterone Levels in Rhesus Monkeys at Various Stages of Development (Mean ± SD)

	Age	*N*	Testosterone (ng/mL)
Neonatal phase	Birth to 4 months	24	2.3 ± 0.6
Neonatal phase (castrated)	Birth to 4 months	NA	<0.27
Infancy phase	Up to 29 months	173	0.58 ± 0.03
Prepubertal phase	Up to 43 months	244	1.03 ± 0.11
Pubertal phase	Greater than 43 months	85	Mean = approx 7 ng/mL

Source: Meusy-Dessolle, N., and Dang, D.C., *J Reprod Fertil,* 74, 347–359, 1985.

comparable to castrated, postnatal males (Robinson and Bridson, 1978). In male chimpanzees, serum testosterone levels increased with age from an average juvenile value of 13 ng/dL at 1–6 years, to an adolescent value of 178 ng/dL at 7–10 years and an adult value of 397 ng/dL (Martin et al., 1977).

Diurnal variations of testosterone, DHT and androstenedione have been described for rhesus monkeys. In general, testosterone levels are significantly lower in the morning and early afternoon as compared to nighttime (Winters et al., 1991; Schlatt et al., 2008; Chambers et al., 1982; Goncharov et al., 1981). However, these diurnal patterns may change to some degree depending on the season of the year (Rose et al., 1978). Testosterone and DHT also have an annual periodicity. The highest levels are typically seen in winter with the lowest levels occurring in the summer (Gordon et al., 1978; Goncharov et al., 1981). Additionally, Schlatt et al. (2008) showed that these diurnal rhythms were enhanced in older rhesus monkeys. The circadian rhythm of androstenedione is characterized by minimum values in the evening, an increase during the night, and a peak in the early morning (Goncharov et al., 1981).

Squirrel monkeys and other NW monkeys have high levels of testosterone as compared to OW monkeys (Wilson et al., 1978). In the owl monkey, the lowest serum levels of testosterone occur during the dark period with fivefold higher levels occurring during the light period, the reverse of patterns reported in diurnal primates (Dixson and Gardner, 1981). During the breeding season, a dramatic rise in testosterone accompanied by more modest elevations in DHT and androstenedione occurred in male squirrel monkeys. The testosterone:DHT level was approximately 7:1 in the nonbreeding season but rose dramatically to 34:1 in the breeding season. In contrast, the testosterone:DHT ratio in humans is approximately 12. In squirrel monkeys, lower 5α-reductase activity during the breeding season may lead to a compensatory increase in androgen production (Gross et al., 2008).

In male vervet African green monkeys, circadian rhythms were demonstrated for androgens, with peak values at 2100 to 0600 hours, and for 17β-estradiol, with peak values at 2400 to 0600 hours (Beattie and Bullock, 1979). In the nocturnal male owl monkey (*A. trivirgatus*), the lowest levels of serum testosterone occurred during the dark period, and approximately fivefold higher levels are present during the light period. This pattern is the reverse of the pattern reported for diurnal primates (Dixson and Gardner, 1981).

Given the importance of monitoring testosterone metabolism in many studies involving NHP, noninvasive methods for quantitating testosterone metabolites are ideal in that they allow repeated sampling without creating significant stress in the animal. Mohle et al. (2002) investigated the feasibility of measuring testosterone metabolites in urine and feces from a chimpanzee, cynomolgus monkey, and common marmoset as a method for studying testosterone metabolism. In all three species, testosterone metabolites were excreted primarily in the urine; however, the quantity of each individual metabolite varied significantly between species and between urine and feces. Thus, noninvasive assessment of testosterone metabolism should be investigated and validated for each species.

6.5.14.2 Estrogen and Progesterone

The major biologically active estrogen varies between NHP species. For example, estrone is the major circulating plasma estrogen in the owl monkey while 17β-estradiol predominates in rhesus monkeys (Bonney et al., 1980). Serum estradiol levels in neonatal male and female macaques did not differ during the first 14 weeks of life and never exceeded 50 pg/mL (Robinson and Bridson, 1978). Many NW monkeys including owl monkeys, tamarins, the common marmoset, and the squirrel monkey have plasma estrogen and progesterone levels that are 50–100 times greater than OW monkeys (Bonney et al., 1979).

Given the many similarities in placentation, pregnancy, menstruation, and the hormonal dynamic, the NHP functions as an important model of human reproduction. Quantitative assessments of estrogens, progesterone, and other reproductive hormones during the menstrual cycle have been described for the chimpanzee (Machatschke et al., 2006), baboon (Koyama et al., 1977), rhesus (Hotchkiss et al., 1982), cynomolgus (Mehta et al., 1986; Goodman et al., 1977), and African green monkeys (Hess et al., 1979). Not surprisingly, these NHP share many similar characteristics with humans. Studies have shown that the hormonal dynamics of chimpanzees are similar to those of women, and levels of estrogen, progesterone, and 17α-hydroxyprogesterone vary throughout the menstrual cycle of rhesus monkey in a similar manner to humans (Hobson et al., 1976; Bosu et al., 1972). However, significant differences between species and humans do exist, and the specific hormonal patterns unique to each species should be established prior to initiation of reproductive studies. In a natural environment, the menstrual cycles of rhesus monkeys are ovulatory in the fall and winter, and anovulatory (with low levels of follicle-stimulating hormone [FSH] and estradiol) in the spring and summer (Walker et al., 1984). The mean levels of estrogen, progesterone, luteinizing hormone (LH) and FSH for female rhesus monkeys throughout the menstrual cycle are provided in Table 6.13.

The owl monkey and other NW monkeys differ from OW monkeys in that they lack a detectable menstrual cycle. Consequently, hormonal assays are often required to index ovarian function. In the owl monkey, a defined peak of 17β-estradiol can be used to time ovulation (Bonney et al., 1980). Owl monkeys and tamarins also differ from OW monkeys and some NW monkey species such as the squirrel monkey and the common marmoset in that they do not have clear hormonal distinctions between the follicular and luteal phases (Bonney et al., 1979).

Postmenopausal rhesus and cynomolgus macaques have low concentrations of 17β-estradiol (Kavanagh et al., 2005). Additionally, low levels of daily urinary estrone conjugate have also been described for postmenopausal rhesus monkeys (Gilardi et al., 1997).

TABLE 6.13
Steroid Hormones and Gonadotropins throughout the Menstrual Cycle in Normal Female Rhesus Monkeys (Mean ± SEM)

	Day of Cycle				
	Day 2	Day 6–9	Day 11–12	3–5 Days after LH Peak	10–15 Days after LH Peak
Number	5	6	4	6	6
Serum estrogens (pg/mL)	54 ± 11	124 ± 11	189 ± 30	51 ± 10	110 ± 27
Serum progesterone (ng/mL)	0.1 ± 0.02	0.2 ± 0.02	0.4 ± 0.2	3.0 ± 0.5	1.9 ± 0.5
Serum LH (ng/mL)	3.1 ± 0.6	4.7 ± 2.0	3.1 ± 0.7	5.5 ± 0.8	3.8 ± 0.4
Serum FSH (ng/mL)	30.6 ± 6.1	23.6 ± 8.5	15.4 ± 2.6	25.1 ± 5.0	30.0 ± 4.7

Source: Hotchkiss, J. et al., *Biol Reprod,* 26, 241–248, 1982.
FSH, follicle-stimulating hormone; LH, luteinizing hormone.

Hormone profiles throughout pregnancy vary between species. Progesterone levels do not show a marked increase during pregnancy in several macaque species and baboons. In the common marmoset and the squirrel monkey, however, progesterone and estrogens increase following ovulation and generally remain high throughout pregnancy (Diamond et al., 1987; Chambers and Hearn, 1979). Many NHPs do not require a decrease in progesterone for the onset of parturition; however, the marmoset does experience a decline in plasma progesterone during the last few weeks of pregnancy (Chambers and Hearn, 1979). The hormonal changes associated with female marmosets show marked diurnal variations in urinary estradiol levels (Bos et al., 1993).

Several reports described changes in hormone levels following spontaneous abortion or fetal death. In Bolivian squirrel monkeys, weekly measurement of chorionic gonadotropin (CG), estradiol, and progesterone was used to characterize animals that aborted (Diamond et al., 1985). The authors demonstrated that a gradual decline in serum hormone concerntrations to levels at or below 20% of peak values occurred in animals undergoing spontaneous abortion. In rhesus monkeys pregnant with live anencephalic fetuses, estradiol was significantly lower than in pregnant normal controls but estrone was not decreased; following fetal death, both estradiol and estrone decreased significantly (Walsh et al., 1979).

Noninvasive methods for evaluating hormonal dynamics are valuable techniques for monitoring pregnancy, menstruation, and reproductive health in female monkeys. Many investigators have successfully quantitated ovarian steroid hormones in feces and urine (Moorman et al., 2002; Bardi et al., 2001). Ovulation and conception were detected by fecal steroid profiles in a group of wild Japanese macaques (Shimizu, 2005). Matsumuro et al. (1999) successfully used a commercially available radioimmunoassay kit to detect estradiol and progesterone levels in fecal samples from cynomolgus monkeys. The excretion of steroids and steroid metabolites was reviewed by Whitten et al. (1998), and a summary of published reports describing validated applications for quantitating excreted steroids as a measurement of ovarian function and pregnancy is provided in Table 6.14.

6.5.14.3 Prolactin

In females, prolactin is an important regulator of maternal behavior. In some NHP species, particularly marmosets, tamarins, and owl monkeys, both sexes demonstrate a high level of paternal behavior. Dixson and George (1982) originally reported that male marmosets carrying their offspring had prolactin levels that were approximately five times higher than males without infants. Subsequent studies of common marmoset and the cotton-top tamarin males have also associated elevated prolactin with various aspects of parenting behavior (Schradin et al., 2003; Ziegler and Snowdon, 2000). Prolactin is typically measured by immunoassay techniques. Although an earlier study in squirrel monkeys reported insufficient cross-reactivity by using antibodies directed at human prolactin, recent studies have successfully used human assays to measure prolactin in the urine from marmosets and tamarins (Scammell, 1992; Ziegler et al., 1996b; Ziegler and Snowdon, 2000; Schradin et al., 2003). Ketamine anesthesia has been shown to greatly increase prolactin levels in rhesus and squirrel monkeys (Scammell, 1992; Puri, 1981).

6.5.14.4 Chorionic Gonadotropin

By contrast to most nonprimate mammals, CG is present in the serum and urine of pregnant female NHPs (Maston and Ruvolo, 2002). The molecule consists of an α and a β subunits. The structure of the α subunit is highly species specific; the β subunit that characterizes CG is immunologically similar among species. An antibody to the β subunit of ovine luteinizing hormone has been used in a hemagglutination inhibition assay and a radioimmunoassay for pregnancy diagnosis in a variety of NHP species. The duration of the reliable positive reaction is brief; in rhesus monkeys, it occurs on days 20–24 of pregnancy, and in cynomolgus monkeys on days 24–28 (Boot and in't Veld, 1981; Lequin et al., 1981; Yoshida, 1983). Use of the hemagglutination inhibition test in rhesus monkeys was evaluated at 19–21 days after breeding. Pregnant females were identified with an accuracy of 73.3%. Of 104 urine samples from non-pregnant intact females, 11.5% yielded a false positive result. Rarely, urine from males or ovariectomized females yielded false positive results (Naqvi and

TABLE 6.14
Excreted Steroid and Steroid Metabolites as Measures of Ovarian Function and Pregnancy in NHPs

	Fecal/Urine Steroid or Metabolite	Reference
Common marmoset	Progesterone	Heistermann (1993)
	Pregnanediol glucuronide	Ziegler (1996a)
	Estrone	
	Estradiol	
Cotton-top tamarin	Progesterone	Heistermann (1993)
	Pregnanediol glucuronide	Ziegler (1996a)
	Estrone	
	Estradiol	
Squirrel monkey	Progesterone	Moorman (2002)
	Estrone	
	Estradiol	
Cynomolgus monkey	Progesterone	Shideler (1993a, b)
	Estradiol	Matsumuro (1999)
	Estrone conjugates	
	Pregnanediol glucuronide	
Rhesus monkey	Progesterone	Stavisky (1994)
	Estradiol	Bardi (2001)
	Estrone conjugates	
Baboon	Progesterone	Wasser (1991)
	Estradiol	Stavisky (1995)
Chimpanzee	Estrone conjugates	Knott (1993)

Source: Adapted from Whitten, P.L. et al., *Am J Phys Anthropol.*, 1–23, 1998.

Lindberg, 1985). Diamond et al. (1987) reported that an increase in CG can be used in the squirrel monkey to distinguish pregnant from nonpregnant females. In chimpanzees, an increase in CG and estrone conjugates are the earliest hormonal changes associated with pregnancy (Shimizu et al., 2003). Human pregnancy tests based on detection of human CG have been used successfully in chimpanzees for early pregnancy detection.

Serum hormone levels for pregnant cynomolgus monkeys have been investigated. Monkey CG rose sharply with a peak at approximately 20 days, which was quickly followed by a return to very low levels throughout the duration of the pregnancy. Serum estradiol levels started to increase at approximately 4 weeks and continued to rise throughout pregnancy with a sharp peak immediately before parturition. Progesterone initially declined until approximately week 7 and then increased steadily until approximately week 21 at which time the levels began to drop until parturition. Prolactin levels remained relatively low until a gradual increase started at approximately 15 weeks and plateaued the last few weeks of gestation. Serum cortisol levels did not change (Hein et al., 1989).

6.5.14.5 Thyroid Hormones

Serum thyroxine (T_4) and triiodothyronine (T_3) may be assayed by standard human immunoassay methods. Although some standardized human assays for thyroid-stimulating hormone (TSH) will cross-react with NHP species, this is not always the case and the method validation for a particular species should always be performed. Cynomolgus monkeys, rhesus monkeys, chimpanzees, and African green monkeys have similar values for total T_4 and total T_3 (Yoshida et al., 1989). Table 6.15 details reference values for thyroid parameters in chimpanzees, rhesus, cynomolgus, African green, owl, and squirrel monkeys.

In male rhesus monkeys, total T_4 levels decline throughout postnatal development, but a transient T_4 elevation occurs immediately prior to puberty and in concert with the peripubertal increase in testicular size and may contribute to the process of sexual development (Mann et al., 2002). An additional study in male rhesus monkeys demonstrated that the low-protein diets affect the thyroid function by decreasing the total T_4 and free T_4 concentrations and elevating the T_3 levels. These changes may indicate a mild hypermetabolic state with increased conversion of T_3 to T_4 (Portman et al., 1985). The administration of estradiol to intact female rhesus monkeys increased their serum TSH by decreasing its degradation (Scammell et al., 1992).

The effects of aging on the TSH, T_3, and T_4 were determined in cynomolgus monkeys. In males, T_3, T_4, and TSH decreased with age. Although T_3 and T_4 decreased with age in females, TSH remained unchanged. Following thyrotropin-releasing hormone (TRH) administration, the TSH concentrations, but not T_3 and T_4, were maximally increased in the oldest group. These results suggested that in aging primates either the sensitivity of the thyroid gland to TSH or the releasing capacities for T_3 and T_4 are decreased (Yoshida et al., 1989). Kaack et al. (1979b, 1980) demonstrated that T_4 progressively decreases in maturing squirrel monkeys, while T_3 does not change. Much higher values for both T_4 and T_3 were observed in the Bolivian subspecies of *S. sciureus* than in the Columbian subspecies. Additionally, male squirrel monkeys displayed higher concentrations of T_3 and T_4 prior to the breeding season when the body weight was at its highest (Kaack et al., 1980). The owl monkey has lower levels of T3 as compared to cynomolgus macaques and many other NHP species. This finding is consistent with the lower metabolic rate of the owl monkeys (Whittow et al., 1979).

Chimpanzees have notable differences in thyroid function as compared to humans. They have lower total T_4 levels but increased free T_4, free T_3, total T_3, and T_3 uptake. Gagneux et al. (2001) hypothesized that a higher affinity of transthyretin and/or T_4-binding globulin for thyroid hormone may account for these differences.

6.6 BRIEF DESCRIPTION OF COMMON PROCEDURES

6.6.1 Evaluation of Hypothalamic–Pituitary–Adrenal Axis Function

ACTH stimulation and dexamethasone suppression tests are commonly performed on NHP to assess hypothalamic–pituitary–adrenal (HPA) function. One published method for performing an ACTH stimulation test in cynomolgus monkeys requires an overnight fast followed by an injection of dexamethasone (0.5 mg/kg) in the morning to suppress the HPA axis. Four hours after this injection, blood is collected for a baseline cortisol, and ACTH is administered (i.e., Cortrosyn® 10 ng/kg intravenously). Additional blood samples are collected 15 and 30 minutes post-ACTH for cortisol determination. A modified dexamethasone suppression test for NHP has also been described. A morning blood sample for cortisol is taken and a low dose of dexamethasone (130 μg/kg intramuscularly) is administered 12–14 hours later. The next morning, a second blood sample for cortisol is collected. The difference between the two cortisol levels is used as an indicator of sensitivity to negative feedback (Shively et al., 1997).

An immunoradiometric assay for plasma ACTH concentration was validated for rhesus monkeys by Norman and Smith (1992). A study by Sarnyai et al. (1995) utilized this method to determine that rhesus monkeys have a high-frequency, low-amplitude micropulsatile ACTH release that is very similar to humans. Recently, a commercial radioimmunoassay kit with 100% cross-reactivity with human and murine ACTH was successfully validated for capuchin monkeys, a NW monkey species closely related to marmosets and tamarins (Torres-Farfan et al., 2008).

6.6.2 Evaluation of Glucose Metabolism and Regulation

Many of the same assays used to evaluate glucose metabolism in humans can be successfully used in NHP. These include (1) fasted insulin and glucose levels, (2) plasma levels of glycated proteins,

TABLE 6.15
Thyroid Parameters in Various NHP Species

	N	Sex	Age	Total T_4 (μg/dL)	Total T_3 (ng/dL)	TSH (μU/mL)	Free T_4 (ng/dL)	T_3 Uptake (%)	Reference
African green monkeys (mean ± SD)	12	Both	Adult	3.7 ± 0.3	84.0 ± 6.0	1.4 ± 0.3	–	–	Morley et al. (1980)
(mean ± SD, range)	9	M	NA	4.85 ± 0.60 (3.9–5.7)	122.0 ± 27.2 (91–178)	–	–	–	Kaack et al. (1979b)
–	9	F	NA	5.39 ± 1.71 (3.0–8.4)	175.9 ± 78.7 (94–350)	–	–	–	–
Rhesus monkey (mean ± SEM)	21–70	Male	Adult	5.06 ± 0.49	103.9 ± 8.9	1.14 ± 0.19	0.84 ± 0.06	27.9 ± 0.45	Portman et al. (1985)
(mean ± SD)	7	M	NA	4.85 ± 0.91 (3.8–6.6)	73.9 ± 20.7 (54–115)	–	–	–	Kaack et al. (1979b)
–	24	F	NA	4.07 ± 1.84 (1.3–7.6)	146.3 ± 54.7 (63–295)	–	–	–	–
Squirrel monkey Bolivian (mean ± SD, range)	9	M	NA	3.02 ± 1.1 (1.7–5.1)	57.1 ± 22.2 (21–83)	–	–	–	Kaack et al. (1979b)
–	13	F	NA	1.99 ± 0.85 (1.0–3.7)	48.8 ± 20.0 (20–86)	–	–	–	–
Squirrel monkey Colombian	6	M	NA	3.42 ± 0.75 (2.6–3.6)	61.4 ± 12.7 (42.5–80.0)	–	–	–	Kaack et al. (1979b)
(mean ± SD, range)	16	F	NA	3.03 ± 1.69 (1.5–7.3)	78.2 ± 34.9 (21–168)	–	–	–	–
Squirrel monkey	12	Both	30 days	6.61 ± 3.70	58.0 ± 30.1	–	–	–	Kaack et al. (1979a, 1979b)
(Mixed strains)	13	Both	6–8.5 months	5.03 ± 2.38	80.4 ± 30.7	–	–	–	–
(mean ± SD)	9	Both	1 year	3.52 ± 2.58	50.6 ± 13.5	–	–	–	–
–	5	Both	2 years	3.32 ± 2.36	59.0 ± 7.90	–	–	–	–
–	54	Both	Adult	2.42 ± 1.26	68.6 ± 30.5	–	–	–	–
Chimpanzee (Mean ± SD, range)	5	Both	NA	4.78 ± 0.78 (3.7–5.9)	109.2 ± 27.0 (87–155)	–	–	–	Kaack et al. (1979b)

(Continued)

TABLE 6.15 (*Continued*)
Thyroid Parameters in Various NHP Species

	N	Sex	Age	Total T_4 (μg/dL)	Total T_3 (ng/dL)	TSH (μU/mL)	Free T_4 (ng/dL)	T_3 Uptake (%)	Reference
Owl monkey (Mean ± SD)	6	Both	Adult	74.59 ± 6.04[a]	3.23 ± 0.4[a]	10.85 ± 3.0[a]	–	–	Whittow et al. (1979)
Cynomolgus monkey (Mean ± SD)	6	Both	Adult	224.11 ± 47.28[a]	4.72 ± 0.55[a]	13.22 ± 4.68[a]	–	–	Whittow et al. (1979)

TSH, thyroid-stimulating hormone.
[a] Units = ng/mL.

(3) the OGTT, (4) the intravenous glucose tolerance test, and (5) the euglycemic clamp. Reference intervals for the glucoregulatory measurements associated with these procedures are provided for baboons, rhesus, and cynomolgus monkeys, in Tables 6.16 through 6.18.

Serum glucose concentration is influenced by numerous factors, including gastrointestinal absorption, insulin, hepatic storage and release, glucagon, somatotropin, epinephrine, and cortisol. Through the latter two hormones, excitement and stress may significantly elevate serum glucose. Variations among primate species with respect to anatomy and transit time of the gastrointestinal tract should be considered in determining the length of fasting required to render an animal nonabsorptive. In monkeys that have cheek pouches, such as macaques, the cheek pouches should be manually emptied or the retention of food in cheek pouches should be considered in determining whether animals are nonabsorptive.

Elevated fasting glucose is often an early indicator of type 2 diabetes mellitus. In humans, overt diabetes is defined as a fasting glucose that exceeds 126 mg/dL. The normal fasting glucose level for most NHP is 20–30 mg/dL lower than humans; consequently, a persistent fasted glucose of 100–126 mg/dL that is not attributable to a stress response is more likely to indicate overt diabetes (Wagner et al., 2006). In fasting rhesus monkeys and baboons, Goodner et al. (1977) observed periodic oscillations of insulin, glucose, and glucagon. Glucose and insulin oscillated in phase with each other and out of phase with glucagon. Once a meal was consumed, these cycles were disrupted; however, anticipation of feeding did not affect serum insulin levels in rhesus monkeys (Natelson et al., 1982; Goodner et al., 1977).

TABLE 6.16
Anthropometric and Glucoregulatory Measurements for Healthy, Nondiabetic Baboons (Mean ± SD)

Measurement	Male	Female
Age (years)	18.2 ± 6.4	20.6 ± 5.9
Weight (kg)	27.7 ± 3.5	22.8 ± 6.4
Crown to heel (cm)	106.8 ± 4.1	94.0 ± 5.3
Waist (cm)	53.6 ± 5.5	59.1 ± 14
Body mass index (kg/m^2)	24.3 ± 3.1	24.6 ± 6.5
% Body fat	6.2 ± 1.5	11.7 ± 2.3
Fasting plasma glucose (mmol/L)	5.6 ± 1.1	5.6 ± 1.1
Hemoglobin A1C (%)	4.6 ± 0.5	4.8 ± 0.7
Cholesterol—total (mg/dL)	78 ± 22	99 ± 30
Cholesterol—HDL (mg/dL)	46 ± 13	45 ± 10
Cholesterol—LDL (mg/dL)	26 ± 10	42 ± 22
Triglycerides (mg/dL)	32 ± 10	62 ± 25.6
Fasting plasma insulin (μU/mL)	8 ± 6	23 ± 14
Fasting c-peptide (ng/mL)	1.6 ± 0.8	2.3 ± 1.1
Fasting free fatty acids (μEq/L)	385 ± 23	697 ± 23
Steady state plasma insulin during euglycemic clamp (μU/mL)	215 ± 60	246 ± 65
Increment in plasma insulin concentration during insulin clamp (μU/mL)	207 ± 60	223 ± 56
Steady state glucose insulin during euglycemic clamp (mg/dL)	89 ± 2	89 ± 4
Free fatty acid$_{90–120}$ (μEq/L)	121 ± 16	358 ± 16
$R_{d90–120}$ (mg·kg^{-1}·min^{-1})[a]	5.7 ± 3.0	6.7 ± 6.4

Source: Chavez, A.O. et al., *Diabetes,* 57, 899–908, 2008.

[a] R_d = insulin sensitivity calculated as the mean rate of insulin-stimulated whole-body glucose disposal.

TABLE 6.17
Anthropometric, and Glucoregulatory Measurements for Rhesus Monkeys

Parameter	Rhesus Male Young Adult $N = 12^{a,b}$	Rhesus Male Adult $N = 12^{a,b}$	Rhesus Male Adult $N = 123^{c,d}$	Rhesus Male Geriatric $N = 297^{c,d}$	Rhesus Female Adult $N = 219^{c,d}$	Rhesus Adult $N = 11^{c,e}$
Age (years)	5.6 ± 0.6 (3.0–8.9)	15.9 ± 1.5 (11.4 ± 27.7)	18.5 ± 3.0 (15–22)	23.2 ± 2.0 (22–28)	19.5 ± 2.0 (17–23)	14 (10–30)
Body weight (kg)	6.3 ± 0.4 (5.0–9.1)	13.2 ± 0.5 (11.1–15.9)	11.9 ± 2.0	11.9 ± 3.0	8.3 ± 2.0	13 ± 3
Body fat (%)	9.7 ± 2.0 (4–16)	25.5 ± 2.0 (22–29)	17.9 ± 9.0	21.5 ± 10.0	19.9 ± 11.0	–
Body mass index (kg/m²)	–	–	41.0 ± 7.0	42.0 ± 9.0	34.6 ± 7.0	–
Abdominal circumference (cm)	–	–	50.1 ± 10.0	51.0 ± 11.0	45.6 ± 9.0	–
Fasting plasma glucose (mmol/L)	3.7 ± 0.1 (3.2–4.2)	3.8 ± 0.1 3.2–4.2	3.6 ± 1.2	3.4 ± 0.4	3.4 ± 0.4	64 ± 10
Fasting plasma insulin (μU/mL)	42 ± 3.0 (23–54)	50 ± 4.2 (23–72)	–	–	–	43 ± 31
Fasting plasma insulin (pmol/L)	–	–	205 ± 195	285 ± 289	254 ± 274	–
Glucose disappearance rate (K_G)	3.6 ± 0.2 4.4–2.90	3.5 ± 0.2 (4.16–2.69)	7.3 ± 4.0	6.4 ± 3.0	10.2 ± 5.0	–
Insulin sensitivity index (10^{-5}/min^{-1}/(pmol/L)	–	–	5.7 ± 5.0	4.6 ± 4.0	7.1 ± 6.0	–
Disposition index (min^{-1})	–	–	526 ± 360	377 ± 282	760 ± 491	–

Sources: Hansen, B.C. and Bodkin, N.L., *Diabetelogia,* 29, 713–719, 1986; Raman, A. et al., *J Gerontol,* 60, 1518–1524, 2005; Najafian, B. et al., *Diabetes Metab Res Rev,* 27, 341–347, 2010.

[a] Mean ± SEM.
[b] Hansen and Bodkin (1986).
[c] Mean ± SD (range).
[d] Raman et al. (2005).
[e] Najafian et al. (2010).

6.6.3 Fructosamine and Glycated Hemoglobin

The measurement of nonenzymatically glycated proteins furnishes a biomarker of long-term glucoregulation that is less subject to artifact than the measurement of blood glucose. Studies have indicated that fructosamine or glycated hemoglobin may provide effective and objective measures for monitoring glycemic control of diabetic animals in both the clinical setting and in research studies (Cefalu et al., 1993; Wagner et al., 1996). Significant species differences exist, however, and it is imperative that species-specific reference ranges be established. Cefalu et al. (1993) concluded that the glycated hemoglobin values for rhesus monkeys were 40% higher than those of cynomolgus monkeys as determined by automated high-pressure liquid chromatography (HPLC). Varied species RBC life span or age-dependent differences in the rates of hemoglobin glycosylation were suggested as possible causes for this discrepancy. Using HPLC, the extra peak for hemoglobin A1c

TABLE 6.18
Clinical Parameters to Assess Glucose Metabolism in Fasted Normal Cynomolgus Monkeys on a High Fructose or Standard Primate Chow Diet

Parameter	High Fructose Diet	Standard Chow Diet
Number	12 (7M, 5F)	24 (24M, 0F)
Body weight (kg)	6.0 ± 0.9	4.8 ± 0.12
Glucose (mg/dL)	55.2 ± 2.4	57.46 ± 1.63
Glucose AUC	8484 ± 349	–
Glucose K-value	5.2 ± 0.3	–
Insulin (μIU/mL)	12.8 ± 2.2	11.42 ± 0.93
Insulin AUC	7283 ± 1178	–
Fructosamine (μmol/L)	–	184.51 ± 8.59
Free fatty acids (mEq/L)	–	0.75 ± 0.04
Leptin (ng/mL)	7.2 ± 2.4	0.64 ± 0.24
Adiponectin (pg/mL)	–	24.8 ± 3.77
Cholesterol (mg/dL)	136 ± 6.9	107 ± 3.8
HDLC (mg/dL)	67 ± 3.9	40 ± 6
Triglycerides (mg/dL)	86 ± 12.1	31 ± 3.8

Source: Wagner, J.D. et al., ILAR J, 47, 259–271, 2006.

(HbA1c) is similar for baboons and humans, and HbA1c can be used effectively to monitor hyperglycemia in baboons (Heffernan et al., 1995). Fructosamine was reportedly increased in diabetic cynomolgus monkeys and along with glycated hemoglobin may play a role in detecting the presence of asymptomatic hyperglycemia in NHPs (Wagner et al., 1996; Cefalu et al., 1993). Normal values for glycated proteins in rhesus and cynomolgus monkeys are provided in Table 6.19.

6.6.4 Intravenous Glucose Tolerance Test

An intravenous glucose tolerance test (IVGTT) can be used effectively in many NHP species to evaluate the effectiveness of glucose-regulating mechanisms following an intravenously administered dose of glucose (Jen and Hansen, 1988; Wagner et al., 2006). For most NHP, this procedure must be performed under anesthesia. Numerous studies have shown that ketamine hydrochloride has minimal effect on the results of an IVGTT in NHP, specifically rhesus, cynomolgus, and African green monkeys (Jen and Hansen, 1988; Brady and Koritnik, 1985; Streett and Jonas, 1982; Kemnitz and Kraemer, 1982; Castro et al., 1981; Fulmer et al., 1984); however, other investigators concluded that both anesthesia and stress had notable effects on glucose regulation in baboons and squirrel monkeys (Lehmann et al., 1997; Ausman and Gallina 1978). In baboons sedated with ketamine, the first phase insulin secretion, basal insulin, and glucose levels, as well as the glucose clearance, were significantly lower during sedation (Lehmann et al., 1997). Both stress and anesthesia reportedly decrease the glucose assimilation rate in squirrel monkeys, whereas manual restraint, but not ketamine sedation, decreases the glucose assimilation in rhesus and African green monkeys (Fulmer et al., 1984; Ausman and Gallina, 1978).

Many additional variables can affect the results of an IVGTT; consequently, it is important to use a standardized approach. To this end, several methods for performing and analyzing the IVGTT in monkeys have been developed and used successfully for research studies and clinical diagnostics. The most common technique involves the determination of basal glucose and insulin levels following a 12-hour fast. An intravenous bolus of 50% glucose solution dosed at 0.5 mg/kg is injected over a short interval (typically 30 seconds to 3 minutes) and followed by serial blood collections at 3, 5, 10, 20, 30, 40, 50, and 60 minutes from the mid-injection time point. Glucose and insulin are

TABLE 6.19
Normal Values for Glycated Proteins in Rhesus and Cynomolgus Monkeys (Mean ± SD)

	Diet	N	Glucose (mg/dL)	Fructosamine (mMol/L)	Total Glycated Hemoglobin (%)	Hemoglobin A1c (%)
Cynomolgus[a]	Standard diet	190	62 ± 13	1.25 ± 0.2	3.4 ± 0.8	–
	Atherogenic	172	70 ± 18	1.32 ± 0.2	3.5 ± 1.2	–
Rhesus[a]	Atherogenic	142	57 ± 13	1.33 ± 0.2	4.9 ± 0.7	–
Rhesus[b]	Standard diet	11	64 ± 10	–	–	4.2 ± 0.1

Sources: Cefalu, W.T. et al., *Lab Anim Sci,* 43, 73–77, 1993; Najafian, B. et al., *Diabetes Metab Res Rev,* 27, 341–347, 2010.

[a] Cefalu et al. (1993).

[b] Najafian et al. (2010).

determined at each of the time points, and several important parameters are derived from the data. Blood glucose decreases exponentially, and the rate of glucose disappearance can be expressed by the fractional turnover rate (K_G). This rate is determined primarily by the deposition of glucose in hepatocytes under the influence of insulin, but it is also affected by the other factors that regulate serum glucose. This rate of decrease can be calculated by two established methods. The first is $K_G = 0.693/t_{1/2} \times 100\%$ per minute, where $t_{1/2}$ (min) equals the time point at which the glucose concentration drops to one-half of the peak value (Jen and Hansen, 1988). Alternatively, K_G can be calculated by the following formula in rhesus monkeys that represents the log-linear decline of glucose levels (Tigno et al., 2004). The area under the curve for insulin can be calculated by the trapezoidal rule, and it provides a useful assessment of insulin resistance:

$$K_G = \frac{[\ln(\text{glucose at 5 minutes}) - \ln(\text{glucose at 20 minutes})]}{15 \text{ minutes}} \times 100\%$$

The minimal model technique is a modified IVGTT that was initially developed in the late 1970s and has been widely used to determine insulin sensitivity and glucose effectiveness through computer modeling (Pacini et al., 1998). Briefly, this technique started with an injection of glucose followed by an injection of tolbutamide to provoke additional endogenous insulin secretion. Insulin and glucose are then measured frequently for up to 3 hours. The values are then entered into a computer program that compares the prediction of the model with measured values and makes adjustments until it is able to calculate glucose effectiveness (S_G) and insulin sensitivity (S_I) (Bergman, 1989). This technique has been utilized effectively in diabetic and nondiabetic rhesus monkeys (Gresl et al., 2003a, 2003b).

6.6.5 Oral Glucose Tolerance Test

The OGTT offers little benefit over the IVGTT in NHP. For the test to be performed successfully without anesthesia, the animals would have to be willing to quickly ingest substantial quantities of fluids containing glucose and allow blood to be collected through manual restraint. The alternative, which is to administer the fluids through a stomach tube while under anesthesia, poses certain risks such as regurgitation and aspiration. Streett and Jonas (1982) concluded that ketamine impaired absorption of glucose from the intestine. Additional disadvantages of the OGTT include the variability of intestinal absorption, the gastric emptying rate, and the influence of enteric hormones on assay results (Lehmann et al., 1997). Only a few studies utilizing the OGTT have been reported. Two obese and one lean chimpanzee had abnormal glucose patterns. One of 17 lean chimpanzees and 2 of 14 obese chimpanzees had significantly abnormal glucose tolerance curves (Steinetz et al., 1996).

6.6.6 Euglycemic Clamp

The euglycemic clamp is considered the gold standard for determining insulin sensitivity as well as determining the amount of glucose metabolized following a controlled hyperglycemic stimulus. It has been widely used in obesity and type II diabetes studies in rhesus monkeys and baboons (Chavez et al., 2008; Bodkin et al., 1989; Pender et al., 2002). At the start of the procedure, the plasma insulin concentration is acutely increased and maintained at a predetermined level by a prime-continuous infusion of insulin. A variable glucose infusion is administered concurrently to maintain a constant basal level of plasma glucose. Under these conditions, the glucose infusion rate equals glucose uptake in the body and provides a measure of tissue sensitivity to exogenous insulin (DeFronzo et al., 1979); the lower the glucose infusion rate, the greater the degree of insulin resistance. Although the euglycemic clamp provides excellent test characteristics, the euglycemic clamp also has several disadvantages. It is time consuming, labor intensive, expensive, and requires an experienced operator to manage technical difficulty. Insulin resistance has been effectively demonstrated and monitored in both rhesus monkeys and baboons with the euglycemic clamp (Chavez et al., 2008; Hotta et al., 2001; Bodkin et al., 1989).

6.6.7 Renal Function Tests and Urinalysis

Measurements of serum urea nitrogen and creatinine are widely used in NHPs, principally to assess renal function. As in other species, extensive renal disease may occur before significant elevations of BUN and creatinine. In addition, nonrenal factors such as diet and dehydration can cause significant increases in both BUN and creatinine. A slight but progressive increase in creatinine signals progressive deterioration of renal function; thus, an animal's own earlier creatinine values may be of greater importance than the historical reference range in detecting renal dysfunction. In humans and baboons, diurnal variations of serum creatinine, glomerular filtration, and renal execration of creatinine occur (Gavellas et al., 1987; Bos et al., 1993).

Normal ranges for the following urine measurements of renal function have been established for cynomolgus monkeys: (1) specific gravity, (2) creatinine clearance, (3) osmolality clearance, (4) fractional excretion of electrolytes, and (5) urine pH (Table 6.20). This study also suggested that a desmopressin response test at 4 hours post injection is preferable to a water deprivation test in assessing urine concentrating ability (Weekley et al., 2003). The desmopressin-induced urine concentration was determined by administering 0.3–0.4 μg/kg of 1-(3-mercaptopropionic acid)-8-D-arginine vasopressin (4 mg/mL) subcutaneously and placing a urinary catheter under ketamine anesthesia. Urine samples were collected prior to and 4 hours following drug administration. Urine-specific gravity and osmolality were evaluated. A baseline pH range of 6.4–8.2 has been reported for cynomolgus monkeys; however, this range should be interpreted with caution. Different dietary management strategies may affect the normal pH range, and it is not uncommon for some macaque colonies to maintain a normal pH range from 8.0 and 8.5. Consequently, it may be prudent to establish normal pH ranges for individual colonies or groups of animals.

In some species, the clearance of endogenous creatinine can be used to approximate glomerular filtration rate (GFR). In other species such as humans and rats, creatinine is primarily filtered by the glomeruli but also secreted through the renal tubules. GFR in male baboons (*Papio hamadryas*) was evaluated by Gavellas et al. (1987) using either 24-hour creatinine clearance or inulin clearance. The 24-hour creatinine clearance was established in awake, chair-restrained baboons by collecting urine through an external condom catheter for 24 hours. Creatinine clearance was measured using the 24-hour excretion of creatinine and the mean serum creatinine concentration established from multiple venous blood samples collected at the beginning and the end of the 24-hour urine collection. Inulin clearance was calculated in anesthetized and awake, chair-restrained baboons. In both settings, the baboons

TABLE 6.20
Renal Function Tests in Cynomolgus Monkeys (Range)

Measurement	Result
Specific gravity Basal	1.005–1.031
Specific gravity Post desmopressin	1.019–1.043
Urine osmolality (mOsm/kg) Basal	182–1081
Urine osmolality (mOsm/kg) Post desmopressin	432–1298
Urine pH Basal	6.4–8.2
Urine pH Post ammonium chloride	4.1–7.1
Creatinine clearance (mL/kg/min)	1.84–2.53
Osmolality clearance (mL/kg/min)	0.03–0.07
Fractional excretion—sodium (%)	0.17–0.77
Fractional excretion—chloride (%)	0.25–1.08
Fractional excretion—potassium (%)	4.46–19.87

Source: Weekley, L.B. et al., *Contemp Top Lab Anim Sci,* 42, 22–25, 2003.

received an intravenous infusion of 0.45% NaCl solution containing inulin (1.3–1.9 mg/min to achieve a blood level of 20–30 mg/dL) with or without creatinine. Three to four urine collections were obtained for clearance measurements after 90–120 minutes of equilibration. Clearance periods were 15 and 60 minutes for anesthetized and awake animals, respectively. Blood was collected at the midpoint of each period. Inulin was measured and renal clearance determined by conventional methods. Through this detailed assessment of GFR, it was found that creatinine clearance overestimated GFR and that the renal mechanisms for excretion of creatinine and inulin are different. Creatinine clearance has also been used to assess kidney function in chimpanzees, and normal ranges are provided in Table 6.21.

6.6.7.1 Urinalysis

In owl monkeys, the urine protein/creatinine (UPC) ratio correlated with 24-hour urine protein loss similar to dogs. Thus, calculating a UPC could replace timed urine collections in most clinical circumstances. In addition, positive linear relationships existed between the following pairs of analytes similar to dogs: (1) urine protein and urine creatinine, (2) urine protein and 24-hour urine protein loss, (3) UPC and 24-hour protein loss, and (5) urine protein and urine-specific gravity. Owl monkeys have a lower urine-specific gravity range (1.002–1.023) as compared to dogs (Weller et al., 1991b). In general, many NHP species including macaques and chimpanzees have a lower urine-specific gravity range as compared to dogs and humans. Reference ranges for normal urinary analytes and selected serum parameters used to assess renal function are provided for *A. nancymae*, *A. vociferans*, and *S. peruviensis*, in Tables 6.22 through 6.25 (Baer, 1994; Weller et al., 1993a, 1993b, 1996).

Weller et al. (1993b) measured urinary alkaline phosphatase (UAP), urinary aspartate aminotransferase (UAST), and N-acetyl-β-D-glucosaminidase (NAG) and calculated enzyme:creatinine ratios. The NAG creatinine ratio was similar to normal values for the dog, man, horse, and cat, whereas UAP and UAST creatinine ratios were significantly higher. These elevations were attributed to either a species difference or a high prevalence of subclinical disease. In addition, the investigators concluded that the measurement of UAP, UAST, and NAG, expressed as $IU/g_{Creatinine}$, is a more sensitive marker for early renal injury than urinary enzymes alone.

TABLE 6.21
Creatinine Clearance in Chimpanzees (5th to 95th percentile)

Measurement	Unit	Median	Result
Age	years	2	1–9
Body surface area	m^2	0.56	0.4–0.94
Height (head to heel)	cm	54.3	38.6–119
Body weight	Kg	29.6	15.0–38.0
Serum creatinine	μmol/L	95.0	64.5–132.6
Volume of urine	mL/24 hours	850	300–1700
Urinary creatinine	mmol/L	3.79	0.66–11.6
Urinary creatinine	mmol/24 hours	2.94	0.6–5.95
Creatinine clearance	mL/min	22.5	4.0–62.5

Source: Eder, G., *Eur J Clin Chem Biochem*, 34, 889–896, 1996.

TABLE 6.22
Normal Urine Parameters in Owl Monkeys

Parameter	Result
Specific gravity	1.010 ± 0.001 (1.002–1.023)
Volume (mL/kg/day)	9–303
Urinalysis—Dipstick	
Protein	0–3+
Glucose	0–1+
Ketones	0–2+
Bilirubin	0
Urobilinogen	0
Occult blood	0–4+
pH	6–8.5
Appearance—color	Light-dark yellow
Appearance—transparency	Clear-cloudy
Urinalysis—Microscopic	
Red blood cells	Rare-few (3–5/hpf)
White blood cells	Rare-occasional
Epithelial cells	Rare-occasional squamous Occasional renal tubular
Casts	Occasional granular
Crystals	Few-moderate triple phosphate Rare-calcium oxalate

Source: Baer, J.F., *Aotus: The Owl Monkey*, Academic Press, San Diego, CL, 1994.

Chimpanzees, like many primate species in captivity, receive a diet of vegetables, fruit, and processed biscuits that contain primarily soy-based proteins. Consequently, it is common to see a urine pH of 8.5 (Kelly et al., 2004). Small levels of hemoglobinuria and protein are frequently found in urine from normal chimpanzees. These findings may be attributable to the highly alkaline urine,

TABLE 6.23
Urinary Enzyme Concentrations in the Owl Monkey (*Aotus nancymae*)

Enzyme	Mean ± SD	Range
Alkaline phosphatase (ALP) (IU/L)	22.48 ± 18.59	2–80
ALP urine creatinine ratio (IU/g Cr)	106.20 ± 168–87	9.5–1000
N-acetyl-β-D-glucosaminidase (NAG) (IU/L)	2.12 ± 1.47	0.1–8
NAG urine creatinine ratio (IU/$g_{Creatinine}$)	7.60 ± 9.00	0.43–60
Aspartate aminotransferase (AST) (IU/L)	15.95 ± 12.85	1–67
AST urine creatinine ratio (IU/$g_{Creatinine}$)	65.14 ± 62.00	7.46–291.30

Source: Weller, R.E. et al., *J Med Primatol,* 22, 340–347, 1993b.

TABLE 6.24
Select Serum and Urine Analytes for Owl Monkeys (*Aotus nancymae* and *Aotus vociferans*) [Mean ± SD (Range)]

	A. nancymae N = 62		*A. vociferans* N = 24	
Measurement	**Mean ± SD**	**Range**	**Mean ± SD**	**Range**
Serum creatinine (mg/dL)	0.91 ± 0.14	0.5–1.2	0.91 ± 0.14	0.6–1.4
Serum calcium (mg/dL)	9.84 ± 0.67	8.6–11.9	9.42 ± 0.48	8.6–10.6
Serum phosphorus (mg/dL)	5.32 ± 1.96	1.8–9.9	4.23 ± 1.23	2.7–7.3
Serum potassium (mEq/L)	3.77 ± 0.7	2.3–6.3	3.33 ± 0.71	2.4–6.0
Serum sodium (mEq/L)	151.89 ± 5.09	129–160	148.08 ± 2.60	143–154
Serum glucose (mg/dL)	147.66 ± 31.48	62–229	136.17 ± 28.57	95–224
Serum urea nitrogen (mg/dL)	17.74 ± 5.28	7–31	13.71 ± 3.71	8–23
Serum protein (g/dL)	7.46 ± 0.68	5.9–8.8	7.40 ± 0.58	6.1–8.6
Serum albumin (g/L)	4.53 ± 0.61	2.5–6.3	4.43 ± 0.58	2.9–5.8
Urine creatinine (mg/dL)	34.74 ± 27.63	6.0–135	37.75 ± 27.67	8–123
Urine calcium (mg/dL)	3.55 ± 2.69	0.3–12.9	6.97 ± 5.00	1.4–22.6
Urine phosphorus (mg/dL)	30.49 ± 23.28	1.2–90.4	24.35 ± 18.02	0.7–63
Urine sodium (mEq/L)	11.34 ± 9.20	0–42	9.50 ± 7.52	1–32
Urine potassium (mEq/L)	29.69 ± 22.19	0–99.9	23.68 ± 13.59	4.4–48.7
Urine glucose (mg/dL)	9.15 ± 8.46	0–54	11.17 ± 9.79	2–32
Urine protein (mg/dL)	41.16 ± 34.15	4.0–147	NA	NA
Urine protein/creatinine (UPC) ratio	1.48 ± 1.49	0.26–9.0	1.97 ± 2.33	0.34–10.33
Urine-specific gravity	1.009 ± 0.005	1.002–1.023	NA	NA
Urine volume (mg/16 hours)	81.94 ± 94.75	15–481	88.42 ± 69.40	15–255
Endogenous creatinine clearance	2.23 ± 0.67	0.97–4.52	2.51 ± 0.72	1.40–4.57
Total Daily Excretion				
Calcium (mg/kg)	3.85 ± 2.89	4.41–12.45	7.39 ± 4.54	1.91–19.38
Phosphorus (mg/kg)	31.90 ± 21.20	1.14–86.45	25.68 ± 17.68	1.63–73.12
Sodium (mEq/kg)	1.17 ± 0.88	0–4.36	1.14 ± 0.80	0.01–3.20
Potassium (mEq/kg)	2.99 ± 1.70	0.78–10.45	2.59 ± 1.32	0.87–5.94
Glucose (mg/kg)	9.45 ± 9.71	0–58.47	10.80 ± 10.92	3.25–54.84
Protein (mg/kg)	45.62 ± 45.36	6.46–256.35	67.66 ± 88.05	12.7–425

(*Continued*)

TABLE 6.24 (*Continued*)
Select Serum and Urine Analytes for Owl Monkeys *(Aotus nancymae* and *Aotus vociferans)* [Mean ± SD (Range)]

Measurement	*A. nancymae* N = 62		*A. vociferans* N = 24	
	Mean ± SD	Range	Mean ± SD	Range
Fractional Excretion (%)				
Calcium	1.24 ± 1.01	0.12–5.30	2.51 ± 2.03	0.73–8.32
Phosphorus	18.43 ± 9.28	1.06–39.80	17.80 ± 12.69	1.63–54.35
Sodium	0.24 ± 0.19	0–0.87	0.21 ± 0.15	0.02–0.69
Potassium	24.61 ± 11.10	2.40–56.55	22.95 ± 12.13	9.80–50.31
Glucose	0.21 ± 0.28	0–1.7	0.34 ± 0.52	0.09–2.58

Sources: Weller, R.E. et al., *J Med Primatol,* 22, 368–373, 1993a; Weller, R.E. et al., *J Med Primatol,* 25, 46–52, 1996.
Mean ± SD (range)

TABLE 6.25
Select Serum and Urine Analytes for Squirrel Monkeys [Mean ± SD (Range)]

Measurement	Saimiri peruviensis N = 20	
	Mean ± SD	Range
Serum creatinine (mg/dL)	0.93 ± 0.18	0.6–1.2
Serum calcium (mg/dL)	9.55 ± 0.27	9.0–10.0
Serum phosphorus (mg/dL)	4.67 ± 1.09	2.4–6.8
Serum potassium (mEq/L)	3.97 ± 0.36	3.4–4.7
Serum sodium (mEq/L)	149.21 ± 3.28	144–155
Serum glucose (mg/dL)	102.47 ± 20.43	57–153
Serum urea nitrogen (mg/dL)	34.89 ± 5.93	24–46
Serum protein (g/L)	6.34 ± 0.56	5.5–7.4
Urine creatinine (mg/dL)	64.68 ± 30.82	14–159
Urine calcium (mg/dL)	8.67 ± 4.23	3.1–20.4
Urine phosphorus (mg/dL)	185.05 ± 79.32	38–360
Urine sodium (mEq/L)	12.32 ± 7.70	2–31
Urine potassium (mEq/L)	88.89 ± 37.47	17–152
Urine glucose (mg/dL)	26.95 ± 33.84	5–142
Urine protein (mg/dL)	21.32 ± 11.01	9–53
Urine protein/creatinine (UPC) ratio	0.43 ± 0.49	0.13–2.36
Urine-specific gravity	1.023 ± 0.006	1.010–1.030
Urine volume (mL/16 hours)	23.21 ± 32.0	8–152
Endogenous creatinine clearance	1.65 ± 0.50	0.78–2.47
Total Daily Excretion		
Calcium (mg/kg)	3.51 ± 2.34	1.04–9.99
Phosphorus (mg/kg)	68.72 ± 29.44	7.73–124.14
Sodium (mEq/kg)	0.50 ± 0.33	0.03–1.25
Potassium (mEq/kg)	3.25 ± 1.37	0.43–6.14
Glucose (mg/kg)	11.29 ± 13.96	1.15–45.33
Protein (mg/kg)	10.53 ± 15.25	2.04–71.24

(*Continued*)

TABLE 6.25 (*Continued*)
Select Serum and Urine Analytes for Squirrel Monkeys [Mean ± SD (Range)]

	Saimiri peruviensis N = 20	
Measurement	**Mean ± SD**	**Range**
Fractional Excretion (%)		
Calcium	1.69 ± 1.07	0.51–4.40
Phosphorus	55.59 ± 19.25	16.46–87.36
Sodium	0.14 ± 0.09	0.02–0.34
Potassium	35.74 ± 13.75	11.74–60.51
Glucose	0.51 ± 0.64	0.09–2.64

Source: Weller, R.E. et al., *J Med Primatol,* 25, 46–52, 1996.
Mean ± SD (range)

TABLE 6.26
Urine Electrolyte Values in Pregnant Female Baboons (*N* = 13)

Parameter	Mean ± SD	Range
Serum sodium (mEq/L)	137.08 ± 2.29	133–140
Serum potassium (mEq/L)	3.15 ± 0.32	2.7–3.8
Urine sodium (mEq/L)	69.15 ± 10.36	51–82
Urine potassium (mEq/L)	29.37 ± 8.85	15–44

Source: Cissik, J.H. et al., *Am J Primatol,* 11, 277–284, 1986.

which can lead to false-positive proteinuria and hemoglobinuria. Additionally, false proteinuria may result from the contamination inherent in voided samples (Kaur and Huffman, 2004). Chimpanzees undergo a monthly menstrual cycle, and erythrocytes and hemaglobinuria are commonly noted in females during menstruation. The amount of creatinine excreted in the urine of chimpanzees is significantly less than that in the urine of humans. This finding may be an important consideration when following human dosages for drugs that are excreted through the kidneys. The potential for prolonged serum concentration as compared to humans exists (Eder, 1996).

Urine electrolyte values for pregnant female baboons are provided in Table 6.26. Very little information exists in the literature on normal urinalysis findings for marmosets and tamarins. Physiological glycosuria reportedly occurs in normal tamarins (Gatesman, 1986).

6.6.8 Miscellaneous

A noninvasive method was recently developed for measuring urinary levels of two additional hormones associated with lactation and parturition, oxytocin and arginine vasopressin (AVP), in squirrel monkeys. This assay utilized HPLC separation of urine followed by a radioimmunoassay to demonstrate that measurable levels of oxytocin and AVP are present and that these levels may alter with changing social conditions (Seltzer and Ziegler, 2007). Luteinizing and FSHs are high in male rhesus monkeys during the first 3 months of life, decreasing thereafter to low or undetectable levels (Frawley and Neill, 1979).

6.7 SERUM REFERENCE INTERVALS/RANGES FOR SELECT NHP SPECIES

Tables 6.27 through 6.35 illustrate reference intervals/ranges for select NHP species.

TABLE 6.27
Reference Intervals for Baboons Expressed as [Mean ± SD (Range), 10th to 90th Percentile]

Reference	Year	Species/Strain	Sex	Age	*N*	BUN mg/dL	Creatinine mg/dL	ALT IU/L	AST IU/L	ALP IU/L	LDH IU/mL	T. Prot g/dL	Albumin g/dL	Globulin g/dL	Glucose mg/dL
Havill et al.	2003	*Papio hamadryas*	Both	Infant	47–106	12.1 ± 6.1	0.67 ± 0.13	32.8 ± 14.7	46.3 ± 14.3	1221.1 ± 414.4	–	6.26 ± 0.47	3.79 ± 0.35	2.46 ± 0.42	–
Hack and Gleiser	1982	*Papio* spp.	M	Adult	15	19 ± 2	1.6 ± 0.2	34 ± 13	27 ± 4	130 ± 36	181 ± 52	6.8 ± 0.5	3.4 ± 0.4	3.4 ± 0.4	82 ± 16
–	–	–	F	Adult	16	16 ± 6	1.4 ± 0.2	34 ± 13	23 ± 7	152 ± 48	199 ± 68	6.9 ± 0.5	2.8 ± 0.5	4.0 ± 0.5	93 ± 30
–	–	–	Both	Juv	43	17 ± 4	1.0 ± 0.2	26 ± 11	24 ± 6	626 ± 233	250 ± 89	6.8 ± 0.5	3.7 ± 0.3	3.1 ± 0.4	80 ± 16
Renquist et al.	1977	*Papio hamadryas* (Sacred baboon)	M	N/A	8–18	15.8 ± 3.1	0.90 ± 0.19	25.72 ± 9.31	19.39 ± 7.08	–	171.6 ± 44.5	6.83 ± 0.41	–	–	82.1 ± 5.0
–	–		F	N/A	10–59	16.2 ± 4.2	0.88 ± 0.19	38.02 ± 20.23	25.02 ± 9.98	–	193.1 ± 104.8	7.29 ± 0.51	–	–	83.7 ± 18.7
Steyn et al.	1975	*Papio ursinus* (Chacma baboon)	Both	>3 years	35–64	48.0 ± 10.9 (19–80)	–	14.0 ± 6.8 (5–36)	16 ± 6.2 (6–35)	555 ± 398 (145–1548)	266 ± 101 (133–759)	6.43 ± 0.74 (4.4–8.7)	3.43 ± 0.59 (1.49–4.34)	–	96.46 ± 27.03 (43–160)

Reference	Year	Species/Strain	Sex	Age	*N*	T. Bili mg/dL	D. Bili mg/dL	Calcium mg/dL (mEq/L)	Phosphorus mg/dL (mEq/L)	Cholesterol mg/dL	Triglycerides mg/dL	Uric Acid mg/dL	Sodium mEq/L	Potassium mEq/L	Chloride mEq/L	CO_2 mEq/L
Havill et al.	2003	*Papio hamadryas*	Both	Infant	47–106	–	–	–	–	135.0 ± 39.5	–	–	144.1 ± 2.8	4.3 ± 0.7	110.7 ± 2.6	20.7 ± 3.9
Hack and Gleiser	1982	*Papio* spp.	M	Adult	15	0.4 ± 0.0	–	9.0 ± 0.9	3.5 ± 1.0	91 ± 13	45 ± 18	–	150 ± 2	4.2 ± 0.3	104 ± 2	–
	–	–	F	Adult	16	0.3 ± 0.1	--	8.8 ± 0.9	2.6 ± 1.3	101 ± 22	78 ± 54	–	151 ± 4	4.3 ± 0.4	107 ± 2	–
			Both	Juv	43	0.5 ± 0.1	--	8.7 ± 0.5	6.8 ± 0.8	123 ± 34	40 ± 14	–	150 ± 4	3.7 ± 0.3	109 ± 3	–
Renquist et al.	1977	*Papio hamadryas* (Sacred baboon)	M	N/A	8–18	0.10 ± 0.08	0.03 ± 0.02	–	–	90.7 ± 13.0	–	1.08 ± 0.94	–	–	–	–
			F	N/A	10–59	0.12 ± 0.07	0.04 ± 0.03	–	–	99.4 ± 16.8	–	1.28 ± 0.56	–	–	–	–

(Continued)

TABLE 6.27 (*Continued*)
Reference Intervals for Baboons Expressed as [Mean ± SD (Range), 10th to 90th Percentile]

Reference	Year	Species/Strain	Sex	Age	*N*	T. Bili mg/dL	D. Bili mg/dL	Calcium mg/dL (mEq/L)	Phosphorus mg/dL (mEq/L)	Cholesterol mg/dL	Triglycerides mg/dL	Uric Acid mg/dL	Sodium mEq/L	Potassium mEq/L	Chloride mEq/L	CO_2 mEq/L
Steyn et al.	1975	*Papio ursinus* (Chacma baboon)	Both	>3 years	35–64	–	–	[5.16 ± 0.52] (4.3–6.2)	[1.63 ± 0.6] (0.3–3.1)	127 ± 47.8 (46–408)	–	–	144 ± 4.7 (135–156)	3.75 ± 0.43 (3.10–4.80)	104 ± 3.95 (90–110)	28 ± 5.27 (9.8–40.1) 9

Reference	Year	Species/Strain	Sex	Age	*N*	Iron µg/dL	TIBC µg/dL	Magnesium mg/dL	Amylase IU/L	Lipase IU/mL
Hack and Gleiser	1982	*Papio* spp.	M	Adult	15	–	–	–	402 ± 106	19 ± 21
	–	–	F	Adult	16	–	–	–	264 ± 64	56 ± 56
	–	–	Both	Juv	43	–	–	–	286 ± 86	25 ± 18
Renquist et al.	1977	Papio hamadryas	M	N/A	–	–	–	–	184.0 ± 71.1	0.62 ± 0.45
	–	–	F	N.A	–	–	–	–	217.3 ± 101.9	0.47 ± 0.60
de la Pena et al.	1970	*Papio* spp.	M	Adult	40	152 ± 53 (54–268)	281 ± 84 (134–434)	1.7 ± 0.3 (1.3–2.6)	233 ± 80 (110–454)	–
	–	–	F	Adult	98	147 ± 55 (44–363)	260 ± 78 (92–490)	1.6 ± 0.2 (1.2–2.3)	220 ± 64 (61–476)	–

ALT, alanine aminotransferase; ALP, alkaline phosphatase; AST, aspartate aminotransferase; BUN, blood urea nitrogen; D. Bili, direct bilirubin; T. Bili, total bilirubin; T. Prot, total protein; on binding capacity.

TABLE 6.28
Reference Intervals for African Green Monkeys (Expressed as Mean ± SD [Range])

Reference	Year	Sex	Age	*N*	BUN mg/dL	Creatinine mg/dL	ALT IU/L	AST IU/L	ALP IU/L	CK IU/L	GGT IU/L	T. Prot g/dL	Albumin g/dL	Globulin g/dL	Glucose mg/dL
Liddie et al.	2010	M[a]	Not given	92–206	19.8 ± 4.4 (10.9–28.7)	0.9 ± 0.2 (0.5–1.4)	46.1 ± 22.6 (0.9–91.3)	48.0 ± 23.5 (0.9–95.1)	163.9 ± 135.0 (32.0–433.8)	1510 ± 1667 (193–4843)	41.8 ± 16.3 (9.2–74.3)	6.9 ± 0.5 (5.9–8.0)	4.1 ± 0.4 (3.3–4.9)	2.9 ± 0.6 (1.6–4.1)	82 ± 18 (46–118)
–	–	F[a]	Not given	90–121	20.1 ± 5.1 (9.9–30.3)	0.7 ± 0.2 (0.3–1.1)	47.5 ± 19.6 (8.3–86.6)	62.2 ± 26.5 (9.2–115.2)	273.3 ± 163.5 (56.0–600.2)	2858 ± 1872 (140–6603)	40.3 ± 16.7 (6.9–73.7)	6.9 ± 0.5 (5.8–8.0)	4.0 ± 0.5 (3.1–4.9)	2.9 ± 0.7 (1.6–4.3)	80 ± 19 (43–118)
Casaco et al.	2010	M[b]	2–3 years	9–33	–	0.75 ± 0.13	59.0 ± 54.8	64.9 ± 41.7	1038.4 ± 328.4	–	57.0 ± 13.1	6.51 ± 0.63	4.67 ± 0.48	–	108 ± 41
–	–	F[b]	2–3 years	9–33	–	0.74 ± 0.13	39.9 ± 18.9	59.6 ± 26.1	923.1 ± 309.7	–	57.9 ± 17.1	6.74 ± 0.54	4.79 ± 0.48	–	113 ± 55
Sato	2005	F	1 year	8	23 ± 2	0.7 ± 0.1	61 ± 11	59 ± 13	628 ± 127	863 ± 356	35 ± 16	6.6 ± 0.5	4.4 ± 0.3	2.3 ± 0.4	56 ± 9
–	–	F	2–3 years	14	19 ± 4	0.8 ± 0.1	52 ± 10	53 ± 14	495 ± 169	903 ± 593	30 ± 10	6.9 ± 0.4	4.1 ± 0.2	2.8 ± 0.4	56 ± 26
–	–	F	4–6 years	24	18 ± 4	0.9 ± 0.2	55 ± 13	58 ± 16	147 ± 65	1131 ± 621	31 ± 14	6.8 ± 0.3	3.9 ± 0.4	2.9 ± 0.2	43 ± 24
–	–	F	7–10 years	24	16 ± 4	0.8 ± 0.2	62 ± 24	50 ± 9	107 ± 36	793 ± 293	32 ± 10	7.0 ± 0.5	3.7 ± 0.4	3.3 ± 0.3	58 ± 24
–	–	F	11–14 years	5	20 ± 5	0.8 ± 0.1	88 ± 36	51 ± 13	97 ± 20	886 ± 415	37 ± 12	6.9 ± 0.6	3.6 ± 0.4	3.3 ± 0.4	72 ± 40
–	–	F	>15 years	5	19 ± 4	0.9 ± 0.2	54 ± 10	48 ± 18	99 ± 17	729 ± 345	33 ± 6	6.9 ± 0.5	3.6 ± 0.3	3.2 ± 0.6	60 ± 19
–	–	M	1 year	7	23 ± 4	0.7 ± 0.2	57 ± 11	52 ± 12	661 ± 98	457 ± 182	38 ± 18	6.5 ± 0.3	4.2 ± 0.3	2.3 ± 0.4	69 ± 30
–	–	M	2–3 years	14	19 ± 2	0.8 ± 0.1	66 ± 21	50 ± 10	647 ± 131	929 ± 977	31 ± 9	6.8 ± 0.3	4.3 ± 0.3	2.5 ± 0.4	66 ± 11

(Continued)

TABLE 6.28 (*Continued*)
Reference Intervals for African Green Monkeys (Expressed as Mean ± SD [Range])

Reference	Year	Sex	Age	*N*	BUN mg/dL	Creatinine mg/dL	ALT IU/L	AST IU/L	ALP IU/L	CK IU/L	GGT IU/L	T. Prot g/dL	Albumin g/dL	Globulin g/dL	Glucose mg/dL
–	–	M	4–6 years	7	17 ± 3	0.9 ± 0.1	68 ± 23	65 ± 14	118 ± 23	1149 ± 741	30 ± 12	6.9 ± 0.3	4.3 ± 0.4	2.6 ± 0.5	51 ± 13
–	–	M	7–10 years	16	17 ± 4	0.9 ± 0.2	69 ± 24	53 ± 21	104 ± 32	1108 ± 804	36 ± 9	6.9 ± 0.3	3.9 ± 0.3	3.0 ± 0.3	56 ± 22
–	–	M	11–14 years	10	19 ± 4	0.8 ± 0.2	66 ± 13	53 ± 31	109 ± 44	554 ± 357	31 ± 18	7.1 ± 0.4	3.7 ± 0.4	3.4 ± 0.6	83 ± 43
–	–	M	>15 years	6	24 ± 6	0.9 ± 0.3	75 ± 23	53 ± 23	116 ± 42	1118 ± 1117	31 ± 3	6.6 ± 0.3	3.4 ± 0.5	3.2 ± 0.4	75 ± 9

Reference	Year	Sex	Age	*N*	BUN mg/dL	Creatinine mg/dL	ALT IU/L	AST IU/L	ALP IU/L	CK IU/L	GGT IU/L	T. Prot g/dL	Albumin g/dL	Globulin g/dL	Glucose mg/dL
Liddie et al.	2010	M[a]	Not given	92–206	0.8 ± 0.6 (0.1–1.9)	–	9.1 ± 0.6 (7.8–10.3)	5.3 ± 1.6 (2.1–8.5)	114.9 ± 18.4 (78.0–151.8)	152 ± 5 (142–162)	3.5 ± 0.5 (2.4–4.6)	105 ± 7 (91–118)	–	473 ± 133 (208–738)	73 ± 34 (6–141)
–	–	F[a]	Not given	90–121	0.4 ± 0.5 (0.1–1.3)	–	9.1 ± 0.7 (7.7–10.4)	5.2 ± 1.6 (2.0–8.4)	131.7 ± 18.9 (94.0–169.5)	151 ± 5 (141–160)	3.8 ± 0.7 (2.5–5.1)	107 ± 7 (93–120)	–	430 ± 139 (151–709)	74 ± 30 (14–135)
Casaco et al.	2010	M[b]	2–3 years	9–33	0.29 ± 0.22	–	9.6 ± 0.76	7.0 ± 1.6	139 ± 20	–	3.93 ± 0.24	105.3 ± 2.0	–	–	–
–	–	F[b]	2–3 years	9–33	0.27 ± 0.14	–	9.6 ± 1.0	6.5 ± 2.0	140 ± 30	–	3.69 ± 0.24	105.3 ± 2.2	–	–	–
Sato	2005	F	1 year	8	0.2 ± 0.10	0.1 ± 0.05	8.9 ± 0.3	3.9 ± 0.9	139 ± 28	153 ± 1	3.6 ± 0.6	110 ± 2	19.7 ± 6.8	–	–
–	–	F	2–3 years	14	0.2 ± 0.05	0.1 ± 0.05	8.8 ± 0.2	3.2 ± 1.2	131 ± 17	151 ± 2	3.4 ± 0.3	108 ± 3	17.8 ± 5.6	–	–
–	–	F	4–6 years	24	0.2 ± 0.05	0.1 ± 0.04	8.2 ± 0.4	3.1 ± 1.2	128 ± 17	149 ± 2	3.5 ± 0.4	107 ± 2	17.3 ± 6.6	–	–

(*Continued*)

TABLE 6.28 (*Continued*)
Reference Intervals for African Green Monkeys (Expressed as Mean ± SD [Range])

–	–	F	7–10 years	24	0.2 ± 0.07	0.1 ± 0.05	8.3 ± 0.6	3.2 ± 1.0	134 ± 36	151 ± 2	3.4 ± 0.3	109 ± 1	19.8 ± 6.5	–	–
–	–	F	11–14 years	5	0.2 ± 0.06	0.1 ± 0.04	8.5 ± 0.4	2.6 ± 0.7	144 ± 30	151 ± 2	3.5 ± 0.3	108 ± 2	17.0 ± 7.2	–	–
–	–	F	>15 years	5	0.3 ± 0.12	0.1 ± 0.05	8.1 ± 04	3.3 ± 1.1	154 ± 26	151 ± 2	3.6 ± 0.4	109 ± 4	17.8 ± 7.0	–	–
–	–	M	1 year	7	0.2 ± 0.08	0.1 ± 0.05	8.6 ± 0.5	4.9 ± 1.4	134 ± 21	150 ± 3	3.7 ± 0.8	106 ± 3	15.9 ± 6.8	–	–
–	–	M	2–3 years	14	0.2 ± 0.11	0.1 ± 0.04	8.9 ± 0.3	3.7 ± 1.0	143 ± 24	152 ± 3	3.5 ± 0.4	108 ± 2	21.4 ± 6.9	–	–
–	–	M	4–6 years	7	0.3 ± 0.08	0.1 ± 0.04	8.6 ± 0.4	3.8 ± 1.0	135 ± 17	151 ± 3	4.2 ± 0.3	108 ± 2	25.2 ± 2.9	–	–
–	–	M	7–10 years	16	0.3 ± 0.10	0.1 ± 0.06	8.7 ± 0.4	4.5 ± 1.0	125 ± 18	152 ± 3	4.1 ± 0.4	106 ± 3	26.1 ± 6.8	–	–
–	–	M	11–14 years	10	0.3 ± 0.08	0.1 ± 0.04	8.7 ± 0.7	4.5 ± 1.1	147 ± 17	151 ± 5	5.0 ± 15	104 ± 4	25.2 ± 9.9	–	–
–	–	M	>15 years	6	0.3 ± 0.15	0.1 ± 0.04	8.7 ± 05	5.7 ± 1.3	140 ± 28	152 ± 2	4.0 ± 0.5	105 ± 3	29.2 ± 3.4	–	–

ALT, alanine aminotransferase; ALP, alkaline phosphatase; AST, aspartate aminotransferase; BUN, blood urea nitrogen; CK, creatine kinase; D. Bili, direct bilirubin; GGT, gamma glutamyl transferase; T. Bili, total bilirubin; T. Prot, total protein.

[a] All monkeys resided on St. Kitts in the Caribbean.

[b] Born in Cuba.

TABLE 6.29

Reference Intervals for Owl Monkeys [Expressed as Mean ± SD]

Reference	Year	Species/ Strain	Sex	Age	*N*	BUN mg/dL	Creatinine mg/dL	ALT IU/L	ALP IU/L	GGT IU/L	T. Prot g/dL	Albumin g/dL	Glucose mg/dL
Malaga et al.	1991	*Karyotype I*	F	Adult	124	15.4 ± 5.3	0.99 ± 0.27	50 ± 43.6	527 ± 461	16.1 ± 10	8.4 ± 1.0	4.4 ± 0.5	143 ± 36
–	–	–	M	Adult	130	15.2 ± 5.5	1.03 ± 0.44	43.0 ± 31.1	462 ± 477	18 ± 13.8	8.2 ± 0.7	4.3 ± 0.4	135 ± 34
Baer	1994	Karyotype I	Both	Adult	254	15 ± 5.4	1.0 ± 0.4	47 ± 37	494 ± 469	17 ± 14	8.3 ± 0.9	4.4 ± 0.5	139 ± 35
–	–	Karyotype II	Both	Adult	57	15 ± 6.7	1.0 ± 0.2	44 ± 34	183 ± 151	20 ± 14	8.0 ± 0.7	3.8 ± 0.5	153 ± 39
–	–	Karyotype III	Both	Adult	53	17 ± 11	1.1 ± 0.4	49 ± 35	143 ± 87	23 ± 18	8.1 ± 1.1	3.7 ± 0.5	150 ± 47
–	–	Karyotype V	Both	Adult	35	15 ± 8.9	1.0 ± 0.3	59 ± 34	364 ± 381	26 ± 21	8.2 ± 0.5	4.6 ± 0.4	172 ± 40

Reference	Year	Species/Strain	T. Bili mg/dL	Calcium	Phosphorus	Cholesterol mg/dL	Sodium mEq/L	Potassium mEq/L
Malaga et al.	1991	*Karyotype I*	0.8 ± 0.5	10.6 ± 1.1	4.1 ± 1.6	140 ± 39	–	–
–	–	–	0.8 ± 0.3	10.2 ± 0.9	3.9 ± 1.4	161 ± 53	–	–
Baer	1994	Karyotype I	0.8 ± 0.4	10.4 ± 1.0	4.0 ± 1.5	150 ± 46	152 ± 5	3.8 ± 0.7
–	–	Karyotype II	0.5 ± 0.2	9.3 ± 0.9	4.4 ± 1.5	91 ± 34	156 ± 9	4.6 ± 1.6
–	–	Karyotype III	0.5 ± 0.2	9.2 ± 0.9	4.6 ± 1.5	111 ± 44	154 ± 6	4.8 ± 2.0
		Karyotype V	0.7 ± 0.2	9.6 ± 0.7	4.8 ± 1.5	99 ± 34	148 ± 3	3.3 ± 0.7

ALT, alanine aminotransferase; ALP, alkaline phosphatase; AST, aspartate aminotransferase; BUN, blood urea nitrogen; GGT, gamma glutamyl transferase; T. Bili, total bilirubin; T. Prot, total protein.

TABLE 6.30

Reference Intervals for Squirrel Monkeys [Expressed as Mean ± SD]

Reference	Year	Species/ Strain	Sex	Age	*N*	BUN mg/dL	Creatinine mg/dL	ALT IU/L	AST IU/L	ALP IU/L	LDH IU/L	GGT IU/L	T. Prot g/dL	Albumin g/dL	Globulin g/dL
Williams	2006	*Saimiri boliviensis*	M	Infant	2–83	–	0.66 ± 0.11	49.8 ± 42.1	121.2 ± 37.8	1391 ± 289	164 ± 55	15.6 ± 3.4	5.81 ± 0.93	3.54 ± 0.22	2.43 ± 0.29
–	–	–	F	Infant	12–94	–	0.60 ± 0.08	75.4 ± 40.2	132.3 ± 23.3	1148 ± 349	146 ± 31	15.2 ± 5.6	5.84 ± 0.79	3.54 ± 0.17	2.06 ± 0.52
Beland et al.	1979	Non-colony bred	M	Adult	6	31 ± 6	–	–	–	46 ± 21	50 ± 27	–	6.7 ± 1.6	2.8 ± 0.8	–
–	–	–	F	Adult	38	30 ± 9	–	–	–	127 ± 49	46 ± 29	–	7.3 ± 1.2	3.1 ± 0.5	–
–	–	Colony bred	M	Adult	23	46 ± 12	–	–	–	255 ± 134	50 ± 27	–	6.6 ± 0.5	4.2 ± 0.4	–
–	–	–’	F	Adult	27	48 ± 12	–	–	–	325 ± 131	59 ± 27	–	6.4 ± 0.5	4.2 ± 0.4	–

Reference	Year	Species/ Strain	T. Bili mg/dL	Calcium	Phosphorus	Cholesterol mg/dL	Triglycerides mg/dL	Uric acid mg/dL	Amylase IU/dL	Sodium mEq/L	Potassium mEq/L	Chloride mEq/L	CO_2 mEq/L	Glucose mg/dL
Williams	2006	*S. boliviensis*	0.35 ± 0.23	9.23 ± 0.54	7.0 ± 0.8	162.1 ± 31.9	–	–	–	145.2 ± 2.1	4.7 ± 0.7	–	–	93 ± 16
–	–	–	0.63 ± 0.41	9.53 ± 0.35	7.0 ± 0.7	200.7 ± 28.2	–	–	–	145.3 ± 1.9	5.1 ± 0.6	–	–	106 ± 17
Beland et al.	1979	Non-colony bred	0.25 ± 0.18	8.2 ± 0.3	5.5 ± 1.8	176 ± 43	–	1.5 ± 0.4	–	148 ± 4	3.7 ± 0.9	111 ± 1	–	93 ± 54
–	–	–	0.31 ± 0.23	9.1 ± 0.7	4.4 ± 2.2	159 ± 39	–	1.2 ± 0.4	–	148 ± 4	3.5 ± 0.7	110 ± 5	–	76 ± 22
–	–	Colony bred	0.24 ± 0.14	10.3 ± 0.6	5.7 ± 1.8	137 ± 29	–	2.2 ± 0.9	–	149 ± 6	4.8 ± 0.6	104 ± 4	–	134 ± 51
–	–	–	0.26 ± 0.12	10.1 ± 0.7	6.0 ± 2.1	144 ± 24	–	2.0 ± 0.7	–	150 ± 6	4.9 ± 0.9	105 ± 5	–	141 ± 49

ALT, alanine aminotransferase; ALP, alkaline phosphatase; AST, aspartate aminotransferase; BUN, blood urea nitrogen; GGT, gamma glutamyl transferase; LDH, lactate dehydrogenase; T. Bili, total bilirubin; T. Prot, total protein.

TABLE 6.31
Reference Intervals for Marmosets [Expressed as Mean ± SD (Range)]

Reference	Year	Species/ Strain	Sex	Age	*N*	BUN mg/dL	Creatinine mg/dL	ALT IU/L	AST IU/L	ALP IU/L	GGT IU/L	SDH IU/L	LDH IU/mL	T. Prot g/dL	Albumin g/dL
Yarbrough	1984	*Callithrix*	M	Adult	31–82	22 ± 7	0.6 ± 0.2	55 ± 17	151 ± 45	61 ± 27	–	–	218 ± 110	7.2 ± 0.8	5.1 ± 0.7
et al.		*jacchus*				(11–43)	(0.1–1.1)	(14–99)	(76–292)	(22–158)			(7–775)	(4.9–10.7)	(2.1–6.8)
–	–	–	F	Adult	2–34	22 ± 7	0.6 ± 0.2	54 ± 23	146 ± 43	58 ± 17	–	–	216 ± 104	6.6 ± 0.8	4.4 ± 0.7
						(14–34)	(0–0.9)	(17–104)	(70–279)	(23–88)			(115–562)	(4.8–7.6)	(1.7–5.3)
–	–	–	M	Juv	8–28	27 ± 5	0.6 ± 0.3	61 ± 17	161 ± 61	182 ± 88	–	–	275 ± 139	6.3 ± 0.8	4.5 ± 0.7
						(18–39)	(0–1.0)	(35–96)	(72–280)	(60–411)			(120–549)	(5.0–8.3)	(2.7–5.6)
–	–	–	F	Juv	4–15	25 ± 3	0.6 ± 0.3	60 ± 18	152 ± 51	151 ± 46	–	–	233 ± 81	6.3 ± 0.5	4.5 ± 0.5
						(21–30)	(0–1.0)	(31–97)	(63–219)	(82–228)			(148–487)	(5.7–7.2)	(3.7–5.3)
Davy et al.	1984	*C. jacchus*	Both	1–2 years	114–142	--	--	0–14	51–201	164–794	0–19	0.7–9.1	175–787	6.0–8.4	3.5–5.1

Reference	Year	Species/ Strain	T. Bili mg/dL (μmol/L)	Calcium	Phosphorus	Cholesterol mg/dL	Triglycerides mg/dL	Amylase IU/dL	Lipase IU/mL	Sodium mEq/L	Potassium mEq/L	Chloride mEq/L	Iron μmol/L	Glucose mg/dL
Yarbrough	1984	*C. jacchus*	0.48 ± 0.54	10.4 ± 1.3	5.6 ± 1.4	185 ± 49	136 ± 73	930 ± 593	33.0 ± 32.4	161 ± 8	4.1 ± 0.6	107 ± 14	–	172 ± 48
et al.			(0.02–4.41)	(1.5–15.7)	(1.6–10.4)	(100–275)	(48–319)	(445–2871)	(2.5–150.8)	(144–175)	(3.1–5.5)	(99–118)		(74–323)
	–	–	0.25 ± 0.22	9.6 ± 1.5	5.2 ± 1.6	155 ± 47	94 ± 42	1057 ± 720	16.8 ± 11.6	155 ± 4	3.9 ± 0.3	106 ± 4	–	192 ± 52
			(0–0.95)	(1.8–11.2)	(2.1–9.1)	(54–251)	(51–214)	(94–2597)	(1.7–57.0)	(152–158)	(3.7–4.1)	(100–113)		(97–294)
	–	–	0.51 ± 0.45	9.5 ± 2.9	7.7 ± 1.6	150 ± 57	144 ± 125	1531 ± 609	43.0 ± 29.2	159 ± 4	4.2 ± 0.8	–	–	230 ± 45
			(0–1.45)	(1.4–12.1)	(5.0–11.5)	(44–264)	(74–671)	(453–2554)	(1.7–79.8)	(151–164)	(3.4–5.5)			(139–337)
	–	–	0.55 ± 0.50	10.0 ± 2.4	7.9 ± 2.2	135 ± 46	105 ± 23	1394 ± 681	35.3 ± 25.1	166 ± 9	4.7 ± 0.8	–	–	243 ± 43
			(0–1.36)	(1.5–11.6)	(3.8–11.5)	(111–180)	(59–148)	(619–2485)	(7.5–76.3)	(160–180)	(4.0–5.7)			(181–321)
Davy et al.	1984	*C. jacchus*	0–3	–	–	–	–	–	–	–	–	–	6–45	–

ALT, alanine aminotransferase; ALP, alkaline phosphatase; AST, aspartate aminotransferase; BUN, blood urea nitrogen; GGT, gamma glutamyl transferase; LDH, lactate dehydrogenase; T. Bili, total bilirubin; T. Prot, total protein; SDH, sorbitol dehydrogenase.

TABLE 6.32
Reference Intervals for Tamarins [Expressed as Mean ± SD (Range)]

Reference	Year	Species/Strain	Sex	Age	*N*	BUN mg/dL	Creatinine mg/dL	ALT IU/L	AST IU/L	ALP IU/L	T. Prot g/dL	Albumin g/dL	Glucose mg/dL
Poleschuk et al.	1996	*Saguinus mystax* (Moustached)	M	A	49–70	1.5 ± 0.1[a] (1.2–2.2)	–	13.8 ± 0.9 (9.0–18.0)	122.0 ± 7.8 (90.0–214.0)	–	8.4 ± 0.4 (6.9–10.6)	4.3 ± 0.18 (3.1–5.8)	8.1 ± 0.4[a] (5.2–9.3)
–	–	–	F	A	49–70	1.4 ± 0.1[a] (1.1–1.7)	–	19.0 ± 1.7 (12.0–18.0)	131.6 ± 11.7 (82.0–190.0)	–	8.3 ± 0.2 (7.7–9.2)	4.9 ± 0.13 (4.3–5.5)	6.9 ± 0.4[a] (4.8–8.7)
Wadsworth et al.	1982	*Saguinus labiatus* (Red-bellied)	M	Juv/A[b]	20	8.5 ± 2.4[a] (4.8–13.6)	83 ± 8.2[c] (70–97)	32 ± 14.6 (11–62)	184 ± 42.0 (132–291)	674 ± 832 (149–3790)	7.1 ± 0.42 (6.4–7.9)	3.9 ± 0.47 (2.8–4.8)	8.6 ± 2.5[a] (3.9–13.4)
–	–	–	F	Juv/A[a]	19	8.8 ± 1.9[a] (5.0–11.5)	74 ± 9.4[c] (66–91)	33 ± 14.1 (12–60)	179 ± 41.4 (131–289)	519 ± 280 (182–1148)	7.2 ± 0.76 (5.7–8.9)	4.0 ± 0.42 (3.4–5.1)	8.0 ± 2.4[a] (4.0–11.0)
Ramer et al.	1995	*Saguinus oedipus* (Cotton-top)	N/A	N/A	10	15 ± 2.4	0.49 ± 0.03	36 ± 13	164 ± 34	119 ± 37	6.2 ± 0.3	3.4 ± 0.3	188 ± 43

Reference	Year	Species/Strain	T. Bili mg/dL	CKIU/L	Calcium mg/dL	Phosphorus	Cholesterol mmol/L	Triglycerides mmol/L	Sodium mEq/L	Potassium mEq/L	Chloride mEq/L	CO_2 mEq/L
Poleschuk et al.	1996	*S. mystax* (Moustached)	–	–	–	–	4.5 ±0.4 (2.7–6.3)	1.0 ± 0.1 (0.9–1.5)	–	–	–	–
–	–	–	–	–	–	–	2.8 ± 0.1 (2.3–3.7)	1.4 ± 0.1 (0.7–1.9)	–	–	–	–
Wadsworth et al.	1982	*Saguinus labiatus* (Red-bellied)	10 ± 5.7[c] (0–19)	973 ± 1381 (116–4480)	2.5 ± 0.20[a] (2.2–2.8)	–	–	–	159 ± 5.0 (153–170)	4.0 ± 0.95 (3.2–6.7)	–	–
–	–	–	9 ± 6.5[c] (0–22)	617 ± 1056 (104–4290)	2.6 ± 0.17[a] (2.3–2.8)	–	–	–	156 ± 6.3 (141–168)	4.5 ± 0.78 (3.5–6.0)	–	–
Ramer et al.	1995	*S. oedipus* (Cotton-top)	0.27 ± 0.07	874 ± 337	9.0 ± 0.3	3.8 ± 0.7	90 ± 23	–	151 ± 3.5	3.4 ± 0.3	107 ± 3.0	20 ± 4.0

ALT, alanine aminotransferase; ALP, alkaline phosphatase; AST, aspartate aminotransferase; BUN, blood urea nitrogen; CK, creatine kinase; T. Bili, total bilirubin; T. Prot, total protein.

[a] mmol/L.

[b] Mixture of juveniles and adults, mean age = 21 months.

[c] μmol/L.

TABLE 6.33
Reference Intervals for Rhesus Macaques (Expressed as Mean ± SD)

Reference	Year	Sex	Age	*N*	BUN mg/dL	Creatinine mg/dL	ALT IU/L	AST IU/L	GGT IU/L	ALP IU/L	CK IU/L	LDH IU/mL	T. Prot g/dL	Albumin g/dL	Globulin g/dL
Buchl and Howard	1997	F	<1 year	27	18 ± 5	0.6 ± 0.2	39 ± 9	48 ± 11	75 ± 18	646 ± 136	386 ± 220	467 ± 186	7.1 ± 0.3	4.3 ± 0.3	2.8 ± 0.3
–	–	M	<1 year	27	20 ± 5	0.7 ± 0.2	42 ± 9	47 ± 10	77 ± 14	727 ± 148 578	366 ± 147	427 ± 116	7.3 ± 0.5	4.5 ± 0.2	2.8 ± 0.5
–	–	F	1–2 years	77[a]	21 ± 6	0.7 ± 0.1	37 ± 10	49 ± 13	71 ± 16	578 ± 149	436 ± 227	443 ± 180	7.2 ± 0.8	4.5 ± 0.3	2.8 ± 0.7
–	–	M	1–2 years	30	21 ± 5	0.7 ± 0.1	38 ± 9	47 ± 13	67 ± 19	527 ± 146	507 ± 297	422 ± 198	7.0 ± 0.6	4.5 ± 0.3	2.6 ± 0.5
–	–	F	2–3 years	50[a]	21 ± 4	0.7 ± 0.1	37 ± 10	44 ± 15	59 ± 13	479 ± 136	446 ± 289	434 ± 211	7.1 ± 0.3	4.5 ± 0.4	2.6 ± 0.3
–	–	M	2–3 years	27	24 ± 5	0.7 ± 0.1	35 ± 11	51 ± 13	72 ± 13	529 ± 177	423 ± 276	542 ± 173	7.0 ± 0.4	4.7 ± 0.4	2.2 ± 0.5
–	–	F	3–4 years	25	19 ± 3	0.8 ± 0.2	36 ± 14	43 ± 12	47 ± 7	384 ± 121	544 ± 289	372 ± 129	7.3 ± 0.4	4.5 ± 1.4	2.8 ± 0.4
–	–	M	3–4 years	30	18 ± 3	0.9 ± 0.1	37 ± 9	40 ± 13	57 ± 20	541 ± 144	491 ± 250	427 ± 222	7.3 ± 0.4	4.6 ± 0.3	2.7 ± 0.4
–	–	F	4–5 years	13	21 ± 3	0.9 ± 0.1	31 ± 8	38 ± 10	49 ± 9	288 ± 71	447 ± 163	404 ± 139	7.6 ± 0.4	4.6 ± 0.3 ±0.4	2.9 ± 0.6
–	–	M	4–5 years	44[a]	19 ± 5	1.0 ± 0.2	41 ± 12	39 ± 13	63 ± 17	456 ± 115	425 ± 184	381 ± 265	7.5 ± 0.4	4.6 ± 0.4	2.8 ± 0.4
–	–	F	5–10 years	30	19 ± 3	0.9 ± 0.1	35 ± 7	32 ± 8	45 ± 7	180 ± 63	446 ± 187	297 ± 83	7.7 ± 0.5	4.5 ± 0.5	3.3 ± 0.4
–	–	M	5–10 years	21	20 ± 3	1.1 ± 0.1	33 ± 8	38 ± 10	55 ± 16	203 ± 84	413 ± 162	363 ± 173	7.8 ± 0.5	4.5 ± 0.4	3.3 ± 0.5

(Continued)

TABLE 6.33 (*Continued*)
Reference Intervals for Rhesus Macaques (Expressed as Mean ± SD)

Reference	Year	Sex	Age	*N*	BUN mg/dL	Creatinine mg/dL	ALT IU/L	AST IU/L	GGT IU/L	ALP IU/L	CK IU/L	LDH IU/mL	T. Prot g/dL	Albumin g/dL	Globulin g/dL
–	–	F	> 10 years	29[a]	21 ± 4	0.9 ± 0.2	40 ± 12	41 ± 11	41 ± 6	118 ± 40	442 ± 231	393 ± 171	7.8 ± 0.4	4.4 ± 0.6	3.4 ± 0.6
Fernie et al.	1994	F	Adult	120–210	13.0–26.0	0.7–1.2	14–59	29–59	33–71	72–179	30–298	143–352	6.5–8.1	3.5–4.7	–
–	–	M	Adult	40–100	10.8–28.8	0.8–1.7	14–170	32–72	42–136	58–290	113–4500	147–889	5.7–7.9	2.3–4.6	–
–	–	B	Infant	29–162	17.0–41.0	0.4–1.0	8–37	33–86	63–152	363–1076	49–776	206–889	5.6–7.8	3.9–5.1	–
Kessler et al.	1983	M	15–28 years	7	25.7 ± 3.8	1.3 ± 0.3	29 ± 18	37 ± 15	–	65 ± 16	–	259 ± 57	7.2 ± 0.9	3.1 ± 0.5	4.1 ± 0.7
–	–	F	16–25 years	17	24.9 ± 4.6	1.3 ± 0.3	44 ± 31	42 ± 26	–	66 ± 30	–	383 ± 243	7.9 ± 1.1	3.1 ± 0.5	4.9 ± 1.3
–	–	M	6–14 years	10	25.3 ± 5.3	1.3 ± 0.1	31 ± 13	35 ± 11	–	59 ± 27	–	276 ± 54	7.5 ± 0.5	4.0 ± 0.5	3.5 ± 0.5
–	–	F	4–10 years	24	23.5 ± 4.0	1.3 ± 0.3	34 ± 13	46 ± 32	–	107 ± 48	–	425 ± 235	7.5 ± 0.5	3.5 ± 0.5	4.0 ± 0.6

Reference	Year	Sex	Age	D. Bili mg/dL	T. Bili mg/dL	Calcium mg/dL	Phosphorus	Glucose mg/dL	Cholesterol mg/dL	Triglycerides mg/dL	Amylase IU/L	Sodium mEq/L	Potassium mEq/L	Chloride mEq/L	CO_2 mEq/L
Buchl and Howard	1997	F	<1 year	–	0.2 ± 0.2	10.5 ± 1.0	5.5 ± 1.2	82 ± 16	165 ± 30	44 ± 14	–	148 ± 3	4.3 ± 0.6	112 ± 3	–
–	–	M	<1 year	–	0.2 ± 0.2	10.6 ± 0.8	6.4 ± 1.1	88 ± 20	179 ± 29	52 ± 35	–	148 ± 3	4.3 ± 0.6	113 ± 2	–
–	–	F	1–2 years	–	0.1 ± 0.1	10.5 ± 1.0	5.3 ± 1.0	74 ± 15	165 ± 30	43 ± 11	–	148 ± 3	3.8 ± 0.6	113 ± 4	–
–	–	M	1–2 years	–	0.2 ± 0.1	10.3 ± 0.5	5.1 ± 0.7	74 ± 12	161 ± 30	41 ± 14	–	148 ± 3	4.0 ± 0.5	114 ± 2	–
–	–	F	2–3 years	–	0.2 ± 0.1	10.1 ± 0.7	5.6 ± 1.0	64 ± 14	146 ± 27	44 ± 16	–	148 ± 2	3.8 ± 0.4	113 ± 2	–

(*Continued*)

TABLE 6.33 (*Continued*)
Reference Intervals for Rhesus Macaques (Expressed as Mean ± SD)

Reference	Year	Sex	Age	D. Bili mg/dL	T. Bili mg/dL	Calcium mg/dL	Phosphorus	Glucose mg/dL	Cholesterol mg/dL	Triglycerides mg/dL	Amylase IU/L	Sodium mEq/L	Potassium mEq/L	Chloride mEq/L	CO_2 mEq/L
–	–	M	2–3 years	–	0.1 ± 0.1	9.7 ± 0.7	6.2 ± 0.7	60 ± 10	151 ± 22	46 ± 11	–	148 ± 2	3.7 ± 0.3	112 ± 2	–
–	–	F	3–4 years	–	0.2 ± 0.1	10.4 ± 1.6	5.1 ± 0.9	67 ± 14	141 ± 20	45 ± 16	–	147 ± 2	4.0 ± 0.3	114 ± 2	–
–	–	M	3–4 years	–	0.2 ± 0.1	10.7 ± 0.6	5.2 ± 0.6	73 ± 16	138 ± 20	50 ± 16	–	148 ± 3	4.0 ± 0.3	113 ± 2	–
–	–	F	4–5 years	–	0.2 ± 0.1	10.4 ± 0.5	4.4 ± 1.1	76 ± 18	152 ± 30	55 ± 23	–	147 ± 3	3.9 ± 0.2	116 ± 3	–
–	–	M	4–5 years	–	0.2 ± 0.1	10.8 ± 0.8	4.7 ± 0.9	77 ± 13	143 ± 23	45 ± 14	–	148 ± 3	4.0 ± 0.4	113 ± 3	–
–	–	F	5–10 years	–	0.2 ± 0.1	10.7 ± 0.9	3.9 ± 0.9	66 ± 13	150 ± 34	45 ± 19	–	148 ± 3	4.0 ± 0.5	115 ± 3	–
–	–	M	5–10 years	–	0.2 ±0.2	10.4 ± 0.9	3.6 ± 0.9	67 ± 16	155 ± 22	43 ± 18	–	148 ± 3	3.9 ± 0.3	113 ± 2	–
–	–	F	>10 years	–	0.1 ± 0.1	10.2 ± 1.1	3.5 ± 1.1	74 ± 15	180 ± 42	58 ± 34	–	150 ± 2	4.0 ± 0.4	116 ± 3	–
Fernie et al.	1994	F	Adult	0–0.1	0–0.4	9.3–11.4	–	56–99	103–246	32–190	289–744	143–155	3.2–4.5	104–117	9.9–22.3
–	–	M	Adult	0	0.1–0.5	8.5–10.9	–	34–104	103–228	38–186	223–600	140–158	3.3–4.7	105–116	13.0–27.0
–	–	B	Infant	0–0.1	0.2–0.4	9.4–11.6	–	39–116	153–266	40–118	284–645	147–162	3.6–5.6	101–118	9.2–22.3
Kessler et al.	1983	M	15–28 years	0.06 ± 0.02	0.19 ± 0.10	–	–	58 ± 7	142 ± 50	124 ± 33	–	–	–	–	–
–	–	F	16–25 years	0.10 ± 0.08	0.27 ± 0.20	–	–	NA	143 ± 38	144 ± 67	–	–	–	–	–
–	–	M	6–14 years	0.04 ± 0.01	0.13 ± 0.02	–	–	67 ± 12	128 ± 28	73 ± 29	–	–	–	–	–
–	–	F	4–10 years	0.04 ± 0.03	0.19 ± 0.16	–	–	56 ± 9	151 ± 21	117 ±76	–	–	–	–	–

[a] The number of samples includes replicates on the same animals.

ALT, alanine aminotransferase; ALP, alkaline phosphatase; AST, aspartate aminotransferase; BUN, blood urea nitrogen; CK, creatine kinase; CRP, C-reactive protein; D. Bili, direct bilirubin; GGT, gamma glutamyl transferase; LDH, lactate dehydrogenase; T. Bili, total bilirubin; T. Prot, total protein

TABLE 6.34
Reference Intervals for Cynomolgus Macaques (Expressed as Mean ± SD)

Reference	Year	Species/ Strain	Sex	Age	*N*	BUN mg/dL	Creatinine mg/dL	ALT IU/L	AST IU/L	ALP IU/L	GGT	LDH IU/L	CK IU/L
Bonfanti et al.	2009	*Mauritian* Purpose-bred	M	2 years	15	48 ± 8.3	0.85 ± 0.09	38 ± 12.4	43 ± 4.4	2731 ± 763.2	182 ± 31.6	790 ± 198.1	252 ± 155.5
–	–	*Mauritian* Captured	M	2 years	15	47 ± 7.8	0.95 ± 0.11	53 ±23.7	46 ±10.8	2379 ± 539.8	185 ±39.1	786 ± 221.6	223 ± 104.2
–	–	*Mauritian* Purpose-bred	F	2 years	15	40 ± 8.6	0.83 ± 0.07	34 ± 7.5	45 ± 6.4	2134 ± 482.9	140 ± 29.2	1001 ± 410.3	171 ± 78.4
–	–	*Mauritian* Captured	F	2 years	15	43 ± 9.3	1.06 ± 0.11	54 ± 33.3	37 ± 7.8	941 ± 252.9	103 ± 17.0	578 ± 112.6	175 ± 131.8
Kim et al.	2005	Southeast Asia Non-anesthetized	M	3–5 years	19	17.67 ± 2.85	0.85 ± 0.10	40.2 ± 20.1	41.0 ± 7.1	1923.0 ± 371.1	–	–	194.7 ± 53.6
–	–	Southeast Asia Ketamine	M	3–5 years	19	18.33 ± 4.11	0.79 ± 0.13	52.2 ± 11.7	64.9 ± 21.3	1829.2 ± 389.5	–	–	732.2 ± 362.6
–	–	Southeast Asia Non-anesthetized	F	3–5 years	16	15.16 ± 1.69	0.84 ± .0.12	42.5 ± 11.2	36.8 ± 8.7	524.2 ± 199.0	–	–	126.3 ± 44.5
–	–	Southeast Asia Ketamine	F	3–5 years	16	20.06 ± 4.77	0.84 ± 0.11	72.5 ± 51.0	50.8 ± 20.9	479.0 ± 176.9	–	–	236.5 ± 136.6
Schuurman and Smith	2005	NA	M	Adult	53	19.3 ± 3.5	1.25 ±0.17	54 ±37	31 ± 9	–	137 ± 47	350 ± 120	280 ± 330
		NA	F	Adult	53	18.8 ± 2.8	1.02 ± 0.12	68 ± 50	32 ± 14	–	78 ± 27	340 ± 130	200 ± 230
Perretta et al.	1991	Closed colony	M	<1 year	9	42.4 ± 21.3	1.01 ± 0.16	28.0 ± 7.0	57.8 ± 9.6	913 ± 205	240.9 ± 87.8	789 ± 91	503 ± 260
–	–	–	M	1–4 years	23	51.2 ± 10.9	0.94 ± 0.14	25.7 ± 6.9	60.9 ± 23.8	610 ± 168	147.1 ± 64.4	585 ± 160	405 ± 251

(*Continued*)

TABLE 6.34 (*Continued*)
Reference Intervals for Cynomolgus Macaques (Expressed as Mean ± SD)

Reference	Year	Species/ Strain	Sex	Age	*N*	BUN mg/dL	Creatinine mg/dL	ALT IU/L	AST IU/L	ALP IU/L	GGT	LDH IU/L	CK IU/L
–	–	–	M	>5 years	13	38.8 ± 5.3	1.25 ± 0.19	23.2 ± 12.5	40.2 ± 8.9	226 ± 162	105.6 ± 35.2	441 ± 133	320 ± 151
–	–	–	F	<1 year	4	38.7 ± 22.9	0.73 ± 0.06	15.5 ± 2.60	41.7 ± 1.70	973 ± 96	233.8 ± 63.3	639 ± 189	281 ± 39
–	–	–	F	1–4 years	24	46.0 ± 8.3	1.03 ± 0.21	26.9 ± 12.0	49.0 ± 14.9	538 ± 221	131.7 ± 57.7	521 ± 109	447 ± 258
–	–	–	F	>5 years	17	49.5 ± 15.5	1.03 ± 0.3	32.5 ± 22.0	47.9 ± 14.8	230 ± 75	86.8 ± 47.2	559 ± 204	360 ± 196

Reference	Year	Species/ Strain	Sex	Age	*N*	Calcium	Phosphorus	Cholesterol mg/dL	Triglycerides mg/dL	T. Prot g/dL	Albumin g/dL	Globulin g/dL	T. Bili mg/dL	D. Bili mg/dL
Bonfanti et al.	2009	*Mauritian* Purpose-bred	M	2 years	15	11.6 ± 0.43	8.4 ± 0.90	132 ± 22.7	65 ± 14.9	7.9 ± 0.28	4.9 ± 0.29	3.0 ± 0.20	0.39 ± 0.08	0.10 ± 0.03
–	–	*Mauritian* Captured	M	2 years	15	11.6 ± 0.46	7.6 ± 0.67	138 ± 31.1	61 ± 20.6	8.3 ± 0.37	5.0 ± 0.15	3.4 ± 0.33	0.44 ± 0.13	0.10 ± 0.04
–	–	*Mauritian* Purpose-bred	F	2 years	15	12.9 ± 0.53	4.5 ± 0.79	121 ± 25.2	66 ± 27.1	8.0 ± 0.46	5.0 ± 0.29	3.0 ± 0.30	0.25 ± 0.05	0.05 ± 0.02
–	–	*Mauritian* Captured	F	2 years	15	12.9 ± 0.97	4.7 ± 1.03	118 ± 18.7	65 ± 33.2	8.3 ± 0.44	4.9 ± 0.28	3.5 ± 0.29	0.26 ± 0.05	0.05 ± 0.02
Kim et al.	2005	Southeast Asia Non-anesthetized	M	3–5 years	19	–	7.0 ± 0.9	126.1 ± 21.4	25.2 ± 7.2	7.5 ± 0.46	4.6 ± 0.25	–	0.18 ± 0.03	–
–	–	Southeast Asia Ketamine	M	3–5 years	19	–	6.0 ± 0.9	196.9 ± 64.3	14.4 ± 10.2	7.4 ± 0.63	4.5 ± 0.34	–	0.29 ± 0.07	–
–	–	Southeast Asia Non-anesthetized	F	3–5 years	16	9.5 ± 0.52	5.9 ± 0.92	129.7 ± 27.4	32.6 ± 10.4	7.9 ± 0.43	4.5 ± 0.22	–	0.17 ± 0.03	–

(*Continued*)

TABLE 6.34 (*Continued*)
Reference Intervals for Cynomolgus Macaques (Expressed as Mean ± SD)

Reference	Year	Species/ Strain	Sex	Age	*N*	Calcium	Phosphorus	Cholesterol mg/dL	Triglycerides mg/dL	T. Prot g/dL	Albumin g/dL	Globulin g/dL	T. Bili mg/dL	D. Bili mg/dL
–	–	Southeast Asia Ketamine	F	3–5 years	16	9.4 ± 0.5	4.1 ± 1.20	137.6 ± 33.2	34.7 ± 53.0	7.7 ± 0.47	4.4 ± 0.22	–	0.20 ± 0.08	–
Schuurman and Smith	2005	NA	M	Adult	53	10.76 ± 0.63	6.12 ± 0.91	143 ± 23	47 ± 23	8.98 ± 0.63	4.88 ± 0.36	4.10 ± 0.49	0.37 ± 0.13	–
–	–	NA	F	Adult	53	10.27 ± 0.45	4.66 ± 0.80	146 ± 32	65 ± 31	8.85 ± 0.58	4.51 ± 0.29	4.33 ± 0.48	0.47 ± 0.19	–
Perretta et al.	1991	Closed colony	M	<1 year	9	–	–	207.6 ± 71.0	58.4 ± 12.6	7.5 ± 0.4	–	–	–	–
–	–	–	M	1–4 years	23	–	–	144.3 ± 33.3	57.8 ± 16.2	7.6 ± 0.3	–	–	–	–
–	–	–	M	>5 years	13	–	–	133.5 ± 15.5	69.8 ± 17.7	8.3 ± 0.3	–	–	–	–
–	–	–	F	<1 year	4	–	–	181.0 ± 41.7	62.5 ± 25.1	7.4 ± 0.2	–	–	–	–
–	–	–	F	1–4 years	24	–	–	142.9 ± 35.0	56.0 ± 13.8	8.0 ± 0.6	–	–	–	–
–	–	–	F	>5 years	17	–	–	149.8 ± 20.8	77.6 ± 34.5	8.2 ± 0.5	–	–	–	–

Reference	Year	Species/ Strain	Sex	Age	*N*	Glucose mg/dL	Iron μg/dL	Amylase IU/L	Sodium mEq/L	Potassium mEq/L	Chloride mEq/L	CRP μg/mL
Bonfanti et al.	2009	*Mauritian* Purpose-bred	M	2 years	15	73 ± 9.8	97 ± 26.9	–	157.0 ± 3.2	6.3 ± 0.7	–	–
–	–	*Mauritian* Captured	M	2 years	15	76 ± 13.8	110 ± 39.4	–	155.7 ± 2.9	5.9 ± 0.7	–	–
–	–	*Mauritian* Purpose-bred	F	2 years	15	80 ± 13.0	231 ± 54.9	–	160.0 ± 2.8	6.1 ± 0.6	–	–
–	–	*Mauritian* Captured	F	2 years	15	88 ± 16.3	187 ± 24.8	–	160.4 ± 4.9	6.8 ± 0.8	–	–

(Continued)

TABLE 6.34 (*Continued*)
Reference Intervals for Cynomolgus Macaques (Expressed as Mean ± SD)

Reference	Year	Species/Strain	Sex	Age	*N*	Glucose mg/dL	Iron µg/dL	Amylase IU/L	Sodium mEq/L	Potassium mEq/L	Chloride mEq/L	CRP µg/mL
Kim et al.	2005	Southeast Asia Non-anesthetized	M	3–5 years	19	83.6 ± 13.0	–	–	152.5 ± 3.1	5.2 ± 0.5	106.7 ± 2.1	--
–	–	Southeast Asia Ketamine	M	3–5 years	19	63.7 ± 19.6	–	–	147.5 ± 2.9	4.7 ± 0.5	108.8 ± 1.8	--
–	–	Southeast Asia Non-anesthetized	F	3–5 years	16	87.4 ± 18.2	–	–	152.7 ± 3.7	5.3 ± 0.7	107.6 ± 2.4	--
–	–	Southeast Asia Ketamine	F	3–5 years	16	73.6 ± 24.5	–	–	147.8 ± 2.3	4.8 ± 0.7	106.8 ± 2.1	--
Schuurman and Smith	2005	NA	M	Adult	53	77 ± 11	–	510 ± 150	159.9 ± 5.5	5.59 ± 0.73	112.7 ± 3.2	--
–	–	NA	F	Adult	53	82 ± 20	–	380 ± 130	157.1 ± 5.0	5.37 ± 0.54	114.0 ± 3.8	--
Jinbo et al.	1998	*Macaca irus*	NA	NA	–	–	–	–	–	–	–	0.71 ± 0.37
Perretta et al.	1991	Closed colony	M	<1 year	9	63.2 ± 14.5	132.0 ± 40.0	–	–	–	–	--
–	–	–	M	1–4 years	23	57.3 ± 17.7	140.0 ± 36.0	–	–	–	–	--
–	–	–	M	>5 years	13	62.2 ± 18.8	160.0 ± 33.0	–	–	–	–	--
–	–	–	F	<1 year	4	82. ± 10.9	120.0 ± 38.0	–	–	–	–	--
–	–	–	F	1–4 years	24	61.0 ± 19.7	156.0 ± 24.0	–	–	–	–	--
–	–	–	F	>5 years	17	53.6 ± 18.6	118.0 ± 32.0	–	–	–	–	--

ALT, alanine aminotransferase; ALP, alkaline phosphatase; AST, aspartate aminotransferase; BUN, blood urea nitrogen; CK, creatine kinase; CRP, C-reactive protein; D. Bili, direct bilirubin; GGT, gamma glutamyl transferase; LDH, lactate dehydrogenase; T. Bili, total bilirubin; T. Prot, total protein.

TABLE 6.35
Reference Intervals for Chimpanzees

Reference	Year	Sex	Age	*N*	Statistic	ALT IU/L	AST IU/L	ALP IU/L	GGT IU/L	LDH IU/l	CK IU/L	T. Prot g/dL
Howell et al.	2003	M	Infant (0–3 years)	110	Mean ± 2SD	40.1 ± 32.2	22.1 ± 12.7	783.8 ±1153.9	19.6 ± 19.1	489.2 ± 165.2	241.2 ± 307.6	6.7 ± 1.0
–	–	M	Juvenile (3–6 years)	112	Mean ± 2SD	45.8 ± 33.9	21.0 ± 12.0	529.1 ± 286.4	27.8 ± 19.8	435.7 ± 200.3	206.9 ± 270.6	7.0 ± 0.9
–	–	M	Adolescent (6–10 years)	136	Mean ± 2SD	35.9 ± 18.9	21.7 ± 13.5	552.7 ± 489.2	25.5 ± 35.8	390.5 ± 197.9	226.4 ± 270.4	7.2 ± 0.8
–	–	M	Adult (>10 years)	312	Mean ± 2SD	39.4 ± 27.7	30.9 ± 32.4	127.6 ± 157.7	30.0 ± 32.3	401.7 ± 297.7	323.0 ± 489.7	7.4 ± 0.7
–	–	F	Infant (0–3 years)	94	Mean ± 2SD	39.6 ± 36.1	21.6 ± 18.5	707.9 ± 918.0	18.0 ± 16.2	475.0 ± 300.6	190.8 ± 230.3	6.8 ± 1.1
–	–	F	Juvenile (3–6 years)	120	Mean ± 2SD	39.8 ± 21.3	20.5 ± 12.5	619.6 ± 460.5	21.8 ± 14.5	423.2 ± 290.9	203.9 ± 279.0	7.1 ± 0.9
–	–	F	Adolescent (6–10 years)	120	Mean ± 2SD	34.9 ± 23.7	17.5 ± 9.3	380.1 ± 377.8	24.0 ± 23.8	382.8 ± 372.6	168.7 ± 221.8	7.3 ± 0.8
–	–	F	Adult (>10 years)	564	Mean ± 2SD	30.8 ± 20.3	18.1 ± 13.1	114.3 ± 155.5	28.5 ± 43.9	320.8 ± 447.6	229.0 ± 431.2	7.5 ± 1.0
Ihrig et al.[a]	2001	M	Infant (0–3 years)	24–104	5th–95th centile	24.35–54.40	13.70–31.52	393.92–857.51	–	–	--	6.14–7.73
–	–	M	Juvenile (3–6 years)	19–81	5th–95th centile	30.00–69.10	15.70–34.73	361.58–706.70	–	–	--	6.62–7.80
–	–	M	Adolescent (6–10 years)	15–100	5th–95th centile	17.00–47.15	11.57–31.77	145.60–943.93	–	–	--	6.80–8.01
–	–	M	Adult (>10 years)	16–358	5th–95th centile	28.57–61.63	22.28–56.21	56.04–146.07	–	259.0–618.5	173.0–1347.5	7.29–8.35
–	–	F	Infant (0–3 years)	17–87	5th–95th centile	21.00–43.85	12.67–38.10	409.4–1064.55	–	–	--	6.00–7.47

(Continued)

TABLE 6.35 (*Continued*)
Reference Intervals for Chimpanzees

Reference	Year	Sex	Age	N	Statistic	ALT IU/L	AST IU/L	ALP IU/L	GGT IU/L	LDH IU/l	CK IU/L	T. Prot g/dL
–	–	F	Juvenile (3–6 years)	31–91	5th–95th centile	28.50–48.56	13.00–27.25	361.78–671.00	–	–	–	6.30–7.71
–	–	F	Adolescent (6–10 years)	27–109	5th–95th centile	17.63–44.31	10.72–27.93	143.13–533.09	–	–	–	6.73–8.29
–	–	F	Adult (>10 years)	19–529	5th–95th centile	20.17–35.87	11.87–24.73	53.68–205.36	–	192.5–423.8	71.5–850.9	6.70–8.25
Hainsey et al.	1993	M	5–33 years	8	Mean ± 2SD	39 ±14	25 ± 23	363 ± 529	13 ± 8	317 ± 111	171 ± 157	7.2 ± 0.6
		F	5–33 years	18	Mean ± 2SD	38 ± 17	18 ± 7	343 ± 360	13 ± 5	321 ± 177	198 ± 168	7.2 ± 0.8

[a] The number of samples includes replicates on the same animals.

Reference	Year	Sex	Age	N	Statistic	T. Bili mg/dL	BUN mg/dL	Creatinine mg/dL	Cholesterol mg/dL	Triglycerides mg/dL
Howell et al.	2003	M	Infant (0–3 years)	110	Mean ± 2SD	–	11.8 ± 11.1	0.6 ± 0.3	235.2 ±85.0	56.5 ± 44.6
–	–	M	Juvenile (3–6 years)	112	Mean ± 2SD	–	14.3 ± 7.3	0.7 ± 0.3	206.3 ± 54.0	86.5 ± 58.9
–	–	M	Adolescent (6–10 years)	136	Mean ± 2SD	–	12.0 ± 5.8	0.9 ± 0.3	193.0 ± 59.9	97.2 ± 70.5
–	–	M	Adult (>10 years)	312	Mean ± 2SD	–	12.2 ± 5.8	1.1 ± 0.4	179.5 ± 46.6	88.7 ± 74.3
–	–	F	Infant (0–3 years)	94	Mean ± 2SD	–	10.6 ± 7.8	0.7 ± 0.3	227.4 ± 105.4	68.7 ± 81.3
–	–	F	Juvenile (3–6 years)	120	Mean ± 2SD	–	12.2 ± 7.6	0.7 ± 0.3	201.1 ± 78.0	88.8 ± 77.6

(*Continued*)

TABLE 6.35 (*Continued*)
Reference Intervals for Chimpanzees

Reference	Year	Sex	Age	*N*	Statistic	T. Bili mg/dL	BUN mg/dL	Creatinine mg/dL	Cholesterol mg/dL	Triglycerides mg/dL
–	–	F	Adolescent (6–10 years)	120	Mean ± 2SD	–	11.8 ± 5.9	0.8 ± 0.3	196.8 ± 70.6	97.7 ± 71.9
-	–	F	Adult (>10 years)	564	Mean ± 2SD	–	11.5 ± 7.8	1.0 ± 1.2	212.2 ± 83.1	109.2 ± 104.5
Ihrig et al.	2001	M	Infant (0–3 years)	24–104	5th–95th centile	0.10–0.60	7.68–18.65	0.50–0.76	170.0–349.0	38.0–140.0
–	–	M	Juvenile (3–6 years)	19–81	5th–95th centile	0–0.70	10.55–26.25	0.45–0.80	192.8–283.0	54.0–144.0
–	–	M	Adolescent (6–10 years)	15–100	5th–95th centile	0–0.82	8.85–24.10	0.60–1.73	161.0–247.3	45.3–109.0
–	–	M	Adult (>10 years)	16–358	5th–95th centile	0.23–0.61	10.62–17.83	0.90–1.26	167.2–253.8	55.6–141.6
–	–	F	Infant (0–3 years)	17–87	5th–95th centile	0.09–0.60	7.55–19.65	0.49–0.79	177.0–363.7	32.0–135.0
–	–	F	Juvenile (3–6 years)	31–91	5th–95th centile	0–0.70	10.13–19.08	0.50–0.85	179.0–292.0	35.0–118.8
–	–	F	Adolescent (6–10 years)	27–109	5th–95th centile	0.08–0.54	9.43–21.63	0.62–1.32	163.0–333.0	33.0–109.0
–	–	F	Adult (>10 years)	19–529	5th–95th centile	0.20–0.50	8.27–17.16	0.7–1.11	170.0–296.2	56.1–181.6
Hainsey et al.	1993	M	5–33 years	8	Mean ± SD	0.3 ± 0.2	10 ± 5	0.9 ± 0.4	202 ± 67	66 ± 36
–	–	F	5–33 years	18	Mean ±SD	0.2 ± 0.1	14 ± 9	0.7 ± 0.4	233 ± 81	81 ± 52

Reference	Year	Sex	Age	*N*	Statistic	Uric Acid mg/dL	Sodium mEq/L	Potassium mEq/L	Chloride mEq/L	CO_2 mEq/L	Anion Gap
Howell et al.	2003	M	Infant (0–3 years)	110	Mean ± 2SD	2.2 ± 1.1	137.9 ± 6.2	4.0 ± 0.7	104.1 ± 6.7	23.3 ± 6.0	10.6 ± 5.3

(*Continued*)

TABLE 6.35 (*Continued*)
Reference Intervals for Chimpanzees

Reference	Year	Sex	Age	*N*	Statistic	Uric Acid mg/dL	Sodium mEq/L	Potassium mEq/L	Chloride mEq/L	CO_2 mEq/L	Anion Gap
–	–	M	Juvenile (3–6 years)	112	Mean ± 2SD	2.3 ± 1.0	139.5 ± 4.7	4.1 ± 0.7	102.3 ± 5.8	26.4 ± 4.6	10.9 ± 5.6
–	–	M	Adolescent (6–10 years)	136	Mean ± 2SD	2.8 ± 1.0	140.5 ± 3.8	4.0 ± 0.6	101.8 ± 4.6	27.7 ± 4.2	10.9 ± 5.2
–	–	M	Adult (>10 years)	312	Mean ± 2SD	2.4 ± 0.9	141.1 ± 5.4	3.7 ± 0.9	101.0 ± 5.2	30.6 ± 5.8	9.5 ± 5.8
–	–	F	Infant (0–3 years)	94	Mean ± 2SD	2.2 ± 1.3	138.6 ± 4.9	3.9 ± 0.8	103.0 ± 7.3	24.4 ± 6.0	11.4 ± 7.3
–	–	F	Juvenile (3–6 years)	120	Mean ± 2SD	2.2 ± 1.3	139.0 ± 4.6	3.9 ± 0.7	102.4 ± 6.2	25.9 ± 5.9	10.5 ± 6.1
–	–	F	Adolescent (6–10 years)	120	Mean ± 2SD	2.2 ± 1.1	138.7 ± 4.7	3.9 ± 0.7	102.0 ± 5.6	25.9 ±5.8	10.6 ± 6.1
–	–	F	Adult (>10 years)	564	Mean ± 2SD	2.1 ± 1.4	138.4 ± 5.4	3.8 ± 0.8	101.1 ± 10.3	27.5 ± 8.7	9.8 ± 6.2
Ihrig et al.	2001	M	Infant (0–3 years)	24–104	5th–95th centile	–	–	–	–	–	–
–	–	M	Juvenile (3–6 years)	19–81	5th–95th centile	–	–	–	–	–	–
–	–	M	Adolescent (6–10 years)	15–100	5th–95th centile	–	–	–	–	–	–
–	–	M	Adult (>10 years)	16–358	5th–95th centile	1.6–6.0	139.0–150.0	3.2–4.7	92.3–116.0	–	–

(*Continued*)

TABLE 6.35 (*Continued*)
Reference Intervals for Chimpanzees

Reference	Year	Sex	Age	*N*	Statistic	Uric Acid mg/dL	Sodium mEq/L	Potassium mEq/L	Chloride mEq/L	CO_2 mEq/L	Anion Gap
–	–	F	Infant (0–3 years)	17–87	5th–95th centile	–	–	–	–	–	–
–	–	F	Juvenile (3–6 years)	31–91	5th–95th centile	–	–	–	–	–	–
–	–	F	Adolescent (6–10 years)	27–109	5th–95th centile	–	–	–	–	–	–
–	–	F	Adult (>10 years)	19–529	5th–95th centile	0.7–3.0	136.6–145.3	3.3–4.4	94.0–113.0	–	–
Hainsey et al.	1993	M	5–33 years	8	Mean ± SD	–	145 ± 4	4.1 ± 0.8	102 ± -5	25–8	22–6
–	–	F	5–33 years	18	Mean ± SD	–	143 ± 5	4.0 ± 1.0	102 ± -7	24–6	21–9

Reference	Year	Sex	Age	*N*	Statistic	Glucose mg/dL	Iron µg/dL	Amylase IU/L	Lipase IU/L	HDL mg/dL	LDL mg/dL	Calcium (Ca) mg/dL	Phosphorus	CRP µg/mL
Lamperez et al.	2005	All	< 3 years	5	Mean ± 2SD	–	–	–	–	–	–	–	–	0.64 ± 0.48
–	–	M	< 3 years	4	Mean ± 2SD	–	–	–	–	–	–	–	–	0.65 ± 0.55
–	–	F	< 3 years	1	Mean ± 2SD	–	–	–	–	–	–	–	–	0.60
–	–	All	>7 years	32	Mean ± 2SD	–	–	–	–	–	–	–	–	1.02 ± 0.92
–	–	M	>7 years	9	Mean ± 2SD	–	–	–	–	–	–	–	–	0.86 ± 0.74
–	–	F	>7 years	23	Mean ± 2SD	–	–	–	–	–	–	–	–	1.08 ± 0.99
Howell et al.	2003	M	Infant (0–3 years)	110	Mean ± 2SD	83.4 ± 24.7	62.7 ± 50.4	–	–	–	–	9.4 ± 0.9	4.7 ± 1.3	–
–	–	M	Juvenile (3–6 years)	112	Mean ± 2SD	86.3 ± 25.0	93.1 ± 58.6	–	–	–	–	9.4 ± 0.7	4.9 ± 1.4	–

(*Continued*)

TABLE 6.35 (*Continued*)
Reference Intervals for Chimpanzees

Reference	Year	Sex	Age	*N*	Statistic	Glucose mg/dL	Iron µg/dL	Amylase IU/L	Lipase IU/L	HDL mg/dL	LDL mg/dL	Calcium (Ca) mg/dL	Phosphorus	CRP µg/mL
–	–	M	Adolescent (6–10 years)	136	Mean ± 2SD	88.7 ± 25.2	110.0 ± 70.1	–	–	–	–	9.5 ± 0.7	4.7 ± 1.7	–
–	–	M	Adult (>10 years)	312	Mean ± 2SD	94.1 ± 34.4	122.4 ± 76.5	–	–	–	–	9.5 ± 9.5	3.3 ± 1.9	–
–	–	F	Infant (0–3 years)	94	Mean ± 2SD	84.9 ± 33.3	79.0 ± 63.3	–	–	–	–	9.4 ± 0.9	4.7 ± 1.7	–
–	–	F	Juvenile (3–6 years)	120	Mean ± 2SD	87.7 ± 28.1	107.5 ± 75.7	–	–	–	–	9.4 ± 0.8	4.9 ± 1.6	–
–	–	F	Adolescent (6–10 years)	120	Mean ± 2SD	87.2 ± 29.0	116.2 ± 73.8	–	–	–	–	9.3 ± 0.8	4.4 ± 1.7	–
–	–	F	Adult (>10 years)	564	Mean ± 2SD	83.6 ± 30.8	100.8 ± 72.1	–	–	–	–	9.1 ± 0.8	3.5 ± 1.8	–
Ihrig et al.	2001	M	Infant (0–3 years)	24–104	5th–95th centile	69.0–127.0	–	–	–	43.0–116.7	97.0–245.5	–	–	–
–	–	M	Juvenile (3–6 years)	19–81	5th–95th centile	55.0–121.5	–	–	–	44.0–103.0	133.3–179.0	–	–	–
–	–	M	Adolescent (6–10 years)	15–100	5th–95th centile	67.1–115.6	–	–	–	31.7–68.0	129.0–173.0	–	–	–
–	–	M	Adult (>10 years)	16–358	5th–95th centile	68.6–106.2	–	–	–	33.7–67.8	101.7–193.1	7.8–10.0	1.8–4.9	–
–	–	F	Infant (0–3 years)	17–87	5th–95th centile	64.9–121.5	–	–	–	45.0–112.7	99.0–240.3	–	–	–
–	–	F	Juvenile (3–6 years)	31–91	5th–95th centile	66.3–117.7	–	–	–	42.0–104.0	114.3–206.0	–	–	–

(*Continued*)

TABLE 6.35 (*Continued*)
Reference Intervals for Chimpanzees

Reference	Year	Sex	Age	*N*	Statistic	Glucose mg/dL	Iron µg/dL	Amylase IU/L	Lipase IU/L	HDL mg/dL	LDL mg/dL	Calcium (Ca) mg/dL	Phosphorus	CRP µg/mL
–	–	F	Adolescent (6–10 years)	27–109	5th–95th centile	68.6–116.0	–	–	–	33.0–102.0	109.7–174.7	–	–	–
–	–	F	Adult (>10 years)	19–529	5th–95th centile	65.7–117.6	–	–	–	36.0–82.0	102.6–214.0	8.2–10.5	1.5–4.1	–
Hainsey et al.	1993	M	5–33 years	8	Mean ± SD	82 ± −37	–	44 ± 17	18 ± -52	82 ± 62	–	9.3 ± 0.6	4.2 ± 2.2	–
–	–	F	5–33 years	18	Mean ± SD	82 ± −18	–	43 ± 24	12 ± 26	84 ± 36	–	9.3 ± 0.7	4.0 ± 1.6	–

ALT, alanine aminotransferase; ALP, alkaline phosphatase; AST, aspartate aminotransferase; BUN, blood urea nitrogen; CK, creatine kinase; CRP, C-reactive protein; GGT, gamma glutamyl transferase; HDL, high-density lipoprotein; LDH, lactate dehydrogenase; LDL, low-density lipoprotein; T. Bili, total bilirubin; T. Prot, total protein; TIBC, total iron binding capacity.

REFERENCES

Altshuler, H.L. and Stowell, R.E. 1972. Normal serum biochemical values of *Cercopithecus aethiops*, *Cercocebus atys*, and *Presbytis entellus*. *Lab Anim Sci.* 22(5):692–704.

Aouidet, A., Bouissou, H., de La Farge, F., and Valdiguie, P. 1990. Serum reference values of the cynomolgus monkey, a model for the study of atherosclerosis. *J Clin Chem Clin Biochem.* 28(4):251–252.

Apple, F.S., Murakami, M.M., Ler, R., Walker, D., and York, M. 2008. Analytical characteristics of commercial cardiac torponin I and T immunoassays in serum from rats, dogs, and monkeys with induced acute myocardial injury. *Clin Chem.* 54(12):1982–1989.

Arnaud, S.B., Navidi, M., Deftos, L., et al. 2002. The calcium endocrine system of adolescent rhesus monkeys and controls before and after spaceflight. *Am J Physiol Endocrinol Metab.* 282:E514–E521.

Ausman, L.M., and Gallina, D.L. 1978. Response to glucose loading of the lean squirrel monkey in unrestrained conditions. *Am J Phys.* 234(1):R20–R24.

Baer, J.F. 1994. Husbandry and medical management of the owl monkey. In *Aotus: The Owl Monkey*. Ed. J.F. Baer, R.E. Weller, and I. Kakoma. San Diego, CL: Academic Press.

Bahr, N.I., Palme, R., Mohle, U., Hodges, J.K., and Heistermann, M. 2000. Comparative aspects of the metabolism and excretion of cortisol in three individual nonhuman primates. *Gen Comp Endocrinol.* 117:427–438.

Bardi, M., Shimizu, K., Fujita, S., Borgognini-Tarli, S., and Huffman, M.A. 2001. Hormonal correlates of maternal style in captive macaques (*Macaca fuscata* and *Macaca mulatta*). *Int J Primatol.* 22(4):647–662.

Barnhart, K.F. 2008. Iron overload in new world monkeys. In Abstract presented at the *36th Annual Workshop of the Association of Primate Veterinarinas*. Indianapolis, IN.

Baroncelli, S., Negri, D.R., Michelini, Z., and Cara, A. 2008. *Macaca mulatta, fascicularis* and *nemestrina* in AIDS vaccine development. *Expert Rev Vaccines.* 7(9):1419–1434.

Beattie, C.W. and Bullock, B.C. 1979. Diurnal variation of serum androgen and estradiol-17beta in the adult male green monkey (*Cercopithecus* sp.). *Biol Reprod.* 19:36–39.

Beland, M.F., Sehgal, P.K., and Peacock, W.C. 1979. Baseline blood chemistry determinations in the squirrel monkey (*Saimiri sciureus*). *Lab Anim Sci.* 29(2):195–199.

Bennett, J.S., Gossett, K.A., McCarthy, M.P., and Simpson, E.D. 1992. Effects of ketamine hydrochloride on serum biochemical and hematologic variables in rhesus monkeys (*Macaca mulatta*). *Vet Clin Pathol.* 21(1):15–18.

Bentson, K.L., Capitanio, J.P., and Mendoza, S.P. 2003. Cortisol responses to immobilization with telazol or ketamiine in baboons (*Papio cynocephalus/anubis*) and rhesus macaques (*Macaca mulatta*). *J Med Primatol.* 32:148–160.

Bergman, R.N. 1989. Toward physiological understanding of glucose tolerance: Minimal-model approach. *Diabetes.* 38(12):1512–1527.

Bernacky, B.J., Gibson, S.V., Keeling, M.E., and Abee, C.R. 2002. Nonhuman primates. In *Laboratory Animal Medition*. Ed. J.G. Fox, L.C. Anderson, F.M. Loew, and F.W. Quimby, pp. 676–791. San Diego, FL: Academic Press.

Bhattacharyya, A.K. and Eggen, D.A. 1983. Mechanism of variability in plasma cholesterol response to cholesterol feeding in rehsus monkeys. *Artery.* 11:306–326.

Blagbrough, I.S., and Zara, C. 2009. Animal models for target diseases in gene therapy—Using DNA and sirna delivery strategies. *Pharm Res.* 26(1):1–18.

Blank, M.S., Gordon, T.P., and Wilson, M.E. 1983. Effects of capture and venipuncture on serum levels of prolactin, growth hormone, and cortisol in outdoor, compound-housed female rhesus monkeys (*Macaca mulatta*). *Acta Endocrinol.* 102:190–195.

Bodkin, N.L. 2000. The rhesus monkey (*Macaca mulatta*): A unique and valuable model for the study of spontaneous diabetes mellitus and associated conditions. In *Animal Models in Diabetes: A Primer*. Ed. A.F. Sima and E. Shafrir, pp. 309–325. Singapore: Taylor & Francis.

Bodkin, N.L., Hannah, J.S., Ortmeyer, H.K., and Hansen, B.C. 1993a. Central obesity in rhesus monkeys: Association with hyperinsulinemia, insulin resistance and hypertriglyceridemia. *Int J Obes.* 17:53–61.

Bodkin, N.L., Metzger, L., and Hansen, B.C. 1989. Hepatic glucose production and insulin sensitivity preceding diabetes in monkeys. *Am J Physiol.* 256(5):E676–E681.

Bodkin, N.L., Ortmeyer, H.K., and Hansen, B.C. 1993b. Diversity of insulin resistance in monkeys with normal glucose tolerance. *Obes Res.* 1(5):364–370.

Bonfanti, U., Lamparelli, D., Colombo, P., and Bernardi, C. 2009. Hematolgoy and serum chemistry parameters in juvenile cynomolgus monkeys (*Macaca fascicularis*) of Mauritius origin: Comparison between purpose-bred and captured animals. *J Med Primatol.* 38(4):228–235.

Bonney, R.C., Dixson, A.F., and Fleming, D. 1979. Cyclic changes in the circulating and urinary steroids in the adult female owl monkey. *J Repord Fertil.* 56:271–280.

Bonney, R.C., Dixson, A.F., and Fleming, D. 1980. Plasma concentrations of oestradiol-17b, oestrone, progesterone and testosterone during the ovarian cycle of the owl monkey (*Aotus trivirgatus*). *J Repord Fertil.* 60:101–107.

Boot, R. and Huis in't Veld, LG. 1981. Pregnancy diagnosis in *Macaca fascicularis*. *J Med Primatol.* 10:141–148.

Bos, A., Probst, B., and Erkert, H.G. 1993. Urinary estradiol-18b exrection in common marmosets, *Callithrix jacchus*: Diurnal pattern and relationship between creatinine-related values and excreted ammount. *Comp Biochem Physiol.* 105(2): 287–292.

Bosu, W.T.K., Johasson, D.B., and Gemzell, C. 1972. Peripheral plasma levels of oestrogens, Progesterone and 17a-hydroxyprogesterone during the menstrual cycle of the rhesus monkeys. *Acta Endocrinol.* 71:755–764.

Bourgoignie, J.J., Gavellas, G., Sabnis, S.G., and Antonovych, T.T. 1994. Effect of protein diets on the renal function of baboons (*Papio hamadryas*) with remnant kidneys: A 5-year follow-up. *Am J Kid Dis.* 23(2):199–204.

Brady, A.G. 2000. The squirrel monkey in biomedical and behavioral research. *ILAR J.* 41(1):10–18.

Brady, A.G., and Koritnik, D.R. 1985. The effects of ketamine anesthesia on glucose clearance in African green monkeys. *J Med Primatol.* 14:99–107.

Brandl, U., Michel, S., Erhardt, M., et al. 2005. Administration of GAS914 in an orthotopic pig-to-baboon heart transplantation model. *Xenotransplantation.* 2005(12):134–141.

Brass, V., Moradpour, D., and Blum, H.E. 2007. Hepatitis C virus infection: In vivo and in vitro models. *J Viral Hepat.* 14(Suppl 1):64–67.

Braun, J.P., Rico, A.G., Benard, P., and Burgat-Sacaze, V. 1980. Gamma-glutamyl transferase distribution in the organs of *Papio papio* and *Macaca fascicularis*. *J Med Primatol.* 9(3):185–188.

Brizzee, K.R., Ordy, J.M., Dunlap, W.P., Kendrick, R., and Wengenack, T.M. 1988. Phenotype and age differences in blood gas chararcteristics, electrolytes, hemoglobin, plasma glucose and cortisol in female squirrel monkeys. *Lab Anim Sci.* 38(2):200–202.

Buchl, S.J., and Howard, W. 1997. Hematologic and serum biochemical and electrolyte values in clinically normal domestically bred rhesus monkeys (*Macaca mulatta*) according to age, sex, and gravidity. *Lab Anim Sci.* 47(5):528–533.

Bush, M. J., and A.J. Verlangieri. 1985. Diet-induced changes in selected clinical chemistry parameters in *M. fascicularis*. *Res Comm Chem Pathol Pharmacol* 50(2): 267-279.

Cabrera-Abreu, J.C., and Green, A. 2002. Gamma-glutamyltransferase: Value of its measurement in paediatrics. *Ann Clin Biochem.* 39:22–25.

Carter, A.M. 2007. Animal models of human placentation—A review. *Placenta.* 21(Suppl A):S41–S47.

Casaco, A., Beausoleil, I., Gonzalez, B., et al. 2010. Hematological, biochemical, respiratory, cardiovascular and electroneurophysiological parameters in African green monkeys (*Cercopitheicus aethiops sabaeus*). Its use in non-clinical toxicological studies. *J Med Primatol.* 39:177–186.

Casetti, R., Taglioni, A., and Perretta, G. 1995. Baseline blood values in the marmosets (*Callithrix jacchus*): Pregnancy related changes. *Primate Rep.* 42:16.

Castro, M.I., Rose, J., Green, W., Lehner, N., Peterson, D., and Taub, D. 1981. Ketamine-HCL as a suitable anesthetic for endocrine, metabolic, and cardiovascular studies in *Macaca fascicularis* monkeys. *Proc Soc Exp Biol Med.* 168:389–394.

Cefalu, W.T., Wagner, J.D., and Bell-Farrow, A.D. 1993. Role of glycated proteins in detecting and monitoring diabetes in cynomolgus monkeys. *Lab Anim Sci.* 43(1):73–77.

Chambers, K.C., Resko, J.A., and Phoenix, C.H. 1982. Correlation of diurnal changes in hormones with sexual behavior and age in male rehsus macaques. *Neurobiol Aging.* 3:37–42.

Chambers, P.L., and Hearn, J.P. 1979. Peripheral plasma levels of progesterone, oestradiol-17 beta, oestrone, testosterone, androstenedione, and chorionic gonadotropin during pregnancy in the marmoset monkey, *Callithrix jacchus*. *J Repord Fertil.* 12:3–5.

Champoux, M., Kriete, M.F., Higley, J.D., and Suomi, S.J. 1996. CBC and serum chemistry differences between Indian-derived and Chinese-Indian hybrid rhesus monkey infants. *Am J Primatol.* 39:79–84.

Chavez, A.O., Gastaldelli, A., Guardado-Mendoza, R., et al. 2009. Predictive models of insulin resistance derived from simple morphometric and biochemical indices related to obesity and the metabolic syndrome in baboons. *Cardiovasc Diabetol.* 8:22–30.

Chavez, A.O., Lopez-Alvarenga, J.C., Tejereo, M.E., et al. 2008. Physiolgoical and molecular determinants of insulin action in the baboon. *Diabetes.* 57:899–908.

Chen, Y., Ono, F., Yoshida, T., and Yoshikawa, Y. 2002. Relationship between body weight and hematological and serum biochemical parameters in female cynomolgus monkeys (*Macaca fascicularis*). *Exp Anim.* 51(2):125–131.

Chen, Y., Qin, S., Ding, Y., et al. 2009. Reference values of clinical chemistry and hematology parameters in rhesus monkeys (*Macaca mulatta*). *Xenotransplant.* 16:496–501.

Chen, Y., Shimizu, M., Sato, K., et al. 2000. Effects of aging on bone mineral content and bone biomarkers in female cynomolgus monkeys. *Exp Anim.* 49(3):163–170.

Christen, P., Peacock, W.C., Christen, A.E., and Wacker, W.E.C. 1970. Urate oxidase in primate phylogenesis. *Eur J Biochem.* 12:3–5.

Cissik, J.H., Hankins, G.D., Hauth, J.C., and Kuehl, T.J. 1986. Blood gas, cardiopulmonary, and urine electrolyte reference values in the pregnant yellow baboon (*Papio cynocephalus*). *Am J Primatol.* 11:277–284.

Clarke, A.S., Wittwer, D.J., Abbott, D.H., and Schneider, M.L. 1994. Long-term effects of prenatal stress on HPA axis activity in juvenile rhesus monkeys. *Dev Psychobiol.* 27(5):257–269.

Colman, R.J., Kemnitz, J.W., Lane, M.A., Abbott, D.H., and Binkley, N. 1999. Skeletal effects of aging and menopausal status in female rhesus macaqes. *J Clin Endocrinol Metab.* 84(11):4144–4148.

Coleman, K., et al. (2008). Training rhesus macaques for venipuncture using positive reinforcement techniques: a comparison with chimpanzees. *J Am Assoc Lab Anim Sci.* 47(1): 37–41.

Contamin, H., Behr, C., Mercereau-Puijalon, O., and Michel, J.C. 2000. Plasmodium falcipaurm in the squirrel monkey (*Saimiri sciureus*): Infection of non-splenectomised animals as a model for exploring clinical manifestations of malaria. *Microbes Infect.* 2:245–954.

Cornelius, C.E. and Freedland, R.A. 1992. Fasting hyperbilirubinemia in normal squirrel monkeys. *Lab Anim Sci.* 42(1):35–37.

Cowie, J.R. and Evans, G.O. 1985. Plasma aminotransferase measurements in the marmoset (*Callithrix jacchus*). *Lab Anim.* 19:48–50.

Czoty, P.W., Gould, R.W., and Nader, M.A. 2008. Relationship between social rank and cortisol and testosterone concentrations in male cynomolgus monkeys (*Macaca fascicularis*). *J Neuroendocrinol.* 21:68–76.

D'Ovidio, M.C. and Turillazzi, P.G. 1994. Changes in serum protein fractions and specific alpha and beta concentrations during lactation in *Macaca fascicularis*. *Lab Anim Sci.* 44:618–623.

Davy, C.W., Jackson, M.R., and Walker, J.M. 1984a. The effect of haemolysis on some clinical chemistry parameters in the marmoset (*Callithrix jacchus*). *Lab Anim.* 18:161–168.

Davy, C.W., Jackson, M.R., and Walker, J. 1984b. Reference intervals for some clinical chemical parameters in the marmoset (*Callithrix jacchus*): Effect of age and sex. *Lab Anim.* 18:135–142.

De la Pena, A., Matthijssen, C., and Goldzieher, J.W. 1970. Normal values for blood constituents of the baboon (*Papio species*). *Lab Anim Care.* 20(2):251–261.

De Wet, E.H., Oosthuizen, J.M.C., Barnard, H.C., and Potgieter, F. 1994. Stress hormones in primates. *SAMS.* 84(5):302–303.

DeFronzo, R.A., Tobin, J.D., and Andres, R. 1979. Glucose clamp technique: A method for quantifying insulin secretion and resistance. *Am J Physiol.* 237(3):E214–E223.

Diamond, E.J., Askel, S., Hazelton, J.M., Barnet, S.B., Williams, L.E., and Abee, C.R. 1985. Serum hormone patterns during abortion in the Bolivian squirrel monkey. *Lab Anim Sci* 35: 619–23.

Diamond, E.J., Aksel, S., Hazelton, J.M., Wiebe, R.H., and Abee, C.R. 1987. Serum oestradiol, progesterone, chorionic gonadotropin and prolactin concentrations during pregnancy in the Bolivian squirrel monkey (*Saimiri sciureus*). *J Repord Fertil.* 80:373–381.

Diehl, K.H., Hull, R., Morton, D., Pfister, R., Rabemampianina, Y., Smith, D., Vidal, J.M., and van de Vorstenbosch, C. 2001. A good practice guide to the administration of substances and removal of blood, including routes and volumes. *J Appl Toxicol.* 21:15–23.

Dixson, A.F. and Gardner, J.S. 1981. Diurnal variations in plasma testosterone in a male nocturnal primate, the owl monkey (*Aotus trivirgatus*). *J Repord Fertil.* 62:83–86.

Dixson, A.F. and George, L. 1982. Prolactin and parental behaviour in a male New World primate. *Nature.* 299(7):551–553.

Drevon-Gaillot, E., Perron-Lepage, M.F., Clement, C., and Burnett, R. 2006. A review of background findings in cynomolgus monkeys (*Macaca fascicularis*) from three different geographical origins. *Exp Toxicol Pathol.* 58:77–88.

du Plooy, W.J., Schutte, P.J., Still, J., Hay, L., and Kahler, C.P. 1998. Stability of cardiodynamic and some blood parameters in the baboon following intravenous anaesthesia with ketamine and diazepam. *J S Afr Vet Assoc.* 69(1):18–21.

Dubey, A.K., Puri, C.P., Puri, V., and Anand Kumar, T.C. 1983. Day and night levels of hormones in male rhesus monkeys kept under controlled or constant environmental light. *Experientia.* 39:889–896.

Dysko, R.C. and Hoskins, D.E. 1995. Collection of biological samples and therapy administration. In *Nonhuman Primates in Biomedical Research: Biology & Management*. Ed. B.T. Bennett, C.R. Abee, and R. Henrickson, Vol. 1, pp. 270–286. San Diego, FL: Academic Press.

Eder, G. 1996. A longitudinal study of the kidney function of the chimpanzee (*Pan troglodytes*) in comparison with humans. *Eur J Clin Chem Biochem.* 34:889–896.

Elfenbein, H.A., Rosen, R.F., Stephens, S.L., et al.. 2007. Cerebral B-amyloid angiopathy in aged squirrel monkeys. *Histol Histopathol.* 22:155–167.

Ely, J.J., Zavaskis, T., Lammey, M.L., Sleeper, M.M., and Lee, D.R. 2011. Association of brain-type natriuretic protein and cardiac troponin I with incipient cardiovascular disease in chimpanzees (*Pan troglodytes*). *Comp Med.* 61(2):163–169.

Eslamboli, A. 2005. Marmoset monkey models of parkinson's disease: Which model, when and why? *Brain Res Bull.* 68(3):140–149.

Fernie, S., Wrenshall, E., Malcolm, S., Bryce, F., and Arnold, D.L. 1994. Normative hematologic and serum biochemical values for adult and infant rhesus monkeys (*Macaca mulatta*) in a controlled laboratory environment. *J Toxicol Environ Health.* 42(1):53–72.

Fincham, J.E., Wilson, G.R., Belonje, P.C., et al. 1993. Parathyroid hormone, ionised calcium, and potentially interacting variables in plasma of an Old world primate. *J Med Primatol.* 22(4):246–252.

Fortman, J.D., Hewett, T.A., and Bennet, B.T. 2002. *The Laboratory Nonhuman Primate*. Ed. M.A. Suckow. Boca Raton, FL: CRC Press.

Frawley, L.S. and Neill, J.D. 1979. Age-related changes in the serum levels of gonadotropins and testosterone in infantile male rehsus monkeys. *Biol Reprod.* 20:1147–1151.

Fredericks, S., Merton, G.K., Lerena, M.J., Heining, P., Carter, N.D., and Holt, D.W. 2001. Cardiac troponins and creatine kinase content of striated muscle in common laboratory animals. *Clin Chim Acta.* 304:65–74.

Friedman, T.B., Planco, G.E., Appoid, J.C., and Mayle, J.E. 1985. On the loss of uricolytic activity during primate evolution—I. Silencing of urate oxidase in a hominid ancestor. *Comp Biochem Physiol B.* 81(3):653–659.

Fuchs, E., Kirschbaum, C., Benisch, D., and Bieser, A. 1997. Salivary cortisol: A non-invasive measure of hypothalamo–pituitary–adrenocortical activity in the squirrel monkey, *Saimiri sciureus. Lab Anim.* 31(4): 306–11.

Fulmer, R., Loeb, W.F., Martin, D.P., and Gard, E.A. 1984. Effects of three methods of retraint on intravenous glucose tolerance testing in rhesus and African green monkeys. *Vet Clin Pathol.* 13(1):19–25.

Gagneux, P.l, Amess, R., Diaz, S., et al. 2001. Proteomic comparison of human and great ape blood plasma reveals conserved glycosylation and differences in thyroid hormone metabolism. *Am J Phys Anthropol.* 115:99–109.

Garg, S.K., Chhina, G.S., and Singh, B. 1978. Factors influencing plasma cortisol (11-Hydroxycorticoids) levels in rhesus monkeys. *Ind J Exp Biol.* 16:1184–1185.

Gartner, L.M., Lee, K.S., Waisman, S., Lane, D., and Zarafu, I. 1977. Development of bilirubin transport and metabolism in the newborn rhesus monkey. *J Pediatr.* 90(4):513–531.

Gatesman, T.J. 1986. A preliminary study of urine analysis in conjunction with diseases of the urinary tract in tamarins and marmosets (Abstract). *Primate Rep.* 14:168.

Gavellas, G., Disbrow, M.R., Hwang, K.H., Hinkle, D.K., and Bourgoignie, J.J. 1987. Glomerular filtration rate and blood pressure monitoring in awake baboons. *Lab Anim Sci.* 37:657–662.

Gatesman, T. J. 1992. Serum amylase values in callitrichids. *Lab Anim Sci* 42(1): 46-50.

Gilardi, K.V., Shideler, S.E., Valverde, C.R., Roberts, J.A., and Lasley, B.L. 1997. Characterization of the onset of menopause in the rhesus macaque. *Biol Reprod.* 57:335–340.

Giulietti, M., Pace, M., La Torre, R., Ovidio, M.C., Patella, A., and Turillazzi, P.G. 1996. Role of delivery on serum iron-related parameters in *Macaca fascicularis* females. *Comp Biochem Physiol.* 114(2):181–184.

Glenn, K.M., Campbell, J.L., and Rotstein, D. 2006. Retrospective evaluation of the incidence and severity of hemosiderosis in a large captive lemur population. *Am J Primatol.* 68:369–381.

Goncharov, N.P., Tavadyan, D.S., and Voronstov, V.I. 1981. Diurnal and seasonal rhythms of androgen content in the plasma in *Macaca mulatta. Probl Endocrinol (Moscow).* 27:53–57.

Goncharova, N.D. and Lapin, B.A. 2000. Changes of hormonal function of the adrenal and gonadal glands in baboons of different age groups. *J Med Primatol.* 29:26–35.

Goodman, A.L., Descalzi, C.D., Johnson, D.K., and Hodgen, G.D. 1977. Composite pattern of circulating LH, FSH, estradiol, and progesterone during the menstrual cycle in cynomolgus monkeys. *Proc Soc Exp Biol Med.* 155(4):479–481.

Goodner, C.J., Walike, B.C., Koerker, D.J., et al. 1977. Insulin, glucagon, and glucose exhibit synchronous, sustained oscillations in fasting monkeys. *Science.* 195:177–179.

Gordon, T.P., Bernstein, I.S., and Rose, R.M. 1978. Social and seasonal influences on testosterone secretion in the male rhesus monkey. *Physiol Behav.* 21:623–627.

Gore, M.A., Brandes, F., Kaup, F-J., Lenzner, R., Mothes, T., and Osman, A.A. 2001. Callitrichid nutrition and food sensitivity. *J Med Primatol.* 30:179–184.

Gozalo, A.S., Chavera, A., Montoya, E.J., Takano, J., and Weller, R.E. 2008. Relationship of creatine kinase, aspartate aminotransferase, lactate dehydrogenase, and proteinuria to cardiomyopathy in the owl monkey (*Aotus vociferans*). *J Med Primatol.* 37(Suppl 1):29–38.

Gresl, T.A., Colman, R.J., Havighurst, T.C., Allison, D.B., Schoeller, D.A., and Kemnitz, J.W. 2003a. Dietary restriction and beta-cell sensitivity to glucose in adult male rhesus monkeys. *J Gerontol.* 58A(7):598–610.

Gresl, T.A., Colman, R.J., Havighurst, T.C., et al. 2003b. Insulin sensitivity and glucose effectiveness from three minimal models: Effects of energy restriction and body fat in adult male rhesus monkeys. *Am J Physiol Regul Integr Comp Physiol.* 285:R1340–R1345.

Gross, K.L., Westberry, J.M., Hubler, T.R., et al. 2008. Androgen resistance in squirrel monkeys (*Saimiri* spp). *Comp Med.* 58(4):381–388.

Hack, C.A. and Gleiser, C.A. 1982. Hematologic and serum chemical reference values for adult and juvenile baboons (*Papio* sp). *Lab Anim Sci.* 32(5):502–505.

Hainsey, B.M., Hubbard, G.B., Leland, M.M., and Brasky, K.M. 1993. Clinical parameters of the normal baboons (*Papio* species) and chimpanzees (*Pan troglodytes*). *Lab Anim Sci.* 43:236–243.

Hall, R.L. and Everds, N.E. 2003. Factors affecting the interpretation of canine and nonhuman primate clinical-pathology. *Toxicol Pathol.* 31(Supp l):6–10.

Hanley, P. 2009. Personal communication.

Hansen, B.C. and Bodkin, N.L. 1986. Heterogeneity of insulin responses: Phases leading to type 2 (non-insulin-dependent) diabetes mellitus in the rhesus monkey. *Diabetelogia.* 29:713–719.

Hansen, B.C., and Bodkin, N.L. 1993. Primary prevention of diabetes mellitus by prevention of obesity in monkeys. *Diabetes.* 42(12):1809–1811.

Harewood, W.J., Gillin, A., Hennessy, A., Armistead, J., Horvath, J.S., and Tiller, D.J. 1999. Biochemistry and haematology values for the baboon (*Papio hamadryas*): The effects of sex, growth, development and age. *J Med Primatol.* 28(19):19–31.

Harewood, W.J., Gillin, A., Hennessy, A., Armistead, J., Horvath, J.S., and Tiller, D.J. 2000. The effects of the menstrual cycle, pregnancy and early lactation on haematology and plasma biochemistry in the baboon (*Papio hamadryas*). *J Med Primatol.* 29:415–420.

Harewood, W.J., Gillin, A., Mohamed, S., et al. 1996. Cyclical changes in the renin-angiotensin-aldosterone system during the menstrual cycle of the baboon (*Papio hamadryas*). *J Med Primatol.* 25:267–271.

Hargis, G.K., Reynolds, W.A., Williams, G.A., et al. 1978. Radioimmunoassay of calcitonin in the plasma of rhesus monkey and man. *Clin Chem.* 24(4):595–601.

Hargis, G.K., Williams, G.A., Reynolds, W.A., et al. 1977. Radioimmunoassay of parathyroid hormone (parathyrin) in monkey and man. *Clin Chem.* 23(11):1989–1994.

Hassimoto, M., Harada, T., and Harada, T. 2004. Changes in hematology, biochemical values, and restraint ECG of rhesus monkeys (*Macaca mulatta*) following 6-month laboratory acclimation. *J Med Primatol.* 33(4):175–186.

Havill, L.M., Snider, C.L., Leland, M.M., and Hubbard, G.B. 2003. Hematology and blood biochemistry in infant baboons. *J Med Primatol.* 32:131–138.

Hearn, J.P. 1987. Marmosets and tamarins. In *The Ufaw Handbook on the Care and Management of Laboratory Animals*. Ed. T.B. Poole, pp. 568–581. Essex: Longman Scientific & Technical.

Heeney, J.L., Dalgleish, A.G., and Weiss, R.A. 2006. Origins of HIV and the evolution of resistance to AIDS. *Science.* 313:462–466.

Heffernan, S., Phippard, A., Sinclair, A., et al. 1995. A baboon (*Papio hamadryas*) model of insulin-dependent diabetes. *J Med Primatol.* 24:29–34.

Hein, P.R., Schatorje, J.S., Frencken, H.J., Segers, M.F., and Thomas, C.M. 1989. Serum hormone levels in pregnant cynomolgus monkeys. *J Med Primatol.* 18(2):133–142.

Heistermann, M., Palme, R., and Ganswindt, A. 2006. Comparison of different enzymeimmunoassays for assessment of adrenocortical activity in primates based on fecal analysis. *Am J Primatol.* 68:257–273.

Heistermann, M., Tari, S., and Hodges, J.K. 1993. Measurement of faecal steroids for monitoring ovarian function in New World primates, callitrichidae. *J Repord Fertil.* 99:243–251.

Hess, D.L., Hendrickx, A.G., and Stabenfeldt, G.H. 1979. Reproductive and hormonal patterns in the African green monkey (*Cercopithecus aethiops*). *J Med Primatol.* 8(5):273–281.

Higami, Y., Yamaza, H., and Shimokawa, I. 2005. Laboratory findings of caloric restriction in rodents and primates. *Adv Clin Chem.* 39:211–237.

Hobson, W.C., Coulston, F., Faiman, C., Winter, J.S., and Reyes, F.I. 1976. Reproductive endocrinology of female chimpanzees: A suitable model of humans. *J Toxicol Environ Health.* 1(4):657–668.

Hom, G.J., Bach, T.J., Carroll, D., et al. 1999. Comparison of cardiovascular parameters and/or serum chemistry and hematology profiles in conscious and anesthetized rhesus monkeys (*Macaca mulatta*). *Contemp Top Lab Anim Sci.* 38(2):60–64.

Hotchkiss, C.E., and Brommage, R. 2000. Changes in bone turnover during the menstrual cycle in cynomolgus monkeys. *Calcif Tissue Int.* 66:224–228.

Hotchkiss, C.E., and Jerome, C.P. 1998b. Evaluation of a nonhuman primate model to study circadian rhythms of calcium metabolism. *Am J Physiol Endocrinol Metab.* 275:R494–R501.

Hotchkiss, C.E., Brommage, R., Du, M., and Jerome, C.P. 1998a. The anesthetic isoflurane decreases ionized calcium and increases parathyroid hormone and osteocalcin in cynomolgus monkeys. *Bone.* 23(5):479–484.

Hotchkiss, J., Dierschke, D.J., Butler, W.R., Fritz, G.R., and Knobil, E. 1982. Relation between circulating ovarian steroids and pituitary gonadotropion during the menstrual cycle of the rhesus monkey. *Biol Reprod.* 26:241–248.

Hotta, K., Funahashi, T., Bodkin, N.L., et al. 2001. Circulating concentrations of the adipocyte protein adiponectin are decreased in parallel with reduced insulin sensitivity during the progression to type 2 diabetes in rhesus monkeys. *Diabetes.* 50:1126–1133.

Howell, S., Hoffman, K., Bartel, L., Schwandt, M., Morris, J., and Fritz, J. 2003. Normal hematologic and serum clinical chemistry values for captive chimpanzees (*Pan troglodytes*). *Comp Med.* 53(4):413–423.

Hseih, A.T., Anthony, J.C., Diersen-Schade, D.A., Nathanielsz, P.W., and Brenna, J.T. 2008. Biochemical and white blood cell profiles of baboon neonates consuming formulas with moderate and high dietary long-chain polyunsaturated fatty acids. *J Med Primatol.* 37:81–87.

Hukkanen, R.R., Liggitt, H.D., Anderson, D.M., and Kelley, S.T. 2006. Detection of systemic amyloidosis in the pig-tailed macaque (*Macaca nemestrina*). *Comp Med.* 56(2):119–127.

Ihrig, M., Tassinary, L.G., Bernacky, B., and Keeling, M.E. 2001. Hematologic and serum biochemical reference intervals for the chimpanzee (*Pan troglodytes*) categorized by age and sex. *Comp Med.* 51(1):30–37.

Iliff, S.A., Murphy, L.M., Mariano, M.A., Trainor, C.E., Pikounis, B., and Anderson, L.C. 2003. Comparison of laboratory values of blood collected from rhesus macaques using two different techniques (Abstract). *Contemp Top Lab Anim Sci.* 42(4):104.

Izumi, Y., Okatani, H., Shiota, M., et al. 2009. Effects of metoprolol on epinephrine-induced takotsubo-like left ventricular dysfunction in non-human primates. *Hypertens Res.* 32(5):339–346.

Jacob, J.R., Lin, K-C., Tennant, B.C., and Mansfield, K.G. 2004. GB virus B infection of the common marmoset (*Callithrix jacchus*) and associated liver pathology. *J Gen Virol.* 85:2525–2533.

Jen, K-L.C. and Hansen, B.C. 1988. Glucose disapperance rate in rhesus monkeys: Some technical considerations. *Am J Primatol.* 14:153–166.

Jen, I.C., Hansen, B.C., and Metzger, B. 1985. Adiposity, anthropometric measures, and plasma insulin levels of rhesus monkeys. *Int J Obesity.* 9:213–214.

Jinbo, T., Hayashi, S., Iguchi, K., et al. 1998. Development of monkey C-reactive protein (CRP) assay methods. *Vet Immunol Immunopathol.* 61:195–202.

Johnson, Q., Veith, W.J., and Mouton, T. 2001. The impact of dietary protein intake on serum biochemical and haematological profiles in vervet monkeys. *J Med Primatol.* 30:61–69.

Johnson, R.J., Sautin, Y.Y., Oliver, W.J., et al. 2009. Lessons from comparative physiology: Could uric acid represent a physiologic alarm signal gone awry in western society? *J Comp Physiol B.* 170:67–76.

Johnson, R.J., Titte, S., Cade, J.R., Rideout, B.A., and Oliver, W.J. 2005. Uric acid, evoluation and primitive cultures. *Semin nephrol.* 25(1):3–8.

Juompan, L.Y., Hutchinson, K., Montefiori, D.C., Nidtha, S., Villinger, F., and Novembre, F.J. 2008. Analysis of the immune responses in chimpanzees infected with HIV type 1 isolates. *AIDS Res Hum Retrovir.* 24(4):573–586.

Kaack, B., Brizzee, K.R., and Walker, L. 1979a. Some biochemical blood parameters in the developing squirrel monkey. *Folia Primatol.* 32:309–317.

Kaack, B., Walker, L.C., Brizzee, K.R., and Wolf, R.H. 1979b. Comparative normal levels of serum triiodothyronine and thyroxine in nonhuman primates. *Lab Anim Sci.* 29(2):191–194.

Kaack, B., Walker, M., and Walker, L. 1980. Seasonal changes in the thyroid hormones of the male squirrel monkey. *Arch Androl.* 4(2):133–136.

Kamili, S., Sozzi, V., Thompson, G.,et al. 2009. Efficacy of hepatitis B vaccine against antiviral drug-resistant hepatitis B virus mutants in the chimpanzee model. *Hepatology.* 49(5):1483–1491.

Kapeghian, J.C., Bush, M.J., and Verlangieri, A.J. 1984. Changes in selected serum biochemical and EKG values with age in cynomolgus macaques. *J Med Primatol.* 13(5):283–288.

Kaur, T., and Huffman, M.A. 2004. Descriptive urological record of chimpanzees (*Pan troglodytes*) in the wild and limitations associated with using multi-reagent dipstick test strips. *J Med Primatol.* 33(4):187–196.

Kavanagh, K., Williams, J.K., and Wagner, J.C. 2005. Naturally occurring menopause in cynomolgus monkeys: Changes in hormone, lipid, and carbohydrate measures with hormonal status. *J Med Primatol.* 34:171–177.

Kelly, T.R., Sleeman, J.M., and Wranghma, R. 2004. Urinalysis in free-living chimpanzees (*Pan troglodytes schweinfurthii*) in Uganda. *Vet Rec.* 154:729–730.

Kemnitz, J.W., and Kraemer, G.W. 1982. Assessment of glucoregulation in rhesus monkeys sedated with ketamine. *Am J Primatol.* 3:201–210.

Kessler, M.J., Rawlins, R.G., and London, W.T. 1983. The hemogram, serum biochemistry, and electrolyte profile of aged rhesus monkeys (*Macaca mulatta*). *J Med Primatol.* 12(4):184–191.

Kim, C.Y., Lee, H.S., Han, S.C., et al. 2005. Hematological and serum biochemical values in cynomolgus monkeys anesthetized with ketamine hydrochloride. *J Med Primatol.* 34(2):96–100.

Klein, R., Bleiholder, B., Jung, A., and Erkert, H.G. 1985. Diurnal variation of several blood parameters in the owl monkey, *Aotus trivirgatus griseimembra. Folia Primatol (Basel).* 45(3–4):195–203.

Klosterman, L.L., Murai, J.T., and Siiteri, P.K. 1986. Cortisol levels, binding, and properties of corticosteroid-binding globulin in the serum of primates. *Endocrinology.* 118:424–434.

Knott, C.D. 1993. Monitoring of hormonal profiles of free-ranging chimpanzees (*Pan troglodytes*) and orangutans (*Pongo pygmaeus*). *Bull Ecol Soc Am.* 74(2,Suppl.):314.

Koerker, D.J., Goodner, C.J., Hansen, B., Brown, A.C., and Rubenstein, A. 1978. Syncrhonous, sustained oscillation of C-peptide and insulin in the plasma of fasting monkeys. *Endocrinology.* 102(5):1649–1652.

Koyama, T., De La Pena, A., and Hagino, N. 1977. Plasma estrogen, progestin, and luteinizing hormone during the normal menstrual cycle in the baboon: Role of leuteinizing hormone. *Am J Obstet Gynecol.* 127:67–72.

Kuo, M.M., Tran, S., and Everds, N. 2008. Short-term and long-term stability of sorbitol dehydrogenase in cynomolgus monkey serum. *Clin Chem.* 54(6):A71.

Lambeth, S.P., Hau, J., Perlman, J.E., Martino, M., and Schapiro, S.J. 2006. Positive reinforcement training affects hematologic and serum chemistry values in captive chimpanzees (*Pan troglodytes*). *Am J Primatol.* 68:245–256.

Lamperez, A.J., and Rowell, T.J. 2005. Normal C-reactive protein values for captive chimpanzees (*Pan troglodytes*). *Contemp Top Lab Anim Sci.* 44(5):25–26.

Lane, M.A., Reznick, A.Z., Tlimont, E.M., et al. 1999. Aging and food restriction alter some indices of bone metabolism in male rhesus monkeys (*Macaca mulatta*). *J Nutr.* 125:1600–1610.

Lees, C.J., Jerome, C.P., Register, T.C., and Carlson, C.S. 1998. Changes in bone mass and bone biomarkers of cynomolgus monkeys during pregnancy and lactation. *J Clin Endocrinol Metab.* 83:4298–4302.

Legrand, J-J, Fisch, C., Guillaumat, P.O., et al. 2003. Use of biochemical markers to monitor changes in bone turnover in cynomolgus monkeys. *Biomarkers.* 8(1):63–77.

Lehmann, R., Bhargava, A.S., and Gunzel, P. 1993. Serum lipoprotein pattern in rats, dogs and monkeys, including method comparison and influence of menstrual cycle in monkeys. *Eur J Clin Chem Biochem.* 31:633–637.

Lehmann, R., Wagner, J.L., Fernandez, L.A., et al. 1997. Effects of ketamine sedation on glucose clearance, insulin secretion and counterregulatory hormone production in baboons (*Papio hamadryas*). *J Med Primatol.* 26:312–321.

Lemere, C.A., Oh, J., Stanish, H.A., et al. 2008. Cerebral amyloid-beta protein accumulation with agin in cotton-top tamarins: A model of early alzheimer's disease? *Rejuvenation Res.* 11(2):321–332.

Lequin, R.M., Elvens, L.H., and Bertens, A.M. 1981. Early detection of pregnancy in rhesus and stump-tailed macaques (*Macaca mulatta* and *Macaca arctoides*): Evaluation of two radioimmunoassays and a hemagglutination inhibition test. *J Med Primatol.* 10:189–190.

Leshner, A.I., Toivola, P.T.K., and Terasawa, E. 1978. Circadian variations in cortisol concentrations in the plasma of female rhesus monkeys. *J Endocrinol.* 78:155–156.

Leszcyzynski, J.K., Danahey, D.G., Ferrer, K.T., Hewett, T.A., and Fortman, J.D. 2002. Primary hyperparathyroidism in an adult female olive baboon (*Papio anubis*). *Comp Med.* 52(2):563–567.

Leuchte, N., Berry, N., Kohler, B., et al. 2004. MhcDRB-sequences from cynomolgus macaques (*Macaca fascicularis*) of different origin. *Tissue Antigens.* 63:529–537.

Liddie, S., Goody, R.J., Valles, R., and Lawrence, M.S. 2010. Clinical chemistry and hematology values in a Caribbean population of African green monkeys. *J Med Primatol.* 39:389–398.

Lynch, K.M., Seller, T., Ennulat, D., and Schwartz, L. 2004. Evaluation and use of a human elisa method for measuring pepsinogen I in monkey serum (Abstract). *Clin Chem.* 50(6):A36.

Machatschke, I.H., Dittami, J., and Wallner, B. 2006. Morphometric and hormonal changes during the chimpanzee menstrual cycle. *J Med Primatol.* 35:331–340.

Malaga, C.A., Weller, R.E., Buschbom, R.L., and Ragan, H.A. 1991. Serum chemistry of the wild caught karyotype I night monkey (*Aotus nancymai*). *Lab Anim Sci.* 41(2):143–144.

Mann, D.R., Akinbami, M.A., Gould, K.G., and Castracane1, V.D. 2002. Leptin and thyroxine during secual development in male monkeys: Effect of neonatal gonadotropin-releasing hormone antagonist treatment and delayed puberty on the development pattern of leptin and thyroxine secretion. *Europ J Endocrinol.* 146:891–898.

Mansfield, K. 2003. Marmoset models commonly used in biomedical research. *Comp Med.* 53(4):383–392.

Martin, D.E., Swenson, R.B., and Collins1, D.C. 1977. Correlation of serum testosterone levels with age in male chimpanzees. *Steroids.* 29:471–481.

Massacesi, L., Genain, C.P., Lee-Parritz, D., Letvin, N.L., Canfield, D., and Hauser, S.L. 1995. Active and passively induced experimental autoimmune encephalomyeloitis in common marmosets: A new model for multiple sclerosis. *Ann Neurol.* 37(4):519–530.

Maston, G.A. and Ruvolo, M. 2002. Chorionic gonadotropin has a recent origin within primates and an evolutionary history of selection. *Mol Biol Evol.* 19(3):320–335.

Matsumuro, M., Sankai, T., Cho, F., Yoshikawa, Y., and Yoshida, T. 1999. A two-step extraction method to measure fecal steroid hormones in female cynomolgus monkeys (*Macaca fascicularis*). *Am J Primatol.* 48:291–298.

Mattison, J. A., et al. 2017. Caloric restriction improves health and survival of rhesus monkeys. *Nat Commun.* 8: 14063.

McGeachin, R. L. and J. R. Akin. 1982. Amylase levels in the tissues and body fluids of several primate species. *Comp Biochem Physiol A Comp Physiol* 72(1): 267-269.

McGuire, M.T., Brammer, G.L., and Raleigh, M.J. 1986. Resting cortisol levels and the emergence of dominant status among male vervet monkeys. *Horm Behav.* 20:106–117.

Mehta, R.R., Jenco, J.M., Gaynor, L.V., and Chatteron, R.T. 1986. Relationships between ovarian morphology, vaginal cytology, serum progesterone, and urinary immunoreactive pregnanediol during the menstrual cycle of the cynomolgus monkey. *Biol Reprod.* 35:981–986.

Meis, P. J., Kaplan, J.R., Koritnik, D.R., and Rose, J.C. 1982. Effects of gestation on glucose tolerance and plasma insulin in cynomolgus monkeys (Macaca fascicularis). *Am J Obstet Gynecol* 144(5): 543-545.

Meis, P.J., and Rose, J.C. 1983. Plasma cortisol response to feeding in African green vervets. *J Med Primatol.* 12(1):49–52.

Meusy-Dessolle, N., and Dang, D.C. 1985. Plasma concentrations of testosterone, dihydrotestosterone, delta4-androsterone, dehydroepiandrosterone and oestradiol-17b in the crab-eating monkey (*Macaca fascicularis*) from birth to adulthood. *J Reprod Fertil.* 74:347–359.

Miller, G.F., Barnard, D.E., Woodward, R.A., Flynn, B.M., and Bulte, J.W.M. 1997. Hepatic hemosiderosis in common marmosets, *Callithrix jacchus*: Effect of diet on incidence and severity. *Lab Anim Sci.* 47(2):138–142.

Minomo, H., Torikai, Y., Furukawa, T., et al. 2009. Characteristics of troponins as myocardial damage biomarkers in cynomolgus monkeys. *J Toxicol Sci.* 34(6):589–601.

Mohle, U., Hesitermann, M., Palme, R., and Hodges, J.K. 2002. Characterization of urinary and fecal metabolites of testosterone and their measurement for assessing gonadal endocrine function in male nonhuman primates. *Gen Comp Endocrinol.* 129:135–145.

Mohr, J.R., Mattenheimer, H., Holmes, A.W., Deinhardt, F., and Schmidt, F.W. 1971. Enzymology of experimental liver disease in marmoset monkeys. *Enzyme.* 12:99–116.

Moorman, E. A., Mendoza, S.P., Schideler, S.E., and Lasley, B.L. 2002. Excretion and measurement of estradiol and progesterone metabolites in the feces and urine of female squirrel monkeys (*Saimiri sciureus*). *Am J Primatol.* 57:79–90.

Morley, J.E., Raleigh, M.J., Brammer, G.L., Yuwiler, A., Geller, E., Flannery, J., and Hershman, J.M. 1980. Serotonergic and catecholaminergic influene on thyroid function in the vervet monkey. *Eur J Pharmacol.* 67:283–288.

Mott, G.E., and Rogers, M.L. 1978. Enzymatic determination of triglycerides in human and baboon serum triglycerides. *Clin Chem.* 24(2):354–357.

Myers, B.A., Bruss, M.L., George, J.W., and Cornelius, C.E. 1991. Endogenous bilirubin excretion in bolivian squirrel monkeys with a gilbert's like syndrome. *J Med Primatol.* 20(3):97–103.

Najafian, B., Masood, A., Malloy, P.C., et al. 2010. Glomerulopathy in spontaneously obese rhesus monkeys with type 2 diabetes: A stereological study. *Diabetes Metab Res Rev.* 27:341–347.

Nakamura, E., Lane, M.A., Roth, G.S., and Ingram, D.K. 1998. A strategy for identifying biomarkers of aging: Further evaluation of hematology and blood chemistry data from a calories restriction study in rhesus monkeys. *Exp Gerontol* 33(5): 421–43.

Naqvi, R.H. and Lindberg, M.C. 1985. Evaluation of the subhuman primate pregnancy test kit for the detection of early pregnancy in the rhesus monkeys (*Macaca mulatta*). *J Med Primatol.* 14:229–233.

Natelson, B.H., Stokes, P.E., and Root, A.W. 1982. Plasma glucose and insulin levels in monkeys anticipating feeding. *Pavlov J Biol Sci.* 17(2):80–83.

Nino-Vasquez, J.J., Vogel, D., Rodriguez, R., et al. 2000. Sequence and diversity of DRB genes of *Aotus nacymaae*, a primate mode for human malaria parasites. *Immunogenet.* 51:219–230.

Norman, R.L. and Smith, D. 1992. Restraint inhibits luteinizing hormone and testosterone secretion in intact male rhesus macaques: Effects of concurrent naloxone administration. *Neuroendocrinology.* 55(4):405–415.

Nyachieo, A., Chai, D.C., Deprest, J., Mwenda, J.M., and D'Hooghe, T. 2007. The baboon as a research mode for the study of endometrial biology, uterine receptivity and embryo implantation. *Gynecol Obstet Invest.* 64(3):149–155.

Oda, M., Satta, Y., Takenaka, O., and Takahata, N. 2002. Loss of urate oxidase activity in hominids and its evolutionary implications. *Mol Biol Evol.* 19(5):640–653.

Pacini, G., Tonolo, G., Sambataro, M., et al. 1998. Insulin sensitivity and glucose effectiveness: Minimal model analysis of regular and insulin-modified FSIGT. *Am J Phys.* 274(4 Pt 1):E592–599.

Paramastri, Y., Royo, F., Eberova, J., et al. 2007. Urinary and fecal immunoglobulin A, cortisol and 11-17 dioxoandrostanes, and serum cortisol in metabolic cage housed female cynomolgus monkeys (*Macaca fascicularis*). *J Med Primatol.* 36:355–364.

Parks, J.S. and Rudel, L.L. 1985. Alteration of high density lipoprotein subfraction distribution with induction of serum amyloid A protein (SAA) in the nonhuman primate. *J Lipid Res.* 26:82–91.

Patterson, J.L. and Carrion, R. 2005. Demand for nonhuman primate resources in the age of biodefense. *ILAR J.* 1:15–22.

Pender, C., Ortmeyer, H.K., Hansen, B.C., Goldfine, I.D., and Youngren, J.F. 2002. Elevated plasma cell membrane glycoprotein levels and diminished insulin receptor autophosphorylation in obese, insulin-resistant rhesus monkeys. *Metabolism.* 51(4):465–470.

Perretta, G., Violante, A., Scarpulla, M., Beciani, M., and Monaco, V. 1991. Normal serum biochemical and hematological parameters in *Macaca fascicularis*. *J Med Primatol.* 20:345–351.

Pessiglione, M., Guehl, D., Agid, Y., Hirsch, E.C., Feger, J., and Tremblay, L. 2003. Impairment of context-adapted movement selection in a primate model of presymptomatic Parkinson's disease. *Brain.* 126:1392–1408.

Poleschuk, V.F., Balayan, M.S., Titova, I.P., et al. 1996. Some hematological and biochemical values of normal blood in captive moustached tamarins (*Saguinus mystax*). *Primate Rep.* 44:67–70.

Portman, O.W., Alexander, M., and Neuringer, M. 1985. Dietary protein effects on lipoproteins and on sex and thyroid hormones in blood of rhesus monkeys. *J Nutr.* 115:425–435.

Portman, O.W., Chowdhury, J.R., Chowdhury, N.R., Alexander, M., Cornelius, C.E., and Arias, I. 1984. A nonhuman primate model of Gilbert's syndrome. *Hepatology.* 4(2):175–179.

Preus, M., Karsten, B., and Bhargava, A.S. 1989. Serum isoenzyme pattern of creatine kinase and lactate dehydrogenase in various animal species. *J Clin Chem Clin Biochem.* 27:787–790.

Prince, A.M. and Brotman, B. 2001. Perspectives on hepatitis B studies with chimpanzees. *ILAR J.* 42(2):85–88.

Purcell, R.H. and Emerson, S.U. 2001. Animal models of hepatitis A and E. *ILAR J.* 42(2):161–177.

Puri, C. P. 1981. Serum levels of testosterone, cortisol, prolactin, and bioactive luteinizing hormone in adult male rhesus monkeys following cage-restraint or anesthetizing with ketamine hydrochloride. *Acta Endocrinolog (Copenhagen).* 97:118–124.

Quabbe, H.J., Gregor, M., Bumke-Vogt, C., and Hardel, C. 1982. Pattern of plasma cortisol during the 24-hour slee/wake cycle in the rhesus monkey. *Endocrinology.* 110(5):1641–1646.

Raman, A., Coman, R.J., Cheng, Y., et al. 2005. Reference body composition in adult rhesus monkeys: Glucoregulatory and antrhopometric indices. *J Gerontol.* 60(12):1518–1524.

Ramer, J.C., MacWilliams, P., and Paul-Murphy, J. 1995. Effects of hemolysis and frozen storage on serum electrolyte and chemistry values in cotton-top tamarins (*Saguinus oedipus*). *J Zoo Wild Med.* 26(1):61–66.

Redl, H. and Bahrami, S. 2005. Large animal models: Baboons for trauma, shock, and sepsis studies. *Shock.* 24(Suppl 1):88–93.

Renquist, D.M., Montrey, R.D., Hooks, J.E., and Manus, A.G. 1977. Hematologic, biochemical, and physiologic indices of the sacred baboon (*Papio hamadryas*). *Lab Anim Sci.* 27(2):271–275.

Rifai, N. and Warnick, G.R. 2006. Lipids, lipoproteins, apolipoproteins, and other cardiovascular risk factors. In *Tietz Textbook of Clinical Chemistry and Molecular Diagnostics*. Ed. C.A. Burtis, E.R. Ashwood, and D.E. Bruns. St. Lous, MO: Elsevier Saunders.

Robinson, J.A. and Bridson, W.E. 1978. Neonatal hormone patterns in the macaque. I. Steroids. *Biol Reprod.* 19:773–778.

Rose, R.M., Gordon, T.P., and Bernstein, I.S. 1978. Diurnal variation in plasma testosterone and cortisol in rhesus monkeys living in social groups. *J Endocrinol.* 76:67–74.

Rudel, L.L., McMahan, M.R., and Shah, R.N. 1981a. Pregnancy effects on non-human primate lipoprotein. *J Med Primatol.* 10:16–25.

Rudel, L.L., Reynolds, J.A., and Bullock, B.C. 1981b. Nutritional effects on blood lipid and HDL cholesterol concentrations in two subspecies of African green monkeys (*Cercopithecus aethiops*). *J Lipid Res.* 22:278–286.

Rutjens, E., Mazza, S., Biassoni, R., et al. 2010. CD8+ NK cells are predominant in chimpanzees, characterized by high NCR expression and cytokine production, and preserved in chronic HIV-1 infection. *Eur J Immunol.* 40:1440–1450.

Saltzman, W., et al. 2004. Social suppression of cortisol in female marmoset monkeys: role of circulating ACTH levels and glucocorticoid negative feedback. *Psychoneuroendocrinol* 29: 141-161.

Sarnyai, Z., et al. 1995. The concordance of pulsatile ultradian release of adrenocorticoptropin and cortisol in male rhesus monkeys. *J Clin Endocrinol Metab* 80(1): 54-59.

Sato, A., et al. 2005. Effects of age and sex on hematological and serum biochemical values of vervet monkeys (chlorocebus aethiops sabaeus). *Contemp Top Lab Anim Sci* 44(1): 29--34.

Scammell, J. G., et al. 2006. Cortisol metabolism in the bolivian squirrel monkey (*saimiri boliviensis boliviensis*). *Comp Med* 56(2): 128-135.

Scammell, J. G., et al. 1992. An immunoradiometric assay for squirrel monkey prolactin. *Lab Anim Sci* 42(3): 293-296.

Schlatt, S., Pohl, C.R., Ehmcke, J., and Ramaswamy, S. 2008. Age-related changes in diurnal rhythms and levels of gonadotropins, testosterone, and inhibin B in male rhesus monkeys (*Macaca mulatta*). *Biol Reprod.* 79:93–99.

Schradin, C., Reeder, D.M., Mendoza, S.P., and Anzenberger, G. 2003. Prolactin and paternal care: Comparison of three species of monogamous new world monkeys (*Callicebus cupreus*, *Callithrix jachhus*, and *Callimico goeldii*). *J Comp Psychol.* 117(2):166–175.

Schuurman, H.J. and Smith, H.T. 2005. Reference values for clinical chemistry and clinical hematology parameters in cynomolgus monkeys. *Xenotransplantation.* 12(1):72–75.

Scott, S.K., P.C. Kosch, and D.E. Hilmas. 1976. Serum lactate dehydrogenase of normal, stressed, and yellow fever virus-infected rhesus monkeys. *Lab Anim Sci.* 26(3):436–442.

Seltzer, L.J. and Ziegler, T.E. 2007. Non-invasive measurement of small peptides in the common marmoset (*Callithrix jacchus*): A radiolabeled clearance study and endogenous excretion under varying social conditions. *Horm Behav.* 51:436–442.

Shideler, S.E., Ortuno, A.M., Moran, F.M., Moorman, E.A., and Lasley, B.L. 1993a. Simple extraction and enzyme immunoassays for estrogen and progesterone metabolites in the feces of *Macaca fascicularis* during non-conceptive and conceptive ovarian cycles. *Biol Reprod.* 48:1290–1298.

Shideler, S.E., Shackleton, C.H.L., Moran, F.M., Stauffer, P., Lohstroh, P.N., and Lasley1, B.L. 1993b. Enzyme immunoassays for ovarian steroid metabolites in the urine of *Macaca fascicularis*. *J Med Primatol.* 22:301–312.

Shimizu, K. 2005. Studies on reproductive endocrinology in non-human primates: Application of non-invasive methods. *J Reprod Develop.* 51:1–13.

Shimizu, K., Douke, C., Fujita, S., et al. 2003. Urinary steroids, FSH and CG measurements for monitoring the ovarian cycle and pregnancy in the chimpanzee. *J Med Primatol.* 32:15–22.

Shively, C.A., Laber-Laird, K., and Anton, R.F. 1997. Behavior and physiology of social stress and depression in female cynomolgus monkeys. *Biol Psychiatry.* 41:871–882.

Simons, J.N., Pilot-Matias, T.J., Leary, T.P., et al. 1995. Identification of two flavivirus-like genomes in the GB hepatitis agent. *Proc Natl Acad Sci U S A.* 92(8):3401–3405.

Smith, K.M., McAloose, D., Torregrossa, A., et al. 2008. Hematologic iron analyte values as an indicator of hepatic hemosiderosis in Callitrichidae. *Am J Primatol.* 70:629–633.

Smith, T.E., Schaffner, C.M., and French, J.A. 1997. Social and developmental influences on reproductive function in female Wied-S black tufted-ear marmosets (*Callithrix kuhli*). *Horm Behav.* 31:156–168.

Smucny, D.A., Allison, D.B., Ingram, D.K., et al. 2001. Changes in blood chemistry and hematology variables during aging in captive rhesus macaques (*Macaca mulatta*). *J Med Primatol.* 30(3):161–173.

Smucny, D.A., Allison, D.B., Ingram, D.K., et al. 2004. Changes in blood chemistry and hematology variables during aging in captive rhesus macaques (*Macaca mulatta*). *J Med Primatol.* 33(1):48–54.

Soma, L.R., Tierney, W.J., Hogan, G.K., and Satoh, N. 1995. The effects of multiple administrations of sevoflurane to cynomolgus monkeys: Clinical pathologic, hematologic, and pathologic study. *Anesth Analg.* 81:347–352.

Sousa, M.B., Leao, A.C., Coutinho, J.F., and de Oliveira Ramos, A.M. 2008. Histopathology findings in common marmosets (*Callithrix jacchus* Linnaeus, 1758) with chronic weight loss associated with bile tract obstruction by infestation with *Platynosomum* (Loos, 1907). *Primates.* 49(4):283–287.

Spray, B.J., Morgan, T.M., and Clarkson, T.B. 1994. Genetic estimates for plasma lipid and lipoproteins in cynomolgus monkeys under assortive mating. *J Med Primatol.* 23:450–457.

Srinivasan, S.R., McBride, J.R., Radhakrishnamurthy, B., and Berenson, G.S. 1974. Comparative studies on serum lipoprotein and lipid profiles in subhuman primates. *Comp Biochem Physiol.* 47:711–716.

Stavisky, R. 1994. *Socioendocrinology: Noninvasive Techniques for Monitoring Reproductive Function in Captive and Free-Ranging Primates*. Atlanta, GA: Emory University.

Stavisky, R.C., Russell, E., Stallings, J., Smith, E.O., Worthman, C., and Whitten, P.L. 1995. Fecal steroid analysis of ovarian cycles in free-ranging baboons. *Am J Primatol.* 36:285–297.

Steinetz, B.G., Randolph, C., Cohn, D., and Mahoney, C.J. 1996. Lipoprotein profiles and glucose tolerance in lean and obese chimpanzees. *J Med Primatol.* 25:17–25.

Steyn, D.G., Hamilton-Bruce, R.J., Zuurmond, T.J., and Pharo, R. 1975. Standard serum chemical and haematological values in the chacma baboon (*Papio ursinus*). *J S Afr Vet Assoc.* 46(2):191–196.

Stockham, S.L. and Scott, M.A. 2008. *Fundamentals of Veterinary Clinical Pathology*, 2nd edition. Ames, IA: Blackwell Publishing.

Streett, J.W. and Jonas, A.M. 1982. Differential effects of chemical and physical restraint on carbohydrate tolerance testing in nonhuman primates. *Lab Anim Sci.* 32:263–266.

Suzuki, T., Suzuki, N., Shimoda, K., and Nagasawa, H. 1996. Hematological and serum biochemical values in pregnant and postpartum females of the squirrel monkey (*Saimiri sciureus*). *Exp Anim.* 45(1):39–43.

Szymanski, E.S. and Kritchevsky, D. 1980. Serum lipid levels of young and old rhesus monkeys. *Exp Gerontol.* 15:365–367.

't Hart, B.A., van Meurs, M., Brok, H.P.M., et al. 2000. A new primate model for multiple sclerosis in the common marmoset. *Immunol Today.* 21(6):290–297.

Taglioni, A., Casetti, A. R., Bernardini, A., and Perretta, G. 1996. Effects of ketamine hydrochloride on haematological and serum biochemical parameters in *Callithrix jacchus* (Abstract). *Folia Primatol.* 67(2):65.

Tigno, X.T., Gerzanich, G., and Hansen, B.C. 2004. Age-related changes in metabolic parameters of nonhuman primates. *J Gerontol.* 59A(11):1081–1088.

Tobi, M., Chintalapani, S., Kithier, K., and Clapp, N. 2000. Gastrointestinal tract antigenic profile of cotton-top tamarin, *Saguinus oedipus*, is similar to that of humans with inflammatory bowel disease. *Dig Dis Sci.* 45(12):2290–2297.

Torres-Farfan, C., Valenzuela, F.J., Ebensperger, R., et al. 2008. Circadian cortisol secretion and circadian adrenal responses to ACTH are maintained in dexamethasone suppressed capuchin monkeys (*Cebus apella*). *Am J Primatol.* 70:93–100.

Vahle, J.L. 1998. Distribution of creatine kinase and creatine kinase isoenzymes in sera and tissues of cynomolgus monkeys. *Toxicologic Pathology*, in preparation.

Valenza, F.P. and Muchmore, E. 1985. The clinical chemistry of chimpanzees. II. Gamma glutamyl transferase levels in hepatitis studies. *J Med Primatol.* 14:305–315.

Van Calsteren, K., Devlieger, R., De Catte, L., et al. 2009. Feasibility of ultrasound-guided percutaneous samplings in the pregnant baboon: A model for studies on transplacental transport. *Repord Sci.* 16(3):280–285.

Videan, E.N., Fritz, J., and Murphy, J. 2008. Effects of aging on hematology and serum clinical chemistry in chimpanzees (*Pan troglodytes*). *Am J Primatol.* 70:327–338.

Wadsworth, P.F., Hiddleston, W.A., Jones, D.V., Fowler, J.S.L., and Ferguson, R.A. 1982. Haematological, coagulation and blood chemistry data in red-bellied tamarins *Saguinus labiatus*. *Lab Anim.* 16:327–330.

Wagner, J.D., Bagdade, J.D., Litwak, K.N., et al. 1996. Increased glycation of plasma lipoproteins in diabetic cynomolgus monkeys. *Lab Anim Sci.* 46(1):31–35.

Wagner, J.D., Cline, J.M., Shadoan, M.K., Bullock, B.C., Rankin, S.E., and Cefalu, W.T. 2001. Naturally occurring and experimental diabetes in cynomolgus monkeys: A comparison of carbohydrate and lipid metabolism and islet pathology. *Toxicol Pathol.* 29(1):142–148.

Wagner, J.D., Kavanagh, K., Ward, G.M., Auerbach, B.J., Harwood H.J., Jr., and Kaplan, J.R. 2006. Old world nonhuman primate models of type 2 diabetes mellitus. *ILAR J.* 47(3):259–271.

Walker, D.B. 2006. Serum chemical biomarkers of cardiac injury for nonclincial safety testing. *Toxicol Pathol.* 34:94–104.

Walker, M.L., Wilson, M.E., and Gordon, T.P. 1984. Endocrine control of the seasonal occurrence of ovulation in rhesus monkeys housed outdoors. *Endocrinology.* 114:1074–1081.

Walsh, S.W., Kittinger, G.W., and Novy, M.J. 1979. Maternal peripheral concentrations of estradiol, estrone, cortisol, and progesterone during late pregnancy in rhesus monkeys (*Macaca mulatta*) and after fetal anenecephaly and fetal death. *Am J Obstet Gynecol.* 135:37–42.

Wang, X.L., Wang, J., Shi, Q., Carey, K.D., and VandeBerg, J.L. 2004. Arterial wall-determined risk factors to vascular diseases. *Cell Biochem Biophys.* 40:371–388.

Ward, K.W., Coon, D.J., Magiera, D., Bhadresa, S., Nisbett, E., and Lawrence, M.S. 2008. Exploration of the african green monkey as a preclinical pharmacokinetic model: Intravenous pharmacokinetic parameters. *Drug Metab Disopos.* 36(4):715–720.

Ward, K.W., Coon, D.J., Magiera, D., Bhadresa, S., Struharik, M., and Lawrence, M.S. 2009. Exploration of the African green monkey as a preclinical pharmacokinetic model: Oral pharmacokinetic parameters and drug-drug interactions. *Xenobiotica.* 39(3):266–272.

Wasser, S.K., Monfort, S.L., and Wildt, D.E. 1991. Rapid extraction of faecal steroids for measuring reproductive cyclicity and early pregnancy in free-ranging yellow baboons (*Papio cynocephalus*). *J Repord Fertil.* 92:415–423.

Watkins, P.E., Warren, B.F., Stephens, S., Ward, P., and Foulkes, R. 1997. Treatment of ulcerative colitis in the cottontop tamarin using antibody to tumour necrosis factor alpha. *Gut.* 40:628–633.

Weatherford, T., Chavez, D., Brasky, K.M., and Lanford, R.E. 2009. The marmoset model of GB virus-B infections: Adaptation to host phenotypic variation. *J Virol.* 83(11):5806–5814.

Weekley, L.B., Deldar, A., and Tapp, E. 2003. Development of renal function tests for measurement of urine concentrating ability, urine acidification, and glomerular filtration rate in female cynomolgus monkeys. *Contemp Top Lab Anim Sci.* 42(3):22–25.

Weingrill, T., Gray, D.A., Barrett, L., and Henzi, S.P. 2004. Fecal cortisol levels in free-ranging female chacma baboons: Relationship to dominance, reproductive state and environmental factors. *Horm Behav.* 45:259–269.

Weller, R.E., Buschbom, R.L., Malaga, C.A., Kimsey, B.B., and Regan, H.A. 1996. Serum and urine biochemical diversity among wild-caught *Aotus nancymae* and *Saimiri peruviensis*. *J Med Primatol.* 25:46–52.

Weller, R.E., Buschbom, R.L., Malaga, C.A., and Ragan, H.A. 1993a. Comparison of blood and urine analytes between two karyotypes of owl monkey, *Aotus nancymae* and *Aotus vociferans*. *J Med Primatol.* 22(6):368–373.

Weller, R.E., Buschbom, R.L., Martell, S.L., Baer, J.F., Malaga, C.A., and Ragan, H.A. 1991a. Total serum creatine kinase and isozyme concentrations in the owl monkey. *J Med Primatol.* 20:290–294.

Weller, R.E., Buschbom, R.L., Ragan, H.A., Baer, J.F., and Malaga, C.A. 1990. Relationship of serum total calcium and albumin and total protein in owl monkeys (Aotus nancymai). *J Med Primatol.* 19:439–446.

Weller, R.E., Malaga, C.A., Buschbom, R.L., Baer, J.F., and Ragan, H.A. 1991b. Protein concentration in urine of normal owl monkeys. *J Med Primatol.* 20(7):365–369.

Weller, R.E., Malaga, C.A., Buschbom, R.L., and Ragan, H.A. 1993b. Urinary enzyme concentrations in the owl monkey (*Aotus nancymae*). *J Med Primatol.* 22(6):340–347.

Whitten, P.L., Brockman, D.K., and Stavisky, R.C. 1998. Recent advances in noninvasive techniques to monitor hormone-behavior interactions. *Am J Phys Anthropol.* (Suppl 27):1–23.

Whittow, G.C., Guernsey, D.L., and Morishige, W.K. 1979. Thyroid activity in a hypometabolic primate, the owl monkey (*Aotus trivirgatus*). *Arch Int Physiol Biochim.* 87(5):963–967.

Williams, L.E. 2006. Hematology and serum chemistry reference values for mother-reared squirrel monkey (*Saimiri boliviensis boliviensis*) infants. In *Nursery Rearing of Nonhuman Primates in the 21st Century.* Ed. G.P. Sackett, G.C. Ruppenthal, and K. Elias, pp. 593–595. New York, NY: Springer.

Williams-Blangero, S., Butler, T., Brasky, K., and Murthy, K.K. 1994. Heritabilities of clinical chemical traits in chimpanzees. *Lab Anim Sci.* 44(2):141–143.

Wilson, M.E., Brown, G.M., and Wilson, D. 1978. Annual and diurnal changes in plasma androgen and cortisol in adult male squirrel monkeys (*Saimiri sciureus*) studies longitudinally. *Acta Endocrinol.* 87:424–433.

Winters, S.J., Medhamurthy R., Gay, V.L., and Plant, T.M. 1991. A comparison of moment to moment and diurnal changes in circulating inhibin and testosterone concentrations in male rhesus monkeys (*Macaca mulatta*). *Endocrinology.* 129(4):1755–1761.

Wolf, R.F. and White, G.L. 2012. Clinical techniques used for nonhuman primates. In *Nonhuman Priamtes in Biomedical Research: Biology and Management*. Eds. C.R. Abee, K. Mansfield, S. Tardiff, and T. Morris, Vol 1, pp. 323–337. San Diego, CA: Academic Press.

Woller, M.J., Binotto, G.E., Nichols, E., et al. 2002. Aging-related changes in release of growth hormone and luteinizing hormone in female rhesus monkeys. *J Clin Endocrinol Metab.* 87(11):5160–5167.

Wondergem, J., Persons, K., Zurcher, C., Frolich, M., Leer, J.W., and Broerse, J. 1999. Changes in circulating atrial natriuretic peptide in relation to the cardiac status of rhesus monkeys after total-body irradiation. *Radiother Oncol.* 53:67–75.

Wood, C., Fang, S.G., Hunt, A., Streich, W.J., and Clauss, M. 2003. Increased iron absorption in lemurs: Quantitative screening and assessment of dietary prevention. *Am J Primatol.* 61:101–110.

Woodward, R.A. and Weld, K.P. 1997. A comparison of ketamine, ketamine-acepromazine, and tiletamine-zolazepam on various hematologic parameters in rhesus monkeys (*Macaca mulatta*). *Contemp Top Lab Anim Sci.* 36(3):55–57.

Yarbrough, L.W., Tollett, J.L., Montrey, R.D., and Beattii, R.J. 1984. Serum biochemical, hematological and body measurement data for common marmosets (*Callithrix jacchus jacchus*). *Lab Anim Sci.* 34(3):276–280.

Yoshida, T. 1981. The changes of hematological and biochemical properties in cynomolgus monkeys (*Macaca fascicularis*) after importation. *Jpn J Med Sci Biol.* 34:239–242.

Yoshida, T. 1983. Serum gonadotropin levels during the menstrual cycle and pregnancy in the cynomolgus monkeys. *Jpn J Med Sci Biol.* 36:231–236.

Yoshida, T., Sato, M., Ohtoh, K., Cho, F., and Honjo, S. 1989. Effects of aging on the in vivo release of thyrotropin (TSH), triidothyronine, and thyroxine induced by TSH-releasing hormone in the cynomolgus monkey (*Macaca fascicularis*). *Endocrinology.* 124(3):1287–1293.

Zaragoza, C., Li, R.M., Fahle, G.A., et al. 2005. Squirrel monkeys support replication of BK virus more efficiently than simian virus 40: An animal model for human BK virus infection. *J Virol.* 79(2):1320–1326.

Ziegler, T.E., Scheffler, G., and Snowdon, C.T. 1995. The relationship of cortisol levels to social environment and reproductive functioning in female cotton-top tamarins, *Saguinus oedipus*. *Horm Behav.* 29:407–424.

Ziegler, T.E., Scheffler, G., Wittwer, D.J., Schultz-Darken, N.J., Snowdon, C.T., and Abbott, D.H. 1996b. Metabolism of reproductive steroids during the ovarian cycle in two species of callitrichids, *Saguinus oedipus* and *Callithrix jacchus*, and estimation of the ovulatory period from fecal steroids. *Biol Reprod.* 54:91–99.

Ziegler, T.E. and Snowdon, C.T. 2000. Preparental hormone levels and parenting experience in male cotton-top tamarins, *Saguinus oedipus*. *Horm Behav.* 38:159–167.

Ziegler, T.E., Wegner, F.H., and Snowdon, C.T. 1996a. Hormonal responses to parental and nonparental conditions in male cotton-top tamarins, *Saguinus oedipus*, a New World primate. *Horm Behav.* 30:287–297.

Zuehlke, U., Srivastav, S., Stanley, M.A., et al. 2006. Cynomolgus monkeys of mauritian origin: Reference data and comparison to chinese/vietnamese animals. In *Novel Approaches Towards Primate Toxicology*. Ed. G.F. Weinbauer and F. Vogel, pp. 185–201. New York, NY: Waxmann Munster.

Zuhlke, U. and Weinbauer, G. 2003. The common marmoset (*Callithrix jacchus*) as a model in toxicology. *Toxicol Pathol.* 31(Suppl 1):123–127.

7 The Laboratory Hamster

Charles B. Clifford and Joe H. Simmons

CONTENTS

7.1 USE OF HAMSTERS IN BIOMEDICAL RESEARCH

Hamsters comprise approximately 25 species belonging to the class *Mammalia*, order *Rodentia*, suborder *Myomorpha*, superfamily *Muroidea*, family *Cricetidae*, and subfamily *Cricetinae*. The *Cricetinae* include all animals that we recognize as hamsters, often divided among seven genera: *Cricetus*, *Mesocricetus*, *Cricetulus*, *Phodopus*, *Tscherskia*, *Mystromys*, and *Calomyscus*. Syrian, or golden, hamsters (*Mesocricetus auratus*) are the most commonly used in research, representing perhaps 90% of hamsters used in the United States (Hankenson and Van Hoosier, 2002). Essentially, all pet and laboratory Syrian hamsters are descendants of three to four littermates captured in the wild in 1930 (Aharoni, 1932; Gattermann et al., 2001). Other species of hamsters are used in lesser numbers, notably including the Chinese hamster (*Cricetulus griseus*) and the Djungarian, or Siberian, hamster (*Phodopus sungorus*). Use of hamsters in research in the United States has declined almost steadily from a high of approximately 503,590 hamsters reported used for research in 1976 to approximately 172,498 hamsters in 2007, the most recent year for which the annual United States Department of Agriculture (USDA) figures are available (USDA APHIS, 2008). The single most common use of hamsters is in potency testing for leptospirosis vaccines (Stephens et al., 2002). Syrian hamsters are used in leptospirosis research due to their susceptibility to many strains of *Leptospira*, as well as the reproducibility of studies conducted in hamsters (Haake, 2006). Syrian hamsters are a favored model for yellow fever research for both study of the pathogenesis and investigation of candidate therapeutics (Julander et al., 2007; Sbrana et al., 2006). Syrian hamsters also continue to play a key role in research into lipid and glucose metabolism, aging, skeletal and cardiac muscular dystrophy, oral carcinogenesis, and circadian rhythm. Because of the preponderance of Syrian hamsters relative to the other hamster species used in biomedical research in North America, the term hamster refers to Syrian hamsters in this chapter, unless otherwise specified.

Both the Chinese hamster (*Cricetulus griseus*) and the South African hamster (*Mystromys albicaudatus*) are used as spontaneous animal models of noninsulin-dependent diabetes mellitus (McIntosh and Pederson, 1999). Diabetic lines of Chinese hamsters are now well established, originally selected from individuals exhibiting spontaneous disease. Affected Chinese hamsters are hyperglycemic, glucosuric, and hypercholesterolemic and may become ketotic (Chang, 1978, 1981). Insulin levels vary greatly but decrease with time, suggesting eventual insulin exhaustion. The South African hamster also develops diabetes similarly characterized by hyperglycemia, glucosuria, and ketonuria (Packer et al., 1970; Riley et al., 1975; Stuhlman et al., 1975; Yesus et al., 1976).

The Djungarian, or Siberian, hamster (*Phodopus sungorus*) plays a major role in studies of the metabolic and reproductive effects of photoperiod (Braulke et al., 2008; Challet et al., 2000; Dark et al., 1994, 1999; Larkin et al., 2003; Mercer and Tups, 2003; Zysling and Demas, 2007).

Mutant lines of hamsters have been bred for use in at least two areas of research. Mutant Syrian hamsters available for research include cardiomyopathic, also called dystrophic, and tau mutants. As reviewed in Vainzof et al. (2008), the Bio14.6 inbred hamster and sublines have a 30-kb deletion in the δ-sarcoglycan gene (Nigro et al., 1997), resulting in an autosomal recessive form of dilated cardiomyopathy and skeletal muscular dystrophy. Affected animals are reported to have elevated creatine kinase, referred to as phosphocreatine kinase in the older literature. Hamsters have long been used in circadian research, in part because of the daily regularity of their wheel running (Elliott et al., 1972). Hamsters with circadian rhythms shorter than the normal 24-hour circadian period were found to have an autosomal mutation in a gene referred to as *tau*. Animals homozygous for the mutation had 20-hour circadian periods; heterozygotes had 22-hour circadian periods (Ralph and Menaker, 1988). The *tau* gene has more recently been identified as encoding for casein kinase 1 epsilon (Lowrey et al., 2000), which is also important in circadian rhythm in *Drosophila*. No reports of genetically modified hamsters could be found at the time of this publication.

7.2 UNIQUE PHYSIOLOGICAL CHARACTERISTICS OF HAMSTERS

Hamsters are nocturnal, that is, they are active primarily during the night or dark period. Nocturnal behaviors that may influence some clinical chemistry parameters include feeding, food hoarding, and wheel running. Relevant aspects are discussed below under the influence of photoperiod and circadian rhythm. An additional important physiologic feature of hamster species is that they may undergo periods of hypometabolism. Syrian, Turkish, and European hamsters undergo hibernation, whereas the Djungarian hamster undergoes daily torpor (Newcomer et al., 1987). The difference between hibernation and torpor, which is sometimes called daily torpor, is the greater degree of duration and extent of metabolic suppression in hibernation; both are qualitatively similar energy-saving metabolic strategies with lowered body temperatures and decreased metabolic rate. Hibernation results from a combination of decreasing length of photoperiod and low temperatures, whereas torpor follows a circadian rhythm, occurring during the normal resting period, that is, the light period. Hibernation may result in reduction of metabolic rates of more than 95% in the European hamster (Mohr and Ernst, 1987). Torpor in the Djungarian hamster may result in up to a 75% decrease in metabolic rate (Heldmaier et al., 2004). Body temperatures approach ambient temperature for both torpor and hibernation. Despite these changes, the animals are normoglycemic (Newcomer et al., 1987), normoxic, and maintain normal pH (Heldmaier et al., 2004).

During periods of normal physiologic activity, that is, not torpor or hibernation, hamsters have an unusually low half-saturation oxygen tension and Bohr shift (Bivin et al., 1987). Although this might be expected in an animal adapted for hibernation, to permit continued delivery of sufficient oxygen to their tissues, one might also expect high cardiac output. Indeed, hamster has a cardiac output, per kilogram of body weight, which is nearly twice that in the rat.

The cheek pouch of hamsters has traditionally played a role in oncology and carcinogenicity studies. These large buccal pouches, which the hamster uses for transporting food, are easily everted and viewed. Significantly, the pouches lack a lymphatic drainage system and have a decreased number of dendritic cells; thus, they are considered to be "immunologically privileged" and will not reject allografts or xenografts. Formerly, this made hamsters desirable research models for the study of xenografted tumor lines, although this role has been eclipsed by immunodeficient mice. However, chemical induction of squamous cell carcinomas in hamster cheek pouches is still considered among the best models of human oral oncogenesis (Vairaktaris et al., 2008). Hamster cheek pouches are also used to study radiation-induced mucositis (Chung et al., 2009; Sonis et al., 1990).

7.3 METHODOLOGY FOR SAMPLE COLLECTION

7.3.1 Blood Collection

A variety of sites are readily available for blood collection from the laboratory hamster. Choice of site depends on quantity of blood required, frequency of collection, training and expertise of personnel involved, and procedural limitations that might be imposed by the Institutional Animal Care and Use Committee. All procedures for blood collection, as for other procedures in hamsters, should be in accordance with the Animal Welfare Act and the Guide for the Care and Use of Laboratory Animals.

7.3.1.1 Blood Volume Limits and Frequency

Because of the small size of the hamster, particular attention needs to be given to the amount of blood removed at single or recurring time points for survival methods. Guidelines for this amount are often established by the Institutional Animal Care and Use Committee, and these guidelines should be strictly followed. Blood volume in veterinary medicine is often estimated at 10% of body weight, and the general rule of thumb is that 10% of blood volume can be safely removed from a healthy, adult animal in an adequate plane of nutrition without significant health consequences (McGuill and Rowan, 1989). However, because in the hamster, blood volume is only 7.8% of body weight, following the typical rule of thumb would actually remove approximately 13% of the hamster's blood volume. This (13%) would be sufficient blood loss to cause a significant cholinergic release and hemodynamic changes (McGuill and Rowan, 1989; Morton et al., 1993). The current standard of practice is that 10% of the blood volume of a healthy, adult animal can be removed once every 3–4 weeks, and that 1% of its blood volume can be removed once daily (Morton et al., 1993). As a reference, Table 7.1 presents recommendations on sample volumes that can be safely taken from laboratory hamsters.

7.3.1.2 Orbital Plexus

The hamster has a large venous sinus occupying the orbital space deep to, and in the caudal one half to two-thirds, of the orbit (Figure 7.1; Timm, 1980). Blood is supplied to the orbital venous sinus by the external ophthalmic artery and is drained by the external ophthalmic veins (Popesko

TABLE 7.1
Blood Volume That Can Be Safely Removed From a Hamster

Body Weight (G)	Estimated Total Blood Volume[a] (mL)	10% Blood Volume[b] (mL)	1% Blood Volume[c] (mL)
50	3.9	0.39	0.039
75	5.9	0.59	0.059
100	7.8	0.78	0.078
125	9.8	0.98	0.098
150	11.7	1.17	0.117

Source: Morton, D.B. et al., *Lab Anim.*, 27, 1–22, 1993.

[a] Total blood volume based upon 7.8% estimate blood volume for a mature healthy hamster on an adequate plane of nutrition.

[b] 10% of blood volume can be safely removed from a healthy hamster once every 3–4 weeks. This is approximately 0.8% of body weight.

[c] 1% of blood volume can be safely removed from a healthy hamster daily. This is approximately 0.08% of body weight.

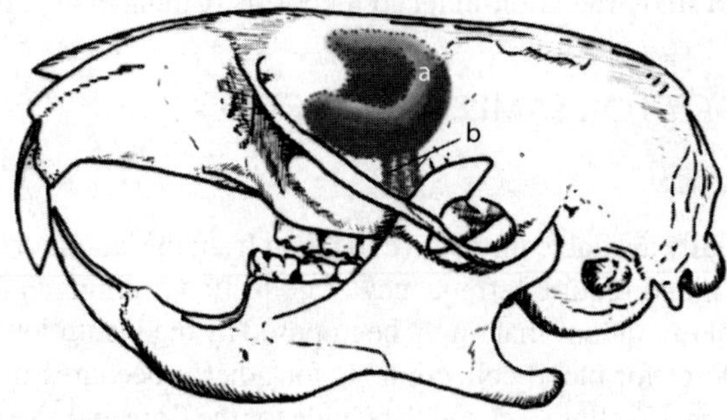

FIGURE 7.1 **(See color insert.)** Hamster skull—showing location of the orbital venous sinus. Since the orbital venous sinus resides in the caudal one-half to two-thirds of the orbit, the microhematocrit tube should be inserted into the lateral canthus of the eye in a posterior and medial direction. (a) Orbital venous sinus. (b) External ophthalmic veins.

et al., 2002). Two techniques have been described for removing small amounts of blood (less than 0.5 mL) from the orbital venous sinus of the Syrian hamster.

7.3.1.2.1 Micropipette Technique

Accessing the orbital sinus of rodents as a site for blood collection was first described by Stone (1954) and later modified by Sorg and Buckner (1964). A detailed description of this technique in the hamster was published by Timm (1980). Briefly, the anesthetized hamster, for example, with 1%–4% isoflurane (Swindle et al., 2002), is grasped by its head and neck with the thumb and index finger of the nondominant hand. Light pressure is applied to the jugular vein with one finger while lifting the upper eye lid dorsally with the other. Since the orbital venous sinus resides in the caudal one-half to two-thirds of the orbit, a microhematocrit tube is inserted into the lateral canthus of the eyelid in a posterior and medial direction. Gentle pressure is applied, and the microhematocrit tube is rotated as it is inserted. The venous sinus will rupture as it is trapped between the orbit and the microhematocrit tube. Once this occurs, the tube is withdrawn slightly and allowed to fill with blood. Up to 0.5 mL of blood, subject to the limits in blood volume limits and frequency discussed below, can be collected by this technique if the free end of the microhematocrit tube is directed downward allowing blood to flow into a microcentrifuge tube. Once a sufficient volume of blood is collected, the microhematocrit tube is withdrawn and gentle pressure is applied to the eye to allow blood clotting to occur and to prevent hematoma formation. Since this technique ruptures the tissues overlying the orbital plexus, it can result in leakage of a number of cellular enzymes which may impact the quality of the sample that is obtained. Significantly higher values for aspartate aminotransferase (AST), lactate dehydrogenase (LDH), and creatine phosphokinase (CPK) have been documented using this technique in rats and hamsters when compared to other commonly used methods of blood sampling, such as from the posterior vena cava, which cause less tissue damage (Izumi et al., 1993). Thus careful consideration should be given to the potential experimental impact of sample contamination before using this technique. Additionally, because of the potential for injury to the eye, this technique should only be performed by trained personnel who perform the technique regularly.

7.3.1.2.2 Syringe

Blood can also be collected from the hamster's orbital venous sinus using a tuberculin syringe fitted with a 1-cm 23-gauge needle (Pansky et al., 1961). For this technique, the hamster should be anesthetized and placed in ventral recumbency on a flat surface. The thumb and forefinger are used to retract the skin behind the orbit thus lifting the upper eyelid and displacing the eye forward. The tip of the needle is inserted at the midway point of the upper eyelid between the lid and the bulb of the eye; the needle and syringe should be held at approximately 20°–40° from vertical and should be directed ventrocaudally into the back of the orbit. After penetrating approximately 4 mm, the needle will contact the boney orbit after which it should be withdrawn slightly. The tip of the needle should then rest within the orbital venous sinus and blood can be withdrawn by gentle pressure on the plunger of the syringe. This technique can be used for multiple 100–400 µL blood collections (Pansky et al., 1961; Breckon and Goy, 1979). Pansky et al. (1961) describe using this technique for repeated sampling at 3–4-hour intervals. As previously noted, because of potential injury to the eye, this technique should only be performed by trained personnel who perform the technique regularly.

7.3.1.3 Saphenous Vein

Small volumes of blood, 50–200 µL, can be obtained from the caudal branch of the lateral saphenous vein, which runs dorsally and then laterally over the tarsal joint in the hamster (Popesko et al., 2002). For this technique, the hamster should either be anesthetized or placed, head first, into a restraining tube. If the hamster is small enough, a 50-mL conical tube with a hole cut in the tip works well, thereby allowing access to the hind limb. Shaving the hair over the lower lateral tibia and applying gentle pressure to the lower thigh with the thumb and forefinger will allow visualization of the caudal branch of the lateral saphenous vein. The tip of a small sterile hypodermic needle (23–25 gauge tuberculin needle works well) is then used like a small lance to rupture the vein by holding the needle, bevel up, at a 45° angle and inserting the tip of the needle through the skin until it punctures the superficial surface of the vein. This results in the accumulation of a drop of blood on the surface of the hamster's leg that is collected using a microhematocrit tube. By directing the tip of the microhematocrit tube downward into a microcentrifuge tube, 50–200 µL of blood can be collected; however, the lesion can clot quickly so anticoagulants should be used in the collection tube (Hem et al., 1998). When blood collection is complete relax the pressure being applied to the thigh and apply gentle pressure to the puncture site with a gauze sponge or cotton ball to potentiate hemostasis and prevent hematoma formation.

7.3.1.4 Cardiocentesis

Cardiocentesis can be performed to obtain blood from hamsters as a terminal procedure; however, blood collected by cardiocentesis may be contaminated with muscle enzymes such as creatine kinase, AST, LDH, or alanine aminotransferase since all of these enzymes, as well as troponins, are found in high levels in cardiac muscle (Thrall et al., 2004). This procedure should only be performed on deeply anesthetized animals. A 20–22 gauge with a 1-inch-long hypodermic needle attached to a 1–5 mL syringe is required, depending upon blood volume to be collected. With the anesthetized hamster in dorsal recumbency, the needle is inserted at a 30° angle just caudal and left lateral to the xyphoid cartilage at the base of the sternum. When the needle is inserted approximately 0.5 inch, gentle aspiration is initiated while insertion of the needle continues. Once blood begins to flow into the syringe, needle insertion is stopped while slow aspiration of blood continues. Depending upon animal size, 2–3 mL of blood can be collected (Donovan and Brown, 2005; Morton et al., 1993). If blood stops flowing, the bevel of the needle should be rotated and the tip redirected until blood flow is reestablished. When blood collection by terminal cardiocentesis is completed, death should be assured by a physical method approved by the Institutional Animal Care and Use Committee, perhaps cervical dislocation or thoracotomy (Morton et al., 1993).

7.3.1.5 Abdominal Aorta or Caudal Vena Cava

Large amounts of blood that is free of contaminating muscle enzymes can be obtained by direct collection from the abdominal aorta or caudal vena cava; however, this is a terminal procedure (Donovan and Brown, 2005; Manning and Giannina, 1966). To perform this procedure, the hamster is anesthetized and placed in dorsal recumbency on a flat surface with the head facing away. A midline incision through the skin, musculature, and peritoneum is made from the xyphoid to the pubis with a scalpel blade or with surgical scissors. With the abdominal cavity opened, the abdominal contents are moved out of the way by reflecting the intestines up and to the left thereby exposing the abdominal aorta and caudal vena cava cranial to the iliac bifurcation and superficial to the lumbar spine (e.g., see Popesko et al., 2002). A 23–25 gauge hypodermic needle or butterfly catheter attached to a 5 mL syringe can then be inserted in a cranial direction, with the needle at a 30°–45° angle, into either the abdominal aorta or vein. For venous collection, a hemostat can be used to occlude the caudal vena cava between to the site of needle insertion and the heart (Manning and Giannina, 1966). For arterial collection, gentle downward pressure at the point of the iliac bifurcation increases the turgor of the aorta (Donovan and Brown, 2005). Gentle pressure is then applied to the plunger to withdraw 3–4 mL of blood, depending upon animal size. At the end of a terminal procedure, death should be assured by a physical method such as cervical dislocation or thoracotomy (Morton et al., 1993).

7.3.1.6 Sample Collection for Blood Gas Analysis

Hamsters are occasionally used for studies that require collection of samples for blood gas analysis. Due to the hamster's small size, direct collection of a sufficient sample for arterial blood gas analysis is difficult; however, samples can be obtained from unrestrained animals by placement of one or more indwelling cannulas. The technique described by Popovic and Popovic, used for cannulation of the aorta, vena cava, or both, in rats and ground squirrels, has been adapted for use in hamsters (Lucey et al., 1980; O'Brien et al., 1979; Popovic and Popovic, 1960). Briefly, the hamster is anesthetized and prepared for aseptic surgery to the left, ventral, cervical region. An incision is made above the left carotid artery, which is then exposed and released from surrounding connective tissue by blunt dissection. The left carotid artery is ligated cranially with a circumferential suture. A caudally directed cannula is then introduced into the artery and advanced until the tip resides within the aortic arch. Next, the cannula is secured to the carotid artery with suture material and the free end of the cannula can be tunneled subcutaneously to the dorsum, exteriorized between the scapulae, and held in place with a suture or wound clip. For a long-term use, the hamster can be fitted with a jacket or harness. The catheter should be flushed and maintained with sterile heparinized saline. A similar procedure can be performed on the right jugular vein to place an indwelling cannula into the right cranial vena cava. Popovic reports that properly maintained cannulae can have a useful lifetime of 40 days and that cannulae have lasted up to 3 months in hibernating animals (Popovic and Popovic, 1960).

7.3.2 Urine Collection

Hamsters produce approximately 5–8 mL of basic (pH 8.5) urine per day. Urine is often turbid due to the presence of triple phosphate and calcium carbonate crystals. As with many other rodents, hamster urine may have high protein levels. As desert-adapted animals, hamsters can conserve water and concentrate their urine to a specific gravity as high as 1.060. There are a variety of techniques available for collection of urine from the laboratory hamster. Choice of method depends upon quality and volume of sample required, frequency of collection, training and comfort level of personnel involved, and procedural limitations that might be imposed by the Institutional Animal Care and Use Committee.

7.3.2.1 Metabolism Cage

Metabolism cages allow for convenient collection of urine and/or feces over an extended period of time and often allow measurement of water consumption as well. While larger sample volumes can usually be collected, they may be contaminated with feces and are often contaminated with bacteria, which must be considered when results are interpreted. Metabolism cages can be homemade, and a variety of cages are described in a review article (Kurien et al., 2004). Several companies produce well-engineered metabolism cages that allow for reliable collection of urine that is minimally contaminated with feces. Commercial manufacturers should be consulted directly for additional information on their products.

7.3.2.2 Microhematocrit Tube

If a small (25–50 μL) urine sample is required, there are several methods that can be used to collect voided urine using a microhematocrit tube. Hamsters do not usually spontaneously urinate upon being picked up and restrained as do many other rodents; however, with patience, hamsters will urinate and a microhematocrit tube can be used to collect the voided urine. Alternatively, the hamster can be anesthetized and the bladder can be digitally palpated and gently expressed manually. A microhematocrit tube can then be used to collect the voided urine. Regardless of which method is used to collect voided urine, it should be considered contaminated with bacteria and analyzed in a timely manner.

7.3.2.3 Cystocentesis

Cystocentesis can be used to collect a sterile urine sample from an anesthetized hamster; however, samples collected by cystocentesis are subject to contamination by small amounts of tissue and red blood cells. After the hamster is anesthetized it should be placed in dorsal recumbency. For male hamsters, testicles should be in a scrotal position and should be moved into the scrotum, if necessary, by gentle digital pressure on the lower abdomen. The urinary bladder should be located by gentle palpation and lightly held between the thumb and forefinger. A small (25–27 gauge) needle attached to a tuberculin syringe or butterfly catheter should be inserted in a craniodorsal direction a safe distance away from the trigone (base) of the bladder near the pelvis, but no more than half the distance to the apex. The tip of the needle should not penetrate more than halfway through the bladder lumen, as guided by palpation. Urine collection can then be initiated by applying gentle traction on the syringe plunger. As urine is withdrawn the bladder wall will begin to collapse and eventually occlude the needle. If this happens, the bevel of the needle can be rotated and the syringe angled slightly more toward the spine. When the bladder is evacuated, or a sufficient sample has been removed, the bladder should be released and the syringe carefully withdrawn along the angle of insertion (Breitweiser, 1992).

7.4 PREANALYTICAL SOURCES OF VARIATION

In general, samples from hamsters are subject to the same sources of preanalytical variation as are those from other laboratory rodents.

7.4.1 Sex

Maxwell et al. (1985) found differences in several serum analytes between male and female Syrian hamsters from two sources, Charles River (CR) and Bio Research Laboratories (BR). In Table 7.2, 30 hamsters were sampled per sex from BR and 32 from CR.

Female BR hamsters had lower glucose values than the other three groups (BR males, CR males, and CR females). Female BR hamsters had lower values for triglycerides and higher values for calcium. The CR female hamsters had higher values for cholesterol. Differences between the two strains, as well as some additional possible limitations of the study, are further discussed below. Female hamsters are reported to have circulating levels of amyloid P of 1–2 mg/mL, which are 100–200-fold those in males (Coe et al., 1981).

7.4.2 Age

As in many mammals, juvenile hamsters have higher serum alkaline phosphatase levels than older animals, 589 ± 105 versus 218 ± 42 in young and mature males, respectively, and 590 ± 75 versus 369 ± 34 in females (Dent, 1977). Young hamsters also have higher serum levels of T3 and T4. Neve et al. (1981) found 3-month-old hamsters to have a mean T4 level of 6.75 ± 0.75 μg/dL, whereas 20-month-old hamsters had 3.59 ± 0.16 μg/dL, $p < 0.01$. For T3, the 3-month-old group had 62 ± 2 ng/dL, whereas the 20-month-old hamsters had 42 ± 3 ng/dL, $p < 0.001$. Evaluation of clinical chemistry results from aging hamsters should also consider the potential for influences from age-related diseases. Principal causes of mortality in geriatric hamsters include amyloidosis and progressive nephritis (Schmidt et al., 1983), as well as typhlocolitis (Feldman et al., 1982; Nambiar et al., 2005, 2006). Amyloidosis is observed more frequently in female hamsters and affects many tissues, but is most often observed in kidney, liver, and adrenal gland. Early in the disease progression, there are increased serum globulins and decreased albumin, followed by renal glomerular amyloid deposition. With advanced renal amyloidosis, a nephrotic syndrome develops with proteinuria, probable hypoproteinemia (as evident by ascites and anasarca), and hypercholesterolemia. Aging hamsters also have a high incidence of age-related nephrosis resembling that in aging rats (Feldman et al., 1982; Percy and Barthold, 2007). Even with severe nephrosis, blood urea nitrogen is elevated only infrequently, and

TABLE 7.2
Summary of Differences in Clinical Chemistry Between Bio Research and Charles River Hamsters

Analyte	Bio Research Laboratories						Charles River					
	Males			Females			Males			Females		
	n	Mean	SD	*n*	Mean	SD	*n*	Mean	SD	*n*	Mean	SD
Glucose	30	124	31	30	104	25	31	120	34	32	134	38
Bilirubin	30	0.5	0.3	28	0.2	0.1	31	0.4	0.2	31	0.3	0.2
Albumin	30	4.0	0.2	30	4.2	0.3	31	4.3	0.3	31	4.1	0.3
Phosphorus	29	7.5	0.9	28	7.0	1.0	31	8.2	1.1	32	8.3	1.2
Alkaline Phosphatase	21	159	17	15	202	23	18	121	17	25	143	22

Source: Maxwell, K.O. et al., *Lab Anim Sci.*, 35, 67–70, 1985.

serum creatinine has been reported to remain within normal limits (Feldman et al., 1982). The chronic proliferative typhlocolitis can be associated with diarrhea, but the expected changes in serum clinical chemistry have not been described. Aging hamsters also have frequent atrial thrombosis (Hubbard and Schmidt, 1987). Effects of the atrial thrombosis on serum coagulation factors have not been described, but might be considered if unusual results are received from aging hamsters.

7.4.3 Strain/Breed

Characteristics of several lines of Syrian hamsters, as well as selected lines of other species, such as the diabetic Chinese hamster, have been described earlier. Differences among Syrian hamsters from different colonies, with regard to various baseline values for clinical analytes, have also been described, as well as differences in response to manipulation. In 1985, Maxwell et al. (1985) compared values for 17 different serum analytes between 64 hamsters from CR and 60 hamsters from BR Laboratories. Hamsters from the two sources were purchased and tested at separate times, but all were approximately 3 months of age and equal numbers of males and females were tested. No health problems were noted, although no laboratory testing for infection was conducted, so differences in obtained values between these sources must be considered carefully. The BR females had higher values for calcium and lower values for glucose and triglycerides than the other groups, and CR females had higher levels of cholesterol. Trautwein et al. (1993) found differences in susceptibility to high-fat-diet-induced gallstones, as well as hepatic cholesterol accumulation and several lipid ratios, among outbred hamsters from CR and Harlan Sprague-Dawley and inbred hamsters from Bio Breeders. Further investigation of changes after feeding a high-fat diet (Dorfman et al., 2003) showed that the outbred CR and the inbred Bio Breeder hamsters had differences in serum total and non-HDL cholesterol, and aortic accumulation of cholesteryl ester.

Only a few examples have been outlined, but they should be sufficient to demonstrate that hamsters obtained from different sources should not be assumed to have the same baseline values or experimental responses. In addition to this caveat, the reader should note that many of the comparisons are old; any divergence between colonies at the time of those studies may not represent variation between the populations with current generations of hamsters, and current equipment may also give somewhat different results. Contemporary control values are strongly encouraged in preference to reliance on decades-old published values.

7.4.4 Nutritional Status

Four-week-old male Syrian hamsters fed a diet containing processed corn starch or rice bran (all diets had the same levels of dietary fiber, fat, and cholesterol) had significantly lower total plasma cholesterol. Diets containing rice bran, in the same study, also lowered low-density lipoprotein cholesterol (Kahlon and Chow, 2000). Although baseline cholesterol levels in hamsters are higher than those in other laboratory rodents, levels increase further with high triglyceride diets (Sullivan et al., 1993). Feeding a diet with 60% carbohydrate as fructose for 2 weeks resulted in significant increases in low density lipoprotein-triglyceride and a corresponding decrease in low density lipoprotein-cholesterol ester. The median diameter of very low density lipoprotein particles was increased, and all high density lipoprotein fractions were elevated. These changes mirror those in humans with an atherogenic lipoprotein profile (Wang and Walzem, 2008). In a lifetime study of the effect of varying levels of dietary protein on the development of age-related nephritis in male and female Syrian hamsters, no differences were found in blood urea nitrogen or serum creatinine, regardless of dietary protein level, 6%, 12%, 18%, or 24% (Feldman et al., 1982). Whether the increased sensitivity of currently available equipment might detect differences, if a similar contemporary study were performed, is unknown.

No specific discussion of the short-term effects of acute fasting is available in the literature. Food deprivation for 27 hours in combination with wheel running markedly reduced plasma glucose in

Syrian hamsters, although plasma glucose was increased by wheel-running in non-fasted animals (Mistlberger et al., 2006).

Feeding a 25% energy-restricted diet to hamsters previously fed a high-fat diet for 7 weeks resulted in significant decreases in serum glucose, cholesterol, and triacylglycerols (Lasa et al., 2007). No influence of long-term dietary restriction on common clinical chemistry parameters without previous manipulation of diet or light cycle is available in the literature, although moderate dietary restriction has been reported to alter adaptability to changes in light cycle in Siberian but not in Syrian hamsters (Challet et al., 2000).

7.4.5 Housing Environment (Caging Materials, Lighting, Temperature, etc.)

Hamsters, typically bred by vendors with 14 hours of light and 10 hours of dark, are strongly affected by photoperiod. With decreasing daylight, or with steady day length of 12 hours or less, males undergo testicular atrophy and have decreases in circulating testosterone, gonadotropins, and thyroid hormones (Ottenweller et al., 1987). The effects of photoperiod changes on body weight are mediated through the hypothalamus by several neuropeptides (Morgan et al., 2003). Increasing photoperiod results in weight gain as a result of hyperphagia mediated by neuropeptide Y (NPY) and Agouti-related peptide (AGRP). In contrast, exposing hamsters to a short photoperiod (8 hours) results in loss of body weight due to anorexia; cocaine and amphetamine-regulated transcript (CART) is one neuropeptide thought to play a key role in this physiologic response.

Group-housed hamsters on an atherogenic diet had higher cholesterol and triglyceride levels than did individually housed hamsters on a similar diet (Yoganathan et al., 1998), although another study found a similar effect only in young hamsters (Smith et al., 1997).

7.4.6 Circadian Rhythm—Time of Collection

Because hamsters have played an important role in investigation of the circadian clock in mammals, a brief review of the understanding of the clock's mechanism is appropriate. Light interacts with photoreceptors in the retina, which transmits nerve impulses via the retino-hypothalamic tract directly to the suprachiasmatic nucleus (SCN), with glutamate as a neurotransmitter. The SCN is thought to function as the central circadian clock, although peripheral clocks may also play a role. Activation of the glutamate receptors in the SCN leads to a calcium influx and activation of signal transduction pathways that eventually modify clock proteins and expression of genes such as *cfos*, NGF1–A, and the clock genes *Dec1*, *Per1*, and *Per2*. As the central clock, the SCN communicates with peripheral clocks by diffusible factors, of which TGFα and prokineticin 2 have been identified (Albrecht, 2004). Melatonin release from the pineal gland, which was previously thought to be important in circadian rhythm, is not currently considered to play a major role. The effects of circadian rhythm on several serum analytes have been reported in hamsters maintained at standard temperatures, that is, without torpor or hibernation. The hamster adrenal is able to secrete both cortisol and corticosterone, and Albers et al. (1985) found that both glucocorticoids varied significantly over a 24-hour period in hamsters maintained on a cycle of 14 hours light and 10 hours dark. Both hormones rose late in the light phase, reached their acrophase (peak) near the beginning of the dark phase, stayed high until late in the dark phase, then decreased to a nadir early in the light phase. However, corticosterone levels exceeded cortisol when both hormones were at low levels (light phase), whereas cortisol predominated during the daily (dark phase) increases. Chelini et al. (2006) assessed fecal cortisol in 10 mature hamsters for 5 days before and 5 days after the ovariectomy. They found more than 40-fold variation among individuals which may have obscured any changes in fecal cortisol in the days following surgery. They also make the point that total fecal output should be considered in addition to merely evaluating fecal cortisol concentration; that "changes in fecal output, either stress-related or not, affect the concentration of fecal metabolites." As a consequence, they did not feel that fecal concentrations of cortisol, *per se*, were very useful (Chelini et al., 2006). Experimental manipulation of cortisol levels had no effect on circadian wheel-running rhythm (Albers et al., 1985). Vaughan et al. (1994), found that in male hamsters maintained with 14.5 hours of daylight (6:30 AM–9 PM), serum gonadotropins, T3, T4, and cholesterol all demonstrated significant circadian rhythms, with acrophase occurring at different times for each analyte. Thus, time of collection should be standardized within a study.

7.4.7 Estrous Cycle, Pregnancy, or Lactation

Female hamsters have a 4-day estrous cycle, with development and regression of corpora lutea within a single cycle. In contrast, rats and mice retain corpora lutea for several subsequent cycles (Bivin et al., 1987). Gestation in the hamster is 15–18 days, with parturition usually occurring on the 16th day. Pregnant females have mild hepatomegaly late in gestation, possibly related to reduced bile flow, with a 37% reduction reported at 8 days of gestation and 62% reduction at 14 days. Additionally, decreased cholic acid secretion during pregnancy causes reduced secretion of total bile acids (Bivin et al., 1987).

7.4.8 Stress

Even mild stressors, such as novelty, may alter sensitive analytes. For example, placing hamsters in an unfamiliar (novel) cage for 15 minutes or more resulted in significant increases in plasma cortisol (Weinberg and Wong, 1986); plasma corticosterone was not measured but both hormones are considered stress-responsive in hamsters, neither is predominant. Being placed in a cage with a large ovariectomized female for 15 minutes (nonreceptive female hamsters will attack males placed into their cage) induced significant increases in ACTH, cortisol, corticosterone, and β-endorphin in submissive males, but not in dominant males. Foot shock induced larger increases than did the novel cage for all of these hormones (Huhman et al., 1990). In contrast to these studies, King-Herbert et al. (1997) found no difference in serum cortisol or corticosterone on the second day, or thereafter, in hamsters immobilized daily for 6 hours in plastic restraint tubes relative to unrestrained hamsters. No serum analytes were assessed prior to the second day. The time of blood collection, from the orbital sinus, during the restraint period was not given. Restrained hamsters did, however, eat and drink less and have lower body weights relative to the unrestrained controls, suggesting some level of stress (King-Herbert et al., 1997).

7.4.9 Infection and Disease

Relatively little is known about prevalent infectious diseases of contemporary laboratory hamsters, and even less about effects of these diseases, especially subclinical infections, on clinical chemistry results. A thorough review by Baker (2003) of the effects on research of infectious disease in laboratory rodents reported no specific alterations of clinical chemistry parameters by infectious disease in hamsters. However, Baker frequently referred readers to chapters dealing with more commonly used laboratory species, such as rats and mice. He advises of the possibility that many pathogens, including those that cause subclinical infections, would have similar effects in hamsters as in other laboratory rodents. A number of diseases of infectious or possibly infectious origin may still occur in laboratory hamsters, although prevalence data are not available. These diseases include enteritis including that caused by *Lawsonia intracellularis*, typhlitis, possibly caused by *Helicobacter* (Nambiar et al., 2005, 2006), and demodicosis (Percy and Barthold, 2007). In addition, several *Helicobacter* spp. have been detected in hamsters (Simmons et al., 2000). One of these, *Helicobacter cholecystus* has been associated with lesions of the liver and biliary tree (Franklin et al., 1996) and could possibly alter levels of enzymes, bile acids, and other analytes with a hepatobiliary origin or metabolism. Chronic hepatitis of undetermined cause in Syrian hamsters has been reported to result in increased cholesterol, alanine aminotransferase, and alkaline phosphatase, but not bile acids (preprandial or postprandial) or LDH (Brunnert and Altman, 1991).

A variety of noninfectious diseases are also common in hamsters, including amyloidosis, glomerulonephritis, atrial thrombosis, and polycystic liver disease (Hankenson and Van Hoosier, 2002;

Schmidt et al., 1983; Percy and Barthold, 2007). Effects of these conditions on clinical chemistry parameters are rarely reported, but should be considered when evaluating data from aging hamsters. In addition, many potentially confounding factors can have additive or synergistic influences. For example, age, chronic stress, and cardiomyopathy combine to depress testosterone levels in male hamsters (Ottenweller et al., 1988).

7.4.10 Anesthesia

Barbiturate anesthesia in hamsters is reported to elevate glucose for up to 5 hours. Hamsters anesthetized with thiobarbiturate (Inactin®) had significantly higher mean blood glucose, 300.1 ± 15.6 mg/dL, than unanesthetized hamsters, 144.8 ± 7.7 mg/dL, ($p < 0.0005$) (Turner and Howards, 1977). Anesthetics are also reported to alter blood gases and blood pH (Reid et al., 1989). A variety of injectable and inhalant anesthetic regimens for hamsters is summarized in Swindle et al. (2002). No specific reports could be found of effects in hamsters of commonly used contemporary anesthetics such as isoflurane gas or ketamine in combination with other drugs on clinical chemistry values. However, one might expect and should be alert to the potential for anesthetics to alter clinical chemistry values in a fashion similar to their effects in other rodent species. For more detail, please see the chapters devoted to mice and rats.

7.4.11 Specimen Collection/Handling Artifact

No specific effects of hemolysis or lipemia on clinical chemistry parameters in hamsters have been reported. It is likely, however, that hemolysis can lead to artifactually increased measured levels of serum potassium, phosphorus, and some enzymes and that lipemia can artifactually decrease serum electrolytes in hamsters as in other species of laboratory animals.

As noted in Table 7.1, serial sampling of blood is recommended to be limited to a volume equivalent to more than approximately 0.8% of body weight every 3–4 weeks, or approximately 0.08% daily.

As noted in Section 7.3.1, and consistent with observations in other species, blood collection by cardiac puncture may result in sample contamination with enzymes present in cardiac muscle, specifically CPK, AST, LDH, and alanine aminotransferase (Maxwell et al., 1985; Thrall et al., 2004).

7.5 BRIEF DESCRIPTION OF COMMON PROCEDURES

7.5.1 Glucose Tolerance Tests

Syrian hamsters are widely used as models of experimental pancreatic cancer and diabetes, so glucose tolerance tests are commonly performed in Syrian hamsters. A number of factors including animal age, method of glucose administration, and whether the procedure is performed on awake or anesthetized animals can have a significant effect on results. In one study that compared the oral glucose tolerance test (OGTT) to the intraperitoneal glucose tolerance test (IPGTT), it was noted that saline-administered control hamsters had a significant increase in plasma glucose (McCullough et al., 1987). This effect, likely due to the stress of handling and saline administration, appeared to decrease with age in the OGTT but not the IPGTT treatment group (McCullough et al., 1987). A study comparing IPGTT to OGTT in nonanesthetized hamsters found that OGTT provided more consistent results that varied with the dose of glucose administered (McCullough et al., 1987). Since so many factors can affect the results of the glucose tolerance test in hamsters, it is strongly recommended that the procedure be performed in all animals in a standardized and consistent manner. Animals should be fasted for approximately 18 hours before starting the study, although water should be provided *ad libitum*. A baseline blood sample should be taken followed by glucose administration. Nonanesthetized hamsters should be given 0.75–1.0 gm/kg glucose by oral gavage. Blood sampling should be performed in the least stressful manner possible, for example, using an indwelling catheter, although consistent results have been obtained by orbital venous puncture. Follow-up blood samples should be taken at 30, 60, and 120 minutes (McCullough et al., 1987).

7.5.2 Adrenocorticotropic Hormone Stimulation Assays

Adrenocorticotropic hormone (ACTH) stimulation assays are typically performed in the hamster to probe the adrenal pituitary axis as a part of study protocols for stress, cortisol, and carbohydrate metabolism. The hamster possesses adrenal 17α-hydroxylase activity and thus responds to ACTH stimulation by producing cortisol (LeHoux et al., 1992). In a basal state, blood corticosterone concentrations were three to four times higher than cortisol concentrations; however, with ACTH stimulation this difference disappeared (Ottenweller et al., 1985). Furthermore, the authors demonstrated that ACTH administration and the application of acute stress elevated plasma cortisol and corticosterone concentrations but only cortisol was increased following chronic stress. They recommended that both cortisol and corticosterone be evaluated when assessing adrenocortical function in the hamster. ACTH stimulation assays can be performed using both short- and long-acting synthetic ACTH. In studies using short-acting ACTH, 2.5 IU of a short-acting ACTH such as Cortrosyn™ is injected intraperitoneally and a blood sample is collected 30 minutes later for analysis (Ottenweller et al., 1985). Synacthen®, a synthetic depot preparation of ACTH, has been used in longer term ACTH stimulation assays in hamsters (LeHoux et al., 1992). In this procedure, 1 IU of Synacthen® is administered intramuscularly every 5 hours until the study is completed (LeHoux et al., 1992).

7.6 SUMMARY

Relative to rats and mice, the number of hamsters used annually in biomedical research is small and declining. Nonetheless, unique characteristics, many of which are related to physiologic adaptations associated with torpor and hibernation, with lipid metabolism and with susceptibility to a few infectious diseases, continue to make the hamster valuable.

REFERENCES

Aharoni, B. 1932. Die Muriden von Palästina und Syrien. *Z Säugetierkd.* 7:166–240.

Albers, H.E., Yogev, L., Todd, R.B., and Goldman, B.D. 1985. Adrenal corticoids in hamsters: Role in circadian timing. *Am J Physiol.* 248(4 Pt 2):R434–R438.

Albrecht, U. 2004. The mammalian circadian clock: A network of gene expression. *Front Biosci.* 9:48–55.

Baker, D.G. 2003. Pathogens of hamsters. In *Natural Pathogens of Laboratory Animals: Their Effects on Research.* Washington, DC: ASM Press.

Bivin, W.S., Olsen, G.A., and Murray, K.A. 1987. Morphophysiology. In *Laboratory Hamsters.* Ed. G.L. Van Hoosier, and C.W. McPherson. Orlando, FL: Academic Press.

Braulke, L.J., Klingenspor, M., DeBarber, A., et al. 2008. 3-Iodothyronamine: A novel hormone controlling the balance between glucose and lipid utilisation. *J Comp Physiol B.* 178(2):167–177.

Breckon, G. and Goy, P. 1979. Routine chromosome screening in Syrian hamsters (Mesocricetus auratus) using orbital sinus blood. *Lab Anim.* 13(4):301–304.

Breitweiser, B. 1992. Practical approach to hamster urinary analysis. *J Small Exotic Anim Med.* 1:104–105.

Brunnert, S.R. and Altman, N.H. 1991. Laboratory assessment of chronic hepatitis in Syrian hamsters. *Lab Anim Sci.* 41(6):559–562.

Challet, E., Kolker, D.E., and Turek, F.W. 2000. Metabolic influences on circadian rhythmicity in Siberian and Syrian hamsters exposed to long photoperiods. *J Neuroendocrinol.* 12(1):69–78.

Chang, A.Y. 1978. Spontaneous diabetes in animals. *Gen Pharmacol.* 9(6):447–450.

Chang, A.Y. 1981. Biochemical abnormalities in the Chinese hamster (*Cricetulus griseus*) with spontaneous diabetes. *Int J Biochem.* 13(1):41–43.

Chelini, M.O., Souza, N.L, Cortopassi, S.R.G., Felippe, E.C.G., and Oliveira, C.A. 2006. Assessment of the physiologic stress response by quantification of fecal corticosteroids. *J Am Assoc Lab Anim Sci.* 45(3):8–11.

Chung, Y.L., Lee, M.Y., and Pui, N.N. 2009. Epigenetic therapy using the histone deacetylase inhibitor for increasing therapeutic gain in oral cancer: Prevention of radiation-induced oral mucositis and inhibition of chemical-induced oral carcinogenesis. *Carcinogenesis.* 30(8):1387–1397.

Coe, J.E., Margossian, S.S., Slayter, H.S., and Sogn, J.A. 1981. Hamster female protein. A new Pentraxin structurally and functionally similar to C-reactive protein and amyloid P component. *J Exp Med.* 153(4):977–991.

Dark, J., Lewis, D.A., and Zucker, I. 1999. Hypoglycemia and torpor in Siberian hamsters. *Am J Physiol.* 276(3 Pt 2):R776–R781.

Dark, J., Miller, D.R., and Zucker, I. 1994. Reduced glucose availability induces torpor in Siberian hamsters. *Am J Physiol.* 267(2 Pt 2):R496–R501.

Dent, N.J. 1977. The use of Syrian hamsters to establish its clinical chemistry and hematology profile. In *Clinical Toxicology*. Ed. W.A. Duncan, and B.J. Leonard. Amsterdam: Excerpta Medica.

Donovan, J. and Brown, P. 2005. Blood collection. *Curr Protoc Neurosci* Appendix 4:Appendix 4G.

Dorfman, S.E., Smith, D.E., Osgood, D.P., and Lichtenstein, A.H. 2003. Study of diet-induced changes in lipoprotein metabolism in two strains of Golden-Syrian hamsters. *J Nutr.* 133(12):4183–4188.

Elliott, J.A., Stetson, M.H., and Menaker, M. 1972. Regulation of testis function in golden hamsters: A circadian clock measures photoperiodic time. *Science.* 178(62):771–773.

Feldman, D.B., McConnell, E.E., and Knapka, J.J. 1982. Growth, kidney disease, and longevity of Syrian hamsters (*Mesocricetus auratus*) fed varying levels of protein. *Lab Anim Sci.* 32(6):613–618.

Franklin, C.L., Beckwith, C.S., Livingston, R.S., et al. 1996. Isolation of a novel Helicobacter species, *Helicobacter cholecystus* sp. nov., from the gallbladders of Syrian hamsters with cholangiofibrosis and centrilobular pancreatitis. *J Clin Microbiol.* 34(12):2952–2958.

Gattermann, R., Fritzsche, P., Neumann, K., et al. 2001. Notes on the current distribution and the ecology of wild golden hamsters (*Mesocricetus auratus*). *J Zool.* 254(03):359–365.

Haake, D.A. 2006. Hamster model of leptospirosis. *Curr Protoc Microbiol.* Chapter 12:Unit 12E 2.

Hankenson, F.C. and Van Hoosier, G.L. 2002. Biology and diseases of hamsters. In *Laboratory Animal Medicine*. Eds. J.G. Fox, L.C. Anderson, F.M. Loew, and F.W. Quimby. New York, NY: Academic Press.

Heldmaier, G., Ortmann, S., and Elvert, R. 2004. Natural hypometabolism during hibernation and daily torpor in mammals. *Respir Physiol Neurobiol.* 141(3):317–329.

Hem, A., Smith, A.J., and Solberg, P. 1998. Saphenous vein puncture for blood sampling of the mouse, rat, hamster, gerbil, guinea pig, ferret and mink. *Lab Anim.* 32(4):364–368.

Hubbard, G.B. and Schmidt, R.E. 1987. Noninfectious diseases. In *Laboratory Hamsters*. Ed. G.L. Van Hoosier, and C.W. McPherson. Orlando, FL: Academic Press.

Huhman, K.L., Bunnell, B.N., Mougey, E.H., and Meyerhoff, J.L. 1990. Effects of social conflict on POMC-derived peptides and glucocorticoids in male golden hamsters. *Physiol Behav.* 47(5):949–956.

Izumi, Y., Sugiyama, F., Sugiyama, Y., and Yagami, K. 1993. Comparison between the blood from orbital sinus and heart in analyzing plasma biochemical values—Increase of plasma enzyme values in the blood from orbital sinus. *Jikken Dobutsu.* 42(1):99–102.

Kahlon, T.S. and Chow, F.I. 2000. Lipidemic response of hamsters to rice bran, uncooked or processed white and brown rice, and processed corn starch. *Cereal Chem.* 77:673–678.

King-Herbert, A.P., Hesterburg, T.W., Thevenaz, P.P., et al. 1997. Effects of immobilization restraint on Syrian golden hamsters. *Lab Anim Sci.* 47(4):362–366.

Kurien, B.T., Everds, N.E., and Scofield, R.H. 2004. Experimental animal urine collection: A review. *Lab Anim.* 38(4):333–361.

Larkin, J.E., Yellon, S.M., and Zucker, I. 2003. Melatonin production accompanies arousal from daily torpor in Siberian hamsters. *Physiol Biochem Zool.* 76(4):577–585.

Lasa, A., Simon, E., Churruca, I., Fernandez-Quintela, A., Rodriguez, V.M., and Portillo, M.P. 2007. Adiposity and serum parameters in hamsters fed energy restricted diets supplemented or not with trans-10,cis-12 conjugated linoleic acid. *J Physiol Biochem.* 63(4):297–304.

LeHoux, J.G., Mason, J.I., and Ducharme, L. 1992. In vivo effects of adrenocorticotropin on hamster adrenal steroidogenic enzymes. *Endocrinology.* 131(4):1874–1882.

Lowrey, P.L., Shimomura, K., Antoch, M.P., et al. 2000. Positional syntenic cloning and functional characterization of the mammalian circadian mutation tau. *Science.* 288(5465):483–492.

Lucey, E.C., O'Brien, J.J., Jr., Pereira, W., Jr., and Snider, G.L. 1980. Arterial blood gas values in emphysematous hamsters. *Am Rev Respir Dis.* 121(1):83–89.

Manning, J.P. and Giannina, T. 1966. A simple method for obtaining blood from hamsters in terminal experiments. *Lab Anim Care.* 16(6):523–525.

Maxwell, K.O., Wish, C., Murphy, J.C., and Fox, J.G. 1985. Serum chemistry reference values in two strains of Syrian hamsters. *Lab Anim Sci.* 35(1):67–70.

McCullough, P.J., Rogers, D.H., and Bell, R.H. 1987. Glucose tolerance in Syrian hamsters. *Lab Anim Sci.* 37(3):361–364.

McGuill, M.W. and Rowan, A.N. 1989. Biological effects of blood loss: Implication for sampling volumes and techniques. *ILAR J.* 31(4):5–18.

McIntosh, C.H.S. and Pederson, R.A. 1999. Noninsulin-dependent animal models of diabetes mellitus. In *Experimental Models of Diabetes*. Ed. J.H. McNeill. Boca Raton, FL: CRC Press.

Mercer, J.G. and Tups, A. 2003. Neuropeptides and anticipatory changes in behaviour and physiology: Seasonal body weight regulation in the Siberian hamster. *Eur J Pharmacol.* 480(1–3):43–50.

Mistlberger, R.E., Webb, I.C., Simon, M.M., Tse, D., and Su, C. 2006. Effects of food deprivation on locomotor activity, plasma glucose, and circadian clock resetting in Syrian hamsters. *J Biol Rhythms.* 21(1):33–44.

Mohr, U. and Ernst, H. 1987. Biology, care and use in research. In *Laboratory Hamsters*. Eds. G.L. Van Hoosier, and C.W. McPherson. Orlando, FL: Academic Press, Inc.

Morgan, P.J., Ross, A.W., Mercer, J.G., and Barrett, P. 2003. Photoperiodic programming of body weight through the neuroendocrine hypothalamus. *J Endocrinol.* 177(1):27–34.

Morton, D.B., Abbot, D., Barclay, R., et al. 1993. Removal of blood from laboratory mammals and birds: First report of the BVA/FRAME/RSPCA/UFAW Joint Working Group on refinement. *Lab Anim.* 27(1):1–22.

Nambiar, P.R., Kirchain, S.M., Courmier, K., et al. 2006. Progressive proliferative and dysplastic typhlocolitis in aging syrian hamsters naturally infected with Helicobacter spp: A spontaneous model of inflammatory bowel disease. *Vet Pathol.* 43(1):2–14.

Nambiar, P.R., Kirchain, S., and Fox, J.G. 2005. Gastritis-associated adenocarcinoma and intestinal metaplasia in a Syrian hamster naturally infected with Helicobacter species. *Vet Pathol.* 42(3):386–390.

Neve, P., Authelet, M., and Golstein, J. 1981. Effect of aging on the morphology and function of the thyroid gland of the cream hamster. Further evidence for two different mechanisms of hormone secretion. *Cell Tissue Res.* 220(3):499–509.

Newcomer, C.E., Fitts, D.A., Goldman, B.D., et al. 1987. Experimental biology: Other research uses of Syrian hamsters. In *Laboratory Hamsters*. Eds. G.L. Van Hoosier and C.W. McPherson. Orlando, FL: Academic Press.

Nigro, V., Okazaki, Y., Belsito, A., et al. 1997. Identification of the Syrian hamster cardiomyopathy gene. *Hum Mol Genet.* 6(4):601–607.

O'Brien, J.J., Jr., Lucey, E.C., and Snider, G.L. 1979. Arterial blood gases in normal hamsters at rest and during exercise. *J Appl Physiol.* 46(4):806–810.

Ottenweller, J.E., Tapp, W.N., Burke, J.M., and Natelson, B.H. 1985. Plasma cortisol and corticosterone concentrations in the golden hamster (*Mesocricetus auratus*). *Life Sci.* 37(16):1551–1558.

Ottenweller, J.E., Tapp, W.N., Creighton, D., and Natelson, B.H. 1988. Aging, stress, and chronic disease interact to suppress plasma testosterone in Syrian hamsters. *J Gerontol.* 43(6):M175–M180.

Ottenweller, J.E., Tapp, W.N., Pitman, D.L., and Natelson, B.H. 1987. Adrenal, thyroid, and testicular hormone rhythms in male golden hamsters on long and short days. *Am J Physiol.* 253(2 Pt 2):R321–R328.

Packer, J.T., Kraner, K.L., Rose, S.D., Stuhlman, R.A., and Nelson, L.R. 1970. Diabetes mellitus in *Mystromys albicaudatus*. *Arch Pathol.* 89(5):410–415.

Pansky, B., Jacobs, M., House, E.L., and Tassoni, J.P. 1961. The orbital region as a source of blood samples in the golden hamster. *Anat Rec.* 139(3):409–412.

Percy, D.H. and Barthold, S.W. 2007. Hamster. In *Pathology of Laboratory Rodents & Rabbits*. Ames, IA: Blackwell Publishing.

Popesko, P., Rajtova, V., and Horak, J. 2002. *A Colour Atlas of Anatomy of Small Laboratory Animals. Vol. II. Rat, Mouse, and Golden Hamster*. London: Saunders.

Popovic, V. and Popovic, P. 1960. Permanent cannulation of aorta and vena cava in rats and ground squirrels. *J Appl Physiol.* 15:727–728.

Ralph, M.R. and Menaker, M. 1988. A mutation of the circadian system in golden hamsters. *Science.* 241(4870):1225–1227.

Reid, W.D., Davies, C., Pare, P.D., and Pardy, R.L. 1989. An effective combination of anaesthetics for 6-h experimentation in the golden Syrian hamster. *Lab Anim.* 23(2):156–162.

Riley, T., Stuhlman, R.A., Van Peenen, H.J., Esterly, J.A., and Townsend, J.F. 1975. Glomerular lesions of diabetes mellitus in *Mystromys albicaudatus*. *Arch Pathol.* 99(3):167–169.

Sbrana, E., Xiao, S.-Y., Popov, V.L., Newman, P.C., and Tesh, R.B. 2006. Experimental yellow fever virus infection in the golden hamster (*Mesocricetus auratus*) III. Clinical laboratory values. *Am J Trop Med Hyg.* 74(6):1084–1089.

Schmidt, R.E., Eason, R.L., Hubbard, G.B., Young, J.T., and Eisenbrandt, D.L. Eds. 1983. *Pathology of Aging Syrian Hamsters.* Boca Raton, FL: CRC Press.

Simmons, J.H., Riley, L.K., Besch-Williford, C.L., and Franklin, C.L. 2000. *Helicobacter mesocricetorum* sp. nov., A novel Helicobacter isolated from the feces of Syrian hamsters. *J Clin Microbiol.* 38(5):1811–1817.

Smith, D., Pedro-Botet, J., Cantuti-Castelvetri, I., Schaefer, E.J., and Ordovas, J.M. 1997. Influence of age, diet, and laboratory caging on lipid profile among F1B hamsters. *Nutr Res.* 17:1569–1575.

Sonis, S.T., Tracey, C., Shklar, G., Jenson, J., and Florine, D. 1990. An animal model for mucositis induced by cancer chemotherapy. *Oral Surg Oral Med Oral Pathol.* 69(4):437–443.

Sorg, D.A. and Buckner, B. 1964. A simple method of obtaining venous blood from small laboratory animals. *Proc Soc Exp Biol Med.* 115:1131–1132.

Stephens, M.L., Alvino, G.M., and Branson, J.B. 2002. Animal pain and distress in vaccine testing in the United States. *Dev Biol (Basel).* 111:213–216.

Stone, S.H. 1954. Method for obtaining venous blood from the orbital sinus of the rat or mouse. *Science.* 119(3081):100.

Stuhlman, R.A., Packer, J.T., Doyle, R.E., Brown, R.V., and Townsend, J.F. 1975. Relationship between pancreatic lesions and serum glucose values in *Mystromys albicaudatus. Lab Anim Sci.* 25(2):168–174.

Sullivan, M.P., Cerda, J.J., Robbins, F.L., Burgin, C.W., and Beatty, R.J. 1993. The gerbil, hamster, and guinea pig as rodent models for hyperlipidemia. *Lab Anim Sci.* 43:575–578.

Swindle, M.M., Vogler, G.A., Fulton, L.K., and Pipilskis, S. 2002. Preanesthesia, anesthesia, analgesia, and euthanasia. In *Laboratory Animal Medicine*. Eds. J.G. Fox, L.C. Anderson, F.M. Loew, and F.W. Quimby, 2nd edition, pp. 955–1033. San Diego, CA: Academic Press.

Thrall, M.A., Baker, D.C., Campbell, T.W., et al. 2004. *Veterinary Hematology and Clinical Chemistry.* Philadelphia, PA: Lippincott Williams & Wilkins.

Timm, K.I. 1980. Peri-orbital bleeding technique for the mouse, hamster, and rat—Anatomical consideration. *Synapse.* 13:14–16.

Trautwein, E.A., Liang, J., and Hayes, K.C. 1993. Cholesterol gallstone induction in hamsters reflects strain differences in plasma lipoproteins and bile acid profiles. *Lipids.* 28(4):305–312.

Turner, T.T. and Howards, S.S. 1977. Hyperglycemia in the hamster anesthetized with Inactin [5-ethyl-5-(-methyl propyl)-2-thiobarbiturate]. *Lab Anim Sci.* 27(3):380–382.

USDA APHIS. 2008. Animal care annual report of activities: Fiscal year 2007.

Vainzof, M., Ayub-Guerrieri, D., Onofre, P.C., et al. 2008. Animal models for genetic neuromuscular diseases. *J Mol Neurosci.* 34(3):241–248.

Vairaktaris, E., Spyridonidou, S., Papakosta, V., et al. 2008. The hamster model of sequential oral oncogenesis. *Oral Oncol.* 44(4):315–324.

Vaughan, M.K., Menendez-Pelaez, A., Buzzell, G.R., Vaughan, G.M., Little, J.C., and Reiter, R.J. 1994. Circadian rhythms in reproductive and thyroid hormones in gonadally regressed male hamsters exposed to natural autumn photoperiod and temperature conditions. *Neuroendocrinology.* 60(1):96–104.

Wang, L., Yu, J., and Walzem, R.L. 2008. High-carbohydrate diets affect the size and composition of plasma lipoproteins in hamsters (*Mesocricetus auratus*). *Comp Med.* 58(2):151–160.

Weinberg, J. and Wong, R. 1986. Adrenocortical responsiveness to novelty in the hamster. *Physiol Behav.* 37(5):669–672.

Yesus, Y.W., Esterly, J.A., Stuhlman, R.A., and Townsend, J.F. 1976. Significant muscle capillary basement membrane thickening in spontaneously diabetic *Mystromys albicaudatus. Diabetes.* 25(5):444–449.

Yoganathan, S., Wilson, T.A., and Nicolosi, R.J. 1998. Housing conditions effect plasma lipid concentrations and early atherogenesis independent of treatment in hamsters. *Nutr Res.* 18(1):83–92.

Zysling, D.A. and Demas, G.E. 2007. Metabolic stress suppresses humoral immune function in long-day, but not short-day, Siberian hamsters (*Phodopus sungorus*). *J Comp Physiol B.* 177(3):339–347.

8 The Laboratory Guinea Pig

Patrick Sharp

CONTENTS

8.1 USE IN BIOMEDICAL RESEARCH

The guinea pig (*Cavia porcellus*) has historically been considered a hystricomorph mammal belonging to a family of burrowing rodents (Caviidae) native to the Western Hemisphere. More recently, sequencing of the mitochondrial genome and molecular analysis has indicated the guinea pig should be considered in a separate taxonomic group currently of intermediate rank (Frederiksen and Heeno-Andersen, 2003; Adkins et al., 2000; Konno et al., 1999; D'Erchia et al., 1996; Li et al., 1992). In the wild, guinea pigs live in small groups in the open grasslands of Bolivia, Western Peru, Argentina, Uruguay, and Brazil (Weir, 1974). They have been domesticated and are used as food animals in several South American countries. Guinea pigs were first brought to Europe in the early 1600s, where they were bred for food and as pets. In the early 1900s, they were first used as laboratory animals, primarily in genetic research. Since then, they have proved useful laboratory animal models for research in areas including nutrition, immunology, gastroenterology, cardiovascular disease, audiology, toxicology (including teratology and reproductive toxicology), pharmacology, and infectious disease research, including tuberculosis, listeriosis, and Q-fever.

Since the first addition of this text in 1989, guinea pig use for biomedical research in the United States has declined approximately 64% from 481,712 to 172,864 in 2015, the last year for which figures are available from the United States Department of Agriculture (USDA, 2016). Even though the popularity of guinea pigs in research has declined from a peak in the 1930s, their use as pets has increased.

8.2 UNIQUE PHYSIOLOGIC CHARACTERISTICS

8.2.1 Gastrointestinal System

Guinea pigs are monogastric and have a completely glandular stomach in contrast to other rodents such as mice and rats which have glandular and nonglandular gastric components (Hargaden and Singer, 2012). The guinea pig gut flora is predominantly Gram-positive and they are very sensitive antibiotic-induced enterotoxemia (Manning et al., 1984). Like other rodents, guinea pigs practice coprophagy and this activity could result in the recirculation of an array of factors potentially impacting a variety of clinical pathology parameters.

In the guinea pig, as in humans, the intestine is the principal site of cholesterol synthesis, whereas the liver is the principal site in other species. Swann et al. (1975) showed the liver-to-ileum ratio of acetate incorporation into cholesterol is 0.061 in the guinea pig and 1.57 in the rat. All cholesterologenic tissues in the guinea pig are subject to feedback inhibition (Swann et al., 1975; Wriston, 1984).

8.2.2 Cardiovascular System

Brewer and Cruise (1994) outlined the comparative aspects of guinea pig cardiovascular physiology, including the low basal and peak coronary blood flow. There are extensive intracoronary collaterals present in the guinea pigs making it difficult to elicit a coronary infarct compared with other species. The guinea pig's electrocardiogram differs from other rodents in that they have longer S-T segments. Guinea pigs are very sensitive to adenosine and their cardiac tissue is unaffected by vasoactive intestinal peptide, unlike other mammals.

Guinea pigs serve as a model of the circulatory form of pregnancy toxemia, where the aorta caudal to the renal vessels undergoes fetal compression due to the relatively large size of the conceptus as guinea pigs are precocious at birth compared to other rodents. Sequelae-to-fetal compression of the caudal aorta is reduced blood pressure to the uterine vasculature, placental necrosis, ketosis, and death (Percy and Barthold, 2007).

8.2.3 Respiratory System

Brewer and Cruise (1997) outlined the comparative aspects of the guinea pigs respiratory system. Alveolar development is nearly complete at birth compared to other rodents. Guinea pigs have a complex pharyngeal anatomy common in hystricomorphs, highlighted by the presence of a palatial ostium which is a small opening in the continuation of the soft palate to the base of the tongue. The palatial ostium makes endotracheal intubation and oral gavage a challenge (Hargaden and Singer, 2012). Access is easily gained to the eustachian tube complex in the guinea pig. Compared to other mammals, guinea pigs have very prominent smooth muscle in the distal bronchi which is arranged spirally (Brewer and Cruise, 1997). Pulmonary serous cells are absent in the guinea pig unlike the rat, whereas goblet cells are common in the guinea pig and rare in other small rodents (Hargaden and Singer, 2012). In the pulmonary capillaries of guinea pigs, neutrophils, not macrophages, adhere to endothelial cells and capture intravascular foreign bodies up to the size of red blood cells (Terada, 1993; Brewer and Cruise, 1997). The neuroendocrine bodies found in the lungs of guinea pigs appear to be a modification associated with their evolutionary development at the high altitude of the Andes Mountains. Percy and Barthold (2007) highlighted unique histological aspects of the respiratory architecture in the guinea pig, such as pulmonary arterial and arteriolar medial thickening, prevalent Clara cells, perivascular lymphoid nodules, and osseous metaplasia in the lungs. Physiologically, the guinea pig offers a well-characterized airway hyperresponsiveness and reaction model of asthma.

8.2.4 Endocrine System

The guinea pig does not require growth hormone for growth, as is the case for other mammals. Pituitary gland removal does not impact growth in this species. Insulin-like growth factor I and II are responsible for growth in guinea pigs (Harkness et al., 2002; Adkins et al., 2000). Guinea pig growth hormone is functional in other species, as it will support growth in hypophysectomized rats. Both growth hormone and the growth hormone receptor have a single amino acid replacement at a functionally significant location, but it is unclear what role this plays.

The alpha (α-) subunit of glycoprotein hormones such as follicle stimulating hormone, luteinizing hormone, thyroid stimulating hormone, and chorionic gonadotropin is produced by the pituitary gland. The guinea pig's common α-subunits of these glycoprotein hormones are not homologous to those in other rodents. Suzuki et al. (2002) speculated that the differences in the guinea pig's common α-subunits was a primary reason that the guinea pig fails to ovulate when treated with human or equine chorionic gonadotropin (hCG or eCG) as routinely used in mice (Suzuki et al. 2002). Instead, they found that ovulation could be induced with human menopausal gonadotropin (hMG) when administered at the appropriate phase of the estrous cycle (Suzuki et al., 2003).

Gonadotropin-releasing hormone (GnRH) is produced in hypothalamus and regulates many aspects of sexual development and reproduction. The guinea pig GnRH receptor differs from most other rodent species in terms of amino acid composition and ligand sensitivities (Fujii et al., 2004). In the female guinea pig (*Cavia aperea*), onset of puberty was dramatically affected by changes in photoperiod (Trillmich et al., 2009). The authors concluded that this effect was due to the ability of melatonin to block GnRH as had been demonstrated in numerous other mammalian species (Jimenez-Linan et al., 1997). Melatonin serves an important function in guinea pigs due to the longer gestation period compared to other rodents. It is believed that this can function as a prenatal mechanism to delay maturity from the pregnant dam to the female offspring in utero (Trillmich et al., 2009). As seen with many other hormones, guinea pig melatonin differs in amino acid structure compared to other mammalian species.

Produced by the mammalian kidney in response to tissue hypoxia, erythropoietin is an essential hormone that controls erythrocyte production. While there is a high degree of sequence homology evidence demonstrating biological cross-reactivity between humans and numerous other species (Wen et al., 1993), guinea pig erythropoietin failed to stimulate mouse or human erythroid differentiation in vitro; however, guinea pig erythroid progenitors were stimulated by human or mouse erythropoietin, suggesting differences in erythropoietin or erythropoietin receptors (Stopka et al., 1998).

Insulin is a highly conserved hormone in numerous species (Jukes, 1979; Smith, 1966). Insulin from hystricomorphs, including guinea pigs, differs from most other species in at least one-third of its amino acid sequence (Beintema and Campagne, 1987; Blundel and Wood, 1975; Jukes, 1979; Smith, 1966). Circulating, guinea pig insulin possess between 1% and 5% of the biological activity of insulin from other mammalian species (Zimmerman and Yip, 1974). Circulating guinea pig insulin reacts poorly with standard anti-insulin antibodies, does not dimerize at high concentrations, does not form crystals, and does not bind zinc (Zimmerman and Yip, 1974). The review article by Beintema and Campagne (1987) provides an overview of the molecular evolution of rodent insulin, highlighting the uniqueness of guinea pig.

Guinea pigs produce insulin in small quantities in extrapancreatic tissues; however, this insulin appears to be confined to the cells in which it is produced and has not been detected in the plasma (Rosenzweig et al., 1980). This insulin is as active metabolically as other mammalian insulin but does not appear to be responsible for controlling variations in plasma glucose levels (Rosenzweig et al., 1980), which is controlled by the less active, pancreatic insulin. Rosenzweig et al. (1983, 1985) proposed that two insulin genes existed in the guinea pig genome; one producing the typical guinea pig insulin in the pancreatic beta cells and the second producing a protein similar to the more conserved mammalian insulin. Chan et al. (1984) contended there is but a single gene. Commercially available insulin radioimmunoassay kits are not valid for measuring plasma insulin levels in the guinea pig but can be used to measure tissue levels of nonpancreatic guinea pig insulin. Some commercial plasma insulin kits utilize anti-insulin antibodies produced in guinea pigs, which further limits their utility in this species. To further complicate the ability to measure guinea pig insulin, de Pablo et al. (1986) determined that protozoa contain materials which can interfere with the guinea pig's insulin radioimmunoassay.

Cortisol is the principal glucocorticoid produced by the guinea pig, in contrast to the rat and mouse, which predominately produce corticosterone. The guinea pig has a high rate of interconversion between cortisol and cortisone (Manin et al., 1982). Garris (1979) described a diurnal cycle with plasma cortisol concentrations increasing from their dark-phase lows, starting at 4 hours prior to the onset of the light phase of the light:dark (14 hours:10 hours) photoperiod, peaking between 4 and 8 hours after the onset of the light phase then followed by a steady decline until reaching basal concentrations prior to the onset of the dark phase. The author suggested that the diurnal cycle of plasma cortisol in the guinea pig resembled what was observed for humans but was in contrast with that seen rats.

Transcortin, or corticosteroid-binding globulin, has been identified in many species and can bind both cortisol and progesterone. The pregnant guinea pig has a second steroid binding protein, progesterone-binding globulin that specifically binds progesterone but not cortisol. Guinea pig transcortin has a much higher affinity for cortisol than for progesterone, in contrast to human transcortin, which has a similar affinity for both steroids. Progesterone-binding globulin appears to be unique to hystricomorph rodents (Wriston, 1984). Guinea pigs, like humans, are able to maintain a pregnancy following ovariectomy in contrast to mice, rats, and rabbits (Zarrow et al., 1963).

Rodriguez et al. (2008) outlined the concept of uterine progesterone receptor localization and its role in various components of parturition, including pubic symphysis relaxation. The article explores the interaction of various hormones involved with the initiation of parturition, including oxytocin, progesterone, relaxin, and estrogen.

Relaxin is a steroid hormone, secreted by the uterus, responsible for interpubic ligament relaxation permitting lengthening of the cartilaginous nonsynovial joint and, in turn, facilitates delivery of the relatively large, precocious young (Hisaw et al., 1944; Rodriguez et al., 2003; Zarrow, 1947). Rodriguez et al. (2008) remarks that the guinea pig interpubic ligament relaxes so markedly that it permits fetal passage where the average head diameter is twice the average pelvic canal diameter. Zarrow (1948) evaluated the role of other hormones in the pubic symphysis relaxation, and Rodriguez et al. (2003) postulated on relaxin's role (and other hormones including estradiol) in the underlying cellular response, a response that resembles inflammation. Relaxin affects corpus luteum function and plays a role in permitting ovulation (Jagiello, 1967), and inhibits guinea pig's myometrial activity; however, total suppression of uterine activity does not occur and myometrial activity is inversely related to serum relaxin levels (Porter, 1971a, b). Furthermore, relaxin has little effect on oxytocin's ability to initiate intrauterine pressure (Porter, 1972).

Zarrow (1947) evaluated relaxin levels in serum, urine, and other tissues. Relaxin was detected in the serum of all guinea pigs by day 21 of pregnancy, peaked by day 28, where it was maintained through gestational day 63 when a sharp drop was noted. A further drop was detected at parturition, most likely due to decreased placenta output. Relaxin's falling serum levels paralleled relaxin's urine levels. Larkin and Reneger (1986) used light microscopy to perform immunolocalization of relaxin. Endometrial gland cells demonstrated high numbers of granules staining positively for relaxin from mid- to late-gestation in the guinea pig.

8.2.5 Hematopoeitic System

Guinea pigs have a lower red blood cell count and the largest erythrocyte of the commonly used rodents in biomedical research (Hargaden and Singer, 2012). Lymphocytes are the predominant peripheral blood leukocyte in the guinea pig and they are resistant to the lymphopenic effects of exogenous corticosteroids compared to other mammals.

Foa-Kurloff or Kurloff cells are mononuclear cells containing lymphocyte and monocyte properties (Eremin et al., 1980) and are observed regularly in blood smears of guinea pigs. These cells contain intracytoplasmic periodic acid Schiff (PAS) positive material found in all guinea pigs (rare in newborn animals) with higher numbers seen in females (and estrogen exposed males) they are thought to be the equivalent of natural killer cells. They are believed to prevent maternal rejection of the fetal placenta during pregnancy and have a role in the increased cancer resistance observed in guinea pigs. Kurloff cells are seen in high numbers in the trophoblast region of the placenta during pregnancy.

As mentioned in Section 8.2.3, guinea pig neutrophils adhere to endothelial cells and capture intravascular foreign bodies the size of red blood cells (Brewer and Cruise, 1997). Calcium ions play an important role in normal guinea pig neutrophil functions, including chemotaxis, superoxide anion generation, and granule enzyme release. Azuma et al. (1986) demonstrated that calcium antagonists (including verapamil and nifedipine) interfered with these important neutrophil functions.

8.3 METHODOLOGY FOR SAMPLING COLLECTION

8.3.1 Blood Collection

Data regarding the clinical chemistry of the laboratory guinea pig remains sparse. This may be due to the relatively small number of guinea pigs used in research and the difficulty in obtaining blood samples from their peripheral veins, as their deep vessels are often covered with many layers of fat. Methods of obtaining repeated blood samples have been described (see Table 8.1), in addition to

TABLE 8.1
Methods for Obtaining Blood Samples from Guinea Pigs

Method	Comments
Cutting nail bed	Small quantities of blood (<1 mL); may be contaminated
Marginal ear vein	Small quantities of blood (<1 mL); may be contaminated
Dorsal metatarsal vein	Small quantities of blood (<1 mL); may be contaminated
Saphenous vein	Small quantities of blood (<1 mL); may be contaminated
Interdigital vein	Small quantities of blood (<1 mL); may be contaminated
Orbital sinus	Moderate quantities of blood (>2 mL); little contamination; requires anesthesia
Jugular vein	Moderate quantities of blood (>2 mL); not contaminated
Lateral metatarsal vein (vacuum assisted)	Moderate quantities of blood (>2 mL); may be contaminated
Femoral vein	Moderate quantities of blood (>2 mL); not contaminated
Cardiocentesis (cardiac puncture)	Large quantities of blood (>5 mL); not contaminated; cardiac or pulmonary laceration may cause death; must be performed under anesthesia as a terminal procedure
Vena cava or other large internal vessels	Large quantities of blood (>5 mL); not contaminated; must be performed surgically under anesthesia; usually a terminal procedure
Decapitation	Large quantities of blood (>5 mL); usually contaminated; terminal procedure

Source: Shomer et al. (1999) *Contemp Top Lab Anim Sci.* 38(5):32–35. (jugular vein); Clifford, C.B. and White, W.J., In W.F. Loeb and F.W. Quimby [ed.], *The Clinical Chemistry of Laboratory Animals*, Philadelphia, PA, Taylor & Francis, 1999 (all other sites).

single-sample terminal methods such as decapitation or surgical intervention (see Huneke, 2012). With the exception of cardiocentesis (cardiac puncture), femoral venopuncture, and orbital sinus bleeding, sample volumes are usually low and often contaminated; however, cardiocentesis, femoral venopuncture, and orbital sinus bleeding have a low degree of repeatability and may be stressful to the animal. Although the blood volume obtained may be low, advancing analyte technologies makes it possible to obtain more data from smaller volumes. As highlighted in Section 8.5.1, select hormone determination can be made from feces versus plasma, thereby reducing stress and the need to collect blood for some parameters.

Blood and plasma volumes of the guinea pig average 6.96 and 3.88 mL per 100 g of body weight, respectively; although these figures vary considerably with age (Green et al., 1976; Sisk, 1976). They are highest at birth and steadily trend downward until 900 g of body weight is reached, at which point they tend to level out. It is generally considered that not more than 10% of the total blood volume should be collected once every 3–4 weeks and daily collections of no more than 1% can occur without adverse effects. In their publication, Terril and Clemmons (1998) indicated that the guinea pig blood volume averaged 75 mL/kg, thus, 7.5 mL of blood/kg body could be removed once every 3–4 weeks. As a general guideline, the author uses 1.25% (1.25 mL/100 g of body weight) once every 2 weeks for blood collection. However, readers are advised to consult their Institutional Animal Care and Use Committee (IACUC) or Ethics Committee for institutional guidelines on permissible collection volumes and frequency.

When preparing guinea pig serum in plastic rather than glass collection tubes or vials, clotting occurs much more slowly. Since potassium is released from platelets during clotting, the use of plastic tubes, such as the Microtainer® (Becton Dickinson, Franklin Lakes, NJ), results in reduced serum potassium levels and minimizes sample dilution due to the Microtainer's® use of lyophilized or freeze-dried anticoagulants (Caisey and King, 1980; Dyer and Cervasio, 2008). During clotting, guinea pig blood cellular elements release lactate dehydrogenase and gamma glutamyl transferase (GGT) into the serum (Campbell, 2012). The release of GGT into the serum is in sharp contrast to many other mammalian species where GGT release does not occur. Of the common laboratory animal species, only the guinea pig, rabbit, and nonhuman primate had detectable serum levels of GGT; cats, dogs, rats, and mice do not. Guinea pig serum GGT levels are approximately one-sixth of those reported for nonhuman primates, and the release may be associated with blood clotting. The source of both elevated GGT and lactate dehydrogenase in blood clot formation must be considered when evaluating these analytes in guinea pigs. The lymphocytes and granulocytes of guinea pigs and man have alkaline phosphatase (ALP) activity (Sisk, 1976).

8.3.2 Urine Collection

Guinea pig urine is typically yellow to orange in color, with the color dependent on the dietary phytocompounds (as observed in rabbits). Care should be taken not to confuse darker urine caused by these dietary phytocompounds with hematuria. Like other herbivores, the urine pH is normally more alkaline, frequently 8.0–9.0. Crystaluria is uncommon and if found warrants further investigation for urinary calculi.

Urinalysis provides a powerful adjunct to clinical chemistry and other diagnostic modalities in guinea pigs. Urine collection techniques parallel those used in other species and include free catch, ventral midline cystocentesis (25-gauge needle), metabolic caging, or a simple, clean, empty cage (Hrapkiewicz et al., 1998; Riggs, 2009; Fisher, 2006). Clearly, the cleaner the sample, the more profound and robust the urinalysis results, especially when bacterial culture is needed in cases of suspected urinary tract infections. Cystocentesis may be facilitated with sedation and ultrasound. At least 4–6 mL of urine is required for urinalysis; with urinalysis results varying depending on factors such as sex, age, stock/strain, and so on.

8.4 PREANALYTICAL SOURCES OF VARIATION

8.4.1 Anesthesia

Anesthesia can be a confounding factor in the interpretation of clinical chemistry analyses of most species including the guinea pig. Inhalant anesthetics are widely used with laboratory animal species. While rarely used now, a large number of publications have demonstrated the hepatotoxic effects of halothane anesthesia (Lind et al., 1987, 1992) including elevated isocitrate dehydrogenase (Lunam et al., 1985). This hepatoxicity appears to be due to cell-mediated immune mechanisms (Furst et al., 1997). Lunam et al. (1986) identified a genetic predisposition for liver damage (serum alanine aminotransferase, ALT) in guinea pigs but did not exclude the possibility that other factors may be involved. Lunam et al. (1985, 1986, 1989) described a variable percentage of animals affected (~20%–50%), provided a description of the histopathology observed, and compared this with human halothane hepatopathology. Bourdi et al. (2001) linked outbred (Hartley) guinea pig hepatotoxicity to an enhanced hepatic halothane metabolism which formed relatively high levels of trifluoroacetylated protein adducts; cytochrome P450 proteins may have a role in catalyzing the formation of these proteins. Durak et al. (1999) evaluated blood urea nitrogen (BUN) and creatinine levels in animals following exposure with 2% isoflurane (in oxygen) and found no significant alterations over the course of the study. Zheng et al. (2001) evaluated the effects of sevoflurane and its degradation product, fluoromethyl-2,2-difluoro-1-(trifluoromethyl)vinyl ether (Compound A), in guinea pigs and found no significant alteration in BUN, ALT, or creatinine after a 4-hour exposure but did note a humoral immune response by 14 days postexposure.

Injectable anesthetic agents can pose similar concerns. Dang et al. (2008) compared five anesthetic regimens and evaluated blood collected from the anterior vena cava of Hartley guinea pigs. Although complete blood count values did not differ between the regimens, serum clinical chemistry values did; specifically glucose, BUN, phosphorus, and creatine phosphokinase varied between anesthetic regimens. The authors concluded that intraperitoneal ketamine–xylazine was preferred for vena cava blood collection. D'Alleinne and Mann (1982) determined that ketamine–xylazine anesthesia might impact toxicologic parameters. They observed elevations in BUN, creatinine, and ALT for up to 5 days following anesthesia; however, these elevations were not significant. Kim et al. (2006) determined that the reversible cardiac depression seen with ketamine was due to increases of intracellular ionized magnesium concentration and total magnesium efflux.

Etomidate is a safe, short-acting, nonbarbiturate anesthetic agent used for anesthetic induction or constant rate infusion maintenance. Etomidate does not provide adequate analgesia, and guinea pigs had the lowest ED_{50} of any species studied (Wauquier, 1983; Calvo et al., 1979; Janssen et al., 1975). Use of etomidate is associated with cortisol depletion (Addison's disease), and Boidin et al. (1986) suggested a role for cytochrome P450 and ascorbic acid (vitamin C). Lambert et al. (1983, 1984, 1985, 1986) evaluated various compounds, including etomidate, *in vitro* with respect to biopotency and sites of action of compounds affecting adrenal steroidogenesis. Lambert's group determined etomidate was the most potent of the 12 compounds studied, which included propofol and thiopentone. Etomidate's site of action was the enzyme 11β-hydroxylase (as is thiopentone's) and propofol acts between adrenocorticotrophin (ACTH) binding and pregnenolone production.

Brown et al. (1989) recently compared blood gas values between resting nonanesthetized guinea pigs and those anesthetized for 30 minutes using various anesthetics. The animals were not intubated but allowed to breathe room air unassisted. As expected, animals became hypercapneic and hypoxic; the effect was slight with ketamine/xylazine anesthesia and pronounced with diazepam/alphaxalone–alphadolone anesthesia. Anesthesia with pentobarbital/fentanyl–droperidol or diazepam/fentanyl resulted in an intermediate degree of respiratory depression.

8.4.2 Age

Age-related changes in clinical chemistry endpoints have been demonstrated. For example, serum ALP levels in the guinea pig have been shown to decrease with increasing body weight and age during the first year of life, similar to the decrease with maturation in other species (Kitagaki et al., 2005).

Also similar to other species, total protein continues to rise in guinea pigs until it reaches its adult value by 200 days of age; followed by a long steady decline (Kitagaki et al., 2005). In addition, triglyceride levels display a long steady rise between 200 and 800 days of age in guinea pigs (Kitagaki et al., 2005).

Serum cholesterol, BUN, and creatinine levels in guinea pigs demonstrated a rapid increase to ~150 days of age followed by a slow but progressive increase in Weiser–Maples guinea pigs (Kitagaki et al., 2005). Chloride levels decrease briskly over the life of female Weiser–Maples guinea pigs, and sodium levels trend toward a slight increase over the life of male Weiser–Maples guinea pigs (Kitagaki et al., 2005).

Malinowska and Nathanielsz (1974) evaluated plasma aldosterone in neonatal and adult guinea pigs via radioimmunoassay. Neonates (between 6 and 24 hours of age) had peak aldosterone values of 552 pg/mL compared to adult male levels of 72 pg/mL (when collected by cardiocentesis). Interestingly, peak aldosterone levels in adult males were found to be 126 pg/mL when collected via an indwelling arterial catheter. There was no relationship found between aldosterone and glucocorticoid levels in either the adults or neonates.

Rigaudiere et al. (1976) determined testosterone and androstenedione in the plasma and testes of Dunkin–Hartley guinea pigs via gas chromatography in animals that ranged from newborns to animals who were 35 months of age. The authors identified four periods of androgenic activity over this wide temporal range of animal life span:

1. Neonatal period from birth to postnatal day (PND) 16
2. Pubertal period from PND 16 to PND 90
3. Adulthood from 3 to 6 months of age through 24 months of age
4. Senescence between 24 and 28 months of age

The peak testosterone concentration associated with the neonatal period occurs at days 2 and 3 of age and as described in Section 8.2.4, readers are reminded that testosterone is a potent pituitary–adrenocortical inhibitor. Pelardy and Delost (1977, 1978) also observed a transient neonatal testosterone peak and determined light, in addition to testes, played a role in the testosterone peak's occurrence.

8.4.3 Strain

Waner et al. (1996) compared the clinical chemistry values of euthymic, normal (haired), and hairless Dunkin–Hartley guinea pigs and demonstrated significant differences in many serum chemistry analytes (Table 8.2).

Kunzl and Sachser (1999) have prepared a review comparing hormonal (cortisol and testosterone) and behavioral differences between the domestic and wild guinea pig.

It is interesting to note that the wild Andean guinea pig hemoglobin oxygen affinity is greater than that observed in either laboratory guinea pigs or rats, yet comparable to the Andean chinchilla, *Chinchilla brevicaudata* (Winslow, 2007; Ostojic et al., 2002).

8.4.4 Diet or Nutritional Status

Dietary constituents and/or the nutritional status of the animal can have notable effects on clinical chemistry parameters in guinea pigs.

TABLE 8.2
Serum Chemistry Differences in Euthymic Hairless Compared to Normal (Haired) Dunkin–Hartley Guinea Pigs[a]

Analyte	Significant Changes, Increase or Decrease, in Euthymic Hairless vs. Normal (Reported Means)
Alanine aminotransferase (ALT)	↑ (90 vs. 37 IU/L)
Albumin	↑ (3.6 vs. 2.9 g/dL)
Alkaline phosphatase (ALP)	↓ (342 vs. 45 IU/L)
Amylaset	↑ (2,257 vs. 1,117 IU/L)
Asparate aminotransferase (AST)	↑ (83 vs. 183 IU/L)
Blood urea nitrogen (BUN)	↑ (103 vs. 56 mg/dL)
Calcium	↑ (10.7 vs. 10.3 mg/dL)
Creatine kinase (CK)	↑ (412 vs. 183 IU/L)
Creatinine	↑ (0.7 vs. 0.5 mg/dL)
Magnesium	↑ (4.9 vs. 3.8 mg/dL)
Phosphorous	↑ (10.8 vs. 7.1 mg/dL)
Potassium	↑ (6.2 vs. 4.0 mEq/dL)
Sodium	↓ (131.5 vs. 134.2 mEq/dL)
Total protein (TP)	↑ (5.3 vs. 4.7 g/dL)

Source: Adapted from Waner, T. et al., *Vet Clin Pathol.*, 25, 61–64, 1996.

Mammals generally differ in the way they react to dietary cholesterol. For example, in species such as rats, dogs, nonhuman primates, and humans, diets high in cholesterol (1%–2%) do not cause extensive or rapid expansion of body cholesterol pools, and hypercholesterolemia is uncommon in these species (Chantuin and Ludewig, 1933; Wilson and Lindsey, 1965). This is not the case in the guinea pig, rabbit, and prairie dog (Green et al., 1976; Prior et al., 1961; Wagner, 1976). In the guinea pig, hypercholesterolemia is often accompanied by fatty infiltration of many tissues, including the liver. Further, high dietary cholesterol may induce hemolytic anemia in the guinea pig. This anemia is accompanied by splenic enlargement and bone marrow hyperplasia and may lead to death before atherogenic plaque formation (Ostwald and Shannon, 1964; Yamanaka and Ostwald, 1968; Yamanaka et al., 1967). Dietary protein sources impact serum cholesterol levels. For example, soy-based protein sources lower serum cholesterol in contrast to casein sources (Atwal et al., 1997). Furthermore, amino acid supplementation of casein sources may positively impact serum cholesterol and serum cholesterol fractions.

As mentioned in Section 8.4.2, age-related cholesterol changes observed in Weiser–Maples guinea pigs showed a rapid increase in serum cholesterol to ~150 days of age with a slow but progressive increase when fed a standard guinea pig diet (Kitagaki et al., 2005). Guinea pigs fed a normal diet have little if any high-density lipoprotein (HDL) until they are fed cholesterol. The cholesterol bound to this HDL is predominantly nonesterfied (Yamanaka et al., 1967). In guinea pigs, as in humans, low-density lipoproteins (LDL) are the predominant lipoprotein fraction, and changes in dietary fiber predominately affect LDL (Fernandez et al., 1997). Similarities to humans in both the "normal" lipid profiles and in the response to dietary modifications have led guinea pigs to be proposed as the most appropriate model for human hypercholesterolemia (Sullivan et al., 1993). However, because dietary cholesterol as low as 0.1% may induce biochemical changes and lesions in the guinea pig, dietary consideration should always be taken into account in interpreting serum levels of lipids and lipoproteins in the guinea pig (Ostwald and Shannon, 1964; Yamanaka et al., 1967).

Guinea pigs are one of a few species that have lost the capability to synthesize Vitamin C (ascorbic acid) and must obtain daily requirements via the diet (Drouin et al., 2011). Conflicting results have been obtained in guinea pigs on the effect of ascorbic acid on serum ALP activity. Degkwitz (1982) demonstrated ascorbic acid deficiency did not increase ALP activity in the guinea pig compared to controls. Whereas, Mahmoodian et al. (1996) demonstrated an 80%–90% decrease in serum ALP activity in scorbutic guinea pigs, specifically due to a loss of bone ALP activity. Fasting and inanition have also been shown to decrease ALP activity (Tsuchiya and Bates, 1994).

Similar conflicting effects on ALP activity have been demonstrated in studies in which guinea pigs were fed diets either deficient in magnesium or zinc. Everson et al. (1959) found no differences in ALP activity in guinea pigs fed a manganese-deficient diet compared to control diet. Everson et al. (1959) also found no differences in ALP activity in preweanling guinea pigs whose dams were fed a magnesium-deficient or control diet, a finding also observed in developing rats (Hurley et al., 1959). In contract, ALP activity dramatically increased in guinea pigs fed either zinc-deficient (<20 ppm) or magnesium-deficient diets (Alberts et al., 1977; Underwood, 1971).

8.4.5 Stress

Glucocorticoids are essential for normal neural development. Since guinea pigs give birth to young with advanced neural development and a large proportion of neuroendocrine maturation occurring in utero (similar to humans, and, compared to rats or mice, which have significant postnatal neural development), they have been used in studies examining the effects of glucocorticoids (i.e., stress-related) on hypothalamo–pituitary–adrenal function in prenatal manipulations (Kapoor et al., 2006). Kapoor and Matthews (2005) reported that maternal, gestational stress (and cortisol secretion) impacts male guinea pig testosterone levels (and behavior). Moderate maternal stress (2 hours over 3 days at gestational day 50 and day 60) results in increased basal cortisol level in male offspring and decreased testosterone levels. Kapoor and Matthews (2008) evaluated moderate maternal stress (2 hours over 3 days at gestational day 50 and day 60) in female offspring following prenatal stress exposure. Timing of the gestational, maternal stress exposure, as in males, varied according to when the stress occurred during gestation and elicited a sex bias. Cortisol measurements in this study were salivary cortisol levels versus plasma levels in the Kapoor and Matthews (2005) study. There was no prenatal stress effect regarding basal cortisol levels or an effect related to the reproductive cycle stage. Females exposed at gestational day 50 and 60 had lower salivary cortisol stressor responses during estrous. Gestational day 60 stress-exposed female offspring had lower estradiol levels during the luteal and diminished ovarian weight. Females, as in males, lacked a diurnal cortisol response. In another study, juvenile guinea pigs (both male and female) born to dams exposed to an "adverse event" every other day through the second half of gestation (chronic maternal stress) had elevated basal salivary cortisol levels at PND 25 (Emack et al., 2008).

Sachser and Lick (1989), Sachser and Kaiser (1996), and Kaiser and Sachser (1998) evaluated social stress in guinea pigs and the impact on hormonal activities and animal behavior. Sachser and Lick (1996) determined confrontational stress resulted in extremely high plasma glucocorticoids, creatinine, urea nitrogen, and decreased testosterone in confrontational losers, whereas the confrontational winners did not differ from control animals. Sachser and Kaiser (1996) determined gestational social stress (unstable social environment) masculinized female offspring characterized by male-typical courtship and play behavior, whereas social stress during lactation did not alter behavior. Kaiser and Sachser (1998) determined social instability impacted behavior and hormonal levels. Male-like behavior was once again observed in female offspring exposed to gestational environmental instability with corresponding higher serum testosterone levels and bilateral adrenal tyrosine hydroxylase activity.

8.4.6 Sex

Sexual dimorphism in the plasma cortisol levels of the guinea pig have been observed after 30 days of age, with males having higher levels than females. These differences are related to differences in metabolism and binding of cortisol by transcortin (El Hani et al., 1980). In guinea pigs between 90 and 120 days of age, basal and stress plasma cortisol levels are the same for both sexes, but sexual dimorphism reappears in adult guinea pigs. These changes seem to correspond to changes in testosterone levels.

8.4.7 Disease

Shapiro (1993) demonstrated in a chronic renal failure model (one- and two-thirds nephrectomy) that guinea pigs develop abnormal LDL catabolism, related not only to clearance mechanisms, but also suggested functional LDL differences develop in the uremic guinea pigs.

In evaluating a series of serum cytokines using the Hartley guinea pig model of osteoarthritis, the serum level of 18 cytokines was evaluated. Cytokine levels were evaluated for correlation with histopathologic findings. For this condition, it was determined that IL-6 and G-CSF correlated most closely with the histopathologic findings (Huebner et al., 2007).

Collins (2008) indicated ovarian cysts are the most common form of endocrine disease encountered in guinea pigs; cysts (5–7 mm in diameter) are observed in >75% of cavies between 1.5 and 5 years of age. These cysts are frequently bilateral and if functional result in secreting estrogen or progesterone and a bilaterally symmetrical nonpruritic flank to lumbosacral alopecia.

New Zealand guinea pigs exposed to toxic oil (canola oil) experienced elevated urinary protein excretion, creatinine clearance, and urine creatinine concentration compared with control animals over a 28-day period of exposure (Sanchez-Bernal et al., 1993).

Bret et al. (1993) evaluated kidney tubule enzymes in urine sequentially in a mercuric chloride nephrotoxicity model in guinea pigs. Urine was collected in metabolic chambers, centrifuged, and analysis executed on the supernatant. GGT and ALP were released first, indicative of cell membrane/brush border damage. Lactate dehydrogenase emergence is later indicating cellular disruption. Lastly, DNA detection is evidence of cell death resulting from tubule cell necrosis.

Although urolithiasis is rare in guinea pigs, Okewole et al. (1991) described calcium oxalate urolithiasis associated with an outbreak of *Streptococcus pyogenes*. Other reports of urolithiasis in the literature include Sprink (1978) and Stuppy et al. (1979). Holowaychuk (2006) offered a case report where a guinea pig had ingested oxalate-containing plants and was presented for renal failure; however, oxalate crystals were not found in the urine. When the animal was ultimately euthanized the owners declined a diagnostic necropsy.

8.5 METHODOLOGY FOR COMMON PROCEDURES

8.5.1 Adrenocorticotrophin Stimulation Test

Kapoor and Matthews (2005) and Liu and Matthews (1999) described an Adrenocorticotrophin (ACTH) stimulation test in guinea pigs in which carotid artery catheters were surgically placed and maintained for 3 days after surgery before initiating the ACTH stimulation test. ACTH was administered intra-arterially (2 μg/kg) to male guinea pigs at 1300 hours and blood samples (plasma) collected for cortisol measurements at –30, 0, 30, 60, and 120 minutes. The –30 and 0 time samples were averaged to determine a baseline cortisol level.

Bauer et al. (2008) described an ACTH stimulation test which measured fecal cortisol levels. Guinea pigs were injected subcutaneously with 20 IU Synacthen® depot at 1200 hours. Fecal samples were collected every 2 hours during the first 24 hours, every 6 hours during the subsequent 24 hours, and every 12 hours during the third 24-hour period. Peak cortisol metabolite levels occur ~18 hours following ACTH administration and are dependent on gastrointestinal transit time. Over the 20-hour gastrointestinal transit time, it is believed the peaks and valleys seen with blood adrenocortical activity are blunted.

8.5.2 Corticotrophin Releasing Hormone Stimulation Test

Liu and Matthews (1999) described a corticotrophin releasing hormone (CRH) stimulation test using surgically catheterized (carotid artery and jugular vein), adult, female guinea pigs. Animals were administered human CRH via the jugular vein catheter at 0.2 and 2.0 µg/kg between 1300 and 1400 hours and blood samples (plasma) were collected via the carotid artery catheter at –30, –10, 0, 5, 15, 30, 60, 90, and 120 minutes for both serum ACTH and cortisol measurements via radioimmunoassay. Peak serum levels were observed at 30 (ACTH) and 60 (cortisol) minutes post-CRH.

8.5.3 Oral Glucose Tolerance Test

Banerjee and Ghosh (1946) described a technique for the oral glucose tolerance test (OGTT) where after an overnight fast, a (fasting) blood glucose level is obtained and animals are fed 200 mg of glucose per 100 g of body weight of a 50% solution. Blood samples are then taken (45-minute intervals for 280 minutes) for glucose determination. Everson and Shrader's (1968) technique varied slightly in that it is specified the animals are fasted for 20 hours and animals were given the glucose in a 20% solution, fed by a dropper and consumed over 2 minutes. Animals were subsequently anesthetized with pentobarbital and sampled at 30 minutes, 1, 2, 3, and 4 hours.

8.5.4 Intravenous Glucose Tolerance Test

Everson and Shrader (1968) described an intravenous glucose tolerance test (IVGTT) in the guinea pig using a surgical aortic cannula placement via the carotid artery for serial blood collection. Following 5–10 days recovery (based on the animal's return to normal body weight), animals were fasted 18 hours and a (fasting) blood sample was collected. Over 3 minutes, animals were administered 100 mg per 100 g of body weight of a sterile 40% glucose solution in physiologic saline. Samples were obtained from unrestrained animals at 15, 30, and 45 minutes and 1, 2, 3, and 4 hours, and serum glucose measured.

Kind et al. (2003) described a similar IVGTT whereby jugular vein and carotid artery catheters were placed and approximately 11 days later animal were fasted for 16 hours and 50% dextrose solution (diluted in 0.9% saline) was administered via the jugular catheter (over a 2-minute period) at 500-mg dextrose/kg body weight in a total volume of 2.5 mL followed by 2 mL of 0.9% saline. Plasma was collected for glucose measurements via carotid artery at 2, 5, 10, 20, 30, 40, 60, 80, 120, 150, 180, and 210 minutes.

8.6 CLINICAL CHEMISTRY REFERENCE RANGES FOR THE GUINEA PIG

Data for clinical chemistry serum reference ranges for several guinea pig strains and urine analytes in the guinea pig are shown in Tables 8.3 and 8.4, respectively.

TABLE 8.3
Clinical Chemistry Serum Reference Ranges for Several Guinea Pig Strains

Analyte	Units	Stock/Strain	Sex	Weight (g)	*N*	Age (weeks)	Fed/Fasted	Mean	SD	Reference
Albumin	g/L	Hartley	F	500–800	95	–	–	24.2	1.4	Loeb and Quimby (1999), Mitruka and Rawnsley (1981)
		Hartley	M	500–800	110	–	–	27.3	3.0	Loeb and Quimby (1999), Mitruka and Rawnsley (1981)
		Dunkin-Hartley	M/F	–	10	3	–	16	–	Loeb and Quimby (1999), Caisey and King (1980)
		Dunkin–Hartley Hairless	M	520–546	12	8	–	35.6	1.4	Waner et al. (1996)
		Dunkin–Hartley	M	520–546	10	8	–	28.7	1.4	Waner et al. (1996)
		–	M	150–200	–	–	–	32.9	1.57	Guler et al. (2007)
ALP	IU/L	Hartley	F	500–800	95	–	–	65.80	5.46	Loeb and Quimby (1999), Mitruka and Rawnsley (1981)
		Hartley	M	500–800	110	–	–	74.20	6.92	Loeb and Quimby (1999), Mitruka and Rawnsley (1981)
		Hartley	–	–	10	3	–	876	—	Loeb and Quimby (1999), Caisey and King (1980)
		Dunkin–Hartley Hairless	M	520–546	12	8	–	342	45	Waner et al. (1996)
		Dunkin–Hartley	M	520–546	10	8	–	455	67	Waner et al. (1996)
		–	M	150–200	–	–	–	143.02	24.41	Guler et al. (2007)
ALT	IU/L	Hartley	F	500–800	95	–	–	38.80	7.15	Loeb and Quimby (1999), Mitruka and Rawnsley (1981)
		Hartley	M	500–800	110	–	–	44.60	6.75	Loeb and Quimby (1999), Mitruka and Rawnsley (1981)
		Hartley	–	–	10	3	–	47	—	Loeb and Quimby (1999), Caisey and King (1980)
		Dunkin–Hartley Hairless	M	520–546	12	8	–	90	23	Waner et al. (1996)
		Dunkin–Hartley	M	520–546	10	8	–	37	11	Waner et al. (1996)
		–	M	150–200			–	38.11	4.20	Guler et al. (2007)
Amylase	IU/L	Dunkin–Hartley Hairless	M	520–546	12	8	–	2,257	407	Waner et al. (1996)
		Dunkin–Hartley	M	520–546	10	8	–	1,117	122	Waner et al. (1996)

(Continued)

TABLE 8.3 (*Continued*)
Clinical Chemistry Serum Reference Ranges for Several Guinea Pig Strains

Analyte	Units	Stock/Strain	Sex	Weight (g)	*N*	Age (weeks)	Fed/Fasted	Mean	SD	Reference
AST	IU/L	Hartley	F	500–800	95	–	–	45.50	7.00	Loeb and Quimby (1999), Mitruka and Rawnsley (1981)
		Hartley	M	500–800	110	–	–	48.20	9.50	Loeb and Quimby (1999), Mitruka and Rawnsley (1981)
		Hartley	–	–	10	3	–	45	—	Loeb and Quimby (1999), Caisey and King (1980)
		Dunkin–Hartley Hairless	M	520–546	12	8	–	83	35	Waner et al. (1996)
		Dunkin–Hartley	M	520–546	10	8	–	183	5	Waner et al. (1996)
Bicarbonate	mmol/L		–	–	12	–	–	22.10	1.90	Loeb and Quimby (1999), Barzago et al. (1994)
		–	–	–	6	–	–	22.00	1.80	Loeb and Quimby (1999), Bar-Ilan and Marder (1980)
		–	–	–	69	–	–	24.40	2.80	Loeb and Quimby (1999), Brown et al. (1989)
Bilirubin	μmol/L	Hartley	F	500–800	–	–	–	5.47	1.20	Loeb and Quimby (1999), Mitruka and Rawnsley (1981)
		Hartley	M	500–800	–	–	–	5.13	1.368	Loeb and Quimby (1999), Mitruka and Rawnsley (1981)
		Dunkin–Hartley Hairless	M	520–546	12	8	–	1.20	0.17	Waner et al. (1996)
		Dunkin–Hartley	M	520–546	10	8	–	1.37	0.51	Waner et al. (1996)
BUN	mmol/L	Hartley	F	500–800	95	–	–	7.68	2.08	Loeb and Quimby (1999), Mitruka and Rawnsley (1981)
		Hartley	M	500–800	110	–	–	9	2.27	Loeb and Quimby (1999), Mitruka and Rawnsley (1981)
		Pigmented		350–500	7	–	–	5.14	0.50	Loeb and Quimby (1999), Song et al. (1997)
		Dunkin–Hartley Hairless	M	520–546	12	8	–	36.7	8.70	Waner et al. (1996)
		Dunkin–Hartley	M	520–546	10	8	–	20.0	2.30	Waner et al. (1996)
		–	M	150–200	–	–	–	6.29	1.66	Guler et al. (2007)

(*Continued*)

TABLE 8.3 (*Continued*)
Clinical Chemistry Serum Reference Ranges for Several Guinea Pig Strains

Analyte	Units	Stock/Strain	Sex	Weight (g)	*N*	Age (weeks)	Fed/Fasted	Mean	SD	Reference
Calcium	mmol/L	Hartley	F	500–800	95	–	–	2.67	0.15	Loeb and Quimby (1999), Mitruka and Rawnsley (1981)
		Hartley	M	500–800	110	–	–	2.40	0.16	Loeb and Quimby (1999), Mitruka and Rawnsley (1981)
		Hartley	F	–	10	3	–	2.66	—	Loeb and Quimby (1999), Caisey and King (1980)
		Dunkin–Hartley Hairless	M	520–546	12	8	–	2.68	0.11	Waner et al. (1996)
		Dunkin–Hartley	M	520–546	10	8	–	2.58	0.08	Waner et al. (1996)
Chloride	mmol/L	Hartley	F	500–800	95	–	–	96.50	1.19	Loeb and Quimby (1999), Mitruka and Rawnsley (1981)
		Hartley	M	500–800	110	–	–	92.30	1.04	Loeb and Quimby (1999), Mitruka and Rawnsley (1981)
		Hartley	–	–	10	3	–	105	—	Loeb and Quimby (1999), Caisey and King (1980)
Cholesterol	mmol/L	Hartley	F	500–800	95	–	–	0.69	0.29	Loeb and Quimby (1999), Mitruka and Rawnsley (1981)
		Hartley	M	500–800	110	–	–	0.83	0.27	Loeb and Quimby (1999), Mitruka and Rawnsley (1981)
		Dunkin-Hartley	M/F	–	10	3	–	0.59	—	Loeb and Quimby (1999), Caisey and King (1980)
		Hartley	F	653	7	–	–	1.06	0.18	Loeb and Quimby (1999), Arbeeny et al. (1989)
		Hartley	M	900	10	–	–	1.01	0.26	Loeb and Quimby (1999), Arbeeny et al. (1989)
		Hartley	F	–	12	–	Fasted	1.32	0.31	Loeb and Quimby (1999), Sullivan et al. (1993)
		Hartley	F	–	4	–	Fed	0.80	0.10	Loeb and Quimby (1999), Sullivan et al. (1993)
		Dunkin–Hartley Hairless	M	520–546	12	8	–	0.87	0.31	Waner et al. (1996)

(*Continued*)

TABLE 8.3 (*Continued*)
Clinical Chemistry Serum Reference Ranges for Several Guinea Pig Strains

Analyte	Units	Stock/Strain	Sex	Weight (g)	*N*	Age (weeks)	Fed/Fasted	Mean	SD	Reference
		Dunkin–Hartley	M	520–546	10	8	–	0.96	0.32	Waner et al. (1996)
		–	M	150–200		–	–	3.81	0.69	Guler et al. (2007)
CK	IU/L	Hartley	F	500–800	95	–	–	110	20	Loeb and Quimby (1999), Mitruka and Rawnsley (1981)
		Hartley	M	500–800	110	–	–	95	15	Loeb and Quimby (1999), Mitruka and Rawnsley (1981)
		Dunkin-Hartley	M/F	–	10	3	–	176	—	Loeb and Quimby (1999), Caisey and King (1980)
		Dunkin–Hartley Hairless	M	520–546	12	8	–	412	200	Waner et al. (1996)
		Dunkin–Hartley	M	520–546	10	8	–	183	50	Waner et al. (1996)
Creatinine	mmol/L	Hartley	F	500–800	95	–	–	123.94	30.94	Loeb and Quimby (1999), Mitruka and Rawnsley (1981)
		Hartley	M	500–800	110	–	–	121.99	34.48	Loeb and Quimby (1999), Mitruka and Rawnsley (1981)
		Pigmented	–	350–500	7	–	–	26.52	—	Loeb and Quimby (1999), Song et al. (1997)
		Dunkin–Hartley Hairless	M	520–546	12	8	–	58.3	7.10	Waner et al. (1996)
		Dunkin–Hartley	M	520–546	10	8	–	44.2	4.42	Waner et al. (1996)
GGT	IU/L	Hartley	–	–	10	3	–	10	—	Loeb and Quimby (1999), Caisey and King (1980)
		Dunkin–Hartley Hairless	M	520–546	12	8	–	11.28	4.68	Waner et al. (1996)
		Dunkin–Hartley	M	520–546	10	8	–	13.50	3.40	Waner et al. (1996)
		–	M	150–200	–	–	–	16.285	5.741	Guler et al. (2007)
Globulin	g/L	Dunkin–Hartley Hairless	M	520–546	12	8	–	17.1	1.6	Waner et al. (1996)
		Dunkin–Hartley	M	520–546	10	8	–	18.1	1.8	Waner et al. (1996)
Glucose	mmol/L	Hartley	F	500–800	95	–	–	4.94	0.53	Loeb and Quimby (1999), Mitruka and Rawnsley (1981)

(*Continued*)

TABLE 8.3 (*Continued*)
Clinical Chemistry Serum Reference Ranges for Several Guinea Pig Strains

Analyte	Units	Stock/Strain	Sex	Weight (g)	*N*	Age (weeks)	Fed/Fasted	Mean	SD	Reference
		Hartley	M	500–800	110	–	–	5.19	0.66	Loeb and Quimby (1999), Mitruka and Rawnsley (1981)
		Hartley	F	653	8	–	–	7.77	1.55	Loeb and Quimby (1999), Arbeeny et al. (1989)
		Hartley	M	900	7	–	–	8.16	0.78	Loeb and Quimby (1999), Arbeeny et al. (1989)
		–	M	150–200	–	–	–	10.60	3.50	Guler et al. (2007)
HDL	mmol/L	–	M	150–200	–	–	–	1.45	0.37	Guler et al. (2007)
Iron	mmol/L	Dunkin–Hartley	–	–	10	3	–	55.30	—	Loeb and Quimby (1999), Caisey and King (1980)
LDH	IU/L	Hartley	F	500–800	95	–	–	52.1	11.2	Loeb and Quimby (1999), Mitruka and Rawnsley (1981)
		Hartley	M	500–800	110	–	–	46.9	9.5	Loeb and Quimby (1999), Mitruka and Rawnsley (1981)
		Hartley	–	–	10	3	–	103	—	Loeb and Quimby (1999), Caisey and King (1980)
		Dunkin–Hartley Hairless	M	520–546	12	8	–	97	48	Waner et al. (1996)
		Dunkin–Hartley	M	520–546	10	8	–	132	85	Waner et al. (1996)
		–	M	150–200	–	–	–	170.01	42.61	Guler et al. (2007)
LDL	mmol/L		M	150–200		–	–	2.14	0.41	Guler et al. (2007)
Magnesium	mmol/L	Hartley	F	500–800	95	–	–	1.01	0.11	Loeb and Quimby (1999), Mitruka and Rawnsley (1981)
		Hartley	M	500–800	110	–	–	0.97	0.10	Loeb and Quimby (1999), Mitruka and Rawnsley (1981)
		Dunkin–Hartley Hairless	M	520–546	12	8	–	2.02	0.12	Waner et al. (1996)
		Dunkin–Hartley	M	520–546	10	8	–	1.55	0.13	Waner et al. (1996)
Phosphorus, inorganic	mmol/L	Hartley	F	500–800	95	–	–	1.71	0.36	Loeb and Quimby (1999), Mitruka and Rawnsley (1981)

(*Continued*)

TABLE 8.3 (*Continued*)
Clinical Chemistry Serum Reference Ranges for Several Guinea Pig Strains

Analyte	Units	Stock/Strain	Sex	Weight (g)	*N*	Age (weeks)	Fed/Fasted	Mean	SD	Reference
		Hartley	M	500–800	110	–	–	1.71	0.37	Loeb and Quimby (1999), Mitruka and Rawnsley (1981)
		Dunkin–Hartley	–	–	10	3	–	2.36	—	Loeb and Quimby (1999), Caisey and King (1980)
		Dunkin–Hartley Hairless	M	520–546	12	8	–	3.50	0.40	Waner et al. (1996)
		Dunkin–Hartley	M	520–546	10	8	–	2.29	0.16	Waner et al. (1996)
Potassium	mmol/L	Hartley	F	500–800	95	–	–	5.06	0.93	Loeb and Quimby (1999), Mitruka and Rawnsley (1981)
		Hartley	M	500–800	110	–	–	4.87	0.80	Loeb and Quimby (1999), Mitruka and Rawnsley (1981)
		Hartley	–	–	10	3	–	5.50	—	Loeb and Quimby (1999), Caisey and King (1980)
		Dunkin–Hartley Hairless	M	520–546	12	8	–	6.24	1.28	Waner et al. (1996)
		Dunkin–Hartley	M	520–546	10	8	–	4.03	0.43	Waner et al. (1996)
Protein	g/L	Hartley	F	500–800	95	–	–	48	3.4	Loeb and Quimby (1999), Mitruka and Rawnsley (1981)
		Hartley	M	500–800	110	–	–	56	2.8	Loeb and Quimby (1999), Mitruka and Rawnsley (1981)
		Dunkin-Hartley	M/F		10	3	–	46	—	Loeb and Quimby (1999), Caisey and King (1980)
		Dunkin–Hartley Hairless	M	520–546	12	8	–	52.7	2.8	Waner et al. (1996)
		Dunkin–Hartley	M	520–546	10	8	–	46.8	2.2	Waner et al. (1996)
		–	M	150–200	–	–	–	51.3	3.64	Guler et al. (2007)
TIBC	mmol/L	Dunkin–Hartley		–	10	3	–	58.39	—	Loeb and Quimby (1999), Caisey and King (1980)
OCT	IU/L	–	F	262–333	40	–	–	6.9	4.9	Arp and Richard (1981)
SDH	IU/L	–	F	262–333	40	–	–	95.7	22.5	Arp and Richard (1981)
		–	M	350–400	6	–	–	20.09[a]	7.97	Sharma et al. (1982)

(*Continued*)

TABLE 8.3 (*Continued*)
Clinical Chemistry Serum Reference Ranges for Several Guinea Pig Strains

Analyte	Units	Stock/Strain	Sex	Weight (g)	*N*	Age (weeks)	Fed/Fasted	Mean	SD	Reference
Sodium	mmol/L	Hartley	F	500–800	95	–	–	125	0.96	Loeb and Quimby (1999), Mitruka and Rawnsley (1981)
		Hartley	M	500–800	110	–	–	122	0.98	Loeb and Quimby (1999), Mitruka and Rawnsley (1981)
		Hartley	–	–	10	3	–	136	—	Loeb and Quimby (1999), Caisey and King (1980)
		Dunkin–Hartley Hairless	M	520–546	12	8	–	131.50	1.60	Waner et al. (1996)
		Dunkin–Hartley	M	520–546	10	8	–	134.20	1.00	Waner et al. (1996)
Total iron binding capacity (TIBC)	mmol/L	Dunkin–Hartley	–	–	10	3	–	58.39	—	Loeb and Quimby (1999), Caisey and King (1980)
Triglycerides	mmol/L	Hartley	F	653	8	–	–	0.49	0.30	Loeb and Quimby (1999), Arbeeny et al. (1989)
		Hartley	M	900	7	–	–	0.68	0.18	Loeb and Quimby (1999), Arbeeny et al. (1989)
		Hartley	F	360	5	–	Fasted	0.69	0.15	Loeb and Quimby (1999), Sullivan et al. (1993)
		Hartley	F	360	5	–	Fed	0.35	0.05	Loeb and Quimby (1999), Sullivan et al. (1993)
		Dunkin–Hartley Hairless	M	520–546	12	8	–	0.64	0.14	Waner et al. (1996)
		Dunkin–Hartley	M	520–546	10	8	–	0.67	0.21	Waner et al. (1996)
		–	M	150–200			–	1.01	0.33	Guler et al. (2007)
Uric acid	µmol/L	Dunkin–Hartley Hairless	M	520–546	12	8	–	55.32	13.68	Waner et al. (1996)
		Dunkin–Hartley	M	520–546	10	8	–	48.18	11.9	Waner et al. (1996)
		–	M	150–200	–	–	–	333.68	33.84	Guler et al. (2007)
VLDL	mmol/L	–	M	150–200	–	–	–	0.40	0.15	Guler et al. (2007)

[a] ×102 Sigma Units/L.

TABLE 8.4
Urine Analytes in the Guinea Pig

Analyte	Results	Reference
Urinary volume	63 ± 8	Duan et al. (1996) and Huerkamp et al. (1996)
Color	Yellow (reddish)	Kraft and Dürr (2005)
Turbidity	Clear-slightly turbid	Kraft and Dürr (2005)
Odor	n.s.	Kraft and Dürr (2005)
Blood	Negative	Kraft and Dürr (2005)
Urobilinogen	Neg-weak positive	Kraft and Dürr (2005)
Bilirubin	Negative	Kraft and Dürr (2005)
Protein	Negative	Kraft and Dürr (2005)
Nitrite	Negative	Kraft and Dürr (2005)
Ketone	Negative	Kraft and Dürr (2005)
Glucose	Negative	Kraft and Dürr (2005)
pH	8.0–9.0	Kraft and Dürr (2005)
Specific gravity	1.000–1.040	Kraft and Dürr (2005)
Leukocytes	Negative	Kraft and Dürr (2005)

ACKNOWLEDGMENTS

I wish to thank Dr. Charles B. Clifford and Dr. William J. White, the previous authors of this chapter, for their vision and contributions to this chapter.

REFERENCES

Adkins, R.M., Vandeberg, J., and Li, W.H. 2000. Molecular evolution of growth hormone and receptor in the guinea-pig, a mammal unresponsive to growth hormone. *Gene.* 246:357–363.

Alberts, J., Lang, L., Reyes, P., and Griggs, G. 1977. Zinc requirements of the young guinea pig. *J Nutr.* 107:1517–1527.

Arbeeny, C.M., Nordin, C., Edelstein, D., Stram, N., Gibbons, N., and Eder, H.A. 1989. Hyperlipoproteinemia in spontaneously diabetic guinea pigs. *Metabolism.* 38:895–900.

Arp, L.H. and Richard, J.L. 1981. Experimental intoxication of guinea pigs with multiple doses of the mycotoxin, penitrem A. *Mycopathologia.* 73:109–113.

Atwal, A.S., Kubow, S., and Wolynetz, M.S. 1997. Effects of protein source and amino acid supplementation on plasma cholesterol in guinea pigs. *Inter J Vit Nutr Res.* 67:192–195.

Azuma, Y., Tokunaga, T., Takeda, Y., Ogawa, T., and Takagi, N. 1986. The effect of calcium antagonists on the activation of guinea pig neutrophils. *Jpn J Pharmacol.* 42:243–251.

Banerjee, S. and Ghosh, N.C. 1946. Adrenalin in scurvy. *J Biol Chem.* 166:25–29.

Bar-Ilan, A. and Marder, J. 1980. Acid base status in unanesthetized, unrestrained guinea pigs. *Pflugers Arch.* 384:93–97.

Barzago, M.M., Bortolotti, A., Stellari, F.F., Pagani, C., Marraro, G., and Bonati, M. 1994. Respiratory and hemodynamic functions, blood-gas parameters, and acid-base balance of ketamine-xylazine anesthetized guinea pigs. *Lab Anim Sci.* 44:648–650.

Bauer, B., Palme, R., Machatschke, I.H., Dittami, J., and Huber, S. 2008. Non-invasive measurement of adrenocortical and gonadal activity in male and female guinea pigs (Cavia aperea f. porcellus). *Gen Comp Endocrinol.* 156:482–489.

Beintema, J.J. and Campagne, R.N. 1987. Molecular evolution of rodent insulins. *Mol Biol Evol.* 4:10–18.

Blundel, J. and Wood, S. 1975. Is the evolution of insulin Darwinian or due to selectively neutral mutation? *Nature.* 257:198–203.

Boidin, M.P., Erdmann, W.E., and Faithfull, N.S. 1986. The role of ascorbic acid in etomidate toxicity. *Eur J Anesthesiol.* 3:417–422.

Bourdi, M., Amouzadeh, H.R., Rushmore, T.H., Martin, J.L., and Pohl, L.R. 2001. Halothane-induced liver injury in outbred guinea pigs: Role of trifluroacetylated protein adducts in animal susceptibility. *Chem Res Toxicol.* 14:362–370.

Bret, L., Hasim, M., Lefebvre, H., Fournie, G.J., and Braun, J.P. 1993. Kidney tubule enzymes and extracellular DNA in urine as markers for nephrotoxicity in the guinea pig. *Enzyme Protein.* 47:27–36.

Brewer, N.R. and Cruise, L.J. 1994. The guinea pig heart—Some comparative aspects. *Contemp Top Lab Anim Sci.* 33:64–67.

Brewer, N.R. and Cruise, L.J. 1997. The respiratory system of the guinea pig: Emphasis on species differences. *Contemp Top Lab Anim Sci.* 36:100–108.

Brown, J.N., Thorne, P.R., and Nuttall, A.L. 1989. Blood pressure and other physiological responses in awake and anesthetized guinea pigs. *Lab Anim Sci.* 39:142–148.

Caisey, J. and King, D. 1980. Clinical chemical values for some common laboratory animals. *Clin Chem.* 26:1877–1879.

Calvo, R., Carlos, R., and Erill, S. 1979. Etomidate and plasma esterase activity in man and experimental animals. *Pharmacology.* 18:294–298.

Campbell, TW. 2012. Clinical chemistry of mammals; laboratory animals and miscellaneous species. In *Veterinary Hematology and Clinical Chemistry*. Ed. M.A. Thrall, G. Veiser, R. Allison, and T.W. Campbell, pp. 571–581. Ames, IA: John Wiley and Sons.

Chan, S.J., Episkopou, V., Zeitlin, S., et al. 1984. Guinea pig preproinsulin gene: An evolutionary compromise? *Proc Nat Acad Sci US.* 81:5056–5050.

Chantuin, A. and Ludewig, S. 1933. The effects of cholesterol ingestion on the tissue lipids of rats. *J Biol Chem.* 102:57–65.

Clifford, C.B. and White, W.J. 1999. The guinea pig. In *The Clinical Chemistry of Laboratory Animals.* Eds. W.F. Loeb and F.W. Quimby, 2nd edition, pp. 65–70. Philadelphia, PA: Taylor & Francis.

Collins, B.R. 2008. Endocrine diseases of rodents. *Vet Clin North Am Exot Anim Pract.* 11:153–162.

Conboy, G.A. and Stromberg, B.E. 1991. Hematology and clinical pathology of experimental *Fascioloides magna* infection in cattle and guinea pigs. *Vet Parasitol.* 40(3–4):241–255.

Dang, V., Bao, S., Ault, A., et al. 2008. Efficacy and safety of five injectable anesthetic regimens for chronic blood collection from the anterior vena cava of Guinea pigs. *J Am Assoc Lab Anim Sci.* 47:56–60.

D'Alleinne, C.P. and Mann, D.D. 1982. Evaluation of ketamine/xylazine anesthesia in the guinea pig: Toxicological parameters. *Vet Hum Toxicol.* 24:410–412.

de Pablo, F., Lesniak, M.A., Hernandez, E.R. LeRoit, D., Shiloach, J., and Roth, J. 1986. Extracts of protozoa contain materials that react specifically in the immunoassay for guinea pig insulin. *Horm Metab Res.* 18:82–87.

Degkwitz, E. 1982. Activity of alkaline phosphatase in the serum of normal and ascorbic acid-deficient guinea pigs. *Zeitschrift fur Ernahrungswissenschaft.* 21:51–56.

D'Erchia, A.M., Gissi, C., Pesole, G., Saccone, C., and Arnason, U. 1996. The guinea pig is not a rodent. *Nature.* 381:597–600.

Drouin, G., Godin, J-R., and Page, B. 2011. The genetics of vitamin C loss in vertebrates. *Curr Genomics.* 12(5):371–378.

Duan, J., Jaramillo, J., Jung, G.L., McLeod, A.L., and Fernandes, B.H. 1996. A novel renal hypertensive guinea pig model for comparing different inhibitors of the renin-angiotensin system. *J Pharmacol Toxicol Methods.* 35:83–89.

Durak, I., Ozturk, H., Dikmen, B., et al. 1999. Isoflurane impairs antioxidant defense system in guinea pig kidney. *Can J Anesth.* 46:797–802.

Dyer, S.M. and Cervasio, E.L. 2008. An overview of restraint and blood collection techniques in exotic pet practice. *Vet Clin Nor Am Exot Anim Prac.* 11:423–443.

El Hani, A., Dalle, M., and DeLost, P. 1980. Sexual dimorphism in binding and metabolism of cortisol during puberty in guinea pigs. *J Physiol (Paris).* 76:25–28.

Emack, J., Kostaki, A., Walker, C., and Matthews, T. 2008. Chronic maternal stress affects growth, behavior, and hypothalamo-pituitary-adrenal function in juvenile offspring. *Horm Behav.* 54:514–520.

Eremin, O., Wilson, AB., Coombs, R.R.A., Plumb, D., and Ashby, J. 1980. Antibody-dependent cellular cytotoxity in the guinea pig: The role of the Kurloff cells. *Cellular Immunol.* 55:312–327.

Everson, G.J., Hurley, L.S., and Geiger, J.P. 1959. Manganese deficiency in the guinea pig. *J Nutr.* 68:49–56.

Everson, G.J. and Shrader, R.E. 1968. Abnormal glucose tolerance in magnesium-deficient guinea pigs. *J Nutr.* 94:89–94.

Fernandez, M.L., Vergara-Jimenez, M., Conde, K., Behr, T., and Abdel-Fattah, G. 1997. Regulation of apolipoprotein B-containing lipoproteins by dietary soluble fiber in guinea pigs. *Am J Clin Nutr.* 65:814–822.

Fisher, P.G. 2006. Exotic mammal renal disease: Diagnosis and treatment. *Vet Clin Nor Am Exot Anim Prac.* 9:69–96.

Frederiksen, S. and Heeno-Andersen, J. 2003. The external promoter in the guinea pig 5S rRNA gene is different from the rodent promoter. *Hereditas.* 139:156–160.

Fujii, Y., Enomoto, M., Ikemoto, T., et al. 2004. Molecular cloning and characterization of a gonadotropin-releasing hormone receptor in the guinea pig, *Cavia porcellus. Gen Comp Endocr.* 136:208–216.

Furst, S.M., Luedke, D., Gaw, H.H., Reich, R., and Gandolfi, A.J. 1997. Demonstration of a cellular immune response in halothane-exposed guinea pigs. *Toxicol Appl Pharmacol.* 143:245–255.

Garris, DR. 1979. Diurnal fluctuation of plasma cortisol levels in the guinea pig. *Acta Endocrinol (Copenh).* 90:622–625.

Green, M., Crim, M., Traber, M., and Ostwald, R. 1976. Cholesterol turnover and tissue distribution in the guinea pig in response to dietary cholesterol. *J Nutr.* 106:515–528.

Güler, G. et al. 2007. Electric field effects on guinea pig serum: the role of free radicals. *Electromagn Biol Med.* 26(3):207–223.

Hargaden, M. and Singer, L. 2012. Anatomy, physiology, and behavior. In *The Laboratory Rabbit, Guinea Pig, Hamster, and Other Rodents*. Eds. M.A. Suckow, K.A. Stevens, and R.P. Wilson, pp. 575–602. San Diego, CA: Academic Press.

Harkness, J.E., Murray, K.A., and Wagner, J.E. 2002. *Laboratory Animal Medicine*. Eds. J. Fox, L.C. Anderson, F.M. Loew, and F.W Quimby, 2nd edition, pp. 203–246. New York, NY: Academic Press.

Hisaw, F.L., Zarrow, M.X., Money, W.L., Talmage, R.V.N., and Abramowitz, A. 1994. Importance of female reproductive tract in the formation of relaxin. *Endocrinology.* 34:122.

Holowaychuk, M.K. 2006. Renal failure in a guinea pig (*Cavia porcellus*) following ingestion of oxalate containing plants. *Can Vet J.* 47:787–789.

Hrapkiewicz, K., Medina, L., Holmes, D. 1998. *Clinical Laboratory Animal Medicine: An Introduction*. Ames, IA: Wiley-Blackwell.

Huerkamp, M.J., Murray, K.A., and Orosz, S.E. 1996. Guinea pigs. In *Handbook of Rodent and Rabbit Medicine*. Eds. K. Laber-Laird, M.M., Swindle, and P.A. Fleckell, pp. 91–149. Tarrytown, NY: Pergamon Press.

Huebner, J.L., Seifer, D.R., and Kraus, V.B. 2007. A longitudinal analysis of serum cytokines in the Hartley guinea pig model of osteoarthritis. *Osteoar Cartilage.* 15:354–356.

Huneke, R.B. 2012. Basic experimental methods. In *The Laboratory Rabbit, Guinea Pig, Hamster, and Other Rodents*. Eds. Suckow, M.A., Stevens, K.A., and Wilson, R.P. (eds.), pp. 621–635. New York, NY: Academic Press.

Hurley, L.S., Everson, G.J., and Geiger, J.F. 1959. Serum alkaline phosphatase activity in normal and manganese-deficient developing rats. *J Nutr.* 67:445–450.

Jagiello, G. 1967. The effect of several relaxin preparations on the hysterectomized guinea pig. *J Reprod Fertil.* 13:175–177.

Janssen, P.A.J., Niemegeers, C.J.E., and Marsboom, R.P.H. 1975. Etomidate, a potent non-barbiturate hypnotic. Intravenous etomidate in mice, rats, guinea-pigs, rabbits and dogs. *Arch Int Pharmacodyn Ther.* 214:92–132.

Jimenez-Linan, M., Rubin, B.S., and King, J.C. 1997. Examination of guinea pig luteinizing hormone-releasing hormone gene reveals a unique decapeptide and existence of two transcripts in the brain. *Endrocrinology.* 138:4123–4130.

Jukes, T.H. 1979. Dr. Best, insulin, and molecular evolution. *Can J Biochem.* 59:455–458.

Kaiser, S. and Sachser, N. 1998. The social environment during pregnancy and lactation affects the female offsprings' endocrine status and behaviour in guinea pigs. *Physiol Behav.* 63:361–366.

Kapoor, A. and Matthews, S.G. 2005. Short periods of prenatal stress affect growth, behaviour, and hypothalamo-pituitary-adrenal axis activity in male guinea pig offspring. *J Physiol.* 566:967–977.

Kapoor, A. et al. 2006. Fetal programming of hypothalamo-pituitary-adrenal function: prenatal stress and glucocorticoids. *J Physiol.* 572(Pt 1):31–44.

Kapoor, A. and Matthews, S.G. 2008. Prenatal stress modifies behavior and hypthalmic-pituitary-adrenal function in female guinea pig offspring: Effects of timing of prenatal stress and stage of reproductive cycle. *Endocrinology.* 149:6406–6415.

Kim, S.G., Kang, H.S., Lee, M.Y., et al. 2006. Ketamine-induced cardiac depression is associated with increase in [Mg2+]i and activation of p38 MAP kinase and ERK 1/2 in guinea pig. *Biochem Biophy Res Comm.* 349:716–722.

Kind, K.L., Clifton, P.M., Grant, P.A., et al. 2003. Effect of maternal feed restriction during pregnancy on glucose tolerance in the adult guinea pig. *Am J Physiol-Reg I.* 284:140–152.

Kitagaki, M., Yamaguchi, M., Nakamura, M., Sakurada, K., Suwa, T., and Sasa, H. 2005. Age-related changes in haematology and serum chemistry of Weiser–Maples guinea pigs (Cavia porcellus). *Lab Anim.* 39:321–330.

Konno, R., Kurabayashi, A., Tsuchiya, M., and Niwa, A. 1999. Guinea pig D-amino acid oxidase cDNA and phylogenetic position. *DNA Sequence.* 10:85–91.

Kraft, W. and Dürr, U.M. 2005. *Klinische Labordiagnostik in der Tiermedizin*, 6th edition, pp. 186–203 and 483–484. Stuttgart: Schattauer. From Medi-Test Combi 10® VET promotional literature.

Kunzl, C. and Sachser, N. 1999. The behavioral endocrinology of domestication: A comparison between the domestic guinea pig (*Cavia ampere* f. *porcellus*) and its wild ancestor, the cavy (*Cavia aperea*). *Horm Behav.* 35:28–37.

Lambert, A., Frost, J., Mitchell, R., and Robertson, W.R. 1986. On the assessment of the in vitro biopotency and site(s) of action of drugs affecting adrenal steroidogenesis. *Annal Clin Biochem.* 23:225–229.

Lambert, A., Frost, J., Mitchell, R., Wilson, A.U., and Robertson, W.R. 1984. On the site of action of the anti-adrenal steroidogenic effect of etomidate and megestrol acetate. *Clin Endocrinol.* 21:721–727.

Lambert, A., Mitchell, R., Frost, J., Ratcliffe, J.G., and Robertson, W.R. 1983. Direct *in vitro* inhibition of adrenal steroidogenesis by etomidate. *Lancet.* 5:1085–1086.

Lambert, A., Mitchell, R., and Robertson, W.R. 1985. Effect of propofol, thiopentone and etomidate on adrenal steroidgenesis *in vitro. Br J Anaesth.* 57:505–508.

Larkin, L.H. and Reneger, R.H. 1986. Immunochemical and cytochemical studies of relaxin-containing cells in the guinea pig uterus. *Am J Anat.* 176:353–365.

Li, W.I., Hide, W.A., Zharkikh, A., Ma, D.P., and Graur, D. 1992. The molecular taxonomy and evolution of the guinea pig. *J Hered.* 83:174–181.

Lind, R.C., Gandolfi, A.J., Brown, B.R., and Hall, P. 1987. Halothane hepatotoxicity in guinea pigs. *Anesth Analg.* 66:222–228.

Lind, R.C., Gandolfi, A.J., and Hall, P. 1992. Subanesthetic halothane in hepatotoxic in the guinea pig. *Anesth Analg.* 74:559–563.

Liu, L. and Matthews, S.G. 1999. Adrenocortical response profiles to corticotrophin-releasing hormone and adrenocorticotrophin challenge in the chronically catheterized adult guinea-pig. *Exp Physiol.* 84:971–977.

Loeb, W.F. and Quimby, F.W. 1999. Appendix. In *The Clinical Chemistry of Laboratory Animals, Second Edition.* Eds. W.F. Loeb and F.W. Quimby, pp. 643–7263. Philadelphia, PA: Taylor & Francis.

Lunam, C.A., Cousins, M.J., and Hall, P. 1985. Guinea pig model of halothane-associated hepatotoxicity in the absence of enzyme induction and hypoxia. *J Pharmacol Exper Therap.* 232:802–809.

Lunam, C.A., Cousins, M.J., and Hall, P. 1986. Genetic predisposition to liver damage after halothane anesthesia in guinea pigs. *Anesth Analg.* 65:1143–1148.

Lunam, C.A., Cousins, M.J., and Hall, P. 1989. The pathology of halothane hepatotoxicity in a guinea-pig model: A comparison with human halothane hepatitis. *Br J Exp Pathol.* 70:533–541.

Mahmoodian, F., Gosiewska, A., and Peterkofsky, B. 1996. Regulation and properties of bone alkaline phosphatase during vitamin C deficiency in guinea pigs. *Arch Biochem Biophys.* 336:86–96.

Malinowska, K.W. and Nathanielsz, P.W. 1974. Plasma aldosterone, cortisol and corticosterone concentrations in the new-born guinea-pig. *J Physiol.* 236:83–93.

Manin, M., Tournaire, C., and DeLost, P. 1982. Measurement of the rate of secretion, peripheral metabolism, and interconversion of cortisol and cortisone in adult conscious male guinea pigs. *Steroids.* 39:81–88.

Manning, P.J., Wagner, J.E., and Harkness, J.E. 1984. Biology and diseases of guinea pigs. In *Laboratory Animal Medicine.* Eds. J.G. Fox, B.J. Cohen, and F.M. Loew, pp. 150–181. Orlando, FL: Academic Press.

Mitruka, B.M. and Rawnsley, H.M. 1981. *Clinical Biochemical and Hematological Values in Normal Experimental Animals and Normal Human.* New York, NY: Masson Publishing.

Okewole, P.A., Odeyemi, P.S., Oladunmade, M.A., Ajagbonna, B.O., Onah, J., and Spencer, T. 1991. An outbreak of *Streptococcus pyogenes* infection associated with calcium oxalate urolithiasis in guinea pigs (*Cavia porcellus*). *Lab Anim.* 25:184–186.

Ostojic, H., Cifuentes, V., and Monge, C. 2002. Hemoglobin affinity in Andean rodents. *Biol Res.* 35:27–30.

Ostwald, R. and Shannon, A. 1964. Composition of tissue lipids and anemia of guinea pigs in response to dietary cholesterol. *Biochem J.* 91:146–154.

Pelardy, G. and Delost, P. 1977. Evolution of testosterone metabolism during neonatal life in the guinea pig. *C R Acad Sci Hebd Seances Acad Sci D.* 284(24):2531–2534.

Pelardy, G. and Delost, P. 1977. Plasma, testicular, and adrenal cortex levels of androgens in the perinatal period and determination of neonatal hypertestosteronemia in guinea pigs. *C R Acad Sci*, Series D: 827–830.

Pelardy, G. and Delost, P. 1978. Secretion of the androgens in the male guinea-pig during the perinatal period. *Acta Endocrinol (Copenh)* 89(4):770–779.

Percy, D.H. and Barthold, S.W. 2007. *Pathology of Laboratory Rodents and Rabbits*, 3rd edition. Ames, IA: Blackwell Publishing.

Porter, D.G. 1971a. The action of relaxin on myometrial activity in the guinea-pig *in vivo*. *J Reprod Fertil.* 26:251–253.

Porter, D.G. 1971b. Quantitative changes in myometrial activity in the guinea-pig during pregnancy. *J Reprod Fertil.* 27:219–226.

Porter, D.G. 1972. Myometrium of the pregnant guinea pig: The probably importance of relaxin. *Biol Reprod.* 7:458–464.

Prior, J., Kurtz, D., and Aiegler, D. 1961. The hypercholesterolemic rabbits. *Arch Pathol.* 71:672–684.

Rigaudiere, N., Pelardy, G., Robert, A., and Delost, P. 1976. Changes in the concentrations of testosterone and androstenedione in the plasma and testis of the guinea-pig from birth to death. *J Reprod Fertil.* 48:291–300.

Riggs, S.M. 2009. Guinea pigs. In *Manual of Exotic Pet Practice*. Eds. M.A. Mitchell and N.T. Tully, pp. 456–473. St. Louis, MO: Saunders Elsevier.

Rodriguez, H.A., Ortega, H.H., Ramos, J.G., Munoz-de-Toro, M., and Luque, E.H. 2003. Guinea-pig interpubic joint (symphysis pubica) relaxation at parturition: Underlying cellular processes that resemble an inflammatory response. *Reprod Biol Endocrinol.* 1:113.

Rodriguez, H.A., Ramos, J.G., Ortega, H.H., Munoz-de-Toro, M., and Luque, E.H. 2008. Regional changes in the spatio-temporal pattern of progesterone receptor expression in the guinea-pig genital tract as parturition approaches. *J Steroid Biochem Mol Biol.* 111:247–254.

Rosenzweig, J., Lesniak, M., Samuels, B., Yip, C., Zimmerman, A., and Roth, J. 1980. Insulin in the extrapancreatic tissues of guinea pig differs markedly from the insulin in their pancreas and plasma. *Trans Assoc Am Physicians.* 93:263–278.

Rosenzweig, J.L., Le Roith, D., Lesniak, M.A., MacIntyre, I., Sawyer, W.H., and Roth, J. 1983. Two distinct insulins in the guinea pig: The broad relevance of these findings to evolution of peptide hormones. *Fed Proc.* 42:2608–2614.

Rosenzweig, J.L., Le Roith, D., Lesniak, M.A., et al. 1985. Two distinct insulin-related molecules in the guinea pig: Immunological and biochemical characterization of insulin-like immunoactivity from extrapancreatic tissues of the guinea pig. *Diabetologia.* 28:237–243.

Sachser, N. and Kaiser, S. 1996. Prenatal social stress masculinizes the females' behaviour in guinea pigs. *Physiol Behav.* 60:589–594.

Sachser, N. and Lick, C. 1989. Social stress in guinea pigs. *Physiol Behav.* 46:137–144.

Sanchez-Bernal, C., Sanchez-Martin, M., Sanchez-Llorente, A., Cabezas, J.A., and Perez-Gonzalez, N. 1993. Toxic oil syndrome: A study of renal function in guinea pigs fed toxic oil. *Comp Biochem Physiol.* 104C:463–468.

Shapiro, R.J. 1993. Catabolism of low-density lipoproteins is altered in experimental chronic renal failure. *Metabolism.* 42:162–169.

Sharma, O.P., Makkar, H.P.S., Dawra, R.K., and Negi, S.S. 1982. Changes in blood constituents in guinea pigs in lantana toxicity. *Toxicol Lett.* 11:73–76.

Shomer et al. 1999. Biomethod for obtaining gastric juice and serum from the unanesthetized guinea pig *(Cavia porcellus)*. *Contemp Top Lab Anim Sci.* 38(5):32–35.

Sisk, D. 1976. Physiology. In *The Biology of the Guinea Pig*. Eds. J.E. Wagner and P.J. Manning, pp. 63–98. New York, NY: Academic Press.

Smith, L. 1966. Species variation in the amino acid sequence of insulin. *Am J Med.* 40:662–666.

Song, B.B., Anderson, D.S., and Schacht, J. 1997. Protection from otonycin ototoxicity by iron chelators in guinea pig in vivo. *J Pharmacol Exp Therap.* 282:309–377.

Sprink, R.R. 1978. Urolithiasis in a Guinea Pig *(Cavia porcellanus)*. *Vet Med Small Anim Clin.* 73(4):501–502.

Stopka, T., Zivny, J.H., Goldwasser, E., Prchal, J.F., Necas, E., and Prchal, J.T. 1998. Guinea pig serum erythropoietin (EPO) selectively stimulates guinea pig erythroid progenitors: Human or mouse erythroid progenitors do not form erythroid burst-forming unit colonies in response to guinea pig serum EPO. *Exp Hematol.* 26:910–914.

Stuppy, D.E., Douglass, P.R., and Douglass, P.J. 1979. Urolithiasis and cystotomy in a guinea pig (*Cavia porcellanus*). *Vet Med Small Anim Clin.* 74:565–567.

Sullivan, M.P., Cerda, J.J., Robbins, F.L., Burgin, C.W., and Beatty, R.J. 1993. The gerbil, hamster, and guinea pig as rodent models for hyperlipidemia. *Lab Anim Sci.* 43:575–578.

Suzuki, O., Koura, M., Noguchi, Y., Takano, K., Yamamoto, Y., and Matsuda, J. 2003. Optimization of superovulation induction by human menopausal gonadotropin in guinea pigs based on follicular waves and FSH-receptor homologies. *Mol Reprod Dev.* 64:219–225.

Suzuki, O., Mochida, K., Yamamoto, Y., et al. 2002. Comparison of glycoprotein hormone a-subunits of laboratory animals. *Mol Reprod Dev.* 62:335–342.

Swann, A., Wiley, M.H., and Siperstin, M.D. 1975. Tissue distribution of cholesterol feedback control in the guinea pig. *J Lipid Res.* 16:360–366.

Terada, M. 1993. A novel role in the removal of blood-borne foreign bodies for pulmonary capillaries in the guinea pig. *Virchows Archiv B Cell Path.* 63:147–157.

Terril, L.A. and Clemmons, D.J. 1998. *The Laboratory Guinea Pig.* CRC Press.

Trillmich, F., Mueller, B., Kaiser, S., and Krause, J. 2009. Puberty in female cavies (*Cavia aperea*) is affected by photoperiod and social conditions. *Physiol Behav.* 96:476–480.

Tsuchiya, H. and Bates, C.J. 1994. Ascorbic acid deficiency in guinea pigs: Contrasting effects of tissue ascorbic acid depletion and of associated inanition of status indices related to collagen and vitamin D. *Br J Nutr.* 72:745–752.

United States Department of Agriculture (USDA) – Animal Plant Health Inspection Service (APHIS) – 2016. Annual Report of Research Facilities: Animals Used in Research – Usage by Fiscal Year (2015). Available at: https://www.aphis.usda.gov/animal_welfare/downloads/reports/Annual-Reports-FY2015.pdf (Accessed 17 April, 2017).

Underwood, E. J. 1971. Manganese. In *Trace Elements in Human and Animal Nutrition.* Ed. E.J. Underwood, pp. 177–201. New York, NY: Academic Press.

Wagner, J.E. 1976. Miscellaneous disease conditions of guinea pigs. In *The Biology of the Guinea Pig.* Eds. J.E. Wagner and P.J. Manning, pp. 227–234. New York, NY: Academic Press.

Waner, T., Avidar, Y., Peh, H., Zass, R., and Bogin, E. 1996. Hematology and clinical chemistry values of normal and euthymic hairless adult male Dunkin-Hartley guinea pigs (*Cavia porcellus*). *Vet Clin Pathol.* 25:61–64.

Wauquier, A. 1983. Profile of etomidate. A hypnotic, anticonvulsant and brain protective compound. *Anaesthesia.* 38: Suppl:26–33.

Weir, B. 1974. *The Biology of the Hystricomorph Rodents.* Eds. I. Rowlands and B. Weir, pp. 437–446. London: Academic Press.

Wen, D., Boissel, J.P., Tracy, T.E., et al. 1993. Erythropoietin structure-function relationships: High degree of sequence homology among mammals. *Blood.* 44:1507–1516.

Wilson, J. and Lindsey, C. 1965. Studies on the influence of dietary cholesterol or cholesterol metabolism in the isotopic steady state of man. *J Clin Invest.* 44:1805–1814.

Winslow, R.M. 2007. The role of hemoglobin oxygen affinity in oxygen transport at high altitude. *Respir Physiol Neurobiol.* 158:121–127.

Wriston, J.C. 1984. Comparative biochemistry of the guinea pig: A partial checklist. *Comp Biochem Physiol B.* 77:253–278.

Yamanaka, W. and Ostwald, R. 1968. Lipid composition of heart, kidney, and lung in guinea pigs made anemic by dietary cholesterol. *J Nutr.* 95:381–387.

Yamanaka, W., Ostwald, R., and French, S. 1967. Histopathology of guinea pigs with cholesterol induced anemia. *Proc Soc Exp Biol Med.* 125:303–306.

Zarrow, M.X. 1947. Relaxin content of blood, urine and other tissues of pregnant and postpartum guinea pigs. *Proc Soc Exp Biol Med.* 66:488–491.

Zarrow, M.X. 1948. The role of the steroid hormones in the relaxation of the symphysis pubis of the guinea pig. *Endocrinology.* 42:129–140.

Zarrow, M.X., Anderson, N.C., and Callantine, M.R. 1963. Failure of progestogens to prolong pregnancy in the guinea pig. *Nature.* 198:690–692.

Zheng, X.H., Begay, C., Lind, R.C., and Gandolfi, A.J. 2001. Humoral immune response to a sevoflurane degradation product in the guinea pig following inhalation exposure. *Drug Chem Toxocol.* 24:339–346.

Zimmerman, A. and Yip, C. 1974. Guinea pig insulin. I. Purification and physical properties. *J Biol Chem.* 249:4021–4025.

9 The Laboratory Ferret

Mary M. Patterson and James G. Fox

CONTENTS

9.1 INTRODUCTION

Domestic ferrets (*Mustela putorius furo*) occupy important niches as animal models in biomedical research. As evidenced by the number of citations in a web-based literature search, their eminent use today is in the field of virology, particularly in influenza-related projects. Ferrets have been represented in influenza research since the 1930s (Smith et al., 1933), but their role has expanded dramatically with concern for a human influenza pandemic from influenza A H5N1 ("bird flu") and, more recently, from H1N1 ("swine flu"; Garrett, 2009). Several review articles (Maher and DeStefano, 2004; Luke and Subbarao, 2008; van der Laan et al., 2008; Barnard, 2009; Belser et al., 2011) enumerate ferret attributes that make them desirable models for influenza research; highlights are a natural susceptibility to infection and parallels with humans in regard to clinical presentation and pathogenesis.

Ferrets are permissive hosts for influenza types A and B (Kiupel and Perpinan, 2014; Kim et al., 2009), and, unlike mice, prior animal adaptation of the ferret is not required for disease. Potential transmission between humans and ferrets is well recognized, and animal care technicians with flu-like symptoms are asked to forego working with research ferrets. Ferret-to-ferret passage, as well as ferret-to-human, has been documented. A 2009 outbreak of respiratory disease among a large farm colony of ferrets in Iowa underscores the clinical importance of influenza in these animals (Patterson et al., 2009). In the latter case report, histology, immunohistochemistry, and molecular techniques allowed the etiology to be characterized as an H1N1 influenza strain. In the face of this sensitivity, it is critical that ferrets destined for influenza research be assessed in advance for preexisting antibodies (Matsuoka et al., 2009).

Similar to infected humans, ferrets dosed intranasally with benign or seasonal influenza will exhibit self-limiting signs of upper respiratory disease such as sneezing, coughing, rhinitis, anorexia, malaise, and fever. The ferret body size allows these clinical signs to be easily monitored, including temperature variations via a subcutaneous transponder microchip. Their ciliated upper respiratory epithelium is selectively infected, sloughed, and regenerated in most cases, and hemagglutination inhibition assays can be performed to demonstrate antibodies after recovery. However, when ferrets are young, immunocompromised, or exposed to more pathogenic strains, influenza virus can replicate in the lower airways and lungs, causing interstitial pneumonitis and other sequelae with variable lethality. In ferrets exposed to virulent H5N1 isolates, van Riel et al. (2006) found the virus attached to similar cell types as were observed in infected humans. Secondary bacterial infections, often with *Streptococcus pneumoniae*, can be superimposed and complicate the course of disease in ferrets (Peltola et al., 2006).

Current influenza studies involving ferrets are designed to elucidate viral virulence, pathology, and transmissibility (Zitzow et al., 2002; Jackson et al., 2009; Watanabe et al., 2009; Koster et al., 2012). With early concern regarding its potential global impact, research ferrets were inoculated almost immediately with strains of the novel 2009 A (H1N1) swine influenza virus obtained from human patients (Maines et al., 2009; Munster et al., 2009). Likewise ferrets are suitable for evaluating antiviral therapies and vaccines (Kugel et al., 2009; Shoji et al., 2009). The development of effective vaccine strategies against the H5N1 subtype of avian influenza is a major focus of research using ferrets (Forrest et al., 2009; Middleton et al., 2009; Perrone et al., 2009). An overview of influenza vaccine research by van der Laan et al. (2009) concludes that ferrets will continue to be invaluable experimental subjects, in part because they can be infected with a viral subtype different from that in a subsequent vaccine and develop a heightened response to the vaccine, that is, a "priming" effect, which is a situation analogous to humans. Recent research using genetically modified strains of influenza in ferrets sparked a debate among scientists about whether the published information could be used by bioterrorists (Cohen, 2012; Kuehn, 2012).

Other viruses that attack the human respiratory system are also evaluated in ferrets. Soon after its emergence, ferrets were among the first laboratory animals experimentally infected with the coronavirus responsible for severe acute respiratory syndrome (SARS; Martina et al., 2003). Subsequent reports have validated the ferret SARS infection model (Chu et al., 2008; van den Brand et al., 2008; Danesh et al., 2011). As with influenza-infected ferrets, efficacy of potential treatments and vaccines for SARS has been tested in ferrets (Ter Meulen et al., 2004; Weingartl et al., 2004; Darnell et al., 2007; See et al., 2008). In a summary article concerning animal models for SARS, Roberts et al. (2007) comment that ferrets constitute an outbred species, and the inherent variability between individuals can be a confounding factor in challenge studies. While true, the relative genetic heterogeneity of ferrets is an additional parameter shared with human populations.

Ferrets are exquisitely sensitive to canine distemper virus (Kiupel and Perpinan, 2014) with ongoing, natural infections (Perpinan et al., 2008). Ferrets serve as a model for the related measles virus in humans (Sawatsky et al., 2012). Both morbilliviruses cause respiratory signs, skin rash, fever, neurological sequelae, and severe immunosuppression in their respective hosts. Marine mammal morbilliviruses have also been partially characterized with passage through ferrets (Nielsen et al., 2008). Pillet et al. (2009) provides a review of morbillivirus research applications in ferrets, including the use of ferrets to study the pathogenesis of subacute sclerosing panencephalitis. These authors and others invoke a lack of ferret-specific reagents and adequate knowledge about ferret chemokines and cytokines as a drawback when using ferrets in research areas such as virology; however, investigations have been undertaken that start to address this deficiency (Senchak et al., 2007; Danesh et al., 2008; Ochi et al., 2008; Rutigliano et al., 2008; Svitek et al., 2008).

Other researchers have used ferrets to study henipaviruses (reviewed in Geisbert et al., 2012), respiratory syncytial virus (Colasurdo et al., 1998; Byrd and Prince, 1997), and human metapneumovirus (MacPhail et al., 2004). In addition, aspects of the ferret respiratory system have been exploited for other than viral-based research. For example, ferrets continue to be used as training models for human pediatric intubation (Kircher et al., 2009). Expression of the cystic fibrosis transmembrane conductance regulator (CFTR) gene in ferret airway epithelium and submucosal glands is identical to that in humans (Li and Englehardt, 2003), and researchers have genetically engineered ferrets with a disrupted CFTR (Sun et al., 2008, 2010). This considerable success may lead to cloned ferrets for investigating other genetic diseases. A related technical advance is sequencing of the ferret genome, which has been performed at the Broad Institute (for information see http://www.broadinstitute.org).

With a relatively immature nervous system at birth, especially in contrast to cats, ferrets constitute a useful system to investigate neurological development and the influence of experience, or activity (Weliky, 2000; Sur and Leamey, 2001; Sengpiel and Kind, 2002; Dalva, 2010). As the eyes of ferret kits do not open until they are 32 days old, a popular research paradigm, in "rewired" ferrets, is to induce retinal projections to innervate nonvisual areas of the brain. The effects of lesions created in neural pathways are also studied in adult and immature ferrets (e.g., Fuentes-Santamaria et al., 2007; Gautschi and Clarke, 2007; Allman et al., 2009). Progressive cortical development has been correlated to the appearance of gyri and sulci on the ferret brain surface by using magnetic resonance imaging (Neal et al., 2007), while other neuroscience researchers are using viral vector techniques to label ferret neurons (Jian et al., 2005).

Comparable to *Helicobacter pylori* in humans, *Helicobacter mustelae* (Swennes and Fox, 2014) colonizes the gastric mucosa of ferrets. Ferrets harboring *H. mustelae* can be clinically normal or can exhibit vomiting, weight loss, and other signs associated with gastritis, gastric ulceration, hypergastrinemia, gastric adenocarcinoma, and mucosa-associated lymphoid tissue (MALT) lymphoma. Marini and Fox (1999), Solnick and Schauer (2001), and Whary and Fox (2004) review the use of ferrets as a gastric helicobacter model; Nedrud and Blanchard (2003) present general techniques for infecting ferrets with *H. mustelae*. Due to the high prevalence of *H. mustelae* in ferrets from commercial vendors in the United States, drug therapy to eradicate the organism is required before experimental inoculation. Alternatively, pregnant jills can be treated with antimicrobials and subsequent kits raised *H. mustelae*-free prior to involvement in helicobacter research (Batchelder et al., 1996). Administration of isogenic mutant strains of *H. mustelae* has helped to identify virulence and colonization factors (Andrutis et al., 1997; Patterson et al., 2003). Also, *H. mustelae*-infected ferrets have contributed to efforts in developing a vaccine against *H. pylori* (Sutton and Lee, 2001; Del Giudice et al., 2001).

There are similarities in emesis between ferrets and humans, which has made ferrets suitable as a nonrodent animal in the testing of novel drugs (Ji et al., 2007; Saif et al., 2007; Duffy et al., 2012; Du Sert et al., 2012), as well as for dissecting basic emetic mechanisms (van Sickle et al., 2003; Osinski et al., 2005; Onishi et al., 2007). In nutritional research, the absorption and metabolism of carotenoids in ferrets have been studied (Wang et al., 1993; Lee et al., 1999; Russell, 2004). Ferrets also are used as models for vitamin A metabolism (Raila et al., 2002), including a report on the ability of vitamin A to protect ferrets from clinical disease when exposed to canine distemper virus (Rodeheffer et al., 2007). Ferrets are convenient subjects for reproductive behavior and neuroendocrinology studies; a summary on the importance of olfaction in mate selection among different species, including ferrets, has been published by Baum and Kelliher (2009). Adrenocortical neoplasia in ferrets has been reviewed as a model for the human disease recently (Beuschlein et al., 2012). Cardiovascular researchers have employed ferrets (Morgan, 2014), such as in a comparative study that identifies the extent of collateral coronary circulation (Maxwell et al., 1987). In other instances, cardiac disease is surgically induced in ferrets (Diaz et al., 2004; Graham and Trafford, 2007). Ferrets continue to be used in parasitologic research (Webster and Kapel, 2005); earlier studies are discussed by Eberhard (1998). To a limited extent, ferrets have been exposed during experiments to non-respiratory viruses, such as lyssaviruses (Vos et al., 2004; Hanlon et al., 2005). They have also been shown to be susceptible to the prion that causes chronic wasting disease in cervids (Perrott et al., 2012). Overall it is apparent that, although total animal numbers used per year are less than in certain other laboratory animal species (Ball, 2006), ferrets are highly appropriate small animal models in diverse areas of study.

9.2 UNIQUE PHYSIOLOGICAL CHARACTERISTICS OF FERRETS

As obligate carnivores, ferrets require diets high in meat protein and fats, and low in complex carbohydrates and fiber (Marini et al., 2002). The simple stomach is like that of humans. There is no cecum present, and the transition from ileum to large intestine is indistinct grossly. Transit time through the ferret gastrointestinal tract is relatively rapid, around 3 or 4 hours, and thus the time when an animal is being fasted should be only a few hours. Ferret spleen size can be variable; potential causes for splenomegaly include extramedullary hematopoiesis, lymphoma, and isoflurane administration. The ferret lung capacity is three times larger than predicted for its body size, and its trachea is long and narrow. These and other characteristics, such as more bronchiolar branching and extensive bronchial submucosal glands similar to the human lung, have made the ferret popular in respiratory research, as described in Section 9.1. Reference values for cerebrospinal fluid in healthy adult ferrets reveal a slightly higher protein concentration than found in dogs and cats (Platt et al., 2004). Because ferret sweat glands are poorly developed, it is important that environmental temperatures for ferrets be less than 85°F–90°F. A distinct musky odor is characteristic of adult ferrets, even when the paired anal scent glands have been surgically removed, because of normal sebaceous secretions (Marini et al., 2002). Proteinuria is not unusual in ferrets, especially in males (Fox, 2014), and urine pH is close to 6.0 when animals are provided a high-quality diet (Quesenberry and Orcutt, 2012).

The most common coat color in commercial ferrets is sable, or "fitch"; however, albino animals and other color variants are also available. Breeding animals and pseudopregnant jills with the two former coat types were used to assist identification of cystic fibrosis clones (Sun et al., 2008). Intact adult male ferrets can be twice the size of adult females (1.0–2.0 kg compared to 0.6–1.0 kg, respectively), and seasonal fluctuations in body fat result in concomitant changes in body weight. Sexual maturity is attained at 4–12 months of age, dependent on photoperiod, and gestation length is 41 ± 1 days (Lindeberg, 2008). In general, female ferrets are seasonal breeders and induced ovulators, with estrus persisting until a female is bred or artificially caused to ovulate. Potentially fatal bone marrow suppression and aplastic anemia can result from estrogen toxicity if estrus is allowed to continue a few weeks, causing some researchers to purchase only male ferrets so as to avoid the complications of estrus in females (Ball, 2006). Distinct blood groups have not been detected in ferrets (Manning and Bell, 1990), which has clinical relevance when repeated blood transfusions are necessary.

The lifespan for a ferret is reported to average 6–8 years. Several neoplastic diseases can develop in adult animals (Li et al., 1998; Miwa et al., 2009); of these, insulinomas are the most common, with presenting clinical signs related to hypoglycemia (Chen, 2008). Adrenal gland disease is unique in ferrets because usually adrenal sex hormones (estradiol, 17-hydroxyprogesterone, androstenedione) are elevated rather than glucocorticoids (Rosenthal and Peterson, 1996; Simone-Freilicher, 2008; Rosenthal and Wyre, 2012), albeit there are single case reports of ferrets with hypercortisolism (Schoemaker et al., 2008) and hyperaldosteronism (Desmarchelier et al., 2008).

9.3 METHODOLOGY OF SAMPLE COLLECTION

9.3.1 Blood Collection

Larger blood volumes (1–6 mL) should be collected from the jugular vein or cranial vena cava, using a 1–6-mL syringe attached to a 25–20-gauge needle. Different restraint methods have been described for these venipuncture sites in the conscious ferret (Ko and Marini, 2014; Quesenberry and Orcutt, 2012). For blood collection from the jugular vein with one assistant, the ferret can be wrapped tightly in a towel that restrains the forelimbs caudally (Figure 9.1). The ferret is held in dorsal recumbency by the scruff of its neck while the phlebotomist presses on the thoracic inlet to enhance venous filling and visualization. The jugular veins of ferrets lie between the thoracic inlet and the ear base, and bending the needle slightly can be helpful (Otto et al., 1993). Jugular venipuncture can also be accomplished by holding the ferret in ventral recumbency with its neck extended and forelegs pulled downward over the edge of a table, as is typically done with cats. Some ferret practitioners (Dyer and Cervasio, 2008; Siperstein, 2008) prefer to obtain blood from the cranial vena cava in ferrets, noting that a relatively caudal placement of the heart minimizes the risk of inadvertent cardiac puncture. In this technique, the ferret is placed in dorsal

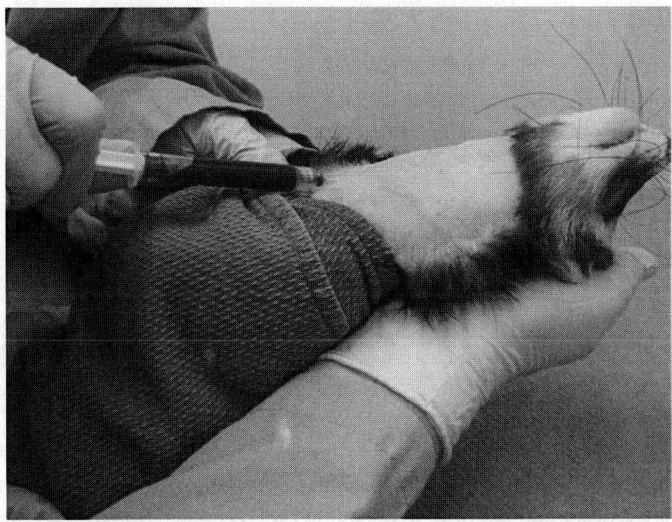

FIGURE 9.1 **(See color insert.)** Restraint for blood collection from right jugular vein in an awake ferret. Clipping the hair at the venipuncture site is recommended.

recumbency as described above. A small gauge, 1-inch needle is inserted at the thoracic inlet, at a 45° angle to the body, and pointed toward the opposite rear leg. With gentle suction applied to the syringe plunger, the needle is withdrawn until blood is visible in the hub. This method should be aborted if the ferret struggles.

Cephalic or lateral saphenous veins are accessible when small amounts of blood are needed; tuberculin or insulin syringes with small gauge needles are appropriate for these sites. A number of other ferret bleeding techniques have been described in the literature but are not routinely used now, such as the use of tail vessels, toenail clipping, and cardiocentesis (Ko and Marini, 2014; Ryland and Bernard, 1983); the latter is only acceptable during a terminal procedure in an anesthetized animal. Disadvantages of these methods include small volumes and/or sample variability (Otto et al., 1993), invasiveness, and concerns for animal welfare.

Additional recommendations when collecting blood from ferrets are prior clipping of the venipuncture site if warranted, distracting the ferret with a food treat (which would elevate blood glucose levels), and considering the use of microfuge tubes. Due to the tough skin of adult ferrets, piercing the skin overlying the vessel beforehand with a 20-gauge needle is helpful. Also sedation for a blood draw can be employed regardless of positioning. Routine injectable agents include intramuscular ketamine hydrochloride (30–60 mg/kg) or intramuscular ketamine/xylazine (20–40 mg/kg, 1–4 mg/kg, respectively); yohimbine (0.5 mg/kg) given intramuscularly after sample collection will reverse xylazine-induced bradycardia and decrease recovery time. Intramuscular ketamine (30 mg/kg) mixed with acepromazine (0.3 mg/kg) has also been used successfully (Otto et al., 1993), whereas isoflurane chamber anesthesia is safe for a pregnant animal. Erythron indices, and to a lesser degree plasma protein values, are reduced during ketamine/xylazine sedation, as well as with isoflurane (Ko and Marini, 2014). Similar to other species, total blood volume in ferrets is estimated to be 5%–7% of body weight, and a maximum of 10% of the total blood volume should be withdrawn at any one time in a normal animal, every 2 weeks; thus a 1-kg male could safely have 6 mL of blood collected at one time. To acquire an adequate amount of plasma or serum, it is suggested that up to three times as much blood volume be collected as plasma or serum volume required, and to spin the blood about 20% longer than for other species (Whary, 2014).

9.3.2 Urine Collection

Cystocentesis of a palpable urinary bladder in a well-restrained ferret can yield one or more milliliters of urine; a small gauge needle is appropriate. Also free catch samples are often adequate and easy to procure. A procedure for urinary bladder catheterization has been described (Ko and Marini, 2014).

9.4 PREANALYTICAL SOURCES OF VARIATION

Earlier authors (Thornton et al., 1979; Lee et al., 1982; Hoover and Baldwin, 1988; Fox, 2014) have reported clinical chemistry data from ferrets. However, comparisons of data are difficult because of different ages and sources of animals, anesthetic regimens, and analytical technology. Nevertheless in previous publications, as well as in current serum chemistry data given below that were obtained from Marshall BioResources, an inverse relationship is suggested between ferret age and values for inorganic phosphorous, alanine transaminase, alkaline phosphatase, and creatine kinase. Intact adult females will have sex hormone levels that reflect their reproductive cycle status, which in turn is affected by photoperiod; for example, a nonstimulatory photoperiod (8 hours light, 16 hours dark) coincides with low estradiol and luteinizing hormone levels (Fox et al., 2014). Progesterone secretion by corpora lutea begins at ovulation, and peak levels are reached at about day 15 of pregnancy or pseudopregnancy (Lindeberg, 2008). Neutered ferrets are expected to have low sex hormone levels, with high hormone levels supporting a diagnosis of adrenal gland disease or an ovarian remnant.

9.5 BRIEF DESCRIPTION OF COMMON PROCEDURES

Functional tests carried out in other animal species are performed rarely in ferrets; to a considerable extent this is because such evaluations are not required to diagnose typical disease syndromes. As stated in Section 9.2, adrenal gland disease in adult ferrets, while fairly frequent, normally affects sex hormone instead of cortisol levels. Primary thyroid, renal, and liver diseases are uncommon in ferrets. Infrequent cases of diabetes mellitus are usually iatrogenic sequelae to islet β cell surgery (Chen, 2008); however, two case reports of diabetes mellitus in ferrets unrelated to pancreatic surgery have been published (Boari et al., 2010, Phair et al., 2011). For research purposes in particular, descriptions of adrenal and thyroid assays (Garibaldi et al., 1988a,b; Heard et al., 1990; Schoemaker

TABLE 9.1
Serum Clinical Chemistry Data for Ferrets

Analyte	Units	Age	Male	Female
ALT	IU/L	Young	327.0 ± 228.1	288.1 ± 203.1
		Adult	89.7 ± 17.3	122.3 ± 19.3
Albumin	g/dL	Young	3.0 ± 0.2	2.9 ± 0.1
		Adult	3.0 ± 0.2	2.7 ± 0.2
AST	IU/L	Young	117.9 ± 66.1	106.7 ± 38.8
		Adult	60.2 ± 8.1	126.7 ± 35.9
ALP	IU/L	Young	162.3 ± 55.7	136.4 ± 60.7
		Adult	48.6 ± 13.0	71.4 ± 22.0
Bilirubin (total)	mg/dL	Young	0.3 ± 0.1	0.3 ± 0.0
		Adult	0.1 ± 0.0	0.2 ± 0.1
BUN	mg/dL	Young	30.7 ± 4.8	34.1 ± 4.0
		Adult	26.6 ± 8.8	28.0 ± 6.1

(Continued)

TABLE 9.1 ***(Continued)***
Serum Clinical Chemistry Data for Ferrets

Analyte	Units	Age	Male	Female
Calcium	mg/dL	Young	9.9 ± 0.5	10.2 ± 0.3
		Adult	9.2 ± 0.3	9.1 ± 0.3
Chloride	mEq/L	Young	115.2 ± 3.1	117.5 ± 2.7
		Adult	113.8 ± 2.2	117.9 ± 2.5
Cholesterol	mg/dL	Young	183.6 ± 25.4	178.0 ± 29.6
		Adult	128.8 ± 22.6	238.2 ± 39.0
Creatinine	mg/dL	Young	0.7 ± 0.2	0.7 ± 0.1
		Adult	0.7 ± 0.1	0.5 ± 0.2
CK	IU/L	Young	286.5 ± 137.6	293.2 ± 143.8
		Adult	128.6 ± 23.5	176.7 ± 54.8
GGT	IU/L	Young	8.0 ± 4.6	6.3 ± 2.3
		Adult	5.6 ± 0.9	14.1 ± 6.2
Globulin	g/dL	Young	3.3 ± 0.3	3.2 ± 0.3
		Adult	2.7 ± 0.2	3.5 ± 0.3
Glucose	mg/dL	Young	109.1 ± 12.3	103.6 ± 10.4
		Adult	110.4 ± 13.8	125.6 ± 16.1
Magnesium	mEq/L	Young	2.8 ± 0.2	2.9 ± 0.2
		Adult	2.9 ± 0.2	2.9 ± 0.2
Phosphorous	mg/dL	Young	9.7 ± 0.8	9.6 ± 0.7
		Adult	6.1 ± 0.5	6.7 ± 1.1
Potassium	mEq/L	Young	5.2 ± 0.2	5.1 ± 0.2
		Adult	5.0 ± 0.3	5.3 ± 0.4
Sodium	mEq/L	Young	151.9 ± 2.5	153.5 ± 2.0
		Adult	147.9 ± 2.0	148.9 ± 2.6
Total protein	g/dL	Young	6.3 ± 0.4	6.1 ± 0.3
		Adult	5.8 ± 0.3	6.2 ± 0.3
Estradiol	pmol/L	Neutered	30–180	103–238
		Intact	109–299	
17-hydroxyprogesterone	nmol/L	Neutered	<0.1–0.8	<0.1–1.9
		Intact	<0.1–20.4	
Androstenedione	nmol/L	Neutered	<0.1–1.5	<0.1–10.8
		Intact	<0.1–30.6	

Note: Values for all analytes except sex hormones (estradiol, 17-hydroxyprogesterone, and androstenedione) are given as mean ± standard deviation. These values were adapted from "The Marshall Ferret Serum Chemistry Data" (Marshall BioResources, Reference Data Guide 2014, available under Reference Data for Ferrets at www.marshallbio.com), as well as unpublished data, using a Vitros 250 analyzer. Young animals (31 males, 31 females) are sexually intact and 12–20 weeks of age; adults (30 males, 30 females) are sexually intact and 1–2 years of age, with females having had at least one litter but "resting" as much as possible, that is, not in visible estrus, pregnant, or lactating, when blood was drawn. All samples were collected under ketamine/xylazine sedation, and were nonhemolyzed.

Ranges for normal sex hormone levels (estradiol, 17-hydroxyprogesterone, and androstenedione) in neutered and *intact ferrets were provided by the Clinical Endocrinology Service, College of Veterinary Medicine, University of Tennessee, and Dr. Jack Oliver (unpublished data). The neutered ferret group consists of animals castrated (13 males) or spayed (13 females) early, with a mean age of 1.5 years when hormone levels were measured. The sexually intact males (40 ferrets) and females (40 ferrets) are 6–9 months of age.*

ALT, alanine aminotransferase; ALP, alkaline phosphatase; AST, aspartate aminotransferase; BUN, blood urea nitrogen; CK, creatine kinase; GGT, gamma glutamyl transferase.

TABLE 9.2
Urinalysis Data for Adult Ferrets

Parameter	Male	Female
Volume[a] (mL/24 h)	26 (8–48)	28 (8–140)
Sodium[a] (mmol/24 h)	1.9 (0.4–6.7)	1.5 (0.2–5.6)
Potassium[a] (mmol/24 h)	2.9 (1.0–9.6)	2.1 (0.9–5.4)
Chloride[a] (mmol/24 h)	2.4 (0.7–8.5)	1.9 (0.3–7.8)
Specific gravity[b]	1.059 ± 0.007	1.047 ± 0.007
Total protein[b] (mg/dL)	9.6 ± 1.4	7.6 ± 1.2
Protein by strip[b] (mg/dL)	30–100	Trace-30
pH by pH meter[b]	6.2 ± 0.1	6.3 ± 0.3
pH by strip[b]	6.0–6.5	6.0–6.5
Leukocytes by strip[b]	Negative	Negative
Nitrite by strip[b]	Negative	Negative
Glucose by strip[b]	Negative	Negative
Ketone by strip[b]	Negative	Negative
Bilirubin by strip[b]	Negative	Negative
Blood by strip[b]	Negative	Negative-2+ hemolyzed (one case)
Urobilinogen by strip[b]	0.2	0.2
Sediment[b]	Urine sediment from all ferrets had amorphous urates present, and most contained mucous strands and/or protein sheaths. The male urine samples had sperm cells and several samples from both sexes had rare RBCs; both sperm and RBCs resulted from sample collection. Squamous epithelial cells, WBCs, cocci, uric acid, and Ca oxalate crystals were rarely seen.	

Source: Fox, J.G., *Biology and Diseases of the Ferret*, 2014.

[a] Values are given as mean (range) and taken from Thornton et al. (1979) (40 males and 24 females).

[b] Urine was collected by cystocentesis from eight males and eight females (sexually intact, 1–2 years of age, sedated with ketamine/xylazine as above), and the samples were evaluated by the Diagnostic Laboratory of the Division of Comparative Medicine, Massachusetts Institute of Technology. A refractometer was used to assess urine-specific gravity and total protein, whereas Multistix 10 SG (Siemens) reagent strips provided semiquantitative results. Values are reported as mean ± standard deviation when warranted.

et al., 2002, 2004), as well as inulin and exogenous creatinine clearance measurements to estimate renal function (Esteves et al., 1994), are available.

9.6 REFERENCE RANGES

Serum clinical chemistry data for ferrets and urinalysis data for adult ferrets are available in Tables 9.1 and 9.2, respectively.

REFERENCES

Allman, B.L., Keniston, L.P., and Meredith, M.A. 2009. Adult deafness induces somatosensory conversion of ferret auditory cortex. *Proc Natl Acad Sci.* 106(14):5925–5930.

Andrutis, K.A., Fox, J.G., Schauer, D.B. et al. 1997. Infection of ferret stomach by isogenic flagellar mutant strains of *Helicobacter mustelae*. *Infect Immun.* 65:1962–1966.

Ball, R.S. 2006. Issues to consider for preparing ferrets as research subjects in the laboratory. *ILAR J.* 47(4):348–357.

Barnard, D.L. 2009. Animal models for the study of influenza pathogenesis and therapy. *Antiviral Res.* 82:A110–A122.

Batchelder, M., Fox, J.G., Hayward, A. et al. 1996. Natural and experimental *Helicobacter mustelae* reinfection following successful antimicrobial eradication in ferrets. *Helicobacter.* 1:34–42.

Baum, M.J. and Kelliher, K.R. 2009. Complementary roles of the main and accessory olfactory systems in mammalian mate recognition. *Ann Rev Physiol.* 71:141–160.

Belser, J.A., Katz, J.M., and Tumpey, T.M. 2011. The ferret as a model organism to study influenza A virus infection. *Dis Model Mech.* 4(5):575–579.

Beuschlein, F., Galac, S., and Wilson, D.B. 2012. Animal models of adrenocortical tumorigenesis. *Mol Cell Endocrinol.* 351:78–86.

Boari, A., Papa, V., DiSilverio, F. et al. 2010. Type 1 diabetes mellitus and hyperadrenocorticism in a ferret. *Vet Res Commun.* 34(Supp 1):S107–S110.

Byrd, L.G. and Prince, G.A. 1997. Animal models of respiratory syncytial virus infection. *Clin Infec Dis.* 25(6):1363–1368.

Chen, S. 2008. Pancreatic endocrinopathies in ferrets. *Vet Clin Exot Anim.* 11:107–123.

Chu, Y.K., Ali, G.D., Jia, F. et al. 2008. The SARS-CoV ferret model in an infection-challenge study. *Virol.* 374(1):151–163.

Cohen, J. 2012. The limits of avian flu studies in ferrets. *Science.* 335:512–513.

Colasurdo, G.N., Hemming, V.G., Prince, G.A. et al. 1998. Human respiratory syncytial virus produces prolonged alterations of neural control in airways of developing ferrets. *Am J Respir Crit Care Med.* 157:1506–1511.

Dalva, M.B. 2010. Remodeling of inhibitory synaptic connections in developing ferret visual cortex. *Neur Develop.* 5:5.

Danesh, A., Cameron, C.M., Leon, A.J. et al. 2011. Early gene expression events in ferrets in response to SARS coronavirus infection versus direct interferon-alpha2b stimulation. *Virol.* 409:102–112.

Danesh, A., Seneviratne, C., Cameron, C.M. et al. 2008. Cloning, expression and characterization of ferret CXCL10. *Mol Immunol.* 45(5):1288–1297.

Darnell, M.E., Plant, E.P., Watanabe, H. et al. 2007. Severe acute respiratory syndrome coronavirus infection in vaccinated ferrets. *J Infec Dis.* 196:1329–1338.

Del Giudice, G., Covacci, A., Telford, J.L. et al. 2001. The design of vaccines against *Helicobacter pylori* and their development. *Ann Rev Immunol.* 19:523–563.

Desmarchelier, M., Lair, S., Dunn, M. et al. 2008. Primary hyperaldosteronism in a domestic ferret with an adrenocortical adenoma. *J Am Vet Med Assoc.* 233:1297–1301.

Diaz, M.E., Graham,, H.K., and Trafford, A.W. 2004. Enhanced sarcolemmal Ca^{2+} efflux reduces sarcoplasmic reticulum Ca^{2+} content and systolic Ca^{2+} in cardiac hypertrophy. *Cardiovas Res.* 62:538–547.

Duffy, R.A., Morgan, C., Naylor, R. et al. 2012. Rolapitant (SCH 619734): A potent, selective and orally active neurokinin NK1 receptor antagonist with centrally-mediated antiemetic effects in ferrets. *Pharmacol Biochem Behav.* 102:95–100.

Du Sert, N.P., Holmes, A.M., Wallis, R. et al. 2012. Predicting the emetic liability of novel chemical entities: A comparative study. *Brit J Pharmacol.* 165:1848–1867.

Dyer, S.M. and Cervasio, D.L. 2008. An overview of restraint and blood collection techniques in exotic pet practice. *Vet Clin Exot Anim.* 11:423–443.

Eberhard, M.L. 1998. Use of the ferret in parasitologic research. In *Biology and Diseases of the Ferret.* Ed. J.G. Fox, 2nd edition, pp. 537–549. Baltimore, MD: Williams & Wilkins.

Esteves, M.I., Marini, R.P., Ryden, E.B. et al. 1994. Estimation of glomerular filtration rate and evaluation of renal function in ferrets (*Mustela putorius furo*). *Am J Vet Res.* 55(1):166–172.

Forrest, H.L., Khalenkov, A.M., Govorkova, E.A. et al. 2009. Single- and multiple-clade influenza A H5N1 vaccines induce cross protection in ferrets. *Vaccine.* 27:4187–4195.

Fox, J.G. 2014. Normal clinical and biologic parameters. In *Biology and Diseases of the Ferret.* Eds. J.G. Fox, and R.P. Marini, 3rd edition. Hoboken, NJ: Wiley.

Fox, J.G, Bell, J.A., and Broome, R. 2014. Growth, reproduction, and breeding. In *Biology and Diseases of the Ferret.* Eds. J.G. Fox, and R.P. Marini, 3rd edition. Hoboken, NJ: Wiley.

Fuentes-Santamaria, V., Alvarado, J.C., Henkel, C.K. et al. 2007. Cochlear ablation in adult ferrets results in changes in insulin-like growth factor-1 and synaptophysin immunostaining in the cochlear nucleus. *Neurosci.* 148:1033–1047.

Garibaldi, B.A., Pecquet-Goad, M.E., Fox, J.G. et al. 1988a. Serum cortisol radioimmunoassay values in the normal ferret and response to ACTH stimulation and dexamethasone suppression tests. Lab Anim Sci. 38(4):452–454.

Garibaldi, B.A., Pecquet-Goad, M.E., Fox, J.G. et al. 1988b. Serum thyroxine and triiodothyroxine radioimmunoassay values in the normal ferret. Lab Anim Sci. 38(4):455–458.

Garrett, L. 11 May, 2009. The path of a pandemic. *Newsweek.* 153(19–20):22–28.

Gautschi, M. and Clarke, P.G. 2007. Neuronal death in the lateral geniculate nucleus of young ferrets following a cortical lesion: Time-course, age dependence and involvement of caspases. *Brain Res.* 1167:20–30.

Geisbert, T.W., Feldman, H., and Broder, C.C. 2012. Animal challenge models of henipavirus infection and pathogenesis. *Curr Top Microbiol Immunol.* 359: 153–177.

Graham, H.K. and Trafford, A.W. 2007. Spatial disruption and enhanced degradation of collagen with the transition from compensated ventricular hypertrophy to symptomatic congestive heart failure. *Am J Physiol Heart Circ Physiol.* 292:H1364–H1372.

Hanlon, C.A., Kuzmin, I.V., Blanton, J.D. et al. 2005. Efficacy of rabies biologics against new lyssaviruses from Eurasia. *Virus Res.* 111(1):44–54.

Heard, D.J., Collins, B., Chen, D.L. et al. 1990. Thyroid and adrenal function tests in adult male ferrets. *Am J Vet Res.* 51(1):32–35.

Hoover, J.P. and Baldwin, C.A. 1988. Changes in physiologic and clinicopathologic values in domestic ferrets from 12 to 47 weeks of age. *Comp Anim Pract.* 2(1):40–44.

Jackson, S., van Hoeven, N., Chen, L. et al. 2009. Reassortment between avian H5N1 and human H3N2 influenza viruses in ferrets: A public health risk assessment. *J Virol.* 83(16):8131–8140. doi:10.1128/JVI.00534-09.

Ji, J., Bunnelle, W.H., Anderson, D.J. et al. 2007. A-366833: A novel nicotinonitrile-substituted 3,6-diazabicyclo(3.2.0)-heptane alpha4beta2 nicotinic acetylcholine receptor selective agonist: Synthesis, analgesic efficacy and tolerability in animal models. *Biochem Pharmacol.* 74(8):1253–1262.

Jian, B.J., Acernese, A.W., Lorenzo, J. et al. 2005. Afferent pathways to the region of the vestibular nuclei that participates in cardiovascular and respiratory control. *Brain Res.* 1044:241–250.

Kim, Y.H., Kim, H.S., Cho S.H. et al. 2009. Influenza B virus causes milder pathogenesis and weaker inflammatory responses in ferrets than influenza A virus. *Viral Immunol.* 22(6):423–430.

Kircher, S.S., Murray, L.E., and Juliano, M.L. 2009. Minimizing trauma to the upper airway: A ferret model of neonatal intubation. *J Am Assoc Lab Anim Sci.* 48(6):780–784.

Kiupel, M. and Perpinan, D. 2014. Viral diseases of ferrets. In *Biology and Diseases of the Ferret.* Eds. J.G. Fox, and R.P. Marini, 3rd edition. Hoboken, NJ: Wiley.

Ko, J. and Marini, R.P. 2014. Anesthesia. In *Biology and Diseases of the Ferret.* Eds. J.G. Fox, and R.P. Marini, 3rd edition. Hoboken, NJ: Wiley.

Koster, F., Gouveia, K., Zhou. Y. et al. 2012. Exhaled aerosol transmission of pandemic and seasonal H1N1 influenza viruses in the ferret. *PLoS One.* 7(4):1–14.

Kuehn, B.M. 2012. International debate erupts over research on potentially dangerous bird flu strains. *J Am Med Assoc.* 307(10):1009–1012.

Kugel, D., Kochs, G., Obojes, K. et al. 2009. Intranasal administration of alpha interferon reduced seasonal influenza A virus morbidity in ferrets. *J Virol.* 83(8):3843–3851.

Lee, C.M., Boileau, A.C., Boileau, T.W. et al. 1999. Review of models in carotenoid research. *J Nutr.* 129:2271–2277.

Lee, E.J., Moore, W.E., Fryer, H.C. et al. 1982. Haematological and serum chemistry profiles of ferrets (*Mustela putorius furo*). *Lab Anim.* 16:133–137.

Li, Z. and Englehardt, J.F. 2003. Progress towards generating a ferret model of cystic fibrosis by somatic cell nuclear transfer. *Reprod Biol Endocrinol.* 1:83.

Li, X., Fox, J.G., and Padrid, P.A. 1998. Neoplastic diseases in ferrets: 574 cases (1968–1997). *J Am Vet Assoc.* 183:1179–1181.

Lindeberg, H. 2008. Reproduction of the female ferret (*Mustela putorius furo*). 2008. *Reprod Dom Anim.* 43(2):150–156.

Luke, C.J. and Subbarao, K. 2008. The role of animal models in influenza vaccine research. In *Influenza Vaccines for the Future.* Eds. R. Rappuoli, and G. del Giudice, pp. 161–202. Basel: Birkhauser Verlag.

MacPhail, M., Schickli, J.H., Tang, R.S. et al. 2004. Identification of small-animal and primate models for evaluation of vaccine candidates for human metapneumovirus (hMPV) and implications for hMPV vaccine design. *J Gen Virol.* 85:1655–1663.

Maher, J.A. and DeStefano, J. 2004. The ferret: An animal model to study influenza virus. *Lab Anim.* 33(9):50–53.

Maines, T.R., Jayaraman, A., Belser, J.A. et al. 2009. Transmission and pathogenesis of swine-origin 2009 A(H1N1) influenza viruses in ferrets and mice. *Science.* 325(5939):484–487. doi: 10.1126/science.1177238.

Manning, D.D. and Bell, J.A. 1990. Lack of detectable blood groups in domestic ferrets: Implications for transfusion. *J Am Vet Assoc.* 197(1):84–86.

Marini, R.P. and Fox, J.G. 1999. Animal models of helicobacter (ferrets). In *Handbook of Animal Models of Infection*. Eds. O. Zak, and M. Sande, pp. 273–284. London: Academic Press.

Marini, R.P., Otto, G., Erdman, S. et al. 2002. Biology and diseases of ferrets. In *Laboratory Animal Medicine*. Eds. J.G. Fox, L.C. Anderson, F.M. Loew, and F.W. Quimby, 2nd edition, pp. 483–517. San Diego: Academic Press.

Marshall BioResources. 2014. Marshall BioResources. Available at: http://www.marshallbio.com. (Accessed 20 January, 2014).

Martina, B.E., Haagmans, B.L., Kuiken, T. et al. 2003. Virology: SARS virus infection of cats and ferrets. *Nature* 425:915.

Matsuoka, Y., Lamirande, E.W., and Subbarao, K. 2009. The ferret model for influenza. *Curr Prot Microbiol.* 15G.2.1–15G.2.29.

Maxwell, M.P., Hearse, D.J., and Yellon, D.M. 1987. Species variation in the coronary collateral circulation during regional myocardial ischaemia: A critical determinant of the rate of evolution and extent of myocardial infarction. *Cardiovas Res.* 21(10):737–746.

Middleton, D., Rockman, S., Pearse, M. et al. 2009. Evaluation of vaccines for H5N1 influenza virus in ferrets reveals the potential for protective single-shot immunization. *J Virol.* 83(15):7770–7778. doi:10.1128/JVI.00241-09.

Miwa, Y., Kurosawa, A., Ogawa, H. et al. 2009. Neoplastic diseases in ferrets in Japan: A questionnaire study for 2000 to 2005. *J Vet Med Sci.* 71(4):397–402.

Morgan, J.P. 2014. Use of the ferret in cardiovascular research. In *Biology and Diseases of the Ferret*. Eds. J.G. Fox, and R.P. Marini, 3rd edition. Hoboken, NJ: Wiley.

Munster, V.J., de Wit, E., van den Brand. J.M. et al. 2009. Pathogenesis and transmission of swine-origin 2009 A(H1N1) influenza virus in ferrets. *Science.* 325(5939):481–483. doi:10.1126/science.1177127.

Neal, J., Takahashi, M., Silva, M. et al. 2007. Insights into the gyrification of developing ferret brain by magnetic resonance imaging. *J Anat.* 210(1):66–77.

Nedrud, J.G. and Blanchard, T.G. 2003. Helicobacter animal models. *Curr Prot Immunol.* Unit 19.8.

Nielsen, O., Smith, G., Weingartl, H. et al. 2008. Use of SLAM transfected Vero cell line to isolate and characterize marine mammal morbilliviruses using an experimental ferret model. *J Wildl Dis.* 44(3):600–611.

Ochi, A., Danesh, A., Seneviratne, C. et al. 2008. Cloning, expression and immunoassay detection of ferret IFN-γ. *Develop Comp Immunol.* 32:890–897.

Onishi, T., Mori, T., Yanagihara, M. et al. 2007. Similarities of the neuronal circuit for the induction of fictive vomiting between ferrets and dogs. *Autonom Neurosci.* 136:20–30.

Osinski, M.A., Uchic, M.E., Seifert, T. et al. 2005. Dopamine D_2, but not D_4, receptor agonists are emetogenic in ferrets. *Pharmacol Biochem Behav.* 81(1):211–219.

Otto, G., Rosenblad, W.D., and Fox, J.G. 1993. Practical venipuncture techniques for the ferret. *Lab Anim.* 27:26–29.

Patterson, A.R., Cooper, V.L., Yoon, K. et al. 2009. Naturally occurring influenza infection in a ferret (*Mustela putorius furo*) colony. *J Vet Diagn Invest.* 21:527–530.

Patterson, M.M., O'Toole, P.W., Forester, N.T. et al. 2003. Failure of surface ring mutant strains of *Helicobacter mustelae* to persistently infect the ferret stomach. *Infec Immun.* 71(5):2350–2355.

Peltola, V.T., Boyd, K.L., McAuley, J.L. et al. 2006. Bacterial sinusitis and otitis media following influenza infection in ferrets. *Infect Immun.* 74:2562–2567.

Perpinan, D., Ramis, A., Tomas, A. et al. 2008. Outbreak of canine distemper in domestic ferrets (*Mustela putorius furo*). *Vet Rec.* 163(8):246–250.

Perrone, L.A., Ahmad, A., Veguilla, V. et al. 2009. Intranasal vaccination with 1918 influenza virus-like particles protects mice and ferrets from lethal 1918 and H5N1 influenza virus challenge. *J Virol.* 83(11):5726–5734.

Perrott, M.R., Sigurdson, C.J., Mason, G.L. et al. 2012. Evidence for distinct chronic wasting disease (CWD) strains in experimental CWD in ferrets. *J Gen Virol.* 93:212–221.

Phair, K.A., Carpenter, J.W., Schermerhorn, T. et al. 2011. Diabetic ketoacidosis with concurrent pancreatitis, pancreatic β islet cell tumor, and adrenal disease in an obese ferret (*Mustela putorius furo*). *J Am Assoc Lab Anim Sci.* 50(4):531–535.

Pillet, S., Svitek, N., and von Messling, V. 2009. Ferrets as a model for morbillivirus pathogenesis, complications, and vaccines. *Curr Top Microbiol Immunol.* 73–87.

Platt, S.R., Dennis, P.M., McSherry, L.J. et al. 2004. Composition of cerebrospinal fluid in clinically normal adult ferrets. *Am J Vet Res.* 65(6):758–760.

Quesenberry, K.E. and Orcutt, C. 2012. Basic approach to veterinary care. In *Ferrets, Rabbits, and Rodents: Clinical Medicine and Surgery*. Eds. K.E. Quesenberry, and J.W. Carpenter, pp. 13–26. St. Louis, MO: Saunders.

Raila, J., Gomez, C., and Schweigert, F.J. 2002. The ferret as a model for vitamin A metabolism in carnivores. *J Nutr.* 132:1787S–1789S.

Roberts, A., Lamirande, E.W., Vogel, L. et al. 2007. Animal models and vaccines for SARS-CoV infection. *Virus Res.* 133(1):20–32.

Rodeheffer, C., von Messling, V., Milot, S. et al. 2007. Disease manifestations of canine distemper virus infection in ferrets are modulated by vitamin A status. *J Nutr.* 137:1916–1922.

Rosenthal, K.L. and Peterson, M.E. 1996. Evaluation of plasma androgen and estrogen concentrations in ferrets with hyperadrenocorticism. *J Am Vet Med Assoc.* 209:1097–1102.

Rosenthal K.L. and Wyre, N.R. 2012. Endocrine diseases. In *Ferrets, Rabbits, and Rodents: Clinical Medicine and Surgery*. Eds. K.E. Quesenberry, and J.W. Carpenter, pp. 86–102. St. Louis, MO: Saunders.

Russell, R.M. 2004. The enigma of ß-carotene in carcinogenesis: What can be learned from animal studies. *J Nutr.* 134:262S–268S.

Rutigliano, J.A., Doherty, P.C., Franks J. et al. 2008. Screening monoclonal antibodies for cross-reactivity in the ferret model of influenza infection. *J Immunol Methods.* 336:71–77.

Ryland, L.M. and Bernard, S.L. 1983. A clinical guide to the pet ferret. *Comp Cont Educ Pract Vet.* 5(1):25–32.

Saif, M.W., Berk, G., Chen Y.C. et al. 2007. IpdR: A novel oral radiosensitizer. *Expert Opin Investig Drugs.* 16(9):1415–1424.

Sawatsky, B., Wong, X., Hinkelmann, S. et al. 2012. Canine distemper virus epithelial cell infection is required for clinical disease but not for immunosuppression. *J Virol.* 86(7):3658–3666.

Schoemaker, N.J., Kuijten, A.M., and Galac, S. 2008. Luteinizing hormone-dependent Cushing's syndrome in a pet ferret (*Mustela putorius furo*). *Domes Anim Endocrinol.* 34:278–283.

Schoemaker, N.J., Mol, J.A., Lumeij, J.T. et al. 2002. Plasma concentrations of adrenocorticotrophic hormone and α-melanocyte-stimulating hormone in ferrets (*Mustela putorius furo*) with hyperadrenocorticism. *Am J Vet Res.* 63(10):1395–1399.

Schoemaker, N.J., Wolfswinkel, J., Mol, J.A. et al. 2004. Urinary glucocorticoid excretion in the diagnosis of hyperadrenocorticism in ferrets. *Domes Anim Endocrinol.* 27:13–24.

See, R.H., Petric, M., Lawrence, D.J. et al. 2008. Severe acute respiratory syndrome vaccine efficacy in ferrets: whole killed virus and adenovirus-vectored vaccines. *J Gen Virol.* 89:2136–2146.

Senchak, A.J., Sato, A.K., Vazquez R. et al. 2007. Characterization of transforming growth factors β1 and 2 in ferrets (*Mustela putorius furo*). *Comp Med.* 57(6):594–596.

Sengpiel, F. and Kind, P.C. 2002. The role of activity in development of the visual system. *Curr Biol.* 12(23):R818–R826.

Shoji, Y., Bi, H., Musiychuk, K. et al. 2009. Plant-derived hemagglutinin protects ferrets against challenge infection with the A/Indonesia/05/05 strain of avian influenza. *Vaccine.* 27:1087–1092.

Simone-Freilicher, E. 2008. Adrenal gland disease in ferrets. *Vet Clin Exot Anim.* 11:125–137.

Siperstein, L.J. 2008. Ferret hematology and related disorders. *Vet Clin Exot Anim.* 11:535–550.

Smith, W., Andrewes, C.H., and Laidlaw, P.P. 1933. A virus obtained from influenza patients. *Lancet* . 222(5732):66–68.

Solnick, J.V. and Schauer, D.B. 2001. Emergence of diverse *Helicobacter* species in the pathogenesis of gastric and enterohepatic disease. *Clin Microbiol Rev.* 14(1):59–97.

Sun, X., Sui, H., Fisher, J.T. et al. 2010. Disease phenotype of a ferret *CRTR*-knockout model of cystic fibrosis. *J Clin Invest.* 120(9):3149–3160.

Sun, X., Yan, Z., Yi, Y. et al. 2008. Adeno-associated virus-targeted disruption of the CFTR gene in cloned ferrets. *J Clin Invest.* 118(4):1578–1583.

Sur, M. and Leamey, C.A. 2001. Development and plasticity of cortical areas and networks. *Nat Rev-Neurosci.* 2:251–262.

Sutton, P. and Lee, A. 2001. *Helicobacter pylori* vaccines—The current status. *Alimen Pharmacol Therap.* 14(9):1107–1118.

Svitek, N., Rudd, P.A., Obojes, K. et al. 2008. Severe seasonal influenza correlates with reduced interferon and increased IL-6 induction. *Virol.* 376:53–59.

Swennes, A.G. and Fox, J.G. 2014. Bacterial and mycoplasmal diseases. In *Biology and Diseases of the Ferret*. Eds. J.G. Fox, and R.P. Marini, 3rd edition, pp.519–552. Hoboken, NJ: Wiley.

Ter Meulen, J., Bakker, A.B., van den Brink, E.N. et al. 2004. Human monoclonal antibody as prophylaxis for SARS coronavirus infection in ferrets. *Lancet.* 363:2139–2141.

Thornton, P.C., Wright, P.A., Sacra, P.J. et al. 1979. The ferret, *Mustela putorius furo*, as a new species in toxicology. *Lab Anim.* 13:119–124.

van den Brand, J.M., Haagmans, B.L., Leijten, L. et al. 2008. Pathology of experimental SARS coronavirus infection in cats and ferrets. *Vet Pathol.* 45:551–562.

van der Laan, J.W., Herberts, C., Lambkin-Williams, R. et al. 2008. Animal models in influenza vaccine testing. *Expert Rev Vacc.* 7(6):783–793.

van Riel, D., Munster, V.J., de Wit, E. et al. 2006. H5N1 virus attachment to lower respiratory tract. *Science.* 312:399.

Van Sickle, M.D., Oland, L.D., Mackie, K. et al. 2003. Δ^9-Tetrahydrocannabinol selectively acts on CB_1 receptors in specific regions of dorsal vagal complex to inhibit emesis in ferrets. *Am J Physiol Gastrointest Liver Physiol.* 285:G566–G576.

Vos, A., Muller, T., Cox, J. et al. 2004. Susceptibility of ferrets (*Mustela putorius furo*) to experimentally induced rabies with European bat lyssaviruses (EBLV). *J Vet Med.* 51:55–60.

Wang, X.D., Russell, R.M., Marini, R.P. et al. 1993. Intestinal perfusion of ß-carotene in the ferret raised retinoic acid level in portal blood. *Biochim Biophys Acta.* 1167:159–164.

Watanabe, T., Watanabe, S., Shinya, K. et al. 2009. Viral RNA polymerase complex promotes optimal growth of 1918 virus in the lower respiratory tract of ferrets. *Proc Natl Acad Sci.* 106(2):588–92.

Webster, P. and Kapel, C.M. 2005. Studies on the vertical transmission of *Trichinella* spp. in experimentally infected ferrets (*Mustela putorius furo*), foxes (*Vulpes vulpes*), pigs, guinea pigs and mice. *Vet Parasitol.* 130:255–262.

Weingartl, H., Czub, M., Czub, S. et al. 2004. Immunization with modified vaccinia virus Ankara-based recombinant vaccine against severe acute respiratory syndrome is associated with enhanced hepatitis in ferrets. *J Virol.* 78(22):12672–12676.

Weliky, M. 2000. Correlated neuronal activity and visual cortical development. *Neuron.* 27(3):427–430.

Whary, M.T. 2014. Physiology of the ferret. In *Biology and Diseases of the Ferret.* Eds. J.G. Fox, and R.P. Marini, 3rd edition. Hoboken, NJ: Wiley.

Whary, M.T. and Fox, J.G. 2004. Natural and experimental *Helicobacter* infections. *Comp Med.* 54:128–158.

Zitzow, L.A., Rowe, T., Morken, T. et al. 2002. Pathogenesis of avian influenza A (H5N1) in ferrets. *J Virol.* 76(9):4420–4429.

10 The Laboratory Zebrafish and Other Fishes

Claudia Harper

CONTENTS

10.1 USE OF FISH IN BIOMEDICAL RESEARCH

The zebrafish, *Danio rerio*, is a freshwater fish originally found in South Asia, with distributions ranging from India, Bangladesh, Nepal, Myanmar, and Pakistan (Lawrence, 2007). They are cyprinids omnivorous poikilothermes and have been used in research for the past 100 years but more extensively since the mid-1970s (Lieschke and Currie, 2007; Sullivan and Kim, 2008). The zebrafish shares many biological attributes with other vertebrates, and it is well suited as a vertebrate integrated organ system model.

Due to the zebrafish's biological attributes and the ability to transfer well-established techniques in embryology, genetics, and molecular biology, researchers have used zebrafish to study a wide range of subjects including genetics, vertebrate development, proteomics, behavior, aging, immunology, toxicology, cancer, neurobiology, drug discovery, and infectious diseases (Berghams et al., 2005; Dovey and Zon, 2009; Drabsch et al., 2016; Bambino and Chu, 2017; Matsui, 2017; Gerhard, 2007; Grunwald and Eisen, 2002; Keller and Murtha, 2004; Onnebo et al., 2004; Trede et al., 2004; Alvarez et al., 2007; Lieschke and Currie, 2007; Nakatani et al., 2007; Schilling and

Webb, 2007; Amatruda and Patton, 2008; Barros et al., 2008; Meeker and Trede, 2008; Sullivan and Kim, 2008; Ellett and Lieschke, 2010; Anderson et al., 2011; Chan and Mably, 2011; Löhr and Hammerschmidt, 2011; Sipes et al., 2011; Gaikwad et al., 2011; Goldsmith and Jobin, 2012; Quaife et al., 2012; Genge et al., 2016; Luderman et al., 2017; Schledgel, 2016). They are used in large-scale genetic screens to identify mutants based on identifying abnormal development and phenotypes (Feitsma and Cuppen, 2008; Hao et al., 2010; Wolman and Granato, 2012). Since the model was originally developed, fundamental progress has been made, making the model even more attractive to researchers. For example, some breakthroughs include the Sanger Institute zebrafish genome sequencing project; availability of full-length cDNAs and DNA microarrays for expression analysis; techniques for generating transgenic lines and targeted mutations; and suitability for functional genomic and phenotypic screens.

The first animal model of congenital sideroblastic anemia was the zebrafish mutant, sauternes (au), which develops microcytic, hypochromic anemia (Brownlie et al., 1998). The zebrafish is the first genetically accurate model of hepatoerythropoietic porphyria that can be used to study the pathogenesis of uroporphyrinogen decarboxylase (UROD) deficiency (Wang et al., 1998). A zebrafish model for the Shwachman–Diamond syndrome (SDS) has been developed (Venkatasubramani and Mayer, 2008). SDS is characterized by exocrine pancreatic insufficiency, neutrophil defect, and skeletal abnormalities. The use of morpholino-mediated gene knockdown technology lead to the loss of nucleolar protein called the Shwachman–Bodian–Diamond syndrome (SBDS) protein in the zebrafish, generating a model system where gene function and novel therapies can be evaluated (Venkatasubramani and Mayer, 2008).

This field is rapidly evolving and provides fundamental information on the formation and function of vertebrate biology, providing insight into mechanisms of human disease (Grunwald and Eisen, 2002; Ingham, 2009; Löhr and Hammerschmidt, 2011; Genge et al., 2017; Matrone et al., 2017). One of the major advantages of working with zebrafish is that they produce a large number of synchronously developing, transparent embryos enabling real-time imaging of developing pathologies. Zebrafish genome has been sequenced; they have a short generation time; they are easily accessible and are amendable to high throughput analysis, making them suitable for large-scale mutagenesis and screening studies, which are not readily available in other vertebrate systems (Wen et al., 2012; Wittmann et al., 2012). The Japanese medaka, *Oryzias latipes*, is another aquatic vertebrate model which is also a small, egg-laying freshwater teleost. Primary research applications of the Japanese medaka include ecotoxicology, developmental genetics, genomics, and evolutionary biology studies. The genome sequence of the medaka inbred strain, Hd-rR, has been completed (Kobayashi and Takeda, 2008; Takeda, 2008).

The cardiovascular system of the zebrafish has been extensively studied since the heart is easily visualized at 72 hours post-fertilization and many of the molecular, cellular, and electrophysiological mechanisms underlying cardiovascular development and function have been conserved in vertebrate evolution (Baker et al., 1997; Milan et al., 2006; Rubinstein, 2006; Arnaout et al., 2007; Milan and Macrae, 2008). As a consequence, many mutations impacting the cardiovascular system have been studied in embryos, and most of the research focusing on the formation, function, anatomy, hemodynamics, and gene expression of the cardiovascular system has been pursued in both the embryo and adult zebrafish (Genge et al., 2016; Matrone et al., 2017; Saffitz, 2017; Burns et al., 2005; Milan et al., 2006). One classic example is the mutation in the slow mo gene in zebrafish where the inwardly directed hyperpolarizing pacemaker current is reduced, leading to bradycardia (Baker et al., 1997; Briggs, 2002).

Zebrafish are oviparous and can easily breed year round in a laboratory setting. Females lay eggs that are then fertilized externally, and the embryos are transparent during organogenesis, enabling visual assessment of their development in real time (Vogt et al., 2009; Yang et al., 2009). Screening for specific phenotypes is possible since embryonic development occurs in full view. Furthermore, they can produce a large number of embryos, and depending on the zebrafish lines, husbandry practices, and diet, their clutch size can range from 100 to 300 embryos per week (Spence et al., 2008). Their generation time is approximately 3 months (Lieschke and Currie, 2007).

Zebrafish eggs and adults are small. At fertilization, the eggs measure approximately 0.7 mm in diameter, and adults measure approximately <120 mm total length (Spence et al., 2008). They are easy to maintain in laboratory settings, can adapt to a wide range of environmental parameters, and require less space than other *in vivo* models and can be housed at higher densities compared to other research animals. It is estimated that the cost of husbandry when working with mice compared to zebrafish is between 1:100 and 1:1000 (Goldsmith, 2004). There are many zebrafish wild type lines used for research and most are described on the Zebrafish Information Network (www.ZFIN.org; Trevarrow and Robison, 2004).

Clinical chemistry is a diagnostic and research tool commonly used in mammals. Clinical chemistry techniques and values have been established in many different fish used for production or environmental conservation program (Ellsaesser and Clem, 1987; Houston, 1990; Bullis, 1993; Axelsson and Fritsches, 1994; Roche and Boge, 1996; Groff and Zinkl, 1999; Jagadeeswaran et al., 1999; Hrubec and Smith, 1999, 2000, 2004; Black, 2000; Congleton and LaVoie, 2001; Dye et al., 2001; Sakomoto et al., 2001; Harms et al., 2002; Greenwell et al., 2003; Murtha et al., 2003; Asadi et al., 2006; Caldwell et al., 2006; Knowles et al., 2006; Reavill, 2006; Elo et al., 2007; Mauel et al., 2007; Tavares-Dias and Moraes, 2007; Zhou et al., 2009). However, the use of clinical chemistry in the research of laboratory fish such as medaka and zebrafish is not common due to the challenges associated with sample collection, small sample size, and lack of procedural standardization.

Zebrafish physiology is affected by stress, disease, water chemistry, and nutrition (Groff and Zinkl, 1999; Bayne and Gerwick, 2001; Briggs, 2002; Evans et al., 2005; Craig et al., 2007; Ramsay et al., 2006, 2009; Harper and Wolf, 2009; Siccardi et al., 2009; Cachat et al., 2010). This chapter reviews current literature focusing on clinical chemistry values, sample collection techniques, as well as preanalytical sources of variation known to impact fish physiology, clinical chemistry, and genetics. Most of the information gathered for this chapter focuses on freshwater fish in an attempt to highlight the need to establish clinical chemistry baselines to promote good research data, minimize variability, and for health monitoring.

Electrolyte values vary between fish species, health status, and water chemistry. Sodium and chloride in conjunction with a hemogram can indicate the hydration status of the fish (Groff and Zinkl, 1999). Sodium and chloride are important in fish osmoregulation and are found in a 1:1 ratio; however, the concentration of sodium is commonly greater than chloride concentration (Groff and Zinkl, 1999).

10.2 METHODOLOGY FOR SAMPLE COLLECTION

Common procedures used in other mammalian models have not yet been standardized or developed in zebrafish, since the model has been primarily developed to study genetics and gene function in embryos and larvae. Very few articles have been published on clinical chemistry of zebrafish and to date, no publications were found pertaining to adrenocorticotropin hormone (ACTH) stimulation, bile acids, bromosulphthalein (BSP) clearance, insulin clearance, thyroid-stimulating hormone (TSH) stimulation, ammonia tolerance, and dexamethasone suppression test in zebrafish. There are several important reviews which focus on clinical chemistry and procedures in fish (Ellsaesser and Clem, 1987; Houston, 1990; Groff and Zinkl, 1999; Greenwell et al., 2003). Groff and Zinkl (1999) wrote a review of clinical chemistry of cyprinid fish focusing on koi, carp, and goldfish. Since zebrafish are cyprinids, this review highlights some similar patterns between gold fish and carp which are also cyprinids. A review of blood collection techniques for biochemical analysis in adult zebrafish has been published (Pedroso et al., 2012).

10.2.1 Blood Collection

Fish clinical chemistry is a valuable tool in disease diagnosis but lacks the nomenclature and procedural standardization that exist with mammalian clinical chemistry. Compared to other mammalian species, clinical chemistry is not routinely performed in fish species; however, significant research has been done to develop the knowledge necessary to collect samples in fish (Ellsaesser and Clem, 1987; Houston, 1990; Bullis, 1993; Axelsson and Fritsches, 1994; Roche and Boge, 1996; Groff and Zinkl, 1999; Hrubec and Smith, 1999, 2000, 2004; Jagadeeswaran et al., 1999; Black, 2000; Congleton and LaVoie, 2001; Dye et al., 2001; Sakomoto et al., 2001; Harms et al., 2002; Greenwell et al., 2003; Murtha et al., 2003; Asadi et al., 2006; Caldwell et al., 2006; Reavill, 2006; Tavares-Dias and Moraes, 2007; Elo et al., 2007; Borges et al., 2007; Pedroso et al., 2012). Although laboratory fish such as medaka and zebrafish are small, phlebotomy can be performed (Jagadeeswaran et al., 1999; Murtha et al., 2003; Onnebo et al., 2004; Elo et al., 2007; Pedroso et al., 2012).

Clinical chemistry in fish can be performed using either serum or plasma. Serum and plasma are the fluid component of blood and the clotting factors are found in plasma and not in serum (Hrubec and Smith, 1999). In mammals, clinical chemistry results from serum or plasma are very similar when samples are handled in a standardized manner. Evaluating the similarity and differences between the use of plasma and serum on the effect on measured blood analytes has not been studied in zebrafish, though. However, it has been assessed in rainbow trout *Oncorhynchus mykiss*, channel catfish *Ictalurus punctatus*, hybrid tilapia *Oreochromis* spp., and hybrid striped bass to name a few (Hrubec and Smith, 1999; Hrubec et al., 2000). Further details pertaining to the differences between plasma and serum on clinical chemistry are discussed in Section 10.3.

10.2.1.1 Primary Sites for Collection

Blood samples can be collected in fish from the dorsal aorta, heart, and caudal vein. The primary site of collection should be determined based on the size of the fish and the sample volume required. In smaller fish such as medaka and zebrafish, blood sampling is a terminal procedure and the common blood collection sites include the dorsal aorta, heart, and caudal vein (Eames et al., 2010; Pedroso et al., 2012). In larger fish, such as salmon, trout, or tilapia, the most common blood collection sites are the caudal vein and heart (Noga, 1996; Jagadeeswaran et al., 1999; Black, 2000).

In zebrafish, blood collection from the dorsal aorta requires anesthesia as discussed in Section 10.2.1.2. The anesthetized fish is placed on a flat surface or restrained in one's hand. A transverse incision measuring 0.3–0.5 cm in depth is made posterior to the dorsal fin by using a sharp pair of scissors (Jagadeeswaran et al., 1999; Murtha et al., 2003; Pedroso et al., 2012). The blood pools from the incision site and it is collected with a micropipette tip or a capillary tube. The risk with this technique is sample contamination from the incision site or a perforated gastrointestinal tract (Jagadeeswaran et al., 1999; Murtha et al., 2003).

In larger fish, collecting blood from the caudal vein is the most commonly used technique and the least traumatic (Noga, 1996; Groff and Zinkl, 1999; Black, 2000). The caudal vessels can be accessed using a ventral or a lateral approach using a 25 or 22 G needle depending on the size of the animal. Pretreating the needle with heparin can minimize coagulation (Reavill, 2006). The needle is inserted ventrally through the skin near the base of the caudal peduncle until firm resistance is felt and then the needle is redirected ventrally and laterally while gently aspirating (Noga, 1996). Depending on the size of the animal, the blood sample can be collected into a syringe or transferred into a heparinized capillary tube from the hub of the needle (Groff and Zinkl, 1999). In contrast, due to the small diameter of the zebrafish caudal vein, the vessel cannot be accessed using a syringe and needle. However, it can be accessed by severing the base of the tail with a scalpel blade in deeply anesthetized or euthanized zebrafish. A heparinized capillary tube is applied on the caudal vessels and blood sample collection is enabled by capillary action (Noga, 1996). Tissue fluid contamination and dilution may impact results if the sample is used for clinical chemistry

(Ikeda and Ozaki, 1981; Noga, 1996; Congleton and LaVoie, 2001). In zebrafish, the blood volume collected from the caudal vein is very small due to rapid clotting.

Black (2000) described a technique for blood collection in very small fish such as medaka or mosquitofish. The fish are anesthetized with MS-222 and submerged with 70% ethanol (Iwama and Ackerman, 1994). The caudal peduncle is severed with sterile scissors. The fish is immediately placed head-up in a 10 mm × 75 mm polyethylene tube (PE) tube with 1 mL sterile physiological saline solution. The blood pools at the bottom of the tube as the tube is delicately swirled. After cessation of the blood flow, the fish is removed with sterile forceps. The content of the tube is then transferred into a conical microcentrifuge tube and centrifuged at 16,000 rpm for 1 minute (Black, 2000). The physiological saline is decanted and the red blood cells (RBCs) are resuspended in 1 mL of physiological saline and centrifuged again at 16,000 rpm. After centrifugation, the supernatant is decanted and the RBC can be used for biochemical analyses such as DNA strand length determination (Black, 2000).

Cardiocentesis (also referred to as cardiac puncture) is another method of blood collection, which has been used to collect blood in small and large fish. This technique should only be used for terminal blood sample collection (Noga, 1996; Black, 2000; Eames et al., 2010; Harper and Lawrence, 2010). The heart is located in the posterior edge of the gills and cardiocentesis is performed in anesthetized animals which are positioned in dorsal recumbancy to access the heart ventrally. Cardiocentesis in larger fish such as catfish and trout can be performed using a 23 G needle attached to a syringe, which is inserted on the linea alba on the ventral midline between the pectoral fins directly into the heart (Black, 2000). Zebrafish hearts are very small. For example, a 1-year-old fish with body length ranging from 3 to 4 cm have hearts 1–2 mm in length with a diameter of 1 mm (Sun et al., 2008).

In small fish, the heart can be exposed by performing a ventral incision between the pectoral fins using scissors (Groff and Zinkl, 1999). This helps in visualizing the heart, minimizes the risk of excessive tissue damage, and reduces contamination of the blood sample with epidermal cells and body fluids that may impact clinical chemistry results. For zebrafish, a micropipette tip is then directly inserted in the ventricle. The blood sample can become hemolysed if the ventricle collapses and air is suctioned into the tip while the sample is being collected (Reavill, 2006).

Alternatively, whole blood can be collected in anesthetized or euthanized zebrafish by decapitation by transecting through the pectoral girdle with scissors. The incision is made immediately anterior to the articulation of the pectoral fin with the girdle that severs the heart, and blood is collected by holding a microcapillary tube adjacent to the heart (Eames et al., 2010).

Serial sampling techniques can be used in large fish species such as salmon, trout, and catfish. Blood can be collected from either restrained or free-swimming fish. In addition to repetitive individual collection of blood samples, several blood vessels in fish can be cannulated for long-term studies which require serial blood collection. Some of the most commonly cannulated vessels include the dorsal aorta, the ventral aorta, and caudal vein (Houston, 1990; Sohlberg et al., 1996; Black, 2000).

10.2.1.2 Methods of Restraint

Optimization of fish blood sampling techniques may require either immobilization under anesthesia and/or the use of physical restraint. Although fish can be restrained physically without anesthesia, the stress associated with the capture, handling, and restraint can affect physiological responses and clinical chemistry values (Torres et al., 1986; Ellsaesser and Clem, 1987; Bullis, 1993; Groff and Zinkl, 1999; Greenwell et al., 2003; Dror et al., 2006; Crosby et al., 2006; Ramsay et al., 2006, 2009; Gravel and Vijayan, 2007; Alsop and Vijayan, 2008; Liu et al., 2008; Cachat et al., 2010). Therefore, the use of anesthesia during phlebotomy is recommended in order to reduce clinical chemistry variables associated with stress.

Fish can be restrained manually or with a device which stabilizes the position of the anesthetized fish by maintaining the animal in dorsal or ventral recumbancy. Depending on the size of the fish, a sponge or piece of styrofoam with a V-shaped groove can be used to stabilize the fish (Wooster et al., 1993; Harms, 2005; Harper and Lawrence, 2010).

There is a large body of literature which indicates that the use of anesthetics can impact the physiology of teleost fish and clinical chemistry (Randall, 1962; King et al., 2005; Rothwell and Forster, 2005; Rothwell et al., 2005; Crosby et al., 2006; Palić et al., 2006). Further details pertaining to the impact of anesthetics on clinical chemistry are discussed in the "Anesthesia" section of this chapter.

The most commonly used anesthetic in fish is Finquel (Argent Chemical Laboratories, Inc., Redmond, Washington) which is commercially available as TMS. Finquel is also known as MS-222, MESAB, Tricaine, 3-amino benzoic acid ethyl ester, and ethyl 3-aminobenzoate (Brown, 1993; Iwama and Ackerman, 1994). MS-222 is the only anesthetic and sedative agent approved for use with food fish by the US Food and Drug Administration and is recommended by the American Veterinary Medical Association (AVMA) Guidelines on Euthanasia. Although there are many other anesthetics used in fish, they will not be discussed in this chapter (Iwama and Ackerman, 1994; Noga, 1996; AVMA, 2007; NIH, 2009).

A large portion of this section will focus on providing background on MS-222 since it is used by most zebrafish laboratories when collecting blood samples. MS-222 is a benzocaine derivative with an additional sulphonate radical which makes it water soluble and also acidic. It is sold as a white crystalline powder and needs to be reconstituted in water. When working with MS-222 in the powder form, caution must be taken to prevent inhaling the powder, or exposing mucous membranes and eyes. The action of the benzoic acid derivative is affected by both water temperature and water hardness (Houston and Woods, 1976). Its action is decreased in cooler temperatures and in soft water conditions (low alkalinity). MS-222 is absorbed across the gills. In salmonids, MS-222 is metabolized by acetylation and excreted in urine 24 hours after administration and no residues are detectable (Houston, 1990; Burka et al., 1997).

According to the manufacturer (Argent Chemical Laboratory), reconstituted MS-222 stored at room temperature showed no significant loss of potency after 3 days but the potency decreases after 10 days. Many research laboratories reconstitute MS-222 in water and make a concentrated stock solution which is then aliquoted into small vials and frozen, although no published information was found regarding impact of freezing on potency/activity of stock solution. The stock solution should not be buffered with sodium bicarbonate unless it is used immediately as this can cause dissociation of the sulfonate group (Houston, 1990; Noga, 1996). MS-222 is light sensitive, and the solution may change color if it is exposed to light. If this is noted, the solution should be discarded (Iwama and Ackerman, 1994; Noga, 1996). The unbuffered MS-222 stock solution should be stored in an opaque container and then frozen.

One of the critical factors when using MS-222 is managing the buffering capacity of the water. Distilled water and reverse osmosis water have little or no buffering capacity and should not be used when reconstituting MS-222. Water with no buffering capacity has zero alkalinity. Alkalinity is needed to neutralize acid and maintain a neutral pH. Because MS-222 is acidic, water solutions with $CaCO_3$ levels <50 mg/L should be buffered with sodium bicarbonate. Otherwise the anesthetic or euthanasia solution can lead to acidosis in fish as the water pH can decrease to 5 (Houston, 1990; Noga, 1996). This has a direct impact on the animal's welfare and physiology.

Different buffering agents are suitable and include sodium bicarbonate and sodium hydroxide (Noga, 1996; Rombough, 2007). Sodium bicarbonate should be added to the solution at a ratio of 2:1 [sodium bicarbonate (wt):tricaine (wt)] and adjusted to a pH of 7 (Noga, 1996). The fish are immersed in buffered water with dissolved MS-222, and the water concentration of MS-222 is usually higher than the levels in the fish (Allen and Hunn, 1986; Burka et al., 1997). MS-222 is readily absorbed across the gills and cannot be administered by injection since the MS-222 will be eliminated via the gills (Burka et al., 1997).

Induction and recovery times are inversely correlated with body weight where the effect is greater in smaller fish (Houston and Woods, 1976; Iwama and Ackerman, 1994).

The most common method of euthanasia in zebrafish embryos, larvae, and adults is by immersing the animals in a buffered solution of MS-222. The MS-222 concentration needed for anesthesia or euthanasia in fish is both species and age dependent (Brown, 1993; Bullis, 1993; Stoskopf, 1993; Iwama and Ackerman, 1994; Massee et al., 1995; Noga, 1996; Rombough, 2007; Westerfield, 2007). The age, species, and duration of anesthetic exposures must be taken into account when using commonly recommended anesthetics in fish (Gilderhus and Marking, 1987; Rombough, 2007; Macova et al., 2008). Euthanasia methods used with laboratory zebrafish should be consistent with the latest AVMA Guidelines on Euthanasia (2007) which recommend a concentrated solution of buffered MS-222 (e.g., 200–500 mg/L) for adult fish for 5–10 minutes following the cessation of opercular movement.

The National Institutes of Health (NIH) has provided a comprehensive review of age-specific euthanasia guidelines for zebrafish (NIH, 2009). For zebrafish older than 8 days post-fertilization (dpf), an overdose of MS-222 (200–300 mg/L) by prolonged immersion for non-survival procedures can be used. The fish should be left in the solution for at least 10 minutes following cessation of opercular movement (NIH, 2009). Necropsy can be initiated 5–10 minutes after cessation of opercular movement.

Another protocol recommended for zebrafish ≥8 dpf is anesthetizing the fish with MS-222 (168 mg/L) followed by rapid freezing in liquid nitrogen (NIH, 2009). Zebrafish ≥8 dpf can be immobilized for euthanasia by submersion in ice water (5 parts ice/1 part water, 0–4°C) for at least 10 minutes following cessation of opercular movement (NIH, 2009). In any fish where it is difficult to visualize opercular movement, fish should be left in the ice water for at least 20 minutes after cessation of all movement to ensure death by hypoxia. For zebrafish 4–7 dpf, immobilization for euthanasia by submersion in ice water (5 parts ice/1 part water, 0–4°C) for at least 20 minutes can be used to ensure death by hypoxia (NIH, 2009). Another protocol recommended by the NIH (2009) for zebrafish 4–7 dpf is the addition of bleach solution (sodium hypochlorite 6.15%) to the culture system water at 1 part bleach to 5 parts water. They should remain in this solution at least 5 minutes prior to disposal to ensure death. As detailed in the scientific background section of the NIH guidelines, pain perception has not developed at these earlier stages so this is not considered a painful procedure (NIH, 2009). For zebrafish embryos ≤3 dpf, development should be terminated using bleach as described with for zebrafish 4–7 dpf (NIH, 2009).

There are other references specific for zebrafish anesthesia and euthanasia. The commonly used MS-222 stock solution concentrations is 4 g/L, and the anesthetic dose is 4 mL of stock solution in 100 mL of water or 40 μg/mL (Westerfield, 2007). The euthanasia dose for adult zebrafish recommended by Westerfield is 10–20 mL of stock solution in 100 mL water (Westerfield, 2007). Research has showed that zebrafish larvae are more tolerant to the affect of MS-222 than adult fish (Rombough, 2007). The recommended dose for euthanasia for 3–9 dpf zebrafish larvae is 1800 mg/L (Rombough, 2007).

10.2.1.3 Blood Volume—Collection Volume Limits

The blood volume in bony fish (*Osteichthyes*) is small compared to other vertebrates. The total blood volume in fish ranges between 1.5% and 5% of body weight (Conte et al., 1963; Groff and Zinkl, 1999). In carp, blood volume is approximately 5% of body mass, and conservative estimates of blood volumes that can be collected from a 100 g fish is 1.0 mL (Groff and Zinkl, 1999).

Depending on the size of the animal, blood sampling technique, and technical proficiency of the phlebotomist, blood volume collected from one adult zebrafish can range from 1 to 10 μL (Jagadeeswaran et al., 1999; Murtha et al., 2003; Eames et al., 2010). With most blood collection methods in zebrafish, the quantity of blood is most commonly 5 μL, and sample volumes of 10 μL are less uncommon. Blood samples are usually pooled from several zebrafish for analysis. Although small volumes are collected from adult zebrafish, researchers have applied different technologies to meet their research needs. For example, blood glucose in zebrafish has been measured by using glucose meters with various test strip sample volumes (Elo et al., 2007; Eames et al., 2010). These include the following:

- OneTouch Ultra, 1 μL sample (LifeScan)
- FreeStyle Lite, 0.3 μL sample (Abbott)

- Accu-Chek Aviva, 0.6 μL sample (Roche Diagnostics)
- Accu-Chek Compact Plus, 1.5 μL sample (Roche Diagnostics)

10.2.1.4 Blood Storage Recommendations

Fish blood is known to coagulate rapidly and the rate of coagulation increases with stress (Groff and Zinkl, 1999). One of the critical factors when preparing samples for analysis and storage is to process the sample immediately since clinical chemistry values can be altered if blood is kept at room temperature for ≥1 hour or after being refrigerated from 1 to 3 hours (Korcock et al., 1988; Houston, 1990; Groff and Zinkl, 1999). Once the blood sample is collected, it should be centrifuged at low temperatures (Houston, 1990; Groff and Zinkl, 1999).

When working with zebrafish or other small fish, whole blood can be pooled from multiple fish. Blood can be pooled in 0.5 mL microcentrifuge tube (OS-pl microcentrifuge tube) and allowed to clot, and spun for 10 minutes at 2,500 rpm. Centrifugation above 2,500 rpm may lead to hemolysis (Murtha et al., 2003). The serum is then pipetted off the top. Serum biochemical values were obtained from the pooled serum of five groups of approximately 50 zebrafish, using the VetScan Diagnostic Profile II (Abaxis. Inc., Union City, California) (Murtha et al., 2003).

The risk of hemolysis increases at room temperature and during storage of sample (Houston, 1990).

10.2.2 Urine Collection

Zebrafish do not have a urinary bladder (Lieschke and Currie, 2007; Harper and Lawrence, 2010). Therefore, there are no easily accessible methods to collect urine in zebrafish. However, urine collection to assess renal function and urinary excretion has been performed in various fish species such as trout, salmon, and catfish using a urethral or urinary bladder catheters (Curtis and Wood, 1991; Black, 2000; McDonald et al., 2002). Many different types of catheters have been used to collect urine in fish. Black (2000) provides a concise summary of materials and techniques which have been developed. Nephrons from freshwater fish work to counteract hypervolemia and salt depletion by producing significant amounts of dilute urine. In freshwater fish, the urine volume ranges from 2 to 6 mL/kg/h (Greenwell et al., 2003).

10.3 PREANALYTICAL SOURCES OF VARIATION IN CLINICAL CHEMISTRIES

Preanalytical sources of variation have been reviewed in many fish species and numerous studies have shown that factors such as age, sex, strain, anticoagulants, anesthetics, environmental conditions, sampling technique, capturing method, analysis techniques, and diet can influence fish blood values (Groff and Zinkl, 1999; Hrubec and Smith, 1999; Sakomoto et al., 2001; Dutta et al., 2005; Asadi et al., 2006; Ramsay et al., 2006, 2009; Harper and Wolf, 2009; Cachat et al., 2010; Goncalves et al., 2012). Some parameters may be affected by multiple factors. For example, glucose values are sensitive to stress, bacterial infection, fish size, fish age, ambient temperatures, water temperature, oxygen levels, nutritional status, fasting, as well as the reproductive stage of the fish (Groff and Zinkl, 1999; Greenwell et al., 2003; Choi et al., 2008). Very little work has been done on assessing sources of variation affecting biochemical values in zebrafish or medaka. In zebrafish, fasting has been used as a research tool to evaluate its impact on behavior, fin regeneration, and gene expression (Novak et al., 2005; Goldsmith, 2006; Amole and Unniappan, 2009; Moss et al., 2009). One can hypothesize that many of the factors affecting blood chemistry in teleost fish also affect zebrafish.

10.3.1 Plasma versus Serum

In mammals, the use of plasma or serum does not generate significant differences and both samples are interchangeable (NCCLS, 1990; Hrubec and Smith, 1999). This interchangeability does not seem to exist in fish, and in general, fish plasma is preferred over serum when evaluating clinical chemistry (Ellsaesser and Clem, 1987; Hrubec and Smith, 1999). One of the advantages of working with plasma rather than serum is that there is more yield with plasma, which is important when working with small blood volumes (Hrubec and Smith, 1999; Sakomoto et al., 2001).

Although, evaluating the similarities and differences between the use of plasma and serum on the effect on measured blood analytes has not been studied in zebrafish, it has been assessed in rainbow trout (*O. mykiss*), channel catfish (*I. punctatus*), hybrid tilapia (*Oreochromis* spp.), and hybrid striped bass (*Morone saxatilis*) (Hrubec and Smith, 1999). Findings in all species had significant differences between plasma and serum affecting potassium, magnesium, and phosphorus concentrations. Serum samples yielded lower potassium values and higher magnesium and phosphorus values compared to plasma samples (Hrubec and Smith, 1999). Glucose values in the rainbow trout, hybrid striped bass, and channel catfish were lower in the serum compared to plasma levels. Rainbow trout, channel catfish, and hybrid tilapia cholesterol levels were higher in the serum sample. It has been shown that the blood plasma calcium and magnesium concentrations are maintained within definite ranges in the common roach, a fish in the *Cyprinidae* family (Martem'yanov, 2001). The most likely difference between plasma and serum is during the clotting process where blood constituents are being metabolically utilized (Hrubec and Smith, 1999).

In fish, serum and plasma have many similarities; however, some of the major differences include that plasma contains clotting factors and an anticoagulant that are absent in serum (Hrubec and Smith, 1999). The metabolic mechanism for the differences between plasma and serum in fish is not known (Hrubec and Smith, 1999). In general, processes that can cause differences between plasma samples and serum sample include hemolysis and cellular metabolism affecting analyte levels due to update and release of various components in the blood (Hrubec and Smith, 1999).

10.3.2 Coagulation and Anticoagulants

The use of anticoagulants is recommended and many have been evaluated in fish. Examples include heparin, citrate, oxalate, and ethylenediamine tetraacetic acid (EDTA) (Axelsson and Fritsches, 1994; Groff and Zinkl, 1999; Jagadeeswaran et al., 1999; Murtha et al., 2003). Selection of the most appropriate anticoagulant in fish will vary depending on the purpose of the sample. Coagulation is less likely to occur when a plastic syringe is used as opposed to using a glass syringe (Houston, 1990).

Heparin is a commonly used antigoagulant in fish and it is available in different salt forms including sodium, calcium, ammonium, or lithium (Black, 2000). The effective concentrations range from 50 to 100 USP units/mL or 0.30–0.75 mg/mL of sample (Houston, 1990; Groff and Zinkl, 1999). The blood sample acid–base status is not affected by the use of heparin. When evaluating plasma electrolyte levels, sodium or potassium heparin is recommended (Groff and Zinkl, 1999). If calcium ions are being measured from plasma stored in heparin, the concentration should not exceed 100 USP units/mL (Axelsson and Fritsche, 1994; Black, 2000;). Due to low biological levels of lithium, some researchers prefer to use heparin lithium salt as opposed to the ammonium, calcium, sodium salt, which are readily available (Houston, 1990). When evaluating plasma electrolyte levels, sodium or potassium heparin is recommended as an anticoagulant (Groff and Zinkl, 1999). EDTA was the anticoagulant used and serum electrolytes are listed in Table 10.1 (Murtha et al., 2003).

Although heparin has been used as an anticoagulant in glucose studies in zebrafish (Eames et al., 2010), fluoride anticoagulant has been recommended for determining glucose levels in other fish if samples are not processed within 30 minutes of collection since fluoride slows down glycolysis

TABLE 10.1
Clinical Chemistry Data for Zebrafish

	Nonspecified	
Strain	**Mean ± SD**	**Range**
Albumin (g/dL)	3.0 ± 0.2	2.7–3.3
Alkaline phosphatase (IU/L)	2.0 ± 4.5	0.0–10.0
Alanine aminotransferase (IU/L)	367.0 ± 25.3	343.0–410.0
Amylase (IU/L)	2331.4 ± 520.6	1898.0–3195.0
Total bilirubin (mg/dL)	0.38 ± 0.1	0.2–0.6
BUN (mg/dL)	3.2 ± 0.4	3.0–4.0
Calcium (mg/dL)	14.7 ± 2.3	12.3–18.6
Phosphorus (mg/dL)	22.3 ± 1.5	20.3–24.3
Creatinine (mg/dL)	0.7 ± 0.2	0.5–0.9
Glucose (g/dL)	82.2 ± 12.0	62.0–91.0
Potassium (mEq/L)	6.8 ± 1.0	5.2–7.7
Total protein (g/dL)	5.2 ± 0.5	4.4–5.8
Globulins (g/dL)	2.1 ± 0.6	1.3–2.8

Source: Murtha, J.M. et al., *Comp Med.*, 53, 37–41, 2003.

in blood. The disadvantage for using fluoride is that it can affect other enzymatic processes in the serum (Stoskopf, 1993). The recommended anticoagulant for evaluating enzymatic activities and electrolyte levels is ammonium heparin or lithium heparin (Stoskopf, 1993). EDTA should be avoided if the fish are being anesthetized or euthanized with MS-222 since it can often lead to hemolysis. Hemolysis affects clinical chemistry parameters, especially if colorometric tests are used to quantify blood parameters (Noga, 1996).

The use of EDTA or heparin can impact the potassium and sodium levels in serum and calcium levels in plasma. These changes occur due to the calcium binding activity of EDTA and due to the potassium and sodium salts found in this anticoagulant (Stoskopf, 1993). EDTA should not be used to determine the concentration of plasma calcium levels in fish (Groff and Zinkl, 1999). EDTA can alter blood–gas tension and can also decrease blood pH (Groff and Zinkl, 1999).

10.3.3 Sex and Age

Age-related changes in clinical chemistry has been reported in fish (Groff and Zinkl, 1999; Hrubec et al., 2001; Asadi et al., 2006). However, no publications were found pertaining to the impact of age or sex on the clinical chemistry of zebrafish or medaka. In carp and goldfish, values including glucose, serum amylase, chloride, creatinine, and total protein increase with age. Calcium and alkaline phosphatase levels decrease with age. Serum cholesterol, uric acid, and urea nitrogen decrease initially and then increase with age (Groff and Zinkl, 1999; Stoskopf, 1993). Asadi et al. (2006) have demonstrated that male sturgeons have higher glucose, albumin, globulin, and phosphorus levels as compared to females. In cyprinids such as koi and carp, males have lower plasma protein levels than females (Groff and Zinkl, 1999). In striped bass, clinical chemistry values were significantly different among age groups except for creatinine and potassium concentrations, and the changes reported were similar to those noted in mammals as well as rainbow trout (Hrubec et al., 2001).

10.3.4 Diet, Feeding, Fasting, and Starvation

Dietary composition, insufficiency, or overabundance can impact the physiological parameters, growth, reproduction, and behavior in fish (Post, 1993; Stewart, 1993; NRC, 1999). Nutritional imbalances impact fish health, research, and can also affect blood chemistry parameters (Post, 1993; Stewart, 1993; Siccardi et al., 2009; Trenzado et al., 2009). Dietary requirements and formulations are not standardized in most fish species—most of the research has focused on important aquaculture or ornamental fish such as salmonids and cyprinids. Although zebrafish are currently one of the most important fish biomedical research models, the nutritional requirements for the different life stages of this species have not yet been established. This is unfortunate as the major food source of zebrafish is brine shrimp which has minimal nutritional value when it is fed as a food source without enrichment (Conklin, 2000; Astrofsky et al., 2002; Stoskopf, 2002). Furthermore, storage losses, bioavailability of nutrients, nutritional imbalances and potential contaminants, from both human and natural sources, which are known to affect the health, growth, and reproduction of fish are important factors that are not addressed within zebrafish research.

The clinical chemistry of carp and koi has been studied by comparing parameters from fish that were fed a reduced ration of food with fish that receive a complete ration of food (Groff and Zinkl, 1999). Parameters such as whole blood ammonia, lipids, plasma protein, and glucose differed between groups where fish receiving a complete ration had elevated glucose, lipid, whole blood ammonia, and plasma protein compared to the fish fed a smaller amount of food (Groff and Zinkl, 1999). Starvation can also lead to increased lipid levels (Groff and Zinkl, 1999). This information indicates that food ratio can impact some clinical chemistry parameters in fish.

10.3.5 Stress

Many different stress factors are known to impact fish such as handling, housing density, capture, restraint, hypoxia, anesthesia, air exposure, disease, and sampling technique. All these factors may therefore impact fish clinical chemistry values (Mazeaud et al., 1977; Ellsaesser and Clem, 1987; Bullis, 1993; Groff and Zinkl, 1999; Bayne and Gerwick, 2001; Greenwell et al., 2003; Dror et al., 2006; Gbore et al., 2006; Ramsay et al., 2006, 2009; Fast et al., 2007; Scott and Ellis, 2007). There are three different phases that occur during a stress response in fish (Barton, 2002). The first phase is a generalized neuroendocrine response where catecholamines (epinephrine and norepinephrine) are released from the chromaffin cells and corticosteroids are released from the interrenal cells (Harrell and Moline, 1992). Increased circulating levels of these hormones trigger a secondary response that involves physiologic and metabolic pathways. Examples of the secondary response include hyperglycemia due to enhanced glycogenolysis and gluconeogenesis, vasodilation of arteries in gill filaments, increased cardiac stroke volume, increased urine production, and immune function depression (Gratzek and Reinert, 1984; Harrell and Moline, 1992; Greenwell et al., 2003). The first and second phases have been described as adaptive responses which enable the fish to adjust to the stress factors and maintain homeostasis. In contrast, the third phase can cause systemic changes which may no longer be able to adapt to stress. As a result, the overall health of the animals may be impacted to the extent that their performance, growth, reproduction, disease resistance, and behavior are adversely affected (Barton, 2002).

Bayne and Gerwick (2001) reviewed the acute phase response and innate immunity of fish and explained how tissue trauma and microbial pathogens change protein and macromolecule concentrations of the body fluids of different teleosts, leading to metabolic changes in several organ systems.

Stress-related diuresis can lead an electrolyte imbalance due to the loss of chloride and other ions in the urine (Greenwell et al., 2003). Stress in carp and goldfish causes decreases in sodium and lipid levels and increases in lactate, potassium, and glucose levels (Groff and Zinkl, 1999). Hyperglycemia can persist for 24–48 hours after the stress factor is removed (Chavin and Young,

1970; Groff and Zinkl, 1999). In contrast, chronic stress was shown to decrease glucose levels (Groff and Zinkl, 1999). Due to the increase in catecholamines that lead to vasoconstriction and hypertension, an increase in branchial perfusion and diuresis follows. The increase in branchial perfusion leads to increase in branchial permeability, causing hemodilution due to an increased water gain. This in turn leads to a loss of electrolytes, which decreases plasma osmolarity because of hyponatremia and hypochloremia (Groff and Zinkl, 1999). Hyponatremia and hypochloremia are exacerbated by diuresis (Mazeaud et al., 1977; Groff and Zinkl, 1999). The impact of stress can be minimized with the use of proper anesthetics and optimal research technique and handling.

Different studies have associated fish handling with an increase in plasma glucose and lactic acid as well as cortisol levels (Bullis, 1993; Fast et al., 2007). Clinical chemistry parameters that are affected by transport stress and handling in channel catfish include glucose, lactate dehydrogenase (LDH), and creatinine phosphokinase (Ellsaesser and Clem, 1987). Other serum chemistry variables that are affected by stress in fish include sodium, CO_2, urea nitrogen, direct bilirubin, cholesterol, creatinine, and protein levels (Ellsaesser and Clem, 1987). Acclimatization prior to sample collection is critical for establishing baseline values and minimizing blood chemistry variables (Torres et al., 1986; Ellsaesser and Clem, 1987; Bullis, 1993; Gravel and Vijayan, 2007).

Serial blood sampling is not recommended in fish due to the stress associated with handling fish and the impact on clinical chemistry results (Torres et al., 1986; Ellsaesser and Clem, 1987; Bullis, 1993; Groff and Zinkl, 1999; Gravel and Vijayan, 2007). The effects of stress on blood values in fish can be extensive and of long duration (Houston, 1990).

10.3.6 Water Chemistry

Water chemistry parameters have shown to influence urine and plasma composition in freshwater fish (Scherer et al., 1986; Stoskopf, 1993; Hrubec et al., 1997; Greenwell et al., 2003; Bolner and Baldisserotto, 2007).

The plasma NaCl in freshwater fish is hypertonic to the water environment. The approximate ratio is 150 mM to <1 mM (Greenwell et al., 2003). Their body fluids are hyperosmotic compared to the water and favor the influx of water across the gill epithelium. The amount of water influx across the gill can reach approximately 50% of the total body water per hour (Greenwell et al., 2003). Therefore, freshwater fish risk hypervolemia, overhydration, and salt depletion (Greenwell et al., 2003).

Bolner and Baldisserotto (2007) studies showed that water pH affects urinary excretion and plasma ion levels in silver catfish, *Rhamdia quelen*. Urine flow rate as well as urine and plasma pH increase with the increase of water pH. Urinary sodium excretion rate increases and ammonia urinary excretion rate decreases with elevated water pH (Bolner and Baldisserotto, 2007). Plasma ammonia levels decrease when fish are housed in water pH from 4.0 to 8.0. However, in water pH of 9.0 ammonia levels are elevated. The majority of the plasma ions and urinary excretion changes observed in silver catfish exposed to acidic or alkaline water were consistent with the results seen in rainbow trout *O. mykiss* (Bolner and Baldisserotto, 2007). In addition, the kidney and urinary bladder appears to contribute to acid–base balance in silver catfish, because urine pH changed according to plasma pH (Bolner and Baldisserotto, 2007).

Other changes include a decrease in serum sodium and chloride levels with an increase in cortisol levels when fish are placed in acidic environments (Scherer et al., 1986; Stoskopf, 1993). This leads to a shift where sodium reabsorption is decreased and magnesium is secreted as opposed to being reabsorbed in order to facilitate water excretion from the fish (Stoskopf, 1993).

A major source of calcium in teleost fish is either dietary or from the surrounding water. Changes in environmental calcium impact calcium uptake through the gills. In zebrafish and trout, changes in water calcium concentration have a direct impact on the fish's calcium regulation, and gene expression and protein levels are directly influenced (Radman et al., 2002; Craig et al., 2007).

Amino acid metabolism in teleosts generates nitrogenous waste which is excreted as ammonia and is associated with increased susceptibility to disease (Goncalves et al., 2012; Shih et al., 2008). The gills are the major site for eliminating ammonia in exchange for sodium (Shih, et al., 2008). Ammonia excretion through the gills is influenced by water pH and ammonia levels in the water, therefore affecting zebrafish physiology (Shih et al., 2008).

Ammonia ion is the primary constituent of blood ammonia levels, and toxicity levels in fish can be diagnosed when blood values range from 400 to 500 µg/dL (Groff and Zinkl, 1999). In zebrafish larvae, ammonia is mainly excreted from the yolk sac epithelium (Shih et al., 2008). Elevated ammonia levels from water exposure in zebrafish affects gene expression, whole body cortisol levels, and suppresses the innate immune response (Goncalves et al., 2012).

Zebrafish are commonly acclimated in soft water prior to toxicology studies. Soft water is ion poor similar to reverse osmosis water. Exposing fish to soft water over a 7-day period affects their overall physiology by altering their osmoregulation due to remodeling of the zebrafish gills (Craig et al., 2007). The fish endocrine system may also be influenced by water parameter changes. For example, changes in salinity can upregulate or downregulate endocrine genes such as atrial natriuretic peptide, rennin, prolactin, growth hormone, and parathyroid hormone (Hoshijima and Hirose, 2007).

10.3.7 Temperature and Seasons

The effect of water temperature on physiological, hematological, and clinical chemistry parameters has been evaluated in many different fish species (Ellsaesser and Clem, 1987; Bullis, 1993; Roche and Boge, 1996; Hrubec et al., 1997; Cataldi et al., 1998; Groff and Zinkl, 1999; Little and Seebacher, 2015; Prassack et al., 2001; Sardella et al., 2004; Fiess et al., 2007; Choi et al., 2008). Biochemical parameters which seem to be affected in channel catfish due to seasonal temperature changes include potassium, magnesium, CO_2, glucose, creatinine, albumin, iron, alkaline phosphatase, and glutamate-pyruvate transaminase (Ellsaesser and Clem, 1987). In zebrafish, most of the work has focused on studying the impact of temperature on cardiac activity, metabolism, and circadian rhythms (Jacob et al., 2002; López-Olmeda and Sánchez-Vázquez, 2009). To date, no reports assessed the impact of temperature variations on clinical chemistry of the zebrafish.

It is well established that temperature can affects the immune function and can lead to stress in fish (Stoskopf, 1993; Prophete et al., 2006; Choi et al., 2008). Fish can be stressed by elevated or low water temperatures as well as by rapid temperature fluctuations without acclimation. Rapid temperature decrease limits a fish's ability to produce antibodies integral to an immediate immune response, and a delay in the immune response may provide sufficient advantage for pathogens, enabling them to colonize, reproduce, and establish an infection (Dror et al., 2006). In cyprinids such as koi and carp, an increase in temperature can lead to altered clinical chemistry parameters such as a decrease in plasma sodium, plasma protein, and whole blood ammonia (Groff and Zinkl, 1999). Thermal stress in sea bass led to increases in plasma glucose (Roche and Boge, 1996).

Many different factors have been reported to affect plasma electrolytes in cyprinids (Houston, 1990; Groff and Zinkl, 1999). Examples include seasonal, diurnal, photoperiod variations as well as temperature cycles (Houston, 1990; Groff and Zinkl, 1999). Electrolytes that seem to be mostly affected include sodium and chloride; however, concentrations of potassium, magnesium, and free calcium seem to be less variable (Groff and Zinkl, 1999). Interestingly, although there are differences between goldfish and carp, they maintain a general overall pattern similar to cyprinids (Groff and Zinkl, 1999).

10.3.8 Hypoxia

In aquatic environments, hypoxia can occur under different circumstances. Low oxygen levels are most commonly observed when fish are shipped in insufficiently aerated containers, or when maintained in anoxic conditions where plant and algae overgrow in either natural or captive environments. A decrease in oxygen availability to tissues can lead to necrotic or apoptotic lesions in multiple organs (van der Meer et al., 2005). For example, channel catfish exposed to sublethal hypoxia led to histopathologically evident necrosis, hyperemia (vascular congestion), edema, hemorrhage, hyperplasia, and/or hypertrophy in a variety of anatomic sites including gills, liver, spleen, and anterior and posterior kidney (Scott and Rogers, 1980; Sollid et al., 2003; Almeida et al., 2017).

Certain animals such as some teleost fish, frogs, and insects have the capacity to tolerate or adapt to hypoxia (van der Meer et al., 2005). It has been shown that zebrafish can survive weeks of severe hypoxia as they develop adaptive responses which modulate their behavioral and physical phenotype (van der Meer et al., 2005). Evidence from cDNA microarray technology revealed that hypoxia was associated with changes in gene expression in the gills of zebrafish, in addition to gene repression that impacted protein biosynthesis and metabolic pathways (van der Meer et al., 2005). Chronic hypoxia has been shown to cause various changes in a diverse range of organ systems and fish species, including the hearts of zebrafish and cichlids (*Haplochromis piceatus*) (Marques et al., 2008); the reproductive tracts of Atlantic croaker (*Micropogonias undulatus*) (Thomas et al., 2007); and peripheral blood leukocytes of tilapia (Choi et al., 2008).

Clinical chemistry values of carp and goldfish are affected by hypoxia. Magnesium levels and whole blood ammonia levels are elevated and lipid levels are decreased in hypoxic carp and goldfish (Groff and Zinkl, 1999). Hypoxia increases plasma glucose levels in hypoglycemic fish as well as affects glucose uptake from various organs (MacCormack and Driedzic, 2006). Hypoxia in cyprinids leads to a reduction in glomerular filtration rate which leads to hyperkalemia, hypercalcemia, hypermagnesia, and hyperphosphatemia (Groff and Zinkl, 1999). Although no published work evaluates the impact of hypoxia on clinical chemistry in zebrafish, work has shown that hypoxia in zebrafish alters gene expression and impacts physiology and cell expression in multiple organs (Roesner et al., 2006; Cossins et al., 2009; Martinovic et al., 2008).

Hypoxia and hypercapnia in fish may alter the distribution of the gill cells such as the pavement and chloride cells which impact the gas diffusion distance between the water and the blood affecting gas exchange and thus fish physiology (Evans et al., 2005). Also, changes in gill surface area can lead to physiological changes. For example, in trout, a 30% decrease in gill surface area led to a significant increase in $PaCO_2$, which limits O_2 uptake and CO_2 excretion (Evans et al., 2005).

10.3.9 Anesthesia

The impact of anesthetics on stress, physiology, plasma cortisol levels, and clinical chemistry parameters has been evaluated in fish, and indicate that there can be significant species differences when using anesthetics such as MS-222 (Houston et al., 1971; Groff and Zinkl, 1999; Small, 2004; King et al., 2005; Crosby et al., 2006; Palić et al., 2006). Physiological changes associated with MS-222 can last for several days after the fish have recovered (Houston et al., 1976; Houston and Woods, 1976; Groff and Zinkl, 1999). Acidosis, ionic imbalance, hemoconcentration, and changes in plasma chemistry parameters have all been reported in carp exposed to unbuffered MS-222 (Groff and Zinkl, 1999). These effects can be eliminated by buffering the water with sodium bicarbonate to neutralize the pH (Groff and Zinkl, 1999).

The use anesthetics while handling fish reduces stress levels and influences plasma cortisol levels (Crosby et al., 2006). For example, plasma cortisol levels increase in fathead minnow, sea bass, and catfish following exposure to stress while anesthetized with MS-222 (Small, 2004; King et al., 2005; Crosby et al., 2006; Palić et al., 2006). However, cortisol levels decrease in gourami exposed to stress while anesthetized with MS-222 (Crosby et al., 2006).

Other changes associated with the use of MS-222 include hypoxia, hypercapnia, hyperglycemia, and increased blood lactate levels (Burka et al., 1997; Houston et al., 1971).

10.3.10 Hemolysis

Hemolysis can lead to inaccurate results in serum chemistry and interfere with colorimetric reactions. Hemolysis in fish can lead to increase in serum aspartate aminotransferase (AST), LDH, and potassium levels (Stoskopf, 1993). Hemolysis can be minimized if the samples are not exposed to moisture or water and by minimizing high-pressure transfer from the needle into the collecting tube (Stoskopf, 1993). The use of MS-222 sedation in conjunction with EDTA can lead to hemolysis (Noga, 1996). It has been reported in different fish species that hemolysis can be reduced if the blood is cooled down to 4°C (Noga, 1996; Groff and Zinkl, 1999). Hemolysis can be prevented by using a large needle, a small syringe and preventing negative pressure when removing the barrel of the needle (Houston, 1990). However, using a large needle size is not feasible when working with small fish. However, preventing the introduction of air in the blood when the sample is collected can minimize the risk of hemolysis.

10.3.11 Sampling Site

Sampling technique can impact serum chemistry (Groff and Zinkl, 1999; Bullis, 1993). There is a difference between blood values depending on whether the blood is collected by cardiocentesis or by severing the caudal peduncle. Muscle damage during sample collection can lead to an increase in creatine kinase (CK) and LDH (Groff and Zinkl, 1999). Samples collected from the caudal vein by severing the caudal peduncle in carp lead to higher levels of alanine aminotransferase (ALT), LDH, creatinine, and phosphorus compared to samples collected by cardiocentesis (Ikeda and Ozaki, 1981; Stoskopf, 1993). Another study working with juvenile salmon found that ALT, LDH, AST, CK, triglyceride, and potassium (K^+) were increased when the caudal peduncle was severed compared to cardiocentesis and caudal venipuncture (Congleton and LaVoie, 2001). Na^+ and Cl^- levels were decreased relative to values for samples obtained by caudal vessel puncture. Some enzyme activities (ALT, AST, LDH) and K^+ concentrations were also greater in samples taken by heart puncture than in samples taken by caudal vessel puncture. Of the methods evaluated, caudal vessel puncture had the least effect on blood chemistry values and was the preferred method for blood chemistry studies on juvenile salmonids (Congleton and LaVoie, 2001).

REFERENCES

Allen, J.L. and Hunn, J.B. 1986. Fate and distribution studies of some drugs used in aquaculture. *Vet Hum Toxicol.* 28:21–24.

Almeida, L.Z., Guffey, S.C., Sepúlveda, M.S., and Höök, T.O. 2017. Behavioral and physiological responses of yellow perch (*Perca flavescens*) to moderate hypoxia. *Comp Biochem Physiol A Mol Integr Physiol.* 209:47--55.

Alsop, D. and Vijayan, M.M. 2008. Development of the corticosteroid stress axis and receptor expression in zebrafish. *Am J Physiol Regul Integr Comp Physiol.* 294:711–719.

Alvarez, M.C., Béjar, J., Chen, S., and Hong, Y. 2007. Fish ES cells and applications to biotechnology. *Mar Biotechnol.* 9:117–127.

Amatruda, J.F. and Patton, E.E. 2008. Genetic models of cancer in zebrafish. *Int Rev Cell Mol Biol.* 271:1–34.

Amole, N. and Unniappan, S. 2009. Fasting induces preproghrelin mRNA expression in the brain and gut of zebrafish, Danio rerio. *Gen Comp Endocrinol.* 161:133–137.

Amsterdam, A. and Becker, T.S. 2005. Transgenes as screening tools to probe and manipulate the zebrafish genome. *Dev Dyn.* 234:255–268.

Anderson J.L., Carten, J.D., and Farber, S. A. 2011. Zebrafish lipid metabolism: From mediating early patterning to the metabolism of dietary fat and cholesterol. *Methods Cell Biol.* 101:111–141.

Arnaout, R., Ferrer, T., Huisken, J., et al. 2007. Zebrafish model for human long QT syndrome. Proc Natl Acad Sci. 104:11316–11321.

Asadi, F., Halajian, A., Pourkabir, M., Asadian, P., and Jadidizadeh, F. 2006. Serum biochemical parameters of *Huso huso*. *Comp Clin Pathol.* 15:245–248.

Astrofsky, K.M., Bullis, R.A., and Sagerstrom, C.G. 2002. Biology and management of the zebrafish. In *Laboratory Animal Medicine*, 2nd edition, Chap. 19, pp. 862–882. Amsterdam: Elsevier Science.

AVMA. 2007. AVMA guidelines on euthanasia. *J Am Vet Med Assoc.* 231:1784–1786.

Axelsson, M. and Fritsches, R. 1994. *Biochemistry and Molecular Biology of Fishes*. Eds. P.W. Hochachka and T.P. Mommsen, Vol. 3, pp. 17–36. Amsterdam: Elsevier.

Baker, K., Warren, K.S., Yellen, G., and Fishman, M.C. 1997. Defective "pacemaker" current (Ih) in a zebrafish mutant with a slow heart rate. Proc Natl Acad Sci. 94:4554–4559.

Bambino, K., and Chu, J. 2017. Zebrafish in toxicology and environmental health. *Curr Top Dev Biol.* 124:331--367.

Barros, T.P., Alderton, W.K., Reynolds, H.M., Roach, A.G., and Berghmans, S. 2008. Zebrafish: An emerging technology for in vivo pharmacological assessment to identify potential safety liabilities in early drug discovery. *Br J Pharmacol.* 154:1400–1413.

Barton, B.A. 2002. Stress in fishes: A diversity of responses with particular reference to changes in circulating corticosteroids. *Integr Comp Biol.* 42:517–525.

Bayne, C. J. and Gerwick, L. 2001. The acute phase response and innate immunity of fish. *Dev Comp Immunol.* 25:725–743.

Berghams, S., Jette, C., Langenau, D., et al. 2005. Making waves in cancer research: New models in the zebrafish. *Biotechniques.* 39:227–237.

Black, M.C. 2000. Collection of body fluids. In *The Laboratory Fish*. Ed. G.K. Ostrander, Chap. 30, pp. 513–527. Baltimore, MD: Academic Press.

Bolner, K.C.S. and Baldisserotto, B. 2007. Water pH and urinary excretion in silver catfish *Rhamdia quelen. J Fish Biol.* 70:50–64.

Borges, A., Scotti, L.V., Siqueira, D.R., et al. 2007. Changes in hematological and serum biochemical values in jundiá *Rhamdia quelen* due to sub-lethal toxicity of cypermethrin. *Chemosphere.* 69:920–926.

Briggs, J.P. 2002. The zebrafish: A new model organism for integrative physiology. *Am J Physiol Regul Integr Comp Physiol.* 282:3–9.

Brown, L.A. 1993. Anaesthesia and restraint. In *Fish Medicine*. Ed. M.K. Stoskopf, pp. 79–90. Philadelphia, PA: W.B. Saunders Company, Harcourt Brace Jovanovich Inc.

Brownlie, A., Donovan, A., Pratt, S.J., et al. 1998. Positional cloning of the zebrafish sauternes gene: A model for congenital sideroblastic anaemia. *Nat Genet.* 20:244–250.

Bullis, R.A. 1993. Clinical pathology of temperate freshwater and estuarine fishes. In *Fish Medicine*. Ed. M.K. Stoskopf, pp. 232–239. Philadelphia, PA: W.B. Saunders Company, Harcourt Brace Jovanovich Inc.

Burka, J.F., Hammel, K.L., Horsberg, T.E., Johnson, G.R., Rainnie, D.J., and Spear, D.J. 1997. Drugs in salmonid aquaculture—a review. *J Vet Pharmacol Ther.* 20:333–349.

Burns, C.G., Milan, D.J., Grande, E.J., Rottbauer, W., MacRae, C.A., and Fishman, M.C. 2005. High-throughput assay for small molecules that modulate zebrafish embryonic heart rate. *Nat Chem Biol.* 1:263–264.

Cachat, J., Stewart, A., Grossman, L., et al. 2010. Measuring behavioral and endocrine responses to novelty stress in adult zebrafish. *Nat Protoc.* 11:1786–1799.

Caldwell, S., Rummer, J.L., and Brauner, C.J. 2006. Blood sampling techniques and storage duration: Effects on the presence and magnitude of the red blood cell beta-adrenergic response in rainbow trout (*Oncorhynchus mykiss*). *Comp Biochem Physiol A Mol Integr Physiol.* 144:188–195.

Cataldi, E., Marco, P.D., Mandich, A., and Cataudella, S. 1998. Serum parameters of Adriatic sturgeon *Acipenser naccarii* (Pisces: Acipenseriformes). Effects of temperature and stress. *Comp Biochem Physiol.* 121:351–354.

Chan, J. and Mably, J.D. 2011. Dissection of cardiovascular development and disease pathways in zebrafish. *Prog Mol Biol Transl Sci.* 100:111–153.

Chavin, W. and Young, J.E. 1970. Factors in the determination of normal serum glucose levels of goldfish (*Carassius auratus* L.). *Comp Biochem Physiol.* 33:629–653.

Choi, C.Y., An, K.W., Choi, Y.K., Jo, P.G., and Min, B.H. 2008. Expression of warm temperature acclimation-related protein 65-kDa (Wap65) mRNA, and physiological changes with increasing water temperature in black porgy, *Acanthopagrus schlegeli. J Exp Zool A Ecol Genet.* 309:206–214.

Congleton, J.L. and LaVoie, W.J. 2001. Comparison of blood chemistry values for samples collected from juvenile chinook salmon by three methods. *J Aquat Anim Health.* 13:168–172.

Conklin, D.E. 2000. Diet. In *The Laboratory Fish*. Ed. G.K. Ostrander, Chap. 3, pp. 65–75, Baltimore, MD: Academic Press.

Conte, F.P., Wagner, H.H., and Harris, T.O. 1963. Measurement of blood volume in the fish (*Salmo gairdneri gairdneri*). *Am J Physiol.* 205:533–540.

Cossins, A.R., Williams, D.R., Foulkes, N.S., Berenbrink, M., and Kipar, A. 2009. Diverse cell-specific expression of myoglobin isoforms in brain, kidney, gill and liver of the hypoxia-tolerant carp and zebrafish. *J Exp Biol.* 212:627–638.

Craig, P.M., Wood, C.M., and McClelland, G.B. 2007. Gill membrane remodeling with soft-water acclimation in zebrafish (*Danio rerio*). *Physiol Genomics.* 30:53–60.

Crosby, T.C., Hill, J.E., Watson, C.A., Yanong, R.P.E., and Strange, R. 2006. Effects of tricaine methansulfonate, hypno, aquacalm, quinaldine, and salt on plasma cortisol levels following acute stress in three spot gourami *Trichogaster trichopterus. J Aquatic Anim Health.* 18:58–63.

Curtis, J. and Wood, C.M. 1991. The function of the urinary bladder *in vivo* in the freshwater rainbow trout. *J Exp Biol.* 155:567–583.

Dovey, M.C. and Zon, L.I. 2009. Defining cancer stem cells by xenotransplantation in zebrafish. *Methods Mol Biol.* 568:1–5.

Drabsch, Y., Snaar-Jagalska, B.E., Ten Dijke, P. 2017. Fish tales: The use of zebrafish xenograft human cancer cell models. *Histol Histopathol.* 33(7):673-686.

Dror, M., Sinyakov, M.S., Okun, E., Dym, M., Sredni, B., and Avtalion, R.R. 2006. Experimental handling stress as infection-facilitating factor for the goldfish ulcerative disease. *Vet Immunol Immunopathol.* 109:279–287.

Dutta T., Acharya, S., and Das, M.K. 2005. Impact of water quality on the stress physiology of cultured *Labeo rohita* (Hamilton-Buchanan). *J Environ Biol.* 26:585–592.

Dye, V.A. Hrubec, T.C., Dunn, J.L., and Smith, S.A. 2001. Hematology and serum chemistry values for winter flounder (*Pleuronectes americanus*). *IJRA.* 2:37–50.

Eames, S., Philipson, L., Prince, V., and Kinkel, M. 2010. Blood sugar measurement in zebrafish reveals dynamics of glucose homeostasis. *Zebrafish.* 7:205–213.

Ellett, F. and Lieschke, G.J. 2010. Zebrafish as a model for vertebrate hematopoiesis. *Curr Opin Pharmacol.* 5:563–70.

Ellsaesser, C.F. and Clem, L.W. 1987. Blood serum chemistry measurements of normal and acutely stressed channel catfish. *Comp Biochem Physiol A Mol Integr Physiol.* 88:589–594.

Elo, B., Villano, C.M., Govorko, D., and White, L.A. 2007. Larval zebrafish as a model for glucose metabolism: Expression of phosphoenolpyruvate carboxykinase as a marker for exposure to anti-diabetic compounds. *J Mol Endocrinol.* 38:433–440.

Evans, D.H., Piermarini, P.M., and Choe, K.P. 2005. The multifunctional fish gill: Dominant site of gas exchange, osmoregulation, acid-base regulation, and excretion of nitrogenous waste. *Physiol Rev.* 85:97–177.

Fast, M.D., Hosoya, S., Johnson, S.C., and Afonso, L.O. 2007. Cortisol response and immune-related effects of Atlantic salmon (*Salmo salar Linnaeus*) subjected to short- and long-term stress. *Fish Shellfish Immunol.* 24:194–204.

Feitsma, H. and Cuppen, E. 2008. Zebrafish as a cancer model. *Mol Cancer Res.* 6:685–694.

Fiess, J.C., Kunkel-Patterson, A., Mathias, L., et al. 2007. Effects of environmental salinity and temperature on osmoregulatory ability, organic osmolytes, and plasma hormone profiles in the Mozambique tilapia (*Oreochromis mossambicus*). *Comp Biochem Physiol A Mol Integr Physiol.* 146:252–264.

Gaikwad, S., Stewart, A., Hart P., et al. 2011. Acute stress disrupts performance of zebrafish in the cued and spatial memory tests: The utility of fish models to study stress-memory interplay. *Behav Processes.* 87:224–230.

Gbore, F.A., Oginni, O., Adewole, A.M., and Aladetan, J.O. 2006. The effect of transportation and handling stress on haematology and plasma biochemistry in fingerlings of *Ciarías gariepinus* and *Tilapia zillii. World J Agric Sci.* 2:208–212.

Genge, C.E., Lin, E., Lee, L., Sheng, X., Rayani, K., Gunawan, M., Stevens, C.M., Li, A.Y., Talab, S.S., Claydon, T.W., Hove-Madsen, L., and Tibbits, G.F. 2016. The zebrafish heart as a model of mammalian cardiac function. *Rev Physiol Biochem Pharmacol.* 171:99--136.

Gerhard, G.S. 2007. Small laboratory fish as models for aging research. *Ageing Res Rev.* 6:64–72.

Gilderhus, P.A. and Marking, L.L. 1987. Comparative efficacy of 16 anesthetic chemicals on rainbow trout. *N Am J Fish Manage.* 7:288–292.

Goldsmith, P. 2004. Zebrafish as a pharmacological tool: The how, why and when. *Curr Opin Pharmacol.* 4:504–512.

Goldsmith, M.I., Iovine, M.K., O'Reilly-Pol, T., and Johnson, S.L. 2006. A developmental transition in growth control during zebrafish caudal fin development. *Develop Biol.* 296: 450--457.

Goldsmith, J.R. and Jobin, C. 2012. Think small: Zebrafish as a model system of human pathology. *J Biomed Biotechnol.* 2012:817341.

Goncalves, A.F., Páscoa, I., Neves J.V., et al. 2012. The inhibitory effect of environmental ammonia on *Danio rerio* LPS induced acute phase. *Dev Comp Immunol.* 36:279–288.

Gratzek, J. B. and Reinert, R. 1984. Physiological responses of experimental fish to stressful conditions. *Natl Cancer Inst Monogr.* 65:187–193.

Gravel, A. and Vijayan, M.M. 2007. Salicylate impacts the physiological responses to an acute handling disturbance in rainbow trout. *Aquat Toxicol.* 85:87–95.

Greenwell, M.G., Sherrill, J., and Clayton, L.A. 2003. Osmoregulation in fish mechanisms and clinical implication. *Vet Clin North Am Exot Anim Pract.* 6:169–189.

Groff, J.M. and Zinkl, J.G. 1999. Hematology and clinical chemistry of cyprinid fish. Common carp and goldfish. *Vet Clin North Am Exot Anim Pract.* 3:741–776.

Grunwald, D.J. and Eisen, J.S. 2002. Headwaters of the zebrafish emergence of a new model vertebrate. *Nat Rev Genet.* 3:717–724.

Hao, J., Williams, C.H., Webb, M.E., and Hong, C.C. 2010. Large scale zebrafish-based in vivo small molecule screen. *J Vis Exp.* 30 December (46): pii:2243.

Harms, C.A. 2005. Surgery in fish research: common procedures and postoperative care. *Lab Anim.* 34:28–34.

Harms, C., Ross, T., and Segars, A. 2002. Plasma biochemistry reference values of wild bonnethead sharks, *Sphyrna tiburo*. *Vet Clin Pathol.* 31:111–115.

Harper, C., and Lawrence, C. 2010. *The Laboratory Zebrafish*. CRC Press: Boca Raton, FL.

Harper, C. and Wolf, J.C. 2009. Morphologic effects of the stress response in fish. *ILAR J.* 50:387–397.

Harrell, R.M. and Moline, M.A. 1992. Comparative stress dynamics of brood stock striped bass (*Morone saxatilis*) associated with two capture techniques. *J World Aqua Soc.* 23:58–63.

Hoshijima, K. and Hirose, S. 2007. Expression of endocrine genes in zebrafish larvae in response to environmental salinity. *J Endocrinol.* 193:481–491.

Houston, A.H. 1990. Blood and circulation. In *Methods in Fish Biology*. Eds. C.B. Schreck and P.B. Moyle, pp. 273–334. Bethesda, MD: American Fisheries Society.

Houston, A.H., Corlett, J.T., and Woods, R.J. 1976. Specimen weight and MS-222. *J Fish Res Board Can.* 33:1403–1407.

Houston, A.H., Madden, J.A., Woods, R.J., and Miles, H.M. 1971. Some physiological effects of handling and tricaine methanesulphonate anaesthetization upon the brook trout, *Salvelinus fontinalis*. *J Fish Res Board Can.* 28:625–633.

Houston, A.H. and Woods, R.J. 1976. Influence of temperature upon tricaine methane sulphonate uptake and induction of anesthesia in rainbow trout (Salmo gairdneri). *Comp Biochem Physiol.* 54C:1–6.

Hrubec, T.C., Cardinale J., and Smith, S.A. 2000. Hematology and plasma chemistry reference intervals for cultured tilapia (*Oreochromis hybrid*). *Vet Clin Hematol.* 29:7–12.

Hrubec, T.C., Robertson, J.L., and Smith, S.A. 1997a. Effects of temperature on hematologic and biochemical profiles of sunshine bass (*Morone chrysops* x *Morone saxatilis*). *Am J Vet Res.* 58:126–130.

Hrubec, T.C., Robertson, J.L., and Smith, S.A. 1997b. Effects of ammonia and nitrate concentration on hematologic and serum biochemical profiles of hybrid striped bass (*Morone chrysops* X *Morone saxatilis*). *Am J Vet Res.* 58:131–134.

Hrubec, T.C. and Smith, S. A. 1999. Differences between plasma and serum samples for the evaluation of blood chemistry values in rainbow trout, channel catfish, hybrid tilapias and striped bass. *J Aquat Anim Health.* 11:116–122.

Hrubec, T.C. and Smith, S.A. 2000. Hematology and plasma chemistry values for production tilapia (*Oreochromis hybrid*) raised in a recirculation system. *IJRA.* 1:5–14.

Hrubec, T.C. and Smith, S.A. 2004. Hematology and blood chemistry reference intervals for yellow perch (*Perca flavescens*) raised in recirculation systems. *IJRA.* 5:29–42.

Hrubec, T.C., Smith, S.A., and Robertson, J.L. 2001. Age-related changes in hematology and plasma chemistry values of hybrid striped bass (*Morone chrysops x Morone saxatilis*). *Vet Clin Pathol.* 30:8–15.

Ikeda, Y. and Ozaki, H. 1981. The examination of tail peduncle severing blood sampling method from aspect of observed serum constituent levels in carp. *B Jpn Soc Sci Fish.* 47:147–1453.

Ingham, P.W. 2009. The power of the zebrafish for disease analysis. *Hum Mol Genet.* 18(R1):R107–112.

Iwama, G.K. and Ackerman, P.A. 1994. Anaesthesia. In: *Biochemistry and Molecular Biology of Fishes*. Eds. P.W. Hochachka and T.P. Mommsen, Vol. 3, pp. 1–15. Amsterdam: Elsevier Science B.V.

Jacob, E., Drexel, M., Schwerte, T., and Pelster, B. 2002. Influence of hypoxia and of hypoxemia on the development of cardiac activity in zebrafish larvae. *Am J Physiol Regul Integr Comp Physiol.* 283:911–917.

Jagadeeswaran, P., Liu, Y.C., and Sheehan, J.P. 1999a. Analysis of hemostasis in the zebrafish. *Methods Cell Biol.* 59:337–357.

Jagadeeswaran, P. and Sheehan, J.P. 1999. Analysis of blood coagulation in the zebrafish. Blood Cells Mol Dis. 25:239–249.

Jagadeeswaran, P., Sheehan J.P., Craig, F.E., and Troyer, D. 1999b. Identification and characterization of zebrafish thrombocytes. *Br J Haematol.* 107:731–738.

Ju, Z., Wells, M.C., and Walter, R.B. 2007. DNA microarray technology in toxicogenomics of aquatic models: Methods and applications. *Comp Biochem Physiol C Toxicol Pharmacol.* 145:5–14.

Keller, E.T. and Murtha, J.M. 2004. The use of mature zebrafish (*Danio rerio*) as a model for human aging and disease. *Comp Biochem Physiol C Toxicol Pharmacol.* 138:335–341.

King, W., Hooper, B., Hillsgrove, S., Benton, C., and Berlinsky, D.L. 2005. The use of clove oil, metomidate, tricaine methanesulphonate and 2-phenoxyethanol for inducing anaesthesia and their effect on the cortisol stress response in black sea bass (*Centropristis striata* L.). *Aquacult Res.* 36:1442–1449.

Knowles, S., Hrubec, T.C., Smith, S.A., and Bakal, R.S. 2006. Hematology and plasma chemistry reference intervals for cultured shortnose sturgeon (*Acipenser brevirostrum*). *Vet Clin Pathol.* 35:434–440.

Kobayashi, D. and Takeda, H. 2008. Medaka genome project. *Brief Funct Genomic Proteomic.* 7:415–426.

Korcock, D.E., Houston, A.H., and Gray, J.D. 1988. Effects of sampling conditions on selected blood variables of rainbow trout, *Salmo gairdneri* Richardson. *J Fish Biol.* 33:319–330.

Lawrence, C. 2007. The husbandry of zebrafish (*Danio rerio*): A review. *Aquaculture.* 269:1–20.

Lieschke, G.J. and Currie, P.D. 2007. Animal models of human disease: Zebrafish swim into view. *Nat Rev Genet.* 5:353–367.

Little, A.G. and Seebacher, F. 2015. Temperature determines toxicity: bisphenol A reduces thermal tolerance in fish. *Environ Pollut.* 197:84--89.

Liu, X., Afonso, L., Altman, E., Johnson, S., Brown, L., and Li, J. 2008. O-acetylation of sialic acids in N-glycans of Atlantic salmon (*Salmo salar*) serum is altered by handling stress. *Proteomics.* 8:2849–2857.

Löhr, H. and Hammerschmidt, M. 2011. Zebrafish in endocrine systems: Recent advances and implications for human disease. *Annu Rev Physiol.* 73:183–211.

López-Olmeda, J.F. and Sánchez-Vázquez, F.J. 2009. Zebrafish temperature selection and synchronization of locomotor activity circadian rhythm to ahemeral cycles of light and temperature. Chronobiol Int. 26:200–218.

Luderman, L.N., Unlu, G., and Knapik, E.W. 2017. Zebrafish developmental models of skeletal diseases. *Curr Top Dev Biol.* 2017;124:81--124.

MacCormack, T.J. and Driedzic, W.R. 2006. The impact of hypoxia on in vivo glucose uptake in a hypoglycemic fish, *Myoxocephalus scorpius. Am J Physiol Regul Integr Comp Physiol.* 292:1033–1042.

Macova, S., Dolezelova, P., Pistekova, V., Svobodova, Z., Bedanova, I., and Voslarova, E. 2008. Comparison of acute toxicity of 2-phenoxyethanol and clove oil to juvenile and embryonic stages of *Danio rerio. Neuroendocrinol Lett.* 29:680–684.

Marques, I.J., Leito, J.T.D., Spaink, H.P., et al. 2008. Transcriptome analysis of the response to chronic constant hypoxia in zebrafish hearts. *J Comp Physiol B Biochem Sys Env Physiol.* 178:77–92.

Martem'yanov, V.I. 2001. Ranges of regulation of sodium, potassium, calcium, magnesium concentrations in plasma, erythrocytes and muscle tissue of *Rutilus rutilus* under natural conditions. *J Evol Biochem Physiol.* 37:141–147.

Martinovic, D., Villeneuve, D.L., Kahl, M.D., Blake, L.S., Brodin, J.D., and Ankley, G.T. 2008. Hypoxia alters gene expression in the gonads of zebrafish (*Danio rerio*). *Aquat Toxicol.* 95:258–272.

Massee, K.C., Rust, M.B., Hardy, R.W., and Stickney, R.R. 1995. The effectiveness of tricaine, quinaldine sulfate and metomidate as anesthetics for larval fish. *Aquaculture.* 134:351–359.

Matrone, G., Tucker, C.S., Denvir, M.A. 2017. Cardiomyocyte proliferation in zebrafish and mammals: lessons for human disease. *Cell Mol Life Sci.* 74:1367--1378.

Matsui H. 2017. The use of fish models to study human neurological disorders. *Neurosci Res.* Feb 16

Mauel, M.J., Miller, D.L., Merrill, A.L. 2007. Hematologic and plasma biochemical values of healthy hybrid tilapia (*Oreochromis aureus x Oreochromis nilotica*) maintained in a recirculating system. *J Zoo Wildlife Med.* 38:420–424.

Mazeaud, M.M., Mazeaud, F., and Donaldson, E.M. 1977. Primary and secondary effects of stress in fish: Some new data with a general review. *Trans Am Fish Soc.* 106:201–212.

McDonald, M.D., Walsh, P.J., and Wood, C.M. 2002. Transport physiology of the urinary bladder in teleosts: A suitable model for renal urea handling? *J Exp Zool.* 292:604–617.

Meeker, N.D. and Trede, N.S. 2008. Immunology and zebrafish: Spawning new models of human disease. *Dev Comp Immunol.* 32:745–757.

Milan, D.J., Jones, I.L., Ellinor, P.T., and MacRae, C.A. 2006. In vivo recording of adult zebrafish electrocardiogram and assessment of drug-induced QT prolongation. *Am J Physiol. Heart Circ Physiol.* 291:269–273.

Milan, D.J. and Macrae, C.A. 2008. Zebrafish genetic models for arrhythmia. *Prog Biophy Mol Biol.* 98:301–308.

Moss, J.B., Koustubhan, P., Greenman, M., Parsons, M.J., Walter, I., and Moss, L.G. 2009. Regeneration of the pancreas in adult zebrafish. Diabetes. 58:1844–1851.

Murtha, J.M., Qi, W., and Keller, E.T. 2003. Hematologic and serum biochemical values for zebrafish (*Danio rerio*). *Comp Med.* 53:37–41.

Nakatani, Y., Kawakami, A., and Kudo, A. 2007. Cellular and molecular processes of regeneration, with special emphasis on fish fins. *Dev Growth Differ.* 49:145–154.

National Committee for Clinical Laboratory Standards (NCCLS). 1990. *Procedures for the Handling and Processing of Blood Specimens; Approved Guideline*. Villanova, PA: NCCLS, NCCLS publication H18–A.

National Institutes of Health (NIH). 2009. *Final Report to OLAW on Euthanasia of Zebrafish.*

National Research Council (NRC). 1999. *Nutrient Requirements of Fish. Committee on Animal Nutrition. Board on Agriculture*. Washington, DC: National Academy Press.

Noga, E.J. 1996. *Fish Disease: Diagnosis and Treatment*, p. 378. Ames, IA: Iowa State University Press.

Novak, C.M., Jiang, X., Wang, C., Teske, J.A., Kotz, C.M., and Levine, J.A. 2005. Caloric restriction and physical activity in zebrafish (*Danio rerio*). *Neurosci Lett.* 383:99–104.

Onnebo, S.M., Yoong, S.H., and Ward, A.C. 2004. Harnessing zebrafish for the study of white blood cell development and its perturbation. *Exp Hematol.* 32:789–796.

Palić, D., Herolt, D.M., Andreasen, C.B., Menzel, B.W., and Roth, J.A., 2006. Anesthetic efficacy of tricaine methanesulfonate, metomidate and eugenol: Effects on plasma cortisol concentration and neutrophil function in fathead minnows (*Pimephales promelas* Rafinesque, 1820). *Aquaculture.* 254:675–685.

Pedroso, G.L., Hammes, T.O., Escobar, T.D., Fracasso, L.B., Forgiarini, L.F., and da Silveira, T.R. 2012. Blood collection for biochemical analysis in adult zebrafish. *J Vis Exp.* 63:e3865.

Post, G.W.1993. Nutrition and nutritional diseases of salmonids. In *Fish Medicine*. Ed. M.K. Stoskopf, pp. 343–357. Philadelphia, WB: Saunders Company, Harcourt Brace Jovanovich Inc.

Prassack, S.L., Bagatto, B., and Henry, R.P. 2001. Effects of temperature and aquatic $P(O_2)$ on the physiology and behaviour of *Apalone ferox* and *Chrysemys picta*. *J Exp Biol.* 204:2185–2195.

Prophete, C., Carlson, E.A., Li, Y., et al. 2006. Effects of elevated temperature and nickel pollution on the immune status of Japanese medaka. *Fish Shellfish Immunol.* 21:325–334.

Quaife, N.M., Watson O., and Chico T.J. 2012. Zebrafish: An emerging model of vascular development and remodelling. *Curr Opin Pharmacol.* 31 July, 12(5):608–614.

Radman, D.P., McCudden, C., James, K., Nemeth, E.M., and Wagner, G.F. 2002. Evidence for calcium-sensing receptor mediated stanniocalcin secretion in fish. *Mol Cell Endocrinol.* 186:111--119.

Ramsay, J.M., Feist, G.W., Varga, Z.M., Westerfield, M., Kent, M.L., and Schreck, C.B. 2006. Whole-body cortisol is an indicator of crowding stress in adult zebrafish, *Danio rerio*. *Aquaculture.* 258:565–574.

Ramsay, J.M., Feist, G.W., Varga, Z.M., Westerfield, M., Kent, M.L., and Schreck, C.B. 2009a. Whole-body cortisol response of zebrafish to acute net handling stress. *Aquaculture.* 297:157–162.

Ramsay, J.M., Watral, V., Schreck, C.B., and Kent, M.L. 2009b. Pseudoloma neurophilia infections in zebrafish *Danio rerio*: Effects of stress on survival, growth, and reproduction. Dis Aquat Organ. 88:69–84.

Ramsay, J.M., Watral, V., Schreck, C.B., and Kent, M.L. 2009c. Husbandry stress exacerbates mycobacterial infections in adult zebrafish, *Danio rerio* (Hamilton). *J Fish Dis.* 11:931–941.

Randall, D.J. 1962. Effect of an anaesthetic on the heart and respiration of teleost fish. *Nature.* 195:506.

Reavill, D.R. 2006. Common diagnostic and clinical techniques for fish. *Vet Clin North Am Exot Anim Pract.* 9:223–235.

Roche, H. and Boge, G. 1996. Fish blood parameters as potential tool for identification of stress caused by environmental factors and chemical intoxication. *Mar Environ Res.* 41:27–43.

Roesner, A., Hankeln, T., and Burmester, T. 2006. Hypoxia induces a complex response of globin expression in zebrafish (*Danio rerio*). *J Exp Biol.* 209:2129–2137.

Rombough, P.J. 2007. Ontogenetic changes in the toxicity and efficacy of the anaesthetic MS-222 (tricaine methanesulfonate) in zebrafish (*Danio rerio*) larvae. *Comp Biochem Physiol A Mol Integr Physiol.* 148:463–469.

Rothwell, S.E., Black, S.E., Jerrett, A.R., and Forster, M.E. 2005. Cardiovascular changes and catecholamine release following anaesthesia in Chinook salmon (*Oncorhynchus tshawytscha*) and snapper (*Pagrus auratus*). *Comp Biochem Physiol.* 140:289–298.

Rothwell, S.E. and Forster, M.E. 2005. Anaesthetic effects on the hepatic portal vein and on the vascular resistance of the tail of the Chinook salmon (*Oncorhynchus tshawytscha*). *Fish Physiol Biochem.* 31:11–21.

Rubinstein, A.L. 2006. Zebrafish assays for drug toxicity screening. *Exp Opin Drug Metab Toxicol.* 2:231–240.

Saffitz, J.E. 2017. Molecular mechanisms in the pathogenesis of arrhythmogenic cardiomyopathy. *Cardiovasc Pathol.* 28:51--58.

Sakomoto, K., Lewbart, G.A., and Smith, T.M. 2001. Blood chemistry values of juvenile red pacu (*Piaractus brachypomus*). *Vet Clin Pathol.* 30:50–52.

Sardella, B.A., Cooper, J., Gonzalez, R.J., and Brauner, C.J. 2004. The effect of temperature on juvenile Mozambique tilapia hybrids (*Oreochromis mossambicus* x *O. urolepis hornorum*) exposed to full-strength and hypersaline seawater. *Comp Biochem Physiol A Mol Integr Physiol.* 137:621–629.

Scherer, E., Harrison, S.E., and Brown, S.B. 1986. Locomotor activity and blood plasma parameters of acid-exposed lake whitefish, *Coregonus clupeaformis*. *Can J Fish Aquat Sci.* 43:1556–1561.

Schilling, T.F., and Webb, J. 2007. Considering the zebrafish in a comparative context. *J Exp Zool B Mol Dev Evol.* 308:515–522.

Scott, A.L. and Rogers, W.A. 1980. Histological effects of prolonged sublethal hypoxia on channel catfish *Ictalurus punctatus* (Rafinesque). *J Fish Dis.* 3:305–316.

Scott, A.P. and Ellis, T. 2007. Measurement of fish steroids in water—A review. *Gen Comp Endocrinol.* 153:392–400.

Shih, T.H., Horng, J.L., Hwang, P.P., and Lin, L.Y. 2008. Ammonia excretion by the skin of zebrafish (*Danio rerio*) larvae. *Am J Physiol Cell Physiol.* 295:C1625–1632.

Siccardi, A.J., Garris, H.W., Jones, W.T., Moseley, D.B., D'Abramo, L.R., and Watts, S.A. 2009. Growth and survival of zebrafish (*Danio rerio*) fed different commercial and laboratory diets. *Zebrafish.* 6(3):275–280.

Sipes, N.S., Padilla, S., and Knudsen, T.B. 2011. Zebrafish: As an integrative model for twenty-first century toxicity testing. *Birth Defects Res C Embryo Today Rev.* 93:256–267.

Small, B.C. 2004. Effect of isoeugenol sedation on plasma cortisol, glucose, and lactate dynamics in channel catfish *Ictalurus punctatus* exposed to three stressors. *Aquaculture.* 238:469–481.

Sohlberg, S., Martinsen, B., Horsberg, T.E., and Søli, N.E. 1996. Evaluation of the dorsal aorta cannulation technique for pharmacokinetic studies in Atlantic salmon (*Salmo salar*) in sea water. *J Vet Pharmacol Ther.* 19:460–465.

Sollid, J., De Angelis, P., Gundersen, K., and Nilsson, G.E. 2003. Hypoxia induces adaptive and reversible gross morphological changes in crucian carp gills. *J Exp Biol.* 206:3667–3673.

Spence, R., Ashton, R.L., and Smith, C. 2007a. Adaptive oviposition decisions are mediated by spawning site quality in the zebrafish, *Danio rerio*. *Behaviour.* 144:953–966.

Spence, R., Fatema, M.K., Ellis, S., Ahmed, Z.F., and Smith, C. 2007b. The diet, growth and recruitment of wild zebrafish (*Danio rerio*) in Bangladesh. *J Fish Biol.* 71:304–309.

Spence, R., Gerlach, G., Lawrence, C., and Smith, C. 2008. The behaviour and ecology of the zebrafish, Danio rerio. *Biol Rev Camb Philos Soc.* 83:13–34.

Stewart, L.J. 1993. Nutrition and of koi, carp and goldfish. In *Fish Medicine*. Eds. M.K. Stoskopf, pp. 461–470. Philadelphia, PA: W.B. Saunders Company, Harcourt Brace Jovanovich Inc.

Stoskopf, M.K. 2002. Biology and health of laboratory fish. In: *Laboratory Animal Medicine*, 2nd edition, Chap. 20. Amsterdam: Elsevier Science.

Stoskopf, M.K. Ed. 1993. *Fish Medicine*, pp. 127–130. Philadelphia, PA: WB Saunders Co.

Sullivan, C. and Kim, C.H. 2008. Zebrafish as a model for infectious disease and immune function. *Fish Shellfish Immunol.* 25:341–350.

Sun, L., Lien C.L., and Shung, K.K.. 2008. In vivo cardiac imaging of adult zebrafish using high frequency ultrasound (45–75 MHz). *Ultrasound Med Biol.* 34:31–39.

Takeda, H. 2008. Draft genome of the medaka fish: A comprehensive resource for medaka developmental genetics and vertebrate evolutionary biology. *Dev Growth Differ.* 50(1):S157–S166.

Tavares-Dias, M. and Moraes, F.R. 2007. Haematological and biochemical reference intervals for farmed channel catfish. *J Fish Biol.* 71:383–388.

Thomas, P., Rahman, M.S., Khan, I.A., and Kummer, J.A. 2007. Widespread endocrine disruption and reproductive impairment in an estuarine fish population exposed to seasonal hypoxia. *Proc Royal Soc B Biol Sci.* 274:2693–2701.

Torres, P., Duthie, G.G., and Tort, L. 1986. Statistical relations of some blood parameters along recovery from imposed stress in dogfish. *Rev Esp Fisiol.* 42:7–14.

Trede, N.S., Langenau, D.M., Traver, D., Look, A.T., and Zon, L.I. 2004. The use of zebrafish to understand immunity. *Immunity.* 20:367–379.

Trenzado, C.E., Morales, A.E., Palma J.M., and de la Higuera, M. 2009. Blood antioxidant defenses and hematological adjustments in crowded/uncrowded rainbow trout (*Oncorhynchus mykiss*) fed on diets with different levels of antioxidant vitamins and HUFA. *Comp Biochem Physiol C Toxicol Pharmacol.* 149:440–447.

Trevarrow, B. and Robison, B. 2004. Genetic backgrounds, standard lines, and husbandry of zebrafish. *Methods Cell Biol.* 77:599–616.

van der Meer, D.L., van den Thillart, G.E., Witte, F., et al. 2005. Gene expression profiling of the long-term adaptive response to hypoxia in the gills of adult zebrafish. *Am J Physiol Regul Integr Comp Physiol.* 289:1512–1519.

Venkatasubramani, N. and Mayer, A.N. 2008. A zebrafish model for the Shwachman–Diamond syndrome (SDS). *Pediatr Res.* 63:348–352.

Vogt, A., Cholewinski, A., Shen, X., et al. 2009. Automated image-based phenotypic analysis in zebrafish embryos. *Dev Dyn.* 238:656–663.

Wang, H., Long, Q., Marty, S.D., Sassa, S., and Lin, S. 1998. A zebrafish model for hepatoerythropoietic porphyria. *Nat Genet.* 20:239–243.

Wen, D., Liu, A., Chen, F., Yang, J., and Dai, R. 2012. Validation of visualized transgenic zebrafish as a high throughput model to assay bradycardia related cardio toxicity risk candidates. *J Appl Toxicol.* 29 Jun, 32:834–842.

Westerfield, M. 2007. T*he Zebrafish Book: A Guide for the Laboratory Use of Zebrafish (Danio rerio)*, 5th edition. Eugene, OR: University of Oregon Press.

Wittmann, C., Reischl, M., Shah, A.H., Mikut, R. Liebel, U., and Grabher, C. 2012. Facilitating drug discovery: An automated high-content inflammation assay in zebrafish. *J Vis Exp.* 65:e4203.

Wolman, M. and Granato, M. 2012. Behavioral genetics in larval zebrafish: Learning from the young. *Dev Neurobiol.* 72:366–372.

Wooster, G.A., Hsu, H.M., and Bowser, P.R. 1993. Nonlethal surgical procedures for obtaining tissue samples for fish health inspections. *J Aquat Anim Health.* 5:157–164.

Yang, L., Ho, N.Y., Alshut, R., et al. 2009. Zebrafish embryos as models for embryotoxic and teratological effects of chemicals. *Reprod Toxicol.* 28:245–253.

Zhou, X., Li, M., Abbas, K., and Wang, W. 2009. Comparison of haematology and serum biochemistry of cultured and wild Dojo loach *Misgurnus anguillicaudatus. Fish Physiol Biochem.* 35:435–441.

11 Evaluation of Hepatic Function and Injury

Charles E. Wiedmeyer

CONTENTS

11.1 INTRODUCTION

The liver is responsible for many vital physiologic functions essential for the maintenance of normal homeostatic mechanisms. It has a remarkable capacity for storage, synthesis, and regulation of a wide variety of substances. In addition, the liver has substantial functional reserve and regenerative capabilities. Because of its important role in preservation of a biologic system, it is prone to injury from a wide variety of toxic, infectious, and metabolic disturbances. The changes in liver functional capacity or detection of disease or injury can be determined using laboratory tests. This review is designed for highlighting the major functions of the liver and the clinical chemistry endpoints/parameters used for detecting the liver pathology and/or functional capabilities.

11.1.1 Hepatic Microanatomy

The microscopic structure of the tissues and organization of the liver has been reviewed (Krishna, 2013). Hepatocytes are the principle cell type of the liver and constitute at least 70% of its total volume (Tennant, 1997). Hepatocytes are polar epithelial cells and, like other epithelial cells, have an apical and basolateral surface. The basal surface of the hepatocyte meets the space of Disse (SD). The SD is separated from the blood-filled hepatic sinusoid by a lining of endothelial cells and Kupffer cells, and Figure 11.1 is a schematic presentation of the liver microscopic architecture and demonstrates the arrangement of hepatocytes to the sinusoids. Kupffer cells of the monocyte–phagocyte system are attached to the luminal face of the endothelial cells (Crawford, 1999). The sinusoidal domain is equivalent to the basolateral domain of other epithelial cells. Hepatic sinusoids differ from capillaries. In this case, the hepatocytes do not rest on a conventional basement membrane, however, are separated from endothelial cells by the SD. Substances released from the hepatocyte to the sinusoids should cross the SD and endothelial cells to gain access to the blood (Solter, 2005). This is facilitated by fenestrations in the sinusoidal lining endothelial cells. These fenestrations are attenuations of the endothelial cells whose structures can be altered by blood pressure, vasoactive substances, toxins, or xenobiotics (Wisse, 1970; Solter, 2005). The SD and endothelial cells do not pose great impedance to the passage of solubilized hepatic enzymes. It is the endothelial cell fenestrations that are important for the regulation of passage of large proteins, such as liver enzymes, and cells (Solter, 2005). Measurement of hepatocellular enzyme activities in the blood remains one of the most useful methods for detecting and monitoring liver pathology.

In the apical portion of the hepatocytes and between adjacent hepatocytes, the biliary system starts as the bile canaliculi (Nathanson and Boyer, 1991; Crawford, 1999). The bile canaliculi are 1–2 μm in diameter formed by grooves in the plasma membrane of facing hepatocytes (Figure 11.1). These canaliculi are demarcated from the vascular space on the basolateral side of the hepatocyte by tight junctions. The tight junctions prevent movement of substances between the bile and blood. Bile flow is facilitated by intracellular actin and myosin filaments whose pulsatile contractions propel the bile through the biliary network (Watanabe et al., 1991; Crawford, 1999). Hepatic bile formation serves two main functions: (1) promotion of dietary fat absorption in gut lumen and (2) elimination

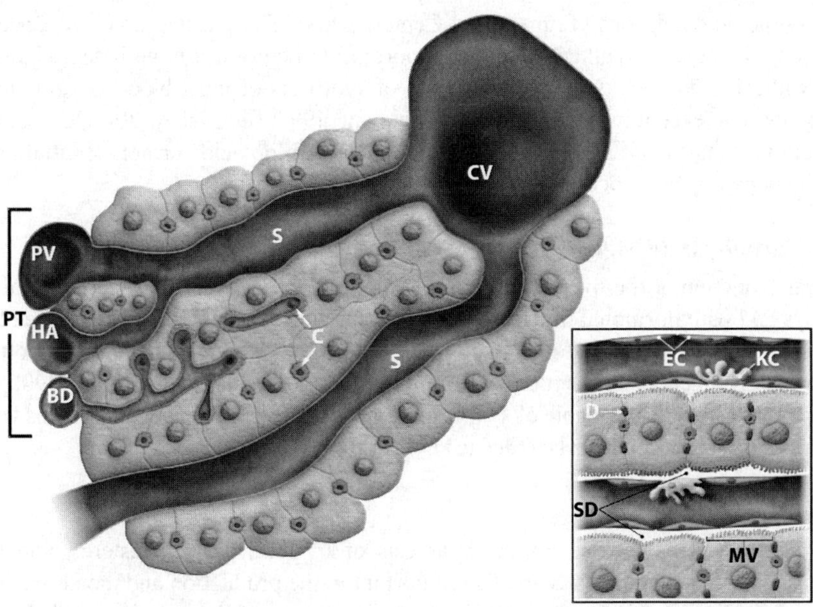

FIGURE 11.1 (See color insert.) Schematic presentation of the liver microanatomy. Hepatic sinusoids (S) are surrounded by one to two layers of cords of hepatocytes. The portal veins (PV), hepatic arterioles (HA), and bile ductules (BD) comprise the portal triad (PT). Blood flows from the portal triad (PV and HA) through the sinusoids to the central vein (CV). Bile flows from the bile canaliculi (C) to the BD of the PT. The inset depicts a close up of the sinusoids lined by fenestrated epithelia (EC) and Kupffer cells (KC). A perisinusoidal space (aka, space of Disse [SD]) is located between the hepatocytes and sinusoids. The basolateral hepatocyte surface has microvilli (MV) that extend into the SD that allows plasma components from the sinusoids to be absorbed by the hepatocytes. Bile canaliculi are formed on the lateral surface of adjacent hepatocytes and the hepatocytes attach to their neighbors with specialized junctions (desmosome; D). Original concept by Chuck Wiedemeyer and Greg Travlos; drawing by David Sabio.

of waste products (Crawford, 1999). Bile flow is the primary method for the elimination of bilirubin, excess cholesterol, and xenobiotics from the liver (Crawford, 1999). Because excretion of bile is one of the main functions of the liver, it is prone to disruption by a variety of hepatic insults. While decreased bile flow, known as cholestasis, can occur as a result of hepatocellular dysfunction, physical obstruction, or other pathologic processes, the exact mechanisms by which biliary constituents enter the blood from the bile are unknown (Solter, 2005). Several laboratory and clinical methods designed for detecting decreases in the bile flow (i.e., cholestasis) will be discussed later in this chapter.

11.1.2 Hepatic Function

The liver has many diverse and important physiologic functions. In general, these functions involve storage, synthesis/metabolism, and excretion/transport. The liver plays a large role in the synthesis and metabolism of a wide variety of endogenous and exogenous substances.

11.1.2.1 Protein Synthesis

Hepatocytes are responsible for the synthesis of most plasma proteins including albumin. Albumin is synthesized exclusively in the liver and degradation of albumin occurs in the liver as well as other tissues, including muscle, kidney, and skin (Tennant, 1997; McCuskey, 2006). Degradation of albumin is probably favored in the liver owing to the fenestrated endothelial lining cells that allow access to almost all plasma proteins directly to the SD and to the sinusoidal surface of the hepatocyte under normal physiologic conditions (Tennant and Center, 2008). The plasma albumin concentration is determined by the hepatic synthetic rate that is normally in equilibrium with degradation. Besides albumin synthesis, the liver is the exclusive site of synthesis of most blood coagulation proteins and most globulins (except immunoglobulins) (Tennant, 1997; McCuskey, 2006; Stockham, 2008). Most protein synthesis is *de novo* from essential dietary amino acids or nonessential amino acids produced by hepatocytes (Stockham, 2008).

11.1.2.2 Carbohydrate Metabolism

An important function of the liver is maintaining blood glucose levels. Through several biochemical pathways and with hormonal influence (e.g., insulin, glucagon), the liver is capable of storing or metabolizing glucose. The liver stores glucose in the form of glycogen and can metabolize the glycogen through glycogenolysis in order to maintain blood glucose levels (Voet D, 1990; McCuskey, 2006). Hepatocytes are also capable of synthesizing glucose from other sugars such as fructose and from amino acids (gluconeogenesis) (McCuskey, 2006).

11.1.2.3 Lipid Metabolism

The hepatocytes are responsible for the synthesis of triglycerides, cholesterol, and fatty acids (Stockham, 2008). The hepatocytes are also important in the production and metabolism of plasma lipoproteins (McCuskey, 2006). The liver is the major source of lipoproteins, excluding chylomicrons, which are synthesized in the intestine. The hepatocytes degrade chylomicrons from the systemic and portal blood and remove remnants of lipoproteins from the systemic blood (Stockham, 2008).

11.1.2.4 Detoxification/Bioactivation

Hepatocytes can detoxify, bioactivate, modify, and degrade a wide range of toxic endogenous and exogenous metabolic byproducts through multiple biochemical processes. Hepatocytes have high constitutive activities of phase I enzymes that convert xenobiotics to reactive electrophilic metabolites (Bishoff, 2007). In addition, hepatocytes have phase II enzymes that are capable of yielding a stable, nonreactive metabolite from the xenobiotic. Many compounds are bioactivated or detoxified by this process (Bishoff, 2007). Endogenous byproducts include uric acid, ammonium from protein catabolism, steroid hormones, and hemoglobin (Stockham, 2008). The role of the liver in activation and detoxification of xenobiotics is of great importance when new compounds are being studied (Cattley and Popp, 2002). The complete cellular mechanisms responsible for detoxification or bioactivation of particular compounds are beyond the scope of this chapter and readers are referred to basic toxicologic and hepatology texts.

11.1.2.5 Storage

Besides storing glycogen, as stated previously, the liver is capable of storing triglycerides and elements such as copper and iron and vitamins (Bishoff, 2007; Stockham, 2008).

11.1.2.6 Excretory

Bile is one of the main substances excreted by the liver and one of its major functions (Pineiro-Carrero and Pineiro, 2004). Bile is produced primarily in the hepatocytes and the composition of the bile is modified in the bile ducts (McCuskey, 2006). The hepatocytes synthesize bile acids from cholesterol for excretion in the bile. Bile is composed of bile salts, bilirubin, glutathione (GSH), phospholipids, cholesterol, proteins, organic anions, metals, and conjugated xenobiotics (Pineiro-Carrero and Pineiro, 2004). Bile serves two different but important functions. First, it is one of the primary routes for excretion of many endogenous and exogenous compounds such as drugs, toxins, and waste products. Second, it supplies bile salts to the intestine for emulsification and subsequent digestion and absorption of dietary lipids (McCuskey, 2006).

11.1.2.7 Mononuclear Phagocytic System

Important non-parenchyma cells within the liver are Kupffer cells. Kupffer cells constitute the largest population of fixed macrophages in most vertebrates (McCuskey, 2006). These cells are part of the mononuclear phagocytic system in the liver and have a wide array of functions. Kupffer cells are responsible for filtering the blood, both systemic and portal, of toxicants (such as endotoxins), damaged cells, organisms, and inflammatory mediators (McCuskey, 2006; Stockham, 2008). In addition, once activated, Kupffer cells secrete a variety of mediators (e.g., reactive oxygen species, nitric oxide, eicosanoids, as well as a myriad of cytokines, including TNF-alpha, IL1, IL6, and others) that affect the function of surrounding cells and produce substances that contribute to host defense (McCuskey, 2006).

11.2 HEPATIC ENZYMES

11.2.1 Introduction

Activities of liver enzymes in the plasma or serum are used primarily to identify cholestasis or injury to the hepatocyte (Hall and Nancy, 2008; Ennulat et al., 2010a, b). Often referred to as, "liver function tests," serum or plasma activities of liver enzymes do not provide specific information about liver function. The liver can be markedly dysfunctional without the evidence of increased liver enzyme activity in the plasma. An example would be an animal with liver cirrhosis. An animal with this condition can have severe loss of liver function with concurrent plasma liver enzyme activities within reference intervals. Alternatively, an animal may exhibit very high liver enzyme elevations but still have fully functional hepatic capacity. The reader is referred to Section 11.3.5 for further information.

The degree of liver enzyme activity in serum or plasma is dependent on multiple factors. Most increases in serum liver enzyme activity are caused by increased quantities of the enzymes released into the blood either by leakage from damaged cells or from increased production and release of that enzyme (Thrall, 2004). Other factors that must be considered when interpreting serum liver enzyme activities include liver specificity, intrahepatic, and cellular location of the enzyme, serum half-life, *in vitro* stability, and assay system used for measurement (Hall and Nancy, 2008).

Serum activity of several "liver specific" enzymes is used for detecting and monitoring liver pathology. What makes an enzyme "liver specific" is dependent on the presence of that enzyme in the liver, the concentration of that enzyme in the liver, and the method of release. For example, in dogs, serum alanine aminotransferase (ALT) is a sensitive indicator of hepatocellular damage or leakage because of its high concentrations in hepatocytes (Hoffmann et al., 1999). However, in guinea pigs and large species (e.g., cow and horse) ALT activity in the liver is quite low thus, insensitive indicator of liver damage in those species (Clampitt and Hart, 1978). In addition, the magnitude of increase of a "liver specific" enzyme in serum may not always be a reflection of the quantity of the enzyme in the tissue from which it is derived. The magnitude and rate of enzyme release from the tissue of origin into blood and its subsequent clearance must be considered (Hoffmann et al., 1999; Thrall, 2004). Those tissues with greater concentrations of an enzyme are more likely to contribute more to the serum than those with little or no concentration of that enzyme. However, the magnitude of increase of an enzyme in serum may not entirely reflect the quantity of the enzyme in the tissue from which it is derived. For example, serum γ-glutamyltranspeptidase (GGT) activity can be markedly increased with cholestatic liver disease. However, the greatest concentrations of GGT in the body are found in the kidney and virtually never increased in renal disease (Clampitt and Hart, 1978; Hoffmann et al., 1999; Hall and Nancy, 2008). GGT can be released from damaged tubular epithelial cells but the released enzyme leaks into the urine rather than the serum (Hall and Nancy, 2008).

Another consideration to serum activities of liver enzymes is the normal cellular location of the enzyme within the cell and the mechanisms by which it is released from the damaged cell during a pathologic state. Enzymes that reside within the cytoplasm can be released directly into the blood through compromised cell membranes of damaged or cells going through necrosis or may be released from viable cells by through blebs that release from the membrane (Gores et al., 1990). Some enzymes whose primary location is in the cytoplasm and tissue of origin does not have direct accessibility to the bloodstream may be released first into interstitial fluid and travel through the lymphatics to the bloodstream. Other enzymes such as GGT, which resides on the cell membrane of the biliary epithelial cells and proximal tubular epithelial cells of kidney do not have direct access to the bloodstream and may be lost in bile or urine.

The effects of drugs, endogenous hormones, or changes in physiology may also play an important role in the serum activity of various enzymes in health and disease. For example, serum and tissue activities of alkaline phosphatase (ALP) isoenzymes can increase in dogs when given exogenous glucocorticoids or under conditions of significantly increased endogenous glucocorticoids (e.g., cortisol) (Hoffmann and Dorner, 1975; Hoffmann, 1976; Wiedmeyer et al., 2002a). Furthermore, the performance of hepatobiliary enzyme biomarkers (including ALT, aspartate aminotransferase (AST), ALP, and GGT) related to drug-induced liver injury has been examined (Ennulat et al., 2010a, b).

Other factors that affect serum liver enzyme activity are rate of clearance (or half-life [T½]) of the enzyme and different isoforms/isoenzymes that can be found in the serum or plasma of a particular enzyme. The T½ of an enzyme is important in determining the magnitude and persistence of the enzyme increase. Both T½ and the different isoforms/isoenzymes found in the serum or plasma will ultimately affect the diagnostic and prognostic value of that enzyme increase. The T½ of liver enzymes varies from minutes to days depending on the enzyme, the species, and the tissue source. For example, intestinal ALP in dogs is cleared from the blood rapidly ($T_{1/2}$ < 6 min) thus offering very little diagnostic information (Hoffmann and Dorner, 1977). However, in rats, intestinal ALP has a longer T½ thus making it the predominant ALP isoenzyme in serum (Young et al., 1981). Another liver enzyme, sorbitol dehydrogenase (SDH), is cleared quite rapidly from the blood yet remains in blood long enough to allow for detection of acute hepatocellular damage (Hoffmann et al., 1999). Other enzymes such as ALT, with a T½ in the order of days rather than minutes or hours, offers diagnostic value during and after the initial tissue insult (Ramaiah, 2007; Ozer et al., 2008).

Some liver enzymes exist in plasma in different forms called isoenzymes. These enzymes have identical catalytic activity, however, are produced by different tissues. While commonly referred to as isoenzymes, the term isoform is occasionally used. If different forms of a particular enzyme exist from one gene product, they are referred to as isoforms. Isoenzymes arise from different gene products. For example, the liver, bone, and kidney forms of ALP originate from the same gene (i.e., the tissue nonspecific ALP gene). These isoforms differ only in degree of glycosylation of the core protein. The intestinal ALP form originates from the intestinal ALP gene, and it is considered an isoenzyme when compared to the liver, bone, and kidney forms. Regardless, the isoforms and isoenzymes of ALP have the same fundamental catalytic abilities. Other examples of enzymes that exist as isoenzymes are ALT and lactate dehydrogenase (LDH) (Hoffmann et al., 1999). Although the isoenzymes have the same catalytic abilities, they may or may not differ in T½. This difference in T½ usually determines the clinical utility of the isoenzyme.

11.2.2 Hepatocellular Leakage Enzymes

11.2.2.1 Alanine Aminotransferase

ALT, formerly known as serum glutamic pyruvic transaminase (SGPT) catalyzes the reductive transfer of amino groups from alanine to α-ketoglutarate to yield glutamate and pyruvate (Hoffmann et al., 1999; Ozer et al., 2008). Enzyme activity can be found in many tissues but the greatest concentration is found within the hepatocyte cytosol (Boyd, 1983; Amacher, 1998). In general, ALT is the most useful enzyme for the detection of hepatocellular necrosis in many species and is the most relied upon liver enzyme to indicate hepatotoxic effects (Amacher, 1998, 2002). However, serum ALT activity is of little value in the large domestic animals (pig, horse, cow, and sheep) and guinea pigs owing to relatively low hepatocyte concentrations (Clampitt and Hart, 1978). In marmosets, the liver has the highest activity of ALT; cardiac muscle and kidney also had substantial amounts (Mohr et al., 1971).

Both soluble (i.e., cytoplasmic) and mitochondrial isoenzymes of ALT exist. The soluble cytosolic and mitochondrial isoenzymes have been separated by isoelectric focusing (Ruscak et al., 1982). The isoelectric point of the soluble enzyme from rat, guinea pig, human liver, and rat and pig kidney differ dramatically from the mitochondrial ALT from the same organ. Additional differences in the physicochemical and kinetic properties of the two isoenzymes have been reported, which indicate that ALT from mitochondria and cytoplasm are two different proteins (DeRosa and Swick, 1975). The similarity of the cytoplasmic enzyme obtained from different organs indicates that the isoenzymes have no organ specificity but rather are specific for the cell compartment from which they are derived. The differentiation between these isoenzymes may therefore be useful in determination of mechanism of cellular injury.

11.2.2.1.1 Isoenzymes

Two ALT isoforms (ALT1 and ALT2) have been identified in humans, mice, rats, and dogs (Yang et al., 2002; Jadhao et al., 2004; Rajamohan et al., 2006). In humans, ALT1 is mainly expressed in kidney, liver, fat, and cardiac tissues and ALT2 is the predominant form in muscle and fat (Yang et al., 2002). It appears the isoforms are conserved across species and display similar tissue distribution. The mouse ALT isoenzymes, ALT1 and ALT2, are highly homologous to the human proteins and show similar tissue distribution (Jadhao et al., 2004). In mice, ALT2 has been proposed as a marker of hepatic steatosis (Jadhao et al., 2004). A novel immunoassay capable of discriminating human ALT1 and ALT2 activities has been developed (Lindblom et al., 2007). To date, assays that discriminate between the different isoforms are not widely available for use in laboratory animals. In the future, ALT isoform specific assays may add information to serum ALT activities and organ specific pathology.

11.2.2.1.2 Causes of Increased Serum ALT Activity

11.2.2.1.2.1 Hepatocellular Damage By far the main cause for an increase in serum ALT activity is damage to hepatocytes. In fact, increase in serum ALT activity is considered the gold standard clinical chemistry marker for liver injury (Ramaiah, 2007; Ozer et al., 2008). Hepatocyte injury can be caused by a variety of insults such as inflammation, toxicity, hypoxia, or trauma (Stockham, 2008). As stated previously, the largest pool of ALT activity in most species is found within the cytosol of hepatocytes (Clampitt and Hart, 1978; Boyd, 1983). Therefore, simple leakage of cytosolic ALT from compromised hepatocyte membranes or overt hepatocyte necrosis can result in increases in serum ALT activity. Besides leakage and cell necrosis, other mechanisms responsible for the appearance of ALT in the serum have been well described such as induction and cytoplasmic blebbing (Gores et al., 1990; Solter et al., 1994; Solter, 2005). Cytoplasmic blebs are reported to detach from the damaged hepatocyte and allow the cell membrane to reseal without cell death (Lemasters et al., 1983; Gores et al., 1990; Kristensen, 1994). Cell membrane bleb formation has been described in hepatocytes following hypoxic events (Gores et al., 1990; Kristensen, 1994). After detachment, the cytoplasmic blebs reportedly rupture within the SD releasing ALT into the sinusoid (Kristensen, 1994; Solter, 2005). Regardless of the mechanism involved with enzyme release, the magnitude of serum ALT activity is typically proportional to the number of affected hepatocytes damaged (Hall and Nancy, 2008). The greatest elevations result from severe lesions affecting a large portion of the liver. Despite this observation, increases in serum ALT activity have been noted without evidence of histopathologic changes to the liver (Van Vleet and Alberts, 1968; Ozer et al., 2008). The causes for increased serum ALT activity without correlating histopathologic liver lesions may be related to enzyme induction by the particular xenobiotic being studied (Pappas, 1986). Finally, increased serum ALT can be observed with biliary disease or bile duct obstruction

(Hall and Nancy, 2008). Theoretically, the increase in ALT is due in part to the effects of retained bile salts on the hepatic cell membranes and leakage of cytosolic enzymes.

11.2.2.1.2.2 Muscle Damage Besides liver, which has the greatest activity of ALT on a per gram basis in most species, heart, and skeletal muscle have been shown to have significant ALT activity (Clampitt and Hart, 1978). Therefore, muscle damage, when severe and diffuse, can result in increased serum ALT activity in the absence of hepatocellular damage (Watkins et al., 1989; Valentine et al., 1990a; Swenson and Graves, 1997). For example, dogs in a colony with canine X-linked muscular dystrophy and ongoing muscle necrosis all had increased serum ALT activity with no biochemical evidence of hepatocellular damage (Valentine et al., 1990b). Both of these observations support the conclusion that ALT is not truly liver specific and that severe muscle necrosis can contribute to serum ALT activity.

11.2.2.1.2.3 Drug Induction There are numerous drugs that cause hepatocellular damage and release of ALT into serum and the effects of xenobiotics causing liver damage, which are closely monitored through measurement of serum ALT activity. However, there are drugs that cause alterations in ALT activity in liver and/or serum without causing hepatocellular damage. Glucocorticoids have been the most often studied class of drug with regard to induction of ALT, causing an increase in ALT in rat liver tissue following treatment (Rosen et al., 1959a, b; Patnaik and Kanungo, 1977). There is general agreement that glucocorticoids induce the cytoplasmic isoenzyme of ALT. In dogs, increases in serum ALT activity following glucocorticoid administration are commonly observed (DeNovo and Prasse, 1983; Solter et al., 1994). Other studies have shown an association between drugs (e.g., anticonvulsants) and toxins and increases in serum ALT activity due in part to increase in intracellular activity (Solter, 2005; Hall and Nancy, 2008). The increases of ALT activity in the serum from these various compounds is believed to be from *de novo* ALT synthesis but a damaging effect to the hepatocytes could not be ruled out. Finally, low protein diets have been shown to increase serum ALT activity, and the cause is unclear (Rao, 1996).

11.2.2.1.3 Causes of Decreased Serum Alt Activity

Typically, decreases in the serum activity of ALT are insignificant and noted infrequently in toxicologic studies. There have been reports of compounds causing decreased in the liver and serum activities of ALT. It has been reported that microcystin-LR administration can result in significant inhibition of the ALT protein in the liver (Solter, 2000). Moreover, it has been shown that vitamin B6 deficiency can lead to artifactual decreased serum transaminase activity (Ono et al., 1995). In addition, cefazolin treatment of rats results in lowered serum ALT activity, which is associated with lowered ALT activity in the liver, brain, and kidney (Dhami et al., 1979).

11.2.2.1.4 Other Influencing Factors

In monkeys, the use of ALT as a marker of hepatocellular damage can be complicated by the presence of subclinical, enzootic hepatitis A infection (Slighter, 1988). The increase in serum ALT activity appears to be transient and occurs concurrently with seroconversion to the virus. Serum values of up to 300 U/L can be observed in individual monkeys from this phenomenon (Slighter, 1988). Imported cynomolgus monkeys (*Macaca fascicularis*) have displayed increases in serum ALT activities but the cause is unknown (Yoshida, 1981). In addition, multiple administrations of sevoflurane, a rapid-acting halogenated either, has been shown to increased serum ALT activity in a dose-related manner (Soma et al., 1995). Increases in serum ALT activity in individual mice have been observed including control animals. The cause for sporadically high serum ALT levels in individual mice is suspected to be from physical damage to the liver during handling (Swaim et al., 1985). These spurious findings of high serum ALT activity in mice may complicate interpretation of results of toxicologic studies.

11.2.2.2 Aspartate Aminotransferase

AST, formerly known as serum glutamic oxaloacetic transaminase (SGOT) catalyzes the transamination of L-aspartate and 2-oxoglutatarate to oxaloacetate and glutamate (Hoffmann, 2008). AST plays a role in amino acid synthesis and degradation, gluconeogenesis, and serves as a link between the urea and tricarboxylic acid cycles. AST activity is found primarily in heart, skeletal muscle, and liver (Ozer et al., 2008). In rats and marmosets, AST activity can be found in the brain comparable to activity found in the muscle (Mohr et al., 1971; Boyd, 1983). Other soft tissue organs such as kidney and intestine have less AST activity in nearly all laboratory species. Within the cell, AST activity can be found in the cytosol and mitochondria (Ramaiah, 2007; Ozer et al., 2008). In rat hepatocytes, 81%–85% of the total AST activity is found in mitochondria and 15%–19% in cytoplasm (Pappas, 1980, 1986). Nearly 30%–40% of canine liver AST activity is of mitochondrial origin (Keller, 1981). In serum from normal rats, cytoplasmic AST activity accounts for approximately 82% of the total AST activity, and mitochondrial AST activity for approximately 18% (Pappas, 1986). The use of AST activity as a diagnostic enzyme was first reported in 1954–1955, when increases in serum AST activity were described in people with myocardial infarction and viral hepatitis (Keil, 1990; Hoffmann et al., 1999). The lack of organ specificity of AST activity limits its usefulness in diagnostic medicine, but when used in conjunction with other enzymes, it has clinical utility.

11.2.2.2.1 Isoenzymes

The cytoplasmic and mitochondrial isoenzymes of AST are the products of different genes and are therefore separable by immunologic means (Rej, 1980; Pappas, 1986). Both cytoplasmic and mitochondrial AST activity increase significantly until adulthood (Patnaik et al., 1987).

11.2.2.2.2 Causes of Increased Serum AST Activity

11.2.2.2.2.1 Hepatocellular Damage AST activity in serum can increase with hepatocellular damage or leakage from many of the same etiologies as noted with increased ALT (i.e., inflammation, toxicity, hypoxia, or trauma). Increased serum AST activity with liver disease is due to necrosis of hepatocytes and the release of cytoplasmic and mitochondrial AST into lymph and blood (Hoffmann et al., 1999). It has been suggested that because the greatest activity for AST is found in the mitochondria in rats, more severe liver necrosis is necessary for serum AST activity increases when compared to ALT (Ramaiah, 2007). Leakage of AST through the cell and mitochondrial membranes has long been suggested as the mechanism of appearance in blood. However, like ALT, membrane injury sufficiently severe to allow the leakage of proteins from viable cells would surely disrupt cellular electrolyte balance and lead to cell death. The alternative to leakage of enzyme is the formation of cytoplasmic blebs, like ALT (Gores et al., 1990; Solter, 2005). Release of AST into the serum from hepatocytes may also occur during reparative processes of liver disease (Stockham, 2008).

11.2.2.2.2.2 Muscle Damage Because of the high concentration of AST in the skeletal and cardiac muscle, a variety of insults to the muscle can result in increased serum AST levels. General etiologic categories include trauma, degenerative changes as a result of hypoxia, metabolic, neoplastic, nutritional, inherited, or inflammatory insults. In short, many of the same etiologies that can result in an increase in ALT serum activity can cause an increase in serum AST.

11.2.2.2.2.3 Other Causes *In vitro* hemolysis or delayed removal of serum from a clotted sample may result in mild to moderate increases in AST activity (Stockham, 2008). It has been shown that adrenalectomy can result in decreases in hepatic AST activity and hydrocortisone administration increases the hepatic cytoplasmic AST activity in rats (Patnaik et al., 1987). Treatment of rats with glucocorticoids increases cytosolic AST mRNA and activity but has no effect on mitochondrial AST (Pave-Preux et al., 1988). Cytosolic AST activity and mRNA have shown increases of approximately twofold with no change in mitochondrial AST in rats fed high-protein diets (Horio et al., 1988a). Likewise, an increase in liver cytoplasmic AST activity and mRNA were observed following both feeding of a high-protein diet and glucagon injections with no increase in mitochondrial AST or AST in skeletal muscle and kidney (Horio et al., 1988b). Fasting of rats for 16 hours can result in mild increases in serum AST activity (Matsuzawa, 1994).

11.2.2.2.3 Causes of Decreased Serum AST Activity

Like ALT, decreases in AST are usually rarely observed and most likely insignificant.

11.2.2.3 Sorbitol Dehydrogenase

SDH, also known as iditol dehydrogenase, catalyzes a reversible reaction involving conversion of fructose to sorbitol. SDH is a cytosolic enzyme in all cells with the highest concentration of activity on a per gram basis is found in the liver followed by the kidney (Boyd, 1983). SDH mRNA has been detected in all tissues except the small intestine in the rat, with highest concentrations found in the testis, liver, and kidney (Estonius et al., 1993; Lee et al., 1995). Measurement of serum SDH is particularly useful in species whereby serum ALT activity is not liver specific, such as in swine or guinea pigs (Hoffmann et al., 1999). Serum SDH activity has also been demonstrated to be useful in the detection of chemical-induced liver damage in fish (Dixon et al., 1987; Webb and Gagnon, 2007). In rats, plasma SDH activity has demonstrated seasonal variations (Petrovich et al., 2007). Furthermore, excessive dietary intake of the sugar substitute sorbitol induced increased activity of SDH in the liver and plasma (Petrovich et al., 2007). In dogs, serum SDH activity can be used in combination with ALT activity to determine if there is persistent hepatic injury. If serum SDH activity is not increased while ALT activity is markedly increased, it suggests that ongoing liver insult is present (Hoffmann, 2008). This is related to the short T½ of SDH compared to ALT but proper interpretation of this type of change requires repeated monitoring.

11.2.2.3.1 Isoenzymes

Isoenzymes of SDH have not been described.

11.2.2.3.2 Causes of Increased Serum SDH Activity

Increases in serum SDH are always related to hepatocellular injury. Administration of certain compounds that cause hepatocellular necrosis results in increased serum SDH activity in a dose-related manner (Blazka et al., 1996; Brondeau et al., 1986; Carakostas et al., 1986; Rikans and Moore, 1988). Because of the short half-life (less than 12 hours in most species), increased serum SDH activity appears early in the course of toxicity and usually returns to baseline levels in a matter of days, depending on the magnitude of the SDH activity increase, the persistence of the toxicity, and the species affected (Hoffmann, 2008). In dogs, SDH activity is less favored for detection of hepatocellular damage than ALT. However, it may be useful in determining if there concurrent hepatocellular damage in cases of traumatic muscle injury where there is also increased serum ALT activity (Hoffmann, 2008). Moreover, the SDH activity measurement in conjunction with ALT may be useful in dogs when attempting to determine if there persists hepatocellular damage. If ALT is markedly increased and SDH activity is not, recovery is likely (Hoffmann, 2008). In mice exposed to certain hepatotoxins, ALT and SDH activities first increase then decrease in parallel (Chapman et al., 1988; Blazka et al., 1996). A review of the results of several toxicologic studies performed in rats found an association between increased ALT and SDH activity and histopathological changes, with SDH activity showing greater positive and negative predictive value than ALT (Travlos et al., 1996). It was found that the SDH activity predicted morphological hepatic change with 75% accuracy. Combining the results of serum SDH activity with ALT activity increased diagnostic accuracy to 100% by 2–3 weeks in repeated dose studies. Nephrotoxicity has not been shown to be a cause for increased serum SDH.

11.2.2.3.3 Causes for Decreased Serum SDH Activity

Decreases in SDH activity may occur but are rare, the cause is unknown and most likely insignificant.

11.2.2.4 Glutamate Dehydrogenase

Glutamate dehydrogenase (GDH) is a key mitochondrial enzyme in amino acid oxidation and urea production (O'Brien et al., 2002). The enzyme is highly conserved in tissue distribution and function across a wide species range (Schmidt and Schmidt, 1988; O'Brien et al., 2002). The liver has the highest concentration of GDH with lesser amounts in the kidney and small intestine. In the kidney, the activity is found in the proximal and distal tubular epithelium (Kaneko et al., 1997; Ozer et al., 2008). Because of liver has the highest concentration, the serum activity originates solely from this organ.

11.2.2.4.1 Isoenzymes

Isoenzymes of GDH have not been described.

11.2.2.4.2 Causes for Increased Serum GDH Activity

Similar to ALT and SDH, increases in serum GDH activity are due to hepatocellular damage (Gopinath et al., 1980). Serum activity of GDH is more liver specific than ALT and is not substantially affected by skeletal muscle damage. When compared to ALT activity, GDH elevations under certain hepatocellular damaging events were of greater magnitude and persisted longer in rats (O'Brien et al., 2002). Moreover, in rats, GDH has been used as a plasma marker of alcohol-induced liver injury (Murayama et al., 2009). GDH is not inhibited by compounds that interfere with pyridoxal-5′-phosphate such as isoniazid and lead (O'Brien et al., 2002). Furthermore, GDH activity does not appear to be induced by certain compounds associated with ALT induction (e.g., dexamethasone) (O'Brien et al., 2002). It has been shown that activity of GDH in the serum is more stable than SDH and has a longer half-life in some species (Collis et al., 1979). Use of GDH as a serum biomarker for hepatic injury has been criticized in the past due to technical difficulties with assay procedures (Carakostas et al., 1986). However, advances in commercial assay availability have led to more clinical use (O'Brien et al., 2002; Ozer et al., 2008).

11.2.2.4.3 Causes for Decreased Serum GDH Activity

Decreases in GDH activity are most likely insignificant.

11.2.2.5 Lactate Dehydrogenase

LDH is a cytoplasmic enzyme that catalyzes the reaction that converts pyruvate to lactate at the end of anaerobic glycolysis (Hoffmann et al., 1999). Although this reaction is reversible, the reduction of pyruvate to lactate is favored and this will generate NAD^+ under anaerobic conditions so glycolysis can continue. LDH is found in all cells and present in all organs. Liver, heart, skeletal muscle, and kidney contain the highest activity per gram (Clampitt and Hart, 1978; Keller, 1981; Boyd, 1983). While LDH activity can be found in most tissues, the distribution among species varies. In dogs, heart muscle has the highest LDH activity per gram of tissue, followed by skeletal muscle (53%) and liver (41%). Rabbits have a similar distribution, while rats have the highest LDH activity in skeletal muscle followed by heart muscle (77%) and liver (41%). Pigs are somewhat unique in that heart muscle (10%) and liver (5%) have very low activity compared to skeletal muscle (Hoffmann et al., 1999). In laboratory animals, the lack of specificity without isoenzyme analysis and lack of sensitivity for detection of liver disease have reduced the utilization of LDH as part of diagnostic enzyme profiles.

11.2.2.5.1 Isoenzymes

Mammals have two different LDH subunits, the H type (heart subunits) and M type (muscle subunits) (Boyd, 1983). These combine randomly to form five tetrameric isoenzymes: H_4, H_3M, H_2M_2, HM_3, and M_4. The electrophoretically slow moving LDH4 and LDH5 (or HM_3, M_4 respectively) isoenzymes are found primarily in skeletal muscle while the fast moving LDH1 and LDH2 (or H_4, H_3M) predominate in cardiac muscle in laboratory animals (Boyd, 1983). Liver is similar to skeletal muscle in that it contains primarily LDH5 and LDH4 in laboratory animals, but interestingly, in sheep and cattle, liver has an LDH isoenzyme profile more like heart rather than skeletal muscle. In laboratory animals, it is difficult or impossible to differentiate the liver or skeletal muscle as the source of increased LDH5 and LDH4. Use of increased LDH1 and LDH2 to identify experimentally induced myocardial infarction is feasible (Preus et al., 1988). LDH1 and LDH2 isoenzymes predominate in erythrocytes of all the species except the rat, which shows a predominance of LDH5 (Boyd, 1983). LDH1 and LDH2 predominate in the normal serum of all the species except the dog, cat, and rat (Boyd, 1983). Cynomolgus monkeys have five LDH isoenzymes. Isoenzymes 1–3 are the most prevalent, and similar quantities of each are found in serum (~22%–28%); isoenzyme 5 is the least prevalent. The activity of isoenzymes 1 and 2 is high in the myocardium, kidneys, and brain; monkeys also have a high amount of these isoenzymes in red blood cells (Preus et al., 1988). In mice affected with the LDH virus, the infection alters the macrophage population and prevents rapid clearance of LDH5 (Rowson and Mahy, 1985). The macrophages that clear LDH5 have no action of clearance on LDH4 (Rowson and Mahy, 1985). Macrophage clearance of other enzymes such as ALP is not affected with virus infection.

11.2.2.5.2 Causes for Increased Serum LDH Activity

Since LDH is a cytoplasmic enzyme and found in all organs it lacks specificity and sensitivity for assessment of hepatocellular damage, although damage to hepatocytes or muscle is the main reasons for increased serum LDH activity. In laboratory animals, LDH has been used for the detection of experimentally induced myocardial injury (Asha and Radha, 1985; Preus et al., 1988; Takami et al., 1990). To increase the specificity of LDH activity for detection of myocardial injury, determining particular isoenzyme activity (i.e., LDH1 activity) can be determined (Boyd, 1983). LDH activity is increased after exercise in rats with higher activity in males compared to females (Van der Meulen et al., 1991). Mice infected with the lactate dehydrogenase elevating virus (LDEV) can have increases of 3-10-fold in serum LDH activity (Rowson and Mahy, 1985). Serum enzyme levels are not directly related to the level of viral infectivity but are dependent on the rate of clearance of the enzymes (Rowson and Mahy, 1985). Clearance rate depends on the activity of macrophages. This virus is thought to destroy or block a population of macrophages that remove LDH from circulation, resulting in a marked reduction in clearance of either endogenous LDH or exogenously administered LDH (Rowson and Mahy, 1985; Hayashi et al., 1988).

11.2.2.5.3 Causes for Decreased Serum LDH Activity

Decreases in LDH activity are most likely insignificant.

11.2.2.6 Glutathione *S*-Transferase

The glutathione *S*-transferases (GST) are a complex family of proteins that display various biological functions. The main purpose of GST is the phase II detoxification of xenobiotics (Giffen et al., 2002). GST is capable of the reaction between GSH and electrophilic compounds and carcinogens allowing for their detoxification (Boyer, 1989). The family of GST enzymes is found predominately in the cytoplasm, and consists of isoforms (alpha, mu, pi, and theta) and a microsomal form (DePierre and Morgenstern, 1983; Morgenstern and DePierre, 1983; Giffen et al., 2002). GST is found in all species and in virtually every organ. In the rat and other species, the liver contains the greatest GST activity (Clarke et al., 1997; Giffen et al., 2002). In the rat, the hepatic GST activity is low at birth and increases progressively until adulthood (Eidne et al., 1984; Harman and Henry, 1987). Erythrocytes of dogs, rats, and mice contain GST activity, which is higher than erythrocyte GST activity found in pigs and rabbits (Vodela and Dalvi, 1997). GST is typically a dimeric enzyme that can be found as a trimer and monomer (Mannervik, 1985; Boyer, 1989).

11.2.2.6.1 *Isoenzymes*

There have been numerous subunits identified and hence numerous isoenzymes. In the rat, the isoenzymes are dimeric hybrids of identical or dissimilar subunits (Mannervik, 1985). The isoenzymes are grouped into classes referred to as alpha, mu, and pi, based on their isoelectric points, structural, and functional similarities (Jensson et al., 1985; Mannervik, 1985; Mannervik et al., 1985). Rat liver expresses primarily alpha and mu classes of GST, while pi classes are present in minimal quantities (Robertson et al., 1985). The pi class is more prevalent in kidney and pancreas.

11.2.2.6.2 *Causes for Increased Serum GST Activity*

11.2.2.6.2.1 Hepatocellular Damage In the rat, alpha-GST has been shown to be a valid serum marker of hepatotoxicity (Giffen et al., 2002). Following carbon tetrachloride administration to rats, serum GST increases either in parallel with ALT activity or preceding the increase of ALT and AST activity (Adachi et al., 1981; Aniya and Anders, 1985; Igarashi et al., 1988; Clarke et al., 1997). In addition, when compared to serum ALT and AST activity, GST activity rapidly returns to pretreatment activity, which is consistent with the shorter half-life of GST activity in blood (Adachi et al., 1981). Administration of other hepatotoxic compounds also results in increases of serum GST activity (Aniya and Anders, 1985; Giffen et al., 2002). A marked increase in serum GST activity in the absence of a significant increase of serum ALT activity is observed in baboons following shock-induced hepatic injury, suggesting that serum GST activity may be used as an early marker of posttraumatic hepatic injury (Redl et al., 1995). Unlike ALT and AST, GST is found in high concentrations in the centrilobular cells in the liver and thus may be a more sensitive indicator to injury in the metabolic zone of the liver (Ozer et al., 2008). In most instances, measurement of serum GST offers no advantages over measurement of ALT and AST in detecting either the time of onset, recovery, or severity of hepatic injury (Giffen et al., 2002).

11.2.2.6.2.2 Drug Induction Administration of phenobarbital and several other compounds (e.g., 3-methylcholanthrene, propylthiouracil, and butylated hydroxyanisole) induce increases of hepatic GST activity in rats of all ages (Eidne et al., 1984; Brondeau et al., 1986; Boyer, 1989).

11.2.2.6.3 *Causes for Decreased Serum GST Activity*

Decreases in GST activity are most likely insignificant.

11.2.2.7 Ornithine Carbamyltransferase

Ornithine carbamyltransferase (OCT) is a mitochondrial enzyme that catalyzes a step in the urea cycle in the liver (Bondy et al., 2000). OCT is an abundant protein found almost exclusively in the liver with very slight activity in the gastrointestinal tract and kidney in dogs and rats (Reichard, 1959; Curtis et al., 1972; Hoffmann et al., 1999; Amacher, 2002). Serum OCT activity in these species is minute (Plaa, 2008). Therefore, serum OCT activity can be considered of hepatic origin. Isoenzymes of OCT have not been described. Methods for determining OCT activity in serum have been developed but may not be available for routine use (Ohshita et al., 1976; Murayama et al., 2006).

11.2.2.7.1 *Causes for Increased Serum OCT Activity*

Because OCT is found almost exclusively in the liver, it is considered a highly specific serum marker of hepatocellular necrosis and hepatotoxicity (Bondy et al., 2000; Amacher, 2002). Past studies have shown that mitochondria-derived serum markers of carbon tetrachloride hepatotoxicity are less sensitive than cytoplasmic enzymes (i.e., ALT and AST) (Baumann and Berauer, 1985). The cause for this finding is believed to be a result of mitochondrial dysfunction causing cell death rather than a consequence of cell death (Murayama et al., 2008). This suggests that some mitochondria are destroyed prior to plasma membrane disturbances resulting in less activity of OCT in the serum following administration of certain hepatotoxins. Several recent reports suggest that changes in serum OCT activity may be more rapid than traditional markers of hepatocellular necrosis from administration of hepatotoxins and alcohol-induced injury (Murayama et al., 2007, 2008, 2009). In spite of these encouraging results, OCT does not appear to be used routinely for diagnostic purposes. This is due in part to analytical assay requirements required for routing screening (Bondy et al., 2000). However, recent developments of ELISA make analysis more practical (Murayama et al., 2006).

Induction of urea cycle enzymes, including OCT, has been shown to occur by glucagon (Snodgrass et al., 1978). De novo synthesis of OCT is induced in rats by increases in protein consumption or administration of the substrate for OCT (Hoffmann et al., 1999). It is likely that OCT can be induced with the need for urea synthesis from ammonia by drugs that cause protein catabolism.

11.2.2.7.2 Causes for Decreased Serum OCT Activity

As mentioned previously, it has been suggested that mitochondria destruction prior to disruptions in plasma membrane may not result in increases in serum OCT activity with administration of certain hepatotoxins (Murayama et al., 2008). However, decreases in OCT serum activity are most likely insignificant.

11.2.2.8 Other Hepatic Leakage Markers

11.2.2.8.1 Arginase I

Arginase I is a hydrolase that catalyzes the hydrolysis of arginine to urea and ornithine (Ashamiss et al., 2004). The enzyme is highly liver specific with most activity noted in the organ with trace amounts found in kidney and erythrocytes (Ashamiss et al., 2004). Serum increases in arginase I have been shown to occur with acute and chronically induced hepatic injury in rats (Murayama et al., 2007, 2008). In comparison to traditional measures of hepatic injury (i.e., ALT and AST), arginase I showed the greatest and earliest increase in the serum in response to acute injury in rats (Ikemoto et al., 2001b; Murayama et al., 2008). Despite the encouraging findings of arginase I as an early marker of acute liver injury the lack of commercially available assays for measurement are lacking. An ELISA for the detection of serum arginase I has been developed and may enhance the use of this enzyme in future studies (Ikemoto et al., 2001a).

11.2.2.8.2 Malate Dehydrogenase

Malate dehydrogenase (MDH) is an enzyme involved with the citric acid cycle and catalyzes the reaction of malate to oxaloacetate (Zelewski and Swierczynski, 1991). MDH is a mitochondrial and cytosolic enzyme with its greatest activity found in the liver followed by heart, muscle, and brain (Ozer et al., 2008). Because activity is found in the cytosol of hepatocytes, the damage to these cells results in release to the serum much like ALT and AST. Increases in serum MDH activity has been shown after dosing rats with hepatotoxins (Korsrud et al., 1972; Zieve et al., 1985). The sensitivity of MDH in detecting hepatocellular necrosis compared to more traditional markers has not been performed to date.

11.2.2.8.3 Purine Nucleoside Phosphorlyase

Purine nucleoside phosphorlyase (PNP) is an enzyme in the purine salvage pathway (Ozer et al., 2008). PNP is a cytoplasmic enzyme with the greatest activity found in liver with lesser activity in the heart and muscle. In the liver, PNP is found in the cytoplasm of endothelial cells, hepatocytes, and Kupffer cells. Damage to these cells results in the release of PNP into the serum much like the other hepatocellular necrosis markers (Ohuchi et al., 1995). It was shown that dosing rats with endotoxin causes increases in serum PNP activity earlier than increases in ALT activity (Mochida et al., 1999). Because PNP is found in the cytoplasm of endothelial cells in the liver, it has been proposed as a marker of endothelial cell damage in the hepatic sinusoids (Fukuda et al., 2004). The wide spread use of PNP in laboratory animal species as a suitable marker of hepatocellular damage has not been established.

11.2.2.8.4 Serum F Protein

Serum F protein is a 44-kDa protein involved in tyrosine catabolism. The protein is produced in large amounts in the liver with minor amounts in the kidney and is found in the cytosol (Oliveira, 1986; Foster et al., 1989). Serum contains very little serum F protein in a normal subject. In humans, the measurement of serum F protein in the serum appears to be a more sensitive indicator of hepatic injury than aminotransferases and serum concentrations correlate with histologic lesions in the liver (Foster et al., 1989). Serum F protein is produced by a wide variety of animals (Oliveira and Vindlacheruvu, 1987). However, correlation of increased serum F protein and histologic lesions in laboratory animals has not been performed. The lack of practical, high-throughput assays for the measurement of serum F protein limit its use as a marker of hepatocellular damage in laboratory animal species.

11.2.3 Hepatic Cholestatic Enzymes

11.2.3.1 Alkaline Phosphatase

ALP is an enzyme that hydrolyzes a wide range of monophosphates and pyrophosphates at an alkaline pH and physiologic pH but at a lesser rate. ALP activity has been described in a wide variety of organisms from bacteria to mammals (Fernandez and Kidney, 2007). In mammals, ALP activity can be found in most tissues of the body. The organs with the greatest ALP activity on a per gram basis are the intestine and kidney in most species (Nagode et al., 1969; Clampitt and Hart, 1978; Boyd, 1983). Other major organs with ALP activity include the liver, bone, and placenta (Clampitt and Hart, 1978; Boyd, 1983). Despite the relative organ activities of ALP, the total serum ALP activity may not offer a clear reflection of disease states involving a particular organ. For example, in dogs, the liver has less than 1% of the ALP activity of intestine, but most of the serum activity of ALP is from the liver (Hoffmann, 2008). On the contrary, the intestine in the dog has the highest ALP activity on a per gram basis but offers no contribution to serum activity.

Despite being widely studied, the *in vivo* function of ALP is not entirely understood but the role of some isoenzymes has been suggested. ALP found on the canalicular membranes of hepatocytes and luminal surface of the biliary epithelium may be involved in choline transport across cell membranes (Fernandez and Kidney, 2007). On the brush border of the intestinal epithelial cells, ALP may be responsible for absorption of dietary phosphates (Harris, 1990). In humans, a point mutation in the bone isoenzyme of ALP leads to hypophosphatasia, markedly defective bone mineralization, and early death of children. This finding strongly suggests a role of ALP in mineralization of bone (Whyte et al., 1996). The role in of ALP in bone mineralization has been confirmed using knockout mice to create hypophosphatemia resulting in impaired bone development (Anderson et al., 2004). One of the more interesting proposed functions of ALP suggest that the enzyme dephosphorylates bacterial endotoxin and diminishes its toxic effects (Poelstra et al., 1997a, b). Other functions of ALP in different organs have been proposed. However, despite the poor understanding of the physiologic function of ALP isoenzymes, their diagnostic importance for the detection of disease has been recognized for many years. ALP can be found attached to the cell surface anchored by a hydrophobic phosphatidylinositol glycan within the membrane. In the small intestine, ALP is located on the tips of mucosal villi and in the kidney, it is found on the brush border of proximal convoluted tubules (Watanabe and Fishman, 1964; Wachstein and Bradshaw, 1965). In the bone, ALP is found on the surface of osteoblasts and on matrix vesicles produced by osteoblasts (Leach et al., 1995). The liver displays different cellular patterns of ALP activity. In a normal animal, ALP is found located primarily on the bile canalicular surface of hepatocytes. During disease states or induction by various drugs, both the sinusoidal and lateral surfaces of the hepatocyte show considerable ALP activity (Sanecki et al., 1987; Ogawa et al., 1990; Solter et al., 1997).

11.2.3.1.1 Isoenzymes

In humans, four gene loci encode four different ALP isoenzymes, which are named for the primary tissue of expression: (1) the tissue nonspecific isoenzyme that is found in the liver, kidney, bone, and most other tissues, (2) the intestinal ALP found on the brush border of the intestine, (3) a placental isoenzyme expressed in trophoblasts during gestation, and (4) a germ cell or placenta-like isoenzyme expressed in small amounts in the testes and thymus (Harris, 1990). In nonhuman primates, all ALP isoenzymes are expressed except the germ cell isoenzyme (Harris, 1990; Hoffmann, 2008). In other mammalian species, there are two genes expressed for ALP isoenzymes: the tissue nonspecific ALP isoenzyme expressed in liver, bone, kidney, and placenta and the intestinal ALP that is generally specific to that tissue (Harris, 1990). The ALP isoenzymes result from the expression of different gene loci and differ antigenically, enzymatically, and biochemically (Hoffmann, 2008). Different ALP isoforms result from the expression from the same gene, have posttranslational modifications of the enzyme but are antigenically and enzymatically similar (Hoffmann, 2008).

Numerous techniques describing the detection, separation, and characterization of the ALP isoenzymes and isoforms have been published. The primary purpose of these techniques is to enhance the diagnostic usefulness of increases in serum ALP activity or gain an understanding of the mechanisms of ALP activity increase in tissues. The general techniques used for identifying the ALP isoenzymes include electrophoresis, isoelectric focusing, inhibition of enzymatic activity by chemicals and heat, selective recognition by lectins, immunochemistry, and cloning and sequencing of the genes (Fernandez and Kidney, 2007; Hoffmann, 2008). Use of these various techniques enhances the diagnostic utility of ALP isoenzymes and isoforms.

The liver alkaline phosphatase (LALP) isoform is moderately heat labile at 56°C, extremely sensitive to inhibition by levamisole, and relatively insensitive to the inhibition by L-phenylalanine, and the carbohydrate portions of the enzyme are terminated with sialic acid, causing the enzyme to migrate rapidly on electrophoresis (Hoffmann, 2008). In rabbits, liver ALP is composed of two isoenzymes separable by diethylaminoethyl (DEAE)-cellulose chromatography that reflects the expression of both the tissue nonspecific gene and the intestinal gene in the liver (Noguchi and Yamashita, 1987). This pattern of expression of two ALP isoenzymes in the liver has been observed in dogs when treated with glucocorticoids (Wiedmeyer et al., 2002a, b). Expression of an intestinal mRNA in rat liver following fat feeding has also been reported (Goseki-Sone et al., 1996). Bone alkaline phosphatase (BALP) isoform, a product of the tissue nonspecific ALP gene like LALP, has a different carbohydrate composition than LALP. Because of this difference, BALP can be distinguished from LALP by a slower anodal migration on cellulose acetate electrophoresis and susceptibility to heat inactivation (Nagode et al., 1969; Hoffmann and Dorner, 1975). In rats and dogs, BALP is also more susceptible to precipitation by wheat germ lectin than LALP (Sanecki et al., 1993; Hoffmann et al., 1994). Use of wheat germ lectin precipitation or heat inactivation with other techniques allows for determining activity of BALP and LALP in serum. Under normal conditions, the BALP makes up approximately 30% of the total serum ALP activity but a very small percentage of rat serum ALP activity (Hoffmann et al., 1994; Allen et al., 1998). Kidney ALP (KALP), like LALP and BALP, is a product of the tissue nonspecific ALP gene, although KALP can display heterogeneity due to variations in the carbohydrate composition especially sialic acid (Saini and Saini, 1978). In the rabbit, both the tissue nonspecific and intestinal genes are expressed in the kidney (Noguchi and Yamashita, 1987). Activity of KALP is not seen in serum, which is likely due to a short circulating half-life and a proximal tubular location (Hoffmann et al., 1999). Intestinal alkaline phosphatase (IALP) isoenzyme, unlike the tissue nonspecific products, is more heat stable, less sensitive to inhibition by levamisole, and readily inhibited by L-phenylalanine (Nagode et al., 1969; Eckersall and Nash, 1983; Eckersall et al., 1986). IALP has a very low carbohydrate composition compared to the tissue nonspecific products and considered asialoglycoprotein (though dog IALP does contain a small amount of sialic acid) (Hoffmann and Dorner, 1975). Because of this low carbohydrate composition, IALP does not migrate to the same extent on cellulose acetate or agarose electrophoresis as does LALP (Hoffmann and Dorner, 1975; Sanecki et al., 1990). In rabbits, IALP may be the product of both the intestinal and tissue nonspecific genes (Noguchi and Yamashita, 1987). In rats, two cDNAs have been identified that code for rat IALP: IALP-1 and IALP-2, which produce a 69-kDa and 93-kDa protein, respectively (Engle and Alpers, 1992; Engle et al., 1995). Under normal conditions, IALP comprises the major portion of total ALP serum activity in the rat (Righetti and Kaplan, 1971; Hoffmann et al., 1994). In adult cynomolgus monkeys, the majority of ALP activity in the serum is LALP representing 56%–94% of the total activity (Wiedmeyer et al., 1999). In addition, male monkeys have a higher ALP activity in serum than females (Wiedmeyer et al., 1999). Placental ALP is a product of the tissue nonspecific gene in laboratory species (Goldstein et al., 1982). In dogs, placental ALP appears to be an asialoglycoprotein since it has little anodal migration on cellulose acetate electrophoresis and is unaffected by neuraminidase treatment (Hoffmann et al., 1999). Increases in placental ALP activity in the serum of pregnant cats and cows has been observed but not in other domestic species (Fernandez and Kidney, 2007). A unique ALP isoenzyme can be found in dogs referred to as the corticosteroid-induced alkaline phosphatase (CIALP). CIALP activity can be found in the serum and liver of dogs during conditions of glucocorticoid treatment and cases of hyperadrenocorticism (Dorner et al., 1974; Sanecki et al., 1990; Wiedmeyer et al., 2002a). The isoenzyme is actually a highly glycosylated form of intestinal ALP, since it has been shown to be antigenically similar to IALP with both polyclonal and monoclonal antibody, responds to heat, levamisole, and L-phenylalanine inhibition in the same manner as IALP, and has an identical N-terminal amino acid sequence (Hoffmann, 2008). CIALP has not been reported in any other species.

11.2.3.1.2 Causes for Increased Serum ALP Activity

11.2.3.1.2.1 Hepatobiliary disease/Cholestasis One of the most common disorders in laboratory animals that can cause an increase in serum ALP activity, more specifically LALP, is cholestasis. In dogs and rats with experimentally induced cholestasis through bile duct ligation, there was a marked increase in serum LALP (Noonan and Meyer, 1979; Guelfi et al., 1982; Kaplan et al., 1983). However, the magnitude and time to peak serum LALP activity differ between the two species. In dogs, marked increases in serum ALP activity do not occur until approximately 24 hours following bile duct ligation with maximum increases at 4–7 days (Noonan and Meyer, 1979; Shull and Hornbuckle, 1979; Guelfi et al., 1982). In rats though, significant increases of serum ALP activity occur approximately 6–7 hours following bile duct ligation with maximum increases of 7–10-fold greater than normal at 12–24 hours (Kryszewski et al., 1973; Kaplan et al., 1983). The difference in time of response between the dog and rat is probably a reflection of the absence of a gall bladder in the rat. Cholestasis secondary to other diseases such as hepatic lipidosis, pancreatitis, neoplasia, nodular regeneration, enteric diseases, or hypotension can also result in increases in serum ALP activity (Fernandez and Kidney, 2007). Increases in serum LALP activity either experimentally or from natural disease occur due to increased synthesis or presumably increased shuttling of ALP to the sinusoidal membrane of hepatocytes (Solter et al., 1997; Fernandez and Kidney, 2007). However, the exact mechanism in which LALP activity increases with these conditions and gains access to the blood remains controversial and is most likely multifactorial. Serum LALP isoenzyme activity can be mildly increased with instances of hepatocellular necrosis, but are considered of little predictive value in detecting either centrilobular or periportal hepatocellular necrosis (Noonan, 1981; Guelfi et al., 1982; Carakostas et al., 1986). More appropriate markers of hepatocellular necrosis are ALT and SDH activity. Marked increases in serum LALP activity can also occur with glucocorticoid administration in the absence of other indicators of cholestasis (Solter et al., 1994, 1997; Syakalima et al., 1997; Wiedmeyer et al., 2002b). The effects of other compounds on serum ALP activity shall be discussed later.

11.2.3.1.2.2 Bone Disease Increased osteoblastic activity from osteogenesis or bone pathology can result in increased serum ALP activity, specifically BALP. Thus measurement of serum BALP is considered a marker of metabolic activity of the bone in dogs, cats, and rats and most likely in other species as well (Allen et al., 1998; DeLaurier et al., 2002; Powers et al., 2007). Besides a metabolic marker of bone activity, increases in serum BALP activity can occur from pathologic bone conditions. In dogs, increases in serum BALP can be observed in dogs with hyperparathyroidism, fracture healing, and osteosarcoma (Ehrhart et al., 1998; Komnenou et al., 2005; Hoffmann, 2008). Of these pathologic conditions, the highest observed serum BALP activity has been in dogs with osteosarcoma (Ehrhart et al., 1998). In some cases, serum BALP activity reached 50 times the normal reference range, but being near normal activity in other cases. This suggests that the measurement of serum BALP activity has poor sensitivity for the diagnosis of osteosarcoma. However, it was shown that serum BALP activity is an important prognostic marker for canine appendicular osteosarcoma (Ehrhart et al., 1998; Garzotto et al., 2000; Kirpensteijn et al., 2002). Finally, familial hyperphosphatasemia in a family of Siberian huskies in which the increased serum ALP is a result of increased BALP isoenzyme activity has been observed (Lawler et al., 1996).

11.2.3.1.2.3 Endocrine Diseases In dogs, serum ALP activity can be increased in endocrine disorders such as hyperadrenocorticism, diabetes mellitus, hypothyroidism, and hyperparathyroidism (Fernandez and Kidney, 2007). Dogs with hyperadrenocorticism or following treatment with exogenous glucocorticoids, display increased serum ALP activity that is dominated by the CIALP isoenzyme (Dorner et al., 1974; Badylak and Van Vleet, 1981; Solter et al., 1994). Most clinically normal dogs have serum CIALP activity that is either nonexistent or represents only a few units of the total serum ALP activity. It has been shown that use of serum CIALP activity for the diagnosis of hyperadrenocorticism has high sensitivity but poor specificity (Teske et al., 1989; Solter et al., 1993). Most dogs with diabetes mellitus display an increase in serum ALP activity (Hess et al., 2000). The reason for the increased serum ALP activity with diabetes has not been determined. However, it is suspected that secondary hepatic lipidosis may be responsible (Hess et al., 2000). Moreover, which ALP isoenzyme predominates in the serum of dogs with diabetes is unknown but some studies have shown 40%–80% of these dogs have an increase in CIALP (Oluju et al., 1984). Like diabetes mellitus, the predominant ALP isoenzyme in the serum of dogs with hypothyroidism or hyperparathyroidism is not entirely known.

11.2.3.1.2.4 Diet In adult rats, IALP isoenzyme is the major ALP isoenzyme in the serum and it increases after feeding a fat-laden meal (Eliakim et al., 1991; Alpers et al., 1994; Hoffmann et al., 1994; Yamagishi et al., 1994). A similar finding was observed in humans (Cho et al., 2005). Reduced serum ALP activity, presumably from decreased IALP activity, has been observed in fasted rats or rats with decreased food consumption from illness or toxicity (Waner and Nyska, 1994; Travlos et al., 1996).

11.2.3.1.2.5 Pregnancy Increases in serum ALP activity, specifically placental ALP, have been observed in pregnant cats but not pregnant dogs (Fernandez and Kidney, 2007). Typically, in normal cats, placental ALP activity is nonexistent in the serum. In cats, in late pregnancy, there is detectable placental ALP activity (Everett et al., 1977). In late stage pregnant rats, a decrease in serum ALP activity has been observed but higher serum ALP compared to nonpregnant females in the early stages of pregnancy (Liberati et al., 2004; Honda et al., 2008). It is unknown in these studies if the changes in serum ALP activity are due to changes in placental ALP.

11.2.3.1.2.6 Age In young puppies, serum BALP activity can be up to 10-fold greater than in adult dogs but the activity wanes as the dog matures (Sanecki et al., 1993). An increase in serum BALP activity in young animals can be observed in many laboratory species. In rats, serum IALP activity is greater in young rats than mature rats (Hoffmann et al., 1994). Increases in serum CIALP activity may occasionally be observed in dogs with chronic and/or inflammatory disease. This appearance in inflammatory conditions is more often observed in older dogs (Teske et al., 1989; Solter et al., 1993, 1997). The cause of increased CIALP activity in dogs with chronic inflammatory disease is not clear. Young healthy dogs used for toxicologic studies usually have no CIALP activity, but serum should still be evaluated for the presence of the isoenzyme prior to the initiation of a study, and those animals with CIALP should be eliminated since they may have underlying disease or possibly skew the data for the study.

11.2.3.1.2.7 Drug Induction Numerous compounds such as cortisol, phenobarbital, theophylline, caffeine, and retinoic acid, and many others have been shown to increase serum ALP activity in rats (Hixson et al., 1979; Hoffmann et al., 1999). Of these many compounds, drugs such as anticonvulsants and glucocorticoids have been shown to induce ALP activity without evidence of pathology (Gaskill et al., 2004; Hall and Nancy, 2008). The effects on ALP of these drugs can be blocked by inhibitors of RNA and protein synthesis (Hoffmann et al., 1999). In dogs, the increased synthesis of both CIALP and LALP in dogs treated with glucocorticoids has been well documented (Dorner et al., 1974; Hoffmann and Dorner, 1975; Solter et al., 1994). Treatment with glucocorticoids induces the presence of CIALP activity in liver and serum but the initial response is a dramatic increase in LALP activity, followed by the appearance of CIALP in 7–10 days after initiation of treatment (Solter et al., 1994). The regulation of both CIALP and LALP is at the gene level (Wiedmeyer et al., 2002b). The cause for the delay in CIALP activity in the serum is unknown. In most cases of compound induced serum ALP activity, an isoenzyme analysis has been done; thus, the tissue of origin of most serum ALP increases is unknown.

11.2.3.1.3 Causes for Decreased Serum ALP Activity

Like most other serum enzymes, decreases in ALP activity are of no diagnostic value (Wolf, 1986). However, decreases in serum total ALP, IALP, and BALP have been observed following hypophysectomy in rats (Yeh et al., 1984). In addition, decreases in serum ALP activity has been observed in rats fasted for approximately 16 hours (Apostolou et al., 1976; Matsuzawa, 1994).

11.2.3.2 Gamma-Glutamyltransferase

GGT has multiple functions including catalytic transfer of γ-glutamyl groups to amino acids (Goldberg, 1980b). It is one of the six enzymes that function in the γ-glutamyl cycle, and GGT is the only one in this cycle that is membrane bound. It plays a major role in the regulation of intracellular GSH which is a major antioxidant. GGT also functions in the GSH transferase/GGT pathway that cleaves γ-glutamyl moieties from GSH conjugates. The role of this pathway is detoxification of xenobiotics and carcinogens by rendering them more water soluble and excreted.

GGT is found in all species with activity in the kidney, pancreas, liver, spleen, lung, intestine, seminal vesicles, mammary gland, and ciliary body (Albert et al., 1964; Clampitt and Hart, 1978). The kidney has by far the greatest activity on a per gram basis (Albert et al., 1964; Clampitt and Hart, 1978). The other tissues have varying activities depending on the species. In guinea pigs, kidney tissue has 15 times the activity of GGT as found in the liver; whereas, the activity in the rat kidney is 200–875 times higher than in the rat liver (Albert et al., 1964; Fiala and Fiala, 1973; Hinchman and Ballatori, 1990). Dogs, mice, hamsters, and rats are similar in that they have lower liver GGT activity than guinea pigs and rabbits (Milne and Doxey, 1985; Sulakhe and Lautt, 1985; Hinchman and Ballatori, 1990). This is most likely the cause for lower serum GGT activity in these species.

GGT is generally membrane bound found on the surface of cells. In rats, the biliary epithelial cells in the portal spaces of the liver display histochemical evidence of GGT activity (Daoust, 1982). In addition, GGT activity has been identified on both bile canalicular and sinusoidal surfaces of rat and guinea pig hepatocytes (Huseby, 1979; Lanca and Israel, 1991). When isolated parenchymal, Kupffer, and biliary cells were examined, it was shown that the biliary epithelial cells displayed approximately 200 times higher GGT activity than hepatocytes (Huseby, 1979; Parola et al., 1990). In the kidney, GGT is found on the brush border of epithelial cells lining the proximal convoluted tubules (Albert et al., 1964). Because of this location, GGT from the kidney is shed into the urine with proximal tubular damage. In the pancreas, the luminal border of cells lining the acini and the pancreatic ducts display GGT activity (Albert et al., 1964). Serum increases in serum GGT are not generally associated with renal or pancreatic pathology.

11.2.3.2.1 Isoenzymes

Isoenzymes of GGT have not been found but changes in the carbohydrate composition of GGT (i.e., isoforms) have been described. Electrophoretic separation and isoelectric focusing of GGT from the kidney and liver from rats resulted in upward of 12 different bands (Jaken and Mason, 1978). GGT extracted from rat hepatomas and hyperplastic liver nodules have shown to be immunologically identical to rat kidney GGT but have varying sialic acid concentrations (Fischer et al., 1986). Varying sialic acid content has been demonstrated for human liver GGT as well (Mortensen and Huseby, 1997). The existence of a single gene for liver GGT in mice has been shown but with at least seven different promoters (Rajagopalan et al., 1993; Sepulveda et al., 1994). Similar observations have been made in rats, though the number of gene promoters is unknown (Darbouy et al., 1991; Brouillet et al., 1994; Okamoto et al., 1994).

11.2.3.2.2 Causes for Increased Serum GGT Activity

11.2.3.2.2.1 Hepatobiliary Disease/Cholestasis Because GGT is found primarily in the liver on bile epithelium, the serum activity increases are mainly due to cholestatic diseases or biliary epithelial necrosis in all species studied (Leonard et al., 1984; Braun et al., 1987; Boone et al., 2005; Ramaiah, 2007). The serum increases with cholestatic disorders may be secondary to membrane solubilization from increased bile acid concentrations (Braun et al., 1987). In experimental models using bile duct ligation, there are moderate differences in the timeframe of appearance of increased GGT serum activity. Bile duct ligation in dogs and rats consistently causes increased serum GGT activity (Wootton et al., 1977; DeNovo and Prasse, 1983). The initial response to bile duct ligation is an increased serum GGT activity with a corresponding decrease in liver GGT activity. In guinea pigs, bile duct ligation results in a pattern of increased serum GGT activity as well (Huseby and Vik, 1978). However, the rate and sustainable increase in serum GGT activity in guinea pigs is different from the dog and rat. This difference in serum GGT activity between guinea pigs and rats or dogs is most likely due to guinea pigs having much higher liver GGT activities normally than the other two species. Therefore, more GGT is available for release into the serum. Generalized hepatocellular necrosis caused by administration of carbon tetrachloride and dibromobenzene or hepatic trauma result in minimal or no increases in serum GGT activity (Noonan and Meyer, 1979; Guelfi et al., 1982; Leonard et al., 1984; Szymanska et al., 1996). In addition to hepatobiliary/cholestatic diseases, chemical-induced hepatocarcinogenesis has been shown to increase tissue GGT activity (Fiala and Fiala, 1973; Manson and Smith, 1984; Fischer et al., 1986). In general, substantial increases in serum GGT activity is considered a specific diagnostic indicator of cholestatic disease.

Despite the kidney having the highly tissue activity of GGT, there is no evidence to support that renal disease causes an increase in serum GGT activity. The absence of kidney GGT activity in the serum is most likely related to the very rapid clearance of kidney GGT activity from blood by the galactose receptor system and the location of GGT on the brush border of the renal proximal tubular epithelium (Hoffmann, 2008). Under pathologic conditions affecting the renal proximal tubules, the GGT is readily shed into the urine. Hence, urine GGT activity has been used as an indicator of nephrotoxicity.

11.2.3.2.2.2 Drug Induction Increases in the GGT activity in liver and serum as a result of induction of enzyme synthesis have been associated with barbiturate treatment and glucocorticoid administration in multiple species (Tazi et al., 1980; Badylak and Van Vleet, 1981; Roomi and

Goldberg, 1981; Solter et al., 1994). The changes in GGT activity from inducing drugs varies among species. Rabbits respond to phenobarbital with a greater increase in liver and serum GGT activity than do guinea pigs and rats (Roomi and Goldberg, 1981). Additionally, rats show an increase in liver GGT activity with phenobarbital administration but no increase in serum GGT activity (Roomi and Goldberg, 1981). In dogs treated with glucocorticoids, an increase in serum and liver GGT was observed (Solter et al., 1994).

11.2.3.2.3 Causes for Decreased Serum GGT Activity

Decreases in GGT activity are insignificant.

11.2.3.3 5′-Nucleotidase

The enzyme 5′-nucleotidase (5NT) is a glycoprotein that hydrolyzes 5′-nucleotides to their corresponding nucleosides (Sunderman, 1990). More specifically, it hydrolyzes nucleoside 5′-monophosphates to adenosine. The exact role of 5NT in the liver is not completely known. In other tissues and cells, the function of 5NT is varied (Sunderman, 1990; Le Hir and Kaissling, 1993). Activity of 5NT is an ectoenzyme predominantly located in the plasma membrane. 5NT activity can be found in numerous tissues including the liver, kidney, brain, lung, intestine, neutrophils, lymphocytes, and muscle (Hardonk and BDe Boer, 1968). The highest activity is found in kidney and intestinal mucosa (Hardonk and BDe Boer, 1968). Despite the varied tissue distribution of 5NT, serum concentrations are specific for hepatobiliary disease (Bodansky and Schwartz, 1968). In the liver, 5NT activity is located primarily on the bile canalicular and sinusoidal membrane of hepatocytes and on connective tissue in the portal triad (Schmid et al., 1994). In mouse and rat tissues, five different bands of 5NT have been identified by agarose gel electrophoresis (Hardonk and BDe Boer, 1968). However, partially purified 5NT from several tissues from the rat exhibits identical enzymatic characteristics (Sunderman, 1990). These findings suggest that the different electrophoretic bands of 5NT most likely represent isoforms and not distinct isoenzymes. There is no indication that separation of 5NT isoforms improves its diagnostic value.

11.2.3.3.1 Causes for IncWreased Serum 5NT Activity

Increases in serum 5NT activity occur in animals with hepatobiliary disease or cholestasis (Carakostas et al., 1990; Ramaiah, 2007). The serum changes in 5NT activity in experimental induction of cholestasis are similar to the serum changes in ALP and GGT (Kryszewski et al., 1973). Thus, it is perceived that the measurement of 5NT offers no advantages in diagnosing hepatobiliary disease over the measurement of ALP or GGT. However, one advantage 5NT has over ALP is the fact that 5NT does not increase with osseous growth or lesions suggesting that it has a higher specificity for hepatic disease than ALP (Pagani and Panteghini, 2001). However, the routine use of 5NT has not gained popularity due to the lack of acceptable methodologies for convenient measurement (Ramaiah, 2007).

Compounds such as thyroxin and chronically administered ethanol have been shown for increasing the serum activity of 5NT (Drozdz et al., 1975; Nishmura and Teschke, 1982). In contrast, 5NT did increase in the serum of dogs treated with glucocorticoids unlike ALP and GGT (Rutgers et al., 1995).

11.2.3.3.2 Causes for Decreased Serum 5NT Activity

Decreases in serum 5NT activity are most likely insignificant.

11.3 ANALYSIS OF HEPATIC FUNCTION

As described previously, the liver has many diverse physiologic functions. Disturbances in those functions as a result of disease or toxic insult can alter specific serum parameters that are routinely measured by laboratory methods. It is important to note that individual test results may not be specific for liver functional abnormalities. Other disease processes may cause similar abnormalities. Thus, it is important to assess liver function using multiple laboratory test results, clinical findings, histopathology, and other ancillary parameters such as imaging. It is also important to note that increases in serum activities of liver specific enzymes do not directly indicate the loss of liver function. Liver function can be markedly reduced without increases in serum liver enzyme activities.

11.3.1 Bilirubin

Bilirubin is the product of catabolism of the heme molecule within the cells of the mononuclear phagocyte system (Hall and Nancy, 2008). Approximately 85% of serum bilirubin comes from the breakdown of hemoglobin from senescent erythrocytes destroyed by macrophages found in the liver, spleen, and bone marrow (Nuttall, 2001). The remaining 15% is produced from erythrocyte precursors destroyed in the bone marrow or catabolism of other heme-containing proteins such as myoglobin, cytochromes, and catalase (Nuttall, 2001). Bilirubin, released from the macrophages into the circulation where it binds covalently to albumin, is water insoluble and referred to as indirect, unconjugated, or prehepatic bilirubin (Hall and Nancy, 2008; Stockham, 2008). The unconjugated bilirubin is removed from circulation by the hepatocytes that prepare it for removal from the body. Removal of bilirubin from the serum is a stepwise process involving uptake, conjugation, secretion, and excretion (Hall and Nancy, 2008). Uptake of unconjugated bilirubin by the hepatocyte occurs after it dissociates from albumin. Once dissociated, uptake is facilitated across the sinusoidal membrane by an organic anion transport polypeptide, which is a sodium and energy independent process (Tennant and Center, 2008). Upon entry into the hepatocyte, bilirubin binds to ligandin, a cytosolic protein that has transport and detoxification functions. Through binding of the bilirubin to ligandin, efflux back into the plasma is prevented (Tennant and Center, 2008). The bilirubin within the hepatocyte is then conjugated to glucuronic acid producing monoglucuronide and diglucuronide to be excreted into the bile (Nuttall, 2001). Secretion of water-soluble conjugated bilirubin into the bile is an energy-dependent process and the rate-limiting step of the whole process (Hall and Nancy, 2008). Small amounts of conjugated (also known as direct or hepatic) bilirubin escape into the serum. The conjugated bilirubin does not bind to albumin, and it can be freely filtered through the glomerulus (Hall and Nancy, 2008). Most of the conjugated bilirubin filtered through the glomerulus is reabsorbed in the proximal tubules. Conjugated bilirubin is excreted in the bile and stored in the gall bladder or directly into the intestines. When bilirubin enters the intestine, it is minimally resorbed, degraded to urobilinogen, and excreted in the feces (Stockham, 2008).

Serum unconjugated (indirect) and conjugated (direct) bilirubin can be differentiated by using the Van den Bergh assay (Nuttall, 2001). By distinguishing the predominant bilirubin in the serum, clinical judgments as to the cause for the increase in bilirubin may be possible. However, this information needs to be additive to clinical observations, other laboratory data, and gross and histologic pathology findings. Laboratory determination of conjugated and unconjugated bilirubin is not usually necessary or recommended as part of routine toxicologic studies (Hall and Nancy, 2008), and Table 11.1 demonstrates previously expected values for total serum bilirubin of a variety of healthy experimental and domestic species and humans. This is due in part to variation in metabolism of bilirubin among different species (Ramaiah, 2007). Nonhuman primates and mice typically have the highest total serum bilirubin concentrations, while other species have considerably less total serum bilirubin concentrations (Tennant, 1999). In addition, it has been demonstrated that male nonhuman primates (specifically vervet monkeys) have a higher total and direct bilirubin serum concentration compared to females (Sato et al., 2005). If the situation originates where there is an increase in serum bilirubin without evidence of hemolysis or histologic changes consistent with cholestasis, determining the ratio of conjugated to unconjugated bilirubin in serum may be helpful (Ramaiah, 2007).

TABLE 11.1
Total Serum Bilirubin of Experimental Species, Domestic Species, and Humans

Species	Total Serum Bilirubin (mg/dL) ± SD	Reference
Dog	0.1 ± 0.1	Klaus (1958)
Cat	0.18 ± 0.06	Mitruka and Rawnsley (1981)
Rat	0.2 ± 0.2	Laird (1974)
Hamster	0.4 ± 0.1	Tomson and Wardrop (1987)
Guinea pig	0.31 ± 0.07	Mitruka and Rawnsley (1981)
Rabbit	0.19 ± 0.10	Tennant et al. (1981)
Mouse	0.4 ± 0.5	Williams et al. (1966)
Cow	0.2 ± 0.1	Berger (1956)
Sheep	0.1 ± 0.01	Berger (1956)
Horse	1.1 ± 0.4	Berger (1956)
Pig	0.2 ± 0.2	Berger (1956)
Rhesus monkey	0.4 ± 0.3	Anderson (1966)
Howler monkey	0.75 ± 0.06	Katz et al. (1968)
Marmoset	0.2 (range: 0.0–0.4)	Deinhardt and Deinhardt (1966)
Human	0.4 ± 0.2	Powell et al. (1967)

11.3.1.1 Causes for Increased Serum Bilirubin

Conditions that cause increases in serum bilirubin concentration (hyperbilirubinemia) can be classified into those that result in the elevation of primarily the unconjugated form of bilirubin and those that are associated with an elevation of the conjugated or both conjugated and unconjugated forms (Table 11.2). Increases of predominantly unconjugated bilirubin have been related to the overproduction of bilirubin, impaired bilirubin uptake by the liver, or deficiencies of bilirubin conjugation. Increases of conjugated or both unconjugated and conjugated bilirubins have been related to biliary obstruction, hepatocellular diseases/injury, and defective canalicular excretion.

11.3.1.1.1 Decrease in Functional Hepatic Mass

A reduction in functioning hepatocytes can affect several steps in the processing of bilirubin. With a loss of hepatocyte function, alterations in uptake and conjugation of unconjugated bilirubin, as well as, secretion of conjugated bilirubin results in hyperbilirubinemia. Often with impaired hepatic function, conjugated bilirubin is the predominant bilirubin fraction found increased in the serum. However, it is possible with decrease in function to result in serum increases in both conjugated and unconjugated bilirubin. Therefore, it is recommended that increased serum bilirubin information be combined with other laboratory or pathologic data. As stated previously, the use of serum liver enzyme activities may not be appropriate for determining liver functional capabilities. Hereditary defects in bilirubin processing resulting in increases in the unconjugated bilirubin similar to that detailed for Crigler–Najjar syndrome, Type I (Chowdhury et al., 1993; Yamazaki et al., 1995) or conjugated bilirubin similar to what occurs in Dubin–Johnson syndrome (Chowdhury et al., 1993; Yamazaki et al., 1995) have been described in rats.

11.3.1.1.2 Cholestasis

Pathologic conditions that impair bile fluid through the bile canaliculi, bile ducts, or gall bladder can result in hyperbilirubinemia. Typically, conjugated bilirubin is increased over unconjugated bilirubin concentrations. Over time, the increase in conjugated bilirubin can lead to increases in unconjugated bilirubin (Stockham, 2008). The pathologic causes for impaired bile flow are varied

TABLE 11.2
Pathophysiologic Mechanisms Responsible for Hyperbilirubinemia

	Plasma Bilirubin		Urine	Urine
	Unconjugated	Conjugated	Bilirubin	Urobilinogen
Increased bilirubin production: hemolytic anemia,resorption from hemorrhage, hematoma	↑	N	0	↑
	–	–	–	–
Impaired hepatic uptake of unconjugated bilirubin:	↑	N	0	↓ or N
neonatal hyperbilirubinemia, fasting hyperbilirubinemia, benign unconjugated hyperbilirubinemia of horses, congenital photosensitivity (Southdown sheep)	–	–	–	–
	–	–	–	–
Impaired conjugation of bilirubin: glucuronyl transferase deficiency (Gunn rat), neonatal hyperbilirubinemia	↑	N	0	↓ or N
Impaired biliary excretion of bilirubin: intrahepatic cholestasis, black liver disease (Corriedale sheep), congenital photosensitivity (Southdown sheep), biliary cirrhosis, bile duct obstruction	↑	↑	↑	↑ or 0

N = normal; 0 = absent; ↑ = increased; ↓ = decreased.

and measurement of serum bilirubin usually does not define the pathologic condition. As stated previously, other laboratory and clinical findings are important for determining the exact cause for hyperbilirubinemia. Other clinical laboratory findings that may be altered with cholestatic disease include serum ALP and GGT activities (Fujii, 1997).

11.3.1.1.3 Intravascular or Extravascular Hemolysis

Disorders that result in red cell lysis can cause abrupt increases in serum bilirubin. Destruction of RBC by macrophages in the spleen, liver, and bone marrow cause increases in production of unconjugated bilirubin. If the increase in production and delivery of unconjugated bilirubin to the liver exceeds the uptake capacity of the hepatocyte, hyperbilirubinemia, dominated by unconjugated bilirubin, will occur. The increase delivery of unconjugated bilirubin to the liver with hemolytic disorders can cause increased bilirubin conjugation and secretion. If the formation of conjugated bilirubin exceeds secretion, the conjugated bilirubin can be released into the circulation. Thus, hemolytic disorders can result in hyperbilirubinemia from both unconjugated and conjugated bilirubin. Typically, the concentration of unconjugated bilirubin is markedly increased with hemolytic events.

11.3.1.2 Causes for Decreased Serum Bilirubin

Decreases in total bilirubin are rarely observed but has been associated with test compounds that induce microsomal enzyme production (Goldberg, 1980a).

11.3.1.3 Influencing Factors

Free hemoglobin in a serum/plasma sample from hemolysis and precipitation of immunoglobulins in the sample can falsely increase bilirubin results (Stockham, 2008). In addition, ultraviolet light can degrade bilirubin in a sample and decrease results.

11.3.2 Bile Acids

Bile acid metabolism is a major function of the liver and an important component of cholesterol homeostasis (Tolman, 2001). Primary bile acids are synthesized from cholesterol by hepatocytes, conjugated to glycine and/or taurine and secreted into the biliary system (Tennant, 1999; Tolman, 2001; Russell, 2003). In general, two primary bile acids (chenodeoxycholic and cholic acid) are produced by most vertebrate species. However, a variety of molecular forms of bile acids can be synthesized by different species (Hoffmann et al., 2010). For example, while cholic acid commonly occurs as a primary bile acid of mammals, chenodeoxycholic acid (found in rat, human, and hamster) can be replaced to muricholic acid (mouse) or hyocholic and hyodeoxycholic acid (pig) (Russell, 2003; Kandrac et al., 2006). A leading form of bile acids in mice, muricholic acids differ from the more common bile acids, cholic acid or chenodeoxycholic, by having a hydroxyl group at the 6-position instead of the 7-position. Bile acid conjugates to taurine primarily in the dog and rat but in the cat, bile acids conjugate to taurine exclusively (Tennant, 1999). In the rabbit, the conjugating appears to be almost completely specific for glycine (Tennant, 1999). The conjugate bile acids are secreted into the bile canalicular system, transported through the bile ducts and stored in the gall bladder. In those species that lack a gall bladder, the bile containing bile acids is continually secreted into the duodenum (Ramaiah, 2007). In the colon, the actions of bacteria modify the structure of primary bile acids to into secondary bile acids. For example, by removal of an α-hydroxyl group at position seven converts the primary bile acids, chenodeoxycholic and cholic acid, to their secondary bile acids, lithocholic and deoxycholic acid, respectively. Figure 11.2 represents the formation of primary and secondary bile acids. Movement of bile acids into the biliary system is an osmotically active process (Handler et al., 1994). Bile acids are considered to be the primary organic solutes responsible for bile flow (Handler et al., 1994). Once deposited in the duodenum, either directly as in the rat or contraction of the gall bladder under the influence of cholecystokinin, bile acids play an important role in the digestion and absorption of dietary fat and other lipids. This digestion process occurs in both the duodenum and jejunum (Tennant and Center, 2008). In the terminal ileum, most of the bile acids are reabsorbed by a highly efficient transport system in the epithelium, and they enter the portal circulation. The portal circulation returns the bile acids to the liver for removal by the hepatocytes and

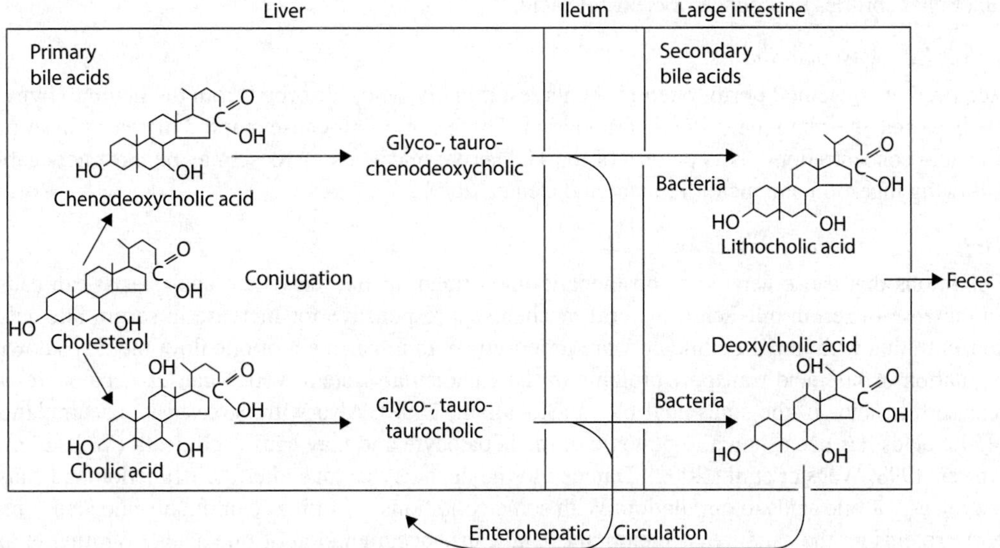

FIGURE 11.2 Schematic representation of bile acid metabolism in the liver and intestinal tract. Primary bile acids are synthesized in the liver and the secondary bile acids are formed by microbial modification of the primary bile acids in the large intestine.

recycling. A small portion of the bile acids is excreted in the feces. This system is known as enterohepatic circulation and is the method for conserving the bile acid pool of the body (Tolman, 2001).

The predominant bile acid found in bile differs between the species. In mice and rats, the predominant bile acid is taurocholate (Tennant and Center, 2008). In dogs, the predominant bile acid is cholic acid and chenodeoxycholic acid in nonhuman primates (Ramaiah, 2007). In most species, serum bile acids can be easily measured by spectrophotometric assays (Tennant and Center, 2008). In addition, the performance of the bile acids test differs among the species depending on the presence of a gall bladder. In those species with a gall bladder, a serum sample for bile acids analysis is taken after a 12-hour fast. After this baseline sample (i.e., prebile acid) is taken, the animal is fed a meal or injected with cholecystokinin as a method to contract the gall bladder and release of a bolus of bile acids into the duodenum. After a set amount of time (typically 30 minutes to 2 hours) another serum sample is taken for bile acids measurement (i.e., postbile acid) (Bridger et al., 2008; Stockham, 2008). Using this method, hepatic functional ability is assessed by exposing the hepatocytes to an influx of endogenous bile acids (Stockham, 2008). Performance of the serum bile acids test using a pre and postprandial bile acids method increases the diagnostic sensitivity and specificity of the test in the dog (Center et al., 1991). In those species that lack a gall bladder, such as a rat, a serum sample after fasting and measured for bile acid content is valid for diagnostic utility.

11.3.2.1 Causes for Increased Serum Bile Acids

11.3.2.1.1 Decrease in Functional Hepatic Mass

Since serum bile acid processing is dependent upon hepatocellular function, bile excretion, and portal blood flow, these processes can be assessed using serum bile acid concentrations. Increased serum bile acids have a high sensitivity for the detection of hepatobiliary dysfunction (Stockham, 2008). However, the cause for the decrease in hepatic function may not be definitively determined and the functional abnormalities can be from primary or secondary insults. Liver toxicity secondary to administration of xenobiotics has the potential to alter multiple steps in the process of bile acid formation and excretion thus causing an increase in serum bile acid concentration (Hall and Nancy, 2008). Other diffuse hepatic pathologic conditions (i.e., chronic or acute inflammation, degenerative disease, metabolic disturbances) can cause sufficient damage to the hepatocytes and alter their functional abilities to produce or clear bile acids.

11.3.2.1.2 Vascular Shunts

Acquired or congenital portosystemic shunts result in bile acids absorbed from the ileum to bypass the liver and enter into the systemic circulation. These conditions cause marked increases in serum bile acid concentrations. This pattern of marked serum bile acids increase may be most noticeable following ingestion of a meal (Tennant and Center, 2008).

11.3.2.1.3 Impaired Bile Flow

Conditions that cause hepatic or posthepatic impairment of bile flow (i.e., cholestasis) can cause an increase in serum bile acids. Several mechanisms responsible for increase in serum bile acids concentration with impaired bile flow are proposed. With impairment of bile flow, there is a downregulation of bile acid transport proteins in the canalicular system, which causes hepatocytes to release bile acids in the sinusoidal blood (Stockham, 2008). Also with cholestasis, accumulation of bile acids has been shown to be toxic to the hepatocyte and may cause cell death (Webster and Anwer, 1998; Webster et al., 2002). Damage to the hepatocytes may alter their function and cause the release of bile acids to circulation. With some conditions, cytokines can impair bile acid transport proteins on the canalicular membranes and cause accumulation of bile acids (Whiting et al., 1995; Moseley et al., 1996). As expected with impairment of bile flow, a concurrent decrease in bilirubin excretion is expected but may not be profound enough to result in increases in serum bilirubin (Stockham, 2008).

Despite the clinical utility of using serum bile acid concentrations to identify hepatic disease, its use has not proven effective for the identification of hepatotoxicity (Cheng-long et al., 1992). It does not appear to have advantages over the use of serum liver enzyme activity measurement for monitoring hepatotoxicity (Hall and Nancy, 2008).

11.3.2.2 Causes for Decreased Serum Bile Acids

In humans, approximately 95% of the bile acids secreted during a single pass through enterohepatic circulation are recirculating bile acids (Tolman, 2001). Therefore, a disruption in this cycle can result in a decrease in serum bile acids. In most instances, it is ileal malabsorption of the bile acids that are the cause for abnormal enterohepatic circulation and thus decreased serum bile acid concentrations (Tolman, 2001).

11.3.2.3 Influencing Factors

Free hemoglobin or excessive lipids in the plasma/serum sample can have a negative effect on the spectrophotometric assay (Stockham, 2008). Other factors that may provide unequivocal results, especially with the bile acid challenge test, are spontaneous contraction of the gall bladder prior to feeding, delayed emptying of gastric contents, increased intestinal transit time, and abnormal bile acid absorption in the ileum (Stockham, 2008).

11.3.3 Ammonium

The catabolism of proteins and nucleic acids results in the formation of nonprotein nitrogenous metabolites for which one is ammonium (NH_4^+). The majority of the circulating NH_4^+ is produced in the gastrointestinal tract by metabolism of dietary protein by bacteria. The NH_4^+ is transported to the liver via the portal vein and hepatic artery where it is converted to urea in the hepatocytes by the Krebs–Henseleit urea cycle (Newman and Price, 2001). The urea diffuses into the sinusoidal blood or bile canaliculi to be excreted through the kidney or gastrointestinal tract, respectively (Stockham, 2008). NH_4^+ can be excreted through the kidney as well. Typically, ammonium (NH_4^+) is the predominate form found in the plasma compared to relatively little ammonia (NH_3). The ratio of NH_4^+ to NH_3 in the plasma at physiologic pH (i.e., 7.4) is approximately 30:1 (Stockham, 2008). Ammonium does not diffuse across cell membranes whereby ammonia is lipid soluble and rapidly diffuses across cell membranes. As the plasma pH increases, there is a shift of ammonium to ammonia and the rate of entry of ammonia into the cell increases. Therefore, the rate of entry of ammonia into the cells is proportional to the plasma concentration. This shift to ammonia and rapid entry into the cells is most profound in the central nervous tissue whereby ammonia has a toxic effect (i.e., hepatic encephalopathy).

11.3.3.1 Causes for Increased Serum Ammonium

The two main reasons for increase in serum NH_4^+ are similar to those causes for increased bile acids: decrease in functional hepatic mass and portal blood shunting. Intestinal bacteria produce large quantities of ammonium daily that requires clearance from the blood (Stockham, 2008). Those conditions that cause diffuse hepatocellular disease (e.g., necrosis, cirrhosis, toxic) can greatly diminish the liver's capacity to clear ammonium from the blood and convert it to urea. Typically, a loss of 70% of hepatic functional mass is required before baseline ammonium levels are increased (Bain, 2003; McCuskey, 2006). Moreover, as expected, congenital or acquired shunting of portal blood away from the liver can cause marked increases in serum levels of ammonium. Other possible causes for increased serum ammonium levels are congenital deficiencies in urea processing (rare), postprandial increase production of NH_4^+ and strenuous exercise (observed in dogs) (Stockham, 2008).

11.3.3.2 Causes for Decreased Serum Ammonium

Decreases in serum NH_4^+ do not appear to be of clinical significance.

11.3.3.3 Influencing Factors

Timely analysis for serum NH_4^+ is important for gaining accurate values. Once collected into the proper tubes (EDTA or heparin), the samples should be cooled to 4°C and analysis performed within 1 hour of collection. Inadequate sampling handling or delay in analysis can result in altered values (Stockham, 2008). In addition, heme pigment from hemolysis can falsely increase NH_4^+ values (Stockham, 2008).

11.3.3.4 Ammonium Tolerance Test

If a decrease in hepatic function is suspected and other laboratory tests (i.e., bile acids, bilirubin, etc.) are equivocal, an ammonia tolerance test may be performed. The principle of this test is to challenge the liver with a large dose of NH_4^+ via administration of NH_4Cl (either rectally or orally) or feeding a high-protein meal. The methodologies for each are described elsewhere (Stockham, 2008). In conditions of loss of hepatic function or portosystemic shunting of blood, an excessive increase in serum NH_4^+ is observed when the tolerance test is performed accordingly. The ammonium tolerance test is contraindicated when resting hyperammonemia is present as it may contribute to furthering of clinical abnormalities (i.e., hepatic encephalopathy). These tests are performed mostly in dogs but can be used with other species such as the rat (Mito et al., 1979; Sutherland, 1989).

11.3.4 Dye Excretion Tests

Hepatic function can be assessed by excretion tests using two organic anions: indocyanine green (ICG) or bromosulfophthalein (BSP). The use of BSP to assess liver function in humans was introduced over 80 years ago and has been used in animals since the 1950s (Flatland et al., 2000). BSP is administered intravenously and circulates bound to primarily albumin (Cornelius, 1991; Thrall, 2004). The bound BSP is then removed from circulation by the hepatocytes, conjugated and excreted in the bile. Therefore, the BSP excretion test is useful for assessing hepatic blood flow, hepatocellular function, and the biliary system (Cornelius, 1991). A straightforward spectrophotometric to determine plasma concentrations is used to measure BSP plasma concentration to determine clearance. Use of the BSP excretion test has been used in many laboratory species to assess liver function (Cornelius, 1991). However, the test is prone to negative influences by nonhepatic processes such as edema and hypoalbuminemia (Thrall, 2004). In addition, BSP is no longer commercially available and other liver tests that assess liver function (i.e., bile acids, ammonia, bilirubin) have proven to be more sensitive for detecting liver abnormalities (Center, 1990; Flatland et al., 2000). Like BSP, ICG is administered intravenously, protein-bound (primarily albumin and β-lipoprotein), and removed from circulation by hepatocytes (Cornelius, 1991; Thrall, 2004). ICG is excreted in bile in an unconjugated form. Also similar to BSP, the ICG excretion test is capable of assessing liver function, hepatic flow, and the patency of the biliary system. ICG excretion can be influenced by nonhepatic abnormalities, which requires numerous timed samples and is expensive (Thrall, 2004). Therefore, ICG offers no advantage over other hepatic function tests (Thrall, 2004). With the advent of bile acids and other measures of hepatic function such as bilirubin and ammonium, the use of dye excretion tests is infrequently used today.

11.3.5 Other Tests to Assess Liver Function

Because of the diverse physiologic roles of the liver, the changes in the concentrations of several plasma analytes may offer clues to the overall assessment of liver function.

11.3.5.1 Albumin

Albumin is the most abundant serum protein and is produced solely in the liver (Eckersall, 2008). As expected, the loss of functional capacity of the liver can result in a decrease in serum albumin concentrations. Typically, 60%–80% of hepatic function must be lost before hypoalbuminemia is noted (Thrall, 2004).

11.3.5.2 Cholesterol

The liver is the chief organ for cholesterol synthesis and catabolism (Bruss, 2008). Bile is the major route of excretion for cholesterol. Therefore, with decreases in bile flow (i.e., cholestasis), increases in serum cholesterol can occur. Since the liver is the main organ for cholesterol synthesis, a loss of function can result in decrease in serum cholesterol (Thrall, 2004). Since the decrease in bile flow and loss of function can occur simultaneously, serum cholesterol may be variable with severe hepatic disease (Thrall, 2004).

11.3.5.3 Urea Nitrogen

As stated previously, the liver converts ammonium from catabolism of proteins to urea via the Krebs–Henseleit urea cycle (Newman and Price, 2001). Subjects with liver failure lack the ability to convert the ammonium to urea thus increasing serum ammonium and decreasing urea concentrations (Newman and Price, 2001).

11.3.5.4 Coagulation proteins

The liver is responsible for the synthesis of most of the coagulation proteins (Stockham, 2008). If any of the clotting factors decrease by less than 30% of normal, a prolongation in coagulation times can be observed (Thrall, 2004).

11.3.5.5 Glucose

The liver plays a key role in glucose metabolism; thus, loss of hepatocellular function can result in decreased serum glucose (Stockham, 2008). However, it should be recognized that numerous nonhepatic conditions can cause hypoglycemia. Therefore, evaluation of glucose for the detection of liver failure should be accompanied by other liver function tests.

11.3.5.6 Triglycerides

The *de novo* synthesis of triglycerides and incorporation into lipoprotein particles is done in the liver in most laboratory animals. Because of this hepatic function, studies have shown that serum triglyceride levels decrease following the experimental toxic insults to the liver in rats (Provost, 2003). The decrease in the serum triglycerides have been suggested to occur due to the increase in the catabolism of the lipids or impairment of synthesis of transport of the triglycerides in the liver (Provost, 2003). Therefore, triglycerides may be used as an early biomarker of toxic liver insults.

11.3.5.7 Cholinesterases

Not considered a traditional enzyme biomarker of hepatic injury or function, cholinesterases (ChEs) have demonstrated some utility evaluating liver impairment. In general, the mammalian liver contains ChEs, catalytic enzymes involved in the hydrolysis of choline esters. There are two main ChEs, acetylcholinesterase (which, most notably, terminates the action of acetylcholine postsynaptically) and butyrylcholinesterase, also known as nonspecific ChE or pseudocholinesterase, (with no clear physiological function). They differ in their substrate specificities and inhibition by selective inhibitors (Chatonnet and Lockridge, 1989).

Clinically, serum and erythrocyte ChEs have demonstrated utility in identifying exposures to anti-ChE agents, some liver disorders, and congenital abnormalities (Wills and Dubois, 1972;

Witter, 1963). In humans, reduced serum butyrylcholinesterase activity has been linked to chronic liver diseases, including cirrhosis, inflammation, injury and infections, and malnutrition (Brown et al., 1981; Santarpia et al., 2013). In laboratory animals, however, evaluation of ChE activity traditionally has been used as a marker of neurotoxicity to examine products or compounds containing organophosphates or carbamates (Hoffmann et al., 1999). Nevertheless, there are studies demonstrating the use of ChE as a marker of altered hepatic function. For example, in rats, García-Ayllón et al. (2006), demonstrated a marked decrease in the acetylcholinesterase levels in rat livers with bile duct ligation- or CCl_4-induced cirrhosis. Furthermore, plasma from the bile duct ligation-induced cirrhosis rats had approximately 45% lower AChE activity than controls. Since liver butyrylcholinesterase was apparently unaffected, the authors suggested this change was specific for acetyl-cholinesterase. In mice experimentally infected with *Toxoplasma gondii*, Da Silva et al. (2013) demonstrated a significant reduction in serum and liver butyrylcholinesterase activity and an increase in serum ALT activity during the acute phase of the infection. The authors concluded that the reduced butyrylcholinesterase activity was related to the liver damage caused by the parasitism. In dogs, Tvarijonaviciute et al. (2012) demonstrated that serum butyrylcholinesterase decreased during experimentally induced endotoxemia and that choline administration attenuated the response. The reader is referred to Hoffmann et al. (1999) for a detailed discussion of ChEs, their evaluation and substrate specificities in laboratory animals.

REFERENCES

Adachi, Y., Horii, K., Suwa, M., Tanihata, M., Ohba, Y., and Yamamoto, T. 1981. Serum glutathione S-transferase in experimental liver damage in rats. *Gastroenterol Jpn.* 16:129–133.

Albert, Z., Orlowska, J., Orlowski, M., and Szewczuk, A. 1964. Histochemical and biochemical investigations of gamma-glutamyl transpeptidase in the tissues of man and laboratory rodents. *Acta Histochem.* 18:78–89.

Allen, M.J., Hoffmann, W.E., Richardson, D.C., and Breur, G.J. 1998. Serum markers of bone metabolism in dogs. *Am J Vet Res.* 59:250–254.

Alpers, D.H., Mahmood, A., Engle, M., Yamagishi, F., and DeSchryver-Kecskemeti, K. 1994. The secretion of intestinal alkaline phosphatase (IAP) from the enterocyte. *J Gastroenterol.* 29(Suppl 7):63–67.

Amacher, D.E. 1998. Serum transaminase elevations as indicators of hepatic injury following the administration of drugs. *Regul Toxicol Pharmacol.* 27:119–130.

Amacher, D.E. 2002. A toxicologist's guide to biomarkers of hepatic response. *Hum Exp Toxicol.* 21:253–262.

Anderson, D.R. 1966. Normal values for clinical blood chemistry tests of the *Macaca mulatto* monkey. *Am J Vet Res.* 27:1484–1489.

Anderson, H.C., Sipe J.B., Hessle, L., et al. 2004. Impaired calcification around matrix vesicles of growth plate and bone in alkaline phosphatase-deficient mice. *Am J Pathol.* 164:841–847.

Aniya, Y. and Anders, M.W. 1985. Alteration of hepatic glutathione S-transferases and release into serum after treatment with bromobenzene, carbon tetrachloride, or N-nitrosodimethylamine. *Biochem Pharmacol.* 34:4239–4244.

Apostolou, A., Saidt, L., and Brown, W.R. 1976. Effect of overnight fasting of young rats on water consumption, body weight, blood sampling, and blood composition. *Lab Anim Sci.* 26:959–960.

Asha, S. and Radha, E. 1985. Effect of age and myocardial infarction on serum and heart lactic dehydrogenase. *Exp Gerontol.* 20:67–70.

Ashamiss, F., Wierzbicki, Z., Chrzanowska, A., et al. 2004. Clinical significance of arginase after liver transplantation. *Ann Transplant.* 9:58–60.

Badylak, S.F. and Van Vleet, J.F. 1981. Sequential morphologic and clinicopathologic alterations in dogs with experimentally induced glucocorticoid hepatopathy. *Am J Vet Res.* 42:1310–1318.

Bain, P. 2003. Liver. In *Duncan & Prasse's Veterinary Laboratory Medicine—Clinical Pathology.* Eds. K.S. Latimer, E.A. Mahaffey, and K.W. Prasse, pp. 193–214. Ames, IA: Iowa State Press.

Baumann, M. and Berauer, M. 1985. Comparative study on the sensitivity of several serum enzymes in detecting hepatic damage in rats. *Arch Toxicol Suppl.* 8:370–372.

Berger, H.J. 1956. Quantitative analysis of "direct" and "indirect" bilirubin in the serum of domestic animals. *Zentralbl Veterinärmed.* 3:273–280.

Bishoff, K.S.R. 2007. Liver toxicity. In *Veterinary Toxicology—Basic and Clinical Principles*. Ed.R.C. Gupta, pp. 145–160. San Diego, CA: Academic Press.

Blazka, M.E., Elwell, M.R., Holladay, S.D., Wilson, R.E., and Luster, M.I. 1996. Histopathology of acetaminophen-induced liver changes: Role of interleukin 1 alpha and tumor necrosis factor alpha. *Toxicol Pathol.* 24:181–189.

Bodansky, O. and Schwartz, M.K. 1968. 5'-Nucleotidase. *Adv Clin Chem.* 11:277–328.

Bondy, G.S., Armstrong, C.L., Curran, I.H., Barker, M.G., and Mehta, R. 2000. Retrospective evaluation of serum ornithine carbamyltransferase activity as an index of hepatotoxicity in toxicological studies with rats. *Toxicol Lett.* 114:163–171.

Boone, L., Meyer, D., Cusick, P., et al. 2005. Selection and interpretation of clinical pathology indicators of hepatic injury in preclinical studies. *Vet Clin Pathol.* 34:182–188.

Boyd, J.W. 1983. The mechanisms relating to increases in plasma enzymes and isoenzymes in diseases of animals. *Vet Clin Pathol.* 12:9–24.

Boyer, T.D. 1989. The glutathione S-transferases: An update. *Hepatology.* 9:486–496.

Braun, J.P., Siest, G., and Rico, A.G. 1987. Uses of gamma-glutamyltransferase in experimental toxicology. *Adv Vet Sci Comp Med.* 31:151–172.

Bridger, N., Glanemann, B., and Neiger, R. 2008. Comparison of postprandial and ceruletide serum bile acid stimulation in dogs. *J Vet Intern Med.* 22:873–878.

Brondeau, M.T., Ban, M., Bonnet, P., Guenier, J.P., and De Ceaurriz, J. 1986. Concentration-related changes in blood and tissue parameters of hepatotoxicity and their interdependence in rats exposed to bromobenzene and 1,2-dichlorobenzene. *Toxicol Lett.* 31:159–166.

Brouillet, A., Darbouy, M., Okamoto, T., et al. 1994. Functional characterization of the rat gamma-glutamyl transpeptidase promoter that is expressed and regulated in the liver and hepatoma cells. *J Biol Chem.* 269:14878–14884.

Brown, S.S., Kalow, W., Pilz, W., Whittaker, M., and Woronick, C.L. 1981. The plasma cholinesterases: A new perspective. *Adv Clin Chem.* 22:1–123.

Bruss, M. 2008. Lipids and ketones. In *Clinical Biochemistry of Domestic Animals*. Eds. J. Kaneko, J.W. Harvey, and M.L. Bruss, pp. 81–116. San Diego, CA: Elsevier.

Carakostas, M.C., Gossett, K.A., Church, G.E., and Cleghorn, B.L. 1986. Evaluating toxin-induced hepatic injury in rats by laboratory results and discriminant analysis. *Vet Pathol.* 23:264–269.

Carakostas, M.C., Power, R.J., and Banerjee, A.K. 1990. Serum 5'nucleotidase activity in rats: A method for automated analysis and criteria for interpretation. *Vet Clin Pathol.* 19:109–113.

Cattley, R.C. and Popp, J. 2002. *Liver*, 2nd edition. San Diego, CA: Academic Press.

Center, S.A. 1990. Liver function tests in the diagnosis of portosystemic vascular anomalies. *Semin Vet Med Surg (Small Anim).* 5:94–99.

Center, S.A., ManWarren, T., Slater, M.R., and Wilentz, E. 1991. Evaluation of twelve-hour preprandial and two-hour postprandial serum bile acids concentrations for diagnosis of hepatobiliary disease in dogs. *J Am Vet Med Assoc.* 199:217–226.

Chapman, D.E. et al. 1988. Acute toxicity of helenalin in BDF1 mice. *Fundam Appl Toxicol.* 10:302–312.

Chatonnet, A. and Lockridge, O. 1989. Comparison of butyrylcholinesterase and acetylcholinesterase. *Biochem J.* 260:625–634.

Cheng-long, B., Canfield, P.J., and Stacey, N.H. 1992. Individual serum bile acids as early indicators of carbon tetrachloride- and chloroform-induced liver injury. *Toxicology.* 75:221–234.

Cho, S.R., Lim, Y.A., and Lee, W.G. 2005. Unusually high alkaline phosphatase due to intestinal isoenzyme in a healthy adult. *Clin Chem Lab Med.* 43:1274–1275.

Chowdhury, J.R., Kondapalli, R., and Chowdhury, N.R. 1993. Gunn rat: A model for inherited deficiency of bilirubin glucuronidation. *Adv Vet Sci Comp Med.* 37:149–173.

Clampitt, R.B. and Hart, R.J. 1978. The tissue activities of some diagnostic enzymes in ten mammalian species. *J Comp Pathol.* 88:607–621.

Clarke, H., Egan, D. A, Heffernan, M., et al. 1997. Alpha-glutathione s-transferase (alpha-GST) release, an early indicator of carbon tetrachloride hepatotoxicity in the rat. *Hum Exp Toxicol.* 16:154–157.

Collis, K.A., Symonds, H.W., and Sansom, B.F. 1979. The half-life of glutamate dehydrogenase in plasma of dry and lactating dairy cows. *Res Vet Sci.* 27:267–268.

Cornelius, C.E. 1991. Liver function tests in the differential diagnosis of hepatotoxicity. In *Hepatotoxicity*. Eds. R. Meeks, S.D. Harrison, and R.J. Bull, pp. 181–214. Boca Raton, FL: CRC Press.

Crawford, J. 1999. The liver and biliary tract. In *Pathologic Basis of Disease*. Ed. K.V. Cotran RS and T. Collins, pp. 846–848. Philadelphia, PA: WB. Saunders.

Curtis, S.J., Moritz, M., and Snodgrass, P.J. 1972. Serum enzymes derived from liver cell fractions. I. The response to carbon tetrachloride intoxication in rats. *Gastroenterology*. 62:84–92.

Daoust, R. 1982. The histochemical demonstration of gamma-glutamyl transpeptidase activity in different populations of rat liver during azo dye carcinogenesis. *J Histochem Cytochem*. 30:312–316.

Darbouy, M., Chobert, M.N., Lahuna, O., et al. 1991. Tissue-specific expression of multiple gamma-glutamyl transpeptidase mRNAs in rat epithelia. *Am J Physiol.* 261:C1130–C1137.

Da Silva, A.S., Tonin, A.A., Thorstenberg, M.L., et al. 2013. Relationship between butyrylcholinesterase activity and liver injury in mice acute infected with Toxoplasma gondii. *Pathol Res Pract.* 209(2):95–98.

Deinhardt, F. and Deinhardt, J. 1966. The use of platyrrhine monkeys in medical research. *Symp Zool Soc Lond* 17:127–150.

DeLaurier, A. Jackson, B., Ingham, K., Pfeiffer, D., Horton, M.A., and Price, J.S. 2002. Biochemical markers of bone turnover in the domestic cat: Relationships with age and feline osteoclastic resorptive lesions. *J Nutr*. 132:1742S–1744S.

DeNovo, R.C. and Prasse, K.W. 1983. Comparison of serum biochemical and hepatic functional alterations in dogs treated with corticosteroids and hepatic duct ligation. *Am J Vet Res*. 44:1703–1709.

DePierre, J.W. and Morgenstern, R. 1983. Comparison of the distribution of microsomal and cytosolic glutathione S-transferase activities in different organs of the rat. *Biochem Pharmacol*. 32:721–723.

DeRosa, R. and Swick, R.W. 1975. Metabolic implications of the distribution of the alanine aminotransferase isoenzymes. J Biol Chem. 250: 7961–7967.

Dhami, M.S., Drangova, R., Farkas, R., Balazs, T., and Feuer, G. 1979. Decreased aminotransferase activity of serum and various tissues in the rat after cefazolin treatment. *Clin Chem*. 25:1263–1266.

Dixon, D.G., Hodson, P.V., and Kaiser, K.L.E. 1987. Serum sorbitol dehydrogenase activity as an indicator of chemically induced liver damage in rainbow trout. *Environ Toxicol Chem.* 6:685–696.

Dorner, J.L., Hoffmann, W.E., and Long, G.B. 1974. Corticosteroid induction of an isoenzyme of alkaline phosphatase in the dog. *Am J Vet Res*. 35:1457–1458.

Drozdz, M., Kucharz, E., and Kozlowski, A. 1975. Studies on 5'-nucleotidase activity in blood serum, tissues and liver mitochondrial fraction of normal, hypo- and hyperthyroid rats. *Endokrinologie*. 65:328–332.

Eckersall, P.D. 2008. Proteins, proteomics and the dysproteinemias. In *Clin Biochem Domestic Animals*. Eds. J. Kaneko, J.W. Harvey, and M.L. Bruss, pp. 117–156. San Diego, CA: Elsevier.

Eckersall, P.D. and Nash, A.S. 1983. Isoenzymes of canine plasma alkaline phosphatase: An investigation using isoelectric focusing and related to diagnosis. *Res Vet Sci*. 34:310–314.

Eckersall, P.D., Thomas, A., Marshall, G.M., and Douglas, T.A. 1986. The effect of neuraminidase on the molecular weight and the isoelectric point of the steroid induced alkaline phosphatase of dogs. *J Comp Pathol*. 96:587–591.

Ehrhart, N., Dernell, W.S., Hoffmann, W.E., Weigel, R.M., Powers, B.E., and Withrow, S.J. 1998. Prognostic importance of alkaline phosphatase activity in serum from dogs with appendicular osteosarcoma: 75 cases (1990–1996). *J Am Vet Med Assoc*. 213:1002–1006.

Eidne, K.A., Bass, N.M., Sherman, M., Millar, R.P., and Kirsch, R.E. 1984. Ligandin concentrations in the steroidogenic tissues of the rat during development. *Biochim Biophys Acta*. 801:424–428.

Eliakim, R., Mahmood, A., and Alpers, D.H. 1991. Rat intestinal alkaline phosphatase secretion into lumen and serum is coordinately regulated. *Biochim Biophys Acta*. 1091:1–8.

Engle, M.J. and Alpers, D.H. 1992. The two mRNAs encoding rat intestinal alkaline phosphatase represent two distinct nucleotide sequences. *Clin Chem.* 38:2506–2509.

Engle, M.J., Mahmood, A., and Alpers, D.H. 1995. Two rat intestinal alkaline phosphatase isoforms with different carboxyl-terminal peptides are both membrane-bound by a glycan phosphatidylinositol linkage. *J Biol Chem.* 270:11935–11940.

Ennulat, D., Magid-Slav, M., Rehm, S., and Tatsuoka, K.S. 2010a. Diagnostic performance of traditional hepatobiliary biomarkers of drug-induced liver injury in the rat. *Toxicol Sci.* 116(2):397–412.

Ennulat, D., Walker, D., Clemo, F., et al. 2010b. Effects of hepatic drug-metabolizing enzyme induction on clinical pathology parameters in animals and man. *Toxicol Pathol.* 38:810–828.

Estonius, M., Danielsson, O., Karlsson, C., Persson, H., Jörnvall, H., and Höög, J.O. 1993. Distribution of alcohol and sorbitol dehydrogenases. Assessment of mRNA species in mammalian tissues. *Eur J Biochem.* 215:497–503.

Everett, R.M., Duncan, J.R., and Prasse, K.W. 1977. Alkaline phosphatases in tissues and sera of cats. *Am J Vet Res.* 38:1533–1538.

Fernandez, N.J. and Kidney, B.A. 2007. Alkaline phosphatase: Beyond the liver. *Vet Clin Pathol.* 36:223–233.

Fiala, S. and Fiala, E.S. 1973. Activation by chemical carcinogens of gamma-glutamyl transpeptidase in rat and mouse liver. *J Natl Cancer Inst.* 51:151–158.

Fischer, G., Lilienblum, W., Ullrich, D., and Bock, K.W. 1986. Immunohistochemical differentiation of gamma-glutamyltranspeptidase in focal lesions and in zone I of rat liver after treatment with chemical carcinogens. *Carcinogenesis.* 7:1405–1410.

Flatland, B., Leib, M.S., Warnick, L.D., and Sponenberg, D.P. 2000. Evaluation of the bromosulfophthalein 30-minute retention test for the diagnosis of hepatic disease in dogs. *J Vet Intern Med.* 14:560–568.

Foster, G.R., Goldin, R.D., and Oliveira, D.B. 1989. Serum F protein: A new sensitive and specific test of hepatocellular damage. *Clin Chim Acta.* 184:85–92.

Fujii, T. 1997. Toxicological correlation between changes in blood biochemical parameters and liver histopathological findings. *J Toxicol Sci.* 22:161–183.

Fukuda, M., Yokoyama, H., Mizukami, T., et al. 2004. Kupffer cell depletion attenuates superoxide anion release into the hepatic sinusoids after lipopolysaccharide treatment. *J Gastroenterol Hepatol.* 19:1155–1162.

García-Ayllón, M.S., Silveyra, M.X., Candela, A., et al. 2006. Changes in liver and plasma acetylcholinesterase in rats with cirrhosis induced by bile duct ligation. *Hepatology.* 43(3):444–453.

Garzotto, C.K., Berg, J., Hoffmann, W.E., and Rand, W.M. 2000. Prognostic significance of serum alkaline phosphatase activity in canine appendicular osteosarcoma. *J Vet Intern Med.* 14:587–592.

Gaskill, C.L., Hoffmann, W.E., and Cribb, A.E. 2004. Serum alkaline phosphatase isoenzyme profiles in phenobarbital-treated epileptic dogs. *Vet Clin Pathol.* 33:215–222.

Giffen, P.S., Pick, C.R., Price, M.A., Williams, A., and York, M.J. 2002. Alpha-glutathione S-transferase in the assessment of hepatotoxicity—its diagnostic utility in comparison with other recognized markers in the Wistar Han rat. *Toxicol Pathol.* 30:365–372.

Goldberg, D.M. 1980a. The expanding role of microsomal enzyme induction, and its implications for clinical chemistry. *Clin Chem.* 26:691–699.

Goldberg, D.M. 1980b. Structural, functional, and clinical aspects of gamma-glutamyltransferase. *CRC Crit Rev Clin Lab Sci.* 12:1–58.

Goldstein, D.J., Rogers, C., and Harris, H. 1982. A search for trace expression of placental-like alkaline phosphatase in non-malignant human tissues: Demonstration of its occurrence in lung, cervix, testis and thymus. *Clin Chim Acta.* 125:63–75.

Gopinath, C., Prentice, D.E., Street, A.E., and Crook, D. 1980. Serum bile acid concentration in some experimental liver lesions of rat. *Toxicology.* 1980;15(2):113–127.

Gores, G.J., Herman, B., and Lemasters, J.J. 1990. Plasma membrane bleb formation and rupture: A common feature of hepatocellular injury. *Hepatology.* 11:690–698.

Goseki-Sone, M., Oida, S., Iimura, T., et al. 1996. Expression of mRNA encoding intestinal type alkaline phosphatase in rat liver and its increase by fat-feeding. *Liver.* 16:358–364.

Guelfi, J.F., Braun, J.P., Benard, P., Rico, A.G., and Thouvenot, J.P. 1982. Value of so called cholestasis markers in the dog: An experimental study. *Res Vet Sci.* 33:309–312.

Hall, R.L., and Nancy, E. 2008. Principles of clinical pathology for toxicology studies. In *Principles and Methods of Toxicology*. Ed. A.W. Hayes, pp. 1317–1358. Boca Raton, FL: CRC Press.

Handler, J.A., Kossor, D.C., and Goldstein, R.S. 1994. Assessment of hepatobiliary function in vivo and ex vivo in the rat. *J Pharmacol Toxicol Methods.* 31:11–19.

Hardonk, M.J. and BDe Boer, H.G. 1968. 5'-nucleotidase. 3. Determinations of 5'-nucleotidase isoenzymes in tissues of rat and mouse. *Histochemie.* 12:29–41.

Harman, A.W. and Henry, C.A. 1987. Differences in glutathione synthesis and glutathione-S-transferase activities in hepatocytes from postnatal and adult mice. *Biochem Pharmacol.* 36:177–179.

Harris, H. 1990. The human alkaline phosphatases: what we know and what we don't know. *Clin Chim Acta.* 186:133–150.

Hayashi, T., Salata, K., Kingman, A., and Notkins, A.L. 1988. Regulation of enzyme levels in the blood. Influence of environmental and genetic factors on enzyme clearance. *Am J Pathol.* 132:503–511.

Hess, R.S., Saunders, H.M., Van Winkle, T.J., and Ward, C.R. 2000. Concurrent disorders in dogs with diabetes mellitus: 221 cases (1993–1998). *J Am Vet Med Assoc.* 217:1166–1173.

Hinchman, C.A. and Ballatori, N. 1990. Glutathione-degrading capacities of liver and kidney in different species. *Biochem Pharmacol.* 40:1131–1135.

Hixson, E.J., Burdeshaw, J.A., Denine, E.P., and Harrison, S.D., Jr. 1979. Comparative subchronic toxicity of all-trans- and 13-cis-retinoic acid in Sprague—Dawley rats. *Toxicol Appl Pharmacol.* 47:359–365.

Hoffmann, W.E. 1976. Alkaline phosphatase isoenzymes in the dog. *Vet Clin Pathol.* 5:9–10.

Hoffmann, W. 2008. Diagnostic enzymology of domestic animals. In Eds. J. Kaneko, J.W. Harvey, and M.L. Bruss, *Clinical Biochemistry of Domestic Animals,* 6th edition, pp. 351–378. San Diego, CA: Academic Press.

Hoffmann, W.E. and Dorner, J.L. 1975. A comparison of canine normal hepatic alkaline phosphatase and variant alkaline phosphatase of serum and liver. *Clin Chim Acta.* 62:137–142.

Hoffmann, W.E. and Dorner, J.L. 1977. Disappearance rates of intravenously injected canine alkaline phosphatase isoenzymes. *Am J Vet Res.* 38:1553–1556.

Hoffmann, W.E., Everds, N., Pignatello, M., and Solter, P.F. 1994. Automated and semiautomated analysis of rat alkaline phosphatase isoenzymes. *Toxicol Pathol.* 22:633–638.

Hofmann, A.F., Hagey, L.R., and Krasowski, M.D. 2010. Bile salts of vertebrates: Structural variation and possible evolutionary significance. *J Lipid Res.* 51(2):226–246.

Hoffmann, W., Solter, P.F., and Wilson, B.W. 1999. Clinical enzymology. In *The Clinical Chemistry of Laboratory Animals*. Eds. F.W. Quimby and F.W. Loeb, pp. 399–454. Philadelphia, PA: Taylor & Francis.

Honda, T., Honda, K., Kokubun, C., et al. 2008. Time-course changes of hematology and clinical chemistry values in pregnant rats. *J Toxicol Sci.* 33:375–380.

Horio, Y., Nishida, Y., Sakakibara, R., Inagaki, S., Kamisaki, Y., and Wada, H. 1988a. Induction of cytosolic aspartate aminotransferase by a high-protein diet. *Biochem Int.* 16:579–586.

Horio, Y., Tanaka, T., Taketoshi, M., Uno, T., and Wada, H. 1988b. Rat cytosolic aspartate aminotransferase: regulation of its mRNA and contribution to gluconeogenesis. *J Biochem.* 103:805–808.

Huseby, N.E. 1979. Subcellular localization of gamma-glutamyltransferase activity in guinea pig liver. Effect of phenobarbital on the enzyme activity levels. *Clin Chim Acta.* 94:163–171.

Huseby, N.E. and Vik, T. 1978. The activity of gamma-glutamyltransferase after bile duct ligation in guinea pig. *Clin Chim Acta.* 88:385–392.

Igarashi, T., Muramatsu, H., Ohmori, S., Ueno, K., Kitagawa, H., and Satoh, T. 1988. Plasma glutathione S-transferase in carbon tetrachloride treated rats and its association to hepatic cytosolic isozymes. *Jpn J Pharmacol.* 46:211–216.

Ikemoto, M., Tsunekawa, S., Awane, M., et al. 2001a. A useful ELISA system for human liver-type arginase, and its utility in diagnosis of liver diseases. *Clin Biochem.* 34:455–461.

Ikemoto, M., Tsunekawa, S., Toda, Y., and Totani, M. 2001b. Liver-type arginase is a highly sensitive marker for hepatocellular damage in rats. *Clin Chem.* 47:946–948.

Jadhao, S.B., Yang, R.Z., Lin, Q., et al. 2004. Murine alanine aminotransferase: cDNA cloning, functional expression, and differential gene regulation in mouse fatty liver. *Hepatology.* 39:1297–1302.

Jaken, S. and Mason, M. 1978. Differences in the isoelectric focusing patterns of gamma-glutamyl transpeptidase from normal and cancerous rat mammary tissue. *Proc Natl Acad Sci USA.* 75:1750–1753.

Jensson, H., Alin, P., and Mannervik, B. 1985. Glutathione transferase isoenzymes from rat liver cytosol. *Methods Enzymol.* 113:504–507.

Kandrac, J., Kevresan, S., Gu, J. K, Mikov, M., Fawceti, J.P., and Kuhajda, K. 2006. Isolation and determination of bile acids. *Eur J Drug Metab Pharmacokinet.* 31(3):157–177.

Kaneko, J., Harvey, J.W., Bruss, M.L. Eds. 1997. *Clinical Biochemistry of Domestic Animals*. San Diego, CA: Academic Press, p. 932.

Kaplan, M.M., Ohkubo, A., Quaroni, E.G., and Sze-Tu, D. 1983. Increased synthesis of rat liver alkaline phosphatase by bile duct ligation. *Hepatology.* 3:368–376.

Katz, S., Gilardoni, A., Genovese, N., Wilkinski, R.W., Cornelius, C.E., and Malinow, M.R. 1968. Liver function studies in free ranging howler monkeys with hepatic pigmentation. *Lab Anim Care.* 18:626–630.

Keil, E. 1990. Determination of enzyme activities in serum for the detection of xenobiotic effects on the liver. *Exp Pathol.* 39:157–164.

Keller, P. 1981. Enzyme activities in the dog: tissue analyses, plasma values, and intracellular distribution. *Am J Vet Res.* 42:575–582.

Kirpensteijn, J., Kik, M., Rutteman, G.R., and Teske, E. 2002. Prognostic significance of a new histologic grading system for canine osteosarcoma. *Vet Pathol.* 39:240–246.

Klaus, H. 1958. Studies on the bilirubin metabolism of horses, sheep, calves, and rabbits. *Arch Exp Veterinärme.* 12:725–740.

Komnenou, A., Karayannopoulou, M., Polizopoulou, Z.S., Constantinidis, T.C., and Dessiris, A. 2005. Correlation of serum alkaline phosphatase activity with the healing process of long bone fractures in dogs. *Vet Clin Pathol.* 34:35–38.

Korsrud, G.O., Grice, H.C., and McLaughlan, J.M. 1972. Sensitivity of several serum enzymes in detecting carbon tetrachloride-induced liver damage in rats. *Toxicol Appl Pharmacol.* 22:474–483.

Krishna, M. 2013. Microscopic anatomy of the liver. *Clin Liver Dis.* 2:S4–S7.

Kristensen, S.R. 1994. Mechanisms of cell damage and enzyme release. *Dan Med Bull.* 41: 423–433.

Kryszewski, A.J., Neale, G., Whitfield, J.B., and Moss, D.W. 1973. Enzyme changes in experimental biliary obstruction. *Clin Chim Acta.* 47:175–182.

Laird, C.W. 1974. Clinical pathology: Blood chemistry. In *Handbook of Laboratory Animal Science,* Eds. E.C. Melby, Jr. and N.H. Altman, Vol. 2, pp. 347–436. Cleveland: CRC Press.

Lanca, A.J. and Israel, Y. 1991. Histochemical demonstration of sinusoidal gamma-glutamyltransferase activity by substrate protection fixation: Comparative studies in rat and guinea pig liver. *Hepatology.* 14:857–863.

Lawler, D.F., Keltner, D.G., Hoffman, W.E., et al. 1996. Benign familial hyperphosphatasemia in Siberian huskies. *Am J Vet Res.* 57:612–617.

Le Hir, M. and Kaissling, B. 1993. Distribution and regulation of renal ecto-5'-nucleotidase: implications for physiological functions of adenosine. *Am J Physiol.* 264:F377–F387.

Leach, R.J. Schwartz, Z., Johnson-Pais, T.L., Dean, D.D., Luna, M., and Boyan, B.D. 1995. Osteosarcoma hybrids can preferentially target alkaline phosphatase activity to matrix vesicles: evidence for independent membrane biogenesis. *J Bone Miner Res.* 10:1614–1624.

Lee, F.K., Lee, A.Y., Lin, C.X., Chung, S.S., and Chung, S.K. 1995. Cloning, sequencing, and determination of the sites of expression of mouse sorbitol dehydrogenase cDNA. *Eur J Biochem.* 230:1059–1065.

Lemasters, J.J., Stemkowski, C.J., Ji, S., and Thurman, R.G. 1983. Cell surface changes and enzyme release during hypoxia and reoxygenation in the isolated, perfused rat liver. *J Cell Biol.* 97:778–786.

Leonard, T.B., Neptun, D.A., and Popp, J.A. 1984. Serum gamma glutamyl transferase as a specific indicator of bile duct lesions in the rat liver. *Am J Pathol.* 116:262–269.

Liberati, T.A., Sansone, S.R., and Feuston, M.H. 2004. Hematology and clinical chemistry values in pregnant Wistar Hannover rats compared with nonmated controls. *Vet Clin Pathol.* 33:68–73.

Lindblom, P., Rafter, I., Copley, C., et al. 2007. Isoforms of alanine aminotransferases in human tissues and serum—differential tissue expression using novel antibodies. *Arch Biochem Biophys.* 466:66–77.

Mannervik, B. 1985. The isoenzymes of glutathione transferase. *Adv Enzymol Relat Areas Mol Biol.* 57:357–417.

Mannervik, B., Alin, P., Guthenberg, C., et al. 1985. Identification of three classes of cytosolic glutathione transferase common to several mammalian species: Correlation between structural data and enzymatic properties. *Proc Natl Acad Sci U S A.* 82:7202–7206.

Manson, M.M. and Smith, A.G. 1984. Effect of hexachlorobenzene on male and female rat hepatic gamma-glutamyl transpeptidase levels. *Cancer Lett.* 22:227–234.

Matsuzawa, T. and Sakazume, M. 1994. Effects of fasting on haematology and clinical chemistry values in the rat and dog. *Comp Haematol Int.* 4:152–156.

McCuskey, R. 2006. Anatomy of the liver. In *Hepatology: A Textbook of Liver Disease No. 1.* Eds. T.D. Boyern and M.P. Manns. Philadelphia, PA: Elsevier.

Milne, E.M. and Doxey, D.L. 1985. Gamma-glutamyl transpeptidase and its multiple forms in the tissues and sera of normal dogs. *Res Vet Sci.* 39:385–387.

Mitruka, B.M. and Rawnsley, H.M. 1981. *Clinical Biochemical and Hematological Reference Values in Normal Experimental Animals*, p. 413. New York, NY: Masson Publishing.

Mito, M., Ebata, H., Kusano, M., Onishi, T., Saito, T., and Sakamoto, S. 1979. Morphology and function of isolated hepatocytes transplanted into rat spleen. *Transplantation.* 28:507–515.

Mochida, S., Arai, M., Ohno, A., et al. 1999. Deranged blood coagulation equilibrium as a factor of massive liver necrosis following endotoxin administration in partially hepatectomized rats. *Hepatology.* 29:1532–1540.

Mohr, J.R., Mattenheimer, H., Holmes, A.W., Deinhardt, F., and Schmidt, F.W. 1971. Enzymology of experimental liver disease in marmoset monkeys. I. Patterns of enzyme activity in liver, other organs and serum of marmosets, compared to man and other mammals. *Enzyme.* 12:99–116.

Morgenstern, R. and DePierre, J.W. 1983. Microsomal glutathione transferase. Purification in unactivated form and further characterization of the activation process, substrate specificity and amino acid composition. *Eur J Biochem.* 134:591–597.

Mortensen, B. and Huseby, N.E. 1997. Clearance of circulating gamma-glutamyltransferase by the asialoglycoprotein receptor. Enzyme forms with different sialic acid content are eliminated at different clearance rates and without apparent desialylation. *Clin Chim Acta.* 258:47–58.

Moseley, R.H., Wang, W., Takeda, H., et al. 1996. Effect of endotoxin on bile acid transport in rat liver: a potential model for sepsis-associated cholestasis. *Am J Physiol.* 271:G137–G146.

Murayama, H., Igarashi, M., Mori, M., Fukuda, Y., Ikemoto, M., and Nagata, A. 2006. A sensitive ELISA for serum ornithine carbamoyltransferase utilizing the enhancement of immunoreactivity at alkaline pH. *Clin Chim Acta.* 368:125–130.

Murayama, H., Ikemoto, M., Fukuda, Y., and Nagata, A. 2008. Superiority of serum type-I arginase and ornithine carbamyltransferase in the detection of toxicant-induced acute hepatic injury in rats. *Clin Chim Acta.* 391:31–35.

Murayama, H., Ikemoto, M., Fukuda, Y., Tsunekawa, S., and Nagata, A. 2007. Advantage of serum type-I arginase and ornithine carbamoyltransferase in the evaluation of acute and chronic liver damage induced by thioacetamide in rats. *Clin Chim Acta.* 375:63–68.

Murayama, H., Ikemoto, M., and Hamaoki, M. 2009. Ornithine carbamyltransferase is a sensitive marker for alcohol-induced liver injury. *Clin Chim Acta.* 401:100–104.

Nagode, L.A., Koestner, A., and Steinmeyer, C.L. 1969. Organ-identifying properties of alkaline phosphatases from canine tissues. *Clin Chim Acta.* 26:45–54.

Nathanson, M.H. and Boyer, J.L. 1991. Mechanisms and regulation of bile secretion. *Hepatology.* 14:551–566.

Newman, D. and Price, C.P. 2001. Nonprotein nitrogen metabolites. In *Tietz Fundamentals of Clinical Chemistry*. Eds. C. Burtis and E.R. Ashwood, pp. 414–426.. Philadelphia, PA: W.B. Saunders.

Nishmura, M. and R. Teschke. 1982. Effect of chronic alcohol consumption on the activities of liver plasma membrane enzymes: Gamma-glutamyltransferase, alkaline phosphatase and 5'-nucleotidase. *Biochem Pharmacol.* 31:377–381.

Noguchi, T. and Y. Yamashita. 1987. The rabbit differs from other mammalian in the tissue distribution of alkaline phosphatase isoenzymes. *Biochem Biophys Res Commun.* 143:15–19.

Noonan, N.E. 1981. Variations of plasma enzymes in the pony and the dog after carbon tetrachloride administration. *Am J Vet Res.* 42:674–678.

Noonan, N.E. and D.J. Meyer. 1979. Use of plasma arginase and gamma-glutamyl transpeptidase as specific indicators of heptocellular or hepatobiliary disease in the dog. *Am J Vet Res.* 40:942–947.

Nuttall, K. and Klee, G.G. 2001. Analytes of hemoglobin metabolism-porphyrins, iron and bilirubin. In *The Fundamentals of Clinical Chemistry*. Eds. C. Burtis and E.R. Ashwood, pp. 584–607. Philadelphia, PA: W.B. Saunders.

O'Brien, P.J., Slaughter, M.R., Polley, S.R., and Kramer, K. 2002. Advantages of glutamate dehydrogenase as a blood biomarker of acute hepatic injury in rats. *Lab Anim.* 36:313–321.

Ogawa, H., Mink, J., Hardison W.G., and Miyai, K. 1990. Alkaline phosphatase activity in hepatic tissue and serum correlates with amount and type of bile acid load. *Lab Invest.* 62:87–95.

Ohshita, M., Takeda, H., Kamiyama, Y., Ozawa, K., and Honjo, I. 1976. A direct method for the estimation of ornithine carbamoyltransferase activity in serum. *Clin Chim Acta.* 67:145–152.

Ohuchi, T., Tada, K., and Akamatsu, K. 1995. Endogenous ET-1 contributes to liver injury induced by galactosamine and endotoxin in isolated perfused rat liver. *Am J Physiol.* 268:G997–1003.

Okamoto, T., Darbouy, M., Brouillet, A., Lahuna, O., Chobert, M.N., and Laperche, Y. 1994. Expression of the rat gamma-glutamyl transpeptidase gene from a specific promoter in the small intestine and in hepatoma cells. *Biochemistry.* 33:11536–11543.

Oliveira, D.B. 1986. Bulk immunopurification and development of a radioimmunoassay for human and murine F liver protein. *J Immunol Methods.* 91:99–105.

Oliveira, D.B. and Vindlacheruvu, S. 1987. The phylogenetic distribution of the liver protein F antigen. *Comp Biochem Physiol B.* 87:87–90.

Oluju, M.P., Eckersall, P.D., and Douglas, T.A. 1984. Simple quantitative assay for canine steroid-induced alkaline phosphatase. *Vet Rec.* 115:17–18.

Ono, K., Ono, T., and Matsumata, T. 1995. The pathogenesis of decreased aspartate aminotransferase and alanine aminotransferase activity in the plasma of hemodialysis patients: the role of vitamin B6 deficiency. *Clin Nephrol.* 43:405–408.

Ozer, J., Ratner, M., Shaw, M., Bailey, W., and Schomaker, S. 2008. The current state of serum biomarkers of hepatotoxicity. *Toxicology.* 245:194–205.

Pagani, F. and Panteghini, M. 2001. 5'-Nucleotidase in the detection of increased activity of the liver form of alkaline phosphatase in serum. *Clin Chem.* 47:2046–2048.

Pappas, N.J., Jr. 1980. Increased rat liver homogenate, mitochondrial, and cytosolic aspartate aminotransferase activity in acute carbon tetrachloride poisoning. *Clin Chim Acta.* 106:223–229.

Pappas, N.J., Jr. 1986. Source of increased serum aspartate and alanine aminotransferase: cycloheximide effect on carbon tetrachloride hepatotoxicity. *Clin Chim Acta.* 154:181–189.

Parola, M., Cheeseman, K.H., Biocca, M.E., Dianzani, M.U., and Slater, T.F. 1990. Biochemical studies on bile duct epithelial cells isolated from rat liver. *J Hepatol.* 10:341–345.

Patnaik, S.K. and Kanungo, M.S. 1977. Age-related expression of alanine aminotransferase isoenzymes in normal & hydrocortisone-treated rats. *Indian J Biochem Biophys.* 14:245–246.

Patnaik, S.K., Sharma, R., and Patnaik, R. 1987. Differential effects of hydrocortisone on aspartate aminotransferase isoenzymes of the liver of rats during growth, development, and senescence. *Biochem Int.* 15:611–617.

Pave-Preux, M., Ferry, N., Bouguet, J., Hanoune, J., and Barouki, R. 1988. Nucleotide sequence and glucocorticoid regulation of the mRNAs for the isoenzymes of rat aspartate aminotransferase. *J Biol Chem.* 263:17459–17466.

Petrovich, Y.A., Volozhin, A.I., Zubtsov, V.A., and Kichenko, S.M. 2007. Biorhythms of activities of liver and blood dehydrogenases and changes in body weight of the rats feeding normal diet or excess of sugar substitutes. *Bull Exp Biol Med.* 144(6):835–839.

Pineiro-Carrero, V.M. and Pineiro, E.O. 2004. Liver. *Pediatrics.* 113:1097–1106.

Plaa, G.L. and Charbonneau, M. 2008. Detection and evaluation of chemically induced liver injury. In *Principles and Methods of Toxicology.* Ed. A.W. Hayes, pp. 1465–1507. Boca Raton, FL: CRC Press.

Poelstra, K., Bakker, W.W., Klok, P.A., Hardonk, M.J., and Meijer, D.K. 1997a. A physiologic function for alkaline phosphatase: Endotoxin detoxification. *Lab Invest.* 76:319–327.

Poelstra, K., Bakker, W.W., Klok, P.A., Kamps, J.A., Hardonk, M.J., and Meijer, D.K. 1997b. Dephosphorylation of endotoxin by alkaline phosphatase in vivo. *Am J Pathol.* 151:1163–1169.

Powell, L.W., Hemingway, E., Billing, B.H., and Sherlock, S. 1967. Idiopathic unconjugated hyperbilirubinemia (Gilbert's syndrome). A study of 42 families. *N Engl J Med.* 277:1108–1112.

Powers, C.S., Schultze, A.E., Krishnan, V., Sato, M., and Hoffmann, W.E. 2007. Comparison of results from the semiautomated serum bone alkaline phosphatase isoenzyme assay with the periosteal alkaline phosphatase assay for use in rat models. *Vet Clin Pathol.* 36:285–287.

Preus, M., Bhargava, A.S., Khater, A.E., and Gunzel, P. 1988. Diagnostic value of serum creatine kinase and lactate dehydrogenase isoenzyme determinations for monitoring early cardiac damage in rats. *Toxicol Lett.* 42:225–233.

Provost, J.P., Hanton, G., Le Net, J.L. 2003. Plasma triglycerides: An overlooked biomarker of hepatotoxicity in the rat. *Comp Clin Path.* 12:95–101.

Rajagopalan, S., Wan, D.F., Habib, G.M., et al. 1993. Six mRNAs with different 5' ends are encoded by a single gamma-glutamyltransferase gene in mouse. *Proc Natl Acad Sci U S A.* 90:6179–6183.

Rajamohan, F., Nelms, L., Joslin, D.L., Lu, B., Reagan, W.J., and Lawton, M. 2006. cDNA cloning, expression, purification, distribution, and characterization of biologically active canine alanine aminotransferase-1. *Protein Expr Purif.* 48:81–89.

Ramaiah, S.K. 2007. A toxicologist guide to the diagnostic interpretation of hepatic biochemical parameters. *Food Chem Toxicol.* 45:1551–1557.

Rao, G.N. 1996. New diet (NTP-2000) for rats in the National Toxicology Program toxicity and carcinogenicity studies. *Fundam Appl Toxicol.* 32:102–108.

Redl, H., Schlag, G., Paul, E., and Davies, J. 1995. Plasma glutathione S-transferase as an early marker of post-traumatic hepatic injury in non-human primates. *Shock.* 3:395–397.

Reichard, H. 1959. Ornithine carbamyl transferase in dog serum on intravenous injection of enzyme, choledochus ligation, and carbon tetrachloride poisoning. *J Lab Clin Med.* 53:417–425.

Rej, R. 1980. An immunochemical procedure for determination of mitochondrial aspartate aminotransferase in human serum. *Clin Chem.* 26:1694–1700.

Righetti, A.B. and Kaplan, M.M. 1971. The origin of the serum alkaline phosphatase in normal rats. *Biochim Biophys Acta.* 230:504–509.

Rikans, L.E. and Moore, D.R. 1988. Acetaminophen hepatotoxicity in aging rats. *Drug Chem Toxicol.* 11:237–247.

Robertson, I.G., Jensson, H., Guthenberg, C., Tahir, M.K., Jernström, B., and Mannervik, B. 1985. Differences in the occurrence of glutathione transferase isoenzymes in rat lung and liver. *Biochem Biophys Res Commun.* 127:80–86.

Roomi, M.W. and Goldberg, D.M. 1981. Comparison of gamma-glutamyl transferase induction by phenobarbital in the rat, guinea pig and rabbit. *Biochem Pharmacol.* 30:1563–1571.

Rosen, F., Roberts, N.R., Budnick, L.E., and Nichol, C.A. 1959a. Corticosteroids and transaminase activity: The specificity of the glutamic-pyruvic transaminase response. *Endocrinology.* 65:256–264.

Rosen, F., Roberts, N.R., and Nichol, C.A. 1959b. Glucocorticosteroids and transaminase activity. I. Increased activity of glutamicpyruvic transaminase in four conditions associated with gluconeogenesis. *J Biol Chem.* 234(3):476–480.

Rowson, K.E. and Mahy, B.W. 1985. Lactate dehydrogenase-elevating virus. *J Gen Virol.* 66(Pt 11):2297–2312.

Ruscak, M., Orlicky, J., and Zubor, V. 1982. Isoelectric focusing of the alanine aminotransferase isoenzymes from the brain, liver and kidney. *Comp Biochem Physiol.* 71: 141–144.

Russell, D.W. 2003. The enzymes, regulation, and genetics of bile acid synthesis. *Annu Rev Biochem.* 72:137–174.

Rutgers, H.C., Batt, R.M., Vaillant, C., and Riley, J.E. 1995. Subcellular pathologic features of glucocorticoid-induced hepatopathy in dogs. *Am J Vet Res.* 56:898–907.

Saini, P.K. and Saini, S.K. 1978. Origin of serum alkaline phosphatase in the dog. *Am J Vet Res.* 39:1510–1513.

Sanecki, R.K., Hoffmann, W.E., Dorner, J.L., and Kuhlenschmidt, M.S. 1990. Purification and comparison of corticosteroid-induced and intestinal isoenzymes of alkaline phosphatase in dogs. *Am J Vet Res.* 51:1964–1968.

Sanecki, R.K., Hoffmann, W.E., Gelberg, H.B., and Dorner, J.L. 1987. Subcellular location of corticosteroid-induced alkaline phosphatase in canine hepatocytes. *Vet Pathol.* 24:296–301.

Sanecki, R.K., Hoffmann, W.E., Hansen, R., and Schaeffer, D.J. 1993. Quantification of bone alkaline phosphatase in canine serum. *Vet Clin Pathol.* 22:17–23.

Santarpia, L., Grandone, I., Contaldo, F., and Pasanisi, F. 2013. Butyrylcholinesterase as a prognostic marker: A review of the literature. *J Cachexia Sarcopenia Muscle.* 4(1):31–39.

Sato, A., Fairbanks, L.A., Lawson, T., and Lawson, G.W. 2005. Effects of age and sex on hematologic and serum biochemical values of vervet monkeys (*Chlorocebus aethiops sabaeus*). *Contemp Top Lab Anim Sci.* 44:29–34.

Schmid, T.C., Loffing, J., Le Hir, M., and Kaissling, B. 1994. Distribution of ecto-5'-nucleotidase in the rat liver: effect of anaemia. *Histochemistry.* 101:439–447.

Schmidt, E.S. and Schmidt, F.W. 1988. Glutamate dehydrogenase: Biochemical and clinical aspects of an interesting enzyme. *Clin Chim Acta.* 173:43–55.

Sepulveda, A.R., Carter, B.Z., Habib, G.M., Lebovitz, R.M., and Lieberman, M.W. 1994. The mouse gamma-glutamyl transpeptidase gene is transcribed from at least five separate promoters. *J Biol Chem.* 269:10699–10705.

Shull, R.M. and Hornbuckle, W. 1979. Diagnostic use of serum gamma-glutamyltransferase in canine liver disease. *Am J Vet Res.* 40:1321–1324.

Slighter, R., Kimball, J.P., Barbolt, T.A., Sherer, A.D., and Drobeck, H.P. 1988. Enzootic hepatitis A infection in cynomolgus monkeys (*Macaca fascicularis*). *Am J Primatolo.* 14:73–81.

Snodgrass, P.J., Lin, R.C., Muller, W.A., and Aoki, T.T. 1978. Induction of urea cycle enzymes of rat liver by glucagon. *J Biol Chem.* 253:2748–2753.

Solter, P.F. 2005. Clinical pathology approaches to hepatic injury. *Toxicol Pathol.* 33:9–16.

Solter, P.F., Hoffmann, W.E., Chambers, M.D., Schaeffer, D.J., and Kuhlenschmidt, M.S. 1994. Hepatic total 3 alpha-hydroxy bile acids concentration and enzyme activities in prednisone-treated dogs. *Am J Vet Res.* 55:1086–1092.

Solter, P.F., Hoffmann, W.E., Chambers, M.D., and Schaeffer, D.J. 1997. CCK-8 infusion increases plasma LMW alkaline phosphatase coincident with enterohepatic circulation of bile acids. *Am J Physiol.* 273:G381–G388.

Solter, P.F., Hoffmann, W.E., Hungerford, L.L., Peterson, M.E., and Dorner, J.L. 1993. Assessment of corticosteroid-induced alkaline phosphatase isoenzyme as a screening test for hyperadrenocorticism in dogs. *J Am Vet Med Assoc.* 203:534–538.

Solter, P.F., Liu, Z., and Guzman, R. 2000. Decreased hepatic ALT synthesis is an outcome of subchronic microcystin-LR toxicity. *Toxicol Appl Pharmoacol.* 164: 216–220.

Soma, L.R., Tierney, W.J., Hogan, G.K., and Satoh, N. 1995. The effects of multiple administrations of sevoflurane to cynomolgus monkeys: clinical pathologic, hematologic, and pathologic study. *Anesth Analg.* 81:347–352.

Stockham, S. and Scott, M.A. 2008. *Fundamentals of Veterinary Clinical Pathology*. 2nd edition. Ames, IA: Iowa: Blackwell Publishing.

Sulakhe, S.J. and Lautt, W.W. 1985. The activity of hepatic gamma-glutamyltranspeptidase in various animal species. *Comp Biochem Physiol B.* 82:263–264.

Sunderman, F.W., Jr. 1990. The clinical biochemistry of 5'-nucleotidase. *Ann Clin Lab Sci.* 20:123–139.

Sutherland, R.J. 1989. Biochemical evaluation of the hepatobiliary system in dogs and cats. *Vet Clin North Am Small Anim Pract.* 19:899–927.

Swaim, L.D., Taylor, H.W., and Jersey, G.C. 1985. The effect of handling techniques on serum ALT activity in mice. *J Appl Toxicol.* 5:160–162.

Swenson, C.L. and Graves, T.K. 1997. Absence of liver specificity for canine alanine aminotransferase (ALT). *Vet Clin Pathol.* 26:26–28.

Syakalima, M., Takiguchi, M., Yasuda, J., and Hashimoto, A. 1997. The age dependent levels of serum ALP isoenzymes and the diagnostic significance of corticosteroid-induced ALP during long-term glucocorticoid treatment. *J Vet Med Sci.* 59:905–909.

Szymanska, J.A., Bruchajzer, E., and Sporny, S. 1996. Comparison of hepatotoxicity of 1,2-, 1,3- and 1,4-dibromobenzenes: The dynamics of changes of selected parameters of liver necrosis in acute poisoning in mice. *J Appl Toxicol.* 16:35–41.

Takami, H., Matsuda, H., Kuki, S., et al. 1990. Leakage of cytoplasmic enzymes from rat heart by the stress of cardiac beating after increase in cell membrane fragility by anoxia. *Pflugers Arch.* 416:144–150.

Tazi, A., Galteau, M.M., and Siest, G. 1980. gamma-Glutamyltransferase of rabbit liver: Kinetic study of phenobarbital induction and in vitro solubilization by bile salts. *Toxicol Appl Pharmacol.* 55:1–7.

Tennant, B.C. 1997. Hepatic function. In *Clinical Biochemistry of Domestic Animals*. Eds. J. Kaneko, J.W. Harvey, and M.L. Bruss, pp. 327–352. San Diego, Academic Press.

Tennant, B.C. 1999. Assessment of hepatic function. In *The Clinical Chemistry of Laboratory Animals*. Eds. F. Quimby and F.W. Loeb, pp. 501–518. Philadelphia, PA: Taylor & Francis.

Tennant, B., Balazs, T., Baldwin, B.H., et al. 1981. Assessment of hepatic function in rabbits with steroid-induced cholestatic liver injury. *Fundam Appl Toxicol.* 1:329–333.

Tennant, B. and Center, S.A. 2008. Hepatic function. In *Clinical Biochemistry of Domestic Animals*. Eds. J. Kaneko, J.W. Harvey, and M.L. Bruss, pp. 379–412. San Diego, CA: Elsevier.

Teske, E., Rothuizen, J., de Bruijne, J.J., and Rijnberk, A. 1989. Corticosteroid-induced alkaline phosphatase isoenzyme in the diagnosis of canine hypercorticism. *Vet Rec.* 125:12–14.

Thrall, M. 2004. *Veterinary Hematology and Clinical Chemistry*, 1st edition. Baltimore, MD: Lippincott Williams & Wilkins.

Tolman, K. and Rej, R. 2001. Liver function. In *Tietz Fundmentals of Clinical Chemistry*. Eds. C. Burtis and E.R. Ashwood, pp. 747–770. Philadelphia, PA: W.B. Saunders.

Tomson, F.N. and Wardrop, K.J. 1987. Clinical chemistry and hematology. In *Laboratory Hamsters*. Eds. G.L. Van Hoosier and C.W. McPherson, pp. 43–59. Orlando, FL: Academic Press.

Travlos, G.S., Morris, R.W., Elwell, M.R., Duke, A., Rosenblum, S., and Thompson, M.B. 1996. Frequency and relationships of clinical chemistry and liver and kidney histopathology findings in 13-week toxicity studies in rats. *Toxicology.* 107:17–29.

Tvarijonaviciute, A., Kocaturk, M., Cansey, M., Tecles, F., Ceron, J.J., and Yilmaz, Z. 2012. Serum butyrylcholinesterase and paraoxonase 1 in a canine model of endotoxemia: Effects of choline administration. *Res Vet Sci.* 93(2):668–674.

Valentine, B.A., Blue, J.T., Shelley, S.M., and Cooper, B.J. 1990a. Increased serum alanine aminotransferase activity associated with muscle necrosis in the dog. *J Vet Intern Med.* 4:140–143.

Valentine, B.A., Cooper, B.J., Cummings, J.F., and de Lahunta, A. 1990b. Canine X-linked muscular dystrophy: Morphologic lesions. *J Neurol Sci.* 97:1–23.

Van der Meulen, J.H., Kuipers, H., and Drukker, J. 1991. Relationship between exercise-induced muscle damage and enzyme release in rats. *J Appl Physiol.* 71:999–1004.

Van Vleet, J.F. and Alberts, J.O. 1968. Evaluation of liver function tests and liver biopsy in experimental carbon tetrachloride intoxication and extrahepatic bile duct obstruction in the dog. *Am J Vet Res.* 29:2119–2131.

Vodela, J.K. and Dalvi, R.R. 1997. Erythrocyte glutathione-S-transferase activity in animal species. *Vet Hum Toxicol.* 39:9–11.

Voet D, V.J. 1990. *Biochemistry*. New York, NY: John Wiley & Sons.

Wachstein, M. and Bradshaw, M. 1965. Histochemical localization of enzyme activity in the kidneys of three mammalian species during their postnatal development. *J Histochem Cytochem.* 13:44–56.

Waner, T. and Nyska, A. 1994. The influence of fasting on blood glucose, triglycerides, cholesterol, and alkaline phosphatase in rats. *Vet Clin Pathol.* 23:78–80.

Watanabe, K. and Fishman, W.H. 1964. Application of the stereospecific inhibitor L-phenylalanine to the enzymorphology of intestinal alkaline phosphatase. *J Histochem Cytochem.* 12:252–260.

Watanabe, N., Tsukada, N., Smith, C.R., and Phillips, M.J. 1991. Motility of bile canaliculi in the living animal: Implications for bile flow. *J Cell Biol.* 113:1069–1080.

Watkins, J.R., Gough, A.W., and McGuire, E.J. 1989. Drug-induced myopathy in beagle dogs. *Toxicol Pathol.* 17:545–548.

Webster, C.R. and Anwer, M.S. 1998. Cyclic adenosine monophosphate-mediated protection against bile acid-induced apoptosis in cultured rat hepatocytes. *Hepatology.* 27:1324–1331.

Webster, C.R., Usechak, P., and Anwer, M.S. 2002. cAMP inhibits bile acid-induced apoptosis by blocking caspase activation and cytochrome c release. *Am J Physiol Gastrointest Liver Physiol.* 283:G727–G738.

Webb, D. and Gagnon, M.M. 2007. Serum sorbitol dehydrogenase activity as an indicator of chemically induced liver damage in black bream (*Acanthopagrus butcheri*). *Environ Bioindic.* 2:172–182.

Whiting, J.F., Green, R.M., Rosenbluth, A.B., and Gollan, J.L. 1995. Tumor necrosis factor-alpha decreases hepatocyte bile salt uptake and mediates endotoxin-induced cholestasis. *Hepatology.* 22:1273–1278.

Whyte, M.P., Walkenhorst, D.A., Fedde, K.N., Henthorn, and Hill, C.S. 1996. Hypophosphatasia: Levels of bone alkaline phosphatase immunoreactivity in serum reflect disease severity. *J Clin Endocrinol Metab.* 81:2142–2148.

Wiedmeyer, C.E., Morton, D.G., Cusick, P.K., Wright, T., Solter, P.F., and Hoffmann, W.E. 1999. Semiautomated analysis of alkaline phosphatase isoenzymes in serum of normal cynomolgus monkeys (*Macaca fascicularis*). *Vet Clin Pathol.* 28:2–7.

Wiedmeyer, C.E., Solter, P.E., and Hoffmann, W.E. 2002a. Alkaline phosphatase expression in tissues from glucocorticoid-treated dogs. *Am J Vet Res.* 63:1083–1088.

Wiedmeyer, C.E., Solter, P.E., and Hoffmann, W.E. 2002b. Kinetics of mRNA expression of alkaline phosphatase isoenzymes in hepatic tissues from glucocorticoid-treated dogs. *Am J Vet Res.* 63:1089–1095.

Williams, J.S., Meroney, F.C., Hutt, G., and Sadun, E.H. 1966. Serum chemical components in mice determined by use of ultramicrotechniques. *J Appl Physiol.* 21:1026–1030.

Wills, J.H. and Dubois, K.P. 1972. The measurement and significance of changes in the cholinesterase activities of erythrocytes and plasma in man and animals. *CRC Crit Rev Toxicol.* 1:153–199.

Wisse, E. 1970. An electron microscopic study of the fenestrated endothelial lining of rat liver sinusoids. *J Ultrastruct Res.* 31:125–150.

Witter, R.F. 1963. Measurement of blood cholinesterase. *Arch Environ Health.* 6:537–563.

Wolf, P.L. 1986. Clinical significance of increased or decreased serum alkaline phosphatase isoenzymes. *Clin Lab Med.* 6:525–532.

Wootton, A.M., Neale, G., and Moss, D.W. 1977. Enzyme activities of cells of different types isolated from livers of normal and cholestatic rats. *Clin Sci Mol Med.* 52:585–590.

Yamagishi, F., Komoda, T., and Alpers, D.H. 1994. Secretion and distribution of rat intestinal surfactant-like particles after fat feeding. *Am J Physiol.* 266:G944–G952.

Yamazaki, K., Mikami, T., Hosokawa, S., et al. 1995. A new mutant rat with hyperbilirubinuria (hyb). *J Hered.* 86:314–317.

Yang, R.Z., Blaileanu, G., Hansen, B.C., Shuldiner, A.R., and Gong, D.W. 2002. cDNA cloning, genomic structure, chromosomal mapping, and functional expression of a novel human alanine aminotransferase. *Genomics.* 79:445–450.

Yeh, J.K., Aloia, J.F., Vaswani, A.N., and Semla, H.M. 1984. Effects of hypophysectomy on tissue alkaline phosphatase in the rat. *Enzyme.* 32:149–156.

Yoshida, T. 1981. The changes of hematological and biochemical properties in cynomolgus monkeys (*Macaca fascicularis*) after importation. *Jpn J Med Sci Biol.* 34:239–242.

Young, G.P., Friedman, S., Yedlin, S.T., and Allers, D.H. 1981. Effect of fat feeding on intestinal alkaline phosphatase activity in tissue and serum. *Am J Physiol.* 241:G461–G468.

Zelewski, M. and Swierczynski, J. 1991. Malic enzyme in human liver. Intracellular distribution, purification and properties of cytosolic isozyme. *Eur J Biochem.* 201:339–345.

Zieve, L., Anderson, W.R., Dozeman, R., Draves, K., and Lyftogt, C. 1985. Acetaminophen liver injury: Sequential changes in two biochemical indices of regeneration and their relationship to histologic alterations. *J Lab Clin Med.* 105:619

12 Evaluation of Renal Function and Injury

Denise Bounous and Ernie Harpur

CONTENTS

12.1 INTRODUCTION

The kidney is a complex organ that is responsive to the changes in the whole organism. As such, kidney function is affected by various hormones, food intake and diet, shifts in acid–base status, and changes in blood pressure and fluid volume. The functional unit of the kidney is the nephron, consisting of two functionally distinct units: the glomerulus, which is basically a vascular bed

TABLE 12.1
Function Specific Regions of the Kidney

Component of Nephron	Action
Glomerulus	Passive formation of ultrafiltrate of plasma devoid of most protein
Bowman's capsule	Collection of glomerular filtrate
Proximal tubule	Active reabsorption of glucose, proteins, and amino acids, vitamins, ascorbic acid, acetoacetate, hydroxybutyrate, uric acid, sodium, potassium, calcium (by PTH), phosphate (by PTH), sulfate, and bicarbonate
	Passive reabsorption of: chloride, water, and urea
	Active secretion of hydrogen ion
	Production of calcitriol
Henle's loop	Generation of medullary hyperosmolality
Descending limb	Passive reabsorption of water
	Passive secretion of sodium, urea
Thin ascending limb	Passive reabsorption of urea and sodium; impermeable to water
Thick ascending limb	Active reabsorption of chloride and calcium
	Passive reabsorption of sodium, impermeable to water, potassium
Distal tubule	Active reabsorption of sodium (by aldosterone), calcium, bicarbonate, and small amounts of glucose
	Passive reabsorption of chloride, water (by ADH)
	Active secretion of hydrogen ions, ammonia, and uric acid
	Passive secretion of potassium
Collecting ducts	Active reabosorption of sodium (by aldosterone)
	Passive reabsorption of chloride and water (by ADH)
	Active secretion of hydrogen ion
	Passive secretion of potassium

ADH, antidiuretic hormone; PTH, parathyroid hormone.

serving as a diffusion membrane, and the renal tubule, which selectively processes the glomerular ultrafiltrate and maintains homeostasis of the organism. The renal system accomplishes this function by three general processes: (1) glomerular filtration and tubular secretion of toxins such as blood urea nitrogen (BUN), creatinine, and metabolic waste products, (2) reabsorption and secretion of water, electrolytes, and solutes from the glomerular filtrate to maintain homeostasis and acid–base balance, and (3) biosynthesis involving formation of a variety of hormones and other chemicals which have both local and systemic effects (Table 12.1).

Detailed descriptions of renal anatomy and physiology are beyond the scope of this chapter. However, knowledge of normal renal function is necessary to understand the pathophysiology and to adequately interpret any changes seen in serum and urine analytes resulting from nephrotoxicity or renal disease. Reviews of renal anatomy and physiology are available in the literature (Pooler and Eaton, 2009; Rennke and Denker, 2010; Rose, 2001).

12.2 INTERDEPENDENCY OF RENAL FUNCTION WITH OTHER ORGAN SYSTEMS

Primary or secondary changes in renal function may affect other organs in the body or may result from dysfunction of these other organs. For example, chronic kidney disease (CKD) can result in inadequate formation of erythropoietin (EPO) and 1,25-dihydroxycholecalciferol. EPO is produced by the kidney and acts on the bone marrow to stimulate the production of red blood cells (RBCs), and synthesis of EPO and its constitutive release into the circulation are controlled by the transcriptional activity of the EPO gene. A key regulator of EPO is the hypoxia-inducible transcription factor (HIF), which essentially triggers EPO production from the cortical interstitial fibroblasts in the kidney (Castrop and Kurtz, 2010). The clinical effect of failure to produce EPO is the nonregenerative anemia of CKD, whereas the clinical impact of inadequate renal production of 1,25-dihydroxycholecalciferol is development of renal osteodystrophy and renal secondary hyperparathyroidism. Both kidney and lungs play major roles in acid–base regulation in vertebrates so that a significant renal tubular defect with loss of electrolytes can result in systemic disease if untreated and/or the respiratory system is unable to correct the imbalance (Rose, 2001; Rothstein et al., 1990). Natriuretic peptides, synthesized in the heart and prostaglandin E2 (PGE2), synthesized in the kidneys facilitate renal excretion of sodium and water (Bonvalet et al., 1987; Farman et al., 1987). Several other hormones have specific effects on the kidney and its functions. Renin is produced in the kidneys from specialized cells (e.g., granular cells) of the juxtaglomerular apparatus in response to renal sympathetic activity, decreased intrarenal blood pressure at the juxtaglomerular cells, or decreased delivery of sodium and chloride to the macula densa (Kumar and Fansto, 2010). When less sodium is sensed by the macula densa, the juxtaglomerular cells increase renin release. Renin cleaves the peptide bond between the leucine (Leu) and valine (Val) residues on angiotensinogen, creating the 10-amino acid peptide (des-Asp) angiotensin I. Angiotensin I is converted to angiotensin II (AII) through removal of two C-terminal residues by the enzyme angiotensin-converting enzyme (ACE) within the kidney. AII increases blood pressure by stimulating the Gq protein in vascular smooth muscle cells (which in turn activates contraction by an inositol 1,4,5-trisphosphate [IP_3]-dependent mechanism, leading to vasoconstriction).

Aldosterone is the major mineralocorticoid hormone secreted by the adrenal cortex. In the kidney, aldosterone promotes retention of sodium and bicarbonate, excretion of potassium and hydrogen ions, and secondary retention of water. Aldosterone synthesis is stimulated by several factors, including an increase in the plasma concentration of (1) angiotensin III (a metabolite of AII), (2) AII (regulated by angiotensin I, which is in turn regulated by the hormone renin), (3) adrenocorticotropic hormone (ACTH), or (4) potassium levels, which are present in proportion to plasma sodium deficiencies. Increased potassium regulates aldosterone synthesis by depolarizing the cells in the zona glomerulosa, which opens the voltage-dependent calcium channels. As such, potassium levels are the most sensitive stimulator of aldosterone (Williams and Dluhy, 1972).

Endothelin-1 (ET-1) together with endothelin-2 (ET-2) and endothelin-3 (ET-3) comprise the endothelin family of 21-amino acid peptides produced in various cells and tissues, especially endothelial and epithelial lineages. ET-1 is a key mediator of vascular tone and renal homeostasis through antagonistic vasoactive effects. ET-1 is a vasoconstrictor, but it also induces the production of the potent vasodilator, nitric oxide (NO). Consequently, dysfunctions of ET-1 signaling are associated with cardiovascular, renal, and respiratory diseases, such as high blood pressure, atherosclerosis, and systemic and pulmonary hypertension (Hynynen and Khalil, 2006).

Arginine vasopressin (AVP), also known as vasopressin, argipressin, or antidiuretic hormone (ADH), is a neurohypophysial hormone found in most mammals. Vasopressin is responsible for increasing water absorption in the kidney by inducing translocation of aquaporin–collecting duct (CD) water channels in the plasma membrane of CD epithelial cells of the nephron (Caldwell and Young, 2006; Nielsen et al., 1995). Vasopressin additionally increases peripheral vascular resistance, which in turn increases arterial blood pressure and plays a key role in homeostasis via regulation of water, glucose, and salts in the blood (Loeb, 1998). Renal disease, which can result in imbalances in these hormones, can invoke plasma volume expansion, hypertension, and peripheral edema.

12.3 LABORATORY TESTS OF RENAL FUNCTION AND INJURY

12.3.1 Routine Urinalysis

Routine urinalysis is an essential part of the laboratory evaluation, and the results should be interpreted along with the results of a chemistry panel. Ideally, urine should be collected at the same time, or as close as possible to the time of blood collection for hematology and clinical chemistry. This allows for accurate interpretation of renal-associated parameters from the clinical chemistry and/or hematology panel by correlation with findings in urinalysis. For example, a BUN of 100 mg/dL in a dog may be interpreted differently when the urine specific gravity (USG) is 1.006 (polyuric renal failure) versus 1.080 (renal or potential prerenal effects). Alternatively, a nonregenerative anemia (no reticulocytes) may be explained by renal injury affecting EPO production.

12.3.1.1 Urine Sample Collection

Urine collection from animals can be difficult, but many urinary analytes are affected by the method of collection, processing, or storage (i.e., lack of preservation of urine during and after collection). Proper collection is required for quality results. Urine should be collected under refrigeration into a clean, dry, and sterile container that is free of any disinfecting or cleaning chemicals. If urine is allowed to remain in shallow containers at room temperature (RT), evaporation occurs with resultant increases in specific gravity and bacteria, changes in pH, and deterioration of formed elements such as casts and crystals, so that the sample is not useful for evaluation.

Urine can be collected as a timed free-catch collection, via catheterization, or by cystocentesis. The collection procedure that is most commonly used in toxicology studies is a free-catch, timed collection (Kurien et al., 2004). Monkeys, dogs, and rodents are housed in individual cages, frequently metabolism cages, and urine is collected over a certain period of time. This may be referred to as an overnight collection, but is most usually for a period of 12–18 hours. The use of metabolism cages is optimal for collection of urine from rodents, as variations in design of these cages enhance the quality of sample collection by eliminating water spillage and decreasing contact with feces while permitting urine to flow down an incline into a collecting vessel. Several styles are commercially available and Nalgene® has optimized rodent metabolism cages with reusable individual refrigeration units that keep the specimens at an acceptable cool temperature overnight. Both rat and mouse cages are available, and there is a measurable difference in both the urine volume and quality when appropriately sized cages are used for the different species (Matandos and Franz, 1980). For example, when mice are placed in rat metabolism cages for urine collection, the volume produced by mice is so small that much of it can evaporate. Proprietary collection containers could also be used, for example, styrofoam shipping containers can be modified to accommodate the urine collection tubes through a hole cut in the container lid. Crushed ice is packed tightly around the collection tube and the lid is placed over the container. However, no system totally eliminates contact between urine and feces or urine and food, and some may potentially permit some spilling of the drinking water that could cause dilution of the urine specimen. It is therefore essential that experienced animal care staff carefully set up and inspect the metabolic units to be certain the tips of the watering devices allow ready access to water by the animals, but minimize spillage of water and contamination of the urine sample. In most cases, the animals should not have access to food during a timed urine collection in order to avoid food contamination of the urine. The use of preservatives can also affect the measurement of urine parameters and their use is generally discouraged. Sodium azide, however, is frequently used in samples that are being collected for metabolomic analysis and this does not appear to adversely affect routine urinalysis parameters.

Urethral catheterization may be performed in most species, but is more frequently used in larger animal species such as dogs, cats, miniature swine, and nonhuman primates (Ragan and Gillis, 1975). While chemical restraint may be required with some species, gentle physical restraint is generally sufficient for catheterization in many situations. This technique has been described for use in the rabbit, dog, cat, and monkey (Kirk and Bistner, 1969; Loeb, 1964; Moreland, 1965), as well as the rat (Kraus, 1980). Catheterized samples have less contamination from the distal urogenital tract; however, contamination from the urethra may still occur resulting in increased epithelial cells or RBCs. And poor catheterization technique may lead to trauma or, less commonly, infection (Zinkl et al., 1999; Osbourne et al. 1972; Chew and DiBarola, 1998).

Random urine samples may be obtained from many species by cystocentesis and can be performed in most animals without sedation, tranquilization, or a local anesthetic. The animal is usually placed in lateral recumbency, with the hind legs extended caudally. For larger or obese animals, the animal may be positioned in dorsal recumbency with the hind legs extended straight back from the body. Cystocentesis may also be performed with the animal standing. The bladder is located by palpation, and if the bladder is empty or small, then cystocentesis should be delayed until the bladder contains more urine. Alternatively, ultrasonography may be used to guide cystocentesis of small bladders or bladders that cannot be manually located (e.g., obese or tense animals). Hair may be clipped from the proposed entry site of the needle or simply spread apart by wetting with alcohol. If the hair is clipped, then the skin may be prepared using sterile technique. A 3–12-cc syringe attached to a 1.5-inch, 22-gauge needle is guided to penetrate through the paralumbar fossa, with the bladder trapped against the body wall or fixed between the thumb and forefingers when the animal is in lateral recumbency or through the ventral, caudal abdominal midline and directed toward the most bulbous part of the bladder when the animal is in dorsal recumbency. Needle penetration through either location can be used when the animal is standing. If possible, the needle is directed into the ventral or ventrolateral aspect of the bladder at a 45°–90° angle. Aspiration on the syringe should yield urine. If no urine is retrieved, the needle is withdrawn almost to the body wall and carefully redirected.

Alternatively, a random, free-catch urine sample may be collected and many small rodents, such as rats, mice, and hamsters, will often urinate spontaneously when handled allowing collection of small quantities (5–250 μL) of urine.

Urine should be stored refrigerated (approximately 4°C) after collection, but allowed to return to RT before analysis. Warming to RT allows for any crystals that may have formed under the refrigerated temperature to dissolve and enables the enzymatic assay reactions to proceed at the required temperature. Urinalysis should be performed on samples from individual animals. Pooling of routine urine samples is not generally an acceptable method, as any alteration in analytes cannot be correlated with alterations in individual animal serum parameters. Stability testing should be performed for various analytes that are assessed in urine samples in order to ensure proper storage conditions and testing limitations. Some stability data may be available on the technical insert sheet proved for each assay. However, when possible, it is optimal for each laboratory to establish stability data for all assays conducted. A general guide for stability information (as determined by one laboratory) for many of the most common urinalysis parameters is listed in Table 12.2.

Sample handling for some nonroutine analytes may require special conditions and in order to obtain reliable results, these conditions should be identified and followed. For example, urine for analysis of *N*-acetyl-β-D-glucosaminidase (NAG) in dogs should not be frozen. The recommended storage conditions for analysis of NAG from dog urine is refrigeration of urine samples at 2°C–8°C for up to 72 hours. However, urine for analysis of NAG from rat urine can be frozen at -80°C for up to 90 days, or aliquots can be refrigerated at 2°C–8°C for up to 72 hours (see Table 12.3). Urine collection for assessment of many of the more novel biomarkers should be performed under similar conditions as for the more routine analytes, for example, clean collection and refrigeration during the collection period. However, stability and storage conditions may be specific for different analytes. One consideration is that proteins are, in general, more stable than enzymes. So it is best to analyze urine samples for enzymes within 24 hours or to establish stability and then follow those criteria.

12.3.1.2 Physical Characteristics

12.3.1.2.1 Volume

Accurate measurement and documentation of urine volume are critical to the assessment of renal function. Volume is often utilized in calculating total output or may be used in normalizing the concentration or activity of many urinary constituents. Measurement of volume is also important in

TABLE 12.2
Urine Specimen Stability Reference Guides (Bristol-Myers Squibb)

Species	Storage Condition	Routine Urine Analysis (Volume, Color, Clarity, pH, Sediment Examination)	Urine Chemistry(Na, K, Cl, Ca, Mg, CREA, UTP, PHOS)	Osmolality(Serum and Urine)
Rat	Room temperature	N/A	N/A	≤5 hours
	2°C–8°C	Analytes: ≤48 hours Sediment: ≤4 hours	Perform same day	≤72 hours
	−80°C	*Note: Do not freeze*	≤90 days	≤30 days
Dog	Room temperature	N/A	N/A	≤5 hours
	2°C–8°C	Analytes ≤48 hours Sediment ≤6 hours	Perform same day	≤30 days
	−80°C	*Note: Do not freeze*	≤90 days	≤30 days
Monkey	Room temperature	N/A	N/A	Not tested
	2°C–8°C	Analytes ≤48 hours Sediment ≤ 6 hours	Perform same day	Not tested
	−80°C	*Note: Do not freeze*	≤85 days Exception: UMTP and PHOS not tested	Not tested

Time period listed for each analyte indicates stability limit at specified temperature. Ca, calcium; Cl, Chloride; CREA, creatinine; K, potassium; Mg, magnesium; Na, sodium; PHOS, phosphorus; UMTP, urine total protein; N/A, not applicable; UA, urinalysis.

TABLE 12.3
Urine Specimen Stability—Duration of Recorded Stability

Species	Storage Condition	Urine Chemistry (UUN)	Urine Chemistry (GLU)	Urine Chemistry (GGT)	Urine Chemistry (NAG)	Urine Chemistry (ALP)
Rat	Room temperature	24 hours	2 hours	6 hours	up to 6 hours	2 hours
	2°C–8°C	72 hours	6 hours	72 hours	up to 72 hours	72 hours
	−20°C	7 days	7 days	Unstable	7 days	Unstable
	−80°C	90 days	90 days	90 days	90 days	Unstable
Dog	Room temperature	24 hours	6 hours	24 hours	24 hours	24 hours
	2°C–8°C	72 hours	72 hours	72 hours	72 hours	72 hours
	−20°C	7 days	7 days	Unstable	Unstable	Unstable
	−80°C	90 days	90 days	90 days	Unstable	90 days

ALP, alkaline phosphatase; GGT, gamma glutamyl transferase; GLU, glucose; NAG, *N*-acetyl-β-D-glucosaminidase; UUN, urine urea nitrogen.

determining potential polyuria associated with polydipsia and/or lack of concentrating ability in the animal. Occasionally, urine is contaminated with drinking water and a very dilute specific gravity or osmolality will result. This abnormality can usually be confirmed by the clinical observations.

Because the reference values for urine sediment evaluation are semiquantitative, it is optimal to start with a standard volume of urine to spin down for microscopic examination. Otherwise, the numbers of cells, casts, or crystals, and so on seen per microscopic field would be diluted or concentrated resulting from variations in the volume of urine that is used for examination. In humans, 10 mL of urine is generally used as the standard volume. Because this volume is not practical for most laboratory animals, particularly rodents, the volume obtained from the "overnight" collection can be standardized to 2–3 mL for small animals (i.e., rats) and 5 mL for larger animals. Using this type of standardization, the investigator can be assured that comparisons among animals are being performed in a consistent manner.

12.3.1.2.2 Color and Clarity

Observations of color and clarity should be made on the well-mixed urine specimen. Normal mammalian urine ranges from pale yellow to amber, primarily due to the pigment urochrome (a degradation product of heme) (Finco, 1989; Free and Free, 2012), and the degree of color is reflective of urine volume and concentration. Abnormal urine color may result from the presence of blood, bilirubin, myoglobin, hemoglobin, or certain drugs and this abnormal color can obscure some urine test strip results. Normal freshly voided urine is clear, but may become cloudy due to precipitation of salts if allowed to stand or if refrigerated. Microscopic examination is necessary to determine the cause of cloudy urine

12.3.1.2.3 pH

The kidneys play a vital role in maintaining acid–base status by regulating blood bicarbonate and hydrogen ion concentrations. The pH of urine is due to many chemical constituents, primarily inorganic phosphates, sulfates, citrate, ammonium salts, bicarbonate, and carbonic acid. These result from metabolic processes that produce nonvolatile acids filtered through the glomerulus in association with cations, such as sodium. In the renal tubules, sodium is selectively reabsorbed and exchanged for hydrogen ions, which are secreted. Processes involving renal tubular excretion and reabsorption affecting pH are covered in more detail in texts of renal physiology (Rose, 2001; Ganong, 2010; Guyton and Hall, 2011; Osborne et al., 1983).

The pH of urine varies considerably with the species, with the animal's diet, and with acid–base status. For example, animals with diets composed primarily of high protein (meat-based) will have acidic urine due to the production of more sulfates and phosphates. Urine from animals whose diet is more vegetable-based will be more alkaline or neutral (Latimer et al., 2011; Chew and DiBarola, 1998). The pH should be measured on fresh urine, as the urine becomes more alkaline on standing due to the conversion of urea to ammonia by bacteria (if present), and loss of CO2 (Latimer et al., 2011). Measurement of urinary pH alone is not generally diagnostic, but should be considered in the context of other findings.

Causes of more acidic urine (lower pH) include excessive catabolic states, as with fever, starvation, ketosis, diabetic mellitus, systemic acidosis, or hypochloridemia. Administration of acidifying agents such as D-, L-methionine or ammonium chloride for the treatment of urolithiasis also will effectively lower urine pH (Osborne et al., 1972; Chew and DiBarola, 1998). Urine with high concentrations of glucose may have a lower pH due to bacterial metabolism of glucose and production of ammonia (Latimer et al., 2011). Fanconi syndrome is a disease of the proximal renal tubules of the kidney where glucose, amino acids, uric acid, phosphate, and bicarbonate are passed into the urine, instead of being reabsorbed, and can result in acid urine. This disease may be inherited or caused by drugs or heavy metals. Additionally, various forms of Fanconi syndrome can affect other functions of the proximal tubule resulting in different complications. The loss of bicarbonate results in type 2 Fanconi syndrome or proximal renal tubular acidosis. Alternatively, the loss of phosphate results in the bone disease rickets even with adequate vitamin D and calcium (Magen et al., 2010).. Causes of alkaline urine (higher pH) include bacterial infection with urease-producing bacteria, systemic alkalosis, and administration of alkalizing agents such as sodium bicarbonate (Osborne et al., 1972; Chew and DiBarola 1998). Urinary obstruction will also potentially raise urine pH due to prolonged retention of urine in the bladder and decomposition of urea to ammonia while urine exposed to room air for an extended time may be artificially more alkaline due to loss of CO2 (Latimer et al., 2011; Osborne et al., 1972; Chew and DiBarola, 1998).

Urine pH additionally impacts the formation of urinary crystals and renal calculi. Uric acid, cystine, and calcium oxalate crystals all tend to form in acidic urine. Struvite, calcium carbonate, calcium phosphate, ammonium biurate, and amorphous phosphate crystals tend to form in alkaline urine (Chew and DiBarola, 1998). Certain drug crystals also may be more likely to form at a specific pH.

For a more accurate assessment of urine pH, a pH meter may be used; however, the precision of a pH meter is not usually required for routine analysis, and the use of a urine test strip is generally satisfactory.

12.3.1.2.4 Solute Concentration

The ability of the kidneys to concentrate urine is a measure of renal function, and loss of urine concentrating ability is often the earliest sign of renal insufficiency. Urine entering the proximal tubule is at approximately the same osmolality as plasma. Water is reabsorbed at the proximal tubules by osmotic action following sodium, glucose, and other solutes, so that upon entering the loop of Henle, urine is isoosmotic. Urine osmolality then increases in the descending loop of Henle, which is permeable to water, but not solute. The reverse occurs in the ascending loop of Henle, where active transport of chloride occurs, so that urine entering the distal tubule is then hypoosmotic relative to plasma. Water is reabsorbed in the distal and collecting tubules in excess of solute under control of ADH.

Specific gravity and osmolality are often used as measures of the urine-concentrating ability of an animal. USG is dependent on particle size, number, and weight. It is the ratio of the density of urine to that of distilled water, which has a density of 1 g/mL at 4°C (Watts, 1971). Current refractometers use a scale that is corrected for refractive index, so that USG can be read directly. Using urine or centrifuged supernatant from a urine sample, USG is read on the refractometer rather than taken from the urine test strip because there is a limited range of specific gravity on urine test strips. Rodent urine frequently exceeds the upper limit of the specific gravity on urine test strips. Osmolality is dependent on particle numbers in s olution and is considered the definitive method for determining the concentration or solute-to-solvent ratios in urine. It is usually measured by freezing point depression and expressed as millimoles per kilogram of water. Both USG and osmolality can be measured using microliter volumes of urine.

12.3.1.3 Chemical Analysis

Urine test strips (also referred to as dipsticks) contain pads of various chemical reagents that provide a color change when a particular analyte is present in urine. This color change is converted to a semiquantitative result for the analyte being measured. Urine test strips are available in various configurations, but for animals, the urine test strip may be used to assess pH, protein, glucose, ketones, bilirubin (primarily the conjugated form), and proteins containing a heme group (iron). Protein quantification is most sensitive to albumin, while ketone measurement is most sensitive to acetoacetic acid. USG, nitrate, leukocytes, and urobilinogen pads are also available on urine test strips, but are either not accurate in animals (leukocytes) or do not provide much additional information in animals and are seldom, if ever, reported. Urine test strip analysis should be performed on uncentrifuged urine, unless there is marked hematuria (which may affect interpretation of the color changes on the test strip). If marked hematuria is present, it may be necessary to centrifuge the urine and perform the urine test strip analysis on the supernatant. The package insert contains useful information about test limitations and interfering substances.

12.3.1.3.1 Protein

The glomerular membrane normally prevents large molecular weight proteins from passage into the filtrate, but the size, shape, and charge of proteins also influence their ability to pass through the glomerulus. Urine test strip measurement of protein is most sensitive for albumin, although the high anion content of alkaline urine may result in false positive results using this method. Positive protein results must be evaluated in relationship to clinical observations, method of urine collection, USG, and microscopic sediment examination. Proteinuria may be due to hemorrhage, infection of the lower urinary tract, intravascular hemolysis, or renal disease (Latimer et al., 2011; Osborne et al., 1972; Chew and DiBarola, 1998), and fever and strenuous exercise may produce transient proteinuria. Microscopic examination of the sediment can help determine the source of protein. Hemorrhage is confirmed by a positive occult blood reaction on the urine test strip and the presence of RBCs in the sediment, and intravascular hemolysis will result in hemoglobinuria leading to a positive occult blood test. A urinary infection or cystitis can be confirmed by observing bacteria and white blood cells (WBCs) on sediment examination (Latimer et al., 2011; Osborne et al., 1972; Chew and DiBarola, 1998).

Proteinuria of renal disease may be due to glomerular and/or tubular lesions. While tubular disease may result in decreased reabsorption of intermediate or low molecular weight proteins such as albumin (66 kDa) or β2-microglobulin (12 kDa), respectively, and may cause increases in levels of these proteins in urine filtrate, overt glomerular disease can also result in large increases in low-, mid- and high-molecular weight proteins in the urine due to increased permeability of the glomerular membrane. If the proteinuria is due to renal disease, the sediment may or may not contain casts. Nephrotic syndrome is caused by various disorders that damage the kidneys, particularly the basement membrane of the glomerulus. This damage causes abnormal excretion of protein in the urine with resultant hypoproteinemia, hypercholesterolemia, hypertriglyceridemia, and generalized edema. Enhanced hepatic synthesis of lipoproteins containing apolipoprotein B and cholesterol is thought to account for most of the increase in cholesterol levels (Appel, 1991; Joven et al., 1990). Protein results must be analyzed with respect to the USG, as "trace" proteinuria (as determined on urine test strips) may represent significant protein loss with low specific gravity but may not be significant when associated with high specific gravity.

Proteinuria is common and considered normal in male rats and mice, due to major urinary proteins such as α2-microglobulins (small monomeric proteins with a molecular weight of approximately 18,000) that are filtered through the glomerulus (Cavaggioni and Mucignat-Caretta, 2000; Finlayson et al., 1965; Lane and Neuhaus, 1972; Saito et al., 1996; Swenberg, 1993). Proteinuria in rats increases with age and is related to the spontaneous conditions of chronic progressive nephropathy and hyaline droplet formation in the proximal tubules (Hard and Khan, 2004; Casadevall et al., 2005; Corman et al., 1985; Corman and Michel, 1987).

12.3.1.3.2 Glucose

Glucose is freely filtered by the glomerulus but is almost completely reabsorbed by active transport in the proximal renal tubules. Therefore, glucose is usually not detectable in the urine of healthy animals. However, transient glucosuria can be associated with stress. Glucosuria is most often a function of hyperglycemia where urine glucose values exceed the capacity of tubular transport and can be due to diabetes mellitus, diabetogenic drugs, or inborn errors of carbohydrate metabolism. Glucosuria may also be the result of renal tubular damage, with loss of reabsorptive capacity in the proximal tubules. Urine test strips measure glucose levels semiquantitatively using the glucose oxidase method, which can be affected by large amounts of ascorbic acid in the urine of some species, specifically dog and mouse. For precise measurement, which is sometimes necessary in toxicology studies, urine glucose can be measured using the enzymatic reactions on chemistry analyzers.

12.3.1.4 Sediment Examination

Microscopic analysis of the urine sediment for formed elements in the urine including cells, crystals, and bacteria is considered part of the routine urinalysis and can potentially yield additional

TABLE 12.4
Formed Elements of Urinary Sediment

Cells	• WBCs
	• RBCs
	• Epithelial
	  • Squamous
	  • Transitional
	  • Renal tubular
	• Neoplastic	

Casts	• Hyaline • Granular • RBC • WBC • Epithelial	• Waxy • Fatty • Mixed • Broad • Pseudocasts

Crystals	• Triple phosphate
	• Uric acid
	• Calcium oxalate
	  • Monohydrate
	  • Dihydrate
	• Calcium carbonate
	• Amorphous phosphates
		• Amorphous urates
		• Bilirubin
		• Ammonium biurate
		• Tyrosine
		• Cystine
		• Cholesterol
		• Drugs

Infectious agents	• Bacteria • Yeast • Parasites and ova	
Miscellaneous	• Lipids • Chyle • Mucus threads • Fibrin threads • Spermatozoa	
External contaminants	• Pollens • Hair • Starch granules • Fibers from clothing	

information that may help explain changes in other parameters (Schumann, 1980) (see Table 12.4). However, proper analysis and interpretation of sediment findings may require specialized training and is not always performed for routine urinalysis. For this examination, the standard volume of urine is centrifuged at a low speed, the supernatant is decanted, and the urine is gently resuspended, placed on a slide, and examined under a microscope at low and high dry objectives. Depending on preference, the slide may or may not be stained with methylene blue or a variety of commercial stains for urinary sediment.

A minimum of 10 microscopic fields are viewed at low (10×) and high (40×) magnification and the number of formed elements are quantified and reported as the average number per field. Casts and sperm are reported as the average number per low-power field and other elements are reported as average number per high-power field (Tables 12.5 and 12.6).

12.3.1.4.1 Cells

Blood cells may be observed in urinary sediment and can be of diagnostic importance. The number of erythrocytes or leukocytes in "normal" urine is generally considered to be less than five cells per high-power field (Schumann and Colon, 1980). An increased number of blood cells in the urine

TABLE 12.5
Formed Elements Graded at Low Magnification (10×)

Formed Elements	Observation/Grade	Additional Instructions
Casts	None = "-" (NF) 1+ = 1–2/lpf (MIN) 2+ = 3–10/lpf (MILD) 3+ = 11–50/lpf (MOD) 4+ = >50/lpf (MKD)	Identify types of casts in comment section
Sperm	None = "-" (NF) 1+ = 1–2/lpf (MIN) 2+ = 3–10/lpf (MILD) 3+ = 6–20/lpf (MOD) 4+ = >20/lpf (MKD)	
Mucus Strands Flagellates Ova	1+ = 1–2/lpf (MIN) 2+ = 3–10/lpf (MILD) 3+ = 6–20/lpf (MOD) 4+ = >20/lpf (MKD)	Grade and describe in comments section if observed

lpf, low-power field; MN, minimal; MOD, moderate; MKD, marked.

TABLE 12.6
Formed Elements Graded at High Magnification (40×)

Formed Element	Observation/Grade	Additional Instructions
Leukocytes (WBC) Erythrocytes (RBC) Epithelial Cells	None = "-" (NF) 1+ = 1–5/hpf (MIN) 2+ = 6–15/hpf (MILD) 3+ = 16–50/hpf (MOD) 4+ = >50/hpf (MKD)	Grade WBC clumps (if seen) in comments section as MIN, MILD, MOD, or MKD.
Renal or Transitional Epithelial Cells	1+ = 1–2/hpf (MIN) 2+ = 3–10/hpf (MILD) 3+ = 11–50/hpf (MOD) 4+ = >50/hpf (MKD)	Grade and describe in comments section if observed.
Crystals and Bacteria (grade using % of field as the guide)	None = "-" (NF) 1+ = 1%–10%/hpf (MIN) 2+ = 11=25%/hpf (MILD) 3+ = 26%–50%/hpf (MOD) 4+ = >50%/hpf (MKD)	Grade and describe types of other (OTH) crystals in comments section if observed.
Yeast	1+ = 1–2/hpf (MIN) 2+ = 3–10/hpf (MILD) 3+ = 11–20/hpf (MOD) 4+ = >20/hpf (MKD)	Grade and describe in comments section if observed.

hpf, high-power field; lpf, low-power field; MN, minimal; MOD, moderate; MKD, marked; NF, none found; RBC, red blood cell; WBC, white blood cell.

is indicative of renal and/or lower urinary tract disease and, when combined with other urinalysis parameters, may help localize the area of disease.

Hemorrhage from the urinary bladder or urethra is the most common source of hematuria in most preclinical species, and is often related to cystitis/urethritis or urolithiasis. In primates, hematuria may also be due to menses. Although the mechanism whereby intact erythrocytes enter the urinary system from the kidney is not clear (Schumann and Colon, 1980), blood may occur in urine without increased permeability of glomerular membranes or without evidence of renal hemorrhage. Increased erythrocytes in urine of renal origin may occur with acute or chronic inflammatory disease, neoplasms, or renal calculi. Increased leukocytes in the urine may result from the same mechanism as increased erythrocytes. Of these, pyelonephritis is a common renal cause while bacterial cystitis or urolithiasis are predisposing factors for the presence of leukocytes in the lower urinary tract.

Epithelial cells from any segment of the urinary tract may be observed in urinary sediment. Large, flattened squamous epithelial cells with a high cytoplasm-to-nucleus ratio may exfoliate from the urethra, vulva, or vagina while transitional epithelial cells line the urinary tract distal to the renal pelvis. Identification of renal tubular epithelial (RTE) cells in the urinary sediment should be distinguished from epithelial cells of the lower urinary tract (transitional or squamous), because the presence of RTE cells may reflect injury or disease in the renal tubules.

Various benign or malignant cells may be observed in the urinary sediment and the same cytologic features used in differentiating benign from malignant cells in other exfoliative cytologic specimens are used in evaluating cells in the urine. Most carcinomas of the lower urinary tract epithelium are transitional cell carcinomas and these cells may be detected in urinary sediment with appropriate staining (Koss, 1968; Schumann and Colon, 1980). Although most tumor cells found in urine arise from the urinary tract, metastatic malignant cells may also be observed and metastatic tumors of the urinary tract infrequently exfoliate into the urine (Schumann and Colon, 1980). These tumors may also be associated with increased erythrocytes and/or WBCs in the sediment.

12.3.1.4.2 Casts

Accurate identification of casts can be important in the diagnosis and prognosis of renal disease. Fresh urine should be examined for the presence of casts because they may disintegrate after a few hours, particularly in alkaline urine. Casts are more readily detected with phase-contrast microscopy than with bright-field microscopy, but phase-contrast is not routinely employed for urine analysis. Renal casts are shaped by the tubules of the nephrons and are formed when proteins (mucoprotein and glycocalyx) gel in the renal tubules. A primary component of the matrix of renal casts is Tamm-Horsfall glycoprotein (Serafini-Cessi et al., 2003). This protein is present in the urine of several species and, though normally in solution, may precipitate and gel under conditions of altered urine flow, pH, and/or electrolyte concentrations within the kidney. Various cellular constituents may be incorporated when the protein gel forms. In kidney disease, blood protein may be present in the glomerular filtrate and may be incorporated into the mucoprotein and glycocalyx matrix. Renal casts vary considerably in size and composition and may be of significance in detecting active renal parenchymal disease. It is important to distinguish among the various types of casts, particularly those containing cells, as cellular casts are early indicators of tubular toxicity. Hyaline casts are basically protein casts that may form in cases of decreased urine flow, low pH, high solute concentration, or high protein concentration. Granular casts may be either fine or coarse, and although the source of the granules has not been well established, they are probably aggregated plasma proteins or the remnants of disintegrated cells. Although the "normal" number of casts is not well established, a few hyaline or granular casts per low-power field is not considered pathologic. More than a few granular casts per low-power field is probably indicative of renal parenchymal disease and would not be considered physiologic. Casts are relatively frequent findings in aged rodents and are related to the chronic progressive nephropathies.

RBC casts either indicate glomerular damage sufficient to permit erythrocytes to enter the renal tubules or bleeding from the renal parenchyma due to damage to the tubular basement membrane. With either type of injury, fibrinogen and other proteins also escape into the tubules and trap the erythrocytes in a fibrin matrix to form the cast. These casts may be made of degenerated red cells and hemosiderin, resulting in an orange-colored granular cast in unstained wet mounts. In addition to acute glomerulonephritis, red cell casts may be present in acute tubular necrosis, chronic nephritis, renal infarction, or renal hemorrhage of traumatic origin.

Leukocyte casts are indicative of bacterial infections of the kidney, such as pyelonephritis. Neutrophils probably gain access to the renal tubules by their own motility between and through renal epithelial cells rather than through the glomerulus. Leukocyte casts may occur in glomerular disease but generally are associated with tubulointerstitial disease.

Fatty casts are those in which lipid material is encased in a hyaline matrix. Such casts are associated primarily with acute renal diseases and tubular degeneration.

Casts of RTE cells may form any time there is damage to the epithelium with subsequent exfoliation of a large number of cells. Thus, tubular epithelial casts may be observed in acute tubular necrosis, interstitial nephritis, renal amyloidosis, and renal allograft rejection.

Waxy casts represent the ultimate stage in cellular degeneration. They are believed to be the end stage of granular casts that have been retained for a time in the tubules due to localized nephron obstruction (Schumann and Colon, 1980). They are associated with tubular degeneration and are most commonly observed in chronic nephritis.

Casts that contain a combination of various cells and other material are described as mixed casts.

Bacteria or crystals may become trapped within the protein matrix of a hyaline cast. If such inclusions are numerous, the cast is described as a bacterial or crystal inclusion cast.

Pseudocasts composed of fibrin or mucous threads and aggregates of crystals or cells may be confused with casts. True casts are the result of extrusion or formation within a tube, and as such, have the characteristic shape of defined parallel sides, whereas pseudocasts do not have these characteristics. However, mucous threads and squamous epithelial cells that have a cylindrical shape may occasionally be misinterpreted as casts.

12.3.1.4.3 Crystals

Various types of crystals may appear in the urinary sediment. Most are formed from normal constituents of urine and are of no specific diagnostic significance. Others are considered "pathologic" crystals and originate from exogenous compounds, defective metabolism, or abnormal excretion and their presence may reflect the composition of coexistent uroliths.

Crystals that form in normal urine are usually the result of an excessively high concentration of a relatively insoluble substance (e.g., calcium oxalate, uric acid, triple phosphate, calcium phosphate, amorphous phosphates or urates, or certain drugs and their metabolites) that precipitate out in urine. The type of crystals formed in such cases correlates with the urine pH (Bradley and Benson, 1974) or may occur with refrigeration and then dissolve upon warming to RT.

Abnormal or pathologic crystals may be of diagnostic significance and should always be reported. Cystine urinary crystals may be due to a defect in renal tubular reabsorption, even though plasma cystine levels are normal. Genetic defects in amino acid metabolism or severe liver disease interfering with normal amino acid metabolism may result in amino acidemia, with urinary precipitation of cystine, tyrosine, or leucine. Crystals of cholesterol can form in the tubules and may be indicative of renal disease. Multiple drug therapies also have been associated with crystal formation (Fogazzi, 1996). Sulfonamide crystals have historically been observed in urinary sediment after therapy, but the incidence is now lower due to the introduction of more soluble sulfonamides. Ampicillin may occasionally precipitate in urine following large parenteral doses, and crystals of investigative pharmaceutical compounds that are excreted or metabolized in the kidney may be observed in laboratory animals on studies. Use of the x-ray contrast media, meglumine diatriazoate, may also result in compound-related crystals appearing in the urine.

12.3.1.4.4 Infectious Agents

Normal urine is sterile and devoid of microorganisms. However, some bacteria are present in most urine specimens, unless appropriate and exacting techniques, such as catheterization, are employed to exclude contaminants present in the lower genitourinary tract. Even then, positive cultures may be obtained unless the specimen was cultured immediately or refrigerated. The presence of a large number of bacteria in the sediment of a fresh urine sample when leukocytes are also present should raise the suspicion of a urinary tract infection. The observance of bacteria in an uncentrifuged, fresh urine specimen is presumptive evidence of a urinary tract infection and usually indicates greater than 100,000 organisms/mL (Schumann and Colon, 1980). In such cases, Gram stains and urine cultures are indicated.

Fungi may occasionally be observed in urinary sediment and may be either saprophytes or pathogens. *Candida* species are the most commonly observed yeast form in human urine specimens. Yeast infection may occur in animals with genetic or acquired immunodeficiency or immunosuppressive chemotherapy. Diabetes also predisposes to yeast infections of the urinary tract.

Only a few parasites or ova are specific to the urinary tract of laboratory animals. However, unless care is taken in obtaining the urine sample, it may contain ova and/or parasites from the gastrointestinal (GI) tract, and some ova (e.g., *Capillaria* and *Trichuris vulpis* ova) may be confused with those of urinary tract parasites.

Diocotophyma renale is a kidney parasite that may live in the renal pelvis of the dog and mink. *Stephanurus dentatus* is a kidney worm found in swine and is relatively common in some parts of the United States. *Capillaria* species are nematode parasites found in the urinary bladder and sometimes in the renal pelvis of dogs, cats, and rats. *Capillaria* species are relatively nonpathogenic and rarely, if ever, found in purpose-bred laboratory animals (Flynn, 1973). *Trichosomoides crassicauda* may be present in the urinary bladder wall, ureters, and renal pelvis of rats, but is usually of low pathogenicity (Flynn, 1973; Owen, 1992). *Klossiella* sp. may also be present in guinea pigs and mice (Seibold and Thorson, 1955). Diagnosis of urinary tract parasitism is made by identification of the characteristic ova in the urine sediment.

12.3.1.4.5 Miscellaneous

Lipid or fat droplets may be observed in urine specimens. They are round, highly refractile bodies that must be distinguished from erythrocytes. Under polarized microscopy, they may exhibit anisotropism. Care must be taken in collecting urine specimens to be certain that contaminating fatty substances are not introduced from lubricating agents or unclean glassware. Lipid of urinary tract origin may indicate degenerative tubular disease, pyelonephritis, acute glomerulonephritis, renal carcinoma, or acute nephritis. Lipiduria may also occur in diabetes mellitus.

Chyluria may rarely occur with obstructions of the lymphatic system (Schumann and Colon, 1980). Elevated urine protein levels and lymphocytes in the sediment and a milky appearance of the urine specimen may be important clues in diagnosing chyluria.

Mucus or fibrin threads are commonly observed in urine. Mucus threads, which are composed of precipitated mucoproteins, may form in most urine as it cools. Fibrin threads are the result of glomerular leakage or hemorrhage into the urinary tract.

Fibers from extraurinary sources may contaminate urine specimens and must be differentiated from casts and mucus or fibrin threads. These contaminants may be cotton, wool, synthetic fibers, or hair. Starch granules from surgical gloves may also contaminate urine specimens. Starch crystals may appear round or oval and highly refractive and corn starch is almost always hexagonal with an irregular indentation in the center.

Spermatozoa are common in the urine of males and may be observed in females following mating. Tailless spermatozoa may be confused with bacteria, yeast, or cell nuclei.

12.3.2 Serum Markers of Renal Injury

12.3.2.1 Creatinine and BUN

Creatinine and BUN are the classic serum markers of renal function. Serum markers generally report changes in glomerular filtration rate (GFR) and reflect functional nephron mass. As the kidney has a large functional reserve, such serum biomarkers only change when there is greater than two-thirds renal compromise. Characteristically, these serum markers are small enough to be freely filtered (nonprotein bound) by the glomerulus, released to the plasma at a constant rate, generally neither secreted nor reabsorbed from the tubule, and minimally influenced by extrarenal disease/physiology. However, the influence by extrarenal changes, such as a change in muscle mass, increased dietary protein, dehydration, or GI hemorrhage, (GFR depends primarily on renal blood flow) does produce some limitations to their use and can result in a wide baseline variation. In addition, plasma levels also are influenced by tubular secretion or reabsorption. Most of the assays for these parameters are also vulnerable to interference, as many are colorimetric and drugs or endogenous substances can interfere with assay performance.

BUN, a product of ammonia metabolism (excretion), is primarily produced by the liver, and >90% is excreted via glomerular filtration. BUN generally underestimates GFR due to reabsorption or equilibration between the intra- and extravascular space as it readily crosses cell membranes/tubules, and significant (up to 70%) tubular reabsorption is possible. Greater reabsorption occurs at low flow rates/decreased renal perfusion (i.e., when function is compromised). Reabsorption from postrenal sources (e.g., peritoneum, urinary bladder) can also be a source for plasma BUN in cases of bladder rupture. Synthesis and plasma release of BUN are not constant and plasma levels also reflect protein intake, liver function, and protein catabolic states including muscle wasting, GI hemorrhage, and corticosteroid administration.

Muscle is the primary source for plasma creatinine, which is nonenzymatically formed from phosphorylcreatine at a rate of approximately 1.6%–2.0%/day (Wyss and Kaddurah-Daouk, 2000). Feedback control of synthesis provides reasonably consistent baseline plasma levels, so that plasma creatinine is less reflective of protein catabolic states than is BUN. Baseline plasma levels of BUN or creatinine, as well as clearance of either endogenous or exogenous creatinine can be used to estimate GFR. However, creatinine concentrations can overestimate GFR, as there is significant tubular secretion in many species (mice, rats, dogs) and frequently in males with larger muscle mass, particularly at low tubular flow rates (i.e., low GFR) (Eisner et al., 2010; O'Connell et al., 1962). It should also be noted that creatinine secretion can be inhibited by some drugs (i.e., cimetidine, trimethoprim, salicylates) resulting in nonrenal increases in plasma levels. In addition, drugs and endogenous substances may also interfere with colorimetric assay methods.

Azotemia occurs when BUN and/or creatinine increase above reference plasma levels. Azotemia can be classified as prerenal, renal, or postrenal. Prerenal azotemia results from dehydration or decreased renal blood flow (e.g., decreased GFR), but the concentrating ability of the kidney is intact. Renal azotemia results in inadequate concentration of the urine secondary to dysfunction of the kidney. Postrenal azotemia occurs from a blockage of urine flow in an area below the kidneys. The urea nitrogen:creatinine ratio is sometimes used to assist in determining which type of azotemia is occurring. If the baseline for both analytes is elevated, renal azotemia is most likely. If the ratio is extremely high, it is more likely of prerenal or postrenal origin. A high ratio due to increased BUN alone is more indicative of GI hemorrhage, a high-protein diet, or tissue catabolism. A low ratio could suggest that an underlying liver disease, low-protein diet, or tissue anabolic states may coexist.

12.3.2.2 Electrolytes

The concentration of serum electrolytes (such as sodium, calcium, potassium, chloride, magnesium, and bicarbonate) can be affected by nutrition, renal disease, and renal response to acid–base status. Tests that measure the concentration of electrolytes are very helpful for the diagnosis and management of renal or endocrine disease, acid–base disturbances, water balance, and many other conditions.

Sodium levels are directly related to the osmotic pressure of the plasma. Because an anion is always associated with sodium (usually chloride or bicarbonate), the plasma osmolality (total dissolved solute concentration) can be estimated. Since water will often follow sodium by diffusion, loss of sodium leads to dehydration and retention of sodium leads to edema. However, conditions that promote hypernatremia do not promote an equivalent gain in water. These conditions include diabetes insipidus (impaired renal water reabsorption), Cushing's disease, and hyperaldosteronism (increased sodium reabsorption) (Wu, 2006). Many other conditions, such as congestive heart failure, cirrhosis of the liver, and renal disease result in renal retention of sodium, but an equivalent amount of water is retained as well. This results in total body sodium excess, which causes hypertension and edema, but not an increased serum sodium concentration. Hyponatremia may result from Addison's disease, excessive diuretic therapy, the syndrome of inappropriate secretion of antidiuretic hormone (SIADH), burns, diarrhea, or vomiting.

Potassium is an important electrolyte associated with renal failure. Like sodium, potassium is freely filtered by the kidney. However, in the distal tubule sodium is reabsorbed and potassium is secreted. In renal failure, the combination of decreased filtration and decreased secretion combine to cause increased plasma potassium. Hyperkalemia is the most significant and life-threatening complication of renal failure, but hyperkalemia can also be caused by hemolytic anemia (release from hemolyzed RBCs), diabetes insipidus, Addison's disease, and digitalis toxicity. Frequent causes of low serum potassium include alkalosis, diarrhea and vomiting, excessive use of thiazide diuretics, Cushing's disease, insufficient dietary intake, intravenous fluid administration, and SIADH (Wu, 2006).

Renal tubular acidosis involves the failure to secrete acid into the urine. The resultant systemic acidosis produces weakness, headache, nausea, and cardiac arrest. Acidemia, as measured by serum bicarbonate and/or blood pH, is also common in individuals with chronic renal failure. Conversely, alkalosis or a decrease in the acid content of the blood can result from low plasma chloride, for example from loss of hydrochloric acid by vomiting. If severe, alkalosis can cause paralysis (tetany) (Edmondson et al., 1975).

Hyperphosphatemia can result from the failure of the kidneys to excrete phosphate into the urine (decreased GFR), causing phosphate to accumulate in the bloodstream. Hyperphosphatemia can also be caused by the impaired action of parathyroid hormone and by phosphate poisoning (associated with sodium phosphate enemas). Severe hyperphosphatemia can cause paralysis, convulsions, and cardiac arrest. These symptoms result because the phosphate, occurring in elevated levels, complexes with free serum calcium, resulting in hypocalcemia.

12.3.3 Urine Markers of Renal Injury

Nephrotoxicity is difficult to monitor noninvasively. As discussed earlier in this chapter, the most widely used parameters to detect and monitor kidney injury include plasma/serum markers such as BUN and serum creatinine (sCr), and urinary markers, such as urinary volume, specific gravity or osmolality, glucose or protein excretion, and sediment examination. Although many of these measurements provide valid indicators of some aspect of kidney function, they lack sensitivity and/or specificity in detecting early stages of injury or disease and in some cases may be influenced by prerenal changes that may confound interpretation.

Over many decades, the potential of a wide variety of urinary proteins to detect and monitor renal injury has been assessed in numerous animal studies. But it is only in recent years that extensive effort involving collaboration among industrial, academic, and regulatory scientists has been applied to the systematic evaluation of the diagnostic utility of these urinary biomarkers. The determination to characterize more reliable renal biomarkers has been given additional impetus by the discovery of a number of potential novel biomarkers through the use of transcriptomic, proteomic, and metabolomic technologies (Amin et al., 2004; Boudonck et al., 2009; Davis et al., 2004; Devarajan et al., 2003; Kharasch et al., 2006; Mendrick, 2008; Thongboonkerd, 2005; Thukral et al., 2005). This has enhanced the prospect of making available a range of sensitive and specific biomarkers which will have real diagnostic utility. These collaborative efforts (Dieterle et al., 2010a; Vaidya et al., 2010; Yu et al., 2010; Harpur et al., 2011) have resulted in the biological qualification of several urinary biomarkers for potential detection of nephrotoxic injury to either the renal tubules or the glomeruli in preclinical safety studies. Some of these biomarkers have been available for years while others are comparatively new. Eight of these biomarkers (albumin, β2-microglobulin, total protein, cystatin C, Kidney Injury Molecule-1 [KIM-1], clusterin, trefoil factor 3 (TFF3), and renal papillary antigen-1 [RPA-1]) were judged by regulatory authorities to be acceptable in specified contexts of nonclinical development for detection of acute drug-induced renal toxicity and to provide additional and complementary information to the currently available standard parameters (EMA, 2009, 2010; FDA, 2008, 2010). There are, however, many gaps in our knowledge to be addressed; thus, more data are required to underpin the current conclusions, to expand the context of use (e.g., to other species including dogs and nonhuman primates), and where necessary to provide additional biomarkers to cover all parts of the nephron. Additionally, an increased understanding of the physiological and pathophysiological roles of the biomarkers as well as their behavior during onset and recovery of injury would enhance their utility.

The following is a summary of those urinary biomarkers regarded by regulators to have the potential for detection of renal injury in animals, as well as more novel biomarkers that have been recently evaluated. Urinary endpoints that have been used over many years to detect and assess renal injury are mostly protein in nature and include measurement of total protein, albumin, and numerous low molecular weight proteins.

The biological role of some proteins found in urine is known to be enzymatic in nature and, therefore, this property has been utilized to determine quantitatively their presence in urine (they can be rapidly and easily measured using standard colorimetric or fluorometric techniques). Hence the term "enzymuria" has been in widespread use for many years. However, other than this historical reason related to their biological properties and the mode of their measurement, there is no logical reason to distinguish them from other proteins in urine. Furthermore, for many of the enzymes of interest, for example, the glutathione S-transferases (GSTs), the enzymatic assays have been replaced by more specific immunological assays which, among other things, allow isoenzymes to be discriminated (e.g., α-GST from μ-GST). Therefore, the term urinary protein biomarker is more appropriate. However, because of the historical importance of "enzymuria" to monitor renal injury as well as the fact that some enzymatic proteins remain useful and enzymatic assays are still used (e.g., NAG), the following discussion includes reference to enzymes as a class of urinary biomarker. However, in order to fully interpret an elevated level of protein in urine, in addition to knowing the biological role of the biomarker, it can be equally important to know the physiology around the biomarker. For example, what is the origin of the biomarker—(extrarenal and/or intrarenal)? If the latter, where is it localized in the nephron or within individual cells? What is the mechanism by which its presence in urine is increased? Does it have a high constitutive presence and leak from injured cells (providing information on acute injury, such as α-GST) or is it induced in response to injury and useful to track onset and recovery from injury (e.g., clusterin)?

Although over 40 enzymes have been identified in urine (Raab, 1972) and have periodically been shown to be sensitive and useful for determining the anatomical location of tubular injury (Stonard, 1990), few have seen widespread acceptance or use as renal biomarkers (Price, 1992a). This is likely related to the fact that these biomarkers do not have diagnostic relevance (Stonard, 1990) that may be attributable to inter- and intrasubject variability resulting from both biological variability (age, sex, time of day, and urine flow rate are contributory factors) and analytical variability (Jung, 1994; Stonard, 1990). With regard to the latter, the majority of enzymes exhibit some degree of instability in urine presenting problems with storage. Another source of variability is the presence of endogenous low molecular weight inhibitors which must be removed by dilution, dialysis, or ultrafiltration. Assay interference can also result from the presence of exogenous substances such as the test (pharmaceutical) compounds (or their metabolites) that have induced the renal injury in toxicity studies. The enzymes are known to have different primary locations along the nephron and within individual cells and those that have attracted most attention are localized in the proximal tubule, the region that is particularly vulnerable to drug toxicity (Bonventre et al., 2010).

The circadian pattern of excretion of some urinary proteins is known to differ but in many cases it is an unknown (Jung, 1994). Thus, it is generally recommended to determine the excretion of urinary analytes as amount/unit time. This requires timed urine collection for the same period each day.

Where accurate and complete timed urine samples cannot be collected (e.g., in an outpatient clinic or in animals where ensuring complete bladder emptying at the beginning and end of the collection period is difficult), the quantity of the analyte of interest can be normalized to the amount of creatinine in urine (dividing the concentration of the analyte by the concentration of creatinine in the same urine sample). In human urine, an excellent correlation between the protein content of a 24-hour urine and the protein/creatinine ratio in a single urine sample has been demonstrated (Ginsberg et al., 1983), and it has become standard clinical practice to normalize urinary excretion of many protein biomarkers to urine creatinine in chronic conditions (Goldstein, 2010). In addition, normalization of urine analytes to creatinine has been shown to correct for incomplete timed urine sample collections in rodents (Haas et al., 1997). In dogs, it has been shown that normalization of urinary enzyme activity per unit of creatinine is reasonably well correlated to 24-hour enzyme activity (Grauer et al., 1995). Normalization to creatinine has the additional advantage of adjusting, at least in part, for alterations in urine flow rate and volume (Jung, 1994). Although urine creatinine is sometimes the preferred approach for normalization of a parameter and is frequently a more convenient factor to obtain than total volume, urine creatinine should not be used when there is significant compromise of renal function, as this will not provide an accurate normalization.

Based on review of the literature, regulatory agencies have agreed that normalization of urinary analytes to creatinine is appropriate in biomarker qualification studies (Dieterle et al., 2010b; Harpur et al., 2011). One case where it is not recommended is when the response to injury results in decrease of a urine biomarker as is the case with TFF3. Yu et al. (2010) stated that dividing a low TFF3 level by a low creatinine level diminishes or masks the information inherent in each biomarker; thus, the signal of TFF3 is "somewhat compromised" if TFF3 is normalized to urinary creatinine. While normalization to urinary creatinine is the most commonly used procedure, it is important to realize that creatinine excretion may be impacted by various factors including age, sex, muscle mass, and diet. As such, control animals on toxicity studies should be matched for these characteristics. In toxicologic studies of renal injury, it should be ensured that creatinine excretion has not been altered by the pharmaceutical agent being investigated (Harpur et al., 2011). Recently, Waikar et al. (2010) cautioned against the normalization of urinary biomarkers to urine creatinine in patients with acute kidney injury where creatinine clearance may be unstable giving rise to misleading results. The authors asserted that actual excretion rate of a biomarker over a timed collection period is the most accurate method of quantification, provided the biomarker was stable over the collection period.

12.3.3.1 *N*-acetyl-β-D-Glucosaminidase

N-acetyl-β-D-glucosaminidase (NAG) is predominantly found in the lysosomes of proximal tubular cells but is also found at lower levels elsewhere in the nephron (Bourbouze et al., 1984). NAG is a widely studied biomarker of proximal tubular injury in both animals and humans (Gibey et al., 1981; Marchewka and Dlugosz, 1998; Price, 1992a, b; Stonard et al., 1987; Westhuyzen et al., 2003). Although NAG is present in plasma, this enzyme is too large (140 kDa) to be filtered at the glomerulus unless there is glomerular damage and the presence of low levels of NAG in normal urine samples results from the pinocytotic and exocytotic activity of the tubular epithelial cells. NAG exists in several isoforms. The A form of NAG is found in solution in the lysosome and may be released during the normal process of exocytosis such that the A form of NAG is the predominant form in normal urine. Thus, an increase in urinary NAG can result from a chemically induced alteration in tubular lysosomal function without renal injury (Bosomworth et al., 1999). The B form of NAG is found on the membrane of the lysosome and may only be released when there is injury to the lysosome and/or cellular necrosis (Sanchez-Bernal et al., 1991). However, increased urinary NAG need not necessarily result from a direct toxic effect on renal tubular cells but may also result from protein overload, provoking increased lysosomal turnover, as seen following chemical induction of glomerulonephrosis and proteinuria (Bosomworth et al., 1999). The measurement of NAG isoenzymes may provide additional diagnostic information, particularly concerning the exact site of injury (Price, 1992a, b). However, it is rarely applied in practice mainly because of the complex analytical methods required for measurement of the isoenzymes and the absence of widely available immunological assays for each isoenzyme. In addition, measurement of NAG isoenzymes does not provide any definitive information on site of injury since (1) no isoenzyme is uniquely located in one tubular segment and (2) the pattern of NAG isoenzymes found in an elevated level of total NAG may reflect the chemical mechanism of renal cell perturbation as much as the site of injury. For example, early increases in the B form of NAG following administration of gentamicin may be attributable to the well-known lysosomotrophic effect of the compound with induction of synthesis of the B form of NAG (Gibey et al., 1984).

Cumulative evidence points to urinary total NAG being a robust and sensitive indicator of acute kidney injury in the clinical setting (Ferguson et al., 2008). It is one of several biomarkers able to both diagnose and predict outcome in patients with acute kidney injury (Coca et al., 2008; Liangos et al., 2007; Parikh et al., 2010). However, urinary NAG activity may be inhibited by endogenous substances (such as urea) and exogenous substances (e.g., industrial solvents and heavy metals) and increased NAG levels may be seen in a variety of conditions unrelated to acute kidney injury such as rheumatoid arthritis, impaired glucose tolerance, and hyperthyroidism (for review, see Ferguson et al., 2008). As a result, insensitivity and nonspecificity may limit the use of NAG as a biomarker of nephrotoxicant-induced renal injury in animal species. Furthermore, in recently reported rodent studies (Harpur et al., 2011), although urinary NAG was increased in the presence of both proximal tubule and CD injury, its diagnostic accuracy was no better than BUN or sCr.

12.3.3.2 Brush Border Membrane Enzymes

There are a number of enzymes located on the brush border membrane (BBM) of the proximal tubular cells including alanine aminopeptidase (AAP), alkaline phosphatase (ALP), and gamma glutamyl transferase (GGT). Occasionally, these have been shown to be sensitive markers of proximal tubular injury in animal studies (for review, see Stonard, 1990), although Gibey et al. (1981) found that AAP (in contrast to NAG) had no prognostic value for development of renal failure in patients treated with gentamicin. Furthermore, neither AAP nor GGT showed increased levels in urine, unlike NAG or β2-microglobulin, in patients treated with the nephrotoxic chemotherapeutic drug cisplatin (Marchewka and Dlugosz, 1998). However, GGT has been advocated as having diagnostic value for renal tubular injury in certain clinical situations, for example, in contrast nephropathy (Donadio et al., 1998) and was found to be an excellent biomarker in clinical acute tubular necrosis (Westhuyzen et al., 2003). Nevertheless, until recently there has been no rigorous analysis of the diagnostic performance of any of the BBM enzymes for detection of nephrotoxic injury in animals using kidney histopathology as the reference standard. Harpur et al. (2011) included GGT in their biological qualification study of renal biomarkers of tubular injury in rats and found no evidence for any diagnostic value of GGT.

12.3.3.3 Glutathione S-Transferases

Until recently, GSTs have rivaled NAG as the most widely used urinary enzymes to monitor renal injury. GSTs are phase II detoxifying enzymes present in the kidney in various isoforms, the distribution and expression of which varies along the nephron and among species (Beckett and Hayes, 1993; Campbell et al., 1991; Harrison et al., 1989; Rozell et al., 1993; Sundberg et al., 1993). In both rats and humans, α-GST is the predominant isoform in the proximal tubule, whereas μ-GST (GSTYb1) and π-GST are the predominant isoforms in the distal tubule of rats and human, respectively. The increased presence of GSTs in the urine after nephrotoxic injury to rats has been known for more than 30 years (Bass et al., 1979) and is attributed to leakage from tubular cells into the lumen, secondary to epithelial cell damage. In studies on the effects of volatile anesthetics on the kidney, Kharasch et al. (1998) reported that urinary excretion of α-GST correlated with the extent of proximal tubular cell necrosis in rats and measurement of the GST isoforms in urine was more sensitive than either BUN or sCr for detection of tubular injury following administration of anesthetics in a study in human volunteers (Eger et al., 1997). Urinary excretion of specific isoforms of GST has been proposed not only as a marker of renal tubular damage in general but also to provide information on the location of the injury along the nephron (Branten et al., 2000; Eger et al., 1997; Sundberg et al., 1994a, b).

Despite their extensive use, only recently has the utility of urinary GSTs as biomarkers of renal tubular injury in rodents been systematically evaluated (Harpur et al., 2011). Harpur et al. (2011) demonstrated that urinary α-GST had superior diagnostic accuracy to BUN, sCr, and NAG for diagnosis of injury to the proximal tubule in the rat and was most evident with early damage (before regeneration was present). This is consistent with the conclusion of Ozer et al. (2010), who found α-GST to be an excellent biomarker for early tubular necrosis. The potential value of α-GST as a biomarker of proximal tubular injury in preclinical toxicology studies is strengthened by the available clinical data suggesting this may be a translatable biomarker across species. Urinary GSTs are reported to be diagnostic and prognostic markers of acute kidney injury in various clinical situations (Coca et al., 2008; Han and Bonventre, 2004; Westhuyzen et al., 2003).

However, confidence in the utility of α-GST as a reliable biomarker of proximal tubular injury in rodents is weakened by a currently unexplained observation that the urinary levels of α-GST were consistently decreased in the presence of CD injury without evidence of any injury to the proximal tubule. Based on these data, regulatory authorities in the United States and Europe concluded that α-GST could not be qualified at this time because of opposing responses (e.g., increases vs. decreases) of this biomarker in response to proximal tubular and CD injury that may confound interpretation (Harpur et al., 2011). Recent studies, in which the diagnostic performance of a number of traditional and novel biomarkers were evaluated in a cisplatin model of nephrotoxicity in rats, have provided disparate evidence for the utility of α-GST. Togashi et al. (2012) demonstrated that α-GST was among the best early markers of cisplatin-induced tubular injury, whereas α-GST did not show any improvement over sCr or BUN in two other studies (Pinches et al., 2012; Vinken et al., 2012). Vinken et al. (2012) found that α-GST did not respond to injury as rapidly as clusterin or KIM-1 and quickly returned to control levels despite continued cisplatin dosing and progression of the injury as assessed by histopathology. Following acute injury induced by short-term (3-day) gentamicin administration, Rouse et al. (2011) found that both α-GST and μ-GST were elevated in urine at the time of maximum injury but rapidly returned to control levels despite the presence of regressing injury alongside regeneration.

In the rat qualification studies by Harpur et al. (2011), no conclusion could be drawn about the utility of μ-GST for the diagnosis of renal injury. There were few diagnoses of injury to the distal tubule, where this isoform is known to be primarily located, and where diagnoses of distal tubule injury occurred, there was concomitant CD injury in most cases. In human patients in an intensive care unit, π-GST (which has the same localization in the distal tubule as μ-GST in the rat), was shown to be comparable to α-GST in its predictive value for acute tubular necrosis (a condition involving injury to both proximal and distal tubules). In theory, demonstrating a lack of change in urinary μ-GST (or π-GST) could also be useful to confirm a diagnosis of proximal tubule-specific injury based on an increase of α-GST. However, because of both functional interdependencies and proximity of different segments within regions of the kidney, collateral and nonspecific injury to adjacent nephron segments can readily occur with severe nephrotoxicity. As a result, μ-GST may be increased in the presence of predominantly proximal tubular injury with no concomitant diagnosis of distal tubular injury based on light microscopic evaluation (Harpur et al., 2011).

12.3.3.4 Total Protein

Urinary total protein levels reflect both glomerular and tubular function in that the glomerular filtration barrier restricts passage of macromolecules into the glomerular filtrate, while receptor mediated endocytosis in the proximal tubular epithelium mediates tubular reabsorption of filtered proteins (for review, see Stonard, 1990). As such, proteinuria may be indicative of disease or injury to either the glomerulus or the proximal tubule (D'amico and Bazzi, 2003). Dieterle et al. (2010a) showed that urine total protein was a more specific and sensitive marker than BUN and creatinine to detect glomerular injury with subsequent impairment of tubular reabsorption in rats. Based on these data, urinary protein has been qualified in rats as a biomarker of glomerular injury and/or impaired tubular reabsorption (EMA, 2009; FDA, 2008). However, urinary total protein has been shown to be less sensitive than urinary albumin for the detection of proximal tubular injury induced in rats by cisplatin (Gautier et al., 2010; Tonomura et al., 2010). Moreover, Harpur et al. (2011) found that measurement of protein in urine offered no diagnostic advantage over BUN or sCr for any of the tubular pathologies that occurred in these rat studies. While the separation of urinary proteins according to molecular weight and the determination of the ratio of high to low molecular weight proteins has been used in clinical practice to discriminate primary tubular disorders from glomerular injury (Stonard, 1990), this is not an established practice in animal studies, especially in rodents where the composition of urine proteins is markedly different from that in humans.

12.3.3.5 Albumin

In the clinical setting, proteinuria is a sign of established kidney damage and plays a pathogenic role in the progression of renal and cardiovascular disease, whereas albuminuria, reflects functional abnormalities that are potentially reversible (Ruggenenti and Remuzzi, 2006). In humans, abnormal albuminuria ranges have been set. Microalbuminuria is excretion of albumin at a rate between 20 and 200 μg/min or between 30 and 300 mg in 24-hour urine collections and is recognized as an early manifestation of renal disease (Ferguson et al., 2008). Macroalbuminuria is defined as urinary albumin excretion of >200 μg/min or >300 mg in 24 hours and identifies the onset of proteinuria and the development of progressive renal and/or cardiovascular disease (Basi et al., 2008; Ruggenenti and Remuzzi, 2006).

Albuminuria is classically considered to arise from damage to the glomerular basement membrane (Haraldsson et al., 2008). However, recent studies have challenged this notion in the rat, demonstrating that albumin is freely filtered through the healthy glomerular basement membrane, and efficiently recycled (and a fraction degraded) by the proximal tubule (Greive et al., 2001; Russo et al., 2007). In experimental glomerulonephritis, albuminuria results not from an increased glomerular sieving coefficient but from inhibition of the uptake of albumin at the BBM of the proximal tubular cells. These studies imply that albuminuria would more commonly reflect proximal tubular damage than glomerular damage. Consistent with that, albuminuria has been reported in humans following administration of nephrotoxic drugs that produce tubular injury (Kern et al., 2000; Koch Nogueira et al., 1998; Tugay et al., 2006). Thus, albuminuria may prove useful as a marker of acute kidney injury and concomitant proximal tubular cell damage (Ferguson et al., 2008).

In rat studies, elevation of urinary albumin has been shown to be a reliable and specific indicator of renal tubular lesions (Yu et al., 2010). Measurement of albumin in urine was shown to have comparable performance to α-GST and clusterin for detection of proximal tubular injury induced by cisplatin in rats (Gautier et al., 2010) and has been qualified as a biomarker of proximal tubular injury in rat studies, outperforming BUN and sCr (Yu et al., 2010). However, the fact that minimal or mild albuminuria can also be a response to a variety of physiological and pathophysiological conditions such as exercise, fever, dehydration, diabetes, or hypertension (Bonventre et al., 2010), or could result from inhibition of albumin uptake by proximal tubule cells without injury (Chana and Brunskill, 2006), complicates the interpretation of urinary albumin as a clinical biomarker of renal tubular injury, particularly in cases where there are only slight changes in urine values.

12.3.3.6 β2-Microglobulin

β2-microglobulin is a 12-kDa polypeptide that is synthesized throughout the body and present in plasma. It is filtered by the glomeruli and almost completely reabsorbed and catabolized in the renal tubules so that only a small amount is normally found in normal urine (Dieterle et al., 2010a). Minimal impairment of uptake in the renal tubules can result in a large increase in β2-microglobulin in urine; thus, measurement of urinary β2-microglobulin has the potential to be a sensitive indicator of impairment of renal tubular function (for review, see Ferguson et al., 2008). It should be noted, however, that increased urinary excretion of β2-microglobulin can result not only from injury to the renal tubules but also from glomerular alterations causing a high protein load in the tubules and competition for tubular uptake. Based on the data of Dieterle et al. (2010a), urinary β2-microglobulin has been qualified as a biomarker of glomerular injury and/or impairment of tubular reabsorption (EMA, 2009; FDA, 2008). A limitation of β2-microglobulin in urine is its instability at acidic pH so that alkalinization of urine is necessary (Trof et al., 2006). This is particularly an issue in human urine where measurement of α1-microglobulin is generally preferred because it is stable at the low pH of human urine (Payn et al., 2002; Weber and Verweibe, 1992). For example, Herget-Rosenthal et al. (2004b) showed that the prognostic accuracy of α1-microglobulin in predicting those patients with acute tubular necrosis who would require renal replacement therapy was much superior to that of β2-microglobulin.

12.3.3.7 Cystatin C

Cystatin C is a low molecular weight protein (approximately 13 kDa) that is produced by all nucleated cells throughout the body (Mussap and Plebani, 2004) and is readily filtered through the glomerulus. As mentioned later in Section 12.3.4.2.2, serum cystatin C has been widely studied for use as an alternative to sCr as an endogenous GFR marker in humans (Madero et al., 2006; Shlipak et al., 2006; Slocum et al., 2012; Westhuyzen, 2006) and has been shown to be superior to sCr as a measure of GFR (Dharnidharka et al., 2002).

In rats, filtered cystatin C is almost completely reabsorbed and catabolized in the tubules (Tenstad et al., 1996). Thus, very low levels of cystatin C are normally present in urine and impairment of tubular reabsorption, either through competition with an increased filtered load of protein (as seen with glomerular injury) or through impaired tubular function (as seen with tubular injury) will result in a large increase in the level of cystatin C in urine (Dieterle et al., 2010a). Based on the results reported by Dieterle et al. (2010a), urinary cystatin C has been qualified as a biomarker of acute drug-induced glomerular damage and/or impaired tubular reabsorption in rats (EMA, 2009; FDA, 2008). However, subsequent studies have provided equivocal results. Ozer et al. (2010) reported results indicating plasma cystatin C was superior to sCr and BUN for the detection of nephrotoxicant-induced injury to various parts of the nephron including tubular injury induced by cisplatin and gentamicin, while Pinches et al. (2012) showed inferiority of plasma cystatin C versus sCr and BUN in a cisplatin model of nephrotoxicity. In addition, Tonomura et al. (2010) found no increase in urinary cystatin C in urine from rats with puromycin-induced glomerular injury. However, in this study the injury was slight and an increase might be anticipated with more marked glomerular injury (Tonomura et al., 2010). Tonomura et al. (2010) also found that urinary cystatin C was insensitive, compared with KIM-1, as a marker of cisplatin-induced tubular injury in rats. In contrast, Togashi et al. (2012) reported that urinary cystatin C had comparable sensitivity to KIM-1 and α-GST for the early detection of tubular injury induced by cisplatin. However, in this model of acute tubular injury plasma cystatin C showed little change, underlining its role as a marker of whole kidney function (glomerular filtration). Collectively, these results indicate that more work is required to establish firmly the utility of measurement of cystatin C, either in serum/plasma or urine, for the detection of glomerular and/or tubular injury in animals.

12.3.3.8 Kidney Injury Molecule-1

KIM-1, a transmembrane glycoprotein with a mucin domain in the extracellular region, has been widely studied in both animals and humans for more than a decade. These studies have shown that KIM-1 has great promise as a sensitive and specific marker of renal tubular injury (for reviews, see Slocum et al., 2012; Vaidya et al., 2008). KIM-1 mRNA and protein levels have been shown to be expressed at a low level in normal kidney tissue but markedly increased in proximal tubular cells following ischemic or toxic injury in rodents (Amin et al., 2004; Ichimura et al., 1998). Following tubular injury from a variety of causes, the mucin ectodomain of KIM-1 is shed into the urine where it is stable for prolonged periods of time (Bonventre, 2008). Following drug-induced or ischemic injury, urinary KIM-1 levels are elevated when other routine urinary or blood-based biomarkers of injury or renal function did not change, showing the potential sensitivity of KIM-1 in monitoring tubular injury (Ichimura et al., 2004; Vaidya et al., 2006). Recent studies have provided evidence that urinary KIM-1 is a highly sensitive and specific biomarker for the early detection of nephrotoxicant-induced proximal tubular injury, regardless of the mechanism underlying that injury (Hoffmann et al., 2010; Ozer et al., 2010; Togashi et al., 2012; Tonomura et al., 2010; Vaidya et al., 2010; Vinken et al., 2012; Zhou et al., 2008). The superior sensitivity of urinary KIM-1 over whole kidney functional assessment by sCr or BUN was shown by Ozer et al. (2010) and Vaidya et al. (2010). Tonomura et al. (2010) found that KIM-1 was the best biomarker for proximal tubular injury based on its early and time-dependent increase as well as the large magnitude of the increase. In addition, the data generated by Vaidya et al. (2010) demonstrated that KIM-1 outperformed traditional markers (sCr and BUN) and enabled regulatory authorities to conclude that KIM-1 was qualified for the detection of acute drug-induced nephrotoxicity in rats (EMA, 2009; FDA, 2008). Changes in urinary KIM-1 may also reflect recovery from tubular injury in rats (Rouse et al., 2011).

Many of the properties of KIM-1 that have been characterized in rodents are also evident in humans. KIM-1 is expressed at high levels in proximal tubular cells and the cleaved ectodomain of KIM-1 can be detected in the urine of patients with acute tubular necrosis (Han et al., 2002). Human studies also indicate the promise of KIM-1 as a diagnostic and prognostic biomarker of acute kidney injury indicating KIM-1 may be a useful translational biomarker for proximal tubular injury (for reviews, see Coca et al., 2008; Slocum et al., 2012; Vaidya et al., 2008).

12.3.3.9 Clusterin

Clusterin, a dimeric glycoprotein, is expressed in the epithelia of many organs (Rosenberg and Silkensen, 1995). In the kidney, it is highly expressed during early stages of development. In contrast, in the healthy mature kidney, clusterin mRNA and protein are not detectable but are upregulated in response to renal tubular injury and in a variety of renal diseases (Rosenberg and Silkensen, 1995). It has been suggested that secreted clusterin suppresses apoptosis and is involved in cell aggregation and attachment (Rosenberg and Silkensen, 1995). Clusterin expression is upregulated in rats following nephrectomy (Correa-Rotter et al., 1992), unilateral ureteral obstruction (Ishii et al., 2007), renal ischemia-reperfusion (Yoshida et al., 2002), or nephrotoxicity (Kharasch et al., 2006; Silkensen et al., 1997) and in dogs with renal papillary necrosis induced by nefiracetam (Tsuchiya et al., 2005). Increased levels of clusterin protein in urine have been detected following ischemic or chemically induced injury in rats (Aulitzky et al., 1992; Dieterle et al., 2010a; Eti et al., 1993; Gautier et al., 2010; Harpur et al., 2011; Hidaka et al., 2002; Hoffmann et al., 2010) and dogs (Tsuchiya et al., 2005). While increased expression of clusterin (mRNA and/or protein) is seen in humans in a variety of renal disorders (Rosenberg and Silkensen, 1995), to date there are no published results demonstrating the use of clusterin as a diagnostic marker of renal injury in humans.

Clusterin was among those urinary proteins shown to outperform BUN and sCr for in the detection of acute chemical-induced tubular injury without specification of the specific segment involved (Dieterle et al., 2010a; FDA, 2008; EMA, 2009). Regulators (EMA, 2010; FDA, 2010) also concluded that the results presented by Harpur et al. (2011) supported the qualification of urinary clusterin by increasing the level of evidence and clarifying the context of its use, namely detection of acute drug-induced renal tubule alterations, particularly when regeneration is present. This is consistent with current understanding of the biological function of clusterin indicating that, in response to injury, clusterin may be involved in cell aggregation and attachment (Rosenberg and Silkensen, 1995). Overall, these results suggest that clusterin may have utility in detecting renal tubular injury and may be particularly useful in monitoring regeneration. This is supported by the finding that urinary levels of both clusterin and NAG rose rapidly following chronic administration of gentamicin over a 2-month period. In contrast, clusterin levels remained significantly elevated over the duration of the experiment while NAG levels were similar to control values within 10 days despite evidence of persistent tubulointerstitial disease (Eti et al., 1993). Furthermore, Ozer et al. (2010) found that increased urinary levels of clusterin (and KIM-1) persist during regeneration. Based on these data, clusterin may add most value in monitoring chronic-active injury and regeneration.

12.3.3.10 Trefoil Factor 3

TFF3 is a small peptide hormone produced by epithelial cells in multiple tissues and is associated with inhibition of apoptosis and migration of epithelial cells toward lesions that could contribute to restoration of injured epithelial tissue (Yu et al., 2010). As shown by mRNA expression, TFF3 is expressed in the kidney and, although its distribution in the nephron is not well characterized, Yu et al. (2010) presented evidence for its presence in the proximal straight tubules. Both the renal presence of TFF3 (mRNA) and the urinary concentration of TFF3 protein (Ozer et al., 2010; Yu et al. 2010) were found to be decreased following treatment with some nephrotoxicants (carbapenem A and gentamicin) but not others (thioacetamide and cyclosporin A). The decreases in urinary TFF3 correlated with the severity of histopathological lesions in the proximal tubule and TFF3 was claimed to be a sensitive and specific biomarker of tubular injury (Yu et al., 2010). This conclusion needs to be confirmed by additional studies in animals; furthermore, at present there is a paucity of information on its potential clinical utility. TFF3 is by far the least studied protein among those evaluated for potential biological qualification for use in rodent toxicology studies. The lack of data on TFF3 is likely related to the lack of a widely available and validated assay as well as the undesirable property (unique among the qualified biomarkers) that its concentration in urine is decreased, rather than increased, in response to renal injury.

12.3.3.11 Renal Papillary Antigen-1

Although the proximal tubule is the most common nephronal segment targeted by nephrotoxic xenobiotics (Bonventre et al., 2010), renal papillary necrosis is caused by an increasing number of pharmaceutical agents, including nonsteroidal anti-inflammatory drugs (Bach and Thanh, 1998). Until recently, there has been no specific urinary biomarker of injury to this region of the kidney. Renal papillary necrosis can be induced experimentally in rats by nonsteroidal anti-inflammatory drugs and chemicals such as 2-bromethanamine or N-phenylanthranilic acid (NPAA), a biphenyl analogue of mefenamic acid (Betton et al., 2005; Price et al., 2010). To develop markers for renal papillary injury, monoclonal antibodies were raised against proteins released in urine from rats treated with nephrotoxicants, and the antibodies were screened for those that correspond to segment specific antigens (Falkenberg et al., 1996; Hildebrand et al., 1999). This procedure identified an antigen, RPA-1, which is specifically expressed in the CD. Price et al. (2010) found RPA-1 particularly difficult to characterize but demonstrated that RPA-1 is a very large membrane-bound glycoprotein located specifically within the CD of the rat kidney. They also showed it to be a good early marker of renal papillary necrosis in the rat. RPA-1 was further evaluated by Betton et al. (2012) and Harpur et al. (2011) as a potential urinary biomarker of CD injury. In these studies, RPA-1 was superior to a number of reference biomarkers (BUN, sCr, protein, and NAG) for diagnosis of injury to the CD in the rat. However, no human equivalent to RPA-1 has yet been identified and thus clinical data are unavailable.

12.3.3.12 Neutrophil Gelatinase-Associated Lipocalin

Human neutrophil gelatinase-associated lipocalin (NGAL), also known as lipocalin-2, is a 25 kDa protein located in neutrophil-specific granules and found in many tissues. In rodents, NGAL gene expression is upregulated in the kidney following ischemic/reperfusion and nephrotoxic injury a response which often occurs in parallel with increases in urinary protein (Hoffmann et al., 2010; Mishra et al., 2003; Rached et al., 2008; Rouse et al., 2011; Sieber et al., 2009). Thus, urinary NGAL has been proposed as an early biomarker for diagnosing acute kidney injury in both animals and humans (for review, see Vaidya et al., 2008). As with other exploratory biomarkers, the results of animal studies have provided discrepant results. Following puromycin administration to rats, urinary NGAL was shown to be increased in the presence of minimal glomerular vacuolation, with no concurrent tubular pathology (Tonomura et al., 2010) and also with glomerular vacuolation accompanied by tubular degeneration (Fuchs et al., 2012). Urinary NGAL increased in response to acute gentamicin-induced tubular injury in rats and was determined to be the most sensitive, together with urinary KIM-1, of a number of novel biomarkers (Sieber et al., 2009). In other studies using gentamicin to induce renal injury in rats, NGAL has been shown to outperform sCr and BUN as a diagnostic biomarker (Hoffmann et al., 2010; Rouse et al., 2011) but it did not prove to be as sensitive as other biomarkers such as KIM-1 or clusterin. Tonomura et al. (2010) found that urinary NGAL was unchanged in rat urine with cisplatin-induced tubular injury. In another study in which rats were given a single injection of various doses of cisplatin and examined over a period of days (Pinches et al. 2012), increases of NGAL in urine were small and seen inconsistently only at the high dose. In a third study in rats, urinary NGAL increased in response to cisplatin (up to 14 doses) but was inconsistent at early time points so that NGAL was judged to show no greater sensitivity compared with standard clinical pathology parameters (Vinken et al., 2012). In contrast, Fuchs et al. (2012) concluded that NGAL had good diagnostic utility based on their observation of a dose-dependent increase in urinary NGAL following administration of cisplatin or vancomycin to rats over 28 days. In summary, these results suggest NGAL may be a useful biomarker in rodents for glomerular injury and, at least some instances, for tubular injury. However, serum levels of NGAL are known to increase in response to infection and inflammation and NGAL filtered by the glomerulus appears in urine. An example of this was observed in a rodent model of carbon tetrachloride liver injury with no injury to the kidney detectable by histopathology (Smyth et al., 2009). Therefore, the specificity of urinary NGAL for diagnosing acute kidney injury has been questioned (Fuchs et al., 2012; Hoffmann et al., 2010; Sieber et al., 2009). However, it needs to be borne in mind that almost all of the animal studies conducted to evaluate the performance of urinary biomarkers did not include measurement of serum or plasma levels of these biomarkers. Furthermore, the growing body of evidence that NGAL is a useful diagnostic and prognostic biomarker for acute kidney injury in humans in a variety of clinical settings (Haase et al., 2009; Mishra et al., 2005; Nickolas et al., 2008; Tuladhar et al., 2009) encourages the prospect that NGAL could be a valuable translational biomarker of kidney injury and merits further study to more fully characterize its behavior in animal models.

12.3.3.13 Experimental Biomarkers

A number of other urinary proteins, such as interleukin-18, cysteine-rich protein, fatty acid-binding protein, and osteopontin, have been proposed as biomarkers of acute kidney injury (for review, see Vaidya et al., 2008). There are variable levels of evidence from human and animal studies for their potential utility as markers of acute kidney injury and these are not established biomarkers for renal injury or disease. Some biomarkers, such as urinary cytokines, may only reflect increased filtration through the glomerulus due to high circulating levels in plasma, and therefore may not actually arise from the site of local renal damage.

12.3.4 Glomerular Filtration Rate (Clearance)

GFR is the most clinically useful index of the severity of renal functional loss and progression (Lane et at., 2009). GFR is defined as the renal clearance of a substance that is neither secreted nor reabsorbed in the tubules, metabolized, or bound to proteins and is nontoxic. GFR is expressed as the volume of plasma cleared of the substance over time and may be evaluated indirectly by measuring serum levels of specific endogenous analytes, or more directly by measuring the clearance of substances removed by the glomeruli and not excreted by the tubules. These substances can be endogenous substances such as creatinine or cystatin C or exogenous substances such as inulin or iohexol.

The most widely used indirect method for measurement of GFR is to determine serum concentrations of creatinine and BUN. As discussed in previous sections, however, creatinine concentrations can overestimate GFR, as there is significant tubular secretion in many species (mice, rats, dogs) (Hackbarth et al., 1981; Eisner et al., 2010; O'Connell et al., 1962), and tubular secretion is greater at low tubular flow rates (i.e., low GFR). BUN generally underestimates GFR due to reabsorption, as it readily crosses cell membranes/tubules and thus significant (40%–70%) reabsorption is possible (Stevens et al., 2006). Greater reabsorption occurs at low flow rates/decreased renal perfusion (i.e., when function is compromised).

Clearance methods are generally more sensitive in estimating GFR than is determination of plasma or urine constituents; however, they are still indirect measurements (Stevens and Levey, 2009). The clearance rate (GFR) of a substance is calculated by the formula (Latimer et al., 2011):

$$Cx = \text{GFR} = \frac{\dfrac{Ux \times Uv}{Px}}{\text{BW}}$$

where Cx = clearance rate of the substance (mL/min/kg), Ux = urine concentration of the substance (mg/mL), Px = plasma concentration of the substance (mg/mL), Uv = minute urine volume (mL/min), and BW = body weight (kg).

As seen from this formula, reliable clearance measurements depend on a stable plasma level of the indicator substance and precisely timed and complete collection of urine.

12.3.4.1 Exogenous Substances Used to Measure GFR

12.3.4.1.1 Inulin

GFR is measured classically as the renal clearance of inulin against which the validity of other substances used to measure GFR is determined. Historically, inulin has been regarded as the substance of choice for reliable determinations of GFR in laboratory species because it is considered to be cleared exclusively by glomerular filtration (Levinski and Lieberthal, 1992). However, the procedures for determining inulin clearance are complex and lack high throughput. As such, inulin clearance is not a useful assay for routine testing of renal function for large-scale screening assays. Because inulin is an exogenous substance, it must be introduced by intravenous infusion to maintain a stable plasma concentration for the test period of about 30–60 minutes. Anesthesia or rigid restraint of the animal is required, as well as complete emptying of the bladder before, during, and at the completion of the test period. The utility of using a single intravenous injection of inulin to estimate GFR has also been explored (Brewer et al., 1990; Brown et al. 1996b; Fettman et al., 1985; Rogers et al., 1991). The use of radiolabeled inulin has simplified the previously demanding chemical assays for inulin (DeWardener, 1985; Thomsen and Olesen, 1981). These radiolabeled materials, ^{14}C-inulin and ^{3}H-inulin, are commercially available. However, it has been reported that within the same rat, clearance of undecomposed [^{3}H]-inulin and [^{14}C]-inulin may differ by 12%, and for this reason should not be used interchangeably as GFR markers (Shalmi et al., 1991).

12.3.4.1.2 Iohexol

Another method for determining GFR uses an x-ray fluorescence technique to measure the disappearance of injected iohexol from plasma (O'Reilly et al., 1986). Iohexol is an iodinated, nonionic, radiographic contrast agent. Sterner et al. (1996) and Lundqvist et al. (1995) have shown that a single sample plasma clearance after single injection of iohexol provides a good estimate of GFR. Studies in dogs and cats administered iohexol at a dose of 300 mg/kg body weight showed that GFR could be measured by using a single compartment model for plasma clearance with three blood samples drawn 3–7 hours after administration (Braselton et al., 1997). Iohexol has been used to estimate GFR in man (Brown and O'Reilly, 1991; Lundqvist et al., 1995; O'Reilly et al., 1986; Sterner et al., 1996), dogs (Braselton et al., 1997; Brown et al., 1996a; Gleadhill and Michell, 1996), cats (Braselton et al., 1997; Brown et al., 1996a), sheep (Nesje et al., 1997), swine (Frennby et al., 1996; Lundqvist et al., 1995, and rats (Masereeuw et al., 1996). The iohexol injection plasma clearance method can substitute for ^{51}Cr-EDTA and inulin for measuring GFR (Brown et al., 1991; Gaspari et al., 1996; Lundqvist et al., 1995). Miyamoto (2001) showed plasma clearance of iohexol can be determined by use of a simple colorimetric assay to provide an estimation of GFR in cats. Inductively coupled plasma-atomic emission spectroscopy and high performance liquid chromatography (HPLC) have also been used to measure serum iodine to determine plasma clearance of iohexol (Braselton et al., 1997; Gaspari et al., 1996).

12.3.4.2 Endogenous Substances Used to Measure GFR

12.3.4.2.1 Creatinine

The most common test used to evaluate glomerular function is the clearance of endogenous creatinine (Rose, 2001). Creatinine levels in plasma are quite constant and not greatly influenced by diet. In addition, GFR estimates using this method do not include the technical issues encountered with inulin clearance studies (Maillard et al., 2010). However, renal tubular secretion of creatinine occurs in some species, such as rats, guinea pigs, and male dogs (Diezi and Biollaz, 1979), and common methods of assaying creatinine also detect noncreatinine chromogens present in plasma that are not present in urine. Tubular secretion of creatinine tends to overestimate GFR, whereas the inclusion of plasma noncreatinine chromogens results in underestimation of GFR. These two opposing effects fortuitously tend to mitigate these effects (Haycock, 1981). Although methods using cimetidine to block renal tubular creatinine secretion are possible, this may be most useful in correction of a particularly high level of creatinine tubular secretion, which possibly could be species-specific (Nickolas et al., 2008; Toto, 1995).

Endogenous creatinine clearance is a relatively easy test to conduct and is adaptable as a screening test for nephrotoxicity following chemical or physical insults. Plasma creatinine is measured at the start and completion of a timed urine collection. The bladder of an adequately hydrated animal should be emptied at the start of the test (discard specimen) and again at the completion of the timed urine collection. It is necessary to accurately measure the collection period, the volume of urine, and the weight of the animal. The creatinine concentration is then determined on an aliquot of the urine and serum samples. The creatinine clearance (mL/min/kg) may be calculated using the following formula where $[\text{creatinine}]_u$ represents creatinine concentration in the collected urine sample, $[\text{creatinine}]_s$ represents creatinine concentration in the collected serum sample, volume_u represents volume of urine collected during the collection period (mL), time represents duration of collection period (minutes), and BW represents body weight (kg) of the animal (Stockham and Scott, 2002):

$$\text{Creatinine clearance rate} = \frac{[\text{Creatinine}]_{\text{urine}}}{[\text{Creatinine}]_{\text{serum}}} \times \text{Volume}_{\text{urine}} \div \text{Time} \div \text{BW}$$

Clearance of exogenous, injected creatinine may also be determined, but it is not well suited for use in large-scale nephrotoxicity studies. In the dog, however, exogenous creatinine clearance correlates more closely to inulin clearance than endogenous creatinine clearance.

A second plasma clearance method that does not require urine collection involves the single intravenous injection of a compound and the clearance from plasma determined from collection of several blood samples. Sapirstein et al. (1955) developed this technique and the calculations necessary to estimate GFR using injected creatinine in the dog. Ohashi et al. (1996) have shown that the plasma clearance of a single injection of iothalamate can be used to estimate GFR in cats. Ronnhedh et al. (1996) have used iothalamate for urine-free estimation of GFR in rats, but the method requires venous and arterial cannulation.

12.3.4.2.2 Cystatin C

A recent marker being utilized for estimating GFR is cystatin C. Cystatin-C is a 13 kDa nonglycosylated protein and cysteine proteinase inhibitor that is used as a clinical marker of kidney function (Stevens et al., 2006). It is released at a constant rate from all nucleated cells, and is freely filtered at the glomerulus, with significant uptake by the epithelial cells of the proximal tubules in the kidney (99% in rats) (Tenstad et al., 1996). Unlike creatinine or BUN, plasma levels of cystatin C are not influenced by gender, age, or diet, so serum levels are considered a more accurate estimate of GFR (Dharnidhark et al., 2002; Herget-Rosenthal et al., 2004a; Madero et al., 2006; Shlipak et al., 2006). Cystatin C is measured using immunoassay methods (i.e., immunoturbidometric or nephelometric methods) with antibodies that generally cross-react across species; however, some species-specific assays are available. Cystatin C can be measured in the blood or urine and an impairment of proximal tubular function can lead to increases in both blood and urine (Collé et al., 1990; Conti et al., 2006; Herget-Rosenthal et al., 2007; Tenstad et al., 1996). With impaired renal tubular function, urine cystatin C concentrations may increase up to 200-fold (Lisoskwa-Myjak, 2010). Cystatin C has been shown to be a sensitive indicator of kidney dysfunction in humans, such that cystatin C-based estimation of GFR has been considered useful for clinical practice (Cha et al., 2010). Cystatin C may be more sensitive to low-level decreases in GFR than either creatinine or BUN, and as such is also used as a potentially sensitive marker of glomerular injury in humans and animals. Cystatin C may, however, be increased in inflammatory disease, cancer, or hypothyroidism.

12.3.5 Tubular Function Tests

The renal tubules are frequently the primary target for nephrotoxic chemicals (Bonventre et al., 2010). For a more detailed account of the points summarized below, see Lote (2010). The physicochemical properties of urine (e.g., volume, osmolality, pH) and the concentration of many substances present in urine such as protein, amino acids, glucose, or electrolytes are influenced by tubular function. For example, normally amino acids and glucose are almost completely reabsorbed in the proximal tubule. For each substance that normally undergoes reabsorption in the tubules, there is a maximum amount that can be absorbed, referred to as the "tubular maximum." If plasma levels of the substance are elevated or the filtered load is increased by some other mechanism, the tubular reabsorptive mechanism may become saturated with a consequent increase in urinary concentration. If plasma levels are normal, then an increased urinary presence of a substance will, in most instances, reflect an impairment of proximal tubule function. Evidence in initial screening for disturbance of one or more of the normal constituents of urine might prompt more detailed investigation of tubular function using specific methodologies. These methods are not employed routinely but generally only used in the research laboratory or to follow up a primary finding where there is a need to understand mechanism. Therefore, the tests to evaluate the tubular functions will be described briefly.

Tubular function can be estimated by determination of the fractional excretion (FE) of endogenous substances that are reabsorbed or secreted through the tubular epithelium. FE is defined as the fraction of filtered load of a substance that is excreted in the urine, usually expressed as a percentage. Thus, percentage FE_a is calculated as

$$\frac{([U_a]\times V)}{([P_a]\times \text{GFR})}\times 100$$

where $[U_a]$ and $[P_a]$ are the concentrations of substance "a" in urine and plasma, respectively, and V is the urine flow rate in the same units as GFR (usually mL/min). Accurate calculation of FE requires carefully timed complete urine collections and a concurrent assessment of GFR. As accurately timed urine collection and measurement of GFR are both difficult in laboratory animals, an approximate FE value can be calculated based on a single isolated urine collection as follows, where P_{cr} and U_{cr} are plasma or urine creatinine, respectively (Rose, 2001):

$$\text{FE}_a = \frac{[U_a]\times[P_{cr}]}{U_{cr}}\times[P_a]$$

Measurement of FE is most commonly applied to electrolytes. A key function of the kidney is maintaining electrolyte and mineral homeostasis in the face of fluctuating dietary intake and body needs. Indeed, because of the large functional reserve of the kidney, a decrease in plasma electrolyte level is usually not detected until the amount of renal functional impairment is marked. Hence, measurement of urinary electrolyte levels together with plasma levels can provide a sensitive index of the functional state of the kidney. In animal studies, the diet is normally controlled thus ensuring a fairly constant intake of electrolytes. Provided there is no compound-induced change in electrolyte intake, for example, through inappetance or loss such as from vomiting or diarrhea, urine electrolyte levels will reflect the effects of the compound on renal electrolyte handling.

FE assessment can be performed for any electrolyte and might be triggered by an observed change in the concentration of an electrolyte in urine or plasma. In humans, measurement of FE of sodium, calcium, and magnesium have been shown to be useful in assessing underlying tubulointerstitial disease in nephrotic patients (Futrakul et al., 1999; Jespersen, 1997), with FE of magnesium being the most sensitive to detect an early abnormality of tubular structure and function. Increases in FE of magnesium and calcium have also been shown to serve as sensitive indices of the effects on renal function caused by aminoglycoside antibiotics without overt renal injury in both rats and humans (Parsons et al., 1997; Elliott et al., 2000). A full examination of the mechanism and site of impairment of tubular absorption of an electrolyte will require specialized techniques such as micropuncture and microperfusion of short lengths of individual nephrons, usually performed in rats (Garland et al., 1992; Parsons et al., 2000).

12.3.6 Concentration/Dilution Tests

The ability of the kidney to concentrate urine above that of the glomerular filtrate is primarily a function of the loop of Henle and the distal tubule. The foundation of testing the ability of the kidney to concentrate the urinary filtrate is based on water deprivation resulting in plasma hyperosmolality. This, in turn, triggers the release of the ADH which acts on the renal tubule cells to cause reabsorption of water and an increase in urine osmolality. Following renal tubular damage, the ability to concentrate urine is variably reduced. A concentration (water deprivation) test may be adapted for use in routine screening studies for adverse effects on the kidney.

The method for the urine concentrating test is to collect a 16–24-hour urine sample for analysis from animals that have free access to water. The animals are then deprived of water and an additional urine collection is made for 12–16 hours. The osmolality of the urine sample is determined and compared with that obtained when the animal was well hydrated.

The ability of the kidney to dilute the urine is also a tubular function. Urine dilution tests require the oral administration of a water load. In man, this test is conducted by ingestion of about 20 mL of water per kilogram of body weight over a 10–20-minute period and collecting urine hourly for 4 hours. With normal renal function, 75% of the ingested volume is excreted during the 4-hour period with a reduced osmolality. The test can also be used in animals by administering a water load by gavage and then making timed urine collections for a period of a few hours. It is generally thought that the dilution test is a less sensitive indicator of renal damage than the urine concentration test.

12.3.7 Measurement of Renal Plasma Flow and Renal Blood Flow

Several techniques are available for determining renal blood flow in laboratory animals. However, none are suitable for routine screening and will not be covered in detail. The techniques are used primarily in laboratories conducting in-depth studies of renal physiology.

Renal blood flow may be determined indirectly by determining the clearance from plasma of a substance that is extensively cleared in a single pass through the kidney and is cleared via the kidney only. The most extensively used compound is para-aminohippurate (PAH), which is both filtered and secreted and has a renal extraction ratio of approximately 1.0. The technique involves infusion of PAH and, in theory, it is necessary to collect samples from the renal artery and vein and assay the concentration of PAH. This provides an estimate of renal plasma flow (RPF) which is calculated as follows:

$$\text{RPF} = \frac{\text{Amount of PAH excreted per unit time}}{\text{Difference in ateriovenous concentration PAH}}$$

Thus

$$\text{RPF} = \frac{[U_{\text{PAH}}] \times V}{\text{RA}_{\text{PAH}} - \text{RV}_{\text{PAH}}}$$

where U_{PAH} is the concentration of PAH in urine, V the urine flow rate, RA_{PAH} and RV_{PAH} the concentrations of PAH in the renal artery and renal vein, respectively.

If the extraction ratio of PAH were truly 1.0, then it would not be necessary to measure the concentration of PAH in the renal vein, since this would be zero. Thus, the equation would simplify to $\text{RPF} = [U_{\text{PAH}}] \times V/\text{RA}_{\text{PAH}}$. In fact, the concentration of PAH in the peripheral venous blood can be substituted for the concentration in the renal artery and this is done in practice (Lote, 2010). It should be noted that because not all of the blood that enters the kidneys perfuses the glomeruli and tubules (the perirenal fat, the capsule, and the deep medulla are also perfused), the extraction ratio of PAH is approximately 0.9. Thus, this measurement is really an estimate of cortical blood flow and is referred to as Effective Renal Plasma Flow (ERPF). PAH clearance, determined by the conventional method of continuous intravenous infusion with peripheral blood and urine sample collections, is the gold standard for estimating RPF (Toto, 1995).

Renal blood flow (RBF) may be calculated indirectly from ERPF as follows:

$$\text{RBF} = \frac{\text{ERPF}}{(1 - \text{VPRC})}$$

where VPRC is the fractional volume of packed red cells (Lote, 2010).

Total RBF may also be measured directly and noninvasively using Doppler ultrasound probes or invasively using implanted Doppler flow probes or electromagnetic flow transducers. While these techniques allow accurate and reproducible measurement of total RBF, they are of limited use in the determination of regional changes in blood flow within the kidney. A wide variety of methods, ranging from use of inert gases, isotopically labeled tracers, radionucleotide-labeled microspheres to computed tomography and positron emission tomography, are available for measurement of intrarenal blood flow (for review see Young et al., 1996). All of these methods are highly specialized, time consuming and not widely available. While most can be applied to animal studies, they are unsuitable for routine application and are generally used only in research studies.

12.4 APPROACH FOR ASSESSMENT OF RENAL INJURY

Routine urinalysis, as described in the beginning sections of this chapter, is the first step in any assessment of the kidney, and accurate interpretation of these screening data can provide helpful guidance toward selection of additional analysis. Any further diagnostic or investigative studies, with additional biomarkers, can then be conducted to determine their correlation with region-specific kidney injury, function, and/or mechanism of injury. A panel of renal biomarkers provides the best approach to this additional assessment because, much like a panel of clinical chemistry biomarkers, a single renal parameter is not always specific to a particular injury. The choice of which assay(s) to use for this second phase of testing should be based on the screening findings, location of the lesion as determined by histopathology, and other pathophysiology that may be accompanying the renal findings, for example, bone, hematopoietic, metabolic.

REFERENCES

Amin, R.P., Vickers, A.E., Sistare, F., et al. 2004. Identification of putative gene based markers of renal toxicity. *Environ Health Perspect.* 112:465–479.

Appel, G. 1991. Lipid abnormalities in renal disease. *Kidney Int.* 39:169–183.

Aulitzky, W.K., Schlegel, P.N., Wu, D.F., et al. 1992. Measurement of urinary clusterin as an index of nephrotoxicity. *Proc Soc Exp Biol Med.* 199:93–96.

Bach, P.H. and Thanh, N.T.K. 1998. Renal papillary necrosis—40 years on. *Toxicol Pathol.* 26:73–91.

Basi, S., Fesler, P., Mimran, A., and Lewis, J.B. 2008. Microalbuminuria in type 2 diabetes and hypertension: A marker, treatment target, or innocent bystander? *Diabetes Care.* 31(Suppl 2):S194–S201.

Bass, N.M., Kirsch, R.E., Tuff, S.A., Campbell, J.A., and Saunders, J.S. 1979. Radioimmunoassay measurement of urinary ligandin excretion in nephrotoxin-treated rats. *Clin Sci (Lond).* 56:419–426.

Beckett, G.J. and Hayes, J.D. 1993. Glutathione S-transferases: Biomedical applications. *Adv Clin Chem.* 30:281–380.

Betton, G.R., Ennulat, D., Hoffman, D., Gautier, J.C., Harpur, E., and Pettit, S. 2012. Biomarkers of collecting duct injury in Han-Wistar and Sprague-Dawley rats treated with N-phenylanthranilic acid. *Toxicol Pathol.* 40:682–694.

Betton, G.R., Kenne, K., Somers, R., and Marr, A. 2005. Protein biomarkers of nephrotoxicity; a review and findings with cyclosporin A, a signal transduction kinase inhibitor and N-phenylanthranilic acid. *Cancer Biomark.* 1:59–67.

Bonvalet, J.P., Pradelles, P., and Farman, N. 1987. Segmental synthesis and actions of prostaglandins along the nephron. *Am J Physiol.* 253:F377–F387.

Bonventre, J.V. 2008. Kidney Injury Molecule-1 (KIM-1): A specific and sensitive biomarker of kidney injury. *Scand J Clin Lab Invest Suppl.* 241:78–83.

Bonventre, J.V., Vaidya, V.S., Schmouder, R., Feig, P., and Dieterle, F. 2010. Next-generation biomarkers for detecting kidney toxicity. *Nat Biotechnol.* 28:436–440.

Bosomworth, M.P., Aparicio, S.R., and Hay, A.W. 1999. Urine N-acetyl-beta-D-glucosaminidase—A marker of tubular damage? *Nephrol Dial Transplant.* 14:620–626.

Boudonck, K.J., Mitchell, M.W., Nemet, L., et al. 2009. Discovery of metabolomics biomarkers for early detection of nephrotoxicity. *Toxicol Pathol.* 37:280–292.

Bourbouze, R., Baumann, F.C., Bonvalet, J.P., and Farman, N. 1984. Distribution of N-acetyl-beta-D-glucosaminidase isoenzymes along the rabbit nephron. *Kidney Int.* 25:636–642.

Bradley, G. and Benson, E.S. 1974. Examination of the urine. In *Tod-Sanford Clinical Diagnosis by Laboratory Methods*. Eds. I. Davidsohn and J.B. Henry. Philadelphia, PA: W.B. Saunders.

Branten, A.J., Mulder, T.P., Peters, W.H., Assmann, K.J., and Wetzels, J.F. 2000. Urinary excretion of glutathione S transferases alpha and pi in patients with proteinuria: Reflection of the site of tubular injury. *Nephron.* 85:120–126.

Braselton, W.E., Stuart, K.J., and Kruger, J.M. 1997. Measurement of serum iohexol by determination of iodine with inductively coupled plasma-atomic emission spectroscopy. *Clin Chem.* 43:1429–1435.

Brewer, B.D., Clement, S.F., Lotz, W.S., and Gronwall, R. 1990. A comparison of inulin, para-aminohippuric acid, and endogenous creatinine clearances as measures of renal function in neonatal foals. *J Vet Intern Med.* 4:301–305.

Brown, S.A., Finco, D.R., Boudinot, F.D., Wright, J., Taver, S.L., and Cooper, T. 1996a. Evaluation of a single injection method, using iohexol, for estimating glomerular filtration rate in cats and dogs. *Am J Vet Res.* 57:105–110.

Brown, S.A., Haberman, C., and Finco, D.R. 1996b. Use of plasma clearance of inulin for estimating glomerular filtration rate in cats. *Am J Vet Res.*, 57:1702–1705.

Brown, S.C. and O'Reilly, P.H. 1991. Iohexol clearance for the determination of glomerular filtration rate in clinical practice: evidence for a new gold standard. *J Urol.* 146:675–679.

Brown, S.C. et al. 1991. *J Urol.* 146(3):675–679.

Caldwell, H.K. and Young, W.S., III. 2006. Oxytocin and vasopressin: Genetics and behavioral implications. In *Handbook of Neurochemistry and Molecular Neurobiology: Neuroactive Proteins and Peptides*. Eds. A. Lajtha and R. Lim, 3rd edition, pp. 573–607. Berlin: Springer.

Campbell, J.A., Corrigall, A.V., Guy, A., and Kirsch, R.E. 1991. Immunohistologic localization of alpha, mu, and pi class glutathione S-transferases in human tissues. *Cancer.* 67:1608–1613.

Castrop, H. and Kurtz, A. 2010. Functional evidence confirmed by histological localization: Overlapping expression of erythropoietin and HIF-2alpha in interstitial fibroblasts of the renal cortex. *Kidney Int.* 77:269–271.

Cavaggioni, A. and Mucignat-Caretta, C. 2000. Major urinary proteins, alpha(2U)-globulins and aphrodisin. *Biochim Biophys Acta.* 1482:218–228.

Cha, R.H., Lee, C.S., Lim, Y.H., et al. 2010. Clinical usefulness of serum cystatin C and the pertinent estimation of glomerular filtration rate based on cystatin C. *Nephrology (Carlton).* 15:768–776.

Chana, R.S. and Brunskill, N.J. 2006. Thiazolidinediones inhibit albumin uptake by proximal tubular cells through a mechanism independent of peroxisome proliferator activated receptor gamma. *Am J Nephrol.* 26:67–74.

Chew, D.J. and DiBarola, S.P. 1998. *Interpretation of Canine and Feline Urinalysis*. St. Louis, MO: Ralston Purina.

Coca, S.G., Yalavarthy, R., Concato, J., and Parikh, C.R. 2008. Biomarkers for the diagnosis and risk stratification of acute kidney injury: A systematic review. *Kidney Int.* 73:1008–1016.

Collé, A., Tavera, C., Laurent, P., Leung-Tack, J., and Girolami, J.P. 1990. Direct radioimmunoassay of rat cystatin C: Increased urinary excretion of this cysteine proteases inhibitor during chromate nephropathy. *J Immunoassay.* 11:199–214.

Conti, M., Moutereau, S., Zater, M., et al. 2006. Urinary cystatin C as a specific marker of tubular dysfunction. *Clin Chem Lab Med.* 44:288–291.

Corman, B. and Michel, J.B. 1987. Glomerular filtration, renal blood flow, and solute excretion in conscious aging rats. *Am J Physiol.* 253:R555–R560.

Corman, B., Pratz, J., and Poujeol, P. 1985. Changes in anatomy, glomerular filtration, and solute excretion in aging rat kidney. *Am J Physiol.* 248:R282–R287.

Correa-Rotter, R., Hostetter, T.H., Manivel, J.C., Eddy, A.A., and Rosenberg, M.E. 1992. Intrarenal distribution of clusterin following reduction of renal mass. *Kidney Int.* 41:938–950.

D'Amico, G. and Bazzi, C. 2003. Pathophysiology of proteinuria. *Kidney Int.* 63:809–825.

Davis, J.W., Goodsaid, F.M., Bral, C.M., et al. 2004. Quantitative gene expression analysis in a nonhuman primate model of antibiotic-induced nephrotoxicity. *Toxicol Appl Pharmacol.* 200:16–26.

Devarajan, P., Mishra, J., Supavekin, S., Patterson, L.T., and Potter, S.S. 2003. Gene expression in early ischemic renal injury: Clues towards pathogenesis, biomarker discovery, and novel therapeutics. *Mol Genet Metab.* 80:365–376.

DeWardener, H.E. 1985. *The Kidney: An Outline of Normal and Abnormal Function*. New York, NY: Churchill Livingstone.

Dharnidharka, V.R., Kwon, C., and Stevens, G. 2002. Serum cystatin C is superior to serum creatinine as a marker of kidney function: A meta-analysis. *Am J Kidney Dis.* 40:221–226.

Dieterle, F., Perentes, E., Cordier, A., et al. 2010a. Urinary clusterin, cystatin C, beta2-microglobulin and total protein as markers to detect drug-induced kidney injury. *Nat Biotechnol.* 28:463–469.

Dieterle, F., Sistare, F., Goodsaid, F., et al. 2010b. Renal biomarker qualification submission: A dialog between the FDA-EMEA and Predictive Safety Testing Consortium. *Nat Biotechnol.* 28:455–462.

Diezi, J. and Biollaz, J. 1979. Renal function tests in experimental toxicity studies. *Pharmacol Ther B.* 5:135–145.

Donadio, C., Tramonti, G., Lucchesi, A., et al. 1998. Gamma-glutamyltransferase is a reliable marker for tubular effects of contrast media. *Ren Fail.* 20:319–324.

Edmondson J.W., Brashear, R.E., and Li, T.K. 1975. Tetany: Quantitative interrelationships between calcium and alkalosis. *Am J Physiol.* 228:1082–1086.

Eger, E.I., Koblin, D.D., Bowland, T., et al. 1997. Nephrotoxicity of sevoflurane versus desflurane anesthesia in volunteers. *Anesth Analg.* 84:160–168.

Eisner, C., Faulhaber-Walter, R., Wang, Y., et al. 2010. Major contribution of tubular secretion to creatinine clearance in mice. *Kidney Int.* 77:519–526.

Elliott, C., Newman, N., and Madan, A. 2000. Gentamicin effects on urinary electrolyte excretion in healthy subjects. *Clin Pharmacol Ther.* 67:16–21.

EMA. 2009. Final Conclusions on the Pilot Joint EMEA/FDA VXDS Experience on Qualification of Nephrotoxicity Biomarkers. Available at: http://www.ema.europa.eu/docs/en_GB/document_library/Regulatory_and_procedural_guideline/2009/10/WC500004205.pdf.

EMA. 2010. Qualification Opinion ILSI/HESI Submission of Novel Renal Biomarkers for Toxicity. Available at: http://www.ema.europa.eu/docs/en_GB/document_library/Regulatory_and_procedural_guideline/2010/11/WC500099359.pdf.

Eti, S., Cheng, C.Y., Marshall, A., and Reidenberg, M.M. 1993. Urinary clusterin in chronic nephrotoxicity in the rat. *Proc Soc Exp Biol Med.* 202:487–490.

Falkenberg, F.W., Hildebrand, H., Lutte, L., et al. 1996. Urinary antigens as markers of papillary toxicity. I. Identification and characterization of rat kidney papillary antigens with monoclonal antibodies. *Arch Toxicol.* 7:80–92.

Farman, N., Pradelles, P., and Bonvalet, J.P. 1987. PGE2, PGF2 alpha, 6-keto-PGF1 alpha, and TxB2 synthesis along the rabbit nephron. *Am J Physiol.* 252:F53–F59.

FDA. 2008. Seven Biomarkers of Drug-Induced nephrotoxicity in Rats. Predictive Safety Testing Consortium. Available at: http://www.fda.gov/Drugs/DevelopmentApprovalProcess/DrugDevelopmentToolsQualificationProgram/ucm284076.htm.

FDA. 2010. Non-Clinical Qualification of Urinary Biomarkers of Nephrotoxicity: HESI Nephrotoxicity Qualification. Available at: http://www.fda.gov/Drugs/DevelopmentApprovalProcess/DrugDevelopmentToolsQualificationProgram/ucm284076.htm.

Ferguson, M.A., Vaidya, V.S., and Bonventre, J.V. 2008. Biomarkers of nephrotoxic acute kidney injury. *Toxicology.* 245:182–193.

Fettman, M.J., Allen, T.A., Wilke, W.L., Radin, M.J., and Eubank, M.C. 1985. Single-injection method for evaluation of renal function with 14C-inulin and 3H-tetraethylammonium bromide in dogs and cats. *Am J Vet Res.* 46:482–485.

Finco, D.R. 1989. Kidney function. In *Clinical Biochemistry of Domestic Animals.* Ed. J.J. Kaneko. San Diego, CA: Academic Press.

Finlayson, J.S., Asofsky, R., Potter, M., and Runner, C.C. 1965.Major urinary protein complex of normal mice: Origin. *Science.* 149:981–982.

Flynn, R.J. 1973. *Parasites of Laboratory Animals*. Ames, IA: Iowa State University.

Fogazzi, G.B. 1996. Crystalluria: A neglected aspect of urinary sediment analysis. *Nephrol Dial Transplant.* 11:379–387.

Free, A.H. and Free, H.M. 2012. *Urinalysis in Clinical Laboratory Practice*. West Palm Beach, FL: CRC Press.

Frennby, B., Sterner, G., Almen, T., et al. 1996. Clearance of iohexol, chromium-51-ethylenediaminetetraacetic acid, and creatinine for determining the glomerular filtration rate in pigs with normal renal function: Comparison of different clearance techniques. *Acad Radiol.* 3:651–659.

Fuchs, T.C., Frick, K., Emde, B., et al. 2012. Evaluation of novel acute urinary rat kidney toxicity biomarker for subacute toxicity studies in preclinical trials. *Toxicol Pathol.* 40:1031–1048.

Futrakul, P., Yenrudi, S., Futrakul, N., et al. 1999. Tubular function and tubulointerstitial disease. *Am J Kidney Dis.* 33:886–891.

Ganong, W.F. 2010. *Review of Medical Physiology*, 23rd edition. Los Altos, CA: Lange Medical Publications.

Garland, H.O., Phipps, D.J., and Harpur, E.S. 1992. Gentamicin-induced hypercalciuria in the rat: Assessment of nephron site involved. *J Pharmacol Exp Ther.* 263:293–297.

Gaspari, F., Guerini, E., Perico, N., et al. 1996. Glomerular filtration rate determined from a single plasma sample after intravenous iohexol injection: Is it reliable? *J Am Soc Nephrol.* 7:2689–2693.

Gautier, J.C., Riefke, B., Walter, J., et al. 2010. Evaluation of novel biomarkers of nephrotoxicity in two strains of rat treated with cisplatin. *Toxicol Pathol.* 38:943–956.

Gibey, R., Dupond, J.L., Alber, D., et al. 1981. Predictive value of urinary N-acetyl-beta-D-glucosaminidase (NAG), alanine-aminopeptidase (AAP) and beta-2-microglobulin (beta 2M) in evaluating nephrotoxicity of gentamicin. *Clin Chim Acta.* 116:25–34.

Gibey, R., Dupond, J.L., and Henry, J.C. 1984. Urinary N-acetyl-beta-D-glucosaminidase (NAG) isoenzyme profiles: A tool for evaluating nephrotoxicity of aminoglycosides and cephalosporins. *Clin Chim Acta.* 137:1–11.

Ginsberg, J.M., Chang, B.S., Matarese, R.A., and Garella, S. 1983. Use of single voided urine samples to estimate quantitative proteinuria. *N Engl J Med.* 309:1543–1546.

Gleadhill, A. and Michell, A.R. 1996. Evaluation of iohexol as a marker for the clinical measurement of glomerular filtration rate in dogs. *Res Vet Sci.* 60:117–121.

Goldstein, S.L. 2010. Urinary kidney injury biomarkers and urine creatinine normalization: A false premise or not? *Kidney Int.* 78:433–435.

Grauer, G.F., Greco, D.S., Behrend, E.N., et al. 1995. Estimation of quantitative enzymuria in dogs with gentamicin-induced nephrotoxicosis using urine enzyme/creatinine ratios from spot urine samples. *J Vet Intern Med.* 9:324–327.

Greive, K.A., Nikolic-Paterson, D.J., Guimaraes, M.A., et al. 2001. Glomerular permselectivity factors are not responsible for the increase in fractional clearance of albumin in rat glomerulonephritis. *Am J Pathol.* 159:1159–1170.

Guyton, A.C. and Hall, J.E. 2011. The kidney and body fluids. In *Textbook of Medical Physiology*. Philadelphia, PA: W.B. Saunders.

Haas, M., Kluppel, A.C., Moolenaar, F., et al. 1997. Urine collection in the freely moving rat: Reliability for measurement of short-term renal effects. *J Pharmacol Toxicol Methods.* 38:47–51.

Haase, M., Bellomo, R., Devarajan, P., Schlattmann, P., and Haase-Fielitz, A. 2009. Accuracy of neutrophil gelatinase-associated lipocalin (NGAL) in diagnosis and prognosis in acute kidney injury: A systematic review and meta-analysis. *Am J Kidney Dis.* 54:1012–1024.

Hackbarth, H., Baunack, E., and Winn, M. 1981. Strain differences in kidney function of inbred rats: 1. Glomerular filtration rate and renal plasma flow. *Lab Anim.* 15:125–128.

Han, W.K., Bailly, V., Abichandani, R., et al. 2002. Kidney Injury Molecule-1 (KIM-1): A novel biomarker for human renal proximal tubule injury. *Kidney Int.* 62:237–244.

Han, W.K. and Bonventre, J.V. 2004. Biologic markers for the early detection of acute kidney injury. *Curr Opin Crit Care.* 10:476–482.

Haraldsson, B., Nyström, J., and Deen, W.M. 2008. Properties of the glomerular barrier and mechanisms of proteinuria. *Physiol Rev.* 88:451–487.

Hard, G.C. and Khan, K.N. 2004. A contemporary overview of chronic progressive nephropathy in the laboratory rat, and its significance for human risk assessment. *Toxicol Pathol.* 32:171–180.

Harpur, E., Ennulat, D., Hoffman, D., et al. 2011. Biological qualification of biomarkers of chemical-induced renal toxicity in two strains of male rat. *Toxicol Sci.* 122:235–252.

Harrison, D.J., Kharbanda, R., Cunningham, D.S., McLellan, L.I., and Hayes, J.D. 1989. Distribution of glutathione S-transferase isoenzymes in human kidney: Basis for possible markers of renal injury. *J Clin Pathol.* 42:624–628.

Haycock, G.B. 1981. Old and new tests of renal function. *J Clin Pathol.* 34:1276–1281.

Herget-Rosenthal, S., Marggraf, G., Husing, J., et al. 2004a. Early detection of acute renal failure by serum cystatin C. *Kidney Int.* 66:1115–1122.

Herget-Rosenthal, S., Poppen, D., Husing, J., et al. 2004b. Prognostic value of tubular proteinuria and enzymuria in nonoliguric acute tubular necrosis. *Clin Chem.* 50:552–558.

Herget-Rosenthal, S., van Wijk, J.A., Brocker-Preuss, M., and Bokenkamp, A. 2007. Increased urinary cystatin C reflects structural and functional renal tubular impairment independent of glomerular filtration rate. *Clin Biochem.* 40:946–951.

Hidaka, S., Kranzlin, B., Gretz, N., and Witzgall, R. 2002. Urinary clusterin levels in the rat correlate with the severity of tubular damage and may help to differentiate between glomerular and tubular injuries. *Cell Tissue Res.* 310:289–296.

Hildebrand, H., Rinke, M., Schluter, G., Bomhard, E., and Falkenberg, F.W. 1999. Urinary antigens as markers of papillary toxicity. II: Application of monoclonal antibodies for the determination of papillary antigens in rat urine. *Arch Toxicol.* 73:233–245.

Hoffmann, D., Adler, M., Vaidya, V.S., et al. 2010. Performance of novel kidney biomarkers in preclinical toxicity studies. *Toxicol Sci.* 116:8–22.

Hynynen, M. and Khalil, R. 2006. The vascular endothelin system in hypertension—recent patents and discoveries. *Recent Pathol Cardiovasc Drug Discov.* 1: 95–108

Ichimura, T., Bonventre, J.V., Bailly, V., et al. 1998. Kidney injury molecule-1 (KIM-1), a putative epithelial cell adhesion molecule containing a novel immunoglobulin domain, is up-regulated in renal cells after injury. *J Biol Chem.* 273:4135–4142.

Ichimura, T., Hung, C.C., Yang, S.A., Stevens, J.L., and Bonventre, J.V. 2004. Kidney injury molecule-1: A tissue and urinary biomarker for nephrotoxicant-induced renal injury. *Am J Physiol Renal Physiol.* 286:F552–F563.

Ishii, A., Sakai, Y., and Nakamura, A. 2007. Molecular pathological evaluation of clusterin in a rat model of unilateral ureteral obstruction as a possible biomarker of nephrotoxicity. *Toxicol Pathol.* 35:376–382.

Jespersen, B. 1997. Regulation of renal sodium and water excretion in the nephrotic syndrome and cirrhosis of the liver. *Dan Med Bull.* 44:191–207.

Joven, J., Villabona, C., Vilella, E., et al. 1990. Abnormalities of lipoprotein metabolism in patients with the nephrotic syndrome. *N Engl J Med.* 323:579–584.

Jung, K. 1994. Urinary enzymes and low molecular weight proteins as markers of tubular dysfunction. *Kidney Int Suppl.* 47:S29–S33.

Kern, W., Braess, J., Kaufmann, C.C., et al. 2000. Microalbuminuria during cisplatin therapy: Relation with pharmacokinetics and implications for nephroprotection. *Anticancer Res.* 20:3679–3688.

Kharasch, E.D., Hoffman, G.M., Thorning, D., Hankins, D.C., and Kilty, C.G. 1998. Role of the renal cysteine conjugate beta-lyase pathway in inhaled compound A nephrotoxicity in rats. *Anesthesiology.* 88:1624–1633.

Kharasch, E.D., Schroeder, J.L., Bammler, T., Beyer, R., and Srinouanprachanh, S. 2006. Gene expression profiling of nephrotoxicity from the sevoflurane degradation product fluoromethyl-2, 2-difluoro-1-(trifluoromethyl) vinyl ether ("compound A") in rats. *Toxicol Sci.* 90:419–431.

Kirk, R.W. and Bistner, S.L. 1969. *Handbook of Veterinary Procedures and Emergency Treatment.* Philadelphia, PA: W.B. Saunders.

Koch Nogueira, P.C., Hadj-Aissa, A., Schell, M., et al. 1998. Long-term nephrotoxicity of cisplatin, ifosfamide, and methotrexate in osteosarcoma. *Pediatr Nephrol.* 12:572–575.

Koss, L. 1968. Urine sediment cell identification. *In Hematology and Clinical Microscopy Glossary*, 4th edition.

Kraus, A.L. 1980. Research applications. In *Research Methodology In the Laboratory Rat.* Eds. H.J. Baker, J.R. Lindsey, and S.H. Weisbroth, Vols, 11. New York, NY: Academic Press.

Kumar, A. and Fausto, A. 2010. Aldosterone biosynthesis. Inter-relationship of regulatory factors. In *Pathologic Basis of Disease,* 8 edition.

Kurien, B, Everds, N., and Scofield, R. 2004. Experimental animal urine collection: A review. *Lab Anim.* 38:333–361.

Lane, B.R., Poggio, E.D., Herts, B.R., Novick, A.C., and Campbell, S.C. 2009. Renal function assessment in the era of chronic kidney disease: Renewed emphasis on renal function centered patient care. *J Urol.* 182:435–444.

Lane, S.E. and Neuhaus, O.W. 1972. Multiple forms of 2 u, a sex-dependent urinary protein of the adult male rat. *Biochim Biophys Acta.* 263:433–440.

Latimer, K.S., Mahaffey, E.A., and Prasse, K.W. 2011. *Duncan and Prasse's Veterinary Laboratory Medicine: Clinical Pathology*, 4th edition. Ames, IA: Iowa State University Press.

Levinski, N.G. and Lieberthal, W. 1992. Clearance techniques. In *Handbook of Physiology*. Ed. E.E. Windhager, Section 8, Vol. 1, pp. 226–247. Oxford: Oxford University Press.

Liangos, O., Perianayagam, M.C., Vaidya, V.S., et al. 2007. Urinary N-acetyl-beta-(D)-glucosaminidase activity and kidney injury molecule-1 level are associated with adverse outcomes in acute renal failure. *J Am Soc Nephrol.* 18:904–912.

Lisoskwa-Myjak, B. 2010. Serum and urinary biomarkers of acute kidney injury. *Blood Purificat.* 29:357–365.

Loeb, W.F. 1964. The clinical examination: Laboratory procedures. In *Feline Medicine and Surgery*. Ed. E.J. Catcott. Santa Barbara, CA: American Veterinary Publishers.

Loeb, W.F. 1998. The measurement of renal injury. *Toxicol Pathol.* 26:26–28.

Lote, C. 2010. *Principles of Renal Physiology*. Dordrecht: Kluwer Academic Publishers.

Lundqvist, S., Hietala, S.O., and Karp, K. 1995. Experimental studies comparing iohexol and 51Cr-EDTA for glomerular filtration rate measurements. *Acta Radiol.* 36:58–63.

Madero, M., Sarnak, M.J., and Stevens, L.A. 2006. Serum cystatin C as a marker of glomerular filtration rate. *Curr Opin Nephrol Hypertens.* 15:610–616.

Magen, D., Berger, L., Coady, M.J., et al. 2010. A loss-of-function mutation in NaPi-IIa and renal Fanconi's syndrome. *N Engl J Med.* 362:1102–1109.

Maillard, N., M. Mehdi, L. Thibaudin et al. 2010. Creatinine-based GFR predicting equations in renal transplantation: reassessing the tubular secretion effect. *Nephrol Dial Transplant.* 25:3076–3082.

Marchewka, Z. and Dlugosz, A. 1998. Enzymes in urine as markers of nephrotoxicity of cytostatic agents and aminoglycoside antibiotics. *Int Urol Nephrol.* 30:339–348.

Masereeuw, R., Moons, M.M., Smits, P., and Russel, F.G. 1996. Glomerular filtration and saturable absorption of iohexol in the rat isolated perfused kidney. *Br J Pharmacol.* 119:57–64.

Matandos, C.K. and Franz, D.R. 1980. Collection of urine from caged laboratory cats. *Lab Anim Sci.* 30:562–564.

Mendrick, D.L. 2008. Genomic and genetic biomarkers of toxicity. *Toxicology.* 245:175–181.

Mishra, J., Dent, C., Tarabishi, R., et al. 2005. Neutrophil gelatinase-associated lipocalin (NGAL) as a biomarker for acute renal injury after cardiac surgery. *Lancet.* 365:1231–1238.

Mishra, J., Ma, Q., Prada, A., et al. 2003. Identification of neutrophil gelatinase-associated lipocalin as a novel early urinary biomarker for ischemic renal injury. *J Am Soc Nephrol.* 14:2534–2543.

Miyamoto, K. 2001. Use of plasma clearance of iohexol for estimating glomerular filtration rate in cats. *Am J Vet Res.* 62 4:572–575.

Moreland, A.F. 1965. *Methods of Animal Experimentation.* Ed. W.L. Gay, Vol. 1. New York, NY: Academic Press.

Mussap, M. and Plebani, M. 2004. Biochemistry and clinical role of human cystatin C. *Crit Rev Clin Lab Sci.* 41:467–550.

Nesje, M., Flaoyen, A., and Moe, L. 1997. Estimation of glomerular filtration rate in normal sheep by the disappearance of iohexol from serum. *Vet Res Commun.* 21:29–35.

Nickolas, T.L., O'Rourke, M.J., Yang, J., et al. 2008. Sensitivity and specificity of a single emergency department measurement of urinary neutrophil gelatinase-associated lipocalin for diagnosing acute kidney injury. *Ann Intern Med.* 148:810–819.

Nielsen, S., Chou, C., Marples, D., Christensen, E., Kishore, B., and Knepper, M. 1995. Vasopressin increases water permeability of kidney collecting duct by inducing translocation of aquaporin-CD water channels to plasma membrane. *Proc Natl Acad Sci.* 92:1013–1017.

O'Connell, B., Romeo, J.M., and Mudge, G.H. 1962. Renal tubular secretion of creatinine in the dog. *Am J Physiol.* 203:985–990.

O'Reilly, P.H., Brooman, P.J., Martin, P.J., et al. 1986. Accuracy and reproducibility of a new contrast clearance method for the determination of glomerular filtration rate. *Br Med J (Clin Res Ed).* 293:234–236.

Ohashi, F., Kuroda, K., Shimada, T., Shimada, Y., and Ota, M. 1996. The iothalamate clearance in cats with experimentally induced renal failure. *J Vet Med Sci.* 58(8):803–804.

Osborne, C.A., Finco, D.R., and Low, D.G. 1983. Pathophysiology of renal disease. Renal failure and uremia. In *Textbook of Veterinary Internal Medicine*. Ed. S.J. Ettinger. Philadelphia, PA: W.B. Saunders.

Osborne, C.A., Low, D.G., and Finco, D.R. 1972. *Canine and Feline Urology*. Philadelphia, PA: W.B. Saunders.

Owen, D.G. 1992. *Parasites of Laboratory Animals*. London: Royal Society of Medicine Services Ltd.

Ozer, J.S., Dieterle, F., Troth, S., et al. 2010. A panel of urinary biomarkers to monitor reversibility of renal injury and a serum marker with improved potential to assess renal function. *Nat Biotechnol.* 28:486–494.

Parikh, C.R., Lu, J.C., Coca, S.G., and Devarajan, P. 2010. Tubular proteinuria in acute kidney injury: A critical evaluation of current status and future promise. *Ann Clin Biochem.* 47:301–312.

Parsons, P.P., Garland, H.O., and Harpur, E.S. 2000. Localization of the nephron site of gentamicin-induced hypercalciuria in the rat: A micropuncture study. *Br J Pharmacol.* 130:441–449.

Parsons, P.P., Garland, H.O., Harpur, E.S., and Old, S. 1997. Acute gentamicin-induced hypercalciuria and hypermagnesiuria in the rat: Dose-response relationship and role of renal tubular injury. *Br J Pharmacol.* 122:570–576.

Payn, M.M., Webb, M.C., Lawrence, D., and Lamb, E.J. 2002. Alpha1-microglobulin is stable in human urine ex vivo. *Clin Chem.* 48:1136–1138.

Pinches, M., Betts, C., Bickerton, S., et al. 2012. Evaluation of novel renal biomarkers with a cisplatin model of kidney injury: Gender and dosage differences. *Toxicol Pathol.* 40:522–533.

Pooler, J. and Eaton, D. 2009. *Vander's Renal Physiology*, 7th edition. New York, NY: McGraw-Hill Medical.

Price, R.G. 1992a. The role of NAG (N-acetyl-beta-D-glucosaminidase) in the diagnosis of kidney disease including the monitoring of nephrotoxicity. *Clin Nephrol.* 38(Suppl 1):S14–S19.

Price, R.G. 1992b. Measurement of N-acetyl-beta-glucosaminidase and its isoenzymes in urine methods and clinical applications. *Eur J Clin Chem Clin Biochem.* 30:693–705.

Price, S.A., Davies, D., Rowlinson, R., et al. 2010. Characterization of renal papillary antigen 1 (RPA-1), a biomarker of renal papillary necrosis. *Toxicol Pathol.* 38:346–358.

Raab, W.P. 1972. Diagnostic value of urinary enzyme determinations. *Clin Chem.* 18:5–25.

Rached, E., Hoffmann, D., Blumbach, K., et al. 2008. Evaluation of putative biomarkers of nephrotoxicity after exposure to ochratoxin a in vivo and in vitro. *Toxicol Sci.* 103:371–381.

Ragan, H.A. and Gillis, M.F. 1975. Restraint, venipuncture, endotracheal intubation, and anesthesia of miniature swine. *Lab Anim Sci.* 25:409–419.

Rennke H.G. and Denker, B.M. 2010. *Renal Pathophysiology: The Essentials,* 3rd edition. Philadelphia, PA: Lippincott Williams and Wilkins.

Rogers, K.S., Komkov, A., Brown, S.A., et al. 1991. Comparison of four methods of estimating glomerular filtration rate in cats. *Am J Vet Res.* 52:961–964.

Ronnhedh, C., Jaquenod, M., and Mather, L.E. 1996. Urineless estimation of glomerular filtration rate and renal plasma flow in the rat. *J Pharmacol Toxicol Methods.* 36:123–129.

Rose, B.D. 2001. *Clinical Physiology of Acid-Base and Electrolyte Disorders.* New York, NY: McGraw Hill Book Company.

Rosenberg, M.E. and Silkensen, J. 1995. Clusterin: Physiologic and pathophysiologic considerations. *Int J Biochem Cell Biol.* 27:633–645.

Rothstein, M., Obialo, C., and Hruska, K.A. 1990. Renal tubular acidosis. *Endocrinol Metab Clin North Am.* 19:869–887.

Rouse, R.L., Zhang, J., Stewart, S.R., et al. 2011. Comparative profile of commercially available urinary biomarkers in preclinical drug-induced kidney injury and recovery in rats. *Kidney Int.* 79:1186–1197.

Rozell, B., Hansson, H.A., Guthenberg, C., Tahir, M.K., and Mannervik, B. 1993. Glutathione transferases of classes alpha, mu and pi show selective expression in different regions of rat kidney. *Xenobiotica.* 23:835–849.

Ruggenenti, P. and Remuzzi, G. 2006. Time to abandon microalbuminuria? *Kidney Int.* 70:1214–1222.

Russo, L.M., Sandoval, R.M., McKee, M., et al. 2007. The normal kidney filters nephrotic levels of albumin retrieved by proximal tubule cells: Retrieval is disrupted in nephrotic states. *Kidney Int.* 71:504–513.

Saito, K., Uwagawa, S., Kaneko, H., and Yoshitake, A. 1996. Behavior of alpha 2u-globulin accumulating in kidneys of male rats treated with D-limonene: Kidney-type alpha 2u-globulin in the urine as a marker of D-limonene nephropathy. *Toxicology.* 70:173–183.

Sanchez-Bernal, C., Vlitos, M., Cabezas, J.A., and Price, R.G. 1991. Variation in the isoenzymes of N-acetyl-beta-D-glucosaminidase and protein excretion in aminoglycoside nephrotoxicity in the rat. *Cell Biochem Funct.* 9:209–214.

Sapirstein, L.A., Vidt, D.G., Mandel, M.J., and Hanusek, G. 1955. Volumes of distribution and clearances of intravenously injected creatinine in the dog. *Am J Physiol.* 181:330–336.

Schumann, G.B. 1980. *Urine Sediment Examination.* Baltimore, MA: Williams and Wilkins.

Schumann, G.B. and Colon, V.F. 1980. Urine cytology. Part II: renal cytology. *Am Fam Physician.* 21:102–106.

Seibold, H.R. and Thorson, R.E. 1955. *Klossiella equi* n. sp. (Protozoa: Klossiellidae) from the kidney of an American Jack. *J Parasitol.* 41:285–288.

Serafini-Cessi, F., Malagolini, N., and Cavallone, D. 2003. Tamm-Horsfall glycoprotein: Biology and clinical relevance. *Am J Kidney Dis.* 42:658–676.

Shalmi, M., Lunau, H.E., Petersen, J.S., Bak, M., and Christensen, S. 1991. Suitability of tritiated inulin for determination of glomerular filtration rate. *Am J Physiol.* 260:F283–F289.

Shlipak, M.G., Praught, M.L., and Sarnak, M.J. 2006. Update on cystatin C: New insights into the importance of mild kidney dysfunction. *Curr Opin Nephrol Hypertens.* 15:270–275.

Sieber, M., Hoffmann, D., Adler, M., et al. 2009. Comparative analysis of novel noninvasive renal biomarkers and metabonomic changes in a rat model of gentamicin nephrotoxicity. *Toxicol Sci.* 109:336–349.

Silkensen, J.R., Agarwal, A., Nath, K.A., Manivel, J.C., and Rosenberg, M.E. 1997. Temporal induction of clusterin in cisplatin nephrotoxicity. *J Am Soc Nephrol.* 8:302–305.

Slocum, J.L., Heung, M., and Pennathur, S. 2012. Marking renal injury: Can we move beyond serum creatinine? *Transl Res.* 159:277–289.

Smyth, R., Lane, C.S., Ashiq, R., et al. 2009. Proteomic investigation of urinary markers of carbon-tetrachloride-induced hepatic fibrosis in the Hanover Wistar rat. *Cell Biol Toxicol.* 25:499–512.

Sterner, G., Frennby, B., Hultberg, B., and Almen, T. 1996. Iohexol clearance for GFR-determination in renal failure—Single or multiple plasma sampling? *Nephrol Dial Transplant.* 11:521–525.

Stevens, L.A., Coresh, J., Greene, T., and Levey, A.S. 2006. Assessing kidney function—Measured and estimated glomerular filtration rate. *N Engl J Med.* 354:2473–2483.

Stevens, L.A. and Levey, A.S. 2009. Measured GFR as a confirmatory test for estimated GFR. *J Am Soc Nephrol.* 20:2305–2313.

Stockham, S.L. and Scott, M.A. 2002. Urinary system. In *Fundamentals of Veterinary Clinical Pathology.* Ames, IA: Iowa State Press.

Stonard, M.D. 1990. Assessment of renal function and damage in animal species. A review of the current approach of the academic, governmental and industrial institutions represented by the Animal Clinical Chemistry Association. *J Appl Toxicol.* 10:267–274.

Stonard, M.D., Gore, C.W., Oliver, G.J., and Smith, I.K. 1987. Urinary enzymes and protein patterns as indicators of injury to different regions of the kidney. *Fundam Appl Toxicol.* 9:339–351.

Sundberg, A., Appelkvist, E.L., Dallner, G., and Nilsson, R. 1994a. Glutathione transferases in the urine: Sensitive methods for detection of kidney damage induced by nephrotoxic agents in humans. *Environ Health Perspect.* 102(Suppl 3):293–296.

Sundberg, A.G., Appelkvist, E.L., Backman, L., and Dallner, G. 1994b. Urinary pi-class glutathione transferase as an indicator of tubular damage in the human kidney. *Nephron.* 67:308–316.

Sundberg, A.G., Nilsson, R., Appelkvist, E.L., and Dallner, G. 1993. Immunohistochemical localization of alpha and pi class glutathione transferases in normal human tissues. *Pharmacol Toxicol.* 72:321–331.

Swenberg, J.A. 1993. Alpha 2u-globulin nephropathy: Review of the cellular and molecular mechanisms involved and their implications for human risk assessment. *Environ Health Perspect.* 101(Suppl 6):39–44.

Tenstad, O., Roald, A.B., Grubb, A., and Aukland, K. 1996. Renal handling of radiolabelled human cystatin C in the rat. *Scand J Clin Lab Invest.* 56:409–414.

Thomsen, K. and Olesen, O.V. 1981. Effect of anaesthesia and surgery on urine flow and electrolyte excretion in different rat strains. *Ren Physiol.* 4:165–172.

Thongboonkerd, V. 2005. Proteomic analysis of renal diseases: Unraveling the pathophysiology and biomarker discovery. *Expert Rev Proteomics.* 2:349–366.

Thukral, S.K., Nordone, P.J., Hu, R., et al. 2005. Prediction of nephrotoxicant action and identification of candidate toxicity-related biomarkers. *Toxicol Pathol.* 33:343–355.

Togashi, Y., Sakaguchi, Y., Miyamoto, M., and Miyamoto, Y. 2012. Urinary cystatin C as a biomarker for acute kidney injury and its immunohistochemical localization in kidney in the CDDP-treated rats. *Exp Toxicol Path.* 64:797–805.

Tonomura, Y., Tsuchiya, N., Torii, M., and Uehara, T. 2010. Evaluation of the usefulness of urinary biomarkers for nephrotoxicity in rats. *Toxicology.* 273:53–59.

Toto, R.D. 1995. Conventional measurement of renal function utilizing serum creatinine, creatinine clearance, inulin and para-aminohippuric acid clearance. *Curr Opin Nephrol Hypertens.* 4:505–509.

Trof, R.J., Di Maggio, F., Leemreis, J., and Groeneveld, A.B. 2006. Biomarkers of acute renal injury and renal failure. *Shock.* 26:245–253.

Tsuchiya, Y., Tominaga, Y., Matsubayashi, K., Jindo, T., Furuhama, K., and Suzuki, K.T. 2005. Investigation on urinary proteins and renal mRNA expression in canine renal papillary necrosis induced by nefiracetam. *Arch Toxicol.* 79:500–507.

Tugay, S., Bircan, Z., Caglayan, C., Arisoy, A.E., and Gokalp, A.S. 2006. Acute effects of gentamicin on glomerular and tubular functions in preterm neonates. *Pediatr Nephrol.* 21:1389–1392.

Tuladhar, S.M., Puntmann, V.O., Soni, M., Punjabi, P.P., and Bogle, R.G. 2009. Rapid detection of acute kidney injury by plasma and urinary neutrophil gelatinase-associated lipocalin after cardiopulmonary bypass. *J Cardiovasc Pharmacol.* 53:261–266.

Vaidya, V.S., Ferguson, M.A., and Bonventre, J.V. 2008. Biomarkers of acute kidney injury. *Annu Rev Pharmacol Toxicol.* 48:463–493.

Vaidya, V.S., Ozer, J.S., Dieterle, F., et al. 2010. Kidney injury molecule-1 outperforms traditional biomarkers of kidney injury in preclinical biomarker qualification studies. *Nat Biotechnol.* 28:478–485.

Vaidya, V.S., Ramirez, V., Ichimura, T., Bobadilla, N.A., and Bonventre, J.V. 2006. Urinary kidney injury molecule-1: A sensitive quantitative biomarker for early detection of kidney tubular injury. *Am J Physiol Renal Physiol.* 290:F517–F529.

Vinken, P., Starckx, S., Barale-Thomas, E., et al. 2012. Tissue kim-1 and urinary clusterin as early indicators of cisplatin-induced acute kidney injury in rats. *Toxicol Pathol.* 40:1049–1062.

Waikar, S.S., Sabbisetti, V.S., and Bonventre, J.V. 2010. Normalization of urinary biomarkers to creatinine during changes in glomerular filtration rate. *Kidney Int.* 78:486–494.

Watts, R.H. 1971 A simple capillary tube method for the determination of the specific gravity of 25 and 50 microliter quantities of urine. *J Clin Pathol.* 24:667–668.

Weber, M.H. and Verwiebe, R. 1992. Alpha 1-microglobulin (protein HC): Features of a promising indicator of proximal tubular dysfunction. *Eur J Clin Chem Clin Biochem.* 30:683–691.

Westhuyzen, J. 2006. Cystatin C: A promising marker and predictor of impaired renal function. *Ann Clin Lab Sci.* 36:387–394.

Westhuyzen, J., Endre, Z.H., Reece, G., et al. 2003. Measurement of tubular enzymuria facilitates early detection of acute renal impairment in the intensive care unit. *Nephrol Dial Transplant.* 18:543–551.

Williams, G.H. and Dluhy, R.G. 1972. Aldosterone biosynthesis. Interrelationship of regulatory factors. *Am J Med.* 53:595–605.

Wu, A.H.B. 2006. *Tietz Clinical Guide to Laboratory Tests*, 4th edition. St. Louis, MO: Saunders Elsevier.

Wyss, M. and Kaddurah-Daouk, R. 2000. Creatine and creatinine metabolism. *Physiol Rev.* 80:1107–1213.

Yoshida, T., Kurella, M., Beato, F., et al. 2002. Monitoring changes in gene expression in renal ischemia-reperfusion in the rat. *Kidney Int.* 61:1646–1654.

Young, L.S., Regan, M.C., Barry, M.K., Geraghty, J.G., and Fitzpatrick, J.M. 1996. Methods of renal blood flow measurement. *Urol Res.* 24:149–160.

Yu, Y., Jin, H., Holder, D., et al. 2010. Urinary biomarkers trefoil factor 3 and albumin enable early detection of kidney tubular injury. *Nat Biotechnol.* 28:470–477.

Zhou, Y., Vaidya, V.S., Brown, R.P., et al. 2008. Comparison of kidney injury molecule-1 and other nephrotoxicity biomarkers in urine and kidney following acute exposure to gentamicin, mercury, and chromium. *Toxicol Sci.* 101:159–170.

Zinkl, J.G, 1999. Urinary sediment and cytology of the urinary tract. In *Diagnostic Cytology and Hematology of the Dog and Cat,* 2nd edition. Cowell, R.L., Tyler, R.D. and Meinkoth, J.H. (eds.) St, Louis, MO: Mosby.

13 Evaluation of Cardiovascular and Pulmonary Function and Injury

Peter O'Brien

CONTENTS

13.1 THE HEART

The cardiovascular system is comprised of three circulatory systems (Stephenson, 2007). The systemic circulation nourishes the body, except for the lungs and heart, which have their own pulmonary and coronary circulations, respectively. Muscular arteries leave the aorta, and branch and narrow into arterioles of the microcirculation. These arterioles branch, narrow, and simplify even further into capillaries whose walls are formed by only the inner vascular lining of the endothelial cells. Here, the passage of blood is slowed and restricted to one blood cell at a time, thereby facilitating nutrient delivery and waste removal. Oxygen is exchanged for carbon dioxide, or vice versa in the lung. Moreover, there is exchange of metabolic substrate and water from metabolic waste products, such as lactic acid. The capillaries then coalesce into venules, which exit the microcirculation by fusing into elastic veins that return blood to the heart by the vena cava for the systemic circulation, or by the pulmonary vein. The high elasticity and low muscularity of veins, compared to arteries, allow them to have approximately 20-fold greater capacity for distension with increasing pressure and to store approximately two-thirds of blood volume.

Blood pressure is the pressure exerted by blood on the vessel walls. It is the potential energy that causes blood flow and is determined by the product of two variables: the cardiac output and the resistance. The former is the product of heart rate and the amount of blood ejected from the ventricle with each beat, the stroke volume. Resistance is largely dependent on arteriolar lumenal diameter, which, like cardiac output, is regulated by innervation from the autonomic nervous system and by various circulating hormones. These contract the circumferential, smooth muscle of arteries. An artery's resistance increases inversely with the fourth power of its radius. In a dog, a typical mean arterial pressure is approximately 100 mmHg, the vena caval pressure is approximately 3 mmHg, and the cardiac output is approximately 2.5 L/min. Thus, the total peripheral resistance is approximately 40 mmHg for each L/min of systemic blood flow (Stephenson, 2007).

The renin–angiotensin–aldosterone system (RAAS) is one of the most important regulators of the cardiovascular system (Stephenson, 2007; Bader, 2010). The renal macula densa produces the plasma protease renin, which hydrolyzes angiotensinogen from the liver to release the decapeptide angiotensin I (Ang I), which in turn is hydrolyzed by endothelial, angiotensin-converting enzyme (ACE) to the octapeptide angiotensin II (Ang II). ACE is also known to hydrolyze kinins. Ang II increases blood volume and pressure by multiple actions. It binds primarily type 1 angiotensin II (1AT1) receptors to cause blood vessel constriction, sodium, and water retention by the proximal renal tubules, increased thirst, activation of the sympathetic nervous system (SNS), and zona glomerulosa production of aldosterone in the adrenal cortex. The latter acts on renal collecting ducts and enhances sodium retention along with chloride and excretion of potassium.

Local RAAS also occurs in heart, kidney, brain, and vessels enhancing the effects of the circulating RAAS (Bader, 2010). RAAS has important regulatory roles in cardiovascular physiology, but have also been shown to be involved in the pathogenesis of hypertension and of heart failure. Mediators, such as Ang I and II, directly act on cardiomyocytes, cause renal and cardiac fibrosis, and are considered key drug targets for the treatment of cardiovascular disease.

Ang II also binds to type 2 angiotensin II (AT2) receptors that are found only sparsely in healthy vascular, myocardial, or neuronal tissues but are markedly up-regulated following injury. Activation of AT2 receptors antagonizes many of the pathophysiological effects of AT1 receptor activation such as oxidative stress, inflammation, fibrosis, vasoconstriction, and myocardiocyte hypertrophy.

The natriuretic peptides, primarily produced by the cardiomyocytes, are critical in the regulation of fluid balance (van Kimmenade and Januzzi, 2009). Atrial natriuretic peptide (ANP), synonymous with atrial natriuretic factor and atriopeptin, is produced and stored by atria in granules and released in response to increased tension in the atrial walls, owing to increased volume or pressure. Natriuresis and diuresis are produced by an increase in glomerular filtration rate (GFR), affected by dilation of the afferent, with simultaneous constriction of the efferent, glomerular arterioles. These effects are largely due to receptor-mediated activation of guanylate cyclase causing increases in cyclic guanosine monophosphate (cGMP). The diuretic and natriuretic actions are also due to inhibition of sodium resorption in the proximal convoluted tubule and cortical collecting ducts, and of renin, aldosterone, and norepinephrine secretion. ANP has relaxing effects on vascular and myocardial muscle. If the increase in tension in the atrial wall is prolonged, there is marked induction of ventricular synthesis for further increasing the atrial ANP effects.

B-type (formerly called brain-type) natriuretic peptide is largely produced by ventricles in response to myocardial stretch and anoxia. Neuroendocrine factors also provoke its release, such as Ang II, interleukin (IL) 1β, and adrenergic agents. It has similar effects as ANP on natriuresis and diuresis by glomerular actions and by inhibition of RAAS and the SNS. It also has antiproliferative and antifibrotic effects on the heart, which are protective in heart disease.

There are local or autocrine or paracrine natriuretic peptides. One, structurally similar to ANP, urodilatin, is produced by distal renal tubules and has similar but locally restricted effects on the kidney and adrenals. There is a C-type natriuretic peptide (CNP) found in blood vessels, kidney, central nervous system (CNS), and the pituitary (Archer, 2003). This lacks direct diuretic effect but retains vascular relaxation effects. Moreover, it may serve as a central neurotransmitter and reproductive factor, and may be involved in bone growth. One isoform of CNP is considered the ancestral origin of the natriuretic peptides. CNP is also expressed in macrophages in response to inflammatory mediators and is increased with sepsis (DeClue et al., 2011).

13.1.1 Cardiac Function

The heart is a specialized muscle whose primary function is to pump blood through the body with sufficient pressure and volume to provide oxygen for aerobic metabolism (Stephenson, 2007). It does this in a cyclical process of contraction and relaxation during which blood is expelled from, and enters into, respectively, its muscular ventricles. The heart must respond to widely changing demands for oxygen delivery for tissue metabolism. For immediate response to these demands, the heart has high reserve capacity for adjusting the rate and volume of blood ejected. This is highly regulated by a complex, neuroendocrine system. For longer term changes in demand, the heart can additionally adapt its mass and its regulatory system. Thus, the heart rate, stroke volume, and heart-to-body weight ratio vary according to differences in functional demand that are related to species, breed or strain, age, gender, physical activity, nutritional state, endocrine state, and as well, a wide range of pathologies (Martin et al., 1993; O'Brien, 1998).

Across a wide range of mammalian species, logarithms of (log) heart size and stroke volume are proportional to log body size; whereas, log resting heart rate is inversely proportional to log body size (West et al., 1997). However, additional capacity is observed in more athletic species and strains or breeds than would be predicted by this relationship (Weibel et al., 2004; Painter, 2005). In contrast, diminished capacity is found with pathology (Van Vleet and Ferrans, 2007). For example, in healthy, adult, laboratory animals, heart-to-body weight ratio (%) varies from 0.24 in rats, 0.27 in rabbits, 0.35 in cynomolgus monkeys, 0.42 in guinea pigs, 0.46 in cats, 0.58 in mice, to 0.75 in dogs (Joseph, 1908; Gray, 1945; Drevon-Gaillot et al., 2006). Most exceptional of these data is that for the mouse, the smallest of these laboratory animals; it has a considerably higher heart weight than would be predicted by the allometric relationship between heart weight and body size for mammals Normal heart rates vary substantially. In dogs, normal heart rates vary from 90 beats per minute (bpm) at rest to 270 bpm at maximal exercise, and in mice normal heart rates vary from 160 bpm during fasting-induced torpor to 500–600 bpm at rest and 840 bpm with maximal exercise (Swoap and Gutilla, 2009). Even greater ranges are achieved in racing greyhounds owing to a significantly greater heart-to-body weight ratio as compared with other dog breeds. Greyhounds can increase resting heart rates from 30 to over 400 bpm (Gunn, 1989; Engleking, 2009).

Capacity for physiological performance of the heart correlates with the activities of three subcellular biochemical systems for contraction, metabolism, and intracellular calcium regulation (Martin et al., 1993). The timing, rate, and degree of the contraction and relaxation cycle of the heart are determined by the timing, rate, and degree of the contraction and relaxation cycle of the contractile myofilaments within the cardiomyocyte (Stephenson, 2007). These in turn are determined by the timing, rate, and magnitude of the intracellular cycle of calcium release and sequestration by the sarcoplasmic reticulum (Martin et al., 1993; O'Brien et al., 1988). An incremental increase in the heart rate of various etiologies is associated with a similar increment in sarcoplasmic reticulum Ca-ATPase activity (O'Brien et al., 1988). Mitochondria provide the energy necessary for these calcium and contraction cycles. Biomarker activities for all three subcellular systems are proportional to cardiac performance across a wide range of species, with adaptation to physiologically increased, functional demand, and with deterioration during various pathological states (Martin et al., 1993; O'Brien and Gwathmey, 1995; O'Brien, 1998).

13.1.2 Cardiac Injury

Cardiac injury may arise from a wide diversity of causes including those that affect the heart primarily, but also those that affect other organs or systems and result in secondary injury to the heart (O'Brien, 2006, 2008; Serra et al., 2010). Etiologies for primary cardiac injury include the following: genetic, nutritional, physical trauma, inflammation, neoplasia, infectious organisms, xenobiotics, hemodynamic overload, severe exertion, ischemia and anoxia, old age, or marked stress. Cardiac injury may also occur secondarily to disease affecting another tissue, organ, or system. Secondary causes include various endocrinopathies (e.g., hyperthyroidism, uncontrolled and marked hypercortisolism, or Addison's disease), marked anemia, pancreatitis, renal disease, and metastatic tumors (Serra et al., 2010).

13.1.2.1 Primary Cardiac Injury

Inherited cardiomyopathy is one type of primary cardiac injury. The Sprague–Dawley rat is commonly affected by an age-dependent and gender-modified spontaneous cardiomyopathy (Kemi et al., 2000; O'Brien et al, 2006). This cardiomyopathy is evident from the finding that at 6–8 months of age, Sprague–Dawley male rats have approximately 10-fold greater levels of serum cardiac troponin I (cTnI), a biomarker of cardiac injury, as compared to age-matched female rats and male rats 3 months of age (O'Brien et al., 2006). These age-dependent cTnI increases correlated with minimal-to-mild, degenerative histopathological change. Spontaneous cardiomyopathy is well described in the Syrian hamster and recently described in the cynomolgus monkey (Recchia and Lionetti, 2007, Zabka et al., 2009) while idiopathic cardiomyopathy affects more than half of chimpanzees (Seiler et al., 2008). There are spontaneous hypertensive rats and the Dahl salt-sensitive strain of rats that develop pathological hypertension leading to pressure overload and cardiac failure (Balakumar et al., 2007). Aging also produces cardiac injury, apparently in association with oxidative stress and the formation of lipofucsin pigment, which may cause a brown discoloration of the myocardium and may be observed at necropsy. Moreover, cardiac injury may occur due to primary neoplasia in the heart such as with hemangiosarcoma or heart base tumors (e.g., chemodectomas), as well occurring secondarily owing to metastasis of neoplasia from another organ, such as with lymphoma (Maxie and Robinson, 2007; Van Vleet and Ferrans, 2007).

Primary cardiac injuries are not only characterized by their etiology, but by the associated morphological or functional cardiac changes. For example, cardiomyopathies may be dilated, hypertrophic, or arrhythmogenic. Other categories include ventricular arrhythmia, pericardial effusion, valvular disease (mitral, aortic insufficiency jet lesions), subaortic stenosis, infarct, and third degree heart block (Serra et al., 2010).

13.1.2.2 Spontaneous Myocarditis

Spontaneous myocarditis is found in preclinical toxicology studies at necropsy in all species, but especially in nonhuman primates. As natural infectious causes of myocarditis are uncommon in nonhuman primates, it is suspected that it may be secondary to stress-induced cardiac injury (Chamanza et al., 2006, 2010). Proinflammatory cytokines such as ILs 1β and 6, tumor necrosis factor (TNF-α), and interferon-γ impair cardiac function by causing myocardiocyte apoptosis, and cardiac remodeling, hypertrophy, and dilation. These cytokines regulate the expression of matrix metalloproteinases (MMPs) and the tissue inhibitors of MMP (TIMP), as well as the cardiac fibroblast production of collagen and fibronectin (Rutschow et al., 2006).

In nonhuman primates, the incidence of spontaneous myocarditis is approximately 20%, compared to approximately 1% for pericarditis or endocarditis (Chamanza et al., 2006, 2010). Males were about 50% more frequently affected than females, and rhesus monkeys were twice as frequently affected as marmosets and cynomolgus monkeys. Inflammatory infiltrates were predominantly mononuclear cells in the primates, especially lymphocytes, and frequently associated with myocardial degeneration and edema or fibrin deposition. In beagles, the incidence of spontaneous myocarditis is approximately 5% for males and 2% for females (Greaves, 2007). In rats, only occasional cases are seen, and in mice even less (Greaves, 2007).

13.1.2.3 Trauma

Blunt trauma may occur during handling and restraint, especially with small animals, and could cause release of biomarkers of myocardial injury. For example, mild mechanical trauma produced by rotating mice in a drum caused cardiac dysfunction, myocardial cell apoptosis, and mild increases in cTnI, a biomarker of cardiac injury (Tao et al., 2005). Direct, physical injury also occurs during blood sampling by cardiac puncture, and as this is associated with, increases in cardiac injury biomarkers in the sampled blood, it is not recommended as a sampling technique for samples to be analyzed for cardiac biomarkers (O'Brien et al., 1997a). The increase in serum troponin may occur because of contamination of myocardial tissue in the bore of the needle. Presumably, the injury produced by cardiac puncture could also increase circulating injury biomarkers.

13.1.2.4 Infectious Disease

Cardiac injury from infectious or parasitic disease is not common in laboratory animals, but it may occur (Wells and Sleeper, 2008; Serra et al., 2010). For example, in young dogs, parvovirus infection may cause focal myocardial inflammation followed by fibrosis (Gagnon et al., 1980). Myocarditis induced by parvovirus in man causes increased serum cardiac troponin (Baig et al., 2006). Heartworm infections are well described in dogs and cats. Babesiosis (Lobetti et al., 2002), leishmaniasis (Silvestrini et al., 2010), ehrlichiosis (Diniz et al., 2008), leptospirosis (Mastrorilli et al., 2007), foot-and-mouth disease (Tunca et al., 2008), endotoxemia (Peek et al., 2008) have all been identified as causes of myocardial injury, with increases in serum cardiac troponin.

13.1.2.5 Cardiotoxicity

Numerous classes of drugs have been demonstrated to directly produce cardiac injury (O'Brien, 2008). Anticancer drugs are widely associated with cardiotoxicity, including alkylating agents, anthraquinones, anthracyclines, antimetabolites, various monoclonal antibody treatments, and IL-2. Other drug classes causing cardiotoxicity are the sympathomimetics such as adrenergic agonists and phosphodiesterase inhibitors (PDEi), antiretroviral drugs such as the nucleoside reverse transcriptase inhibitors and protease inhibitors, and peroxisomal-proliferator-activated receptor alpha (PPARα) agonists (Pruimboom-Brees et al., 2006). It is noteworthy, that the latter toxicity is only known to occur in mice and rats. Increased oxidative stress and mitochondrial injury are frequently involved in the pathogenesis of myocardial toxicity, although the overstimulatory effects of suprapharmacologic doses of sympathomimetics (e.g., ephedrine) may disrupt myocardial perfusion and cause ischemic necrosis. Significant myocardial injury causes necrosis leading to inflammation followed by fibrosis and mineralization. If these changes are extensive, they may lead to compromised cardiac function and heart failure.

13.1.2.6 Hemodynamic Overload

Functional overload of the heart, if excessive and prolonged, may overwhelm adaptive capacity and cause development of cardiac failure (Muders and Elsner, 2000). The overload may be due to increased preload, which occurs with increased volume of blood, or due to increased afterload, which occurs with increased arterial pressure. Less commonly, it may occur due to a chronically increased cardiac rate (O'Brien et al., 1994). The ventricles respond to a chronically increased hemodynamic burden with progressive hypertrophy. With volume overload, hypertrophy is eccentric. Moreover, it occurs with dilatation of the ventricular cavity and an increase in myocardial mass such that the ratio between wall thickness and ventricular cavity size remains relatively constant. With chronic pressure overload, hypertrophy is concentric; it occurs such that the ratio between wall thickness and ventricular cavity size increases (Maxie and Robinson, 2007). Fluid retention and volume overload occur with chronic treatment with thiazolidinedione insulin sensitizers (i.e., glitazones, PPARγ agonists) and rarely with insulin, producing cardiac hypertrophy that can progress to cardiac failure (Kalambokis et al., 2004; Bas et al., 2010; Chaggar et al., 2009). Systemic hypertension and pressure overload occur with hypercortisolism, and produce cardiac hypertrophy (Reini et al., 2008).

13.1.2.7 Endocrinopathy

Excessive endocrine stimulation may also cause cardiac injury (Van Vleet and Ferrans, 2007). Stress, which occurs with unaccustomed handling or restraint, especially in nonhuman primates, produces cardiac injury owing to the excessive stimulation of SNS and catecholamine release by a mechanism similar to that described above for the sympathomimetics (Akashi et al., 2010). As thyroid and growth hormones are critical growth factors for the heart, hypertrophic cardiomyopathy with progression to heart failure may occur with chronic hyperthyroidism or excessive secretion of growth hormone as seen in acromegaly (Clayton, 2003). Surprisingly, growth hormone releasing hormone may have direct cardioprotective effects after cardiac injury (Kanashiro-Takeuchi et al., 2010). As indicated above, hypercortisolism occurring with Cushing's disease also has a cardiotrophic effect, in part by activation of the mineralocorticoid receptor (Reini et al., 2008). Hypoaldosteronism occurring with Addison's disease results in impaired sodium and water retention and excretion of potassium. The resultant hypovolemia and hyperkalemia and acidosis may result in impaired cardiac activity, brown atrophy, and ischemic injury (Goodof and Macbryde, 1944; Fallo et al., 1999).

13.1.2.8 Nutrient Deficiency

Cardiac atrophy occurs in parallel with body weight loss during inanition due to deficient caloric and protein intake (Keys et al., 1947). Dietary insufficiency of various macrominerals such as calcium, magnesium, phosphate, and potassium has adverse effects on cardiac performance because of the critical role these ions play in regulating activity. For example, calcium influx during the action potential activates myocardium. Its deficiency has negative inotropic effects with compensatory positive chronotropic effects mediated by the neuroendocrine system (Stephenson, 2007). Chronic hypocalcemia, with untreated hypoparathyroidism or vitamin D deficiency, can cause dilated cardiomyopathy (Sung et al., 2010). The action of calcium is opposed by magnesium. Magnesium, along with phosphate, has a critical role in energy metabolism. Potassium is important in maintaining the resting and action potentials, as well as activating key regulatory enzymes of metabolic pathways. In severe potassium deficiency due to decreased intake or pharmacologic antagonists of potassium homeostasis, cardiac output may be impaired and arrhythmias may develop and lead to heart failure

(Serebruany, 2006) and myocardial necrosis (Allen, 1955). Vitamin E and selenium play critical roles in protection from oxidative stress, and deficiencies of these micronutrients are well known to be associated with cardiomyopathy (Green and Lemckert, 1977; Maxie and Robinson, 2007). Thiamin deficiency, because of its critical role in oxidative metabolism, also impairs cardiac function. Moreover, severe deficiency causes wet beriberi with heart failure (Tran, 2006).

13.1.2.9 Ischemia and Hypoxia

Ischemia and hypoxia are common causes of cardiac injury and necrosis and occur with a wide range of pathologies including myocardial infarct, coronary thrombosis, hypovolemia occurring with marked hypoalbuminemia or shock, anesthesia and depression of the respiratory system, or gastric dilation and volvulus (Maxie and Robinson, 2007; Van Vleet and Ferrans, 2007; Serra et al., 2010). The mineralocorticoid receptor is thought to induce cardiac hypertrophy and fibrosis in response to ischemia. Systemic administration of blockers of this receptor has been shown to reduce markers of inflammation and fibrosis (Fallo et al., 1999). Marked anemia, with hematocrits less than 20% are typically associated with myocardial injury, as indicated by increases in blood troponin in dogs and cats (Serra et al., 2010). The cardiac injury is reasonably attributed to anoxia.

13.1.2.10 Pancreatitis

Pancreatitis and the subsequent release of a wide range of degradative enzymes and myocardial depressant factor cause cardiac injury and is associated with impaired cardiac performance and release of myocardial biomarkers into the peripheral blood (Serra et al., 2010).

13.1.2.11 Renal Disease

In human renal failure, myocardial injury occurs with increased short-term mortality (Martin et al., 1998). Apparently, uremia occurring with renal failure causes accumulation of toxic substances in the blood that produce cardiac injury. Recent studies demonstrate that myocardial injury also occurs in dogs that have severe renal disease (Sharkey et al., 2009; Serra et al., 2010).

13.1.2.12 Marked Stress or Exertion

Marked stress may increase catecholamine levels to the point that myocardial necrosis occurs. This has been well described in the stress-susceptible pig (O'Brien and Ball, 2006), but is well known to occur in man (Akashi et al., 2010) and laboratory animals (O'Brien, 2008). Exertional rhabdomyolysis may occur with unaccustomed or extreme levels of exertion such as in racing or capture myopathy; this is a well-known syndrome associated with cardiac injury and is likely associated with tachycardia, hypercatecholemia, and anoxia, all of which can individually cause cardiac necrosis (Wells et al., 2009).

13.1.3 Impact of Cardiac Injury on Other Organ Systems

Failure of the heart causes underperfusion and limited function of various viscera and skeletal muscle. There is loss of muscle mass and aerobic capacity with exercise intolerance (Minotti et al., 1991; Miller et al., 2010). Hepatic passive congestion occurs with impairment of liver function and hepatocyte injury that releases intracellular enzymes, such as alanine and aspartate transaminases (O'Brien et al., 1993). Renal underperfusion causes decreased GFR with increases in urea and creatinine, and other metabolites and ions normally filtered by the kidney.

The decreased cardiac output stimulates activation of central and peripheral mechanisms to restore output and maintains tissue perfusion. Initially, the compensatory mechanisms maintain circulatory homeostasis. There is a balance of salt and water retention by the RAAS and antidiuretic hormone (ADH) with diuresis produced by ANP. There is also a balance of endogenous mechanisms for vasoconstriction, such as the RAAS, SNS, ADH, endothelin, and thromoboxanes, and for vasodilation, such as the parasympathetic nervous system (PNS), prostacyclin, ANP, and nitric oxide. However, in the later phase, there is excessive vasoconstriction, which inhibits left ventricular outflow to reduce cardiac output. The degree of activation of the compensatory mechanisms correlates with prognosis and life expectancy with plasma norepinephrine concentration having one of the highest predictive values (Cohn et al., 1984).

13.1.4 Biomarkers of Cardiac Injury

13.1.4.1 Historical Biomarkers (Creatine Kinase and Lactate Dehydrogenase)

Historically, myocardial injury has been assessed by electrophoretic measurement of cardiac-specific isozymes (multiple forms of an enzyme that catalyze the same reaction) of lactate dehydrogenase (LD) and creatine kinase (CK), enzymes important in intermediary metabolism (Archer, 2003; O'Brien et al., 1997a; O'Brien, 2009). Recently, immunoassays have been developed for the assay of the human CK isozyme that is the most specific biomarker for cardiac injury, CK-MB, although these assays are usually not effective for laboratory animal use because of poor cross-species reactivity (O'Brien et al., 1997a). Each of these two enzymes, LD and CK, is coded by two different genes, although CK is a dimer comprised of only two gene products and LD is a tetramer comprised of four gene products. The different isozymes are formed by the random association of transcripts of two genes that are differentially expressed depending on the tissue type. Cardiac muscle expresses far more of its B than its M gene for CK, and far more of its H than its M gene for LD than occurs in skeletal muscle. Consequently, CK-MB and LD-H_4 (i.e., LD1), and LDH_3M_1 (i.e., LD2) are useful biomarkers of cardiac injury. Cardiac disease apparently further increases the myocardial expression of the B gene. The cardiac isozyme of LD can be measured as hydroxybutyrate dehydrogenase (HBDH) by automated assay based on its substrate specificity for hydroxybutyrate. In a study of blunt trauma in dogs, this was found to be more sensitive than CK-MB (Schober et al., 1999).

Several factors have limited the use of CK and LD isozymes as cardiac biomarkers in animals. First, their tissue specificity is not absolute. For example, slow twitch muscle may express cardiac isozymes. Furthermore, in commonly used laboratory animals, liver, erythrocytes, leukocytes, and platelets may express cardiac LD isozymes, so that liver injury, hemolysis and clotting may confound the diagnosis of cardiac injury (O'Brien et al., 1997a; Walker, 2006). In erythrocytes, LD-1 predominates in guinea pigs, LD-4 or LD-5 predominates in rats and mice, and an intermediate LD isozyme predominates in the hamster (Yasuda et al., 1990). In liver, LD-5 predominates for mice, rats, and hamsters, but not for guinea pigs, where intermediate isozymes predominate (Yasudas, 1990). In the rat, platelets contain mostly LD-5 at a similar level of activity as in erythrocytes, but CK in platelets was approximately 30-fold higher than in erythrocytes and found to be exclusively CK-BB (Beck et al., 1997). Leukocytes of dog and rabbit, but not cat, preferentially express cardiac over skeletal muscle LD isozymes (Washizu et al., 2002). Secondly, and more importantly, these isozymes have poor sensitivity. This reflects significant background levels in the blood and relatively low levels in myocardium of the tissue-specific form compared to the total activity (Aktas et al., 1993). Consequently, their release usually causes less than an order of magnitude increase in the blood. Furthermore, the kinetics of their release and clearance are insufficient to cause early and prolonged increases in the blood. For example, after cardiac injury in man, there is a rapid rise of plasma CK-MB levels reaching a peak within 12 hours and baseline levels within 1–2 days due to rapid clearance. Increases in plasma LD levels are slower, peaking within 48 hours and clearing within several days (Babuin and Jaffe, 1995). Finally, species-specific immunoassays for CK-MB and LD isozymes are not commercially available for use in nonhuman species.

13.1.4.2 Myoglobin and Fatty Acid Binding Protein 3

Myoglobin and fatty acid binding protein 3 (FABP3) are important cytosolic proteins in intermediary metabolism of striated muscle and are small proteins that leak out of cardiac muscle rapidly after injury with plasma levels peaking within 6 hours. Because of rapid release from damaged tissue and high cardiac concentrations, myoglobin and FABP3 have the potential to be used as sensitive biomarkers of acute injury (Mion et al., 2007). However, these biomarkers are cleared by the kidney within 12–24 hours of injury and their effective use as cardiac biomarkers is substantially limited because of their lack of specificity. For example, myoglobin is found in high concentration in aerobic striated muscle (O'Brien et al., 1992). Although FABP3 is preferentially found in cardiac tissue, it is also found in skeletal muscle and kidney. As such, injury to these other tissues should be excluded before they could be used as cardiac biomarkers and their use may be restricted to negative prediction (i.e., exclusion) of peracute myocardial injury. Finally, the use of myoglobin and FABP3 as biomarkers is also limited by the absence of commercially available, species-specific immunoassays.

13.1.4.3 Ischemia-Modified Albumin

Ischemia-modified albumin (IMA) forms in blood of capillaries within minutes of onset of myocardial ischemia due to oxidative stress (van Belle et al., 2010). This causes changes in the amino end of plasma albumin that decreases its cobalt binding activity, which can be measured by an automated clinical chemistry analyzer method. Plasma levels of IMA peak in a couple of hours and return to baseline within 6 hours (Gaze, 2009). In man, it has been recently demonstrated to be increased with myocardial ischemia (Bar-Or et al., 2000), and, in combination with other cardiac biomarkers, it has been demonstrated to provide additional prognostic information for myocardial ischemic patients (Anwaruddin et al., 2005; van Belle et al., 2010). However, despite high sensitivity for myocardial ischemia, IMA lacks specificity, being also elevated with cerebral, mesenteric, skeletal, and pulmonary ischemia, with severe renal and liver disease, and certain neoplasms. Similar to FABP3 and myoglobin, it may also be useful as a negative or rule-out biomarker of peracute myocardial injury. However, its effective use in laboratory animals has not been proven.

13.1.4.4 Cardiac Troponin

Cardiac troponin (cTn) is currently the gold standard biomarker for acute cardiac injury in man (Daubert and Jeremias, 2010). It is extensively used for detection and assessment of active and ongoing cardiac injury in heart disease (Babuin and Jaffe, 2005). In addition, it has been extensively used for clinical assessment and monitoring of cardiac toxicity in humans being treated for cancer (Shakir and Rasul, 2009).

Troponin regulates the interaction of thin and thick contractile muscle filaments comprised of actin and myosin, respectively (Solaro et al., 2008). Troponin is a complex of three, small globular proteins: C that binds calcium (cTnC), I that inhibits actin and myosin interaction (cTnI), and T that binds tropomyosin (cTnT). These proteins have molecular weights of 23, 18, and 37 kDa, respectively. Calcium binding causes sequential conformation changes in cTnC, cTnI, and tropomyosin that cause cTnI to detach from actin and tropomyosin and to roll out of the way of the myosin cross-bridges that pull on the actin filaments to contract muscle (Metzger and Westfall, 2004).

The high sensitivity and near absolute specificity of cTn have made it the preferred biomarker for myocardial infarct in humans (Daubert and Jeremias, 2010). It is used in man for the identification of myocardial injury and risk stratification, as its elevation correlates with clinical severity and life expectancy (Babuin and Jaffe, 2005). Troponin is now used as a biomarker in a wide range of cardiac injuries, including unstable angina and minimal infarct, left ventricular hypertrophy, congestive heart failure, pulmonary embolism, blunt trauma, sepsis, moderate renal disease and renal failure, diabetes mellitus, and cardiotoxicity associated with anticancer drugs and sympathomimetics. Initially, the delayed onset to peak plasma concentrations (up to 12 hours) following cardiac infarct limited the early use of cTn; however, recent high sensitivity assays have been introduced and preliminary studies in humans using these newer assays demonstrate earlier increases in plasma cTn levels following cardiac injury (Keller et al., 2009).

In the last 10 years, several dozen preclinical published studies have directly confirmed the effectiveness of cTn in laboratory animals for the assessment of cardiotoxicity, including identification, quantitation, and prognosis of cardiotoxicity (O'Brien et al., 1997a; Wallace et al., 2004; O'Brien, 2006, 2008; Serra et al., 2010). The cTn response in animal models in which cardiac muscle injury is induced is similar to the human cTn response to cardiac muscle injury with respect to cardiac tissue specificity, association with cardiac histological change, and the onset, magnitude, and duration of cTn response. cTn is a dose-responsive biomarker of cardiac injury that correlates with severity of injury at the cellular, tissue, physiological, and clinical levels (O'Brien, 2008).

In veterinary medicine, cTn is rapidly emerging as the preferred biomarker for the detection of myocardial injury in more than a dozen mammalian species. There have been approximately 100 reports of its effective use in various disease states, including a wide range of primary cardiac diseases, numerous infectious diseases, severe respiratory disease, trauma, exertion, anemia, pancreatitis, uncontrolled Cushings and Addisons, hyperthyroidism, sepsis, systemic neoplasia, old age, severe colic, and renal failure (O'Brien, 2008; Wells and Sleeper, 2008; Serra et al., 2010).

Cardiac troponin, predominantly cTnI, has essentially replaced all other biomarkers of myocardial injury over the last decade, first in humans and now in veterinary medicine and preclinical and clinical safety studies. This reflects not only its unique and extraordinary myocardial specificity and diagnostic sensitivity for myocardial injury but also its robustness as a biomarker, and the simplicity and accessibility of assays (Table 13.1; O'Brien, 2006, 2008).

The troponins are released from cardiac tissue during the active phase of cell lysis and return to baseline following termination of active pathogenesis. In situations of progressive cell injury, there is a long-sustained increase in serum troponins. In human and animal studies, cTn has been demonstrated to be the first released within minutes of myocardial injury with peak plasma levels occurring as early as 2–6 hours depending on the duration and severity of the cardiac injury. In experimental models of myocardial infarct in dogs in which coronary occlusion was restricted to 90 minutes, peak plasma cTn levels are seen in 3–4 hours (O'Brien, et al., 1997a). In rats treated with a single, subcutaneous toxic dose of isoproterenol, plasma concentrations of cTnI and cTnT peaked within 2–6 hours. In these rat and dog models, cTnI increases correlated with the severity of histopathological cardiac lesions and infarct size at 3 hours (O'Brien et al., 2006). With naturally occurring myocardial infarct in humans, plasma cTn levels typically rise within 4–6 hours and peak at 18–24 hours. At 72 hours, plasma concentrations correlated with scintigraphic measurement of infarct size. In a rat study with cardiotoxicity induced by a single dose of isoproterenol, cTnI was found to increase almost 800 times the minimal detectable concentration and to decrease with a half-life of 6 hours, resulting in an expected return to baseline of 2.5 days (O'Brien et al., 2006).

TABLE 13.1
Advantage of cTn over Other Cardiac Injury Biomarkers

- Tissue specificity—near absolute discrimination from skeletal muscle and other tissue injury
- Cross-species immunoreactivity—highly conserved epitopes
- Diagnostic sensitivity—can detect background levels, minor injury
- Correlation with cytopathologic and histopathologic biomarkers of acute injury, physiological performance indicators, clinical severity
- Prognostic value
- Effective assays and analyzers widely available
- Microvolume assays available (25 μL sample)
- Kinetics of release and plasma clearance characterized and appropriate: time to peak, half-life
- Inexpensive
- Robust with good storage stability
- Dose responsive
- Translational across species and into humans
- Widely used and characterized—hundreds of publications
- Candidate for qualification by regulatory agencies

Source: O'Brien, P.J., *Expert Rev Mol Diagn*, 6, 685–702, 2006; O'Brien, P.J., *Toxicology*, 245, 206–218, 2008.

Several reports indicate that cTnT may be more sensitive immediately after injury (Christenson et al., 1998; O'Brien, 2006), possibly because the cytoplasmic pool of cTnT is approximately 7%, which is twice that of cTnI, and the cytoplasmic cTn pool is considered to be released earlier than the myofibrillar pool (Bleier et al., 1998). However, approximately 6 hours after injury both troponins provided equivalent information. Furthermore, cTn is released as a ternary complex, consisting of binary complexes of cTnI and cTnC, and as free cTnT.

As for other organ biomarkers, the amount of cTnI release is affected by tissue content. Partial depletion of tissue cTn (as seen with prior injury, inanition and weight loss, and heart failure) may be associated with decreased amounts of release. Body and cardiac weight loss of approximately 25% in rats produced an approximately 50% decrease in cTn content of myocardium (O'Brien, 2006). In heart failure, loss of myofibrillar volume fraction is indicated by an approximately 30% loss of troponin (O'Brien, 1997; O'Brien et al., 1997a).

Cardiac troponin serves as a biomarker of myofibrillar volume fraction not only in cardiac atrophy but also in cardiac hypertrophy (Slaughter et al., 2004). Pressure overload increased myofibrillar density by up to 30%, whereas volume overload decreased myofibrillar density by up to 15%. Growth factor-induced hypertrophy was confirmed to occur by a mixture of processes; while myofibrillar density had increased by 31% at 1 week, it had normalized by 4 weeks. Minoxidil-induced hypertrophy occurred by a mixture of the processes, with myofibrillar density first decreased by 15% at 1 week before normalizing by 4 weeks. Progressive, pathological hypertrophy, as modeled with spontaneous hypertension, was confirmed to be associated with abnormally increased myocardial, myofibrillar density.

Commercially available assays for cTn are robust, simple, accurate, reproducible, inexpensive, and widely available. The analytical performance for most has been recently evaluated for application in laboratory animals and those with insufficient precision, dynamic range, or cross-species reactivity have been identified (O'Brien et al., 2006; Apple et al., 2008). Effective cTn assays have good cross-species reactivity, reflecting the high degree of conservation of cTn structure, although some assays are species restricted because their antibodies target epitopes that are not well conserved (O'Brien et al., 1997b). Also identified were several highly sensitive assays that were able to detect background levels of cTn in laboratory animals. Four cTnI assays (from Abbott, Bayer, Beckman, and Dade analyzers) gave good responses across multiple species (O'Brien et al., 2006; Apple et al., 2008). More recently, a supersensitive assay that uses capillary flow technology and detects single troponin molecules has been described (Todd et al., 2007) and applied successfully in preclinical toxicology studies (Mikaelian et al., 2009; Schultze et al., 2009). It has sensitivity at least an order of magnitude greater than previous assays, and it has been used for detecting drug-induced injury at levels that have not produced histopathological effects on myocardium (Mikaelian et al., 2011).

Whereas there are numerous cTnI assays, patent restrictions limit cTnT assays to one assay for clinical use (Roche Diagnostics, Basel, Switzerland) and one assay for research and preclinical use (MesoScale Discovery, Gaithersburg, Maryland, USA). Recent reports indicate that as cTnT assays have been developed for sensitivity and tissue specificity, and are now in their third and fourth generations, these assays have lost some cross-species reactivity and significant effectiveness for animal applications (Serra et al., 2010).

In a recent comparative study using numerous models of cardiac injury, a new, high-sensitivity generation of one of the four above-mentioned cTnI assays demonstrated the performance across six species (Centaur cTnI Ultra; Serra et al., 2010). This assay generation was found to be an order of magnitude that is more sensitive than the previous assay version (O'Brien et al., 2006), and had higher precision at low cTnI concentrations. The concentration of cTnI in the blood highly correlated with loss of cardiac function, and outperformed other assays tested. It had a dynamic range (maximum divided by minimum value) of almost 7000 and was able to detect cTnI at concentrations as low as 0.006 μg/L (Serra et al., 2010).

Despite the effectiveness of cTnI as a biomarker of cardiotoxicity, there are caveats to the use of cTnI as a biomarker (Table 13.2). Further, similar to other leakage biomarkers used in clinical

TABLE 13.2
Caveats for Use of cTn in Safety Assessment Studies for Detection of Cardiac Effects

1. Detection of acute and active ongoing injury causing release of intracellular constituents; does not detect past injury, or loss of cardiac function
2. Causes of Increased Background
   - Cardiac pacing of pharmacological studies
   - Blood collection by cardiac puncture
   - Ischemic injury during anesthesia and euthanasia
   - Excessive handling stress, restraint or exertion, or trauma
   - Spontaneous cardiomyopathy, especially male Sprague–Dawley rat
3. Causes of Blunted Increases
   - Choice of assay with insufficient sensitivity, dynamic range, or tissue specificity, or cross-species reactivity
   - Decreased tissue concentration due to past cardiac injury, inanition, heart failure
   - Inappropriate timing of blood collection

Source: O'Brien, P.J., *Expert Rev Mol Diagn*, 6, 685–702, 2006; O'Brien, P.J., *Toxicology*, 245, 206–218, 2008.

chemistry for detection of organ damage, cTnI does not directly measure tissue function nor does it reflect previous tissue injury. There are preanalytical causes of changes in serum cTn. It may be increased by background cardiomyopathy or by procedures used during sample collection, such as extreme stress, ischemic injury, cardiac puncture, or cardiovascular instrumentation. In addition, cTn may be decreased if there is decreased tissue concentration as may occur with previous cardiac injury, inanition, or heart failure (O'Brien, 2006, 2008).

13.1.4.5 Natriuretic Peptides

Congestive heart failure is associated with numerous neuroendocrine changes. Several of these have been utilized effectively as biomarkers of the severity of the cardiac dysfunction. The characteristic increase in peripheral vascular resistance seen with heart failure has been attributed to increases in sympathetic tone, norepinephrine, Ang II, ADH, and endothelin-1 (ET-1). The increased venous pressure is associated with atrial distension that stimulates production and release of ANP and brain natriuretic peptides (BNPs) that are normally produced primarily in the atria (although BNP is produced primarily in the ventricles in heart disease). ANP is stored in atrial granules, whereas BNP is primarily produced on demand by *de novo* synthesis.

The natriuretic peptides of the atria and ventricles, ANP and BNP, are produced as pre–prohormones and released as prohormones. Both forms are inactive. The pre–pro form is converted to the pro form, which is subsequently converted to the active hormone and then to multiple, inactive, degradative products. This conversion process is mediated by various serum proteinases. In the first step, a small signal peptide is cleaved in the myocardial cell from the pre–pro form to generate pro-ANP or pro-BNP. Both peptides are cleared from the blood by multiple pathways. They are bound to their clearance receptor (natriuretic peptide receptor C [NPR-C]), internalized, and hydrolyzed by lysosomal enzymes. They are also cleaved by nephrilysin, a membrane-bound, neutral endopeptidase, and metalloproteinase. Propeptides are converted to active peptides by corin and furin. Corin is a transmembrane cardiac serine protease that cleaves pro-ANP to form ANP and NT-proBNP. Both corin and furin cleave pro-BNP into BNP and the twofold larger N-terminal fragment, NT-proBNP (van Kimmenade and Januzzi, 2009). The NT-pro forms of the natriuretic peptides are inactive and cleared passively more than half by the kidney, and a quarter by the liver (Thygesen et al., 2011).

The atrial and ventricular natriuretic peptides produce their effects by binding to natriuretic peptide receptors A and B (NPR-A, NPR-B) that are coupled to guanylate cyclase. BNP mostly binds NPR-A, which increases cGMP that regulates ion channels, protein kinases, and phosphodieserases.

Both natriuretic peptides act similarly, to promote natriuresis and diuresis, cause vasodilation, and antagonize the effects of the RAAS and SNS (Thygesen et al., 2011). Furthermore, ANP and BNP are neurotransmitters in the CNS, decreasing sympathetic tone and reducing ACTH and ADH secretion thereby reducing salt appetite and drinking. Accordingly, increases in ANP and BNP may accelerate the development of heart failure.

BNP and NT-proBNP have become important cardiovascular biomarkers in humans, especially in diagnosis, prognosis, and monitoring of heart failure, and a wide spectrum of cardiovascular diseases (Thygesen et al., 2011). The use of BNP and NT-proBNP as cardiac biomarkers in humans is affected by noncardiac factors that affect their blood concentration, such as age, gender, decreases with obesity, and increases with renal dysfunction. However, body weight, age, and gender have not been found to be complicating factors in animals (van Kimmenade and Januzzi, 2009). BNP may be early biomarker of the left ventricular dysfunction developing with doxorubicin cardiotoxicity or congestive heart failure or occult dilated cardiomyopathy (van Kimmenade and Januzzi, 2009).

In rats, species-specific BNP and NT-proBNP assays have been used effectively as biomarkers of cardiac dysfunction. Plasma BNP increased approximately twofold within 6 weeks of weekly doses of doxorubicin and correlated with development of cardiomyopathy and deterioration of fractional shortening of the left ventricle (Koh et al., 2004). Drug-induced cardiomyopathy developing over 2 weeks was associated with a threefold increase in NT-proBNP and a one-third increase in cardiac size (Berna et al., 2008). With infarct-induced heart failure, rats progressively developed cardiac dysfunction, which correlated with up to tenfold increases in NT-proBNP (Fu et al., 2009).

Veterinary application of natriuretic peptide biomarkers has been substantially complicated by several factors. The effectiveness of their use in humans has only partially transferred across species. First, there is considerably more rapid clearance of natriuretic peptides in animals as compared with humans. For example, the plasma half-life of BNP is approximately 90 seconds in dogs but approximately 20 minutes in man (Thomas and Woods, 2003). Second, clearance of BNP biomarkers is markedly inhibited in dogs by decreased GFR and azotemia and this decreases in GFR may increase the natriuretic peptides to similar plasma concentrations associated with heart disease or heart failure (Raffan et al., 2009; Schmidt et al., 2009). There is additionally a lack of cross-species homology in peptide structure, especially for canine BNP, whose pre–pro peptide has only half the sequence homology with man as for canine ANP (approximately 45% vs. approximately 90%; Oikawa et al., 1985). Finally, natriuretic peptides have poor storage stability in serum. Approximately 70% deterioration of natriuretic peptides occurs within 24 hours at room temperature; however, the addition of 0.1% formic acid stabilizes the natriuretic peptides for at least 3 months at 4°C (Berna et al., 2008). Thus, BNP assays developed for use in humans, typically do not work effectively in animals, contrasting remarkably with the cross-species reactivity of those cTnI assays that target antigenic epitopes with high sequence homology. There are, however, ANP assays developed for use in humans that are sufficiently cross-reactive for use in dogs (Prosek et al., 2007).

However, species-specific assays have emerged for cardiovascular peptides (Schellenberg et al., 2008) and are showing similar applications as for humans, although with more blunted differences in concentration (Hori et al., 2008). NT-proBNP has been especially successful in differentiating cardiac disease, compared to BNP, or ANP or its precursors (Oyama et al., 2008).

The atrial peptides, ANP and NT-proANP, were first found to be effective biomarkers for heart failure in dogs, being increased up to sixfold in dogs with heart failure as compared to plasma levels in normal dogs. In the same model of heart failure in dogs, BNP was increased only twofold. Concentration of NT-proANP was 40-fold higher than ANP, and both atrial peptides were almost threefold greater in concentration than the ventricular peptide, BNP (Häggström et al., 2000). In another study, BNP was shown to be much more diagnostically effective, being substantially increased in dogs with advanced heart disease, and even more in heart failure (MacDonald et al., 2003). Mean BNP concentration in dogs with congestive heart failure was 10-fold higher than for dogs with noncardiac causes of cough or dyspnea (DeFrancesco et al., 2007). Although, BNP was found to be increased significantly only in dogs with advanced heart disease, NT-proBNP had greater diagnostic sensitivity and correlated with cardiac dysfunction, cardiomegaly, and heart failure (Oyama et al., 2008). Using a dog model of acute volume overload, it was shown that NT-proBNP was a considerably weaker and slower responder to overload (Hori et al., 2010) than was ANP.

In dogs with heart failure and associated dyspnea, ANP, BNP, and endothelin are significantly higher than occurs with noncardiac causes of dyspnea (Prosek et al., 2007). Highest sensitivity and specificity for differentiating cardiac and noncardiac dyspnea in dogs, is found with a human proANP assay, followed by canine-specific BNP assay, and human ET-1 assay. In cats, NT-proBNP also accurately distinguishes between cardiac and noncardiac causes of dyspnea (Fox et al., 2009). Widespread clinical application of these biomarkers in veterinary cardiology awaits further assay development and characterization of their effectiveness (Boswood, 2009; Sisson, 2009). So far, only a fraction of the success obtained by adopting human cardiac injury biomarkers (i.e., cTn) for use in animals has been obtained by adopting the new human cardiac functional biomarkers (i.e., natriuretic peptides).

13.2 THE VASCULAR SYSTEM

Interest in biomarkers for vasculitis has developed rapidly in recent years primarily owing to the occurrence of mesenteric vasculitis in rats with phosphodiesterase type 4 (PDE4) inhibitors characterized by medial necrosis and hemorrhage with perivascular edema and inflammation (Daguès et al., 2007a,b). This enzyme is the major inactivator of cAMP in inflammatory and immune cells and is important in regulating airway smooth muscle tone. It is targeted for the treatment of asthma and chronic obstructive pulmonary disease. Absence of biomarkers to identify and monitor the possible occurrence of PDE4 inhibitor-induced vasculitis in man has limited the progression of this drug class.

13.2.1 Vascular Physiology and Function

The primary function of the vascular system is to transport blood to and away from the cells throughout the body. Although the driving force for this is the heart, the blood vessels control the amount, rate, and direction of blood flow to the various tissues. Blood vessels accomplish this by the massive number and surface area of capillaries that reach within 20–30 μm of all cells. This high surface area is critical since it is proportional to the rate of diffusion (Sherwood, 2012).

In a medium-sized dog, one aorta of approximately 2 cm diameter branches out to 50 thousand arteries with an average diameter of approximately 140 μm and subsequently into 20 million arterioles with approximately 30 μm average diameter. These arterioles in turn divide into the 2 billion capillaries from which most chemical exchange between blood and tissue occurs. The capillaries are only slightly wider than an erythrocyte and are about 50 μm long. The capillaries condense into 130 million venules from 70 thousand veins that ultimately flow into the vena cava (Stephenson, 2007).

Tissue blood flow is controlled by the capillary density, and by the degree of contraction of arterial and arteriolar walls and of precapillary sphincters. This capacity for regulating flow is well demonstrated during vigorous exercise. For example, visceral blood flow is reduced by more than a half, while skeletal muscle flow increases by more than 10-fold to support metabolism and contraction, and the blood flow in skin increases several fold to dissipate metabolic heat. The role of the transported blood is to distribute nutrients and their waste products, respiratory gases, regulatory factors for cellular and tissue activity, and protective substances (e.g., cells and factors involved in hemostasis and immunity).

Capillaries are the site for intestinal mucosal absorption or renal reabsorption of fluid and nutrients, and for exchange of nutrients for waste products at capillary beds of metabolic tissues. The exchange is mediated by diffusion along the concentration gradients between capillary blood plasma and tissues. Fluid ultrafiltration through the capillary wall is based mostly on size and is dependent on the semipermeability of the glycocalyx of the endothelial cell membrane. This filtration is produced by the steric hindrance and electrostatic charge repulsion of the glycocalyx (Reitsma et al., 2007).

Starling's law of the capillaries indicates that transendothelial fluid flux is driven by hydraulic fluid pressure from the arteriolar end of the capillary and by osmotic pressure generated by the substantial plasma protein that has leaked into the interstitium. These pressures are counteracted by the plasma protein osmotic pressure and by the interstitial fluid pressure. Since capillary fluid pressure falls from arteriolar to venous ends of the capillary, fluid is predicted by this model to flow out the arteriolar end and back in at the venous end. Normally, the amount of fluid leaving the arteriolar end of the capillary bed is equivalent to that entering the venule side. Excess filtered fluid is returned to the circulatory system via the lymphatics (Sherwood, 2012).

This model explains the observation of fluid movement from tissue to blood when the vascular compartment volume is reduced, for example, owing to hemorrhage, sweating, or diarrhea. It apparently explains that fluid moves from blood to tissue when there is decreased oncotic pressure from hypoproteinemia, increased capillary permeability, such as with inflammation or trauma, or increased tissue hydrostatic pressure such as with venous or lymphatic obstruction, or congestive heart failure. However, more recently, Starling's principle has been revised based on experimental evidence indicating that the interstitial osmotic pressure effect is overestimated and glycocalyx effects and microenvironment are more important (Levick and Michel, 2010). Furthermore, in inflammation, lowering of interstitial fluid pressure was found to be of greater importance than permeability increase. This decrease in pressure was due to a change in extracellular matrix leading to up take of water by the glycosaminoglycan ground substance (Reed and Rubin, 2010).

Capillaries are of three basic types. The continuous type is uninterrupted with fluid movement only through intercellular clefts at the tight junctions. Fenestrated capillaries have small pores of about 70 nm diameter that are covered by a diaphragm of radial fibers that will allow small molecules and limited amounts of proteins to diffuse. Sinusoidal capillaries have considerably larger pores with 30–40 μm and allow cell and protein movement.

Leukocytes exit the vasculature by diapedesis through gaps between endothelial cells, usually at postcapillary venules, where blood pressure is reduced. This process is controlled by attractant and activating cytokines and chemokines, and cell surface receptors. These cause cell binding, shape change, and transmigration.

The glycocalyx is a carbohydrate-rich layer that lines the lumen of the vascular endothelium. It is comprised of membrane-bound and soluble components. In capillaries, it is 0.5 μm thick, but up to 5 μm thick in arteries. Bound and projecting from the cell membrane are glycoproteins with short, branched carbohydrate side chains, and proteoglycans with long, unbranched glycosaminoglycan side chains. On top of these are plasma and endothelial-derived soluble components, including hyaluronic acid, thrombomodulin, extracellular superoxided dismutase, and antithrombin III (Reitsma et al., 2007).

The glycocalyx has multiple functions. First, it restricts solutes and cells from reaching the endothelium, thereby providing protective and filtrative roles. It also transmits shear stress of blood flow into biochemical cell signaling that regulates nitric oxide production and vascular tone, cytoskeletal reorganization, and production of glycocalyx components. This layer is also important as a docking station to concentrate specific plasma constituents, for example, growth factors, lipoprotein lipase, and anticoagulants such as antithrombin III, thrombomodulin, tissue factor pathway inhibitor, and heparin cofactor II (Reitsma et al., 2007).

The countercurrent exchange is used for maximizing the transfer of blood constituents by diffusion gradients over vascular circuits in which blood vessels are adjacent but have blood flowing in opposite directions (Robinson, 2007). It is commonly found in various vertebrate, physiological systems in order to conserve one constituent, such as water, heat, or oxygen, while excreting an unwanted constituent, such as nitrogenous waste or salt. This mechanism is found in various organs including the mammalian kidney to concentrate urine, the placenta, the avian salt gland to distill seawater, and fish gills to extract oxygen from water.

13.2.2 Endothelium

Vascular endothelium dysfunction is an early event in vascular disorders, reflecting its critical role in regulation of vascular tone, antithrombosis, leukocyte trafficking, and oncotic pressure by production and release or surface expression of various factors (Tesfamariam and DeFelice, 2007). As described below, vascular injury is associated with activation or increase of numerous factors that can be used as biomarkers.

13.2.3 Vasculitis

Vasculitis is characterized by inflammation and fibrinoid necrosis of blood vessel walls. It may be primary, or secondary to infection, malignancy, or immune disease (Guillevin and Dorner, 2007). There are several possible mechanisms by which drugs can cause vasculitis (Louden et al., 2006). Immunologic and vasoactive mechanisms are most commonly implicated. For example, antineutrophil cytoplasmic autoantibody (ANCA) vasculitis is caused by autoantibodies to neutrophil cytoplasm, resulting in neutrophilic attack of small vessel walls, causing purpura in skin, pulmonary hemorrhage, neuropathy, redness and itching of the eyes, and renal disease with hematuria and proteinuria. Necrotizing angitis occurs in drug abusers and is considered to be produced by an immune mechanism possibly in association with toxic injury or infection. Vasoactive drugs may also cause vasculitis. For example, cerebral vasculitis may be produced by sympathomimetics in humans. Furthermore, vascular-targeting drugs used in cancer treatment may have cardiovascular effects.

In laboratory animals, vasculitis is known to be produced by various mechanisms including immune, infection, particles, cytotoxicity, hypertension, and renal failure (Louden et al., 2006). Spontaneous necrotizing vasculitis occurs with aging in rodents, usually sporadically affecting smaller arteries. Although its cause is unknown, its prevalence is affected by nutrition, hypertension, and gender. Vasculitis may also be induced by various substances, including cytotoxins, foreign proteins and immunosuppressive drugs, and antibiotics. Inotropic vasodilators and PDEi produce medial artery necrosis and inflammation in rats apparently by exaggeration of their pharmacologic vasoactivity resulting in injury of smooth muscle of medium-sized arteries of the pancreas, stomach, mesentery, intestine, and kidney (Joseph, 2000; Louden and Morgan, 2001). These targets are also affected by age, hypertension, and renal failure in rats.

In dogs and rats, inotropic amines, PDE3 inhibitors, adenosine agonists, cardiac glycosides, and ET-1 receptor antagonists produce extramural, coronary, segmental, medial necrosis, and inflammation, apparently, because of their exaggerated hemodynamic effect locally or on heart rate and blood pressure (Joseph, 2000; Louden et al., 2006). Similar coronary changes are seen in monkeys with many of the same cardiovascular drugs.

13.2.4 Vascular Analytes and Laboratory Tests

Blood biomarkers that have been investigated and proposed for the identification of vasculitis include those associated with inflammation or endothelial cell injury (Brott et al., 2005; Louden1 2006) (Table 13.3). For example, mesenteric vasculitis in rats owing to PDE4 inhibition produces significant increases in injury biomarkers such as plasma concentrations of tissue inhibitor of metalloproteinase-1 (TIMP-1), vascular endothelial growth factor (VEGF), thrombomodulin, and in inflammatory biomarkers α1-acid glycoprotein (AGP), C-reactive protein (CRP), haptoglobin, and IL-1 and IL-6 (Daguès et al., 2007a,b; Weaver et al., 2008). Inflammatory biomarkers are also increased in dogs treated with the same PDE4 inhibitor (Hanton et al., 2008).

13.2.4.1 Cytokines

Cytokines can be valuable biomarkers of inflammation, especially IL-6; however, their role is limited by their short half-life compared to acute phase proteins (APPs) (Shaikh, 2011). Cytokines are

TABLE 13.3
Biomarkers for Vasculitis: Acute Phase Proteins (APP) and Endothelial Proteins

Biomarker	MW (kDa)	Species		Major Role
		Acute Phase Response		
		Major APP	Moderate APP	–
IL-1	12–15	–	–	Early proinflammatory cytokine
TNF-α	17	–	–	Early proinflammatory cytokine
IL-6	21–29	–	–	Chemoattractant
TIMP	24–31	–	–	Tissue remodeling
C-reactive protein (CRP)	100	C, P, H	–	Opsonin
Serum amyloid A (SAA)	14	E, B, O, H	M	Apolipoprotein
Haptoglobin (Hp)	81	B, O	D, P, M, R	Bind hemoglobin
α2 macroglobulin (A2M)	720	R	–	Antiprotease
α1 acid glycoprotein (AGP)	44	–	C, F, B, O, R	Bind drugs
Serum amyloid P (SAP)	230	M	–	Opsonin, amyloidosis
Fibrinogen	340	–	all	Coagulation
		Adhesion Molecules		
Von Willebrand factor (vWF)	500–20,000	–	–	Hemostasis
vWF pro-peptide		–	–	Hemostasis
Caveolin-1	21	–	–	Flow sensor
				Coagulation and fibrinolysis
NO	0.03	–	–	Vasodilator
Endothelin	2.5	–	–	Vasoconstrictor
Circulating endothelial cell (CEC)	–	–	–	Exfoliated cells

Species: C, canine; F, feline; P, porcine; E, equine; B, bovine; O, ovine; M, murine; NHP, nonhuman primate; H, human.

cell signaling and modulating peptides of the immune system and are produced and released by macrophages and lymphocytes, as well as epithelial and endothelial cells. ILs are produced primarily by T helper cells and macrophages. In injury or infection, extracellular and blood concentrations of cytokines may increase up to a 1000-fold. Chemokines act as chemotactic factors and include erythropoietin for red blood cells, thrombopoeitin for platelets, IL-8 for neutrophils, eotaxin for eosinophils, and RANTES (CCL5) for leukocytes.

13.2.4.2 Acute Phase Proteins

APPs are produced and released into the blood primarily by hepatocytes in response to the proinflammatory cytokines, IL-1 and IL-6, and TNF-α (Paltrinieri, 2007). APPs are produced and released by macrophages when exposed to foreign antigen at sites of inflammation. Both IL-1 and IL-6 increase the hypothalamic thermostat. IL-1 increases the endothelial adhesion factors for leukocyte migration, stimulates hematopoiesis, and stimulates the adrenocortical axis to produce glucocorticoids. IL-6 is also important in lymphocyte differentiation and proliferation. TNF-α induces peripheral proteolysis in order to increase hepatic supply of amino acids. IL-1 inhibits the synthesis of negative APP, and stimulates positive APP production in the presence of glucocorticoids (Paltrinieri, 2007).

There are four major classes of APPs based on the magnitude of change in blood concentration in response to inflammation (Watterson et al., 2009): (1) major—increasing rapidly 10–1000 folds and decreasing rapidly; includes CRP in man, dog, pig, and mink, serum amyloid A (SAA) in dog, cat, pig, and ruminants, α2-macroglobulin (A2M) in rats, serum amyloid P (SAP) in mice, and haptoglobin in ruminants, (2) moderate—increasing 2–10 folds at slower rate but persisting longer in the blood; includes fibrinogen in all species, haptoglobin in dog, rat, mouse, and pig, AGP in dogs and cats and ruminants, (3) minor—increasing slowly to less than twofold but persisting the longest, and (4) negative—decreasing slowly and mildly; includes albumin and binding proteins for thyroid hormone, cortisol, and retinol in all species.

The multiple APP has different properties and functions, and species distribution (Ceron et al., 2005). CRP is a cyclic pentameric pentraxin that exhibits calcium-dependent binding to bacteria and intracellular antigen of damaged cells to facilitate phagocytosis. It also induces anti-inflammatory cytokines and inhibits neutrophil chemotaxis and function. SAP is a pentraxin glycoprotein homologue of CRP that neutralizes lipopolysaccharide of Gram negative bacteria and has been shown to be involved in the pathogenesis of reactive amyloidosis. SAA is a highly conserved apolipoprotein involved in cholesterol transport. It is precursor to amyloid protein A that is found in α-amyloid, which is deposited in amyloidosis. SAA is also chemotactic for inflammatory cells and inhibits myeloperoxidase release and lymphoproliferation. Haptoglobin is a glycosylated tetramer that binds free hemoglobin, thereby reducing its oxidative stress and proinflammatory effects, and restricting availability of iron for bacterial growth. It antagonizes receptor-ligand activation of the immune system and inhibits granulocyte chemotaxis and phagocytosis. Haptoglobin may be increased with hyperadrenocorticism and certain anthelminthics in dogs and guinea pigs (Boretti et al., 2009). A2M is a tetrameric, irreversible protease inhibitor that is adsorbed to the surface of peripheral blood lymphocytes. It traps proteinase within a cavity thereby exposing sites for receptor-mediated endocytosis by macrophages. AGP is a highly glycosylated protein that binds numerous basic and neutral lipophilic drugs and acidic drugs such as phenobarbital. It has antineutrophil and anticomplement activity and increases secretion of IL-receptor antagonist by macrophages.

13.2.4.3 Caveolin

A potential mechanistically linked biomarker of vascular injury is caveolin-1, which is released from endothelial cells into blood with vascular injury (Louden et al., 2006). This protein is a component of caveolae, which are important contributors to the regulation of vascular permeability and blood flow. Caveolae are microscopic, flask-shaped invaginations of cell surface membrane that are found especially in endothelial cells. They have lipid rafts that are enriched in (1) cholesterol for maintaining their structure, (2) sphingolipid for cell signaling, (3) the integral membrane protein, caveolin-1, for structure and for sequestering and inactivating endothelial nitric oxide synthase (eNOS), and (4) albondin, a 60 kDa albumin-binding glycoprotein. Caveolae detect changes in blood flow by mechanosensing shear stress and play a key role in transcellular movement (important in the activation of eNOS, exposing endothelial leukocyte adhesion molecules, transcellular movement of albumin to maintain the oncotic pressure gradient). Caveolae are additionally considered to participate in regulation of adherins junctions between endothelial cells and hence in paracellular movement.

Caveolin-1 inhibits eNOS conversion of L-arginine into nitric oxide (NO), which is an important cause of vascular injury (Govers et al., 2002). Endothelial nitric oxide synthase is induced by preinflammatory cytokines and acts as a messenger in modulating inflammatory responses. This enzyme also has several other functions including vasodilation, inhibition of platelet aggregation, thrombus formation, leukocyte adhesion, smooth muscle cell proliferation, and low density lipoprotein oxidation. Reaction of NO with superoxide anion forms peroxynitrite, a reactive nitrogen species implicated in oxidative stress-induced vascular injury during inflammation. There is rapid, spontaneous inactivation of NO by conversion into nitrite and nitrate (Tesfamariam and DeFelice, 2007).

13.2.4.4 Endothelins

Endothelins are a family of vasoconstrictor peptides produced by endothelial cells. They are key mediators in regulating vascular function, counterbalancing vasodilators such as nitric oxide and prostacyclin. In cardiovascular diseases such as cardiac failure and pulmonary arterial hypertension, endothelial cell dysfunction occurs causing vasodilator concentrations to decrease and endothelin concentration to increase. Endothelins also produce proinflammatory effects (Kedzierski and Yanagisawa, 2001; Maguire and Davenport, 2014) and have been reported to activate polymorphonuclear cell secretion and adhesion and macrophage activity. Endothelins contributes to extracellular matrix remodeling during tissue repair and thus may participate in intimal damage in vascular diseases. Increased blood concentration of ET-1 and its inactive prohormone, big endothelin-1 (Big-ET) have been found to have prognostic value in cardiac disease in humans (Barton and Yanagisawa, 2008). There is relatively high cross-species homology for these peptides. Assays for these biomarkers in humans have been validated for use in rats and dogs. ET-1 increased several folds during the development of heart failure in rats and dogs (Tonnessen et al., 1997; Prosek et al., 2007). Thus, endothelins have been shown to have similar effectiveness for detection of cardiovascular diseases in dogs as in humans (Schellenberg et al., 2008). Moreover, human endothelins have nearly identical sequence homology with those of dogs, rats, and mice (Biondo et al., 2003).

13.2.4.5 Thrombomodulin

Thrombomodulin has been shown to be mildly increased in vasculitis (Weaver et al., 2008). Thrombomodulin is a cell surface receptor found on and synthesized by vascular endothelial cells (Califano et al., 2000). Its major role is as an inhibitor of coagulation and fibrinolysis. Thrombomodulin functions as a cell surface receptor and an essential cofactor for active thrombin, with which it binds in a 1:1 stoichiometric complex. This complex activates and increases protein C activity by up to a 1000-fold by removing a small peptide by proteolytic cleavage. Thrombomodulin catalyzes the thrombin activation of fibrinolysis inhibitor (TAFI), also known as carboxypeptidase B2. Thrombomodulin is found in plasma and urine after endothelial injury and may predict thrombotic crisis. It is used as a specific biomarker of microvascular endothelial injury and thrombotic events, such as in disseminated intravascular coagulation (DIC) and vasculitis.

13.2.4.6 Adhesion Molecules

Inflammatory cell migration from the vascular space is mediated by adhesion molecules on inflammatory cells and endothelium including vascular cell adhesion molecule-1 (VCAM-1), E-selectin, and intercellular adhesion molecule-1 (ICAM-1) (Lukas and Dvorak, 2004). They are released into the blood following leucocyte and/or endothelial cell activation in various diseases, including autoimmune disease and vasculitis.

13.2.4.7 von Willebrand Factor

von Willebrand factor (vWF) has also been evaluated as a potential biomarker of vascular injury. Hemostatic, platelet-plug formation requires vWF to bridge from platelet glycoprotein IB to exposed collagen in the subendothelium. vWF is also important in the one-to-one stoichiometric transport and stabilization of factor VIII by protecting it from rapid degradation, cellular uptake or from binding to the surface of activated platelets or endothelial cells (De Meyer et al, 2009). The carbohydrate surface of vWF protects it from proteolysis.

A proteolytic, cleavage product of a precursor of vWF may be an effective biomarker of vascular injury. vWF is a polymeric glycoprotein synthesized by endothelial cells and megakaryocytes in a precursor form, pre–pro-vWF. The precursor has a signal peptide that identifies vWF as a protein for secretion. This peptide is removed from pre–pro-vWF by proteolytic cleavage to form pro-vWF. This then forms dimers, and after glycosylation, polymerizes into multimers. Within endothelial cells, these multimers undergo further proteolysis to yield mature vWF multimers and propeptide dimers (vWFpp), both of which are either released constitutively or else stored together in Weibel–Palade bodies. Endothelial vWFpp and VWF are secreted in equimolar amounts, although they are cleared from the blood at several-fold different rates. This differential clearance rate results in their ratio reflecting the time-course of their release (de Wit and van Mourik, 2001). Furthermore, vWFpp is specific for endothelial cell origin, as it is not cleaved from the pro-vWF precursor in platelets. Blood concentration of vWFpp may increase 100-fold with vascular injury, although it is with a half-life of only hours (Louden et al., 2006).

13.2.4.8 Circulating Microparticles

Circulating microparticles are membranous fragments 0.1–1 μm in diameter that are released from circulating white blood cells and endothelial cells during cell activation or apoptosis (Azevedo et al., 2007). Increased microparticles are found in a wide variety of conditions and are not pathology-specific, including heart failure, sepsis, diabetes, hypertension, renal failure, embolism, and vasculitis. They retain the antigenic signature of the parent cell, and they are formed by the disruption of cytoskeletal structure with formation of the plasma membrane evaginations in a process referred to as budding or blebbing. They are distinct from the larger apoptotic bodies, which are considerably larger cell fragments, and from the small exosomes (0.06–0.1 μm), which are preformed vesicles from the endocytic-lysosomal system and play a role in immune activation and antigen presentation (Azevedo et al., 2007).

Microparticles produce multiple effects from signaling to activation because of their containing surface membrane and cytoplasmic contents of their parent cell. Many of these are proinflammatory, by activating complement, causing chemotaxis and endothelial adherence of leukocytes, and by stimulating cytokine release. They are also procoagulant, by providing phospholipid surface for assembly of clotting complexes or providing activating factors such as tissue factor and factor V.

13.2.4.9 Circulating Endothelial Cells

Circulating endothelial cells (CECs) appear in the blood after injury and in response to inflammatory, immune, and infectious disease. CECs were first described decades ago in rabbits, pigs, rodents, and dogs and have been demonstrated to be increased in shock, endotoxemia, myocardial infarction, hypertension, immunosuppression, and with prostaglandin E inhibition (Erdbruegger et al., 2006; Wills et al., 2009; Burger and Touyz, 2012). They are now considered to be sensitive and specific indicators of endothelial cell injury in humans and can be assayed by fluorescence-activated cell sorting (FACS) based on cell surface markers. CECs arise from detachment from the underlying matrix because of impaired adhesion via vitronectin, fibronectin, and vascular endothelial cadherin, which is an endothelial-specific adhesion molecule located at the junctions between endothelial cells. Detachment occurs due to the action of proteases, (as from neutrophils), due to oxidative stress from reactive oxygen and nitrogen species, or by mechanical injury. The CECs are large (10–100 μm) and are intact or anucleate remnants of cells or sheets of multiple cells. They characteristically express wWF and thrombomodulin as well as cluster differentiation antigens CD-31 and CD-146. Endothelial progenitor cells from the bone marrow may be confused with CECs as they have similar cell surface makers. These progenitor cells are involved in vascular repair.

13.2.4.10 Matrix Metalloproteinases

An inhibitor of MMP has been identified as one of the more effective biomarkers of vasculitis (Daguès et al., 2007b). These MMP function in tissue remodeling during diverse physiological and pathological states including morphogenesis, angiogenesis, tissue repair, inflammation, fibrosis, tumor metastasis, and aneurysm (Spinale, 2007). In these processes, they have roles in cell proliferation, migration, differentiation, angiogenesis, apoptosis, and host defense. Their effect is attributable to their endopeptidase activity, which requires zinc as a cofactor at the active site. This degrades extracellular matrix proteins, modulates cell surface receptors and cytokines, and releases ligands (e.g., apoptotic FAS). The MMP are inhibited by one-to-one stoichiometric complexing with specific endogenous TIMP.

13.3 THE RESPIRATORY SYSTEM

13.3.1 Pulmonary Function and Injury

The respiratory system has air conducting and air exchanging zones, served by bronchiolar and pulmonary circulatory systems, respectively (Robinson, 2007). The former zone begins with the nasal cavity and associated sinuses, extends into the pharynx, larynx, and trachea, and ends with the bronchi. The tracheobronchial portion has cartilage for support, and submucosal glands with mucus and serous fluid producing cells. The tracheobronchial lining consists of pseudostratified epithelium, where all cells reach the basement membrane in contrast to stratified epithelium. The lining cells form a mucociliary layer comprised mostly of columnar ciliated epithelial cells, goblet cells, and a mucus layer. This layer moves inhaled particles sized between 2 and 10 μm that are trapped in the mucus by the beating action of the cilia (Lopez, 2007).

There is a transitional zone between the air conducting and exchanging zones that is comprised of the bronchioles. They lack cartilage and glands but have a thick, circumferential layer of smooth muscle in their walls. These bronchioles are lined by ciliated, cuboidal epithelium, and secretory Clara cells, which are not ciliated. They metabolize inhaled xenobiotics by their cytochrome P450 system and produce a bronchiolar lining fluid comprised of glycosaminoglycans, lysozymes, and Clara cell secretory protein (uteroglobin), which has antioxidant, anti-inflammatory, and immunomodulatory functions. Clara cells are also mitotically active and can differentiate into ciliated bronchial cells during repair.

Bronchiolar smooth muscle and therefore bronchiolar diameter, is controlled by opposing signals (Panettieri et al., 2008). SNS norepinephrine activates β2 receptors and adenylate cyclase to increase cAMP and cause bronchodilation. Increased cAMP may also occur with PDE inhibitors, or by H2 receptor agonists such as histamine. Decreased cAMP occurs with α-receptor agonists such as phenylephrine, leukotrienes, prostaglandins, or thromboxane. PNS acetylcholine activates M3 muscarinic receptors and guanylate cyclase to increase cGMP, thereby causing resting tone and bronchoconstriction. Increased cGMP also occurs with H1 receptor agonists such as histamine, platelet activating factor, or serotonin. Agonists for the H2 receptor stimulate mucus secretion whereas H1 receptor agonists stimulate serous secretion (Shimura, 2000).

The respiratory zone contains the respiratory bronchioles that terminate in alveolar ducts that form multiple alveoli lined by the respiring, membranous type I pneumocytes and surfactant-producing, granular type II pneumocytes. Smooth muscle extends down the respiratory tract only to the level of the alveolar ducts. The adjacent alveoli are supported and interfaced with capillaries by a network of connective tissue fibers. To facilitate gaseous exchange, cytoplasm of the type I pneumocytes and endothelial cells of the pulmonary capillaries are on either side of a fused basement membrane over >90% of the alveolar surface area. Adjacent alveoli are connected by pores of Kohn through the septa, which function as collateral ventilation during partial lung expansion and allow the passage of other materials such as fluid and bacteria (Weibel, 2008). The type I cells are thin and flat with a large surface area covering 95% of the alveolar surface. They are replenished by differentiation of the mitotically active type II cells. The type II cells are large and cuboidal, and protrude into the alveoli and have cytoplasmic multilamellar bodies that store phospholipid-rich surfactant. Type II cells are also known to secrete alkaline phosphatase (ALP) along with surfactant (Henderson et al., 1995).

Pulmonary alveolar macrophages (PAMs) are found within the alveolar lumen or on the capillary side with extensions protruding across the intercellular space of the alveolar lining into its lumen (Robinson, 2007). They derive from migrating blood monocytes that have adapted to aerobic metabolism and for phagocytosis of inhaled bacteria, particles less than 2 μm in diameter, erythrocytes from hemorrhage, or neutrophils from inflammation. PAM may also play a role in clearance of surfactant as demonstrated by the accumulation of surfactant with defective PAM, as seen in pulmonary alveolar proteinosis. PAM has abundant, vacuolated cytoplasm rich with mitochondria, and antioxidant and detoxification enzymes. They migrate with phagocytosed material to the mucociliary layer which traps and moves them up and out of the respiratory tract.

The pleural cavity is the potential space between the parietal pleura lining the inner wall of the thoracic cage and the visceral pleura lining the lungs (Robinson, 2007). It normally contains a small amount of pleural fluid to allow close and effortless sliding of pleural against each other during ventilation, thereby allowing optimal alveolar inflation. The pleura also transmit the chest wall movements during ventilation to the lung. The parietal pleura have sensory innervations and are highly sensitive to pain.

13.3.2 Bronchoalveolar Lavage Fluid

The biochemistry, cytological changes and microbiological changes associated with respiratory disease may be examined by a bronchoalveolar lavage (BAL) in which warmed, sterile, physiological saline is infused and then retrieved from a tube inserted into a bronchus (Henderson, 2005). Although, the BAL is the most reliable method for sampling the lower respiratory tract, it is an invasive technique requiring sedation, limiting its clinical use. Most BAL fluid (BALF) cells are PAM, with smaller numbers of lymphocytes in large animals, and only small numbers of neutrophils and eosinophils (except cats) and few mast cells (Mathers et al., 2007; Burkhard and Millward, 2010; Picinin et al., 2010). The presence of PAM indicates the alveolar origin of the recovered material and the correct interpretation of cell profile, whereas the presence of large numbers of epithelial cells indicates bronchial, nonalveolar material, which hinders the interpretation of total and differential cell distribution. Squamous epithelial cells with bacteria (e.g., *Simonsiella*) indicate oropharyngeal contamination. Changes in differential cell counts on BALF samples may be indicative of different types of disease: (1) Increases in eosinophils in BALF indicate allergic or parasitic disease, (2) increases in neutrophils indicate bacterial or viral infection or cough, (3) increases in mast cells indicate type I hypersensitivity, and (4) increases in erythrocytes and/or PAMs containing eyrthrocytes or blue-green to black hemosiderin indicate hemorrhage (Burkhard and Millward, 2010).

Toxicological testing of various chemicals and nanoparticles has occasionally included BALF biomarkers for cytotoxicity, inflammation, and oxidative stress (Table 13.4). For example, lung exposure to nanoparticles (particle size <100 nm in one dimension) produces increases in lactate dehydrogenase or decreases in mitochondrial activity due to cytotoxicity, inflammatory mediators and cells due to inflammation, and antioxidant enzymes due to oxidative stress (Carter et al., 2006; Sayes et al., 2007, Warheit et al., 2008).

During collection of BALF samples, recovery of instilled fluid is typically approximately 80% when the dwell times of the lavage fluid are limited to approximately half a minute. However, this recovery can be quite variable, depending on sample handling, lavage volume, number of lavage aliquots, and pulmonary dwell time. Thus, concentrations of endogenous urea or albumin or of dyes added to the instillate, compared to plasma concentration have been used for estimating the degree of dilution of epithelial lining fluid by the instillate (Mills and Lister, 2005). The increased permeability of the plasma-to-airway during pathological conditions can, however, increase the movement of constituents into or out of the instillate causing significant underestimates using the measurement of endogenous substances or overestimates using exogenous substances.

Increases in BALF biomarkers can be used as quantitative and dose-responsive indicators of injury to the respiratory system (Carter et al., 2006). An increase in a BALF biomarker frequently precedes clinical signs and morphological alterations in the lung. Lavages may be repeated to follow a disease process. There are specific biomarkers for inflammation including its early signaling, chemotaxis of the cells involved, and the type and severity of inflammation. Additionally, there are biomarkers for the associated changes including increased capillary permeability, PAM activation, cell lysis, pneumocyte secretion, and oxidative stress.

After cellular elements, inflammatory biomarkers are the most well studied BALF biomarkers. Following stimulation, activated PAM release early proinflammatory cytokines, as described in the

TABLE 13.4
Biomarkers for Pulmonary Disease in BALF

Biomarker	MW (kDa)	Assay	Role
Neutrophils	–	AHA	Inflammation, infection
Eosinophils	–	AHA	Allergy
GSH	0.37	ACCA	Oxidative stress—antioxidant
O_2^-, H_2O_2, NO	0.3	Spec	Oxidative stress—oxidants
GPx, GRx, SOD	84, 100, 33	ACCA	Oxidative stress—enzymatic antioxidants
8-isoprostane	–	ELISA	Oxidative stress—macromolecular (DNA) injury
LD	230	ACCA	Cytotoxicity
ALP	150	ACCA	Increased type II cell secretion or injury
Protein	–	ACCA	Alveolar capillary permeability
Fibronectin	440	ELISA	Chemoattract fibroblasts, endothelial cells, monocytes; acts as fibroblast growth factor
B-glucuronidase	130	ACCA	Lysosomal; macrophage activation
IL1, TNFα	12–17	ELISA	Early proinflammatory cytokines from PAM
IL-6, IL-8	25, 11	ELISA	Chemoattract/activate neutrophils, lymphocytes
MIP-2, MCP-1	8. 12	ELISA	chemoattract and activate PAM
Total phospholipids	–	Spec	Surfactant production

ACCA, automated clinical chemistry analyzer; AHA, automated hematology analyzer; ALP, alkaline phosphatase; ELISA, enzyme-linked immunosorbent assay; GPx, glutathione reductase; GRx, glutathione reductase; GSH, glutathione; H_2O_2, hydrogen peroxide; IL, interleukin; LD, lactate dehydrogenase; MCP-1, monocyte chemoattractant protein-1; MIP-2, macrophage inflammatory protein-2; NO, nitric oxide; O_2^-, superoxide; PAM, pulmonary alveolar macrophage; SOD, superoxide dismutase; Spec, spectrophotometric; TNFa, tumor necrosis factor alpha.

vasculitis section. These proinflammatory cytokines serve as chemoattractants for inflammatory cells. For example, IL-8 causes chemotaxis and activation of neutrophils, induces the full pattern of responses observed in chemotactically stimulated neutrophils, and is a potent angiogenic factor. Monocyte chemoattractant protein-1 (MCP-1) is chemotactic and is produced by endothelial cells after exposure to cytokines (IL-1ß, TNF-α) and oxidized lipoproteins. MCP-1 attracts and activates monocytes and T cells and regulates the proliferation of vascular smooth muscle cells. Macrophage inflammatory protein (MIP-2) causes leukocyte chemotaxis (Ishida et al., 2006; Carter et al., 2006; Sayes et al., 2007).

Activated PAM also plays a role in chronic lung disease and the development of fibrosis. This reflects their production of growth factors such as transforming growth factor (TGF)-β, a potent fibrogenic growth factor that promotes pulmonary fibrosis by enhancement of transcription for collagen genes, and platelet-derived growth factor (PDGF) that is chemotactic for fibroblasts and stimulates their proliferation.

Oxidative stress plays a major role in pulmonary pathology, especially provided the high oxygen tensions and the heavy use of oxidants in the defensive mechanisms of inflammatory cells. *Ex vivo* production of superoxide, hydrogen peroxide, and nitric oxide from BAL cells is an indicator of inflammatory cell activation and oxidative stress (Jackson et al., 2007). Antioxidant capacity is also a biomarker for oxidative stress and can be assessed by the measurement of several parameters (Tsai et al., 2006; Carter et al., 2006). Glutathione (GSH) is a key component of the antioxidant system by providing a reducing environment. There are also several enzymes that play key roles in oxidative stress including (1) superoxide dismutase (SOD) that detoxifies superoxide, converting it into hydrogen peroxide; (2) glutathione reductase (GR), which maintains GSH in its reduced state; and (3) glutathione peroxidase (GPx), which detoxifies hydrogen peroxide and nitric oxide. These parameters can be readily measured using automated clinical chemistry analyzers (Slaughter et al., 2002).

In chronic inflammation, there is reversible airway obstruction, nonspecific bronchial hyperresponsiveness, and airway remodeling due to basement membrane thickening due to collagen and fibronectin deposition, fibroblast proliferation, airway smooth muscle thickening as a result of both smooth muscle cell hyperplasia and hypertrophy, and excessive production of mucus glycoproteins.

Fibronectin concentration in BALF has been used effectively as a biomarker of lung remodeling and pulmonary fibrosis, with its concentration increasing up to 100-fold (Trifilieff et al., 2000; Tsai et al., 2003). Fibronectin is a dimeric glycoprotein found in the epithelial surface of airways and in the interstitial parenchyma of the lung. It is chemotactic for fibroblasts, endothelial cells, and monocytes and is apparently a growth factor for fibroblasts. Fibronectin is a major component of extracellular matrix, binding collagen, fibrin, and heparan sulfate proteoglycans and mediating the attachment of fibroblasts to the extracellular matrix.

Total phospholipid content of BALF is an indication of surfactant production. Total phospholipid content may be decreased with chronic inflammatory disease and increased with acute disease (Russo et al., 2002); however, the cause of an increase or decrease in total phospholipid content is not always clear.

In contrast, mucus hypersecretion and mucus metaplasia of airways apparently contribute to structural changes occurring in chronic disease. Mucus production is increased by Th2 cells largely by an IL-13-mediated pathway. The Th2 cells also increase eosinophils in allergic airway disease and they in turn produce cytokines that stimulate mucus production.

REFERENCES

Akashi, Y.J., Nef, H.M., Mollmann, H., et al. 2010. Stress cardiomyopathy. *Annu Rev Med.* 61:271–286.

Aktas, A., Auguste, D., and Lefebrve, E. 1993. Creatine kinase in the dog: A review. *Vet Res Comm.* 17:353–369.

Allen, P.M. 1955. Myocardial changes occurring in potassium deficiency. *Br Heart J.* 17:5–15.

Anwaruddin, S., Januzzi, J.L., Baggish, A.L., et al. 2005. Ischemia-modified albumin improves the usefulness of standard cardiac biomarkers for the diagnosis of myocardial ischemia in the emergency department setting. *Clin Chem.* 123:140–145.

Apple, F.S., Murakami, M.-A.M., Ler, R., et al. 2008. Analytical characteristics of commercial cardiac troponin I and T immunoassays in serum from rats, dogs, and monkeys with induced acute myocardial injury. *Clin Chem.* 54:1982–89.

Archer, J. 2003. Cardiac biomarkers: A review. *Comp Clin Path.* 12:1211–1218.

Azevedo, L.C.P., Pedroc, M.A., and Laurindoc, F.R.M. 2007. Circulating microparticles as therapeutic targets in cardiovascular diseases. *Rec Patents Cardiovasc Drug Disc.* 2:41–51.

Babuin, L. and Jaffe, A.S. 2005. Troponin: The biomarker of choice for the detection of cardiac injury. *Can Med Assoc J.* 173:1191–1202.

Bader, M. 2010. Tissue renin-angiotensin-aldosterone systems: Targets for pharmacologic therapy. *Annu Rev Pharmacol Toxicol.* 50:439–465.

Baig, M.A., Ali, S., Khan, M.U., et al. 2006. Cardiac troponin I release in non-ischemic reversible myocardial injury from parvovirus B19 myocarditis. *Inter J Cardiol.* 113:e109–e110.

Balakumar, P., Singh, A.P., and Singh, M. 2007. Rodent models of heart failure. *J Pharmacol Toxicol Meth.* 56:1–10.

Bar-Or, D., Lau, E., and Winkler, J.V. 2000. A novel assay for cobalt-albumin binding and its potential as a marker for myocardial ischemia: A preliminary report. J Emerg Med. 19:311–315.

Barton, M. and Yanagisawa, M. 2008. Endothelin: 20 years from discovery to therapy. *Can J Physiol Pharmacol.* 86:485–498.

Bas, V.N., Cetinkaya, S., Agladioglu, S.Y., Kendirici, N.N.P., Bilgili, H., Yildirim, N., and Aycan, Z. 2010. Insulin oedema in newly diagnosed type 1 diabetes mellitus. J Clin Res Pediatr Endocrinol. 2(1):46–48.

Beck, M.L., Dameron, G.W., and O'Brien, P.J. 1997. Effects of storage, platelet lysis, and hemolysis on blood determinations of CK-MB, LDH-1, and cardiac troponin T in rats. *Clin Chem.* 43:S192.

Berna, M., Ott, L., Engle, S., et al. 2008. Quantification of NTproBNP in rat serum using immunoprecipitation and LC/MS/MS: A biomarker of drug-induced cardiac hypertrophy. *Anal Chem.* 80:561–566.

Biondo, A.W., Wiedmeyer, C.E., Sisson, D.D., and Solter, P.F. Comparative sequences of canine and feline endothelin-1. 2003. *Vet Clin Pathol.* 32:188–194.

Bleier, J., Vorderwinkler, K.P., Falkensammer, J., et al. 1998. Different intracellular compartmentations of cardiac troponins and myosin heavy chains: A causal connection to their different early release after myocardial damage. *Clin Chem.* 44:1912–1918.

Boretti, F.S., Buehler, P.W., D'Agnillo, F. et al. 2009. Sequestration of extracellular hemoglobin within a haptoglobin complex decreases its hypertensive and oxidative effects in dogs and guinea pigs. *J Clin Invest.* 119:2271–2280.

Boswood, A. 2009. Biomarkers in cardiovascular disease: Beyond natriuretic peptides. *J Vet Cardiol.* 11:S2–S32.

Brott, D., Gould, S., Jones, H., et al. 2005. Biomarkers of drug-induced vascular injury. *Toxicol Appl Pharmacol.* 207:441–445.

Burger, D. and Touyz, R.M. 2012. Cellular biomarkers of endothelial health: Microparticles, endothelial progenitor cells, and circulating endothelial cells. *J Amer Soc Hypertens.* 6:85–99.

Burkhard, M.J. and Millward, L.M. 2010. Respiratory tract. In *Canine and Feline Cytology. A Color Atlas and Interpretation Guide.* Eds. R.E. Raskin and D.J. Meyer, 2nd edition, pp. 123–170. St. Louis, MO: Saunders Elsevier.

Califano, F., Giovanniello, T., Pantone, P., et al. 2000. Clinical importance of thrombomodulin serum levels. *Eu Rev Med Pharmacol Sci.* 4:59–66.

Carter, J.M., Corson, N., Driscoll, K.E., et al. 2006. A comparative dose-related response of several key pro- and anti-inflammatory mediators in the lungs of rats, mice, and hamsters after subchronic inhalation of carbon black. *J Occup Environ Med.* 48:1265–1278.

Ceron, J.J., Eckersall, P.J., and Martınez-Subiela, S. 2005. Acute phase proteins in dogs and cats: Current knowledge and future perspectives. *Vet Clin Path.* 34:85–99.

Chaggar, P.S., Shaw, S.M., and Williams, S.G. 2009. Thiazolidinediones and heart failure. *Diabetes Vasc Dis Res.* 6:146–152.

Chamanza, R., Marxfeld, H.A., Blanco, A.I., et al. 2010. Incidences and range of spontaneous findings in control cynomolgus monkeys (Macaca fascicularis) used in toxicity studies. *Toxicol Pathol.* 38:642–657.

Chamanza, R., Parry, N.M., Rogerson, P., et al. 2006. Spontaneous lesions of the cardiovascular system in purpose-bred laboratory nonhuman primates. *Toxicol Pathol.* 34:357–363.

Christenson, R.H., Duh, S.-H., Newby, L.K., et al. 1998. Cardiac troponin I and cardiac troponin T: Relative values in short-term risk stratification of patients with acute coronary syndromes. *Clin Chem.* 44:494–501.

Clayton, R.N. 2003. Cardiovascular function in acromegaly. *Endoc Rev.* 24:272–277.

Cohn, J.N., Levine, T.B., Olivari, M.T., et al. 1984. Plasma norepinephrine as a guide to prognosis in patients with chronic congestive heart failure. *New Eng J Med.* 311:819–823.

Dagùes, N., Pawlowsk, V., Guigon, G., et al. 2007a. Altered gene expression in rat mesenteric tissue following *in vivo* exposure to a phosphodiesterase 4 inhibitor. *Toxicol Appl Pharmacol.* 218:52–63.

Dagùes, N., Pawlowski, V., and Sobry, C. 2007b. Investigation of the molecular mechanisms preceding PDE4 inhibitor-induced vasculopathy in rats: Tissue inhibitor of metalloproteinase 1, a potential predictive biomarker. *Toxicol Sci.* 100:238–247.

Daubert, M.A. and Jeremias, A. 2010. The utility of troponin measurement to detect myocardial infarction: Review of the current findings. *Vasc Health Risk Manag.* 6:691–699.

DeClue, A.E., Osterbur, K., Bigio, A., et al. 2011. Evaluation of serum NT-pCNP as a diagnostic and prognostic biomarker for sepsis in dogs. *J Vet Intern Med.* 25:453–459.

DeFrancesco, T.C., Rush, J.E., Rozanski, E.A., et al. 2007. Prospective clinical evaluation of an ELISA B-type natriuretic peptide assay in the diagnosis of congestive heart failure in dogs presenting with cough or dyspnea. *J Vet Intern Med.* 21:243–550.

De Meyer, S.F., Deckmyn, H., and Vanhoorelbeke, K. 2009. von Willebrand factor to the rescue. *Blood.* 113:5049–5057.

De Wit, T.R. and van Mourik, J.A. 2001. Biosynthesis, processing and secretion of von Willebrand factor: Biological implications. *Best Pract Res Clin Haematol.* 14:241–255.

Diniz, P.P.P.V., de Morais, H.S.A., Breitschwerdt, E.B., et al. 2008. Serum cardiac troponin I concentration in dogs with ehrlichiosis. *J Vet Int Med.* 22:1136–1143.

Drevon-Gaillot, E., Perron-Lepage, M-F., Clement, C., and Burnett, R. 2006. A review of background findings in cynomolgus monkey (Macaca fascicularis) from three different geographical origins. *Exp Toxicol Pathol.* 58:77–88.

Engleking, L.R. 2009. *Textbook of Veterinary Physiological Chemistry.* Deer Park: Linus Publications.

Erdbruegger, U., Haubitz, M., and Woywodt, A. 2006. Circulating endothelial cells: A novel marker of endothelial damage. *Clin Chim Acta.* 373:17–26.

Fallo, F., Betterle, C., Budano, S., et al. 1999. Regression of cardiac abnormalities after replacement therapy in Addison's disease. *Eur J Endocrinol.* 140:425–428.

Fox, P.R., Oyama, M.A., Reynolds, C., et al. 2009. Utility of plasma N-terminal pro-brain natriuretic peptide (NT-proBNP) to distinguish between congestive heart failure and non-cardiac causes of acute dyspnea in cats. *J Vet Cardiol.* 11: S51–S61.

Fu, Y.H., Lin, Q.X., Li, X.H., et al. 2009. A novel rat model of chronic heart failure following myocardial infarction. *Meth Find Exp Clin Pharmacol.* 31:367–373.

Gagnon, A.N., Crowe, S.P., Allen, D.G., et al. 1980. Myocarditis in puppies: Clinical, pathological and virological findings. *Can Vet J.* 21:195–197.

Gaze, D.C. 2009. Ischemia modified albumin: A novel biomarker for the detection of cardiac ischemia. *Drug Metab Pharmacokinet.* 24:333–341.

Goodof, I.I. and Macbryde, C.M. 1944. Heart failure in Addison's disease with myocardial changes of potassium deficiency. *J Clin Endocrinol.* 4:30–34.

Govers, R., van der Sluijs, P., van Donselaar, E., et al. 2002. Endothelial nitric oxide synthase and its negative regulator caveolin-1 localize to distinct perinuclear organelles. *J Histochem Cytochem.* 50:779–788.

Gray, H. 1945. Heart-weight and body-weight in rodents. *J Mammalogy.* 26:285–299.

Greaves, P. 2007. Cardiovascular system. In *Histopathology of Preclinical Toxicity Studies*, 3rd edition, pp. 270–333. Hanover: Elsevier.

Green, P.D. and Lemckert, J.W.H. 1977. Vitamin E and selenium responsive myocardial degeneration in dogs. *Can Vet J.* 18:290–291.

Guillevin, L. and Dorner, T. 2007. Vasculitis: Mechanisms involved and clinical manifestations. *Arthritis Res Ther.* 9:S1–S9.

Gunn, H.M. 1989. Heart weight and running ability. *J Anat.* 167:225–233.

Häggström, J., Hansson, K., Kvart, C., et al. 2000. Relationship between different natriuretic peptides and severity of naturally acquired mitral regurgitation in dogs with chronic myxomatous valve disease. *J Vet Cardiol.* 2:7–16.

Hanton, G. Sobry, C., Dagués, N., et al. 2008. Characterisation of the vascular and inflammatory lesions induced by the PDE4 inhibitor CI-1044 in the dog. *Toxicol Lett.* 179:15–22.

Henderson, RF. 2005. Use of bronchoalveolar lavage to detect respiratory tract toxicity of inhaled material. *Exp Toxicol Path.* 57:155–159.

Henderson, R.F., Scott, G.G., and Waide, J.J. 1995. Source of alkaline phosphatase activity in epithelial lining fluid of normal and injured F344 rat lungs. *Toxicol Appl Pharmacol.* 134:170–174.

Hori, Y., Sano, N., Kanai, K., et al. 2010. Acute cardiac volume load-related changes in plasma atrial natriuretic peptide and N-terminal pro-B-type natriuretic peptide concentrations in healthy dogs. *Vet J.* 185:317–321.

Hori, Y., Tsubaki, M., Katou, A., et al. 2008. Evaluation of NT-Pro BNP and CT-ANP as markers of concentric hypertrophy in dogs with a model of compensated aortic stenosis. *J Vet Intern Med.* 22:1118–1123.

Ishida, Y., Takayasu, T., Kimura, A., et al. 2006. Gene expression of cytokines and growth factors in the lungs after paraquat administration in mice. *Leg Med (Tokyo).* 8:102–109.

Jackson, A.S., Sandrini, A., Campbell, C., et al. 2007. Comparison of biomarkers in exhaled breath condensate and bronchoalveolar lavage. *Am J Respir Crit Care Med.* 175:222–227.

Joseph, D.R. 1908. The ratio between the heart-weight and body-weight in various animals. *J Exp Med.* 10:521–528.

Joseph, E.C. 2000. Arterial lesions induced by phosphodiesterase III (PDE III) inhibitors and DA(1) agonists. *Toxicol Lett.* 112–113:537–546.

Kalambokis, G.N., Tsatsoulis, A.A., Tsianos, E.V. 2004. The edematogenic properties of insulin. Am *J Kidney Dis.* 44:575–590.

Kanashiro-Takeuchi, R.M., Tziomalos, K., Takeuchi, L.M., et al. 2010. Cardioprotective effects of growth hormone-releasing hormone agonist after myocardial infarction. *Proc National Acad Sci.* 107:2604–2609.

Kedzierski, R.M. and Yanagisawa, M. 2001. Endothelin system: The double-edged sword in health and disease. *Ann Rew Pharmacol Toxicol.* 41:851–876.

Keller, T., Zeller, T., Peetz, D., et al. 2009. Sensitive troponin I assay in early diagnosis of acute myocardial infarction. *New Engl J Med.* 361:868–877.

Kemi, M., Keenan, K.P., McCoy, C., et al. 2000. The relative protective effects of moderate dietary restriction versus dietary modifications on spontaneous cardiomyopathy in male Sprague-Dawley rats. *Toxicol Pathol.* 28:285–296.

Keys, A., Henschel, A., and Taylor, H.L. 1947. The size and function of the human heart at rest and in semi-starvation and in subsequent rehabilitation. *Am J Physiol.* 150:153–169.

Koh, E., Nakamura, T., and Takahashi, H. 2004. Troponin-T and brain natriuretic peptide as predictors for adriamycin-induced cardiomyopathy in rats. *Circ J.* 68:163–167.

Levick, J.R. and Michel, C.C. 2010. Microvascular fluid exchange and the revised Starling principle. *Cardiovasc Res.* 87:198–210.

Lobetti, R., Dvir, E., and Pearson, J. 2002. Cardiac troponins in canine babesiosis. *J Vet Intern Med.* 18:831–839.

Louden, C., Brott, D., Katein, A., et al. 2006. Biomarkers and mechanisms of drug-induced vascular injury in non-rodents. *Toxicol Pathol.* 34:19–26.

Louden, C. and Morgan, D.G. 2001. Pathology and pathophysiology of drug-induced arterial injury in laboratory animals and its implications on the evaluation of novel chemical entities for human clinical trials. *Pharmacol Toxicol.* 89:158–170.

Lopez, A. 2007. Respiratory system. In *Pathologic Basis of Veterinary Disease*. Eds. M.D. McGavin and J.F. Zachary, pp. 463–558. St Louis, MO: Mosby Elsevier.

Lukas, Z. and Dvorak, K. 2004. Adhesion molecules in biology and oncology. *Acta Vet Brno.* 73:93–104.

MacDonald, K.A., Kittleson, M.D., Munro, C., and Kass, P. 2003. Brain natriuretic peptide concentration in dogs with heart disease and congestive heart failure. *J Vet Intern Med.* 17:172–177.

Maguire, J.J. and Davenport, A.P. 2014. Endothelin@25—new agonists, antagonist, inhibitors and emerging research frontiers. *Br J Pharmacol.* 171:5555–5572.

Martin, G.S., Becker, B.N., and Schulman, G. 1998. Cardiac troponin-I accurately predicts myocardial injury in renal failure. *Nephrol Dial Transplant.* 13:1709–1712.

Martin, V., McCutcheon, L.J., Poon, L., et al. 1993. Comparative mammal model of chronic rate overload: Relationship of myocardial Ca-cycling to heart, metabolic and lipoperoxidation rates. *Comp Biochem Physiol.* 106B:453–461.

Mastrorilli, C., Dondi, F., Agnoli, C., et al. 2007. Clinicopathologic features and outcome predictors of Leptospira interrogans Australis serogroup infection in dogs: A retrospective study of 20 cases (2001–2004). *J Vet Intern Med.* 21:3–10.

Mathers, R.A., Evans, G.O., Bleby, J., and Tornow, T. 2007. Total and differential leucocyte counts in rat and mouse bronchoalveolar lavage fluids using the Sysmex XT-2000iV. *Comp Clin Pathol.* 16:29–39.

Maxie, M.G. and Robinson, W.F. 2007. Cardiovascular system. In *Jubb, Kennedy, and Palmer's Pathology of Domestic Animals*. Ed. M.G. Maxie, Vol. 2, 5th edition. Toronto: Saunders Elsevier.

Metzger, J.M. and Westfall, M.V. 2004. Covalent and noncovalent modification of thin filament action. The essential role of troponins in cardiac muscle regulation. *Circ Res.* 94:146–158.

Mikaelian, I., Buness, A., Hirkaler, G., et al. 2011. Serum cardiac troponin I concentrations transiently increase in rats given rosiglitazone. *Toxicol Lett.* 201:110–115. doi:10.1016/j.toxlet.2010.12.012

Mikaelian, I., Coluccio, D., Hirkaler, G., et al. 2009. Assessment of the cardiotoxicity of hydralazine using an ultrasensitive flow-based troponin immunoassay. *Toxicol Pathol.* 37:878–881.

Miller, M.S., VanBuren, P., LeWinter, M.M., et al. 2010. Chronic heart failure decreases cross-bridge kinetics in single skeletal muscle fibers from humans. *J Physiol.* 588(Pt 20):4039–4053. published on line: doi:10.1113/jphysiol.2010.191957

Mills, P.C. and Lister, A.L. 2005. Using urea dilution to standardise components of pleural and bronchoalveolar lavage fluids in the dog. *New Zealand Vet J.* 53:423–427.

Minotti, J.R., Christoph, I., Oka, R., et al. 1991. Impaired skeletal muscle function in patients with congestive heart failure. Relationship to systemic exercise performance. *J Clin Invest.* 88:2077–2082.

Mion, M.M., Novello, E., Altinier, S., et al. 2007. Analytical and clinical performance of a fully automated cardiac multimarkers strategy based on protein biochip microarray technology. *Clin Biochem.* 40:1245–1251.

Muders, F. and Elsner, D. 2000. Animal models of chronic heart failure. *Pharmacol Res.* 41:605–612.

O'Brien, P.J. 1997. Deficiencies of myocardial troponin-T and creatine kinase MB isoenzyme in dogs with idiopathic dilated cardiomyopathy. *Amer J Vet Res.* 58:11–16.

O'Brien, P.J. 1998. Correlation of sarcoplasmic reticulum Ca2+-cycling activity and physiological performance of mammalian cardiac and skeletal muscle in health and disease. *Trends Comp Biochem Physiol.* 5:1–15.

O'Brien, P.J. 2006. Blood cardiac troponin in toxic myocardial injury: Archetype of a translational, safety biomarker. *Expert Rev Mol Diagn.* 6:685–702.

O'Brien, P.J. 2008. Cardiac Troponin is the most effective translational safety biomarker for myocardial injury in cardiotoxicity. *Toxicology.* 245:206–218.

O'Brien, P.J. 2009. Assessment of cardiotoxicity and myotoxicity. In *Animal Clinical Chemistry: A Practical Handbook for Toxicologists and Biomedical Researchers.* Ed. G.O. Evans, pp.145–158. Abingdon: CRC Press.

O'Brien, P.J. and Ball, R.O. 2006. Porcine stress syndrome. In *Diseases of Swine. Diseases of Swine.* Eds. B.E. Straw, J.J. Zimmerman, S. D'Allaire, and D.J. Taylor, pp. 945–963. Hoboken, NJ: Wiley Blackwell.

O'Brien, P.J., Dameron, G.W., Beck, M.L., et al. 1997a. Cardiac troponin T is a sensitive and specific biomarker of cardiac injury in laboratory animals. *Lab Anim Sci.* 47:486–495.

O'Brien, P.J., and Gwathmey, J.K. 2005. Myocardial $Ca2^+$- and ATP-cycling imbalances in end-stage dilated and ischemic cardiomyopathies. *Cardiovasc Res.* 30:394–404.

O'Brien, P.J., Landt, Y., and Ladenson, J.H. 1997b. Comparative reactivity and specificity of cardiac troponin I immunoassay in cardiac and skeletal muscle from different species. *Clin Chem.* 43:2333–2338.

O'Brien, P.J., Ling, E., Williams, H., et al. 1988. Compensatory increase of myocardial sarcoplasmic reticulum Ca-ATPase activity in response to chronic metabolic overload. *Can J Cardiol.* 4:243–250.

O'Brien, P.J., Moe, G.W., Nowack, L.M., et al. 1994. Sarcoplasmic reticulum Ca-release channel and ATP synthesis activities are early myocardial markers of heart failure produced by rapid ventricular pacing in dogs. *Can J Physiol Pharmacol.* 72:999–1006.

O'Brien, P.J., O'Grady, M., Lumsden, J.H., et al. 1993. Clinical pathology profiles of dogs with congestive heart failure, either noninduced or induced by rapid ventricular pacing, and turkeys with furazolidone toxicosis. *Am J Vet Res.* 54:60–68.

O'Brien, P.J., Shen, H., McCutcheon, L.J., et al. 1992. Rapid, simple and sensitive microassay for skeletal and cardiac muscle myoglobin and hemoglobin: Use in various animals indicates functional role of myohemoproteins. *Molec Cell Biochem.* 112:45–52.

O'Brien, P.J., Smith, D.E.C., Knechtel, T.J., et al. 2006. Cardiac troponin I is a sensitive, specific biomarker of cardiac injury in laboratory animals. *Lab Anim.* 40:153–171.

Oikawa, S., Imai, M., Inuzuka, C., Tawaragi, Y., Nakazato, H., and Matsuo, H. 1985. Structure of dog and rabbit precursors of atrial natriuretic polypeptides deduced from nucleotide sequence of cloned cDNA. *Biochem Biophys Res Commun.* 132:892–899.

Oyama, M.A., Fox, P.R., Rush, J.E., Rozanski, E.A., and Lesser, M. 2008. Clinical utility of serum N-terminal pro-B-type natriuretic peptide concentration for identifying cardiac disease in dogs and assessing disease severity. *J Am Vet Med Assoc.* 232:1496–1503.

Painter, P.R. 2005. Allometric scaling of the maximum metabolic rate of mammals: Oxygen transport from the lungs to the heart is a limiting step. *Theor Biol Med Modelling.* 2:31–39.

Paltrinieri, S. 2007. Early biomarkers of inflammation in dogs and cats: The acute phase proteins. *Vet Res Commun.* 31:125–129.

Panettieri, R.A., Kotlikoff, M.I., Gerthoffer, W.T., et al. 2008. Airway smooth muscle in bronchial tone, inflammation, and remodeling: Basic knowledge to clinical relevance. *Am J Respir Crit Care Med.* 177:248–252.

Peek, S.F., Apple, F.S., Murakami, M.A., et al. 2008. Cardiac isoenzymes in healthy Holstein calves and calves with experimentally induced endotoxemia. *Can J Vet Res.* 72:356–361.

Picinin, I.F. de, M., Camargos, P.A.M., and Marguet, C. 2010. Cell profile of BAL fluid in children and adolescents with and without lung disease. *J Bras Pneumol.* 36:372–391.

Prosek, R., Sisson, D.D., Oyama, M.A., et al. 2007. Distinguishing cardiac and noncardiac dyspnea in 48 dogs using plasma atrial natriuretic factor, B-type natriuretic factor, endothelin, and cardiac troponin-I. *J Vet Intern Med.* 21:238–342.

Pruimboom-Brees, I., Haghpassand, M., Royer, L., et al. 2006. A critical role for PPAR alpha nuclear receptors in the development of cardiomyocyte degeneration and necrosis. *Am J Pathol.* 169:750–760.

Raffan, E., Loureiro, J., Dukes-McEwan, J., et al. 2009. The cardiac biomarker NT-proBNP is increased in dogs with azotemia. *J Vet Intern Med.* 23:1184–1189.

Recchia, F.A. and Lionetti, V. 2007. Animal models of dilated cardiomyopathy for translational research. *Vet Res Commun.* 31:35–41.

Reed, R.K. and Rubin, K. 2010. Transcapillary exchange: Role and importance of the interstitial fluid pressure and the extracellular matrix. *Cardiovasc Res.* 87:211–217.

Reini, S.A., Dutta, G., Wood, C.E., et al. 2008. Cardiac corticosteroid receptors mediate the enlargement of the ovine fetal heart induced by chronic increases in maternal cortisol. *J Endocrinol.* 198:419–427.

Reitsma, S., Slaaf, D.W., Vink, H., et al. 2007. The endothelial glycocalyx: Composition, functions and visualization. *Pflugers Arch.* 454:345–359.

Robinson, N.E. 2007. Respiratory Function. In *Veterinary Physiology.* Eds. J.G. Cunningham and B.G. Klein, pp. 565–618. St. Louis, MO: Saunders.

Russo, T.A., Bartholomew, L.A., Davidson, B.A., et al. 2002. Total extracellular surfactant is increased but abnormal in a rat model of gram-negative bacterial pneumonia. *Am J Physiol Lung Cell Mol Physiol.* 283:L655–L663.

Rutschow, S., Li, J., Schultheiss, H.P., and Pauschinger, M. 2006. Myocardial proteases and matrix remodeling in inflammatory heart disease. *Cardiovasc Res.* 69:646–656.

Sayes, C.M., Reed, K.L., and Warheit, D.B. 2007. Assessing toxicity of fine and nanoparticles: Comparing *in vitro* measurements to *in vivo* pulmonary toxicity profiles. *Toxicol Sci.* 97:163–180.

Schellenberg, S., Grenacher, B., Kaufmann, K., et al. 2008. Analytical validation of commercial immunoassays for the measurement of cardiovascular peptides in the dog. *Vet J.* 178:85–90.

Schmidt, M.K., Reynolds, C.A., Estrada, A.H., et al. 2009. Effect of azotemia on serum N-terminal proBNP concentration in dogs with normal cardiac function: A pilot study. *J Vet Cardiol.* 11: S81–S86.

Schober, K.E., Kirbach, B., and Oechtering, G. 1999. Non invasive assessment of myocardial cell injury in dogs with suspected cardiac contusions. *J Vet Cardiol.* 1:17–25.

Schultze, A.E., Carpenter, K.H., Wians, F.H., et al. 2009. Longitudinal studies of cardiac troponin-I concentrations in serum from male Sprague Dawley rats: Baseline reference ranges and effects of handling and placebo dosing on biological variability. *Toxicol Pathol.* 37:754–760.

Seiler, B.M., Dick Jr, E.J., Guardado-Mendoza, R., et al. 2009. Spontaneous heart disease in the adult chimpanzee (pan troglodytes). *J Med Primatol.* 38:51–58.

Serebruany, V.L. 2006. Hypokalemia, cardiac failure, and reporting NXY-059 safety for acute stroke. *J Cardiovasc Pharmacol Ther.* 11:229–231.

Serra, M., Papakonstantinou, S., Adamcova, M., et al. 2010. Veterinary and toxicological applications for the detection of cardiac injury using cardiac troponin. *Vet J.* 185:50–57.

Shaikh, P.Z. 2011. Cytokines and their physiologic and pharmacologic functions in inflammation: A review. *Inter J Pharmacy Life Sci.* 2:1247–1263.

Shakir, D.K. and Rasul, K.I. 2009. Chemotherapy induced cardiomyopathy: Pathogenesis, monitoring and management. *J Clin Med Res.* 1:8–12.

Sharkey, L.C., Berzina, I., Ferasin, L., et al. 2009. Evaluation of serum cardiac troponin I concentration in dogs with renal failure. *J Am Vet Med Assoc.* 234:767–770.

Sherwood, L. 2012. *Human Physiology From Cells to Systems*, 8th edition. Belmont, CA: Brooks/Cole Cengage Learning.

Shimura, S. 2000. Signal transduction of mucous secretion by bronchial gland cells. *Cell Signal.* 12:271–277.

Silvestrini, P., Piviani, M., Alberola, J., et al. 2010. Serum cardiac troponin I concentration in dogs with Leishmaniasis. *J Vet Intern Med.* 24:7075

Sisson, E. 2009. B-type natriuretic peptides. *J Vet Cardiol.* 1:55–57.

Slaughter, M.R.S., Campbell, S., and O'Brien, P.J. 2004. Myocardial concentration of cardiac troponin T as an early discriminator of mechanisms of cardiac hypertrophy. *Comp Clin Path.* 13:59–64.

Slaughter, M.R., Thakkar, H., and O'Brien, P.J. 2002. Effect of diquat on the antioxidant system and cell growth in human neuroblastoma cells. *Tox Appl Pharmacol.* 178:63–70.

Solaro, R.J., Posevear, P., and Kobayashi, T. 2008. The unique functions of cardiac troponin I in the control of cardiac muscle contraction and relaxation. *Biochem Biophys Res Commun.* 369:82–87.

Spinale, F.G. 2007. Myocardial matrix remodeling and the matrix metalloproteinases: Influence on cardiac form and function. *Physiol Rev.* 87:1285–1342.

Stephenson, R.B. 2007. Cardiovascular physiology. In *Veterinary Physiology.* Eds. J.G. Cunningham and B.G. Klein, pp. 178–299. St. Louis, MO: Saunders.

Sung, J.K., Kim, J.-Y., Ryu, D.-W., et al. 2010. A case of hypocalcemia-induced dilated cardiomyopathy. *J Cardiovasc Ultrasound.* 18:25–27.

Swoap, S.J. and Gutilla, M.J. 2009. Cardiovascular changes during daily torpor in the laboratory mouse. *Am J Physiol Regul Integr Comp Physiol.* 297(3):R769–R774.

Tao, L., Liu, H.-R., Gao, F., et al. 2005. Mechanical traumatic injury without circulatory shock causes cardiomyocyte apoptosis: Role of reactive nitrogen and reactive oxygen species. *Am J Physiol Heart Circ Physiol.* 288:H2811–H2818.

Tesfamariam, B. and DeFelice, A.F. 2007. Endothelial injury in the initiation and progression of vascular disorders. *Vascular Pharmacol.* 46:229–237.

Thomas, C.J. and Woods, R.L. 2003. Haemodynamic action of B-type natriuretic peptide substantially outlasts its plasma half life in conscious dogs. *Clin Exp Pharmacol Physiol.* 30:369–375.

Thygesen, K., Mair, J., Mueller, C., et al. 2011. Recommendations for the use of natriuretic peptides in acute cardiac care. A position statement from the Study Group on Biomarkers in Cardiology of the ESC Working Group on Acute Cardiac Care. *Eur Heart J.* 33(16):2001–2006.

Todd, J., Freese, B., Lu, A., et al. 2007. Ultrasensitive flow-based immunoassays using single-molecule counting. *Clin Chem.* 53:1990–1995.

Tonnessen, T., Christensen, G., Oie, E., et al. 1997. Increased cardiac expression of endothelin-1 mRN in ischemic heart failure in rats. *Cardiovasc Res.* 33:601–610.

Tran, H.A. 2006. Increased troponin I in "wet" beriberi. *J Clin Pathol.* 59:555.

Trifilieff, A., El-Hashim, A., and Bertrand, C. 2000. Time course of inflammatory and remodeling events in a murine model of asthma: Effect of steroid treatment. *Am J Physiol Lung Cell Mol Physiol.* 279:L1120–L1128.

Tsai, S.F., Liu, B.L., Liao, J.W., et al. 2003. Pulmonary toxicity of thuringiensin administered intratracheally in Sprague-Dawley rats. *Toxicology.* 186:205–16.

Tsai, S.F., Yang, C., Liu, B.L., et al. 2006. Role of oxidative stress in thuringiensin-induced pulmonary toxicity. *Toxicol Appl Pharmacol.* 216:347–353.

Tunca, R., Sozmen, M., Erdogan, H., et al. 2008. Determination of cardiac troponin I in the blood and heart of calves with foot and mouth disease. *J Vet Diagnostic Invest.* 20:598–605.

Van Belle, E., Dallongeville, J., Vicaut, E., et al. 2010. Ischemia-modified albumin levels predict long-term outcome in patients with acute myocardial infarction. The French Nationwide OPERA study. *Am Heart J.* 159:570–576.

Van Kimmenade, R.R.J. and Januzzi, J.L. 2009. The evolution of the natriuretic peptides—current applications in human and animal medicine. *J Vet Cardiol.* 11: S9–S21.

Van Vleet, J.E. and Ferrans, V.J. 2007. Cardiovascular system. In *Pathologic Basis of Veterinary Disease*. Eds. M.D. McGavin and J.F. Zachary, pp. 559–611. St Louis, MO: Mosby Elsevier.

Walker, D.B., 2006. Serum chemical biomarkers of cardiac injury for nonclinical safety testing. *Toxicol Pathol.* 34:94–104.

Wallace, K.B., Hausner, E., Herman, E., et al. 2004. Serum troponins as biomarkers of drug-induced cardiac toxicity. *Toxicol Pathol.* 32:106–121.

Warheit, D.B., Sayes, C.M., Reed, K.L., et al. 2008. Health effects related to nanoparticle exposures: Environmental, health and safety considerations for assessing hazards and risks. *Pharmacol Therapeut.* 120:35–42.

Washizu, T., Nakamura, M., Izawa N., et al. 2002. The activity ratio of the cytosolic MDH/LDH and the isoenzyme pattern of LDH in the peripheral leukocytes of dogs, cats and rabbits. *Vet Res Commun.* 26:341–346.

Watterson, C., Lanevschi, A., Horner, J., et al. 2009. A comparative analysis of acute-phase proteins as inflammatory biomarkers in preclinical toxicology studies: Implications for preclinical to clinical translation. *Toxicol Pathol.* 37:28–33.

Weaver, J.L., Snyder, R., Knapton, A., et al. 2008. Biomarkers in peripheral blood associated with vascular injury in Sprague-Dawley rats treated with the phosphodiesterase IV inhibitors SCH 351591 or SCH 534385. *Toxicol Pathol.* 36:840–849.

Weibel, E.R. 2008. How to make an alveolus. *Eur Respir J.* 31:483–485.

Weibel, E.R., Bacigalupe, L.D., Schmitt, B., et al. 2004. Allometric scaling of maximal metabolic rate in mammals: Muscle aerobic capacity as determinant factor. *Resp Physiol Neurobiol.* 140:115–117.

Wells, R.J., Sedacca, C.D., Aman, A.M., et al. 2009. Successful management of a dog that had severe rhabdomyolysis with myocardial and respiratory failure. *J Amer Vet Med Assoc.* 234:1049–1054.

Wells, S.M. and Sleeper, M. 2008. Cardiac troponins. *J Vet Emerg Crit Care.* 18:235–245.

West, G.B., Brown, J.H., and Enquist, B.J. 1997. A general model for the origin of allometric scaling laws in biology. *Science.* 276:122–126.

Wills, T.B., Heaney, A.M., Wardrop, K.J., and Haldorson, G.J. 2009. Immunomagnetic isolation of canine circulating endothelial and endothelial progenitor cells. *Vet Clin Pathol.* 38:437–442.

Yasuda, J., Tateyama, K., Syuto, B., et al. 1990. Lactate dehydrogenase and creatine phosphokinase isoenzymes in tissues of laboratory animals. *Jpn J Vet Res.* 38:19–29.

Zabka, T. S., Irwin M., and Albassam, M.A. 2009. Spontaneous cardiomyopathy in cynomolgus monkeys (macaca fascicularis). *Toxicol Pathol.* 37:814–818.

14 Evaluation of Skeletal Muscle Function and Injury

Carol B. Grindem, Jennifer A. Neel, and Carolina Escobar

CONTENTS

14.1 INTRODUCTION

Skeletal muscle is a complex organ composed of an intricate array of specialized contractile proteins, conductile membranes with ion channels, and pumps, together with their associated vascular and nerve supply. It represents approximately 40%–50% of the body's weight, and besides its general function in body movement and posture, skeletal muscle contraction is important in heat production, temperature homeostasis, and metabolism. Because skeletal muscle participates in the function of virtually all organ systems in the body, its function should not be overlooked when evaluating other body organs or systemic disorders (Dukes and Reece, 2004; Valberg, 2008). For example, skeletal muscle plays a critical role in the control of diabetes. By increasing the production of glucose transporter protein (GLUT4), the uptake of glucose into muscle cells is improved by exercise and so the progression of the disease may be retarded (Stehno-Bittel et al., 2008). Also, muscle-derived cytokines called myokines appear to have important anti-inflammatory, metabolic, and physiologic roles, which may explain how regular exercise helps to protect against chronic disorders such as cardiovascular disease, type 2 diabetes, dementia, and depression (Pedersen et al., 2007; Pedersen and Febbraio, 2005). Myokines released from contracting skeletal muscle play important roles in lipid and glucose metabolism in other metabolically active tissue such as liver and adipose tissue and can decrease body fat mass and improve whole body metabolism, which may be valuable in the treatment of obesity and cardiovascular-related disorders (Febbraio and Pedersen, 2005; Hittel et al., 2009; Izumiya et al., 2008; Walsh, 2009).

The regulatory pathways, hormones, growth factors, and key molecules that signal skeletal muscle growth or atrophy or satellite stem cell self-renewal are being deciphered (Carlson et al., 2009; Evans, 2010; Lee, 2007; Welle, 2009; Zammit, 2008). Knowledge of these factors is critical to the development of therapeutic approaches to hereditary muscle diseases such as Duchenne's muscular dystrophy, muscle repair, and muscle loss from cachexia, sarcopenia, and inactivity.

14.2 MUSCLE STRUCTURE

Skeletal muscle is composed of extremely elongated multinucleated cells (up to 30 cm) referred to as muscle fibers or myofibers. A whole muscle consists of a bundle of longitudinally arranged muscle fibers that are made up of myofibrils formed from thick (myosin) and thin (actin) myofilaments organized into repeating subunits along the length of the myofibril. These repeating subunits are called sarcomeres and form the basic contractile unit of muscle. Muscle fibers are filled with numerous myofibrils, mitochondria, sarcoplasmic reticulum (SR), Golgi apparatus, and liposomes. The sarcoplasm is the cytoplasm and the SR is a structure that is similar to the endoplasmic reticulum in other cells. Variation in skeletal muscles results from their different constituent myofiber populations and the vascular and nerve supply.

14.3 SUBCELLULAR MUSCLE PROTEINS

Myofibrils are made up of still finer thick and thin myofilaments. The thick filaments consist almost exclusively of myosin molecules (molecular weight 460,000 Da), whereas the thin filaments are composed of actin (molecular weight 43,000 Da), tropomyosin (molecular weight 70,000 Da), and troponin (Hill et al., 2008; Ruckebusch et al., 1991). Troponin is composed of three subunits (troponin I, troponin T, and troponin C) with a molecular weight ranging from 18,000 to 35,000 Da.

Each myofibril consists of a series of sarcomeres that run parallel to each other on the long axis of the cell. Sarcomeric subunits of one myofibril are almost perfectly aligned with those of the myofibrils next to it. The optical properties of this alignment result in the striped or striated appearance of skeletal muscle (see Figures 14.1 and 14.2).

The characteristic cross-striations of skeletal muscle caused by differences in the refractive indexes of various parts of the muscle fiber are identified by letters referring to the optical properties of living muscle as demonstrated using polarized light microscopy. I (isotropic) bands appear lighter because these sarcomeric regions contain mainly thin actin filaments, whose smaller diameter allows the passage of light between them, whereas A (anisotropic) bands contain mostly larger diameter myosin filaments that restrict the passage of light. The Z line (from the German *zwischenscheibe*, the band in between the I bands) is a dark line found in the center of the I band. Within the A band is a brighter central region called the H zone from the German *helle*, meaning bright. No actin–myosin overlap occurs in this zone in a relaxed muscle. Finally, the M-line (from the German *mittel* meaning middle) is a dark central line that bisects the A band (see Figure 14.1). The heads of myosin molecules projecting from the ends of the thick filaments contain catalytic sites that hydrolyze adenosine triphosphate (ATP) and sites that cross-link to actin. A sarcomere is defined as the area between two adjacent Z lines and functions as a contractile unit. Nebulin and titin are structural proteins that help stabilize the actin and myosin filaments in the sarcomeres, whereas the dystrophin–glycoprotein complex strengthens the muscle by connecting the fibrils to the extracellular environment (Hill et al., 2008).

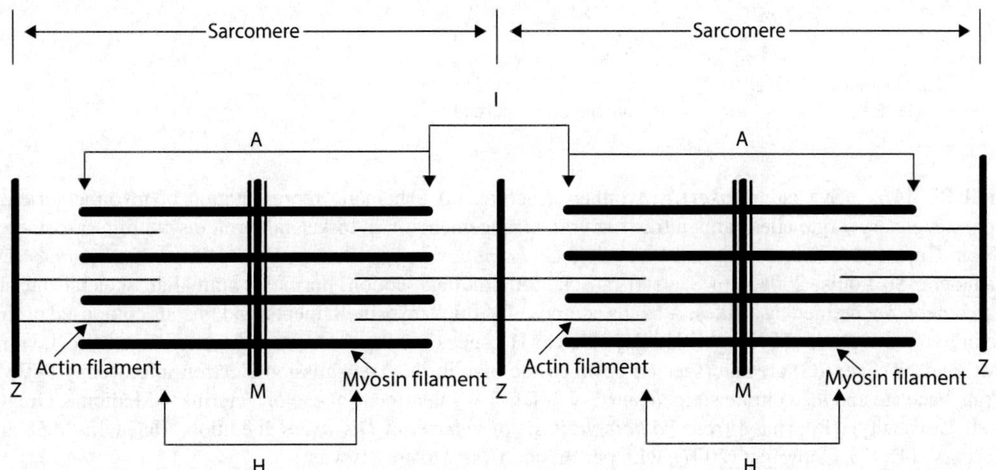

FIGURE 14.1 Diagram of two relaxed sarcomeres of skeletal muscle. The arrangement of the thick myosin and thin actin filaments is identified by letters. The light I band is divided by a dark Z line to which the actin filaments are attached. The dark A band has a lighter H band in the center that is transected by an M line. A sarcomere is defined as the area between two adjacent Z lines. (Courtesy of Cari Grindem-Corbett.)

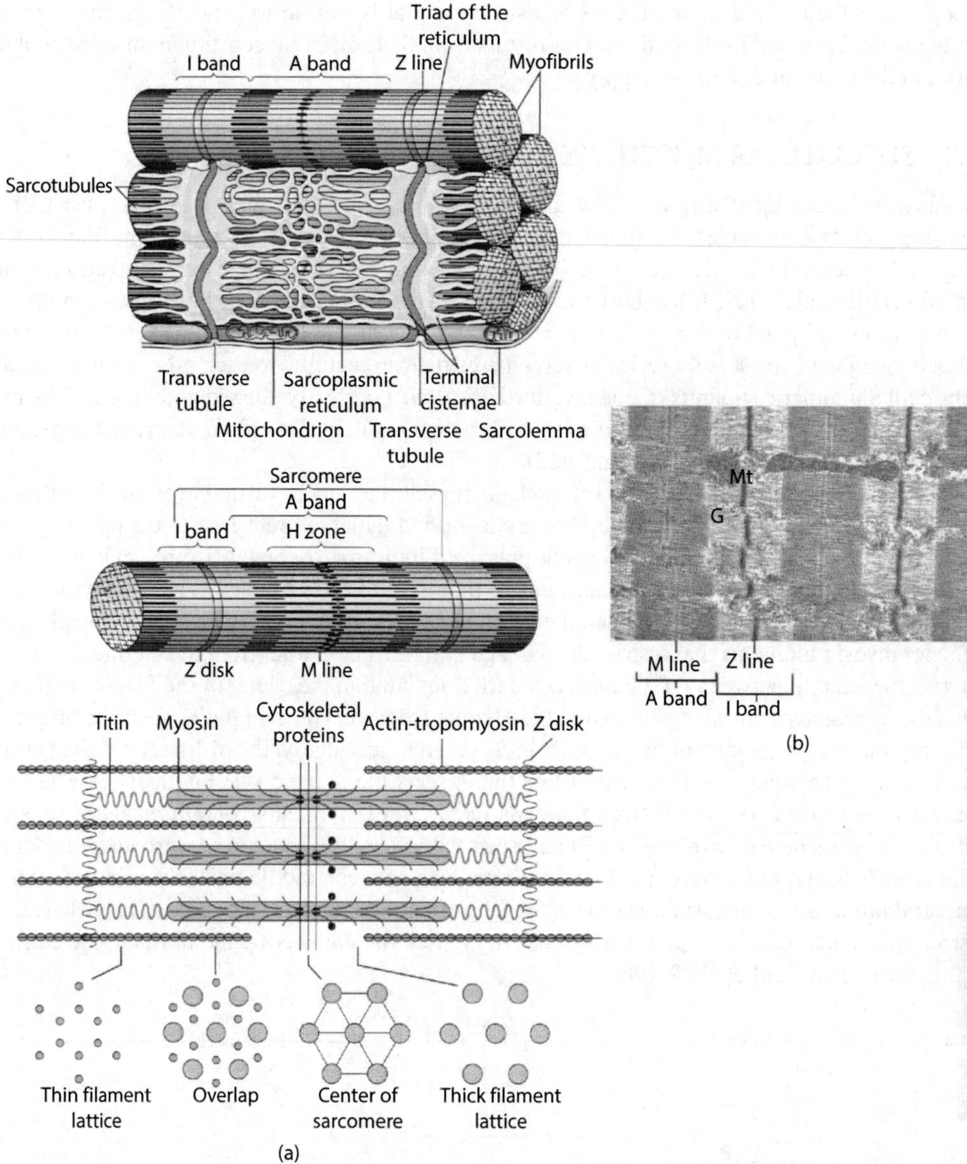

FIGURE 14.2 (See color insert.) Myofiber structure. (a) Schematic representation of myofiber orientation, secondary organelles, and ultrastructural arrangement of cytoskeletal proteins within sarcomeres. (From Copstead-Kirhorn, L.E. and Banasik, J.L., *Pathophysiology Biological and Behavioral Perspective*, Saunders, St. Louis, 2005.) (b) Skeletal muscle, longitudinal section, normal mammalian skeletal muscle. Sarcomeres are defined by Z lines, A bands composed of thick myosin filaments, and I bands composed of thin actin filaments. Dense M lines with adjacent clear H zones occur in the center of the A band. Mitochondria (Mt) and glycogen (G) are interspersed between the myofibrils. Transmission electron microscopy (TEM). Uranyl acetate and lead citrate stain. (Courtesy of Dr. BA Valentine, College of Veterinary Medicine, Oregon State University). (Reprinted from *Pathologic Basis of Veterinary Disease*, 4th edition, McGavin, M.D. and Zachary, J.F, 976, Copyright (2007), with permission from Mosby Elsevier.)

14.4 SARCOLEMMA AND TUBULAR SYSTEM

The sarcolemma surrounding each muscle fiber is a specialized plasma membrane that contains ion channels along its length and is designed to receive and conduct stimuli. It is composed of two layers, an inner plasma membrane proper and an outer basement membrane rich in glycoprotein and thin collagen fibrils. T tubules are tubular extensions of the sarcolemma that penetrate the myofibers at the junction of the A and I bands (mammals and reptiles) or at the level of the Z line (amphibians) allowing rapid penetration of the wave of depolarization into the muscle fiber (Hill et al., 2008).

The basement membrane consists of two layers, the outer *reticular lamina* and the inner *basal lamina*. The outermost layer of the sarcolemma (the *reticular lamina*) is composed of the proteins fibronectin, type I collagen, and a high-salt soluble protein, and it fuses with the tendon fibers that form tendons at the ends of the muscle. The tendons, in turn, are attached to the bone. The inner basal lamina contains the proteins laminin, fibronectin, and type IV collagen. Surrounding each individual muscle fiber is the endomysium, a dense connective tissue layer composed of collagen fibrils. A similar thick connective tissue layer called the perimysium divides the muscle fibers into large bundles; this layer also contains loose connective tissue through which arterioles, venules, and nerve branches run. The epimysium is a thick, dense connective tissue layer that covers the entire muscle belly and separates it from other muscles. The reticular lamina and endomysium blend with the perimysial sheaths at the myotendious joints. Pericytes (satellite cells), located within the basal lamina, may represent precursors of muscle cells, differentiating in response to muscle damage (Dukes and Reece, 2004; McGavin and Zachary, 2007). Alterations in the sarcolemma membrane stability can result in muscular dystrophy. For example, muscular dystrophy results from a lack or defective function of dystrophin. Dystrophin is a cytoplasmic protein that is a critical part of a protein complex (dystropin-associated protein complex), which connects the myofibrils to the extracellular matrix through the sarcolemma.

The sarcotubular system is made up of the SR and the transverse tubular or T system. The T system functions in the rapid transmission of the action potential from the cell membrane to all fibrils in the muscle. The SR is a complex network of channels that completely surrounds the muscle fiber and is related to calcium movement and muscle metabolism. It functions in the uptake and storage of calcium within its lumina and in the release of calcium into the sarcoplasma bathing the myofilaments and organelles. The T tubules form narrow, perpendicular channels around the muscle fiber, and where the T tubules intersect the SR, the SR forms sac-like structures called terminal cisternae on either side, which serve primarily to store and release calcium. This structure of the T tubule with two terminal cisternae is called a triad.

14.5 MOTOR UNIT AND NEUROMUSCULAR JUNCTION

A motor unit is defined as one motor neuron with all of its branches and all the muscle fibers that it innervates. The ratio of nerve-to-muscle fibers varies with muscle function.

Muscles requiring fine movement have a higher nerve-to-muscle ratio. Motor axons terminate at skeletal muscle sites called neuromuscular junctions. At these locations (usually near the middle of the muscle fiber), the sarcolemma is modified to form a motor end plate, which contains numerous surface folds indenting the muscle fiber. Motor neuron axon terminals lie in these folds and have numerous transmitter vesicles containing acetylcholine (ACh) (see Figure 14.3). Selective and nonselective transport of Na^+, K^+, Ca^{2+}, and Cl^- across neuromuscular membranes is essential to initiation and propagation of action potentials. Action potentials in the motor axon result in activation of voltage-gated Ca ion channels in the presynaptic membrane. The Ca influx initiates a calcium-dependent release of ACh by exocytosis into the synaptic cleft between the presynaptic axon terminal of the motor neuron and the postsynaptic skeletal myofiber. The synaptic cleft is filled with basal lamina containing acetycholinesterase (AChE) (Hill et al., 2008). The ACh diffuses across the sarcolemma of the motor end plate and attaches to phasic ACh receptors (AChR) initiating increased membrane permeability to Na^+, K^+, and Cl^-. The increased diffusion of ions depolarizes the motor end plate membrane. When the amplitude of depolarization exceeds the threshold, depolarization of adjacent sarcolemma produces a muscle action potential (MAP).

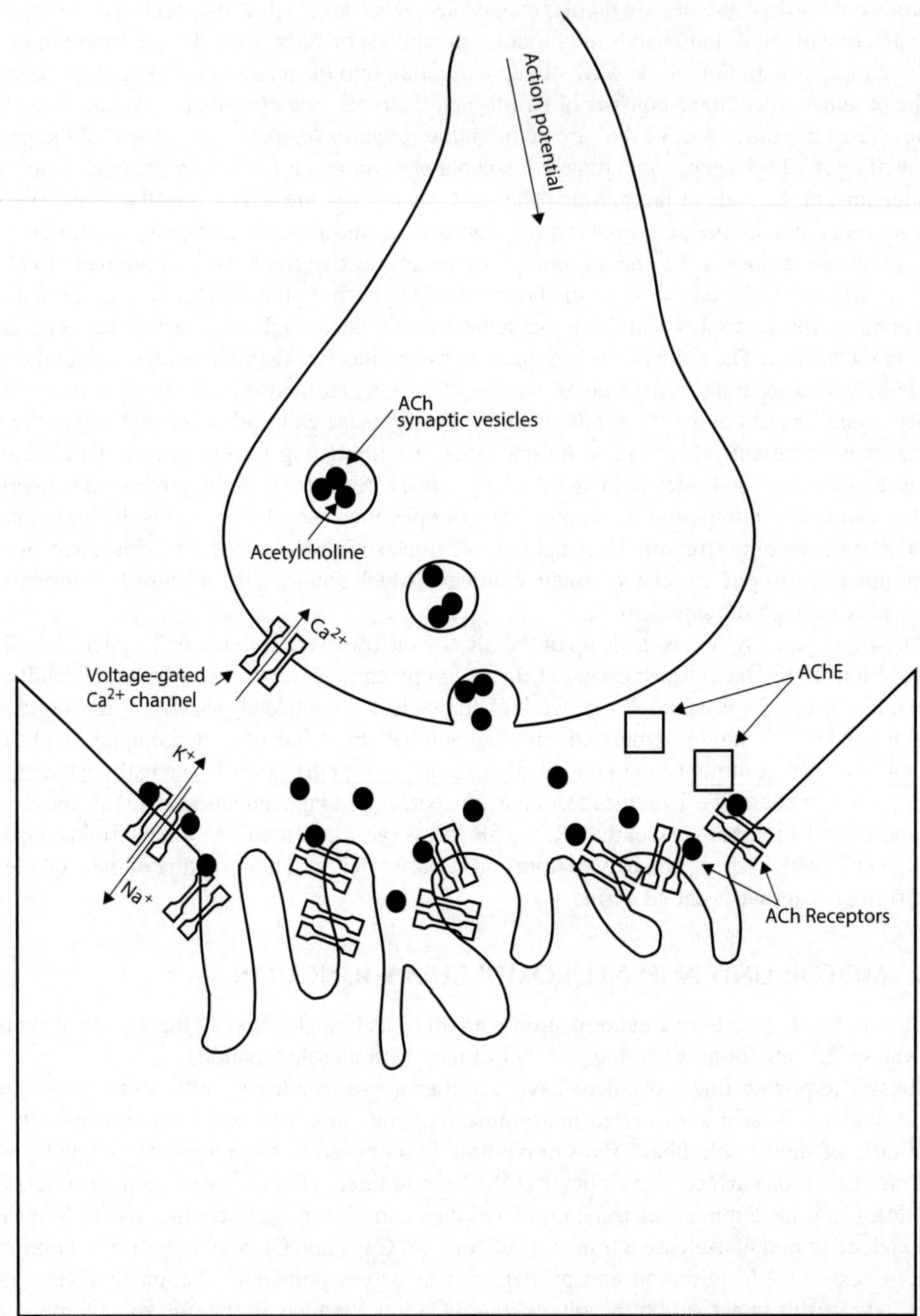

FIGURE 14.3 Transmission of an action potential at a neuromuscular junction. An action potential depolarizes the presynaptic axon terminal and opens voltage-gated Ca^{2+} channels resulting in vesicle fusion and release of acetylcholine (ACh) into the synaptic cleft. ACh diffuses across the synaptic cleft and binds to ligand-gated channels (ACh receptors) in the postsynaptic membrane. Receptor channels open allowing ion exchange. Na^{2+} influx results in an action potential that spreads causing depolarization and initiation of muscle contraction. Acetylcholine esterase (AChE) in the synaptic cleft and at the postsynaptic membrane hydrolyzes ACh into choline and acetate terminating the action potential. Choline is actively transported into the motor neuron for resynthesis of ACh. (Courtesy of Cari Grindem-Corbett.)

The action of ACh is terminated by enzymatic degradation by AChE in the sarcolemma of the motor end plate. AChE hydrolyzes ACh into acetate and choline. Choline is actively transported back into the motor axon terminal for the synthesis of ACh.

The action potential can be inhibited at multiple stages. Magnesium or other divalent cations can partially block the voltage-gated Ca ion channels in the presynaptic membrane. *Clostridium botulinum* toxin attaches to axon terminals and prevents release of ACh resulting in skeletal muscle paralysis. In contrast, the neurotoxin alpha latrotoxin found in the venom of black widow spiders (*Latrodectus*) stimulates the release of ACh from motor nerve terminals resulting in depletion of ACh and skeletal muscle paralysis (Dukes and Reece, 2004; McGavin and Zachary, 2007).

14.6 MUSCLE CONTRACTION

Skeletal muscle contraction is initiated by release of acetylcholine resulting in depolarization of the muscle cell that spreads across the entire muscle cell membrane (sarcolemma). T tubules transmit this potential down deep into the myofilaments. The T tubules form an intimate and complex association with the adjacent terminal cisternae of the SR (triads) (see Figure 14.4). A quaternary protein complex composed of ryanodine receptor (the major mediator of calcium-induced calcium release from the SR) together with triadin, junctin, and calsequestrin proteins (important regulators of ryanodine receptor function) in the SR interacts with a voltage-sensitive dihydropyridine receptor (DHPR) in the sarcolemma at the junctional triads to regulate Ca^{2+} storage and release. Simplistically, depolarization results in the release of Ca^{2+} from the terminal cisternae of the SR into the sarcoplasma, which triggers muscle contraction. The released Ca^{2+} binds to troponin causing a conformational shape change of the troponin molecule. This results in an orientation change of the tropomyosin molecule exposing a myosin-binding site on the actin filament. Cross-bridging of myosin to actin pulls the thick and thin filaments toward each other shortening the length of the sarcomere and causing the muscle to contract. Additionally, ATP is released. It is the cleavage of the high-energy phosphate bonds of ATP that provides the energy required for muscle contraction. Muscle contraction ceases as the calcium ions are rapidly pumped back into the sarcomplasmic reticulum by an active calcium-ATPase membrane pump located in the SR.

14.7 ENERGY METABOLISM

Hydrolysis of ATP provides the energy required for muscle contraction. ATP must be continually resynthesized by muscle fibers because only small amounts can be stored. Creatine phosphate (CP—phosphorylcreatine), another high-energy compound present in small amounts, supplies the energy for resynthesis of ATP. Muscle utilizes free fatty acids for energy during periods of rest or light exercise. Carbohydrates become the predominant energy source during times of intense exercise. During aerobic glycolysis, pyruvate is formed by degradation of glucose and glycogen and enters the citric acid cycle where it is metabolized to CO_2 and H_2O generating large quantities of ATP from adenosine diphosphate (ADP). Insufficient O_2 supplies result in anaerobic glycolysis; pyruvate must then be converted to lactate rather than entering the citric acid cycle. This results in the production of only small quantities of ATP.

Muscle fatigue results when the body is unable to supply sufficient energy or metabolites to the contracting muscles to meet the increased demands of the muscle. Metabolic acidosis develops, which further disrupts metabolic pathways. Lactic acid build-up was once believed to cause muscle fatigue but currently its role in muscle fatigue is uncertain and it may actually help to reduce muscle fatigue (Cairns, 2006). Although lactate production is a good indirect marker for exercise-induced metabolic acidosis, the cause of the metabolic acidosis appears to be increased nonmitochondrial ATP turnover (Robergs et al., 2004).

14.8 MUSCLE ADAPTATION

Muscle is remarkably adaptive to a wide range of physiologic and pathologic stimuli. Responses include atrophy, hypertrophy, necrosis, regeneration, elongation, shortening, and fiber-type conversion (Charge and Rudnicki, 2004; McGavin and Zachary, 2007). Muscle cells regenerate by

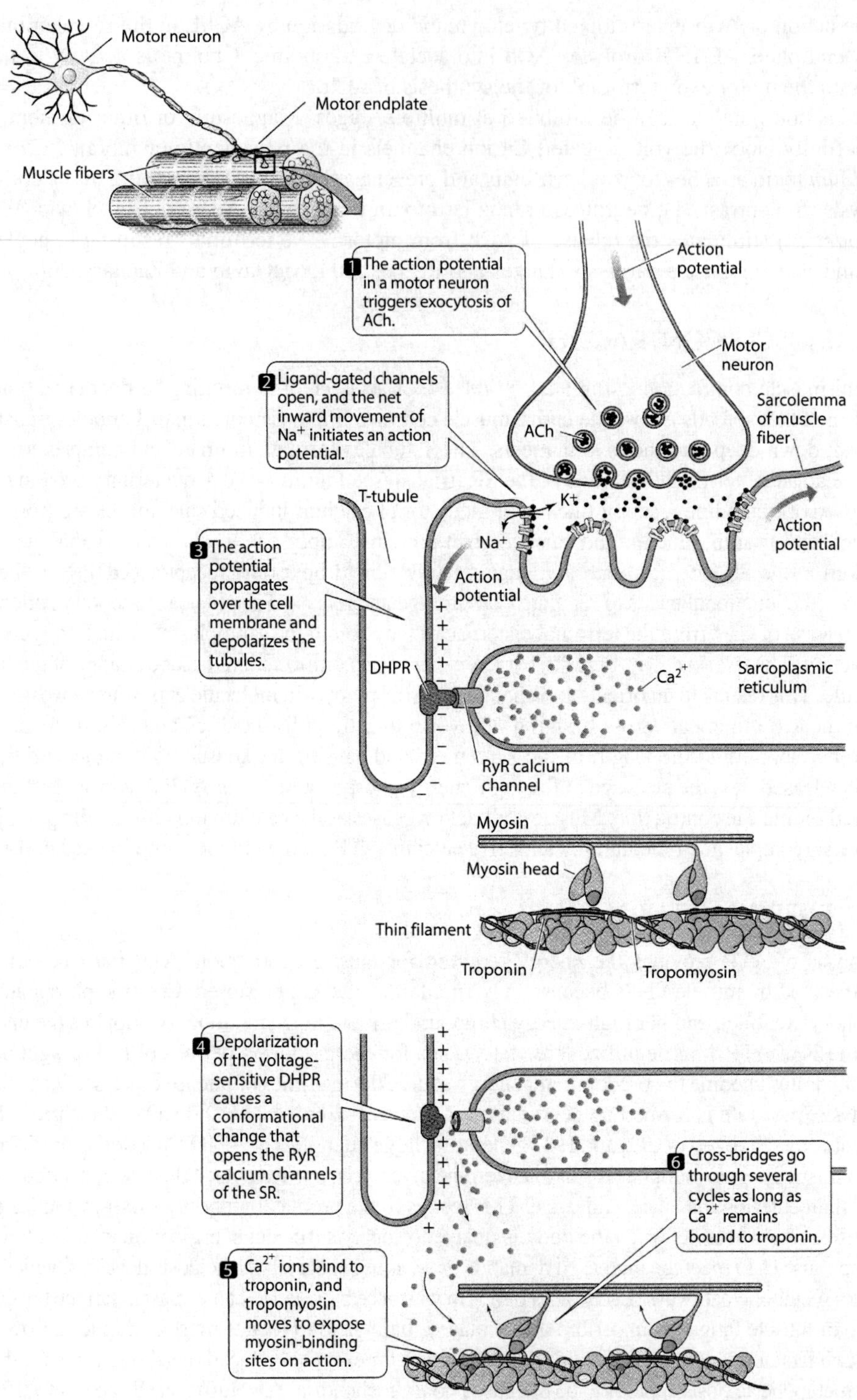

FIGURE 14.4 **(See color insert.)** Excitation–contraction coupling is accomplished by the interactions of components in two intimately associated membrane systems: the transverse tubular system and the sarcoplasmic reticulum. (After Silverthorn, D.U., *Human Physiology: An Integrated Approach*, Pearson/Benjamin Cummings, San Francisco, 2004; Reprinted from Hill, R.W. et al., *Animal Physiology* Sinauer Associates, Sunderland, 2004, 471. With permission.)

activation of a quiescent population of undifferentiated muscle stem (satellite) cells. Mechano growth factor (MGF) derived from alternate splicing of the insulin-like growth factor-I gene is expressed by active muscle cells and appears to be important in the activation of satellite cells (Hill et al., 2008). Although muscle stem cells are relatively resistant to aging, they are strongly influenced by aging changes in their microenvironment. Exposure of old satellite cells to young systemic factors enhances their regenerative capacity (Carlson et al., 2009). The pathways and factors that regulate muscle stem cells and regeneration are complex but are being delineated and include Wnt, Notch, transforming growth factor-beta (TGF-β), phospho Smad3 (pSmad3), and pair box protein Pax-7 (Carlson et al., 2009; Zammit, 2008). If the basal lamina remains intact, muscle regeneration is orderly and forms a cylindrical structure; otherwise the regenerative process is more disorganized and includes more fibrosis. Lack of a viable blood supply or intact motor nerves will inhibit optimal regeneration. Areas of severe muscle damage or large devascularized areas will heal by scar tissue formation.

Exercise-induced skeletal muscle adaptation varies with training duration, intensity, and frequency and is also influenced by nutritional state, age, and degree of physical fitness. The major metabolic change that exercise induces is an increase in the oxidative capacity to utilize fat, carbohydrate, and ketones (Ruckebusch, Phaneuf, and Dunlop, 1991; Bruss, 2008). Endurance training elicits mitochondrial biogenesis (increased mitochondrial density and enzyme activity), fast-to-slow fiber-type transformation, and changes in substrate metabolism. This contrasts with heavy resistance training, which stimulates the synthesis of contractile proteins responsible for muscle hypertrophy and increases the maximal contractile force output. The molecular and genetic mechanisms of adaptation are distinctly different between these diverse exercise modes (Coffey and Hawley, 2007).

By increasing fat oxidation, enhancing lactate kinetics, and inducing greater type 1 fiber (slow twitch) volume, endurance training results in increased muscle glycogen stores and glycogen sparing. It also increases capillary and mitochondrial density. Additionally, altered gene expression results in altered muscle phenotype with improved resistance to fatigue. In skeletal muscle, mitochondria are the main subcellular structure determining oxidative capacity and resistance to fatigue. Mitochondrial protein can be increased 50%–100% with continuous endurance training; however, with a protein half-life of about 1 week, continuous training is necessary to maintain elevated mitochondrial content (Coffey and Hawley, 2007).

Improved endurance is mainly associated with mitochondrial biogenesis, although enhanced oxygen kinetics, substrate transport, and buffering capacity are contributing factors. Mitochondrial biogenesis is complex, but upregulation of peroxisome proliferator-activated receptor γ coactivator-1α (PGC-1α), a coactivator of the peroxisome proliferator-activated receptor (PPAR), is a critical regulator. Increased PGC-1α-PPAR–mediated transcription is important for establishing an endurance, but not a resistance, training phenotype. Increased gene expression of metabolic proteins (hexokinase, lipoprotein lipase, and carnitine palmitoyltransferase) also promotes an endurance phenotype (Coffey and Hawley, 2007). Ras-extracellular signal regulated mitogen-activated protein kinase (MAPK/Erk), phosphatidylinositol 3′ kinase (P13K)-Akt1, p38 MAPK, and calcineurin pathways are the key signaling cascades for skeletal muscle phenotype. Functional genomics using microarray technology and proteomics are increasing our understanding of the molecular determinants of muscle phenotype (Chang, 2007).

Resistance exercise increases muscle cross-sectional area and alters neural recruitment patterns. Adaptation changes induced by resistance training include increased protein synthesis and production of muscle cells. Compensatory hypertrophy increases ribosomal protein synthesis and induces activation and differentiation of nonspecialized satellite cells into new muscle cells.

Muscle loss occurs with aging (sarcopenia), inactivity (atrophy), and disease (cachexia) and is characterized by protein degradation in excess of protein resynthesis (Cohen et al., 1999, Evans, 2010). Proteolysis is regulated by at least three systems: ubiquitin-proteasome, lysosomal, and calpain (Jackman and Kandarian, 2004; Kandarian and Jackman, 2006). Two recently characterized markers of skeletal muscle atrophy are muscle-specific E3 ubiquitin ligases muscle RING-finger 1 (MuRF1) and muscle atrophy F-box (MAFbx; also called atrogin-1), which are upregulated in rodent and human models of skeletal muscle atrophy (Trendelenburg et al., 2009). Myostatin is a negative regulator of skeletal muscle size and inhibits muscle cell differentiation (Lee, 2007; Trendelenburg et al., 2009; Welle, 2009). Elevated circulating levels of myostatin observed with obesity and insulin resistance may contribute to the systemic metabolic deterioration of skeletal muscles in type 2 diabetes (Hittel et al., 2009). Animals treated with follistatin, a myostatin inhibitor, or animals lacking myostatin have increased muscle mass (Lee, 2007). The capacity of exercise to delay, reverse, or exacerbate atrophy is unclear. Swim training in one rat study did not minimize the deleterious effects of immobilization (Nascimento et al., 2008).

14.9 CLASSIFICATION OF SKELETAL MUSCLE

Mammalian skeletal muscles are composed of different muscle fiber types, which express distinct sets of structural proteins and metabolic enzymes. Myofibers have been classified by both histochemical and immunohistochemical methods. Because the methods are different, the classification schemes are not identical, which can cause some confusion.

Skeletal muscle fibers can be broadly grouped into type I and type II fibers based on histochemical myosin ATPase staining. Type I fibers are slow contracting and slow fatiguing, and have oxidative metabolism, numerous mitochondria, and low myosin ATPase. Type II fibers are fast contracting and more easily fatigable, and have glycolytic metabolism, fewer mitochondria, and higher myosin ATPase. Type II fibers can be further subdivided based on ATPase activity following preincubation in acid and alkaline media into type IIA, IIB, and IIC (see Tables 14.1 and 14.2). Most muscles contain both type I and type II fibers. Red muscles (slow, oxidative, and more vascular) contain many type I fibers and are primarily associated with muscles that maintain posture and slow locomotion. White muscles (fast, glycolytic, and less vascular) contain mostly type II fibers and are used for sprinting. The proportion of these muscle fibers varies among animal species and even between breeds (Burke et al., 1971; Dickinson and LeCouteur, 2002; Valberg, 2008). For example, the proportion of type I fibers is 3% in greyhound dogs, 31% in mongrel dogs, and 12% in thoroughbred horses (Ruckebusch et al., 1991).

TABLE 14.1
Characteristics of Skeletal Muscle Fibers

Factor	Type I	Type IIA	Type IIx
Contraction rate	Slow	Intermediate	Fast
Oxidative capacity	High	Intermediate	Low
Fatigue resistance	High	Intermediate	Low
Glycolytic capacity	Low	Intermediate	High
Vascularity (redness)	High	Intermediate	Low
Myoglobin content	High	Intermediate	Low
Nuclei location	Peripheral	Peripheral	Central
Mitochondrial density	High	High	Low
Fiber diameter	Small	Intermediate	Large
ATPase pH 4.5	High	None	Low
ATPase pH 9.4	None	High	Low
Major storage fuel	Triglycerides	Creatine phosphate, glycogen	Creatine phosphate, glycogen
Function	Aerobic (posture)	Long-term anaerobic (walking, standing, repetitive movements)	Short-term anaerobic (burst of high-speed locomotion)

TABLE 14.2
Selected Histologic and Histochemical Stains Employed in the Evaluation of Muscle Biopsy Specimens

Histologic or Histochemical Stain	Normal Features	Disease Features
Hematoxylin eosin	• General histopathologic features	• Basophilia of degenerating/regenerating fibers • Necrotic fibers pale
Modified trichrome	• General histopathologic features • Contents of intermyofibrillar space (red) (sarcoplasmic reticulum, mitochondria, lysosomes, lipid, glycogen) • Intrafascicular nerve branches (myelin red) • Muscle fibers (blue) • Connective tissue (blue green)	• Aggregates and vacuoles, "ragged red" fibers, nemaline rods • Loss of myelinated nerve fibers • Fibrosis

Myofibrillar adenosine triphosphatase (ATPase) pH 9.8	• Differentiation of type 1 and 2 myofibers
	• Dog Type 1 Light
	  • Type 2A Dark
	  • Type 2C Dark
	• Cat Type 1 Light
	  • Type 2A Dark
	  • Type 2B Dark
	  • Type 2C Dark
		• Type 1 and 2 myofiber atrophy in denervation
		• Selective myofiber type atrophy (various)
		• Fiber type grouping

ATPase preincubation pH 4.3 (reversal)	• Differentiation of Type 2A, 2B, and 2C myofibers
	• Dog Type 1 Dark
	  • Type 2A Light
	  • Type 2C Intermediate
	• Cat Type 1 Dark
	  • Type 2A Light
	  • Type 2B Light
	  • Type 2C Intermediate	

ATPase preincubation pH 4.6	Differentiation of Type 2A and 2B myofibers
	Cat Type 1 Dark
	  • Type 2A Light
	  • Type 2B Intermediate
	  • Type 2C Intermediate
		Not required in dog because of lack of type 2B fibers

Periodic acid–Schiff–hematoxylin	External lamina, glycogen, and myelin are positively stained (magenta)	Glycogen storage disease (vacuoles/accumulations) Loss of myelinated nerve fibers
Oil red O	Intermyofibrillar lipid inclusions and fat cells in mysial connective tissue (orange/red)	Lipid storage myopathies Increased staining, often predominantly type 1 myofibers
Nicotinamide adenine dinucleotide–tetrazolium reductase	Mitochondrial oxidative enzyme	Mitochondrial and sarcoplasmic reticulum aggregates Pyknotic nuclear clumps stain darkly Atrophied myofibers may stain darkly Target myofibers
Succinate dehydrogenase	Mitochondrial oxidative enzyme	As for nicotinamide adenine dinucleotide, mitochondrial specific

(*Continued*)

TABLE 14.2 (*Continued*)
Selected Histologic and Histochemical Stains Employed in the Evaluation of Muscle Biopsy Specimens

Histologic or Histochemical Stain	Normal Features	Disease Features
Acid phosphatase	Lysosomes, predominantly in macrophages, stain red	Macrophages (inflammation and necrotic myofibers) Increased lysosomal activity in myofibers
Alkaline phosphatase	No staining in normal tissues	Positive staining of myofibers in dermatomyositis Subset of degenerating/ regenerating fibers maybe stained
Staphylococcal protein A-horseradish peroxidase	No staining in normal tissues	Immunoglobulin deposition in immune-based disease (nuclear, sarcolemmal, diffuse, neuromuscular junction) Stains eosinophils black, artifactually stains necrotic fibers
Esterase	Localization of myoneural junction (acetylcholine) Lysosomes in macrophages	Stains lysosomes of macrophages (inflammation and necrotic myofibers) Angular atrophied fibers may stain darkly

Source: Reprinted from Dickinson, P.J. and LeCouteur, R.A., *Small Anim Pract* 32, 63–102, 2002. With permission.

Immunohistochemical staining using antibodies against myosin heavy chain (MHC) has identified 10 isoforms of MHC in mammalian muscle, each with its own characteristic mATPase activity (Dickinson and LeCouteur, 2002; Peter et al., 1972; Smerdu et al., 2009; Weiss and Leinwand, 1996; Weiss et al., 1999). Myosin isoforms include slow-twitch M I (type I), several specialized isoforms (neonatal, jaw muscle, and extraocular muscle), and three or four major fast-twitch MHC adult mammalian isoforms (IIa, IIx [also known as IId], IIb). The fast-twitch isoforms expressed vary with species and within different muscles. Small mammals like rodents and lagomorphs, in addition to domestic pigs and llamas, express MHC IIa, IIx, and IIb. Humans and some other domestic animals such as dogs, cats, goats, and horses express only two, MHC IIa and IIx (Brooke and Kaiser, 1970; Schiaffino and Reggiani, 1994; Smerdu et al., 2009).

In general, the histochemically classified type I and IIa fibers correspond to MHC I and IIa (see Table 14.1). The histochemical type IIB fibers express MHC IIx. Hybrid fibers coexpress more than one MHC isoform simultaneously, for example, IIC express MHC I and IIa isoforms. MHC isoforms correlate with mATPase activity, fatigability, and also maximum shortening velocity. Different fast and developmental MHC isoforms can be coexpressed in muscle fibers in development, regeneration, transformation, and some normal adult muscles (Smerdu et al., 2009; Schiaffino and Reggiani, 1994).

14.10 LABORATORY EVALUATION

Routine laboratory evaluation of neuromuscular disorders primarily focuses on the measurement of serum enzyme levels as indicators of myocyte damage or necrosis. The activity or concentration of the muscle enzymes in serum is usually low because of their intracellular location within healthy myofibers. Necrosis of myofibers with disruption of cell membranes results in diffusion of cellular contents, including enzymes, into lymphatics or circulation. Other factors that may influence the activity of muscle enzymes include permeability of the cell membrane, rate of enzyme production, alternate sources of enzyme excretion or degradation, and variation in enzyme removal or inactivation (Dunlop and Malbert, 2004; Latimer et al., 2003). Leakage of enzymes, especially cytosolic enzymes, does not require cell death and, therefore, does not indicate irreversible damage. However, the magnitude of the enzyme elevation generally relates to the number of cells damaged. Magnitude and persistence of enzyme elevation are important parameters in monitoring myocyte injury. Decreased muscle enzyme levels are usually of no clinical significance but may occur with decreased muscle mass, interfering substances, and laboratory errors.

Creatine kinase (CK) is the most commonly used, muscle-specific enzyme to detect and monitor muscle damage. However, it is limited by its relatively short half-life (0.6–9 hours) in most species (Boyd, 1983; Stockham and Scott, 2008; Walker, 2006). Other enzymes such as aspartate aminotransferase (AST), lactate dehydrogenase (LDH), and alanine aminotransferase (ALT) have longer half-lives but lack the specificity of CK. Therefore, if these later enzymes are used to evaluate muscle damage, they must be used in combination with other tests, clinical information, and/or histopathologic evaluation that rule-out nonmuscle causes of enzyme elevation. For example, AST could be used in combination with CK and sorbitol dehydrogenase (SDH) or glutamate dehydrogenase (GLDH) to conclude that an elevation in AST is from muscle rather than liver. Aldolase (ALD) is also used as a biomarker for skeletal muscle injury, especially in the rat. Use of CK isoenzymes also increases muscle specificity but this has limited availability and limited application especially regarding skeletal muscle. Serum CK isoenzyme profiling, most often used for evaluating cardiac injury, has largely been replaced by cardiac troponins (Apple et al., 2008; O'Brien, 2008; Panteghini and Bais, 2008; Walker, 2006). In certain diseases such as progressive muscular dystrophies, tissues may fail to mature normally or maintain normal state of isoenzymes. The distribution of isoenzymes of CK, LDH, and ALD in muscle of progressive muscular dystrophy patients is similar to fetal muscle. The abnormalities of the isoenzymes in this disease are interpreted as a failure to reach or maintain a normal degree of differentiation. Isoenzyme patterns of regenerative muscle may also have fetal distribution patterns (Panteghini and Bais, 2008; Wilson, 2008).

Additional tests to evaluate muscle include proteins (troponin, myoglobin, fatty acid binding protein-Fabp3), antibody titers (immune-mediated diseases such as myasthenia gravis [MG] and masticatory myositis, and infectious diseases), lactate and pyruvate levels, electrolytes, hormones (thyroid, adrenal, sex), metabolic testing, and genetic testing. Of these, troponin and myoglobin are of limited value for investigating skeletal muscle disorders as their use is more applicable to cardiac muscle. "Omics" is a rapidly growing technology that focuses on large-scale and holistic data to understand life through the various "omes." For example, transcriptomics is the study of the entire set of mRNA in an organism, tissue, or cell and is becoming an integral tool for research as well as for the identification and potential therapy of neuromuscular disorders. Specialized electrodiagnostic tests include electromyography (EMG), evaluation of sensory and motor nerve conduction velocity measurements, and evoked MAPs.

Myofibers can be dysfunctional without exhibiting elevations in serum muscle enzyme concentrations. Therefore, histopathology, immunohistopathology, and/or ultrastructure of skeletal muscle and nerve biopsies are necessary for the investigation of neuromuscular conditions lacking enzyme changes or for a definitive morphologic diagnosis. The focus of this chapter is the basic clinical pathology tests used to diagnose and monitor muscular disorders. Some newer technologies or technologies used less frequently will be briefly discussed.

14.11 PREANALYTICAL AND ANALYTICAL VARIABLES

Identifying or controlling preanalytical variables is important for the interpretation and reproducibility of laboratory data. This is especially critical for research of neuromuscular disorders, testing the myotoxicity of different drugs, or evaluating therapeutic responses (emerging gene therapy). Individuals interpreting data from animals in neuromuscular studies or with neuromuscular disorders should be aware of the following: sample type (plasma or serum, whole blood); how and into what type of tube was the sample collected; specimen handling prior to analysis (stored at room, refrigerator or freezer temperature; separated immediately, within X hours); bleeding site;

recent handling of the animals and their level of acclimation to handling; any history of recent surgery or injections; any confounding factors (lipemia, hemolysis, icterus, drugs); and use of species specific assays and/or reference intervals (Hall, 2007; O'Brien, 2008). Serum or plasma can be used for many of the tests, but the results will vary slightly, and the anticoagulant can make a difference. Platelets, which contain CK and potassium in some animals, may also influence results (Aktas et al., 1993; Stockham and Scott, 2008). Age, sex, and breed/strain may affect the reference interval (Aktas et al., 1993; Honda et al., 2008; Matsuzawa et al., 1993; Walker, 2006; Waner et al., 1991). If anesthesia is used to collect the sample, it may have an effect, especially if any injections or recent surgeries (such as placement of catheters) have been performed. Research animals should be acclimated to handling techniques prior to study initiation. The need for acclimating laboratory animals to handling techniques is well documented in muscle research (Hall, 2007; Goicoechea et al., 2008; Lefebvre et al., 1992). For example, handling mice increases their serum ALT, AST, and LDH levels (Hall, 2007). Many examples of the effect of conditioning of animals exist. Aerobic exercise (swimming) protected the heart from ischemic/reperfusion injury in research rats and was associated with lower CK and LDH values after injury compared with sedentary rats (Zhang et al., 2007). Similarly, endurance training (swimming) in mice was protective for doxorubicin injury and decreased the elevation in cardiac troponin (Ascensao et al., 2005). Conditioned dogs, such as sled dogs, field trial dogs, and racing greyhounds, also appear to have fewer changes in analytes with exercise (McKenzie et al., 2007; Steiss and Wright, 2008).

Sample handling is very important for the accurate interpretation of both neuromuscular biopsies and serum enzyme levels. Serum is the preferred sample for enzyme analysis. Some enzymes, especially AST and LDH, can escape from erythrocytes, and if the serum is left in contact with the clot for a long time or if hemolysis occurs, AST and LDH levels can increase significantly.

For accurate interpretation, reference intervals must be established for each laboratory (Evans, 1996; Mitruka and Rawnsley, 1981). Additional recommendations are necessary for animal toxicologic and safety studies. Kinetic spectrophotometric assays are often preferred over colorimetric, end point, or flurometric methods for measuring enzymes in experimental safety studies. Better linearity and less interference with endogenous pyruvate or drugs, metabolites, or other chemicals have been reported (Dooley, 1979, 1984). Reference intervals for each strain, sex, and age group or a matched control group are usually required (Keller, 1981; Loeb and Quimby, 1989). For example, genetic variation of CK, LDH, and ALD occurs in mice; and CK and LDH isoenzyme profiles change as gestation progresses. CKBB (CK_1) and LDH_5:MMMM predominate in the embryonic mouse heart muscle, whereas CKMB (CK_2) and $LDH_{1\ \mathrm{and}\ 2}$ (HHHH and HHHM) predominate at birth (Loeb and Quimby, 1989). Routine measurement of CK and LDH activities has not been recommended for animal toxicology and safety studies (Weingand et al., 1992, 1996).

14.12 PROTEINS AND ENZYME MARKERS

14.12.1 Creatine Kinase

CK (EC 2.7.3.2; ATP:creatine *N*-phosphotransferase) catalyzes the reversible phosphorylation of creatine by ATP.

$$\text{Creatine} + \text{ATP} \xleftrightarrow{\text{CK}} \text{creatinine phosphate} + \text{ADP}$$

14.12.1.1 Tissue Distribution and Isoenzymes

In all species including cat, dog, horse, ox, man, marmoset, pig, rabbit, rat, and sheep, CK is in the highest concentration in skeletal muscle followed by cardiac muscle, brain, and intestine (Boyd, 1983; Wyss and Kaddurah-Daouk, 2000). CK consists of three dimeric cytoplasmic isoenzymes (CKBB-CK_1, CKMB-CK_2, and CKMM-CK_3) and one mitochondrial isoenzyme (CK-Mt). The molecular weight for all four isoenzymes is approximately 80,000 Da (Panteghini and Bais, 2008). The cytosolic isoenzymes are dimers of two subunits called M and B. CKBB predominates in the nervous tissue but is also found in the thyroid, kidney, intestines, and smooth muscle of the lungs; CKMB is mainly found in heart muscle where it represents 10%–20% of total CK, but is also present in the diaphragm and esophagus. In skeletal muscle, this isoenzyme represents only 2%–5% of total CK (Panteghini and Bais, 2008). CK-Mt is in mitochondria from many tissues (Stockham and Scott, 2008).

CKMM is the most common isoenzyme and is present in all tissues, especially skeletal muscle. Skeletal muscle from dogs has nearly 100% CKMM; heart muscle has about 98% CKMM and 2% CKMB; brain has about 8% CKMM and 90% CKBB; and intestine has approximately 12% CKMM, 35% CKMB, and 53% CKBB (Kikuta and Onishi, 1986), CK activity in skeletal muscle varies depending on breed (greyhounds > mongrels) and muscle type (fast acting muscles > slow) (Guy and Snow, 1981; Lindena et al., 1982). Dog plasma contains 30%–86% (usually 40%–55%) CKMM, 4%–45.5% (usually 30%–45%) CKBB, and 0%–18% CKMB (Loeb and Quimby, 1999; Voss et al., 1995). Rat myocardium has about 67% CKMM, 16% mitochondrial CK, 15% CKMB, and 2% CKBB. In rat plasma, 5%–10% of CK activity is CKBB with virtually no CKMB (Loeb and Quimby, 1999; Fontanet et al., 1988). In pigs, 4%–5% of the total myocardial CK activity is CKMB (Thoren-Tolling and Jonsson, 1983). Similar to humans, CKMB comprises about 20% of the total CK activity in the myocardium of baboon making baboons potentially a better model for human cardiac disease than dogs, which have only 2%–3% CKMB (Yasmineh et al., 1976). CK isoenzyme distribution patterns change with gestational development, disease states, and training, but the CKMM isoenzyme remains the predominant isoenzyme (Loeb and Quimby, 1999; Schultz et al., 1996).

On electrophoresis, the CKBB isoenzyme migrates most rapidly and is consequently found in the prealbumin area, CKMB has intermediate mobility and migrates to the $\alpha 2$-globulin region, and CKMM is the slowest and migrates to the γ-globulin zone. CKMB is relatively specific for myocardial infarction but measurements of CKBB and CKMM are of little clinical utility. Techniques for isoenzyme separation include electrophoresis or immunoassay using specific antibodies (Panteghini and Bais, 2008; Wilson, 2008).

CKMB and CKMM isoforms have been described in the dog and have been studied in experimental acute myocardial infarction (AMI). Proportions of the various isoforms have been used to estimate duration and progression of the lesion (Billadello et al., 1989; George et al., 1984).

14.12.1.2 Effect of Disorders and Exercise

Elevations in CK can be caused by skeletal and cardiac muscle damage, intramuscular (IM) injections, exercise, shivering, seizures, hypokalemia, or hypothyroidism (Valberg, 2008; Chanoit et al., 2001). Intramuscular injections can cause variable to marked increases in CK activity, peaking at 4 hours and persisting for 24–72 hours (Aktas et al., 1995; Klein et al., 1973; Lewis and Rhodes, 1978). CK activity can increase secondary to myocardial disease in dogs with dirofilariasis and parvovirus but may remain unchanged in dogs with hypertrophic cardiomyopathy (Loeb and Quimby, 1999). In contrast to humans and dogs, hypothyroid rats do not have elevated CK activity (Nuttall, 1968; Rossmeisl et al., 2009). Low CK values probably have no meaning but may reflect either small muscle mass, and/or sedentary lifestyle or marked muscle atrophy. Lack of CK elevation does not rule out muscle disease. Because of the relatively short half-life (0.6–9 hours), persistent elevations indicate ongoing injury or decreased clearance. Monkeys infected with simian immunodeficiency virus can have 10–15-fold increase in CK early in the disease but during the chronic cachectic phase muscle phosphocreatine levels are decreased (Dalakas, 1993; Hack et al., 1997). Syrian hamsters with hereditary myopathy have increased CK (Eppenberger et al., 1964).

Exercise-induced increases in CK have been reported in dogs (13-fold increase in greyhounds and huskies) and rats especially males or ovarectomized females (Amelink et al., 1988; Ilkiw et al., 1989; McKenzie et al., 2007; Ready and Morgan, 1984).

Serum CKMB has been used as an indicator of myocardial injury in experimental rodent models of AMI (Loeb and Quimby, 1999). Severe skeletal muscle injury (trauma, surgery, etc.) can also elevate serum CKMB. Persistent elevations of total CK and CKMB are diagnostic challenges and occur in muscular dystrophy, end-stage renal disease, or polymyositis, and in healthy subjects undergoing extreme exercise or physical activities, but cardiac troponin should be normal if the myocardium is not injured (Panteghini and Bais, 2008). Cardiac troponin I or T has largely replaced CKMB testing in the human field.

CKBB has been used as a marker of intestinal infarction in an experimental rat model, in which total CK activity increased 14-fold and CKBB activity increased 12-fold (Loeb and Quimby, 1999; Roth et al., 1989).

14.12.1.3 Diagnostic Testing and Sample Handling

Serum or heparinized plasma is the preferred sample. CK activity is unstable; if samples cannot be analyzed immediately (<4 hours), they should be refrigerated (5–7 days) or frozen (1–2 months, possibly longer at –80°C). The addition of sulfhydryl agents restores the original activity but the mechanism is unknown (Aktas et al., 1993; Panteghini and Bais, 2008).

Interferences include hemolysis (>39 mg/dL due to adenylate kinase), exposure to direct sunlight, or fluorescent light (due to loss of CO_2 which causes a slight decrease in CK), very high or low Mg levels, and contamination with oxidizing agents such as hypochlorite (cause slight decrease in CK). Drugs reported to cause interference include amphotericin B, ampicillin, anticoagulants, aspirin, dexamethasone, furosemide, lithium, morphine, and anesthetic agents (Wilson, 2008). Bilirubin, lipemia, and heparin cause little to no interference (Aktas et al., 1993; Wilson, 2008).

CK can elevate with restraint and handling animals for sample collection. Therefore, in some species like mice and monkeys, CK may be an insensitive test with wide reference intervals. Fasting can increase CK in pigs (Baetz and Mengeling, 1971). Male rats have higher CK values than females, whereas a sex difference is controversial in dogs but larger dogs have lower CK activity (Aktas et al., 1993, 1994; Goicoechea et al., 2008). CK activity decreases with age (Aktas et al., 1993; Shibata and Kobayashi, 1978). During the first few months it decreases dramatically then stabilizes during adulthood (Aktas et al., 1993). Platelets are a source of CK and contribute to the higher serum than plasma levels of CK (Aktas et al., 1994; Shibata and Kobayashi, 1978).

14.12.1.4 Serum Half-Life

In general, CK has a short half-life of 2–4 hours; elevates in 4–6 hours and peaks in 12 hours (Stockham and Scott, 2008). Half-life of total CK in the dog has been reported as <2 hours (Rapaport, 1975), 2.6 hours (Aktas et al., 1993, 1994), 4.7 hours (Boyd, 1983), and 0.6–16.2 hours (Lindena, et al., 1986); 9 hours in the rabbit (Lefebvre et al., 1993); 34 minutes in rats (Friedel et al., 1975; Lindena et al., 1986), and 5.2 hours in pigs (Boyd, 1983). In the dog, the half-life of CKMB is 1.3–8.1 hours (Lindena et al., 1986). In humans, the CK half-life is slightly longer at 13–20 hours (Janssen et al., 1989).

14.12.2 Aspartate Aminotransferase

AST (EC 2.6.1.1; L-aspartate:2 oxoglutarate aminotransferase) catalyzes the transamination of L-aspartate and 2-oxoglutarate to oxalacetate and glutamate.

$$\text{L-aspartate} + \text{2-oxoglutararte} \xrightarrow{\text{AST}} \text{oxalacetate} + \text{L-glutamate}$$

Addition of pyridoxal-5′-phosphate (P5P) is recommended for the measurement of total enzyme activity. Both AST and ALT can occur in apoenzyme forms that have no catalytic activity. Addition of exogenous P5P activates any available apoenzyme and therefore may increase measured AST and ALT activity (Mesher et al., 1998; Stokol and Erb, 1998; Wan et al., 1993; Waner and Nyska, 1991).

14.12.2.1 Tissue Distribution and Isoenzymes

AST is located in the cytoplasm and mitochondria of hepatocytes, skeletal myocytes, cardiac myocytes, and erythrocytes. It has two isoenzymes, one mitochondrial and one cytosolic with 50% identity and 80% identity, respectively, between different species (Pavé-Preux et al., 1988). Both isoenzymes play a role in amino acid synthesis and degradation, as well as in the link between the urea and the tricarboxylic acid cycles (Pavé-Preux et al., 1988). AST has a molecular weight of 100 Da.

14.12.2.2 Effect of Disease or Tissue Injury

AST is a nonspecific analyte; serum values are increased mainly with liver, muscle, and erythrocyte damage. It can increase up to eight times the upper reference value with muscular dystrophy and dermatomyositis, but is usually within reference interval in neurogenic muscle disorders (Panteghini and Bais, 2008; Wilson, 2008). Its half-life is longer than CK but shorter than ALT. AST should be interpreted together with CK or ALD (as well as liver enzymes) for the evaluation of muscle damage, although, in the absence of liver disease (elevations in liver enzymes and/or histopathologic findings) and hemolysis, increased AST is indicative of muscle damage. In laboratory animals, muscle injury is more likely to elevate AST than ALT, whereas ALT is generally preferred over AST for the evaluation of liver injury.

14.12.2.3 Diagnostic Testing and Sample Handling

AST is stable at room, refrigeration, and freezer temperatures (Latimer et al., 2003). Hemolysis causes an increase in AST levels. Apoenzyme and P5P levels have also influenced AST activity in dogs and rats (Mesher et al., 1998; Stokol and Erb, 1998; Wan et al., 1993; Waner and Nyska, 1991). Addition of P5P to an AST assay resulted in a median decrease of –6.3% (range –33.3% to 25%) in 80 dogs (Mesher et al., 1998). Site of venipuncture in rats also has an impact on the enzyme activity and is markedly elevated in the serum from retroorbital and ventral aorta venipuncture compared with activity in serum obtained from jugular vein and heart (Friedel et al., 1975). AST levels may be increased by the following drugs: acetaminophen, allopurinol, antibiotics, ascorbic acid, methyldopa, morphine, phenothiazines, pyridoxine, salicylates, sulfonamides, and vitamin A. Drugs that can decrease AST levels include metronidazole and trifluoperazine (Wilson, 2008). Cephalosporin treatment in rats also resulted in decreased AST activity (Dhami et al., 1979).

14.12.2.4 Serum Half-Life

AST has a short half-life; less than 12 hours in cats (Nilkumhang and Thornton, 1979), 12 hours in dogs (Boyd, 1983), 3.3–4.4 hours (Evans, 1996) and 18 hours in pigs (Massarrat, 1965), 1.6 hours (Friedel et al., 1979) and 2.3 hours in rats (Evans, 1996), and 2.5 hours in rabbits (Amelung, 1960; Boyd, 1983).

14.12.3 Alanine Aminotransferase

ALT (EC 2.6.1.2; L-alanine:2-oxoglutarate aminotransferase) catalyzes the reversible reaction of deamination of L-alanine to pyruvate. Pyridoxal-5-phosphate (P-5′-P) is the main cofactor for ALT and affects its activity (Stockham and Scott, 2008).

$$\text{L-alanine} + \text{2-oxoglutarate} \xrightarrow{\text{ALT}} \text{pyruvate} + \text{L-glutamate}$$

ALT activity is measured by absorbance of NADH, which is directly proportional to ALT activity. It is recommended that P-5′-P is added to the reaction so that all of the enzyme activity is measured. Adding P-5′-P resulted in an increase in ALT activity in dogs (median of 9.6%, range –7.1% to 46.5%) and in manatees (Mesher et al., 1998; Harr et al., 2008).

14.12.3.1 Tissue Distribution and Isoenzymes

ALT is a nonspecific analyte abundantly expressed in liver, but is also present in muscle. ALT has two isoenzymes: ALT_1, which is a cytoplasmic protein, and ALT_2, which is located in the mitochondria. ALT_1 has a longer half-life (about 36 hours) than ALT_2 (about 3 hours) in humans, dogs and Sprague–Dawley rats (Dooley, 1984) ALT_1 appears widely expressed in different tissues, whereas ALT_2 expression is more restricted and mainly found in muscle and liver. ALT_2 gene expression is higher in male than in female rats (Yang et al., 2009). In rats and pigs, ALT_1 is the predominant isoenzyme in skeletal and cardiac muscle, but the cytosolic ALT concentration varies from species to species (DeRosa and Swick, 1975).

Tissue distribution of ALT within organs can also vary. For example, periportal hepatocytes in rats may contain five times more ALT activity than centrolobular hepatocytes but unfortunately this cannot be used clinically to localize intrahepatic lesions (Dooley, 1984).

14.12.3.2 Effect of Disease

ALT is primarily used to identify liver disease or injury, but it can increase with severe muscle damage, especially in pigs where its activity is higher in cardiac and skeletal muscle than in liver (Markert, 1984). In mice, handling them by the body compared to the tail resulted in a fourfold increase in ALT activity (Swain et al., 1985). Increased serum ALT can also be induced by anticonvulsants (phenobarbital, phenytoin and primidone), glucocorticoids (prednisone, prednisolone), and thiacetarsemide (Latimer et al., 2003).

In horses, ruminants, pigs, and birds, hepatic ALT is very low and serum increases are the result of muscle damage. In dogs, cats, and most laboratory animals, ALT increases are usually associated with liver disease but can increase with some muscle diseases including muscular dystrophy and acute rhabdomyolysis (Stockham and Scott, 2008). Up to 25-fold increases in serum ALT have been reported in dogs with muscular disorders (Swenson and Graves, 1997; Valentine et al., 1990). In the guinea pig, rabbit, monkey, and baboon, ALT has little to no organ specificity with similar tissue concentrations in heart muscle and liver (Hall, 2007; Loeb and Quimby, 1989; Clampitt and Hart, 1978). Decreased serum activity of ALT and/or AST are occasionally observed in toxicology studies and may relate to decreased hepatocellular production or release, assay interferences, enzyme inhibition, or decreased coenzyme (P-5′-P) activity. Decreased ALT activity does not appear to be pathologically significant. Many drugs are reported to cause increases or decreases in ALT levels in humans (Fischbach and Dunning, 2004). Cephalosporin treatment in rats resulted in decreased ALT activity (Dhami et al., 1979).

14.12.3.3 Diagnostic Testing and Sample Handling

Serum is the preferred sample. Some anticoagulants such as citrate and fluoride should be avoided because they can inhibit the enzyme activity. ALT is stable for 2 days at 25°C, 1 week at 4°C, and unstable at –25°C; –70°C is recommended for longer storage. Up to a 25% decrease in activity was observed in manatee plasma stored for 1 month at –70°C (Harr et al., 2008). Interestingly, rat erythrocytes contain significant ALT activity but hemolysis does not cause a problem, possibly because ALT binds more strongly to erythrocyte membranes than other enzymes (Dooley, 1984). Icterus does not interfere with ALT measurements but lipemia can decrease ALT values. Diet and sex can influence ALT activity in rats. Female rats fed NIH-07 diet had lower ALT values than female rats fed NTP-2000 or male rats fed either diet (Rao, 1996). In rats, ALT is slightly increased when serum is obtained from the retro-orbital venous plexus and markedly increased when obtained from the ventral aorta, as compared with jugular vein and heart (Friedel et al., 1975). Numerous drugs may increase ALT levels and include acetaminophen, anticonvulsants, antibiotics, nonsteroidal anti-inflammatory drugs (NSAIDs), lipid-lower agents, salicylates, and thiazine (Wilson, 2008).

14.12.3.4 Serum Half-Life

The clearance half-life in dogs is 60 hours, increasing 12 hours postinsult and peaking at 1–2 days and then declining (Latimer et al., 2003) and has also been reported as 2.5–60.9 hours (Evans, 1996). In rats, the clearance *t*½ has been reported as 4.5–8 hours (Loeb and Quimby, 1989), 3 hours (Boyd, 1983), and 4.4 hours (Evans, 1996); in rabbits 5 hours (Amelung, 1960) and 5.1 hours (Boyd, 1983); and in pigs 51 hours (Boyd, 1983).

14.12.4 Lactate Dehydrogenase

LDH (EC 1.1.1.27; (S)-lactate:NAD$^+$oxidoreductase; LD) is a cytoplasmic hydrogen transfer enzyme that catalyzes the reversible conversion of L-lactate to pyruvate with mediation of NAD as a hydrogen acceptor (Panteghini and Bais, 2008).

$$\text{L-lactate} + \text{NAD}^+ \xrightarrow{\text{LDH}} \text{pyruvate} + \text{NADH} + \text{H}^+$$

LDH activity is measured spectrophotometrically at 340 nm by following either the oxidation of NADH with pyruvate or reduction of NAD$^+$.

14.12.4.1 Tissue Distribution and Isoenzymes

LDH is a tetramer and has two subunits, M for muscle and H for heart. The DNA encoding these subunits are LD-A and LD-B, respectively (Rossignol et al., 2003). There are five recognized isoenzymes, based on their electrophoretic mobility:

- LDH_1: HHHH
- LDH_2: HHHM
- LDH_3: HHMM
- LDH_4: HMMM
- LDH_5: MMMM

LDH_5 or electrophoretically slow moving isoenzyme is the main isoenzyme in skeletal muscle. Isoenzyme patterns vary between species but LDH_5 and LDH_4 are the primary isoenzymes in serum with lesser but variable amounts of the other isoenzymes (Preus et al., 1989). LDH_1 and LDH_2 are the main isoenzymes in the heart and may be helpful in monitoring cardiac damage in experimental models of heart disease (Preus et al., 1989).

14.12.4.2 Effect of Disease

Serum LDH has been used for diagnostic purposes for many years. Increased levels are associated with many diseases, in particular those involving the heart or skeletal muscles, liver, erythrocytes, and tumors (Skillen, 1984). LDH activity can be found in all tissues, but the main serum sources are muscle, liver, and erythrocytes. Without isoenzyme analysis, the measurement of LDH is not organ specific. The arterivirus, mouse LDH elevating virus (LDEV or LDV) is associated with chronic elevations of LDH, AST, isocitric dehydrogenase, malic dehydrogenase, and phosphohexase isomerase in infected mice (Notkins, 1965; Riley, 1974). The increased enzyme activity in these mice is due to a decreased rate of endogenous clearance. Any disorder, infection, or chemical that damages cells and releases endogenous enzyme will result in prolonged enzyme elevations. Decreased plasma protein turnover has also been observed in these LDEV mice (Riley, 1974).

14.12.4.3 Diagnostic Testing and Sample Handling

The preferred specimen is serum. Platelets contain high concentrations of LDH and serum values of LDH are higher than plasma (Shibata and Kobayashi, 1978). Hemolysis can contribute significantly to elevations in serum LDH. Ethylenediaminetetraacetic acid (EDTA) inhibits the enzyme, perhaps by binding Zn^{2+}(Panteghini and Bais, 2008). LDH is stable for 3 days at room temperature, stable in refrigeration, and unstable when frozen (Panteghini and Bais, 2008). Drugs that may increase LDH include anabolic steroids, anesthetics, antibiotics, aspirin, and NSAIDs, whereas ascorbic acid and oxalates may decrease LDH levels (Wilson, 2008).

14.12.4.4 Serum Half-Life

The half-life is different for each isoenzyme, but it is approximately 1.6 hours in dogs (Evans, 1996). LDH_5 has a half-life of 0.6 hours in rats (Friedel et al., 1979) and 2.5 hours in rabbits. In pigs, the half-lives for $LDH_{1, 2, 3, 4, \text{ and } 5}$ are 40, 27, 12, 5, and 3 hours, respectively (Boyd, 1983). In dogs, the half-lives for $LDH_{1 \text{ and } 5}$ are 3.3 and 0.8 hours, respectively (Bär et al., 1972/1973). In rats, the site of venipuncture has an impact on LDH activity and is markedly elevated in serum from retro-orbital and ventral aorta venipuncture compared with activity in serum obtained from jugular vein and heart (Friedel et al., 1975).

14.12.5 Aldolase

ALD (EC 4.1.2.13 D-fructose-1, 6-bisphosphate D-glyceraldehyde-3-phosphate-lyase) catalyzes

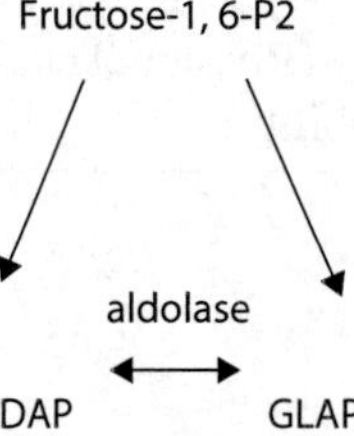

the reversible reaction that splits D-fructose-1, 6 diphosphate to D-glyceraldehyde-3-phospate (GLAP) and dihydroxyacetone-phosphate (DAP) in the glycolytic breakdown of glucose to lactate (Panteghini and Bais, 2008; Sherawat et al., 2008).

14.12.5.1 Tissue Distribution and Isoenzymes

ALD is present in skeletal muscle, liver, and cardiac muscle. In addition to its enzymatic activity, ALD plays a structural role in binding and polymerization of actin in the cytoskeleton (Kao et al., 1999). ALD is a tetramer with numerous isoenzymes. ALD-A_4 is found primarily in skeletal muscle, ALD-B hybrids in liver, ALD-A-C hybrids in heart muscle, and ALD-C_4 in brain and embryonic tissue (Andrews et al., 1961; Loeb and Quimby, 1989).

14.12.5.2 Effect of Disease or Tissue Injury

ALD activity has been used to help distinguish neuromuscular atrophies from myopathies in combination with CK and AST. Generally, there is no advantage in measuring ALD compared to more readily available enzyme assays such as CK, AST, and LDH. However, ALD was once the muscle-specific serum enzyme of choice and is still used in some toxicology studies (Dare et al., 2002; Loeb and Quimby, 1989).

14.12.5.3 Diagnostic Testing and Sample Handling

ALD is stable for 2 days at 25°C and 4°C and unstable at –25°C. A sex and age differences have been reported in human reference intervals (Panteghini and Bais, 2008). Hemolysis may falsely increase ALD. Drugs that may increase ALD levels are corticotrophin, cortisone acetate, and hepatotoxic drugs. Phenothiazines may decrease levels (Wilson, 2008).

14.12.5.4 Serum Half-Life

A muscle half-life of 20 days has been reported in the rat (Segal and Kim, 1963).

14.12.6 Troponin

Troponin is the contractile regulatory protein of skeletal muscle. Three troponin subunits form a complex that regulates interactions of actin and myosin in muscle contraction. Troponin C is the calcium-binding component, troponin I is the inhibitory component, and troponin T is the tropomyosin-binding component. Troponin is located primarily in myofibrils (94%–97%) with a small cytoplasmic fraction (3%–7%). Cardiac troponin (cTn) subunits I and T are encoded by different genes and have amino acid sequences that differ from troponins found in skeletal muscle (Panteghini et al., 2008). cTnT is not expressed in normal or diseased skeletal muscles; however, in regenerating rat skeletal muscle, a small amount of cTnT is expressed and has been reported in fetal and diseased human skeletal muscle (muscular dystrophy, polymyositis, dermatomyositis, and end-stage renal disease) (Panteghini and Bais, 2008). cTnT produced by these aberrant skeletal muscles does not react with newer generations of cardiac troponin diagnostic immunoassays (Wilson, 2008). Troponin C is not specific for heart muscle and, therefore, is not used as a cardiac marker. Cardiac troponin levels are generally not affected by skeletal muscle damage, that is, intramuscular injections, trauma, strenuous exercise, or medications. Human cardiac troponin I (cTnI) and T (cTnT) immunoassays have been used with variable success in animals (Burgener et al., 2006). Species-specific differences exist but it is apparent that cardiac troponin can be used as a marker of myocardial damage in large and small mammals and possibly birds (Apple et al., 2008; Fredericks et al., 2001; O'Brien, 1998). CTnI is a more sensitive and specific marker of myocardial ischemic injury than CKMB or myoglobin (Feng et al., 1998).

Troponin I increases in 3–6 hours, peaks at 14–20 hours, and returns to normal at 5–7 days (Wilson, 2008). Recently, drug-induced skeletal muscle injury in the rat was assessed through The Critical Path Institute's (C-Path) Predictive Safety Testing Consortium Skeletal Muscle Working Group (Burch et al., 2016). Evaluations determined through this consortium demonstrated that, for the diagnosis of drug-induced skeletal muscle injury, the biomarkers skeletal troponin I (sTnI), myosin light chain 3 (Myl3), CKMM, and fatty acid binding protein 3 outperformed assays of AST and CK with greater sensitivity and specificity in rat toxicology studies. Further, in the dog, findings have demonstrated that sTnI, Myl3, CKMM were sensitive early leakage biomarkers of skeletal muscle injury showing their translational utility beyond the rat in preclinical studies (Vlasakova et al., 2017).

14.12.7 Myoglobin

Myoglobin is a heme and oxygen-containing cytoplasmic protein in skeletal and cardiac muscle and resembles a single hemoglobin subunit containing one heme per molecule (Drabkin, 1950; Kagen, 1978; Lawrie, 1950; Poel, 1949). Myoglobin can function as an oxygen carrier and can use the bound oxygen for mitochondrial function during hypoxia, but does not display the property of cooperative binding seen in hemoglobin due to the single binding site. It is a 17,800-Da protein with rapid plasma clearance. Gene-knockout mice lacking myoglobin exhibit normal exercise capacity and response to hypoxia indicating adaptation (Ordway and Garry, 2004).

Serum increases in myoglobin occur after injury to either skeletal or cardiac muscle, and myoglobin molecules from both tissues are identical. Myoglobin appears to increase earlier than CKMB after AMIs; this may relate to its low molecular weight and cytoplasmic location. However, even minor injury to skeletal muscle can result in increased serum myoglobin, and this can be mistaken for myocardial injury. Myoglobin is rapidly (8.9 ± 1.5 minutes) cleared by the kidney (Klocke et al., 1982). In humans, serum concentrations usually increase with age and men have higher concentrations than women. Myoglobin concentrations also can vary with the different fiber type composition of muscle and variation among species and ages of animals is reported (Meng et al., 1993). Rapid and quantitative commercial assays that incorporate monoclonal antibodies are available, but results vary with different assays. Test validation is necessary for each species for these commercial myoglobin assays due to the use of species-specific reference material (Walker, 2006). Myoglobin lacks specificity as an indicator of cardiac injury, but because it rises as early as 1 hour after myocardial infarction, it may be useful in the early detection of myocardial infarction before CK_2 or cardiac troponin increase. Therefore, myoglobin could be used as an early negative predictor of cardiac injury (Panteghini and Bais, 2008).

Myoglobin is readily filtered by the kidney at concentrations >15–20 mg/dL. Myoglobinuria is associated with brown colored urine and elevated serum CK levels. Although both myoglobinuria and hemoglobinuria can cause grossly brown urine with a positive occult blood reaction on the urine dipstick, lack of red cells in the urine sediment and lack of a pink colored serum help to distinguish myoglobinuria from hemoglobinuria. Additionally, myoglobinuria can be differentiated from hemoglobinuria by the ammonium sulfate precipitation test; hemoglobin, but not myoglobin, will precipitate out with the addition of saturated ammonium sulfate. Other methods such as ultrafiltration and isoelectric focusing in polyacrylamide gel have been used to differentiate the two. Myoglobin and hemoglobin may contribute to the impairment of renal function.

Hemolysis will interfere with myoglobin testing and drugs such as statins and theophylline will increase myoglobin levels (Panteghini and Bais, 2008).

Myoglobin increases in 2–5 hours, peaks at 8–12, and is back to normal within 24 hours in humans with muscle damage and has a reported half-life of 20 minutes to 20 hours (Panteghini and Bais, 2008). Statins and theophylline may increase myoglobin levels (Wilson, 2008). In dogs, the peak activity after artery occlusion was reported as 20–40 minutes with a half-life of 38 ± 3 minutes (Klocke et al., 1982; Ellis et al., 1985).

14.12.8 Carbonic Anhydrase III

Carbonic anhydrase III is a cytosolic enzyme released from injured skeletal muscle in a fixed ratio with myoglobin. Unlike myoglobin, CA-III is not found in cardiac muscle (McGavin and Zachary, 2007). The combination of myoglobin and CA-III increases the specificity of myoglobin for the early detection of AMI. In one study, MYO-CAIII was significantly more sensitive than CK-MB but equally specific for the early diagnosis of AMI (Brogan et al., 1996; Mion et al., 2007).

14.12.9 Fatty Acid Binding Protein 3

Fatty acid binding protein 3 (Fabp3) is a member of the family of carrier proteins for fatty acids and other lipophilic substances. These proteins are thought to facilitate the transfer of fatty acids between intra- and extracellular membranes. Fabp3 is in the highest concentration in cardiac and skeletal muscles with type I fibers. Skeletal muscle necrosis can be an adverse reaction from drugs (statins) used to treat hyperlipidemia. Compared to CK, AST, and ALT, in one rat study Fabp3 had a higher concordance, sensitivity, positive, and negative predicative values and false negative rate for skeletal muscle necrosis. Additionally, Fabp3 and AST were found to be more specific biomarkers of skeletal muscle damage than CK_3 and AST (Pritt et al., 2008). Heart-type fatty acid-binding protein has been used in the early detection of AMI (Pritt et al., 2008).

14.12.10 Myokines

Myokines are muscle-derived cytokines that are released with muscle contraction. Myokines possess important metabolic and anti-inflammatory properties and can act in an autocrine, paracrine, or endocrine way (Brandt and Pedersen, 2010; Scheele et al., 2009). IL-6 was the first and most extensively described myokine. Data suggest that exercise-induced acute increases in IL-6 are beneficial by increasing lipolysis, glucose availability, and being anti-inflammatory (Brandt and Pedersen, 2010). Regular exercise appears to offer protection against such chronic disorders as cardiovascular disease, type 2 diabetes, dementia, and depression; myokines may provide an explanation on how regular muscle activity positively influences mood, performance, and cognitive function (Pedersen and Febbraio, 2005). Brain-derived neurotrophic factor (BDNF), IL-8, IL-15, leukemia inhibitory factor (LIF), fibroblast growth factor 21 (FGF21), and follistatin-like-1 (FSTL1) are members of the growing list of myokines (Brandt and Pedersen, 2010).

14.13 MISCELLANEOUS TESTS OR MARKERS

14.13.1 Antiacetylcholine Receptor Antibody Test

Antiacetylcholine receptor antibodies are antibodies against the nicotinic AChR. Elevation of these antibodies is diagnostic for acquired MG (Le Panse et al., 2008). MG is a disease that displays fluctuating muscle weakness. Muscles most often involved include those of the eyes, face, neck, and limbs, and those used for chewing, swallowing, vocalization, and breathing. There is minimal muscle atrophy and no sensory abnormalities (Shelton, 2002). Acquired and congenital forms of naturally occurring MG exist but the congenital forms are rare. Experimental models of the disease have also been described in rodents and rabbits (Shelton, 1999). Acquired MG is the most common neuromuscular disorder diagnosed in dogs and can occur, but is less common, in cats. Acquired MG results from autoantibody-mediated destruction of AChR at the neuromuscular junction. Clinical presentations vary from focal MG associated with regurgitation, to generalized weakness with or without associated megaesophagus or thymoma, to acute fulminating MG. The disease course is variable and unpredictable (Shelton, 2002).

The gold standard test for the diagnosis of acquired MG is the immunoprecipitation radioimmunoassay for the detection of antibodies against AChR. About 98% of dogs with generalized MG are seropositive. A serum sample collected prior to corticosteroid therapy is the specimen of choice. Antibody titers greater than 0.6 and 0.3 nmol/L are considered diagnostic of acquired MG in the dog and cat, respectively. Potential causes for negative titers in MG patients include corticosteroid therapy, antibodies directed at other areas of the neuromuscular junction (muscle-specific kinase—MuSK), and low-affinity anti-AChR antibodies (Eymard, 2009).

A pharmacological test (Tensilon® also known as edrophonium chloride) can be used as a presumptive diagnosis of MG. This drug is a rapidly acting, reversible AChE inhibitor with a short duration of action. It functions by competitively inhibiting AChE thereby increasing the available supply of acetylcholine at sites of cholinergic transmission. A positive test result is a dramatic increase in muscle strength after an intravenous (IV) injection (0.1–0.2 mg/kg) (Shelton, 2002).

14.13.2 Antitype 2M Antibody Test

Antitype 2M antibody testing is used to confirm masticatory muscle myositis, which is an autoimmune inflammatory myopathy characterized by jaw pain or inability to open the jaw (trismus).

Limb muscles are unaffected (Shelton, 2007). Historically, this disease has been called eosinophilic myositis or atrophic myositis, which probably represents the acute and chronic phase of the disease, respectively. The masticatory muscle (temporalis, masseter, pterygoid, and digastricus) has a unique isoform of myosin (type 2M fibers). In masticatory myositis, antibodies are produced specifically against these myofibers. A specific (100%) and sensitive (85%–90%) enzyme-linked immunoabsorbent assay (ELISA) test measures the antibody titers from serum samples collected prior to corticosteroid therapy (Melmed et al., 2004).

14.13.3 Lactate and Pyruvate

Lactate and pyruvate concentrations are recommended for the evaluation of muscle disorders especially those with exercise intolerance and a suspected underlying metabolic myopathy such as mitochondrial abnormalities. Pyruvate is produced from the aerobic metabolism of glucose. Under aerobic conditions, it is converted into acetyl-coenzyme A and enters the Krebs cycle but under anaerobic conditions lactate is produced. Lactic acidosis can be associated with a variety of conditions including systemic disorders (severe hypotension, shock, malignant hyperthermia), extreme muscular activity, or a primary enzyme defect (e.g., pyruvate dehydrogenase, pyruvate decarboxylase, enzymes of the respiratory chain or enzymes of the Krebs cycle). Concurrent measurement of lactate and pyruvate and comparing the ratio of the two can help differentiate various enzyme defects (Houlton and British Small Animal Veterinary Association, 2006; Matwichuk et al., 1999). For example, a defect in pyruvate dehydrogenase has elevations in both lactate and pyruvate with a normal ratio, whereas pyruvate carboxylase deficiency or mitochondrial electron transport chain defects have increased lactate and an increased lactate to pyruvate ratio. Pre- and postexercise lactate and pyruvate samples are ideal for evaluation of metabolic myopathies. Collection techniques and sample handling can affect results of lactate and pyruvate measurements. Therefore, contacting the laboratory for correct specimen handling is recommended (Pang and Boysena, 2007). Lactate samples should be analyzed immediately. Alternatively, samples for lactate can be collected into sodium fluoride/potassium oxalate anticoagulant tubes, cooled, and centrifuged within 15 minutes and analyzed immediately or plasma can be stored at –20°C for up to 30 days. Point of care testing has made lactate measurements more readily available in the clinical setting (Matwichuk et al., 1999; Karagiannis et al., 2006). Pyruvate is more difficult to handle as samples must be diluted with an equal volume of 10% perchloric acid prior to centrifugation. Immediate analysis is preferred but plasma can be frozen at –20°C until analyzed (Olby, 2005).

14.13.4 Metabolic Testing

Metabolic testing of urine and plasma can be performed to identify inborn errors of metabolism that result in impaired energy production. Metabolic myopathies are a heterogeneous group of muscle disorders characterized by defects in glycogen, lipid, adenine nucleotide, and mitochondrial metabolism (Preedy and Peters, 2002; Shelton et al., 1998). Mitochondrial myopathies, fatty acid oxidation defects (FAODs), and glycogen storage diseases (GSDs) are the three main categories. Although many medications can impair muscle intermediary metabolism (e.g., statins), they are generally grouped with the toxic myopathies category. Many metabolic disorders result from carnitine deficiency (van Adel and Tarnopolsky, 2009).

14.13.5 Genetic Tests

Genetic testing to detect mutant alleles is available for a variety of muscle diseases and can be used to identify both carriers and affected animals. DNA for analysis can be collected from blood, cheek swabs, or hair. Polymerase chain reaction technology is the basis for many genetic tests.

Molecular defects have been identified and animal models are available for many muscular disorders (Shelton and Engvall, 2005; Wells, 2005). Genetic testing is becoming more available. For example, in dogs, genetic testing is available for the following muscular disorders: phosphofructokinase deficiency (Smith et al., 1996), pyruvate dehydrogenase I deficiency (Cameron et al., 2007), centronuclear myopathy disease (Pelé et al., 2005), Duchenne's muscular dystrophy (Collins and Morgan, 2003; Feron et al., 2009), and myotonia congenital (Finnigan et al., 2007).

14.13.6 Electrolytes and Hormones

Containing approximately 60%–75% of total body potassium, skeletal muscle is the largest single pool of K+ in the body (DiBartola, 2005). Potassium is the major or primary intracellular cation and is critical in the maintenance of polarized muscle and nerve membranes. Both hyper- and hypokalemia can have significant effects on muscle function. Hyperkalemia decreases the resting potential of muscles and initially makes the cell hyperexcitable; conversely hypokalemia increases the resting potential and hyperpolarizes the cell. Extensive muscle necrosis in conditions such as exertional rhabdomyolysis or arterial thromboembolism can cause dangerous elevations in serum potassium. Hypokalemia (2–3.0 mEq/L) can also cause generalized muscle weakness, elevations in CK, and rhabdomyolysis. Hypokalemia can occur with dietary insufficiency, renal loss, diuretics, diabetic ketoacidosis, and as an inherited disease (Stockham and Scott, 2008). Flame photometry and ion-selective potentiometry are methods commonly used to measure electrolytes. Hyperlipemia or hypergammaglobulinemia can cause errors (i.e., pseudohypokalemia) in flame photometry and indirect potentiometry by exclusion of electrolytes from the solid (lipid and protein) portion of plasma. Depending on the species and breed, hemolysis may cause pseudohyperkalemia. Pigs, rabbits, guinea pigs, hamsters, rats, some breeds of dogs (Asian breeds such as Akita and Shiba Inu), and humans have high intracellular potassium (Hall, 2007; Harvey, 2008). Potassium can also leak from platelets and leukemic cells (Stockham and Scott, 2008).

Ionized calcium affects the threshold potential of membranes. Ionized hypocalcemia lowers the threshold and increases membrane excitability while ionized hypercalcemia increases the threshold. Therefore, hypercalcemia counteracts hyperkalemia but hypocalcemia exacerbates the effects of hyperkalemia on membrane excitability (DiBartola, 2005).

Epinephrine, norepinephrine insulin, and thyroid hormones all influence the basal activities of skeletal muscle Na^+-K^+-ATPase (Dukes and Reece, 2004). Myopathies associated with hypothyroidism and hyperadrenocorticism result from reduced repair and replacement of muscle protein, and progressive loss of skeletal muscle from enhanced catabolism and inhibition of myofibrillar protein synthesis, respectively (Shelton and Cardinet, 1987). Additionally, impaired insulin action that occurs in hypothyroidism and glucocorticoid excess may contribute to muscle atrophy as insulin is a potent anabolic hormone in muscle (Shelton and Cardinet, 1987).

14.14 HISTOPATHOLOGY, HISTOCHEMISTRY, AND IMMUNOHISTOCHEMISTRY

Muscle and nerve biopsy is often the best way to definitively identify a neuromuscular disorder. Conventional muscle biopsies using formalin fixation provides limited information. Frozen unfixed muscle biopsies are the "gold-standard" for evaluation of muscle disorders (Dickinson and LeCouteur, 2002). Specialized immunohistochemical and histochemical techniques using frozen skeletal muscle biopsies have greatly enhanced our understanding of muscle physiology and pathology. Histochemistry or immunohistochemistry stains used on muscle biopsies include hematoxylin and eosin (H&E), modified Gomori's trichrome, PAS, alizarin red S, alkaline phosphatase, acid phosphatase, nonspecific esterase, lipid stains (i.e., oil red O), nicotinamide adenine dinucleotide dehydrogenase tetrazolium reductase (NADH-TR), succinate dehydrogenase (SDH), ATPase at pH 9.8, 4.3, and 4.6, and cytochrome oxidase (Dickinson and LeCouteur, 2002; see Table 14.2). Staphylococcal protein A and horseradish peroxidase (SPA-HRPO) can be used to localize immune complexes associated with muscle disorders (Shelton et al., 1985).

Immunohistochemistry is available for the detection of many proteins that result in muscular dystrophy including dystrophin, sarcoglycans, laminin α2, dysferlin, α- and β-dystroglycans, utrophin, and spectrin (Shelton and Engval, 2002).

Frozen muscle biopsies require meticulous handling. Briefly, the muscle of interest is biopsied, the specimen trimmed to 0.5-cm blocks and mounted on thin cork squares with muscle fibers vertical to the cork (facilitating transverse sectioning), snap frozen in isopentane precooled with liquid nitrogen, sectioned in 10-μm consecutive sections with a cryostat, and stored at –80°C (Dickinson and LeCouteur, 2002).

14.15 OMIC TECHNOLOGY

Omics refers to a field of biologic study ending in the suffix -omics, such as genomics (de koning et al., 2007), proteomics (Doran et al., 2007, 2009), transcriptomics, interactomics, localizomics, metabolomics (O'Connell et al., 2008), and glycomics (Mahoney and Tarnopolsky, 2008). These studies assay an entire level of biological information; for example, transcriptomics evaluates the mRNA complement of an entire organism, tissue type, or cell. The advantage of omics is that it allows scientists to make thousands or even tens of thousands of measurements in a single experiment that would take months to years to generate using more conventional techniques.

Transcriptomic technology has been the major omic in the study of muscle damage. A transcriptional stimulus from muscle damage alters the expression of many genes. These genes are primarily involved in recovery from and adaptation to the damage. Adaptation can be divided into repeated-bout effect and training-induced adaptation. Two broad categories of transcriptomic technology offer rapid, efficient whole-genome transcriptional profiling. Closed techniques (complementary DNA [cDNA] and oligonucleotide arrays) have become the assay of choice because of increased availability of sequence information from major genomic studies. Closed techniques require sequence knowledge of the genome under study but are less expensive and less labor intensive than open techniques that do not require previous genomic sequence information. Open techniques include differential display (DD), serial analysis of gene expression (SAGE), and massively parallel signature sequencing (MPSS) (Mahoney and Tarnopolsky, 2008).

Proteomic profiling of animal models of skeletal muscle disorders has been valuable in understanding the molecular pathogenesis, and the effectiveness of drugs, genetic modifications, or cell-based therapies on disease progression (Doran et al., 2007). Proteomics of aging skeletal muscle is valuable in identifying the major pathophysiological pathways responsible for fiber aging and may translate into better treatment options (Doran et al., 2009). Age-related muscle wasting can be partially, but not fully, counterbalanced by exercise programs and nutritional supplements. Therefore, once these pathways are known, alternative or additional therapeutic strategies based on pharmacological interventions, cellular therapies, or gene transfer techniques can be considered for our aging population.

Omic technology combined with nonomic technology will allow researchers unprecedented knowledge to understand muscle damage, repair, recovery, adaptation, and response to therapy (Patterson et al., 2008).

14.16 ULTRASOUND, MAGNETIC RESONANCE IMAGING, ELECTROMYOGRAMS

Ultrasound and magnetic resonance imaging (MRI) are noninvasive diagnostic tools that are being used for the early diagnosis, evaluation of disease extent, therapeutic monitoring, and guidance for biopsies in skeletal muscle disease. Although histopathology is necessary for a definitive diagnosis, ultrasound and MRI have assumed a major role in the evaluation and management of many disorders such as the inflammatory myopathies. MRI is sensitive in detecting acute muscle inflammation, edema and fatty infiltration (Curiel et al., 2009). Contrast-enhanced ultrasound, which can measure perfusion, is a useful diagnostic tool in diagnosing acute inflammation in idiopathic inflammatory myopathies (Weber, 2009).

TABLE 14.3
Selected Myopathies in Animals

Classification of Disease	Examples	Animals Affected or Models
Ion channel myopathies	Acetylcholine ion channel—myasthenia gravis	Dog
	Sodium channels—periodic paralysis (HyPP)	Horse
	Chloride channels—congenital myotonia	Adr mouse, miniature schnauzer dogs
	Chloride channels—myotonic dystrophy	Various transgenic mice, horse
	Calcium channels—malignant hyperthermia	Pigs, dogs, horses
Muscular dystrophy	Dystrophin deficiency (Duchenne muscular dystrophy—DMD)	Mdx mouse, golden retriever and other dogs, cat
	Limb girdle muscular dystrophy	Various knockout mice
Disorders of glyco (geno)lysis	α-1,4 glucosidase deficiency (GSDII), Pompe's disease	Knockout mice, cattle, Japanese quail, sheep, cat, turkey
	Debranching enzyme deficiency (GSD III)	Dog
	Branching enzyme deficiency (GSD IV)	Cat, horse
	Myophosphorylase deficiency (GSD V), McArdle's disease	Cattle, sheep
	Phosphofructokinase deficiency (GSD VII)	Dog
	Polysaccharide storage myopathy	Horse
Mitochondrial myopathies	Respiratory chain complex 1 (NADH ubiquinone oxidoreductase deficiency)	Horse
	Cytochrome *c* oxidase deficiency	Dog
	Lipid storage disorders	Dog
	Adenine nucleotide translocator (Ant 1) deficiency	Knockout mice
	Transcription factor A disorder	Tfam knockout mice
Toxic/iatrogenic myopathies	Drugs—zidovudine (AZT), chloroquine, ethanol, statins (cerivastatin), monensin, snake venom, toxic plants	
Immune-mediated myopathies	Immune-mediated canine masticatory myositis	Dog
	Acquired autoimmune myasthenia gravis	Dog
	Experimental autoimmune myositis (EAM)	Transgenic mice

(*Continued*)

TABLE 14.3 (*Continued*)
Selected Myopathies in Animals

Classification of Disease	Examples	Animals Affected or Models
Infectious myopathy	Bacterial—*Clostridial* spp., *Pasteurella* spp., *Leptospira* spp.	
	Protozoal—*Toxoplasma gondii*, *Neosporum caninum*, *Hepatozoon canis*, *Trypanosoma cruzi*, *Sarcocystis* spp., *Hammondia* spp.	
	Nematode—*Trichina spiralis*, nematode larva migrans	
	Cestode—*Taenia solium* (cysticercosis)	
	Rickettsial—*Ehrlichia canis*	
	Viral—Simian immunodeficiency virus (SIV), feline immunodeficiency virus (FIV)	
Endocrine myopathies	Hyper/hypoadrenocorticism myopathy	Dog
	Hyper/hypothyroid myopathy	Dog
Nutritional myopathies	Selenium/vitamin E deficiency	
Miscellaneous/second myopathies	Renal disease	
	Collagen IV deficiency (Bethlem myopathy)	Mice
	Malignant hyperthermia	Pig
	Ischemia—vascular, thromboembolism, hypotension	
	Rhabdomyolysis (trauma, exertion, malignant hyperthermia)	
	Electrolyte disorders—hypo/hyperkalemia, hypocalcemia, hypomagnesemia	

Sources: Dalakas, M.C., *Baillière's Clin Neurol*, 2, 659–691, 1993; Dickinson, P.J. and LeCouteur, R.A., *Vet Clin North Am Small Anim Pract*, 32, 63–102, 2002; Shelton, G.D., *Neuromuscul Disord*, 17, 663–670, 2007; Shelton, G.D. and Engvall, E. *Neuromuscul Disord*, 15, 127–138, 2005; Shelton, G.D. and Engvall, E., *Vet Clin North Am Small Anim Pract,* 32, 103–124, 2002; *Clinical Biochemistry of Domestic Animals,* Valberg, S.J, Skeletal muscle function, 419–484, Copyright (2008), Elsevier; Wells, D.J., *Handbook of Laboratory Animal Science*, CRC Press, Boca Raton, 2005.

GSD, glycogen storage disease.

14.17 NEUROMUSCULAR DISORDERS AND ANIMAL MODELS

A variety of neuromuscular diseases have been reported in animals (McGavin and Zachary, 2007; de Sousa-e-Silva et al., 2003; Evans, 2004; Shelton and Engvall, 2005). Neuromuscular diseases are disorders of muscle, motor, or sensory nerves or both muscle and nerves. Myopathies are due directly to skeletal muscle abnormalities. Neuropathies are disorders of the nerve innervating the muscle but they can produce secondary changes in the skeletal muscle such as atrophy. A select list of some of the more common diseases with a focus on myopathies is presented in Table 14.3. Diagnostic tests useful in distinguishing these disorders include genetic testing, metabolic testing for enzyme defects, antibody titers for infectious, and immune-mediated diseases, endocrine testing, evaluation of calcium, magnesium, and potassium concentrations, and muscle and nerve histopathologic biopsies (Olby, 2005; Shelton and Cardinet, 1987).

Animal models for myopathies provide vital information related to the pathophysiology of muscular diseases, the physiologic effects of exercise and aging on muscle and the efficacy and toxicity of therapeutic modalities (Shelton and Engvall, 2005; Warren and Palubinskas, 2008; Wells, 2005). Duchenne's muscular dystrophy is the most common inherited myopathy of children and two good animal models that lack dystrophin are the mdx mouse and the golden retriever muscular dystrophy dog (GRMD also known as CXMD) (Shelton and Engvall, 2005; Wells, 2005). Myotonic dystrophy is the most common human inherited adult myopathy. It is due to expansion of a triplet (CTG) repeat in the 3′ untranslated region of a protein kinase gene called dystrophia myotonica protein kinase (DMPK). Transgenic mice have enhanced our understanding of this disease. Spontaneous and genetically engineered animal models are available for many of the ion channel, mitochondrial and metabolic myopathies (Coulton et al., 1988; Wells, 2005; see Table 14.3). An experimental autoimmune myositis produced by injecting homogenates of skeletal muscle and adjuvant into animals is a model of human inflammatory muscle disease. Animal testing has enhanced our understanding and reduced the risk of toxic myopathies in humans. Drugs such zidovudine (AZT), chloroquine, ethanol, and some statins can produce skeletal myopathy (Sieb and Gillessen, 2003; Wells, 2005).

Rodents are and will continue to be extremely important models for basic research into the pathophysiology and treatment of muscle disorders. Additionally, intermediate to larger animal models are emerging as desirable models for preclinical drug trials.

REFERENCES

Aktas, M., Auguste, D., Concordet, D., et al. 1994. Creatine-kinase in dog plasma-preanalytical factors of variation, reference values and diagnostic-significance. *Res Vet Sci.* 56:30–36.

Aktas, M., Auguste, D., Lefebvre, H.P., et al. 1993. Creatine-kinase in the dog—A review. *Vet Res Commun.* 17:35–369.

Aktas, M., Vinclair, P., Lefebvre, H.P., et al. 1995. In-vivo quantification of muscle damage in dogs after intramuscular administration of drugs. *Br Vet J.* 15:189–196.

Amelink, G.J., Kamp, H.H., and Bar, P.R. 1988. Creatine kinase isoenzyme profiles after exercise in the rat: Sex-linked differences in leakage of CK-MM. *Pflugers Arch.* 412:417–421.

Amelung, D. 1960. Studies on the magnitude of the elimination speed of enzymes from rabbit serum. *Hoppe-Seyler's Z Physiol Chem.* 318:219–228.

Andrews, M.F., McIlwain, P.K. and Eveleth, D. F. 1961. Serum transaminase and aldolase during migration of larval ascaris suum in swine. *Am J Vet Res.* 22:1026–1029.

Apple, F.S., Murakami, M.M., Ler, R., et al. 2008. Analytical characteristics of commercial cardiac troponin I and T immunoassays, in serum from rats, dogs, and monkeys with induced acute myocardial injury. *Clin Chem.* 54:1982–1989.

Ascensao, A., Magalhaes, J., Soares, J., et al. 2005. Endurance training attenuates doxorubicin-induced cardiac oxidative damage in mice. *Int J Cardiol.* 10:45–60.

Baetz, A.L. and Mengeling. W.L. 1971. Blood constituent changes in fasted swine. *Am J Vet Res.* 32:1491–1499.

Bär, U., Friedel, R., Heine, H., et al. 1972/1973. Studies on enzyme elimination. III. Distribution, transport, and elimination of cell enzymes in the extracellular space. *Enzyme.* 14:133–156.

Billadello, J.J., Fontanet, H.L., Strauss, A.W. and Abendschein, D.R. 1989. Characterization of MB creatine kinase isoform conversion in vitro and in vivo in dogs. *J Clin Invest.* 83:1637–1643.

Boyd, J.W. 1983. The mechanisms relating to increases in plasma enzymes and isoenzymes in diseases of animals. *Vet Clin Pathol.* 12:9–24.

Brandt, C. and Pedersen, B.K. 2010. The role of exercise-induced myokines in muscle homeostasis and the defense against chronic disease. *J Biomed Biotechnol.* 2010:6. Article ID 520258, doi:10.1155/2010/520258

Brogan, G.X., Jr., Vuorl, J., Friedman, S., et al. 1996. Improved specificity of myoglobin plus carbonic anhydrase assay versus that of creatine kinase-MB for early diagnosis of acute myocardial infarction. *Ann Emerg Med.* 27:22–28.

Brooke, M.H. and Kaiser, K.K. 1970. Muscle fiber types—How many and what kind. *Archv Neurol.* 23:369–379.

Bruss, M.L. 2008. Lipids and ketones. In *Clinical Biochemistry of Domestic Animals.* Eds. J.J. Kaneko, J.W. Harvey and M. Bruss, 6th edition, pp. 81–116. Amsterdam; Boston, MA: Academic Press/Elsevier.

Burch, P.M., Greg Hall, D., Walker, E.G., Bracken, W., Giovanelli, R., Goldstein, R., Higgs, R.E., King, N.M., Lane, P., Sauer, J.M., Michna, L., Muniappa, N., Pritt, M.L., Vlasakova, K., Watson, D.E., Wescott, D., Zabka, T.S., and Glaab, W.E. 2016. Evaluation of the relative performance of drug-induced skeletal muscle injury biomarkers in rats. Toxicol Sci. 150(1):247--256.

Burgener, I.A., Kovacevic, A., Mauldin, G.N., and Lombard, C.W. 2006. Cardiac troponins as indicators of acute myocardial damage in dogs. *J Vet Int Med.* 20:277–283.

Burke, R.E., Levine, D.N., and Zajac, F.E. 3rd. 1971. Mammalian motor units: Physiological-histochemical correlation in three types in cat gastrocnemius. *Science.* 174:709–712.

Cairns, S.P. 2006. Lactic acid and exercise performance: Culprit or friend? *Sports Med.* 36:279–291.

Cameron, J.M., Maj, M.C., Levandovskiy, V., et al. 2007. Identification of a canine model of pyruvate dehydrogenase phosphatase 1 deficiency. *Mol Genet Metab.* 90:15–23.

Carlson, M.E., Suetta, C., Conboy, M.J., et al. 2009. Molecular aging and rejuvenation of human muscle stem cells. *EMBO Mol Med.* 1:381–391.

Chang, K.C. 2007. Key signaling factors and pathways in the molecular determination of skeletal muscle phenotype. *Animal.* 1:1681–1698.

Chanoit, G.P., Lefebvre, H.P., Orcel, K., et al. 2001. Use of plasma creatine kinase pharmacokinetics to estimate the amount of exercise-induced muscle damage in beagles. *Am J Vet Res.* 62:1375–1380.

Charge, S.B.P. and Rudnicki, M.A. 2004. Cellular and molecular regulation of muscle regeneration. *Physiol Rev.* 84:209–238.

Clampitt, R.B. and Hart, R.J. 1978. Tissue activities of some diagnostic enzymes in 10 mammalian-species. *J Comp Pathol.* 88:607–621.

Coffey, V.G. and Hawley, J.A. 2007. The molecular bases of training adaptation. *Sports Med.* 37:737–763.

Cohen, I., Bogin, E., Chechick, A., and Rzetelny, V. 1999. Biochemical alterations secondary to disuse atrophy in the rat's serum and limb tissues. *Arch Orthop Trauma Surg.* 119:410–417.

Collins, C.A. and Morgan, J.E. 2003. Duchenne's muscular dystrophy: Animal models used to investigate pathogenesis and develop therapeutic strategies. *Int J Exp Pathol.* 84:165–172.

Copstead-Kirhorn, L.E.and Banasik, J.L. 2005. *Pathophysiology Biological and Behavioral Perspective*, 3rd edition. St. Louis, MO: Saunders.

Coulton, G.R., Morgan, J.E., Partrideg, T.A. and Sloper, J.C.1988. The MDX mouse skeletal-muscle myopathy. 1. A histological, morphometric and biochemical investigation. *Neuropathol Appl Neurobiol.* 14:53–70.

Curiel, R.V., Jones, R., and Brindle, K. 2009. Magnetic resonance imaging of the idiopathic inflammatory myopathies structural and clinical aspects. *Ann N Y Acad Sci.* 1154:101–114.

Dalakas, M.C. 1993. Retroviruses and inflammatory myopathies in humans and primates. *Baillière's Clin Neurol.* 2:659–691.

Dare, T.O., Davies, H.A., Turton, J.A., Lomas, L., et al. 2002. Application of surface-enhanced laser desorption/ionization technology to the detection and identification of urinary parvalbumin-alpha: A biomarker of compound-induced skeletal muscle toxicity in the rat. *Electrophoresis.* 23:3241–3251.

De Koning, D.J., Archibald, A., and Haley, C.S. 2007. Livestock genomics: Bridging the gap between mice and men. *Trends Biotechnol.* 25:483–491.

de Sousa-e-Silva, M.C., Tomy, S.C., Tavares, F.L., et al. 2003. Hematological, hemostatic and clinical chemistry disturbances induced by crotalus durissus terrificus snake venom in dogs. *Hum Exp Toxicol.* 22:491–500.

DeRosa, G. and Swick, R.W. 1975. Metabolic implications of the distribution of the alanine aminotransferase isoenzymes. *J Biol Chem.* 250:7961–7967.

Dhami, M.S., Drangova, R., Farkas, R., et al. 1979. Decreased aminotransferase activity of serum and various tissues in the rat after cefazolin treatment. *Clin Chem.* 25:1263–1266.

DiBartola, S.P. 2005. *Fluid, Electrolyte and Acid-Base Disorders in Small Animal Practice*, 3rd edition. Philadelphia, PA: Elsevier Saunders.

Dickinson, P.J. and LeCouteur, R.A. 2002. Muscle and nerve biopsy. *Vet Clin North Am Small Anim Pract.* 32:63–102.

Dooley, J.F. 1979. The role of clinical chemistry in chemical and drug safety evaluation by use of laboratory animals. *Clin Chem.* 25:345–347.

Dooley, J.F. 1984. The role of alanine aminotransferase for assessing hepatotoxicity in laboratory animals. *Lab Anim.* 13:20 and 23.

Doran, P., Donoghue, P., O'Connell, K., et al. 2009. Proteomics of skeletal muscle aging. *Proteomics.* 9:983–1003.

Doran, P., Gannon, J., O'Connell, K., and Ohlendieck, L. 2007. Proteomic profiling of animal models mimicking skeletal muscle disorders. *Proteomics.* 1:1169–1184.

Dossin, O., Rives, A., and Germain, C., et al. 2005. Pharmacokinetics of liver transaminases in healthy dogs: Potential clinical relevance for assessment of liver damage. *J Vet Int Med.* 19:442.

Drabkin, D.L. 1950. The distribution of the chromoproteins, hemoglobin, myoglobin, and cytochrome-C, in the tissues of different species, and the relationship of the total content of each chromoprotein to body mass. *J Biol Chem.* 182:317–333.

Dukes, H.H. and Reece, W.O. 2004. *Dukes' Physiology of Domestic Animals*, 12th edition. Ithaca, NY: Comstock Pub./Cornell University Press.

Dunlop, R.H. and Malbert, C.H. 2004. *Veterinary Pathophysiology*, 1st edition. Ames, IA: Blackwell Publishing.

Dunn, M.E., Coluccio, D., Hirkaler, G., Mikaelian, I., Nicklaus, R., Lipshultz, S.E., Doessegger, L., Reddy, M., Singer, T., and Geng, W. 2011. The complete pharmacokinetic profile of serum cardiac troponin I in the rat and the dog. *Toxicol Sci.* 123(2):368–373.

Ellis, A.K., Little, T., Masud, Z., and Klocke, F.J. 1985. Patterns of myoglobin release after reperfusion of injured myocardium. *Circulation.* 72:639–647.

Ellis, A.K. and Saran, B.R. 1989. Kinetics of myoglobin release and prediction of myocardial myoglobin depletion after coronary artery reperfusion. *Circulation.* 80:676–683.

Eppenberger, M., Nixon, C.W., Baker, J.R., and Homburger, F.1964. Serum phosphocreatine kinase in hereditary muscular dystrophy and cardiac necrosis of Syrian golden hamsters. *Proc Soc Exp Biol Med.* 117:465–468.

Evans, G.O. 1996. *Animal Clinical Chemistry: A Primer for Toxicologists.* Ed. G.O. Evans, pp. 59–70 and 147–154. London; Bristol, PA: Taylor & Francis.

Evans, J. 2004. Canine inflammatory myopathies: A clinicopathologic review of 200 cases. *J Vet Int Med.* 18:679–691.

Evans, W.J. 2010. Skeletal muscle loss: cachexia, sarcopenia, and inactivity. *Am J Clin Nutr.* 91:11235–11275.

Eymard, B. 2009. Antibodies in myasthenia gravis. *Rev Neurol.* 165:137–143.

Febbraio, M.A. and Pedersen, B.K. 2005. Contraction-induced myokine production and release: Is skeletal muscle an endocrine organ? *Exerc Sport Sci Rev.* 33:114–119.

Feng, Y.J., Chen, C., Fallon, J.T., et al. 1998. Comparison of cardiac troponin I, creatine kinase-MB, and myoglobin for detection of acute ischemic myocardial injury in a swine model. *Am J Clin Pathol.* 110:70–77.

Feron, M., Guevel, L., Rouger, K., et al. 2009. PTEN contributes to profound PI3K/Akt signaling pathway deregulation in dystrophin-deficient dog muscle. *Am J Pathol.* 174:1459–1470.

Finnigan, D.F., Hanna, W.J. Poma, R., and Bendall, A.J. 2007. A novel mutation of the CLCN1 gene associated with myotonia hereditaria in an Australian cattle dog. *J Vet Int Med.* 21:458–463.

Fischbach, F.T. and Dunning, M.D. 2004. *A Manual of Laboratory and Diagnostic Tests*, 7th edition. Philadelphia, PA: Lippincott Williams & Wilkins.

Fontanet, H., Billadello, J.J., and Abendschein, D.R. 1988. The nature of MB creatine-kinase isoforms in plasma. *Clin Res.* 36:A275.

Fredericks S., Merton, G.K., Lerena, M.J., et al. 2001. Cardiac troponins and creatine kinase content of striated muscle in common laboratory animals. *Clin Chim Acta.* 304:65–74.

Friedel, R.F., Diederichs, J., and Lindena, J., 1979. Release and extracellular turnover of cellular enzymes. In *Advances in Clinical Enzymology.* Ed. E. Schmidt, pp. 70–105. Basel; New York, NY: S. Karger.

Friedel, R., Trautschold, I., Gärtner, K., et al. 1975. Effects of blood-sampling on enzyme-activities in serum of small laboratory-animals. *Z Klin Chem Klin Biochem.* 13:499–505.

George, S., Ishikawa, Y., Perryman, M.B., and Roberts, R. 1984. Purification and characterization of naturally-occurring and in vitro induced multiple forms of MM creatine-kinase. *J Biol Chem.* 259:2667–2674.

Goicoechea, M., Cía, F., San José, C., et al. 2008. Minimizing creatine kinase variability in rats for neuromuscular research purposes. *Lab Anim.* 42:19–25.

Guy, P.S. and Snow, D.H. 1981. Skeletal muscle fiber composition in the dog and its relationship to athletic ability. *Res Vet Sci.* 31:244–248.

Hack, V., Gross, A., Bohme, A., et al. 1997. Decrease in phosphocreatine level in skeletal muscle of SIV-infected rhesus macaques correlates with decrease in intracellular glutathione. *AIDS Res Hum Retroviruses.* 13:1089–1091.

Hall, R.L. 2007. Clinical pathology of laboratory animals. In *Animal Models in Toxicology.* Ed. S.C. Gad, 2nd edition, pp. 787–830. Boca Raton, FL: CRC/Taylor & Francis.

Harr, K.E., Allison, K., Bonde, R.K., et al. 2008. Comparison of blood aminotransferase methods for assessment of myopathy and hepatopathy in Florida manatees (trichechus manatus latirostris). *J Zoo Wildl Med.* 39:180–187.

Harvey, J.W. 2008. The erythrocyte: Physiology, metabolism, and biochemical disorders. In *Clinical Biochemistry of Domestic Animals*. Ed. J.J. Kaneko, J.W. Harvey, and M. Bruss, 6th edition, pp. 173–240. Amsterdam; Boston, MA: Academic Press/Elsevier.

Hill, R.W., Wyse, G.A., and Anderson, M. 2008. *Animal Physiology*, 2nd edition. Sunderland, MA: Sinauer Associates.

Hittel, D.S., Berggren, J.R., Shearer, J., et al. 2009. Increased secretion and expression of myostatin in skeletal muscle from extremely obese women. *Diabetes.* 58:30–38.

Honda, T., Honda, K., Kokubun, C., et al. 2008. Time-course changes of hematology and clinical chemistry values in pregnant rats. *J Toxicol Sci.* 33:375–380.

Houlton, J. E. F. British Small Animal Veterinary Association. 2006. *BSAVA Manual of Canine and Feline Musculoskeletal Disorders*. BSAVA manual series. Quedgeley: British Small Animal Veterinary Association.

Ilkiw, J.E., Davis, P.E. and Church, D.B. 1989. Hematologic, biochemical, blood-gas, and acid-base values in greyhounds before and after exercise. *Am J Vet Res.* 50:583–586.

Izumiya, Y., Hopkins, T., Morris, C., et al. 2008. Fast/glycolytic muscle fiber growth reduces fat mass and improves metabolic parameters in obese mice. *Cell Metab.* 7:159–172.

Jackman, R. W. and Kandarian, S.C. 2004. The molecular basis of skeletal muscle atrophy. *Am J Physiol Cell Physiol.* 287:C834–C843.

Janssen, G.M., Kuipers, H., Willems, G.M., et al. 1989. Plasma activity of muscle enzymes: Quantification of skeletal muscle damage and relationship with metabolic variables. *Int J Sports Med.* 10:S160–S168.

Kagen, L.J. 1978. Myoglobin: Methods and diagnostic uses. *CRC Crit Rev Clin Lab Sci.* 9:273–302.

Kandarian, S.C. and Jackman, R.W. 2006. Intracellular signaling during skeletal muscle atrophy. *Muscle Nerve.* 33:155–165.

Kao, A.W., Noda, Y., Johnson, J.H., et al. 1999. Aldolase mediates the association of F-actin with the insulin-responsive glucose transporter GLUT4. *J Biol Chem.* 274:17742–17747.

Kaneko, J.J., Harvey, J.W., and Bruss, M. 2008. *Clinical Biochemistry of Domestic Animal*, 6th edition. Amsterdam, Boston, MA: Academic Press/Elsevier.

Karagiannis, M.H., Remker, N., Kerl, M.E., and Mann, F.A. 2006. Lactate measurement as an indicator of perfusion. *Compend Contin Educ Pract Vet.* 28:287–298.

Keller, P. 1981. Enzyme-activities in dogs—Tissue-analyses, plasma values, and intracellular-distribution. *Am J Vet Res.* 42:575–582.

Kikuta, Y. and Onishi, T. 1986. The contribution of intestinal creatine kinase to serum creatine kinase activity and its isoenzymes in dogs. *Jpn J Vet Sci.* 4:547–551.

Klein, M.S., Shell, W.E., and Sobel, B.E. 1973. Serum creatine phosphokinase (CPK) isoenzymes after intramuscular injections, surgery, and myocardial infarction. experimental and clinical studies. *Cardiovasc Res.* 7:412–418.

Klocke, F.J., Copley, D.P., Krawczyk, J.A., and Reichlin, M. 1982. Rapid renal clearence of immunoreactive canine plasma myoglobin. *Circulation.* 65:1522–1528.

Latimer, K.S., Mahaffey, E.A., Prasse, K.W., and Duncan, J.R. 2003. *Duncan & Prasse's Veterinary Laboratory Medicine: Clinical Pathology*, 4th edition. Ames, IA: Iowa State Press.

Lawrie, L.A. 1950. Some observations on factors affecting myoglobin concentrations in muscle. *J Agr Sci.* 40:356–366.

Le Panse, R., Cizeron-Clairac, G., Cuvelier, M., et al. 2008. Regulatory and pathogenic mechanisms in human autoimmune myasthenia gravis. *Ann N Y Acad Sci.* 1132:135–142.

Lee, S-J. 2007. Quadrupling muscle mass in mice by targeting TGF-β signaling pathways. *PLoS ONE.* 2(8):e789. doi:10.1371/journal.pone.0000789

Lefebvre, H.P., Jaeg, J.P., Rico, A.G., et al. 1992. Variations of plasma creatine-kinase in rabbits following repetitive blood-sampling effects of pretreatment with acepromazine, carazolol and dantrolene. *Eur J Clin Chem Clin Biochem.* 30:425–428.

Lefebvre, H.P., Toutain, P.L., Bret, L., et al.1993. Compared kinetics of plasma creatine kinase activity in rabbits after intravenous injection of different preparations of skeletal muscle. *Vet Res.* 24:468–476.

Lewis, H.B. and Rhodes, D.C. 1978. Effects of I.M. injections on serum creatine phosphokinase (CPK) values in dogs. *Vet Clin Pathol.* 7:11–13.

Lindena, J., Diederichs, F., Wittenberg, H., and Trautschold, I. 1986. Kinetic of adjustment of enzyme catalytic concentrations in the extracellular space of the man, the dog and the rat. Approach to a quantitative diagnostic enzymology, V. Communication. *J Clin Chem Clin Biochem.* 24:61–71.

Lindena, J., Kupper, W., and Trautschold, J. 1982. Effect of transient hypoxia in skeletal muscle on enzyme activities in lymph and plasma. *J Clin Chem Clin Biochem.* 20:95–102.

Loeb, W.F. and Quimby, F.W. 1989. *The Clinical Chemistry of Laboratory Animals*. New York, NY: Pergamon Press.

Loeb, W.F. and Quimby, F.W. 1999. *The Clinical Chemistry of Laboratory Animals*, 2nd edition, p. 753. Philadelphia, PA: Taylor & Francis.

Mahoney, D.J. and Tarnopolsky, M.A. 2008. Emerging molecular trends in muscle damage research. In *Skeletal Muscle Damage and Repair*. Ed. P.M. Tiidus, pp. 89–102. Champaign, IL: Human Kinetics.

Markert, C.L. 1984. Lactate dehydrogenase. Biochemistry and function of lactate dehydrogenase. *Cell Biochem Funct*. 2:131–134.

Massarrat, S. 1965. Enzyme kinetics half-life and immunological properties of iodine-131-labelled transaminases in pig blood. *Nature*. 206:508–509.

Matsuzawa, T., Nomura, M., and Unno, T. 1993. Clinical pathology reference ranges of laboratory animals. *J Vet Med Sci*. 55:351–362.

Matwichuk, C.L., Taylor, S., Shmon, C.L., et al. 1999. Changes in rectal temperature and hematologic, biochemical, blood gas, and acid-base values in healthy Labrador retrievers before and after strenuous exercise. *Am J Vet Res*. 60:88–92.

McGavin, M.D. and Zachary, J.F. 2007. *Pathologic Basis of Veterinary Disease*, 4th edition. St. Louis, MO: Elsevier Mosby.

McKenzie, E.C., Jose-Cunilleras, E., Hinchcliff, K.W., et al. 2007. Serum chemistry alterations in Alaskan sled dogs during five successive days of prolonged endurance exercise. *J Am Vet Med Assoc*. 230:1486–1492.

Melmed, C., Shelton, G.D., Bergman, R., and Barton, C. 2004. Masticatory muscle myositis: Pathogenesis, diagnosis, and treatment. *Comp Cont Edu Pract Vet*. 1:590–605.

Meng, H., Bentley, T.B., and Pittman, R.N. 1993. Myoglobin content of hamster skeletal-muscles. *J Appl Physiol*. 74:2194–2197.

Mesher, C.I., Rej, R., and Stokol, T. 1998. Alanine aminotransferase apoenzyme in dogs. *Vet Clin Pathol*. 27:26–30.

Mion, M.M., Novello, E., Altinier, S., et al. 2007. Analytical and clinical performance of a fully automated cardiac multi-markers strategy based on protein biochip microarray technology. *Clin Biochem*. 40:1245–1251.

Mitruka, B.M. and Rawnsley, H.M. 1981. *Clinical Biochemical and Hematological Reference Values in Normal Experimental Animals and Normal Humans*, 2nd edition. New York, NY: Masson Pub. USA.

Nascimento, C.C., Padula, N., Milani, J.G., et al. 2008. Histomorphometric analysis of the response of rat skeletal muscle to swimming, immobilization and rehabilitation. *Braz J Med Biol Res*. 41:818–824.

Nilkumhang, P. and Thornton, J.R. 1979. Plasma and tissue enzyme-activities in the cat. *J Small Anim Pract*. 20:169–174.

Notkins, A.L. 1965. Lactic dehydrogenase virus. *Bacteriol Rev*. 29:143–160.

Nuttall, F. 1968. Tissue and serum creatine kinase in hypothyroid cats. *J Endocrinol*. 42:495–499.

O'Brien, P.J. 2008. Cardiac troponin is the most effective translational safety biomarker for myocardial injury in cardiotoxicity. *Toxicology* 245:206–216.

O'Brien, P.J., Dameron, G.W., Beck, M.L., and Brandt, M. 1998. Differential reactivity of cardiac and skeletal muscle from various species in two generations of cardiac troponin-T immunoassays. *Res Vet Sci*. 65:135–137.

O'Brien, P.J., Smith, D.E., Knechtel, T.J., Marchak, M.A., Pruimboom-Brees, I., Brees, D.J., Spratt, D.P., Archer, F.J., Butler, P., Potter, A.N., Provost, J.P., Richard, J., Snyder, P.A., and Reagan, W.J. 2006. Cardiac troponin I is a sensitive, specific biomarker of cardiac injury in laboratory animals. *Lab Anim*. 40(2):153–171.

O'Connell, T.M., Ardeshirpour, F., Asher, S., et al. 2008. Metabolomic analysis of cancer cachexia reveals distinct lipid and glucose alterations. *Metabolomics*. 4:216–225.

Olby, N. 2005. Laboratory evaluation of muscle disorders. In *BSAVA Manual of Canine and Feline Clinical Pathology*. Eds. E. Villiers and L. Blackwood, 2nd edition, pp. 364–372. Quedgeley, Gloucester: British Small Animal Veterinary Association.

Ordway, G.A. and Garry, D.J. 2004. Myoglobin: An essential hemoprotein in striated muscle. *J Exp Biol*. 207:3441–3446.

Pang, D.S. and Boysen, S. 2007. Lactate in veterinary critical care: Pathophysiology and management. *J Am Anim Hosp Assoc*. 43:270–279.

Panteghini, M. and Bais, R. 2008. Enzymes. In *Tietz Fundamentals of Clinical Chemistry*. Eds. C.A. Burtis, E.R. Ashwood, and D.E. Bruns, 6th edition, pp. 317–336. St. Louis, MO: Saunders Elsevier.

Panteghini, M., Bunk, D.M., Christenson, R.H., et al. 2008. Review: Standardization of troponin I measurements: An update. *Clin Chem Lab Med*. 46:1501–1506.

Patterson, E.E., Minor, K.M., Tchernatynskaia, A.V., et al. 2008. A canine DNM1 mutation is highly associated with the syndrome of exercise-induced collapse. *Nat Genet.* 40:235–239.

Pavé-Preux, M., Ferry, N., Bouguet, J., et al. 1988. Nucleotide sequence and glucocorticoid regulation of the mRNAs for the isoenzymes of rat aspartate aminotransferase. *J Biol Chem.* 263:17459–17466.

Pedersen, B.K. and Febbraio, M. 2005. Muscle-derived interleukin-6—A possible link between skeletal muscle, adipose tissue, liver, and brain. *Brain Behav Immun.* 19:371–376.

Pedersen, B.K., Åkerström, T.C., Nielsen, A.R., and Fischer, C.P. 2007. Role of myokines in exercise and metabolism. *J Appl Physiol.* 103:1093–1098.

Pelé, M., Tiret, L., Kessler, J.L., et al. 2005. SINE exonic insertion in the PTPLA gene leads to multiple splicing defects and segregates with the autosomal recessive centronuclear myopathy in dog. *Hum Mol Genet.* 14:1417–1422.

Peter, J.B., Barnard, R.J., Edgerton, V.R., et al. 1972. Metabolic profiles of three fiber types of skeletal muscle in guinea pigs and rabbits. *Biochemistry.* 11:2617–2633.

Poel, W. 1949. Effect of anoxic anoxia on myoglobin concentration in striated muscle. *Am J Physiol.* 156:44–51.

Preedy, V.R. and Peters, T.J. 2002. *Skeletal Muscle: Pathology, Diagnosis and Management of Disease.* London; San Francisco, CA: Greenwich Medical Media.

Preus, M., Karsten, B., and Bhargava, A.S. 1989. Serum isoenzyme pattern of creatine kinase and lactate dehydrogenase in various animal species. *J Clin Chem Clin Biochem.* 27:787–790.

Pritt, M.L., Hall, D.G., Recknor, J., et al 2008. Fabp3 as a biomarker of skeletal muscle toxicity in the rat: Comparison with conventional biomarkers. *Toxicol Sci.* 103:382–396.

Rao, G.N. 1996. New diet (NTP-2000) for rats in the national toxicology program toxicity and carcinogenicity studies. *Fund Appl Toxicol.* 32:102–108.

Rapaport, E. 1975. The fractional disappearance rate of the separate isoenzymes of creatine phosphokinase in the dog. *Cardiovasc Res.* 9:473–477.

Ready, A.E. and Morgan, G. 1984. The physiological-response of Siberian husky dogs to exercise-effect of interval training. *Can Vet J.* 25:86–91.

Riley, V. 1974. Persistence and other characteristics of the lactate dehydrogenase-elevating virus (LDH-virus). *Prog Med Virol.* 18:198–213.

Robergs, R.A., Ghiasvand, F., and Parker, D. 2004. Biochemistry of exercise-induced metabolic acidosis. *Am J Physiol Regul Integr Comp Physiol.* 287:R502–R516.

Rossignol, F., Solares, M., Balanza, E., et al. 2003. Expression of lactate dehydrogenase A and B genes in different tissues of rats adapted to chronic hypobaric hypoxia. *J Cell Biochem.* 89:67–79.

Rossmeisl, J.H., Duncan, R.B., Inzana, K.D., et al. 2009. Longitudinal study of the effects of chronic hypothyroidism on skeletal muscle in dogs. *Am J Vet Res.* 70:879–889.

Roth, M., Jaquet, P.Y., and Rohner, A. 1989. Increase of creatine-kinase and lactate-dehydrogenase in the serum of rats submitted to experimental intestinal infarction. *Clin Chim Acta.* 183:65–69.

Ruckebusch, Y., Phaneuf, L.P., and Dunlop, R. 1991. *Physiology of Small and Large Animals.* Philadelphia, PA: Decker.

Scheele, C., Nielsen, S, and Pedersen, B.K. 2009. ROS and myokines promote muscle adaptation to exercise. *Trends Endocrinol Metab.* 20:95–99.

Schiaffino, S. and Reggiani, C. 1994. Myosin isoforms in mammalian skeletal-muscle. *J Appl Physiol.* 77:493–501.

Schultz, D., Su, X., Bishop, S.P., et al. 1996. Myocyte stretch induces creatine kinase isoform switching by selective induction of the creatine kinase B gene in chronic volume overload hypertrophy. *Circulation.* 94:1795.

Segal, H.L. and Kim, Y.S. 1963. Glucocorticoid stimulation of the biosynthesis of glutamic-alanine transaminase. *Biochemistry.* 50:912–918.

Shelton, G.D. 1999. Acquired myasthenia gravis: What we have learned from experimental and spontaneous animal models. *Vet Immunol Immunopathol.* 69:239–249.

Shelton, G.D. 2002. Myasthenia gravis and disorders of neuromuscular transmission. *Vet Clin North Am Small Anim Pract.* 32:189–206.

Shelton, G.D. 2007. From dog to man: The broad spectrum of inflammatory myopathies. *Neuromuscul Disord.* 17:663–670.

Shelton, G.D. and Cardinet, G.H. 3rd. 1987. Pathophysiologic basis of canine muscle disorders. *J Vet Int Med.* 1:36–44.

Shelton, G.D. and Engvall, E. 2002. Muscular dystrophies and other inherited myopathies. *Vet Clin North Am Small Anim Pract.* 32:103–124.

Shelton, G.D. and Engvall, E. 2005. Canine and feline models of human inherited muscle diseases. *Neuromuscul Disord.* 15:127–138.

Shelton, G.D., Cardinet, G.H., 3rd., Bandman, E., et al 1985. Fiber type-specific autoantibodies in a dog with eosinophilic myositis. *Muscle Nerve.* 8:783–790.

Shelton, G.D., Nyhan, W.L., Kass, P.H., et al 1998. Analysis of organic acids, amino acids, and carnitine in dogs with lipid storage myopathy. *Muscle Nerve.* 21:1202–1205.

Sherawat, M., Tolan, D.R., and Allen, K.N. 2008. Structure of a rabbit muscle fructose-1, 6-bisphosphate aldolase A dimer variant. *Crystallogr D Biol Crystallogr.* 64:543–550.

Shibata, S. and Kobayashi, B. 1978. Blood-platelets as a possible source of creatine-kinase in a rat plasma and serum. *Thromb Haemost.* 39:701–706.

Sieb, J.P. and Gillessen, G.T. 2003. Iatrogenic and toxic myopathies. *Muscle Nerve.* 27:142–156.

Silverthorn, D.U. 2004. *Human Physiology: An Integrated Approach.* San Francisco: Pearson/Benjamin Cummings.

Skillen, A.W. 1984. Clinical biochemistry of lactate dehydrogenase. *Cell Biochem Funct.* 2:140–144.

Smerdu, V., Cehovin, T., Strbenc, M., and Fazarinc, G. 2009. Enzyme- and immunohistochemical aspects of skeletal muscle fibers in brown bear (*Ursus arctos*). *J Morphol.* 270:154–161.

Smith, B.F., Stedman, H., Rajpurohit, Y., et al. 1996. Molecular basis of canine muscle type phosphofructokinase deficiency. *J Biol Chem.* 271: 20070–20074.

Stehno-Bittel, L., Al-Jarrah, M., and Williams, S.J. 2008. Diabetes. In *Skeletal Muscle Damage and Repair.* Ed. P.M. Tiidus, pp. 135–145. Champaign, IL: Human Kinetics.

Steiss, J.E. and Wright, J.C. 2008. Respiratory alkalosis and primary hypocapnia in labrador retrievers participating in field trials in high-ambient-temperature conditions. *Am J Vet Res.* 69:1262–1267.

Stockham, S.L. and Scott, M.A. 2008. *Fundamentals of Veterinary Clinical Pathology*, 2nd edition. Ames, IA: Blackwell Publishing.

Stokol, T. and Erb, H. 1998. The apo-enzyme content of aminotransferases in healthy and diseased domestic animals. *Vet Clin Pathol.* 27:71–78.

Swaim, L.D., Taylor, H.W., and Jersey, G.C. 1985. The effect of handling techniques on serum ALT activity in mice. *J Appl Toxicol.* 5:160–162.

Swenson, C.L. and Graves, T.K. 1997. Absence of liver specificity for canine alanine aminotransferase (ALT). *Vet Clin Pathol.* 26:26–28.

Thoren-Tolling, K. and Jonsson, L. 1983. Creatine-kinase isoenzymes in serum of pigs having myocardial and skeletal-muscle necrosis. *Can J Comp Med.* 47:207–216.

Trendelenburg, A.U., Meyer, A., Rohner, D., et al. 2009. Myostatin reduces Akt/TORC1/p70S6K signaling, inhibiting myoblast differentiation and myotube size. *Am J Physiol Cell Physiol.* 296:C1258–C1270.

Valberg, S.J. 2008. Skeletal muscle function. In *Clinical Biochemistry of Domestic Animals.* Eds. J.J. Kaneko, J.W. Harvey, and M. Bruss, 6th edition, pp. 419–484. Amsterdam; Boston, MA: Academic Press/Elsevier.

Valentine, B.A., Blue, J.T., Shelley, S.M., and Cooper, B.J. 1990. Increased serum alanine aminotransferase activity associated with muscle necrosis in the dog. *J Vet Int Med.* 4:140–143.

van Adel, B. and Tarnopolsky, M. 2009. Metabolic myopathies: Update 2009. *J Clin Neuromuscul Dis.* 10:97–121.

Vlasakova, K., Lane, P., Michna, L., Muniappa, N., Sistare, F.D., and Glaab, W.E. 2017. Response of novel skeletal muscle biomarkers in dogs to drug-induced skeletal muscle injury or sustained endurance exercise. *Toxicol Sci.* 156(2):422–427.

Voss, E.M., Sharkey, S.W., Gernert, A.E., et al. 1995. Human and canine cardiac troponin-T and creatine kinase distribution in normal and diseased myocardium—Infarct sizing using serum profiles. *Arch Pathol Lab Med.* 119:799–806.

Walker, D.B. 2006. Serum chemical biomarkers of cardiac injury for nonclinical safety testing. *Toxicol Pathol.* 34:94–104.

Walsh, K. 2009. Adipokines, myokines and cardiovascular disease. *Circ J.* 73:13–18.

Wan, D.Y., Cerklewski, F.L., and Leklem, J.E. 1993. Increased plasma pyridoxal-5′-phosphate when alkaline phosphatase activity is reduced in moderately zinc-deficient rats. *Biol Trace Elem Res.* 39:203–210.

Waner, T. and Nyska, A. 1991. The toxicological significance of decreased activities of blood alanine and aspartate aminotransferase. *Vet Res Commun.* 15:73–78.

Waner, T., Nyska, A., and Chen, R. 1991. Population distribution profiles of the activities of blood alanine and aspartate-aminotransferase in the normal F344 inbred rat by age and sex. *Lab Anim.* 25:263–271.

Warren, G.L. and Palubinskas, L.E. 2008. Human and animal experimental muscle injury models. In *Skeletal Muscle Damage and Repair.* Ed. P.M. Tiidus, pp. 13–35. Champaign, IL: Human Kinetics.

Weber, M.A. 2009. Ultrasound in the inflammatory myopathies. *Ann N Y Acad Sci.* 1154:159–170.
Weingand, K., Bloom, J., Carakostas, M., et al. 1992. Clinical pathology testing recommendations for nonclinical toxicity and safety studies. *Toxicol Pathol.* 20:539–543.
Weingand, K., Brown, G., Hall, R., et al. 1996. Harmonization of animal clinical pathology testing in toxicity and safety studies. *Fundam Appl Toxicol.* 29:198–201.
Weiss, A. and Leinwand, L.A. 1996. The mammalian myosin heavy chain gene family. *Ann Rev Cell Dev Biol.* 12:417–439.
Weiss, A., Schiaffino, S., and Leinwand, L.A. 1999. Comparative sequence analysis of the complete human sarcomeric myosin heavy chain family: Implications for functional diversity. *J Mol Biol.* 290:61–75.
Welle, S.L. 2009. Myostatin and muscle fiber size. Focus on "Smad2 and 3 transcription factors control muscle mass in adulthood" and "Myostatin reduces Akt/TORC1/p70S6K signaling, inhibiting myoblast differentiation and myotube size". *Am J Physiol Cell Physiol.* 296:C1245–C1247.
Wells, D.J. 2005. Animal models for muscular disorders. In *Handbook of Laboratory Animal Science.* Eds. J. Hau, G.L. Van Hoosier, and Inc NetLibrary, 2nd edition, pp. 225–239. Boca Raton, FL: CRC Press.
Wilson, D. 2008. *McGraw-Hill's Manual of Laboratory & Diagnostic Tests.* New York, NY: McGraw-Hill Medical.
Wyss, M. and Kaddurah-Daouk, R. 2000. Creatine and creatinine metabolism. *Physiol Rev.* 80:1107–1213.
Yang R.Z., Park, S., Reagan, W.J., et al. 2009. Alanine aminotransferase isoenzymes: Molecular cloning and quantitative analysis of tissue expression in rats and serum—Elevation in liver toxicity. *Hepatology.* 49:598–607.
Yasmineh, W.G., Pyle, R.B., and Nicoioff, D.M. 1976. Rate of decay and distribution volume of MB isoenzyme of creatine-kinase, intravenously injected into baboon. *Clin Chem.* 22:1095–1097.
York, M.J. 2017. 14. Clinical pathology. In *A Comprehensive Guide to Toxicology in Preclinical Drug Development*, 2nd edition, A.S. Faqi (ed.), p. 359. Amsterdam: Elsevier, Inc. Academic Press.
Zammit, P.S. 2008. All muscle satellite cells are equal, but are some more equal than others? *J Cell Sci.* 121:2975–2982.
Zhang, K.R., Liu, H.T., Zhang, H.F., et al. 2007. Long-term aerobic exercise protects the heart against ischemia/reperfusion injury via PI3 kinase-dependent and akt-mediated mechanism. *Apoptosis.* 12:1579–1588.
Zinkl, J.G., Bush, B.M., Cornelius, C.E., et al. 1971. Comparative studies on plasma and tissue sorbital, glutamic, lactic and hydroxybutyric dehydrogenase and transaminase. *Res Vet* Sci. 12:211–214.

APPENDIX 14.1

Tissue Source and Species Half-Life Comparison

Tissue Source (Cellular/Subcellular Location) and Species Half-Life Comparison for Skeletal Muscle Analytes[a]

			Circulating half-life				
Analyte	**Tissue Source(s)**	**Cellular Location**	**Rat**	**Mouse**	**Dog**	**Rabbit**	**Pig**
Aldolase	Skeletal and cardiac muscle, liver		20 days[b]				
ALT	Liver, skeletal muscle	Cytosol, mitochondria (minor)	4.5-8 h[c] 0.9-3 h[d]		48-72 h[e] 149 min^{-1} [f] 59 ± h[g] 3-60 h[f,h]	5 h[i] 5.1 h[d]	
AST	Liver, skeletal and cardiac muscle, RBCs	Cytosol, mitochondria	1.6 h[d,j]		263 min[f,k] 22 ± 1.6 h[f,g,h] 12 h[j]	2.5 h[d,j]	18 h[j]
CK	Skeletal, cardiac and smooth (minor) muscle	Cytosol, mitochondria	0.5-1 h[l] Biphasic: 0.2 h and 0.6 h[d,m]		< 2 h[e] 2.61 h[n] 1-3 h[l] 4.7 h[d]	9 h[l]	5.2 h[d,o]
CK isoenzymes	MM – Skeletal muscle MB and MM – Cardiac muscle BB – Brain				CKMM: 77 min[p]		

(Continued)

APPENDIX 14.1 (*Continued*)

Tissue Source and Species Half-Life Comparison

Tissue Source (Cellular/Subcellular Location) and Species Half-Life Comparison for Skeletal Muscle Analytes[a]

			Circulating Half-Life				
Analyte	**Tissue Source(s)**	**Cellular Location**	**Rat**	**Mouse**	**Dog**	**Rabbit**	**Pig**
LDH	Liver, skeletal and cardiac muscle, RBCs		0.6 h[d]			2.5 h[d]	
LDH isoenzymes	LDH-1: Cardiac muscle, RBCs and brain LDH-2: Reticuloendothelial system LDH-3: Lung LDH-4: Kidney, LDH-5: Liver and skeletal muscle			LDH-1: 3.3 h[o,q] LDH-5: 0.8 h[o,q]	LDH-5: 0.8 h[d]		LDH-5: 3 h[q]
Myoglobin	Skeletal and cardiac muscle; not found in smooth muscle				8.9 ± 1.5 min[r] 5.5 ± 0.2 min[p]		
Troponin	Skeletal and cardiac isoforms; not found in smooth muscle		Cardiac troponin I: 6 h[s] 0.8 h[t] Skeletal troponin I is thought to have similar characteristics as cardiac-type[u]	Cardiac troponin I: 1.9 h[t]			

APPENDIX 14.1 (*Continued*)

Tissue Source and Species Half-Life Comparison

Tissue Source (Cellular/Subcellular Location) and Species Half-Life Comparison for Skeletal Muscle Analytes[a]

[a] Values are given for adult animals.
[b] Segal and Kim (1963).
[c] Loeb and Quimby (1999).
[d] Boyd (1983).
[e] Stockham and Scott (2008).
[f] Kaneko et al. (2008, p. 391).
[g] Dossin (2005).
[h] Kaneko et al. (2008, p. 356).
[i] Loeb and Quimby (1999, p. 402).
[j] Loeb and Quimby (1999, p. 406).
[k] Zinkl et al. (1971).
[l] Loeb and Quimby (1999, p. 428).
[m] Loeb and Quimby (1999, p. 42).
[n] Kaneko et al. (2008, p. 369).
[o] Loeb and Quimby (1999, p. 119).
[p] Ellis and Saran (1989).
[q] Loeb and Quimby (1999, p. 430).
[r] Klocke et al. (1982).
[s] O'Brien et al. (2006).
[t] Dunn et al. (2011).
[u] York (2017).

15 Evaluation of Bone Function and Injury

Holly L. Jordan and Bruce E. LeRoy

CONTENTS

15.1 GENERAL CONCEPTS

The skeleton has a key role in locomotion, protecting vital organs, and regulating calcium and phosphorus metabolism. A wide range of disorders may perturb bone metabolism and/or affect mineral ion concentrations, particularly nutritional, renal, endocrine, or neoplastic etiologies. Markers of bone status are valuable not only for clinical appraisal in human and veterinary medicine, but also as endpoints in the experimental animal models of human bone disorders, such as osteoporosis, metastatic bone disease, and fracture healing, and in identifying the toxic effects of novel xenobiotics on bone during preclinical evaluations.

Biochemical assessment of skeletal system injury may include quantification of serum and urine mineral ions such as calcium, phosphorus, and magnesium; evaluation of circulating hormones involved in bone metabolism, such as parathyroid hormone (PTH) and vitamin D; and evaluation of other biological molecules reflecting the balance of bone formation and resorption, the so-called "bone turnover biomarkers," for example, bone alkaline phosphatase (BALP), osteocalcin (OC), and collagen telopeptides (Herrmann, 2011). In clinical practice, fluid markers provide useful adjuncts to more cumbersome or invasive measures of bone health, such as bone density measurement by dual-energy x-ray absorptiometry (DEXA) and bone biopsy. However, because fluid biomarkers tend to reflect the whole-body balance between bone formation and resorption only at the time of sampling, serial measurements may be necessary to detect progression of disease or response to interventions. Bone turnover markers are available for use in humans and many other species; most are measured in serum, plasma, and/or urine by immunoassay methods, for example, ELISA, RIA, and/or chemiluminescence. It is essential to verify that the biomarkers of interest are validated for the species under consideration, as not all markers or reagents are appropriate across species. In addition to species-specific factors, application of these markers requires consideration of preanalytical factors, such as sample handling, gender, age, diet, and cyclical influences (Cremers and Garnero, 2006).

15.2 CELLULAR AND MOLECULAR MECHANISMS OF BONE PHYSIOLOGY AND PATHOPHYSIOLOGY

Bone is a dynamic tissue. Even in adult animals, the skeletal system undergoes constant remodeling. Basic multicellular units (also called bone remodeling units) intricately regulate the formation and resorption of bone in response to load stresses and metabolic demands (Seeman and Delmas, 2006). In people, resorption requires approximately 3 weeks per site and rebuilding bone requires 3-4 months (Rodan and Martin, 2000). At the start of the resorptive phase, osteoclasts are recruited from hematopoietic stem cell precursors. Under the influence of macrophage colony stimulating factor and receptor activator of nuclear factor kappa B ligand (RANK-ligand or RANK-L), these precursor cells differentiate, mature, and fuse into multinuclear osteoclasts with ruffled borders that form sealed resorption lacuna. Into these spaces, osteoclasts secrete hydrochloric acid, cathepsin K (CTSK), and other factors that dissolve mineral and degrade the extracellular matrix. With cessation of resorption, osteoclasts undergo apoptosis and bone formation is initiated by osteoblasts recruited from mesenchymal stem cells. Osteoblasts produce collagen type I, alkaline phosphatase, OC, and other components, leading to the formation of an extracellular matrix that subsequently mineralizes. After bone formation, the osteoblasts undergo apoptosis or they become incorporated within bone as osteocytes, which function as mechanosensors (Herrmann, 2011; Sorensen et al., 2007).

The specific molecular mechanisms regulating bone remodeling are very complex, and this field is rapidly evolving. Three important mediators are members of the tumor-necrosis factor family: RANK, RANK-L, and osteoprotegerin (OPG) (Boyce et al., 2008). Upon stimulation by PTH, the active form of vitamin D (1,25$(OH)_2$D also called calcitriol), parathyroid hormone-related protein (PTHrP), and other cytokines and hormones, the osteoblasts upregulate the expression of RANK-L, which stimulates the resorption by mature osteoclasts and the recruitment of osteoclast precursors (Ralston, 2009). Matrix-embedded osteocytes and chondrocytes are also a major, if not the major, source of RANK-L in bone and can stimulate osteoclastogenesis as well (Xiong et al., 2011). OPG is a decoy or "pseudo-receptor" for RANK-L. It is secreted by osteoblasts and acts as an osteoprotector or negative regulator of bone resorption (Boyce et al., 2008; Herrmann, 2011). Soluble OPG captures and inactivates RANK-L in the osteoblast membrane, preventing it from coupling with RANK on osteoclasts. This leads to inhibition of osteoclast function and survival (Capen and O'Brien, 2004). Osteoclasts, in turn, promote bone formation by modulating osteoblast function through the release of bone matrix-embedded growth factors during resorption, such as insulin-like growth factors, transforming growth factor-β, fibroblast growth factors, and bone morphogenetic proteins, which stimulate differentiation and activation of osteoblast precursors (Kraenzlin and Seibel, 2006).

While PTH and 1,25$(OH)_2$D upregulate bone resorption and circulating calcium concentrations, other mediators, such as calcitonin, inhibit osteoclastogenesis and reduce free calcium. Both PTH and calcitonin modulate 1,25(OH)$_2$D concentrations through regulation of the renal 25-hydroxyvitamin D$_3$ 1α-hydroxylase gene. During normocalcemic states, calcitonin predominates, whereas PTH predominates in hypocalcemic states (Zhong et al., 2009). Both factors as well as fibroblast growth factor 23 (FGF23), decrease renal resorption of phosphorus (Capen and O'Brien, 2004).

Maintaining whole-body bone mass depends not only on healthy function of the skeletal system, but also on coordinate pathways in other systems and organs, including the nervous system and adipose tissue. For example, the adipose hormone, leptin causes bone loss via a hypothalamic/sympathetic nervous system signaling pathway, which inhibits osteoblast proliferation and stimulates RANK-L-mediated osteoclastic bone resorption (Karsenty, 2006). Hyperinsulinemia due to impaired hepatic insulin clearance is associated with decreased bone turnover in mice (Huang et al., 2010). Bone tissue can mediate metabolic pathways as well via the osteoblast-derived uncarboxylated form of OC, which modulates insulin production and glucose metabolism (Wei and Ducy, 2010). The full implications of the complex interactions between bone, adipose, pancreas, and other tissues are still being defined.

15.3 BIOCHEMICAL INDICATORS OF BONE FORMATION AND RESORPTION

Perturbations in some bone turnover markers may correlate with the presence of histologic changes in many bone diseases, such as osteoporosis and bone malignancies (Allen, 2003; Cremers and Garnero, 2006; Brown and Chow, 2009), although the premonitory value of currently available bone markers has been somewhat limited. In many instances, these markers are not sufficiently sensitive or specific to serve as independent diagnostic endpoints and must be combined with additional disease markers, functional parameters, and/or imaging modalities (Coleman et al., 2011). Serum and urine markers have been used to monitor responses to therapeutics, to identify patients at risk of fracture, and to identify patients that are most likely to benefit from antiresorptive therapy. Table 15.1 outlines key characteristics of commonly used biomarkers of bone formation and resorption. Select markers have been used for prognosticating bone metastasis with some success, for example, procollagen type I N propeptide (PINP) and BALP (Joerger and Huober, 2012; Selvarajah and Kirpensteijn, 2010).

Concentrations of bone formation markers may vary with the stage of bone formation. For example, BALP is a characteristic marker of osteoblast proliferation; PINP and procollagen type I C propeptide (PICP) characterize the matrix maturation phase; and OC is primarily expressed during mineralization (Herrmann, 2011). Therefore, evaluation of bone turnover should include at least one marker of bone formation and one marker of bone resorption (Herrmann, 2011). Bone resorption is characterized by constituents synthesized by osteoclasts (i.e., tartrate-resistant acid phosphatase 5b [TRACP5b] and CTSK) or released from the extracellular matrix by osteoclasts (i.e., cross-linked N-telopeptide [NTX-1] and C-telopeptide [CTX-1]). Indeed TRAP5b and CTSK concentrations correlate with osteoclast numbers, while CTX-1 and NTX-1 reflect resorptive activity (Herrmann, 2011).

Variability in bone biomarkers owing to factors such as age and cyclical rhythms have been investigated in some common laboratory animals (Allen et al., 1998). Similar to humans, nonhuman primates have high intra- and interindividual variability for most bone markers (Legrand et al., 2003). Diurnal variation in bone turnover markers has been described in rats (Muhlbauer and Fleisch, 1990), mice (Tonna et al., 1987), rabbits (Hansson et al., 1974), and dogs (Ladlow et al., 2002). Dogs show significant diurnal variation in serum concentrations of OC, BALP, pyridinoline cross-linked carboxyterminal telopeptide of type I collagen (ICTP), and urinary deoxypyridinoline (DPD) (Ladlow et al., 2002). Interestingly, there is no significant difference in bone marker concentrations between normal toy and giant breed dogs (Breur et al., 2004). Owing to dynamic changes in bone markers during growth, age and gender-specific reference intervals are essential. Human reference intervals for serum OC, BALP, PINP, and collagen degradation products are highest during childhood and gradually decline with age (Huang et al., 2011). Legrand et al. (2003) reported

TABLE 15.1
Bone Turnover Biomarkers

Bone Formation	Abbreviation	Comments	Species for Which Assays Are Available
Bone isoenzyme of alkaline phosphatase	BALP (serum)	Produced by osteoblasts; marker of osteoblast differentiation	ELISA: mouse, rat, dog, and monkey Wheat-germ lectin precipitation: dog and monkey
Osteocalcin	OC (serum)	Osteoblast-derived protein released into the bone matrix and the circulation; fragments released during bone resorption from the extracellular matrix, thus reflects bone turnover rather than simply formation, unless assay measures the intact form. Also important in energy metabolism	Mouse, rat, dog, monkey, rabbit, and guinea pig
Procollagen type I C or N propeptide	PICP, PINP (serum)	Released from newly synthesized preprocollagen prior to incorporation of collagen into bone matrix; marker also of collagen type I formation	Mouse, rat, dog, monkey, rabbit, guinea pig, and pig
Bone Resorption			
C-terminal cross-linking telopeptide of collagen type I collagen	CTX-1 (serum or urine)	Released during osteoclastic bone resorption by cathepsin K	Mouse, rat, dog, monkey, rabbit, guinea pig, and pig
N-terminal cross-linking telopeptide of type I collagen	NTX-1 (urine)	Released during osteoclastic bone resorption by cathepsin K	Mouse, rat, dog, monkey, rabbit, guinea pig, and pig
C-terminal cross-linking telopeptide of type 1 collagen generated by MMPs	CTX-MMP	Released during pathologic bone resorption by matrix metalloproteases	Mouse, rat, dog, and sheep
Urinary hydroxyproline	Urine HYP	Released from collagen triple helix during bone resorption	Not species specific
Urinary pyridinoline and deoxypyridiniolinie	Urine PYD Urine DPD	Released from mature collagen during bone resorption	Mouse, rat, dog, monkey, rabbit, guinea pig, pig, and sheep
Cathepsin K	CTSK	Essential protease for collagen degradation that is mainly produced by osteoclasts; marker of osteoclast number	Mouse, rat, dog, rabbit, and pig
Tartrate-resistant acid phosphatase 5b	TRACP5b	Enzyme produced by osteoclasts that is involved in intracellular processing of degraded organic bone matrix; marker of osteoclast number, bone resorption	ELISA: mouse, and rat Enzymatic test (TRAP): all species

Source: With kind permission from Springer Science + Business Media: *Osteoporosis Research,* Methods in bone biology in animals: Biochemical markers, 2011, Herrmann, M., Springer-Verlag, London Limited, 2011, p. 59, Herrmann, M. 2011, *see also* Delmas (2001).

similar trends in cynomolgus monkeys. In addition, concentrations in males are generally higher than female monkeys.

Sample handling can be an important factor with more labile markers such as OC, which requires rapid processing and freezing for long-term storage. To avoid the effect of transient changes in urine concentration or dilution, urine marker concentrations should be normalized to urine creatinine concentration as a ratio (i.e., urine NTX-1/creatinine) or urine markers can be measured from samples collected over an extended period and reported as the total amount excreted during that collection period (i.e., urine volume × urine NTX-1 concentration = total amount of NTX-1 excreted/collection period). Indeed, total excretion/collection period may be more accurate in situations where urine creatinine is altered by significant renal injury or changes in muscle mass. For analytes that can be measured in both serum and urine "spot" samples collected simultaneously (usually calcium, phosphorus, or electrolytes), fractional excretion (FE) calculations based on serum and urine creatinine may be applied when overnight collections are not feasible (Stockham and Scott, 2008b). While the routine clinical use of FE tests is limited in veterinary medicine, they have shown value in evaluating mineral deficiencies, in toxicology studies, and in endocrine/renal research (Lefebvre et al., 2008).

15.4 BIOCHEMICAL MARKERS OF BONE INJURY

15.4.1 Calcium

Physiology, function, and half-life: The majority of the body's calcium is in the inorganic portion of the skeleton, which serves as a reservoir for maintaining circulating free (ionized) calcium within a very narrow critical range (approximately 1.1–1.6 mmol/L depending on species) under the influence of mediators such as PTH, vitamin D, and calcitonin (Capen and O'Brien, 2004). Maintenance within this range is essential given the central role that free calcium plays in signal transduction throughout the body and the detrimental effects that can result from dysregulation, such as seizures, tetany, and heart dysfunction. Blood calcium is present in three forms. In mammalian species tested to date, approximately 50% is in the free form (the biologically active ionized form or iCa), 40%–45% is bound to serum proteins (pCa), principally albumin, and the remainder is complexed with citrates, lactate, and other diffusible anions (cCa) (Stockham and Scott, 2008a). Although complete fractionation data is limited for most laboratory animals, serum calcium fractions have been evaluated in healthy dogs, cats, and horses: in these species, pCa is 56%, 40%, and 47%, respectively; iCa is 34%, 52%, and 49%, respectively; and cCa is 10%, 8% and 4%, respectively (Schenck et al., 1996; Schenck et al., 2005; Lopez et al., 2006).

Circulating calcium is maintained via ingestion and uptake in the intestine and through resorption from bone and renal tubules. This relies on a complex network of receptors and transporters (O'Toole, 2011). Within the gut of most mammals, $1,25(OH)_2D$ is required to induce intestinal epithelial cell uptake of calcium (Perez et al., 2008). Calcitonin and PTH act indirectly on the intestine by stimulating 1α-hydroxylase in the kidney, which increases $1,25(OH)_2D$ production. It has been suggested that calcitonin is the predominant mediator during normocalcemia and PTH predominates during hypocalcemia (Zhong et al., 2009); PTH also stimulates calcium resorption from bone and distal renal tubules in response to hypocalcemia. $1,25(OH)_2D$ stimulates calcium release from bone by inducing osteoclastogenesis. In the kidney, nonprotein-bound calcium is freely filtered at the glomerulus and most is passively resorbed in the proximal tubules and thick ascending loop of Henle via paracellular pathways. Active uptake occurs primarily in the distal tubules under the influence of PTH (Allgrove, 2009; O'Toole, 2011).

Total calcium is commonly measured in serum, lithium heparinized plasma, and urine by spectrophotometric methods using metallochromic dyes. Atomic absorption methods are more accurate, but less accessible for most laboratories. Plasma anticoagulants containing chelators, such as EDTA or citrate, should not be used because these will falsely decrease calcium concentrations. To avoid the effects of urine concentration or dilution, it is best to normalize urine calcium concentration to urine creatinine concentration as a ratio (calcium in mmol/L/creatinine in mmol/L). Total urine calcium excreted over a defined collection period (usually 12–24 hours) may also be used to assess renal handling of calcium.

As it is the biologically active form, the measurement of iCa by ion-specific electrode is often recommended for accurately assessing the abnormalities in blood total calcium (Schenck and Chew, 2005). Concentrations of iCa are influenced by temperature and pH (iCa concentration and pH are inversely related) and there is debate on optimal sample and handling regimes. Each laboratory should determine the appropriate handling and storage conditions for the species of interest in the context of their specific methodology. In general, serum or lithium heparinized whole blood is preferred over plasma (Krahn and Lou, 2008; Unterer et al., 2004). Samples should be collected anerobically to prevent pH changes; some investigators recommend placing whole blood samples on ice until analysis (Boink et al., 1992). Serum should be separated immediately to prevent lactic acid production by erythrocytes, which can cause artifactual increase in iCa. Analysis should be performed within 8 hours, if samples are at room temperature (Unterer et al., 2004), although Schenck et al. (1995) found canine serum samples were stable for up to 72h. If necessary, serum can be stored at –20°C for up to 6 weeks (Boink et al., 1992).

Because of the close correlations between blood concentrations of total calcium, iCa, and albumin, formulae have been proposed for some species in an attempt to adjust or "normalize" total calcium results that are low due to decreased albumin concentrations and to attempt to predict iCa status without performing direct measurements (Meuten et al., 1982; Siggaard-Andersen et al., 1983). Studies have refuted the accuracy of this practice (Schenck and Chew, 2005). While the interpretation of total calcium changes should take into consideration qualitative changes in serum albumin and protein concentrations, strict reliance on calculated/adjusted values for total calcium or for prediction of iCa is discouraged (Schenck and Chew, 2005).

Significance of increased concentration/activity: Causes of elevated serum calcium (hypercalcemia) include elevated PTH or PTHrP (i.e., primary hyperparathyroidism, paraneoplastic hypercalcemia), hypervitaminosis D (i.e., dietary supplementation, toxic plants containing vitamin D_2, rodenticides containing cholecalciferol, paraneoplastic hypervitaminosis D, granulomatous disease), decreased renal excretion of calcium (i.e., renal insufficiency, diuretic drugs, hypoadrenocorticism), hypomagnesemia, steroid hormones, and hyperproteinemia (Lumachi et al., 2011; Stockham and Scott, 2008a; Raisz et al., 1977). High serum calcium concentrations can lead to organ dysfunction secondary to mineralization of soft tissues, particularly in the kidney and cardiovascular system. Hypercalcemia may also interfere with normal receptor-mediated cell signaling and cause loss of urine concentrating ability and clinical changes such as altered mentation, and constipation. In people, hypercalcemia is most frequently due to increased secretion of PTH or PTHrP (Lumachi et al., 2011). PTH-secreting parathyroid adenomas are the most common cause in human outpatients (Gopinath and Mihai, 2011). PTHrP is a hormone secreted by tumor cells that mimics PTH. In canine patients, common etiologies of hypercalcemia are paraneoplastic secretion of PTHrP (most commonly associated with lymphoma and apocrine gland carcinomas of the anal sacs), renal failure, hyperparathyroidism, and hypoadrenocorticism (Messinger et al., 2009; Rosol and Capen, 1992). In Fisher 344 rats, hypercalcemia has been associated with testicular interstitial tumors (Rice et al., 1975). Activated macrophages expressing extrarenal 1α-hydroxylase can produce hypercalcemia due to hypervitaminosis D (Christakos et al., 2010). Thus, hypercalcemia may be observed with granulomatous disorders such as sarcoidosis and disseminated fungal infections (Jacobs and Bilezikian, 2005).

Hypercalciuria occurs with a variety of conditions, including congenital defects in calcium-sensing receptors and transporters (Stechman et al., 2009), primary hyperparathyroidism, renal tubular acidosis, hypervitaminosis D, diabetes, and with certain drugs, such as, furosemide, acetazolamide, ammonium chloride, and others (Ordóñez et al., 1998; Foley and Boccuzzi, 2010).

Unlike most laboratory animals, rabbits normally excrete large amounts of calcium in their urine with mean fractional excretion of approximately 45%, compared with <2% in most other species (Buss and Bourdeau, 1984).

Significance of decreased concentration/activity: Decreased serum calcium (hypocalcemia) can be caused by hypoalbuminemia (factitious), decreased PTH activity (i.e., primary hypoparathyroidism, pseudohypoparathyroidism, hypomagnesemia), insufficient mobilization of calcium from bone or intestinal absorption (i.e., hypovitaminosis D, vitamin D receptor abnormalities, lipid malabsorption, exocrine pancreatic insufficiency, pregnancy, lactation, hypercalcitoninism, nutritional hypocalcemia, oxalate toxicity), excess renal calcium excretion, calcium-binding anions (i.e., EDTA, citrate, oxalate, tetracycline), renal failure, myopathies, and urinary tract obstruction [Stockham and Scott, 2008a]). Clinically, hypocalcemia can result in diseases such as rickets with attendant lameness and deformity, altered myocardial contractility, dystocia, tetany, and/or seizures, depending on the species. The threshold for manifestation of clinically evident signs varies in dogs, although signs usually manifest when serum free calcium is <0.8 mmol/L and include muscle tremors, fasciculations, facial rubbing, cramping, aggression, stiff gait, and seizures (Schenck and Chew 2008).

Low serum protein, particularly hypoalbuminemia (80% of protein-bound calcium binds albumin versus 20% to globulins) is a very common cause of low total calcium concentration. Thus, disorders associated with loss or impaired synthesis of serum proteins (i.e., renal injury, protein-losing enteropathy, malabsorption, hepatic failure, etc.) may be accompanied by low serum total calcium. Because iCa is unaffected by decreased serum albumin alone, animals with low serum/plasma albumin do not manifest clinical signs of hypocalcemia. PTH deficiency is a cause of hypocalcemia and may be observed with parathyroid gland injury (i.e., inflammation, trauma, surgery, neoplasia) or due to inadequate release of PTH. Aberrant PTH receptor activity on target tissues, or pseudohypoparathyroidism, is a rare cause of hypocalcemia. Hypomagnesemia can result in hypocalcemia due to apparent refractoriness of bone and kidney to PTH (Yamamoto et al., 2011). Hypocalcemia due to hypovitaminosis D can have multiple underlying causes, including renal injury, fat malabsorption, dietary deficiency, and protein-losing enteropathy. For example, dogs with inflammatory bowel disease may become hypocalcemic (Gow, et al., 2011). Minipigs subjected to subtotal gastrectomy develop transient decreases in serum calcium, which normalizes by 12 months postoperatively (Maier et al., 1997). Primates fed diets low in vitamin D, housed indoors and not provided artificial sunlight, or fed diets with high phosphorus content may develop hypocalcemia and nutritional secondary hyperparathyroidism (commonly referred to as cage paralysis, simian bone disease, or osteomalacia) (Capen and O'Brien, 2004). Rats administered a calcium-deficient diet have decreased serum total calcium, although iCa is usually normal due to heightened serum vitamin D and PTH concentrations leading to increased bone resorption (D'Amour et al., 2011). Decreases in blood calcium concentrations may also occur with excess urinary calcium loss secondary to metabolic alkalosis, antidiuretics (e.g., furosemide), and renal toxins (e.g., ethylene glycol) (Stockham and Scott, 2008a).

Influencing factors (sources of error, interferences, dietary/fasting, etc.): Sources of error in total or iCa determination include using an inappropriate anticoagulant, such as those containing EDTA, oxalate, or citrate. Even heparin, which is an anion, binds calcium to some extent and heparin concentrations should be limited to 15 U/mL of blood when measuring iCa (Stockham and Scott, 2008a). Analytical errors in iCa measurement occur if pH is altered through excessive exposure to air (a vacutainer or capped syringe is recommended) or due to lactic acid from erythrocytes, which occurs when serum is not separated from the clot within 1 hour of collection. Fasting is recommended to limit effects of dietary calcium intake and postprandial alkalosis (Stockham and Scott, 2008). Serum separator tubes are not recommended for determination of iCa due to the presence of calcium-containing material and acidifying products. However, the clinical impact is small; iCa is approximately 0.02 mmol/L higher than when collected in plain serum tubes (Larsson and Ohman, 1985). When measuring calcium concentrations in urine, it has been recommended that samples be acidified to dissolve precipitated calcium (Foley and Boccuzzi, 2010). However, the difference between calcium concentrations in acidified and nonacidified samples from human volunteers is actually quite small (Feres et al., 2011) and in the absence of clinical impact, some investigators refute this requirement, unless urine samples must be stored 12 hours or more at 4°C prior to analysis (Sodi et al., 2009).

Age, gender, and strain differences in serum total and ionized calcium have been observed in mice (Frith et al., 1980; Leiben et al., 2012; Barrett et al., 1975; Tordoff et al., 2007; Champy et al., 2008; Mazzaccara et al., 2008). Serum free calcium increases with age in rats and is higher in females than males (D'Amour et al., 2011). Pregnant rats have higher total calcium than nonpregnant cohorts (Liberati, 2004). Lactation reportedly lowers total calcium in sows (Lauridsen et al., 2010). Circadian rhythm in total but not free calcium concentration has been noted in macaques likely due to albumin fluctuation (Hotchkiss and Jerome, 1998). Fasting may decrease not only free calcium, but also total calcium concentrations in some species, such as the pig (Baetz and Mengeling, 1971). In rabbits, increased dietary calcium can markedly increase serum total calcium concentration (Redrobe, 2002) while calcium restriction initially causes an increase, followed by decreases, in intestinal calcium absorption (Barr, 1991).

15.4.2 Phosphorus

Physiology, function, and half-life: Phosphorus is the second most abundant mineral in the body next to calcium and the majority of phosphorus (85%) is complexed with calcium in hydroxyapatite in the skeleton (Khoshniat et al., 2011). In soft tissue, phosphate has a structural role in cell membranes, nucleoproteins, and nucleic acids. It is also vital in cellular energetics, cell signaling, muscle and nerve function, tissue oxygenation, and lipid metabolism (Khoshniat et al., 2011). In plasma, inorganic phosphate is present as monovalent ($H_2PO_4^-$) and divalent (HPO_4^{2-}) anions; the ratio of the monovalent and divalent forms is pH-dependent varying from 1:1 in acidosis, 1:4 at pH 7.4 to 1:9 in alkalosis. In people, most plasma phosphate is free (55%), 35% is complexed with sodium, calcium, or magnesium and 10% is protein-bound. Serum phosphate reference intervals for adult humans are in the range of 0.8–1.5 mmol/L (Penido and Alon, 2012); for adult dogs, the range is 0.8–1.8mmol/L (Bates, 2008). Primary mediators of phosphate homeostasis include dietary phosphate, 1,25$(OH)_2$D, PTH, and phosphate regulating factors or phosphatonins, such as, secreted frizzled related protein-4, matrix extracellular phosphoglycoprotein, and particularly FGF23. Although, it is found in many tissues, FGF23 is primarily expressed in bone where it is produced by osteocytes and to a lesser extent, osteoblasts. Its expression is triggered by hyperphosphatemia, increased dietary phosphate concentrations, and increased 1,25$(OH)_2$D concentrations (Prié et al., 2009; Alon, 2011). Upon ingestion, phosphate is absorbed primarily in the ileum. Intestinal uptake is regulated by dietary phosphate content and 1,25$(OH)_2$D, although it is also affected by epidermal growth factor, glucocorticoids, estrogens, metabolic acidosis, FGF23, and other phosphatonins (Marks et al., 2010). Excretion occurs via the kidney where phosphate is freely filtered by the glomerulus and can be resorbed in the proximal tubule via sodium-dependent phosphate cotransporters under the tight regulation of PTH and FGF23, which act as phosphaturic agents (Lee and Partridge, 2009). In concert with its cofactor, Klotho, a transmembrane protein highly expressed in the kidney and to a lesser extent in the parathyroid glands, FGF23 stimulates proximal renal tubule cells to downregulate phosphate reabsorption and vitamin D production and suppresses PTH secretion by the parathyroid glands (Alon, 2011). In the skeleton, phosphorus mobilization is promoted by PTH, vitamin D, and FGF23. Increased plasma inorganic phosphate concentration in turn inhibits osteoclast differentiation and bone resorption (Khosniat et al., 2011).

Significance of increased concentration/activity: General causes of increased phosphate concentrations in blood (hyperphosphatemia) include decreased urinary phosphate excretion, increased phosphate absorption from the intestine, and shift of intracellular phosphate to the extracellular fluid. Common etiologies of reduced renal excretion include prerenal, renal, and postrenal conditions that reduce glomerular filtration rate, such as dehydration, kidney injury, urinary bladder obstruction or rupture, primary hypoparathyroidism, pseudohypoparathyroidism, and acromegaly (Bates, 2008). Elevated intestinal uptake of phosphate is seen with phosphate-containing laxatives or enemas, phosphate-containing therapeutics, conditions associated with excess vitamin D, and diets with a low Ca:P ratio. Myopathies and tumor lysis syndrome can cause increased blood phosphate concentrations due to release of intracellular phosphate. Lactic acidosis, respiratory acidosis, untreated diabetic ketoacidosis, and hyperadrenocorticism may also be associated with elevated serum phosphate (Burtis et al., 2006; Stockham and Scott, 2008a). Clinically, a rapid rise in plasma phosphate may be associated with a concomitant decrease in calcium and manifestations of hypocalcemia (tetany, seizures, etc.). Protracted hyperphosphatemia can lead to secondary hyperparathyroidism and soft-tissue mineralization.

Significance of decreased concentration/activity: General causes of decreased phosphate concentrations in blood (hypophosphatemia) include increased urinary phosphate excretion, decreased intestinal phosphate absorption, shift of phosphate from the extracellular compartment to the intracellular compartment, and defective mobilization of phosphate from bone. Excessive urinary phosphate loss occurs with prolonged diuresis due to therapeutics or tubular defects, genetic defects, and increased PTH or PTHrP activity (Aono et al., 2009). Uptake of phosphate can be limited by malabsorption, vomiting/diarrhea, vitamin D deficiency, phosphate-binding agents, and phosphate-deficient diets. Hyperinsulinemia, glucose infusion, hyperalimentation, and respiratory alkalosis result in decreased phosphate blood concentrations due to a shift of phosphate from the extracellular fluid into cells. Insulin promotes transport of phosphate and glucose into cells. Respiratory alkalosis causes increased intracellular CO_2 and pH, which stimulates the glycolytic pathway, particularly phosphofructokinase and the production of increased intracellular sugar phosphates drives phosphate into cells from the circulation (Amanzadeh and Reilly, 2006). Severe catabolic states (e.g., thermal injury, diabetic ketoacidosis, and severe emaciation) have been associated with hypophosphatemia. Severe hypophosphatemia (<1.0 mg/dL or 0.3 mmol/L) can cause hemolysis due to ATP depletion and increased red blood cell fragility. Low phosphorus concentrations may also lead to decreased production of erythrocyte 2,3-bisphosphoglycerate resulting in exacerbation of tissue hypoxia (Harvey, 1997). Although rare, prolonged dietary phosphorus deficiency can cause rickets due to resorption of both calcium and phosphorus from bone stores (Capen and O'Brien, 2004).

Influencing factors (sources of error, interferences, dietary/fasting, etc.): Serum inorganic phosphate concentration is often referred to as "phosphorus" concentration, although phosphorus actually circulates in the form of inorganic and organic phosphate, not the elemental form. The concentration of circulating phosphate is usually expressed in terms of circulating inorganic phosphorus concentration (mg/dL; 1 mg/dL of inorganic phosphorus is equal to 0.32 mmol/L of phosphate) (Stockham and Scott, 2008a). Most assays use ammonium molybdate, which reacts with inorganic phosphate in serum, heparinized plasma, or urine to form a colored phosphomolybdate complex that is detected by spectrophotomer. Some methods use vandate–molybdate and enzymes (Burtis et al., 2006). Anticoagulants containing EDTA, citrate, and oxalate should not be used due to interference with complex formation. When measuring inorganic phosphorus in the urine, samples should be acidified to solubilize precipitated forms. Hemolysis, icterus, and lipemia can cause interference with these assays. Hemolysis releases intracellular phosphate in some species and can falsely elevate measurements (Capen and O'Brien, 2004). High serum immunoglobulins concentrations may also give falsely elevated results with some methods due to precipitation of the immunoglobulins (Bowles et al., 1994). Serum phosphate concentrations may be influenced by age, strain, gender, and pregnancy (Barrett et al., 1975; Champy et al., 2008; Mazzaccara et al., 2008; Liberati et al., 2004). Generally, growing animals have higher concentrations that decrease with age (Wolford et al., 1986; Russo and Nash, 1980; Buchl and Howard, 1997; Penido and Alon, 2012) and concentrations decrease during pregnancy and lactation. In rats, serum phosphate decreases with age and is higher in males than females (D'Amour et al., 2010). Seasonal variation in serum phosphate has been reported in dogs (Southern et al., 1993). Concentrations may be increased postprandially depending on the diet (Shuto et al., 2009). High-meat diets may increase serum phosphate due to phosphate content; whereas, high-carbohydrate diets are associated with lower concentrations due to intracellular shift in response to glycolysis (Capen and O'Brien, 2004).

15.4.3 Magnesium

Physiology, function, and half-life: Bone contains approximately two-thirds of the body's magnesium: 20% is in muscle and 11% in other soft tissues. High concentrations are present in the cytosol of most cells (second only to potassium), reflecting its role as a cofactor for ATP and glycolytic enzyme function as well as for proper functioning of ion channels. Similar to circulating calcium, there are three magnesium fractions in blood: protein-bound (albumin and globulins), free (biologically active form), and complexed to anions (i.e., citrate and phosphate). Only free magnesium concentrations represent overall magnesium status (Alfrey et al., 1974; Arnold et al., 1995; Fiser et al., 1998).

In healthy dogs, these fractions are approximately 31%, 63%, and 6%, respectively (Schenck et al., 2005). Normal total serum magnesium concentration in people is 0.7–0.9 mmol/L (Kaplinsky and Alon, 2013); in 2–6 month old rats, it is approximately 0.8 ± 0.08 mmol/L (Rude and Gruber, 2004); in normal adult dogs, it is approximately 0.8–1.0 mmol/L (Martin et al., 1994); and in adult (5 month old) pigs, it is approximately 1.2 mmol/L (Ullrey et al., 1967). Plasma free magnesium concentrations in dogs are in the range of 0.25–0.41 mmol/L (Fincham et al., 2004). Dietary magnesium is absorbed primarily in the jejunum, ileum, and colon down an electrochemical gradient via passive paracellular pathways and to a lesser extent, regulated transcellular pathways. Paracellular absorption is affected by water reabsorption and chronic diarrhea results in malabsorption of magnesium (Kaplinsky and Alon, 2013). Steatorrhea also reduces absorption due to formation of nonabsorbable magnesium lipid salts. Transcellular transport is mediated by the transient receptor potential melastatin (TRPM)-6 channel on the apical intestinal epithelium. TRPM-7 and members of the solute carrier family 41 also play a role in magnesium transport (Arnaud, 2008a). Absorption is enhanced by PTH, vitamin D and high dietary calcium or phosphate (Stockham and Scott, 2008). In people, the majority of plasma magnesium is filtered by the glomerulus and in health, 15% is reabsorbed by the kidney, mostly by the thick ascending loop of Henle (Saris et al., 2000). PTH, antidiuretic hormone, glucagon, aldosterone, calcitonin, and β-adrenergic agonists promote renal magnesium resorption (Stockham and Scott, 2008). Very little is known regarding the molecular basis of magnesium storage or mobilization in the skeletal system. It is unclear if transporters such as TRPM-6 and 7 are also expressed in bone cells.

Significance of increased concentration/activity: Causes of elevated circulating magnesium (hypermagnesemia) include decreased renal excretion, which can occur with renal injury and other causes of reduced glomerular filtration rate, increased PTH, and increased ingestion of magnesium-containing foods, de-icing chemicals, or drugs such as laxatives and antacids. Renal disease must be severe to cause hypermagnesemia as the normal kidney is capable of rapid excretion of large amounts of magnesium. High concentrations of magnesium interfere with neuromuscular transmission and release of acetylcholine, which results in symptoms of weakness, decreased reflexes, hypotension, cardiac arrhythmias, and decreased alertness, and if severe, it can result in respiratory paralysis, CNS depression, and coma (Fung et al., 1995; Schaer, 1999). In experimental situations, supraphysiologic concentrations of magnesium result in marked increases in calcitonin secretion similar to the release induced by hypercalcemic states (Capen and O'Brien, 2004).

Significance of decreased concentration/activity: For human patients, Kaplinsky and Alon (2013) recommend measuring the fractional excretion of magnesium [FEMg: (urine Mg/urine creatinine) × (serum creatinine/serum Mg) × 100] to obtain an indication of the source of low blood magnesium concentrations (hypomagnesemia). Causes include extra-renal etiologies (FEMg < 2%: e.g., hypoalbuminemia/hypoproteinemia, dietary deficiency, malabsorption syndromes, enteric disease, chronic diarrhea, and protein-losing enteropathy) and renal etiologies (FEMg = 2%: e.g., impaired renal tubular resorption, osmotic diuresis, and loop diuretics) (Bush et al., 2001; Stockham and Scott, 2008b; Kaplinsky and Alon, 2013). Hypomagnesemia is not uncommon in hospitalized human patients, especially those in intensive care (Herroeder et al., 2011) and many conditions have been associated with low magnesium in veterinary patients as well (Bateman, 2008). Dogs with diabetic ketoacidosis have lower plasma ionized magnesium concentrations than healthy dogs or dogs with uncomplicated diabetes mellitus (Fincham et al., 2004). Functionally, rodent models of severe dietary magnesium deficiency manifest decreased bone magnesium content, abnormalities of growth plate and cartilage, as well as reduced bone strength and trabecular bone mass (Rude et al., 2009). Reductions of dietary magnesium in rats and mice causes decreased osteoblast function and bone formation, which is reflected by reductions in serum and bone ALP activities and serum calcium, vitamin D, PTH, and OC concentrations. However, osteoclast activity and numbers are increased (Rude and Gruber, 2004) suggesting an uncoupling of bone formation and resorption. In most species, including humans, magnesium deficiency causes impaired PTH secretion and/or resistance to PTH (Rude and Gruber, 2004).

Influencing factors (sources of error, interferences, dietary/fasting, etc.): Similar to calcium, total magnesium is measured by spectrophotometric methods using metallochromic dyes. Atomic absorption can also be performed. Free magnesium is measured by ion-specific electrodes, although is rarely done clinically. Calcium ions interfere with magnesium-ISEs, and correction for this must be taken into account (Rayana et al., 2008). Erythrocyte magnesium content has been used as a surrogate of magnesium status; however, this is discouraged due to inaccuracies (Basso et al., 2000). Serum or heparinized plasma samples are preferred; some anticoagulants cause false reductions (i.e., EDTA, citrate, oxalate). Fasting can reduce serum magnesium in pigs (Baetz and Mengeling, 1971). Hemolysis leads to release of intracellular magnesium from erythrocytes and may falsely increase serum magnesium concentrations (Stockham and Scott, 2008a).

15.4.4 Parathyroid Hormone

Physiology, function, and half-life: Derived from its precursor, preproPTH, the 84-amino acid active PTH peptide is secreted by parathyroid chief cells in response to decreases in circulating free calcium or increases in circulating phosphate. In humans, PTH has a half-life of 2–3 minutes (Gopinath and Mihai, 2011). PTH maintains calcium and phosphate homeostasis on a minute-by-minute basis by acting at two primary sites, the kidney and bone, and secondarily in the intestine (Capen and O'Brien, 2004). Calcium-sensing receptors on chief cells are activated when circulating free calcium declines. When circulating calcium concentrations are high, intracellular calcium rises inhibiting the secretion of preformed PTH from storage granules. Magnesium is important for normal secretion of PTH due to the magnesium dependency of the adenylate cyclase pathway that facilitates PTH secretion (Allgrove, 2009). Magnesium deficiency can lead to hypoparathyroidism and secondary hypocalcemia (see Section 15.4.3).

In response to hypocalcemia, PTH restores circulating free calcium by mobilizing calcium from bone, increasing renal tubular calcium resorption, and accelerating formation of vitamin D in the kidney, which enhances calcium absorption in the gut. PTH also decreases phosphate resorption in the kidney. Circulating phosphate in turn affects PTH secretion, in part via hypocalcemia that results when serum becomes saturated with the two ions (Capen and O'Brien, 2004), and Khoshniat et al. (2011) proposed the presence of a phosphorus-sensing mechanism that is independent of serum calcium. PTH has direct effects on osteoblasts and renal tubular epithelial cells through the G-protein coupled receptor, PTH receptor type 1 or PTHR (also called PTH/PTHrP receptor)

(Gensure et al., 2005). In the skeleton, PTH demonstrates biphasic activity: under continuous infusion, it catabolizes bone; whereas, intermittent injection results in anabolic bone formation by a mechanism that is unclear (Lee and Partridge, 2009). Administration of intermittent low dose PTH has been utilized to treat osteoporosis (Canalis et al., 2007).

There are multiple circulating forms of PTH; intact PTH (1–84) is the primary active form in blood (Capen and O'Brien, 2004). Recent studies with PTH fragments, such as C-terminal PTH, suggest these may play a role in renal failure and other disease states (D'Amour et al., 2011). PTHrP is a paracrine hormone with actions similar to PTH, including stimulating bone and renal calcium resorption. Although PTHrP binds the N-terminal of PTHR in tissues, it does not cross-react with native PTH and it is not detected by endogenous PTH immunoassays. PTHrP has a high level of sequence homology across species. It is involved in normal fetal development and in development of bone, heart, and mammary gland, however very little is produced by healthy cells after birth. Excessive production of PTHrP by tumor cells is a common mechanism of humoral hypercalcemia of malignancy (Capen and O'Brien, 2004).

Significance of increased concentration: Elevated PTH concentration (hyperparathyroidism) may be caused by primary disorders of the parathyroid gland that result in excessive PTH secretion (primary hyperparathyroidism) or secondary conditions, such as calcium-restricted or deficient diets (nutritional secondary hyperparathyroidism), renal disease or hypovitaminosis D (Gow et al., 2011). Hyperparathyroid gland lesions are usually chief cell adenomas, although chief cell hyperplasia or carcinoma can also occur. In chronic kidney disease, increased serum concentrations of PTH and accompanying decreases in vitamin D 1,25-dihydroxyvitamin D3 can lead to renal osteodystrophy. Data suggests that PTH (7–84) may interfere with expression of the PTHR and with binding of the intact form (1–84), leading to a state of functional PTH resistance. Increased serum PTH develops in growing rabbits fed a calcium-deficient diet (Gilsanz et al., 1991). Dogs with hypocalcemia and vitamin D deficiency due to inflammatory bowel disease also develop high serum PTH (Gow et al., 2011). Marmosets given bisphosphonates show increased PTH likely secondary to decreased serum calcium (Angeliewa et al., 2004). Clinical changes in hyperparathyroidism are attributed to skeletal weakening and calcium imbalance: lameness, loose teeth, vertebral compression fractures with motor or sensory dysfunction, anorexia, vomiting, constipation, depression, and muscle weakness.

Significance of decreased concentration: Low circulating PTH (hypoparathyroidism) may be caused by primary hypoparathyroidism, hypercalcemic conditions, hypovitaminosis D, or hypomagnesemia. Primary hypoparathyroidism can result from parathyroid gland inflammation, damage (i.e., as a result of thyroid surgery), or metastasis/neoplastic invasion. Idiopathic lymphocytic parathyroiditis occurs in dogs and is considered to have an immune basis. Agenesis of the glands is a rare defect in dogs and humans (Thakker et al., 1990; Capen and O'Brien, 2004). Clinically, hypoparathyroid animals may be nervous, restless, or ataxic, eventually developing tetany and seizures. Laboratory abnormalities may include hypocalcemia due to decreased bone resorption and hyperphosphatemia as a result of reduced renal excretion.

Influencing factors (sources of error, interferences, dietary/fasting, etc.): Two-site immunoassays are recommended to measure serum intact PTH and to avoid cross-reaction with PTH peptide fragments (Capen and O'Brien, 2004). The relative concentrations and functions of PTH fragments, especially in renal failure, is an active area of research (D'Amour et al., 2011). For PTHrP measurement, a similar platform (2-site IRMA) is recommended using EDTA plasma samples with protease inhibitors, such as aprotinin (Capen and O'Brien, 2004). Age and gender can influence circulating concentrations of PTH. In rats, plasma PTH concentration increases with age in males and females, although PTH concentrations do not change with age in female and male rhesus monkeys (Black et al., 2001) or in dogs (Lawler et al., 2007). PTH concentrations tended to decrease in female Gottingen minipigs over time (Scholz-Ahrens et al., 2007). Gender influences PTH fragment ratios in growing rats (D'Amour et al., 2010). PTH concentrations may also vary with strain. For example, F344 rats have considerably higher PTH concentrations than Wistar or Sprague-Dawley rats (Kalu and Hardin, 1984).

15.4.5 Vitamin D

Physiology, function, and half-life: Vitamin D is a seco-steroid (steroid with an open B-ring) that is essential for uptake of dietary calcium and phosphorus and for normal bone formation and growth. It is also involved in such diverse processes as regulation of cell proliferation and differentiation, maintaining immune system homeostasis, and regulation of non-bone-related hormone secretion (Bikle, 2009). Vitamin D is obtained by ingestion of vitamin D_2 (ergocalciferol) and D_3 (cholecalciferol) and synthesized endogenously in the skin via the ultraviolet-light dependent conversion of 7-dehydrocholesterol into vitamin D_3. Vitamin D_3 is converted to 25-hydroxyvitamin D_3 (25(OH)D_3) in the liver by cytochrome P_{450} and a second hydroxylation step by 1α-hydroxylase (CYP27B1) occurs in the kidney. The resulting form, 1,25-dihydroxyvitamin D_3 [1,25 $(OH)_2D_3$ or calcitriol] binds the vitamin D nuclear receptor and is biologically active. There are species differences in these processes. Unlike rats, ultraviolet light exposure does not significantly increase vitamin D_3 in the skin of dogs. Consequently, dogs do not show seasonal variation in serum vitamin D concentrations (Laing et al., 1999).

Rabbits normally have higher serum total calcium concentrations than most other mammals and excrete significant quantities of calcium in their urine. Still, they have less reliance on vitamin D for intestinal uptake of calcium, as feeding a vitamin D-deficient diet has minimal effect on serum calcium concentrations (Eckermann-Ross, 2008). In contrast, C3H/HeJ mice, which have high tibial mineral bone density compared to C57BL/6 mice, are considered to have enhanced calcium transport/availability due to increased sensitivity of intestinal cells to vitamin D activity (Armbrecht et al., 2002; Chen and Kalu, 1999). There is some evidence that female mice have enhanced intestinal vitamin D-mediated calcium absorption and gene expression compared to males (Song and Fleet, 2004).

Significance of increased concentration/activity: Increased circulating vitamin D (hypervitaminosis D) may be caused by excessive vitamin D intake through over-supplementation or ingestion of vitamin D-containing rodenticides, granulomatous disease, and paraneoplastic secretion by various cancers. Cholecalciferol has been used in rodenticides and ingestion causes increased absorption of calcium and phosphorus with subsequent hypercalcemia and hyperphosphatemia. Vitamin D-induced skeletal disease is infrequent since calcium and phosphorus are derived primarily from the intestine and not through bone resorption; however, soft-tissue mineralization, cardiac effects, and renal failure can be life threatening. Although total calcium concentrations are not different, vitamin D (calcitriol) concentrations are increased 1.5-fold higher in growing rabbits fed a calcium-deficient diet relative to those consuming a calcium-replete diet (Gilsanz et al., 1991). New world monkeys have higher plasma concentrations of vitamin D, versus other animals, which may indicate a natural degree of vitamin D resistance. As such, they require exposure to artificial sunlight and/or dietary supplementation with vitamin D3 (Lowenstein, 2003; Adams et al., 2003).

Significance of decreased concentration/activity: Low circulating vitamin D (hypovitaminosis D) may be caused by dietary vitamin D deficiency, severe renal disease [due to decreased activity of renal 25(OH)D-1α-hydroxylase], insufficient exposure to sunlight in some species, and genetic diseases. Vitamin D deficiency causes impaired mineralization during endochondral ossification resulting in osteomalacia or rickets. Animal models of rickets have been reviewed by Dittmer and Thompson (2011), including mouse knockouts for 1 alpha-hydroxylase, vitamin D receptor and vitamin D-binding protein. Rats fed a vitamin D-deficient diet have low serum 1,25(OH)2D, decreased total and free calcium, normal phosphate, and high PTH (D'Amour et al., 2011); growing animals develop irregular thickened epiphyses due to failure of the cartilaginous matrix to mineralize properly. Deficiency of 1α-hydroxylase can also cause rickets (type 1) and congenital defects in this enzyme have been described in pigs and humans (Capen and O'Brien, 2004). Type II rickets is found in some New World primates, such as the common marmoset and is due to calcitriol resistance or to overexpression of vitamin D response element-binding protein, which interferes with vitamin D transactivation (Dittmer and Thompson, 2011). These animals develop osteomalacia, hypocalcemia, and secondary hyperparathyroidism in the presence of high calcitriol concentrations. Dogs with inflammatory bowel disease may have low 25-hydroxyvitamin D concentrations (Gow et al., 2011). Genetically modified mice that either lack the vitamin D receptor (VDR) and have elevated calcitriol concentration, or that lack renal 25-hydroxyvitamin D-1α-hydroxylase and have increased concentrations of 25(OH)D3 and low calcitriol concentration become hypocalcemic, and develop elevated serum PTH concentration and elevated serum ALP activity (Hendy et al., 2006).

Influencing factors (sources of error, interferences, dietary/fasting, etc.): Excessive exposure of the sample to ultraviolet light may result in falsely decreased measured concentrations. Concentrations are influenced by age, gender, and diet. In rats, vitamin D increases with age and is higher in females than males (D'Amour et al., 2010). Black et al. (2001) found that serum 25-hydroxyvitamin D concentration decreases with age in female rhesus macaques while PTH and 1,25(OH)2D concentrations did not change. A similar age-related change in 25-hydroxyvitamin D concentration was not evident in males (Black et al., 2001; Colman et al., 1999).

Vitamin D enhances calcium uptake in the intestine by upregulation of the epithelial calcium channel, transient receptor potential vanilloid 6 (TRPV6), and the intracellular transporter, calbindin D. In concert with PTH, it accelerates calcium retention by the kidney through TRPV5 and calbindin transport in the distal tubule. It also promotes phosphate absorption by the intestine and kidney and suppresses PTH synthesis and secretion by the parathyroid gland. In bone, $1,25(OH)_2D_3$ mediates osteoclastogenesis and calcium mobilization by stimulating RANKL (receptor activation of NF-kB ligand) on osteoblasts. RANKL then binds RANK on osteoclast progenitor cells inducing their differentiation and maturation (Dittmer and Thompson, 2011).

15.4.6 Calcitonin

Physiology, function, and half-life: Calcitonin is a member of the functionally diverse calcitonin gene-related peptide superfamily. This superfamily includes amylin, adrenomedullin, calcitonin receptor-stimulating peptide, and other peptides (Katafuchi et al., 2009). Calcitonin is a 32-amino acid calcitropic peptide hormone produced primarily by the medullary C (parafollicular) cells of the thyroid gland in response to high calcium concentrations (de Paula and Rosen, 2010). It can also be triggered by pentagastrin, growth hormone releasing hormone, beta adrenergic agonists, gastrointestinal peptides, and other factors (Elisei, 2008). Calcitonin receptors are located on mature osteoclasts, epithelial cells in the distal nephron, the placenta, and other tissues (Zhong et al., 2009).

Although its functions have yet to be fully defined, it has been proposed that calcitonin protects against hypercalcemia or "calcemia stress" during such physiologic states as pregnancy, lactation, and during early development (Zhong et al., 2009). It suppresses bone resorption by osteoclasts and decreases calcium resorption in the renal tubules. It also inhibits prolactin secretion and affects the maternal–fetal calcium exchange (Zhong et al., 2009). Thus, during normocalcemic states, calcitonin serves as a primary regulator of renal 25-hydroxyvitamin D3 1α-hydroxylase gene expression, whereas PTH is the predominant mediator during hypocalcemia (Zhong et al., 2009). Indeed dogs with drug-induced renal failure, secondary hyperparathyroidism, and low serum calcium exhibit normal calcitonin concentrations (García-Rodríguez et al., 2003). Despite limited sequence homology within the calcitonin gene-related peptide family across species (Katafuchi et al., 2009), there are some shared functional domains. For example, oral salmon calcitonin has been used to treat osteoporosis in postmenopausal women (Karsdal et al., 2011). Interestingly, this oral form has recently been shown to improve glucose homeostasis and weight in a rat model of obesity (Feigh et al., 2011) indicating that calcitonin has effects beyond bone and calcium metabolism.

Significance of increased concentration/activity: In normal individuals, circulating calcitonin is usually low to undetectable. Increased serum calcitonin concentration has been associated with medullary thyroid carcinomas, nonthyroidal neoplasms, C-cell hyperplasia, thyroid nodules, , hypercalcemia, renal failure, and chronic administration of some drugs (i.e., beta-blockers, glucorticoids, and potential secretagogues) (Toledo et al., 2009). In bulls, particularly those ingesting a high-calcium diet, C-cell neoplasms are not uncommon (Capen, 2007). C-cell tumors have also been described in Fisher 344 rats and Balb/c mice (Haseman, 1998; Van Zwieten et al., 1983). Interestingly, humans and dogs with medullary thyroid carcinoma and hypercalcitoninemia, show minimal effect on calcium concentrations (Elisei, 2008; Feldman and Nelson, 2003). Sepsis upregulates calcitonin gene expression in multiple tissues in hamsters (Müller B et al., 2001). Supraphysiologic doses of magnesium can result in marked increases in calcitonin secretion (Capen and O'Brien, 2004). Calcium or pentagastrin administration can be used as a provocative test to stimulate calcitonin release in patients suspected of having medullary thyroid neoplasia (Elisei, 2008).

Significance of decreased concentration/activity: normal animals usually have undetectable circulating calcitonin. Animals with hypocalcemia or lacking a thyroid gland have undetectable serum calcitonin. Knockout mice lacking calcitonin or calcitonin receptor show increased bone formation due to inhibition of osteoclast activation (Martin et al., 2009).

Influencing factors (sources of error, interferences, dietary/fasting, etc.): Calcitonin is typically measured by immunoassay. False elevations can occur due to heterophilic antibodies. For assays that lack sufficient specificity, calcitonin precursors may cross-react causing false increases (Elisei, 2008). Serum calcitonin increases with age in rats, in contrast to humans in which it decreases with aging. Strain differences in baseline calcitonin have been reported in rats (Peng et al., 1976). Kmieć et al. (2001) reported no difference in serum calcitonin in fed and fasted rats, although refeeding resulted in elevated concentrations in aged rats and reduced concentrations in young rats.

15.4.7 Alkaline Phosphatase, Bone Isoenzyme

Physiology, function, and half-life: Alkaline phosphatases catalyze the alkaline hydrolysis of many naturally occurring and synthetic substrates. The bone isoenzyme of alkaline phosphatase (BALP; also referred to as bone-specific ALP or BSAP) is produced by osteoblasts through posttranslational modification of the tissue nonspecific ALP gene product (TNSALP), which is also the source of the intestinal and liver ALP isoenzymes. Several isoforms of BALP with distinct glycosylation and catalytic properties have been identified in the circulation of humans and there is some evidence that their expression may be influenced by disorders such as chronic kidney disease (Linder et al., 2009). In bone, BALP mediates hydrolysis of pyrophosphate (a potent inhibitor of mineralization), which releases inorganic phosphorus for incorporation into hydroxyapatite and generates extracellular inorganic phosphate (Harmey, et al., 2004; Coulibaly et al., 2010). Thus, BALP is essential for normal mineralization of skeletal osteoid and mutations of the TNSALP gene can result in bone disorders such as the osteomalacic disease hypophosphatasia (Whyte, 2008).

Circulating (serum or plasma) BALP can serve as a marker of bone formation in humans and many laboratory animal species, including dogs (Sanecki et al., 1993), rats (Hoffmann et al., 1994;

Powers et al., 2007), mice (Huang et al., 2010), minipigs (Scholz-Ahrens et al., 2007), guinea pigs (Li et al., 2005), rabbits (Southwood et al., 2003), cynomolgus macaques (Wiedmeyer et al., 1999), and rhesus macaques (Kramer and Hoffman, 1997). It has been used as a bone turnover marker in assessment of osteoporosis, fractures, antiresorptive therapy, osteomyelitis, malignancy, and other bone disorders (Coleman et al., 2011; Liesegang et al., 2007; Philipov et al., 1995; Southwood et al., 2003; Vasikaran et al., 2011b). The half-life of BALP in human serum is approximately 40 hours (Seibel et al., 2006). The half-life of canine serum BALP is approximately 72 hours, similar to that of the hepatic and corticosteroid isoenzymes (Kramer and Hoffman, 1997). In most species, BALP activity may be influenced by factors such as circadian rhythm, age, gender and hormonal status (Seibel et al., 2006).

Significance of increased concentration/activity: increased BALP activity is associated with bone formation and osteoblastic activity, that is, growth in young animals, metabolic bone disease (i.e., osteomalacia), bone neoplasms (i.e., osteosarcoma or metastasis to bone), endocrine diseases (i.e., hyperparathyroidism), traumatic bone injury, and inflammatory bone disease (i.e., osteomyelitis) (Fernandez and Kidney, 2007). Congenitally increased BALP activity (benign familial hyperphosphatasemia) has been identified in Scottish Terriers (Nestor et al., 2006) and Siberian Huskies (Fernandez and Kidney, 2007). BALP is highly correlated with periosteal ALP activity, a tissue-based marker of bone formation, in a rat model of orchiectomy-induced bone loss (Powers et al., 2007). BALP is considered a useful marker of bone metastasis in men with castration-resistant prostate cancer (Coleman et al., 2011). BALP and total ALP were significantly increased by 1 week after experimental radial fracture in dogs and remained elevated 4 weeks postsurgery (Mohamadnia et al., 2007).

Significance of decreased concentration/activity: Decreased serum BALP is associated with reduced bone formation and osteoblastic activity. An alkaline phosphatase knockout mouse model with mutations in TNSALP recapitulates many of the features of human infants with congenital hypophosphatasia, including growth deformities and osteomalacia (Fedde et al., 1999). In an ovariectomy-induced bone loss model in cynomolgus monkeys, decreases in both total and bone-specific alkaline phosphatase were highly correlated with decreased bone mineral density (Legrand et al., 2003).

Influencing factors (sources of error, interferences, dietary/fasting, etc.): BALP activity can be measured by physicochemical methods such as heat or urea inactivation, levamisole inhibition, differential binding to wheat germ lectin or electrophoresis (Itoh et al., 2002). Less cumbersome immunoassays are now available to measure BALP protein in some species. Cross-reactivity with the liver isoenzyme has been reported in some human immunoassays (Vasikaran et al., 2011a). BALP is influenced by many factors, including age, gender, hormonal status, and diet. In rats and mice, BALP shows little circadian variation (Herrmann, 2011). BALP is generally higher in immature animals than older animals (Hatayama et al., 2012; Legrand et al., 1993; Tsutsumi et al., 2004 a and b). Indeed, BALP is the predominant isozyme in rat serum through at least 19 weeks of age (Hatayama et al., 2012). BALP declined in female minipigs tested for up to 76 months after birth (Tsutsumi et al., 2004a). Itoh et al. (2002) found that BALP represents 65% of total ALP activity in dogs less than 1 year, 31% in dogs 1–7 years and 16% in dogs >7 years. Male cynomolgus monkeys have slightly higher BALP activities than females (Wiedmeyer et al., 1999). Significant diurnal variation in serum BALP occurs in dogs (Ladlow et al., 2002), but not female Göttingen minipigs (Tsutsumi et al., 2004b). Relative to non-lactating females, lactating cynomolgus monkeys have increased BALP, as well as increased OC, PYD, and DPD likely due to mobilization of bone calcium (Lees et al., 1998). Marked increases in total ALP activity were found in juvenile rhesus macaques with nutritional metabolic bone disease, presumably due to elevated BALP (Wolfensohn, 2003).

15.4.8 Osteocalcin

Physiology, function, and half-life: OC is a small (5.8 kD) peptide produced by osteoblasts, hypertrophic chondrocytes, and odontoblasts. It is the most abundant noncollagenous protein in bone matrix (Coulibaly et al., 2010). OC is also known as bone γ-carboxyglutamic acid (Gla) protein due to the presence of three Gla residues, which bind calcium. Similar to coagulation factors II, VII, IX, and X, the formation of the glutamic acid residues on OC is vitamin K-dependent. OC has carboxylated and uncarboxylated forms that have unique properties. The carboxylated form has a high affinity for minerals, such as calcium, binds hydroxyapatite and is incorporated into the extracellular bone matrix. The uncarboxylated form released into the circulation mediates energy metabolism through effects on insulin and insulin sensitivity (Confavreux, 2011) and plays a role in vascular calcification (Kapustin and Shanahan, 2011). Mice deficient in OC have increased cortical bone thickness and density with improved mechanical properties, but they also develop hyperglycemia, hypoinsulinemia, low beta cell mass, increased fats mass, and decreased energy expenditure (Ducy et al., 1996; Ducy, 2011).

During bone formation, osteoblasts secrete OC and measurement of serum concentration can be a sensitive and specific indicator of bone formation. Intact OC is susceptible to proteolysis, and there can be considerable variability in interlaboratory results (Seibel, 2005). In resorptive states, OC fragments may be released into the plasma, and the measurement of individual fragments may provide information on the status of bone resorption (Kraenzlin and Seibel, 2006). Thus, if an assay does not measure intact OC, OC is more appropriately considered to be a marker of generalized bone turnover rather than either formation or resorption specifically. Serum OC has been used as a bone turnover marker in osteoporosis and fracture, but it is also influenced by nonbone disorders, such as diabetes, stress, corticosteroids, heart disease, and renal disease (Ducy, 2011; Olmos et al., 2006).

The half-life of OC in human beings is approximately 20 minutes. When stored at room temperature, serum OC concentration may decrease by 20% within a few hours due to protein degradation. This may be avoided by assays that measure intact OC as well as OC fragments. The addition of protease inhibitors may prevent degradation of the intact molecule. OC has been measured in rats, mice, dogs, cynomolgus macaques, rhesus macaques, rabbits, and minipigs. It has been used as a marker of bone turnover in disorders such as osteoporosis (Garnero, 2008), bone lengthening (Theyse et al., 2006), and osteomyelitis (Philipov et al., 1995). It is influenced by age, gender, hormonal status, renal function, and other factors.

Significance of increased concentration/activity: Serum OC increases with bone formation, osteoblastic activity, and bone resorption. As OC is eliminated via glomerular filtration, circulating concentrations may increase in renal failure in the absence of bone formation (Seibel, 2005). OC increases in rats given daily PTH injections (Han et al., 2007). It rises with progression of osteoporosis in women and in some animal models of the disease: ovariectomy causes increased serum concentrations in rhesus monkeys (Keller et al., 2000); transient elevations were seen in an orchidectomized marmoset model (Seidlov-Wuttke et al., 2008). Osteomyelitis was associated with increased OC in dogs (Philipov et al., 1995). Concentrations are typically higher in younger animals than older animals (Colman et al., 1999).

Significance of decreased concentration/activity: OC is decreased with decreased bone formation during physiologic and pathologic conditions. From postweaning to adulthood, rats may experience an approximately 50% decrease in serum OC concentration. This decrease is associated with increasing bone mineral deposition (Horton et al., 2008). In pregnant animals, placental clearance of OC can result in falsely decreased concentrations (Rodin et al., 1989). In rabbits, lower serum OC concentrations were associated with infected fractures when compared with rabbits with noninfected fractures. The rabbits with infected fractures also had decreased BALP and higher DPD concentrations than the noninfected controls (Southwood et al., 2003). Glucocorticoids lower OC concentrations as evidenced by decreased plasma OC concentration in piglets following dexamethasone treatment (Weiler et al., 1995) and in rats given prednisolone (Han et al., 2007). In a mouse model of glucocorticoid-induced osteoporosis, decreases in serum OC concentrations mirrored the reduction in bone formation rate observed microscopically (McLaughlin et al., 2002). In an ovariectomy-induced model of bone loss in cynomolgus monkeys, decreased OC was highly correlated with decreased bone mineral density (Legrand et al., 2003). Serum OC was decreased in streptozotocin-induced diabetic rats, and correlated with decreased ALP activity in femoral bone sections consistent with decreased osteoblast activity/bone formation in this model (Hie et al., 2007). OC is decreased with heart injury, including myocardial infarction and coronary heart disease (Ducy, 2011).

Influencing factors (sources of error, interferences, dietary/fasting, etc.): OC is measured by immunoassays and because it circulates as intact and fragmented forms, results are affected by the specific epitopes identified by the assay. Epitopes in the midfragment are most stable and assays detecting this region tend to be most consistent. Detection may be compromised due to degradation resulting from inadequate storage. Serum should be promptly processed and analyzed. If not assayed within 1 hour, samples should be stored frozen (–20 to −80°C) (Allen, 2003; Herrmann, 2011). Variability in sample quality and/or assay differences may explain the conflicting results sometimes observed with this analyte. For example, Theyse et al. (2006) found that OC concentrations were lowest in dogs with the highest amount of bone formation in a bone distraction study. This is in contrast to a distraction study performed by Lammens et al. (1998) in which OC concentrations were increased dogs with the most bone formation. Serum OC concentrations are higher in smaller strains of mice such as C57BL/6 mice than large-sized mice such as SENCAR mice likely as a reflection of favoring bone growth over remodeling (Murray et al., 1993). Interestingly, C3H/HeJ mice have increased mineral bone density and high bone OC content, but decreased serum OC concentration, relative to other strains (Li et al., 2002). When conducting studies with the OC, it is important to take samples at consistent times, during the day, since serum OC exhibits circadian rhythms in dogs (Ladlow et al., 2002) and mice (Liesegang et al., 1999; Srivastava et al., 2001). Female Gottingen minipigs have significant diurnal variation in OC concentration (Tsutsumi et al., 2004a). Minimal changes in serum OC concentrations were noted in female Sprague-Dawley rats during estrous cycle, pregnancy, and lactation (Sengupta et al., 2005). Serum OC concentrations declined with age in male rhesus macaques, but not females (Black et al., 2001). Cahoon et al. (1996) found that OC declined in both genders in rhesus up to 20 years, then plateaued or increased slightly in animals >25 years. In cynomolgus monkeys, OC is higher in young versus old females (Legrand et al., 2003). OC declined in female minipigs tested for up to 76 months after birth (Tsutsumi et al., 2004a). Calorie restriction in young male rhesus macaques was associated with lower OC at 1 month relative to animals on an unrestricted diet, but concentrations normalized by 6 months (Black et al., 2001).

15.4.9 Molecules Associated with Collagen Maturation and Degradation: Propeptides; Cross-Linked C- and N-Telopeptides; Pyridinoline, Deoxypyridinoline

Physiology, function, and half-life: Collagen type I is the principal organic constituent of the extracellular bone matrix. Proteolytic processing of the precursor, procollagen type I, during bone formation results in the release of free peptides (propeptides) from the amino (N-) and carboxy (C)-termini before incorporation of collagen type I into new bone. These terminal peptides, called procollagen type I N-propeptide and C-propeptide (PINP and PICP), serve as indicators of newly formed collagen type I and active bone formation. They are cleared from the circulation primarily by sinusoidal endothelial cells in the liver (Melkko et al., 1994). The smaller PINP molecule is also cleared by the kidney (Melkko et al., 1994). Thus, both peptides are measurable in serum, but only PINP can be measured in urine.

Collagen type I has a triple helix structure and in bone, the helices are covalently cross-linked by short peptides (known as telopeptides) at the amino- and carboxy ends. The telopeptides are further linked via pyridinium or pyrrole to neighboring collagen helices (Herrmann and Seibel, 2008). During bone resorption, the degradation of mature type I collagen by CTSK and matrix metalloproteases frees these terminal peptides known as N- and C-Terminal cross-linking telopeptide of type I collagen. In addition, "Crosslaps" is a commercial assay that measures specific CTX-1 degradation products called collagen C-Terminal extension peptides, as well as the related molecule, C-terminal cross-linking telopeptide of type I collagen generated by metalloproteinases (CTX-MMP) (Cremers and Garnero, 2006). CTX-MMP resists further degradation and is released into serum (Eriksen et al., 1993) where it can serve as a sensitive marker of pathological bone resorption in conditions such as metastatic bone disease (Herrmann, 2011). NTX-1 and CTX-1 are sufficiently small to be cleared by renal mechanisms and can therefore be quantified in urine. Results are generally normalized to urine creatinine concentration, for example, urine NTX-1/Cr. However, telopeptides present in many tissues and non–bone-related processes (i.e., cardiac disease, cancer) may influence urine and serum concentrations (Herrmann, 2011).

Unlike CTX-MMP, NTX-1 and CTX-1 are subject to enzymatic digestion resulting in amino acids and free or peptide-bound pyridinoline (PYD) or DPD, the small trivalent linking molecules. Thus, the release of PYD and DPD into serum and urine also signifies degradation of mature (cross-linked) collagen. PYD is found in cartilage, ligaments, and vessels, and DPD is also found in dentin. However, these sources contribute very little to serum or urine concentrations, and PYD and DPD are considered specific markers of bone resorption (Herrmann, 2011). Hydroxylysylpyridinoline and lysylpyridinoline are non-reducible collagen cross-links that stabilize collagen fibrils by increasing tissue resistance to proteolytic resorption, decreasing the tissue's solubility, and providing proper spacing of bone collagen alpha-chains for normal function (Martinez et al., 2008). Hydroxylysylpyridinoline and lysylpyridinoline serve as markers of mature collagen. Urine concentrations of hydroxylysylpyridinoline and lysylpyridinoline increased in rhesus monkeys exposed to chronic hypergravity (Martinez et al., 2008). Urinary hydroxyproline has been used as a marker of collagen degradation; concentrations increase in humans with reduced weight-bearing conditions such as during spaceflight or during prolonged bedrest (Martinez et al., 2008). It is not specific to bone, however, and can be affected by connective tissue disorders.

Assays for collagen degradation products are frequently antibody-based ([e.g., enzyme-linked immunosorbent assay (ELISA) or radioimmunoassay (RIA)]), although HPLC methods may be used (Martinez et al., 2008). PINP and PICP are relatively stable in serum (Herrmann, 2011). Rat and mouse PINP share homology in some regions, but differ considerably from the human peptide. Therefore, specific-assays are important for this endpoint (Han et al., 2007). Serum PINP has been used in rat models of osteoporosis as a marker of bone turnover. In contrast, pyridinolines are highly conserved across species, and there is significant cross-reactivity between human and animal assays (Allen et al., 2000). There is also high cross-reactivity of human and canine assays for urinary DPD, NTX-1, and CTX-1.

Significance of increased concentration/activity: Circulating PICP and PINP increase with bone formation and posttranslational modification of procollagen I. PINP offers a significant advantage in specificity over OC for assessment of bone formation as OC fragments may be released during bone resorption (Ivaska et al., 2004). PINP increases following PTH treatment of in rats, and correlates with increased bone formation/bone mineral density (Han et al., 2007; Hale et al., 2007).

Increased NTX-1, CTX-1, CTX-MMP, urine PYD, and urine DPD are associated with bone resorption and osteoclastic activity. NTX-1 is considered one of the more useful predictors of bone metastasis in people with multiple myeloma and breast cancer (Coleman et al., 2011). Lucas et al. (2008) found that dogs with osteosarcoma have increased serum and urine concentrations of

NTX-1compared to dogs with osteoarthritis and healthy controls. In contrast, serum CTX-MMP does not discriminate dogs with osteosarcoma from healthy dogs (Hintermeister et al., 2008), although serum CTX-MMP was increased in an experimental canine model of septic osteomyelitis (Philipov et al., 1995). Urinary PYD:Cr was increased following 15 days of dexamethasone treatment of 3 to 5-day-old piglets (Weiler et al., 1995). Urine NTX-1 and DPD were high at birth, but decreased with age in female minipigs. There is a strong negative correlation between bone markers and bone mineral content and mineral bone density measured with DEXA (Tsutsumi et al., 2004b). Serum CTX-1 is higher in older rats compared with younger rats in a model of ageing osteoporosis (Pietschmann et al., 2007). Urinary excretion of DPD and NTX-1 is increased in streptozotocin-induced diabetic rats (Hie et al., 2007). Urinary DPD excretion is markedly increased in rats with cirrhosis-induced osteopenia (Cemborain et al., 1998).

Significance of decreased concentration/activity: Prednisolone administration in rats is associated with decreased serum PINP (Han et al., 2007). Inhibition of CTSK in normal and ovariectomized cynomolgus monkeys results in reduced serum CTX-1 and serum and urine NTX-1 concentrations, consistent with an osteoclast-mediated decrease in bone resorption (Kumar et al., 2007). In a murine model of collagen-induced osteoarthritis, inhibition of CTSK resulted in decreased urinary excretion of DPD (Svelander et al., 2009), which correlated with microscopic evidence of reduced bone erosion. However, serum CTX-1 concentration was increased in this study, which was attributed to augmented matrix metalloprotease activity secondary to inhibition of CTSK. Urinary DPD excretion was not different between control and ovariectomized aged (> 10 years) cynomolgus monkeys (Legrand et al., 2003). Serum NTX-1 and DPD were decreased in cynomolgus monkeys treated with osteoprotegerin, reflecting its ability to inhibit osteoclast differentiation/activity (Smith et al., 2003). Serum CTX-1 and PINP decreased in marmosets given bisphosphonates (Angeliewa et al., 2004).

Influencing factors: CTX-1, NTX-1, CTX-MMP are generally measured by immunoassays, although chromatographic techniques such as HPLC may be used, particularly for urine PYD and DPD. After the age of 50 years, these peptides are elevated in men and women, but more so in women, particularly until late menopause. Immunoassays for these markers may not cross-react across species. Rat PINP shares little homology with the human molecule. Consequently, Han et al. (2007) optimized a mass spectrometry-based assay to measure rat PINP. Pyridinolines in urine samples are subject to photodynamic breakdown and should be protected from light (Allen, 2003). CTX-MMP may lose significant activity if subjected to prolonged storage at room temperature (Kraenzlin and Seibel, 2006). Concentrations may be influenced by age, gender, diurnal variation, and circadian rhythm. Macaques exhibit circadian rhythm in serum PICP (Hotchkiss and Jerome, 1998). Urinary cross-links increase with age in male rhesus macaques, but not females (Black et al., 2001). Cahoon (1996) found that urine PYD, DPD, and hydroxyproline decreased with age in rhesus in both genders up to 20 years, then increased slightly in animals >25 years. Cahoon did not observe gender differences in PYD or DPD in rhesus. Urine NTX-1/Cr and DPD/Cr declined in female minipigs tested for up to 76 months after birth (Tsutsumi et al., 2004a). In a rat ovariectomy model of osteoporosis, serum PINP concentration correlated more closely with histologic parameters of bone formation than either OC or CTX-1 (Rissanen et al., 2008). Diurnal variation can be significant for NTX-1 and CTX-1 concentrations in serum and urine (Hermann, 2011) and collection times should be standardized. Urinary NTX-1 concentrations exhibit diurnal variation in female Gottingen minipigs (Tsutsumi et al., 2004a). CTX-1 exhibits circadian variation in C3H/HeJ mice (Srivastava et al., 2001). Dogs show significant diurnal variation in serum concentrations of CTX-MMP and urinary DPD, but not urine NTX-1 (Ladlow et al., 2002). Circadian rhythms also exist for PYD and DPD in dogs (Liesegang et al., 1999). Despite diurnal changes, Ladlow et al. (2002) found no significant longer-term (up to 12 weeks) variability in these turnover markers in dogs. Diet may influence telopeptide concentrations through alterations in net acid or base intake. Collecting samples from fasted animals is recommended (Hermann, 2011), although diet reportedly has no effect on urine PYD or

DPD concentrations (Cahoon et al., 1996). Age and gender are important preanalytical variables. Growing animals tend to have higher urinary CTX-1 and NTX-1 (Allen et al., 2000). Urinary CTX-1, serum CTX-1, DPD, and PICP were higher in young male cynomolgus macaques versus young females (Legrand et al., 2003); urinary NTX-1 and CTX-MMP were not different between genders. Serum CTX-MMP, urine DPD, and urine PYD decrease with age in dogs (Allen et al., 2000) during the first 7 years of age. Urine PYD and DPD are high in rhesus monkeys less than 3 years of age, and these values decline until late in life (>25 years) when they rise (Cahoon et al., 1996). PINP is higher in young rats versus older animals (Han et al., 2007); these investigators found that assay sensitivity may need to be optimized for lower concentrations in older animals. Impaired renal function may result in increased CTX-1 and NTX-1 due to decreased clearance.

15.4.10 Tartrate-Resistant Acid Phosphatase Isoform 5b

Physiology, function, and half-life: TRACPs are produced primarily by macrophages, dendritic cells, and osteoclasts, although detectable concentrations are present in many tissues (Hayman, 2008). Six isoenzymes have been elucidated by electrophoresis. Isozyme 5 is tartrate-resistant and has two isoforms (a and b). TRACP5a is produced by macrophages and dendritic cells, and 5b is secreted by osteoclasts. Functionally, TRACP5b cleaves type I collagen fragments liberated by CTSK and matrix metalloproteases (Cremers and Garnero, 2006) and circulating TRACP5b is considered a marker of osteoclast number and function (Herrmann, 2011). In human serum, TRACP5b circulates complexed with alpha-2-macroglobulin (and likely other molecules), but the biological significance of this is unclear. In rat serum, TRACP5b is found as a free molecule (Ylipahkala et al., 2003). TRACP5b can be measured by enzymatic methods, although these lack specificity for the 5b isoform and immunoassays are preferred to detect 5b alone. Serum TRACP5b activity has been evaluated in healthy dogs by an enzymatic method (Sousa et al., 2011). In beagle dogs with surgically induced osteoarthritis, Lee et al. (2008) found no effect on serum TRACP5b activity, however synovial fluid activity was elevated. In genetically modified rodents, decreased TRACP5b activity results in mild osteopetrosis due to decreased resorption (Hayman et al., 1996), while overexpression leads to osteoporosis due to increased resorption that is partly compensated by increased bone synthesis (Angel et al., 2000).

Significance of increased concentration/activity: increased serum concentrations of TRACP5b indicate increased osteoclast numbers and bone resorption. Pathologic conditions leading to increased serum TRACP5b activity include renal secondary hyperparathyroidism (e.g., chronic renal failure), osteoporosis, metastatic bone disease, hyperparathyroidism, and Paget's disease (Halleen et al., 2006). Because TRACP5b is not eliminated by renal mechanisms, it can be useful in the assessment of metabolic bone disease in animals with kidney failure (Cremers et al., 2008a and b). In a rat model of ovariectomy-induced bone loss, serum TRACP5b activity closely paralleled *in vivo* bone resorption as indicated by increased osteoclasts per bone surface/tissue area, suggesting that serum TRACP5b may be a useful surrogate for histomorphometric analysis of osteoclast numbers in tissue sections (Rissanen et al., 2008). In this model, total osteoclast numbers were decreased due to an overall loss of bone, but their activity was increased, suggesting that an increased CTX-1/TRACP5b ratio may indicate whole-body bone resorption. Mammary and ovarian carcinomas, and malignant melanoma, upregulate TRACP expression, which may play a role in the development of bone metastases (Hayman, 2008). Selective estrogen receptor modulator treatment in a cynomolgus monkey model of osteoporosis is associated with decreased TRACP5b activity, ALP, BALP, urinary CrossLaps, and OC and greater bone mass indicating reduced bone turnover (Hotchkiss et al., 2001; Lee et al., 2002).

Significance of decreased concentration/activity: TRACP5b knockout animals exhibit osteopetrosis caused by reduced osteoclast activity. These mice also have impaired macrophage function and abnormal immunomodulatory cytokine responses (Hayman and Cox, 2003; Bune et al., 2001).

In a rat model of age-related osteoporosis, serum TRACP5b concentration was decreased in older rats compared with younger rats (Pietschmann et al., 2007).

Influencing factors (sources of error, interferences, dietary/fasting, etc.): High concentrations of bilirubin may interfere with colorimetric TRACP assays (Alvarez et al., 1999). Serum TRACP5b is stable for up to 48 hours at room temperature, and up to 3 days if refrigerated. Frozen TRACP5b is stable for years; however, re-freezing samples may result in marked decreases in activity (Halleen et al., 2006). In normal Sprague-Dawley rats, serum TRACP5b concentrations remained relatively unchanged from weaning to 20 weeks of age (Horton et al., 2008). Serum TRACP5b activity does not exhibit diurnal variation, and is not affected by feeding (Rissanen et al., 2008).

15.4.11 Cathepsin K

Physiology, function, and half-life: The cysteine protease, CTSK, is secreted by osteoclasts into the resorption lacuna. There it cleaves triple-helical collagens at multiple sites into small peptides and degrades noncollagenous termini releasing end products (and markers), such as NTX, CTX, PYD, and DPD. CTSK also regulates TRAP release from osteoclasts, which further digests collagen remnants (Henriksen et al., 2007). Because of its key role in bone resorption, CTSK is a therapeutic target for the treatment of osteoporosis (Deaton and Tavares, 2005). Protein sequences vary across species: rodent CTSK has low homology with the human peptide, while rabbit and primate CTSK exhibit 96% and 100% homology, respectively (Pennypacker et al., 2009). Indeed, CTSK was first cloned from rabbit osteoclasts (Lecaille et al., 2008). The enzyme is expressed by many types of nonbone cells, for example, synovial fibroblasts, a variety of epithelial cells, cartilage, white adipose tissue, macrophages, etc. (Pietschmann et al., 2007), however circulating concentrations are considered to be indicative of osteoclast activity (Herrmann, 2011).

Significance of increased concentration/activity: Increased serum CTSK denotes increased osteoclastic activity and bone resorption. It has been utilized more frequently as a circulating bone marker in humans than animals: concentrations are elevated in people with chronic rheumatoid arthritis (Skoumal M, Haberhauer G, Kolarz G, Hawa G, Woloszczuk W, Klingler A. Serum cathepsin K levels of patients with longstanding rheumatoid arthritis: correlation with radiological destruction. Nov 2004; 7:R65-R70), osteoporosis, and Paget's disease (Meier et al., 2006). Genetically modified mice overexpressing CTSK have decreased trabecular bone due to excessive resorption (Lecaille et al., 2008).

Significance of decreased concentration/activity: Pycnodysosotosis is a rare autosomal recessive disorder resulting from CTSK deficiency. Defective osteoclast activity causes osterosclerosis and short stature in affected individuals (Lecaille et al., 2008). CTSK-deficient mice have similar lesions. CTSK concentrations decrease with age in humans and rats. Serum CTSK declines in elderly women during calcium carbonate supplementation (Zhao et al., 2010) and in osteoporotic women administered alendronate (Muñoz-Torres et al., 2009). CTSK was slightly decreased in aged rats used as a model of senile osteoporosis (Pietschmann et al., 2007).

Influencing factors (sources of error, interferences, dietary/fasting, etc.): Serum or plasma CTSK can be measured by immunoassay (Skoumal et al., 2005). Concentrations of CTSK decrease with age in people.

15.4.12 Matrix Metalloproteinases and Tissue Inhibitor of Metalloproteinases

Physiology, function, and half-life: Matrix metalloproteinases (MMPs) are a large family of calcium or zinc-dependent proteases that cleave a wide variety of substrates in extracellular matrix, as well as nonstructural proteins throughout the body (Nagase et al., 2006; Shiomi et al., 2010). MMP activity is directly controlled by specific inhibitors called tissue inhibitors of matrix metalloproteases (TIMPs). MMPs and TIMPs are involved in diverse physiologic and pathophysiologic pathways, including tissue growth and repair, inflammation, tumor metastasis, and fibrosis in many organ systems (van der Jagt et al., 2010; Shiomi et al., 2010). In the skeletal system, MMPs and TIMPs are expressed by osteoblasts, osteoclasts, osteocytes, chondrocytes, and other cells (Hatori et al., 2004). MMPs and TIMPs are involved in skeletal remodeling, endochondral and intramembranous ossification, and vascular invasion/calcification (Andersen et al., 2004; Aiken and Khokha, 2010). They are highly conserved among species (Aiken and Khokha, 2010). While many MMPs and TIMP-1 are secreted and some can be measured in serum and body fluids by immunoassays, their use as clinical markers of skeletal disorders has been hampered by inferior specificity and sensitivity relative to other markers. Serum and synovial concentrations of MMPs and TIMPs have shown some modest value in assessment of conditions such as REF (Keyszer et al., 1999; Hegemann et al., 2002) and osteoporosis (Luo et al., 2006). For example, Hegemann et al. (2003) found that dogs with chronic REF have an increased ratio of synovial MMP-3 to TIMP-1.

15.5 GENERAL PATTERNS OF THE CHANGES IN LABORATORY TESTS RELATED TO SPECIFIC ETIOLOGIES

Markers of bone formation and/or enhanced osteoblastic activity include BALP, OC, PICP, and PINP and markers of bone resorption and/or enhanced osteoclastic activity include NTX-I, CTX-I, PYD, DPD, TRACP5b, and metalloproteases. Because of the complex interrelationships between osteoblasts and osteoclasts, these classifications are somewhat artificial and the markers are probably more accurately applied as a panel as indicators of bone turnover or remodeling. The outcome of changes in bone turnover (i.e., increased bone mass or decreased bone mass) is the balance between bone synthesis and bone resorption processes. Table 15.2 provides general guidelines for several disorders of bone metabolism and the expected findings in widely-available laboratory tests.

15.5.1 Osteoporosis Models

In people, osteoporosis is characterized by low bone mass and microarchitectural deterioration of bone leading to enhanced bone fragility and increased risk of fracture (Vasikaran et al., 2011a).

TABLE 15.2
Conditional Alterations in Bone Biomarkers

	Calcium	Phosphorus	PTH	Vit D3	Other
Primary hyperparathyroidism	Increased	Normal to decreased	Increased	Normal to increased	Increased urine calcium; BALP and OC may be increased
Secondary hyperparathyroidism	Normal to decreased	Increased	Increased	Decreased	–
Hypoparathyroidism	Decreased	Increased	Decreased	Decreased	–
Vitamin D3 excess	Increased	Increased	Decreased to normal	Increased	Normal to increased urine calcium
Vitamin D3 deficiency	Decreased	–	Increased	Decreased	–
Hypercalcemia of malignancy	Increased	Decreased	Normal to low	Normal to increased (inappropriate for concentration of Ca)	PTHrP increased, hypercalciuria

While some species develop osteopenia with age naturally, most experimental animal models of osteoporosis rely on deprivation of reproductive hormones or administration of glucocorticoids for closely approximating the human disease (Herrmann, 2011). Nonetheless, these models have been very important in the discovery of effective therapies. Ovariectomy in females (e.g., mice, rats, sheep, cynomolgus macaques, and rhesus macaques) and orchidectomy in males (e.g., rodents, nonhuman primates) cause increases in both bone formation and resorption with progressive resorption predominating (Reinwald and Burr, 2008; Sorensen et al., 2007). Other *in vivo* models include dietary interventions, immobilization, retinoic acid-induced hypercalcemia in thyroparathyroidectomized rats, and genetically modified rodents (i.e., osteoprotegerin knockout mice) (Sorensen et al., 2007; Levolas et al., 2008; Reinwald and Burr, 2008). Female aged (>10 years) cynomolgus monkeys develop osteopenia after ovariectomy and have been frequently used to evaluate new treatments, particularly biopharmaceuticals. Many bone turnover markers can be measured in this species (e.g., BALP, OC, PICP, CTX-MMP, CTX-1, NTX-1, urine DPD, and serum PYD) in concert with densitometry, bone histology/histomorphometry, or dynamic histomorphological endpoints. With progression of osteopenia in monkeys, markers such as serum BALP, serum OC, and urine NTX-1/Cr increase significantly reflecting increased bone turnover (Legrand et al., 2003). Ominsky et al. (2011) showed that administration of a RANKL antibody reduced BALP and CTX-1 indicative of decreased bone turnover. CTSK inhibition results in reduced urinary NTx (Stroup et al., 2009) and selective estrogen receptor modulators (i.e. raloxifene, levormeloxifene) lower BALP, TRACP, OC, and urinary collagen degradation products (CrossLaps) (Lees et al., 2002; Hotchkiss et al., 2001). There is considerable interest in applying bone turnover markers in predicting fracture risk in people, although the field is currently hampered by insufficient quality control, assay differences, and limited correlative data (Vasikaran et al., 2011a). There are no standardized bone turnover markers for osteoporosis animal studies. However, an evaluation of markers by the International Osteoporosis Foundation and the International Federation of Clinical Chemistry and Laboratory Medicine concluded that a marker of bone formation (particularly serum PINP) and a marker of bone resorption (particularly serum CTX-1) should be used as reference bone turnover markers in human clinical practice (Vasikaran et al., 2011a, b).

15.5.2 Primary Hyperparathyroidism

Primary hyperparathyroidism presents as hypercalcemia in concert with inappropriately normal or high PTH concentrations and usually results from increased secretion of PTH by chief cell adenomas, less common causes are parathyroid carcinoma and parathyroid hyperplasia. Prolonged high PTH concentration leads to excessive calcium resorption in the bone and kidney, which results in elevated circulating free and total calcium concentrations and increased urine calcium excretion. PTH inhibits reabsorption of phosphate by the kidney so serum phosphorus concentrations may be normal to low. Most humans are asymptomatic at the time of diagnosis when it is typically recognized during routine laboratory testing (Gopinath and Mihai, 2011). If not diagnosed early—as is more likely to occur in animals—clinical changes related to skeletal weakening and progressive hypercalcemia develop, including lameness, loose teeth, vertebral compression fractures with motor or sensory dysfunction, anorexia, vomiting, constipation, depression, fatigue, and muscle weakness. Although severe skeletal changes are rare in modern clinical practice, untreated patients do exhibit increased bone turnover, decreased bone mineral density, and increased fracture risk (Gopinath and Mihai, 2011). HPTH patients tend to have higher serum BALP and OC compared with healthy controls (Cortet et al., 2000). Trends in other markers are less consistent, that is, CTX-MMP, PICP, and PINP may be similar or increased, and CTX-1/Cr is not different from controls (Cortet et al., 2000). In a rat model of primary hyperparathyroidism, thyroparathroidectomized animals administered excess PTH for 6 days develop high serum total calcium and 1,25(OH)2D, low serum phosphorus, and unchanged serum magnesium. Histologic assessment confirmed the presence of nephrocalcinosis and increased numbers of osteoclasts (Jaeger et al., 1987); bone markers were not evaluated.

15.5.3 Secondary Hyperparathyroidism

Secondary hyperparathyroidism may be of nutritional or renal origin. Nutritional hyperparathyroidism occurs when diets contain insufficient calcium or vitamin D or when phosphorus is excessive and calcium content is normal or low. "Cage paralysis" and "simian bone disease" are terms that have been applied to this disorder in New World monkeys, which is due to inadequate vitamin D due to lack of sufficient sunlight exposure or poor diet. Most modern commercial animal diets adhere to species-specific mineral and vitamin requirements, but improper storage or formulation errors can occur. Renal secondary hyperparathyroidism is a multifactorial disorder resulting from the failing kidney's inability to maintain normal excretion of phosphorus in conjunction with reduced calcitriol concentrations due to decreased activity of renal 1-α-hydroxylase. As serum phosphorus rises, FGF23 is upregulated, which further suppresses 1-α-hydroxylase activity. In early kidney failure, declining serum calcitriol and free calcium enhance synthesis and secretion of PTH, which maintains osteoblast activity and stable bone turnover. With disease progression, the parathyroid gland becomes more resistant to calcitriol and to free calcium due to reduced expression of vitamin D receptor and calcium receptor. PTH concentration may actually exceed that observed in primary hyperparathyroidism due to reduced renal degradation of the PTH peptide. Dogs with drug-induced renal failure show increased PTH concentrations within 12 weeks; serum calcium and phosphorus increase after 24 weeks (García-Rodríguez et al., 2003). High dietary phosphorus also exacerbates chief cell hyperplasia and PTH synthesis; indeed, restriction of phosphorus intake can return PTH concentrations toward normal, despite persisting chief cell hyperplasia (Slatopolsky et al., 2001).

With progression, secondary hyperparathyroidism causes severe disturbances in bone metabolism that can lead to fibrous osteodystrophy or osteomalacia. Affected animals may be inactive, less resistant to handling, and may have difficulty in chewing ("rubber jaw") due to osteoid deposition and fibrous connective tissue proliferation of the jaw. Bones are susceptible to deformity, bowing, and fracture without mineralized calluses. Microscopic lesions include cortical thinning with severe peritrabecular and marrow fibrosis. Soft-tissue mineralization may be evident in the kidneys, cardiovascular system, and intestinal tract. The calcium–phosphorus product (Ca × P) has been traditionally used as a marker portending soft-tissue mineralization, but this has been challenged (O'Neill, 2007). Renal failure can be induced in rats by 5/6th nephrectomy. Moderately affected rats have normal total and free calcium, normal phosphorus, low 1,25(OH)2D, and increased PTH. With increased severity, hypocalcemia develops, but serum phosphate rises only slightly (D'Amour et al., 2011). This model has been used to study the effects of uremia on bone. Treated rats have increased osteoid and changes in bone turnover markers including increased serum concentrations of OC and TRACP and increased urinary PYD and DPD (Oste et al., 2007).

15.5.4 Hypercalcemia of Malignancy

Animals with humoral hypercalcemia of malignancy or pseudohyperparathyroidism have high serum total and free calcium that is often accompanied by hypophosphatemia, hypercalciuria, and normal or low PTH. Vitamin D may be normal or increased, which is inappropriate in the presence of hypercalcemia. This disorder is caused by autonomous production of PTHrP by neoplastic cells, although other factors (IL-1, TGF-alpha and -beta, vitamin D, TNFa) may play synergistic roles. In dogs, lymphoma is the most common neoplasm associated with hypercalcemia followed by adenocarcinoma of the apocrine gland of the anal sac. In the skeleton, demineralization with increased osteoclasts, decreased trabecular bone, and increased resorptive surface are evident. Mineralization may be seen in soft tissues such as kidney, stomach, or endocardium. Animals exhibit anorexia, vomiting, and constipation due to diminished smooth muscle contractility, weakness, behavioral changes, lameness, bone pain, polyuria and polydipsia, and renal failure (Capen and O'Brien, 2004). Urine NTX-I, Crosslaps, and DPD concentrations are increased in human patients with this disorder (Vinholes et al., 1997).

15.5.5 Future Markers of Bone Turnover

As investigators discover new insights into the pathophysiology of bone disorders, potential novel biomarkers have been identified that may provide greater sensitivity and/or specificity relative to current markers. Examples of proposed markers include posttranslationally modified collagen type 1, for example, alpha–alpha CTX, beta–beta-CTX, and advanced glycation end products; novel noncollagenous proteins, such as bone sialoprotein, osteopontin, and periostin; and Wnt signaling molecules, including Dickkopf-1 and sclerostin (Cremers et al., 2008).

ACKNOWLEDGMENTS

Special thanks to Dr. Ray Hamel, director of the Jacobsen Library at the Wisconsin Primate Center.

REFERENCES

Adams, J.S., Chen, H., Chun, R.F., et al. 2003. Novel regulators of vitamin D action and metabolism. *J Cell Biochem.* 88:308–314.

Aiken, A. and Khokha, R. 2010. Unraveling metalloproteinase function in skeletal biology and disease using genetically altered mice. *Biochem Biophys Acta.* 1803:121–132.

Alfrey, A.C., Miller, N.L., and Butkus, D. 1974. Evaluation of body magnesium stores. *J Lab Clin Med.* 84:153–162.

Allen, M.J. 2003. Biochemical markers of bone metabolism in animals: Uses and limitations. *Vet Clin Pathol.* 32:101–113.

Allen, M.J., Allen, L.C.V., Hoffmann, W.E., et al. 2000. Urinary markers of type I collagen degradation in the dog. *Res Vet Sci.* 69:123–127.

Allgrove, J. 2009. Physiology of calcium, phosphate and magnesium. *Endrocr Dev.* 16:8–31.

Alon, U.S. 2011. Clinical practice. Fibroblast growth factor (FGF)23: A new hormone. *Eur J Pediatr.* 170:545–554.

Alvarez, L., Peris, P., Bedini, J.L., et al. 1999. High bilirubin concentrations interfere with serum tartrate-resistant acid phosphatase determination: Relevance as a marker of bone resorption in jaundiced patients. *Calcif Tissue Int.* 64:301–303.

Amanzadeh, J. and Reilly, R.F. 2006. Hypophosphatemia: An evidence-based approach to its clinical consequences and management. *Nature Clin Pract Nephrol.* 2:136–148.

Andersen, T.L., del Carmen Ovejero, M., Kirkegaard, T., et al. 2004. A scrutiny of matrix metalloproteinases in osteoclasts: Evidence for heterogeneity and for the presence of MMPs synthesized by other cells. *Bone.* 35:1107–1119.

Angel, N.Z., Walsh, N., Forwood, MR., et al. 2000. Transgenic mice overexpressing tartrate-resistant acid phosphatase exhibit an increased rate of bone turnover. *J Bone Miner Res.* 15:103–110.

Angeliewa, A., Budde, M., Schlachter, M., Hoyle, N.R., and Bauss, F. 2004. Biochemical bone turnover markers are useful tools to assess changes in bone metabolism in marmosets. *J Bone Miner Metab.* 22:192–197.

Aono, Y., Yamazaki, Y., Yasutake, J., et al. 2002. Differences in intestinal calcium and phosphate transport between low and high bone density mice. *Am J Physiol Liver Physiol.* 282:G130–G136.

Armbrecht, H.J., Boltz, M.A., Hodam, T.L. 2002. Differences in intestinal calcium and phosphate transport between low and high bone density mice. *Am J Physiol Gastrointest Liver Physiol.* 282(1):G130–136.

Arnaud, M.J. 2008. Update on the assessment of magnesium status. *Br J Nutr.* 99(Suppl 3):S24–S36.

Arnold, A., Tovey, J., Mangat, P., et al. 1995. Magnesium deficiency in critically ill patients. *Anaesthesia.* 50:203–205.

Baetz, A.L. and Mengeling, W.L. 1971. Blood constituent changes in fasted swine. *Am J Vet Res.* 32:1491–1499.

Barr, R.D., Sadowski, D.L., Hu, J., et al. 1991. Characterization of the renal and intestinal adaptations to dietary calcium deprivation in growing female rabbits. *Miner Electrolyte Metab.* 17:32–40.

Barrett, C.P., Donati, E.J., Volz, J.E., et al. 1975. Variations in serum calcium between strains of inbred mice. *Lab Anim Sci.* 25:638–640.

Basso, L.E., Ubbink, J.B., and Delport, R. 2000. Erythrocyte magnesium concentration as an index of magnesium status: A perspective from a magnesium supplementation study. *Clin Chem Acta.* 291:1–8.

Bateman, S.W. 2008. Magnesium: A quick reference. *Vet Clin Small Anim Pract.* 38:467–470.

Bates, J.A. 2008. Phosphorus: A quick reference. *Vet Clin Small Anim Pract.* 38:471–475.

Bikle, D. 2009. Nonclassical actions of vitamin D. *J Clin Endocrinol Metab.* 94:26–34.
Black, A., Tilmont, E.M., Scott, W.W., Shapses, S.A., Ingram, D.K., Roth, G.S., Lane, M.A. 2001. A nonhuman primate model of age-related bone loss: A longitudinal study in male and premenopausal female rhesus monkeys. *Bone* 28:295–302.
Boink, A.B.T.J., Buckely, B.M., Christiansen, T.F., et al. 1992. Recommendation on sampling transport, and storage for the determination of the concentration of ionized calcium in whole blood, plasma and serum. *J Int Fed Clin Chem.* 4:147–152.
Bowles, S.A., Tait, R.C., and Jefferson, S.G. et al. 1994. Characteristics of monoclonal immunogloblulins that interfere with serum inorganic phosphate measurement. *Ann Clin Biochem.* 31:249–254.
Boyce, B.F. and Xing, L. 2008. Functions of RANKL/RANK/OPG in bone modeling and remodeling. *Arch Biochem Biophys.* 473(2):139–146.
Brown, J.E. and Chow, E. 2009. Bone biomarkers in research and clinical practice. In *Bone Metastases: A Translational and Clinical Approach.* Kardamakis, D., Vassoliou, V., and Chow, E. (eds.), pp. 93-116. Springer.
Buchl, S.J. and Howard, B. 1997. Hematologic and serum biochemical and electrolyte values in clinically normal domestically bred rhesus monkeys (*Macaca mulatta*) according to age, sex, and gravidity. *Lab Anim Sci.* 47:528–533.
Bune, A.J., Hayman, A.R., Evans, M.J., et al. 2001. Mice lacking tartrate-resistant acid phosphatase (Acp 5) have disordered macrophage inflammatory responses and reduced clearance of the pathogen, *Staphylococcus aureus. Immunology.* 102:103–113.
Burtis, C.A., Ashwood, E.R., and Bruns, D.E. 2006. Mineral and bone metabolism. In *Tietz Textbook of Clinical Chemistry and Molecular Diagnostics* Burtis, C.A., Ashwood, E.R., and D.E. Bruns (eds.), pp. 1891–1965. St. Louis, MO: Elsevier Saunders.
Bush, W.W., Kimmel, S.E., Wosar, M.A., and Jackson, M.W. 2001. Secondary hypoparathyroidism attributed to hypomagnesemia in a dog with protein-losing enteropathy. *J Am Vet Med Assoc.* 219:1732–1734.
Buss, S.L. and Bourdeau, J.E. 1984. Calcium balance in laboratory rabbits. *Mine Electrolyte Metab.* 10:127–132.
Cahoon, S., Boden, S.D., Gould, K.G., and Vailas, A.C. 1996. Noninvasive markers of bone metabolism in the rhesus monkey: Normal effects of age and gender. *J Med Primatol.* 25:333–338.
Canalis, E., Giustina, A., and Bilezikian, J.P. 2007. Mechanisms of anabolic therapies for osteoporosis. *N Engl J Med.* 357:905–916.
Capen, C.C. 2007. Parathyroid glands and calcium-regulating hormones. In *Pathology of Domestic Animals*, Ed. G.H. Maxie, pp. 357–358. Philadelphia, PA: Elsevier.
Capen, C.C. and O'Brien, T.D. 2004. Pathophysiology of endocrine homeostasis. In *Veterinary Pathophysiology.* Eds. R.H. Dunlop and C.-H. Malbert, pp. 401–443. Ames, IA: Blackwell Publishing.
Cemborain, A., Castilla-Cortázar, I., García, M., et al. 1998. Osteopenia in rats with liver cirrhosis: Beneficial effects of IGF-I treatment. *J Hepatol.* 28:122–131.
Champy, M.F., Selloum, M., Zeitler, V., et al. 2008. Genetic background determines metabolic phenotypes in the mouse. *Mamm Genome.* 19:318–331.
Chen, C. and Kalu, D.N. 1999. Strain differences in bone density and calcium metabolism between C3H/HeJ and C57BL/6J mice. *Bone.* 25:413–420.
Christakos, S., Ajibade, D.V., Dhawan, P., Fechner, A.J., and Mady, L.J. 2010. Vitamin D: Metabolism. *Endocrin Metab Clin NA.* 39:243–253.
Coleman, R., Costa, L., Saad, F., et al. 2011. Consensus on the utility of bone markers in the malignant bone disease setting. *Crit Rev Oncol Hematol.* 80:411–432.
Colman, R., Kemnitz, J.W., Lane, M.A., Abbott, D.H., and Binkley, N. 1999. Skeletal effects of aging and menopausal status in female rhesus macaques. *J Clin Endocrinol Met.* 84:4144–4148.
Confavreux, C.B. 2011. Bone: From a reservoir of minerals to a regulator of energy metabolism. *Kidney Int.* 79 (Suppl 121):S14–S19.
Cortet, B., Cortet, C., Blanckaert, F., et al. 2000. Bone ultrasonometry and turnover markers in primary hyperparathyroidism. *Calcified Tissue Intl.* 66:11–15.
Coulibaly, M.O., Sietsema, D.L., Burgers, T.A., et al. 2010. Recent advances in the use of serological bone formation markers to monitor callus development and fracture healing. *Crit Rev Eukaryot Gene Expr.* 20:105–127.
Cremers, S., Bilezikian, J.P., and Garnero, P. 2008b. Bone markers—new aspects. *Clin Lab.* 54:461–471.
Cremers, S. and Garnero, P. 2006. Biochemical markers of bone turnover in the clinical development of drugs for osteoporosis and metastatic bone disease. *Drugs.* 66(16):2031–2058.
Cremers, S., Garnero, P., Seibel, M.J. 2008a. Biochemical markers of bone metabolism. In *Principles of Bone Biology.* Eds. J. Bilezikian, L. Raisz, T.J. Martin, pp. 1857–1881. Philadelphia, PA: Elsevier.

D'Amour, P., Rousseau, L., Hornyak, S., et al. 2010. Rat parathyroid hormone (rPTH) ELISAs specific for regions (2–7), (22–34) and (40–60) of the rat PTH structure: Influence of sex and age. *Gen Comp Endocrinol.* 168:312–317.

D'Amour, P., Rousseau, L., Hornyak, S., Yang, Z., and Cantor, T. 2011. Influence of secondary hyperparathyroidism induced by low dietary calcium, vitamin D deficiency, and renal failure on circulating rat PTH molecular forms. *Intl J Endocrinol.* 2011:469783. doi:10.1155/2011/469783. Epub 2011 Jun 22.

Deaton, D.N., and Tavares, F.X. 2005. Design of cathepsin K inhibitors for osteoporosis. *Curr Top Med Chem.* 5:1639–1675.

Delmas, P.D. 2001. Standardization of bone marker nomenclature. *Clin Chem.* 47:1497.

de Paula, F.J. and Rosen, C.J. 2010. Back to the future: Revisiting parathyroid hormone and calcitonin control of bone remodeling. *Horm Metab Res.* 42:299–306.

Dittmer, K.E. and Thompson, K.G. 2011. Vitamin D metabolism and rickets in domestic animals. *Vet Pathol.* 48:389–407.

Ducy, P. 2011. The role of osteocalcin in the endocrine cross-talk between bone remodelling and energy metabolism. *Diabetologia.* 54(6):1291–1297.

Ducy, P., Desbois, C., Boyce, B., et al. 1996. Increased bone formation in osteocalcin-deficient mice. *Nature.* 382:448–452.

Eckermann-Ross, C. 2008. Hormonal regulation and calcium metabolism in the rabbit. *VCNA Exotic Ani Prac.* 11:139–152.

Elisei, R. 2008. Routine serum calcitonin measurement in the evaluation of thyroid nodules. *Best Pract Res Clin Endocrinol Metab.* 22:941–953.

Eriksen, E.F., Charles, P., Melsen, F., et al. 1993. Serum markers of type I collagen formation and degradation in metabolic bone disease: correlation with bone histomorphometry. *J Bone Mineral Res.* 8:127–132.

Fedde, K.N., Blair, L., Silverstein, J., et al. 1999. Alkaline phosphatase knock-out mice recapitulate the metabolic and skeletal defects of infantile hypophosphatasia. *J Bone Miner Res.* 14:2015–2026.

Feigh, M., Henriksen, K., Andreassen, K.V., et al. 2011. A novel oral form of salmon calcitonin improves glucose homeostasis and reduces body weight in diet-induced obese rats. *Diabetes Obesity Metabol.* 13:911–920.

Feldman, E.C. and Nelson, R.W. 2003. Hypocalcemia and primary hypoparathyroidism. In *Canine and Feline Endocrinology and Reproduction.* Eds. E.C. Feldman and R.W. Nelson, pp. 247–248. Philadelphia, PA: Saunders.

Feres, M.C., Bini, R., De Martino M.C., et al. 2011. Implications for the use of acid preservatives in 24-hour urine for measurements of high demand biochemical analytes in clinical laboratories. *Clin Chim Acta.* 412:2322–2325.

Fernandez, N.J. and Kidney, B. 2007. Alkaline phosphatase: Beyond the liver. *Vet Clin Path.* 36:223–233.

Fincham, S.C., Drobatz, K.J., Gillespie, T.N., et al. 2004. Evaluation of plasma-ionized magnesium concentration in 122 dogs with diabetes mellitus: A retrospective study. *J Vet Intern Med.* 18:612–617.

Fiser, R.T., Torres, A., Jr., Butch, A.W., et al. 1998. Ionized magnesium concentrations in critically ill children. *Crit Care Med.* 26:2048–2052.

Foley, K.V. and Boccuzzi, L. 2010. Urine calcium: Laboratory measurement and clinical utility. *Lab Med.* 41:683–686.

Fractionation of calcium and magnesium in equine serum. *Am J Vet Res.* 67:463–466.

Frith, C.H., Suber, R.L., and Umholtz, R. 1980. Hematologic and clinical chemistry findings in control BALB/c and C57BL/6 mice. *Lab Anim Sci.* 30:835–840.

Fung, M.C., Weintraub, M., and Bowen, D.L. 1995. Hypermagnesemia: Elderly over-the-counter drug users at risk. *Arch Fam Med.* 4:718–723.

García-Rodríguez, M.B., Pérez-García, C.C., Ríos-Granja, M.A., et al. 2003. Renal handling of calcium and phosphorus in experimental renal hyperparathyroidism in dogs. *Vet Res.* 34:379–387.

Garnero, P. 2008. Biomarkers for osteoporosis management: utility in diagnosis, fracture risk prediction and therapy monitoring. *Mol Diagn Ther.* 12:157–170.

Gensure, R.C., Gardella, T.J., and Jüppner, H. 2005. Parathyroid hormone and parathyroid hormone-related peptide and their receptors. *Biochem Biophys Res Commun.* 328:666–678.

Gilsanz, V., Roe, T.F., Antunes. J., et al. 1991. Effect of dietary calcium on bone density in growing rabbits. *Am J Physiol.* 260:E471–E476.

Gopinath, P. and Mihai, R. 2011. Hyperparathyroidism. *Surgery.* 29:451–458.

Gow, A.G., Else, R., Evans, H., Berr, J.L., Herrtage, M.E., and Mellanby, R.J. 2011. Hypovitaminosis D in dogs with inflammatory bowel disease and hypoalbuminemia. *J Sm Anim Pract.* 52:411–418.

Hale, L.V., Galvin, R.J., Risteli, J., et al. 2007. PINP: A serum biomarker of bone formation in the rat. *Bone.* 40:1103–1109.

Halleen, J.M., Tiitinen, S.L., Ylipajkala, H., et al. 2006. Tartrate-resistant acid phosphatase 5b as a marker of bone resorption. *Clin Lab.* 52:499–509.

Hansson, L.I., Stenstrom, A., and Thorngren, K.G. 1974. Diurnal variation of longitudinal bone growth in the rabbit. *Acta Orthop Scand.* 45:499–507.

Harmey, D., Hessle, L., Narisawa, K., et al. 2004. Concerted regulation of inorganic pyrophosphate and osteopontin by Akp2, Enpp1, and Ank. *Am J Pathol.* 164:1199–1209.

Harvey, J.W. 1997. The erythrocyte. In *Clinical Biochemistry of Domestic Animals.* Eds. J.J. Kaneko, J.W. Harvey, and M.W. Bruss, pp. 178–181. San Diego, CA: Academic Press.

Haseman, J.K. 1998. Spontaneous neoplasm incidences in Fischer 344 rats and B6C3F1 mice in two-year carcinogenicity studies: A National Toxicology Program update. *Tox Pathol.* 26:428–441.

Hatayama, K., Ichikawa, Y., Nishihara, Y., et al. 2012. Serum alkaline phosphatase isoenzymes in SD rats detected by polyacrylamide-gel disk electrophoresis. *Toxicol Mech Meth.* 22:289–295.

Hatori, K., Sasano, Y., Takahashi, I., Kamakura, S., Kagayam, M., and Sasaki, K. 2004. Osteoblasts and osteocytes express MMP2 and -8 and TIMP1, -2, -3 along with extracellular matrix molecules during appositional bone formation. *Anatomical Rec Part A.* 277:262–271.

Hayman, A.R. 2008. Tartrate-resistant acid phosphatase and the osteoclast/immune cell dichotomy. *Autoimmunity.* 41(3):218–223.

Hayman, A.R. and Cox, T.M. 2003. Tartrate-resistant acid phosphatase knockout mice. *J Bone Mineral Res.* 18:1905–1907.

Hayman, A.R., Jones, S.J., Boyde, A., et al. 1996. Mice lacking tartrate-resistant acid phosphatase (Acp 5) have disrupted endochondral ossification and mild osteopetrosis. *Development.* 122:3151–3162.

Hegemann, N., Kohn, B., Brunnberg, L., and Schmidt, M.F. 2002. Biomarkers of joint tissue metabolism in canine osteoarthritic and arthritic joint disorders. *Osteoarthr Cartilage.* 10 (9):714–721.

Hegemann, N., Wondimu, A., Ullrich, K., and Schmidt, M.F. 2003. Synovial MMP-3 and TIMP-1 concentrations and their correlation with cytokine expression in canine rheumatoid arthritis. *Vet Immunol Immunopathol.* 91(3–4):199–204.

Hendy, G.N., Hruska, K.A., Mathew, S., et al. 2006. New insights into mineral and skeletal regulation by active forms of vitamin D. *Kidney Int.* 69:218–223.

Henriksen, K., Tanko, L.B., Qvist, P., et al. 2007. Assessment of osteoclast number and function: Application in the development of new and improved treatment modalities for bone diseases. *Osteoporos Int.* 18:681–685.

Herrmann, M. 2011. Methods in bone biology in animals: Biochemical markers. In *Osteoporosis Research.* Eds. G. Duque and K. Watanabe, pp. 57–82. London: Springer-Verlag.

Herrmann, M. and Seibel, M. 2008. The amino- and carboxyterminal cross-linked telopeptides of collagen type I, NTX-1 and CTX-1: A comparative review. *Clin Chem Acta.* 393:57–75.

Herroeder, S., Schonherr, M.E., De Hert, S.G., and Hollmann, M.W. 2011. Magnesium—essentials for anesthesiologists. *Anesthesiology.* 114:971–993.

Hie, M., Shimono, M., Fujii, K., et al. 2007. Increased cathepsin K and tartrate-resistant acid phosphatase expression in bone of streptozotocin-induced diabetic rats. *Bone.* 41:1045–1050.

Hintermeister, J.G., Jones, P.D., Hoffmann, W.E., Siegel. A.M., Dervisis, N.G., and Kitchell, B.E. 2008. Measurement of serum carboxyterminal cross-linked telopeptide of type I collagen concentration in dogs with osteosarcoma. *Am J Vet Res.* 69:1481–1486.

Hoffmann, W.E., Everds, N., Pignatello, M. and Solter, P.F. 1994. Automated and semiautomated analysis of rat alkaline phosphatase isoenzymes. *Toxicol Pathol.* 22:633–638.

Hollis, B.W. 2010. Assessment and interpretation of circulating 25-hydroxyvitamin D and 1,25-dihydroxyvitamin D in the clinical environment. *Endocrinol Metab Clin North Am.* 39(2):271–286.

Horton, J.A., Bariteau, J.T., Loomis, R.M., et al. 2008. Ontogeny of skeletal maturation in the juvenile rat. *The Anat Rec.* 291:283–292.

Hotchkiss, C.E. and Jerome, C.P. 1998. Evaluation of a nonhuman primate model to study circadian rhythms of calcium metabolism. *Am J Physiol.* 275:R494–R501.

Hotchkiss, C.E., Tavisky, S., Nowak, J., Brommage, R., Lees, C.H., and Kaplan, J. 2001. Levormeloxifene prevents increased bone turnover and vertebral bone loss following ovariectomy in cynomolgus monkeys. *Bone.* 29:7–15.

Huang, Y., Eapen, E., Steele, S., and Grey, V. 2011. Establishment of reference intervals for bone markers in children and adolescents. *Clin Biochem.* 44:771–778.

Huang, S., Kaw, M., Harris, M.T., et al. 2010. Decreased osteoclastogenesis and high bone mass in mice with impaired insulin clearance due to liver-specific inactivation to CEACAM1. *Bone.* 46:1138–1145.

Itoh, H., Kakuta, T., Genda, G.,Sakonju, I., and Takase, K. 2002. Canine serum alkaline phosphatase isoenzymes detected by polyacrylamide gel disk electrophoresis. *J Vet Med Sci.* 64:35–39.

Ivaska, K.K., Hentunen, T.A., Vääräniemi, J., et al. 2004. Release of intact and fragmented osteocalcin molecules from bone matrix during bone resorption *in vitro*. *J Biol Chem.* 279:18361–18369.

Jacobs, T.P. and Bilezikian, J.P. 2005. Clinical review: Rare causes of hypercalcemia. *J Clin Endocrinol Metab.* 90:6316–6322.

Jaeger, P., Jones, W., Kashgarian, M. et al. 1987. Animal model of primary hyperparathyroidism. *Am J Physiol.* 252:E790–98.

Joerger, M. and Huober, J. 2012. Diagnostic and prognostic use of bone turnover markers. *Recent Results Cancer Res.* 192:197–223.

Kalu, D.N. and Hardin, R.R. 1984. Age, strain and species differences in circulating parathyroid hormone. *Horm Metab Res.* 16:654–657.

Kaplinsky, C. and Alon, U.S. 2013. Magnesium homeostasis and hypomagnesemia in children with malignancy. *Pediatr Blood Cancer.* 60:734–740.

Kapustin, A.N. and Shanahan, C.M. 2011. Osteocalcin: A novel vascular metabolic and osteoinductive factor? *Arterioscler Thromb Vasc Biol.* 31:2169–2171.

Karsdal, M.A., Henriksen, K., Bay-Jensen, A.C., et al. 2011. Lessons learned from the development of oral calcitonin: The first tablet formulation of a protein in phase III clinical trials. *J Clin Pharmacol.* 51:460–471.

Karsenty, G. 2006. Convergence between bone and energy homeostasis. *Cell Metab.* 4:341–348.

Katafuchi, T., Yasue, H., Osaki, T., and Minamino, N.. Calcitonin receptor-stimulating peptide: Its evolutionary and functional relationship with calcitonin/calcitonin gene-related peptide based on gene structure. *Peptides.* 30:1753–1762.

Keller, E.T., Binkley, N.C., and Stebler, B.A. et al. 2000. Ovariectomy does not induce osteopenia through interleukin-6 in rhesus monkeys *(Macaca mulatta)*. *Bone* 26:55–62.

Keyszer, G., Lambiri, I., Nagel, R., et al. 1999. Circulating levels of matrix metalloproteinases MMP-3 and MMP-1, tissue inhibitor of metalloproteinases 1 (TIMP-1), and MMP-1/TIMP-1 complex in rheumatic disease. Correlation with clinical activity of rheumatoid arthritis versus other surrogate markers. *J Rheumatol.* 26(2):251–258.

Khoshniat, S., Bourgine, A., Julien, M., et al. 2011. The emergence of phosphate as a specific signaling molecule in bone and other cell types. *Cell Mol Life Sci.* 68:205–218.

Kleerekoper, M. 2011. Clinical applications for vitamin D assays: What is known and what is hoped for. *Clin Chem.* 57:1227–1232.

Kmieć, A., Myśliwski, A., Wyrzykowska, M., and Hoppe, A. 2001. The effects of fasting and refeeding on serum parathormone and calcitonin concentrations in young and old male rats. *Horm Metab Res.* 33:276–280.

Kraenzlin, M.E. and Seibel, M.J. 2006. Measurement of biochemical markers of bone resorption. In *Dynamics of Bone and Cartilage Metabolism*. Ed. M.J. Seibel, S.P. Robins, and J.P. Bilezikian, pp. 541–563. San Diego, CA: Academic Press.

Krahn, J. and Lou, H. 2008. Ionized calcium: Whole blood, plasma or serum? *Clin Lab.* 54:185–189.

Kramer, J.W. and Hoffman, W.E. 1997. Clinical enzymology. In *Clinical Biochemistry of Domestic Animals*. Eds. J.J. Kaneko, J.W. Harvey, M.L. Bruss, pp. 316–317. San Diego, CA: Academic Press.

Kumar, S., Dare, L., Vasko-Moser, J.A., et al. 2007. A highly potent inhibitor of cathepsin K (relacatib) reduces biomarkers of bone resorption both *in vitro* and in an acute model of elevated bone turnover *in vivo* in monkeys. *Bone.* 40:122–131.

Ladlow, J.F., Hoffman, W.F., Breur, G.J., et al. 2002. Biological variability in serum and urinary indices of bone formation and resorption in dogs. *Calcif Tissue Int.* 70:186–193.

Laing, C.J., Malik, R., Wigney, D.I., and Fraser, D.R. 1999. Seasonal vitamin D status of greyhounds in Sydney. *Aust Vet J.* 77:35–38.

Lammens, J., Liu, Z., Aerssens, J., Dequeker, J., and Fabry, G. 1998. Distraction bone healing versus osteotomy healing: A comparative biochemical analysis. *J Bone Miner Res.* 13(2):279–286.

Larsson, L. and Ohman, S. 1985. Effect of silicone-separator tubes and storage time on ionized calcium in serum. *Clin Chem.* 31:169–170.

Lauridsen, C., Halekoh, U., Larsen, T., and Jensen, S.K. 2010. Reproductive performance and bone status markers of gilts and lactating sows supplemented with two different forms of vitamin D. *J Anim Sci.* 88:202–213. Lawler, D.F., Ballam, J.M., Meadows, R., Larson, B.T., Li, Q., Stowe, H.D., and Kealy, R.D. 2007. Influence of lifetime food restriction on physiological variables in Labrador retriever dogs. *Exp Gerontol.* 42(3):204–214.

Lecaille, F., Bromme, D., and Lalmanach, G. 2008. Biochemical properties and regulation of cathepsin K activity. *Biochimie.* 90:208–226.

Lee, H.B., Alam, M.R., Seol, J.W., and Kim, N.S. 2008. Tartrate-resistant acid phosphatase, matrix metalloproteinase-2 and tissue inhibitor of metalloproteinase-2 in early stages of canine osteoarthritis. *Vet Med.* 53:214–220.

Lee, M. and Partridge, N.C. 2009. Parathyroid hormone signaling in bone and kidney. *Curr Opin Nephrol Hypertens.* 18:298–302.

Lees, C.J., Jerome, C.P., Register, T.C., et al. 1998. Changes in bone mass and bone biomarkers of cynomolgus monkeys during pregnancy and lactation. *J Clin Endocrinol Metab.* 83:4298–4302.

Lees, C.J., Register, T.C., Turner, C.H., Want, T., Stancill, M., and Jerome, C.P. 2002. Effects of raloxifene on bone density, biomarkers, and histomorphometric and biomechanical measures in ovariectomized cynomolgus monkeys. *Menopause.* 9:320–328.

Lefebvre, H.P., Dossin, O., Trumel, C., and Braun, J.P. 2008. Fractional excretion tests: A critical review of methods and applications in domestic animals. *Vet Clin Pathol.* 37:4–20.

Legrand, J.-J., Fisch, C., Guillaumat, P.O., et al. 2003 Use of biochemical markers to monitor changes in bone turnover in cynomolgus monkeys. *Biomarkers.* 8:63–77.

Levolas, P.P. Xanthos, T.T., and Thoma, S.E. et al. 2008. The laboratory rat as an animal model for osteoporosis research. *Comp Med.* 58:424–430.

Li, X., Srivastava, A.K., Gu, W., et al. 2002. Opposing changes in osteocalcin levels in bone vs serum during the acquisition of peak bone density in C3H/HeJ and C57BL/6J mice. *Calcif Tissue Int.* 71:416–420.

Li, Z.-B., Kai, L.-S., and Zhao, Y.C. 2005. Changes in bone metabolism in early stage following spinal cord injury in guinea pig: Value of related biochemical indices in risk assessment for osteoporosis. *Chinese J Clin Rehab.* 9:157–159.

Liberati, T.A., Sansone, S.R., and Feuston, M.H. 2004. Hematology and clinical chemistry values in pregnant Wistar Hannover rats compared with nonmated controls. *Vet Clin Pathol.* 33:68–73.

Liesbet, L., Masuyama, R., and Torrekens, S. et al. 2012. Normocalcemia is maintained in mice under conditions of calcium malabsorption by vitamin D–induced inhibition of bone mineralization. *J Clin Invest.* 122:1803–1815.

Liesegang, A., Limacher, S., and Sobek, A. 2007. The effect of carprofen on selected markers of bone metabolism in dogs with chronic osteoarthritis. *Schweiz Arch Tierheilkd.* 149:353–362.

Liesegang, A., Reutter, R., Sassi, M.L., et al. 1999. Diurnal variation in concentrations of various markers of bone metabolism in dogs. *Am J Vet Res.* 60:949–953.

Linder, C.H., Narisawa, S., Millán, J.L., and Magnusson, P. 2009. Glycosylation differences contribute to distinct catalytic properties among bone alkaline phosphatase isoforms. *Bone.* 45:987–993.

Lopez, I., Estepa, J.C., Mendoza, F.J., Mayer-Valor, R., and Aguilera-Tejero, E. 2006. Serum concentrations of calcium, phosphorus, magnesium and calciotropic hormones in donkeys. *Am J Vet Res.* 67: 1333–1336.

Lowenstein, L. 2003. A primer of primate pathology: Lesions and nonlesions. *Toxicol Pathol.* (Suppl 31):92–102.

Lucas, P.W., Fan, T.M., Garrett, L.D., et al. 2008. A comparison of five different bone resorption markers in osteosarcoma-bearing dogs, normal dogs, and dogs with orthopedic diseases. *J Vet Intern Med.* 22:1008–1013.

Lumachi, F., Motta, R., Cecchin, D., et al. 2011. Calcium metabolism and hypercalcemia in adults. *Curr Med Chem.* 18:3529–3536.

Luo, X.H., Guo, L.J., Shan, P.F., et al. 2006. Relationship of circulating MMP-2, MMP-1, and TIMP-1 levels with bone biochemical markers and bone mineral density in postmenopausal Chinese women. *Osteoporos Int.* 17(4):521–526. Epub 2005 Dec 20.

Maier, G.W., Kreis, M.E., Zittel, T.T., et al. 1997. Calcium regulation and bone mass loss after total gastrectomy in pigs. *Ann Surg.* 225:181–192.

Marks, J., Debnam, E.S., and Unwin, R.J. 2010. Phosphate homeostasis and the renal-gastrointestinal axis. *Am J Physiol Renal Physiol.* 299:F285–F296.

Martin, L.G., Matteson, V.L., Wingfield, W.E., Van Pelt, D.R., and Hackett, T.B. 1994. Abnormalities of serum magnesium in critically ill dogs: Incidence and implications. *J Vet Emerg Crit Care.* 4:1476–4431.

Martin, T.J., Gooi, J.H., and Sims, N.H. 2009. Molecular mechanisms in coupling of bone formation to resorption. *Crit Rev Eukaryot Gene Expr.* 19:73–88.

Martinez, D.A., Patterson-Buckendahl, P.E., Lust, A., et al. 2008. A noninvasive analysis of urinary musculoskeletal collagen metabolism markers from rhesus monkeys subject to hypergravity. *J Appl Physiol.* 105:1255–1261.

Mazzaccara, C., Labruna, G., Cito, G., et al. 2008. Age-related reference intervals of the main biochemical and hematological parameters in C57BL/6J, 129SV/EV and C3H/HeJ mouse strains. *PLOS ONE.* 3:e3772.

McLaughlin, F., Mackintosh, J., Hayes, B.P., et al. 2002. Glucocorticoid-induced osteopenia in the mouse as assessed by histomorphometry, microcomputed tomography, and biochemical markers. *Bone.* 30:924–930.

Meier, C., Meinhardt, U., Greenfield, J.R., et al. 2006. Serum cathepsin K concentrations reflect osteoclastic activity in women with postmenopausal osteoporosis and patients with Paget's disease. *Clin Lab.* 52:1–10.

Melkko, J., Hellevik, T., Risteli, L., et al. 1994. Clearance of NH2-terminal propeptides of types I and III procollagen is a physiological function of the scavenger receptor in liver endothelial cells. *J Exp Med.* 179:405–412.

Messinger, J.S., Windham, W.R., and Ward, C.R. 2009. Ionized hypercalcemia in dogs: A retrospective study of 109 cases (1998–2003). *J Vet Intern Med.* 23:514–519.

Meuten, D.J., Chew, D.J., Capen, C.C., and Kociba, G.J. 1982. Relationship of serum total calcium to albumin and total protein in dogs. *J Am Vet Med Assoc.* 180:63–67.

Mohamadnia, A.R., Shahbazkia, H.R., Sharifi, S., and Shafaei, I. 2007. Bone-specific alkaline phosphatase as a good indicator of bone formation in sheepdogs. *Com Clin Pathol.* 16:265–270.

Muhlbauer, R.C. and Fleisch, H. 1990. A method for continual monitoring of bone resorption in rats: Evidence for a diurnal rhythm. *Am J Physiol.* 259:R679–R689.

Muñoz-Torres, M., Reyes-García, R., Mezquita-Raya, P., et al. 2009. Serum cathepsin K as a marker of bone metabolism in postmenopausal women treated with alendronate. *Maturitas.* 64:188–192.

Murray, E.J., Song, M.K., Laird, E.C., et al. 1993. Strain-dependent differences in vertebral bone mass, serum osteocalcin, and calcitonin in calcium-replete and -deficient mice. *Proc Soc Exp Biol Med.* 203:64–73.

Müller, B., White, J.C., Nylén, E.S., et al. 2001. Ubiquitous expression of the calcitonin-I gene in multiple tissues in response to sepsis. *J Clin Endocrinol Metab.* 86:396–404.

Nagase, H., Visse, R., and Murphy, G. 2006. Structure and function of matrix metalloproteinases and TIMPs. *Cardiovasc Res.* 69:562–573.

Nestor, D.D., Holan, K.M., Johnson, C.M., et al. 2006. Serum alkaline phosphatase activity in Scottish Terriers versus dogs of other breeds. *JAVMA.* 228:222–224.

O'Toole, J.F. 2011. Disorders of calcium metabolism. *Nephron Physiol.* 118:22–27.

Olgaard, K. and Lewin, E. 2001. Prevention of uremic bone disease using calcimimetic compounds. *Annu Rev Med.* 52:203–220.

Ominsky, M.S., Stouch, B. Schroeder, J. et al. 2011. Denosumab, a fully human RANKL antibody, reduced bone turnover markers and increased trabecular and cortical bone mass, density, and strength in ovariectomized cynomolgus monkeys. *Bone.* 49:162–173.

O'Neill, W.C. 2007. The fallacy of the calcium–phosphorus product. *Kidney Int.* 72:792–796.

Ordóñez, F.A., Fernández, P., Rodríguez, J., et al. 1998. Rat models of normocalcemic hypercalciuria of different pathogenic mechanisms. *Pediatr Nephrol.* 12:201–205.

Oste, L., Behets, G.J., Dams, G., et al. 2007. Role of dietary phosphorus and degree of uremia in the development of renal bone disease in rats. *Ren Fail.* 29:1–12.

Oxlund, H., Ortoft, G., Thomsen, J.S. et al. 2006. The anabolic effect of PTH on bone is attentuated by simultaneous glucocorticoid treatment. *Bone* 29:244–252.

Peng, T.C., Cooper, C.W., and Garner, S.C. 1976. Thyroid and blood thyrocalcitonin concentrations and C-cell abundance in two strains of rats at different ages. *Proc Soc Exp Biol Med.* 152:268–272.

Penido, M.G.M.G. and Alon, U.S. 2012. Phosphate homeostasis and its role in bone health. *Pediatr Nephrol.* 27:2039–2048.

Pennypacker, B., Shea, M., Liu, Q., et al. 2009. Bone density, strength, and formation in adult cathepsin K (– /–) mice. *Bone.* 44:199–207.

Perez, A.V., Picotto, G., Carpentieri, A.R., Rivoira, M.A., Lopez, M.E.P., and de Talamoni, N.G. 2008. Minireview on regulation of intestinal calcium absorption. *Digestion.* 77:22–34.

Philipov, J.P., Pascalev, M.D., Aminkov, B.Y., et al. 1995. Changes in serum carboxyterminal telopeptide of type I collagen in an experimental model of canine osteomyelitis. *Calcif Tissue Int.* 57:152–154.

Pietschmann, P., Skalicky, M., Kneissel, M., et al. 2007. Bone structure and metabolism in a rodent model of male senile osteoporosis. *Exp Gerontol.* 42:1099–1108.

Powers, C.S., Schultze, A.E., Krisnan, V., et al. 2007. Comparison of results from the semiautomated serum bone alkaline phosphatase isoenzyme assay with the periosteal alkaline phosphatase assay for use in rat models. *Vet Clin Path.* 36:285–287.

Prié, D., Ureña Torres, P., and Friedlander, G. 2009. Latest findings in phosphate homeostasis. *Kidney Int.* 75:882–889.

Raisz, L.G., Mundy, G.R., Dietrich, J.W., and Canalis, E.M. 1977. Hormonal regulation of mineral metabolism. *Int Rev Physiol.* 16:199–240.

Ralston, S.H. 2009. Bone structure and metabolism. *Medicine.* 37:46–474.

Rayana, M.C., Burnett, R.W., Covington, A.K., et al. 2008. IFCC guideline for sampling, measuring and reporting ionized magnesium in plasma. *Clin Chem Lab Med.* 46:21–26.

Redrobe, S. 2002. Calcium metabolism in rabbits. *Sem Av Exotic Pet Med.* 11:94–101.

Reinwald, S. and Burr, D. 2008. Review of nonprimate, large animal models for osteoporosis research. *J Bone Miner Res.* 23:1353–1368.

Rice, B.F., Roth, L.M., Cole, F.E., et al. 1975. Hypercalcemia and neoplasia. Biologic, biochemical, and ultrastructural studies of a hypercalcemia-producing Leydig cell tumor of the rat. *Lab Invest.* 33:428–439.

Rissanen, J.P., Suominen, M.I., Peng, Z., et al. 2008. Secreted tartrate-resistant acid phosphatase 5b is a marker of osteoclast number in human osteoclast cultures and the rat ovariectomy model. *Calcif Tiss Int.* 82:108–115.

Rodan, G.A. and Martin, T.J. 2000. Therapeutic approaches to bones diseases. *Science.* 289:1508–1514.

Rodin, A., Duncan, A., Quartero, H.W., et al. 1989. Serum concentrations of alkaline phosphatase isoenzymes and osteocalcin in normal pregnancy. *J Clin Endocrinol Metab.* 68:1123–1127.

Rosol, T.J. and Capen, C.C. 1992. Mechanisms of cancer-induced hypercalcemia. *Lab Invest.* 67:680–702.

Rude, R.K. and Gruber, H.E. 2004. Magnesium deficiency and osteoporosis: Animal and human observations. *J Nutr Biochem.* 15:710–716.

Rude, R.K., Singer, F.R., and Gruber, H.E. 2009. Skeletal and hormonal effects of magnesium deficiency. *J Am Coll Nutr.* 28:131–141.

Russo, J.C. and Nash, M.A. 1980. Renal response to alterations in dietary phosphate in the young beagle. *Biol Neonate* 38:1–10.

Sanecki, R.K., Hoffmann, W.E., Hansen, R., and Schaeffer, D.J. 1993. Quantification of bone alkaline phosphatase in canine serum. *Vet Clin Pathol.* 22:17–23.

Saris, N.E., Mervaala, E., Karppanen, H., et al. 2000. Magnesium. An update on physiological, clinical and analytical aspects. *Clin Chem Acta.* 294:1–26.

Schaer, M. 1999. Disorders of serum potassium, sodium, magnesium and chloride. *J Vet Emerg Crit Care.* 9:209–217.

Schenk, P.A. 2005. Fractionation of canine serum magnesium. *Vet Clin Pathol.* 34:137–139.

Schenck, P.A., Chew, D.J., and Behrend, E.N. 2005. Updates on hypercalcemic disorders. In *Consultations in Feline Internal Medicine*. Ed. J. August, Vol. 5, pp. 157–168. St. Louis, MO: Elsevier.

Schenck, P.A. and Chew, D.J. 2008. Hypocalcemia: A quick reference. *Vet Clin NA Small Anim Pract.* 38:455–458.

Schenck, P.A., Chew, D.J., and Brooks, C.L. 1995. Effects of storage on serum ionized calcium and pH values in clinically normal dogs. *Am J Vet Res.* 56:304–307.

Schenck, P.A., Chew, D.J., and Brooks, C.L. 1996. Fractionation of canine serum calcium, using a micropartition system. *Am J Vet Res.* 57:268–271.

Schenk, P.A. and Chew, D.J. 2005. Prediction of serum ionized calcium concentration by use of serum total calcium concentration in dogs. *Am J Vet Res.* 66:1330–1336.

Schneider, H.G. and Lam, Q.T. 2007. Procalcitonin for the clinical laboratory: A review. *Pathology.* 39:383–390.

Scholz-Ahrens, K.E., Delling, G., Stampa, B., et al. 2007. Glucocorticosteroid-induced osteoporosis in adult primiparous Göttingen miniature pigs: Effects on bone mineral and mineral metabolism. *Am J Physiol Endocrin Metabol.* 293:E385–E395.

Seeman, E. and Delmas, P. 2006. Bone quality—The material and structural basis of bone strength and fragility. *N Engl J Med.* 354:2250–2261.

Seibel, M.J. 2005. Biochemical markers of bone turnover part I: Biochemistry and variability. *Clin Biochem Rev.* 26:97–122.

Seibel, M.J., Robins, S.P., and Bilezikian, J.P. 2006. *Dynamics of Bone and Cartilage Metabolism*, p. 533. Burlington, MA: Elsevier Inc.

Seidlová-Wuttke, D., Schlumbohm, C., and Jarry, H. et al. 2008. Orchidectomized (orx) marmoset (Callithrix jacchus) as a model to study the development of osteopenia/osteoporosis. *Am J Primatol.* 70:294–300.

Selvarajah, G.T. and Kirpensteijn, J. 2010. Prognostic and predictive biomarkers of canine osteosarcoma. *Vet J.* 185:28–35.

Sengupta, S., Arshad, M., Sharma, S., et al. 2005. Attainment of peak bone mass and bone turnover rate in relation to estrous cycle, pregnancy and lactation in colony-bred Sprague-Dawley rats: Suitability for studies on pathophysiology of bone and therapeutic measures for its management. *J Steroid Biochem Mol Biol.* 94:421–429.

Shetty, S., Kapoor, N., and Bondu, J.D. et al. 2016. Bone turnover markers: emerging tool in the management of osteoporosis. *Indian J Endocrinol Metab.* 20:846–852.

Shiomi, T., Lemaître, V., D'Armiento, J., Okada, Y. 2010. Matrix metalloproteinases, a disintegrin and metalloproteinases, and a disintegrin and metalloproteinases with thrombospondin motifs in non-neoplastic diseases. *Pathol Int.* 60(7):477–496.

Shuto, E., Taketani, Y., Tanaka, R., et al. 2009. Dietary phosphorus acutely impairs endothelial function. *J Am Soc Nephrol.* 20:1504–1512.

Siggaard-Andersen, O., Thode, J., and Fogh-Andersen, N. 1983. Nomograms for calculating the concentration of ionized calcium of human blood plasma from total calcium, total protein and/or albumin, and pH. *Scand J Clin Lab Invest Suppl.* 165:57–64.

Skoumal, M., Haberhauer, G., Kolarz, G., et al. 2004. Serum cathepsin K levels of patients with longstanding rheumatoid arthritis: Correlation with radiological destruction. *Arthritis Res Ther.* 7:R65–R70.

Slatopolsky, E., Brown, A., and Dusso, A. 2001. Role of phosphorus in the pathogenesis of secondary hyperparathyroidism. *Am J Kidney Dis.* 37(1 Suppl 2):S54–S57.

Smith, B.B., Cosenza, M.E., Mancini, A., et al. 2003. A toxicity profile of osteoprotegerin in the cynomolgus monkey. *Int J Toxicol.* 22:403–412.

Sodi, R., Bailey, L.B., Glaysher, J., et al. 2009. Acidification and urine calcium: Is it a preanalytical necessity? *Ann Clin Biochem.* 46:484–487.

Song, Y. and Fleet, J.C. 2004. 1,25 dihydroxycholecalciferol-mediated calcium absorption and gene expression are higher in female than in male mice. *J Nutr.* 134:1857–1861.

Sorensen, M.G., Henriksen, K., Schaller, S., and Karsdal, M.A. 2007. Biochemical markers in preclinical models of osteoporosis. *Biomarkers.* 12:266–286.

Sousa, C.P., Nery, F., Azevedo, J.T., Viegas, C.A., Gomes, M.E., and Dias, I.R. 2011. Tartrate-resistant acid phosphatase as a biomarker of bone turnover in dog. *Arq Bras Med Vet Zootec.* 63:40–45.

Southern, R.B., Farber, M.S., and Gruber, S.A. 1993. Circannual variations in baseline blood values of dogs. *Chronobiol Int.* 10:364–382.

Southwood, L.L., Frisbie, D.D., Kawcak, C.E., et al. 2003. Evaluation of serum biochemical markers of bone metabolism for early diagnosis of nonunion and infected nonunion fractures in rabbits. *Am J Vet Res.* 64:727–735.

Srivastava, A.K., Bhattacharyya, S., Li, X., et al. 2001. Circadian and longitudinal variation of serum C-telopeptide, osteocalcin, and skeletal alkaline phosphatase in C3H/HeJ mice. *Bone.* 29:361–367.

Stechman, M.J., Loh, N.Y., and Thakker, R.V. 2009. Genetic causes of hypercalciuric nephrolithiasis. *Pediatr Nephrol.* 24:2321–2332.

Stockham, S.L. and Scott, M.A. (eds.) 2008a. Calcium, phosphorus, magnesium and their regulatory roles. In *Fundamentals of Veterinary Clinical Pathology*, pp 593–638. Ames, IA: Blackwell Publishing.

Stockham, S.L. and Scott, M.A. (eds.) 2008b. Urinary system. In *Fundamentals of Veterinary Clinical Pathology*, pp 415–494. Ames, IA: Blackwell Publishing.

Stroup, G.B., Kumar, S., and Jerome, C.P. 2009. Treatment with a potent cathepsin K inhibitor preserves cortical and trabecular bone mass in ovariectomized monkeys. *Calcif Tissue Int.* 85:344–355.

Svelander, L., Erlandsson-Harris, H., Astner, L., et al. 2009. Inhibition of cathepsin K reduces bone erosion, cartilage degradation and inflammation evoked by collagen-induced arthritis in mice. *Eur J Pharmacol.* 613:155–162.

Thakker, R.V., Davies, K.E., Whyte, M.P., Wooding, C., and O'Riordan, J.L. 1990. Mapping the gene causing X-linked recessive idiopathic hypoparathyroidism to Xq26-Xq27 by linkage studies. *J Clin Invest.* 86:40–45.

Theyse, L.F., Mol, J.A., Voorhout, G., Terlou, M., and Hazewinkel, H.A. 2006. The efficacy of the bone markers osteocalcin and the carboxyterminal cross-linked telopeptide of type-I collagen in evaluating osteogenesis in a canine crural lengthening model. *Vet J.* 171(3):525–531.

Toledo, S.P.A., Lourenco, Jr., D.M., and Santos, M.R. et al. 2009. Hypercalcitoninemia is not pathognomonic of medullary thyroid carcinoma. *Clinics (Sao Paulo).* 64:699–706.

Tonna, E.A., Singh, I.J., and Sandhu, H.S. 1987. Autoradiographic investigation of circadian rhythms in alveolar bone periosteum and cementum in young mice. *Histol Histopathol.* 2:129–133.

Tordoff, M.G., Bachmanov, A.A., and Reed, D.R. 2007. Forty mouse strain survey of voluntary calcium intake, blood calcium, and bone mineral content. *Physiol Behav.* 91:632–643.

Tsutsumi, H., Katagiri, K., Morimoto, M., et al. 2004a. Diurnal variation and age-related changes of bone turnover markers in female Göttingen minipigs. *Lab Anim.* 38:439–446.

Tsutsumi, H, Katagiri, K., Takeda, S., et al. 2004b. Standardized data and relationship between bone growth and bone metabolism in female Göttingen minipigs. *Exp Anim.* 53:331–337.

Ullrey, D.E., Miller, E.R., Brent, B.E., Bradley, B.L., and Hoefer, J.A. 1967. Swine hematology from birth to maturity IV. Phosphorus, magnesium, sodium, potassium, copper, zinc and inorganic phosphorus. *J Anim Sci.* 26:1024–1029.

Unterer, S., Lutz, H., Gerber, B., Glaus, T.M., Hässig, M., and Reusch, C.E. 2004. Evaluation of an electrolyte analyzer for measurement of ionized calcium and magnesium concentrations in blood, plasma, and serum of dogs. *Am J Vet Res.* 65(2):183–187.

van der Jagt, M.F.P., Wobbes, T., Strobbe, L.J.A., Sweep, F.G.C.J., and Span, P.N. 2010. Metalloproteinases and their regulators in colorectal cancer. *J Surg Oncol.* 101(3):259–269.

Van Zwieten, M.J., Frith, C.H., Nooteboom, A.L., et al. 1983. Medullary thyroid carcinoma in female BALB/c mice. A report of 3 cases with ultrastructural, immunohistochemical, and transplantation data. *Am J Pathol.* 110:219–229.

Vasikaran, S., Cooper, C., Eastell, R., et al. 2011a. International Osteoporosis Foundation and International Federation of Clinical Chemistry and Laboratory Medicine position on bone marker standards in osteoporosis. *Clin Chem Lab Med.* 49:1271–1274.

Vasikaran, S., Eastell, R., Bruyère, O., et al. 2011b. Markers of bone turnover for the prediction of fracture risk and monitoring of osteoporosis treatment: A need for international reference standards. *Osteoporos Int.* 22:391–420.

Vinholes, J., Guo, C.Y., Purohit, O.P. et al. 1997. Evaluation of new bone resorption markers in a randomized comparison of Pamidronate or Clodronate for hypercalcemia of malignancy. *J Clin Oncol.* 15:131–138.

Wei, J. and Ducy, P. 2010. Co-dependence of bone and energy metabolisms. *Arch Biochem Biophys.* 503:35–40.

Weiler, H.A., Wang, Z., and Atkinson, S.A. 1995. Dexamethasone treatment impairs calcium regulation and reduces bone mineralization in infant pigs. *Am J Clin Nutr.* 61:805–811.

Whyte, M.P. 2008. Hypophosphatasia: Nature's window on alkaline phosphatase function in humans. In *Principles of Bone Biology*. Eds. J.P. Bilezikian, L.G. Raisz, and T.J. Martin, pp. 1573–1598. San Diego, CA: Elsevier.

Wiedmeyer, C.E., Morton, D.G., Cusick, P.K., et al. 1999. Semiautomated analysis of alkaline phosphastas isoenzymes in serum of normal cynomolgus monkeys. *Vet Clin Path.* 28:2–7.

Wolfensohn, S.E. 2003. Case report of a possible familial predisposition to metabolic bone disease in juvenile rhesus macaques. *Lab Anim.* 37:139–144.

Wolford, S.R., Schroer, R.A., Gohs, F.X., et al. 1986. Reference range data base for serum chemistry and hematology values in laboratory animals. *J Toxicol Environ Health.* 18:161–188.

Xiong, J., Onal. M., Jilka, R.L., Weinstein, R.S., Manolagas, S.C., and O'brien, C.A. 2011. Matrix-embedded cells control osteoclast formation. *Nat Med.* 17:1235–1241.

Yamamoto, M., Yamaguchi, T., Yamauchi, M., Yano, S., and Sugimoto, T. 2011. Acute-onset hypomagnesemia-induced hypocalcemia caused by the refractoriness of bones and renal tubules to parathyroid hormone. *J Bone Mineral Metab.* 29:752–755.

Ylipahkala, H., Halleen, J.M., Kaija, H., et al. 2003. Tartrate-resistant acid phosphatase 5B circulates in human serum in complex with alpha2-macroglobulin and calcium. *Biochem Biophys Res Commun.* 308:320–324.

Zhao, Y., Cao, R., Ma, D., et al. 2011. Efficacy of calcium supplementation for human bone health by mass spectrometry profiling and cathepsin K measurement in plasma samples. *J Bone Miner Metab.* 29:552–560.

Zhong, Y., Armbrecht, H.J., and Christakos, S. 2009. Calcitonin, a regulator of the 25-hydroxyvitamin D3 1alpha-hydroxylase gene. *J Biol Chem.* 284:11059–11069.

16 Biochemistry of Immunoglobulins

Barbara R. von Beust and Gregory S. Travlos

CONTENTS

16.1 GENERAL CONSIDERATIONS

The immune system is a collection of multiple, interconnected and active, and adaptive mechanisms that together are essential for the body's defense against invasion by microbes and other organisms (a thorough review can be found in Tizard, 2013). Immunoglobulin (Ig) proteins or antibodies are an indispensable component of the immune system in vertebrates, including fish, linking the innate with the antigen-specific defense against invading pathogens such as viruses, bacteria, and parasites. Antibodies are produced by B-lymphocytes and plasma cells, which exclusively transcribe and translate Ig genes by a complex mechanism of recombination. Clonal selection or deletion depending on the affinity of the naturally occurring antibodies produced by their respective lymphocytes to a particular self or foreign antigen results in increasing antigen specificity and affinity, and enhanced efficacy of antigen neutralization or elimination. Aberrant or uncontrolled antibody production against self-antigens can contribute to or cause autoimmune diseases, such as lupus erythematosus. Finally, overproduction of certain antibody classes such as IgE in response to nonpathogenic antigens or allergens can lead to allergic conditions.

Ig can be quantitated either as a protein group in serum analysis or, more specifically, as antigen specific entities. Antibody concentrations vary according to age and are in general absent or lower in neonates, and increase with adulthood and the exposure to naturally occurring antigens in a normal, non-germ-free, environment.

Importantly, Ig can be partially or totally absent in gene-deficient animals (e.g., nude mice). As a consequence, antibody deficiency leads to increased incidence of infectious diseases and debilitating infections with agents of normally low virulence.

Ig diversity, critical for the development of the antigen specific antibody response, is generated through several processes (e.g., V(D)J recombination) that guide somatic rearrangements and mutations of DNA sequences of antigen receptor genes. The processes of simultaneous affinity increase for a particular antigen, and quantitative upgrading of antibody production by specialized plasma cells are unique. For example, through a complex sequence of somatic hypermutation in the Ig gene transcription and translation process, as well as highly regulated mechanisms of clonal expansion of selected B lymphocytes, over a million different antibody specificities with different functions and of variable classes can be identified in one individual. Likewise, clonal deletion of B-lymphocytes with unwanted specificities (e.g., self-recognition) grants protection from self-directed immune reactions in normal individuals. Finally, aberrant regulation of DNA-based recombination events can result in neoplastic geno- and phenotypes of B lymphocytes. There are two types of B lymphocytes (Table 16.1).

Antibody types and concentrations change and increase, respectively, throughout infancy and childhood unless the individual lives in a germ-free environment. Serum levels depend on synthetic rate and degradation or catabolic rate. Antibody secretion by a specialized plasma cell can reach up to several 1000 antibody molecules per second. The half-life depends on the antibody isotype and is longest in the IgG (up to 3 weeks) and shortest in IgD and IgE isotypes. While memory antibodies

TABLE 16.1
B-Lymphocyte Types Contributing to Protective Antibody Titers

	B1	**B2**
Antibody location	Membrane bound	Secreted, present in blood and tissues
Effect of antigen binding	B-lymphocyte activation, hypermutation, proliferation, antibody secretion, immunoregulation	Effector function: neutralization, complement binding, antibody-dependent cytotoxicity, mast cell degranulation
	Blood, mucosal surfaces	Blood, tissues
Isotypes	IgM, IgA, IgG	IgG, IgA, IgE
Location in lymph node	Marginal zone (naive cells)	Follicle (memory cells)
Affinity to antigen	Low	High
Antigen secretion rate, titers	Low	High, persistent, immunologic memory
CD5 expression	+	–

Source: Adapted from Manz, R.A. et al., *Annu Rev Immunol*, 23, 367–386, 2005.

can persist in serum for years, IgE will disappear within 2–3 days. It follows that the determination of "normal" Ig levels in different laboratory animal species should be accompanied by detailed documentation of health, respectively, infectious pathogen screening programs.

Ig typing and quantification require specific antibodies. Depending on the significance of a particular species to serve as a model of human disease, the qualitative and quantitative analysis of the different isotypes is more or less well documented to date.

Normal antibody levels from a biologic functional point of view cover a certain range. When below this range, increased incidence and severity of infectious diseases are anticipated and seen, including with organisms in general considered of low or no pathogenic potential. On the other side, persistent antibody levels above a certain range can become harmful by formation of immune complexes, leading for instance to glomerular disease in the kidneys.

For reviews concerning maintenance of antibody levels, see Manz et al. (2005); for specifics concerning mucosal antibody production, see Mage et al. (2006); and for details on V(D)J recombination, class switch recombination, and somatic hypermutation, see Xu et al. (2005), Dudley et al. (2005), and Cannon et al. (2004).

16.2 BASIC BIOCHEMISTRY AND GENETIC REGULATION

Most of the initial structural and genetic studies on Ig were performed in the murine and human species. Therefore, much information provided in this chapter is based on these studies to present a general overview of the structure and function of these proteins. However, it is recognized that there is a great diversity of Ig and Ig genes among the different species, and direct extrapolations from mouse and human immune systems are not always possible when studying other species. Some of the structural differences in the Ig of other species, particularly the rabbit, rat, nonhuman primate, and dog will be addressed, and special studies in swine are reviewed below.

Ig from all species possessing such molecules share some common structural features (for a review, see Tizard, 2013). The basic functional unit consists of four polypeptide chains, two light [L], and two heavy [H] chains, linked by interchain disulfide bridges. Each chain can further be subdivided into structural domains, containing at least one intrachain disulfide bond. The domain containing the amino-terminus of each polypeptide chain is termed the variable-region domain, and the domains adjacent to this are referred to as constant-region domains. The ligand-binding ability of Ig resides within the variable portion of the polypeptide chains. The diversity of amino acid sequences found within this region of the polypeptide chains (both H and L) accounts for the great variability of antigen-binding specificities exhibited by Ig. In contrast, the constant-region domains, so named due to their relatively constant amino acid composition among Ig of different specificities, mediate other effector functions associated with the Ig molecule, such as neutralization, complement fixation, protein A binding, opsonization, placental/intestinal transport, immediate hypersensitivity reactions, and antibody-dependent cellular cytotoxicity.

Ig heavy chains are composed of four to five domains, including the variable-region domain. Heavy chains have been further classified based on different structural determinants located in the constant-region domains. In contrast, Ig light chains are composed of only two structural domains and have been classified as being of the kappa (κ) or lambda (λ) isotype chain, again based on determinants found in the constant region of the polypeptide chain. The distribution among different species is shown in Table 16.2. The molecular weight of the light chains from a variety of species has been calculated to be between 20 and 25 kDa. Cross-reactivities between primate species have been noted using light chain inhibition of radioimmunoprecipitation assays (Spiegelberg, 1972).

Much of the information on the structural aspects of Ig molecules comes from molecular genetic studies of the Ig gene. Most of the work in this area was originally done on either mouse or human lymphocytes. Since the findings in the human system (Honjo et al., 1981; Rabbitts et al., 1981) corroborate principles found in the mouse, the murine system will be discussed here (Adams et al., 1981) as a general example of the structure of Ig genes. More recent molecular genetic and structural

TABLE 16.2
Expression of κ and λ Immunoglobulin Light Chain Isotypes in the Sera of Various Species

		Percentage of Light Chains in the Serum	
Order	**Species**	**κ**	**λ**
Lagomorpha	Rabbit	70–90	10–30
Rodentia	Mouse	95	5
	Rat	95	5
	Guinea pig	70	30
Carnivora	Dog	10	90
	Cat	10	90
Primates	Human	70	30
	Rhesus	50	50
	Baboon	50	50

studies of Ig have been conducted on other species and are discussed later (also reviewed in Eason et al., 2004).

Although Ig are composed of only two different polypeptide chains (heavy and light), the genes encoding these polypeptides are highly segmented at the genetic level (Figure 16.1). One should notice that each domain is coded for by one or more segments of DNA with special purpose areas, such as the hinge region or the hydrophobic tail of Ig (allowing insertion into the cell membrane), also encoded by separate gene segments. The heavy chain variable-region domain is encoded by three separate minigene segments (VH, D, and JH) in the germ-line DNA. The VH and D regions of DNA contain many different minigene segments that can be used to construct the variable-region domain, while the JH region contains only four possible segments. During maturation of the B lymphocyte, a recombinational event occurs at the level of the DNA joining one VH segment with one D segment and one JH segment to form a functional VDJ minigene adjacent to the mu

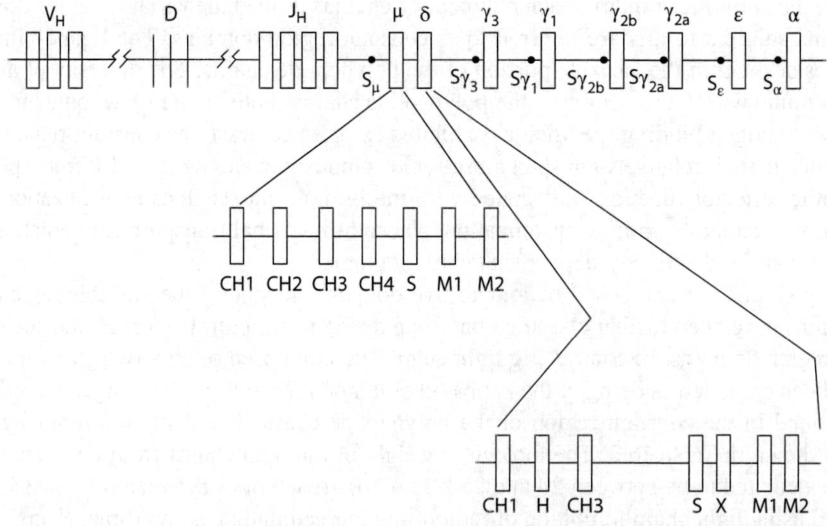

FIGURE 16.1 Diagram of murine Ig heavy chain gene loci. The variable (VH), diversity (D), junction (JH), and constant region genes (μ, δ, γ, ε, α) are shown within these loci. The μ and δ constant region portions are expanded to show individual coding segments for the protein domains (CH1–CH3, 4), hinge (H) region and membrane (M1, M2), and secreted (S, γ) tail pieces of the Ig molecule. Also shown are the switch sites (Sμ/Sγ3), which allow placement of VDJ gene segments adjacent to the various heavy chain gene regions.

minigene segment (Figure 16.2). Other rearrangements of the genome can also occur to place the VDJ segment in close proximity to other heavy chain constant region minigenes (isotype switching). The VDJ and constant region segments are joined at the level of transcription by RNA splicing to remove the intervening sequences of RNA between individual segments.

The light chain genes have a similar structural basis, with the exception that a D-region segment has not been described, so that only a VJ recombination occurs at the DNA level (Bernard et al., 1978; Sakano et al., 1979; Seidman et al., 1979; Valbuena et al., 1978). Five basic classes, or isotypes, have been defined (IgM, IgG, IgA, IgE, and IgD), and the various aspects of these heavy and light chain isotypes as they pertain to individual species of laboratory animals will be discussed below.

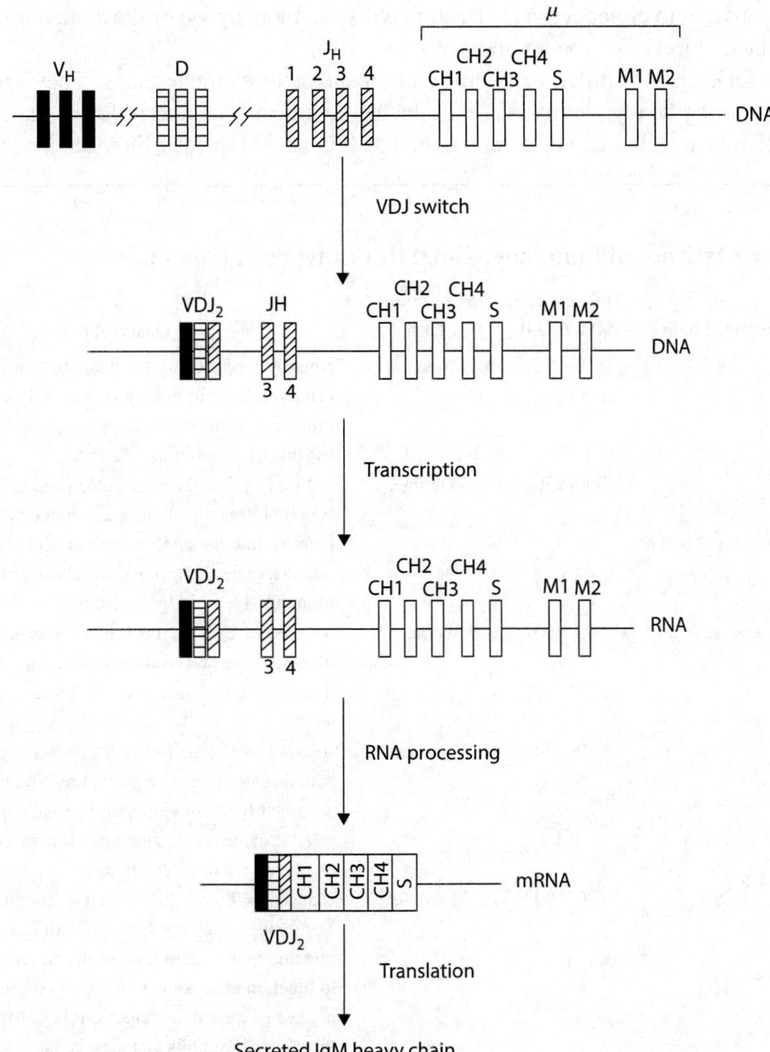

FIGURE 16.2 Diagram of IgM molecule formation (DNA and RNA level). Nascent DNA undergoes a rearrangement early in the development of B cells to yield a VDJ gene combination. The DNA is then transcribed into a precursor RNA molecule, which undergoes further processing and removal of intervening sequences between the VDJ gene segment and the various constant region genes. The mRNA product is then translated into its protein product, in this case a secreted IgM heavy chain molecule.

16.2.1 Immunoglobulin Isotypes

As mentioned previously, Ig come in different classes known as isotypes. In mammals, there are five antibody isotypes related to the different types of heavy chains the antibody contains, with each heavy chain class named alphabetically: α, γ, δ, ε, and μ (known as IgA, IgG, IgD, IgE, and IgM, respectively). Each isotype has different biologic and functional properties (Table 16.3). The classes and subclasses of Ig from a variety of species are shown in Table 16.4, arranged for comparison with their human Ig counterparts. In general, structural and functional correlates of the human Ig subclasses can be found in most other species, although some species appear to lack specific subclasses that can be correlated with their human IgG counterparts.

16.2.1.1 Immunoglobulin G

IgG is the most abundant Ig isotype found in mammalian serum. The central role of IgG is to bind to target antigens and to either activate effector cells (e.g., monocytes) or the complement system to destroy Ig-coated objects (Schroeder and Cavacini, 2010).

All of the IgGs share similar structural and biochemical characteristics. They are composed of two light and two heavy chains and exist in the serum in monomeric form. Interchain disulfide bridges join heavy chains. For example, mouse IgG has three such linkages among the heavy

TABLE 16.3
General Characteristics of Immunoglobulin (Ig) Isotypes in Mammals

Ig Isotype	Heavy Chain	Approximate MW (kDa)	Functional Unit	Description
IgG	γ	150–180	Monomer	Primarily produced by B cells in the spleen and LN, it is the primary circulating Ig responsible for humoral immunity against invading pathogens. The only Ig capable of crossing the placenta.
IgM	μ	900–950	Pentamer	Produced by B cells in the spleen and LN, it is found on B-cell plasma membranes as a monomer, but is secreted into the circulation as a pentamer. Acts as a first responder Ig during the early stages of humoral immunity (prior to IgG secretion).
IgA	α	350–400	Dimer	Produced by B cells; it is found associated with the mucosa of gut, respiratory, and urinary tracts, prevents microbial colonization; also in breast milk, saliva, and tears.
IgE	ε	180–200	Monomer	Produced by B cells found in LN draining sites of antigen entry (e.g., the gut and respiratory tracts); least abundant Ig in circulation, it is usually bound to mast cells. Provides protection against parasites and is involved in allergic reactions.
IgD	δ	170–180	Monomer	Produced by B cells, it is found on B-cell plasma membranes often coexpressed with IgM. It is also secreted in low amounts into the circulation. It appears to function as an antigen receptor on B cells that have not been exposed to antigens. It has also been shown to activate basophils and mast cells.

Source: Adapted from Pier, G.B. et al., *Immunology, Infection, and Immunity*, ASM Press, Washington, 2004; Geisberger, R. et al., *Immunology*, 118, 889–898, 2006; Chen, K. et al., *Nat Immunol*, 10, 889–898, 2009; Tizard, I., *Veterinary Immunology*, Elsevier, St. Louis, 2013.

LN, lymph node.

TABLE 16.4
Immunoglobulin Classes and Subclasses in Different Species

Species	Immunoglobulin Class and Subclass				
Human	IgG1, IgG2, IgG3, IgG4	IgA1, IgA2	IgM1, IgM2	IgE	IgD
Ape	IgG[a]	IgA	IgM	IgE	IgD
Monkey	IgG[b]	IgA	IgM[c]	IgE	IgD
Mouse	IgG2a, IgG2b, IgG3, IgG1	IgA1, IgA2	IgM	IgE	IgD
Rat	IgG2a, IgG2b, IgG2c, IgG1	IgA	IgM	IgE	IgD
Rabbit	IgG2, IgG1	IgA1, IgA2	IgM	IgE	IgD
Dog	IgG1, IgG2, IgG3, IgG4	IgA	IgM	IgE	IgD
Swine[d]	IgG1, IgG2, IgG3, IgG4, IgG5, IgG6	IgA	IgM	IgE	IgD

[a] Using antisera specific for human subclasses, four corresponding subclasses have been identified in the chimpanzee, gorilla, and orangutan.
[b] Four subclasses have been identified in the baboon based on γ-chain differences, though these determinants are not shared with the human subclasses.
[c] Two distinct types have been reported in the rhesus monkey after immunization.
[d] According to Butler et al. (2009a).

chains, while the rabbit IgG has only a single disulfide link similar to that found in human IgM and IgD. IgG from other species, however, may be more variable in the number of interchain disulfide bridges, as evidenced from the human IgG subclasses, which have 2–15 such linkages among the chains.

The IgG isotype exhibits the greatest degree of diversity with respect to the number of subclasses defined for each species. Four subclasses have been defined for human, dog, mouse, and rat IgG. In nonhuman primates, the cross-reactivity of five different rabbit polyclonal antibodies to human IgG and IgG subclasses (IgG1, IgG2, IgG3, and IgG4) was examined for several apes, including New and Old World monkeys (Asada et al., 2002). The authors demonstrated that, similar to previous reports, the level of reactivity of antihuman IgG antibody with plasma IgG from different primate species was related to the phylogenic distance from humans. Antisera specific for the four human subclasses identified similar molecules in the sera of chimpanzees, gorillas, and orangutans (Alepa, 1968; Alepa and Terry, 1965). Based on antigenic differences in the Fc region of the Ig-heavy chain molecule, baboons demonstrated four IgG subclasses (Damian et al., 1971). More recently, serum protein A- and protein G-purified human IgG consisted of IgG1, IgG2, IgG3, and IgG4, whereas baboon and macaque IgG demonstrated only IgG1, IgG2, and IgG4 (Shearer et al., 1999).

Cleaved by various enzymes, IgG molecules yield specific peptide fragments. For example, treatment with papain cleaves the IgG molecule into three fragments of approximately equal molecular weight (45–50 kDa). Two of the fragments formed contain an intact antigen-binding region (light chain plus two heavy chain domains) and are termed the Fab portion of the molecule. The third fragment, termed the Fc portion, is composed entirely of heavy chain domains from the carboxyl-terminal end of the molecule. The isolated Fc portion of rabbit Ig was found to crystallize from solution, indicating the homogeneity of the isolate (Porter, 1959). However, Fc regions from other species, including the dog, mouse, and rat, do not crystallize easily from solution. In contrast, rabbit IgG is composed almost entirely of a single IgG subclass (IgG1) and therefore would yield a very homogeneous preparation of Fc fragments for crystallization.

Pepsin treatment of IgG from most species, including rabbits (Nisonoff et al., 1960a, b) and people (Nisonoff et al., 1975a), yields a single large fragment termed $F(ab')_2$ (MW 95 kDa), which includes the hinge region of the original molecule and some smaller fragments of the Fc portion of the molecule that are nonfunctional and not recognized by Fc-specific antisera. However, mouse

IgG has been shown to be sensitive to treatment with pepsin, although not yielding many $F(ab')_2$ fragments; instead, the molecule is digested into smaller fragments. This sensitivity to pepsin digestion is presumed to reflect unfolding or denaturation of the molecule caused by the low pH required for proteolytic activity of the enzyme (Gorini et al., 1969).

The various IgG subclasses have been defined using subclass-specific antisera; however, they differ in their functional (to be discussed later) and some of their biochemical properties. The IgG1 (IgGd) subclass of the dog differs from IgG of other species in that this molecule will not cause precipitation of multideterminant antigens from solution. Structural analysis of both molecules does not show any commonality that could account for this property (Grant et al., 1972).

16.2.1.2 Immunoglobulin M

Immunoglobulin M is the second most abundant and largest Ig isotype found in mammalian serum (Tizard, 2013). Due to its size, IgM is predominantly found in plasma; it does not cross the placenta and is found in tissue fluids in small amounts. Dubbed the "natural antibody," IgM has been isolated from serum bound to specific antigens without prior immunization (Jayasekera et al., 2007). It is the first antibody to appear in response to initial exposure to an antigen and is superior to IgG at complement activation (i.e., 1000-fold higher binding affinity for C1q than IgG, see Ehrenstein and Notley, 2010). On its own, IgM is not an effective opsonin (Wellek et al., 1976); however, with the activation of complement, it does amplify opsonization by inducing antigen binding by C3b. IgM is also primarily responsible for the erythrocyte agglutination that occurs as result of an incompatible blood transfusion.

IgM has been found in virtually all vertebrates tested and is thought to be the most evolutionarily conserved Ig class. Generally, this class does not show any subclass diversity; however, human IgM is known to exist in two forms (IgM1 and IgM2), and there has been a suggestion that the rhesus monkey may also have two forms of IgM (Lakin et al., 1969).

Secreted IgM from all species exists primarily as a pentamer of the basic 7S subunit characteristic of Ig. This 19S molecule has a molecular weight in the range of 900–1000 kDa (Bours et al., 2005; Tizard, 2013). The 7S chains are linked by a J chain disulfide bonded to the penultimate half-cystine residue of the heavy chains (Mestecky and Schrohenloher, 1974). The J chain is associated with IgM molecules from most species, including people, dogs, rabbits, mice, and rats. The molecular weight of the J chain is between 14 and 16 kDa, depending upon the species from which it was isolated and the procedure used for analysis. The J chain has also been shown to be a highly conserved molecule among the vertebrates. There is a high degree of sequence homology and cross-reactivity of anti-J chain antisera between widely divergent species.

Classically, the IgM pentameric structure can be disintegrated into its components by the reduction of the J chain disulfide links with 2-mercaptoethanol. The 7S unit of IgM is characteristically heavier than its IgG counterpart, having a molecular weight of 190 kDa (Arnason et al., 1964; Fahey et al., 1964a; Lakin et al., 1969). This is due in part to the IgM molecule containing an extra heavy chain domain (four heavy chain domains in IgG, five in IgM) and to the higher proportion of carbohydrate groups associated with the heavy chain (10%–11% carbohydrate for IgM, vs. 2%–3% for IgG). This higher content of carbohydrate allows separation of IgM from IgG by using a lentil-lectin affinity column preferentially binding the IgM molecules. Proteolytic digestion of IgM with papain or pepsin will yield Fab and $F(ab')_2$ fragments, respectively, as found for IgG; however, the Fc portion is usually digested and cannot be isolated as an intact fraction as with IgG (Richerson et al., 1968).

As mentioned above, the polymerization of the IgM molecules results most commonly in secretion of a pentamer. However, though not abundant, a hexameric form of IgM also exists in people and animals (Hughey et al., 1998; Wiersma et al., 1998). While the J chain is found in the pentameric form of IgM, it is not found in the hexameric form (Kownatzki, 1973). Additionally, while its physiologic function/relevance has not been characterized, hexameric IgM has a higher activity of complement fixation than pentameric IgM (Randall et al., 1990). This increased activity can range between 2- and >100-fold depending on species of the complement source (Randall et al., 1990; Collins et al., 2002).

16.2.1.3 Immunoglobulin A

The structure and function of IgA in people and other species have been reviewed (Kerr, 1990; Woof and Russell, 2011; Snoeck et al., 2006; Rogier et al., 2014). This Ig class and the respective B lymphocytes are primarily found in tissues associated with mucosal surfaces, their glands and their secretions, respectively. This includes salivary gland and saliva, liver and bile, mammary gland, colostrum and milk, lacrimal gland and tears, and the intestine. Stability to protease activity is provided by a polymeric structure and the association with the secretory component. While IgA typically will not contribute to agglutination or opsonization, it is an important mediator of antibody-dependent cytotoxicity, and a process called immune exclusion on mucosal surfaces. In terms of immunomodulation, fetal IgA has been found to be able to bind potentially harmful maternal autoreactive antibodies. Typically, activated natural IgA producing B lymphocytes will migrate from the mucosa-associated immune tissue (MALT) through the blood and lymph to high endothelial venules and subepithelial stroma, where potential pathogens will be bound and transported back to the lumen of the gut. An exception to this process was found in rodents and lagomorphs, where polymeric serum IgAs are directly secreted from bile and hepatocytes to the gut.

The secreted form of IgA is typically a dimer (or larger polymer) of the 7S monomer linked by both a J chain and a secretory component (SC, MW 70 kDa). The J chain is structurally the same as that associated with IgM and binds the IgA molecule at the penultimate half-cystine on the heavy chains. The secretory component, which has high carbohydrate content (15%–20%), is also associated with the heavy chains. This association includes both noncovalent and covalent interactions of the secretory component with the IgA heavy chain. The noncovalent interactions occur between the N-terminal SC1 portion of the secretory component and the $C\alpha3$ domains of IgA. The covalent associations are the disulfide bonds forming between the SC5 of the secretory component and the cysteine at position 311 of the IgA heavy chain (Mestecky et al., 1991). The secretory component is derived from a transmembrane protein called polymeric Ig receptor expressed on the surface of epithelial cells (Mostov et al., 1980; Mostov and Bloebel, 1982). This protein has structural homologies with the Ig molecule (Mostov et al., 1984) and is used to transport IgA or IgM from the basolateral surface of the cell, across the intracellular matrix (as an endocytotic vesicle), and to the luminal surface, where a proteolytic event cleaves the protein, yielding the soluble secretory piece in association with the polymeric Ig molecules (Mullock et al., 1979; Nagura et al., 1979; Renston et al., 1980; Simionescu, 1979; Sztul et al., 1983).

In most species, the secretory component is disulfide bonded to the IgA molecule, which is supported by biochemical evidence (i.e., a larger sedimentation coefficient and resistance to reduction with 2-mercaptoethanol) would suggest that IgA from these species contains a secretory component as well. Polymers of the basic 7S molecules have been demonstrated in the secretions of rats. Dog, mouse, pig, and primate (baboon, rhesus monkey) IgA appear to have properties similar to human IgA, both structurally and in the heterogeneity of electrophoretic patterns.

Serum IgA cannot bind to complement component C1q and thus cannot activate the classical pathway; however, activation of the alternate pathway seems possible.

16.2.1.4 Immunoglobulin E

Immunoglobulin E or reaginic (homocytotropic) antibody has been reported in people and in current laboratory animal species, either in their own right as in dogs (clinically relevant skin and food allergies) or as models for the study of allergic syndromes such as asthma, or the treatment thereof, including pigs (reviewed in Hammerberg, 2009; Rupa et al., 2009). IgE plays a crucial role in the type I hypersensitivity response and in the body's defense against parasites (Gould et al., 2003; Erb, 2007; Fitzsimmons et al., 2007; Duarte et al., 2007; Keir et al., 2011). The least abundant isotype found in the circulation, IgE is capable of provoking a robust inflammatory response (Winter et al., 2000). The functional properties of IgE are discussed in Section 16.3.9 and have been reviewed by Prussin and Metcalfe (2006).

The IgE molecule exists in the serum of most species as a four-chain monomer with a sedimentation coefficient of 8S, corresponding to a MW of 185–200 kDa. IgE molecules are not transferred through the placenta, do not activate complement, and are heat labile, losing their reaginic activity after exposure to 56°C for 1 hour. In blood, the half-life is between 1 and 5 days, in the skin IgE molecules persist for relatively long periods (>6 days) after passive transfer. IgE levels are lowest at birth and gradually increase up to the age of about 20 years in people, thereafter the levels decline steadily. IgE levels increase in response to infection with parasites or in conditions that include skin disease, neoplasias, and immune deficiencies. The low concentration of IgE in serum has precluded direct isolation and characterization of this molecule; therefore, most of what is known about the structure of IgE has been obtained from IgE myeloma proteins as found in certain people, dogs, mice, and rats with specific gammopathies. However, the physical and functional properties that are known for each species appear to be similar to the model IgE molecules isolated from people and mice. For a review, see Kelly and Grayson (2016).

16.2.1.5 Immunoglobulin D

This Ig represents an oddity among the isotypes in that no clear effector functions had been assigned to the IgD molecule for a long time. This is due to the extremely low concentrations of IgD found in the serum (<1 μg/mL). However, the availability of IgD myeloma proteins from mouse and people as well as the comparative study of Ig genotypes in different species has revealed recently that IgD is present in all jawed vertebrates (see reviews by Chen et al., 2009 and Sun et al., 2011).

Being expressed together with IgM as one of the first Ig in ontogeny, but also in the development of B-cell mediated immune responses, IgD is now considered an important link between native resistance to infection and the antigen-specific immune response (Chen et al., 2009). Considering that IgD-producing mature but naïve B lymphocytes mainly home to aerodigestive mucosal structures such as tonsils, adenoids, salivary and lacrimal glands, as well as the nasal mucosa undermines the importance of IgD as an early mediator in response to invading pathogens. High concentrations of IgD have also been found in mammary gland, bronchial and pancreatic secretions, in cerebrospinal and amniotic fluid, and it has been found to be produced in the fetus. In serum, the half-life of IgD is 2.8 days, with a catabolic rate comparable to IgM. IgD also exists as a transmembrane Ig receptor involved in B-lymphocyte signaling, where it complements IgM. After secretion, it can bind to myeloid cells such as basophils and mast cells, which in turn will release B-cell stimulatory mediators, such as IL-4 and IL-13. In cases of allergic skin disease, binding of IgD to neutrophils has been observed. Secreted IgD contains mostly λ light chains, which is in contrast to other Ig isotypes, and membrane bound IgD (Chen and Cerutti, 2010, 2011).

However, the exact function of membrane bound as well as secreted IgD is not yet clear. Mice deficient in IgD showed a slightly delayed antibody response and lower numbers of peripheral mature B cells, suggesting a role in B-cell homeostasis. Interestingly, IgD binds to virulence relevant antigens in pathogenic viruses and bacteria. Also, some studies showed that IgD levels were increased during infections in general, and in individuals with IgA deficiency in particular. For a detailed review, see Chen and Cerutti (2010). Finally, an age-dependent drop in IgD correlates with the reduced immunity in older individuals.

Based on current knowledge, IgD is in summary considered an important mediator for adaptive B-cell responses and antimicrobial activation of myeloid cells such as basophils (Chen et al., 2010).

The structure and biochemistry of mouse and human IgD have been extensively studied. In addition, significant advances in animal genome availability and gene identification strategies allowed lining up the respective gene sequences of the putative protein sequence of the mammalian IgD light and heavy chains in different species (see Chen and Cerutti, 2010; Ohta and Flajnik, 2006; Sun et al., 2011). Primate IgD appears to be structurally similar to human IgD, which is composed of four heavy chain domains and two light chain domains. The first and second constant-region domains are separated by a hinge region similar to that found in IgG and IgA molecules. However, IgD is unique in that this region is highly extended (64 amino acid residues) in people (Putnam et al., 1982), which makes the hinge more susceptible to proteolytic enzymes. In contrast, mouse IgD has been shown to lack an extended hinge region and also is missing the second constant-region domain (Tucker et al., 1982). However, the molecular weight of the heavy chain reported for mouse IgD (70,000 Da) is comparable to human IgD (70,000 Da), due to a larger content of carbohydrates (Pearson et al., 1977; Sitia et al., 1977). The human IgD molecule is also known to have a single disulfide link between each of the heavy and light chain portions, as well as one disulfide link between the two heavy chains in the lower half of the hinge region. Since this region is absent from mouse IgD, Putnam et al. (1982) have hypothesized that mouse IgD does not contain an interheavy chain disulfide bridge and may exist as an HL monomer. However, strong noncovalent bonds may form a stable H2L2 molecule as well. For a review on structure and functional properties of IgD in different species, see Preud'homme et al. (2000).

16.2.2 Immunoglobulin Allotypes and Idiotypes

While the basic structural characteristics of Ig are very similar, there is a substantial heterogeneity in amino acid sequences in both the constant and variable regions of the light and heavy chains. These differences often reflect only one or a few amino acid substitutions, and are most commonly detected by appropriate antisera that contain antibodies (i.e., anti-antibodies) able to recognize subtle differences among molecules. There are three major serologically and structurally defined determinants that are found on Ig of most of the species that have been studied. These markers are isotypes, allotypes, and idiotypes. Since isotypes are presented in Section 16.2.1, this section focuses on the latter two components of Ig.

16.2.2.1 Immunoglobulin Allotypes

Allotypes are inherited variants of Ig light and heavy chains that segregate in a simple Mendelian fashion among members of an outbred species. As a result, the allelic amino acid sequence of Ig can vary between individuals within a population. Many of the currently studied Ig allotypes are analogous in many respects to the allelic forms of other proteins, such as the hemoglobin chains. However, there are some interesting exceptions that have a very complex pattern of inheritance and expression. These more complex systems will be discussed later as we consider individual species differences. Several good reference articles on allotypes are available (Pandey and Li, 2013).

The genetically determined antigenic differences in the serum Ig of all of the species to be covered here are attributed to amino acid substitutions caused by mutations in the corresponding structural genes. Unlike genetic variants of other proteins, allotype variations do not appear to affect antibody specificity or any known biologic function of Ig. The fact that allotypy does not affect antibody specificity is not surprising, since most allotypic determinants are located completely within the constant region of the light or heavy chain, and the antibody combining site is, of course, completely within the variable region. The rabbit is one exception to the generalization regarding the placement of the allotypic determinant since it is now well established that several allotypes are found in the variable region of rabbit Ig heavy chains.

When animals are bred, each expressing a different allele at a given locus, the heterozygous offspring expresses both allotypes in the serum Ig. This codominant expression of allotypes is seen in all species studied and occurs with both heavy and light chain allotypes. Thus, in an animal that is heterozygous for both heavy and light chain alleles, all four alleles are seen in the serum. Since it is generally agreed that an antibody-producing cell expresses only one of two possible parental heavy chain alleles and one of two parental light chain alleles (allelic exclusion), the serum contains a mixture of symmetric Ig molecules, that is, both heavy chains have the same allotypic determinant and both light chains have the same allotypic determinant on any given antibody molecule. Genetic studies using Ig allotypes as markers revealed that genes coding for heavy chains and light chains were not linked, and that κ and λ light chain genes were also unlinked. Further, studies with rabbit heavy chain allotypes led investigators to hypothesize that the variable and constant region genes represent a gene family on the same chromosome. These conclusions based solely upon studies with allotypes have subsequently been verified by somatic cell geneticists and molecular biologists.

16.2.2.1.1 Methods of Detecting Allotypes

Allotypes are typically identified by antibodies that are able to recognize individual allotypic determinants. Antiallotypic antibodies are generally elicited by injecting the Ig (or antibody–antigen complexes) of a donor individual bearing the allotype into a recipient of the same species lacking the allotype. While antiallotypic antibodies can be raised by immunizing across species (i.e., mouse Ig into rabbit), one must then adsorb the rabbit antisera with mouse sera that do not contain the reference allotype. Prolonged immunization is frequently required to elicit allotype-specific antibodies, but the response can be enhanced by immunization with antibody–antigen complexes in Freund's complete adjuvant. Antisera specific for human allotypes are obtained from multiparous women, patients who have received blood transfusions, or patients recovering from various diseases.

Immunoprecipitation tests in agar gel (Oudin, 1960) can be employed for the detection of allotypic specificities in some species, particularly rabbits. Since some allotypes are manifested by only minor structural changes in the polypeptide chain, anti-allotypic antisera often detect only one or two unique antigenic determinants. In such cases, there is an insufficient development of a lattice formation that is required for an allotype–antiallotype precipitate to form. Therefore, other detection methods such as hemagglutination inhibition and radioimmunoassays (RIAs) using solid-phase adsorption or fluid phase second antibody precipitations are used (Gilman et al., 1964; Landucci-Tosi and Mage, 1970). The RIAs have a distinct advantage in that they are quantitative and one can detect the proportions of allotypic markers in test sera. Several typical RIAs have been described (Gilman et al., 1964; Landucci-Tosi and Mage, 1970).

16.2.2.1.2 Rabbit Allotypes

Allotypic determinants in the rabbit were first discovered in 1956. Since this original discovery, numerous allotypes have been identified and characterized (Kindt, 1975). The allotype gene loci are designated by small italicized letters (*a*, *b*, *c*, etc.), and the individual determinants (allotypes) at each locus are designated by nonitalicized letters and numbers (al, a2, a3, etc.). The numbers are assigned consecutively in order of their discovery, regardless of the positions of the loci coding for the determinant. Each species has a different nomenclature that will be covered as each is discussed. A representative list of the rabbit allotypes and their location within a particular heavy or light chain of Ig is presented in Table 16.5. Note that allotypes have been found in the constant region of κ (*b*) (Dray et al., 1962) and λ (*c*) (Dray et al., 1963) light chains, and the constant regions of γ (*d* and *e*, these may be identical), α1, (*f*), α2 (*g*), and μ (*n*) heavy chains. It is of particular interest that a few loci code for allotypic determinants detected in the variable region (*a*, *x*, *y*) of the rabbit heavy chain. These variable region allotypes are found on Ig of all isotypes.

The *a* and *b* loci constitute an exceptional case. These are so-called complex allotypes, since when the chains carrying these allotypes were sequenced, no single allotype-specific residue could be identified. This was the case with most other allotypes as well. The determinants coded for by the *a* and *b* loci consisted of a multitude of amino acid residues. The *a*l, *a*2, and *a*3 and *b*4, *b*5, *b*6, and *b*9 loci may represent in a tightly linked cluster. If *b*4, *b*5, *b*6, and *b*9 were alleles, a single individual should not possess more than two of them, and this is true. However, several investigators have reported rabbits transiently expressing three alleles. This may occur with greater frequency after hyperimmunization with a single antigen such as ovalbumin. While the transitory and latent allotypes may be explained by regulatory genes that alter the expression of structural genes within a cluster, the issue remains currently unresolved.

Rabbits heterozygous for the *a* and *b* loci exhibit a preferential expression of each allele, that is, *a*101 > *a*l > *a*3 > *a*2 > *a*100 and *b*4 > *b*6 > *b*5 > *b*9. This order may change in the face of an infectious disease or after immunization with different antigens. Nearly all molecules of rabbit IgG are precipitated by a combination of anti-*b* or anti-*c* locus allotypes, indicating that if another light chain locus exists, it must code for a very small proportion of rabbit light chains (Vice et al., 1970). Since these two genes segregate independently, it was correctly speculated that they exist on separate chromosomes (Gilman-Sachs et al., 1969). It was also noted that the genes coding for the light

TABLE 16.5
Rabbit Immunoglobulin Allotypes

Locus	Chain Location	Alleles
A	Variable Heavy H Chain	*a*1, *a*2, *a*3, *a*100–*a*103
x	Variable Heavy H Chain	x32, x
y	Variable Heavy H Chain	y33, y
n	Constant μ H Chain	Ms16, Ms17
d	Constant γ H Chain	D11, d12
e	Constant γ H Chain	e14, e15
f	Constant α1 H Chain	F69–f73
g	Constant α2 H Chain	g74–g77
t	Secretory Component of IgA	t61, t62
b	Constant κ L Chain	b4, b5, b6, b9
c	Constant λ L Chain	c7, c21

chain allotypes were not linked to the genes controlling markers on rabbit heavy chains (Dray et al., 1963; Kelus and Gell, 1967; Oudin, 1960).

16.2.2.1.3 Mouse and Rat Allotypes

The recommended nomenclature for allotypes in mice designates the loci by Igh or Igl (h and l for heavy and light chains, respectively) with a number assigned in the order of discovery (Igh-1, Igh-2, Igh-3, etc.). The allotypic determinants are also designated consecutively in order of their discovery and are separated from the locus by a period (Igh-1.1, Igh-1.2, Igh-1.3, etc.). Mouse heavy chain allotypes and their isotype association are listed in Table 16.6. All of the loci listed here code for determinants found in the constant region of the molecule. Most of the allotypic determinants in the mouse, however, are on the constant region, and they are restricted to a single Ig class and subclass. As noted in Table 16.7, there are exceptions, for example, determinant four is shared by IgG2a and IgG2b, and determinant eight is shared by IgG1 and IgG2a.

The heavy chain allotype loci in the mouse are closely linked genes. Specific combinations of alleles at these loci (haplotypes) are designated in Table 16.7, and the distribution of the alleles among selected inbred strains is illustrated in Table 16.8. The mouse Igh-1 locus is unusually polymorphic with 12 alleles (see Table 16.8). The allotypes at this locus are very complex and resemble those of the rabbit *a* and *b* loci.

No serologically defined allotypic variants have been identified in the κ light chains, but intraspecies differences of V-regions have been detected by other means (i.e., isoelectric focusing and peptide mapping). Allotypes similar to those of inbred strains have been observed in wild mice. The wild mice, however, exhibit new haplotypes suggesting that recombinational events have occurred within the Igh locus.

Contrary to the lack of allotypic variants in the mouse κ light chain, rats exhibit two alleles of this gene. The locus in the rat is termed RI-1, and there are two allotypes: RI-la is found in the DA-inbred strain, and RI-lb is found in the LEW strain (Gutman and Weissman, 1971). These two markers are also considered to be complex allotypes, since they differ by 11 amino acid substitutions (Gutman et al., 1975).

16.2.2.1.4 Nonhuman Primate Allotypes

The first human allotype was discovered using an indirect method based upon the inhibition of hemagglutination similar to the one previously described (Grubb, 1956). The genetic locus was termed Gm, since the determinant was found on the gammaglobulins. Six human heavy chain loci

TABLE 16.6
Mouse and Rat Immunoglobulin Allotypes

Locus	Chain	Alleles	Allotypic Determinants
Mouse Allotypes			
Igh-1	γ2a	1a–1h; 1j–1m	1–8; 26–30
Igh-2	α	2a–2d; 2f	12, 13, 14, 15, 17, 35
Igh-3	Γ2b	3a, 3b, 3d–3g	4, 9, 11, 16, 22, 23, 31–34
Igh-4	γ1	4a, 4b, 4d	18, 19, 42
Igh-5	δ	5a, 5b	36, 37
Igh-6	μ	6a, 6b, 6e	38–41
Rat Allotypes			
RI-1	κ	1a, 1b	

TABLE 16.7
Igh Haplotypes of Mice

Prototype Strain	Igh Haplotype	Gene Loci Encoding Allotypic Determinants (Ig Chain in Parentheses) Igh-1 (γ2a)	Igh-2(a)	Igh-3(γ2b)	Igh-4(γ1)	Igh-5(δ)	Igh-6(μ)
BALB/c	a	1, 6, 7, 8, 26, 28, 29, 30	12, 13, 14	9, 11, 22, 31, 33, 34	8, 19	36	38, 39
C57BL	b	2, 27, 29	15	9, 16, 22, 33, 34	42	37	40, 41
DBA/2	c	3, 8, 29	35	9, 11, 22, 31, 33, 34	8, 19	36	–
AKR	d	4, 6, 7, 8, 26, 29	13, 17	4, 23, 31, 32, 33, 34	8, 19	36	–
A	e	4, 6, 7, 8, 26, 28, 29, 30	13, 17	4, 23, 31, 32, 33	8, 19	36	39, 41
CE	f	5, 7, 8, 26, 30	14	9, 11, 31, 32	8, 19	36	–
RIII	g	3, 8, 26	35	9, 11, 31	8, 19	36	–
SEA	h	1, 6, 7, 8, 28, 29	12, 13, 14	9, 11, 22, 31, 33, 34	8, 19	36	38, 39
CBA	j	1, 6, 7, 8, 28, 29, 30	12, 13, 14	9, 11, 22, 31, 33, 34	8, 19	36	38, 39
KH-1	k	3, 5, 7, 8	35	9, 11, 25	8, 19	–	–
KH-2	l	3, 5, 8	35	9, 11, 22	8, 19	–	–
Ky	m	1, 2, 6, 7, 8	15	9, 16, 22	8, 19	–	–
NZB	n	4, 6, 7, 8, 26, 28, 24, 30	13, 17	4, 23, 31, 32, 33	8, 19	36	39, 41

have been identified: G1m, G2m, G3m, Mm, A2m, and Km, encoding allotypes on γ1, γ2, γ3, μ, α2, and κ chains, respectively. In his review, Dugoujon (1993) presented findings for Ig allotypes (Gm, Am, and Km) in nonhuman primates belonging to 72 species and subspecies of the Hominoidea, Cercopithecoidea, Ceboidea, Lorisoidea, and Tupaoidea superfamilies. The distribution of human allotypes was also presented. There were allotypes that were exclusive to people. Hominoidea,

TABLE 16.8
Distribution of Alleles (Igh Haplotypes) at the Igh Loci in Different Mouse Strains

		Locus (Chain)					
Igh Haplotype	**Prototype Strain**	**Igh-1 (γ2a)**	**Igh-2 (α)**	**Igh-3 (γ2b)**	**Igh-4 (l)**	**Igh-5 (δ)**	**Igh-6 (μ)**
a	BALB/c	a	a	a	a	a	a
b	C57BL	b	b	b	b	b	b
c	DBA/2	c	c	a	a	a	•
d	AKR	d	d	d	a	a	•
e	A	e	d	e	a	e	e
f	CE	f	f	f	a	a	•
g	RIII	g	c	g	a	a	•
h	SEA	h	a	a	a	a	•
j	CBA/H	j	a	a	a	a	a
k	KH-1 (wild)	k	c	a	a	•	•
l	KH-2 (wild)	l	c	a	a	•	•
m	Ky	m	b	b	b	•	•
n	NZB	e	d	e	a	a	e

however, demonstrated the most Gm allotypes with relatively few reported for Cercopithecoidea and Prosimians; no allotypes were reported for platyrrhinian species.

16.2.2.2 Immunoglobulin Idiotypes

Idiotypes are a group of structural variants that result from variations in the amino acid sequence of the antigenic determinants located exclusively in the variable region of the light and heavy chains. In contrast to the allotypes that are typically found on all Ig of a given isotype, the idiotypic determinants represent individual and specific markers, with each antibody or myeloma protein having its own unique set of idiotypic determinants. One may think of idiotypes on Ig as being analogous to the fingerprints of an individual, since both can be used to distinguish unique entities.

While Ig represent a relatively homogenous group of glycoproteins when compared between and within species, the heterogeneity of the amino acid sequences in the amino-terminal (variable region) of the molecule results in almost unsurpassed heterogeneity. This variability called idiotypic determinants is responsible for the almost unlimited possibility for selecting and adapting idiotypes to suit the recognition of all possible antigens an individual is confronted with. Specifically, each antibody-producing cell secretes an antibody with a single defined idiotype. Only through the unique mechanisms of preexisting gene sequence recombination in the different V, D, and J regions of the Ig gene, this almost unlimited diversity is possible. This activity is controlled by recombination-activating genes RAG-1 and RAG-2 and a cellular repair mechanism. In Table 16.9, the estimated diversity levels for each V, D, and J regions are summarized. The almost unlimited combined diversity grants for the recognition of virtually any possible antigen. Through selective proliferation (clonal expansion), triggered by repeated immunization of an animal with a defined antigen, the number of specific B lymphocytes will increase and the respective titer of this particular antibody will rise.

Several excellent review articles documenting the molecular structure, the genetic regulation and the biologic and functional significance of idiotypes are available (Eichman, 1978; vanLoghem and Litwin, 1972). Therefore, our focus in this section will be limited to a few generalizations about idiotypes and anti-idiotype antibodies that apply to all of the species that produce antibodies.

TABLE 16.9
Diversification of B-Lymphocyte Antigen Receptor Idiotype Elements

	Immunoglobulin	
Element	**Heavy Chain**	**κ and λ**
V segments	65	70
D segments	27	–
J segments	6	5κ and 4λ
Number of V region combinations	3.4×10^6	3.4×10^6
Junctional diversity	3×10^7	3×10^7
Total diversity	10^{14}	10^{14}

Source: Adapted from Market, E., and Papavasiliou, F.N., *PLoS Biol*, 1, e16, 2003.

The best characterized idiotypes are those reported in mice. It has been demonstrated with conventional and monoclonal antibodies (usually by direct or indirect quantitative precipitation and RIA) that some preparations of idiotype-specific reagents can recognize a single amino acid interchange within the variable region. In spite of this exquisite resolving power of anti-idiotype antibodies, one cannot draw conclusions regarding structural identity of antibodies based solely upon the binding of the antibody to two separate antibody samples. Remarkably, antibodies of different isotypes may share a common idiotype, and antibodies with the same isotype may share only partial identity with any particular idiotype (i.e., microheterogeneity within the V-region).

Idiotypes have been divided into private and public idiotypes, based upon their distribution within a species. Originally, it was thought that an idiotype was unique and restricted to a single antibody clone derived from a single individual. This type of idiotype also referred to as a minor, individual, or private idiotype, does exist, at least in principle. However, it is now recognized that other idiotypes can be shared among individuals, called public, major, or cross-reactive idiotypes. The private idiotype may represent a single clonal product, whereas a public idiotype may be a manifestation of an entire family of related antibodies that differ at various positions throughout the V-region of the light or heavy chain. Both private and public idiotypes may be inherited from generation to generation. Idiotype sharing among individuals is therefore much more frequent within inbred strains than within outbred animals. All animals of a given strain may produce antibodies, a portion of which cross-reacts idiotypically in response to a given antigen, but antibodies from another strain specific for the same antigen may show little or no cross-reactivity.

The concept of idiotypy has led to a number of valuable contributions regarding the genetics and biology of antibodies and antibody-producing cells. These contributions include (1) their use as markers, with which one can quantitatively follow the expression of an individual clone or a family of related clones of antibody producing cells within a heterogeneous population of antibody-producing cells, (2) the recognition that a clone of cells can switch from IgM to IgG secretion (isotype switching), (3) the broad range of idiotypic specificities of antibody directed against a single antigen or hapten has reflected a great diversity within the antibody repertoire, (4) alterations in the degree of idiotype cross-reactivity in an antibody population as a function of time after immunization has led to the recognition that somatic mutations occur during an immune response, and (5) B- or T-lymphocyte recognition of idiotypes displayed on the membrane of immunocompetent cells plays a role in immune regulation (clonal deletion) (Nemazee and Hogquist, 2003; Nemazee, 2006).

16.2.2.3 Structural and Genetic Studies of Immunoglobulins in Swine

Significant progress has been made in recent years to understand immune system ontogeny in swine, not lastly due to its suitability as a model for a number of experimental systems to study xenotransplantation, cystic fibrosis, and developmental immunity including allergenicity (reviewed in Butler et al., 2009; Dearman and Kimber, 2009). A particular focus is on the mechanisms of maternal transfer and development of mucosal immunity (Butler et al., 2009 a and b, 2011; Cervenak and Kacskovics, 2009).

Like other vertebrate species, swine have all five isotypes of Ig (Butler et al., 2009a). Their concentrations in various body fluids, the location of the respective secreting plasma cells throughout the body, and their transport to lacteal secretions and absorption by the gut of the newborn piglet have been well studied (Butler et al., 2011; Butler and Brown, 1994). Like people, swine have both κ and λ light chains. Nucleotide sequencing of cDNA's encoding κ and λ light chains revealed a high degree of homology with other species (Lammers et al., 1991). The constant region lengths are 105 amino acids for λ and 108 amino acids for κ light chains. The frequency of κ and λ expression in swine is similar to that observed in people.

IgG comprises about 88% of serum Igs, and recent molecular genetic studies reveal that swine have the largest number of IgG subclass genes of all species tested so far. Sequences of six different IgG subclasses IgG1(a), IgG2(a), IgG3(a), IgG4(a), IgG5(a), and IgG(a), and their respective predicted functional properties in terms of C1q or Protein A binding are now available (Kloep et al., 2012; Butler and Brown, 1994; Butler et al., 1996), and as many as 11 copies of the Cγ gene have been recognized (Butler et al., 2009a). Swine have only a single gene for IgA that occurs in two allelic forms that differ in hinge length. Swine also contain single genes encoding the constant regions of Cμ (Bosch et al., 1992) and Cε. IgG3 accounts for about 80% of the Ig in neonates but <5% in adults, whereas IgG1 is high in adults (with IgG4 being the lowest) (Kloep et al., 2012).

Newborn piglets are virtually agammaglobulinemic as the epitheliochorial placenta of sows does not allow Ig transfer. Consequently, passive transfer of Ig from colostrum and milk by subsequent uptake in the neonatal gut is indispensable for the offspring (Butler et al., 2009; Salmon et al., 2009; see also Section 16.3.3). Ig G comprises about 80% of all Igs in colostrum (Rejnek et al., 1965, 1966). Importantly, the composition of the lacteal secretions changes dramatically during the first week, as IgG is substituted by IgA. Thus, mature milk in both swine and people transfers the local (mucosal) immunologic experience of the mother, that is, IgA, to the neonate, while the colostrum of swine is also the vehicle for transfer of maternal systemic immunity, that is, IgG antibodies (Butler and Brown, 1994).

Swine represent a valuable model for the hypothesis-based study of immunoontogeny in general and mucosal immunity in particular. Both the influences of maternal regulatory factors as well as intestinal gut flora can be experimentally controlled. Thus, instead of extrapolating from mice to human beings, swine represent a species deserving further studies in its own right and also as a very valuable model for human disease (Butler et al., 2009a and b).

16.3 PHYSIOLOGY AND EFFECTOR ACTIVITY OF IMMUNOGLOBULINS

The function of antibodies has been investigated for over 100 years and their importance in protection from infectious pathogens has been known since the very beginning. Fundamental mechanisms of Ig functions and their correlation to Ig structural components were established with a number of models in vitro and in vivo. The following sections reflect these conventional antibody functions in health and disease. More recently, more complex aspects in antibody-mediated immunity have emerged. For a review, see Casadevall and Pirofski (2012).

16.3.1 Neutralization of Virulence

One of the key effector functions of antibodies is the neutralization of virulence-related proteins or components in toxins (e.g., tetanus toxin), viruses (e.g., rabies), bacteria, and parasites (Bachmann and Zinkernagel, 1997; Childers et al., 1989; Norrby-Teglund et al., 2006). By binding to such antigenic determinants, the toxic invader is prevented from binding to target surfaces and cells, from eliciting pathophysiologic reactions and from killing target cells. Ultimately, this will inhibit successful multiplication of an infectious organism and prevent the actual infectious process as such. Further functions of antibodies listed below will assist the primary goal of the antigen-specific defense reaction mediated by antibodies.

16.3.2 Cytophilic and Opsonizing Activity

Antibodies that are cytophilic for macrophages presumably function to focus on the phagocytic activities of macrophages on the intruding organism or particle (opsonic activity) (Childers et al., 1989; Ravetch and Clynes, 1998; Tizard, 2013). IgG2 exhibits more opsonic activity than the IgG1 subclass. In contrast, only the IgG2 subclass of mice is cytophilic for macrophages (Boyden, 1964), while all four human IgG subclasses (Huber and Fudenberg, 1968) bind to macrophages (IgG1, IgG3 > IgG2, IgG4). The murine and human IgM isotype has also been shown to have opsonic activity when complexed with complement.

16.3.3 Placental/Gut Transfer of Immunoglobulins

Passive transfer of Ig from the mother to the fetus or the newborn is an important mechanism of protection from infectious disease. Ig may be transferred either prenatally, postnatally, or both. Ig transfer differs among species due to the different types of placenta. In addition, Ig isotypes and their transfer mechanisms vary according to the stage of pregnancy and lactation. Ig transfer occurs through the yolk sac in rabbits, whereas it is transplacental in the other listed species including people. Only postnatal transfer occurs in swine (reviewed in Salmon et al., 2009).

The transport of IgG from mother to fetus depends on a specific transport protein in the placenta, termed the neonatal Fc receptor (FcRn). Although the structure of FcRn is closely related in structure to MHC Class I molecules (Raghavan and Bjorkman, 1996; Simister et al., 1997), the binding to FC is different. Essentially, two molecules of FcRn bind to one molecule of IgG, enabling its transport across the placenta into the vascular space in the fetus.

Postnatal transfer of maternal IgG across the intestinal epithelium occurs in rat, mouse, and dog up to 21, 16, and 10 days following birth, respectively (Brambell, 1966; Halliday, 1955; Morris, 1964). Again, the postnatal transfer of maternal IgG is mediated by binding to the FcRn on the brush border of the proximal small intestine. After delivery to the vascular circulation and tissues of the neonate, it can be recycled to the gut lumen for mucosal protection. The FcRn is found only in the fetus (suggesting also uptake of IgG from amniotic fluid) and in early postnatal life in rodents, whereas in people it is also expressed in adults (Israel et al., 1997; Shah et al. 2003; reviewed by Roopenian and Akilesh, 2007). Besides IgG, there is also transfer of IgA (people, piglets) and IgM (rabbits) from mother to offspring (Waldmann and Strober, 1969; Butler et al., 2009). There are likely differences in the transfer efficiency of certain IgG subclasses, depending upon the species investigated (Cervenak and Kacskovics, 2009). Mouse IgG3 is transferred much more readily than the other IgG subclasses (Grey et al., 1971), while all IgG subclasses are transferred equally well in people (Spiegelberg, 1974). Importantly, FcRn is expected to play a role in the development of the induction of oral tolerance and immune surveillance (Israel et al., 1997; Bailey et al., 2005).

16.3.4 Complement Fixation

Fixation of complement by Ig is an important property of antibody molecules that may lead to cell lysis, Arthus reaction, and/or enhanced opsonic activity and cytophilic binding. The classic pathway for complement activation uses all nine components (1, 4, 2, 3, 5–9, respectively), while the alternative pathway involves activation of the third and fifth to ninth components, respectively (for review on these pathways, see Sarma and Ward, 2011). The IgG and IgM isotypes of all species appear to fix complement by the classic pathway, though there may be subclass differences. Complement fixation requires Ig to be either polymeric (as IgM) or complexed with antigen. Human IgG4 and mouse IgG1 and IgG3 do not fix complement via this pathway. In addition, a subpopulation of noncomplement-fixing IgM has been described for people and the rabbit (Spiegelberg, 1974). The IgA, IgE, and IgD isotypes also do not fix complement via the classic pathway for any of the species considered here.

The alternative pathway of complement activation in people involves only the two IgA subclasses, while the other isotypes are not able to fix complement via this pathway. In contrast, IgG1 in mice and rabbits can fix complement via the alternative pathway (Spiegelberg, 1974). Aggregated IgD and IgE in many species also activate the alternative pathway.

16.3.5 Antibody-Dependent Cell-Mediated Cytotoxicity

Stimulated by Ig binding, antibody-dependent cell-mediated cytotoxicity (ADCC) is the killing of antibody-coated target cells by cytotoxic effector cells (e.g., natural killer cells, neutrophils, eosinophils, monocytes, macrophages) using nonphagocytic processes involving the release of cytotoxic granules or the expression and release of mediators of cell death (e.g., tumor necrosis factor, reactive oxygen species, perforin) (Teillaud, 2012). ADCC of virus-infected cells has been shown in HIV-infected patients (Ahmad and Menezes, 1996). Furthermore, ADCC is an important mechanism in the area of therapeutic antibodies and also in the area of organ transplantation (Alderson and Sondel, 2011; Singh et al., 2009).

16.3.6 Protein A Binding

Staphylococcal protein A has been shown to bind to IgG from a variety of mammalian species (Langone, 1978). The protein A molecule is known to have four binding sites available for interaction with the Fc portion of Ig molecules, and can therefore form immune complexes of protein A and antibody in the serum. These immune complexes have been shown to fix complement as well as classic antigen–antibody complexes in serum (Forsgren and Sjoquist, 1966, 1967). The relative effectiveness of protein A binding to IgG from different species is shown in Table 16.10. In addition to IgG, the IgA2 subclass of human Ig and IgM from human, rabbit, mouse, and rat also exhibit low levels of binding to protein A (Goding, 1978). Within the IgG subclasses of different species, there may also be heterogeneity in the affinity of binding to protein A. The murine IgG1 subclass and human IgG3 subclass do not bind to protein A. Presumably, protein A binding can play a physiologic role in protection against disease, though there is no direct evidence for this.

16.3.7 Monoclonal and Therapeutic Antibodies

An excellent review on the development and types of therapeutic antibodies is the one by Nissim and Chernajovsky (2008). The concept of monoclonal antibodies, based on hybridoma formation of mouse myeloma cells with clonal antigen-specific lymphocytes almost 40 years ago by Milstein and Köhler set the ground for a rapidly growing number of biologic therapeutic modalities, especially in oncology but also in the area of chronic debilitating diseases such as

TABLE 16.10
Relative Binding Affinity of IgG Antibody to Protein A

Species	Relative Binding Affinity of IgG Antibody to Protein A[a]
Human	1
Rabbit	1
Dog	0.21
Mouse	1.33×10^{-2}
Rat	$<6.0 \times 10^{-4}$

[a] Numbers based on the amount of IgG required to inhibit binding of 125I-labeled protein A to immobilized rabbit IgG.

Source: Reported by Langone, J.J., *J Immunol Methods*, 24, 269–285, 1978.

rheumatoid arthritis. Advanced molecular biology technologies and transgenic mouse models are being used to develop an ever growing number of chimeric or humanized therapeutic antibodies that target growth receptors, cytokines or their receptors, and other biologically relevant key determinants (for reviews, see also Bodey et al., 2000; Majidi et al., 2009; and Mauerer and Gruber, 2012).

16.3.8 Immunomodulation by FCγ-Receptors

The long-term outcome of multiple minor and major immune responses taking place in an organism over time is regulated by checks and balances at every step of the process. The binding of antibody–antigen complexes (or immune complexes) to the different types of Fc receptors by the Fc portion of the antibody component is considered an important link between the antigen-specific response and effector cells of nonspecific defense functions, that is, granulocytes, monocytes, mast cells, and macrophages (reviewed by Nimmerjahn and Ravetch, 2007). Essentially, studies with human and murine IgG have shown two important variables. One is the Fcγ—receptor-binding affinity (FcγRI = high affinity, FcγRII, FcγRIII, and FcγRIV = low affinity), the other one is the nature of the signals transferred to the respective target cells. Signal transduction is influenced by the (cytokine) environment, where TGF-β and interleukin-4 (IL-4) are inhibitory while IFN-γ, TNF-α, and molecules such as lipopolysaccharide (LPS) or C5a are activating. In addition, the types of sugar residues on the Fc part of the IgG molecule play a role, and the complexity of the FCγR-regulated system is underscored by the presence of over 30 different types of IgG Fc—glycovariants in human serum.

Importantly, the balance between activating and inhibitory signals will influence for instance, the tolerance to autoantigens and can thus contribute to antibody-mediated autoimmune diseases such as arthritis, multiple sclerosis, and systemic lupus erythematosus (Nimmerjahn and Ravetch, 2007).

Finally, the neonatal Fc receptor FcRn has been shown to play an important role in antibody metabolization in people, including adults (but not rodents). Whether this is true for other species has so far mostly been addressed in neonates. For a review, see Roopenian and Akilesh (2007).

IgG and IgG-receptor (i.e., Fc receptor) interactions demonstrate differences between primate species. For example, there are cynomolgus monkey IgG subclasses that have greater Fc receptor-binding affinity and a more pronounced effector function than human IgG (Warncke et al., 2012).

16.3.9 Hypersensitivity Reactions

Hypersensitivity-type reactions are a collection of unwanted, harmful, and potentially life-threatening responses that occur in an affected individual or animal as a sequela of the normal function of the immune system. There are essentially four classes, or groups, of hypersensitivity reactions (labeled as type I through type IV). A fifth type (Type V) has been described but may be more appropriately considered a subclassification of Type II hypersensitivity (Rajan, 2003). Types I, II, III (and V) are mediated through the binding of antigens to Ig that, in general, either stimulate the release of vasoactive compounds (type I), induces cytotoxicity (type II) or results in immune complex-induced inflammatory reactions (type III); type IV reactions occur through an Ig-independent, cell-mediated mechanism.

16.3.9.1 Type I Hypersensitivity

Immediate type I hypersensitivity, or allergic reactions, is mediated through the action of IgE and can be further subclassified as "early-" or "late-phase" reactions. This class of hypersensitivity reactions is mediated by IgE bound to high-affinity IgE receptors called FcεRI on the surface of mast cells and basophilic granulocytes. After crosslinking of surface-bound IgE by an antigen (also known as allergen) or an anti-IgE antibody, FcεRI-mediated signaling results in exocytosis or degranulation of histamine, eicosanoids, and other cytokines from such activated mast cells. Early-phase type I responses occur within seconds to minutes; the late-phase response occurs within 8–12 hours. Depending on the location of the immediate-type response, there will be itching, reddening (due to vasodilation), and swelling (due to increased vascular permeability) in the skin, airway constriction due to smooth muscle contraction resulting in wheezing and shortness of breath in the lung, while systemic reactions can ultimately result in shock due to a rapid hypotonic vascular crisis. Peanut-induced food anaphylaxis of people is an example of an IgE-mediated type I reaction.

Reaginic or IgE antibody can be demonstrated by the prick test, that is an epidermal application of an allergen after a superficial needle prick. Alternatively, serum IgE can be determined by enzyme-linked immunosorbent assay (ELISA), either with anti-IgE antibodies or a specific allergen. However, serum levels of IgE may not correlate with the local presence of allergen-specific reactivity, respectively, the real allergy status of an individual.

IgE is heat labile at 56°C in the skin, but it is long lived (11–15 days), as was demonstrated after passive transfer. Besides of people, all laboratory animal species exhibit reaginic reactivity.

Mast cells have also a receptor for IgG, called FcγRIII, a low-affinity receptor. Local IgG is heat stable but has a short half-life (<1 day) in the skin after passive transfer. In the rat and mouse, this antibody belongs to the IgG1 subclass (Spiegelberg, 1974). For a review of IgE and its interaction with basophils, mast cells, and eosinophils, see Prussin and Metcalfe (2006). For a review on different animal models of protein allerginicity, see Dearman and Kimber (2009).

16.3.9.2 Type II Hypersensitivity

Type II hypersensitivity (or cytotoxic hypersensitivity) occurs as a consequence of antibody binding to membrane-bound antigen resulting in a complement-mediated cytotoxicity or opsonization/inflammation (Tizard, 2013; Baldo and Pham, 2013). Type II reactions can occur within minutes to hours and are mediated through IgM or IgG, either by complement fixation or ADCC mechanisms. Immune-mediated hemolytic anemia is an example of a type II hypersensitivity response.

16.3.9.3 Type III Hypersensitivity

Type III reactions (or immune complex hypersensitivity) occur when Ig (primarily IgG, but occasionally IgM) bind to soluble antigens to form immune complexes (Tizard, 2013; Baldo and Pham, 2013). The soluble antigen–antibody immune complexes are deposited and accumulate in tissues resulting in the induction of a localized inflammatory process, including recruitment of leukocytes.

This type of response can occur within hours and is typified by the intradermal Arthus reaction in rabbits or farmer's lung (an Arthus-type response in people).

16.4 CIRCULATING CONCENTRATIONS OF IMMUNOGLOBULINS

16.4.1 Normal Levels

Reported normal serum concentrations and half-life of immunoglobulins are presented for a number of laboratory animals (Tables 16.11 through 16.15). The differences in serum concentrations among species reflect differences of Ig synthesis and catabolism in these animals. In a normal antigenic environment, Ig synthesis in people (Birke et al., 1963; Solomon et al., 1963) ranges from 25 to 35 mg/kg/day, while mice (Bell and Fahey, 1964; Fahey et al., 1965; Humphrey and Fahey, 1961), rats (Kekki and Eisalo, 1964), and rabbits (Andersen and Bjorneboe, 1964; Catsoulis et al., 1964) synthesize from 50 to 130 mg/kg/day. In addition, the half-life of IgG in serum appears to be more variable among species than other isotypes. The reported half-time survival of IgG in mouse serum (Bell and Fahey, 1964; Humphrey and Fahey, 1961) is 4.5 days, 5.5 days in rats (Kekki and Eisalo, 1964), 6 days in rabbits (Catsoulis et al., 1964), 6.6 days in

TABLE 16.11
Properties of Rat Immunoglobulins

		Immunoglobulin Class/Subclass							
		IgG1	**IgG2a**	**IgG2b**	**IgG2c**	**IgA**	**IgM**	**IgE**	**IgD**
Sedimentation coefficient		7S	7S	7S	7S	7S–19S[a]	19S	8S	8S
Molecular weight		150K	150K	150K	150K	≥150K	900K	185K	190K
Electrophoretic mobility		Fast γ	Slow γ[b]	Slow γ	Slow γ	β	–	–	–
Half-life in serum (in days)		5	5	5	5[c]	–	–	–	–
Concentrations	Serum (mg/mL)	0.5[d]	7	0.9	–	0.2	N.D.[e]	–	–
	Colostrum (mg/mL)	–	0.7	0.3	–	1.2	N.D.	–	–
	Saliva (mg/mL)	–	0.05	N.D.	–	0.1–0.2	N.D.	–	–
Placental transfer (prenatal)		+	+	+	–	N.D.	N.D.	–	–
Intestinal transfer (postnatal)		+	++	+	–	N.D.	N.D.	+	–
PCA reaction[f]	Homologous	+[g]	N.D.[h]	N.D.[h]	N.D.[h]	–	–	+	–
	Heterologous[i]	N.D.	+[h]	+[h]	+[h]	N.D.	N.D.	N.D.	–
Protein A binding[j]		+	+	+	+	N.D.	+	–	–

[a] The predominant form in serum is 7S, while polymeric forms of IgA can be found in the secretions.
[b] Electrophoretic mobility increases slightly from G2a to G2c.
[c] The half-life was determined for rat IgG only and therefore mainly reflects catabolism of the predominant IgG subclass (G2a).
[d] The serum concentration of this subclass is highly variable and may reach levels 10 times those reported after immunization or appear naturally in certain strains (i.e., Wistar).
[e] N.D. means not detected by the assay procedure used.
[f] Passive cutaneous anaphylaxis.
[g] There appears to be a controversy as to the ability of this subclass to mediate a homologous PCA reaction, though it does compete with IgE for cellular binding.
[h] These three subclasses were not separated when assayed and were simply referred to as IgG2.
[i] The heterologous reaction was performed using guinea pigs as recipients.
[j] Rat IgG as a whole exhibits only weak binding, and no distinction is made between the subclasses. IgM binds more weakly than IgG.

TABLE 16.12
Properties of Rabbit Immunoglobulins

		Immunoglobulin Class/Subclass					
		IgG1	IgG2	IgA[a]	IgM	IgE	IgD
Sedimentation coefficient		7S	7S	–	19S	8S	8S
Molecular weight		150K	150K	>150K[b]	900K	180K	190K
Electrophoretic mobility		–	γ	–	–	–	–
Half-life in serum (days)		–	7–9	–	34	–	–
Concentration:serum (mg/mL)		minor	9–12	<1	<1	<0.01	–
Complement fixation	Classical	N.D.[c]	+	N.D.	+	N.D.	–
	Alternate	+	N.D.	–	N.D.	–	–
Placental transfer (prenatal)		–	+	N.D.	+	N.D.	–
Cytophilic	Basophil	N.D.	N.D.	–	N.D.	+	–
	Mast cells	N.D.	N.D.	–	N.D.	+	–
PCA reaction[d]	Homologous	N.D.	N.D.	N.D.	N.D.	+	–
	Heterologous[e]	N.D.	+	N.D.	N.D.	N.D.	–
Protein A binding		–	+	N.D.	+[f]	–	–

[a] Two subclasses of IgA have been described in the rabbit (IgA1, IgA2) as in people.
[b] Polymeric forms of IgA are found similar to other species.
[c] N.D. means not detected in the assay procedure used.
[d] Passive cutaneous anaphylaxis.
[e] The heterologous reaction was performed using guinea pigs as recipients.
[f] IgM binding is much weaker than IgG binding

rhesus monkeys (Dixon et al., 1952), 8 days in dogs (Dixon et al., 1952), 12 days in baboons (Cohen, 1956), and 20–25 days in humans (Birke et al., 1963; Solomon et al., 1963). Differences in metabolism also exist among the various classes and subclasses of immunoglobulin. IgM has a predominantly intravascular distribution and a decreased survival rate in the serum (1/10–1/2 the half-time survival rate of IgG). Similarly, IgA in mice has a half-time survival rate 1/4 that of IgG (Fahey and Sell, 1965). Subclass variations in the serum survival rate of mouse IgG (Fahey and Sell, 1965), similar to that found within the human IgG subclasses, also exist in other species. In general, reference ranges of Ig levels in normal healthy animals should preferably be determined in a defined environment in a particular species and strain and with validated laboratory methods. Additionally, Stein et al. (1977) have described statistical methods utilizing tolerance limits instead of the familiar but considered incorrect confidence limits, for the determination of the range of normal values of serum Ig in any population, including the conversion of those values or ranges from milligram per milliliter (mg/mL) to World Health Organization International Units.

One factor that can alter the catabolic rate of Ig is the preexisting serum concentration (Bell and Fahey, 1964; Fahey and Robinson, 1963; Fahey and Sell, 1965; Humphrey and Fahey, 1961; Lippincott et al., 1960; Rogentine et al., 1966; Solomon et al., 1963; Wiener, 1951). For instance, the catabolic rate of IgG class of Ig in both people and mice goes up with increasing serum levels, while for IgA there is no correlation between serum level and catabolism (Barth et al., 1964; Fahey and Sell, 1965; Solomon and Tomasi, 1964; Spiegelberg et al., 1968; Strober et al., 1968). In contrast, the catabolic rate of human IgD has been found to be inversely proportional to its serum concentration (Rogentine et al., 1966). Thus, as the concentration of IgD increases, the catabolic rate decreases.

TABLE 16.13
Properties of Nonhuman Primate Immunoglobulins

		Immunoglobulin Class/Subclass				
		IgG	**IgA**	**IgM**	**IgE**	**IgD**
Sedimentation coefficient		7S	7S–13S[a]	19S	8S	8S
Number of subclasses		4[b]	–	2[c]	–	–
Half-life in serum (days)	Rhesus monkey	6.6	–	–	–	–
	Baboon	12	–	–	–	–
Serum concentration (mg/mL)	Chimpanzee	8–13	0.8–2.9	0.2–0.8	–	–
	Orangutan	11–13	0.9–1.9	0.2–0.9	–	–
	Baboon	11–14	1.1–4.1	0.3–1.8	–	–
	Rhesus monkey	12–30	0.3–0.9	0.8–2.0	–	–
	Vervet monkey	10	4	1.5	–	–
Placental transfer (prenatal)		+	N.D.[d]	N.D.	–	–
Cytophilic	Basophils	N.D.	N.D.	N.D.	+	–
	Mast cells	N.D.	N.D.	N.D.	+	–
PCA reaction[e]	Homologous	N.D.	N.D.	N.D.	+	–
	Heterologous[f]	+	N.D.	N.D.	+	–

[a] Polymeric forms of IgA can be found as in human serum and secretions.
[b] Four subclasses have been identified in apes using antihuman IgG subclass antiserum. In the baboon, determinants cross-reactive with the antihuman antisera were not identified, though four structural forms of IgG could be identified using antibaboon IgG antisera.
[c] Two subclasses have been defined in the rhesus monkey.
[d] N.D. means not detected by the assay procedure used.
[e] Passive cutaneous anaphylaxis.
[f] The heterologous reaction was performed using guinea pigs as recipients.

Catsoulis et al. (1964) reported an increased catabolic rate of IgG in hyperimmunized rabbits, while in neonatal rabbits with low levels of serum IgG, the survival time of this isotype in their serum was longer when compared with adult values (Humphrey, 1961).

Finally, in people and in contrast to rodents the neonatal Fc receptor FcRn has been shown to play an important role in stabilizing IgG levels by preventing metabolization (reviewed by Roopenian and Akilesh, 2007).

16.4.2 Antigenic Stimulation

The major overall factor affecting the concentrations of serum Ig is antigenic stimulation, while isotype expression is influenced by the type of antigen—presenting cell and potential T-lymphocyte help and the respective cytokines (see below). At one extreme are animals that have been raised in a germ-free environment. These animals are "immunologically virgin" and express very low concentrations of Ig in their serum. At the opposite extreme are animals that have been exposed to an environment high in pathogens, or have been hyperimmunized. These animals may have serum concentrations of Ig that are 5–10 times the concentrations found in normal animals.

Specific classes or subclasses of Ig may be preferentially elicited by different antigenic stimuli or disease states. Expression of the IgG3 subclass in mice and IgG2 subclass in people has been predominantly associated with anticarbohydrate or antibacterial immunity (Perlmutter et al., 1978; Riesen et al., 1976; Yount et al., 1968). The IgG2 isotype found in mice often increases more rapidly

TABLE 16.14
Properties of Dog Immunoglobulins

		Immunoglobulin Class/Subclass						
		IgG1	**IgG2a**	**IgG2b**	**IgG2c**	**IgA**	**IgM**	**IgE**
Sedimentation coefficient		7S	7S	7S	7S	11S[a]	19S	8S
Electrophoretic mobility		Fast γ	Slow γ	Slow γ	Slow γ	β	β	–
Half-life in serum (in days)		8[b]	8[b]	8[b]	–	–	–	–
Concentrations (mg/mL)	Serum	3–6	5–8c	5–8c	1	0.8	1.5	–
	Colostrum	6.9	6.7[c]	6.7[c]	0.9	3.1	2.2	–
	Intestine	3.5	0.6[c]	0.6[c]	0.5	3.0	0.9	–
	Saliva	0.015[b]	0.015[b]	0.015[b]	0.015[b]	0.033	0.51	–
Placental transfer (prenatal)		+[b]	+[b]	+[b]	+[b]	N.D.[d]	N.D.	–
Intestinal transfer (postnatal)		N.D.[b]	N.D.[b]	N.D.[b]	N.D.[b]	+	N.D.	–
Cytophilic for:	Mast cells	N.D.[b]	N.D.[b]	N.D.[b]	N.D.[b]	–	–	+
	Basophils	N.D.[b]	N.D.[b]	N.D.[b]	N.D.[b]	–	–	+
PCA reactione (homologous)		N.D.[b]	N.D.[b]	N.D.[b]	N.D.[b]	N.D.	N.D.	+
Protein A binding		+[b]	+[b]	+[b]	+[b]	–	N.D.	–

[a] Serum IgA has a slightly lower molecular weight than the secreted IgA although similar.
[b] The IgG subclasses were not differentiated in the study; therefore, the values given probably refer mainly to the predominant subclasses IgG1 and IgG2a, b.
[c] No distinction was made between IgG2a and IgG2b.
[d] N.D. means not detected by the assay procedure used.
[e] Passive cutaneous anaphylaxis.

than IgG1 after antigenic stimulation of the animals with protein antigens. IgM antibody typically appears in the serum early and for several weeks following a primary exposure to antigen.

The circulating levels of IgE are often found to be elevated in animals infected with parasites or afflicted with a variety of allergic disorders (for reviews, see Becker, 1971; Bloch, 1967; Patterson, 1969). Protein antigens, when injected with the appropriate adjuvant, will also elicit high titers of reaginic antibody (Vaz et al., 1971).

The mechanism(s) by which different antigens preferentially elicit expression of one isotype over another is mediated by cytokines such as IL-4 and IL-12 (Kaplan et al., 1996; Lee et al., 1999). For a review, see Romagnani (2000). Most of what is known about the regulation of isotype switching by helper T cells (TH) has come from experiments in which mouse B cells are stimulated with LPS and purified cytokines in vitro. These studies suggest that selected cytokines can induce, augment, or inhibit the production of certain heavy chain isotypes. For example, IL-4 induces the production of both IgG1 and IgE, but inhibits IgM, IgG3, and IgG2a (Janeway and Travers, 1997). The inhibitory effect of a cytokine is likely due to the result of directly switching to a different isotype. Another example of a cytokine influence over isotype expression is interferon gamma (INF-γ) inducing IgG3 and IgG2a and inhibiting IgM, IgG1, and IgE. The isotype switching is dependent upon T cells. TH cells include at least two different subsets, that is, TH1 and TH2. TH1 cells produce cytokines such as INF-γ that induces switching to IgG2a and IgG3, while TH2 helper subsets release IL-4 and IL-5, which favor the switch to IgG1, IgA, and IgE isotypes. For reviews on the role of antigenic stimulation and mechanisms of isotype switching and idiotype selection, see Bouvet and Fischetti (1999), Manz et al. (2005), and Borghesi and Milcarek (2006).

TABLE 16.15
Properties of Mouse Immunoglobulins

		Immunoglobulin Class/Subclass							
		IgG1	IgG2a	IgG2b	IgG3	IgA	IgM	IgE	IgD
Sedimentation coefficient		7S	7S	7S	7S	7S–13S[a]	18S	8S	8S
Molecular weight		150K	150K	150K	150K	≥150K	900K	190K	180K
Electrophoretic mobility		Fast γ	Slow γ	Slow γ	Slow γ	β	Mid γ	–	–
Half-life in serum (in days)		4	5	2	4	1	1	–	–
Concentration	Serum (mg/mL)[b]	6.5	4.2	1.2	0.1–0.2	0.7	1	<0.01	<0.01
	Placental transfer (prenatal)		+	+	+	N.D.[c]	N.D.	N.D.	N.D.
Complement fixation	Classical	N.D.	–	+	N.D.	–	+	N.D.	–
	Alternate	+	+	–	–	+	–	–	–
Cytophilic	Macrophages	N.D.	+	–	N.D.	–	–	–	–
	Mast cells	+	N.D.	N.D.	N.D.	N.D.	N.D.	+	N.D.
PCA reaction[d]	Homologous	+	N.D.	N.D.	N.D.	N.D.	N.D.	+	N.D.
	Heterologous[e]	N.D.	+	N.D.	N.D.	N.D.	N.D.	+	N.D.

[a] Monomeric and polymeric forms of IgA exist in the secretions.
[b] Serum concentrations for a normal BALB/c mouse.
[c] N.D. means not detected by the assay procedure used.
[d] Passive cutaneous anaphylaxis.
[e] The heterologous reaction was performed using guinea pigs as recipients.

16.4.3 Gammopathies

The most significant shift in serum immunoglobulin concentration occurs with various monoclonal gammopathies such as multiple myeloma, a common neoplasic condition in people, nonhuman primates, dogs, mice, and rats. Gammopathies result in expansion of a single clone of neoplastic B cells secreting copious amounts of antibody. Often, the monoclonal antibody product may represent >90% of the total Ig present in serum. Monoclonal gammopathy is demonstrated by cellulose acetate electrophoresis of serum proteins. The normally diffuse banding region occupied by Ig will contain a single, darkly stained band (representing the neoplastic product) and a fainter, diffusely stained region (representing the normal Ig in the serum). The large amounts of pure antibody that can be isolated from such serum have allowed a variety of biochemical and functional analyses on specific isotypes that are normally expressed only at low levels (i.e., IgE and IgD) and have thus proven to be extremely useful to immunologists.

16.5 QUANTIFICATION OF IMMUNOGLOBULIN CLASSES AND SUBCLASSES

Numerous protocols for immunologic methods in general and analytic procedures for and with Ig in particular can be found in the series immunology protocols (e.g., immunoblotting and immunodetection, Gallagher et al., 2008). The isolation of IgG and IgM from animal serum has classically been performed using a combination of ion-exchange and gel permeation chromatography, often on an Ig fraction precipitated from the serum with either ammonium or sodium sulfate (Herbert, 1974; Herbert et al., 1973; Williams et al., 2004). A good separation of rabbit IgG/IgM can be obtained by these procedures, including separation of the IgG subclasses. Mouse (Fahey, 1962; Fahey and McLaughlin, 1963) and rat (Binaghi and Boussac-Aron, 1975; McGhee et al., 1975) IgG and IgM can be separated by similar procedures, although incomplete separation of the IgG subclasses may occur, especially with the IgG2a and IgG2b subclasses of the mouse, which are similar in structure (Fahey et al., 1964a, b). The IgA class can also be isolated by similar techniques and elutes later than IgG from a Diethylaminoethylcellulose (DEAE) ion-exchange column. However, due to the low concentration of IgA in the serum, colostrum, milk, or other secretion products are often used as the starting material for IgA isolation (Cebra and Robbins, 1966). IgE and IgD cannot be isolated in pure form from the serum due to their low concentrations, and elution properties from DEAE and gel permeation columns that are common with the other isotypes (Halliwell et al., 1975; Ishizaka et al., 1969; Spiegelberg, 1972). Consequently, these IgE and IgD have been isolated in pure form mostly in cases of specific gammopathies (i.e., IgE or IgD myelomas), where relatively high serum isotype titers occur in affected animals.

Immuno- or γ-globulins can be quantitated by standard electrophoresis. Basically, after measuring the concentration of total proteins in serum, the relative areas of migration occupied by albumin and α-, β-, and γ-globulins are determined, and the final concentrations for each group are then calculated. For the quantitation of classes and subclasses, specific antisera for detecting the various isotypes are necessary. Thus, the ability to quantitate Ig from different species is dependent upon the availability of species-specific anti-Ig antisera. These antisera are prepared by purifying the Ig class or subclass of interest, and immunizing a second species of animal (i.e., a rabbit or goat) with the product. The antisera are made isotype specific by adsorbing the unwanted specificities on an affinity column conjugated with Ig containing all of the known light and heavy chain isotypes except for the relevant isotype. The specificity of these adsorbed antisera is checked against a battery of known isotype standards in the assay system of interest. Often myeloma proteins are used in place of the normal serum Igs, since myeloma proteins are more easily isolated and can be obtained in larger quantities. These proteins have proven to be extremely useful for developing antiserum to the rare isotypes (i.e., IgE and IgD). However, myelomas have not been described in all species for all of the different classes and subclasses of Ig. Complete sets of myeloma proteins have been described for people, mice, and rats (with the exception of an IgD myeloma in rats), while other species of laboratory animals lack more than one myeloma protein representing a specific class or subclass of Ig.

A quantification of the major isotypes (IgG, IgM) in the serum can be accomplished using a variety of immunoassay techniques since the concentration of these isotypes is reasonably high and, therefore, assay sensitivity is not a prime consideration (for the sensitivity range of various techniques, see Table 16.11). Quantitative immunoprecipitation and radial immunodiffusion may be used for the analysis of these Ig isotypes. Of these two assays, radial immunodiffusion is the more sensitive technique, and methods for extending its range of sensitivity by adding a radiolabeled second antibody or enhancing the contrast and intensity of precipitin lines in the gel (Harrington et al., 1971; Sieber and Becker, 1974) have been described. These enhancements have allowed the detection of IgD and IgE in serum. The quantitative precipitation assays are capable of detecting 50–100 μg of Ig per mL. Typically, the radial immunodiffusion is able to detect as little as 1–10 μg/mL. Both assays are far less sensitive than the current RIAs or enzyme immunoassays (EIAs).

Rocket immunoelectrophoresis, another popular technique used for quantitation of antibodies to a variety of different antigens, is a less useful technique for the quantitation of Ig isotypes. This assay involves electrophoresing the antigen preparation into an agar gel containing anti-antigen antibody. The technique relies on selecting an optimal pH of the buffer system, which allows migration of the antigen into the gel while maintaining a neutral net charge on the anti-antigen antibodies and thus preventing their migration into the gel. In this way, precipitin arcs can form in the agar. However, for the quantitation of isotypes, both the antigen and antibody in the assay system are Ig, and thus optimizing conditions for electrophoresis that would allow migration into the gel of one Ig species (i.e., the Ig isotype of interest) while maintaining a neutral charge on the second Ig species (i.e., the anti-isotype antisera in the agar) would be very difficult, if not impossible.

RIAs and EIAs offer more sensitivity in detecting the various Ig classes and subclasses than the previously discussed techniques. This increase in sensitivity may be necessary when assaying for the presence of certain Ig isotypes (i.e., IgE, IgD) that are normally present in very low concentration in the serum. These assays are also advantageous when a large number of different samples are to be assayed. As with the previously mentioned assays, the quality and sensitivity of the RIA and EIA are dependent upon the specificity and affinity of the isotype-specific antisera used in the assay and also the detecting label (Fan et al., 2009). These include new color and enzymatic reagents as they are being used with chemoluminescence platforms. These not only allow enhanced sensitivity but also the simultaneous analysis of multiple isotypes in very small sample volumes in a high throughput format. Basically, the isotype of interest is quantitated by assaying the ability of an unknown isotype sample to inhibit the binding between a labeled Ig isotype standard and an anti-isotype antiserum. These results are then compared with a standard curve to obtain the quantity of isotype in the assay sample. Both the RIA and EIA are able to detect Ig in the low nanogram per milliliter range (ng/mL) (Fan et al., 2009).

As many new technologies such as chemoluminescence-related methods are evolving rapidly the importance of proper method validation cannot be overstated. Specifically, testing formats must previously be checked for their precision, accuracy, and bias with well-established reference methods for each species in question. Availability for species-specific Ig isotype reagents has to be checked with current commercial providers (Findlay et al., 2000).

ACKNOWLEDGMENT

We wish to thank Richard B. Bankert and Paul K. Mazzaferro, authors of this chapter from the second edition of this book, for their vision and contributions to this chapter.

REFERENCES

Adams, J.M., Kemp, D.J., Bernard, O., et al. 1981. Organization and expression of murine immunoglobulin genes. *Immunol Rev.* 59:5–32.

Ahmad, A. and Menezes, J. 1996. Antibody-dependent cellular cytotoxicity in HIV infections. *FASEB J.* 10(2):258–266.

Alderson, K.L. and Sondel, P.M. 2011. Clinical cancer therapy by NK cells via antibody-dependent cell-mediated cytotoxicity. *J Biomed Biotechnol.* 2011:379123.

Alepa, F.P. 1968. Antigenic factors characteristic of human immunoglobulin G detected in sera of non-human primates. *Primates in Med.* 1:1–9.

Alepa, F.P. and Terry, W.D. 1965. Genetic factors and polypeptide chain subclasses of human immunoglobulin G detected in chimpanzee serums. *Science.* 150:1293–1294.

Andersen, S.B. and Bjorneboe, M. 1964. Gamma globulin turnover in rabbits before and during hyperimmunization. *J Exp Med.* 119:537–546.

Arnason, B.G., DeVaux, S.C., and Relyveld, E.H. 1964. Role of the thymus in immune reactions in rats. IV. Immunoglobulins and antibody formation. *Int Arch Allergy Appl Immunol.* 25:206–224.

Asada, Y., Kawamoto, T., Shotake, T., and Terao, K. 2002. Molecular evolution of IgG subclass among nonhuman primates: Implication of differences in antigenic determinants among Apes. *Primates.* 43(4):343–349.

Bachmann, M.F. and Zinkernagel, R.M. 1997. Neutralizing antiviral B cell responses. *Annu Rev Immunol.* 15:235–270.

Bailey, M., Haverson, K., Inman, C., et al. 2005. The development of the mucosal immune system pre- and post-weaning: Balancing regulatory and effector function. *Proc Nutr Soc.* 64(4):451–457.

Baldo, B.A. and Pham, N.H. 2013. Classification and descriptions of allergic reactions to drugs. In *Drug Allergy: Clinical Aspects, Diagnosis, Mechanisms, Structure-Activity Relationships*. New York, NY: Springer.

Barth, W.F., Wochner, R.D., Waldman, T.A., and Fahey, J.L. 1964. Metabolism of human gamma macroglobulins. *J Clin Investig.* 43:1036–1048.

Becker, E.L. 1971. Nature and classification of immediate type allergic reactions. *Adv Immunol.* 13:267–313.

Bell, S. and Fahey, J. 1964. Relationship between γ-globulin metabolism and low serum γ-globulin in germ free mice. *J Immunol.* 93:81–87.

Bernard, O., Hozumi, N., and Tonegawa, S. 1978. Sequences of mouse immunoglobulin light chain genes before and after somatic changes. *Cell.* 15:1133–1144.

Binaghi, R. A. and Boussac-Aron, Y. 1975. Isolation and properties of a 7S rat immunoglobulin different from IgG. *European J Immunol.* 5:194–197.

Birke, G., Liljedahl, S.D., Olhagen, B., Plantin, L.O., and Ahlinder, S. 1963. Catabolism and distribution of gamma-globulin. A preliminary study with 131I-labeled gammaglobulin. *Acta Med Scand.* 173:589–603.

Bloch, K.J. 1967. The anaphylactic antibodies of mammals including man. *Prog Allergy.* 10:84–150.

Bodey, B., Bodey, B., Jr., Siegel, S.E., and Kaiser, H.E. 2000. Genetically engineered monoclonal antibodies for direct anti-neoplastic treatment and cancer cell specific delivery of chemotherapeutic agents. *Curr Pharm Des.* 6(3):261–276.

Borghesi, L. and Milcarek, C. 2006. From B cell to plasma cell: Regulation of V(D)J recombination and antibody secretion. *Immunol Res.* 36(1–3):27–32.

Bosch, B.L., Beaman, K.D., and Kim, Y.B. 1992. Characterization of a cDNA clone encoding for a porcine immunoglobulin mu chain. *Dev Comp Immunol.* 16:329–337.

Bours, J., Reitz, C., Strobel, J., and Breipohl, W. 2005. Detection of secretory IgM in tears during rhino-conjunctivitis. *Graefes Arch Clin Exp Ophthalmol.* 243(5):456–463.

Bouvet, J.P. and Fischetti, V.A. 1999. Diversity of antibody-mediated immunity at the mucosal barrier. *Infect Immun.* 67(6):2687–2691.

Boyden, S.V. 1964. Cytophilic antibody in guinea pigs with delayed-type hypersensitivity. *Immunology.* 7:474–483.

Brambell, F.W.R. 1966. The transmission of immunity from mother to young and the catabolism of immunoglobulins. *Lancet.* 2:1087–1093.

Butler, J.E. and Brown, W.R. 1994. The immunoglobulins and immunoglobulin genes of swine. *Vet Immunol Immunopathol.* 43:5–12.

Butler, J.E., Santiago-Mateo, K., Sun, X.Z., Wertz, N., Sinkora, M., and Francis, D.H. 2011. Antibody repertoire development in fetal and neonatal piglets. XX. B cell lymphogenesis is absent in the ileal Peyer's patches, their repertoire development is antigen dependent, and they are not required for B cell maintenance. *J Immunol.* 187(10):5141–5149.

Butler, J.E., Sun, J., Kacskovics, I., Brown, W.R., and Navarro, P. 1996. The VH and CH immunoglobulin genes of swine: Implications for repertoire development. *Vet Immunol Immunopathol.* 54:7–17.

Butler, J.E., Wertz, N., Deschacht, N., and Kacskovics, I. 2009a. Porcine IgG: Structure, genetics, and evolution. *Immunogenetics.* 61(3):209–230.

Butler, J.E., Zhao, Y., Sinkora, M., Wertz, N., and Kacskovics, I. 2009b. Immunoglobulins, antibody repertoire and B cell development. *Dev Comp Immunol.* 33(3):321–333.

Cannon, J.P., Haire, R.N., Rast, J.P., and Litman, G.W. 2004. The phylogenetic origins of the antigen-binding receptors and somatic diversification mechanisms. *Immunol Rev.* 200:12–22.

Casadevall, A. and Pirofski, L.A. 2012. A new synthesis for antibody-mediated immunity. *Nat Immun.* 13(1):21–28.

Catsoulis, E.A., Franklin, E.C., Oratz, M., and Rothschild, M.A. 1964. Gamma globulin metabolism in rabbits during the anamnestic response. *J Exp Med.* 119:615–631.

Cebra, J.J. and Robbins, J.B. 1966. γA-immunoglobulin from rabbit colostrum. *J Immunol.* 97:12–24.

Cervenak, J. and Kacskovics, I. 2009. The neonatal Fc receptor plays a crucial role in the metabolism of IgG in livestock animals. *Vet Immunol Immunopathol.* 128(1–3):171–177.

Chen, K. and Cerutti, A. 2010. New insights into the enigma of immunoglobulin D. *Immunol Rev.* 237(1):160–179.

Chen, K. and Cerutti, A. 2011. The function and regulation of immunoglobulin D. *Curr Opin Immunol.* 23(3):345–352.

Chen, K., Xu, W., Wilson, M., et al. 2009. Immunoglobulin D enhances immune surveillance by activating antimicrobial, proinflammatory and B cell-stimulating programs in basophils. *Nat Immunol.* 10(8):889–898.

Childers, N.K., Bruce, M.G., and McGhee, J.R. 1989. Molecular mechanisms of immunoglobulin A defense. *Annu Rev Microbial.* 43:503–536.

Cohen, S. 1956. Plasma-protein distribution and turnover in the female baboon. *Biochem J.* 64:286–296.

Collins, C., Tsui, F. W. L., and M. J. Shulman. 2002. Differential activation of human and guinea pig complement by pentameric and hexameric IgM. *Eur. J. Immunol.* 32: 1802–1810.

Damian, R.T., Greene, N.D., and Kalter, S.S. 1971. IgG subclasses in the baboon (Papio cynocephalus). *J Immunol.* 106:246–257.

Dearman, R.J. and Kimber, I. 2009 April. Animal models of protein allergenicity: Potential benefits, pitfalls and challenges. *Clin Exp Allergy.* 39(4):458–468.

Dixon, F.J., Talmage, D.W., Maurer, P.H., and Deichmiller, M. 1952. The half-life of homologous gamma globulin (antibody) in several species. *J Exp Med.* 96:313–318.

Dray, S., Dubiski, S., Kelus, A.S., Lennox, E.S., and Oudin, J. 1962. A notation for allotypy. *Nature (Lond).* 195:785–786.

Dray, S., Young, G.O., and Gerald, L. 1963. Immunochemical identification and genetics of rabbit γ-globulin allotypes. *J Immunol.* 91:403–415.

Duarte, J., Deshpande, P., Guiyedi, V., et al. 2007. Total and functional parasite specific IgE responses in plasmodium falciparum-infected patients exhibiting different clinical status. *Malar J.* 6:1.

Dudley, D.D., Chaudhuri, J., Bassing, C.H., and Alt, F.W. 2005. Mechanism and control of V(D)J recombination versus class switch recombination: Similarities and differences. *Adv Immunol.* 86:43–112.

Dugoujon, J-M. 1993. Immunoglobulin allotypes (Gm, Am and Km) in non-human primates. *Primates.* 34(2):237–250.

Eason, D.D., Cannon, J.P., Haire, R.N., Rast, J.P., Ostrov, D.A., and Litman, G.W. 2004. Mechanisms of antigen receptor evolution. *Semin Immunol.* 16(4):215–226.

Ehrenstein, M.R. and Notley, C.A. 2010. The importance of natural IgM: Scavenger, protector and regulator. *Nat Rev Immunol.* 10:778–786.

Eichman, K. 1978. Expression and function of idiotypes on lymphocytes. *Adv Immunol.* 26:195–254.

Erb, K.J. 2007. Helminths, allergic disorders and IgE-mediated immune responses: Where do we stand?. *Eur J Immunol.* 37(5):1170–1173.

Fahey, J.L. 1962. Chromatographic studies of anomalous γ, β2a, and γ1-macroglobulins and normal γ-globulins in myeloma and macroglobulinemic sera. *J Biol Chem.* 237:440–445.

Fahey, J.L., Barth, W.F., and Law, L.W. 1965. Normal immunoglobulins and antibody response in neonatally thymectomized mice. *J Nat Cancer Inst.* 35:663–678.

Fahey, J.L. and McLaughlin, C. 1963. Preparation of antisera specific for 6.6s γ-globulins, β2a-globulins, γ1-macroglobulins, and for type I and II common γ-globulin determinants. *J Immunol.* 91:484–497.

Fahey, J.L. and Robinson, A.G. 1963. Factors controlling serum γ-globulin concentration. *J Exp Med.* 118:845–868.

Fahey, J.L. and Sell, S. 1965. The immunoglobulins of mice. V. The metabolic (Catabolic) properties of five immunoglobulin classes. *J Exp Med.* 122:41–58.

Fahey, J.L., Wunderlich, J., and Mishell, R. 1964a. The immunoglobulins of mice. I. Four Major classes of immunoglobulins: 7S γ2-, 7S γ1-, γ1a (β2a)-, and 18S γ1 M-globulins. *J Exp Med.* 120:223–242.

Fahey, J.L., Wunderlich, J., and Mishell, R. 1964b. The immunoglobulins of mice. II. Two subclasses of mouse 7S γ2-globulins: γ2 and γ2-globulins. *J Exp Med.* 120:243–251.

Fan, A., Cao, Z., Li, H., Kai, M., and Lu, J. 2009. Chemiluminescence platforms in immunoassay and DNA analyses. *Anal Sci.* 25(5):587–597.

Findlay, J.W.A., Smith, W.C., Lee, J.W., et al. 2000. Validation of immunoassays for bioanalysis: A pharmaceutical industry perspective. *J Pharm Biomed Anal.* 21:1249–1273.

Fitzsimmons, C.M., McBeath, R., Joseph, S., et al. 2007. Factors affecting human IgE and IgG responses to allergen-like Schistosoma mansoni antigens: Molecular structure and patterns of in vivo exposure. *Int Arch Allergy Immunol.* 142(1):40–50.

Forsgren, A. and Sjoquist, J. 1966. "Protein A" from S. aureus. I. Pseudo-immune reaction with human γ-globulin. *J Immunol.* 97:822–827.

Forsgren, A. and Sjoquist, J. 1967. "Protein A" from *Staphylococcus aureus*. III. Reaction with rabbit γ-globulin. *J Immunol.* 99:19–24.

Gallagher, S., Winston, S.E., Fuller, S.A., and Hurrell, J.G. 2008. Immunoblotting and immunodetection. *Protoc Immunol.* Chapter 8:Unit 8.10.

Geisberger, R., Lamers, M., and Achatz, G. 2006. The riddle of the dual expression of IgM and IgD. *Immunology.* 118(4):889–898.

Gilman, A.M., Nisonoff, A., and Dray, S. 1964. Symmetrical distribution of genetic markers in individual rabbit γ-globulin molecules. *Immunochemistry.* 1:109–120.

Gilman-Sachs, A., Mage, R.G., Young, G.O., Alexander, C., and Dray, S. 1969. Identification and genetic control of two rabbit immunoglobulin allotypes at a second light chain locus, the c locus. *J Immunol.* 103:1159–1167.

Goding, J.W. 1978. Use of staphylococcal protein A as an immunological reagent. *J Immunol Methods.* 20:241–253.

Gorini, G., Medgyesi, G.A., and Doria, G. 1969. Heterogeneity of mouse myeloma γG globulins as revealed by enzymatic proteolysis. *J Immunol.* 103:1132–1142.

Gould, H.J., Sutton, B.J., Beavil, A.J., et al. 2003. The biology of IGE and the basis of allergic disease. *Annu Rev Immunol.* 21:579–628.

Grant, J.A., Harrington, J.T., and Johnson, J.S. 1972. Carboxy-terminal amino acid sequences of canine immunoglobulin G subclasses. *J Immunol.* 108:165–168.

Grey, H.M., Hirst, J.W., and Cohn, M. 1971. A new mouse immunoglobulin: IgG3. *J Exp Med.* 133:289–304.

Grubb, R. 1956. Agglutination of erythrocytes coated with "Incomplete" anti-RH by certain rheumatoid arthritic sera and some other sera. *Acta Pathol Microbiol Scand.* 39:195–197.

Gutman, G.A., Loh, E., and Hood, L. 1975. Structure and regulation of immunoglobulins: Kappa allotypes in the rat have multiple amino-acid differences in the constant region. *Proc Natl Acad Sci.* 72(12):5046–5050.

Gutman, G.A. and Weissman, I.L. 1971. Inheritance and strain distribution of a rat immunoglobulin allotype. *J Immunol.* 107(5):1390–1393.

Halliday, R. 1955. The adsorption of antibodies from immune sera by the gut of the young rat. *Proc R Soc Biol.* 143:408–413.

Halliwell, R.E.W., Swartzman, R.M., Montgomery, P.C., and Rockey, J.H. 1975. Physicochemical properties of canine IgE. *Transplant Proc.* 7:537–543.

Hammerberg, B. 2009. Canine immunoglobulin E. *Vet Immunol Immunopathol.* 132(1):7–12.

Harrington, J.C., Fenton, J.W., II., and Pert, J.H. 1971. Polymer-induced precipitation of antigen-antibody complexes: 'Precipilex' reactions. *Immunochemistry.* 8:413–421.

Herbert, G.A. 1974. Ammonium sulfate fractionation of sera: Mouse, hamster, guinea pig, monkey, chimpanzee, swine, chicken, and cattle. *Appl Microbiol.* 27:389–393.

Herbert, G.A., Pelham, P.L., and Pittman, B. 1973. Determination of the optimal ammonium sulfate concentration for the fractionation of rabbit, sheep, horse, and goat antisera. *Appl Microbiol.* 25:26–36.

Honjo, T., Nakai, S., Nishida, Y., et al. 1981. Rearrangements of immunoglobulin genes during differentiation and evolution. *Immunol Rev.* 59:33–67.

Huber, H. and Fudenberg, H.H. 1968. Receptor sites of human monocytes for IgG. *Int Arch Allergy Appl Immunol.* 34:18–31.

Hughey, C.T., Brewer, J.W., Colosia, A.D., Rosse, W.F., and Corley, R.B. 1998. Production of IgM hexamers by normal and autoimmune B cells: Implications for the physiologic role of hexameric IgM. *J Immunol.* 161(8):4091–4097.

Humphrey, J.H. 1961. The metabolism of homologous and heterologous serum proteins in baby rabbits. *Immunology.* 4:380–387.

Humphrey, J.H. and Fahey, J.L. 1961. The metabolism of normal plasma proteins and gamma-myeloma protein in mice bearing plasma-cell tumors. *J Clin Investig.* 40:1696–1705.

Ishizaka, K., Ishizaka, T., and Tada, T. 1969. Immunoglobulin E in the monkey. *J Immunol.* 103:445–453.

Israel, E.J., Taylor, S., Wu, Z., et al. 1997. Expression of the neonatal Fc receptor, FcRn, on human intestinal epithelial cells. *Immunology.* 92:69–74.

Janeway, C. A., Jr. and Travers, P. 1997. *Immunobiology. The Immune System in Health and Disease,* 3rd Edition. New York: Current Biology Limited/Garland Publishing, Inc.

Jayasekera, J.P., Moseman, E.A., and Carroll, M.C. 2007. Natural antibody and complement mediated neutralization of Influenza virus in the absence of prior immunity. *J Virol.* 81(7):3487–3494.

Kaplan, M.H., Schindler, U., Smiley, S.T., and Grusby, M.J. 1996. Stat6 is required for mediating responses to IL-4 and for the development of Th2 cells. *Immunity.* 4:313–319.

Keir, S.D., Spina, D., Douglas, G., Herd, C., and Page, C.P. 2011. Airway responsiveness in an allergic rabbit model. *J Pharmacol Toxicol Methods.* 64(2):187–195.

Kekki, M. and Eisalo, A. 1964. Turnover of 35S-labeled serum albumin and gamma globulin in the rat: Comparison of the resolution of plasma radioactivity curve by graphic means (manually) and by computer. *Ann Med Exp Fenn.* 42:196–208.

Kelly, BT. and Grayson, M.H. 2016. Immunoglobulin E, what is it good for?. *Ann Allergy Asthma Immunol.* 116(3):183–187.

Kelus, A.S. and Gell, P.G.H. 1967. Immunoglobulin allotypes of experimental animals. *Prog Allergy.* 11:141–184.

Kerr, M.A. 1990. The structure and function of human IgA. *Biochem J.* 271:285–296.

Kindt, T.J. 1975. Rabbit immunoglobulin allotypes: Structure, immunology, and genetics. *Adv Immunol.* 21:35–86.

Kloep, A., Wertz, N., Mendicino, M., Ramsoondar, J., and Butler, J.E. 2012 June. Linkage haplotype for allotypic variants of porcine IgA and IgG subclass genes. *Immunogenetics.* 64(6):469–473.

Kownatzki, E. 1973. Reassociation of IgM subunits in the presence and absence of J chain. *Immunol Commun.* 2:105–113.

Lakin, J.D., Patterson, R., and Pruzansky, J.J. 1969. Immunoglobulins of the rhesus monkey (*Macaca mulatta*). III. Structure and activity of rhesus IgG and IgM antibodies synthesized in the primary response and in the hyperimmune state. *J Immunol.* 102:975–985.

Lammers, B.M., Beaman, K.D., and Kim, Y.B. 1991. Sequence analysis of porcine immunoglobulin light chain cDNAs. *Mol Immunol.* 28:877–880.

Landucci-Tosi, S. and Mage, R.G. 1970. A method for typing rabbit sera for the A14 and A15 allotypes with cross-linked antisera. *J Immunol.* 105:1046–1048.

Langone, J.J. 1978. [125I] protein A: A tracer for general use in immunoassay. *J Immunol Methods.* 24:269–285.

Lee, T-S., Yen, H-C., Pan, C-C., and Chau, L-Y. 1999. The role of interleukin 12 in the development of atherosclerosis in ApoE-deficient mice. *Arterioscler Thromb Vasc Biol.* 19:734–742.

Lippincott, S.W., Korman, T., Fong, C., Stickley, E., Wolins, W., and Hughes, W.L. 1960. Turnover of labelled normal gamma globulin in multiple myeloma. *J Clin Investig.* 39:565–572.

Mage, R.G., Lanning, D., and Knight, K.L. 2006. B cell and antibody repertoire development in rabbits: The requirement of gut associated lymphoid tissues. *Dev Comp Immunol.* 30(1–2):137–153.

Majidi, J., Barar, J., Baradaran, B., Abdolalizadeh, J., and Omidi, Y. 2009. Target therapy of cancer: Implementation of monoclonal antibodies and nanobodies. Hum Antibodies. 18(3):81–100.

Manz, R.A., Hauser, A.E., Hiepe, F., and Radbruch, A. 2005. Maintenance of serum antibody levels. *Annu Rev Immunol.* 23:367–386.

Market, E. and Papavasiliou, F.N. 2003. V(D)J recombination and the evolution of the adaptive immune system. *PLoS Biol.* 1(1):e16.

Mauerer, R. and Gruber, R. 2012. Monoclonal antibodies for the immunotherapy of solid tumours. *Curr Pharm Biotechnol.* 13(8):1385–1398.

McGhee, J.R., Michalek, S.M., and Ghanta, V.K. 1975. Rat immunoglobulins in serum and secretions: Purification of rat IgM, IgA, and IgG, and their quantitation in serum, colostrum, milk and saliva. *Immunochemistry.* 12:817–823.

Mestecky, J., Lue, C., and Russell, M.W. 1991. Selective transport of IgA. Cellular and molecular aspects. *Gastroenterol Clin North Am.* 20:441–471.

Mestecky, J. and Schrohenloher, R.E. 1974. Site of attachment of J chain to human immunoglobulin M. *Nature.* 249:650–652.

Morris, I.G. 1964. The transmission of antibodies and normal γ-globulins across the young mouse gut. *Proc R Soc Biol.* 160:276–292.

Mostov, K.E. and Bloebel, G. 1982. A transmembrane precursor of secretory component. The receptor for transcellular transport of polymeric immunoglobulins. *J Biol Chem.* 257:11816–11821.

Mostov, K.E., Friedlander, M., and Blobel, G. 1984. The receptor for transepithelial transport of IgA and IgM contains multiple immunoglobulin-like domains. *Nature.* 308:37–43.

Mostov, K.E., Kraehenbuhl, J.-P., and Blobel, G. 1980. Receptor-mediated transcellular transport of immunoglobulin: Synthesis of secretory component as multiple and larger transmembrane forms. *Proc Natl Acad Sci USA.* 77:7257–7261.

Mullock, B.P.M., Hinton, R.H., Dobrota, M., Peppard, J., and Orlans, E. 1979. Endocytic vesicles in liver carry polymeric IgA from serum to bile. *Biochim Biophys Acta.* 587:381–391.

Nagura, H., Nakane, P., and Brown, W.R.J. 1979. Translocation of dimeric IgA through neoplastic colon cells in vitro. *J Immunol.* 123:2359–2368.

Nemazee, D. 2006. Receptor editing in lymphocyte development and central tolerance. *Nat Rev Immunol.* 6(10):728–740.

Nemazee, D. and Hogquist, K.A. 2003. Antigen receptor selection by editing or downregulation of V(D)J recombination. *Curr Opin Immunol.* 15(2):182–189.

Nimmerjahn, F. and Ravetch, J.V. 2007. Fc-receptors as regulators of immunity. *Adv Immunol.* 96:179–204.

Nisonoff, A., Wissler, F.C., and Lipman, L.N. 1960a. Properties of the major component of a peptic digest of rabbit antibody. *Science.* 132:1770–1771.

Nisonoff, A., Wissler, F.C., Lipman, L.N., and Woernley, D.C. 1960b. Separation of univalent fragments from the bivalent rabbit antibody molecule by reduction of disulfide bonds. *Arch Biochem Biophy.* 89:230–244.

Nissim, A. and Chernajovsky, Y. 2008. Historical development of monoclonal antibody therapeutics. *Handb Exp Pharmacol.* 181:3–18.

Norrby-Teglund, A., Haque, K.N., and Hammarström, L. 2006. Intravenous polyclonal IgM-enriched immunoglobulin therapy in sepsis: A review of clinical efficacy in relation to microbiological aetiology and severity of sepsis. *J Int Med.* 260(6):509–516.

Ohta, Y. and Flajnik, M. 2006 July. IgD, like IgM, is a primordial immunoglobulin class perpetuated in most jawed vertebrates. *Proc Natl Acad Sci USA.* 103(28):10723–10728.

Oudin, J. 1960. Allotypy of rabbit serum proteins. I. Immunochemical analysis leading to the individualization of seven main allotypes. *J Exp Med.* 112:107–124.

Pandey, J.P. and Li, Z. 2013. The forgotten tale of immunoglobulin allotypes in cancer risk and treatment. *Exp Hematol Oncol.* 2:6.

Patterson, R. 1969. Laboratory models of reaginic allergy. *Prog Allergy.* 13:332–407.

Pearson, T., Galfre, G., Ziegler, A., and Milstein, C. 1977. A myeloma hybrid producing antibody specific for an allotypic determinant on IgD-like molecules of the mouse. *Eur J Immunol.* 7:684–690.

Perlmutter, R.M., Hansburg, D., Briles, D.E., Nicolotti, R.A., and Davie, J.M. 1978. Subclass restriction of murine anticarbohydrate antibodies. *J Immunol.* 121:566–572.

Pier, G.B., Lyczak, J.B., and Wetzler, L.M. 2004. *Immunology, Infection, and Immunity.* Washington, DC: ASM Press.

Porter, R.R. 1959. The Hydrolysis of rabbit γ-globulin and antibodies with crystalline papain. *Biochem J.* 73:119–126.

Preud'homme, J.L., Petit, I., Barra, A., Morel, F., Lecron, J.C., and Lelièvre, E. 2000. Structural and functional properties of membrane and secreted IgD. *Mol Immunol.* 37(15):871–887.

Prussin, C., and Metcalfe, D.D. 2006. IgE, mast cells, basophils, and eosinophils. *J Allergy Clin Immunol.* 117(2 Suppl Mini-Primer):S450–S456.

Putnam, F.W., Takahashi, N., Tetaert, D., Lin, L-C., and Debuire, B. 1982. The last of the immunoglobulins: Complete amino acid sequence of human IgD. *Ann N Y Acad Sci.* 399:41–68.

Rabbitts, T.H., Bentley, D.L., and Milstein, C.P. 1981. Human antibody genes: V gene variability and CH gene switching strategies. *Immunol Rev.* 59:69–91.

Raghavan, M. and Bjorkman, P.J. 1996. Fc receptor and their interactions with immunoglobulins. *Ann Rev Dev Biol.* 12:181–220.

Rajan, T.V. 2003. The Gell–Coombs classification of hypersensitivity reactions: A re-interpretation. *Trends Immunol.* 24(7):376–379.

Randall, T.D., King, L.B., and Corley, R.B. 1990. The biological effects of IgM hexamer formation. *Eur J Immunol.* 20:1971.

Ravetch, J.V. and Clynes, R.A. 1998. Divergent roles for Fc receptors and complement in vivo. *Ann Rev Immunol.* 16:421–432.

Rejnek, J., Kostka, J., and Travnicek, J. 1966. Studies on the immunoglobulin spectrum or porcine serum and colostrum. *Folia Microbiol (Prague).* 11:173–178.

Rejnek, J., Kotynek, O., and Kostka, J. 1965. Contribution to the structural characterization of gamma globulin from pig colostrum. *Folia Microbiol (Prague).* 10:327–334.

Renston, R.H., Jones, A.L., Christiansen, W.D., Hradek, G.T., and Underdown, B.J. 1980. Evidence for a vesicular transport mechanism in hepatocytes for biliary secretion of immunoglobulin A. *Science.* 208:1276–1278.

Richerson, H.B., Ching, H.F., and Seebohm, P.M. 1968. Heterogeneity of rabbit anti-ovalbumin antibodies sensitizing human, guinea pig, and rabbit skin. *J Immunol.* 101:1291–1299.

Riesen, W.F., Skvaril, F., and Braun, D.J. 1976. Natural infection of man with group A streptococci. Levels, restriction in class, subclass and type, and clonal appearance of polysaccharide group-specific antibodies. *Scand J Immunol.* 5:383–390.

Rogentine, G.N., Jr., Rowe, D.S., Bradley, J., Waldman, T.A., and Fahey. J.L. 1966. Metabolism of human immunoglobulin D (IgD). *J Clin Investig.* 45:1467–1478.

Rogier E.W., Frantz, A.L., Bruno, M.E., et al. 2014. Secretory antibodies in breast milk promote long-term intestinal homeostasis by regulating the gut microbiota and host gene expression. *Proc Natl Acad Sci USA.* 111(8):3074–3079.

Romagnani, S. 2000. T-cell subsets (Th1 versus Th2). *Ann Allergy Asthma Immunol.* 85(1):9–18; quiz 18, 21.

Roopenian, D.C. and Akilesh, S. 2007. FcRn: The neonatal Fc receptor comes of age. *Nat Rev Immunol.* 7(9):715–725.

Rupa, P., Schmied, J., and Wilkie, B.N. 2009. Porcine allergy and IgE. *Vet Immunol Immunopathol.* 132(1):41–45.

Sakano, H., Huppi, K., Heinrich, G., and Tonegawa, S. 1979. Sequences at the somatic recombination sites of immunoglobulin light chain genes. *Nature.* 280:288–294.

Salmon, H., Berri, M., Gerdts, V., and Meurens, F. 2009. Humoral and cellular factors of maternal immunity in swine. *Dev Comp Immunol.* 33(3):384–393.

Sarma, J.V. and Ward, P.A. 2011. The complement system. *Cell Tissue Res.* 343(1):227–235.

Schroeder, H.W. and Cavacini, L. 2010. Structure and function of immunoglobulins. *J Allergy Clin Immunol.* 125(2 Suppl 2):S41–52.

Seidman, J.G., Max, E.E., and Leder, P. 1979. A κ-immunoglobulin gene is formed by site-specific recombination without further somatic mutation. *Nature.* 280:370–375.

Shah, U., Dickinson, B.L., Blumberg, R.S., Simister, N.E., Lencer, W.I., and Walker, W.A. 2003 February. Distribution of the IgG Fc receptor, FcRn, in the human fetal intestine. *Pediatr Res.* 53(2):295–301.

Shearer, M.H., Dark, R.D., Chodosh, J., and Kennedy, R.C. 1999. Comparison and characterization of immunoglobulin G subclasses among primate species. *Clin Diagn Lab Immunol.* 6(6):953–958.

Sieber, A. and Becker, W. 1974. Quantitation determination of IgE by single radial immunodiffusion. A comparison of three different methods for intestification of the precipitates. *Clin Chim Acta.* 50:153–159.

Simionescu, N. 1979. The microvascular endothelium: Segmental differentiations, transcytosis, selective distribution of anionic sites. *Adv Inflamm Res.* 1:61–70.

Simister, N.E., Jacobowitz Israel, E., Ahouse, J.C., and Story, C.M. 1997. New functions of the MHC class I-related Fc receptor, FcRn. *Biochem Soc Int.* 25:481–486.

Singh, N., Pirsch, J., and Samaniego, M. 2009. Antibody-mediated rejection: Treatment alternatives and outcomes. *Transplant Rev (Orlando).* 23(1):34–46.

Sitia, R., Corte, G., Ferrarini, M., and Bargellesi, A. 1977. Lymphocyte membrane immunoglobulins: Similarities between human IgD and mouse IgD-like molecules. *Eur J Immunol.* 7:503–507.

Snoeck, V., Peters, I.R., and Cox, E. 2006. The IgA system: A comparison of structure and function in different species. *Vet Res.* 37(3):455–467.

Solomon, A. and Tomasi, T.B., Jr. 1964. Metabolism of IgA (foA) globulin. *Clin Res.* 12:452.

Solomon, A., Waldman, T.A., and Fahey, J. 1963. Metabolism of normal 6.6s γ-globulin in normal subjects and in patients with macroglobulinemia and multiple myeloma. *J Lab Clin Med.* 62:1–17.

Spiegelberg, H.L. 1972. γD immunoglobulin. *Contemp Top Immunochem.* 1:165–180.

Spiegelberg, H.L. 1974. Biological activities of immunoglobulins of different classes and subclasses. *Adv Immunol.* 19:259–294.

Stein, S.F., Ware, J.H., and Woods, R. 1977. Serum immunoglobulins: Methods for the determination of normal values in international units. *J Immunol Methods.* 16(4):371–384.

Strober, W., Wochner, R.D., Barlow, M.H., McFarlin, D.E., and Waldmann, T.A. 1968. Immunoglobulin metabolism in ataxia telangiectasia. *J Clin Investig.* 47:1905–1915.

Sun, Y., Wei, Z., Hammarstrom, L., and Zhao, Y. 2011. The immunoglobulin δ gene in jawed vertebrates: A comparative overview. *Dev Comp Immunol.* 35(9):975–981.

Sztul, E.S., Howell, K., and Palada, G.E. 1983. Intracellular and transcellular transport of secretory component and albumin in rat hepatocytes. *J Cell Biol.* 97:1582–1591.

Teillaud, J.-L. 2012. *Antibody-Dependent Cellular Cytotoxicity (ADCC).* Chichester: John Wiley & Sons Ltd. doi: 10.1002/9780470015902.a0000498.pub2

Tizard, I. 2013. *Veterinary Immunology*, 9th edition. St. Louis, MO: Elsevier.

Tucker, P.W., Cheng, H.-L., Richards, J.E., Fitzmaurice, L., Mushinski, J.F., and Blattner, F.R. 1982. Genetic aspects of IgD expression: III. Functional implications of the sequence and organization of the C6 gene. *Ann N Y Acad Sci.* 399:26–40.

Valbuena, O., Marcu, K.B., Weigert, M., and Perry, R.P. 1978. Multiplicity of germline genes specifying a group of related mouse κ-chains with implications for the generation of immunoglobulin diversity. *Nature.* 276:780–784.

vanLoghem, E. and Litwin, S.Dt. 1972. Antigenic determinants on immunoglobulins of non-human primates. *Transplant Proc.* 4:129–135.

Vaz, E.M., Vaz, N.M., and Levine, B.B. 1971. Persistent formation of reagins in mice injected with low doses of ovalbumin. *Immunology.* 21:11–15.

Vice, J.L., Hunt, W.L., and Dray, S. 1970. Contribution of the b and c light chain loci to the composition of rabbit γ-G-immunoglobulin. *J Immunol.* 104:38–44.

Waldmann, T.A. and Strober, W. 1969. Metabolism of immunoglobulins. *Prog Allergy.* 13:1–110.

Warncke, M., Calzascia, T., Coulot, M., et al. 2012. Different adaptations of IgG effector function in human and nonhuman primates and implications for therapeutic antibody treatment. *J Immunol.* 188(9):4405–4411.

Wellek, B., Hahn, H., and Opferkuch, W. 1976. Opsonizing activities of IgG, IgM antibodies and the C3b inactivator-cleaved third component of complement in macrophage phagocytosis. *Agents Actions.* 6(1–3):260–262.

Wiener, A.S. 1951. The half-life of passively acquired antibody globulin molecules in infants. *J Exp Med.* 94:213–221.

Wiersma, E.J., Collins, C., Fazel, S., and Shulman, M.J. 1998. Structural and functional analysis of J chain-deficient IgM. *J Immunol.* 160(12):5979–5989.

Williams, A., Reljic, R., Naylor, I., et al. 2004. Passive protection with immunoglobulin A antibodies against tuberculous early infection of the lungs. *Immunology.* 111(3):328–333.

Winter, W.E., Hardt, N.S., and Fuhrman, S. 2000. Immunoglobulin E: Importance in parasitic infections and hypersensitivity responses. *Arch Pathol Lab Med.* 124(9):1382–1385.

Woof, J.M. and Russell, M.W. 2011. Structure and function relationships in IgA. *Mucosal Immunol.* 4(6):590–597.

Xu, Z., Fulop, Z., Zhong, Y., Evinger, A.J., 3rd., Zan, H., and Casali, P. 2005. DNA lesions and repair in immunoglobulin class switch recombination and somatic hypermutation. *Ann N Y Acad Sci.* 1050:146–162.

Yount, W.J., Dorner, M.M., Kunkel, H.G., and Kabat, E.A. 1968. Studies on human antibodies. VI. Selective variations in subgroup composition and genetic markers. *J Exp Med.* 127:633–646.

17 Complement

Barbara R. von Beust and Gregory S. Travlos

CONTENTS

17.1 INTRODUCTION

The complement system is composed of 30 or more chemically and immunologically distinct proteins capable of interacting with each other, antibodies, certain bacterial products, and cell membranes (Walport, 2001a). Each protein of the complement system is normally present in the circulation as a functionally inactive molecule. Together these proteins make up approximately 15% (wt/wt) of the human plasma globulin fraction. It has been shown, however, that the placenta of human beings, rodents, and ungulates is an effective barrier in preventing the passage of complement either to or from the fetus (Colten, 1976).

Once activated, complement proteins function as part of the innate immune system acting as a primary effector mechanism of antibody-mediated immunity. In general, the complement system has three physiologic activities (Walport, 2001a, b). First, it acts in the host defense against infection (e.g., by facilitating opsonization, leukocyte chemotaxis, and lysis of bacteria). Second, it acts as an interface between innate and adaptive immunity (e.g., by enhancing response to antibodies). Finally, it plays a role in the clearance of waste products of inflammation and apoptotic cells generated during normal cell turnover (e.g., supporting removal of immune complexes) (Merle et al., 2015).

The activation of complement is a highly regulated process consisting of a sequential series of enzymatic reactions resulting in the formation of peptide fragments, or anaphylatoxins (e.g., C3a and C5a), that are potent inducers of multiple physiologic responses ranging from chemoattraction to apoptosis (Sarma and Ward, 2011). Three series of enzymatic activation reactions (aka. complement activation pathways) have been described, specifically, the alternative pathway, the classic pathway, and the lectin pathway. Being elicited by different mechanisms they all lead ultimately to the activation of the terminal, biologically important effector portion of the complement cascade, the membrane attack complex (MAC), unless being abbreviated by inhibitory mechanisms (Merle et al., 2015). Production of the MAC results in the ability to lyse target cell membranes establishing the complement system as a primary mediator of antibody-dependent cellular cytotoxicity (ADCC) (Sarma and Ward, 2011; Tizard, 2013).

Besides its role in innate and adaptive immunity, complement also appears to be involved with tissue regeneration and tumor growth (Qu et al., 2009), and human pathologic states such as atypical hemolytic uremic syndrome and age-related macular degeneration (Wagner and Frank, 2010).

Therefore, the investigation into therapeutic approaches and the interaction with the complement system have become an important area of research and development (Merle et al., 2015).

As mentioned in the Introduction, there are three complement activation pathways that result in the formation of the MAC. These pathways are termed the classic, alternative (or properdin), and lectin pathway, and are triggered by different substances (Sarma and Ward, 2011; Merle et al., 2015). All three pathways have been demonstrated in human beings and mammals in which they have been investigated (Zhang et al., 1999). The activating sequence for complement consists of four steps: triggering, amplification, feedback loop, and lysis (Liszewski et al., 1996; Merle et al., 2015). Amplification is a rapid process, with millions of copies of C3b being deposited on a target membrane in less than 5 minutes. The spread of this reaction into the fluid phase is prevented by feedback and other regulatory mechanisms that include the spontaneous decay of activated proteins, destabilization or inhibition of activation complexes, and proteolytic cleavage of activated components. In addition to their role as effectors of cell membrane lysis, many of the biologically active split products of complement proteins contribute to the pathogenesis of inflammatory reactions (Sundsmo and Fair, 1983; Merle et al., 2015). The physiology, biochemistry, and measurement of these split products, as well as of the specific cellular receptors they are binding to, have been reviewed and will not be covered extensively in this section (see Aegerter-Shaw et al., 1987; Cooper et al., 1983; Dierich and Schultz, 1983; Hugli, 1981; Weigle et al., 1983; Barrington et al., 2001; Ricklin and Lambris, 2013; Merle et al., 2015).

17.1.1 Nomenclature

The nomenclature of the complement cascade-related proteins and receptors has been an evolving process. For example, in 1963, it became generally accepted that the components of complement in serum were to be designated by the letter "C" followed by the prime symbol and the component number (e.g., C′1 for the first component of complement) (Rapp and Borsos, 1963). Further, activated products were designated by the letter "a" added to the symbols (e.g., C′1a). By the late 1960s, the prime symbol was dropped and the importance of proteolytic fragmentation of components was recognized (Karlson et al., 1981). To designate these fragments, letters (e.g., a, b, and c) were added to the native component from which the fragment was generated (e.g., C3a and C3b from component C3). At the time, this fragmentation process resulted in the need to identify the activated components, and the use of a bar over the activated component or complex name was used to indicate that it was in an activated form (e.g., C′1 for C1a and EAC1423 for the activated complex). By 1981, another pathway of complement activation and its component proteins (different from the original or "classical" pathway) had been described. Moreover, a subcommittee of the Nomenclature Committee of the International Union of Immunological Societies formalized the nomenclature for this "alternative" pathway (Alper et al., 1981). Components of the alternative pathway were identified with letters (i.e., B, D, H, I, and P), plus C3 and active complexes were represented as component and fragment combinations (e.g., C3b, Bb or C3b, Bb, C3b, P). With the recognition of the lectin pathway of complement activation in 1990 (Evans-Osses et al., 2013), and the continued discovery of cellular receptors for the different activation fragments, the nomenclature process is still developing. In the continued effort to harmonize nomenclature, a Complement Nomenclature Committee (under the backing of the International Complement Society and the European Complement Network) convened and was charged with conducting the first formal evaluation of complement nomenclature since 1981. Though more progress required, Table 17.1 outlines their initial set of recommendations for the nomenclature of the components of complement cascade.

17.2 COMPLEMENT ACTIVATION PATHWAYS

Recently, the three distinct pathways of complement activation (i.e., classic, alternative, and lectin) have been investigated in detail, and excellent reviews are available (Figure 17.1) (Gál and Ambrus,

TABLE 17.1
Recommended Nomenclature of Complement Pathways, Components and Receptors

Proposed Label	Descriptor (terms in parentheses signify names used previously)
	Pathways
CP	Classic pathway
AP	Alternative pathway
LP	Lectin pathway
TP	Terminal pathway
	Proteins and Protein Complexes of Complement
C1	Complex of C1q, 2C1r, 2C1s
C1q	
C1r	
C1s	
C1-INH	C1 Inhibitor (C1 esterase inhibitor)
C2	
C3	
C3(H_2O)	Thioester-hydrolyzed form of C3
C3a	Anaphylatoxin from C3
C3a-desArg	C3a without C-terminal arginine
C3b	
iC3b	Inactivated C3b
C3d	
C3dg	
C4	
C4a	
C4a-desArg	C4a without C-terminal arginine
C4b	
C4d	
C4BP	C4b binding protein
C5	
C5a	Anaphylatoxin from C5
C5a-desArg	C5a without C-terminal arginine
C5b	
C6	
C7	
C8	
C9	
C5b6	Terminal pathway complex of C5b + C6
C5b-7	Terminal pathway complex of C5b6 + C7
C5b-8	Terminal pathway complex of C5b-7 + C8
C5b-9	Terminal pathway complete complex
sC5b-9	Soluble C5b-9 with Vn or Cn bound
C3bBb	AP C3 convertase
C3bBbP	AP C3 convertase with properdin
C3bBbC3b	AP C3/C5 convertase
C4BP-protein S	C4BP bound to protein S
Vn	Vitronectin (S protein, S40)

(*continued*)

TABLE 17.1 (*Continued*)
Recommended Nomenclature of Complement Pathways, Components and Receptors

Proposed Label	Descriptor (terms in parentheses signify names used previously)
FB	Factor B
FD	Factor D
FH	Factor H
FI	Factor I
MBL	Mannose binding lectin
Ficolin-1	(M-ficolin)
Ficolin-2	(L-ficolin)
Ficolin-3	(H-ficolin)
MASP-1	MBL-associated serine protease 1
MASP-2	MBL-associated serine protease 2
MASP-3	MBL-associated serine protease 3
FHL-1	Factor H-like protein 1
FHR-1	Factor H-related protein 1
FHR-2	Factor H-related protein 2
FHR-3	Factor H-related protein 3
FHR-4	Factor H-related protein 4
FHR-5	Factor H-related protein 5
CD59	(Protectin, homologous restriction factor)
Cn	Clusterin (apolipoprotein J, SP-40,40)
	Receptors of Complement
CR1	CD35 (C3b/C4b receptor)
CR2	CD21 (C3d receptor)
CR3	CD11b/CD18 complex
CR4	CD11c/CD18 complex
C3aR	Requesting CD number
C5aR1	CD88 (C5aR)
C5aR2	(C5L2) Requesting CD number
CRIg	Complement receptor of the Ig family
C1qR	C1q receptor
gC1qR	Recognizes globular C1q domains
cC1qR	Calreticulin, recognizes collagen domain
LHR	Long homologous repeat [within CR1]

Source: Adapted from Kemper, C. et al., *Mol Immunol*, 61, 56–58, 2014.

2001; Walport, 2001a, b; Sarma and Ward, 2011, Barrington et al., 2001; Ricklin and Lambris, 2013; Osses et al., 2013; Merle et al., 2015).

17.2.1 Classic Pathway

The classic pathway (Figure 17.1) is initiated by the pattern recognition molecule C1q produced in immature dendritic cells, macrophages and monocytes, and interacting with a target structure such as immune complexes or pathogen-associated molecular patterns including lipopolysaccharide (LPS) and bacterial porins, and molecules exposed on the surface of dying cells (phosphatidylserine, double stranded DNA, glyceraldehyde-3-phosphate dehydrogenase, annexins A2 and

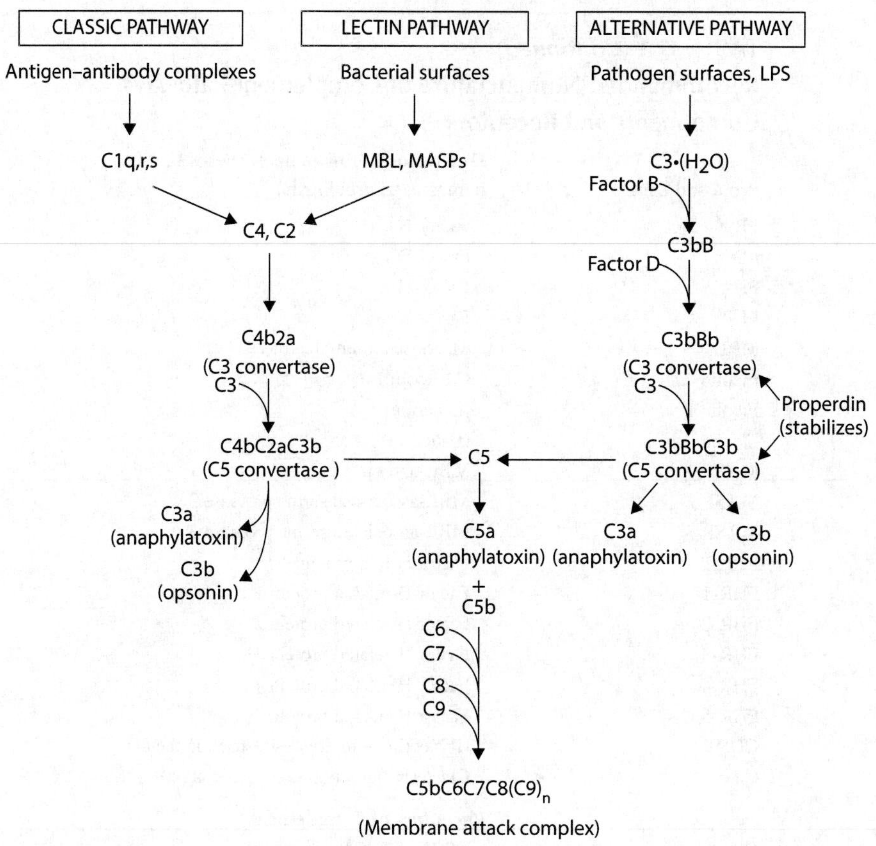

FIGURE 17.1 Illustration of complement activation of classic, lectin, and alternative pathways. (Adapted from Sarma, J.V. and Ward, P.A., *Cell Tissue Res*, 343, 227–235, 2011; Drawing by David Sabio.)

A5, and calreticulin) (Merle et al., 2015). In addition, older studies listed trypsin-like enzymes, staphylococcal protein A, teichoic acids and C-reactive protein (CRP), a number of polyanions, DNA precipitates, heparin, dextran sulfate, kallikrein, plasmin and amyloid β-protein, and certain RNA tumor viruses as initiating recognition structures (Atkinson and Frank, 1980; Burger et al., 1977; Fevereiro et al., 1992; Muller-Eberhard, 1975; Sundsmo and Fair, 1983; Velazquez et al., 1997). Recently, more details on the stoichiometry between C1q and IgM and IgG/antigen complexes have been reviewed (Merle et al., 2015). Essentially, the activation process begins with the binding of the C1q subcomponent of C1 to the Fc portion of antigen-bound IgM or IgG molecules (Sim and Reid, 1991). Once bound, C1q provides a noncovalent binding site for the C1 subcomponents C1r and C1s. A C1 complex consisting of C1q, C1r, and C1s molecules is formed. Ultimately, there is formation of a multimeric, calcium- and magnesium-dependent (Atkinson and Frank, 1980) serine protease tetramer, C1s–C1r–C1r–C1s (Gál and Ambrus, 2001). C1r undergoes self-cleavage and modifies C1s, leading to the active C4-cleavage enzyme. C1, by limited proteolysis of C4 and C2, generates the C3 convertase, named C4b2a. The potential of C1 to split several hundred C4 molecules results in a tremendous amplification process. Activated C4b2a interacts with C3 to generate C4b2a3b named C5 convertase, as well as several biologically active C3 split products such as C3a and C3b. The interaction of C4b2a3b complex with C5 results in cleavage of the C5 molecule into C5a and C5b.

17.2.2 Terminal Complement Pathway

Attachment of C5b to the cell membrane through a C5b membrane-binding site initiates the formation of the MAC by interaction with C6 (forming C5b6, without cleavage of C6), and subsequent assembly of C7, C8, and C9 (without molecular cleavage). The MAC C5b6789 is composed of one molecule each of C5, C6, C7, and C8, with a variable number of C9 molecules. The participating molecules integrate into the membrane lipid bilayer and polymerize into a ring structure forming an inner hydrophilic channel or core, surrounded by a hydrophobic rim (Muller-Eberhard, 1975), permitting water and ions to pass into the cell through this core or hole. The result is cellular swelling and eventually total lysis of the target cell (Hobart, 1984). Depending on membrane fluidity, partial leaks may be initiated by C5b67 or C5b678 (Muller-Eberhard, 1975; Morgan, 1995). Furthermore, liposome and viral membranes, as well as bacterial cell walls, may be disassembled by the MAC independent of the formation of transmembrane channels.

17.2.3 Alternative Pathway

The alternative, or properdin, pathway (Figure 17.1) is characterized by three areas of activity: silent elimination of apoptotic cells (without danger signal), elimination of pathogens (80% of terminal complement activity during pathogen recognition is provided by the alternative pathway), and maintenance of a low level of activated C3 (tick-over) kept in check by complement inhibitors in the absence of need (Merle et al., 2015). The alternative pathway can be initiated directly by a variety of nonimmunologic molecules including proteins, LPS, staphylococcal peptidoglycans, cobra venom factor (CoF), and zymosan (Walport, 2001a; Harboe et al., 2006; Kimura et al., 2008; Spitzer et al., 2007; Xu et al., 2008). In addition, viruses, bacteria, parasites, and certain eukaryotic cells (Gorman, 1984) activate the alternative pathway. Though the alternative pathway does not require specific antibody for its activation, heat-aggregated immunoglobulins and certain monomeric immunoglobulins can initiate alternative pathway activation (Gotze and Muller-Eberhard, 1976), as can IgA immune precipitates in some species (Rits et al., 1987), and under experimental conditions.

The current hypothesis for the activation of the alternative pathway is that certain surfaces, such as bacterial cell walls, fungi, and helminth cuticles, contain carbohydrate-rich polymers that allow binding of C3b but impair the binding of factor H. This allows the rapid formation of surface-bound C3bBb. Other substances containing polyanions bind and sequester factor H directly, allowing the C3bBb complex to develop into C5 convertase. Although the alternative pathway does not require specific antibody for its activation, it appears quite effective in deactivating a wide variety of infectious agents, suggesting it evolved earlier in ontogeny (Egwang and Befus, 1984).

Besides direct triggering, the alternative pathway is slowly and spontaneously activated by hydrolysis of C3 (Harboe and Mollnes, 2008). Native C3 in plasma possesses a thioester bond that spontaneously and continuously hydrolyzes, forming C3a and C3b. Factor C3b binds to the cell surface, where it complexes with factor B. Complex C3bB is split (in the presence of magnesium) by the enzymatic factor D, to form C3bBb, a C3 convertase (Muller-Eberhard and Schreiber, 1980). C3 convertase (C3bBb) self-amplifies the cleavage of C3 and leads to the generation of the C5 convertase, C3bBbC3b. Approximately 10% of the C3b so released may bind activator surfaces, resulting in amplification of the sequence.

The C3Bb complex, however, is unstable, with a reported half-life of 90 seconds (Pangburn and Muller-Eberhard, 1986a, b). Released by activated neutrophils, the protein properdin stabilizes the C3Bb complex; properdin is also found in macrophages and T cells (Kemper et al., 2010). Properdin (P) associates with C3Bb, forming a stable $(C3b)_2BbP$ complex (aka C5 convertase) (Fearon, 1979). This molecular complex recognizes and activates C5 (similar to C4b2a3b complex in the classic pathway). Additionally, the properdin-stabilized complex is protected against spontaneous and factor H-mediated decay and inhibits the cleavage of C3b by factor I. Properdin is the only known regulator of complement that enhances activation (Harboe and Mollnes, 2008).

17.2.4 Lectin Pathway

In the absence of immune complexes, the lectin pathway (Figure 17.1) is initiated by the binding of a lectin pathway activation complex to pathogen-associated molecules (primarily carbohydrate moieties) found on microorganisms such as yeast, bacteria, parasites, and viruses (Fujita, 2002, Petersen et al., 2000, Dahl et al., 2001; Youssif et al., 2012; Zhang et al., 1999). Additionally, irregular glycocalyx structures on apoptotic, necrotic, malignant, or oxygen-deprived cells can activate the lectin pathway (Fujita, 2002; Schwaeble et al., 2002).

Specifically, the pattern recognition molecules of the lectin pathway include the mannose-binding lectin (MBL), collectins, as well as ficolins H, L, and M. The LP-pattern recognition molecules have an N-terminal collagenous region similar to C1q; however, their C-terminal domains differ from gC1q. Collectins contain carbohydrate recognition domains, which recognize sugar patterns frequently expressed on bacteria, viruses, and dying cells, but usually not host cells. MBL, which belongs to the collectin family, recognizes terminal monosaccharide exposing horizontal 3′- and 4′-OH groups (glucose, mannose, and N-acetyl-glucosamine) in a Ca-dependent manner. In general, the lectin pathway is activated when mannan- or MBL, or ficolin bind to the surfaces of microorganisms resulting in neutralization, opsonization, and cytotoxic reactions (Sarma and Ward, 2011; Youssif et al., 2012; Zhang et al., 1999; Merle et al., 2015). Once MBL binds to mannose, it allows for the binding of C1r/C1s with subsequent complement activation (Holmskov et al., 1994; Sato et al., 1994). Both MBL and ficolin circulate in the serum as complexes with MBL-associated proteins, or MASP (Wallis, 2007; Sørensen et al., 2005). In human beings, circulating lectin pathway recognition molecules consist of one MBL (the product of MBL2 gene), collectin-11 (CL-11), collectin kidney 1 (CL-K1), and three ficolins (M-ficolin, or FCN1; L-ficolin, or FCN2; and H-ficolin, or FCN3) (Fujita, 2002; Liu et al., 2005; Hansen et al., 2010). In rodents, four recognition molecules have been described, including two mannan-binding lectins (MBL-A and MBL-C), CL-11, and ficolin A (Schwaeble et al., 2011). A second murine ficolin, ficolin B, linked to monocytes and macrophages, does not activate complement in mice, but may do so in rats (Girija et al., 2011). MASP-1, -2, and -3, and truncated, nonenzymatic products of MASP2 and MASP1/3 genes (i.e., MAp19 and MAp44, respectively) have been reported in human beings and mice (Sørensen et al., 2005; Ali et al., 2012).

Since neither MASP-1 nor MASP-3 can cleave C4, MASP-2 is a vital and required component for the formation of the C3 and C5 convertases (i.e., C4b2a and C4b2a(C3b)n, respectively) by the lectin pathway (Schwaeble et al., 2011; Ali et al., 2012). The binding to pathogens leads to a conformational change resulting in the activation of MASP-2. Similar to C1s, activated MASP-2 cleaves C4 to form C4a and C4b. The C4b attaches to the surface of the pathogen and to C2. The bound C2 is then cleaved by MASP-2 to form C2a and C2b. Together, C4b with the bound C2a forms the enzymatically active C3 convertase (C4bC2a). The exact role of the other MASP is presently unknown although MASP-1 can cleave C2 but not C4 (Wallis, 2007) and thus help in enhancing complement activation by the bound complexes.

17.2.5 Membrane Attack Complex

Formation of the MAC results from activation of the terminal complement pathway and C5 cleavage into C5b by the C5 convertase, inducing a dramatic conformational change. Interaction of C5b with C6, C7, C8, and multiple copies of C9 results in MAC formation. The lipophilic portion of C5b-7 binds to the cell membrane, and C8 is the first component to penetrate the lipid bilayer upon interaction with the forming MAC tubular channel. A single MAC contains up to 18 C9 molecules but one or two C9 molecules are sufficient to form a functional pore. One MAC is sufficient to lyse the membrane of metabolically inert cells, like erythrocytes or liposomes by colloid osmosis, and in coordination with calcium flux and poorly understood signal transduction in target cells can be activated leading to cell proliferation or apoptosis, which is dependent on the targeted cell type and experimental conditions (Merle et al., 2015).

In summary, the described mechanisms of activation of the three complement pathways rely on the versatility of the target pattern recognition molecules (C1q, MBL, and ficolins) that can discriminate between self and nonself and bind to pathogen- or danger-associated molecules. These molecular patterns result from specific conformational changes, such as with IgM or IgG-antigen clustering, CRP, or pathogen-associated carbohydrates. Complement activation is thus driven by conformational changes following a recognition process, leading to the subsequent activation or modulation of downstream complement components (Merle et al., 2015) involved in phagocytosis, opsonization, inflammatory and immune reactions including antibody production, and actual cell/pathogen lysis and elimination (Merle et al., 2015).

17.2.6 Pathway Regulation

While the activation of classic and lectin pathways is, in general, dependent on foreign components, both pathways can be activated under some other situations (e.g., tissue ischemia/reperfusion injury) and cause injury to the host. Further, there are complement-related diseases in which deposition of C3b after activation and amplification of the alternative pathway, without proper regulation, results in host cell injury. Thus, in view of the damage that unchecked complement activation can cause on host cells, it makes biologic sense that mechanisms are in place to limit complement activation (Sarma and Ward, 2001; Noris and Remuzzi, 2013). Consequently, human beings and mammals have a variety of regulatory soluble and membrane-bound proteins that participate in the control of complement activity (Table 17.2 and Figure 17.2).

TABLE 17.2
Complement Regulatory Proteins, and Their Functions, Demonstrated in Plasma or Bound to Cell-Membranes

Plasma	
C1 inhibitor (C1INH)	Inactivates C1r and C1s, MASP-1, and MASP-2
C4 binding protein (C4BP)	Binds to C4b; decay accelerating and cofactor activity
Factor H	Binds to C3b; has decay accelerating activity of the AP C3 and C5 convertases and cofactor activity
Factor I	Degrades C3b and C4b aided by cofactors
S-protein (vitronectin)	Binds to C5b-7 and inhibits C9 polymerization
Clusterin (SP-40,40)	Binds to C5b-7 and inhibits generation of C5b-9
Membrane-Bound	
MCP	Cofactor for factor I-mediated cleavage of C3b and C4b
DAF	Destabilizes C3/C5 convertases of the CP and AP (decay accelerating activity)
CR1	Decay accelerating activity as well as cofactor activity for factor I-mediated cleavage of C3b and C4b
Thrombomodulin	Increases CFH cofactor activity, activates TAFI-mediated C3a and C5a inactivation
Factor I	Degrades C3b and C4b aided by cofactors
CD59	Blocks the C9 association with C5b-8 to prevent C5b-9 formation on host cells

TAFI, thrombin activatable fibrinolysis inhibitor.
Source: Adapted from Noris, M. and Remuzzi, G., *Semin Nephrol*, 33, 479–492, 2013.

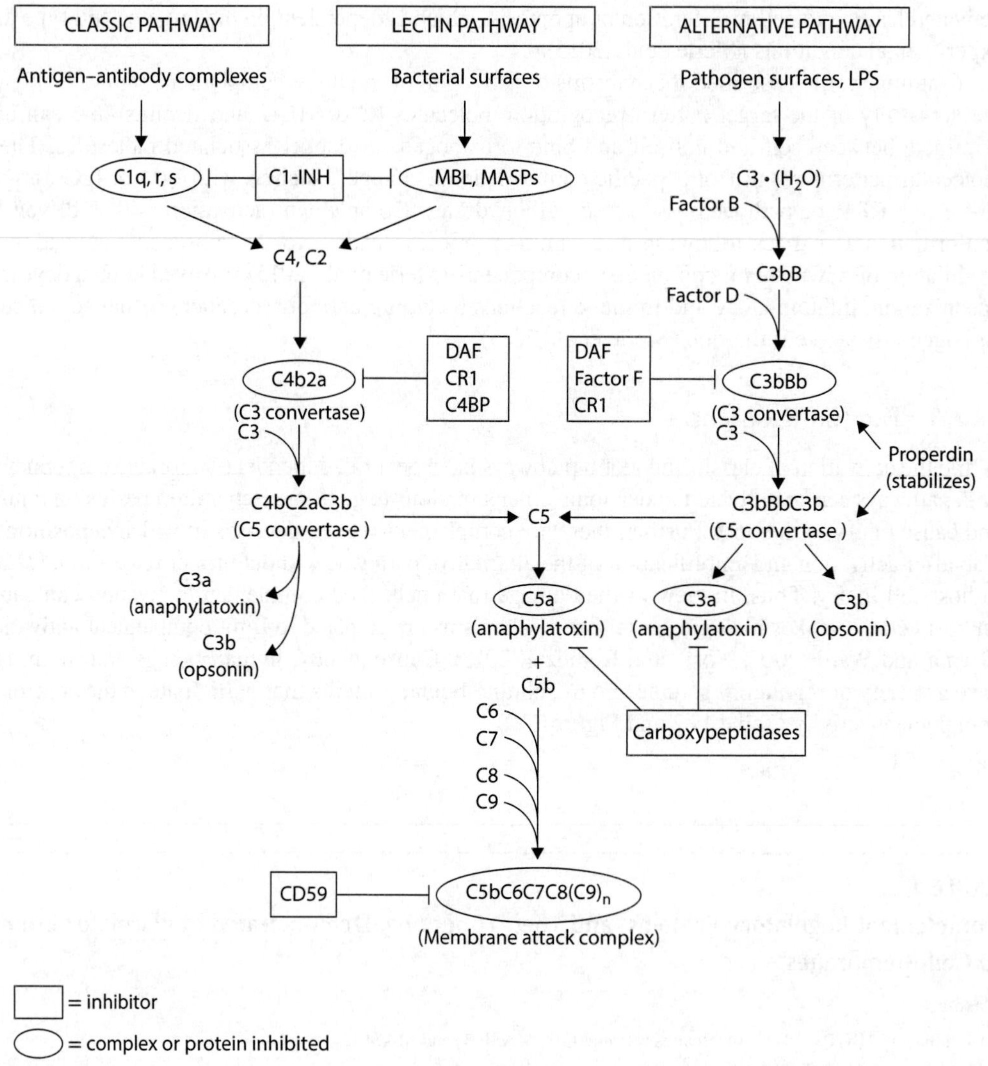

FIGURE 17.2 Illustrated representation of complement pathway regulation involving soluble or cell membrane-bound inhibitory factors. (Adapted from Sarma, J.V. and Ward, P.A., *Cell Tissue Res*, 343, 227–235, 2011; Drawing by David Sabio.)

17.2.6.1 Soluble Factors

Circulating carboxypeptidases, by cleaving the C-terminal Arginine, attenuate the inflammatory capacity of the anaphylatoxins C3a and C5a (Sarma and Ward, 2011). The resulting C3a des-Arg and C5a des-Arg have markedly reduced biologic activity (<10% of their original activity).

C1 inhibitor (C1INH, SERPING1) is a circulating serine protease inhibitor that irreversibly binds to the C1r and C1s of the C1q–C1r–C1s complex of the classic pathway. This binding blocks the active sites of C1r and C1s, allowing dissociation from C1q (Liszewski et al., 1996). Further, C1INH can bind MASP-1 and -2 of the lectin pathway (Noris and Remuzzi, 2013). Thus, the initiating steps of these pathways are inhibited. In addition to its action as an inhibitor of complement activity, C1INH plays a role as an inhibitor of the contact system of coagulation by inhibiting factor

XIIa and kallikrein. A deficiency of C1INH results in excess generation of bradykinin leading to increased vascular permeability, and angioedema (Cugno et al., 2009).

Circulating proteins such as factors H and I both inhibit complement activation (Noris and Remuzzi, 2013). Factor H (FH) is a large glycoprotein (155 kDa) that provides regulatory control of the complement system by multiple mechanisms. Acting as a primary inhibitor of the alternative pathway, the binding of FH to C3b obstructs the interaction of C3b with both Factor B (Pangburn, 2000) and C5 (Isenman et al., 1980), and causes displacement of the Bb fragment of Factor B from active C3 and C5 convertases of the alternative pathway (Weiler et al., 1976). Additionally, FH acts as a cofactor for the serine proteinase factor I (FI), which cleaves C3b into inactive C3b (iC3b), thus inhibiting the action of C3b in all complement pathways (Pangburn et al., 1977). Since FH binds to glycosaminoglycans (molecules generally found on the membranes of mammalian cells), FH protects host cells and surfaces but not the surfaces of pathogens (e.g., viruses and bacteria) (Pangburn, 2000).

As mentioned earlier, FI (aka C3b/C4b inhibitor) is a serine proteinase that, in the presence of cofactors (FH or C4b-binding protein), rapidly inactivates C3b and C4b by proteolytic cleavage into the fragments, inactive C3b (iC3b), C3dg, C3c, C4c, and C4d (Sarma and Ward, 2001; Noris and Remuzzi, 2013). Factor I cleaves C3b in the presence of factor H by hydrolysis of its α-polypeptide resulting in the prevention of C3 convertase formation. The C4b component of complement is cleaved by FI in the presence of the plasma cofactor C4b-binding protein.

C4b-binding protein (C4BP) is a potent circulating soluble inhibitor of the classic and lectin pathways of complement (Blom et al., 2004). Through its interaction with C4b, C4BP acts on the complement system in at least three ways. First, C4BP acts as a cofactor to FI, for the proteolytic inactivation of C4b, preventing the formation of C3 convertase (C4bC2a) (Scharfstein et al., 1978). How C4BP functions as a cofactor to FI is not understood, but it appears to involve a conformational change of C4b following binding to C4BP, thus becoming more susceptible to cleavage by FI. Second, C4BP physically prevents the assembly of C3 convertase by binding nascent C4b. Third, C4BP, accelerates the natural decay of the C3-convertase complex (Gigli et al., 1979). Finally, C4BP can also can act as a cofactor to FI in the cleavage of C3b in the fluid phase thereby providing some inhibition of the alternative pathway of complement activation as well (Blom et al., 2003; Seya et al., 1985; Seya et al., 1995). However, since it does not inhibit the fluid phase C3 convertase of the alternative pathway, it appears that C4BP does not inhibit assembled C3 convertase (Seya et al., 1985). Furthermore, unless it is present in very high concentrations, C4BP does not reduce the hemolytic activity of cell-bound C3b (Blom et al., 2003). Thus, C4BP is not able to fully replace the major fluid phase inhibitor of the alternative pathway, factor H.

Other factors that protect against the fluid phase activation of the MAC include S Protein (vitronectin) and clusterin (SP40, 40, cytolysis inhibitor), both of which inhibit the terminal complement pathway after the formation of C5b-7 (Liszewski et al., 1996).

17.2.6.2 Membrane-Bound Factors

The membrane-bound decay-accelerating factor (DAF, CD55) is named for its ability to accelerate the decay of C3 convertase (C4b2a) of the classic and lectin pathways, and the C3bBb complex of the alternative pathway (Pangburn et al., 1983). It functions by releasing C2a from its binding site on C4b (classic) and Bb from C3b (alternative). Its actions are limited to C3 convertases assembled on the same cell expressing DAF (Medof et al., 1984). DAF is expressed on all hematopoietic cells, endothelial and epithelial cells, at the feto–maternal interface of the placenta, and as a soluble molecule in plasma and other body fluids. Expression of human DAF on swine xenografts protects them against hyperacute rejection by nonhuman primates (McCurry et al., 1995).

Membrane cofactor protein (MCP; also known as CD46, measles virus receptor) is a membrane-bound complement regulator that serves as a cofactor for factor I-induced degradation of C3b and C4b. MCP and its analogs in other species are widely expressed on tissues throughout the body, and its expression on endothelium in transgenic pigs aids in the prevention of acute (antibody-mediated) rejection of swine xenografts (Rooney et al., 1993).

Complement receptors type 1 (CR1; C3b/C4b receptor, immune adherence receptor, CD35) and type 2 (CR2; C3d receptor, Epstein–Barre Virus (EBV) receptor, CD21), found on circulating cell membranes, bind ligands, including derivatives of C3 (CR1 and CR2) and/or C4 (CR1), and immune complexes (Hourcade et al., 1989). While CR1 facilitates both complement regulation and immune complex processing, CR2 interacts only with C3b-derived ligands degraded by other regulators, and as such makes only a minor contribution to complement regulation. Although CR1 has decay accelerating and cofactor activities, its principal role is to reduce complement activity after immune complexes containing C3b/C4b adhere to cells. In the blood, CR1 is found mainly on erythrocytes. Soluble CR1 (recombinant) (SCR1) infused into animal models blocked inflammation and reduced the extent of myocardial necrosis in models of myocardial infarction, suggesting that complement may play an important role in the removal of dead and dying tissues and may promote healing (Moore, 1994). Infusion of SCR1 into rats transplanted with renal allografts delayed complement activation, prolonged graft survival, and down regulated B cell antibody synthesis (Pratt et al., 1997).

MAC-inhibitory protein (CD59, MAC-IP) is a membrane-bound glycoprotein that inhibits the formation of MAC on membranes by inhibiting C9 from associating with C5b-8 and preventing the polymerization of C9 on the membrane (Huang et al., 2006; Liszewski et al., 1996; Noris and Remuzzi, 2013). Analogs of human CD59 have been documented in rats, sheep, and pigs, and appear to be effective in the control of experimental glomerulonephritis and other inflammatory conditions (Hughes et al., 1992; van den Berg and Morgan, 1994).

17.2.7 Atypical Pathways of Complement Activation

Other atypical routes can lead to complement activation. A number of molecules can directly bind and activate C1 without involving antibody, leading to activation by the classic pathway. The acute phase reactants CRP and serum amyloid-P component (SAP) bind to damaged cells and nuclear constituents as well as microorganisms and, once bound, bind C1, allowing for complement activation and enhancing phagocytosis of inflammatory debris (Jiang et al., 1991; Hicks et al., 1992; Vaith et al., 1996). Additionally, damaged mitochondria and myelin (Moore, 1994), proteases from neutrophils and macrophages (Ward and Zvaifler, 1973; Huber-Lang et al., 2002), and coagulation factors resulting from the activation of the coagulation cascade (i.e., kallikrein, plasmin, factors IXa, Xa, XIa, XIIa, plasmin, and thrombin) (Huber-Lang et al., 2006; Sarma and Ward, 2011) can generate complement activation products (Merle et al., 2015).

17.3 METHODS OF ANALYSIS

It has been shown that alterations in the complement system can be part of direct or indirect pathophysiologic mechanisms of a number of diseases and pathologic conditions such as autoimmune disease, infections, cancer, allogeneic and xenogeneic transplantation, and inflammation (Figueroa and Densen, 1991; Nilsson and Ekdahl, 2012; Ricklin and Lambris, 2013; Morgan and Harris, 2015). To characterize the alterations, complement analyses have been performed on these conditions in both prospective and retrospective studies, and in experimental settings in human beings and animals (Figueroa and Densen, 1991; Kirschfink and Mollnes, 2003; Mollnes et al., 2007). Further, it has been considered that the indications for serologic diagnostic complement analysis be divided into three primary types: (a) acquired and inherited complement deficiencies; (b) disorders of complement activation; (c) inherited and acquired C1INH deficiencies (Nilsson and Ekdahl, 2012).

The various components of the complement system are quantitated by assays designed to measure either the functional properties of these proteins or the presence of their antigens. Additionally, functional assays measure the ability of the total classic, lectin or alternative pathway, or individual components to lyse (hemolyze) antibody-coated (sensitized) or noncoated (for alternative pathway) red blood cells in suspension or in agarose gel (Porcel et al., 1993). Functional assays are both precise and sensitive (Atkinson and Frank, 1980). Tests designed to measure complement factor antigens generally are simpler, less subject to error due to mishandling of serum, and less expensive. However, they have the disadvantage of measuring both active and inactive forms of these proteins and therefore may not necessarily correlate well with the functionally active protein concentration. As with most immunologic assays, specificity and sensitivity are enhanced when species-specific antisera are employed. Methods of complement analysis have been comprehensively reviewed (Kirschfink and Mollnes, 2003; Mollnes et al., 2007; Nilsson and Ekdahl, 2012).

17.3.1 Functional Assays

Using functional assays has been a traditional method for the evaluation of the integrity of the complement system. They have proven useful as a screening tool for the detection of complement deficiencies or monitoring dysfunction (Kirschfink and Mollnes, 2003; Nilsson and Ekdahl, 2012). Potential deficiencies can be subsequently analyzed quantitatively for specific components using component-specific immunoassays, with and/or without procedures in which the test sample is reconstituted with the relevant component protein. The addition of this follow-up, confirmatory-type testing provides information as to whether it is an actual or functional deficiency (Kirschfink and Mollnes, 2003).

17.3.1.1 The Hemolytic Assay

Since the 1930s, the complement fixation hemolytic assay has been a useful functional screening test for assessment of complement activity of whole serum or plasma (Atkinson and Frank, 1980; Nilsson and Nilsson, 1984; Porcel et al., 1993, Costabile, 2010). Because calcium and magnesium are required components of the assay buffer, the use of chelating agents such as ethylenediaminetetraacetic acid (EDTA) should be avoided. In general, most complement component assays are performed using serum rather than plasma. In the hemolytic assay, the degree of hemolysis is measured spectrophotometrically as the absorbance of released hemoglobin can be directly related to the number of lysed red blood cells. The hemolytic complement activity is estimated as the amount of complement required to achieve 50% hemolysis and is referred to as the CH_{50}.

17.3.1.1.1 Evaluation of Pathway Activation

As a screening assay for the activation of the classic complement pathway, the CH_{50} is sensitive to the reduction or absence and/or inactivity of any component of the pathway. In general, it tests the functional capability of the complement components in the serum to lyse sheep red blood cells, precoated (sensitized) with rabbit antisheep red blood cell antibody (hemolysin). When antibody-coated sheep red blood cells are incubated with test serum, the classic pathway of complement is activated and hemolysis results.

The amount of complement activity is determined by examining the ability of various dilutions of test serum to lyse the sensitized sheep red blood cells. Thus, a fixed volume of the red blood cells is added to each serum dilution. The mixture is incubated, then centrifuged, and the degree of hemolysis is determined by measuring the absorbance of the hemoglobin released at 540 nm. The percentage of red blood cell lysis in a standardized system follows an S-shaped curve when plotted against increasing amounts of added complement. In the midregion of the curve, there is nearly a linear relationship between the degree of hemolysis and the amount of complement added. The amount of complement required to achieve 50% hemolysis is the CH_{50}. When human or animal serum is submitted to this procedure, a whole complement titer is measured, and the titer is expressed as the reciprocal of the serum dilution that lyses 50% of a standard suspension of erythrocytes.

For the alternative pathway, fresh human serum is capable of lysing unsensitized rabbit erythrocytes in the presence of Mg-EDTA by the alternative pathway (Atkinson and Frank, 1980). This assay has been used to measure alternative pathway components (ACH_{50}) in 25 species of mammals; while rabbit red cells served as targets for alternative pathway activation in 18 of 20 species, the red cells of other mammals were frequently more sensitive. Sialic acid concentration of the red cell membrane correlated with ACH_{50} (Ish et al., 1993; Menger and Aston, 1984; Naka et al., 1997; Olahu-Mukani et al., 1994).

17.3.1.1.2 Measurement of Individual Complement Components

The hemolytic assay can also be used to measure individual complement components. Target red cells with membrane-bound components are prepared by producing antibody-sensitized sheep red cells (EA), and incubating them in purified guinea pig or human C1. This reaction mixture yields EAC1. Incubation of EAC1 with fresh human serum in EDTA yields EAC14 and EAC4. The application of EAC1 to test serum allows for the rapid binding of C4, which in the presence of fresh guinea pig serum, containing C3–C9, will result in hemolysis limited only by the concentration of C4 in the test sample. Likewise, the application of the cellular intermediate EAC14 to test serum allows for the binding of C2 from the test serum, which in the presence of fresh guinea pig serum allows for hemolysis limited only by the concentration of C2 in the test serum.

The use of cellular intermediates and purified components for the measurement of all nine classic pathway components was reviewed for use in human (Gaither and Frank, 1979) and other animal samples (Barta and Barta, 1973a). Testing animal complement components using commercially available reagents for human beings has produced acceptable results for the measurement of C1 and C5 through C9; however, the results obtained when measuring C4, C2, and C3 are generally much lower in domestic animals than in human beings or the guinea pig (Barta and Hubbert, 1978). For this reason, the purification of C4, C2, and C3 from each species and their use in a homologous assay is encouraged. The hemolytic assay for individual components using cellular intermediates was used to measure C1 through C7 in rats (Arroyave et al., 1977; Sakamoto et al., 1981), C1 through C9 in rabbits (Menger and Aston, 1984), C1 through C9 and factor B in nonhuman primates (McMahan, 1982; Schur et al., 1975), C1 through C9 in guinea pigs (Bitter-Suermann et al., 1981; Nelson et al., 1966), and C1 through C6 in the mouse (Nilsson and Muller-Eberhard, 1967).

Several modifications to the hemolytic assay have been made for the measurement of individual components in human beings and animals. In one modification, the EA cells are incubated with test serum or serum from animals that have a genetically related deficiency in one complement component. In addition, a number of animals with genetically related deficiencies of individual complement components including, C2-, C3-, or C4-deficient guinea pigs, C3-deficient dogs, C1q-, C3-, C4-, C5- and factor B-deficient mice, and C6-deficient rats and rabbits have been described (Rother and Rother, 1986; Botto, 1998; Barrington et al., 2001; Tuzun et al., 2003). An often-used assay employs sera from C4-deficient guinea pigs, and has been used to measure C4 in human beings, mice, and rats (Arroyave et al., 1977; Atkinson et al., 1980; Gaither and Frank, 1979). Similarly, human C2-deficient sera and rabbit C6-deficient sera have been used to measure levels of these components in human and animal serum (Atkinson et al., 1980; Bitter-Suermann et al., 1981; Gaither and Frank, 1979). In a second modification, Pepys (1974) measured murine C3 by observing rosette formation where $EAC142^{gp}$ (isolated components of guinea pig origin) bound to C3 on mouse mesenteric lymph node cells.

Yamamoto et al. (1995) developed a liposome-based assay to measure total complement activity in human beings. When liposomes had glucose-6-phosphate dehydrogenase entrapped in their core and dinitrophenyl integrated in the outer membrane, a fully automated complement assay could be quantitated following the binding of anti-DNP as the initiator.

17.3.1.1.3 Testing Sensitivity

Since hemolysis will be lowered proportionally to the consumption of complement, these types of complement evaluations can be used to assess the effect of complement inhibition by a certain substance or agent or as a semiquantitative estimator of complement activation under controlled conditions. If any single component of the classic pathway is missing, hemolysis will not occur. The total absence of a component, however, is rare in most clinical situations. Problems with the assay may include complex mathematical and or technical manipulations, lack of objectivity, and poor sensitivity. These have been addressed somewhat in a modification of the tube assay involving microtiter plates and an enzyme-linked immunosorbant assay (ELISA) reader (measuring hemolysis), and a computer program for calculation of values (Blann et al., 1990; Costabile, 2010).

17.3.1.1.4 Species-Specific Considerations

Though hemolytic assays can be designed for any species, in some instances a comprehensive analysis of complement is limited due to the lack of appropriate reagents and procedures (Kirschfink and Mollnes, 2003). For example, in a previously unstudied species, the selection of a relevant target cell is a considerable factor. Thus, when testing animal serum, determining the optimum conditions for hemolysis for the individual species is critical and factors such as target red cell, buffer pH, buffer ionic strength, and concentration of calcium ions must all be carefully selected (Barta and Barta, 1984). In general, serum for all animal species should be harvested within 60 minutes of blood collection and either tested immediately or stored frozen at –70°C until tested. Swine and chicken complement, however, are relatively unstable even when frozen at –70°C (Barta and Barta, 1984). Since the resultant hemolytic titers are influenced by the source and quality of erythrocyte-specific antibodies, comparison of pathway activity between different species can be difficult to assess (Higgins and Langley, 1985). It appears, however, when the assay has been optimized, activity of the classic and the alternative pathways can be demonstrated in essentially any species of laboratory and domestic animal (Barta, 1978; Ish et al., 1993; Tanaka et al., 1987). Finally, techniques have been thoroughly reviewed for both human (Alper and Rosen, 1975; Gaither and Frank, 1979) and animal assays (Barta and Barta, 1984; Grant, 1977).

Using the basic technique, the total hemolytic complement of animals was measured in dogs (Barta and Barta, 1973a; Madewell, 1978; Trail et al., 1984; Wolfe and Halliwell, 1980), rats (Naka et al., 1997; Sakamoto et al., 1981), mice (Nilsson and Muller-Eberhard, 1967), guinea pigs (Thurston et al., 1980), nonhuman primates (Ellingsworth et al., 1983; Rommel et al., 1980), rabbits (Nelson and Biro, 1968), sheep (Jonas and Stankiewicz, 1981; Stankiewicz and Jonas, 1981), goats (Oyekan and Barta, 1980), swine (Oyekan and Barta, 1980), cats (Barta and Oyekan, 1981), hamsters (Yang et al., 1974), horses (Barta and Barta, 1973b), and chickens (Barta and Barta, 1975). It has been reported that many mouse strains have low complement activity relative to human beings, rats, guinea pigs, and rabbits (Ong and Mattes, 1989). Of 43 mouse strains evaluated, only 8 strains demonstrated complement activity levels comparable to those of other mammals.

Modifications to the hemolytic assay have been made to measure hemolytic complement in bovine milk (Poutrel and Caffin, 1984). A test for measuring cytotoxic complement in rabbits using murine lymphocytes and alloantisera in a microtiter system has been reported (Fox and Cherry, 1978; Fox et al., 1978, 1979).

17.3.1.2 Evaluation of Complement Activation by Immunoassay

Methods using a solid-phase enzyme immunoassay (ELISA or EIA) format have been described for screening the activation of all three (classic, alternative, and lectin) pathways (Fredrikson et al., 1993; Seelen et al., 2005). One assay (Seelen et al., 2005) includes three separate EIA assessing all three activation pathways simultaneously in human samples; it is commercially available (Wieslab, Euro Diagnostica, Malmö, Sweden). For this method, IgM (for the classic pathway), mannan or acetylated bovine serum albumin (for the lectin pathway), and LPS (for the alternative pathway) are used as the specific recognition molecules for the immunoassay. In general, the recognition molecules are coated onto microtiter plate wells. The test serum is added and incubated under conditions in which only one pathway is activated. Complement activation is then detected using a monoclonal antibody against either a C9 neoepitope (classic pathway) or an antibody against properdin (alternative pathway). To create a lectin pathway-specific assay, the other activation pathways must be blocked. This blockade is achieved by the use of a monoclonal anti-C1q antibody inhibiting classic pathway activation (Roos et al., 2005).

The solid-phase immunoassay format has advantages compared with the hemolytic assays. For example, as an EIA, it is easily performed, it is not dependent on erythrocyte availability, and the alternative pathway assay can detect a properdin deficiency. These assays can be used in combination with the measurement of C3 and C4 and, if a complement deficiency is suggested, could be supplemented by measurement of an activation product assay to distinguish primary from secondary complement deficiency (Seelen et al., 2005). Recently, ELISA methods for measuring functional complement pathways in rats, mice and some old world monkeys, similar to the human assays outlined in Section 17.3.1, have been described (TECOmedical Group, 2010; Kotimaa et al., 2014; Kotimaa et al., 2015; van der Pol et al., 2012).

17.3.2 Immunochemical Assays

Individual complement components, irrespective of functional activity, can be measured by a variety of methods that rely on the formation of antigen–antibody complexes as the test principle. For example, antigenic assays including radial immunodiffusion, electroimmunodiffusion (rocket electrophoresis), automated immunoprecipitation (measured nephelometrically), crossed immunoelectrophoresis (Lewis and Picut, 1989; Mancini et al., 1965), time-resolved immunofluorometric assay (Moller Kristensen et al., 2003), radioimmunoassay (Guiguet et al., 1987), and ELISA (Porcel et al., 1993) have all been used to measure complement components in human beings and other animals. A brief description follows for some of the listed methods.

17.3.2.1 Radial Immunodiffusion

A widely used method, radial immunodiffusion, is based on the principle that a quantitative relationship exists between the amount of antigen placed in a well cut in the agar antibody plate and the resulting ring of precipitation. The assay may be conducted using one of two methods. In the Mancini method (Mancini et al., 1965), specific antibody raised against the complement component to be measured is added to agar so that the antibody is in excess (relative to the concentration of the complement component in test sera). In this assay, the incubation time is not critical.

The Fahey method (Fahey and McKelvey, 1965) employs antibody that is not in excess, and therefore, the time of incubation is critical. In both assays, a standard curve is first generated using purified complement components, and the diameter of the precipitin ring is directly related to antigen (complement) concentration through a logarithmic relationship. When universal reference standards or chemically pure components are unavailable, a standard reference serum may be used in which the exact concentration of the specific complement component is known. The radial immunodiffusion assay should be run on fresh or fresh frozen (–70°C) serum and, as in all complement assay methods, bacterial contamination of the test serum must be avoided. Reference standards should be frozen as aliquots because repeated freeze–thawing may influence the results. The radial immunodiffusion assay has been used successfully to measure various complement components in guinea pigs (Thurston et al., 1980), cattle (Table et al., 1983), mice (Ferreira and Nussenzweig, 1975; Karp et al., 1982a), and nonhuman primates (Holmberg et al., 1977).

17.3.2.2 Electroimmunodiffusion

The electroimmunodiffusion (rocket electrophoresis) assay is based on the principle of electrophoresis of antigen (complement) into antiserum-containing agarose. In this assay, the peak heights of rocket-shaped precipitin bands are measured and compared with those of standards used for quantitation of antigen in the test sample. This method is both sensitive and rapid, but it requires some special equipment. Rocket electrophoresis has been used to quantitate complement components in nonhuman primates (Alper et al., 1971; McMahan, 1982), dogs (Feldman et al., 1981), mice (Ferreira and Nussenzweig, 1975; Natsuume-Sakai et al., 1978; Pepys et al., 1977), and guinea pigs (Bitter-Suermann et al., 1981).

A modification of the rocket electrophoresis, used for rapid qualitative assessment of complement components, was described by Natsuume-Sakai et al. (1978). In this procedure, wells are cut from agarose-coated glass slides, and antigen is first isolated by charge using constant voltage. After a period of time, a trough is cut between two wells, and specific antiserum is added. Precipitin bands occur when antigen and antiserum reach equivalence by double diffusion. This technique is useful to detect the presence or absence of a component and to observe charge variation in components. It has been used to evaluate complement in such divergent species as mice (Natsuume-Sakai et al., 1980) and cattle (Table et al., 1983).

17.3.2.3 Crossed Immunoelectrophoresis

Crossed immunoelectrophoresis is a variant of immunoelectrophoresis and is more sensitive. It allows precise measurement of the amount of each antigen present in a mixture. Antigens placed in the sample slot are electrophoresed in agarose. A central strip of agarose containing all of the isolated components is then removed and placed on a second slab of agarose, which contains the antisera (Laurell, 1972). This assay has the advantage of providing quantitative estimations of complement component conversion, and therefore complements activation that occurred *in vivo* (Alper and Rosen, 1975). Crossed immunoelectrophoresis has been used successfully to quantitate complement components in dogs (Gorman et al., 1981a), cats (Gorman et al., 1981b), nonhuman primates (Ziegler et al., 1975b), and mice (Pepys et al., 1977).

17.3.2.4 Quantitative Immunoassays

The availability of monoclonal antibodies that bind neoepitopes present on the split products of individual human complement components allows for the initial binding of the split product (and its removal from serum or plasma), and later quantitation with an enzyme-linked (ELISA-type assay) or radio-labeled (RIA-type assay) secondary antibody. These types of assays can be specific, sensitive, and conducive to automation. Currently, antibodies exist to measure human C4b, C4c, C4d, Ba, Bb, C3dg, and C4BP (Porcel et al., 1993; Coppola et al., 1995; Pavlov et al., 2011). When C4d, Bb, and iC3b (quantitated by ELISA) were compared to levels of C3 and C4 (by radial immunodiffusion) and CH_{50}, good agreement was found between human patients and controls for all levels except iC3b, which was elevated compared to CH_{50}. The authors attributed these elevated iC3b levels in patients to a decreased iC3b clearance, an increased C3 synthesis, or an enhanced C3 cleavage by nonimmune mechanisms (Goldberg et al., 1997).

17.3.2.4.1 Measurement of Anaphylotoxins

Tests for total hemolytic complement and components are indirect measures of activation tests that are capable of directly detecting and quantitating complement activation. In each of these assays, in vitro activation must be prevented, therefore, blood is collected into EDTA tubes containing nafamostat mesylate (to stabilize components), and the plasma should be separated as soon as possible. A sensitive radioimmunoassay was developed to measure the anaphylatoxins C3a, C4a, and C5a (Wagner and Hugli, 1984); however, this procedure first requires precipitation of the native molecules (C3, C4, and C5) from plasma. The detection of false plasma elevations due to complement activation *in vitro* is a major limiting factor in all anaphylatoxin assays. This radioimmunoassay could be used to detect anaphylatoxins in rhesus monkey and baboon serum; however, the test appears to be no more than 10% efficient in measuring C3a in nonhuman primate samples.

17.3.2.4.2 Species Cross-Reactivity

While numerous specific assays have been described for human complement activation, only a few are available for animal studies. Tests developed specifically for animals include assays based on monoclonal antibodies to guinea pig C5a (Link et al., 1999) and C3 activation products (Hawlisch et al., 2000), rabbit C5a (Bergh and Iversen, 1989), and rat C5b-9 (Schulze et al., 1989). A double antibody radioimmunoassay specific for rat C3 was developed and utilized for quantifying C3 in cell culture media (Guiguet et al., 1987). There are examples of human epitope-specific assays that cross-react with other species including baboon C3bc (Hiramatsu et al., 1997); baboon C3bc, C5a, and C5b-9 (Mollnes et al., 1993); baboon C4d, C3a, Bb, and C5b-9 (Fung et al., 2001); and porcine C5b-9 (Jansen et al., 1993). Further, using a human assay of complement activation, potential species cross-reactivity can be assessed by activating the serum from the respective species and comparing it to the nonactivated sample. If the signal is stronger in the activated serum compared to the nonactivated serum, the assay cross-reacts to some level with that species.

17.4 SPECIFIC COMPONENTS OF THE COMPLEMENT CASCADE

The complement system is an indispensable host defense mechanism against external pathogens. However, several perturbations of this defense apparatus are related to a variety of diseases. For example, unregulated activation of complement significantly contributes to inflammation-mediated tissue damage, and inherited or acquired complement deficiencies can contribute to the development of autoimmunity (Markiewski and Lambris, 2007; Ram et al., 2010; Nilsson and Ekdahl, 2012). Additionally, alterations of complement activity can play a role for such pathologic conditions as transplantation reactions, infections, and cancer (Nilsson and Ekdahl, 2012). Moreover, complement analyses including quantification of complement activity and complement activation products, and genetic methods for the detection of deficiencies, mutations, and polymorphisms, have been performed on many of these conditions in human and experimental animal studies (Kirschfink and Mollnes, 2003; Mollnes et al., 2007).

Basic indications for diagnostic complement analysis have been divided into three major categories: (1) acquired and inherited complement deficiencies; (2) disorders with complement activation; (3) inherited and acquired C1INH deficiencies (Nilsson and Ekdahl, 2012). Animal models of acquired complement inhibition (e.g., CoF) have been used (Frank, 1995). Additionally, a variety of animals (e.g., mouse, rat, guinea pig, dog, rabbit, and swine) with spontaneous or genetically engineered overexpression or deficiency of individual components have enabled investigators to study the role of complement in a focused manner (Frank, 1995; Botto et al., 1998; Linton, 2001; Hanafusa et al., 2002; Loeffler, 2004; Markiewski and Lambris, 2007; Ram et al., 2010). The following section highlights some of the information regarding specific components of complement and associated animal models.

17.4.1 THIRD COMPONENT OF COMPLEMENT (C3)

17.4.1.1 Physical, Chemical, and Genetic Properties of C3

The third component of complement (C3) is a secreted glycoprotein with the electrophoretic migration properties of a β-globulin (Colten, 1976). It is present in human serum in concentrations higher than any other component, and was the first isolated in pure form. The molecules of C3,

C4, and C5 have common structural and functional properties, and it has therefore been postulated that they may all have arisen from a common ancestral molecule (Muller-Eberhard, 1975). The molecular weight of secreted human C3 is 180,000 Daltons (Da) (Budzko et al., 1971). It consists of two chains linked by disulfide bonds (Nilsson and Mapes, 1973; Tack and Prahl, 1976). The C3 α-chain weighs 110 kDa, and the C3 β-chain weighs 70 kDa. Both chains are part of a large intracellular polypeptide, pro-C3, which in the mouse and guinea pig has the subunit arrangement NH_2-β-α-COOH (Goldberger et al., 1981). The pro-C3 subunits are linked by four arginine residues that must be cleaved to produce the native two-chain molecule (Fey et al., 1983). The secreted two-chain molecule undergoes extracellular enzymatic cleavage that selectively affects the larger α-chain. Cleavage of the chain leads to generation of the C3a and C3b fragments, each with biologic activity. Further cleavage of the C3b fragment of the α-chain leads to production of C3c, C3d, and C3e (Muller-Eberhard, 1975). Rat C3 has a molecular weight of 187 kDa (Daha et al., 1979) and consists of two polypeptide chains weighing 125 and 73 kDa (Guiguet et al., 1987). Swine C3 α-chain has a molecular weight of 110 kDa and the C3 β-chain is 60 Da (Storm et al., 1992).

Three electrophoretic variants of C3 have been described in the rhesus monkey. The three alleles have been designated $C3^S$, $C3^F$, and $C3^{F1}$, with a gene frequency of 0.66, 0.33, and 0.01 among 81 rhesus monkeys (Alper et al., 1971). Using high voltage electrophoresis, Gorman et al. (1981a, b) described three allotypes of canine C3, designated F, FS, and S. Family studies in dogs demonstrated that the C3F and C3S alleles are codominantly expressed at a single autosomal locus. The canine C3 genetic locus was not linked to the major histocompatibility complex (MHC).

Human C3 α- and C3 β-chains are both glycosylated, whereas only the C3 β-chain is glycosylated in the mouse (Fey et al., 1983). It is also known that the mouse C3 β-chain is 9 kDa smaller than the human C3 β-chain due to a difference in the amino acid chain length. A number of rare variants of the S and F alleles have been described in human beings; however, they are all functionally identical (Colten, 1983b; Colten and Alper, 1972).

The amino acid sequence of the C3 chain is known for the mouse and man (Fey et al., 1983). In addition, the sequence of C3a (anaphylatoxin) is also known for the rat (Jacobs al., 1978) and pig (Corbin and Hugli, 1976). Mouse C3a shares 92% amino acid homology with rat C3a, 70% with rabbit C3a, 67% homology with human C3a, and 65% homology with swine C3a (Becherer et al., 1989; Hugli, 1975; Karp et al., 1982a). All 10 amino acid residues common to the thioester bond region of human C2, C4, and α-macroglobulin (the thioester bond is considered essential for function) are also identical to those in mouse C3. Structural characteristics of cattle, avian, reptilian, amphibian, and fish C3 have been published (Becherer et al., 1989; DiCarlo et al., 1997).

The human and murine C3 gene has been cloned (Hobart, 1984). A single gene in both species codes C3, and strong homologies are seen in the primary structure of each C3 gene. The gene for human C3 is located on chromosome 19, unlinked to the MHC (Fey et al., 1983). The murine C3 gene is linked to the MHC on chromosome 17 but maps outside the MHC, at a recombination distance of 12 centimorgans. Mice have three alleles encoding different electrophoretic variants (da Silva et al., 1978). The C3a allele determines a protein with an isoelectric point (pI) of 6.0 and an intermediate migration rate on cellulose acetate electrophoresis. C3b determines a protein of pI 6.1 and slow(S) migration; it is found in C57BL/6, BALB/c, CBA/J, and many other murine strains. C3c determines a protein with a pI of 6.0 but is antigenically different from the C3a protein; it migrates fast (F) and is found in SWR/J, WB/Re, SF/Cam, SJL and other murine strains (da Silva et al., 1978). The alleles responsible for these variants in both species are codominantly expressed (Natsuume-Sakai et al., 1978), and the allotypic determinants are located on the C3c fragment (as part of the primary structure). Antigenic variants in murine C3 have been demonstrated using specific alloantisera (Natsuume-Sakai et al., 1979). Constitutive and cytokine-induced expression of the C3 gene requires both *cis*- and *trans*-acting elements (Kawamura et al., 1992).

17.4.1.2 Function of C3

Due to its central position in both the alternative and classic pathways, C3 is of paramount importance in the generation of both the MAC and biologically active split products. The initial extracellular enzymatic cleavage of C3 occurs in the α-chain by C3 convertase (either classic or alternative), yielding a small molecular weight (9 kDa) C3a, and the large C3b fragments. The biologic activities of C3a include receptor binding and histamine release from mast cells (Johnson et al., 1975), polymorphonuclear leukocyte chemotaxis (Muller-Eberhard, 1975), and contraction of bronchial smooth muscle and hypotension (Bokisch and Muller-Eberhard, 1970; Regal et al., 1993).

The C3b fragment has a binding site, allowing for its attachment to other acceptor molecules. Once bound, C3b has a second binding site, allowing it to react with the immune adherence receptor on a variety of cells (Morgan, 1995; Muller-Eberhard, 1975). The binding of C3b to these receptors allows polymorphonuclear leukocytes/granulocytes and macrophages to engage in phagocytosis (Gigli and Nelson, 1968). The binding sites of human C3 for properdin, factor H, CR1, CR2, factor B, and MCP have all been identified (Sahu et al., 1998).

The C3b fragment is also subject to enzymatic cleavage by the C3 inactivator, which also occurs on the α-chain (Bokisch et al., 1975). During this cleavage, a small peptide, C3d, remains attached to the cell, while a larger molecule, C3c, is released (Ruddy and Austen, 1971). The C3c fragment maintains an intact β-chain, but during fission from C3b it loses another small fragment (16 kDa), C3e (Bokisch et al., 1975). The membrane-bound C3b combines with classic pathway C3 convertase to yield the trimolecular complex C4b2a3b, which acts as a C5 convertase, cleaves C5, and, initiates the assembly of the MAC, C5b-C9 (Kolb et al., 1972). Likewise, the alternative pathway C3 convertase, C3bBb, may initiate a similar sequence, resulting in the activation of C3–C9 (Fearon et al., 1973). There is some evidence that the C4b2a3b complex of rabbits is a much more efficient C5 convertase than that of human beings or guinea pig (Ong et al., 1996).

Another interesting feature of C3 is that its blood concentrations increase during acute and chronic inflammation, and after tissue injury (Kusher, 1982; Muller-Eberhard, 1975). Although the acute phase reactants CRP and serum amyloid A protein rise rapidly within hours after injury, C3 levels rise more slowly (2–10 days) and often parallel ceruloplasmin concentrations. The concentration of C3 in the blood often increases by 50% during this acute phase response, whereas other acute phase reactants, such as CRP and serum amyloid A protein increase by hundred or thousand folds. Although most acute phase reactants of hepatic origin are induced by interleukin-1, glucocorticoids are the only well-characterized C3 regulators (Fey et al., 1983). Extracellular phosphorylation of C3 occurs under several pathologic conditions and renders C3 less susceptible to cleavage by either the classic or alternative pathways (Ekdahl et al., 1997).

17.4.1.3 Synthesis and Catabolism of C3

Estimates of C3 synthetic rates in human beings range between 0.45 and 2.7 mg/kg/h (Alper and Rosen, 1967; Peters et al., 1972; Sliwinski and Zvaifler, 1972). C3, like most of the C proteins, is synthesized early in fetal life (Hirschfeld and Lunell, 1962). Gitlin and Biasucci (1969) demonstrated fetal C3 synthesis in as early as the fourth week of human gestation. In normal human adults, the liver was shown to be the principal site of C3 synthesis (Alper et al., 1969a). However, small amounts of C3 have been produced in short-term cultures of human monocytes, lymphoid cells, and certain epithelial cells (Fey et al., 1983), and C3 synthesis by glomerular epithelial and mesangial cells in the kidney has been documented during human membranous nephropathy and Heymann nephritis in rats (Sasaki et al., 1997).

Hepatocytes of adult rats and mice failed to synthesize C3 in vitro except after endotoxin stimulation; however, C3 synthesis was easily demonstrated in unstimulated hepatocytes from juvenile animals. In mice, a locus that maps in the MHC locus controls the serum levels of C3 in the newborn, while no significant differences in C3 concentrations are seen in adults (Ferreira and Nussenzweig,

1975, 1976). Induction of hepatic C3 synthesis may be mediated by IL-1, IL-6, or tumor necrosis factor (TNF) (Singer et al., 1994).

Several investigators (Stecher and Thorbecke, 1967; Strunk et al., 1975) have shown that hydrocortisone increases the synthesis of C3 in vitro; however, injection of cortisone acetate into experimental animals has yielded contradictory results (Atkinson and Frank, 1973). In one study, periorbital abscesses secondary to blood sampling procedures abolished the expected depression of the C3–C9 complex (Colten, 1976). C3 expression in the mouse can be suppressed by anti-C3 antibody, and $CD4^+$ and $CD8^+$ T-lymphocytes are required for suppression (Goldman et al., 1992).

C3a is inactivated in serum by carboxypeptidase B, an α-globulin that removes the COOH-terminal arginine residue from C3a and neutralizes its activity. The trimolecular complex C4b2a3b decays with the dissociation of the C2 fragment. C3b inactivator splits cell-bound or soluble C3b into two fragments, C3c and C3d, and the function of C3b is thus abolished (Muller-Eberhard and Gotze, 1972; Tamura and Nelson, 1967). In man, mouse, and several other species, C3 turnover is regulated by CR1, CR2, DAF, and MCP binding proteins (Holers et al., 1992).

17.4.1.4 Analysis of C3

Serum concentrations of C3 were measured by hemolytic assay using cellular intermediates in eight species of nonhuman primates. The hemolytic titers for C3 were equivalent to those in human beings for five species of Old World nonhuman primates; however, both antigenic and functional assays were inadequate in several New World primates (Quimby, 1999). C3 was also measured by rocket electrophoresis in four species of Old World primates (Alper et al., 1971; McMahan, 1982) and by radial immunodiffusion using human antiserum in nine nonhuman primates. In all of these studies, Old World primates had strong cross-reactivity with human reagents (rhesus monkey is nearly identical to human sequence) while prosimians had no detectable reactivity (Holmberg et al., 1977).

In rabbits, rats, guinea pigs, and mice, C3 was measured by immunoelectrophoresis, double diffusion in agar, and immune adherence (Cochrane et al., 1970). Both rocket electrophoresis and crossed electrophoresis were used successfully to quantitate C3 in the mouse (Natsuume-Sakai et al., 1978; Pepys et al., 1977). C3 was also quantitated in dogs, rabbits, and swine using radial immunodiffusion (Kalowski et al., 1975; Molleda et al., 1993; Storm et al., 1992; Ulevitch and Cochrane, 1977). Canine C3 has been measured by rocket electrophoresis (Feldman et al., 1981; Gorman et al., 1981a, b). A double antibody radioimmunoassay has been developed to measure C3 in the rat (Guiguet et al., 1987).

As with all other C-component assays, the lack of universal reference standards in animals makes comparison between laboratories impossible. These and other technical considerations when testing laboratory animal species were reviewed by Barta and Barta (1984).

Assays designed to measure antigenic determinants on the split products of C3 have been developed for human beings and guinea pig (Regal et al., 1993; Sinosich et al., 1982). Cross immunoelectrophoresis of swine C3 does not elucidate the C3b/iC3b/c3c fragments as seen with human C3 (Storm et al., 1992).

17.4.1.5 Clinical Significance of C3 Concentrations

When measured by radial immunodiffusion, the adult levels of C3 in human beings are 1–2 mg/mL (Fey et al., 1983). Levels of serum C3 in women are known to increase during late pregnancy (Propp and Alper, 1968). No differences were reported in the levels of C3 between male and female dogs; however, higher levels were observed in older dogs (Molleda et al., 1993). Human beings with obstructive jaundice have an increase in C3 (Colten, 1976), and patients with membranoproliferative glomerulonephritis have a decrease in serum C3 (Alper et al., 1966; Peters et al., 1972). Because liver samples from two patients with membranoproliferative glomerulonephritis failed to produce C3 in culture, it was postulated that the decrease in C3 seen in this condition is due to both decreased synthesis as well as increased catabolism (Colten et al., 1973). Decreased serum C3 due to increased catabolism is also seen in patients with diseases characterized by circulating immune complexes, such as systemic lupus erythematosus and lupus nephritis (Levo and Pick, 1974; Swaak et al., 1986).

The concentrations of total hemolytic complement (CH_{50}) and C3 were significantly depressed in dogs with acute necrotizing pancreatitis (Feldman et al., 1981) and in rats fed a protein-deficient (0.5%) diet (Schaller et al., 1977). Rabbits developing disseminated intravascular coagulation had significantly depressed levels of C3 and CH_{50}; a relationship between clotting and complement activation was demonstrated, indicating that platelets were partially responsible for complement activation (Kalowski et al., 1975). C3 concentrations are elevated in the cerebrospinal fluid of mice with bacterial meningitis (Stahel et al., 1997). The role of C3 in hyperacute xenograft rejection has been studied in monkeys, rats, guinea pigs, and dogs (Braidley et al., 1994; Cable et al., 1997; McCurry et al., 1995; Tanaka et al., 1996).

CoF has been widely used in experimental animals to evaluate the role of complement in various biologic systems. CoF is composed of two anticomplementary factors: a low molecular weight factor (140 kDa), which activates both C3 and C5, and a high molecular weight factor (10^6 Da), which is anticomplementary for the early complement components only (Ballow and Cochrane, 1969). The effect of CoF has been studied in rats, rabbits, guinea pigs, hamsters, and mice (Cochrane et al., 1970; Roxvall et al., 1990). In these studies, C3, as measured by immunoelectrophoresis, double diffusion, and immune adherence, was depressed to <10% normal in all animals after treatment with CoF. Furthermore, complement-depleted animals undergoing acute nephrotoxic nephritis had fewer neutrophils infiltrating the glomeruli. CoF was also shown to inhibit the Arthus reaction, thus demonstrating an important pathologic effect associated with C3 activation.

Mice depleted of C3 by CoF treatment had no change in the rate of clearance of preformed immune complexes in vivo (Bockow and Mannik, 1981), but had a significantly prolonged survival of *Trypanosoma lewisi* (Albright and Albright, 1985). These investigators concluded that resistance to *T. lewisi* involved activation and binding of C3b by uncoated trypanosomes (Desai et al., 1987).

Rabbits treated with CoF and depleted of C3 (measured by radial immunodiffusion) had rapid C3-dependent depression of platelet function and blood pressure. The hypotensive effects could be blocked by a histamine H2-receptor antagonist (Trail et al., 1984). Mathison and Ulevitch (1981) also showed that thrombocytopenia associated with endotoxemia in rabbits could be abrogated if the animals were depleted of C3. However, despite the abrogation of this early reaction, CoF had no effect on the final development of hypotension and disseminated intravascular coagulation in these animals.

Genetic deficiencies in C3, though rare, have been described in human beings (Alper et al., 1969b), dogs (Winkelstein et al., 1981, 1982), guinea pigs (Burger et al., 1986; Moore, 1919), rabbits (Komatsu et al., 1988), and mice (Pekna et al., 1998; Prodeus et al., 1997; Singer et al., 1994). Total (homozygous) C3 deficiency in human beings is characterized by the complete absence of C3 in the serum, and it is usually associated with recurrent pyogenic infections and the development of membranous glomerulonephritis. Many individuals with total C3 deficiency die in childhood. Transfusion with normal plasma gives patients transient relief from systemic infections. Sera from these patients lack the typical complement-mediated biologic functions, such as hemolytic activity, opsonization of endotoxin-coated particles, and chemotaxic and bactericidal activities (Alper et al., 1972c, 1976). Dogs with total C3 deficiency display similar signs and a lack of normal complement-mediated functions.

In both human beings and dogs, the defect is inherited as an autosomal recessive trait, and heterozygotes have half the normal C3 concentrations. The first report of a complement defect in a laboratory animal was published by Moore (1919). He studied a guinea pig strain whose serum failed to lyse antibody-sensitized horse erythrocytes. This guinea pig serum showed reduced opsonization capacity, and affected guinea pigs were more susceptible to infection with *Bacillus cholerae suis* (*Salmonella cholerae suis*). This colony was decimated by an infectious disease; therefore, the true nature of the defect will never be known. The defect was transmitted as a simple Mendelian recessive trait.

Partial deficiencies also have been described in human beings. These deficiencies may be due to either a partially inactive gene product or partially reduced synthesis of a normal product from at least one defective allele. Carriers of a partial deficiency are generally healthy (Fey et al., 1983).

Burger et al. (1986) also described a colony of guinea pigs with C3 deficiency. Animals homozygous for the deficiency had markedly reduced hemolytic activity, reduced antigenic activity (6% normal), reduced bactericidal activity, and impaired antibody responses (Bottger et al., 1986a, b; Burger et al., 1986). The defect in guinea pigs is inherited in a codominant autosomal fashion and is not linked to the MHC locus (Burger et al., 1986).

Rabbits displaying 6%–12% serum levels of C3 were found in a colony of C8 deficient rabbits (Komatsu et al., 1988). The C3-hypocomplementemic rabbits had no alteration in C3 conversion, antigenicity, or catabolism, and no C3 inhibitors were detected. C3 hypocomplementemia was inherited in a simple codominant fashion, and serum from these rabbits had lower bactericidal activity compared to normal serum. Unlike rabbits with C8 deficiency, C3 hypocomplementemic rabbits had no decrease in body weight; however, they did have poor survival rates (Komatsru et al., 1988).

Mice homozygous for a targeted mutation of the C3 gene have been developed, and they have no detectable levels of circulating C3 (Pekna et al., 1998). C3 deficient mice have increased mortality following cecal perforation and exhibit decreased peritoneal mast cell degranulation, production of TNF-α, neutrophil infiltration, and clearance of bacteria (Prodeus et al., 1997). C3 knockout mice have also been used to demonstrate the critical role of complement in antiglomerular basement membrane-induced nephritis (Sheerin et al., 1997).

17.4.2 Fourth Component of Complement (C4)

17.4.2.1 Physical, Chemical, and Genetic Properties of C4

The fourth component of complement (C4) was first described by Gordon et al. (1926) but was not isolated until 1963 (Muller-Eberhard and Biro, 1963). Human C4 is a glycoprotein weighing 209 kDa and containing 8% carbohydrate residues. It migrates electrophoretically as a β-protein. Human C4 is composed of three unequal, covalently linked polypeptide chains designated as α, β, and γ with molecular weights of 93, 78 and 33 kDa, respectively (Schreiber and Muller-Eberhard, 1974). Guinea pig and mouse C4 have a similar molecular weight and three-chain structure (Hall and Colten, 1977). The mouse has two C4-like molecules, each coded by a separate gene in the S-region of the MHC (Shreffler, 1982); however, only one of these molecules (formerly known as Ss protein) is the functional homologue of guinea pig and human C4 (Ferreira et al., 1977). C4 has been identified in the rat, and amino acid sequence homology (derived from a cDNA clone) was 81.7% and 86.6% for murine and human C4, respectively (Fimmel et al., 1996). A molecule having C4-like functional activity has also been described in the hamster, but this protein has not been isolated and characterized (Arroyave et al., 1977). Canine C4 containing three polypeptide subunit chains has also been described (O'Neill et al., 1984). The order of subunit composition in human beings, mice, and guinea pigs is β–α–γ (Chan et al., 1984; Morris et al., 1982; Odink et al., 1981). In mice and human beings, the carbohydrate moiety is found on the α- and β-chains only (Chan et al., 1984).

There are two C4 structural gene loci in human beings, C4A (acidic) and C4B (basic) (O'Neill et al., 1978), with allelic variants described for each locus (Awdeh and Alper, 1980). Complement 4 variants have been identified in the mouse and are linked to the S-region (Ferreira et al., 1977; Natsuume-Sakai et al., 1980). The product of one locus, *Slp*, is hormone regulated (Shreffler, 1982). There is some evidence that the two C4 loci of human beings and mice arose by gene duplication (Shreffler, 1982). Despite duplication of the C4 gene in mice, only one gene product is hemolytically active (Ss protein). The product of the second C4 gene, *Slp*, contains a thioester site in a different portion of the molecule, preventing it from being cleaved by C1 (Hobart, 1984); however, this gene may regulate the expression of a closely linked *Cyp2 1a1* gene and play a role in a third complement pathway in mice (Milstone et al., 1992; van den Berg et al., 1992).

While only a single C4 gene has been identified in guinea pigs, linked to the MHC (Shevach et al., 1976), three variants of guinea pig C4, called C4-F, C4-S, and C4-S1, have been identified by electrophoresis (Bitter-Suermann et al., 1977). These variants are under the control of three codominant alleles at the single C4 locus (Bitter-Suermann et al., 1977).

The dog appears to have only a single C4 structural gene linked to the MHC/dog leukocyte antigen complex (DLA), which has at least five codominantly expressed alleles (Day et al., 1985). They arise from the combination of two allelic products in both the α- and γ-chains (O'Neill et al., 1984). The two allelic products of the canine C4 α-chain also differ in molecular weight (in contrast to the human gene products, which are of identical molecular weight). As in the mouse, the dog C4 γ-chain variant also shows molecular heterogeneity (Ferreira et al., 1980).

Two structural genes encoding C4 appear to be present in certain nonhuman primates (Mevag et al., 1983). Two isoforms of C4 have been reported in the rat (Galibert et al., 1993).

The structural genes for C4, C2, and factor B have all been mapped to the MHC region in guinea pig, mouse, and human beings and are referred to as MHC *class III genes* (Bitter-Suermann et al., 1981; Kronke et al., 1977; Parker et al., 1979; Roos and Demant, 1982; Shreffler and Owen, 1963). The DNA sequence of the various murine and human complement component genes is 5′-C2-Bf-C4–3′. The Slp gene of mice is closer to Bf than to C4. Similarly, the C4A gene of human beings is closer to the Bf gene than it is to the C4B gene (Hobart, 1984). The observation of frequent gene deletion and variations in the number of C4 genes in both mouse and man suggests that this MHC class III region is not genetically stable and may still be undergoing gene expansion and contraction (Shiroishi et al., 1987).

17.4.2.2 Function of C4

During activation of the classic pathway, C4 is cleaved by C1 to produce two split products, C4a and C4b. In human beings, C4a has a molecular weight of 10 kDa and acts as a weak anaphylatoxin. The human C4b fragment is much larger at 190 kDa and covalently binds the biologic material. This bound C4b fragment combines with activated C2 to form a C3 convertase capable of completing the classic pathway of activation (Morgan, 1995; Muller-Eberhard and Biro, 1963). A similar role has been proposed for functionally active C4 of all other species.

Mouse C4 is known to have poor hemolytic activity compared to other species. Molecular analysis of murine C4 identified a short amino acid segment in the β-chain that differed from the human sequence and was responsible for the compromised C5 convertase subunit activity of mouse C4 (Ebanks and Isenman, 1996).

C4BP regulates the classic pathway of complement activation by binding C4b, enhancing degradation of C4b, and accelerating the decay of C3 convertase. Molecular cloning of rat C4BP and an evaluation of the functional relationships among human, bovine, rabbit, mouse, and rat C4BP have been reviewed (Hillarp et al., 1997).

17.4.2.3 Synthesis and Catabolism of C4

Using immunologic methods, C4 biosynthesis has been demonstrated for macrophages and hepatocytes (Colten, 1976). In vitro production of functionally active guinea pig C4 has been demonstrated using cultures of bone marrow, spleen, and liver (Siboo and Vas, 1965), and again the cell type responsible for production of C4 was a phagocytic cell (Ilgen and Burkholder, 1974; Littleton et al., 1970). In contrast, using allogeneic bone marrow chimeras established in mice, Geng et al. (1986) found that circulating C4 in the blood was not primarily synthesized by descendants of bone marrow cells. Recent studies using cell-free biosynthetic systems have shown that guinea pig (Hall and

Colten, 1977), mouse (Parker et al., 1979), and human (Gigli, 1978) C4 is synthesized from a single stranded precursor protein (pro-C4) (Karp et al., 1981) that undergoes intracellular processing, including the cleavage of two proteolytic bonds, sulfation and glycosylation, subsequent to secretion as native C4 (Whitehead et al., 1983), known as C4s (s designates the secreted form). Approximately 8% of the circulating C4 of mouse and man is C4s (Chan and Atkinson, 1983; Karp et al., 1982b); the remaining C4 circulates as C4p, a molecule produced by extracellular proteolytic cleavage.

Both C4s and C4p are active in the fluid phase of blood and respond to regulatory enzymes. The combination of posttranslational intracellular processing, as well as extracellular cleavage, is responsible for as many as 20 structural variants of plasma C4 in a single human being (Chan et al., 1984). Each of the major intracellular and extracellular cleavage products has also been demonstrated in murine biosynthetic systems.

Control of C4 biosynthesis in guinea pigs has been shown to involve a specific feedback mechanism involving C4 itself (Auerbach et al., 1983). This feedback control of synthesis appears to be directed at the level of transcription or is a function of the stability of C4-specific mRNA. No similar feedback control of C4 biosynthesis, using similar systems, has been detected in mice (Newell and Atkinson, 1983). *In vitro* culture systems have also identified specific antibody and a lymphoid cell as supressors of guinea pig macrophage C4 production (McMannis et al., 1987). Rat hepatic stellate cell cultures have been used to study the induction of C4 mRNA by interferon-γ. *In vivo* stellate cells were induced to transcribe C4 by iron overload. C4 production by hepatocytes was unchanged during this procedure (Fimmel et al., 1996).

In normal human beings, approximately 2% of the plasma pool of C4 turns over each hour; therefore, 50% of the plasma pool must be newly synthesized daily (Atkinson and Frank, 1980). When Ruddy et al. (1975) compared fractional catabolic or synthetic rates for C4 in normal human beings based on serum concentrations, it was concluded that the primary determinant of serum concentrations was the synthetic rate. The turnover rate for other animal species is not known.

17.4.2.4 Analysis of C4

The fourth component of complement may be measured using radial immunodiffusion, electroimmunodiffusion (rocket electrophoresis), automated immunoprecipitation, and sheep red cell hemolysis using C4-deficient guinea pig serum. Electroimmunodiffusion is an extremely sensitive assay for human C4 and requires less total time. Universal reference standards for human C4 are available for calibration of all immunologic methods. When C4-deficient guinea pig serum is available, the hemolytic assay is simple and accurate; however, care must be taken to use only fresh or frozen guinea pig serum to prevent the loss of complement activity (Cooper et al., 1983; Gaither and Frank, 1979; Mancini et al., 1965). One benefit of the hemolytic assay is that unlike immunologic assays, functionally active C4 is measured. Human C4 is measured in a hemolytic assay with antibody-sensitized sheep erythrocytes and C1; however, this cellular intermediate, while commercially available using purified guinea pig or human C1, is unreliable for testing many animal sera for C4. Therefore, purification of homologous C1 is usually necessary (Barta and Barta, 1984).

Rats have been successfully evaluated for C4 using the hemolytic assay and the cellular intermediate $EAC1^{gp}$, and adding human C2. Hemolysis was expressed as a percentage of the maximum hemolysis obtained by substituting purified human C4 in the reaction mixture (Arroyave et al., 1977). Using a similar technique, Sakamoto et al. (1981) expressed the results of C4 as the reciprocal of the end titer serum dilution giving 50% hemolysis. The values for normal rats were 419 ± 93 (SD).

Mouse C4 has been successfully quantitated by a sensitive one-step hemolytic assay with sensitized sheep red blood cells and C4-deficient guinea pig sera in the reaction mixture (Atkinson et al., 1980). Results of this assay were expressed in arbitrary hemolytic units in which B10.D2 mouse serum was used as the positive control. These investigators found that the addition of purified human C2 to the assay increased hemolytic titers twofold. They speculate that the human C2 helped to overcome a partial incompatibility between guinea pig C2 and mouse C4. More recent analyses found that several amino acid substitutions in the mouse C4 β-chain abolished C5 convertase subunit activity, and "humanizing" this segment replenished convertase activity (Ebanks and Isenman, 1996). Murine C4 also has been measured using agarose electrophoresis coupled with immunodiffusion (Natsuume-Sakai et al., 1980). In this case, alloantisera specific for each C4 allotype were prepared by injecting mice that did not express the allotype with purified mouse C4. The method for purification of mouse C4 closely followed the method described for human C4 (Bolotin et al., 1977). Heterologous anti-mouse C4 has also been prepared for immunoprecipitation assays (Passmore and Beisel, 1977).

Immunoprecipitation procedures using heterologous goat antihuman C4 have been described for canine C4 (Kay and Dawkins, 1984).

Taking advantage of the absolute C4 deficiency of C4D guinea pigs (Co-4), Ellman et al. (1970) were able to develop an antiguinea pig C4 antiserum that was effective in precipitating guinea pig C4 by gel diffusion. This principle of immunoprecipitation has been used by others to develop an effective radial immunodiffusion technique for guinea pigs (Thurston et al., 1980). In addition, guinea pig C4 can be quantitated in a hemolytic assay using the cellular intermediate EAC1, with human C1 (Ellman et al., 1970).

Rabbit C4 has been measured in the hemolytic assay using the EAC1 cellular intermediate with C1 of guinea pig origin. After initial incubation of intermediate cells with rabbit test sera, normal guinea pig serum in EDTA is added to complete the reaction (Nelson and Biro, 1968).

The sera of various nonhuman primates have been evaluated for detection of C4 by double immunodiffusion using goat antihuman C4. Although cross-reactivity was observed between rhesus, stumptail, and cynomolgus macaques, as well as Patas and African green monkeys, differences in migration distances, lengths of arcs, and spur formation suggested molecular differences in the proteins among species. Although this method may be useful in detecting genetic polymorphic forms of C4 among nonhuman primates, purified homologous C4 is necessary to quantitate this complement component (McMahan, 1982). Baboon C4 was measured using cellular intermediates prepared with human purified complement components.

In most studies performed to evaluate C4 in various animals, internal laboratory standards rather than commercially available reference standards were used; therefore, a direct comparison between laboratories is often difficult. A more complete discussion of the various methods is presented elsewhere in this chapter, and the technical aspects of the hemolytic assays for various domestic species have previously been reviewed (Barta and Barta, 1984).

As in man, the assays for native C4 have been particularly useful in the detection of genetic C4 deficiency in the guinea pig and rat as well as the quantitative deficiency in mice (Arroyave et al., 1977; Ellman et al., 1970; Kunstmann and Mauff, 1980).

17.4.2.4.1 Analysis of C4 Activation

The fourth component of complement is activated by limited proteolysis to produce a large (C4b) and a small cleavage product (C4a). Because the charge of C4b differs from that of the parent molecule, activation can be detected by immunoelectrophoresis (Cooper et al., 1983). C4b is broken down in human serum to C4d, a smaller fragment that is antigenically different from C4. Immunoelectrophoresis in agarose allows for the simultaneous quantitation of C4 and C4d. This method has been particularly useful in the assessment of such clinical conditions as rheumatoid arthritis, hereditary angioedema, and systemic lupus erythematosus (Milgrom et al., 1980). Extremely sensitive radioimmunoassays have been developed to detect the smaller C4a fragment; however, though as little as 10 ng/mL of C4a can be detected in human plasma, the plasma must first be treated for selective precipitation of the native C4 molecule before application of the radioimmunoassay (Gorski, 1981; Wagner and Hugli, 1984). Measurement of C4a has been a particularly sensitive marker of classic pathway activation in systemic lupus erythematosus (Wagner and Hugli, 1984). ELISA assays for rat, mouse and bovine and possibly other species may be found on the internet (http://www.biocompare.com/pfu/110627/soids/9361/ELISA_Kit/Complement_C4a).

17.4.2.5 Clinical Significance of C4 Concentrations

In human beings, serum C4 concentrations of 200–800 μg/mL (as measured by radial immunodiffusion) are considered normal (Agnello, 1978). However, as previously mentioned, the use of different techniques and the lack of reference standards prevent a comparison of C4 concentrations (in animal species) among the various laboratories. The serum C4 concentrations in human beings and animals increase from birth to sexual maturity, and levels in women increase during pregnancy (Atkinson and Frank, 1980; Barta and Barta, 1984).

In human beings, C4 acts as an acute phase reactant with levels increasing two- to threefold during acute inflammation. Elevations in C4 are also parallel increased corticosteroids. However, C4 levels are decreased during infections associated with the development of antigen–antibody complexes such as malaria and poststreptococcal glomerulonephritis (Atkinson and Frank, 1980). Further, marked depression of C4 is seen during exacerbations of systemic lupus erythematosus in human beings (Swaak et al., 1986). Increased catabolism is the suspected cause of the lower C4 levels seen in hereditary angioedema, systemic lupus erythematosus, and complement-mediated anemias (Alper and Rosen, 1975; Atkinson and Frank, 1980; Swaak et al., 1986).

Few attempts have been made to measure C4 during rheumatic and infectious disease in animals. Whereas total hemolytic complement activity is decreased during certain rheumatic diseases in dogs, the levels of specific components have not been measured (Barta and Barta, 1984; Wolfe and Halliwell, 1980). It is of interest that the inheritance of two disorders in dogs, idiopathic cardiomyopathy and systemic lupus erythematosus, are associated with a particular C4 allele (Day, 1996; Day et al., 1985).

Depression of C4 has been associated with acute aflatoxicosis in guinea pigs (Thurston et al., 1980) and dietary protein restriction in rats (Sakamoto et al., 1981). Sex-limited protein (Slp), the nonfunctional homologue of C4 in mice, has an androgen-dependent inducible synthesis in some strains (Passmore and Shreffler, 1970), and a constitutive, androgen-independent synthesis in others (Hansen and Shreffler, 1976).

Recent studies suggest that hormonal regulation of the Slp gene product is associated with DNase I-hypersensitive sites in the 5′ regions of the Slp gene (Hemenway and Robins, 1987). Strains showing androgen-independent expression of Slp have C4-Slp recombinant genes with the 5′ region derived from the C4 gene (Nakayama et al., 1987). No other differences in circulating C4 have been described in animals of different sexes, in association with natural cycles, or in response to specific drugs.

A genetic deficiency of C4 has been described in guinea pigs, Wistar strain rats, and human beings, and a quantitative reduction in the hemolytic activity of C4 has been described in mice (Karp et al., 1982a). In human beings, guinea pigs and rats, C4 deficiency is inherited as an autosomal recessive trait, with heterozygotes expressing intermediate levels of C4 (Arroyave et al., 1977; Ellman et al., 1970; Ochs et al., 1977; Schaller et al., 1977). Homozygotes in all three species cannot activate complement through the classic pathway.

The deficiency in guinea pigs has been studied extensively. C4 deficiency is thought to have arisen from a mutation in the C4-F allele, which is designated Co-4. Deficient guinea pig cells have no detectable intracellular pro-C4 (Colten and Frank, 1972); however, a C4 precursor RNA was detected using a cDNA probe for the fourth component of complement (Whitehead et al., 1983). These authors speculate that the basis for the C4 deficiency in guinea pigs is a posttranscriptional defect in the processing of C4 precursor RNA to mature C4 mRNA. Affected guinea pigs are more susceptible to experimental infection with *S. cholerae suis* or injection of endotoxin, and they had markedly impaired antibody responses to certain T-lymphocyte-dependent antigens (May et al., 1972; Moore, 1919; Ochs et al., 1978, 1983), serologic evidence for polyclonal B-cell activation (Bottger et al., 1986a), and an absence of glomerulonephritis (Foltz et al., 1994).

Mice expressing the H-2^{w7} MHC haplotype have C4 (Ss), which has only 30% of the functional activity of other strains (24). In affected mice, the C4 α-chain has a lower molecular weight due to a difference in its carbohydrate content (Karp et al., 1982b). This genetic variation in glycosylation was shown to affect the hemolytic activity of the C4 molecule directly. Quantitative differences in the circulating levels of C4 have been demonstrated in certain strains of mice. The Ss locus is directly involved with 20-fold reduced levels of C4 being expressed in low (Ss-L) level mice. These quantitative differences in C4 are linked to the H-2^k haplotype. Despite these low levels of C4, Ss-L mice have an intact classic pathway for the activation of complement, and are not prone to infectious disease (Shreffler and Owen, 1963); however, they do have a greatly prolonged contact sensitivity reaction to picryl chloride (Dieli and Salerno, 1986).

Mice were rendered C4 deficient by homologous recombination and shown to have no circulating C4. When these mice were injected with antiglomerular basement membrane antibody, there was a significant (but not total) attenuation of nephritis, leading the authors to speculate that both classic and alternative complement pathways contributed to this disease (Sheerin et al., 1997).

17.4.3 Second Component of Complement (C2)

17.4.3.1 Physical, Chemical, and Genetic Properties of C2

In human beings, the second component of complement is a single-chain glycoprotein with a molecular weight of 117 kDa (Colten, 1983a). Human C2 migrates as a β_1-globulin with a sedimentation constant of 6S (Colten, 1976). The C2 molecule has two free reactive SH groups that are positioned in close proximity to form an intramolecular disulfide bond on oxidation with iodine. This reaction allows for an extraordinary increase in hemolytic activity (Muller-Eberhard, 1975; Polley and Muller-Eberhard, 1967). Guinea pig C2 has a molecular weight of 130 kDa (Colten, 1976).

Factor B, C2, and C4 are linked with the MHC in human beings, guinea pig, and mouse (Ishikawa et al., 1990). In human beings, C2 and Bf genes are very close and separated from C4 genes by 50 kilobases (Hobart, 1984). Based on the structure of the C2 and factor B genes in mice, it was determined that they had arisen by a duplication that preceded the development of the alternative and classic pathways (Tosi et al., 1985).

Genetic polymorphism of C2 has been described in human beings (Alper, 1976; Hobart and Lachmann, 1976), who have one main C2 allotype and two rare allotypic variants. In contrast, guinea pigs have six C2 phenotypes resulting from three alleles occurring with equal gene frequency. The three allotypic variants are known as C2b (basic), C2a, and C2a1, the latter two both being acidic variants. These variants of a single structural C2 gene behave as autosomal codominant traits (Bitter-Suermann et al., 1981). In mice, studies have established that the multiple transcripts of C2 and factor B are expressed but the molecular mechanisms were not elucidated (Ishikawa et al., 1990).

17.4.3.2 Function of C2

C2 is a serine protease found normally as a trace protein in serum, and it is one of the two precursor molecules of the complex enzyme C3 convertase (Muller-Eberhard, 1975). C3 convertase (C4b2a) is assembled by the enzyme C1s. The cleavage products of C2 are C2a (80 kDa) and C2b (37 kDa). C3 convertase is then capable of activating C3 and continuing the classic pathway (Morgan, 1995).

17.4.3.3 Synthesis and Catabolism of C2

A variety of studies have demonstrated that monocytes and tissue macrophages are the cellular sites of C2 synthesis in human beings and guinea pigs (Colten, 1976). Human monocytes in culture generally require 3 days of incubation in vitro before C2 synthesis is detected. This delay in C2 secretion can be shortened by adding a lymphokine to the culture medium (Littman and Ruddy, 1977). Human bronchoalveolar macrophages incubated in vitro initiate C2 synthesis without this 3-day lag period (Cole et al., 1982). Likewise, differences are seen in the rate of C2 synthesis by guinea pig macrophages; however, in this species, the proportion of tissue macrophages bound to synthesize C2 varies from 2% for bronchoalveolar macrophages to 45% for peritoneal or splenic macrophages (Alpert et al., 1983).

The plasma levels of C2 vary greatly among the strains of mice, and the genes outside the MHC are thought to be involved in the transcriptional control of C2 (Falus et al., 1987; Ishikawa et al., 1990). In addition, exogenous IL-1 has been shown to increase specific C2 mRNA levels in murine kidney and lung (Falus et al., 1987; Perlmutter et al., 1986). In healthy human beings, approximately 2% of the plasma pool of C2 turns over each hour (Atkinson and Frank, 1980). The human C3 convertase, C4b2a, has a half-life of 10 minutes at 37°C.

17.4.3.4 Analysis of C2

Guinea pig C2 may be quantitated using the cellular intermediate EAC14gp and guinea pig serum diluted 1:10 in Veronal Buffered Saline-EDTA as a source of C3–C9 (Bitter-Suermann et al., 1981). Similarly, C2-deficient guinea pig serum may be used in a one-step hemolytic assay. Quantitative estimates for guinea pig C2 have also been conducted by rocket immunoelectrophoresis using homologous antiguinea pig C2 antibody (Bitter-Suermann et al., 1981).

The hemolytic assay using sheep red blood cells sensitized in C4 deficient guinea pig serum was used to quantitate hemolytic rat C2. However, when EAC1gp red blood cells were used to quantitate rat hemolytic complement, much weaker hemolytic activity was observed at 37°C than at 20°C. It was found that at 37°C, the natural decay of rat C2a from C3 convertase was much faster compared to rates of decay for guinea pig or human C2 (Naito and Okada, 1997).

Mouse C2 has been quantitated by hemolytic assay using the cellular intermediate EAC1gp4h (Goldman and Goldman, 1976). Rat and rabbit C2 have been quantitated similarly, with cellular intermediates made from purified guinea pig C1 and C4 (Nelson and Biro, 1968; Sakamoto et al., 1981).

Schur et al. (1975) quantitated the hemolytic activity for individual complement components in eight species of nonhuman primates using cellular intermediates prepared from purified human components. The C2 hemolytic titers of chimpanzees and gibbon ape were roughly the same as those of the human. The C2 hemolytic titers of *Papio anubis* (baboon), *Macaca fascicularis* (crab-eating macaque), *Ateles geoffroyi* (spider monkey), and *Cebus albifrons* (cebus monkey) were all greater than those of the human, and the titer of *Galago crassicaudatus* (greater bush baby), a prosimian, was approximately one tenth that of the human (Schur et al., 1975).

17.4.3.5 Clinical Significance of C2 Concentrations

Healthy human beings have 25 µg/mL of C2 in serum as measured by radial immunodiffusion (Muller-Eberhard, 1975). The hemolytic titer of C2 measured in Old World nonhuman primates and Great Apes is similar to human titers when purified human components are used as intermediates. The concentration of C2 in other species varies with methodology and the laboratory standard used.

Studies of 26 families with homozygous C2 deficiency (C2D) probands demonstrated that 23 of 38 C2D patients had diseases of the autoimmune type. Fourteen (37%) had systemic lupus erythematosus or discoid lupus erythematosus (Agnello, 1978). Only 2 of 38 patients had recurrent infections. As a primary clinical problem, however, an increased susceptibility to infections is thought to occur in all C2D homozygotes. The disease manifestations in C2D patients with systemic lupus erythematosus are different from those of "classic" systemic lupus erythematosus because C2D patients do not have anti-DNA antibodies and have reduced immunoglobulins deposited in skin, a low incidence of renal disease, and an increased frequency of discoid lesions, suggesting that certain genes controlling the disposition to these lesions may be missing in C2D patients. A similar systemic lupus erythematosus-like syndrome has not been described in the C2D guinea pig; however, circulating immune complexes are seen in these animals (Bottger et al., 1986a).

In several cases of C2D in human beings, there has also been a partial deficiency in factor B (Newman et al., 1978). These patients suffer from repeated *Streptococcus pneumoniae* infections. Because clearance of this organism is thought to depend on C3b-induced opsonization, an inability to activate C3 through the alternative pathway appears to predispose these individuals to streptococcal infection.

Human beings affected by autoimmune disorders characterized by antibody–antigen binding and activation of the classic pathway of complement, such as systemic lupus erythematosus and autoimmune hemolytic anemia, characteristically have sharp depressions in serum C2 (and most other classic components). Although not specifically studied, it is assumed that C2 levels are lower in animals that develop spontaneous systemic lupus erythematous and autoimmune hemolytic anemia, similar to markedly decreased total hemolytic complement in susceptible strains of mice exhibiting comparable diseases (Andrews et al., 1978).

In human beings infected with malaria, there is rapid activation of the classic pathway and a resultant sharp decline in serum C1, C4, C2, and C3 levels concomitant with schizont rupture and intravascular release of malaria antigens (Atkinson and Frank, 1980). Patients affected by cutaneous necrotizing vasculitis and disseminated intravascular coagulation also have lower serum C2 levels. A similar reduction may be expected in animals with disseminated intravascular coagulation.

C2, like C1, C4, C3, and factor B, acts as acute phase reactants, increasing two- to fourfold during a systemic inflammatory response in human beings. C2 levels are also elevated in women during pregnancy; however, similar findings in animals have not been reported.

Finally, there has been some speculation that the pathogenesis of the edema in human hereditary angioedema (C1 esterase inhibitor deficiency) is mediated by a cleavage product of C2 with kinin-like activity (Donaldson et al., 1969). Serum C2 levels are also known to be very low during acute episodes of this disease. No equivalent deficiency has been described in animals.

The functional levels of C2 were found to vary among inbred strains of mice (Goldman and Goldman, 1976). Serum C2 levels in mice appear to be controlled by genes closely linked to the Ss locus. Rats maintained on protein-deficient diets (0.5 vs. 18%) for 8 weeks had a 58% depression in serum C2 activity (Sakamoto et al., 1981). In addition, normal Sprague-Dawley pathogen-free rats challenged with an intradermal inoculation of 2×10^9 *Staphylococcus aureus* organisms had a 100% elevation in serum C2, which remained elevated 14 days following inoculation (Sakamoto et al., 1981). An extract of *Ephedra sinica* used in the treatment of nephritis contains a fraction called complement-inhibiting component, which is composed of a polyanionic carbohydrate. Incubation of this fraction with serum from human beings, pig, guinea pig, rat, or rabbit was associated with inhibition of the classic pathway of complement, likely due to carbohydrate binding to C2, thus preventing binding to $EAC1^{hu}4^{hu}$ (Ling et al., 1995).

Deficiency of C2 occurs in 1 in 10,000 individuals, making it the most common human complement deficiency (Glass et al., 1976). Macrophages from C2 deficient human beings function normally but are incapable of secreting C2 (Colten, 1983a). Recently, Cole et al. (1985), using a combination of protein radiolabeling, immunoprecipitation, and Northern and Southern blot analyses, discovered that C2-deficient human beings do not have a major gene deletion or rearrangement, but instead have a specific and selective pretranslational regulatory defect in C2 gene expression. This leads to a lack of detectable C2 mRNA and a lack of C2 synthesis.

The C2D in guinea pigs was the first C2D described in an animal (Hammer et al., 1981). Homozygous deficient guinea pigs have no detectable hemolytic activity, whereas heterozygotes have 50%–70% hemolytic activity (Bitter-Suermann et al., 1981). These C2-deficient guinea pigs show no C1s-induced vascular permeability (Strang et al., 1986), have impaired humoral immunity (Bottger et al., 1985), and demonstrate characteristics of immune complex disease (Bottger et al., 1986a). Guinea pigs homozygous for C2D synthesize a C2-like protein that can be detected immunologically within the cytoplasm of monocytes, but it is not secreted. Extracellular fluid from in vitro cultured C2-deficient macrophages contained reduced amounts of C2 antigen, which consisted of small molecular weight molecules (14–15 kDa). These studies suggested that C2-deficient guinea pig macrophages produce a structurally abnormal C2 protein, but they could not distinguish between a block in secretion or secretion of an instable C2 protein (Goldberger et al., 1982). The $C2^{\circ}$ allele of C2 deficient guinea pigs appears to be a silent $C2^{B}$ allele.

17.4.4 Fifth Component of Complement (C5)

17.4.4.1 Physical, Chemical, and Genetic Properties of C5

Human C5 has a molecular weight of 180 kDa and is a β_1-globulin. The human C5 glycoprotein contains approximately 20% carbohydrate moieties. The C5 molecule is a two-chained structure linked by disulfide bonds (Nilsson and Mapes, 1973). The approximate molecular weights of α- and β-chains are 110 and 70 kDa, respectively (Muller-Eberhard, 1975). A protein immunochemically defined as C5 in the mouse was previously called MuB1. In mice, plasma C5 consists of two chains of unequal size, an α-chain (115 kDa) and a β-chain (82 kDa) structurally similar to those of both human beings and guinea pig C5 (Patel and Minta, 1979).

17.4.4.2 Function of C5

When C5 is subjected to enzymatic attack by C5 convertase (C4b2a3b) or (C3bBb), the resulting product, C5b, serves as the focus for a self-assembling process leading to the stable C5b-9 complex (Kolb et al., 1972). The entire MAC is composed of one molecule each of C5, C6, C7, and C8 and a variable number (8–18) of C9 molecules (Hobart, 1984). This large molecular complex is assembled without the need for enzymatic activity following C5 convertase (Morgan, 1995; Muller-Eberhard, 1975). One report (Kitamura et al., 1984) suggests that C5 may compensate for the lack of C3, at least in some cases of human C3 deficiency. These investigators provide evidence for the direct activation of C5 by the C3 convertase (C4b2a), resulting in the formation of the MAC C5b-9.

C5a biological behavior is very similar to C3a, causing the release of histamine from mast cells, eliciting chemotaxis of neutrophils, and triggering contraction of smooth muscle. The C5a of pig, rat, and guinea pig differs from human C5a in that their COOH-terminus is susceptible to inactivation by serum carboxypeptidase B, which forces a conformational change on this molecule that results in reactivation and resistance to carboxypeptidase B (Hugli et al., 1975; Vogt et al., 1971; Weigle et al., 1983). C5a and C3a bind to specific receptors on lymphocytes and macrophages, and are potent regulators of the immune response (Weigle et al., 1983). Human C5a triggers a wide variety of neutrophil responses after binding to the neutrophil receptor (Hugli, 1981). Murine C5a binds to specific receptors on murine macrophages, but murine lymphocyte C5a receptors have not been identified. Purified C5a, given in physiologic doses, was shown to enhance the primary murine anti-sheep red blood cell response in vitro by induction of cytokine secretion by macrophages (Goodman et al., 1982) including interleukin-1 (Weigle et al., 1983).

17.4.4.3 Synthesis and Catabolism of C5

Evidence from several studies suggests that C5 may be synthesized in many human tissues, including lung, liver, spleen, thymus, placenta, peritoneal cells, bone marrow, and fetal intestine (Colten, 1974; Kohler, 1973). In the mouse, splenic macrophages were shown to be a site of C5 synthesis by one group (Colten, 1976), whereas another group found that circulating C5 was not synthesized by descendants of bone marrow cells (Geng et al., 1986). Studies of murine C5 synthesis in C5-deficient (C5D) strains have demonstrated the presence of a 200 kDa single polypeptide located intracellularly, though no extracellular C5 was detected. These authors suggested that C5D strains produce a nonglycosylated pro-C5 molecule intracellularly that is not secreted (Ooi and Colten, 1979). Studies conducted in mice have shown that C5 is synthesized in the fetus at 10–12 days of gestation, and that passive transfer of C5 from mother to fetus does not occur (Tachibana and Rosenberg, 1966).

C5 convertase (C4b2a3b or C3bBb) cleaves a small fragment (molecular weight 17 kDa) from the α-chain called C5a, leaving a slightly smaller biologically active C5b molecule (molecular weight 163 kDa). The C5b molecule is inactivated by a second enzymatic cleavage also of the α-chain, which yields a small C5d fragment. The biologically active C5a, like C3a and C4b, binds to surface receptors on white blood cells. It has been shown that both human and murine neutrophils and macrophages are capable of degrading C5a following its specific receptor binding (Weigle et al., 1983).

17.4.4.4 Analysis of C5

The hemolytic assay for murine C5 is conducted using the EAC1a,4,^{oxy}2a3b intermediate derived from purified human components. The use of oxidized C2 resulted in 10 times greater stability of the complex (Nilsson and Muller-Eberhard, 1967). The cellular intermediate can also be induced using certain purified guinea pig components (Terry et al., 1964). Qualitative determination for the presence or absence of murine C5 has been assayed using immunodiffusion with antihuman C5 (Parrish et al., 1984).

The hemolytic titers of porcine C5 were very low when measured using cellular intermediates constructed from human components; therefore, the isolation of autologous components for accurate testing is required (Barta and Hubbert, 1978).

Hemolytic titers for C5 can be measured accurately in guinea pigs using cellular intermediates derived from either guinea pig or human purified components (Lachmann, 1970; Nelson and Biro, 1968). Rat C5a has been quantitated using a double antibody ELISA (Schmid et al., 1997).

17.4.4.5 Clinical Significance of C5 Concentrations

The average human serum concentration of C5 is 80 μg/mL as measured by radial immunodiffusion (Muller-Eberhard, 1975). The mouse was once considered to have particularly low amounts of hemolytically active complement until it was realized that many inbred strains and outbred mice are deficient in the C5 (Herzenberg et al., 1963). An early attempt to develop a more sensitive assay using radioactive chromium-labeled sheep erythrocytes was described by Rosenberg and Tachibana (1962). However, the development of cellular intermediates from purified components and specific antisera against C5 has rectified this situation. Many Hc^o homozygous strains have been described (Staats, 1985). Cinader et al. (1964) and Dubiski and Cinader (1966) showed that adult female mice have only two-thirds the concentration of C5 (MuB1) found in adult C5-sufficient males.

The kinin, coagulation, and fibrinolytic systems share important interactions with the complement system. In particular, the activation of the coagulation cascade, for example, in experimental endotoxemia may result in metabolites that activate certain complement proteins, including C5 (Sundsmo and Fair, 1983). Furthermore, conditions leading to the activation of C3 and the production of C5 convertase will result in decreased concentrations of C5 (and other late phase components) in the serum. Direct measurement of C5 concentrations in diseased animals has not been extensively reported; however, it is assumed that changes in C5 concentration in most mammalian species will parallel changes seen in similar human conditions (Agnello, 1978; Alper and Rosen, 1975; Atkinson and Frank, 1980).

In rats, either intrapulmonary deposition of IgG immune complexes or systemic activation of complement by CoF leads to inflammatory lung injury mediated by neutrophil infiltration. While C6-deficient rats were still susceptible, pretreatment of rats with anti-C5a antibody protected against increased pulmonary vascular permeability (Mulligan et al., 1996). Later, it was shown that serum levels of C5a were directly proportional to the amount of CoF infused, and that peak serum C5a correlated with peak neutrophil chemotactic activity and upregulation of CD11b on neutrophil cell membrane. Treatment with anti-C5a was associated with down regulation of pulmonary vascular intercellular adhesion molecule (ICAM). Thus, C5a in the rat appears to upregulate both the pulmonary vascular and neutrophil adhesion molecules, allowing neutrophils to form intravascular aggregates that damage the pulmonary endothelium and cause lung injury (Schmid et al., 1997).

Human beings with both total deficiency of C5 and C5 dysfunction have been described. Related clinical disease is rare, but has been associated with the absence of C5 (immunogenic and hemolytic), and an increased susceptibility to infection, particularly pneumococcal pneumonia, and systemic lupus erythematosus. One patient with C5D and systemic lupus erythematosus had typical serologic and dermal manifestations of systemic lupus erythematosus, but the renal disease was not progressive (Rosenfeld et al., 1976a). In vitro studies with C5D serum demonstrated impaired cytolytic and bactericidal activities. Deficient sera could not generate chemotaxic factor, but they could provide normal opsonization of Baker's yeast (Rosenfeld et al., 1976b). C5D is transmitted as an autosomal trait in which heterozygotes have half-normal levels.

Several reports have described family members with normal antigenic and hemolytic C5 levels that are predisposed to infections. A functional defect in C5 in these individuals is postulated because purified C5 corrects the opsonization defect but C5D serum does not. These patients have Leiner's disease, which is characterized by eczema and secondary infections in infants (Miller and Nilsson, 1970). Because the defect in opsonization is not seen in homozygous C5-deficient serum, another factor may be responsible for the dysfunction.

Mice deficient in the fifth component of complement were first described by Rosenberg and Tachibana (1966), who were able to show that two strains, DBA/2 and B10.D2 (old), were lacking in vitro hemolytic activity. They also demonstrated that the defect was inherited as a single Mendelian recessive trait, the locus of which was designated as Hc (Herzenberg et al., 1963; Tachibana et al., 1963). By immunizing DBA/2 mice with serum from other normal mice, two groups of investigators independently discovered a new serum β-globulin (formerly called MuB1) that was present only in mice with normal hemolytic activity (Cinader and Dubiski, 1963; Erickson et al., 1964). Homologous and heterologous antibody to MuB1 reacted with the serum of many mammalian species, demonstrating common antigenic determinants among them (Cinader and Dubiski, 1964). Later, a protein contaminant of murine β1c, β1F glycoprotein, was characterized as the fifth component of complement (Nilsson and Muller-Eberhard, 1965) and shown to be the same as MuB1 (Nilsson and Muller-Eberhard, 1967). Because purified human C5 was able to reconstitute mice bearing the homozygous Hc^o (deficient) gene, it was concluded that the Hc locus controlled the production of C5 in mice. As in human beings, there is no linkage between the Hc gene and the MHC-H-2 in mice. There is some evidence that the molecular basis for C5 deficiency in mice involves an abnormal primary transcript of the C5 gene, retarding the processing of C5 mRNA and resulting in an abnormal C5 protein (Wheat et al., 1987).

The availability of two coisogenic lines of mice, one deficient in C5 (B10.D2/oSn) and the other (B10.D2/nSn) containing normal levels of C5, has allowed investigations concerning the role of C5 in a variety of experimental situations. The ability to reject large numbers of sarcoma tumor cells was shown to require the presence of C5 (Phillips et al., 1968). Two groups demonstrated that C5D strains of mice were deficient in rejecting skin allografts after treatment with antilymphocyte serum (Cinader et al., 1971; Weitzel and Rother, 1970). Lindberg and Rosenberg (1968) found that C5-sufficient (B10. D2/nSn) strains were at risk of developing experimental nephritis; however, C5D strains of mice were more susceptible to the development of experimental thyroiditis (Nakamura and Weigle, 1968). C5D mice are less susceptible to development of experimental autoimmune myasthenia gravis because the MAC is necessary to destroy acetylcholine receptors (Christadoss, 1988).

The importance of C5 in resistance to experimental bacterial infections has been studied extensively. Killing of *Escherichia coli* but not phagocytosis (Glynn and Medhurst, 1967), in vivo and in vitro defense against *S. pneumoniae* (Shin et al., 1969), opsonization of *S. aureus* (Easmon and Glynn, 1976), and the early attraction of neutrophils against *Listeria monocytogenes* (Lawrence and Schell, 1978) all required C5 for maximum activity. Later studies showed that C5 yields important neutrophil chemotaxins during the early period after intrapulmonary inoculation with *S. pneumoniae,* and that pulmonary clearance of the organism is impaired in C5D mice (Toews and Vial, 1984). Similar findings regarding pulmonary clearance of aerosolized *S. aureus* have also been reported (Cerquetti et al., 1983).

Morelli and Rosenberg (1971) demonstrated that normal mice survived longer than C5D mice after injection with *Candida albicans*. Moreover, infection of C5D mice with *Mycoplasma pulmonis* resulted in a more severe and persistent arthritis than that seen in normal mice (Keystone et al., 1978). Finally, the incidence of pulmonary consolidation and mortality seen in mice inoculated with the influenza virus was much higher in C5D mice (Hicks et al., 1978).

17.4.5 Complement Components of the Terminal Attack Complex (C6–C9)

17.4.5.1 Physical, Chemical, and Genetic Properties of C6–C9

The sixth component of human complement is a β-globulin with a molecular weight of 111 kDa (Podack et al., 1976). Homogenous preparation of C6 from rabbit and guinea pig serum revealed proteins of similar molecular weight and structure (Arroyave and Muller-Eberhard, 1971). Murine C6 is also a single peptide chain with a molecular weight slightly larger than that of human C6 (140 kDa); the PI range of murine C6 is more basic than that of human C6 (Hayakawa et al., 1984). The location of the epitope on human C6 responsible for binding C5b was identified using monoclonal antibody WU6–4. The Src homology domain containing (SHC) is encoded by the third thrombospondin repeat (of C6 α-chain), and a similar epitope is found on rabbit C6 (Wurzner et al., 1995).

Purified human C7 has a molecular weight of 102 kDa and an electrophoretic mobility identical to that of C6. Both C6 and C7 are single polypeptide chains (Podack et al., 1976). Additional investigations showed similarities between C6 and C7 in both amino acid and carbohydrate content, and trypsinization studies suggest similar tertiary structures (Podack et al., 1979).

Both human C6 and C7 show polymorphisms in isoelectric focusing (Hobart et al., 1975). Polymorphisms have also been demonstrated for C6 of rhesus monkey (Hall and Alper, 1977), chimpanzee (Raum et al., 1980), rabbit (Kunstmann and Mauff, 1980), dog (Anderson et al., 1983; Eldridge et al., 1983), and mouse (Hayakawa et al., 1984). Canine C7, like human C7, is polymorphic (Eldridge et al., 1983).

Murine C6 occurs as two major protein bands by isoelectric focusing, with molecular weights of 90 and 100 kDa. All inbred strains belong to one of four haplotypes: *C6A*a encodes the 90 kDa molecule (pI < 6.3), which occurs in A/J, BALB/c, DBA/2, and C57BL/6 strains; *C6A*m̲ encodes a 90 kDa molecule (pI < 6.2), which occurs in *Mus musculus molossinus*; *C6A*a*B*a encodes both 90 and 100 kDa molecules with pIs such as *C6A*[a] and occurs in CBA/Ca; and haplotype *C6A*a*B*b determines both 90 and 100 kDa with the acidic PIs and occurs in AKR mice (Orren et al., 1988). Each protein band is also associated with one wor more minor acidic bands. Two common variants of human C6 were also described by isoelectric focusing, and they are designated as the A and B variants. Individuals may express any of three phenotypes, C6A, C6B, and C6AB, which occur with frequencies 37%, 14%, and 45%, respectively (Hobart et al., 1975). Studies by Hobart et al. (1977a) showed that the gene responsible for C6 deficiency in human beings man is not linked to the human leukocyte antigen (HLA) complex, but is closely linked to the gene for C7. In the rat, the C6 gene has been used to isolate full-length transcripts of rat C6 mRNA (Bhole and Stahl, 2004). Sequence analysis demonstrated that the amino acid sequence for rat C6 was highly homologous to the human and murine sequence.

It has been determined that C7 is a single-chain plasma glycoprotein that is encoded by a gene containing 18 exons and spanning 80 kb (Hobart et al., 1995). Products of three codominant alleles at an autosomal locus, there are three structural forms of C7 in humans (Hobart et al., 1978). In human beings, the genes C6 and C7, along with C9, are closely linked and located on chromosome 5 (Coto et al., 1991). In mice, C7 is encoded by a genetic locus with two alleles. *C7*[b] encodes peptides that display five bands on isoelectric focusing, while *C7*[a] has all five plus an extra cathodal band. AKR mice carry the *C7*[b] allele, while 26 other murine strains each carry the *C7*[a] allele (Orren et al., 1985).

The structure and function of C8 has been reviewed Sodetz (1988). In general, C8 is a serum protein consisting of three nonidentical subunits (α, β, γ) arranged asymmetrically as a C8α-C8γ disulfide-linked dimer noncovalently associated, with a C8β subunit; each subunit is encoded by a different gene (Kolb and Muller-Eberhard, 1976; Ng et al., 1987). The human C8α gene consists of at least 11 exons, spanning approximately 70 kb of DNA, and the genomic organization is very similar to that of C6, C8β, and C9. While the C8 α- and β-chains show an overall sequence homology to

C6, C7, and C9, the C8 γ-chain was found to have a structural homology to the α-1-microglobulin/bikunin precursor, protein HC (Haefliger et al., 1987; Hunt et al., 1987). The crystal structure of the C8α component domain of the MAC perforin demonstrated that it was structurally homologous to the bacterial, pore-forming, cholesterol-dependent cytolysins (Hadders et al., 2007). Two wild-derived strains of mice were found to lack C8, but hemolytic activity could be restored with purified human C8. Backcrosses between DBA and the wild strain (MSM) indicated that inheritance was at a single locus called *C8b*. Mice carrying C8b1 have lytic activity, whereas those carrying C8b0 lack hemolytic activity (Tanaka et al., 1991).

Complement component 9 (C9) is the major constituent of the MAC and, while single molecules of C5b, C6, C7, and C8 are needed for MAC formation, multiple molecules of C9 are recruited and assembled (DiScipio et al., 1984). In contrast to homologous proteins that require the membrane for oligomerisation (e.g., perforin and cholesterol-dependent cytolysins), soluble C9 assembles directly onto the MAC (Dudkina et al., 2016). In a recent report, Dudkina et al. (2016) showed an 8 Å cryo-EM structure of the soluble form of poly-C9. Additionally, they demonstrated a 22-fold symmetrical arrangement of C9 molecules resulting in an 88-strand pore-forming β-barrel. Facilitating this solution-based oligomerisation was an N-terminal thrombospondin-1 (TSP1) domain, and the authors suggested that these TSP1 interactions might explain how additional C9 subunits are recruited to the expanding MAC subsequent to membrane insertion. It has been demonstrated that the genetic locus for C9 is tightly linked to the C6 and C7 loci (Coto et al., 1991). However, while it was determined that the C6 and C7 genes are contained in the same NotI fragment of 500 kb, no evidence was found for a physical linkage between C9 and C6 or C7 (Setien et al., 1993).

17.4.5.2 Function of C6–C9

Regardless of which pathway is activated, C5 convertase cleaves C5 to produce C5b, which attacks the membrane at a third topologically distinct site (Muller-Eberhard, 1975). The final MAC C5–C9 is assembled by the sequential addition of one molecule each of C5b, C6, C7, with C8 attaching to the cell surface, and a variable number of C9 molecules inserting themselves into the lipid bilayer and polymerizing into a ring with a central channel (DiScipio et al., 1984; Hobart, 1984). The attachment of late-acting complement components (C6–C9) takes place spontaneously without the necessity for enzymatic cleavage (Morgan, 1995; Muller-Eberhard, 1975). Following the lytic phase, the soluble C5–C9 complex circulates in the fluid phase with a molecular weight of 10400 kDa (Kolb and Muller-Eberhard, 1973).

17.4.5.3 Synthesis and Catabolism of C6–C9

It is considered that the liver is the major site of synthesis of C6, C8, and C9 (Hobart et al., 1977b; Alper et al., 1980; Adinolfi and Lehner, 1988). However, while C7 cDNA sequence analysis has been successfully performed on liver-derived cDNA (DiScipio et al., 1984), implying that C7 is also synthesized by hepatocytes, the liver does not appear to be the primary site for C7 synthesis. For example, C7 is not an acute phase reactant similar to C6 and C9 (Pepys, 1992). It has also been demonstrated that small amounts of C6 and trace amounts of C8, but not C7, were secreted by a human hepatoma-derived cell line, HepG2 (Morris et al., 1982). Further, in a study of liver transplantation patients, serum C7 evaluations demonstrated that there was a ≤50% contribution of the transplanted liver toward the C7 concentrations at 2–3 weeks posttransplantation (Wurzner et al., 1994). That contribution decreased with time to approximately 10% at 6 weeks after transplantation. The authors concluded that C7 is the only terminal complement component not predominantly synthesized by hepatocytes. Moreover, since cells such as monocytes, peritoneal macrophages, and alveolar macrophages are known to synthesize C7 in vitro, they suggested that C7 synthesis was attributable to the cells of the mononuclear phagocyte lineage. Monocytes also produce C5, C6, C8, and C9 in vitro (Hetland et al., 1986).

The half-life ($t^{1/2}$) of rabbit C6, calculated by infusion of plasma from normal into C6D rabbits, is 30 hours (Biro and Ortega, 1966).

17.4.5.4 Analysis of C6–C9

Hemolytic assays designed to measure C6 in various animals have taken advantage of the availability of human and rabbit C6D serum for simple one-step assays to quantitate C6 activity in the hamster (Yang et al., 1974), dog (Eldridge et al., 1983), rabbit (Goldman et al., 1982), mouse (Nilsson and Muller-Eberhard, 1967), and rat (Van Dixhoorn et al., 1997). The quantitation of both rabbit (Nelson and Biro, 1968) and mouse (Nilsson and Muller-Eberhard, 1967) C6 and C7 using cellular intermediates and purified components has been documented. The details for measuring C6 and C7 in human beings and nine animal species using purified components derived from cellular intermediates were given by Barta and Hubbert (1978). The hemolytic titers for both C6 and C7 for seven nonhuman primate species were published by Schur et al. (1975). Immunologic techniques have been employed for the measurement of C6 in mouse (Hayakawa et al., 1984) and rabbit (Goldman et al., 1982).

17.4.5.5 Clinical Significance of C6–C9 Concentrations

The levels of antigenic C6 and C7 in human serum average 60 μg/mL (Atkinson and Frank, 1980). As with most complement components, the measurement of C6 and C7 in animals varies between laboratories according to the methodology used, therefore direct comparisons between laboratories are difficult.

Deficiency of C6 (C6D) has been described in human beings who lack antigenic and functional levels of C6 in their plasma. The disease is transmitted in families with an autosomal codominant pattern of inheritance (Agnello, 1978). Heterozygotes for the C6D gene have half-normal antigenic levels of C6 but normal CH_{50} levels. Although some C6D patients appear to be normal, others have been described with Raynaud's syndrome, recurrent gonococcal septicemia, and recurrent meningococcal meningitis (Atkinson and Frank, 1980).

A biologically normal individual was found who had a partial genetic deficiency of both C6 and C7. Plasma levels of C6 were low, and the molecular size of the C6 was smaller than normal. A structural mutation in the C6 gene causing hyposynthesis of C6 and C7 was hypothesized (Glass et al., 1978; Lachmann et al., 1978). In most instances, however, human C6 deficiency is not associated with reduced C7 (Leddy et al., 1974; Lim et al., 1976). In addition, C6D rabbits have normal levels of C7 (Nelson and Biro, 1968). A simultaneous deficiency of C6 and C2 occurred in three members of a single family; however, the deficient genes segregated independently, indicating separate genetic events (Delage et al., 1979).

At least three separate instances of spontaneous C6 deficiency have occurred among different strains of rabbits. In each instance, C6D rabbits had little or no hemolytic C6 in their serum. The hemolytic activity of serum was reconstituted in one C6D strain by adding purified human or rabbit C6 (Rother et al., 1966) and purified guinea pig C6 in another C6D strain (Nelson and Biro, 1968). Lachmann (1970) showed that C6D rabbits had no circulating antigenic C6. Given the fact that these deficiencies occurred in different strains of rabbits in England, Mexico, and Germany, it is assumed that the defect in C6 synthesis in this species is fairly common. The defect in C6 synthesis in rabbits was shown to be transmitted as a single autosomal recessive trait with heterozygotes containing half-normal serum levels of C6 (Lachmann, 1970).

C6D rabbits appear to withstand common infections well and have normal antibody production. Abnormal coagulation, as measured by prolonged whole blood clotting time and reduced prothrombin consumption, was observed in C6D rabbits and corrected by adding purified C6 to deficient blood (Zimmerman et al., 1971). Experimental polyneuropathy induced by the injection of IgM antimyelin-associated glycoprotein was abolished in C6D rabbits, suggesting that the MAC acted as effector for the development of disease (Monaco et al., 1995).

In rodents, C6 deficiency has been reported in the rats, mice, and Syrian hamster (Yang et al., 1974; Bhole and Stahl, 2004; Spicer et al., 2007). Rats with complete deficiency of C6 have been identified in the PVG/c strain (Spicer et al., 2007). While a C6 mRNA transcript was found in the liver of deficient rats, its expression was 100-fold less than in sufficient rats. Since Northern blot analysis failed to reveal a large deletion in C6 DNA of C6D rats, the authors attributed deficiency to mRNA instability or a point mutation resulting in aberrant transcription (Van Dixhoorn et al., 1997). In an experimental model of thrombotic microangiopathy, antibodies to glomerular endothelial cells infused in rats produce glomerular endothelial cell injury, platelet aggregation, fibrin deposition, acute renal failure, tubular necrosis, and interstitial inflammation. The C6D rat was protected against this disease (Nangaku et al., 1997). Bhole and Stahl (2004) identified a 31 bp deletion in exon 10 of the C6 gene that leads to C6 deficiency in the PVG rats (PVG/c-) and developed a polymerase chain reaction (PCR)-based genotyping test. An unexpected finding from this study was a coagulation defect in the C6 deficient mice and rats.

In the Syrian hamster, serum from C6D hamsters could not reconstitute C6D serum from human beings or rabbits (Yang et al., 1974). However, normal hamster serum could. Although no differences between C6D and normal hamster sera were noted in induction of immune adherence or phagocytosis, this colony was extremely susceptible to proliferative enteritis and was subsequently lost.

While a rare occurrence in western countries, a high incidence of C9 deficiency has been observed in Korea and is the most common complement deficiency in Japan (Kang et al., 2005; Miura et al., 2011). It has been linked with immune complex-associated glomerulonephritis, but not systemic lupus erythematosus, and is related to an Arg95Stop mutation of the C9 gene (Kanemitsu et al., 2000; Miura et al., 2011).

17.4.6 Alternate Pathway Components (Factors B and H)

17.4.6.1 Physical, Chemical, and Genetic Properties of Factors B and H

In human beings, factor B is a single chain glycoprotein with a molecular weight of 95 kDa (Christie et al., 1980) migrating as a β-globulin (Muller-Eberhard and Schreiber, 1980). This thermolabile glycoprotein is composed of 7.3% carbohydrate (Curman et al., 1977), and its amino acid composition is known (Lesavre et al., 1979). Murine factor B has a molecular weight of approximately 100 kDa (Natsuume-Sakai et al., 1983; Roos and Demant, 1982).

The intact human factor B is cleaved by factor D into Ba and Bb fragments of 30 kDa and 61 kDa molecular weight, respectively (Morgan, 1995). The Ba and Bb fragments of murine factor B have similar molecular weights (Roos and Demant, 1982).

Multiple alleles of *Bf* (the factor B structural gene) have been described in human beings (Alper et al., 1972b), mouse (Natsuume-Sakai et al., 1983; Roos and Demant, 1982), guinea pig (Bitter-Suermann et al., 1977), and rhesus monkey (Ziegler et al., 1975a). Multiple alleles in all species are codominantly expressed. Four allelic variants have been found in mice (Natsuume-Sakai et al., 1983), two variants in guinea pigs (Bitter-Suermann et al., 1977), and six in the rhesus monkey (Ziegler et al., 1975b).

The gene for human factor B is closely linked to the gene for C2 (Alper et al., 1972a; Bitter-Suermann et al., 1977), C4 (Awdeh and Alper, 1980), and the MHC locus (Allen, 1974; Raum et al., 1981). Linkage between Bf, C2, C4, and the MHC has also been demonstrated for the rhesus monkey (Ziegler et al., 1975a), guinea pig (Kronke et al., 1977), and mouse (Natsuume-Sakai et al., 1980; Roos and Demant, 1982). Restriction map analysis of the genomic clone and total genomic DNA have elucidated a single Bf gene (per haploid) spanning more than 5.5 kb. Using a human factor B cDNA probe, a murine cDNA clone that has 85% homology with the human cDNA was isolated (Colten, 1983a). Restriction enzyme analysis of multiple human and murine cDNA clones failed to reveal differences in the DNA sequence among members of the same species.

In mice, the structural gene for factor H, *cfh*, is found on chromosome 1 and has two alleles, *cfh* and *cfh*[2] (formerly called *Sas*[1] and *Sas*[0] or Mudl and Mud2 [D'Eustachio et al., 1986]). Polymorphisms of factor H identified by electrophoresis and alloantisera were determined by the *cfhe* locus where allele cfhe[a] occurs in BALB/c, A/J, and C57BL/10 (and most other) strains and allele cfhe[b] occurs in the STR strain. Another allele cfhe[c] has been identified on the BFM/2Ms strain derived from European wild mice (Natsuume-Sakai et al., 1985). The *cfhe* locus maps to chromosome 2. Three allotypes of mouse factor H have been purified and their functional properties investigated (Okada et al., 1993).

17.4.6.2 Function of Factors B and H

As mentioned previously, when factor B (bound to C3b) is cleaved by factor D (in the presence of Mg^{2+}), it generates C3bBb, an unstable C3 cleaving enzyme. This cleaving enzyme is stabilized by the addition of properdin (P) to form C3 and C5 convertases (Colten, 1983a). Because Bb can hydrolyze the synthetic ester, acetyl-glycyl-lysine methyl ester, in a form unassociated with C3b, it is classified as a serine protease (Cooper, 1971). Two short consensus repeat (SCR) regions, SCR-2 and SCR-3, were shown to impart the ability of factor B to bind fluid phase C3b (Hourcade et al., 1995). Control over the amplification of convertases in the fluid phase is mediated in part by C4BP, which acts as a cofactor (with factor I) in the cleavage of C3b in the convertase (Morgan, 1995).

Schreiber et al. (1979) found that the mixture of isolated alternative pathway proteins and the isolated membrane attack pathway proteins constitutes an intact cytolytic pathway capable of killing bacteria in the absence of antibody. The activated alternative pathway appears to be effective in the lysis of some virus-infected cells (Schreiber et al., 1980), inactivation of viruses (Cooper, 1979), killing of certain parasites (Flemmings and Diggs, 1978), and influencing many host cellular functions. Guinea pig Ba has neutrophil chemotaxic activity (Hamuro et al., 1978); however, human Ba does not (Lesavre et al., 1979).

17.4.6.3 Synthesis and Catabolism of Factors B and H

Human factor B is synthesized by macrophages (Brade et al., 1978; Whaley, 1980), fibroblasts (Watanabe et al., 1995), and lymphocytes (Halbwachs and Lachmann, 1976), and it accounts for 0.1% of the total protein synthesized by the liver (Hobart and Lachmann, 1976). Similarities between factor B and C2 have been seen in biosynthesis, postsynthetic processing, and secretion (Matthews et al., 1982). Like C2, factor B synthesis may be induced by interferon-γ via a protein kinase c dependent pathway (Watanabe et al., 1995).

Factor B is activated by enzymatic cleavage into fragments Ba (the N-terminal component that behaves electrophoretically as an α-globulin) and Bb, which behaves as a γ-globulin. Under physiologic activation, Bb remains complexed to C3b (forming an alternative pathway C3 convertase), and Ba is released. The maintenance of stable C3bBb and the formation of C3/C5 convertase require an activator that prevents the interaction of C3b with factor H. Many such activators are known, including LPS, viruses, fungi, bacteria, parasites, and some animal cells; however, the critical feature of their structure that inhibits the C3b-factor H interaction is not known. Increased catabolism of factor B has been observed in human patients with immune complex-mediated diseases (Charlesworth et al., 1974).

Factor H can be synthesized by a variety of tissues, including liver and skeletal muscle. Unlike most complement components, where synthesis is induced by interleukin-1, TNF, and interferon-γ. IL-1 is not involved with the synthesis of factor H (Legoedec et al., 1995).

17.4.6.4 Analysis of Factors B and H

In man, factor B is routinely measured using the radial immunodiffusion assay (Gaither and Frank, 1979). Erythrocytes of some animal species are sensitive to alternative complement pathway-mediated lysis by fresh heterologous sera in the presence of magnesium and ethyleneglycol-bis-(2-aminoethyl)-tetra-acetic acid (EGTA). The proper target red cell for 12 animal species has been reported (Van Dijk et al., 1983). Antigenic analysis using specific antifactor B antisera has been published for guinea pig (Bitter-Suermann et al., 1977) and mice (Natsuume-Sakai et al., 1983).

Factor B has been measured in cattle using a hemolytic diffusion plate assay and radial immunodiffusion, with poor concordance between these assays (Table et al., 1983). The investigators suggest that because hemolytic activity depends on the concentration of other complement components, it is not as reliable as radial immunodiffusion. Rocket immunoelectrophoresis has been developed for measuring consumption of factor B after activation with zymosan (Table et al., 1983).

Schur et al. (1975) demonstrated lines of identity between factor B of six nonhuman primate species and antihuman factor B. This observation was confirmed by McMahan (1982) and used as a basis for crossed electrophoresis to measure rhesus monkey factor B (Ziegler et al., 1975a).

Factor H has been measured in human beings both by double antibody ELISA and by their capacity to cleave ^{125}I-labeled C3b analyzed by electrophoresis and autoradiography (Legoedec et al., 1995).

17.4.6.5 Clinical Significance of Factors B and H Concentrations

The serum concentrations of factor B in healthy human beings average 200 µg/mL (Muller-Eberhard and Schreiber, 1980) and range from 180 to 230 µg/mL (Adinolfi and Beck, 1975; Nagaki et al., 1980). In cattle, mean factor B levels in serum were 34 mg/dL (Table et al., 1983). In mice, sexual dimorphism is seen in the expression of factor B variants, with female mice lacking several anodal bands present in males; however, no differences in total factor B were seen using radial immunodiffusion or rocket immunoelectrophoresis (Roos and Demant, 1982). Strain-specific differences in plasma levels of factor B have been documented with 10-fold differences seen between B10.WR and B10.SM strains (Falus et al., 1987). Factor B levels are commonly elevated in inflammatory disorders, leaving some to classify factor B as an acute phase reactant (Atkinson and Frank, 1980). In both man and mouse, interleukin-1 has been shown to modulate factor B gene expression, resulting in increased mRNA levels in tissues and factor B in plasma (Falus et al., 1987; Perlmutter et al., 1986).

Membranoproliferative glomerulonephritis occurs in factor H-deficient human beings (Rougier et al., 1998). Similarly, an inherited deficiency in factor H has been described in Yorkshire pigs. In these pigs, there is continuous activation of C3 through the alternative pathway, resulting in renal deposition and complement-mediated kidney injury (Frank, 1995; Jansen et al., 1993). Pickering et al. (2002) demonstrated that mice, deficient in factor H (*Cfh*$^{-/-}$ mice), spontaneously developed a membranoproliferative glomerulonephritis and were highly susceptible to developing immune complex-related renal injury. With the addition of a second mutation in the gene encoding complement factor B, thereby, preventing the in vivo turnover of C3, the authors abrogated the phenotype of *Cfh*$^{-/-}$ mice. Thus, they demonstrated that uncontrolled C3 activation was essential for the development of renal injury associated with factor H deficiency.

17.5 CONCLUSIONS

Complement is a powerful immune modulating system that is not only based on lytic activities, but also on pathogen recognition components and important interactions with antigen-specific and nonspecific inflammatory host components. Recent elucidation of pathogenic hereditary deficiencies and dysfunctions have also lead to potential therapeutic interventions, by affecting the unique enzymatic reactions and the resulting conformational changes thus limiting the potential harmful host pathology such as that encountered in Lupus erythematosus, cancer, transplantation medicine, and atypical hemolytic uremic syndrome (Merle et al., 2015).

ACKNOWLEDGMENT

I wish to thank Fred W. Quimby, the author of this chapter from the second edition of this book, for his vision and contributions to the current chapter.

REFERENCES

Adinolfi, M. and Beck, S. 1975. Human complement C7 and C9 in fetal and newborn serum. *Arch Dis Child.* 50:562–564.

Adinolfi, M. and Lehner, T. 1988. C9 and factor B as acute phase proteins and their diagnostic and prognostic value in disease. *Exp Clin Immunogenet.* 5:I23–I132.

Aegerter-Shaw, M., Cole, J.L., Klickstein, L.B., et al. 1987. Expansion of the complement receptor gene family. *J Immunol.* 138:3488–3494.

Agnello, V. 1978. Complement deficiency states. *Medicine.* 57:1–23.

Albright, J.W. and Albright, J.F. 1985. Murine natural resistance to *Trypanosoma lewisi* involves complement component C3 and radiation-resistant, silica dust-sensitive effector cells. *Infect Immun.* 47:176–182.

Ali, Y.M., Lynch, N.J., Haleem, K.S., et al. 2012. The lectin pathway of complement activation is a critical component of the innate immune response to pneumococcal infection. *PLOS Pathog.* 8(7):e1002793. doi:10.1371/journal.ppat.1002793.

Allen, F.H. 1974. Linkage of HLA and GBG. *Vox Sanguinis.* 27:382–384.

Alper, C.A. 1976. Inherited structural polymorphism in human C2: Evidence of genetic linkage between C2 and Bf. *J Exp Med.* 144:1111–1115.

Alper, C.A., Austen, K.F., Cooper, N.R., et al. 1981. Nomenclature of the alternative activating pathway of complement. *J Immunol.* 127:1261–1262.

Alper, C.A., Beonisch, T., and Watson, L. 1972a. Genetic polymorphism in human glycine-rich beta-glycoprotein. *J Exp Med.* 135:68–80.

Alper, C.A., Colten, H.R., Gear, J.J.S., Rabson, A.R., and Rosen, F.S. 1976. Homozygous human C3 deficiency. *J Clin Invest.* 57:222–229.

Alper, C.A., Colten, H.R., Rosen, F.S., Rabson, A.R., MacNab, G.M., and Gear, J.S.S. 1972c. Homozygous deficiency of C3 in a patient with repeated infections. *Lancet.* II:1179–1181.

Alper, C.A., Goodofsky, I., and Lepow, I.H. 1972b. The relationship of glycine rich B glycoprotein to factor B in the properdin system and to cobra factor binding protein of human serum. *J Exp Med.* 137:424–437.

Alper, C.A., Johnson, A.M., Birtch, A.G., and Moore, F.D. 1969a. Human C3: Evidence for the liver as the primary site of synthesis. *Science.* 163:286–288.

Alper, C.A., Levin, A.S., and Rosen, F.S. 1966. Beta-IC-Globulin: Metabolism in glomerulonephritis. *Science.* 153:180–182.

Alper, C.A., Propp, R.P., Klemperer, M.R., and Rosen, F.S. 1969b. Inherited deficiency of the third component of human complement (C3). *J Clin Invest.* 48:553–557.

Alper, C.A, Raum, D., Awdeh, Z.L., Petersen, B.H., Taylor, P.D., and Starzl, T.E. 1980. Studies of hepatic synthesis *in vivo* of plasma proteins, including orosomucoid, transferrin, a-antitrypsin, C8 and factor B. *Clin Immunol Immunoputhol.* 16:84–89.

Alper, C.A., Robin, N.I., and Refetoff, S. 1971. Genetic polymorphism in rhesus C3 and Gc globulin. *J Immunol.* 107:96–98.

Alper, C.A. and Rosen, F.S. 1967. Studies of the *in vivo* behavior of human C3 in normal subjects and patients. *J Clin Invest.* 46:2021–2034.

Alper, C.A. and Rosen, F.S. 1975. Complement in laboratory medicine. In *Laboratory Diagnosis of Immunologic Disorders*. Eds. G.N. Vyas, D.P. Stites, and G. Brecher, pp. 47–68. New York, NY: Grune & Stratton.

Alpert, S.E., Auerbach, H.S., Cole, F.S., and Colten, H.R. 1983. Macrophage maturation: Differences in complement secretion by marrow, monocyte, and tissue macrophages detected with an improved hemolytic plaque assay. *J Immunol.* 130:102–107.

Anderson, J.E., Ladiges, W.C., Giblett, E.R., Weiden, P., and Storb, R. 1983. Polymorphism of the sixth component of complement (C6) in the dog. *Biochem Genet.* 21:155–160.

Andrews, B.S., Eisenberg, R.A., Theofilopoulos, A.N., et al. 1978. Spontaneous murine lupus-like syndromes. Clinical immunopathological manifestations in several strains. *J Exp Med.* 148:1198–1215.

Arroyave, C.M., Levy, R.N., and Johnson, J.S. 1977. Genetic deficiency of the fourth component of complement (C4) in Wistar rats. *Immunology.* 33:453–459.

Arroyave, C.M. and Muller-Eberhard, J.H. 1971. Isolation of the sixth component of complement from human serum. *Immunochemistry.* 8:995–1006.

Atkinson, J.P. and Frank, M.M. 1973. Effects of cortisone therapy on serum complement components. *J Immunol.* 111:1061–1070.

Atkinson, J.P. and Frank, M.M. 1980. Complement. In *Clinical Immunology*. Ed. C.W. Parker, Vol. 1, pp. 219–271. Philadelphia, PA: W.B. Saunders.

Atkinson, J.P., McGinnis, K., Brown, L., Peterein, J., and Shreffler, D. 1980. A murine C4 molecule with reduced hemolytic efficiency. *J Exp Med.* 151:492–497.

Auerbach, H.S., Lalande, M.E., Lalande, M.E., Latts, S., and Colten, H.R. 1983. Isolation of guinea pig macrophages bearing surface C4 by fluorescence activated cell sorting: Correlation between surface C4 antigen and C4 protein secretions. *J Immunol.* 131:2420–2426.

Awdeh, Z.L. and Alper, C.A. 1980. Inherited structural polymorphism of the fourth component of complement (C4). *Proc Natl Acad Sci USA.* 77:3576–3580.

Ballow, M. and Cochrane, C.G. 1969. Two anticomplementary factors in cobra venom: Hemolysis of guinea pig erythrocytes by one of them. *J Immunol.* 103:944–952.

Barrington, R., Zhang, M., Fischer, M., and Carroll, M.C. 2001. The role of complement in inflammation and adaptive immunity. *Immunol Rev.* 180:5–15.

Barta, O. 1978. Testing of hemolytic complement components in domestic animals. *Am J Vet Res.* 39:1303–1308.

Barta, O. and Barta, V. 1973a. Canine hemolytic complement: Optimal conditions for its titration. *Am J Vet Res.* 34:653–657.

Barta, O. and Barta, V. 1973b. A method for titrating equine haemolytic complement. *Immunobiology.* 146:114–122.

Barta, O. and Barta, V. 1975. Chicken (Gallus gallus) hemolytic complement: Optimal conditions for its titration. *Immunol Commun.* 4:337–351.

Barta, O. and Barta, V. 1984. *Laboratory Techniques of Veterinary Clinical Immunology*. Ed. O. Barta, pp. 138–155. Springfield, IL: Charles C. Thomas.

Barta, O. and Hubbert, N.L. 1978. Testing of hemolytic complement components in domestic animals. *Am J Vet Res.* 39:1303–1308.

Barta, O. and Okyean, P.P. 1981. Feline (Cat) hemolytic complement optimal testing conditions. *Am J Vet Res.* 42:378–381.

Becherer, J.D., Alsenz, J., and Lambris, J.D. 1989. Molecular aspects of C3 interactions and structural/functional analysis of C3 from different species. *Curr Topics Microbiol Immunol.* 115:47–72.

Bergh, K. and Iversen, O.J. 1989. Measurement of complement activation in rabbit plasma or serum using monoclonal antibodies against C5a. *Scand J Immunol.* 29:333–341.

Bhole, D. and Stahl, G.L. 2004. Molecular basis for complement component 6 (C6) deficiency in rats and mice. *Immunobiology.* 209(7):559–568.

Biro, C.E. and Ortega, M.L. 1966. Algunas Caracteristicas del Sexto Componente del Complemento. *Arch Inst Cardiol Mex.* 36:166–168.

Bitter-Suermann, D., Hoffman, T., Burger, R., and Hadding, U. 1981. Linkage of total deficiency of the second component (C2) of the complement system and the genetic C2-polymorphism to the major histocompatibility complex of the guinea pig. *J Immunol.* 127(2):608–612.

Bitter-Suermann, D., Kronke, M., Brade, V., and Hadding, U. 1977. Inherited polymorphism of guinea pig factor B and C4: Evidence for genetic linkage between the C4 and Bf Loci. *J Immunol.* 118:1822–1826.

Blann, A.D., Lewin, I., and Bacon, P.A. 1990. Development and evaluation of a rapid, semi-automatic micromethod for CH50 estimation using a computer program. *Immunol Invest.* 19:109–118.

Blom, A.M., Kask, L., and Dahlback, B. 2003. Structural requirements for the complement regulatory activities of C4BP. *J Biol Chem.* 276:27136–27144.

Blom, A.M., Villoutreix, B.O., and Dahlback, B. 2004. Complement inhibitor C4b-binding protein—Friend or foe in the innate immune system? *Mol Immunol.* 40:1333–1346.

Bockow, B. and Mannik, M. 1981. Clearance and tissue uptake of immune complexes in complement-depleted and control mice. *Immunology.* 42:497–604.

Bokisch, V.A. and Muller-Eberhard, H.J. 1970. Anaphylatoxin inactivator of human plasma: Its isolation and characterization as a carboxypeptidase. *J Clin Invest.* 49:2427–2436.

Bokisch, V.A., Muller-Eberhard, H.J., and Dierich, M.P. 1975. Third component of complement (C3): Structural properties in relation to functions. *Proc Natl Acad Sci USA.* 72:1989–1993.

Bolotin, C.G., Morris, S., Tack, B., and Prahl, J. 1977. Purification and structural analysis of the fourth component of human complement. *Biochemistry.* 16:2008–2015.

Bottger, E.C., Hoffmann, T., Hadding, U., and Bitter-Suermann, D. 1985. Influence of genetically inherited complement deficiencies on humoral immune response in guinea pigs. *J Immunol.* 135:4100–4107.

Bottger, E.C., Hoffmann, T., Hadding, U., and Bitter-Suermann, D. 1986a. Guinea pigs with inherited deficiencies of complement components C2 or C4 have characteristics of immune complex disease. *J Clin Invest.* 78:689–695.

Bottger, E.C., Metzger, S., Bitter-Suermann, D., Stevenson, G., Kleindienst, S., and Burger, R. 1986b. Impaired humoral immune response in complement C3-deficient guinea pigs: Absence of secondary antibody response. *Eur J Immunol.* 16:1231–1235.

Botto M, Dell'Agnola C, Bygrave AE, et al. 1998. Homozygous C1q deficiency causes glomerulonephritis associated with multiple apoptotic bodies. *Nat Genet.* 19:56–59.

Botto, M. 1998. C1q knock-out mice for the study of complement deficiency in autoimmune disease. *Exp Clin Immunogenet.* 15(4):231–234.

Brade, V., Fries, W., and Bentley, C. 1978. Identification of properdin B, D, and C_3 as biosynthetic products of guinea pig peritoneal macrophages and influence of culture conditions on their secretion (Abstr). *J Immunol.* 120:1766.

Braidley, P.C., Dunning, J.J., Wallwork, J., and White, D.J.D. 1994. Prolongation of survival of rat heart xenografts in C3-deficient guinea pigs. *Transplant Proc.* 26:1259–1260.

Budzko, D.B., Bokisch, V.A., and Muller-Eberhard, H.J. 1971. A fragment of the third component of human complement with anaphylatoxin activity. *Biochemistry.* 10:1166–1172.

Burger, R., Bitter-Suermann, D., Loos, M., and Hadding, U. 1977. Insoluble polyanions as activators of both pathways of complement. *Immunology.* 33:827–837.

Burger, R., Gordon, J., Stevenson, G., et al. 1986. An inherited deficiency of the third component of complement, C_3, in guinea pigs. *Eur J Immunol.* 16:7–11.

Cable, D.G., Hisamochi, K., Hartzell, V., and Schaff, M.D. 1997. Complement mediates attenuation of endothelium-dependent relaxations in canine coronary arteries after porcine serum exposure. *Circulation.* 96:58–63.

Cerquetti, M.C., Sordelli, D.O., Ortegon, R.A., and Bellanti, J.A. 1983. Impaired lung defenses against *Staphylococcus aureus* in mice with hereditary deficiency of the fifth component of complement. *Infect Immun.* 41:1071–1076.

Chan, A.C. and Atkinson, J.P. 1983. Identification and structural characterization of two incompletely processed forms of the fourth component of human complement. *J Clin Invest.* 72:1639–1649.

Chan, A.C., Karp, D.R., Shreffler, D.C., and Atkinson, J.P. 1984. The 20 faces of the fourth component of complement. *Immunol Today.* 5:200–203.

Charlesworth, J.A., Williams, D.G., Sherington, E., Lachmann, P.J., and Peters, D.K. 1974. Metabolic studies of the third component of complement and the glycine rich beta glycoprotein in patients with hypocomplementemia. *J Clin Invest.* 53:1578–1587.

Christadoss, P. 1988. C5 gene influences the development of murine myasthemia gravis. *J Immunol.* 140:2589–2592.

Christie, D.L., Gagnon, J., and Porter, R.R. 1980. Partial sequence of human complement component factor B: Novel type of serine esterase. *Proc Natl Acad Sci USA.* 77:4923–4927.

Cinader, B. and Dubiski, S. 1963. An alpha-globulin allotype in the mouse (MuB1). *Nature.* 200:781.

Cinader, B. and Dubiski, S. 1964. Effects of autologous protein on the specificity of the antibody response: Mouse and rabbit antibody to MuB1. *Nature.* 202:102–103.

Cinader, B., Dubiski, S., and Wardlow, A.C. 1964. Distribution, inheritance and properties of an antigen, MuB1, and its relation to hemolytic complement. *J Exp Med.* 120:879–924.

Cinader, B., Jeejeebhoy, H.F., Koh, S.W., and Rabbat, A.G. 1971. Immunosuppressive and Graft-rejecting antibodies in heteroloqous antilymphocyte serum. *J Exp Med.* 133:81–99.

Cochrane, C.G., Muller-Eberhard, H.J., and Aikin, B.S. 1970. Depletion of plasma complement *in vivo* by a protein of cobra venon: Its effect on various imtnunologic reactions. *J Immunol.* 105:55–69.

Cole, F.S., Schneeberger, E.E., Lichtenberg, N.A., and Colten, H.R. 1982. Complement biosynthesis in human breast milk macrophages and blood monocyktes. *Immunology.* 46:429–441.

Cole, F.S., Whitehead, A.S., Auerbach, H.S., et al. 1985. The molecular basis for genetic deficiency of the second component of human complement. *N Engl J Med.* 313:11–16.

Colten, H.R. 1974. Synthesis and metabolism of complement proteins. *Transplant Proc.* 6:33–38.

Colten, H.R. 1976. Biosynthesis of complement. *Adv Immunol.* 22:67–118.

Colten, H.R. 1983a. Molecular biology and biosynthesis of the complement proteins. In *Progress in Immunology.* Eds. Y. Yamamura and T. Tada, Vol. 5, pp. 397–406. Tokyo: Academic Press.

Colten, H.R. 1983b. Molecular genetics of the major histocompatibility linked complement genes. *Springer Semin Immunopathol.* 6:149–158.

Colten, H.R. and Alper, C.A. 1972. Hemolytic efficiencies of genetic variants of human C3. *J Immunol.* 108:1184–1198.

Colten, H.R. and Frank, M.M. 1972. Biosynthesis of the second (C2) and fourth (C4) components of complement in vitro by tissues isolated from guinea pigs with genetically determined C4 deficiency. *Immunology.* 22:991–999.

Colten, H.R., Levy, R.H., Rosen, F.S., and Alper, C.A. 1973. Decreased synthesis of C3 in membranoproliferative glomerulonephritis (Abstract). *J Clin Invest.* 52:20.

Cooper, N.R. 1971. Enzymes of the complement system. *Prog Immunol.* 1:567–577.

Cooper, N.R. 1979. Humoral immunity to viruses. *Compr Virol.* 15:123–170.

Cooper, N.R., Nemerow, G.R., and Mayes, J.T. 1983. Methods to detect and quantitate complement activation. *Springer Semin Immunopathol.* 6:195–212.

Coppola, R., Tombesi, S., Cristilli, P., Bergamaschini, L., and Mannucci, P.M. 1995. Comparison of two immunoassays for the complement protein C4b-binding protein in health and disease. *Intl J Clin Lab Res.* 25(2):88–92.

Corbin, N.C. and Hugli, T.E. 1976. The primary structure of porcine C3a anaphylatoxin. *J Immunol.* 117:990–995.

Costabile M. 2010. Measuring the 50% haemolytic complement (CH50) activity of serum. *J Vis Exp.* 37:1923. doi:10.3791/1923.

Coto, E., Martinez-Naves, E., Dominguez, O., DiScipio, R.G., Urra, J.M., and Lopez-Larrea, C. 1991. DNA polymorphism and linkage relationship of the human complement component C6, C7, and C9 genes. *Immunogenetics.* 33:184–187.

Cugno, M., Zanichelli, A., Foieni, F., Caccia, S., and Cicardi, M. 2009. C1-inhibitor deficiency andangioedema: Molecular mechanisms and clinical progress. *Trends Mol Med.* 15:69–78.

Curman, B., Sandberg-Tragardh, K., and Peterson, P.A. 1977. Chemical characterization of human factor B of the alternate pathway of complement activation. *Biochemistry.* 16:5368–5375.

D'Eustachio, P., Kristensen, T., Wetsel, R.A., Riblet, R., Taylor, B.A., and Tack, B.F. 1986. Chromosomal location of the genes encoding complement components C5 and factor H in the mouse. *J Immunol.* 137:3990–3995.

da Silva, F.P., Hoecker, G.F., Day, N.K., Vienne, K., and Rubinstein, P. 1978. Murine complement component 3: Genetic variation and linkage to H-2. *Proc Natl Acad Sci USA.* 75:963–965.

Daha, M.R., Stuffers-Heiman, M., Kijlstra, A., and vanEst, L.A. 1979. Isolation and characterization of third component of rat complement. *Immunology.* 36:63–70.

Dahl, M.R., Thiel, S., Matsushita, M., et al. 2001. MASP-3 and its association with distinct complexes of the mannan-binding lectin complement activation pathway. *Immunity.* 15(1):127–135.

Day, M.J. 1996. Inheritance of serum autoantibody, reduced serum IgA, and autoimmune disease in a canine breeding colony. *Vet Immunol Immunopathol.* 53:207–219.

Day, M.J., Kay, P.H., Clark, W.T., Shaw, S.E., Penhale, W.J., and Dawkins, R.L. 1985. Complement C4 allotype association with and serum C4 concentration in an autoimmune disease in the dog. *Clin Immunol Immunopathol.* 35:85–91.

Delage, J.M., Lehner-Netsch, G., LaFleur, R., and Simard, J. 1979. Simultaneous occurrence of hereditary C6 and C2 deficiency in a French-Canadian family. *Immunology.* 37:419–428.

Desai, B.B., Albright, J.W., and Albright, J.F. 1987. Cooperative action of complement component C3 and phagocytic effector cells in innate murine resistance to *Trypanosoma lewisi*. *Infect Immun.* 55:358–363.

DiCarlo, A.L., Paape, M.J., Hellman, J., and Lilius, E.-M. 1997. Purification and Characterization of bovine complement component C3 and its cleavage products. *Am J Vet Res.* 58:585–589.

Dieli, F. and Salerno, A. 1986. Role of the fourth complement component (C4) in the regulation of contact sensitivity. *Cell Immunol.* 105:386–396.

Dierich, M.P. and Schultz, T. 1983. The nature and function of complement receptors. *Prog Immunol.* 5:407–418.

DiScipio, R.G., Gehring, M.R., Podack, E.R., Kan, C.C., Hugli, T.E., and Fey, G.H. 1984. Nucleotide sequence of cDNA and derived amino acid sequence of human complement component C9. *Proc Nat Acad Sci.* 81:7298–7302.

Donaldson, V.H., Rafnoff, O.D., and da Silva, W. 1969. Permeability-increasing activity in hereditary angioneurotic edema plasma II. Mechanism of formation and partial characterization. *J Clin Invest.* 48:642–653.

Dubiski, S. and Cinader, B. 1966. Gene dosage effect of serum concentration of a complement component, MuB1. Proc Soc Exp Biol Med. 122:775–778.

Dudkina, N.V., Spicer, B.A., Reboul, C.F., et al. 2016. Structure of the poly-C9 component of the complement membrane attack complex. *Nat Commun.* 7:10588. doi:10.1038/ncomms10588.

Easmon, C.S. and Glynn, A.A. 1976. Comparison of subcutaneous and intraperitoneal staphylococcal infections in normal and complement deficient mice. *Infect Immun.* 13:399–406.

Ebanks, R.O. and Isenman, D.E. 1996. Mouse complement component C4 is devoid of classical pathway C5 convertase subunit activity. *Mol Immunol.* 33:297–309.

Egwang, T.G. and Befus, A.D. 1984. The role of complement in the induction and regulation of immune responses. *Immunology.* 51:207–224.

Ekdahl, K.N., Ronnblom, L., Sturfett, G., and Nilsson, B. 1997. Increased phosphate content in complement component C3, fibrinogen, vitronectin, and other plasma proteins in systemic lupus erythematosus. *Arthritis Rheum.* 40:2178–2186.

Eldridge, P.R., Hobart, M.J., and Lachmann, P.J. 1983. The genetics of the sixth and seventh components of complement in the dog: Polymorphism, linkage, locus duplication, and silent alleles. *Biochem Genet.* 21:81–91.

Ellingsworth, L.R., Holmberg, C.A., and Osburn, B.I. 1983. Hemolytic complement measurement in eleven species of nonhuman primates. *Vet Immunol Immunopathol.* 5:141–149.

Ellman, L., Green, I., and Frank, M. 1970. Genetically controlled total deficiency of the fourth component of complement in the guinea pig. *Science.* 170:74–75.

Erickson, R.P., Tachibana, D.K., Herzenberg, L.A., and Rosenberg, L.T. 1964. A single gene controlling hemolytic complement and a serum antigen in the mouse. *J Immunol.* 92:611–615.

Evans-Osses, I., de Messias-Reason, I., and Ramirez, M.I. 2013. The emerging role of complement lectin pathway in trypanosomatids: Molecular bases in activation, genetic deficiencies, susceptibility to infection, and complement system-based therapeutics. *ScientificWorldJournal.* 2013:675898.

Fahey, J.L. and McKelvey, E.M. 1965. Quantitative determination of serum immunoglobulins in antibody agar plates. *J Immunol.* 94:84–90.

Falus, A., Beuscher, H.U., Auerbach, H.S., and Colten, H.R. 1987. Constitutive and IL 1-regulated murine complement gene expression is strain and tissue specific. *J Immunol.* 138:856–860.

Fearon, D.T. 1979. Activation of the alternative complement pathway. *CRC Crit Rev Immunol.* 1:1–32.

Fearon, D.T., Austen, K.F., and Ruddy, S. 1973. Formation of a haemolytically active cellular intermediate by the interaction between properdin factors B and D and the activated third component of complement. *J Exp Med.* 138:1305–1313.

Feldman, B.F., Attix, E.A., Strombeck, D.R., and O'Neill, S. 1981. Biochemical and coagulation changes in a canine model of acute necrotising pancreatitis. *Am J Vet Res.* 42:805–809.

Ferreira, A., Michaelson, J., and Nussenzweig, V. 1980. A polymorphism of the γ-chain of mouse C4 controlled by the S region of the major histocompatibility complex. *J Immunol.* 125:1178–1182.

Ferreira, A. and Nussenzweig, V. 1975. Genetic linkage between serum levels of the third component of complement and the H-2 complex. J Exp Med. 141:513–517.

Ferreira, A. and Nussenzweig, V. 1976. Control of C3 levels in mice during ontogeny by a gene in the central region of the H-2 complex. *Nature.* 260:613–614.

Ferreira, A., Takahashi, M., and Nussenzweigh, V. 1977. Purification and characterization of mouse serum protein with specific binding affinity for C4 (Ss protein). *J Exp Med.* 146(4):1001–1018.

Fevereiro, M., Roneker, C., and deNoronha, F. 1992. Enhanced neutralization of feline immunodeficiency virus by complement viral lysis. *Vet Immunol Immunopathol.* 36:191–206.

Fey, G., Domdey, H., Wiebauer, K., Whitehead, A.S., and Odink, K. 1983. Structure and expression of the C3 gene. *Springer Semin Immunopathol.* 6:119–147.

Figueroa, J.E. and Densen, P. 1991. Infectious diseases associated with complement deficiencies. *Clin Micro Rev.* 4(3):359–395.

Fimmel, C.J., Brown, K.E., O'Neill, R., and Kladney, R.D. 1996. Complement C4 protein expression by rat hepatic stellate cells. *J Immunol.* 157:2601–2609.

Flemmings, B. and Diggs, C. 1978. Antibody-dependent cytotoxicity against *Trypanosoma rhodesiense* mediated through an alternate complement pathway. *Infect Immun.* 19:928–933.

Foltz, C.J., Cork, L.C., and Winkelstein, J.A. 1994. Absence of glomerulonephritis in guinea pigs deficient in the fourth component of complement. *Vet Pathol.* 31:201–206.

Fox, R.R. and Cherry, M. 1978. Effect of rabbit strain on activity level and cytotoxicity of serum complement. II. Comparison of 5 murine target cells. J Hered. 69:331–336.

Fox, R.R., Cherry, M., and Schultz, K.L. 1978. Effect of rabbit strain on activity level and cytotoxicity of serum complement. *J Hered.* 69:107–112.

Fox, R.R., Cherry, M., Shultz, K.L., and Salvatore, K.J. 1979. Effect of rabbit strain on activity level and cytotoxicity of serum complement. III. Comparison of 4 tumor target cells. *J Hered.* 70:109–114.

Frank, M.M. 1995. Animal models for complement deficiencies. *J Clin Immunol.* 15(Suppl 6):*S113–S121.*

Fredrikson, G.N., et al. 1993. New procedure for the detection of complement deficiency by elisa. analysis of activation pathways and circumvention of rheumatoid factor influence. *J Immunol Methods 166 (2): 263–270.*

Fujita, T. 2002. Evolution of the lectin–complement pathway and its role in innate immunity. *Nat Rev Immunol.* 2:346–353.

Fung, M., Loubser, P.G., and Undar, A., et al. 2001. Inhibition of complement, neutrophil, and platelet activation by an anti-factor D monoclonal antibody in simulated cardiopulmonary bypass circuits. *J Thorac Cardiovasc Surg.* 122:113–122.

Gaither, T.A. and Frank, M.M. 1979. Complement. In *Clinical Diagnosis and Management by Laboratory Methods.* Ed. J.B. Henry, Vol. 2, pp. 1245–1261. Philadelphia, PA: W.B. Saunders.

Gál, P. and Ambrus, G. 2001. Structure and function of complement activating enzyme complexes: C1 and MBL-MASPs. *Curr Protein Pept Sci.* 2(1):43–59.

Galibert, M.-D., Miyagoe, Y., and Meo, T. 1993. E-box activator of the C4 promoter is related to but distinct from the transcription factor upstream stimulating factor. *J Immunol.* 151:6099–6103.

Geng, L., Iwabuchi, K., Sakai, S., et al. 1986. Analysis of synthetic sites of fourth and fifth components of serum complement system in allogenic bone marrow chimaeras. *Immunology.* 58:453–457.

Gigli, I. 1978. A single chain precursor of C4 in human serum. *Nature.* 272:836–837.

Gigli, I., Fujita, T., and Nussenzweig, V. 1979. Modulation of the classical pathway C3 convertase by plasma protein C4b binding and C3b inactivator. *Proc Natl Acad Sci USA.* 76:6596–6600.

Gigli, I. and Nelson, R.A. 1968. Complement dependent immune phagocytosis I. requirements for C1, C4, C2, C3. *Exp Cell Res.* 51:45–67.

Girija, U.V., Mitchell, D.A., Roscher, S., and Wallis, R. 2011. Carbohydrate recognition and complement activation by rat ficolin-B. *Eur J Immunol.* 41:214–223.

Gitlin, D. and Biasucci, A. 1969. Development of γG, γA, γM, BIC/BIA, C1 esterase inhibitor, cerulpolasmin, transferrin, hemopexin, haptoglobin, fibrinogen, plasminogen, α1-antitrypsin, orosomuscid, β-Lipoprotein, macroglobulin, and prealbumin in the human conceptus. *J Clin Invest.* 48:1433–1446.

Glass, D., Raum, D., Balavitch, D., et al. 1978. Inherited deficiency of the sixth component of complement. A silent or null gene. *J Immunol.* 120:538–541.

Glass, D., Raum, D., Gibson, D., Stillman, J.S., and Schur, P.H. 1976. Inherited deficiency of the second component of complement: Rheumatic disease associations. *J Clin Invest.* 58:853–861.

Glynn, A.A. and Medhurst, F.A. 1967. Possible extracellular and intracellular bactericidal actions of mouse complement. *Nature.* 213:608–610.

Goldberg, B., Lad, P., Ghekierre, L., and Wolde-Tsadik, G. 1997. Comparison between assays for complement fragments and total hemolytic complement in the routine assessment of complement activation. *J Clin Ligand Assay.* 20:212–215.

Goldberger, G., Cole, S.F., Einstein, L.P., Auerbach, H.S., Bitter-Suermann, D., and Colten, H.R. 1982. Biosynthesis of a structurally abnormal C2 complement protein by macrophages from C2-deficient guinea pigs. *J Immunol.* 129:2061–2065.

Goldberger, G., Thomas, M.L., Tack, B.R., Williams, J., Colten, H.R., and Abraham, G.N. 1981. NH-2-terminal structure and cleavage of guinea pig pro C3, the precursor of the third component of complement. *J Biol Chem.* 256:12617–12619.

Goodman, M.G., Chenoweth, D.E., and Weigle, W.O. 1982. Potentiation of the primary humoral immune response in vitro by C5a anaphlatoxin. *J Immunol.* 129:70–75.

Goldman, M.B., Cohen, C., Stronski, K., Banaglore, S., and Goldman, J.N. 1982. Genetic control of C6 polymorphism and C6 deficiency in rabbits. *J Immunol.* 128:43–48.

Goldman, M.B. and Goldman, J.N. 1976. Relationship of functional levels of early components of complement to the H-2 complex of mice. *J Immunol.* 117:1584–1588.

Goldman, M.B., Knovich, M.A., and Goldman, J.N. 1992. T lymphocytes mediate immunologic control of C3 gene expression. *Eur J Immunol.* 22:3103–3109.

Gordon, J., Whitehead, H.R., and Wormall, A. 1926. The action of ammonia on complement. The fourth component. Biochem J. 20:1028–1035.

Gorman, N.T. 1984. Activation of the alternative complement pathway by lymphoblasts isolated from canine thymic lymphomas. *Vet Immunol Immunopathol.* 7:213–225.

Gorman, N.T., Hobart, M.J., and Lachmann, P.J. 1981a. Polymorphism of the third component of canine complement. *Vet Immunol Immunopathol.* 2:301–307.

Gorman, N.T., McConnell, I., and Lachmann, P.J. 1981b. Characterization of the third component of canine and feline complement. *Vet Immunol Immunopathol.* 2:309–320.

Gorski, J.P. 1981. Quantitation of human complement fragment C4ai in physiological fluids by competitive inhibition of radioimmune assay. *J Immunol Methods.* 47:61–62.

ZGrant, C.K. 1977. Complement "specificity" and interchangeability. Measurement of hemolytic complement levels and use of the complement-fixation test with sera from common domesticated animals. *Am J Vet Res.* 38:1611–1617.

Guiguet, M., Dethieux, M.C., Exilie-Frigere, M.F., Bidan, Y., Lautissier, J.L., and Mack, G. 1987. Third component of rat complement. Purification from plasma and radioimmunoassay in culture media from cell lines. *J Immunol Methods.* 96:157–164.

Hadders, M.A., Beringer, D.X., and Gros, P. 2007. Structure of C8-alpha-MACPF reveals mechanism of membrane attack in complement immune defense. *Science.* 317:1552–1554.

Haefliger, J.-A., Jenne, D., Stanley, K.K., and Tschopp, J. 1987. Structural homology of human complement component C8-gamma and plasma protein HC: Identity of the cysteine bond pattern. *Biochem Biophys Res Commun.* 149:750–754.

Halbwachs, L. and Lachmann, P.J. 1976. Factor B of the alternative complement pathway on human lymphocytes. *Scand J Immunol.* 5:697–704.

Hall, J.R., Jr. and Alper, C.A. 1977. Genetic polymorphism of the sixth component of complement (C6) in the rhesus monkey. *J Immunol.* 119:253–255.

Hall, R.E. and Colten, H.R. 1977. Cell-free synthesis of the fourth component of guinea pig complement (C4): Identification of a precursor of serum C4 (Pro-C4). *Proc Natl Acad Sci USA.* 74:1707–1710.

Hammer, C.H., Gaither, T., and Frank, M.M. 1981. Complement deficiencies in laboratory animals. In *Immunologic Defects in Laboratory Animals*. Eds. M.E. Gershaw and B. Merchant, Vol. 2, pp. 207–240. New York, NY: Plenum Press.

Hamuro, J., Hadding, U., and Bitter-Suermann, D. 1978. Fragments Ba and Bb derived from guinea pig factor B of the properdin system: Purification, characterization, and biologic activities. *J Immunol.* 120:438–444.

Hanafusa, N., Sogabe, H., Yamada, K., Wada, T., Fujita, T., and Nangaku, M. 2002. Contribution of genetically engineered animals to the analyses of complement in the pathogenesis of nephritis. *Nephrol Dial Transplant.* 17(Suppl 9):34–36.

Hansen, S., Selman, L., Palaniyar, N., et al. 2010. Collectin 11 (CL-11, CL-K1) is a MASP-1/3-associated plasma collectin with microbialbinding activity. *J Immunol.* 185:6096–6104.

Hansen, T.H. and Shreffler, D.C. 1976. Characterization of a constitutive variant of the murine serum protein allotype, Slp. *J Immunol.* 117:1507–1513.

Harboe, M., Garred, P., Borgen, M.S., Stahl, G.L., Roos, A., and Mollnes, T.E. 2006. Design of a complement mannose-binding lectin pathway-specific activation system applicable at low serum dilutions. *Clin Exp Immunol.* 144:512–520.

Harboe, M. and Mollnes, T.E. 2008. The alternative complement pathway revisited. *J Cell Mol Med.* 12:1074–1084.

Hawlisch, H., Vilsendorf, M.A.Z., Bautsch, W., Klos, A., and Kohl, J. 2000. Guinea pig C3 specific rabbit single chain Fv antibodies from bone marrow, spleen and blood derived phage libraries. *J Immunol Methods.* 236:117–131.

Hayakawa, J., Nikaido, H., and Koizumi, T. 1984. Genetic polymorphism of the sixth component of complement (C6) in mice. *Immunogenetics.* 20:633–638.

Hemenway, C. and Robins, D.M. 1987. DNase I-hypersensitive sites associated with expression and hormonal regulation of mouse C4 and Spl genes. *Proc Natl Acad Sci USA.* 84:4816–4820.

Herzenberg, L.A., Tachibana, D.K., Herzenberg, L.A., and Rosenberg, L.T. 1963. A gene locus concerned with hemolytic complement in *Mus musculus. Genetics.* 48:711–715.

Hetland, G., Johnson, E., Falk, R.J., and Eskeland, T. 1986. Synthesis of complement components C5, C6, C7, C8 and C9 in vitro by human monocytes and assembly of the terminal complement complex. *Scand J Immunol.* 24:421–428.

Hicks, J.T., Ennis, F.A., Kim, E., and Verbonita, M. 1978. The importance of an intact complement pathway in recovery from a primary viral infection: Influenza in decomplemented and C5-deficient mice. *J Immunol.* 121:1437–1445.

Hicks, P.S., Saunero-Nava, L., and DuClos, T.W. 1992. Serum amyloid P component binds to histones and activates the classical complement pathway. *J Immunol.* 149:3689–3694.

Higgins, D.A. and Langley, D.J. 1985. A comparative study of complement activation. *Vet Immunol Immunopathol.* 9:37–51.

Hillarp, A., Wiklund, H., Thern, A., and Dahlback, B. 1997. Molecular cloning of rat C4b binding protein α- and β-Chains. *J Immunol.* 158:1315–1323.

Hiramatsu, Y, Gikakis, N., Gorman III, J.H., et al. 1997. A baboon model for hematologic studies of cardiopulmonary bypass. *J Lab Clin Med.* 130:412–420.

Hirschfeld, J. and Lunell, N.O. 1962. Serum protein synthesis in foetus. Haptoglobins and group-specific components. *Nature.* 196:1220.

Hobart, M. 1984. The biochemistry and genetics of complement component: Agreement now the norm. *Immunol Today.* 5:121–125.

Hobart, M.J., Cook, P.J.L., and Lachmann, P.J. 1977a. Linkage studies with C6. *Immunogenetics.* 4:423–428.

Hobart, M.J., Fernie, B.A., and DiScipio, R.G. 1995. Structure of the human C7 gene and comparison with the C6, C8A, C8B, and C9 genes. *J Immun.* 154:5188–5194.

Hobart, M.J., Joysey, V., and Lachmann, P.J. 1978. Inherited structural variation and linkage relationships of C7. *J Immunogenet.* 5:157–163.

Hobart, M.J. and Lachmann, P.J. 1976. Allotypes of complement components in man. *Transplant Rev.* 32:26–42.

Hobart, M.J., Lachmann, P.J., and Alper, C.A. 1975. Polymorphism of human C6. In *Protides of the Biological Fluids.* Ed. H. Peeters, pp. 575–580. Oxford: Pergamon Press.

Hobart, M.J., Lachmann, P.J., and Calne, R.Y. 1977b. C6: Synthesis by the liver *in vivo*. *J Exp Med.* 146:629–630.

Holers, V.M., Kiroshita, T., and Molina, H. 1992. The evolution of mouse and human complement C3-binding proteins: Divergence of form but conservation of function. *Immunol Today.* 13:231–236.

Holmberg, C.A., Ellingsworth, L., Osburn, B.I., and Grant, C.K. 1977. Measurement of hemolytic complement and the third component of complement in non-human primates. *Lab Anim Sci.* 27:993–998.

Holmskov, U., Malhotra, R., and Sim, R.B. 1994. Collections, collagenous C-type lectins of the innate immune system. *Immunol Today.* 15:67–74.

Hourcade, D., Holers, V.M., and Atkinson, J.P. 1989. The regulators of complement activation (RCA) gene cluster. *Adv Immunol.* 45:381–416.

Hourcade, D.E., Wagner, L.M., and Oglesby, T.J. 1995. Analysis of the short consensus repeats of human complement factor B by site-directed mutagenesis. *J Biol Chem.* 270:19716–19722.

Huang, Y., Qiao, F., Abagyan, R., Hazard, S., and Tomlinson, S. 2006. Defining the CD59–C9 binding interaction. *J Biol Chem.* 281(37):27398–27404.

Huber-Lang, M., Sarma, J.V., Zetoune, F.S., et al. 2006. Generation of C5a in the absence of C3: A new complement activation pathway. *Nat Med.* 12(6):682–687.

Huber-Lang, M., Younkin, E.M., Sarma, J.V., et al. 2002. Generation of C5a by phagocytic cells. *Am J Pathol.* 161(5):1849–1859.

Hughes, T.R., Piddlesden, S.J., Williams, J.D., Harrison, R.A., and Morgan, B.P. 1992. Isolation and characterization of a membrane protein from rat erythrocytes, which inhibits lysis by the membrane attack complex of rat complement. *Biochem J.* 284:169–176.

Hugli, T.E. 1975. Human anaphylatoxin (C3a) from the third component of complement: Primary structure. *J Biol Chem.* 250:8293–8301.

Hugli, T.E. 1981. The structural basis for anaphylatoxin and chemotaxic functions of C3a, C4a, and C5a. *CRC Crit Rev Immunol.* 2:321–366.

Hugli, T.E., Vallota, E.H., and Muller-Eberhard, H.J. 1975. Purification and partial characterization of human and porcine C3a anaphylatoxin. *J Biol Chem.* 250:1472.

Hunt, L.T., Elzanowski, A., Barker, W.C. 1987. The homology of complement factor C8 gamma chain and alpha-1-microglobulin. *Biochem Biophys Res Commun.* 149:282–288.

Ilgen, C.L. and Burkholder, P.M. 1974. Isolation of C4 synthesizing cells from guinea pig liver by Ficoll density gradient centrifugation. *Immunology.* 26:197–203.

Isenman, D.E., Podack, E.R., and Cooper, N.R. 1980. The interaction of C5 with C3b in free solution: A sufficient condition for cleavage by a fluid phase C3/C5 convertase. *J Immunol.* 124:326–331.

Ish, C., Ong, G.L., Desai, N., and Mattes, M.J. 1993. The specificity of alternative complement pathway-mediated lysis of erythrocytes: A survey of complement and target cells from 25 species. *Scand J Immunol.* 38:113–122.

Ishikawa, N., Nonaka, M., Wetsel, R.A., and Colten, H.R. 1990. Murine complement C2 and factor B genomic and cDNA cloning reveals different mechanisms for multiple transcripts of C2 and B. *J Biol Chem.* 265:19040–19046.

Jacobs, J.W., Rubin, J.S., Hugli, T.E., et al. 1978. Purification, characterization, and amino acid sequence of rat anaphylatoxin (C3a). *Biochemistry.* 17:5031–5038.

Jansen, J.H., Hogasen, K., and Mollnes, T.E. 1993. Extensive complement activation in hereditary porcine membranoproliferative glomerulonephritis type II (porcine dense deposit disease). *Am J Pathol.* 143:1356–1365.

Jiang, H.X., Siegel, J.N., and Gewurz, H. 1991. Binding and complement activation by C-reactive protein via the collagen-like region of C1q and inhibition of the reactions by monoclonal antibodies to C-reactive protein and C1q. *J Immunol.* 146:2324–2330.

Johnson, A.E., Hugli, T.E., and Muller-Eberhard, H.J. 1975. Release of histamine from fat mast cells by the complement peptides C3a and C5a. *Immunology.* 28:1069–1080.

Jonas, W. and Stankiewicz, M. 1981. Haemolytic activity of sheep complement for two assay systems. *Vet Immunol Immunopathol.* 2:393–400.

Kalowski, S., Howes, E.L., Margaretten, W., and McKay, D.G. 1975. Effects of intravascular clotting on the activation of the complement system. *Am J Pathol.* 78:525–536.

Kanemitsu, S.I., hara, K., Kira, R., et al. 2000. Complement component 9 deficiency is not a susceptibility factor for SLE. *Lupus.* 9(6):456–457.

Kang, H.J., Kim, H.S., Lee, Y.K., and Cho, H.C. 2005. High incidence of complement C9 deficiency in Koreans. *Ann Clin Lab Sci.* 35(2):144–148.

Karlson, P., Bielka, H., Liebecq, C., et al. 1981. Enzyme nomenclature. Recommendations 1978. Supplement 2: Corrections and addition. *Eur J Biochem.* 16:423–435.

Karp, D.R., Atlinson, J.P., and Shreffler, D.C. 1982a. Genetic variation in glycosylation of the fourth component of murine complement. *J Biol Chem.* 257:7330–7335.

Karp, D.R., Parker, K.L., Shreffler, D.C., and Capra, J.D. 1981. Characterization of the murine C4 precursor (pro-C4): Evidence that the carboxy-terminal subunit is the C4-γ-chain. *J Immunol.* 126:2060–2061.

Karp, D.R., Parker, K.L., Shreffler, D.C., Slaughter, C., and Capra, J.D. 1982b. Amino acid sequence homologies and glycosylation differences between the fourth component of murine complement and sex-limited protein. *Proc Natl Acad Sci USA.* 79:6347–6349.

Kawamura, N., Singer, L., Wersel, R.A., and Colten, H.R. 1992. *Cis-* and *trans-*acting elements required for constitutive and cytokine-regulated expression of the mouse complement C3 gene. *Biochem J.* 283:705–712.

Kay, P.H. and Dawkins, R.L. 1984. Genetic polymorphism of complement C4 in the dog. *Tissue Antigens.* 23:151–155.

Kemper, C., Atkinson, J.P., and Hourcade, D.E. 2010. Properdin: Emerging roles of a pattern-recognition molecule. *Annu Rev Immunol.* 28:131–155.

Kemper, C., Pangburn, M.K., and Fishelson, Z. 2014. Complement nomenclature 2014. *Mol Immunol.* 61(2):56–58.

Keystone, E., Taylor-Robinson, D., Pope, C., Taylor, G., and Furr, P. 1978. Effect of inherited deficiency of the fifth component of complement on artritis induced in mice by *Mycoplasma pulmonis*. *Arthritis Rheum.* 21:792–797.

Kimura, Y., Miwa, T., Zhou, L., and Song, W.C. 2008. Activator-specific requirement of properdin in the initiation and amplification of the alternative pathway complement. *Blood.* 111:732–740.

Kirschfink, M. and Mollnes, T.E. 2003. Modern complement analysis. *Clin Diag Lab Immunol.* 10(6):982–989.

Kitamura, H., Matsumoto, M., and Nagaki, K. 1984. C3-independent immune hemolysis: Hemolysis of EAC14oxy2 cells by C5–C9 without participation of C3. *Immunology.* 53:575–582.

Kohler, P.F. 1973. Maturation of the human complement system. 1. Onset time and sites of fetal C1q, C4, C3, and C5 synthesis. *J Clin Invest.* 52:671–677.

Kolb, W.P., Haxby, J.A., Arroyave, C.M., and Muller-Eberhard, H.J. 1972. Molecular analysis of the membrane attack mechanism of complement. *J Exp Med.* 135:549–566.

Kolb, W.P. and Muller-Eberhard, H.J. 1973. The membrane attack mechanism of complement verification of a stable C5-9 complex in free solution. *J Exp Med.* 138:438–451.

Kolb, W.P. and Muller-Eberhard, H.J. 1976. The membrane attack mechanism of complement: The three polypeptide chain structure of the eighth component (C8). *J Exp Med.* 143:1131–1139.

Komatsu, M., Yamamoto, K., Nakano, Y., et al. 1988. Hereditary C3 hypocomplementemia in the rabbit. *Immunology.* 64:363–368.

Kotimaa, J., van der Pol, P., Leijtens, S., et al. 2014. Functional assessment of rat complement pathway activities and quantification of soluble C5b-9 in an experimental model of renal ischemia/reperfusion injury. *J Immunol Methods.* 412:14–23.

Kotimaa, J.P., van Werkhoven, M.B., O'Flynn, J.O., et al. 2015. Functional assessment of mouse complement pathway activities and quantification of C3b/C3c/iC3b in an experimental model of mouse renal ischemia/reperfusion injury. *J Immunol Methods.* 419:25–34.

Kronke, M., Hadding, U., Geezy, A.F., DeWeck, A.L., and Bitter-Suermann, D. 1977. Linkage of guinea pig Bf and C4 to the GPLA. *J Immunol.* 119:2016–2018.

Kunstmann, G. and Mauff, G. 1980. Genetic polymorphism of rabbit C6. *Immunology.* 158:30–33.

Kusher, I. 1982. The phenomenon of the acute phase response. *Ann N Y Acad Sci.* 389:39–48.

Lachmann, P.J. 1970. C6-Deficiency in rabbits. In *Protides of the Biological Fluids*. Ed. H. Peeters, pp. 301–309. Oxford: Pergamon Press.

Lachmann, P.J., Hobart, M.J., and Woo, P. 1978. Combined genetic deficiency of C6 and C7 in man. *Clin Exp Immunol.* 33:193–203.

Laurell, C.B. 1972. Electroimmunoassay. *Scand Clin Lab Invest.* 29(Suppl 124):21–37.

Lawrence, D.A. and Schell, R.F. 1978. Susceptibility of C5-deficient mice to listeriosis: Modulation by concanavalin A. *Cell Immunol.* 39:336–344.

Leddy, J.P., Frank, M.M., Gaither, T., Baum, J., and Klemperer, M.R. 1974. Hereditary deficiency of the sixth component of complement in man. I. Immunological, biologic, and family studies. *J Clin Invest.* 53:544–553.

Legoedec, J., Gasque, P., Jeanne, J.F., and Fontaine, M. 1995. Expression of the complement alternative pathway by human myoblasts in vitro: Biosynthesis of C3, factor B., factor H., and factor I. *Eur J Immunol.* 25:3460–3466.

Lesavre, P., Hugli, T.E., Esser, A.F., and Muller-Eberhard, H.J. 1979. The alternative pathway of C3/C5 convertase: Chemical basis of factor B activation. *J Immunol.* 123:529–534.

Levo, Y. and Pick, A.I. 1974. The significance of C3 and C4 complement levels in lupus nephritis. *Intl Urol Nephrol.* 6(3):233–238.

Lewis, R.M. and Picut, C.A. 1989. *Veterinary Clinical Immunology*, p. 267. Philadelphia, PA: Lea & Febiger.

Lim, D., Gewurz, A., Lint, T.F., Chaze, M., Sephein, B., and Gewurz, H. 1976. Absence of the sixth component of complement in a patient with repeated episodes of meningococcal meningitis. *J Pediatr.* 89:42–47.

Lindberg, L.H. and Rosenberg, L.T. 1968. Nephrotoxic serum nephritis in mice with a genetic deficiency in complement. *J Immunol.* 100:34–38.

Ling, M., Piddlesden, S.J., and Morgan, B.P. 1995. A component of the medical herb ephedra blocks activation in the classical and alternative pathways of complement. *Clin Exp Immunol.* 102:582–588.

Link, C., Hawlisch, H., Vilsendorf, A.M.Z., Gyleruz, S., Nagel, E., and Kohl, J. 1999. Selection of phage-displayed anti-guinea pig C5 or C5a antibodies and their application in xenotransplantation. *Mol Immunol.* 36:1235–1247.

Linton, S. 2001. Animal models of inherited complement deficiency. *Mol Biotechnol.* 18(2):135–148.

Liszewski, M.K., Fames, T.C., Lublin, D.M., Rooney, I.A., and Atkinson, J.P. 1996. Control of the complement system. *Adv Immunol.* 61:201–283.

Littleton, C., Keisler, D., and Burkholder, P.M. 1970. Cellular basis for the synthesis of the fourth component of guinea pig complement and determined by a hemolytic plaque technique. *Immunology.* 18:693–704.

Littman, B.H. and Ruddy, S. 1977. Production of the second component of complement by human monocytes: Stimulation by antigen-activated lymphocytes or lymphokines. *J Exp Med.* 145:1344–1352.

Liu, Y., Endo, Y., Iwaki, D., et al. 2005. Human M-ficolin is a secretory protein that activates the lectin complement pathway. *J Immunol.* 175:3150–3156.

Loeffler, D.A. 2004. Using animal models to determine the significance of complement activation in Alzheimer's disease. *J Neuroinflammation.* Open Access, 1:18. doi:10.1186/1742-2094-1-18

Madewell, B.R. 1978. Serum complement level in dogs with neoplastic disease. *Am J Vet Res.* 39:1373–1376.

Mancini, G., Carbonara, A.O., and Heremans, J.F. 1965. Immunochemical quantitation of antigens by single radial immunodiffusion. *Immunochemistry.* 2:235–254.

Markiewski, G.M. and Lambris, J.D. 2007. The role of complement in inflammatory diseases from behind the scenes into the spotlight. *Am J Pathol.* 171:715–727.

Mathison, J.C. and Ulevitch, R.J. 1981. *In vivo* interaction of bacterial lipopolysaccaride (LPS) with rabbit platelets: Modulation by C3 and high density lipoproteins. *J Immunol.* 126:1575–1580.

Matthews, W.J., Jr., Goldberger, G., Marino, J.T., Einstein, L.P., Gasj, D.J., and Colten, H.R. 1982. The major histocompatibility complex linked complement protein C2, C4, and factor B: Effect of glycosylation on their secretion and catabolism. *Biochem J.* 204:839–846.

May, J.E., Kane, M.A., and Frank, M.M. 1972. Host defense against bacterial endotoxemia. Contribution of the early and late components of complement to detoxification. *J Immunol.* 109:893–895.

McCurry, K.R., Kooyman, D.L., Alvarado, C.G., et al. 1995. Human complement regulatory proteins protect swine-to-primate cardiac xenografts from humoral injury. *Nat Med.* 1:423–427.

McMahan, M.R. 1982. Complement components C3, C4, and Bf in six nonhuman primate species. *Lab Anim Sci.* 32:57–59.

McMannis, J.D., Goldman, M.B., and Goldman, J.N. 1987. The role of lymphoid cells in antibody-induced suppression of the fourth component of guinea pig complement. *Cell Immunol.* 106:22–32.

Medof, M.E., Kinoshita, E.T., and Nussenzweig, V. 1984. Inhibition of complement activation on the surface of cells after incorporation of decay-accelerating factor (DAF) into their membranes. *J Exp Med.* 160:1558–1578.

Menger, M. and Aston, W.P. 1984. Factor D of the alternative pathway of bovine complement: Isolation and characterization. *Vet Immunol Immunopathol.* 7:325–336.

Merle, N.S., Church S.E., Fremeaux-Bacchi, V., and Roumenina, L.T. 2015. Complement system Part I—Molecular mechanisms of activation and regulation. Front Immunol. 6:Article 262.

Mevag, B., Olaisen, B., Teisberg, P., and Smith, D.G. 1983. Two C4 loci in *macaca* monkeys (abstr.). *Immunobiology.* 164:276–277.

Milgrom, H., Curd, J.G., Kaplan, R.A., Muller-Eberhard, H.J., and Vaughan, J.H. 1980. Activation of the fourth component of complement (C4): Assessment by rocket immunoelectrophoresis in correlation with the metabolism of C4. *J Immunol.* 124:2780–2785.

Miller, M.E. and Nilsson, U.R. 1970. A familial deficiency of the phagocytosis-enhancing activity of serum related to a dysfunction of the fifth component of complement (C5). *N Engl J Med.* 282:354–358.

Milstone, D.S., Shaw, S.K., Parker, K.L., Szyf, M., and Seidman, J.G. 1992. An element regulating adrenal-specific steroid 21-hydroxylase expression is located with the Slp gene. *J Biol Chem.* 267:21924–21927.

Miura, T., Goto, S., Iguchi, S., et al. 2011. Membranoproliferative pattern of glomerular injury associated with complement component 9 deficiency due to Arg95Stop mutation. *Clin Exp Nephrol.* 15(1):86–91.

Molleda, J.M. Lucena, R. López, R. Novales, M. Moreno, P., and Ginel, P.J. 1993. Effect of age on serum concentrations of the third component of complement in dogs. *Zentralbl Veterinarmed B.* 40(6):409–412.

Moller Kristensen, M., Jensenius, J.C., Jensen, L., et al. 2003. Levels of mannan-binding lectin-associated serine protease-2 in healthy individuals. *J Immunol Methods.* 282:159–167.

Mollnes, T.E., Jokiranta, T.S. Truedsson, L. Nilsson, B. Rodriguez de Cordoba, S., and Kirschfink, M. 2007. Complement analysis in the 21st century. *Mol Immunol.* 44:3838–3849.

Mollnes, T.E., Redl, H., Hogasen, K., et al. 1993. Complement activation in septic baboons detected by neoepitope-specific assays for C3b/iC3b/C3c, C5a and the terminal C5b-9 complement complex (TCC). *Clin Exp Immunol.* 91:295–300.

Monaco, S., Ferrari, S., Bonetti, B., et al. 1995. Experimental induction of myelin changes by anti-MAG antibodies and terminal complement complex. *J Neuropathol Exp Neurol.* 54:96–104.

Moore, H.D. 1919. Complementary and opsonic functions in their relation to immunity. A study of the serum of guinea pigs naturally deficient in complement. *J Immunol.* 4:425–432.

Moore, F.D., Jr. 1994. Therapeutic regulation of the complement system in the acute injury states. *Adv Immunol.* 56:267–299.

Morelli, R. and Rosenberg, L.T. 1971. Role of complement during experimental *Candida* infection in mice. *Infect Immun.* 3:521–529.

Morgan, B.P. 1995. Physiology and pathophysiology of complement: Progress and trends. *Crit Rev Clin Lab Sci.* 32(3):265–298.

Morgan, B.P. and Harris, C.L. 2015. Complement, a target for therapy in inflammatory and degenerative diseases. *Nat Rev Drug Discov.* 14:857–877.

Morris, K.M., Aden, D.P., Knowles, J.F., and Colten, H.R. 1982. Complement biosynthesis by the human hepatoma-derived cell line HepG2. *J Clin Invest.* 70:906–913.

Muller-Eberhard, H.J. 1975. Complement. *Ann Rev Biochem.* 44:697–724.

Muller-Eberhard, H.J. and Biro, C.E. 1963. Isolation and description of the fourth component of human complement. *J Exp Med.* 118:447–466.

Muller-Eberhard, H.J. and Gotze, O. 1972. C3 proactivator convertase and its mode of action. *J Experim Med.* 135:1003–1008.

Muller-Eberhard, H.J. and Schreiber, R.D. 1980. Molecular biology and chemistry of the alternative pathway of complement. *Adv Immunol.* 29:1–53.

Mulligan, M.S., Schmid, E., Beck-Schimmer, B., et al. 1996. Requirement and role of C5a in acute lung inflammatory injury in rats. *J Clin Invest.* 98:503–512.

Nagaki, K., Hiramatsu, S., Inai, S., and Saski, A. 1980. The effect of aging on complement activity (CH_{50}) and complement protein levels. *J Clin Lab Immunol.* 3:45–50.

Naito, A. and Okada, H. 1997. Stability of C3 convertase in rat classical complement pathway. *Microbiol Immunol.* 41:621–624.

Naka, Y., Marsh, H.C., Scesney, S.M., Oz, M.C., and Pinsky, D.J. 1997. Complement activation as a cause for primary graft failure in an isogenic rat model of hypothermic lung preservation and transplantation. *Transplantation.* 64:1248–1255.

Nakamura, R.M. and Weigle, W.O. 1968. Experimental thyroiditis in complement intact and deficient mice following injections of heterologous thyroglobulins without adjuvant. *Proc Soc Exp Biol Med.* 129:412–416.

Nakayama, K., Nonaka, M., Yokoyama, S., Yeul, Y.D., Pattanakitsakul, S.N., and Takahashi, M. 1987. Recombination of two homologous MHC class III genes of the mouse (C4 and Slp) that accounts for the loss of testosterone dependence of sex-limited protein expression. *J Immunol.* 138:620–627.

Nangaku, M., Alpers, C.E., Pippin, J., et al. 1997. Renal microvascular injury induced by antibody to glomerular endothelial cells in mediated by C5b-9. *Kidney Int.* 52:1570–1578.

Natsuume-Sakai, S., Hayakawa, J., and Takahashi, M. 1978. Genetic polymorphism of murine C3 controlled by a single co-dominant locus on chromosome 17. *J Immunol.* 121:491–498.

Natsuume-Sakai, S., Kaidoh, T., Nonaka, M., and Takahashi, M. 1980. Structural polymorphism of murine C4 and its linkage to H-2. *J Immunol.* 124:2714–2720.

Natsuume-Sakai, S., Moriwaki, K., Amano, S., Hayakawa, J., Kaidoh, T., and Takahashi, M. 1979. Allotypes of C3 in laboratory and wild mouse distinguished by alloantisera. *J Immunol.* 123:216–221.

Natsuume-Sakai, S., Moriwaki, K., Migita, S., et al. 1983. Structural polymorphism of murine factor B controlled by a locus closely linked to the H-2 complex and demonstration of multiple alleles. *Immunogenetics* 18:117–124.

Natsuume-Sakai, S., Sudoh, K., Kaidoh, T., Hayakawa, J.-I., and Takahashi, M. 1985. Structural polymorphism of murine complement factor H controlled by a locus located between Hc and the beta 2M locus on the second chromosome of the mouse. *J Immunol.* 134:2600–2606.

Nelson, R.A., Jr. and Biro, C.E. 1968. Complement components of a haemolytically deficient strain of rabbits. *Immunology.* 14:525–540.

Nelson, R.A., Jr., Jensen, J., Gigli, I., and Tamuro, N. 1966. Methods for the separation and measurement of nine components of hemolytic complement in guinea pig serum. Immunochemistry. 3:111–135.

Newell, S.L. and Atkinson, J.P. 1983. Biosynthesis of C4 by mouse peritoneal macrophages: II. Comparison of C4 synthesis by resident and elicited cell populations. *J Immunol.* 130:834–838.

Newman, S.L., Vogler, L.B., Feigin, R.D., and Johnston, R.B. 1978. Recurrent septicemia associated with congenital deficiency of C2 and partial deficiency of B and the alternative complement pathway. *N Engl J Med.* 299:290–292.

Ng, S.C., Rao, A.G., Howard, O.M.Z., and Sodetz, J.M. 1987. The eighth component of human complement: Evidence that it is an oligomeric serum protein assembled from products of three different genes. *Biochemistry.* 26:5229–5233.

Nilsson, B. and Ekdahl, K.N. 2012. Complement diagnostics: Concepts, indications, and practical guidelines. *Clin Dev Immunol.* 2012:11 Article ID 962702. Hindawi Publication Corporation. doi:10.1155/2012/962702.

Nilsson, U. and Mapes, J. 1973. Polyacrylamide gel electrophoresis (PAGE) of reduced and dissociated C3 and C5: Studies of polypeptide chain (PPC) subunits and their modification by trypsin (TRY) and C42–C423 (abstr). *J Immunol.* 111:293–294.

Nilsson, U.R. and Muller-Eberhard, H.J. 1965. Isolation of B1F-globulin from human serum and its characterization as the fifth component of complement. *J Exp Med.* 122:277–298.

Nilsson, U.R. and Muller-Eberhard, H.J. 1967. Deficiency of the fifth component of complement in mice with inherited complement defect. *J Exp Med.* 124:1–16.

Nilsson, U.R. and Nilsson, B. 1984. Simplified assays of hemolytic activity of the classical and alternative complement pathways. *J Immunol Meth.* 72:4–59.

Noris, M. and Remuzzi, G. 2013. Overview of complement activation and regulation. *Semin Nephrol.* 33(6):479–492.

O'Neill, G.J., Lang, M., Nerl, C., and Deeg, H.J. 1984. C4 polymorphism in the dog: Molecular heterogeneity of the C4α and C4γ subunit chains. *Immunogenetics.* 20:649–654.

O'Neill, G.J., Yang, S.Y., and Dupont, B. 1978. Two HLA-linked loci controlling the fourth component of human complement. *Proc Natl Acad Sci USA.* 75:5165–5169.

Ochs, H.D., Jackson, C.G., Heller, S.R., and Wedgewood, R.J. 1978. Defective antibody response to a T-dependent antigen in C4-deficient guinea pigs and its correction by addition of C4. *Fed Proc.* 37:1477.

Ochs, H.D., Rosenfeld, S.I., Thomas, E.D., et al. 1977. Linkage between the fourth component of complement and the major histocompatibility complex. *N Engl J Med.* 296:470–475.

Ochs, H.D., Wedgewood, R.J., Frank, M.M., Heller, S.R., and Hosea, S.W. 1983. The role of complement in the induction of antibody responses. *Clin Exp Immunol.* 53:208–216.

Odink, K.G., Fey, G., Wiebauer, K., and Digglemann, H. 1981. Mouse complement components C3 and C4. Characterization of their messenger RNA and molecular cloning of complementary DNA for C3. *J Biol Chem.* 256:1453–1458.

Okada, M., Kojima, A., Takano, H., et al. 1993. Functional properties of the allotypes of mouse complement regulatory protein, factor H: Difference of compatibility of each allotype with human factor I. *Mol Immunol.* 30(9):841–848.

Olahu-Mukani, W., Nyang'ao, J.N.M., Kimani, J.K., and Omuse, J.K. 1994. Studies on the haemolytic complement of the dromedary camel (*Camelus dromedarius*). II. Alternate complement pathway haemolytic activity in serum. *Vet Immunol Immunopathol.* 48:169–176.

Ong, G.L. and Mattes, M.J. 1989. Mouse strains with typical mammalian levels of complement activity. *J Immunol Methods.* 125:147–158.

Ong, G.L., Shah, P.B., and Mattes, M.J. 1996. Rabbit complement lysis tumor cells without massive C3 deposition. *Immunol Invest.* 25:215–229.

Ooi, Y.M. and Colten, H.R. 1979. Genetic defect in secretion of complement C5 in mice. *Nature.* 282:207–208.

Orren, A., Hayakawa, J., Johnson, J.E., Nash, H.R., and Hobart, M.J. 1988. Allotypes of mouse complement component C6 in inbred strains and some wild populations. *Immunogenetics.* 28:153–157.

Orren, A., Hobart, M.J., Nash, H.R., and Lachman, P.J. 1985. Close linkage between mouse genes determining the two forms of complement component 6 and component 7 and cis action of a C6 regulatory gene. *Immunogenetics.* 21:591–599.

Osses, I.E., de Messias-Reason, I., and Ramirez, M.I. 2013. The emerging role of complement lectin pathway in trypanosomatids: Molecular bases in activation, genetic deficiencies, susceptibility to infection, and complement system-based therapeutics. *Sci World J.* 2013. Article ID 675898. 12 pp. doi:10.1155/2013/675898. Hindawi Publishing Corporation.

Oyekan, P.P. and Barta, O. 1980. Hemolytic assay for goat (caprine) and swine (porcine) complement. *Vet Immunol Immunopathol.* 2:393–400.

Pangburn, M.K. 2000. Host recognition and target differentiation by factor H, a regulator of the alternative pathway of complement. *Immunopharmacology.* 49(1–2):149–157.

Pangburn, M.K., Muller-Eberhard, H.J. 1986a. Complement C3 convertase: Cell surface restriction of beta1H control and generation of restriction on neuraminidase-treated cells. Proc Natl Acad Sci USA. 75(5):2416–2420.

Pangburn, M.K., Muller-Eberhard, H.J. 1986b. The C3 convertase of the alternative pathway of human complement. Enzymic properties of the bimolecular proteinase. Biochem J. 235:723–730.

Pangburn, M.K., Schreiber, R.D., and Muller-Eberhard, H.J. 1983. Deficiency of an erythrocyte membrane protein with complement regulatory activity in paroxysmal nocturnal hemoglobinuria. *Proc Natl Acad Sci USA.* 80:5434.

Pangburn, M.K., Schreiber, R.D., and Muller-Eberhard, H.J. 1977. Human complement C3b inactivator: Isolation, characterization, and demonstration of an absolute requirement for the serum protein beta1H for cleavage of C3b and C4b in solution. *J Exp Med.* 146(1):257–270.

Parker, K.L., Roose, M.H., and Shreffler, D.C. 1979. Structural characterization of the murine fourth component of complement and sex-limited protein and their precursors: Evidence for two loci in the S region of the H-2 complex. *Proc Natl Acad Sci USA.* 76:5853–5857.

Parrish, D.A., Mitchell, B.C., Henson, P.M., and Larsen, G.L. 1984. Pulmonary response in fifth component of complement-sufficient and deficient mice to hyperoxia. *J Clin Invest.* 74:956–965.

Passmore, H.C. and Beisel, K.W. 1977. Preparation of antisera for the detection of the Ss protein and Slp alloantigen. *Immunogenetics.* 4:393–399.

Passmore, H.C. and Shreffler, D.C. 1970. A sex-limited serum protein variant in the mouse: Inheritance and association with the H-2 region. *Biochem Genet.* 4:351–365.

Patel, F. and Minta, J.O. 1979. Biosynthesis of a single chain pro-C5 by normal mouse liver mRNA: Analysis of the molecular basis of C5 deficiency in AKR/J mice. *J Immunol.* 123:2408–2414.

Pavlov, I.Y., De Forest, N., and Delgado, J.C. 2011. Specificity of EIA immunoassay for complement factor Bb testing. *Clin Lab.* 57(3–4):225–228.

Pekna, M., Hietala, A., Rosklint, T., Betsholtz, C., and Pekny, M. 1998. Targeted disruption of the murine gene coding for the third complement component (C3). *Scand J Immunol.* 47:25–29.

Pepys, M.B. 1974. Complement mediated mixed aggregation of murine spleen cells. *Nature.* 249:51–53.

Pepys, M.B. 1992. Acute phase proteins. In *Encyclopedia of Immunology*. Eds. I.M. Roitt and P.J. Delves, pp. 16–18. London: Academic Press,

Pepys, M.B., Dash, A.C., Fielder, A.H.L., and Mirjah, D.D. 1977. Isolation and study of murine C3. *Immunology.* 33:491–499.

Perlmutter, D.H., Goldberger, G., Dinarello, C.A., Mizel, S.B., and Colten, H.R. 1986. Regulation of class III major histocompatibility complex gene products by interleuken-1. *Science*. 232:850–852.

Peters, D.K., Martin, A., Weinstein, A., et al. 1972. Complement studies in membranoproliferative glomerulonephritis. *Clin Exp Immunol*. 11:311–320.

Petersen, S.V. Thiel, S. Jensen, L. Vorup-Jensen, T. Koch, C., and Jensenius, J.C. 2000. Control of the classical and the MBL pathway of complement activation. *Mol Immunol*. 37(14):803–811.

Phillips, M.E., Rother, V., and Rother, K. 1968. Serum complement in the rejection of sarcoma I ascites tumor grafts. *J Immunol*. 100:493–500.

Pickering, M.C., Cook, H.T., Warren, J., et al. 2002. Uncontrolled C3 activation causes membranoproliferative glomerulonephritis in mice deficient in complement factor H. *Nat Genet*. 31:424–428.

Podack, E.R., Kolb, W.P., Esser, A.F., and Muller-Eberhard, H.J. 1979. Structural similarities between C6 and C7 of human complement. *J Immunol*. 123:1071–1078.

Podack, E.R., Kolb, W.P., and Muller-Eberhard, H.J. 1976. Purification of the sixth and seventh component of human complement without loss of hemolytic activity. *J Immunol*. 116:263–269.

Polley, M.J. and Muller-Eberhard, H.J. 1967. Enhancement of the hemolytic activity of the second component of human complement by oxidation. *J Exp Med*. 126:1013–1025.

Porcel, J.M., Peakman, M., Senaldi, G., and Vergani, D. 1993. Methods for assessing complement activation in the clinical immunology laboratory. *J Immunol Methods*. 157:109.

Poutrel, B. and Caffin, J.P. 1984. Determination of hemolytic complement activity in bovine milk. *Vet Immunol Immunopathol*. 5:177–184.

Pratt, J.R., Harmer, A.W., Levin, J., and Sacks, S.H. 1997. Influence of complement on the allospecific antibody response to primary vascularized organ graft. *Eur J Immunol*. 27:2848–2853.

Prodeus, A.P., Zhou, X., Maurer, M., Galli, S.J., and Carroll, M.C. 1997. Impaired mast cell-dependent natural immunity in complement C3-deficient mice. *Nature*. 390:172–175.

Propp, R.P. and Alper, C.A. 1968. C3 synthesis in the human fetus and lack of transplacental passage. *Science*. 162:672–673.

Qu, H., Ricklin, D., and Lambris, J.D. 2009. Recent developments in low molecular weight complement inhibitors. *Mol Immunol*. 47(2–3):185–195.

Quimby, F.W., 1999. Complement. In *Clinical Chemistry of Laboratory Animals, 2nd Edition,* Loeb, W.F. and Quimby F.W. (eds.), pp. 266--308. Philadelphia, PA: Taylor & Francis.

Ram, S., Lewis, L.A., and Rice, P.A. 2010. Infections of human beings with complement deficiencies and patients who have undergone splenectomy. *Clin Microbiol Rev*. 23:740–780.

Rapp, H.J. and Borsos, T. 1963. Complement and hemolysis. *Science*. 141:738–740.

Raum, D., Awdeh, Z.L., Glass, D., Yunis, E., and Alper, C.A. 1981. The location of C2, C4, and Bf relative to HLA-B and HLA-D. *Immunogenetics*. 12:473–483.

Raum, D., Balner, H., Peterson, B.H., and Alper, C.A. 1980. Genetic polymorphism of serum complement components in the chimpanzee. *Immunogenetics*. 10:455–468.

Regal, J.F., Fraser, D.G., and Toth, C.A. 1993. Role of the complement system in antigen-induced bronchoconstriction and changes in blood pressure in the guinea pig. *J Pharmacol Exp Ther*. 267:979–988.

Ricklin, D. and Lambris, J.D. 2013. Complement in immune and inflammatory disorders: Pathophysiological mechanisms. *J Immunol*. 190(8):3831–3838.

Rits, M., Kints, J.P., Bazin, H., and Vaerman, J.P. 1987. Rat C3 conversion by rat anti-2,4, dinitrophenyl (DNP) hapten IgA immune precipitates. *Scand J Immunol*. 25:359–366.

Rommel, F.A., Bendure, D.W., and Kalter, S.S. 1980. Hemolytic complement in nonhuman primates. *Lab Anim Sci*. 30:1026–1029.

Rooney, I.A., Liszewski, M.K., and Atkinson, J.P. 1993. Using membrane-bound complement regulatory proteins to inhibit rejection. *Xeno*. 1:29–35.

Roos, A., Bouwman, L.H., Munoz, J., et al. 1982. Functional characterization of the lectin pathway of complement in human serum. *Mol Immunol*. 39:655–668.

Roos, M.H. and Demant, P. 1982. Murine complement factor B (Bf) sexual dimorphism and H-2 linked polymorphism. *Immunogenetics*. 15:23–30.

Rosenberg, L.T. and Tachibana, D.K. 1962. Activity of mouse complement. *J Immunol*. 89:861–867.

Rosenfeld, S.E., Baum, J., Steigbigel, R.T., and Leddy, J.P. 1976b. Hereditary deficiency of the fifth component of complement in man. II. Biological properties of C5 deficient human serum. *J Clin Invest*. 57:1635–1643.

Rosenfeld, S.E., Kelly, M.E., and Leddy, J.P. 1976a. Hereditary deficiency in the fifth component of complement in man. I. Clinical, immunochemical, and family studies. *J Clin Invest*. 57:1626–1634.

Rother, K. and Rother, U. 1986. Hereditary and acquired complement deficiencies in animals and man. *Prog Allergy*. 39:1–7.

Rother, K., Rother, U., Muller-Eberhard, H.J., and Nilsson, U.R. 1966. Deficiency of the sixth component of complement in rabbits with an inherited complement defect. *J Exp Med.* 124:773–785.

Rougier, N. Kazatchkine, M.D., Rougier, J.P., et al. 1998. Human complement factor H deficiency associated with hemolytic uremic syndrome. *J Am Soc Nephrol.* 9:2318–2326.

Roxvall, L., Sennerby, L., Johansson, B.R., and Heideman, M. 1990. Trypsin-induced vascular permeability and leukocyte accumulation in hamster cheek pouch: The role of complement activation. *J Surg Res.* 49:504–513.

Ruddy, S. and Austen, K.F. 1971. C3b inactivator of man. II. Fragments produced by C3b inactivator cleavage of cell-bound or fluid phase C3b. *Immunology.* 107:742–750.

Ruddy, S., Carpenter, G.B., Chin, K.W., et al. 1975. Human complement metabolism: An analysis of 144 studies. *Medicine.* 54:165–178.

Sahu, A., Sunyer, J.O., Moore, W.T., Sarrias, M.R., Soulika, A.M., and Labbris, J.D. 1998. Structure, functions, and evolution of the third complement component and viral molecular mimicry. *Immunologic Res.* 17:109–121.

Sakamoto, M., Ishii, S., Nisheoka, K., and Shimasa, K. 1981. Level of complement response to bacterial challenge in malnourished rats. *Infect Immun.* 32:553–556.

Sarma, J.V. and Ward, P.A. 2011. The complement system. *Cell Tissue Res.* 343(1):227–235.

Sasaki, O., Zhou, W., Miyazaki, M., et al. 1997. Intraglomerular C3 synthesis in rats with passive heymann nephritis. *Am J Pathol.* 151:1249–1256.

Sato, T., Endo, Y., and Matsuhita, M. 1994. Molecular characterization of a novel serine protease involved in activation of the complement system by mannose-binding protein. *Int Immunol.* 6:665–669.

Schaller, J.G., Gilliland, B.G., Ochs, H.D., Leddy, J.P., Agodoa, L.C.Y., and Rosenfeld, S.I. 1977. Severe systemic lupus erythematosus with nephritis in a boy with deficiency of the fourth component of complement. *Arthritis Rheum.* 20:1519–1525.

Scharfstein, J., Ferreira, A., Gigli, I., and Nussenzweig, V. 1978. Human C4b-binding protein, isolation and characterization. *J Exp Med.* 148:207–222.

Schmid, E., Warner, R.L., Crouch, L.D., et al. 1997. Neutrophil chemotactic activity and C5a following systemic activation of complement in rats. *Inflammation.* 21:325–333.

Schreiber, R.D., Morrison, D.C., Podack, E.R., and Muller-Eberhard, H.J. 1979. Bactericidal activity of the alternative complement pathway generated from 11 isolated plasma proteins. *J Exp Med.* 149:870–882.

Schreiber, R.D. and Muller-Eberhard, H.J. 1974. Fourth component of human complement: Description of three polypeptide chain structure. *J Exp Med.* 140:1324–1335.

Schreiber, R.D., Pangburn, M.K., Medicus, R.G., and Muller-Eberhard, H.J. 1980. Raji cell injury and subsequent lysis by the purified cytolytic alternative pathway of human complement. *Clin Immunol Immunopathol.* 15:384–396.

Schur, P.H., Connelly, A., and Jones, T.C. 1975. Phylogeny of complement components in non-human primates. *J. Immunol.* 114:270–273.

Schulze, M., Baker, P.J., Perkinson, D.T., et al. 1989. Increased urinary excretion of C5b-9 distinguishes passive Heymann nephritis in the rat. *Kidney Int.* 35:60–68.

Schwaeble, W., Dahl, M.R., Thiel, S., Stover, C., and Jensenius, J.C. 2002. The mannanbinding lectin-associated serine proteases (MASPs) and MAp19: Four components of the lectin pathway activation complex encoded by two genes. *Immunobiology.* 205:455–466.

Schwaeble, W.J., Lynch, N.J., Clark, J.E., et al. 2011. Targeting of mannan-binding lectin-associated serine protease-2 confers protection from myocardial and gastrointestinal ischemia/reperfusion injury. *Proc Natl Acad Sci.* 108:7523–7528.

Seelen, M.A., Roos, A., Wieslander, J., et al. 2005. Functional analysis of the classical, alternative, and MBL pathways of the complement system: Standardization and validation of a simple ELISA. *J Immunol Methods.* 296(1–2):187–198.

Setien, F., Alvarez, V., Coto, E., DiScipio, R.G., and Lopez-Larrea, C. 1993. A physical map of the human complement component C6, C7, and C9 genes. *Immunogenetics.* 38:341–344.

Seya, T., Holers, V.M., and Atkinson, J.P. 1985. Purification and functional analysis of the polymorphic variants of the C3b/C4b receptor (CR1) and comparison with H, C4b-binding protein (C4bp), and decay accelerating factor (DAF). *J Immunol.* 135:2661–2667.

Seya, T., Nakamura, K., Masaki, T., Ichihara-Itoh, C., Matsumoto, M., and Nagasawa, S. 1995. Human factor H and C4b-binding protein serve as factor I cofactors both encompassing inactivation of C3b and C4b. *Mol Immunol.* 32:355–360.

Sheerin, N.S., Springall, T., Carroll, M.C., Hartley, B., and Sacks, S.H. 1997. Protection against anti-glomerular basement membrane (GBM)-mediated nephritis in C3- and C4-deficient mice. *Clin Exp Immunol.* 110:403–409.

Shevach, E., Green, I., and Frank, M.M. 1976. Linkage of C4 deficiency to the major histocompatibility locus in the guinea pig. *J Immunol.* 116:1750.

Shin, H.S., Smith, M.R., and Wood, W.B., Jr. 1969. Heat labile opsonins to pneumoccoccus. II. Involvement of C3 and C5. *J Exp Med.* 130:1229–1241.

Shiroishi, T., Sagai, T., Natsuume-Sakai, S., and Moriwaki, K. 1987. Lethal deletion of the complement component C4 and steroid 20-hydroxylase genes in the mouse H-2 class III region, caused by meiotic recombination. *Proc Natl Acad Sci USA.* 84:2819–2823.

Shreffler, D.C. 1982. MHC-linked complement components. In *Receptors and Recognition, Series B.* Eds. P. Parham and J. Strominger, Vol. 14, pp. 187–219. London: Chapman and Hall.

Shreffler, D.C. and Owen, R.D. 1963. A serologically detected variant in mouse serum: Inheritance and association with the histocompatibility-2 locus. *Genetics.* 48:9–25.

Siboo, R. and Vas, S.I. 1965. Studies in vitro antibody production III. Production of complement. *Can J Microbiol.* 11:415–425.

Sim, R.B. and Reid, K.B.M. 1991. C1: Molecular interactions with activating systems. *Immunol Today.* 12:307–311.

Singer, L., Colten, H.R., and Wetsel, R.A. 1994. Complement C3 deficiency: Human, animal, and experimental models. *Pathobiology.* 62:14–28.

Sinosich, M.J., Best, N., Teisner, B., and Grudzinskas, J.G. 1982. Demonstration of antigenic determinants specific for the split products of the third complement factor, C3. *J Immunol Methods.* 51:355–358.

Sliwinski, A.J. and Zvaifler, N.H. 1972. Decreased synthesis of the third component of complement (C3) in hypocomplementemic systemic lupus erythematosus. *Clin Exp Immunol.* 11:21–29.

Sodetz, J.M. 1988. Structure and function of C8 in the membrane attack sequence of complement. *Curr Topics Microbiol Immunol.* 140:19–31.

Sørensen, R., Thiel, S., and Jensenius, J.C. 2005. Mannan-binding-lectin associated serine proteases, characteristics and disease associations. *Semin Immunopathol.* 27(3):299–319.

Spicer, S.T., Tran, G.T., Killingsworth, M.C., et al. 2007. Induction of passive Heymann nephritis in complement component 6-deficient PVG rats. *J Immunol.* 179(1):172–178.

Spitzer, D., Mitchell, L.M., Atkinson, J.P., and Hourcade, D.E. 2007. Properdin can initiate complement activation by binding specific target surfaces and providing a platform for de novo convertase assembly. *J Immunol.* 179:2600–2608.

Staats, A. 1985. Standardized nomenclature for inbred species of mice 8th listing. *Cancer Res.* 45:945–977.

Stahel, P.F., Frein, K., Fontana, A., Eugster, H.-P., Ault, B.H., and Barnum, S.R. 1997. Evidence for intrathecal synthesis of alternative pathway complement activation proteins in experimental meningitis. *Am J Pathol.* 151:897–904.

Stankiewicz, M. and Jonas, W. 1981. Haemolysis of human erythrocytes heavily sensitized with sheep amboceptor by sheep complement chelated with EGTA or Mg^{+2} EGTA. *Vet Immunol Immunopathol.* 2:253–264.

Stecher, V.J. and Thorbecke, G.J. 1967. Sites of synthesis of serum proteins. II. Medium requirements for serum protein production by rat macrophages. *J Immunol.* 99:653–659.

Storm, K.-E., Arturson, G., and Nilsson, U.R. 1992. Purification and characterization of porcine C3. Studies of the biologically active protein and its split products. *Vet Immunol Immunopathol.* 34:47–61.

Strang, C.J., Auerbach, H.S., and Rosen, F.S. 1986. C1s-induced vascular permeability in C2-deficient guinea pigs. *J Immunol.* 137:631–635.

Strunk, R.S., Tashjian, A.H., and Colten, H.R. 1975. Complement biosynthesis in vitro by rat hepatoma cell strains. *J Immunol.* 114:331–335.

Sundsmo, J.S. and Fair, D.S. 1983. Relationships among the complement, kinin, coagulation, and fibrinolytic systems. *Springer Semin Immunol.* 6:231–258.

Swaak, A.J., van Rooyen, A., Vogelaar, C., Pillay, M., and Hack, E. 1986. Complement (C3) metabolism in systemic lupus erythematosus in relation to the disease course. *Rheumatol Int.* 6(5):221–226.

Table, H., Menger, M., Aston, W.P., and Cochran, M. 1983. Alternative pathway of bovine complement: Concentration of factor B, hemolytic activity, and heritability. *Vet Immunol Immunopathol.* 5:389–398.

Tachibana, D.K. and Rosenberg, L.T. 1966. Fetal synthesis of Hc, a component of mouse complement. *J Immunol.* 97:213–215.

Tachibana, D.K., Ulrich, M., and Rosenberg, L.T. 1963. The inheritance of hemolytic complement activity on CF-1 mouse. *J Immunol.* 91:230–232.

Tack, B.F. and Prahl, J.W. 1976. Third component of human complement. Purification from plasma and physico-chemical characterization. *Biochemistry.* 15:4513–4521.

Tamura, N. and Nelson, R.A. 1967. Three naturally-occurring inhibitors of components of complement in guinea pig and rabbit serum. *J Immunol.* 99:582–589.

Tanaka, M., Murase, N., Ye, Q., et al. 1996. Effect of anticomplement agent K76 COOH on hamster-to-rat and guinea pig-to-rat heart xenotransplantation. *Transplantation.* 62:681–688.

Tanaka, S., Kitamura, F., and Suzuki, T. 1987. Studies on the hemolytic activity of the classical and alternative pathway of complement in various animal species. *Complement.* 4(1):33–41.

Tanaka, S., Suzuki, T., Sakaizumi, M., et al. 1991. Gene responsible for deficient activity of the β-Subunit of C8, the eighth component of complement, is located on mouse chromosome 4. *Immunogenetics.* 33:18–23.

TECOmedical Group. 2010. *Complement Diagnostics: Hemocompatibility Testing of Medical Devices, Pharmaceuticals, and Blood Products. Clinical and Technical Review*, pp. 1–80. Switzerland: TECOmedical AG. Sissach.

Terry, W.D., Borsos, T., and Rapp, H. 1964. Differences in serum complement activity among inbred strains of mice. *J Immunol.* 92:576–578.

Thurston, J.R., Baetz, A.L., Cheville, N.F., and Richard, J.L. 1980. Acute aflatoxicosis in guinea pigs: Sequential changes in serum proteins, complement, C4, and liver enzymes and histopathologic changes. *Am J Vet Res.* 41:1272–1276.

Tizard, I. 2013. *Veterinary Immunology*, 9th edition. St. Louis, MO: Elsevier Saunders.

Toews, G.B. and Vial, W.C. 1984. The role of C5 polymorphonuclear leukocyte-recruitment in response to *Streptococcus pneumoniae. Am Rev Respir Dis.* 129:82–86.

Tosi, M., Levi-Strauss, M., Georgatsou, S., Amor, M., and Meo, T. 1985. Duplications of complement and non-complement genes in the H-2S region: Evolutionary aspects of the C4 isotypes and molecular analysis of their variants. *Immunol Rev.* 87:151–183.

Trail, P.A., Yang, T.J., and Cameron, J.A. 1984. Increase in the haemolytic complement activity of dogs affected with cyclic haematopoiesis. *Vet Immunol Immunopathol.* 7:359–368.

Tuzun, E., Scott, B.G., Goluszko, E., Higgs, S., and Christadoss, P. 2003. Genetic evidence for involvement of classical complement pathway in induction of experimental autoimmune myasthenia gravis. *J Immunol.* 171(7):3847–3854.

Ulevitch, R.J. and Cochrane, C.G. 1977. Complement dependent hemodynamic and hematologic changes in the rabbit. *Inflammation.* 2:199–216.

Vaith, P., Prasauska, V., Potempa, L.A., and Peter, H.H. 1996. Complement activation by C-reactive protein on the HEp-2 cell substrate. *Int Arch Allergy Immunol.* 111:107–117.

van den Berg, C.W., Demant, P., Aerts, P.C., and Van Dijk, H. 1992. Slp is an essential component on an EDTA-resistant activation pathway of mouse complement. *Proc Natl Acad Sci USA.* 89:10711–10715.

van den Berg, C.W. and Morgan, B.P. 1994. Complement inhibitory activities of CD59 and analogs from rat, sheep, and pig are not homologously restricted. *J Immunol.* 152:4095–4101.

van der Pol, P., Schlagwein, N., van Gijlswijk, D.J., et al. 2012. Mannan-binding lectin mediates renal ischemia/reperfusion injury independent of complement activation. *Am J Transplant.* 12:877–887.

Van Dijk, H., Heezius, E., Van Kooten, P.J.S., Rademaker, P.M., Van Dam, R., and Willers, J.M.N. 1983. A study of the sensitivity of erythrocytes to lysis by heterologous sera via the alternative complement pathway. *Vet Immunol Immunopathol.* 4:469–477.

Van Dixhoorn, M.G.A., Timmerman, J.J., Van Gijlswijk-Janssen, D.J., et al. 1997. Characterization of complement C6 deficiency in a PVG/C rat strain. *Clin Exp Immunol.* 109:387–396.

Velazquez, P., Cribbs, D.H., Poulos, T.L., and Tenner, A.J. 1997. Aspartate residue 7 in amyloid β-proteins is critical for classical complement pathway activation. Implications for Alzheimer's disease pathogenesis. *Nat Med.* 3:77–79.

Vogt, W., Lieflander, M., Stalder, K.H., Lufft, E., and Schmidt, G. 1971. Functional identity of anaphylatoxin preparations obtained from different species and by different activation procedures. II. Immunological identity. *Eur J Immunol.* 1:139–140.

Wagner, E. and Frank, M.M. 2010. Therapeutic potential of complement modulation. *Nat Rev Drug Discov.* 9(1):43–56.

Wagner, J.L. and Hugli, T.E. 1984. Radioimmunoassay for anaphylatoxins: A sensitive method for determining complement activation products in biological fluids. *Analyt Biochem.* 136:75–88.

Wallis, R. 2007. Interactions between mannose-binding lectin and MASPs during complement activation by the lectin pathway. *Immunobiology.* 212(4–5):289–299.

Walport, M.J. 2001a. Complement First of two parts. *N Engl J Med.* 344(14):1058–1066.

Walport, M.J. 2001b. Complement Second of two parts. *N Engl J Med.* 344(15):1140–1144.

Ward, P.A. and Zvaifler N.J. 1973. Quantitative phagocytosis by neutrophils. II. Release of the C5-cleaving enzyme and inhibition of phagocytosis by rheumatoid factor. *J Immunol.* 111(6):1777–1782.

Watanabe, I., Horiuchi, T., and Fujita, S. 1995. Role of protein kinase C activation in synthesis of complement components C2 and factor B in interferon-γ-stimulated human fibroblasts, glioblastoma, cell line A172, and monocytes. *Biochem J.* 305:425–431.

Weigle, W.O., Goodman, M.G., Morgan, E.L., and Hugli, T.E. 1983. Regulation of immune response by components of the complement cascade and their activated fragments. *Springer Semin Immunopathol.* 6:173–194.

Weiler, J.M., Daha, M.R., Austen, K.F., and Fearon, D.T. 1976. Control of the amplification convertase of complement by the plasma protein beta1H. *Proc Natl Acad Sci USA.* 73(9):3268–3272.

Weitzel, H.K. and Rother, K. 1970. Studies on the role of serum complement in allograft rejection and in immunosuppression by antihymocyte serum. *Eur Surg Res.* 2:310–317.

Whaley, K. 1980. Biosynthesis of the complement components and the regulatory proteins of the alternative complement pathway by human peripheral blood monocytes. *J Exp Med.* 151:501–516.

Wheat, W.H., Wetsel, R., Falus, A., Tack, B.F., and Strunk, R.C. 1987. The fifth component of complement (C5) in the mouse. *J Exp Med.* 165:1442–1447.

Whitehead, A.S., Goldberger, G., Woods, D.E., Markham, A.F., and Colten, H.R. 1983. Use of a cDNA clone for the fourth component of human complement (C4) for analysis of a genetic deficiency of C4 in guinea pig. *Proc Natl Acad Sci USA.* 80:5387–5391.

Winkelstein, J.A., Cork, L.C., Griffin, D.E., Griffin, J.W., Adams, R.J., and Price, D.L. 1981. Genetically determined deficiency of the third component of complement in the dog. *Science.* 212:1169–1170.

Winkelstein, J.A., Johnson, J.P., Swift, A.J., Ferry, R., Yolken, R., and Cork, L.C. 1982. Genetically determined deficiency of the third component of complement in the dog. *In vivo* studies on the complement system and complement mediated serum activities. *J Immunol.* 129:2598–2602.

Wolfe, J.H. and Halliwell, R.E.W. 1980. Total hemolytic complement values in normal and diseased dog populations. *Vet Immunol Immunopathol.* 1:287–298.

Wurzner, R., Joysey, V.C., and Lachmann, P.J. 1994. Assessment of *in vivo* synthesis after liver transplantation reveals that hepatocytes do not synthesize the majority of human C7. *J Immunol.* 152:4624–4629.

Wurzner, R., Mewar, D., Fernie, B.A., Hobart, M.J., and Lachmann, P.J. 1995. Importance of the third thrombospondin repeat of C6 for terminal complement complex assembly. *Immunology.* 85:214–219.

Xu, W., Berger, S.P., Trouw, L.A., et al. 2008. Properdin binds to late apoptotic and necrotic cells independently of C3band regulates alternative pathway complement activation. *J Immunol.* 180:7613–7621.

Yamamoto, S., Kubotsu, K., Kida, M., et al. 1995. Automated homogeneous liposome-based assay system for total complement activity. *Clin Chem.* 41:586–590.

Yang, S.Y., Jensen, R., Folke, L., Good, R.A., and Day, N.K. 1974. Complement deficiency in hamsters. *Fed Proc.* 33:795.

Youssif, M.A., Nicholas, J.L., Kashif, S.H., Teizo, F., Yuichi, E., Soren, H. et al. 2012. The lectin pathway of complement activation is a critical component of the innate immune response to pneumococcal infection. *PLoS.* doi: http://dx.doi.org/10.1371/journal.ppat.1002793.

Zhang, Y., Suankratay, C., Zhang, X.-H., Jones, D.R., Lint, T.F., and Gewurz, H. 1999. Calcium-independent haemolysis via the lectin pathway of complement activation in the guinea-pig and other species. *Immunology.* 97:686–692.

Ziegler, J.B., Alper, C.A., and Balner, H. 1975a. Properdin factor B and histocompatibility loci linked in the rhesus monkey. *Nature.* 254:609–611.

Ziegler, J.B., Watson, L., and Alper, C.A. 1975b. Genetic polymorphism of properdin factor B in the rhesus: Evidence for single subunit structure in primates. *J Immunol.* 114:1649–1653.

Zimmerman, T.S., Arroyave, C.M., and Muller-Eberhard, H.J. 1971. A blood coagulation abnormally in rabbits deficient in the sixth component of complement (C6) and its correction by purified C6. *J Exp Med.* 134:1591–1600.

18 Transport Proteins

Claire L. Parry

CONTENTS

18.1 INTRODUCTION

In most of the animal species, plasma proteins make up approximately 7% of the total plasma. These nitrogenous compounds are often unique and specific for individual species. Most plasma proteins have specific functions as, for example, enzymes, blood coagulation factors, hormones, antibodies, or transport compounds. Most transport proteins in humans and many in animals have been well characterized. The major transport proteins covered in this chapter include albumin, transthyretin (TTR), thyroid hormone-binding proteins, haptoglobin, group-specific components (Gc), hemopexin, transferrin, and corticosteroid-binding globulin. Many of these proteins have multiple roles and can be classified differently depending on the subject matter. In this text, ceruloplasmin has been included in Chapter 19 due to its role in inflammation.

18.2 ALBUMIN

18.2.1 Properties

Serum albumin (SA) is the most abundant protein in the circulation and the most prominent component on electrophoresis. Albumin is a single peptide chain of over 580 amino acid residues. The amino acid composition and sequence of albumin have been determined in many domestic and laboratory animals, including cattle, horse, rat, mouse, pig, and sheep (Brown, 1976; Brown et al., 1971; Carter and Ho, 1994; Peters, 1977; Peters and Reed, 1980). The complete amino acid sequence of human and bovine albumin has been described (Behrens et al., 1975; Brown, 1975; Meloun et al., 1975). The molecular weights of human and bovine albumin calculated from the sequences are 66,500 and 66,210 Da, respectively. The proposed structure for both human and bovine albumin consists of three repeating units or domains (domains I, II, and III). Each domain is composed of two large double loops and one small double loop (loops 1–9) (Behrens et al., 1975; Brown, 1975; Carter and Ho, 1994). The double loops are formed by disulfide bonds between the 34 half-cystine residues. Only 20% of the amino acid residues differ between human and bovine albumin. Sequence homologies between equine and bovine SAs and equine and rat SAs are 73% and 76%, respectively (Carter and Ho, 1994).

18.2.2 Role/Function

Albumin serves many functions. It binds and transports large organic anions that are normally insoluble in aqueous fluid, for example, bilirubin and long-chain fatty acids, poorly soluble hormones, such as steroid and thyroid hormones, and virtually all constituents of plasma not bound and transported by specific proteins. Albumin is a major contributor to the plasma osmotic pressure and accounts for 75% of total osmotic activity. It plays a minor nutritive role, acting as reservoir and contributing approximately 5% of amino acids used in peripheral tissues. It is also involved in the binding of heavy metals (Grant and Kachmar, 1976; Peters, 1977). Ligand-binding locations for several substances have also been reported (Peters, 1977; Reed et al., 1975). Copper and nickel bind at the amino terminus. Cystine and glutathione bind near the first thiol group, and normally two fatty acids bind on loops 4–6 and 7. Furthermore, the efficacy, distribution, and metabolism of many drugs are affected by their affinity to SA. In different species of SA, single changes in relevant sequence were found to significantly alter their binding selectivity (Titlebach and Gilpin, 1995). Structural differences in the binding sites between rat and human SA have been reported (Massolini et al., 1996).

During the acute phase response, the concentration of albumin is decreased due to either, a decrease in its synthesis due to inflammatory cytokines, or by a negative feedback mechanism involving an oncotic pressure receptor on the hepatocytes. Hypoalbuminemia is observed when inflammation has lasted up to 1 week. Four factors are responsible for the reduction in albumin:

- Hemodilution
- Loss into the extravascular space, as vascular permeability increases in the areas of inflammation
- Increased catabolism due to localized cell consumption
- Decreased synthesis as the result of direct inhibition by cytokines, for example, IL-1, IL-6, and TNF-α, and an increased colloidal osmotic pressure (Gentry, 1999; Nassir et al., 2002; Stockham and Scott, 2008)

The synthesis of albumin involves an intracellular precursor form, proalbumin. Rat studies in the rat have shown that proalbumin, formed by the microsomes, contains a basic hexapeptide extension at the amino terminus. Proalbumin binds bilirubin and palminate as effectively as albumin. Although the role of proalbumin is unknown, it has been suggested that the hexapeptide extension on proalbumin serves to channel the nascent albumin through the liver cell and to regulate albumin synthesis (Peters, 1977; Peters and Davidson, 1982, 1986; Peters and Reed, 1980).

Overall rates of albumin catabolism have been determined for various animal species by conventional protein tracer techniques, such as radioiodination (Allison, 1960; Dixon et al., 1953; Mattheeuws et al., 1966). The rate of catabolism varies with the species, and is frequently measured as the time in which one half the serum concentration disappears ($T_{1/2}$). There appears to be a direct correlation between albumin turnover and body size. The $T_{1/2}$ for albumin in various species is listed in Table 18.1.

The tissue sites for albumin catabolism have been studied using nondegradable radioactive tracers that accumulate in tissues following protein degradation. Studies in rabbits using (^{14}C) sucrose-labeled albumin suggested that all tissues catabolized albumin, with no tissue of predominant importance. The most active tissues were those with fenestrated or discontinuous capillary beds, suggesting that exposure to high concentrations of albumin was an important determinant in albumin degradation (Yedgar et al., 1983). Similar studies in rats showed that the major fraction of albumin catabolism occurs in muscle and skin (Baynes and Thorpe, 1981).

18.2.3 Pathophysiological Significance

Genetic polymorphism has been observed in many species, including domestic fowl, pig, cattle, horse, and toad (Tarnoky, 1980). Breeding experiments with inbred lines of brown leghorns, white leghorns, and Rhode Island Red chickens have shown three phenotypes of albumin controlled by

TABLE 18.1
Albumin Turnover in Animals

Species	$T_{1/2}$ (days)	Reference
Mouse	1.9	Allison (1960)
Rat	2.5	Allison (1960)
Guinea pig	2.8	Allison (1960)
Rabbit	5.7	Dixon et al. (1953)
Dog	8.2	Dixon et al. (1953)
Man	15.0	Dixon et al. (1953)
Baboon	16.0	Cohen (1956)

two codominant autosomal alleles: a homozygous fast, a homozygous slow, and a heterozygous fast–slow combination type (McIndoe, 1962). Patterns of albumin polymorphism similar to those of chickens are also observed in turkeys (Quinteros et al., 1964) and horses (Stormont and Suzuki, 1963). In pigs, the genetic control of albumin phenotypes appears to involve three codominant alleles (Kristjansson, 1966). Eleven albumin alleles present in 29 phenotypes were found in the American toad (*Bufo americanus*) (Constans and Viau, 1977). Genetic variants have also been described in cattle (Soos, 1971).

Measurement of SA is of considerable diagnostic value, as it relates to (a) general nutritional status, (b) the integrity of the vascular system, and (c) liver function. SA concentrations for most laboratory animal species are between 2.42 and 4.19 g/dL, and reference values for each laboratory animal species have been reported (Mitruka and Rawnsley, 1977). In man, the rate of albumin synthesis by the liver is approximately 14 g per day (Putman, 1975b). In 5- to 7-week old rats, it is 3.13 mg/100 g of body weight per hour (Peters and Peters, 1972).

Fasting rats for 18 hours caused a 40% reduction in the rate of albumin synthesis (Peters and Peters, 1972). Circadian fluctuation of plasma protein and albumin levels in rats maintained on a 12-hour light-dark cycle has been reported, with highest levels observed at 0100 and 0800 hours, and lowest levels observed at 1800 (Scheving et al., 1968). A significant decrease in SA levels in late gestation has been reported in rhesus monkeys (Golub and Kaaekuahiwi, 1997). The formation of albumin decreases with increasing age (Jeffrey, 1960); however, the properties and composition of SA from adult and aging mice are identical (Schofield, 1980). Increased albumin production, has not been known to occur in animals. An increase in the SA concentration is usually interpreted as consistent with dehydration. Hypoalbuminemia may result from (a) impaired synthesis, as in malnutrition or chronic liver disease; (b) loss through urine and feces, as in renal and intestinal disease; (c) increased catabolism, as in neoplastic conditions and acute phase reaction (albumin is a "negative" acute phase reactant); and (d) changes in distribution between intra- and extravascular compartments (Grant and Kachmar, 1976; Kalberg et al., 1983; Kurosky et al., 1980). Interestingly, a strategy for hepatocyte transplantation, using retrorsine and partial hepatectomy, has been demonstrated to restore albumin synthesis and physiological function of the liver, suggesting its potential use as a method to treat genetic-based or acquired liver diseases (Oren et al., 1999).

18.2.4 Analytical Methods

Currently used procedures for estimation of SA are based on one of the following principles: (a) salt precipitation, (b) dye binding, (c) electrophoretic mobility, and (d) antigenicity (Grant and Kachmar, 1976; Peters, 1977).

The most commonly used salts for precipitation are sodium and ammonium sulfate. Serum globulins can be removed selectively by salt precipitation, and the remaining albumin assayed by the biuret method.

Albumin has the tendency to bind certain dyes, such as BG, methyl orange, and 2-(4′-hydroxyazobenzene) benzoic acid (HABA). This characteristic has been used to measure albumin directly. HABA binds very poorly to albumin of domestic animals and is susceptible to bilirubin interference. The use of BG appears to be quite accurate when compared to electrophoresis and is less affected by pigment interference. For example, measurement of rabbit albumin by unmodified dye binding with either BG or bromcresol purple yields falsely elevated values if human or bovine albumin is used to calibrate the assay. If determined this way, the measured concentration of rabbit albumin may exceed the concentration of total protein. This may be related to the configuration of the binding sites of rabbit albumin. The error may be overcome by using rabbit albumin as the calibrator for the measurement of rabbit albumin. The opposite is true for birds where avian albumin binds BG with less affinity, therefore, if a bovine albumin is used as the standard, all avian values will be falsely decreased (Hall, 1992).

The assay of albumin using electrophoresis and protein staining has frequently been used as the reference against which other procedures are judged. However, there is no convincing evidence that the staining intensity is linear to protein concentration.

Immunochemical techniques for albumin determination such as radial immunodiffusion and immunonephelometry are gaining popularity (Peters, 1977). Immunologic cross-reactivity between SA from various species has been studied and correlated with the phylogenetic relatedness between species. Cross-reactivity between human SA and those of several primate species, as well as cross-reactivity among SAs of various domestic and laboratory animals, has been reported (Kamiyama, 1976; Rangel, 1965; Sakata and Atassi, 1979; Sarich and Wilson, 1966; Weigle, 1961). In these studies, rabbit antibovine SA antibodies will cross-react most strongly with sheep and goat albumin and less so with pig, horse, rodent, and chicken albumin in decreasing order. A species-specific standard if available should be used. If unavailable, alternative standards can be selected and tested for cross-reactivity or alternatively the protein can be measured by serum protein electrophoresis or the biuret method.

18.3 CORTICOSTEROID-BINDING GLOBULIN

18.3.1 Properties

Corticosteroid-binding globulin (CBG), or transcortin, a member of the superfamily of serine protease inhibitors, is a plasma carrier protein of obscure biologic function. Human and animal CBGs are α-globulins of similar size. The amino acid composition and carbohydrate content of CBG in rats, rabbits, and guinea pigs have been reported (Chader and Westphal, 1968a, b; Mickelson and Westphal, 1979; Rosner and Hochberg, 1972). Rat and rabbit CBG has more cystine than does human CBG. Cystine is involved in the maintenance of the conformational structure of CBG; therefore, higher cystine content found in rat CBG may be related to its greater tendency to form polymeric structures after removal of corticosterone (Westphal, 1971). The number of corticosteroid-binding sites per molecule of CBG is one in all species tested (Mickelson and Westphal, 1979; Rosner, 1972; Rosner and Hochberg, 1972). The partial amino acid sequence analysis of mouse CBG shows a low overall homology (60%) to human CBG (Nyberg et al., 1990). Sequence homologies between hamster CBG and rat and human CBGs are 70% and 59%, respectively (Lin et al., 1990). Squirrel monkey (*Saimiri sciureus*) CBG has a molecular weight of approximately 42,000 Da and, as expected, shows high sequence identity (86%) with human CBG (Hammond et al., 1994).

CBG, like other glycoproteins, is synthesized mainly in the liver, but a small amount is probably produced in other tissues such as the kidney, lung, and spleen (Allison, 1960; Scrocchi et al., 1993; Seralini et al., 1990). CBG receptors on plasma membranes of a variety of cells have been shown. CBG, when exposed to a serine protease, is cleaved and releases all or most of its bound cortisol (Rosner, 1991).

18.3.2 Role/Function

It is generally accepted that CBG protects the corticosteroids from peripheral metabolism and loss through the kidney, and therefore helps maintain relatively constant plasma corticosteroid levels; however, firm evidence supporting this hypothesis is lacking. CBG has been found in all vertebrate species examined. The CBG binding capacities of 131 vertebrate species have been determined by Seal and Doe (Seal and Doe, 1963, 1965, 1966). A comprehensive review of the CBG of various animal species was made by Westphal (1971).

18.3.3 Pathophysiological Significance

Normal CBG reference values for practically all vertebrate species have been compiled by Westphal (1971). The female rat has a higher CBG level than does the male; however, there is no change in CBG concentration during estrus or pregnancy (Gala and Westphal, 1965a, b; Grunder, 1966). The CBG activity of female mice is three times that of the male. In contrast to that in rats, pregnancy in mice results in a 13-fold increase in CBG activity (Gala and Westphal, 1967). This increase during pregnancy is also observed in the rabbit, guinea pig, and hamster (Gala and Westphal, 1967; Lin et al., 1990). The rise in guinea pig plasma CBG during gestation is as dramatic as that seen in the mouse, with peak values of 900 μg of CBG/mL of plasma (compared to 75–155 μg/mL in nonpregnant animals) (Goodman et al., 1981). Pregnant baboons have only a moderate increase in CBG during pregnancy (59 ± 6.4 μg of cortisol/100 mL of plasma in pregnant animals compared to 33.4 ± 5.5 μg/100 mL in nonpregnant animals) (Oakey, 1975). The CBG levels in fetuses are higher than those in neonates, and newborn animals have much lower levels of CBG than do adults (Ballard et al., 1982; Beamer et al., 1973; D'Agnostino and Henning, 1982). The development and synthesis of CBG are probably regulated through the pituitary-adrenal and pituitary-thyroid axes (Ballard et al., 1982; D'Agnostino and Henning, 1982; Rosenthal et al., 1974; Sakly and Koch, 1983). Estrogen administration caused a marked increase in CBG activity in rats and monkeys (Barbosa et al., 1970; Cody, 1980; Coe et al., 1986). This effect was not observed in hypophysectomized rats, suggesting that thyroid-stimulating hormone is involved in the estrogen effect, because it is the only pituitary hormone that influences CBG activity. Conversely, testosterone administration depresses CBG activity in the rat. Testosterone also depresses CBG activity in monkeys, though not significantly (Barbosa et al., 1971). Testosterone did not seem to have a depressive effect on CBG in badgers (Audy et al., 1982). In Peking ducks, in which males have higher CBG levels than do females, testosterone was found to stimulate CBG production without altering thyroxine levels (Daniel et al., 1981).

Diurnal variations in CBG levels have been observed in the guinea pig, rat, and mouse. The guinea pig has a maximum CBG binding capacity at 1600 hours (9 hours of light per day cycle, and lights on at 0800 hours) and the lowest binding capacity at 1200 and 2400 hours (Fujieda et al., 1982). Biphasic circadian rhythm for CBG has been observed in the rat. D'Agnostino et al. (1982) observed two distinct peaks, one during the light phase and the other during the dark phase, which were sustained for almost the entire dark period. Other investigators (Ottenweller et al., 1979) found both peaks in the light period. The CBG rhythm in the mouse is monophasic, with peak levels found during the dark phase (Ottenweller et al., 1979).

Pathologic variations in CBG levels in man have been reviewed (Brien, 1981). Altered values have been reported in liver disease, nephrosis, and other protein-losing conditions, thyroid disease, adrenal diseases (including Cushing's syndrome and Addison's disease), mental illness, and stress. Sows and gilts subjected to stress (heat and crowding) during midgestation had lower CBG levels (Kattesh et al., 1980). Acute inflammation induced by subcutaneous injection of turpentine produced an average threefold decrease in serum corticosterone and CBG levels in both pregnant and nonpregnant rats (Savu et al., 1980). CBG may represent one of the "negative" acute phase proteins like transferring and albumin.

18.3.4 Analytical Methods

Plasma CBG can be measured indirectly by determining the cortisol or corticosterone-binding capacity, and is expressed as micrograms of cortisol or of corticosterone per 100 mL of plasma. The most commonly used methods for indirect measurement are equilibrium dialysis, competitive binding analysis, and gel filtration (Westphal, 1971). The CBG can be measured directly using radial immunodiffusion (Van Baelan and De Moor, 1974) and radioimmunoassay (Bernutz et al., 1977). The results obtained by homologous radioimmunoassay for rat CBG were consistently 0.25 μM lower than those obtained by the steroid-binding method (Ramoure and Kuhn, 1983). Chemical alterations of the protein and radioisotope decay are inherent problems in the radioimmunoassay for guinea pig CBG (Rosenthal et al., 1974). The CBG concentrations calculated by radial immunodiffusion are in good agreement with estimates made by equilibrium dialysis (Goodman et al., 1981).

18.4 GROUP-SPECIFIC COMPONENT

18.4.1 Properties

Gc was first discovered in human serum by Hirschfeld in 1959 (Hirschfeld, 1959). It is an α_2-globulin with an electrophoretic mobility similar to but distinct from that of haptoglobin. The protein was later isolated and characterized, and its amino acid composition was determined by various investigators (Cleve et al., 1963; Simons and Bearn, 1967). The total amino acid composition and molecular weight of the major human Gc phenotypes are very similar. They have a molecular weight of about 50,800 Da and appear to be a single polypepide chain. Gc in various animal species, including primate, cattle, pig, horse, rodent, and rabbit, has also been reported (Ashton, 1963b; Cinader and Dubinski, 1963; Cleve and Patutschnick, 1979; Reinskou, 1968; Weitkamp, 1978). Mouse and rat Gc have been well characterized, and their amino acid sequences have been determined (Yang et al., 1990; Borke et al., 1988; Yamamoto et al., 1997). Their molecular weights are estimated at 49,000 and 52,000 Da, respectively. The amino acid sequence of mouse Gc is 78% identical to human and 91% identical to rat Gc.

Variants of human Gc are controlled by some 30 different alleles (Constans, 1976), but the three most common phenotypes are Gc 1-1, Gc 2-1, and Gc 2-2, controlled by codominant alleles Gc 1 and Gc 2. Gc 1 consists of two suballeles, Gc 1F (fast) and Gc 1S (slow) (Cleve and Patutschnick, 1979). Antiserum specific to human Gc was found to cross-react with serum from horse, cow, rhesus monkey, chimpanzee, goat, sheep, rat, and mouse (Daiger et al., 1975; Reinskou, 1968), but not with rabbit and guinea pig serum (Courtoy et al., 1981a). In many species, Gc appears as single-band components on electrophoresis. However, genetic polymorphism of Gc has been observed in cattle (Ashton, 1963b), mouse (Cinader and Dubinski, 1963), horse (Weitkamp, 1978), and primate (Cleve and Patutschnick, 1979). In the horse, Gc polymorphism is apparently under the control of two autosomal codominant alleles, with three different phenotypes found in standard bred, thoroughbred, and Arabian horses as well as the Shetland pony (Weitkamp, 1978). Kitchin and Beam (1965) studied Gc polymorphism in chimpanzees, orangutans, rhesus monkeys, and a gorilla, and found genetic variations only in orangutans. Cleve and Patutschnick (1979) observed two phenotypes in a group of 78 chimpanzees and postulated that two alleles controlled the genetic variation in chimpanzee Gc. Two phenotypes, Gc pan 1-1 and Gc pan 2-1, were found, but the third phenotype, Gc pan 2-2, was not observed.

18.4.2 Role/Function

The Gc system has been used for individual identification and parentage exclusion. Gc has affinity for actin and is known to bind vitamin D and its metabolites (Constans, 1992; Daiger et al., 1975; Daiger and Cavalli-Sforza, 1977; Rodriguez et al., 1997). Additionally, Gc may have a function in vitamin D transport and may also act as a buffer to prevent the toxic effects of vitamin D at the tissue level (Daiger et al., 1975). Data collated by Goldschmidt-Clermont et al. (1988) suggest a crucial role for Gc in the sequestration and clearance of released cellular actin. The biologic function of Gc is largely unknown.

18.4.3 Pathophysiological Significance

Increased levels of Gc were observed in subjects with asthma, therefore the neutralization of the Gc protein could be a therapeutic strategy for asthma (Lee et al., 2011). Also, Gc complexes are drastically increased where tissue necrosis is present, such as in hepatic failure (Goldschmidt-Clermont et al. 1988).

18.4.4 Analytical Methods

Demonstration and quantitation of Gc components can be conducted using various methods, such as electrophoresis, isoelectrofocusing, and immunoprecipitation (Constans, 1976; Reinskou, 1968). High doses of vitamin D, hemolysis, and bacterial contamination may induce modification of the Gc electrophoretic pattern (Constans, 1976).

18.5 HAPTOGLOBIN (SEROMUCOID α2)

18.5.1 Properties

Haptoglobin (Hp) was first identified in 1939 as a serum component responsible for enhancing the peroxidase activity associated with hemoglobin (Hb) (Polonovski and Jayle, 1939). It is a serum α_2-glycoprotein present in man and animals that can bind free Hb, forming a stable complex. This complex has a pink color and can be visualized after electrophoresis or chromatography. Hp is synthesized in the liver and has a plasma half-life of about 3 days (Koj, 1974). Hp appears to exhibit little species specificity in binding to Hb. Human Hp can bind Hb from numerous animals; however, very distantly related Hbs only bind weakly (Cohen-Dix et al., 1973; Makinen et al., 1972). Chicken Hp has a narrow specificity and binds only avian and reptilian Hb (Musquera et al., 1979).

Human Hp has a tetrachain structure with two α chains and two β chains. The α and β chains are covalently linked by disulfide bonds (Kurosky et al., 1980). The covalent disulfide linking of the α and the β chains is observed in most mammals, except in the dog and probably other carnivores, where the two chains are joined by noncovalent interaction (Mominoki et al., 1995). The Hp β subunit shows substantial homology to the chymotrypsinogen family of serine proteases. Evolution from a common ancestral molecule is suggested; however, no proteolytic activity remains in the case of Hp (Kurosky et al., 1980).

The dissociation of Hb tetramers into dimers is a prerequisite for binding to Hp. This suggests that the $\alpha_1\beta_2$ contact region between Hb dimers is the binding site for Hp (Benesch et al., 1976; Makinen et al., 1972). Evidence has also been presented that Hb binds to Hp as intact $\alpha_1\beta_1$ dimers and that the primary region of Hb involved in the intermolecular contact is the $\alpha_1\beta_2$ interface (Hwang and Greer, 1980). Binding sites on the Hb α- and β-subunit interacting surfaces have been localized (Kazim and Atassi, 1981; Yedgar et al., 1983; Yoshioka and Atassi, 1986).

Hp has been found in the sera of all vertebrates studied (Javid, 1978; Putman, 1975a). Hp isolated from most nonhuman species resembles human Hp 1 on gel electrophoresis and appears as a single component. Hp forms similar to human Hp 2 and Hp 2-1 have been observed in members of the Bovidae and Cervidae families, such as goat, sheep, and cattle (Bradshaw et al., 1985; Ritter and Smith, 1971; Runnegar et al., 1997; Tranz et al., 1975; Van Der Walt and van Jaarsveld, 1978). Despite an extensive search in several species of nonhuman primates (Blumberg, 1960; Shim and Bearm, 1965), dogs (Shifrine and Stortmont, 1973), rabbits (Grunder, 1966), and swine (Kristjansson, 1961), there is no convincing evidence that polymorphism exists in any animals other than man (Bowman and Kurosky, 1982; Buettner-Janusch, 1970). Other variations in the Hp structure have been observed in the chicken and dog. Chicken Hp is composed of only two chains with a molecular weight of 3,000 and 54,000 Da (Lombart et al., 1979).

18.5.2 Role/Function

One known function of Hp is to protect the kidneys from tissue destruction by binding free Hb after hemolysis (Bowman and Kurosky, 1982). The formation of Hp-Hb complexes may also be beneficial by decreasing the availability of Hb iron to support bacterial growth at sites of septic inflammation (Eaton et al., 1982; Murata et al., 2004; Mahmud et al., 2007). Another possible role of Hp is stimulation of angiogenesis (Cid et al., 1993).

Hb binds to the β chain of Hp, and the α chain does not directly participate in the binding (Bowman and Kurosky, 1982; Gordon and Beam, 1966). The stable Hp-Hb complex, once formed in the blood stream following hemolysis, is rapidly cleared from the plasma and accumulates in the liver. When cats were injected intravenously with Hb in quantities sufficient to bind all circulating Hp, unbound Hp was not present after 3 hours, and the Hp-Hb complexes were cleared in as little as 6 hours (Harvey and Gaskin, 1978). Studies using solubilization and assay of the hepatic receptor for the Hp-Hb complex suggest that the carbohydrate moiety of haptoglobin did not appear to participate in the binding of the Hp-Hb complex to its receptors (Lowe and Ashwell, 1982). These complexes are also beneficial as they decrease the availability of hemoglobin iron that supports bacterial growth at sites of septic inflammation (Parra et al., 2005; Mahmud et al., 2007). The complexes are recognized and scavenged via CD163, the specific surface receptor on macrophages and scavenged by phagocytes. The immunodulation is partly mediated through binding of haptoglobin to the CD11/CD18 receptor of effector cells (Murata et al., 2004). Hp also inhibits prostaglandin synthesis by blocking catalytic effect of the heme moiety of hemoglobin on the cyclooxygenase enzymes. Furthermore, haptoglobin may also have an important role in the host defense to infections and neoplasms by withholding iron from invading pathogens and tumor cells, by modulating angiogenesis and other local inflammatory processes (Mahmud et al., 2007).

Hp is a major extracellular protein that protects against protein misfolding and assisting in the preservation of cell function. It is elevated in pregnancy, myocardial infarction, and obesity as these conditions are characterized by tissue growth and repair that require anti-inflammatory responses (Quaye, 2008).

18.5.3 Pathophysiological Significance

Genetic studies showed that Hp polymorphism in man is controlled by three codominant alleles coding for the α chain, that is, Hp a 1F (fast), Hp α1S (slow), and Hp α2. These three major alleles are responsible for the six common phenotypes observed (Smithies et al., 1962). Other rare variants of human Hp have also been reported (Bowman and Kurosky, 1982). The simplest phenotypic form, Hp 1-1, is monomeric, whereas phenotypes Hp 2-1 and Hp 2-2 are polymeric and appear as several bands on electrophoresis. Complete amino acid sequences of the α- and β-chains of human haptoglobin type 1-1 have been determined (Kurosky et al., 1980). In humans, haptoglobin is expressed by a genetic polymorphism as three phenotypes: Hp1-1, Hp2-1, and Hp2-2 (Burbea et al., 2004). Structural and functional differences between the three major Hp phenotypes have been demonstrated to have biological consequences, such as hemoglobin binding and antioxidative activity. Purified Hp2-2, in vitro, shows less inhibition of hemoglobin-induced oxidation of low-density lipoprotein than purified Hp1-1, which indicates that Hp2-2 has lower antioxidative activity than Hp1-1 and Hp 2-1. As the neutralization activity of Hp2-2 is weaker than that of the other Hp phenotypes, concentrations of free nonhaptoglobin bound hemoglobin are increased in this phenotype (Lee et al., 2004; Mahmud et al., 2007; Quaye, 2008). Hp is synthesized in the liver during granulocyte differentiation and stored for release when neutrophils are activated. It has a plasma half-life of approximately 3 days and appears to exhibit little species specificity in binding to hemoglobin (Quaye, 2008).

TABLE 18.2
Normal Haptoglobin Levels of Some Animal Species

Species	Serum Haptoglobin mg/100 mL of Serum	Serum Haptoglobin mg Hb bound/100 mL of Serum	References
African green monkey (*Cercopithecus aethiops*)	—	21–105	Barbosa et al. (1973)
Cattle	—	0–50	Bremner (1966)
	2.2–4.7	—	Salonen et al. (1996)
Rabbit	10–30	—	Lombart et al. (1965)
Rat			
Unspecified	10–30	—	Lombart et al. (1965)
Unspecified	30–60	—	Akaiwa (1982)
Unspecified	50	—	Courtoy et al. (1981b)
Sprague-Dawley	100	—	Baglia et al. (1981)
Mouse—DBA/2	—	50–150	Peacock et al. (1967)
	—	45–55	Palmer (1976)
Dog	—	14–252	Harvey (1976)
Cat	—	31–216	Harvey (1976)
Horse	—	19–177	Harvey (1976)

Amino acid compositions of dog, rat, and rabbit Hps have also been reported (Hanley et al., 1983; Kurosky et al., 1979; Lombart et al., 1965). Strain-dependent variation in Hp concentration was reported among 11 strains of mice examined (Peacock et al., 1967). The DBA/2 and AKR strains represent the extremes of this variation, with serum Hp levels of 50–150 and 5–10 mg of hemoglobin-binding capacity (HbBC) per 100 mL, respectively. No reports were found regarding gender-related differences in Hp levels in animals. In contrast to the unchanged concentration reported in pregnant women, Hp was increased in pregnant C57BL/10 mice (Waites et al., 1983). The increase was of greater degree and duration in allogeneic than in syngeneic pregnancy. Levels returned to normal by 8 days postpartum (Waites et al., 1983). Age also has an effect on baseline levels in mice. Normal Hp levels of some animal species are listed in Table 18.2.

Baseline Hp levels in human serum are influenced by genetic factors, gender, and age (Putman, 1975a; Sutton, 1970). Hp is one of the major acute-phase reactants (Koj, 1974). Concentrations in serum increase during inflammation and decrease after hemolysis. Raised levels are noted with acute or chronic inflammatory conditions and with neoplastic disease. Absence or a low level of Hp indicates hemolysis or severe liver diseases (Grant and Kachmar, 1976).

In animals, changes in Hp levels associated with various pathologic processes are similar to those seen in humans. Decreased Hp levels were documented in cats with experimental and spontaneous hemolytic anemias (Harvey and Gaskin, 1978) and in some rats with induced hepatic cirrhosis (Courtoy et al., 1981a). Increased concentrations are seen in bacterial and viral infections, inflammatory conditions (Cid et al., 1993; Eckersall et al., 1996; Francisco et al., 1996; Godson et al., 1996; Salonen et al., 1996), and tissue injuries, including those caused by irradiation (Magic et al., 1995). Absence or a low level of Hp indicates hemolysis or acute hepatocellular damage (Grant and Kachmar, 1976). In newborn DBA/2 mice, serum Hp was about 50% of the adult levels (Polonovski and Jayle, 1939). The levels then dropped quickly and remained at only 10%-30% of the adult range during the first 2 weeks of life.

18.5.4 Analytical Methods

Dog Hp under standard gel electrophoretic conditions appears similar to human Hp 1 in both charge and size, with a molecular weight of approximately 100,000 Da. However, under denaturing conditions employing 6 M urea or 0.1% sodium lauryl sulfate, the molecular weight is that of a Hp $\alpha\beta$ subunit, which is 48,500 Da (Kurosky et al., 1979). Hp typing by vertical electrophoresis conducted on 47 blood samples from three breeds of dogs (Doberman, German shepherd, and pit bullterrier) revealed two common phenotypes that could not be used to differentiate among them (Harrington et al., 1991).

Several methods for purifying and quantitating serum Hp have been described. The quantitating procedures include measuring enhancement of peroxidase activity, changes in electrophoretic mobility, rivanol precipitation, and immunochemical techniques (Young et al., 1995). In most methods, an excess of Hb is added to the serum to saturate the Hp. The amount of Hp-Hb complex is then estimated by peroxidase activity. The complex can also be separated from free Hb by electrophoresis or gel filtration, and the proportion of Hb bound to Hp is then calculated. Immunotechniques may be complicated, depending on the heterogeneity and the degree of polymerization of Hp. Immunochemical methods that have been used to measure Hp in animals include rocket electroimmunoassay (Palmer, 1976; Voelkel et al., 1978), immunonephelometry (Courtoy et al., 1981b), enzyme linked immunosorbent assay (ELISA) (Baker, 1967; Mominoki et al., 1995), radial immunodiffusion (Baglia et al., 1981), and fluoroimmunoassay using monoclonal antibodies (McNair et al., 1995). A high-performance liquid chromatography (HPLC) method has also been described (Salonen et al., 1996). Some degree of interspecies cross-reactivity does occur. Antiserum against human Hp was found to produce clear rockets when used in electroimmunoassay to measure rabbit (Voelkel et al., 1978) and mouse (Waites et al., 1983) haptoglobin. Hemolysis in samples does not affect Hp estimation, but hyperlipidemia may give high results (Bowman and Kurosky, 1982; Grant and Kachmar, 1976).

18.6 HEMOPEXIN

18.6.1 Properties

Hemopexin (Hx) is a β-glycoprotein and is synthesized by the liver. Human and rabbit Hx have been found to be very similar (Hrkal and Muller-Eberhard, 1971; Seery et al., 1972). They both have a molecular weight of approximately 57,000 $\pm$ 3,000 Da and appear to consist of a single polypeptide chain. The carbohydrate content is about 20% and consists of sialic acid, mannose, galactose, and glucosamine. The amino acid composition of both human and rabbit Hx has been determined (Hrkal and Muller-Eberhard, 1971), and complete amino acid sequence of human Hx has been reported (Takahashi et al., 1985b). Pig Hx has been isolated in almost pure form and has a molecular weight ranging from 57,000 to 62,000 daltons (Majuri, 1982; Van Gelder et al., 1995). Mouse Hx was reported as a β-2-III globulin with a molecular weight of approximately 65,000 Da (Witz and Gross, 1965). Bovine Hx migrates as a β_1-globulin (Bremner, 1966). Rat and guinea pig heme-Hx complexes have also been reported to migrate with β-globulins (Hughes-Jones et al., 1961). Rhesus monkey Hx purified by the wheat-germ lectin-sepharose method has a molecular weight of 60,000 Da (Foidart et al., 1982). Sheep Hx has a molecular weight of 56,000 Da, and its chemical composition has been reported (Stratil et al., 1984a).

Studies on the immunologic cross-reactivity of serum Hx from 64 vertebrates representing many different phylogenetic orders revealed that many antigenic determinants are shared by the Eutherian mammals but not by the non-Eutherian mammals and lower animals. The Hx of apes and man appears to be identical (Cox et al., 1978). Rat Hx shows a 76% amino acid sequence homology with human Hx (Nikkila et al., 1991).

18.6.2 Role/Function

During intravascular hemolysis, Hb is released into the circulation and cleared by glomerular filtration or hepatocellular uptake. Hp, albumin, and Hx are the three plasma proteins associated with the transport of circulating Hb and heme (heme in this discussion is defined as ferriprotoporphyrin IX). In man, haptoglobin binds Hb but not heme, and Hx and albumin bind heme but not Hb (Hershko, 1975; Muller-Eberhard, 1970, 1978). Mouse Hx has been reported to bind both heme and Hb (Witz and Gross, 1965).

The Hx molecule has two non–disulfide-linked domains, an N-terminal domain (domain I) that binds heme, and a C-terminal domain (domain II) that does not (Wu and Morgan, 1995). Hx binds heme specifically and carries circulating heme to the liver for uptake and breakdown (Muller-Eberhard, 1978; Wu and Morgan, 1995). Radiolabeled heme-Hx complex given intravenously was found exclusively in the liver parenchymal cells, whereas spleen, kidney, lung, and bone marrow cells remained free of radiolabeled material. This finding suggests that plasma heme is eliminated as a heme-Hx complex by the hepatocyte (Lane et al., 1973; Muller-Eberhard et al., 1970). It appears that the delivery of heme to the liver cells is a receptor-mediated process and that Hx is degraded or returned intact into the circulation, depending on the physiological conditions (Potter et al., 1993; Wu and Morgan, 1995). Hx has also been found in neurons and glial cells, and it is believed to play a role in neuronal iron homeostasis (Morris et al., 1993).

18.6.3 Pathophysiological Significance

Genetic polymorphism of Hx has been described in rabbits, pigs, and sheep. Studies in rabbits (Grunder, 1968; Hagen et al., 1978) suggest that rabbit Hx is controlled by four codominant autosomal alleles and that the Hx locus is located between the color locus (c) and the Hq blood group locus (Linkage Group I). American and European pigs are reported to have a Hx system under the control of seven alleles (Hpx°, Hpx^{1}, Hpx^{1F}, Hpx^{2}, Hpx^{3}, Hpx^{3F}, and Hpx^{4}) (Baker, 1967, 1968). A new allele, Hpx^{5}, was described in East Asian pigs (Ohmini miniature pigs) (Oishi et al., 1980). The Hpx locus in pigs appears to be linked to the K blood group system (Andersen, 1966; Hagen et al., 1968). In sheep and probably goats, Hx is genetically controlled from a single locus by two codominant alleles, and three phenotypes, Hpx A, Hpx AB, and Hpx B, have been described (Stratil et al., 1984a).

The normal plasma concentration of Hx in New Zealand white rabbits is 31–52 mg/100 mL (Lane et al., 1973). As in humans, neonatal rabbits have much lower levels of Hx than adults, and adult rabbit Hx values are reached at about 30–60 days of age (Muller-Eberhard, 1970). Rhesus monkeys have serum Hx levels of 53.3 ± 2.8 U/100 mL (1 unit represents the amount of monkey Hx equivalent to 1.0 mg/mL of human serum) (Foidart et al., 1982).

In man, decreased serum levels of Hx are associated with severe hemolytic diseases or fulminant rhabdomyolysis (Adornato et al., 1978a; Muller-Eberhard et al., 1968; Sears, 1968). Increased Hx levels have been observed in certain heme deficiency and chronic neuromuscular diseases in which small amounts of heme are released from increased circulating myoglobin (Adornato et al., 1978b; Lamon et al., 1978). The most important factor controlling the plasma level of Hx is heme (Muller-Eberhard et al., 1968; Sears, 1968). Unlike haptoglobin and other acute phase reactants, Hx levels are rarely and only minimally affected by nonspecific stimuli such as acute inflammation, connective tissue disease, surgical procedures, and fractures. Hyperoxia has been shown to induce the expression of Hx gene in the liver in vivo (Kietzmann et al., 1995; Nikkila et al., 1991). Serum Hx is probably a more reliable measurement of the severity of hemolysis than haptoglobin or other acute phase reactants (Kusher et al., 1972).

Experiments in calves, however, have shown that turpentine injection produced a marked increase in plasma Hx (Bremner, 1966). The same investigator also reported the disappearance of Hx from the plasma of calves during the hemolytic crisis of babesiosis. In rabbits receiving varying amounts of heme, the level of Hx was lowest 4–6 hours after injection. Thereafter, plasma Hx concentration rose slowly in rabbits injected with large amounts of heme. These observations suggest that the administration of heme may stimulate Hx synthesis, mobilize it from the extravascular site, or both (Muller-Eberhard et al., 1969). Heterologous Hxs from rabbits and man maintain the heme transport function when injected into rats (Liem, 1976). In the rhesus monkey, small doses of heme administered intravenously elevated serum Hx to 150% of control levels with a 76% increase in the net rate of Hx synthesis, whereas large doses of heme caused a 60% decrease in the serum Hx level, and intermediate doses of heme produced no change in the circulating Hx levels (Foidart et al., 1982). The changes observed following heme administration appeared to be specific for Hx, because serum haptoglobin and transferrin levels were unaffected by heme administration.

18.6.4 Analytical Methods

Several methods for Hx purification and serum level determination, including preparative electrophoresis, affinity and ion-exchange chromatography, rivanol precipitation, immunoelectrophoresis, and immunodiffusion, have been described (Foidart et al., 1982; Hrkal and Muller-Eberhard, 1971; Majuri, 1982; Takahashi et al., 1985a; Van Gelder et al., 1995).

18.7 THYROID HORMONE-BINDING PROTEINS

18.7.1 Properties

In plasma, there are three proteins that regulate the circulation of thyroid hormones: (a) thyroxine-binding globulin (TBG), the most important and transports the major part of T_4 in most animals; (b) thyroxine-binding prealbumin (PA) (see TTR); and (c) SA, which usually plays a minor role in thyroid hormone transport (see albumin). In addition, lipoproteins also carry minor quantities of thyroxine, but their importance is unknown. These serum proteins may store thyroxine in a nondiffusible form in the extrathyroidal space, and they may serve to carry thyroxine from the circulation to target cells (Cody, 1980; Horn and Gartner, 1979; Robbins et al., 1978).

Human TBG is a single polypeptide chain with a molecular weight of 54,000–63,000 Da (Horn and Gartner, 1979; Robbins et al., 1978). It is an acidic inter-α-globulin rich in sialic acid and shares a high degree of homology with two serpin antiproteases, alpha-1-antichymotrypsin and alpha-1-antitrypsin (Bartalena et al., 1992). Bovine TBG has a molecular weight of 54,000 Da and a carbohydrate content similar to that of human TBG (Van Der Walt and van Jaarsveld, 1978). TBG is synthesized by the liver (Glinoer et al., 1970, 1977a).

18.7.2 Role/Function

In man, TBG is responsible for the transport of 75% of the thyroxine, thyroxine-binding prealbumin (TBPA) 15%, and albumin, despite its abundance in plasma, transports only about 10% of the plasma thyroxine.

TBG has the highest affinity for T_4 and binds most of the circulating T_4, with over one-third of the binding sites on the protein occupied.

18.7.3 Pathophysiological Significance

In the rhesus monkey, the serum TBG concentration is approximately 20 μg/mL, and the synthesis rate of TBG in the rat is approximately 2 mg/day/kg of body weight (Glinoer et al., 1979; McGuire et al., 1982). The biologic significance of a given serum TBG concentration is not completely understood.

In humans with normal thyroid function, the T_4/TBG ratio remains constant. Elevation in the T_4/TBG ratio is found in hyperthyroidism, and a decreased T_4/TBG ratio is seen in hypothyroidism (Horn and Gartner, 1979). Abnormalities in thyroxine-binding proteins must be suspected when abnormally elevated or diminished total thyroid hormone concentrations are encountered in clinically euthyroid subjects to avoid misinterpretation of the thyroid condition (Bartalena and Robbins, 1993). Many xenobiotics such as dioxan and polychlorinated biphenyls (PCBs) alter the binding of T_4 to carrier proteins. PCBs, specifically 3, 4, 3′, 4′ tetrachlorobiphenyl, bind to and displace rat T_4 from TTR but not albumin (Brouwer, 1989; McKinney and Waller, 1994; Rickenbacher et al., 1986).

18.7.4 Analytical Methods

With the use of agarose gel electrophoresis, rhesus monkey T_4 may be found bound to the interalpha, PA, and albumin zones; T_3 is bound to the interalpha and albumin zones only. The interalpha protein in rhesus monkey migrates slightly more slowly than does human TBG. Baboon and chimpanzee have thyroxine-binding patterns similar to those of rhesus monkey, but TBPA and its polymorphic variations have only been seen in mandrills and macaques (Farer et al., 1962; Refetoff et al., 1970; Weiss et al., 1971). In the dog and cat, T_4 is bound to the interalpha and albumin zones, and there is no binding to a PA area. In the mouse, T_4 is bound to albumin and α-globulin; however, there appears to be some interstrain variation in the electrophoretic mobility of these proteins. Mouse TTR does not bind T_4. In the rat, T_4 is bound to TTR and albumin. Postalbumin TBG was reported by some investigators (Davis et al., 1970) but not confirmed by others (Farer et al., 1962; Refetoff et al., 1970; Shutherland and Brandon, 1976). TTR in the rat was found to be the major T_4 transport protein, carrying 55% of the total T_4 compared to 15% and 18% by albumin and TBG, respectively (Davis et al., 1970). Rabbit T_4 binds similarly to albumin and postalbumin, and a small amount is also bound to TTR (271). In the guinea pig, thyroxine seems to be associated only with albumin. In cattle, sheep, and goat, T_3 and T_4 are bound in postalbumin and albumin zones. In the horse and chicken, a PA zone (in addition to the albumin and postalbumin zones) is also found to bind T_4 (Farer et al., 1962; Refetoff et al., 1970). In many animal species, the thyroxine carrier proteins reported in the literature are unspecific and poorly characterized, and TBG probably does not exist in a number of species, including the cat, rat, rabbit, frog, and chicken (Larsson et al., 1985).

TBG may be isolated and purified using immunoprecipitation, affinity chromatography (throxine-coupled agarose), anion-exchange chromatography, and gel filtration. Serum TBG concentrations can also be measured using radioimmunoassay methodology (Glinoer et al., 1977b, 1979; Horn and Gartner, 1979).

18.8 TRANSFERRIN

18.8.1 Properties

Transferrin (formerly called siderophilin), the major component of β-globulin, is the iron-transporting protein of plasma. The molecular weight of human transferrin ranges from 75,000 to 80,000 Da, as estimated by sedimentation equilibrium and diffusion (Mann et al., 1970; Roberts et al., 1966). The molecular weight of most animal transferrin also falls within this range, whereas turtle and hagfish transferrin have molecular weights of 92,000 and 44,000 Da, respectively (Hudson et al., 1973; Palmour and Sutton, 1971; Schreiber et al., 1979; Spooner et al., 1974; Van Gelder et al., 1995).

The structure and composition of transferrin have been studied in several species. Generally, it is a glycoprotein consisting of a single peptide chain with a varying number of heteropolysaccharide units attached to it (Aisen and Brown, 1977; Greene and Feeney, 1968; Hudson et al., 1973; Palmour and Sutton, 1971; Richardson et al., 1973). Rabbit transferrin was reported to contain two heterosaccharide units per molecule by some investigators (Hudson et al., 1973), and only 1 U by others (Heaphy and Williams, 1978; Leger et al., 1978). Most serum transferrin molecules in the rabbit contain two sialic acid residues. Transferrin isolated from rabbit milk appears to be identical to serum transferrin, except that most milk transferrin molecules contain only one sialic acid residue (Baker et al., 1968). Analysis of pooled plasma from 116 rats revealed that one third of the total transferrin contains three moles of sialic acid, and two-thirds contain 2 mol of sialic acid per mole of transferrin (Schreiber et al., 1979). The N-terminal sequences of rabbit and rat transferrins show clear homology with human transferrin (Heaphy and Williams, 1978; MacGillivray et al., 1977; Schreiber et al., 1979).

Sheep transferrin has an amino acid composition similar to that of cattle. Individual components of two variants of sheep transferrin containing three to four sialic acid residues have been isolated. However, there is no evidence for pairs of bands with the same number of sialic acid residues, as seen in cattle (Spooner et al., 1974). Transferrin in carp (*Cyprinus carpio* L.) contains no sialic acid (Valenta et al., 1976). The sialic acid content may be of importance in transferrin catabolism. The catabolic rate of asialotransferrin in rabbits was found to be higher than the corresponding value for normal transferrin (Regoeczi et al., 1974).

Although transferrin may be synthesized by tissues other than the liver, such as testes, lung, brain, hematopoietic, and mammary tissues, the liver is the major site of transferrin synthesis in adult animals (Bradshaw et al., 1985; Focht et al., 1997; Idzerda et al., 1986; Meek and Adamson, 1985; Yang et al., 1997). In the rat and rabbit, the rate of transferrin production is about 95 and 27 mg/kg of body weight per day, respectively. In the rat, the rate of transferrin synthesis is one-fifth the rate of albumin synthesis (Morgan and Peters, 1971a). In mouse embryos, transferrin can be detected by immunoperoxidase staining in the egg cylinders from the seventh day of gestation onward and in the visceral yolk sac at all gestational stages (Adamson, 1982). Thus, transferrin can be produced by both mature and immature hepatocytes. Fasting decreases transferrin synthesis, while reduced ambient temperature increases it (Gardiner and Morgan, 1981).

Precise information about the site of transferrin catabolism is unavailable. It is probably taken up by the cells of many tissues and enzymatically degraded intracellularly (Aisen and Brown, 1977). Studies of transferrin turnover in 11 mammalian species showed that the turnover rate closely correlated with species size (Regoeczi and Hatton, 1980).

18.8.2 Role/Function

Each transferrin molecule has two active sites for iron binding, with the exception of hagfish transferrin, which has only one (Palmour and Sutton, 1971). Sequence studies of human and rabbit transferrin polypeptide chains revealed two regions of internal homology (MacGillivray et al., 1977; Strickland and Hudson, 1978). This internal homology reflects a doubling of an ancestral structural gene responsible for the production of a transferrin with two metal-binding sites from a precursor with a single metal-binding site (MacGillivray et al., 1977). There are definite physicochemical differences between the two iron-binding sites (Aisen et al., 1978; Delaney et al., 1982); however, it is unclear whether functional differences exist. Several investigators have observed functional heterogeneity of the two iron-binding sites (Awai et al., 1979; Baarlen et al., 1980; Fletcher and Huehns, 1968), whereas others have not (Delaney et al., 1982; Hudson et al., 1973; Young, 1982).

Transferrin carries iron from cells involved with the absorption or storage of iron to cells that utilize iron, as in Hb synthesis (erythroblasts and reticulocytes), the incorporation into cytochromes involved with electron transfer, or as a component of an enzyme system. Transferrin may also play a role in the regulation of iron absorption in the intestine (Forth and Rummel, 1973; Huebers et al., 1982, 1983). More recently, it has been suggested that transferrin may serve as a physiologic regulator of granulocyte maturation (Evans et al., 1986). It is now generally accepted that transferrin is transported across the cell membrane by receptor-mediated endocytosis (Runnegar et al., 1997).

Transferrin receptors on reticulocyte and hepatocyte membranes in rat, rabbit, and mouse have been studied extensively (Van Der Heul et al., 1982; Goodman et al., 1965; Kamiyama, 1976; Massolini et al., 1996; Van Gelder et al., 1995; Weiss et al., 1971). Transferrin receptors of rabbit mammary gland cells and placenta have also been described (Ballard et al., 1982; Moutafchicv et al., 1983; Navab et al., 1977b).

18.8.3 Pathophysiological Significance

Transferrin polymorphism has been observed in man as well as many animal species (Buettner-Janusch, 1970; Giblett et al., 1959; Giblett, 1969). In man, at least 18 genetic variants have been described; however, only 28 phenotypes have been observed (Giblett, 1969). All genetic variants appear to be compatible with good health. In animals, transferrin polymorphism has been observed in many species, including nonhuman primates, cattle, sheep, swine, fish, and toad. Of the nonhuman primates, the chimpanzee has the greatest variation of transferrin phenotypes, while a remarkable number of variants are observed in baboons and macaques. The genus *Macaca* has at least 11 variants; of the 66 possible phenotypes, 34 have been described (Goodman et al., 1965). The transferrins of prosimians are extremely complex, particularly in lemurs, where 22 alleles are described. Some monkeys, such as the *Erythrocebus patas*, appear to have no transferrin variants (Buettner-Janusch, 1970). Certain transferrin variants such as Tf-D and Tf-G in rhesus monkeys may be responsible for or associated with lower infant growth rates and decreased fertility (Smith, 1982).

In cattle, transferrin polymorphism is under the control of four alleles: Tf^{A}, Tf^{D1}, Tf^{D2}, and Tf^{E} (Ashton, 1963a; Kristjansson and Hickman, 1965; Smithies and Hickman, 1958; Spooner and Baxter, 1969). In addition, polymorphic variation in the amount of sialic acid attached to bovine transferrin is believed to be controlled by a recessive epistatic gene with two alleles: Tfs A and Tfs a. Thus, Tfs a/a cattle are lacking the two faster transferrin bands from the four bands normally observed in any Tf allele. Tfs A/a and Tfs A/A animals have a full complement of phenotypes (Spooner et al., 1977). The Tf and Tfs loci are apparently not linked.

There are 10 known transferrin variants in horses (D, F1, F2, F3, G, H, J, M, O, and R), of which the F variant is the most common (Chung and McKenzie, 1985; Stratil and Glasnak, 1981; Stratil et al., 1984b). More new variants have been found recently (Bell et al., 1995). As in cattle, equine transferrin is highly heterogeneous. Transferrin polymorphism has also been observed in Duroc and Hampshire pigs (Baker, 1968), the American toad (*B. americanus*) (Guttman and Wilson, 1973), and carp (*C. carpio*) (Valenta et al., 1976). In the toad, 13 transferrin alleles are present, and 36 phenotypes have been described. Seven variants (A, B, C, D, E, F, and G) are found in the carp. Shifrine and Stormont (1973) studied variants of transferrin in 100 samples of plasma from beagles and found a single phenotype with a three-band pattern. Other transferrin variants in the dog have been reported (Braend, 1966).

The average concentration of transferrin in human plasma is about 290 mg/100 mL (about 30 µmol/L) or, in terms of total iron-binding capacity (TIBC), about 300 µg/100 mL (60 µmol/L) (Grant and Kachmar, 1976). There are no sex differences or diurnal variation, but there is a tendency for the transferrin level to fall with age (Bernat, 1983). Serum transferrin concentrations of many animal species, such as baboon, goat, mouse, rabbit, and sheep, fall within a broad range of 250–350 mg/100 mL. The pig and rat have higher mean concentrations, that is, 593 and 458 mg/100 mL, respectively, whereas the dog and guinea pig have somewhat lower mean levels, that is, 192 and 187 mg/100 mL, respectively (Regoeczi and Hatton, 1980). Adult male hamsters have a TIBC level of 104.5 µmol/ L with 44% transferrin saturation (Rennie et al., 1981). Increased serum transferrin levels have been observed in pregnancy (Grant and Kachmar, 1976; Hofvander, 1968), iron-deficiency anemia (Morton and Tavill, 1975), and cortisol and estrogen administration (Horne et al., 1971; Jeejeebhoy et al., 1972). Low levels, usually accompanied by low albumin, are found in many diseases and are due either to impaired synthesis, as in cirrhosis, starvation, and chronic infection, or to increased excretion as in the nephrotic syndrome (Grant and Kachmar, 1976; Jarnum and Lassen, 1961; Morgan and Peters, 1971b).

18.8.4 Analytical Methods

Bovine transferrin exhibits a very complex heterogeneity on starch-gel electrophoresis. In addition to genetic polymorphism, each homozygous variant of bovine transferrin may exhibit multiple bands that are due, in part, to differing numbers of sialic acid residues (Richardson et al., 1973; Spooner et al., 1970, 1977; Stratil and Spooner, 1971). With high resolution chromatographic and electrophoretic techniques, 12 components (6 pairs) can be visualized in the TfA homozygous variant of bovine transferrin (Stratil and Spooner, 1971). These components have been designated as 0a, 0b, 1a, 1b, 2a, 2b, 3a, 3b, 4a, 4b, 5a, and 5b (in increasing order of mobility). The numeral in each designation reflects the number of residues of sialic acid per mole of transferrin. After complete removal of sialic acid by neuraminidase treatment, all the "a" bands have the same mobility and all the "b" bands have the same mobility. However, the "b" bands have greater mobility than do the "a" bands, in spite of the fact that the "a" and "b" components of a single genetic variant have been shown to have the same molecular weight, amino acid composition, and peptide maps (Richardson et al., 1973). Maeda et al. (1980) have found cleavage in the peptide chain of the "b" component and suggested that the difference in mobility is due to scission of the "b" component peptide chain.

Several methods for isolation and purification of transferrin have been described. Most commonly, methods involve precipitation or fractionation with rivanol or ammonium sulfate, followed by ion-exchange chromatography (Letendre and Holbein, 1981; Palmour and Sutton, 1971; Sawatzki et al., 1981; Spooner et al., 1974; Van Gelder et al., 1995). Serum transferrin may be estimated directly by immunochemical methods, such as radial immunodiffusion or electrodiffusion, or indirectly by measuring the maximum amount of iron the serum can bind. This TIBC includes both bound iron and the unbound or latent iron-binding capacity; therefore, it represents the total amount of apotransferrin in the serum. The indirect method overestimates transferrin by 10%–20% because the metal attaches to proteins other than transferrin when the latter is more than half saturated (Grant and Kachmar, 1976).

18.9 TRANSTHYRETIN (PREALBUMIN)

18.9.1 Properties

TTR, formerly called PA, is a plasma protein of high negative charge when compared with other plasma proteins. Its electrophoretic mobility is greater than that of SA. The PA band is usually visible only by transmitted light on an electrophoretogram (Grant and Kachmar, 1976). The name TTR was recommended to replace PA to avoid confusion with albumin precursors and to indicate its function as a serum transport protein for both thyroxin and retinol-binding protein (RBP) (Nomenclature Committee of IUB [NC-IUB], 1981). The structure and physicochemical properties of TTR in man have been well described (Kanda et al., 1974; Morgan et al., 1971; Robbins et al., 1978). Human TTR has a molecular weight of approximately 55,000 Da and is a stable tetramer of four identical polypeptide subunits. It is high in acidic protein but contains no sialic acid or carbohydrate groups. The complete amino acid sequence has been determined.

Rat TTR is slightly smaller than human TTR and contains four identical subunits. It has a molecular weight of approximately 51,000 Da, as determined by sedimentation equilibrium analysis (Navab et al., 1977a; Peterson et al., 1973). Although rat and human TTRs are immunologically distinct, their amino acid compositions are quite similar. Analysis of the NH_2-terminal 30 amino acid residues of the rat TTR subunit showed only four substitutions from that of the human TTR subunit (Palmour and Sutton, 1971). Homologies between rat and human TTRs and rat and mouse TTRs are 93% and 97%, respectively (Fung et al., 1988). Rhesus and cynomolgus monkey TTRs have molecular weights of approximately 65,000 and 58,000 Da, respectively, and are believed to be a tetramer similar to that of rat and man (Bernstein et al., 1970; Vahlquist and Petersone, 1972). Rabbit TTR contained the same number of amino acid residues and showed 80% homology with rat and human TTR by sequence analysis (Sundelin et al., 1985).

In man, TBPA has been shown to have two binding sites for T4, and though the binding sites are identical, the binding of T4 to one site inhibits the binding to the other (Robbins et al., 1978). Thus, one molecule of TBPA only binds one molecule of thyroxine.

Hepatic secretions of TTR and RBP are believed to be independently regulated processes, and the TTR-RBP complex is formed in the plasma after the independent secretion of the two proteins from liver cells (Navab et al., 1977b). The rate of PA synthesis in the rat was estimated at 3.6 mg/100 g of body weight per day, and the half-life of PA in the blood stream was 29 hours (Dickson et al., 1982). TTR also was reported to be synthesized and secreted by retinal epithelium (Dwork et al., 1990; Ong et al., 1994) and the choroid plexus in many species, including pig, rat, sheep, amphibian, and reptile (Duan et al., 1995; Dwork et al., 1990; Harms et al., 1991; Schreiber et al., 1990).

18.9.2 Role/Function

TTR plays an important role in the plasma transport of thyroid hormones and is also involved in the transport of vitamin A (Kanai et al., 1968; Oppenheimer et al., 1965). In contrast to human TBPA that plays a minor role in transporting thyroid hormones when compared to TBG (Cody, 1980), TBPA in the rat appears to be the major thyroid hormone transport protein (Davis et al., 1970; Peterson et al., 1973; Shutherland and Brandon, 1976). T_4 binding to TBPA has also been reported in the rabbit, rhesus monkey, horse, pigeon, and chicken (Refetoff et al., 1970; Shutherland and Brandon, 1976). T_3 binding to PA has been demonstrated in the pigeon (Reed et al., 1975).

TTR synthesis by the choroid plexus may be important in the transport of thyroxin across the blood-brain barrier (Schreiber et al., 1990). The synthesis of TTR by the liver and the choroid plexus appears to be independently regulated during the acute phase response (Dickson et al., 1985, 1986). It has been proposed that during evolution, TTR synthesis first appeared in the choroid plexus of reptiles, and TTR synthesis in the liver evolved much later (Schreiber and Richardson, 1997). In human, there are over 50 variants of TTR. Most of the mutations in TTR are not compatible with its normal metabolism and lead to its deposition as amyloid.

The electrophoretic mobility of TBPA differs considerably among animal species. In the monkey, horse, and chicken, the protein was found anodal to albumin, but in cattle, swine, dog, cat, rabbit, and frog, it was cathodal to albumin, making the term "PA" even less suitable in these species (Larsson et al., 1985).

Vitamin A normally circulates in plasma as retinol, which is bound to RBP. In turn, RBP strongly interacts with TTR and circulates together with TTR in plasma as a 1- to 1-protein–protein complex. RBP–TTR complex is thought to prevent the glomerular filtration of the low molecular size RBP in the kidney, and play a role in the secretion of RBP from hepatocytes (Wei et al., 1995). TTR knockout mice with a null mutation of TTR locus have low serum RBP and thyroid hormone (Episkopou et al., 1993). In man, purified RBP has α_1 mobility on electrophoresis and a molecular weight of approximately 21,000–22,000 Da (Kanai et al., 1968). The RBP-TTR interactions of rat, cattle, and monkey are similar to those in man (Peterson et al., 1973; Richardson et al., 1994; Vahlquist and Petersone, 1972).

Experiments using rat liver perfusion and hepatocyte culture techniques as well as metabolic studies indicate that the liver is the main site of TTR synthesis and that TTR plays a role in the delivery of retinol to hepatocytes (Dickson et al., 1982; Felding and Fex, 1982; Navab et al., 1977b; Yamamoto et al., 1997).

18.9.3 Pathophysiological Significance

In animals, genetic polymorphism of TTR has been described for the nonhuman primate. *Macaca mulatta* (rhesus monkey) TBPA exists in three forms, and is under the control of two autosomal codominant alleles: the fast PA (designated Pt^1) and the slow PA (designated Pt^2). The homozygous type Pt 1-1 migrates similarly to human TBPA. The two homozygous types Pt 1-1 and Pt 2-2 migrate as single bands on 8.5% polyacrylamide gels when submitted to electrophoresis (pH 8.9). The heterozygote Pt 1-2 is seen as three bands between the two Pt 1-1 and Pt 2-2 bands. PA polymorphism has also been observed in drills and mandrills, but no polymorphism like that seen in macaques has been found in baboons, chimpanzees, or orangutans. There is no evidence that the PA polymorphism affects thyroxine transport or RBP-PA complexing (Alper et al., 1969; Bernstein et al., 1970; Weiss et al., 1971).

TTR has been reported in the nonhuman primate, horse, cattle, rabbit, rat, mouse, chicken, pigeon, and quail (Farer et al., 1962; Heaf et al., 1980; Refetoff et al., 1970; Richardson et al., 1994; Shutherland and Brandon, 1976; Wolf, 1995). In primates, TBPA was found in catarrhini and prosimiae species, but not in platyrrhini (Callithricidae and Cebidae) (Seo et al., 1989). In pig, no clear identification of TTR was achieved in electrophoresis of serum (Larsson et al., 1985), but TTR mRNA has been found in the liver and choroid plexus (Duan et al., 1995). Reptiles have very low levels of TTR, and serum TTR has not been detected in amphibians (Harms et al., 1991).

The serum levels in selected animals are listed in Table 18.3.

Serum TTR concentrations are decreased in liver disease, hyperthyroidism, and protein calorie malnutrition, and is proposed as a nutritional marker (Ingenbleek and Young, 1994). They are unchanged in chronic renal disease (Robbins et al., 1978). Acute inflammation induced by turpentine in rats was shown to decrease the serum TTR level considerably (Dickson et al., 1982). Therefore, TTR is termed a "negative" acute-phase protein. Androgenic steroids markedly increase serum TTR concentrations, whereas estrogenic compounds have much less effect (Barbosa et al., 1970, 1971, 1973). Seasonal changes in TBPA concentrations have been described in quail, being lowest during the summer and highest during midwinter (Heaf et al., 1980).

18.9.4 Analytical Methods

Isolation and purification of TTR is facilitated by the relative abundance of TTR and especially by its high negative charge. For bulk preparation, precipitation methods have been used; however,

TABLE 18.3
Transthyretin Serum Levels of Various Animal Species

	Serum Levels of Transthyretin	
Animal Species	**µg/mL (Reference)**	**mg of T_4 Bound/100 mL (Reference)**
Rat	400–500 (Dickson et al., 1982)	140 (Davis et al., 1970)
	398 ± 50 (Navab et al., 1977b)	—
Rhesus monkey (*Macaca mulatta*)	291 (Robbins et al., 1978)	—
Green monkey (*Cercopithcus aethiops*)	—	203 ± 9 (Barbosa et al., 1970)
Quail		—
1-day old	220 (Heaf et al., 1980)	—
14 days old	430 (Heaf et al., 1980)	—

ion-exchange chromatography, gel filtration, and preparative electrophoresis (Robbins et al., 1978) are more commonly employed for purification. At high ionic strength, TTR complexes with RBP, which has a characteristic green fluorescence; therefore, affinity chromatography on sepharose with covalently bound RBP has also been widely used for TTR purification (Fex et al., 1977; Navab et al., 1977a).

Serum levels of TTR can be measured directly by radioimmunoassay (Benvenga et al., 1986; Navab et al., 1977b) and radial immunodiffusion (Dickson et al., 1982). TTR concentrations can also be determined indirectly and expressed in terms of thyroxine-binding capacity (Barbosa et al., 1971). Serum TTR is relatively stable under various storage conditions (Chen et al., 1986).

ACKNOWLEDGMENTS

I wish to thank Hai T. Nguyen, VMD, MS, author of this chapter in the second edition, for his vision and contributions to this chapter.

REFERENCES

Adamson, E.D. 1982. The location and synthesis of transferrin in mouse embryos and teratocarcinoma cells. *Dev Biol.* 91:227–234.

Adornato, B.T., Engel, W.K., and Foidart-Desalle, M. 1978a. Elevations of hemopexin levels in neuromuscular disease. *Arch Neurol.* 35:577–580.

Adornato, B.T., Kagen, L.J., Garver, F.A., and Engel, W.K. 1978b. Depletion of serum hemopexin in fulminant rhabdomyolysis. *Arch Neurol.* 35:547–548.

Aisen, P. and Brown, E.B. 1977. The iron-binding function of transferrin in iron metabolism. *Semin Hematol.* 14:31–53.

Aisen, P., Liebman, A., and Zweier, J. 1978. Stoichiometric and site characteristics of the binding of iron to human transferrin. *J Biol Chem.* 253:1930–1937.

Akaiwa, S. 1982. Purification of haptoglobin from rat serum. *Anal Biochem.* 123:178–182.

Allison, A.C. 1960. Turnovers of erythrocytes and plasma proteins in mammals. *Nature (London).* 188:37–40.

Alper, C.A., Robin, N.I., and Refetoff, S. 1969. Genetic polymorphism of rhesus thyroxine-binding prealbumin: Evidence for tetrameric structure in primates. *Proc Natl Acad Sci USA.* 63:775–781.

Andersen, E. 1966. Linkage between the K blood group locus and the Hp locus for hematin-binding globulins in pigs. *Genetics.* 54:805–812.

Ashton, G.C. 1963a. Cattle serum transferrins: A balanced polymorphism? *Genetics.* 52:983–997.

Ashton, G.C. 1963b. Polymorphism in the serum post-albumins of cattle. *Nature.* 198:1117–1118.

Audy, M.C., Marin, B., Charron, G., and Bonnin, M. 1982. Steroid-binding proteins and testosterone level in the badger plasma during the animal cycle. *Gen Comp Endocrinol.* 48:239–246.

Awai, M., Chipman, B., and Brown, E.B. 1979. In vivo evidence for the functional heterogeneity of transferrin-bound iron. 1. Studies in normal rats. *J Lab Clin Med.* 85:769–784.

Baarlen, J.V., Brouwer, J.T., Liebman, A., and Aisen, P. 1980. Evidence for the functional heterogeneity of the two sites of transform in vitro. *Br J Haematol.* 46:417–426.

Baglia, F.A., Kwan, S.W., and Fuller, G.M. 1981. Haptoglobin biosynthesis in rats. *Biochim Biophys Acta.* 696:107–113.

Baker, E., Shaw, D.C., and Morgan, E.H. 1968. Isolation and characterization of rabbit serum and milk transferrin. *Evidence for difference in sialic acid contents only. Biochemistry.* 7:1371–1378.

Baker, L.N. 1967. A new allele, Hp^4, in the hemopexin system in pigs. *Vox Sang.* 12:397–400.

Baker, L.N. 1968. Serum protein variation in duroc and hampshire pigs. *Vox Sang.* 15:154–158.

Ballard, P.L., Kitterman, J.A., Bland, R.D., et al. 1982. Ontogeny and regulation of corticosteroid-binding globulin in plasma of fetal and newborn lambs. *Endocrinology.* 110:359–366.

Barbosa, J., Doe, R.P., and Seal, U.S. 1970. Effects of clomiphene on estrogen-induced changes in plasma proteins in monkeys. *J Clin Endocrinol.* 31:654–658.

Barbosa, J., Seal, U.S., and Doe, R.P. 1971. Effects of anabolic steroids on hormone-binding proteins, serum cortisol, and serum non-protein bound cortisol. *J Clin Endocrinol Metabol.* 32:232–240.

Barbosa, J., Seal, U.S., and Doe, R.P. 1973. Anti-estrogens and plasma proteins. I. Clomiphene and isomers, ethamoxytriphetol, U-11, 100A, and U-11, 555A. *J Clin Endocrinol Metabol.* 36:666–678.

Bartalena, L., Farsetti, A., Flink, I.L., and Robbins, J. 1992. Effects of interleukin-6 on the expression of thyroid hormone-binding protein genes in cultured human hepatoblastoma-derived (Hep G2) cells. *Mol Endocrinol.* 6:935–942.

Bartalena, L. and Robbins, J. 1993. Thyroid hormone transport proteins. *Clin Lab Med.* 13:583–598.

Baynes, J.W. and Thorpe, S.R. 1981. Identification of the sites of albumin—Catabolism in the rat. *Arch Biochem Biophy.* 206:372–379.

Beamer, N., Hagemenas, F.C., and Kittinger, G.W. 1973. Development of cortisol-binding in the rhesus monkey. *Endocrinology.* 93:363–368.

Behrens, P.Q., Spikerman, A.M., and Brown, J.R. 1975. Structure of human serum albumin. *Fed Proc.* 34:591.

Bell, K., Arthur, H., and Breen, M. 1995. Mutations in the equine plasma transferrin and esterase systems. *Anim Genet.* 26:407–411.

Benesch, R.E., Ikeda, S., and Benesch, R. 1976. Reaction of haptoglobin with hemoglobin covalently cross-linked between the $\alpha\beta$ dimers. *J Biol Chem.* 251:465–470.

Benvenga, S., Bartalena, L., Antonelli, A., et al. 1986. Radioiummonoassay for human thyroxine-binding prealbumin. *Ann Clin Sci.* 16:231–240.

Bernat, I. 1983. *Iron Metabolism*, p. 82. New York, NY: Plenum Press.

Bernstein, R.S., Robbin, J., and Rail, J.E. 1970. Polymorphism of monkey thyroxine-binding prealbumin (TBPA). Mode of inheritance and hybridization. *Endocrinology.* 86:383–390.

Bernutz, C., Horn, K., and Pickardt, C.R. 1977. Corticosteroid-binding globulin (CBG) isolation and radioimmunological determination in serum. *Acta Endocrinol (Kbh).* 87(Suppl 215):25–26.

Blumberg, B.S. 1960. Biochemical polymorphisms in animals. Haptoglobin and transferrins. *Proc Soc Exp Biol Med.* 104:25–28.

Borke, J.L., Litwiller, R.D., Bell, M.P., Fass, D.N., Mckean, D.J., and Kumar, R. 1988. The isolation, characterization and amino acid terminal sequence of the vitamin D-binding protein (group specific component) from mouse plasma. *Int J Biochem.* 20:1343–1349.

Bowman, B.H. and Kurosky, A. 1982. Haptoglobin: The evolutionary product of duplication, unequal crossing over, and point mutation. *Adv Hum Genet.* 12:189–261.

Bradshaw, J.P., Hatton, J., and White, D.A. 1985. The hormonal control of protein N-glycosylation in the developing rabbit mammary gland and its effect upon transferrin synthesis and secretion. *Biochim Biophys Acta.* 847:344–352.

Braend, M. 1966. *Serum transferrin in dog. In 10th European Conference on Animal Blood Groups and Biochemical Polymorphism.* Paris: Institut National de la Recherche Agronomique, 319–322.

Bremner, K.C. 1966. Studies on haptoglobin and haemopexin in the plasma of cattle. *Aust J Exp Biol Med Sci.* 42:643–656.

Brien, T.G. 1981. Human corticosteroid binding globulin. *Clin Endocrinol.* 14:193–212.

Brouwer, A. 1989. Inhibition of thyroid hormone transport in plasma of rats by polychlorinated biphenyls. *Arch Toxicol Suppl.* 13:440–445.

Brown, J.R. 1975. Structure of bovine serum albumin. *Fed Proc.* 34:591.

Brown, J.R. 1976. Structural origins of mammalian albumin. *Fed Proc.* 35:2141–2144.

Brown, J.R., Lou, T., Behrens, P., Sepulveda, M., Parker, M., and Blakeney, E. 1971 Amino acid sequence of bovine and porcine serum albumin. *Fed Proc.* 30:1241.

Buettner-Janusch, J. 1970. Evolution of serum polymorphisms. *Annu Rev Genet.* 4:47–68.

Burbea, Z., Nakhoul, F., Zoabi, R., et al. 2004. Haptoglobin phenotype as a predicative factor of mortality in diabetic haemodialysis patients. *Ann Clin Biochem.* 41:469–473.

Carter, D.C. and Ho, J.X. 1994. Structure of serum albumin. *Adv Protein Chem.* 45:153–203.

Chader, G.J. and Westphal, U. 1968a. Steroid-protein interactions. XVIII. Isolation and observations on the polymeric nature of the corticosteroid-binding globulin of the rat. *Biochemistry.* 7:4272–4282.

Chader, G.J. and Westphal, U. 1968b. Steroid-protein interactions. XVI. Isolation and characterization of the corticosteroid-binding globulin of the rabbit. *J Biol Chem.* 243:928–939.

Chen, B.H., Turley, C.P., Brewster, M.A., and Arnold, W.A. 1986. Storage stability of serum transthyretin. *Clin Chem.* 32:1231–1232.

Chung, M.C.M. and McKenzie, H.A. 1985. Studies on equine transferrin I. The isolation and partial characterization of the D and R variants. *Comp Biochem Physiol.* 80B:287–297.

Cid, M.C., Grant, D.S., Hoffman, G.S., Auerbach, R., Fauci, A.S., and Kleinman, H.K. 1993. Identification of haptoglobin as an angiogenic factor in sera from patients with systemic vasculitis. *J Clin Invest.* 91:977–985.

Cinader, B. and Dubinski, S. 1963. An alpha-globulin allo-type in the mouse (MuBI). *Nature.* 200:781.

Cleve, H. and Patutschnick, W. 1979. Different pheno types of the group-specific component (Gc) in chimpanzees. *Hum Genet.* 50:217–220.

Cleve, H., Prunier, J.H., and Beam, A.G. 1963. Isolation and partial characterization of the two principal inherited group-specific components of human serum. *J Exp Med.* 118:711–726.

Cody, V. 1980. Thyroid hormone interactions: Molecular conformation protein binding and hormone action. *Endocrinol Rev.* 1:140–166.

Coe, C.L., Murai, J.T., Wiener, S.G., Levine, S., and Siiteri, P.K. 1986. Rapid cortisol and corticosteroid-binding globulin responses during pregnancy and after estrogen administration in the squirrel monkey. *Endocrinology.* 118:435–440.

Cohen, S. 1956. Plasma protein distribution and turnover in the female baboon. *J Biochem.* 64:286–296.

Cohen-Dix, P., Noble, R.W., and Reichlin, M. 1973. Comparative binding studies of the hemoglobin-haptoglobin and hemoglobin-antihemoglobin reactions. *Biochemistry.* 12:3744–3751.

Constans, J. 1976. Group-specific component. Report on the first international workshop. *Hum Genet.* 48:143–149.

Constans, J. 1992. Group-specific component is not only a vitamin D-binding protein. *Exp Clin Immunogenet.* 9:161–175.

Constans, J. and Viau, M. 1977. Group-specific component. Evidence for two subtypes of the Gc1 gene. *Science.* 198:1070–1071.

Courtoy, P.J., Feldman, G., Rogier, E., and Moguilevsky, N. 1981a. Plasma protein synthesis in experimental cirrhosis. *Lab Invest.* 45:67–76.

Courtoy, P.J., Lombart, C., Feldman, G., Moguilevsky, N., and Rogier, E. 1981b. Synchronous increase of four acute phase proteins synthesized by the same hepatocytes during the inflammatory reaction. *Lab Invest.* 44:105–115.

Cox, K.H., Wormley, S., Northway, N.A., Creighton, L., and Muller-Eberhard, U. 1978. Immunological cross-reactions between heterologous hemopexin. *Comp Biochem Physiol B.* 60:473–479.

D'Agnostino, J. and Henning, S.J. 1982. Postnatal development of corticosteroid-binding globulin. Effect of thyroxine. *Endocrinology.* 111:1476–1482.

D'Agnostino, J., Vaeth, G.F., and Henning, S.J. 1982. Diurnal rhythm of total and free concentrations of serum corticosterone in the rat. *Acta Endocrinol.* 100:85–90.

Daiger, S.P., Schanfield, M.S., and Cavalli-Sforza, L.L. 1975. Human group specific component (Gc) proteins bind vitamin D and 25-hydroxy-vitamin D. *Proc Natl Acad Sci USA.* 72:2076–2080.

Daiger, S.P. and Cavalli-Sforza, L.L. 1977. Detection of genetic variation with radioactive ligands. II. Genetic variants of vitamin D-labelled group specific component (Gc) proteins. *Am J Hum Genet.* 29:593–604.

Daniel, J.Y., Malaval, F., and Assenmacher, I. 1981. Evidence of a sex-related difference of transcortin level in adult ducks. *Steroids.* 38:29–34.

Davis, P.J., Spaulding, S.W., and Gregerman, R.I. 1970. The three thyroxine-binding proteins in rat serum. Binding capacities and effect of binding inhibitors. *Endocrinology.* 87:978–986.

Delaney, T.A., Morgan, W.H., and Morgan, E.H. 1982. Chemical, but not functional, differences between the iron-binding sites of rabbit transferrin. *Biochim Biophys Acta.* 701:295–304.

Dickson, P.W., Aldred, A.R., Marley, P.D., Bamister, D., and Schreiber, G. 1986. Rat choroid plexus specializes in the synthesis and the secretion of transthyretin (prealbumin). *J Biol Chem.* 261:3475–3478.

Dickson, P.W., Howlett, G.J., and Schreiber, G. 1982. Metabolism of prealbumin in rats and changes induced by acute inflammation. *Eur J Biochem.* 129:289–293.

Dickson, P.W., Howlett, G.J., and Schreiber, G. 1985. Rat transthyretin (prealbumin). *J Biol Chem.* 260:8214–8219.

Dixon, F.J., Maurer, P.H., and Deichmiller, M.P. 1953. Half-lives of homologous serum albumin in several species. *Proc Soc Exp Biol Med.* 83:287–288.

Duan, W., Richardson, S.J., Kohrle, J., Chang, L., Southwell, B.R., and Harms, P.J. 1995. Binding of thyroxine to pig transthyretin, its cDNA structure, and other properties. *Eur J Biochem.* 230:977–986.

Dwork, A.J., Cavallaro, T., Martone, R.L., Goodman, D.S., Schon, E.A., and Herbert, J. 1990. Distribution of transthyretin in the rat eye. *Invest Ophthalmol Vis Sci.* 31:489–496.

Eaton, J.W., Brandt, P., Mahoney, J.R., and Lee, J.T. 1982. Haptoglobin: A natural bacteriostat. *Science.* 215:691–692.

Eckersall, P.D., Saini, P.K., and McComb, C. 1996. The acute phase response of acid soluble glycoprotein, alpha(1)-acid glycoprotein, ceruloplasmin, haptoglobin, and C-reactive protein in the pig. *Vet Immunol Immunopathol.* 51:377–385.

Episkopou, V., Maeda, S., Nishiguchi, S., et al. 1993. Disruption of the transthyretin gene results in mice with depressed levels of plasma retinol and thyroid hormone. *Proc Natl Acad Sci USA.* 90:2375–2379.

Evans, W.E., Wilson, S.M., and Mage, M.G. 1986. Transferrin induces maturation of neutrophil granulocyte precursors in vitro. *Leuk Res*. 10:429–436.

Farer, L.S., Robbins, J., Blumberg, B.S., and Rall, J.E. 1962. Thyroxine-serum protein complexes in various animals. *Endocrinology*. 70:686–696.

Felding, P. and Fex, G. 1982. Cellular origin of prealbumin in the rat. *Biochim Biophys Acta*. 716:446–449.

Fex, G., Laurell, C.B., and Thulin, E. 1977. Purification of prealbumin from human and canine serum using a two-step affinity chromatographic procedure. *Eur J Biochem*. 75:181–186.

Fletcher, J. and Huehns, E.R. 1968. Function of transferrin. *Nature*. 218:1211–1218.

Focht, S.J., Snyder, B.S., Beard, J.L., Van Gelder, W., Williams, L.R., and Conner, J.R. 1997. Regional distribution of iron, transferrin, ferritin, and oxidatively-modified proteins in young and aged fischer rat brains. *Neuroscience*. 79:255–261.

Foidart, M., Eisman, J., Engel, W.K., Adornato, B.T., and Liem, H.H. 1982. Effect of heme administration on hemopexin metabolism in rhesus monkey. *J Lab Clin Med*. 100:451–460.

Forth, W. and Rummel, W. 1973. Iron absorption. *Physiol Rev*. 53:724–792.

Francisco, C.J., Shryock, T.R., Bane, D.P., and Unverzagt, L. 1996. Serum haptoglobin concentration in growing swine after intranasal challenge with Bordetella bronchiseptica and toxigenic Pasteurelle multocida type D. *Can J Vet Res*. 60:222–227.

Fujieda, K., Goff, A.K., Pugeat, M., and Strott, C.A. 1982. Regulation of the pituitary-adrenal axis and corticosteroid-binding globulin-cortisol interaction in the guinea pig. *Endocrinology*. 111:1944–1950.

Fung, W., Thomas, T., Dickson, P.W., et al. 1988. Structure and expression of the rat transthyretin (prealbumin) gene. *J Biol Chem*. 263:480–488.

Gala, R.R. and Westphal, U. 1965a. Corticosteroid-binding globulin in the rat. Studies on the sex difference. *Endocrinology*. 77:841–851.

Gala, R.R. and Westphal, U. 1965b. Corticosteroid-binding globulin in the rat. Possible role in the initiation of lactation. *Endocrinology*. 76:1079–1088.

Gala, R.R. and Westphal, U. 1967. Corticosteroid-binding activity in serum of mouse, rabbit, and guinea pig during pregnancy and lactation. Possible involvement in the initiation of lactation. *Acta Endocrinol*. 55:47–61.

Gardiner, M.E. and Morgan, E.H. 1981. Effect of reduced atmospheric pressure and fasting on transferrin synthesis in the rat. *Life Sci*. 29:1641–1648.

Gentry, P.A. 1999. Acute phase proteins. In *The Clinical Chemistry of laboratory Animals*. Eds. W.F. Loeb and F.W. Quimby, 2nd edition, pp. 336–398. Philadelphia, PA: Taylor and Francis.

Giblett, E.R. 1969. *Genetic Markers in Human Blood*, pp. 126–159. Oxford: Blackwell Scientific Publications.

Giblett, E.R., Hickman, C.G., and Smithies, O. 1959. Serum transferrins. *Nature*. 183:1589–1590.

Glinoer, D., Gershengorn, M.C., Dubois, A., and Robbins, J. 1977a. Stimulation of thyroxine-binding globulin synthesis by isolated rhesus monkey hepatocytes after in vivo B-estradiol administration. *Endocrinology*. 100:807–813.

Glinoer, D., Gershengorn, M.C., and Robbins, J. 1970. Thyroxine-binding globulin biosynthesis in isolated monkey hepatocytes. *Biochim Biophys Acta*. 418:232–244.

Glinoer, D., McGuire, R.A., Gershengorn, M.C., Robbins, J., and Berman, M. 1977b. Effects of estrogen on thyroxine-binding globulin metabolism in rhesus monkeys. *Endocrinology*. 100:9–17.

Glinoer, D., McGuire, R.A., Cogen, J.P., Robbins, J., and Berman, M. 1979. Thyroxine-binding globulin metabolism in rhesus monkeys. Effects of hyper- and hypothyroidism. *Endocrinology*. 104:175–183.

Godson, D.L., Campos, M., Attah-Poku, S.K., et al. 1996. Serum haptoglobin as an indicator of the acute phase response in bovine respiratory disease. *Vet Immunol Immunopathol*. 51:277–292.

Goldschmidt-Clermont, P.J., Van Balen, H., Boullin, R., et al. 1988. Role of Gc in clearance of actin from circulation in the rabbit. *J Clin Invest*. 81(5):1519–1527.

Golub, M.S. and Kaaekuahiwi, M.A. 1997. Changes in plasma alphal-acid glycoprotein and albumin concentrations during late pregnancy in rhesus monkeys. *Clin Chim Acta*. 262:29–37.

Goodman, M., Kulkarni, A., Poulik, E., and Reklys, E. 1965. Species and geographic differences in the transferrin polymorphism of macaques. *Science*. 147:884–886.

Goodman, W.C., Mickelson, K.E., and Westphal, U. 1981. Immunochemical determination of corticosteroid-binding globulin in the guinea pig during gestation. *J Steroid Biochem*. 14:1293–1296.

Gordon, S. and Bearn, A.G. 1966. Hemoglobin binding capacity of isolated haptoglobin polypeptide chains. *Proc Soc Exp Biol Med*. 121:846–850.

Grant, G.H. and Kachmar, J.F. 1976. The proteins of body fluids. In *Fundamentals of Clinical Chemistry*. Ed. N.W. Tietz, pp. 298–376. Philadelphia, PA: W.B. Saunders.

Greene, F.C. and Feeney, R.E. 1968. Physical evidence for transferrin as single polypeptide chains. *Biochemistry*. 7:1366–1371.

Grunder, A.A. 1966. Inheritance of a heme-binding protein in rabbits. *Genetics*. 54:1085–1093.

Grunder, A.A. 1968. Hemopexin of rabbits. *Vox Sang*. 14:218–223.

Guttman, S.I. and Wilson, K.G. 1973. Genetic variation in the genus Bufo. I. An extreme degree of transferrin and albumin polymorphism in a population of American toad (Bufo americanus). *Biochem Genet*. 8:329–340.

Hagen, K.L., Rasmusen, B.A., and Mittal, K.K. 1968. Further investigations on linkage between the loci for heme-binding globulins and K blood groups in pig. *Vox Sang*. 15:147–151.

Hagen, K.L., Suzuki, Y., Tissot, R., and Cohen, C. 1978. The hemopexin locus. Its assignment to linkage group I in the laboratory rabbit (Oryctolagus cuniculus) and evidence for a fourth allele. *Anim Blood Groups Biochem Genet*. 9:151–159.

Hall, R.E. 1992. Clinical pathology of laboratory animals. In *Animal Models in Toxicology*, Gad, S.C. and Chengelis, C.P. (eds). New York: Marcel Dekker.

Hammond, G.L., Smith, C.L., Lahteenmaki, P., et al. 1994. Squirrel monkey corticosteroid-binding globulin: Primary structure and comparison with the human protein. *Endocrinology*. 134:891–898.

Hanley, J.M., Haugen, T.H., and Heath, E.C. 1983. Biosynthesis and processing of rat haptoglobin. *J Biol Chem*. 258:7858–7869.

Harms, P.J., Tu, G.F., Richardson, S.J., Aldred, A.R., Jaworowski, A., and Schreiber, G. 1991. Transthyretin (prealbumin) gene expression in choroid plexus is strongly conserved during evolution of vertebrates. *Comp Biochem Physiol*. 99:239–249.

Harrington, J., Heaney, H., McSweeney, C., Quarino, L., Schwartz, T., and Versoza, J. 1991. Haptoglobin typing in canine bloods. *J Forensic Sci*. 36:1561–1564.

Harvey, J.W. 1976. Quantitative determinations of normal horse, cat, and dog haptoglobins. *Theriogenology*. 6:133–138.

Harvey, J.W. and Gaskin, J.M. 1978. Feline haptoglobin. *Am J Vet Res*. 39:549–553.

Heaf, D.J., El-Sayed, M., and Glover, J. 1980. Changes in plasma concentrations of thyroxine-binding prealbumin and retinol binding protein in Japanese quail after hatching. *Br J Nutr*. 44:287–293.

Heaphy, S. and Williams, J. 1978. The preparation and partial characterization of N-terminal and C-terminal iron-binding fragments from rabbit serum transferrin. *Biochem J*. 205:611–617.

Hershko, C. 1975. The fate of circulating haemoglobin. *Br J Haematol*. 29:199–204.

Hirschfeld, J. 1959. Immune-electrophoretic demonstration of qualitative differences in human sera and their relation to the haptoglobins. *Acta Pathol Microbiol Scand*. 47:160–168.

Hofvander, Y. 1968. Hematological investigation in ethiopia. *Acta Med Scand*. 185(Suppl 494):1–74.

Horn, K. and Gartner, R. 1979. Thyroxine-binding globulin-structure, assay and function. *Acta Endocrinol*. 225:447–448.

Horne, C.H.W., Mallison, A.C., Ferguson, J., and Goudie, R.B. 1971. Effects of estrogen and progestogen on serum levels of α^2-macroglobulin, transferrin, albumin, and IgG. *J Clin Pathol*. 24:464–466.

Hrkal, Z. and Muller-Eberhard, U. 1971. Partial characterization of the heme-binding serum glycoproteins—Rabbit and human hemopexin. *Biochemistry*. 10:1746–1750.

Hudson, B.G., Ohno, M., Brodeway, W.J., and Castellino, F.J. 1973. Chemical and physical properties of serum transferrin from several species. *Biochemistry*. 12:1047–1053.

Huebers, H.A., Huebers, E., Csiba, E., Rummel, W., and Finch, C.A. 1983. The significance of transferrin for intestinal iron absorption. *Blood*. 61:283–290.

Huebers, H., Urelli, D., Celada, A., Josephson, B., and Finch, C. 1982. Basis of plasma iron exchange in the rabbit. *J Clin Invest*. 70:769–779.

Hughes-Jones, N.C., Gardner, B., and Helps, R. 1961. Observation on the binding of haemoglobin and hematin by serum proteins of the rabbit, rat, and guinea pig. *Biochem J*. 79:220–223.

Hwang, P.K. and Greer, J. 1980. Interaction between hemoglobin subunits in the hemoglobin-haptoglobin complex. *J Biol Chem*. 255:3038–3041.

Idzerda, R.L., Huebers, H., Finch, C.A., and McKnight, G.S. 1986. Rat transferrin gene expression: Tissue-specific regulation by iron deficiency. *Proc Natl Acad Sci*. 83:3723–3727.

Ingenbleek, Y. and Young, V. 1994. Transthyretin (prealbumin) in health and disease: Nutritional implication. *Ann Rev Nutr*. 14:495–533.

Jarnum, S. and Lassen, N.A. 1961. Albumin and transferrin metabolism in infectious and toxic disease. *Scand J Clin Lab Invest*. 13:357–368.

Javid, J. 1978. Human haptoglobins. *Curr Top Hematol*. 1:151–192.

Jeejeebhoy, K.N., Bruce-Robertson, A., Ho, J., and Sodtke, U. 1972. The effect of cortisol on the synthesis of rat plasma albumin, fibrinogen, and transferrin. *Biochem J*. 130:533–538.

Jeffrey, H. 1960. The metabolism of serum proteins. *J Biol Chem*. 235:2352–2356.

Kalberg, H.I., Hern, K.A., and Fischer, J.E. 1983. Albumin turnover in sarcoma-bearing rats in relation to cancer anorexia. *Am J Surg*. 145:95–101.

Kamiyama, T. 1976. Immunological cross reactions and species specificities of cyanogen bromide cleaved fragments of bovine, goat, and sheep serum albumins. *Immunochemistry*. 14:91–98.

Kanai, M., Raz, A., and Goodman, D.S. 1968. Retinol binding protein. The transport protein for vitamin A in human plasma. *J Clin Invest*. 47:2025–2044.

Kanda, Y., Goodman, D.S., Canfield, R.E., and Morgan, F.J. 1974. The amino acid sequence of human plasma prealbumin. *J Biol Chem*. 249:6796–6805.

Kattesh, H.G., Kornegay, E.T., Knight, J.W., Gwazdauskas, F.G., Thomas, H.R., and Notter, D.R. 1980. Glucocorticoid concentrations, corticosteriod binding protein characteristics, and reproduction performance of sows and gilts subjected to applied stress during mid-gestation. *J Anim Sci*. 50:897–905.

Kazim, A.L. and Atassi, M.Z. 1981. Hemoglobin binding with haptoglobin. *Biochem J*. 197:507–510.

Kietzmann, T., Immenschuh, S., Katz, N., Jungermann, K., and Muller-Eberhard, U. 1995. Modulation of hemopexin gene expression by physiological oxygen tensions in primary rat hepatocyte cultures. *Biochem Biophy Res Commun*. 213:397–403.

Kitchin, F.D. and Bearn, A.G. 1965. The serum group specific component in non-human primates. *Am J Hum Genet*. 17:42–50.

Koj, A. 1974. Acute phase reactants. In *Structure and Functions of Plasma Proteins*. Ed. A.C. Allison, pp. 73–133. New York, NY: Plenum Press.

Kristjansson, F.K. 1961. Genetic control of three haptoglobins in pigs. *Genetics*. 46:907–910.

Kristjansson, F.K. 1966. Fractionation of serum albumin and genetic control of two albumin fractions in pigs. *Genetics*. 53:675–679.

Kristjansson, F.K. and Hickman, C.G. 1965. Subdivision of the alleles TfD for transferrin in Holstein and Ayrshire cattle. *Genetics*. 52:627–630.

Kurosky, A., Barnett, D.R., Lee, T.H., et al. 1980. Covalent structure of human haptoglobin—Serine protease homolog. *Proc Natl Acad Sci USA*. 77:3388–3392.

Kurosky, A., Hay, R.E., and Bowman, B.H. 1979. Canine haptoglobin, a unique haptoglobin subunit arrangement. *Comp Biochem Physiol B*. 62:339–344.

Kusher, I., Edington, T.S., Trimble, C., Liem, H.H., and Muller-Eberhard, U. 1972. Plasma hemopexin homeostasis during the acute phase response. *J Lab Clin Med*. 80:18–25.

Lamon, J.M., Sach, J., Zavazal, V., Nozlckova, M., and Mateja, F. 1978. Hematine therapy in acute porphyria and observation on hemopexin. In *Diagnosis and Therapy of Porphyrias and Lead Intoxication*. Ed. M. Doss, p. 285. Berlin: Springer-Verlag.

Lane, R.S., Rangeley, D.M., Liem, H.H., Womsley, S., and Muller-Eberhard, U. 1973. Plasma clearance of 125 I-labelled haemopexin in normal and heme loaded rabbits. *Br J Haematol*. 25:533–540.

Larsson, M., Pettersson, T., and Carlstrom, A. 1985. Thyroid hormone binding in serum of 15 vertebrate species: Isolation of thyroid-binding globulin and prealbumin analogs. *Gen Comp Endocrinol*. 58:360–375.

Lee, S.H., Kim, K.H., Yoo, S.H., et al. 2011. Relationship between Gc and the development of asthma. *Am J Respir Crit Care Med*. 184(5):528–536.

Lee, Y.W., Min, W.K., Chun, S., et al. 2004. Lack of association between oxidized LDL-cholesterol concentrations and haptoglobin phenotypes in healthy subjects. *Assoc Clin Biochem*. 41:485–487.

Leger, D., Tordera, V., and Spik, G. 1978. Structure determination of the single glycan of rabbit sero-transferrin by methylation analysis and 360 MHz 1H NMR spectroscopy. *FEBS Lett*. 93:255–260.

Letendre, E.D. and Holbein, B.E. 1981. A sensitive and convenient assay procedure for transferrin and its application to the purification of mouse transferrin. *Can J Biochem*. 59:906–910.

Liem, H.H. 1976. Catabolism of homologous and heterologous hemopexin in the rat and uptake of hemopexin by isolated perfused rat liver. *Ann Clin Res*. 8(Suppl 17):233–238.

Lin, G.X., Selcer, K.W., Beale, E.G., Gray, G.O., and Leavitt, W.W. 1990. Characterization of corticosteroid-binding globulin messenger ribonucleic acid response in the pregnant hamster. *Endocrinology*. 127:1934–1940.

Lombart, C., Moretti, J., and Jayie, M.F. 1965. Preparation et proprietes physiques des haptoglobines de lapin et de rat. *Biochim Biophys Acta*. 97:262–269.

Lombart, C., Musquera, S., and Delers, F. 1979. Characterization and specific properties of chicken haptoglobin. In *XIth International Congress of Biochemistry*, p. 178. Toronto, Canada: National Research Council of Canada.

Lowe, M.E. and Ashwell, G. 1982. Solubilization and assay of a hepatic receptor for the haptoglobin-hemoglobin complex. *Arch Biochem Biophys*. 216:704–710.

MacGillivray, R.T.A., Mendez, E., and Brew, K. 1977. Structure and evolution of serum transferrin. In *Proteins of Iron Metabolism*. Eds. E.B. Brown, P. Aisen, J. Feilding, and R.R. Crichton, pp. 133–141. New York, NY: Grune & Stratton.

Maeda, K., McKenzie, H.A., and Shaw, D.C. 1980. Nature of the heterogeneity within genetic variants of bovine serum transferrin. *Anim Blood Groups Biochem Genet*. 11:63–75.

Magic, Z., Matic-Ivanovic, S., Savic, J., and Poznanovic, G. 1995. Ionizing radiation-induced expression of the genes associated with the acute response to injury in the rat. *Radiat Res*. 143:187–193.

Mahmud, S.M., Koushik, A., Duarte-Franco, E., et al. 2007. Haptoglobin phenotype and risk of cervical neoplasia: A case control study. *Clin Chim Acta*. 385:67–72.

Majuri, R. 1982. Purification of pig serum haemopexin by haemin-sepharose affinity chromatography. *Biochim Biophys Acta*. 719:53–57.

Makinen, M.W., Milstein, J.B., and Kon, H. 1972. Specificity of interaction of haptoglobin with mammalian hemoglobin. *Biochemistry*. 11:3851–3860.

Mann, K.G., Fis, W.W., Cox, A.C., and Tanford, C. 1970. Single chain nature of human serum transferrin. *Biochemistry*. 9:1348–1354.

Massolini, G., De Lorenzi, E., Ponci, M.C., and Caccialanza, G. 1996. Comparison of drug binding sites on rat and human serum albumins using immobilized-protein stationary phases as a tool for the selection of suitable animal models in pharmacological studies. *Boll Chim Farm*. 135:382–386.

Mattheeuws, D.R.G., Kaneko, J.J., Loy, R.G., Cornelius, C.E., and Wheat, J.D. 1966. Compartmentalization and turnover of 131 I-labelled albumin and gamma globulin in horses. *Am J Vet Res*. 27:699–705.

McGuire, R.A., Glinoer, D., Albert, M.A., and Robbins, J. 1982. Comparative effects of thyroxine (T4) and triiodothyronine on T4-binding globulin metabolism in rhesus monkeys. *Endocrinology*. 110:1340–1346.

McIndoe, W.M. 1962. Occurrence of two plasma albumins in the domestic fowl. *Nature*. 195:353–354.

McKinney, J.D. and Waller, C.L. 1994. Polychlorinated biphenyls as hormonally active analogues. *Environ Health Perspect*. 102:290–297.

McNair, J., Elliott, C.T., and Mackie, D.P. 1995. Development of a sensitive and specific time resolved fluorimetric immunoassay for the bovine acute phase protein haptoglobin (Hp). *J Immunol Methods*. 184:199–205.

Meek, J. and Adamson, E. 1985. Transferrin in foetal and adult mouse tissues: Synthesis, storage, and secretion. *J Embryol Exp Morphol*. 86:205–218.

Meloun, B., Moravek, L., and Kostka, V. 1975. Complete amino acid sequence of human serum albumin. *FEBS Lett*. 58:134–137.

Mickelson, K.E. and Westphal, U. 1979. Purification and characterization of the corticosteroid-binding globulin of pregnant guinea pig serum. *Biochemistry*. 18:2685–2690.

Mitruka, B.M. and Rawnsley, H.M. 1977. Clinical, biochemical, and haematological reference values. In *Normal Experimental Animals*, pp. 117–181. New York, NY: Masson Publishing USA.

Mominoki, K., Nakagawa-Tosa, N., Morimatsu, M., Syuto, B., and Saito, M. 1995. Haptoglobin in carnivora: A unique molecular structure in bear, cat, and dog haptoglobins. *Comp Biochem Physiol B Biochem Mol Biol*. 110:785–789.

Morgan, E.H. and Peters, T. 1971a. Intracellular aspects of transferrin synthesis and secretion in the rat. *J Biolo Chem*. 246:3508–3511.

Morgan, E.H. and Peters, T. 1971b. The biosynthesis of rat serum albumin. V. Effects of protein depletion and refeeding on albumin and transferrin synthesis. *J Biol Chem*. 246:3500–3507.

Morgan, F.J., Canfield, R.E., and Goodman, D.S. 1971. The partial structure of human plasma prealbumin and retinol-binding protein. *Biochim Biophys Acta*. 236:798–801.

Morris, C.M., Candy, J.M., Edwardson, J.A., Bloxham, C.A., and Smith, A. 1993. Evidence for the localization of haemopexin immunoreactivity in neurons in the human brain. *Neurosci Lett*. 149:141–144.

Morton, A.G. and Tavill, A.S. 1975. Studies on the mechanism of iron supply in the regulation of hepatic transferrin synthesis. In *Proteins of Iron Storage and Transport in Biochemistry and Medicine*. Ed. R.R. Crichton, pp. 167–172. Amsterdam: North-Holland.

Moutafchicv, D.A., Shisheva, A.C., and Sirakov, M. 1983. Binding of transferrin-iron to the plasma membrane of a lactating rabbit mammary gland cell. *Int J Biochem*. 15:755–758.

Muller-Eberhard, U. 1970. Hemopexin. *N Engl J Med*. 283:1090–1094.

Muller-Eberhard, U. 1978. Heme transport and properties of hemopexin. In *Transport by Proteins*. Eds. G. Blauer and H. Sund, p. 295. Berlin: Walter de Gruyter.

Muller-Eberhard, U., Bosnian, C., and Liem, H.H. 1970. Tissue localization of the heme-hemopexin complex in the rabbit and the rat as studied by light microscopy with the use of radiosotopes. *J Lab Clin Med.* 76:426–431.

Muller-Eberhard, U., Javid, J., Liem, H.H., Hamstein, A., and Hanna, M. 1968. Plasma concentration of hemopexin, haptoglobin, and heme in patients with various hemolytic diseases. *Blood.* 32:811–815.

Muller-Eberhard, U., Liem, H.H., Hamstein, A., and Saarinen, P.A. 1969. Studies on the disposal of intravascular heme in the rabbit. *J Lab Clin Med.* 73:210–218.

Murata, H., Shimada, N., and Yoshioka, M. 2004. Current research on acute phase proteins in veterinary diagnosis: An overview. *Vet J.* 168(1):28–40.

Musquera, S., Lombart, C., Jayle, M.F., Rogard, M., and Waks, M. 1979. Identification of haptoglobin in chicken serum and specificity of the chicken haptoglobin-hemoglobin complex formation. *Comp Biochem Physiol B.* 62:241–244.

Nassir, F., Zimowska, W., Bayle, D., Gueux, E., Rayssiguier, Y., and Mazur, A. 2002. Hypoalbuminaemia in acute phase response is not related to depressed albumin synthesis: Experimental evidence in magnesium-deficient rat. *Nutr Res.* 22:489–496.

Navab, M., Malliam, A.K., Kanda, Y., and Goodman, D.S. 1977a. Rat plasma prealbumin: Isolation and partial characterization. *J Biol Chem.* 252:5107–5114.

Navab, M., Smith, J.E., and Goodman, D.S. 1977b. Rat plasma prealbumin. *J Biol Chem.* 252:5107–5114.

Nikkila, H., Gitlin, J.D., and Muller-Eberhard, U. 1991. Rat hemopexin: Molecular cloning, primary structural characterization, and analysis of gene expression. *Biochemistry.* 30:823–829.

Nomenclature Committee of IUB [NC-IUB]. 1981. IUBIUPAC Joint Commission on Biochemical Nomenclature newsletter. *J Biol Chem.* 256:12–14.

Nyberg, L., Marekov, L.N., Jones, I., Lundquist, G., and Jornvall, H. 1990. Characterization of the murine corticosteroid-binding: Variations between mammalian forms. *J Steroid Biochem.* 35:61–65.

Oakey, R.E. 1975. Serum cortisol binding capacity and cortisol concentration in the pregnant baboon and its fetus during gestation. *Endocrinology.* 97:1024–1029.

Oishi, T., Tomita, T., and Komatsu, M. 1980. New genetic variants detected in the haemopexin and ceruloplasmin systems of ohmini miniature pigs. *Anim Blood Groups Biochem Genet.* 1:59–62.

Ong, D.E., Davis, J.T., O'Day, W.T., and Bok, D. 1994. Synthesis and secretion of retinol-binding protein and transthyretin by cultured retinal pigment epithelium. *Biochemistry.* 33:1835–1842.

Oppenheimer, J.H., Surks, M.I., Smith, J.C., and Squef, R. 1965. Isolation and charactenzation of human throxine-binding prealbumin. *J Biol Chem.* 240:173–180.

Oren, R., Dabeva, M.D., Petkov, P.M., Hurston, E., Laconi, E., and Shafritz, D.A. 1999. Restoration of serum albumin levels in nagase analbuminemic rats by hepatocyte transplantation. *Hepatology.* 29(1):75--81.

Ottenweller, J.E., Meier, A.H., Russo, A.C., and Frenske, M.E. 1979. Circadian rhythms of plasma corticosteroid binding activity in the rat and the mouse. *Acta Endocrinol.* 91:150–157.

Palmer, W.G. 1976. The serum haptoglobin response to inflammation in neonatal mice and its relationship to phagocytosis. *J Reticuloendothel Soc.* 19:301–309.

Palmour, R.M. and Sutton, H.E. 1971. Vertebrate transferrins. Molecular weights, chemical compositions, and iron-binding studies. *Biochemistry.* 10:4026–4032.

Parra, M., Vaisanen, V., and Ceron, J. 2005. Development of a time resolved fluorometry-based immunoassay for the determination of canine haptoglobin in various body fluids. *Vet Res.* 36:117–129.

Peacock, A.C., Gelderman, A.H., Ragland, R.H., and Hoffman, H.A. 1967. Haptoglobin levels in serum of various strains of mice. *Science.* 158:1703–1704.

Peters, T., Jr. 1977. Serum albumin: Recent progress in the understanding of its structure and biosynthesis. *Clin Chem.* 23:5–12.

Peters, T., Jr. and Davidson, L.K. 1982. The biosynthesis of rat serum albumin. *J Biol Chem.* 257:8847–8853.

Peters, T., Jr. and Davidson, L.K. 1986. The biosynthesis of rat serum albumin. *J Biol Chem.* 261:7242–7246.

Peters, T., Jr. and Peters, J.C. 1972. The biosynthesis of rat serum albumin. VI. Intracellular transport of albumin and rates of albumin and liver protein synthesis in vivo under various physiological conditions. *J Biol Chem.* 247:3858–3863.

Peters, T., Jr. and Reed, R.G. 1980. The biosynthesis of rat serum albumin. *J Biol Chem.* 255:3156–3163.

Peterson, P.A., Rask, L., Ostberg, L., Anderson, L., Kamwendo, F., and Pertoft, H. 1973. Studies on the transport and cellular distribution of vitamin A in normal and vitamin A-deficient rats with special reference to the vitamin A-binding plasma protein. *J Biol Chem.* 248:4009–4022.

Polonovski, M. and Jayle, M.F. 1939. Peroxidases animates. Leur specificities et leur role biologiques. *Bull De La Soc De Chim Biol (Paris).* 21:66–91.

Potter, D., Chroneos, Z.C., Baynes, J.W., et al. 1993. In vivo fate of hemopexin and heme-hemopexin complexes in the rat. *Arch Biochem Biophys.* 300:98–104.

Putman, F.W. 1975a. Haptoglobin. In *The Plasma Proteins: Structure, Function, and Genetic Control*, Vol. 2. Ed. F.W. Putman, pp. 1–50. New York, NY: Academic Press.

Putman, F.W. 1975b. Serum albumin. In *The Plasma Protein: Structure, Function and Genetic Control*. Ed. F.W. Putman, pp. 133–181. New York, NY: Academic Press.

Quaye, K. 2008. Haptoglobin, inflammation and disease. *Trans R Soc Trop Med Hyg*. 102(8):735–742.

Quinteros, I.R., Stevens, S.C., Stormont, C., and Asmundson, V.S. 1964. Albumin phenotypes in turkeys. *Genetics*. 50:579–582.

Ramoure, W.J. and Kuhn, R.W. 1983. A homologous radioimmunoassay for rat corticosteroid-binding globulin. *Endocrinology*. 112:1091–1097.

Rangel, H. 1965. Study of the cross-reaction between rabbit and anti-bovine serum albumin and equine serum albumin. *Immunology*. 8:88–94.

Reed, R.G., Feldhoff, R.C., Clute, O.L., and Peters, T., Jr. 1975. Fragments of bovine serum albumin produced by limited proteolysis. Conformation and ligand binding. *Biochemistry.* 14:4578–4583.

Refetoff, S., Robin, N., and Fang, V.S. 1970. Parameters of thyroid function in serum of 16 selected vertebrate species: A study of PBI, serum T^4, free T^4, and the pattern of T^4 and T^3 binding to serum proteins. *Endocrinology*. 86:793–805.

Regoeczi, E. and Hatton, W.C. 1980. Transferrin catabolism in mammalian species of different body sizes. *Am J Physiol*. 238:R306–R310.

Regoeczi, E., Hatton, M.W.C., and Wong, K.L. 1974. Studies of the metabolism of asialotransferrins: Potentiation of the catabolism of human sialotransferrin in the rabbit. *Can J Biochem*. 52:155–161.

Reinskou, T. 1968. The Gc system. *Ser Haematol*. 1:21–37.

Rennie, J.S., MacDonald, D.G., and Douglas, T.A. 1981. Haemoglobin, serum iron, and transferrin values of adult male Syrian hamsters (Mesocricetus auratus). *Lab Anim*. 15:35–36.

Richardson, S.J., Bradley, A.J., Duan, W., et al. 1994. Evolution of marsupial and other vertebrate thyroxin-binding plasma proteins. *Am J Physiol*. 266:1359–1370.

Richardson, N.E., Buttress, N., Feinstein, A., Stratil, A., and Spooner, R.L. 1973. Structural studies on individual components of bovine transferrin. *Biochem J*. 135:87–92.

Rickenbacher, U., McKinney, J.D., Oatley, S.J., and Blake, C.C.F. 1986. Structurally specific binding of halogenated biphenyls to thyroxine transport protein. *J Med Chem*. 29:641–648.

Ritter, H. and Smith, J. 1971. Hp 2–2 like phenotypes in mammals. *Humangenetik*. 12:351–353.

Robbins, J.R., Cheng, S.Y., Gershengorn, M.C., Glinoer, D., Chanman, H.J., and Edelnoch, H. 1978. Thyroxine transport proteins of plasma. Molecular properties and biosynthesis. *Recent Prog Horm Res*. 34:477–519.

Roberts, R.C., Makey, D.G., and Seal, U.S. 1966. Human transferrin molecular weight and sedimentation properties. *J Biol Chem*. 241:4907–4913.

Rodriguez, J.A., Evans, R.L., Daiger, S.P., and Northrup, H. 1997. Molecular analysis of the human vitamin D-binding protein (group-specific component, Gc) in tuberous sclerosis complex (TSC). *J Med Genet*. 34:509–511.

Rosenthal, H.E., Paul, M.A., and Sandberg, A.A. 1974. Transcortin. A corticosteroid-binding protein of plasma. XII. Immunologic studies on transcortin in guinea pig tissues. *J Steroid Biochem*. 5:219–225.

Rosner, W. 1972. Recent studies on the binding of cortisol in serum. *J Steroid Biochem*. 3:531–542.

Rosner, W. 1991. Plasma steroid-binding proteins. *Endocrinol Metab Clin North Am*. 20:697–720.

Rosner, W. and Hochberg, R. 1972. Corticosteroid-binding globulin in the rat: Isolation and studies of its influence on cortisol action in vivo. *Endocrinology*. 91:626–632.

Runnegar, M., Wei, X., Berndt, N., and Hamm-Alvarez, S.F. 1997. Transferrin receptor recycling in rat hepatocytes is regulated by protein phosphatase 2A, possibly through effects on microtubule-dependent transport. *Hepatology*. 26:176–185.

Sakata, S. and Atassi, M.Z. 1979. Immunochemistry of serum albumin. VI. A dynamic approach to the immunochemical cross-reactions of proteins using serum albumins from various species as models.*Biochim Biophys Acta*. 579:322–332.

Sakly, M. and Koch, B. 1983. Ontogenetical variation of transferrin modulate glucocorticoid receptor function and corticotropic activity in the pituitary gland. *Horm Metab Res*. 15:92–96.

Salonen, M., Hirvonen, J., Pyorala, S., Sankari, S., and Sandholm, M. 1996. Quantitative determination of bovine serum haptoglobin in experimentally induced Escherichia coli mastitis. *Res Vet Sci*. 60:88–91.

Sarich, V.M. and Wilson, A.C. 1966. Quantitative immunochemistry and the evolution of primate albumins: Micro-complement fixation. *Science*. 154:1563–1566.

Savu, L., Lombart, C., and Nunez, E.A. 1980. Corticosteroid-binding globulin: An acutephase "negative" protein in the rat. *FEBS Lett*. 113:102–106.

Sawatzki, G., Anselstetter, V., and Kubanek, B. 1981. Isolation of mouse transferrin using salting out chromatography on Sepharose CL-6B. *Biochim Biophys Acta.* 667:132–138.

Scheving, L.E., Pauly, J.E., and Tsai, T.H. 1968. Circadian fluctation in plasma proteins of the rat. *Am J Physiol.* 215:1096–1101.

Schofield, J.D. 1980. Altered proteins in aging organisms: Purification and properties of serum albumin from adult and aging C57BI mice. *Exp Gerontol.* 15:433–455.

Schreiber, G., Aldred, A.R., Jaworowski, A., Nilsson, C., Achen, M.G., and Segal, M.B. 1990. Thyroxin transport from blood to brain via transthyretin synthesis in choroid plexus. *Am J Physiol.* 258:338–345.

Schreiber, G., Doryburgh, H., Millership, A., et al. 1979. The synthesis and secretion of rat transferrin. *J Biol Chem.* 254:12012–12019.

Schreiber, G. and Richardson, S.J. 1997. The evolution of gene expression, structure, and function of transthyretin. *Comp Biochem Physiol B Biochem Mol Biol.* 116:137–160.

Scrocchi, L.A., Hearn, S.A., Han, V.K., and Hammond, G.L. 1993. Corticosteroid-binding biosynthesis in the mouse liver and kidney during postnatal development. *Endocrinology.* 132:910–916.

Seal, U.S. and Doe, R.P. 1963. Corticosteroid-binding globulin: Species distribution and small scale purification. *Endocrinology.* 73:371–376.

Seal, U.S. and Doe, R.P. 1965. Vertebrate distribution of corticosteroid-binding globulin and some endocrine effects on concentration. *Steroids.* 5:827–841.

Seal, U.S. and Doe, R.P. 1966. Corticosteroid-binding globulin: Biochemistry, physiology, and phylogeny. In *Steroid Dynamics.* Eds. G. Pincus, T. Nakao, and J.F. Tail, p. 63. New York, NY: Academic Press.

Sears, D.A. 1968. Plasma heme-binding in patient with hemolytic disorders. *J Lab Clin Med.* 71:484–494.

Seery, V.L., Hathaway, G., and Muller-Eberhard, U. 1972. Hemopexin of human and rabbit: Molecular weight and extinction coefficient. *Arch Biochem Biophys.* 150:269–272.

Seo, H., Ando, M., Yamaguchi, K., Matsui, N., and Takaneka, O. 1989. Plasma thyroxine-binding proteins and thyroid hormone levels in primate species. Is callithricidae thyroid hormone resistant? *Endocrinol Jpn.* 36:665–673.

Seralini, G.E., Smith, C.L., and Hammond, G.L. 1990. Rabbit corticosteroid-binding globulin: Primary structure and biosynthesis during pregnancy. *Mol Endocrinol.* 4:1166–1172.

Shifrine, M. and Stortmont, C. 1973. Hemoglobins, haptoglobins, and transferrins in beagles. *Lab Anim Sci.* 23:704–706.

Shim, B.S. and Bearn, A.G. 1965. The distribution of haptoglobin subtypes in various populations, including subtype patterns in some non-human primates. *Am J Hum Genet.* 16:477–483.

Shutherland, R.L. and Brandon, M.R. 1976. The thyroxine-binding properties of rat and rabbit serum proteins. *Endocrinology.* 98:91–98.

Simons, K. and Bearn, A.G. 1967. The use of preparative polyacrylamide-column electrophoresis in isolation of electrophoretically distinguishable components of the serum group-specific proteins. *Biochim Biophys Acta.* 133:499–505.

Smith, D.G. 1982. Iron binding and transferrin polymorphism in rhesus monkey (Macaca mulatto). *Lab Anim Sci.* 32:153–156.

Smithies, D., Connel, G.E., and Dixon, G.H. 1962. Inheritance of haptoglobins subtypes. *Am J Hum Genet.* 14:14–21.

Smithies, O. and Hickman, C.G. 1958. Inherited variations in the serum proteins of cattle. *Genetics.* 43:374–385.

Soos, P. 1971. Genetic variants of serum albumin in two Hungarian cattle breeds. *Acta Vet Acad Sci Hung.* 24:341–343.

Spooner, R.L. and Baxter, G. 1969. Abnormal expression of normal transferrin alleles. *Biochem Genet.* 2:371–382.

Spooner, R.L., Land, R.B., Oliver, R.A., and Stratil, A. 1970. Fetal and neonatal transferrin in cattle. *Anim Blood Groups Biochem Genet.* 1:241–246.

Spooner, R.L., Oliver, R.A., Richardson, N., et al. 1974. Isolation and partial characterization of sheep transferrin. *Comp Biochem Physiol B.* 52:515–522.

Spooner, R.L., Oliver, R.A., and Williams, G. 1977. Polymorphic variation in the amount of sialic acid attached to bovine transferrin. *Anim Blood Groups Biochem Genet.* 8:21–24.

Stockham, S.L. and Scott, M.A. 2008. Proteins. In *Fundamentals of Veterinary Clinical Pathology*, 2nd edition, pp. 369–413, Ames, IA: Blackwell Publishing.

Stormont, C. and Suzuki, Y. 1963. Genetic control of albumin phenotypes in horses. *Proc Soc Exp Biol Med.* 114:673–675.

Stratil, A. and Glasnak, V. 1981. Partial characterization of horse transferrin heterogeneity with respect to the atypical type, Tf C. *Anim Blood Groups Biochem Genet.* 12:113–122.

Stratil, A., Glasnak, V., Tomasek, V., Williams, J., and Clamp, J.R. 1984a. Haemopexin of sheep, mouflon, and goat: Genetic polymorphism, heterogeneity, and partial characterization. *Anim Blood Groups Biochem Genet.* 15:285–297.

Stratil, A. and Spooner, R.L. 1971. Isolation and properties of individual components of cattle transferrin: The role of sialic acid. *Biochem Genet.* 5:347–365.

Stratil, A., Tomasek, V., Bobak, P., and Glasnak, V. 1984b. Heterogeneity of horse transferrin: The role of carbohydrate moiety. *Anim Blood Groups Biochem Genet.* 15:89–101.

Strickland, D.K. and Hudson, B.G. 1978. Structural studies on rabbit transferrin: Isolation and characterization of the glycopeptides. *Biochemistry.* 17:3411–3418.

Sundelin, J., Melhus, H., Das, S., et al. 1985. The primary structure of rabbit and rat prealbumin and a comparison with the tertiary structure of human prealbumin. *J Biol Chem.* 260:6481–6487.

Sutton, H.E. 1970. The haptoglobins. In *Progress in Medical Genetics.* Steinburg, A.G. and Bearn, A.G. Vol. 7. New York and London: Grune & Stratton.

Takahashi, M., Takahashi, Y., and Putman, F.W. 1985b. Complete amino acid sequence of human hemopexin, the heme-binding protein of serum. *Proc Natl Acad Sci USA.* 82:73–77.

Takahashi, N., Takahashi, Y., Heiny, M.E., and Putman, F.W. 1985a. Purification of hemopexin and its domain fragments by affinity chromatography and high performance liquid chromatography. *J Chromatogr.* 326:373–385.

Tarnoky, A.L. 1980. Genetic and drug induced variations in serum albumin. *Adv Clin Chem.* 21:101–146.

Titlebach, V. and Gilpin, R.K. 1995. Species dependency of the liquid chromatographic properties of silica-immobilized serum albumins. *Anal Chem.* 67:44–47.

Tranz, J.C., Garza, T., and Sanders, B.G. 1975. Structural characterization of polymeric haptoglobin from goats. *Comp Biochem Physiol B.* 51:93–97.

Vahlquist, A. and Petersone, P.A. 1972. Comparative studies on the vitamin A transporting protein complex in human and cynomolous plasma. *Biochemistry.* 1:4526–4532.

Valenta, M., Stratil, A., Slechtova, V., Kalal, L., and Slechta, V. 1976. Polymorphism of transferrin in carp (*Cyprinus carpio* L.). Genetic determination, isolation, and partial characterization. *Biochem Genet.* 14:27–45.

Van Baelan, H., and De Moor, P. 1974. Immunochemical quantitation of human transcortin. *J Clin Endocrinol Metab.* 39:160–163.

Van Der Heul, C., Froos, M.J., and van Eijk, H.C. 1982. Characterization and localization of the transferrin receptor or rat reticulocytes. *Int J Biochem.* 14:467–476.

Van Der Walt, B.J., and van Jaarsveld, P.P. 1978. Bovine thyroxine-binding globulin. *Biochim Biophys Acta.* 535:44–53.

Van Gelder, W., Huijkes-Heins, M.I., Hukshorn, C.J., de Jeu-Jaspars, C.M., van Noort, W.L., and van Eijk, H.G. 1995. Isolation, purification, and characterization of porcine serum transferrin and hemopexin. *Comp Biochem Physiol B Biochem Mol Biol.* 111:171–179.

Voelkel, E.F., Levine, L., Alper, C.A., and Tashjian, A.H. 1978. Acute-phase reactants ceruloplasmin and haptoglobin and their relationship to plasma prostaglandins in rabbits bearing the VX carcinoma. *J Exp Med.* 147:1078–1088.

Waites, G.T., Bell, A.M., and Bell, S.G. 1983. Acute phase serum proteins in syngeneic and allogeneic mouse pregnancy. *Clin Exp Immunol.* 53:225–232.

Wei, S., Episkopou, V., Piantedosi, R., et al. 1995. Studies on the metabolism of retinol and retinol-binding protein in transthyretin-deficient mice produced by homologous recombination. *J Biol Chem.* 270:866–870.

Weigle, W.O. 1961. Immunochemical properties of the cross-reactions between anti-BAS and heterologous albumins. *J Immunol.* 87:599–607.

Weiss, M.L., Goodman, M., Prychodko, W., and Tanaka, T. 1971. Species and geographic distribution patterns of the macaque prealbumin polymorphism. *Primates.* 12:75–80.

Weitkamp, L.R. 1978. Equine markers genes: Polymorphism for group-specific components (Gc). *Anim Blood Groups Biochem Genet.* 9:123–126.

Westphal, U. 1971. *Steroid Protein Interactions*, pp. 164–350. Berlin: Springer-Verlag.

Witz, I. and Gross, J. 1965. Purification and partial characterization of mouse hemopexin (beta 2-III globulin). *Proc Soc Exp Med.* 118:1003–1006.

Wolf, G. 1995. Retinol transport and metabolism in transthyretin-"knockout" mice. *Nutr Rev.* 53:98–99.

Wu, M.L. and Morgan, W.T. 1995. Thermodynamics of heme-induced conformational changes in hemopexin: Role of domain–domain interaction. *Protein Sci.* 4:29–34.

Yamamoto, Y., Yoshizawa, T., Kamio, S., et al. 1997. Interactions of transthyretin (TTR) and retinol-binding protein (RBP) in the uptake of retinol by primary rat hepatocytes. *Exp Cell Res.* 234:373–378.

Yang, F., Bergeron, J.M., Linehan, L.A., Lalley, P.A., Sakaguchi, A.Y., and Bowman, B.H. 1990. Mapping and conservation of the group-specific component gene in mouse. *Genomics.* 7:509–516.

Yang, F., Friedrichs, W.E., and Coalson, J.J. 1997. Regulation of transferrin gene expression during lung development and injury. *Am J Physiol.* 273:417–426.

Yedgar, S., Carew, T.E., Pittman, R.C., Beltz, W., and Steinberg, D. 1983. Tissue sites of catabolism of albumin in rabbits. *Am J Physiol.* 244:E101–E107.

Yoshioka, N. and Atassi, M.Z. 1986. Hemoglobin binding with haptoglobin. *Biochem J.* 234:453–456.

Young, S. 1982. Evidence for the functional equivalence of the iron-binding sites of rat transferrin. *Biochimica Bio-phys Acta.* 718:35–41.

Young, C.R., Eckersall, P.D., Saini, P.K., and Stanker, L.H. 1995. Validation of immunoassays for bovine haptoglobin. *Vet Immunol Immunopathol.* 49:1–13.

19 Acute Phase Proteins

Claire L. Parry

CONTENTS

19.1 INTRODUCTION

The acute phase response encompasses a broad spectrum of pathophysiological changes that occur in an animal following numerous stimuli such as infection, tissue injury, or trauma. Among the systemic alterations are fever, leukocytosis, activation of complement and coagulation cascades, production and secretion of cytokines and glucocorticoids, and changes in the circulating levels of some plasma proteins (Watterson, 2009; Baumann and Gauldie, 1990; Dowton and Colten, 1988; Eckersall, 1995; Gruys et al., 1994; Heinrich et al., 1990; Titus et al., 1991). These liver-derived plasma proteins are collectively referred to as acute phase reactant (APR) proteins. Alterations in serum levels of individual APR proteins can occur within a few hours after exposure to an inflammatory stimulus (Kushner, 1988). Due to their value as markers of inflammation, they are being increasingly used as a diagnostic aid in both human and veterinary medicine (Watterson et al., 2008; Eckersall, 1995; Gruys et al., 1994; Kent, 1992).

The liver is the principal target of systemic inflammatory mediators; all or most hepatocytes, irrespective of their location in the lobule, are able to respond to these mediators and alter their rate of synthesis and secretion of APR proteins (Feldmann et al., 1989). These APR proteins can be broadly classified into two categories, depending on whether their circulating levels increase (positive APR proteins) or decrease (negative APR proteins) in response to an inflammatory stimulus. Interspecies variations exist in the hepatic response, which is reflected as species variations in serum levels of individual APR proteins (Table 19.1). In general, C-reactive protein (CRP), serum amyloid P (SAP), serum amyloid A (SAA), α_1-acid glycoprotein (α_1-AGP), haptoglobin, α_1-proteinase inhibitor (α_1-PI), α_2-macroglobulin (α_2M), ceruloplasmin (Cer), complement component C3, and fibrinogen (Fib) function as positive APR proteins, while albumin and transferrin respond as negative APRs (Watterson, 2009; Watterson et al., 2008).

TABLE 19.1
Examples of Interspecies Differences in Acute-Phase Reactant Proteins

Species	CRP	SAP	SAA	α_1-AGP	α_1-PI	α_2M	CP	Fib
Human	++++	0	++++	++	++	0	++	++
Mouse	+	+++	++++[a]	0	++[a]	+/−	++	++
Rat	++	0	0	+++	++	++++[a]	++	++
Dog	+++	0	++	++	+/−	+/−	++	++

CRP, C-reactive protein; SAP, serum amyloid P; SAA, serum amyloid A; α_1AGP, α_1-acid glycoprotein; α_1-PI, α_1-proteinase inhibitor; α_2M, $\alpha_2$macroglobulin; CP, ceruloplasmin; Fib, fibrinogen.

[a] Strain-dependent acute phase reponses; +/− = variable results recorded; 0 = not an acute phase reactant.

The overall importance of the positive APRs as a part of the animal's defense mechanism in the early stages of inflammation is reflected in the broad spectrum of their collective activities and the highly evolutionarily conserved nature of members of this group of proteins. These include scavenging free radicals, hemoglobin, and nuclear debris; modulating proteolytic enzyme activity; binding to bacterial components; activating complement; and regulating lipid metabolism (Watterson, 2009; Watterson et al., 2008; Dowton and Colten, 1988; French, 1989; Gruys et al., 1994; Heinrich et al., 1990; Mackiewicz et al., 1988).

Despite the intraspecies and interbreed differences observed for individual proteins, there exists overall a high degree of similarity in the qualitative and quantitative patterns of APR protein responses to inflammation and trauma. The cytokine and hormone specificities of gene regulation and the genetic elements controlling the transcription of genes for specific APR proteins are quite similar for homologous genes among various species. The mediators involved in APR regulation can be divided into four main categories: interleukin-1 (IL-1) type cytokines, IL-6 type cytokines, glucocorticoids, and growth factors (Baumann and Gauldie, 1994; Murata et al., 2004). Cytokines act as primary stimulators of APR protein gene expression, while glucocorticoids and growth factors function more as modulators of cytokine function. In some species, the expression of specific APR proteins is also controlled by steroid hormones, which contributes to the altered levels observed for several of the proteins associated with age, sex, and pregnancy.

The analysis of APR proteins has been facilitated in recent years by the development of molecular biological techniques and advances in the application of immunological procedures. Initially, gross changes in the profile of plasma proteins following inflammation were evaluated by monitoring increased production in α- and β-globulins with either cellulose or agarose electrophoresis (French, 1989). Alterations in individual proteins were generally quantified with biochemical assays that did not always permit precise discrimination between different plasma proteins with related functional activity, for example, antiproteinases (French, 1989). Due to the increasing commercial availability of species-specific antibody reagents to individual APR proteins, immunological assays are now generally used to quantitate the levels of individual APR proteins in animal sera (Watterson et al., 2008).

The information that has accumulated over the past decade on the mediators regulating the hepatic expression of APR proteins in laboratory animals and the extensive studies with laboratory animals on the role of these proteins in ameliorating the extent of tissue damage subsequent to inflammation and trauma have made a significant contribution to expanding the appreciation of the biological role(s) of the individual proteins in mammalian health and disease. This chapter will focus on those APR proteins listed in Table 19.1. Descriptions of the transport proteins, haptoglobin, transferrin, albumin, and complement C3 component are provided in other sections of the text.

19.2 α_1-ACID GLYCOPROTEIN

19.2.1 Properties

α_1-AGP, also referred to as orosomucoid or seromucoid, is a normal constituent of mammalian plasma that has been shown to respond as an APR in humans, rats, mice, and dogs. α_1-AGP is now classified as one of the lipocalins, which are a group of proteins that bind lipophilic substances (Murata et al., 2004; Hochepied et al., 2003).

Human α_1-AGP circulates as a single polypeptide chain consisting of 183 amino acids and two disulphide bonds (Kremer et al., 1988; Schmid, 1975; Schmid et al., 1973, 1974). The molecular weight of native human α_1-AGP varies between 37 and 54 kDa due to (1) microheterogeneity in the carbohydrate moieties, (2) the laboratory procedures used to isolate the protein, and (3) the tissue source of the protein (reviewed in Kremer et al., 1988). The α_1-AGPs isolated from mice, rabbits, and dogs show similar size and carbohydrate profiles as the human protein (Baumann et al., 1984; Charlwood et al., 1976; Dello et al., 1988). Rat hepatocyte cultures secrete two forms of α_1-AGP, a

39-kDa α_1-AGP-1 form and an α_1-AGP-2 form, which exhibit a molecular weight range of 43–60 kDa depending on the carbohydrate content (Andus et al., 1988; Nicollet et al., 1981). Lower molecular weight forms of α_1-AGP (with lower sialic acid content) are preferentially expressed in rats during the inflammatory response (Venembre et al., 1993). The concanavalin A binding patterns of α_1-AGPs isolated from the sera of dogs with and without inflammation indicate that in this species, there is no preferrential expression of a particular form of AGP during an inflammatory response (Dello et al., 1988).

In some strains of mice, such as BALB/c, two distinct α_1-AGP-mRNAs are expressed, which result in the synthesis of two α_1-AGPs of differing size and charge (Baumann et al., 1984; Yiangou and Papaconstantinou, 1993). These mouse proteins are encoded on genes *Apg-1* and *Apg-2*, which are both located on chromosome 4 (Baumann and Berger, 1985). Some inbred mouse strains, such as CE/J, express only one form of α1-AGP as a consequence of gene deletion (Baumann and Berger, 1985). In rats, there appears to be a single α_1-AGP gene (Liao et al., 1985; Reinke and Feigelson, 1985). However, comparison of the complementary DNA (cDNA) sequences among rats and mice indicates significant homology between the deduced amino acid sequences of the respective α_1-AGP proteins (Cooper and Papaconstantinou, 1986). Similarly, there is significant homology between rat and human α_1-AGP (Fournier et al., 2000; Ricca et al., 1981).

Although secretion of α_1-AGP by human T lymphocytes during the acute phase response has been reported (Haston et al., 2002; Fournier et al., 2000; Laurent, 1989), the synthesis of α_1-AGP occurs primarily in the liver (Courtoy et al., 1981; Feldman et al., 1989; Jamieson and Ashton, 1973). Hepatic synthesis of α_1-AGP is induced by a variety of inflammatory agents, including lipopolysaccharide (LPS) and turpentine (Schreiber et al., 1986), thermal injury (Gilpin et al., 1996), hypoxia (Wenger et al., 1995), exposure to heavy metals (Yiangou and Papaconstantinou, 1993; Yiangou et.al., 1991), and phenobarbital administration (Chauvelot-Moachon et al., 1988; Fournier et al., 1994). The mechanism of α_1-AGP induction associated with each inflammatory stimulus is similar but differs from the induction mechanism of phenobarbital, which does not function through an acute phase response mechanism (Fournier et al., 2000, 1994; Gilpin et al., 1996; Kremer et al., 1988; Yiangou and Papaconstantinou, 1993; Yiangou et al., 1991).

The synthesis of α_1-AGP is influenced by both cytokines and glucocorticoids (Baumann et al., 1983, 1990, 1993; Dewey et al., 1990; Koj et al., 1984; Prowse and Baumann, 1989; Richards et al., 1992; Won and Baumann, 1990; Hochepied et al., 2003), and it is regulated at both transcriptional and posttranscriptional levels (Baumann, 1990; Ingrassia et al., 1994; Vannice et al., 1984). Maximal expression of α_1-AGP-mRNA and protein synthesis requires the synergistic action of glucocorticoids and cytokines (Prowse and Baumann, 1989; Vannice et al., 1984). Distal regulatory elements responsive to IL-1, IL-6, tumor necrosis factor-α (TNFα), leukemia inhibitory factor (LIF), and phorbol esters have been located on the cDNA nucleotide sequence upstream from the transcription site (Dewey et al., 1990; Won and Baumann, 1990). A single glucocorticoid response element (GRE) has also been identified. However, in both rats and mice, the GRE alone is not sufficient to activate transcription, and the presence of other transcription factor(s) are required, such as α_1-AGP/enhancer-binding protein (a member of the C/EBP transcription family), α_1-AGP nuclear factor, and NF-κB (Baumann et al., 1991, 1992; De Lorenzo et al., 1991; Ingrassia et al., 1994; Lee et al., 1996; Ratajczak et al., 1992).

The serum half-life of α_1-AGP is 5.5 days in people (Weisman et al., 1961), 3.7 days in dogs (Zeineh et al., 1972), and about 24 hours in rats (Kuranda and Aronson, 1983). Studies of α_1-AGP catabolism in rats indicate that several tissues, including kidney, liver, muscle, and skin, may be active in degrading the protein (Kuranda and Aronson, 1983).

19.2.2 Role/Function

Although the physiological functions of α_1-AGP have yet to be fully defined, available evidence suggests that it may act as a nonspecific immunosuppressant (Laurent, 1989) and that it may also serve as a transporter of cationic compounds (Kremer et al., 1988; Hochepied et al., 2003; Smith et al., 2002). For example, α_1-AGP can suppress human T-cell activation at concentrations below those observed during the human acute phase response (Laurent, 1989). Human α_1-AGP can also suppress the murine lymphocyte mitogenic response and inhibit neutrophil activation (Costello et al., 1984). The effectiveness of the immunosupression is enhanced when the sialic acid content of α_1-AGP is reduced (Bennett and Schtmidt, 1980). While there are conflicting reports on the role of sialic acid in the regulation of the inhibitory effects of α_1-AGP on human platelet aggregation (Andersen and Eika, 1980; Costello et al., 1979), the increased reactivity of desialylated α_1-AGP could have important implications in disease conditions, because in humans and rats, inflammation is associated with a reduction in the sialic acid content of α_1-AGP (Serbource-Goguel Seta et al., 1986; Venembre et al., 1993; Murata et al., 2004; Fournier et al., 2000).

There have been numerous studies on the affinity of neutral and basic drugs for α_1-AGP (Kremer et al., 1988). In people, due to the increased plasma levels of α_1-AGP as a result of disease, drug use, and pregnancy, and due to its greater drug affinity, α_1-AGP is considered a more important drug ligand than albumin (Kremer et al., 1988). Hormones, such as progesterone, cortisol, and testosterone, appear to become associated with human α_1-AGP at a single binding site, while estradiol can interact at several sites (Kerkay and Westphal, 1968). Drugs such as propranolol also appear to bind to α_1-AGP at a single site (Kremer et al., 1988). Indeed, the ability to bind propranolol is a consistent feature of α_1-AGP in dogs, rats, rabbits, and sheep as well as people, and the protein–drug interaction results in alterations in the pharmacokinetics and pharmacodynamics of propranolol (Murata et al., 2004; Fournier et al., 2000; Hochepied et al., 2003; Belpaire et al., 1984; Evans et al., 1973; Hill et al., 1989).

A1AG is a natural anti-inflammatory agent as it inhibits mitogen-induced lymphocyte proliferation, natural killer cell activity, neutrophil activation, and increases the secretion of IL-1 receptor antagonist by macrophages (Murata et al., 2004; Fournier et al., 2000). At low concentrations, A1AG exerts an aggregating effect on neutrophils, while at higher concentrations, it inhibits aggregation. It also inhibits superoxide generation by neutrophils stimulated either by opsonized zymozan or phorbol myristate actetate. The inhibitory effect is dose dependent and inversely proportional to the concentration of the stimulus. This suggests that A1AG acts on the neutrophil membrane, rather than the stimulus itself (Hochepied et al., 2003). A1AG inhibits thrombin-induced platelet aggregation and also aggregation initiated by ADP or adrenalin in a dose-dependent manner. In all cases, inhibition of aggregation is directed against the second wave of platelet aggregation and subsequently as an inhibitor of the release reaction. This suggests that A1AG contributes to the downregulation of the further recruitment of platelets. This function is shared with polymorphonuclear leucocytes, which are in close contact with platelets and serves as an antithrombic function by inhibiting further platelet activation and recruitment. The local production of A1AG by these leucocytes may be one of the mechanisms by which the leucocytes exert their antithrombic function (Hochepied et al., 2003; Kremer et al., 1988; Fournier et al., 2000).

It has been suggested that A1AG is required to maintain capillary permeability by increasing the polyanionic charge selectively of the endothelial barrier. It has also been reported that the partially protective effect of A1AG in different rodent models of shock can be explained by enhancing the capillary barrier function and thereby maintaining the perfusion of vital organs (Fournier et al., 2000; Kremer et al., 1988). In addition, A1AG has also been found to facilitate the passage of erythrocytes through membranes. A1AG increases the bilayer thickness of liposomes and decreases the permeability for ions (Kremer et al., 1988).

19.2.3 Analytical Methods

The various methods used to isolate human α_1-AGP have been reviewed (Kremer et al., 1988), and the influence of different laboratory procedures on the desialylation, denaturation, and polymerization of the molecule documented. Due to poor cross-reactivity, antiserum to human α_1-AGP cannot be used to assess α_1-AGP in sera from other species (Chauvelot-Moachon et al., 1988). One of the characteristics of α_1-AGP is that unlike 98% of plasma proteins, it is nonprecipitable with 1.2 M perchloric acid. Hence, this acid treatment has been used as a means of isolating α_1-AGP from mammalian plasma (Hill et al., 1989). Cation exchange chromatography has also been used for the purification of rat α_1-AGP (Chauvelot-Moachon et al., 1988) as has immunoaffinity chromatography (Drechou et al., 1989).

Various methods that have been employed to evaluate α_1-AGP in mammalian plasma have been reviewed (French, 1989). Currently, immunological methods are the most commonly used procedures in laboratory animal medicine (Chauvelot-Moachon et al., 1988; Gilpin et al., 1996; Ikawa and Shozen, 1990; Koj et al., 1984; Poüs et al., 1990). A commercial radial immunodiffusion kit method has been used for canine plasma (Rikihisa et al., 1994) that yielded a baseline α_1-AGP value of 0.37 ± 0.04 mg/mL in healthy dogs, compared to baseline values of around 0.5 mg/mL reported with a lectin/glycoprotein precipitation method (Conner and Eckersall, 1988).

19.2.4 Pathophysiological Significance

Injection of IL-6 into male Wistar rats produced a 16-fold increase in hepatic α_1-AGP-mRNA within 4 hours, which was considerably faster than the 16–25-hour response time following turpentine injection (Geiger et al., 1988a). Male Buffalo rats also responded to turpentine by expressing increased levels of α_1-AGP-mRNA, but only a moderate increase was observed following administration of IL-1 (De Jong et al., 1988; Schreiber et al., 1986). In cultured rat hepatoma cells, increased expression of α_1-AGP-mRNA could only be induced by a hepatocyte-stimulating factor when dexamethasone was also added to the culture medium (Baumann et al., 1987a). Similarly, the combined action of TNFα and IL-1 had a greater effect on α_1-AGP synthesis in rat hepatoma cells than the individual cytokines, and the response could be further enhanced by inclusion of hepatocyte growth factor (HGF) in the culture medium (Baumann et al., 1993; Poüs et al., 1990). Likewise, in mouse hepatocytes, neither IL-1 nor IL-6 alone stimulated α_1-AGP production above basal levels, and only a 1.5–2.0-fold increase was induced by dexamethasone alone (Prowse and Baumann, 1989). However, when the hepatocytes were exposed to a combination of each cytokine and dexamethasone, a fivefold increase in both α_1-AGP-mRNA and α_1-AGP protein synthesis was observed (Prowse and Baumann, 1989). In both rat and human hepatocyte cultures, insulin (unlike glucagon, growth hormone, or catecholamines) can cause a rapid, nonspecific decrease in the synthesis of α_1-AGP induced by a combination of IL-1, IL-6, and dexamethasone (Campos and Baumann, 1992).

The human range for serum α_1-AGP is accepted to be between 0.5 and 1.0 mg/mL, which increases two- to threefold in many disease conditions (Kremer et al., 1988). For example, in individuals with advanced rheumatoid arthritis, average serum levels of 2.2 mg/mL have been reported compared to 0.4 mg/mL in a healthy control group (Lacki et al., 1994). Using similar assay procedures, average serum α_1-AGP values have been determined as 0.9 mg/mL in Wistar rats (Koj et al., 1984), 0.4 mg/mL in male F344 rats (Poüs et al., 1990), 0.3 mg/mL in Sprague-Dawley rats (Chauvelot-Moachon et al., 1988), and 0.3 g/L in Dark Agouti rats (Chauvelot-Moachon et al., 1988). The extent of the increase observed in serum α_1-AGP levels in rats depends on the strain of the rat and the type of stimulus to which the animals are exposed. For example, in F344 rats that are more susceptible to thermal injury than the Buffalo strain, serum α_1-AGP levels rose 1600-fold following burn injury compared to only 300-fold in the Buffalo strain (Gilpin et al., 1996). In comparison, only a threefold increase in serum α_1-AGP was observed in Fisher rats following treatment with either turpentine or dexamethasone (Koj et al., 1984; Poüs et al., 1990). Phenobarbital administration caused a relatively modest increase in serum α_1-AGP in Sprague-Dawley rats, with levels rising from 0.30 ± 0.04 mg/mL to 0.49 ± 0.05 mg/mL, while it produced a fivefold increase in serum α_1-AGP levels in Dark Agouti rats, a strain that is susceptible to adjuvant-induced arthritis (Chauvelot-Moachon et al., 1988).

In dogs, α_1-AGP values rise in response to endotoxin (Eckersall et al., 1985) and following surgical trauma (Conner and Eckersall, 1988). The serum α_1-AGP values of healthy dogs have been variously reported as 0.37 ± 0.04 mg/mL and 0.47 ± 0.09 mg/mL, which rises to 2.85 ± 0.51 mg/mL during inflammatory reactions (Belpaire et al., 1987; Dello et al., 1988). However, increases as high as 17-fold above baseline have also been reported in dogs with inflammatory diseases (Ganrot, 1973a). The 1.9–8.6-fold increase in serum α_1-AGP levels observed in dogs 4–6 days after inoculation with *Ehrlichia canis* was significantly greater than the elevation recorded for serum CRP levels (Rikihisa et al., 1994).

In most inbred strains of mice, the two forms of α_1-AGP (AGP-1 and AGP-2) are equally inducible by acute inflammation. However, the predominant expression switches to AGP-2 in chronic inflammation (Glibetic and Baumann, 1986). This response is similar to the α_1-AGP induction with heavy metals in BALB/c mice (Yiangou and Papaconstantinou, 1993). Prior to administration of mercury (0.5 mg $HgCl_2$/kg), hepatic AGP-2-mRNA levels were approximately 10-fold higher than AGP-1-mRNA levels, while at the peak of induction with Hg, AGP-2-mRNA was 80–100-fold higher than the AGP-1-mRNA (Yiangou and Papaconstantinou, 1993). Although adrenalectomy had no effect on the induction of AGP-2, the AGP-1 response was delayed in the adrenalectomized animals (Yiangou and Papaconstantinou, 1993). These studies confirm that the α_1-AGP response is mediated by multiple factors and that the mechanism of induction has not yet been fully elucidated.

In rats, as in people, inflammatory stimuli alter the extent of glycosylation of the α_1-AGP molecules secreted into the circulation during the acute phase of the reaction (Koj et al., 1982; Nicollet et al., 1981). In rats, the same type of response is observed in reaction to administration of either phenobarbital or pharmacological doses of estrogen (Diarra-Mehrpour et al., 1985; Monnet et al., 1986). In contrast, in dogs and mice, there is no change in the glycosylation profile of the increased amount of α_1-AGP released into the circulation during the acute phase reaction (Dello et al., 1988; Eckersall et al., 1985; Heegaard, 1992).

Growth and development can also influence the rate of α_1-AGP expression. Both newborn human infants and newborn rats have markedly lower serum α_1-AGP than adult animals (Ganrot, 1972; Glibetic et al., 1992). In fetal rats, though α_1-AGP-mRNA can be detected in the liver, inflammation in the mother does not induce an increase in the fetal hepatic transcription rate (Yiangou and Papaconstantinou, 1993). This differs from the response of fetal α_2M and haptoglobin, which exhibit increased hepatic fetal transcription rates of their respective mRNAs in response to maternal stimulation (Yiangou and Papaconstantinou, 1993).

19.3 α_1-PROTEINASE INHIBITOR

19.3.1 Properties

α_1-PI, also called α_1-antitrypsin, is the prototypical member of the family of serine proteinase inhibitors (Serpins) found in the circulation of all mammals (Goodwin et al., 1996; Potema et al., 1994; Travis and Salveson, 1983). During acute inflammation, the massive release of proteolytic enzymes from injured tissue and inflammatory cells disturbs the dynamic equilibrium between blood and tissue proteinases and their inhibitors (French, 1989; Koj et al., 1988). In laboratory animals, α_1-PI, along with α_2-M, has a critical role in modulating the extent of increased protease activity and hence limiting the extent of tissue damage.

There is considerable structural homology among the α_1-PIs isolated from mammalian plasma. Human, rat, mouse, rabbit, guinea pig, gerbil, canine, and monkey α_1-PIs are all single-chain glycoproteins consisting of 370–390 amino acids with molecular weights ranging from 51 to 60 kDa (Carrell et al., 1982; Goodwin et al., 1996; Goto et al., 1994; Koj et al., 1988; Melgarejo et al., 1996; Poller et al., 1995; Potema et al., 1994; Travis and Salveson, 1983; Verbanac and Heath, 1983). Extensive homology has been found among human, rat, guinea pig, mouse, rabbit, gerbil, and baboon α_1-PI amino acid sequences (Goodwin et al., 1996; Melgarejo et al., 1996; Nakatani et al.,

1995; Saito and Sinohara, 1991, 1995). The arrangement of amino acids in the reactive center of the molecule is critical for recognition and binding to target proteinases and highly conserved among human, rat, rabbit, canine, hamster, and gerbil α_1-PIs (Chao et al., 1990; Goto et al., 1994; Melgarejo et al., 1996; Nakatani et al., 1995; Saito and Sinohara, 1991). An exception is mouse α_1-PI, which exhibits considerable structural variation, not only in comparison to human α_1-PI but also in the amino acid sequences of the α_1-PIs isolated from different domestic and wild-type mouse strains (Goodwin et al., 1996).

In people and rats, a single α_1-PI gene has been identified, while in guinea pigs and rabbits, multigene families are found (Chao et al., 1990; Long et al., 1984; Ray et al., 1994, 1996; Suzuki et al., 1990). In mice, a single gene has been reported for *Mus caroli*, *Mus cooki*, *Mus cervicolor*, *Mus pahari*, and *Mus minutoides*, while three to five genes for α_1-PI are present in *Mus domesticus*, *Mus spretus*, *Mus hortulanus*, and *Mus saxicolo* (Goodwin et al., 1996; Rheaume et al., 1994). In *Mus musculus*, α_1-PI is encoded by two multigene families located on chromosome 12 (Goodwin et al., 1996; Hill et al., 1985).

In addition to microheterogeneity of serum α_1-PIs as a result of variations in carbohydrate content, various isoforms of α_1-PI are also present in many species. These isoforms exhibit both different biological functions and different acute phase responses (Chao et al., 1990; Melgarejo et al., 1996; Nathoo and Finlay, 1986; Sevelius et al., 1994; Verbanac and Heath, 1983). For example, two forms of guinea pig α_1-PI have been identified: a fast moving 61 kDa "F" form and a slower moving 55 kDa "S" form (Suzuki et al., 1990). Both forms exhibit similar substrate specificity, but only the S form, which is present in barely detectable amounts in healthy animals, acts as an acute phase protein (Suzuki et al., 1990). Four isoforms of α_1-PI, designated as F, S-1, S-2, and E, have been identified in rabbits, and as occurs in guinea pigs, the F form is the major form of α_1-PI present in normal serum (Koj et al., 1978; Ray et al., 1994; Saito and Sinohara, 1993, 1995). The rabbit isoforms of α_1-PI exhibit a variety of biological activities (Koj et al., 1978; Ray et al., 1994; Saito and Sinohara, 1988, 1993, 1995). Both S-1 and S-2 can inhibit elastase but not trypsin activity, while the E form does not exhibit proteolytic inhibitory activity despite its capacity to form equimolar complexes with both elastase and trypsin (Ganrot, 1966; Saito and Sinohara, 1988, 1995). A similar pattern of α_1-PI isoform activity has been found in *M. musculus* (Paterson and Moore, 1996). Of the five highly related α_1-PI proteins expressed in this strain, only two are efficient inhibitors of neutrophil elastase, and there is poor correlation between substrate binding and inhibitory activities (Paterson and Moore, 1996).

The cDNA encoding rat α_1-PI shares 70%–80% sequence identity with its human and mouse counterparts (Chao et al., 1990). Similarly, the rabbit liver cDNA coding for the F isoform of α_1-PI exhibits 74% and 64% homology at the nucleotide and amino acid levels, respectively, with human α_1-PI (Saito and Sinohara, 1991). The rabbit F and S isoforms share 95% homology in their complete amino acid sequences, and nine of the twenty amino acid differences that exist are located in the stretch of amino acids encompassing the reactive site region (Saito and Sinohara, 1993).

The hepatocyte is the primary source of serum α_1-PI (Carlson et al., 1984; Hood et al., 1980; Mackiewicz and Kushner, 1989), though low levels of synthesis have also been reported in alveolar epithelial cells, submandibular glands, alveolar macrophages, neutrophils, and activated lymphocytes (Bashir et al., 1992; Carlson et al., 1988; Chao et al., 1990; Du Bois et al., 1991; Takemura et al., 1986; Venembre et al., 1994). Evaluation of human α_1-PI expression in transgenic mice has confirmed that the presence of α_1-PI in extrahepatic tissue is the result of de novo synthesis and not endocytosis of the protein. Studies in rabbits, rats, and mice have demonstrated that expression of α_1-PI is regulated at the transcriptional level through *cis*-regulatory elements (Latimer et al., 1990; Montgomery et al., 1990; Ray et al., 1996; Rheaume et al., 1988). The synthesis of α_1-PI in different tissues is regulated by different factors. For example, in *M. caroli*, which is characterized by the accumulation of α_1-PI-mRNA in the kidneys, the expression of renal but not hepatic mRNA is regulated by testosterone (Latimer et al., 1987). Sexual dimorphism in serum α_1-PI levels has been observed in dogs and mice, with females exhibiting higher values than males (Hughes et al., 1995;

Kueppers and Mills, 1983). In monocytes and macrophages, LPS stimulates α_1-PI synthesis, while in human hepatocyte cultures, exposure to IL-6 alone is sufficient to increase the rate of α_1-PI synthesis (Barbey-Morel et al., 1987; Perlmutter et al., 1989).

Serpins such as α_1-PI are found in the circulation in three forms: (1) active or native, (2) inactive or cleaved, and (3) as stable serpin–enzyme complexes (Travis and Salveson, 1983). The cleavage of human α_1-PI by mouse macrophage elastase, a metalloproteinase, results in the rearrangement and inactivation of the molecule (Banda et al., 1988). The native and inactive α_1-PIs are immunologically identical, and both forms are eliminated from the circulation more slowly than the serpin–enzyme complexes (Mast et al., 1991). The rapid clearance of these α_1-PI-enzyme complexes from the circulation is mediated by the liver through their interaction with the low-density lipoprotein receptor (LDLR) or an LDLR-related protein (LPR) (Kounnas et al., 1996; Poller et al., 1995). Macrophages and fibroblasts also express high concentrations of LPR (Moestrup et al., 1992) that contributes to the selective cellular degradation of the complexed forms of α_1-PI (Kounnas et al., 1996). The affinity of hepatic LPR for α_1-PI complexes is lower than that of the serpin–enzyme complexes formed with α_2-M (Kounnas et al., 1996).

19.3.2 Role/Function

The primary function of α_1-PI is thought to be its role as a modulator of the proteinases released from infiltrating neutrophils and macrophages, as well as from damaged cells, during acute inflammation. In both people and mice genetically deficient in α_1-PI activity, spontaneous emphysematous lesions are associated with a progressive increase in elastase activity in the alveolar interstitium, resulting in the degradation of matrix proteins (De Santi et al., 1995; Martorana et al., 1993; Snider et al., 1991). Examination of pulmonary changes as a consequence of experimentally induced alveolar sepsis in Pallid, C57BL/6J, and NMRI mice, which have low, intermediate, and high levels of serum α_1-PI activity, respectively, demonstrated that the degree of lung destruction was inversely correlated with elastase inhibitory activity levels and hence related to serum α_1-PI activity (Cavarra et al., 1996). The increase in cellular infiltration into alveolar spaces observed in the Pallid and C57BL/6J mice (but not in NMIR mice) was considered to be related to the ability of the inactivated or cleaved form of α_1-PI to act as a chemoattractant (Banda et al., 1988). In addition to its function as an elastase inhibitor, α_1-PI may also have a role in the alveolar metabolism of lung surfactant, possibly through its inhibitory action on the surfactant convertase enzyme, which is a serine protease (Gross et al., 1995). Like α_1-AGP, α_1-PI may also have a more global role in regulating the inflammatory response because Buffalo rats, which are more resistant to thermal injury than F344 rats, exhibit higher hepatic α_1-PI-mRNA levels both before and after burn injury than the F344 strain (Gilpin et al., 1996).

19.3.3 Analytical Methods

The lack of cross-reactivity of α_1-PI between species has hindered the application of immunological methods for the accurate determination of this protein in mammalian sera. For example, a monoclonal antibody against human α_1-PI only cross-reacts with rat and baboon serum, and shows no reaction with serum from rabbits, hamsters, guinea pigs, or dogs (Silvestrini et al., 1990). The isolation procedures described for human, rat, guinea pig, gerbil, and canine α_1-PIs employed a variety of isolation steps, including ion exchange and affinity chromatography (Goto et al., 1994; McGilligan and Thomas, 1991; Melgarejo et al., 1996; Silvestrini et al., 1990; Suzuki et al., 1990). However, dogs, mice, and humans appear to the only species in which α_1-PI has been quantitated by an immunological procedure such as radial immunodiffusion (Baumann et al., 1986; Hughes et al., 1995). A specific enzyme-linked immunosorbent assay (ELISA) method has been developed for the determination of α_1-PI-bound leukocyte elastase in canine plasma and tissue fluids (Axelsson et al.,

1991). Using this procedure, it was determined that 70% of the elastase in canine plasma is bound to α_1-PI, while the remainder is bound to α_2-M.

Serum α_1-PI levels have usually been quantified with functional assays using chromogenic substrates to evaluate antielastase activity (Cavarra et al., 1996; Conner et al., 1988; Goto et al., 1994; James and Cohen, 1978; Laskowski, 1986; Martorana et al., 1993; Mullins et al., 1984; Schwarzenberg et al., 1987; Suzuki et al., 1990). The use of low-molecular-weight substrates (e.g., benzoyl-arginine-*p*-nitroanilide) rather than larger proteins prevents α_2-M from contributing to the apparent α_1-PI antiproteolytic activity, because only the α_1-PI-enzyme complexes remain active against the smaller synthetic compounds (French, 1989). When bovine trypsin, bovine chymotrypsin, or pancreatic elastase have been used to evaluate serum α_1-PI activity in laboratory animals, the results of the assays have only reflected broad antiprotease inhibitory activity in the sample and not the species-specific interaction between the target enzyme and the α_1-PI inhibitor and, hence, may have overestimated the actual α_1-PI inhibitory activity (French, 1989).

19.3.4 Pathophysiological Significance

The plasma levels of α_1-PI in most species are normally 1–4 mg/mL, with levels rising three- to fourfold under inflammatory conditions (French, 1989; Koj et al., 1988). In people, rats, rabbits, and guinea pigs, α_1-PI responds as a typical APR (French, 1989; Koj and Regoeczi 1978; Nakatani et al., 1995; Suzuki et al., 1990). The response of α_1-PI in mice is strain dependent. Although C57BL/6J mice show no increase in hepatic α_1-PI-mRNA or serum α_1-PI levels following turpentine or LPS administration (Baumann et al., 1986), in Swiss mice (Ha/ICR), a 35%–40% increase above baseline levels was found for both mRNA and serum α_1-PI values 12 hours after turpentine injection (Frazer et al., 1985). This variable response is compatible with the variation in baselines serum levels of α_1-PI found in different strains of mice. For example, in Pallid, C57BL/6J, and BALB/C strains, the serum α_1-PI values are 0.2 ± 0.1 mg/mL, 0.6 ± 0.1 mg/mL, and 0.7 ± 0.1 mg/mL, respectively (Martorana et al., 1993). A strain-dependent acute phase response has also been observed in rats following thermal trauma (Xia et al., 1992). Subsequent to burn injury, the increase in serum α_1-PI values was higher in the more resistant Buffalo rats than in the less resistant F344 rats (Xia et al., 1992).

In species that normally express multiple forms of α_1-PI, there appears to be a selective increase in the circulating levels of the individual isoforms following trauma. In rabbits, turpentine injection induced a 100-fold increase in the transcription rate of α_1-PI S-2 mRNA, while the mRNA transcription rate for the "F" and S-1 forms remains relatively constant (Ray et al., 1994). Similarly, in guinea pigs a significant increase in the circulating levels of the "S" form of α_1-PI occurred 3 days after turpentine injection, with serum levels rising from being barely detectable to approximately 1.3 g/L, while in comparison, the "F" form of α_1-PI only increased from 0.5 to 1.2 g/L (Suzuki et al., 1990).

The observations on the acute phase response of α_1-PI in dogs are contradictory. Serum α_1-PI values have been variously reported to increase (Conner et al., 1986; Lonky et al., 1980; Ohlsson, 1971), remain unchanged (Conner and Eckersall, 1988; Ganrot, 1973a), or decrease (Laurell and Rannevik, 1979; Murtaugh and Jacobs, 1985) as a result of inflammation. Whether the disparity of response is due to breed differences has yet to be determined. It is possible that serum values alone may not accurately reflect the extent of α_1-PI synthesis because, due to its relatively small size, α_1-PI can diffuse from the circulation into the interstitium (Andersen et al., 1994; Hughes et al., 1995). Hence, differences in the extent of extravasation of the protein during an inflammatory response can confound the observation and interpretation of alteration in serum α_1-PI values. Further, in dogs with liver disease, though only a modest elevation was detected in serum α_1-PI levels compared to healthy dogs, immunohistochemical staining of hepatic tissue demonstrated that α_1-PI had accumulated in the cytoplasm as a result of protein precipitation (Sevelius et al., 1994). This type of accumulation was only observed in dogs expressing the "S" isoform of α_1-PI and not in animals expressing only the F isoform of the protein (Sevelius et al., 1994).

The expression of α_1-PI can also be influenced by steroid hormones (Hughes et al., 1995; Kueppers and Mills, 1983). While the mean value for serum α_1-PI has been determined as 2.3 ± 0.4 mg/mL in healthy dogs, the value for intact females was 2.6 ± 0.1 mg/mL compared to 2.1 ± 0.1 mg mL in intact males (Hughes et al., 1995). In spayed females and castrated males, the serum α_1-PI values were 2.2 ± 0.1 mg/mL and 2.1 ± 0.1 mg/mL, respectively (Hughes et al., 1995). Increased serum α_1-PI activity has been reported in human females receiving oral contraceptive therapy (Song et al., 1970). These results suggest that in both dogs and people, α_1-PI production may be regulated by estrogen levels. In *M. caroli*, the developmental pattern of renal α_1-PI-mRNA but not hepatic mRNA appears to be regulated by testosterone levels, because large increases in α_1-PI-mRNA are observed in the kidneys at puberty in male mice (Rheaume et al., 1988). In rats, the rate of α_1-PI mRNA transcription is also regulated, at least in part, by pituitary hormones (Schwarzenberg et al., 1987). In Sprague-Dawley rats that underwent hypophysectomy, the drop in circulating levels of α_1-PI from 14.1 ± 0.8 mg/mL to 3.9 ± 0.4 mg/mL was matched by a 50%–75% drop in hepatic α_1-PI-mRNA levels (Schwarzenberg et al., 1987). The administration of growth hormone alone or the administration of a combination of thyroxine, corticosterone, and dihydrotestosterone failed to reverse the effects of hypophysectomy. However, when all four hormones were administered simultaneously to hypophysectomized rats, serum α_1-PI values rose to 8.8 ± 0.1 mg/mL, and a two- to threefold increase in hepatic α_1-PI mRNA levels was observed (Schwarzenberg et al., 1987).

19.4 α_2-MACROGLOBULIN

19.4.1 PROPERTIES

Protease inhibitors of the α_2M superfamily are all large glycoproteins characterized by their particular mechanism of nonspecific binding with proteinase enzymes (Gauthier and Mouray, 1976; Geiger et al., 1987; Starkey and Barrett, 1982). Amino acid sequence homology suggests that α_2M shares a common evolutionary origin with complement components C3 and C4 (Jensen et al., 2004; Sottrup-Jensen et al., 1984, 1985). In rats, α_2M is considered the prototype APR, though variable responses are observed in some other laboratory animals (French, 1989; Versavel et al., 1983; Weimer and Benjamin, 1965).

Rat α_2M, like human α_2M, consists of four identical 170 kDa subunits joined by disulfide bonds and strong noncovalent interactions (Nieuwenhuizen et al., 1979; Schaeufele and Koo, 1982). It has been estimated that there is 80% homology between the complete rat and human α_2M cDNA and amino acid sequences, and that all 25 cysteine residues in each α_2M subunit between rat α_2M and human α_2M are completely conserved (Beitel et al., 1986; Gehring et al., 1987; Northemann et al., 1985). A tetrameric form of α_2M, homologous with rat and human α_2M, is also found in mice (Overbergh et al., 1991; Umans et al., 1994; Van Leuven et al., 1992). Similiarly, the guinea pig and hamster forms of α_2M exhibit tetrameric structures (Godfrey et al., 1984; Miyake et al., 1993). Antibodies generated against human α_2M yield reactions of partial identity with monkey, cat, dog, and guinea pig plasma (Baker and Valli, 1988; Pellegrini, 1994; Suzuki and Sinohara, 1986). Structurally, hamster α_2M appears to be more loosely packed than native human α_2M and, following activation, undergoes conformation change more slowly than its human and rat counterparts (Miyake et al., 1993).

α_2M is unique as an antiproteinase both in terms of the broad spectrum of enzymes that it can inhibit and the nature of its inhibitory activity. In addition to binding to all types of serine proteases (serine, thiol, aspartic, and metallo), α_2M also possesses cytokine-binding properties through a "trapping" mechanism (Jensen et al., 2004; Barrett and Starkey, 1973). The interaction between α_2M and a protease results in the cleavage of a specific peptide bond within a small "bait" region near the center of each α_2M subunit (Sottrup-Jensen et al., 1989). The α_2M then undergoes a conformational change, trapping the proteinase and forming a nondissociable complex (Jensen et al., 2004; Sottrup-Jensen, 1989). The proteinase enzyme within this complex is protected from degradation by other proteinase inhibitors, while the reactive site of the enzyme retains reactivity toward small molecules, though steric hindrance impedes the enzymatic activity directed toward larger substrates (Andres et al., 1989; Barrett and Starkey, 1973). Similarly, when IL-6 is bound to human α_2M, it retains its biological activity and is resistant to proteolytic degradation (Matsuda et al., 1989). The α_2M molecules isolated from hamsters, guinea pigs, and rabbits exhibit several trypsin susceptible sites, in addition to the "bait" region (Gonias and Pizzo, 1983; Miyake et al., 1993; Suzuki and Sinohara, 1986; Tamamizu et al., 1989). Further, trypsin interacts with human α_2M at a 2:1 molar ratio (Travis and Salveson, 1983) and with rodent α_2Ms at a 1:1 ratio (Godfrey et al., 1984; Nieuwenhuizen et al., 1979; Suzuki and Sinohara, 1986; Van Leuven et al., 1992). In all species, the conformational change associated with the formation of an α_2M-proteinase complex results in alterated electrophoretic mobility of the α_2M molecule on polyacrylamide gel electrophoresis. The activated, or complexed, form of α_2M typically shows increased mobility relative to the native, or noncomplexed, form of the molecule (Barrett et al., 1979; Lamarre et al., 1991).

As a result of the activation-induced conformational change in the α_2M molecule, a latent receptor-binding domain is exposed that facilitates the rapid removal of α_2M-proteinase complexes from the circulation by α_2M-specific receptor-mediated endocytosis (Gonias et al., 1983; Imber and Pizzo, 1981; Lamarre et al., 1991). For example, the half-life of radiolabeled human α_2M-trypsin complexes in rats is only 2 minutes (Davidsen et al., 1985). There appears to be a common pathway for cellular uptake of both constitutive and acute phase macroglobulins in all mammals. Human and mouse α_2M-proteinase complexes are eliminated by the same receptor-mediated route (Gonias et al., 1983), which is compatible with the high degree of amino acid sequence homology observed for α_2M-receptor proteins among the species (Van Leuven et al., 1993). The human α_2M receptor is a single-chain 440 kDa glycoprotein that is identical to the low-density lipoprotein receptor-related protein (Strickland et al., 1990) and only reacts with the activated, or complexed, form of α_2M (Lamarre et al., 1991). Specific activated α_2M receptors are expressed on hepatocytes (Feldman et al., 1985), fibroblasts (Hanover et al., 1983), and macrophages (Khan et al., 1995) and, at least in rabbits, on alveolar and peritoneal macrophages (Debanne et al., 1975). In healthy animals, hepatocytes are the principal cells responsible for clearing α_2M-proteinase complexes from the circulation (Gonias et al., 1983; Lamarre et al., 1990). During an inflammatory reaction, other cell types may also become involved in the clearance of α_2M-proteinase complexes. A comparison of the uptake and distribution of radiolabeled α_2M in Wistar rats demonstrated that the accumulation of radiolabeled material was two to three times greater in inflammed tissue than in healthy tissue and that large amounts of both nondegraded and degraded α_2M accumulated in inflammed renal tissue (Okubo et al., 1984).

In mice, the genes coding for α_2M and the α_2M-receptor have been located on chromosomes 6 and 15, respectively (Hilliker et al., 1992a, 1992b). As has been reported for other acute phase proteins, α_2M synthesis is controlled at the transcriptional level (Baumann et al., 1991; Kurokawa et al., 1987; Pierzchalski et al., 1992). Within the nucleotide sequence, *cis*-acting hormone response elements of the α_2M gene have been identified, which exhibit sequence homology for other APRs, such as α_1-AGP (Baumann et al., 1991). In rat hepatoma, cells exposed to IL-1, IL-6, and dexamethasone, the transcriptional activity for α_2M, like that of α_1-AGP, was delayed 2–4 hours and required ongoing protein synthesis (Baumann et al., 1991; Jensen et al., 2004).

The major source of plasma α_2M is the hepatocyte, though other cell types, such as human fibroblasts (Mosher and Wing, 1976) and human monocytes (Hovi et al., 1977), are also capable of synthesizing and secreting α_2M. In both pregnant rats and mice, α_2M is additionally synthesized in placental tissue (Overbergh et al., 1995; Sarcione and Bohne, 1969) along with the α_2M receptor (Ashcom et al., 1990). In mouse embryos, mRNA for the α_2M receptor is expressed in most organs and mRNA levels for the α_2M protein increase progressively after day 17 of gestation (Lorent et al., 1995). As in the adult animal, the liver is the main site of α_2M synthesis in fetal mice (Van Leuven et al., 1992).

19.4.2 Role/Function

In both Wistar and Buffalo rats, turpentine injection induces an increase in both hepatic α_2M-mRNA and in plasma α_2M levels that peak 16–24 hours after treatment (Geiger et al., 1988b; Glibetic et al., 1992). A more rapid α_2M response is observed when IL-6 is injected into Wistar rats with peak plasma α_2M values appearing within 4 hours of treatment (Geiger et al., 1988b). Exposure of either rat or mouse hepatocyte cultures, or human hepatoma cells, to IL-6 is also sufficient to induce an increase in α_2M synthesis (Koj et al., 1991). In rat hepatoma cells, this effect of IL-6 can be enhanced by the addition of HGF to the culture medium (Koj et al., 1995). In the presence of dexamethasone, HGF alone can induce a selective increase in α_2M-mRNA expression and α_2M protein secretion in cultured rat hepatoma cells (Pierzchalski et al., 1992). When rat hepatoma cells are exposed to a combination of IL-1, IL-6, and dexamethasone, the initiation of α_2M-mRNA transcription, like that of α_1-AGP, is delayed 2–4 hours (Baumann et al., 1991). Other cytokines, including ciliary neurotrophic factor (CNTF), can also stimulate α_2M synthesis in rat hepatocyte and human hepatoma cells (Kurokawa et al., 1987; Schooltink et al., 1992).

The broad spectrum of proteinases with which α_2M interacts suggests that α_2M has a general role in controlling inflammation, coagulation, and fibrinolysis. However, for almost all endogenous proteinases that form complexes with α_2M, there is a more specific and a rapidly acting antiproteinase present in the circulation that confounds the elucidation of the biological function(s) of α_2M (Jensen et al., 2004; Lamarre et al., 1991). In addition, α_2M does not appear to be able to compensate for diseases associated with congenital deficiencies of specific proteinase inhibitors such as α_1-PI. Consequently, it is likely that the major physiological role of α_2M is as a vehicle for the rapid removal of proteinases from the circulation, as opposed to it serving primarily as a proteinase inhibitor. Such a role for α_2M would be compatible with another proposed function, namely, as a binding and carrier protein for several important cytokines, such as IL-6 and TNFα (Jensen et al., 2004; James, 1990; Lamarre et al., 1991). For example, α_2M does not inhibit the biological activity of IL-6 or the binding of IL-6 to its receptor, but it does protect IL-6 from proteolytic degradation (Matsuda et al., 1989). Cytokines, like IL-1 and TNFα, do not bind extensively with the native form of human α_2M, but readily interact with the proteolytically active form (Borth and Luger, 1989; Wollenberg et al., 1991a). Following binding, TNFα/α_2M complexes are removed from the circulation by the α_2M receptor pathway (Wollenberg et al., 1991a). While α_2Ms isolated from several species can interact with both TGFβ_1 and TGFβ_2, α_2M exhibits a 10-fold greater affinity for TGFβ_2 and selectively exerts an inhibitory action only on TGFβ_2 (Danielpour and Sporn, 1990; Lamarre et al., 1990). A combination of dexamethasone and human α_2M enables normal rat hepatocytes to overcome the inhibitory effects of TGFβ_1 and TGFβ_2, which indicates that α_2M may have a role in regulating proliferative responses in hepatocytes (Wollenberg et al., 1991b).

Despite the incomplete understanding of the physiological role of α_2M as an antiprotease, it is apparent that α_2M has a critical role as a host defense factor in septic shock. Not only has α_2M been shown to be the major factor in guinea pig plasma that inhibits elastase activity in vitro (Khan et al., 1994), but it can also ameliorate the development of septic shock in guinea pigs inoculated with an elastase-producing bacterial strain (Khan et al., 1995). In the inoculated guinea pigs, two-thirds of the circulating α_2M was consumed prior to the clinical appearance of symptoms of shock, an observation that may partially explain the consistent failure to observe increases in serum levels of α_2M in some species during inflammation. In vitro studies have demonstrated that α_2M is able to impair cell invasion and has the capacity to enhance the phagocytic and microbicidal actions of macrophages to *Trypanosoma cruzi* (Araujo-Jorge et al., 1990). When BALB/cJ mice were infected with *T. cruzi*, only surviving animals displayed a significant increase in circulating α_2M levels (Araujo-Jorge et al., 1992). This protective effect of α_2M may be related to the observation that both human and rat α_2Ms can form complexes with human fibroblast collagenase in a 1:2 stoichiometric ratio (Sottrup-Jensen and Birkedal-Hansen, 1989). Fibroblast collagenase is a proteinase that has a primary substrate specificity resembling that of the microbial proteinase thermolysin. Hence, α_2Ms can potentially modulate the activity of a broad spectrum of proteinases, including collagenases, of the extracellular matrix (ECM) (Sottrup-Jensen and Birkedal-Hansen, 1989).

In addition to its role as an inhibitor of mitogen-induced stimulation of lymphocytes isolated from humans (Rastogi and Clausen, 1985), rats (Miyanaga et al., 1982), and hamsters (Hart and Stein-Streilein, 1981), α_2M has been shown to suppress T-cell blastogenesis in several species (James, 1980; Mannhalter et al., 1986). Further, activated α_2M (but not native α_2M) can inhibit the stimulation of macrophage by a T-cell dependent inflammatory lymphokine isolated from guinea pig lymph node cells (Godfrey et al., 1984). Consequently, α_2M, like other APRs, may function as an immunosuppressive agent. α_2M has been isolated from both rat and human brain tissue (Dziegielewska et al., 1986; Kodelja et al., 1986), and human, mouse, and equine α_2Ms all exhibit nerve growth factor binding activity (Ronne et al., 1979). The ability of the activated form of α_2M to suppress neurite outgrowth has led to the suggestion that accumulation and activation of α_2M associated with inflammatory neuropathies may inhibit synaptic plasticity (Cavus et al., 1996).

19.4.3 Analytical Methods

The majority of studies evaluating α_2M levels in laboratory animals have employed immunological methods in part due to the availability of species-specific antibodies, because α_2M has been purified from rat, mouse, guinea pig, hamster, and rabbit plasma (Watterson et al., 2008; Barrett et al., 1979; Godfrey et al., 1984; Hirschelmann et al., 1990; Miyake et al., 1993; Okubo et al., 1981; Suzuki and Sinohara, 1986; Tamamizu et al., 1989; Van Leuven et al., 1992). While single peaks are generally observed for α_2M determined with rocket immunoelectrophoretic procedures, multiple bands staining for α_2M are generally observed in polyacrylamide gel electrophoresis because native α_2M and α_2M-proteinase complexes display similar antigenic properties but have different molecular weights (Barrett et al., 1979; Lamarre et al., 1991). Spectrophotometric assays using chromogenic substrates are frequently used to assess the functional activity of α_2M-proteinase complexes. However, this type of assay does not discriminate between the different forms of macroglobulin-type proteinase inhibitors that are present in rat, mouse, guinea pig, rabbit, and hamster plasma (French, 1989; Ganrot, 1973b; Geiger et al., 1987; Miyake et al., 1993; Saito and Sinohara, 1985b). Inactivation of α_2M can occur during sample storage, which can cause disparity between estimations of α_2M determined by immunological and functional procedures (Ganrot, 1966; Gressner and Peltzer, 1984).

19.4.4 Pathophysiological Significance

Circulating α_2M levels are low in healthy rats, with values of 300 μg/mL or less being reported (French, 1989; Geiger et al., 1987; Kurokawa et al., 1987; Okubo et al., 1981). Strain differences in the α_2M response in rats to turpentine as an inflammatory stimulant have been observed. For example, in Wistar rats, circulating α_2M levels rose from approximately 30 to 400 μg/mL within 24 hours of turpentine injection (Okubo et al., 1981). While a ninefold increase was observed in Hans Wistar rats after 4 days of dosing with drug candidate during a preclinical toxicology study (Watterson et al., 2008). In comparison, this treatment only induced a 2.5-fold increase in serum α_2M in male Buffalo rats (Warwas and Osada, 1985). In Wistar:Barby rats, circulating α_2M levels rose from 9 ± 5 mg/mL to 157 ± 55 mg/mL within 3 days of the induction of an inflammatory response (Hirschelmann et al., 1990). Similar differences in the α_2M response have been documented for August and Lewis rats (French, 1989). Although no sex differences have been observed in the response of rat α_2M to turpentine injection, the injection of recombinant human IL-6 into Wistar rats produced an increase in circulating α_2M values only in male animals (Geiger et al., 1988b).

Higher blood α_2M levels are found in pregnant, fetal, and neonatal rats than in mature animals (French, 1989). Throughout gestation days 10–20, the level of α_2M-mRNA in fetal rat liver is twofold higher than that in adult liver, and the fetal liver responds to inflammation in the mother by the transcriptional increase in α_2M (Glibetic et al., 1992). The ability of fetal liver to synthesize large amounts of α_2M is consistent with the observation that α_2M is the major circulating proteinase inhibitor in human newborns (Andrew et al., 1987). During pregnancy in human females, an inducible protein, referred to as *pregnancy zone protein*, with characteristics of a macroglobulin appears in the circulation (Sand et al., 1985).

In mice, normal circulating α_2M levels are around 1–2 mg/mL with similar values being found in pregnant and nonpregnant animals (Van Leuven et al., 1992). No increases in plasma α_2M levels occur in mice treated with *T. cruzi* despite evidence of an inflammatory response being mounted in the animals (Araujo-Jorge et al., 1992). In Syrian hamsters, normal circulating α_2M values are about threefold higher than human values at 6.9 mg/mL and, as was found for mice, no increase in serum α_2M levels was observed during the acute phase reaction (Miyake et al., 1993). In contrast to the decrease in plasma α_2M levels observed in human patients with sepsis, a dose-dependent increase in serum α_2M levels was detected in baboons treated with *Escherichia coli* or *Staphylococcus aureus* (de Boer et al., 1993). Likewise, in rhesus monkeys, administration of IL-6 induced an increase in plasma α_2M values from 2.2 to 4.0 mg/mL (Myers et al., 1995).

19.5 C-REACTIVE PROTEIN

19.5.1 Properties

CRP was the first APR protein to be discovered in people (Tillett and Francis, 1930), and while species variations exist, CRP is now recognized as an APR protein in most laboratory animals, including rabbits, rats, mice, dogs, and cats. Both rabbit and rat CRP have also been referred to as phosphorylcholine-binding protein (PCBP) (Murata et al., 2004; Marnell et al., 2005).

The CRPs isolated from different mammalian species share structural homology in being composed of five identical subunits, each approximately 20–23 kDa, that are arranged in a flat pentameric disk structure with cyclical symmetry (Osmand et al., 1977; Sui et al., 1996; Whitehead, 1989). In rabbit and human CRP, the subunits are noncovalently linked, while rat CRP is unique in containing a covalently linked dimer in its pentameric structure (Murata et al., 2004; Marnell et al., 2005; Nagpurkar and Mookerjea, 1981; Rassouli et al., 1992). In rat CRP, two of the five identical monomeric units are linked by interchain disulfide bonds involving the same cysteine residues that form the intrachain disulfide bonds in the other monomers (Rassouli et al., 1992). Only dog and rat CRPs are glycoproteins (Caspi et al., 1984; Nagpurkar and Mookerjea, 1981; Rassouli et al., 1992). Each mammalian CRP examined to date has been found to contain between 204 and 206 amino acid residues in the native molecule, with a hydrophobic leader consisting of 18 or 19 amino acids in the premolecule (Dowton and Holden, 1991; Rubio et al., 1993; Whitehead, 1989; Whitehead et al., 1990). There is extensive homology in the amino acid sequences among rabbit, human, rat, and mouse CRPs (Hu et al., 1986; Lei et al., 1985; Liu et al., 1987; Ohnishi et al., 1986; Rassouli et al., 1992; Taylor et al., 1984; Whitehead, 1989). For example, there is greater than 71% homology among the amino acid sequences of rabbit and human CRP, which is similar to that found between rat and human CRP (Taylor et al., 1984; Whitehead, 1989).

Both the mouse and human CRP gene are encoded as a single copy on chromosome 1 (Floyd-Smith et al., 1986; Ku and Mortensen, 1993). cDNA and genomic DNA have been cloned and sequenced for human, mouse, rat, hamster, and guinea pig CRP (Dowton and Holden, 1991; Ku and Mortensen, 1993; Rubio et al., 1993; Whitehead et al., 1990). Comparisons among species show that the major differences in the organization of the gene are in the regions that potentially determine the capacity of the CRP gene to be induced during acute inflammation (Dowton and Holden, 1991; Rubio et al., 1993; Taylor et al., 1984; Whitehead et al., 1990). Indeed, the type of response element associated with the CRP gene appears to be critical in regulating CRP synthesis (Li and Goldman, 1996; Lin and Liu, 1993; Rubio et al., 1993; Whitehead, 1989; Zhang et al., 1996). Several *cis*-elements and trans-activators are required for cytokine-induced CRP gene transcription. These include two IL-6 inducible C/EBP family members, whose binding sites are located in the proximal region of the CRP promoter (Ramji et al., 1993), and one of the signal transducer and activators of transcription (STAT) family members, STAT3 (Zhang et al., 1996). The STAT3-IL-6 response element was originally named the acute phase response element (Zhang et al., 1996; Zhong et al., 1994). In cultures of human hepatocytes, IL-6 is the primary cytokine that stimulates CRP gene expression (Marnell et al., 2005; Li et al., 1990). Although the mouse CRP gene also contains an IL-6 response element, neither recombinant human nor mouse IL-6 preparations were found to trigger CRP expression in isolated mouse hepatocytes (Ku and Mortensen, 1993). In mice, IL-1 is the primary cytokine responsible for inducing CRP synthesis. Gene transcription is induced through IL-1 interaction with both a C/EBP element and a hepatocyte nuclear factor-1 (HNF-1) element in the mouse gene (Lobetti et al., 2000; Ku and Mortensen, 1993). Since the HNF-1 element is one of the distinct promoters of liver-specific gene expression, these results may account for the tissue-specific expression of CRP as well as its limited expression as an APR protein in mice relative to other species (Ku and Mortensen, 1993).

The hepatocyte is the major site of CRP synthesis, where the rate of production is regulated at the transcriptional level (Ciliberto et al., 1987; French, 1989; Goldberger et al., 1987; Li and Goldman, 1996; Nunomura et al., 1994). In primary cultures of human hepatocytes, IL-6, in the presence of dexamethasone, stimulates the synthesis and secretion of CRP within 24 hours (Yap et al., 1991). When IL-1 is also included in the culture medium, a further increase in CRP production occurs within 48 hours. The stimulatory effect of IL-1 can be blocked by the inclusion of antibodies to IL-6 in the culture medium, indicating that the effect of IL-1 is mediated through IL-6 (Yap et al., 1991). In human hepatocyte cultures, TNFα by itself acts as an inhibitory cytokine for CRP synthesis, and it can also antagonize the actions of both IL-6 and IL-1 (Yap et al., 1991). In contrast, TNFα, like IL-1 and IL-6, induces the hepatic accumulation of CRP-mRNA in Syrian hamsters (Dowton and Holden, 1991), while in rabbits, neither IL-1 nor TNFα appear to be involved in the expression of hepatic CRP-mRNA and CRP synthesis during the inflammatory response (Mackiewicz et al., 1988).

19.5.2 Role/Function

Based on comparison of the structural similarities among rabbit, human, and *Limulus* CRP (which, unlike the mammalian proteins, consists of a hexameric disc of six subunits [Fernandez-Moran et al., 1986]), two functionally important regions of the molecule have been identified (Liu et al., 1987). One region confers the ability to bind calcium and is one of the most highly conserved regions of the molecule (Liu et al., 1987; Swanson et al., 1991b). The second region is a phosphorylcholine (PC)-binding region (Roux et al., 1983). Although the extent of CRP binding to PC varies between species, calcium-dependent PC binding is considered the common functional characteristic of all CRP molecules (Murata et al., 2004; Marnell et al., 2005; Nunomura, 1992; Oliveira et al., 1980; Pepys and Baltz, 1983; Schwalbe et al., 1992; Swanson and Mortensen, 1990; Swanson et al., 1991a). Interactions between CRP and a variety of ligands can also occur, indicating that CRP may be one of the proteins that serves as a connection between inflammation, immunity, lipid metabolism, and possibly atherosclerosis (Murata et al., 2004; Marnell et al., 2005; Adib-Conquy and Cavaillon, 2007). Human, rat, and rabbit CRPs have all been shown to selectively bind to plasma lipoproteins in a calcium-dependent manner (Cabana et al., 1983; Mookerjea et al., 1994; Rowe et al., 1984a, 1984b; Schwalbe et al., 1995). Further, CRP binding to immune complexes (Motie et al., 1996), basement membrane components such as fibronectin and laminin (Kolb-Bachofen, 1992; Salonen et al., 1984; Swanson et al., 1989; Tseng and Mortensen, 1988), and nuclear material (Dougherty et al., 1991; Du Clos, 1989; Nunomura, 1992) have also been demonstrated.

CRP, like other pentraxin molecules, is highly resistant to proteolytic degradation, especially in the presence of calcium (Ying et al., 1992), but human neutrophil enzymes can digest human CRP

(Shephard et al., 1992; Ying et al., 1992) and rat peritoneal macrophages can digest rat CRP with the generation and release of biologically active peptides (Nagpurkar et al., 1993). Since native CRP appears to have little biological activity unless bound to a ligand (Potempa et al., 1988), it is likely that these CRP degradation products contribute to the anti-inflammatory function of CRP (Murata et al., 2004; Marnell et al., 2005; Adib-Conquy and Cavaillon, 2007; Heuertz et al., 1996).

Based on studies in rabbits, mice, rats, and people, it has been concluded that hepatocytes are the most important site of clearance of serum CRP and that the rate of clearance is independent of plasma CRP levels (Baltz et al., 1985a; French, 1989; Hutchinson et al., 1994; Vigushin et al., 1993; Yang et al., 1992). In healthy rabbits, rats, and mice, the circulating half-life of CRP is short, ranging from 3 to 4.5 hours (Chelladurai et al., 1983; Rowe et al., 1984c). In rats undergoing an acute phase response, CRP is even more rapidly removed from the circulation, with the clearance rate increasing twofold (Rowe et al., 1984c). In transgenic mice programmed to synthesize rabbit CRP, the clearance rate of rabbit CRP from the circulation varies between 30 and 60 minutes under both normal and inflammatory conditions (Lin et al., 1995). The clearance rate of CRP is independent of ligand binding, but removal of sialic acid residues from rat CRP reduces the clearance time to approximately 5 minutes (Baltz et al., 1985a; Yang et al., 1992). The relatively rapid rate of CRP clearance may contribute to the rapid return of serum CRP to basal levels following exposure of an animal to a single inflammatory challenge.

CRP clearly plays an important role in initiating and modulating inflammatory and immune responses (French, 1989; Kushner, 1988). In the early stages of inflammation, CRP functions to stimulate the monophagocytic system through its interaction with several types of white cells. Specific and saturable high- and low-affinity binding sites for CRP have been identified on macrophages, neutrophils, and monocytes (Ballou et al., 1989; Crowell et al., 1991; Kempka et al., 1990; Kolb-Bachofen, 1991; Tebo and Mortensen, 1991; Zahedi et al., 1989) and T lymphocytes but not B lymphocytes (Mortensen et al., 1975). CRP can induce opsonin-like enhancement of phagocytosis (Murata et al., 2004; Marnell et al., 2005; Adib-Conquy and Cavaillon., 2007; Kilpatrick and Volanakis, 1985; Mold et al., 1982), which is considered a factor in the passive protection of mice against lethal challenge of *pneumocci* afforded by increased serum CRP levels (Kolb-Bachofen and Abel, 1991; Mold et al., 1981). Mouse macrophages and human monocytes respond to CRP activation by exhibiting a tumoricidal activity (Barna et al., 1984; Zahedi and Mortensen, 1986; Zahedi et al., 1989) through increased superoxide production (Foldes-Filep et al., 1992; Kolb-Bachofen and Abel, 1991; Nunomura, 1992; Zeller et al., 1986). On the other hand, both neutrophil chemotaxis and expression of adhesion molecules on the surface of activated neutrophils are inhibited by exposure to CRP (Heuertz et al., 1993, 1996; Kew et al., 1990; Webster et al., 1994), as is protein phosphorylation in CRP pretreated activated neutrophils (Buchta et al., 1988). These effects likely contribute to the protective effect that CRP exerts on lung injury in rabbit and mouse models of adult respiratory distress syndrome (Heuertz et al., 1993, 1994, 1996).

Human CRP can depress the in vitro aggregation response in activated mammalian platelets (Cheryk et al., 1996). When human, rabbit, or rat platelet suspensions are exposed to CRP and stimulated with the inflammatory mediator platelet activating factor (PAF), a biologically active phospholipid both the rate and extent of aggregation is depressed compared to untreated platelet suspension (Fiedel and Gewurz, 1976; Nagpurkar et al., 1988; Vigo, 1985). This response is mediated through the direct interaction of CRP with PAF, which reduces the bioavailability of the platelet agonist (Filep et al., 1991; Kilpatrick and Virella, 1985; Randell et al., 1990). The basal rate of removal of low-density lipoproteins (LDLs) from the circulation is enhanced when serum CRP levels rise, because macrophages readily endocytose the complexes formed between CRP and Apo-B and Apo-E-containing lipoproteins (Mookerjea et al., 1994). The CRP-induced increased rate of clearance of LDLs, together with the suppression of platelet aggregation, likely function to retard the activation of the hemostatic system during an inflammatory reaction, thus modulating thrombus formation at sites of tissue damage.

Another biological role for CRP in maintaining homeostasis is its function in facilitating the removal of cellular debris from areas of tissue injury. Not only can CRP bind to one or more components of damaged cells to facilitate their removal or repair (Crowell et al., 1991), but CRP is also deposited at sites of tissue damage through selective calcium-dependent binding to laminin and fibronectin (Salonen et al., 1984; Shephard et al., 1986; Swanson and Mortensen, 1990; Swanson et al., 1989; Tseng and Mortensen, 1988, 1989). At these sites, CRP may act as a scavenger of nuclear debris because human, rat, and rabbit CRPs all have the ability to bind to histones, chromatin, and small ribonuclear proteins (Burlingame et al., 1996; Dougherty et al., 1991; Du Clos, 1989; Du Clos et al., 1988; Shephard et al., 1991). The interaction of CRP with nuclear material may be a contributing factor in the role that CRP has in reducing autoantibody formation and increasing survival time in a mouse model of systemic lupus erythromatosis (Du Clos et al., 1994).

19.5.3 Analytical Methods

The majority of procedures described to isolate CRP are based on its calcium-dependent phospholipid binding and have utilized affinity chromatography with either PC or phosphatidyl ethanolamine substituted agarose beads (Burger et al., 1987; Caspi et al., 1984; Fujise et al., 1992; Macintyre, 1988; Nunomura et al., 1994; Onishi et al., 1994; Pruden et al., 1988; Yamamoto et al., 1992, 1993a). Immunoaffinity chromatography has also been used when species-specific CRP antibodies have been available (Nunomura et al., 1994; Tanaka and Robey, 1983). Numerous assay procedures, based on either immunological or functional properties, have been employed to quantitate serum CRP. Rocket immunoelectrophoresis and ELISA assays have been frequently used for measuring CRP in serum from laboratory animals (Eckersall et al., 1989; French, 1989; Nunomura et al., 1990a; Tanaka and Robey, 1983). The ELISA for canine CRP has an advantage over both the electroimmunoassay and immunodiffusion procedures in being quantitative and sensitive to levels as low as 2.5 μg/mL serum (Yamamoto et al., 1994a); however, the assay is affected by sample hemolysis (Eckersall et al., 1991). A capillary reversed passive latex agglutination test has been developed to quantitate canine serum CRP (Wadsworth et al., 1985; Yamamoto et al., 1994a). The method is rapid and correlates well with a canine ELISA when serum CRP concentrations are >6.9 μg/mL, but it is not sufficiently sensitive to detect CRP in normal sera (Tagata et al., 1996). Other nonimmunological procedures, including an assay based on the calcium-dependent interactions of CRP and lipososomes, have been developed (French, 1989; Umeda and Yasuda, 1994; Umeda et al., 1986).

19.5.4 Pathophysiological Significance

In beagle dogs, the temporal changes in serum IL-6 and TNFα, during the inflammatory response, precede the appearance of increased serum CRP levels (Yamashita et al., 1994), which explains in part the consistent and species-independent delay between an initiating stimulus and the appearance of increased circulating CRP levels (Conner and Eckersall, 1988; Myers and Fleck, 1988).

In mice, rats, and hamsters, the age and sex of the animal can influence both hepatic CRP-mRNA levels and the amount of CRP appearing in the circulation (Murata et al., 2004; Dowton et al., 1991; Nunomura, 1990; Szalai et al., 1995). In both Wistar and August strain rats, serum CRP levels are elevated at birth compared to adult values (De Beer et al., 1982; Nunomura, 1990). The constitutive levels of hepatic CRP-mRNA are significantly lower in fetal rabbits than in adult animals (Rygg et al., 1996). In the fetal Syrian hamster, hepatic CRP-mRNA exhibited an increased response following direct exposure to an inflammatory stimulant compared to the extent of the response in adult liver (Dowton et al., 1991). The role of sex hormones in controlling CRP synthesis has not been fully elucidated. Estradiol administration to male Wistar rats produced a decrease in serum CRP levels without producing any decline in hepatic CRP-mRNA levels (Nunomura, 1990; Nunomura et al., 1994). Testosterone administration to male or ovarectomized female Wistar rats resulted in an increase in serum CRP levels (Nunomura, 1990). These results correlated with the observation that in both Wistar and Hooded strain rats serum CRP levels are significantly higher in males than in females (De Beer et al., 1991; Nunomura, 1990). Further, a direct relationship between CRP synthesis and testosterone secretion has been documented in transgenic mice genetically manipulated to express human CRP (Klein et al., 1995; Szalai et al., 1995).

In normal rabbit hepatocytes, the rate of hepatic secretion of CRP into the blood stream is inhibited due to the retention of the protein in the endoplasmic reticulum (ER) (Macintyre et al., 1994). The binding of CRP to ligands in the ER is reduced during the acute phase response, resulting in the increased secretion efficiency of CRP (Hu et al., 1988; Macintyre et al., 1985). In hepatocyte cultures derived from turpentine-stimulated rabbits, CRP represented 3.9% of the secreted protein, compared to 0.3% of the protein in control cultures (Macintyre et al., 1983).

The normal basal serum concentration of CRP varies among species, as does the acute phase response (French, 1989). Typical species variations are illustrated in Table 19.2. Healthy dogs, rabbits, and people usually exhibit low circulating levels of CRP (Table 19.1). In these species, CRP is one of the major acute phase proteins, with levels rising rapidly within 24 hours of stimulation by up to 1000-fold (Watterson et al., 2008; Caspi et al., 1987; Conner and Eckersall, 1988; French, 1989; Hunneyball et al., 1986; Nunomura, 1992). In a group of 77, clinically ill dogs in which CRP levels were markedly elevated, postmortem diagnosis established that in all the affected dogs, raised CRP values were associated with bacterial infections and pyrometra and that the elevation of CRP reflected the extent of inflammatory damage (Yamamoto et al., 1993b). In this study, the extent of serum CRP levels increased from basal levels of 8.5 ± 0.5 μg/mL in a healthy control group to up to 394 μg/mL in dogs with leptosirosis, while no increases in CRP were observed in dogs with gastrointestinal disorders or nephritis. The association between bacterial infections and elevations in serum CRP levels has also been observed in experimental studies. Leptospira inoculation in dogs resulted in serum CRP rising from <5 to up to 400 μg/mL 2-4 days after inoculation (Caspi et al., 1987). Inoculation of dogs with *Bordetella bronchiseptica* produced a similar response (Yamamoto et al., 1994b), while a slightly reduced response was observed following inoculation with *E. canis* with serum CRP values being increased by 3.3–6.5-fold (Rikihisa et al., 1994). It is likely that the CRP response is mediated (at least in part) by IL-6 because following turpentine injection, the increase in serum CRP from barely detectable levels up to 431.5 ± 31.3 μg/mL was preceded by a dramatic increase in serum IL-6 levels (Yamashita et al., 1994). Elevations of CRP have also been observed in dogs postsurgery (Caspi et al., 1984, 1987; Conner and Eckersall, 1988; Yamamoto et al., 1993b), and the extent of the increases shows a weak but significant correlation with alteration in neutrophil counts (Burton et al., 1994).

In healthy New Zealand white rabbits, basal serum levels of CRP have been reported as being barely detectable to being as high as 31 ± 9 μg/mL (Cabana et al., 1983; Heuertz et al., 1993; Noe et al., 1989). In rabbits, variations in the serum CRP response to different inflammatory stimuli, as well as the response of individual animals, have been observed. For example, the administration of

TABLE 19.2
Interspecies Differences in Basal Serum C-Reactive Protein (CRP) in Healthy Adult Animals and during the Acute Phase Response

	CRP μg/mL	
Species	**Normal Sera**	**Acute Phase Sera**
Human	<1	300–500
Rabbit	0–31	65–350
Dog	3–22	83–720
Rat	180–500	700–1300
Mouse	<2	1–2
Guinea pig	Not detected	Not detected

1% croton oil to rabbits has variously been reported as inducing a twofold increase in serum CRP to a maximum of around 64 μg/mL 24 hours after treatment (Cabana et al., 1983) to producing an increase from barely detectable serum CRP to a peak of 350 ± 70 μg/mL within 48 hours of treatment (Heuertz et al., 1993). When the effects of turpentine, endotoxin, and IL-1 administration in rabbits were compared, only turpentine was found to produce a marked increase in serum CRP with values rising to around 150 μg/mL (Noe et al., 1989). In this study, the serum CRP reponse to endotoxin was 10-fold lower than the turpentine response, and there was no CRP response to IL-1 administration. Transient increases in serum CRP levels have been noted in rabbits with antigen-induced monoarticular arthritis (French, 1989).

Healthy rats exhibit relatively high serum CRP values, and in this species, CRP reacts only as a moderately responsive acute phase protein (Bout et al., 1986; Mookerjea and Hunt, 1995; Nunomura, 1990). A consistent observation in rats is a two- to fourfold increase in serum CRP levels following an inflammatory stimulus such as turpentine (Burger et al., 1987; Myers and Fleck, 1988; Nunomura, 1992; Nunomura et al., 1990b). However, studies carried out by Watterson et al. (2008) discovered that CRP levels in Wistar rats were variable and did not support CRP as a sensitive acute phase protein in rats. In rats, as in people, age-related changes in serum CRP levels have been found. In Wistar strain rats, serum CRP was determined to be 3.6 ± 0.8 μg/mL at birth, and an increase to adult values did not begin until the rats were more than 15 days old (Nunomura, 1990). This is similar to the lower serum CRP values observed in human neonates compared to adults (French, 1989). In both rats and women, increased serum CRP levels are observed around the time of parturition (French, 1989; Nunomura, 1990, 1992). In pregnant rats, two additional serum CRP peaks occur at days 0 and 15 of gestation, with mean values of 770 ± 100 μg/mL being observed for the later peak (Nunomura, 1990). The factors regulating these pregnancy-related changes are unclear. However, estradiol has been shown to exert an inhibitory activity on rat CRP expression while testosterone exerts a stimulatory effect (Nunomura, 1990, 1992).

In both the mouse and guinea pig, CRP is barely detectable (if at all) in the serum of normal animals (Table 19.2), and in neither species does CRP respond as an acute phase protein (French, 1989; Lin et al., 1995; Rubio et al., 1993; Whitehead et al., 1990). The lack of CRP response in the guinea pig has been related to a lack of the appropriate promoter region in the guinea pig CRP gene (Rubio et al., 1993).

19.6 CERULOPLASMIN

19.6.1 Properties

Ceruloplasmin (CP) is a blue multicopper oxidase that is found in all vertebrates. The circulating Cps of all species have similar molecular weights (French, 1989; Ryden, 1972). It is the major plasma copper (Cu) carrying protein in rats and people but not in dogs or mice (Montaser et al., 1992). It has been suggested that in dogs and mice transcuprein is the major Cu transport protein (Montaser et al., 1992).

Ceruloplasmin is a glycoprotein (8%–9% carbohydrate) that migrates as an α_2-globulin and contains six to seven Cu atoms per molecule. Human CP circulates as a single polypeptide chain with a molecular weight of 132 kDa that carries 70%–90% of the circulating Cu (Gutteridge and Stocks, 1981; Harris, 1991; Kingston et al., 1977). The complete amino acid sequence of human CP and rat CP has been determined by protein sequence analysis (Takahashi et al., 1984) and by cDNA cloning (Aldred et al., 1987; Fleming and Gitlin, 1990; Kischinsky et al., 1986; Yang et al., 1986). The amino acid sequence of rat CP is 93% homologous with human CP and contains a 19 amino acid leader peptide plus a 1040 amino acid mature protein (Fleming and Gitlin, 1990). Similarly, the amino acid structure of murine CP deduced from cDNA clones indicates that close homology exists between murine and human CP (Klomp et al., 1996). Despite the similarities in structure, there are obvious physical and enzymatic differences between rat and human CPs. Rat CP is less susceptible to proteolysis and possesses only a fraction of the ferroxidase activity found in human CP (Ryan et al., 1992).

Circulating CP is primarily derived from the liver, though studies using a variety of techniques, such as molecular cloning, gene expression, and immunohistochemical staining, have confirmed that CP can also be synthesized in many other tissues including lung (Bingle et al., 1992; Fleming and Gitlin, 1990; Klomp et al., 1996), brain (Aldred et al., 1987; Kalmovarin et al., 1991; Levin et al., 1984; Thomas et al., 1989), uterus (Thomas and Schreiber, 1988, 1989; Thomas et al., 1995), placenta (Aldred et al., 1987; Thomas and Schreiber, 1989), mammary tissue (Jaeger et al., 1991), testes (Forti et al., 1989; Skinner and Griswold, 1983), and macrophages and lymphocytes (Fleming et al., 1991; Pan et al., 1996). Investigations into the biosynthesis of CP in rat hepatocytes have been facilitated by the availability of Long-Evans Cinnamon (LEC) rats, which display a genetic defect in Cu metabolism, and by studies with rats nutritionally deficient in Cu (Gitlin et al., 1992; Yamada et al., 1993). The Cu-deficient apo-form of CP is immunologically identical to the holo-form of the enzyme and exhibits a similar glycosylation pattern, but the apo-form lacks oxidase activity (Gitlin et al., 1992; Hiyamuta and Takeichi, 1993; Terada et al., 1995; Yamada et al., 1993). The incorporation of Cu into CP occurs in the Golgi apparatus (Terada et al., 1995). Hepatic Cu content appears to have no effect on CP gene expression or the extent of CP biosynthesis, and the rates of secretion of both Cu-containing and Cu-deficient CP from hepatocytes are similar (Bingle et al., 1990; Gitlin et al., 1992; Terada et al., 1995).

The rat CP gene has been cloned, sequenced, and assigned to chromosome 2 (Fleming and Gitlin, 1992; Li et al., 1991). The CP-mRNA isolated from different rat tissues is identical in nucleotide sequence and is the product of a single transcription start site (Fleming and Gitlin, 1992). Although the tissue-specific expression of CP appears to be regulated in the rat by an exacting region 393 base pairs upstream of the transcription start site, the enhancer-binding (C/EBP) consensus elements are not involved in the selective tissue expression of CP (Klomp et al., 1996). In both guinea pigs and humans, in addition to the 3.7 kb mRNA that is expressed in rats, a second larger mRNA also encodes CP (Bingle et al., 1991). The additional CP-mRNA found in guinea pig liver is slightly larger (5.0 kb) than that found in human liver (4.2 kb) (Bingle et al., 1991). In guinea pigs, no hepatic synthesis of CP is detectable before birth, and after birth, there is no clear differential expression of the two mRNA species (Bingle et al., 1991). The expression of guinea pig CP appears to be related to the birth process rather than the gestational age of the animal (Bingle et al., 1992). This contrasts with the situation in rats and humans, where CP-mRNA is detectable in fetuses during the later stages of gestation, though the CP-mRNA levels are lower than those found in adults (Fleming and Gitlin, 1990; Gutteridge and Stocks, 1981). While CP-mRNA is found in the liver of fetal rats after day 15 of gestation, CP is not present in the circulation until later, which suggests that some posttranslational control mechanism is involved in synthesis and secretion of the protein (Bingle et al., 1991). This conclusion is also supported by kinetic studies of CP expression during the acute phase response (Gitlin, 1988).

19.6.2 Role/Function

One of the biological functions of CP is the delivery of Cu to tissues. Specific CP receptors have been identified in a variety of tissues, including aortic and cardiac tissue (Stevens et al., 1984), brain (Crowe and Morgan, 1996), monocytes, granulocytes, and lymphocytes (Kataoka and Tavassoli, 1985), erythrocytes (Barnes and Freiden, 1984; Stern and Freiden, 1993), and hepatic endothelial cells (Kataoka and Tavassoli, 1984, 1985; Tavassoli et al., 1986). The binding of CP to rat erythrocytes is saturable, reversible, specific, and is mediated through a 150 kDa receptor composed of 50 kDa subunits (Stern and Freiden, 1990, 1993). In contrast, the CP receptor isolated from liver endothelium is a 35 kDa protein (Omoto and Tavassoli, 1990). Whether the different molecular weights reflect the existence of different types of tissue-specific receptors has yet to be determined. It is known, however, that the receptors on erythrocytes and hepatic endothelium recognize different parts of the CP molecule. Furthermore, a comparison of the CP receptors on hepatic Kupffer and hepatic endothelial cells indicates that the Kupffer cells can discriminate between the native, physiological conformation of CP and other forms of the protein, such as asialo-CP (Dini et al., 1990). Hepatic endothelial cells not only interact with CP but they can desialate native CP, which is then transferred to hepatocytes, where it is endocytosed via asialoglycoprotein receptors (Dini et al., 1990; Tavassoli, 1985). These galactosyl receptors are likely responsible for the rapid clearance of CP from the circulation that has been observed following removal of sialic acid residues (Gregoriadis et al., 1970; Van den Hamer et al., 1970).

Like other acute phase proteins, CP is a multifunctional protein with one of its primary physiological roles being that of an antioxidant. There are several ways in which CP can fulfill this function: (1) by donating Cu to tissues for the synthesis of Cu-containing enzymes (Campbell et al., 1981), (2) by directly scavenging superoxide anions (Goldstein et al., 1979), and (3) by inhibiting metal-catalyzed lipid peroxidation through the reincorporation of iron back into serum ferritin or transferrin (Osaki et al., 1971; Samokyszyn et al., 1989). In both rats and humans, CP is the major Cu-carrying component in blood (Gubler et al., 1953; Montaser et al., 1992; Sternlieb et al., 1961) and delivers Cu to peripheral cells and tissues, where it is absorbed by specific surface receptors (Goode et al., 1990; Percival and Harris, 1988). In both dogs and mice, CP is less important as a Cu transporter in the circulation, and both these species exhibit lower circulating levels of Cu and CP than either rats or humans (Montaser et al., 1992). It has been suggested that the high levels of gene expression in the lung during fetal development in the rat may serve as a pulmonary antioxidant defense mechanism (Fleming and Gitlin, 1990). This suggestion is compatible with the proposed role for CP during inflammation because CP can function to neutralize free radicals produced by activated leukocytes (Broadley and Hoover, 1989; Gutteridge and Stocks, 1981). Likewise, the increase in CP-mRNA in the mouse uterus at the time of implantation may occur to provide sufficient CP to serve as an effective free radical scavenger that can moderate the uterine inflammatory response and prevent overstimulation of the immune system during pregnancy (Thomas et al., 1995). It has been suggested that at least in the rat, CP may play a role in protecting the fetus and maintaining homeostasis at different stages of reproduction (Thomas and Schreiber, 1988). High levels of CP-mRNA, but not α_2M-mRNA or α_1-AGP-mRNAs, are present in the uterus of both pregnant and nonpregnant rats, further indicating a selective role for CP (Thomas and Schreiber, 1988).

Pulmonary CP gene expression is increased during conditions of both inflammation and hyperoxia (Fleming et al., 1991; Moak and Greenwald, 1984). The antioxidant function of CP in the airways may be related to its ferroxidase activity (Gutteridge, 1991). Relative to the oxidase activity of CP, dog and mouse CPs possess higher levels of ferroxidase activity than rat CP (Montaser et al., 1992). High-affinity iron acquisition from the environment is an essential determinant of bacterial virulence, and hence the presence of CP in alveolar epithelium may represent a host defense by limiting ferrous iron availability (Cornelissen and Sparling, 1994). The expression of CP in astrocytes within the retina and brain, as well as the epithelium of the choroid plexus may also be associated with the role of CP in iron metabolism (Klomp et al., 1996). Human aceruloplasminemia is an autosomal recessive disorder characterized by neurodegeneration of the retina and basal ganglia associated with iron accumulation (Logan et al., 1994; Miyajima et al., 1987). A further link between CP and iron metabolism is apparent in the downregulation of hepatic CP receptors that can be induced in the suckling rat as a result of iron loading (Crowe and Morgan, 1996).

In addition to its role in the inflammatory response as an antioxidant, the expression of CP in immune tissues, such as the spleen and thymus, supports a role for this protein in the activation, effector function, and cytoprotection of immune cells (Kalmovarin et al., 1991; Kojima et al., 1986; Pan et al., 1996; Saenko et al., 1994). Not only is immune system function suppressed in Cu deficiency (Bala and Failla, 1992), but in the macular mutant mouse (which is characterized by reduced CP levels), antibody production against sheep red blood cells is also reduced (Nakagawa et al., 1993). Ceruloplasmin may also influence the innate immune system in animals, because it has been shown that the phagocytosis of *Candida albicans* by human neutrophils and monocytes is stimulated by CP (Saenko et al., 1994).

19.6.3 Analytical Methods

Serum CP levels have been evaluated by both functional and immunological procedures, though both systems are subject to problems of accuracy in distinguishing and quantifying active CP. Ceruloplasmin oxidase in serum deteriorates on sample storage (Gutteridge et al., 1985), and while absolute protein levels are stable, laboratory procedures are frequently inadequate to discriminate between active Cu-containing CP and inactive Cu-depleted CP (Terada et al., 1995). In a denaturing polyacrylamide electrophoretic system, apo- and holo-CP cannot be distinguished, but under non-denaturing conditions, the holo-CP migrates faster than apo-CP (Terada et al., 1995). Monoclonal antibodies generated to the active site of holo-CP and to inactive CP, or apo-CP, have been used to demonstrate that only inactive CP is present in hepatic tissue in LEC rats, while both forms are present in normal rats (Hiyamuta and Takeichi, 1993). While antibodies raised in rabbits to human CP can partially cross-react with CP from dogs and rhesus monkeys (French, 1989; Ganrot, 1973a), the lack of cross-reactivity with rat CP necessitated the development of a noncompetitive ELISA assay (DiSilvestro et al., 1988). Two-dimensional electrophoresis followed by immunofixation has also been used to evaluate serum CP in dogs (Watanabe, 1995). Several methods have been used to isolate CP from serum and appear to yield similar results (Montaser et al., 1992; Ryan et al., 1992; Stern and Freiden, 1990, 1993; Terada et al., 1995). Procedures for the isolation and characterization of CP have been reviewed (Arnaud et al., 1988).

The most commonly used functional assay for serum CP is based on the enzymatic oxidation of p-phenylenediamine (pPD) (French, 1989; Ravin, 1961). If phosphate buffers are used in the assay, there can be nonenzymatic oxidation of iron, which interferes with the apparent CP oxidase activity (Ryan et al., 1992). While this problem can be overcome by the use of a sodium acetate buffering system (Ryan et al., 1992), this does not solve the difficulty of distinguishing the oxidation of the substrate by CP oxidase and the ferroxidase II activity present in some CP species (Montaser et al., 1992). When pPD is used as substrate in the absence of sodium azide, both CP oxidase and ferroxidase activity are determined; while in the presence of sodium azide, only ferroxidase activity is measured. The apparent CP oxidase activity in rat, dog, and mouse serum has been estimated to be reduced by 4.2%, 15.8%, and 46.2%, respectively, when CP ferroxidase activity is discounted (Montaser et al., 1992). Further, the net CP oxidase activity estimated as pPD oxidase $\times 10^{-2}$ nmol/min/mL was 18.6 ± 6, 3.2 ± 0.5, and 2.0 ± 0.4 for rat, dog, and mouse serum, compared to 90 ± 8, 8.2 ± 1.8, and $3.6 \pm 1.1 \times 10^{-2}$ µmol o-dianisidine oxidised /min/mL (Montaser et al., 1992). In addition to different sensitivities toward different substrates, the optimum pH for the CP oxidase reaction also varies among species (Bingley and Dick, 1969). Consequently, when comparing published serum CP values for laboratory animals, the methodologies used by the various researchers should be considered.

19.6.4 Pathophysiological Significance

The exposure of human hepatoma cells to either IL-1 or TNFα induces a time- and dose-dependent increase in both CP-mRNA and CP-protein synthesis (Ramadori et al., 1988). The effects of IL-1 and TNFα on net CP synthesis were comparable with values increasing by 224% and 285% relative to control values, respectively, within 18 hours of treatment (Ramadori et al., 1988). The injection of IL-6 or TNFα into Wistar rats induced a twofold increase in circulating CP values within 12 hours, and this level was sustained for a further 12 hours (Sato et al., 1994). The daily injection of human recombinant IL-6 to marmosets produced a four- to fivefold increase in serum CP levels within 8–24 hours, though the dose of IL-6 that was required to induce this response was approximately 100-fold greater than that required to induce a similar increase in circulating haptoglobin values

(Ryffel et al., 1994). Although the increase in circulating CP values observed in rabbits, rat, and mice following inflammatory stimuli is likely mediated at least in part through cytokine induction, the tissue-specific nature of the response indicates that CP expression is controlled by a complex regulatory system (Fleming et al., 1991; Giclas et al., 1985; Kimura et al., 1994; Kimura-Takeuchi et al., 1992; Milland et al., 1990; Min et al., 1991). For example, in both Sprague-Dawley and Wistar rats, 8 hours after endotoxin injection, an increase in CP-mRNA was only observed in liver and lung tissue with no alterations in CP-mRNA levels being found in other tissues (Fleming et al., 1991). When the rats in this study were exposed to 95% O_2, a five- to sixfold increase in CP-mRNA was only observed in lung tissue (Fleming et al., 1991). When Lewis rats were exposed to 85% O_2 for 19 days, an increase in serum CP levels was observed, and the elevation in serum CP levels correlated with an increase in lung antioxidase activity (Moak and Greenwald, 1984). It is not clear, however, whether the hyperoxic response of serum CP levels is an acute phase reaction or is related to some other type of noninflammatory response because other APR proteins, such as plasma fibrinogen, remained unchanged in oxygen treated Lewis rats (Moak and Greenwald, 1984).

In humans, rats, rabbits, dogs, and primates, the CP responds to inflammatory stimuli as an APR, though the rapidity of the rise, as well as the extent of the increase, is generally lower than that of other acute phase proteins (Burlingame et al., 1996; Eckersall and Conner, 1988; Ganrot, 1973c; Hirschelmann et al., 1990; Solter et al., 1991). For example, following turpentine injection to rabbits, a maximum two- to threefold increase in serum CP levels is observed between 48 and 72 hours, compared to a 50-fold increase in CRP that occurs between 12 and 36 hours (Giclas et al., 1985; Mackiewicz et al., 1988). Similary, in mice, turpentine injection induces a two- to threefold increase in serum CP oxidase activity, which is less than the alteration in either fibrinogen or metallothionein (Min et al., 1991). In a study involving 285 normal dogs, serum CP oxidase activity was determined as 17.1 ± 0.3 IU/L, which increased approximately twofold during inflammation (Solter et al., 1991). Intravenous administration of LPS (1 µg LPS/kg) to rabbits induced a dose-related increase in serum CP with values rising from 26 ± 2 µg/mL to 69 ± 2 µg/mL within 24 hours of treatment (Kimura et al., 1994). In rabbits, serum CP is also responsive to viral challenge. Basal serum CP values rose from 29 ± 2 µg/mL to 47 ± 3 µg/mL within 24 hours of a challenge with influenza virus (Kimura-Takeuchi et al., 1992). The synthetic viral product analogue, polyriboinosinic:polyribocytidylic acid, likewise induced a twofold increase in serum CP levels in rabbits (Kimura et al., 1994). The extent of the increases in serum CP values induced by these inflammatory stimulants is similar to that induced in marmosets following daily IL-6 injections for 7 days. In the marmosets, the IL-6 treatment regime caused serum CP levels to rise from 0.3 to about 1.5 g/L (Ryffel et al., 1994). In contrast, administration of IL-1 to rats did not alter either the serum CP oxidase or serum CP protein levels (Gitlin et al., 1992). It is possible that relatively modest increases in serum CP levels following stimulation do not represent the total increase in CP synthesis during an inflammatory response. For example, in rats, endotoxin treatment can induce an increase in CP-mRNA expression in both the liver and lungs (Moak and Greenwald, 1984), and in turpentine treated rabbits, CP can be detected in the pleural fluid (Giclas et al., 1985). These increases in local tissue expression of CP are not reflected in the extent of change observed in serum CP values.

The largest variation in circulating CP activity is observed in animals with either hereditary- or dietary-induced impairment of Cu metabolism (Li et al., 1991). For example, a serum CP value of 373 ± 37 µg/mL was found in Sprague-Dawley rats maintained on a Cu-adequate diet, compared to values of 29 ± 2 µg/mL in animals maintained on a Cu-deficient diet (Chen et al., 1995). Nutritionally induced Cu deficiency appears to produce a greater decrease in serum CP oxidase activity than in the serum CP protein values as determined by immunological procedures (Gitlin et al., 1992). This is similar to the observation in LEC rats with inherited impairment of Cu metabolism, which exhibit approximately half the serum CP protein values compared to Sprague-Dawley rats despite the apparently identical CP-mRNA levels and the similar levels of intracellular CP synthesis in the two species (Terada et al., 1995). Further, the exposure of Cu-deficient Sprague-Dawley rats to LPS induced an increase in serum CP levels from 110 ± 10 μg/mL to 280 ± 34 μg/mL without inducing a change in serum CP oxidase activity (Gitlin et al., 1992). In contrast, inflammation in normal rats induces a comparable increase in both serum CP oxidase activity and CP protein values (DiSilvestro et al., 1988).

The circulating CP levels in laboratory animals are affected by age, with newborn animals having consistently lower values than adults. In Sprague-Dawley and Wistar rats, serum CP levels are 14 ± 8 μg/mL at birth, rising rapidly to about 200 μg/mL at day 20, with adult levels of 300–350 μg/mL being reached at about 1 year of age (Evans et al., 1970). This is similar to the age profile in guinea pigs (Bingle et al., 1992; Srai et al., 1986) and people (Cox, 1996). In guinea pigs, serum CP level is not detectable before birth, it is 3.1 ± 2.8 ng/mL at birth, and reaches 32.1 ± 11.8 ng/mL by 28 days of age (Bingle et al., 1991). Pregnancy in both rabbits and humans results in an increase in circulating CP values (Ganrot, 1972; Ungar-Waron et al., 1978), which may be related to the increased production of CP in the uterus (Thomas et al., 1995). However, although administration of estradiol increased CP levels by 75% in female rats, there is no evidence that CP-mRNA levels in the rat uterus are directly related to estrogen levels (Meier and MacPike, 1968; Thomas et al., 1995).

19.7 FIBRINOGEN

19.7.1 PROPERTIES

Fibrinogen is a large, poorly soluble β-globulin present in the plasma of all vertebrates. Due to its central role in hemostasis, fibrinogen levels in veterinary medicine are evaluated as one of the parameters included in a routine assessment of a blood coagulation profile.

An increased rate of liver fibrinogenesis represents a uniform response of the liver to hepatocyte damage induced by infectious, toxic, or metabolic agents (Neubauer et al., 1995). This response is translated into hyperfibrinogenemia, which is characteristic of a broad range of bacterial infections and other inflammatory conditions in many animal species (Hawkey and Hart, 1987).

All vertebrates have fibrinogen molecules composed of three nonidentical polypeptide chains, designated as Aα, Bβ, and γ, that are linked by disulfide bridges (Gentry and Downie, 1993; Lord, 1995). Among different species, the three chains share many structural features but vary in size. The human Aα, Bβ, and γ chains have molecular weights of 67.6, 52.3, and 48.9 kDa, respectively, resulting in a total molecular weight of 340 kDa for the complete molecule, which is similar to that of rat fibrinogen (Ichinose and Davie, 1994; VanRuijven and Nieuwenhuizen, 1978). In all species, soluble fibrinogen is cleaved by thrombin to remove short amino-terminal peptides from the Aα and Bβ chains. This allows the resulting fibrin monomers to undergo spontaneous polymerization, followed by their covalent cross-linkage under the catalytic action of a transglutaminase enzyme, Factor XIIIa (Hantgan et al., 1994; Lord, 1995). While there are differences in the molecular weight of the Aα chains, the molecular weights of the Bβ and γ chains are relatively constant among mammals (Crabtree et al., 1985; Doolittle, 1973). For example, there is 80% homology between rat and human γ chains (Frost and Weigel, 1990). The structural diversity of the Aα chain is due to species differences in the terminal two-thirds of the chain, the αC domain (Medved et al., 1985). A comparison of this domain among rhesus monkey, pig, dog, mouse, and Syrian hamster fibrinogen indicates that the greatest variation occurs in the middle region of the αC domain and that the carboxy- and amino-terminal regions are highly conserved (Murakawa et al., 1993). There is also considerable variation among species in the amino acid sequences of the fibrinopeptides A and B released as a result of thrombin cleavage (Penny and Hendy, 1986). Based on both structural evidence and the ability of fibrinogen from various species to selectively bind hyaluronic acid, it has been estimated that the fibrinogen molecule isolated from human, baboon, rabbit, dog, and rat plasma is evolutionarily divergent from that of the fibrinogen molecule found in cow, pig, horse, goat, and sheep plasma (Frost and Weigel, 1990; Henschen et al., 1983).

While the fibrinogen stored in the α-granules of blood platelets is released during blood clot formation, the liver is both the primary site of fibrinogen synthesis and the source of circulating fibrinogen (Handagama et al., 1990; Hantgan et al., 1994). The Aα, Bβ, and γ fibrinogen polypeptides are each encoded by distinct genes that are clustered at a 50 kbase locus on chromosome 4 in people and on chromosome 2 in rats (Ichinose and Davie, 1994; Kant et al., 1985; Lord, 1995; Marino et al., 1986). The nucleotide sequences of the cDNAs that encode for each chain of fibrinogen are quite similar, as are the cDNAs encoding for rat and human proteins (Crabtree et al., 1985; Eastman and Gilula, 1989; Morgan et al., 1987). Because the mRNAs for the Aα, Bβ, and γ subunits of fibrinogen are transcribed by separate genes, efficient control of fibrinogen production requires coordinated expression of the three independent genes (Crabtree and Kant, 1982; Kant et al., 1985; Moshage et al., 1988). In human hepatoma cells, there is an excess of the Aα and γ chains, and hence the synthesis of the Bβ chains is the rate limiting step (Roy et al., 1990; Yu et al., 1983), which is similar to the regulatory step for rabbit fibrinogen synthesis (Alving et al., 1982). In contrast, the formation of the Aα chain is the rate limiting step in the synthesis of rat fibrinogen (Hirose et al., 1988). In all species, the assembly of the complete fibrinogen molecule occurs in the rough ER (Bouma et al., 1975; Kudryk et al., 1982).

19.7.2 Role/Function

Fibrinogen not only has an essential role in hemostasis, but it also contributes to inflammatory and tissue repair processes. The conversion of soluble fibrinogen to insoluble fibrin is required for the formation of the fibril mesh that adheres to damaged vascular endothelial surfaces and constitutes the matrix of the thrombus that stems the loss of blood from the circulation when the vascular endothelium is compromised (Thomas, 2000; Gentry and Downie, 1993). During the initial stage of thrombus formation, platelets are activated, and the glycoprotein IIb–IIIa complex forms on the platelet membrane, which then functions as a receptor for fibrinogen and other adhesive proteins, such as fibronectin and vonWillebrand factor (Charo et al., 1994). These interactions not only promote the adhesion of activated platelets to the damaged vasculature but also facilitate the accumulation of platelet aggregates and the localized release of mitogenic components, such as platelet-derived growth factor, from the platelets at the site of injury (Gentry, 1992). Once wound healing has been initiated, fibrinolytic components, including tissue-plasminogen activator and plasminogen that adhered to the fibrin(ogen) matrix during thrombus formation, facilitate the localized generation of plasmin, a proteolytic enzyme that selectively degrades fibrin and permits the dissolution of the thrombus with the release of proteinaceous and cellular debris, that can be removed from the circulation by phagocytic cells (Murata et al., 2004; Thomas, 2000; Gentry and Downie, 1993). Fibrin deposition can also occur in interstitial fluid because the increased vascular permeability associated with inflammation permits the extravascular accumulation of hemostatic proteins. Fibrin(ogen) can modulate the inflammatory response by enhancing fibroblast migration and proliferation and facilitating leukocyte–endothelial cell adhesion and transmigration (Brown et al., 1993; Ge et al., 1992; Languino et al., 1995; Olman et al., 1996; Senior et al., 1986; Vogels et al., 1993). A small peptide in the γ-chain of fibrinogen, representing <1% of the total molecule, is responsible for the proinflammatory activity of fibrin(ogen) (Tang et al., 1996). In a mouse model, polymerization and cross-linking of extravascular fibrin was found to be spacially and temporally related to the alveolitis and fibroproliferative areas of bleomycin-induced lung injury (Olman et al., 1996).

Induction of fibrinogen synthesis during the acute phase response is primarily transcriptional and mediated in large part by IL-6 (Birch and Schreiber, 1986; Marinkovic et al., 1989; Otto et al., 1987). Exposure of rat hepatocytes to IL-6 induced a 10-fold increase in both mRNA levels and the rates of transcription of each of the three fibrinogen subunit genes (Munck et al., 1984; Otto et al., 1987). Northern blot hybridization analysis demonstrated that IL-6 induced a coordinated increase in the mRNAs of each fibrinogen chain (Nesbitt and Fuller, 1991). An increase in mRNA levels began immediately after the addition of IL-6 to the culture system and reached a maximum between 12 and 18 hours (Andus et al., 1988). Constant exposure of IL-6 was required to maintain the increased mRNA expression (Nesbitt and Fuller, 1991). The rapidity of the response to IL-6 is compatible with the activation of a preexisting inactive DNA binding factor, the acute phase response factor (APRF) (Wegenka et al., 1993). This APRF can bind to the CTGGGA hexanucleotide motif in the IL-6 response elements in both rat and human β fibrinogen genes (Anderson et al., 1993; Baumann et al., 1990; Huber et al., 1990; Wegenka et al., 1993). The IL-6 response element of β fibrinogen has been located close to the promoter region of the fibrinogen gene, which is similar to the organization of other IL-6 regulated rat and human genes (Baumann et al., 1987b, 1990; Marinkovic and Baumann, 1990). In rats, administration of either turpentine or human recombinant IL-6 induces an almost identical increase in hepatic β-fibrinogen-mRNA levels (De Jong et al., 1988; Gauldie et al., 1990).

Dexamethasone administration to primary cultures of *Xenopus* hepatocytes induced a dramatic increase in fibrinogen synthesis with the low basal Bβ-mRNA levels increasing 20-fold (Bhattacharya et al., 1991). In contrast, in rat and human hepatocytes, variable increases in fibrinogen-mRNA levels and in fibrinogen secretion are observed in response to glucocorticoids in the absence of IL-6 (Huber et al., 1990; Otto et al., 1987). This variable response is also observed in intact animal studies. For example, administration of adrenocorticotrophic hormone (ACTH) consistently produces an elevation in circulating fibrinogen levels in rabbits but not in calves (Gentry et al., 1992). It is now well established that the full gene expression of fibrinogen, like that of α_1-AGP and haptoglobin, requires the combined action of IL-6 and glucocorticoid (Baumann et al., 1989; Castell et al., 1988; Crabtree and Kant, 1982; Geiger et al., 1988a; Otto et al., 1987). The β-fibrinogen GRE functions similarly to that of α_1-AGP (Baumann et al., 1990).

Other members of the IL-6 cytokine family, including CNTF, LIF, and cardiotrophin-1 (which all share the common signaling subunit gp 130), also induce increased β-fibrinogen-mRNA and protein expression in a dose- and time-dependent manner (Baumann and Schendel, 1991; Fuller et al., 1985; Nesbitt et al., 1993; Peters et al., 1995). Both IL-11 and LIF, in the absence of dexamethasone, induce an increase in fibrinogen synthesis equivalent to that of IL-6, but, in the presence of dexamethasone, the synergistic effect of either of these cytokines is lower than that observed for the stimulatory effect of the combination of IL-6 and dexamethasone (Baumann and Schenel, 1991; Baumann and Wong, 1989). In contrast, neither IL-1 nor TNFα, even in the presence of dexamethasone, has any effect on fibrinogen synthesis, even at concentrations that induce a 20-fold increase in α_1-AGP (Andus et al., 1983). Furthermore, in hepatic cell cultures, IL-1 not only inhibits the basal expression of rat fibrinogen but also suppresses the stimulatory effect of IL-6, LIF, and IL-11 (Baumann and Gauldie, 1990; Baumann and Schendel, 1991). Although the injection of IL-1 into male Buffalo rats appeared to induce an increase in β-fibrinogen-mRNA expression within 24 hours of treatment, the response was indirect because heat-inactivated IL-1 also induced a similar response (De Jong et al., 1988). Further, antibodies to IL-6 but not IL-1 suppress the approximately threefold increase in fibrinogen induced by exposure of rat hepatocyte cultures to LPS (Lanser and Brown, 1989).

In human liver, the steady-state synthetic rate of fibrinogen is between 1.7 and 5.0 g/day (Hantgan et al., 1994). Hypofibrinogenemia due to decreased fibrinogen synthesis is uncommon in animals, not only due to the synthetic reserve capacity of hepatic tissue but also to fibrinogen's relatively long circulating half-life, which has been estimated as 3–5 days (Hantgan et al., 1994).

19.7.3 Analytical Methods

Three types of laboratory procedures can be used to quantify fibrinogen: biological, physicochemical, and immunological. The biological assay based on the rate of formation of insoluble fibrin in citrated plasma in the presence of excess thrombin is the most widely used procedure for laboratory animals. Commercial reagents kits, formulated for human fibrinogen determinations, have been used successfully for laboratory animals, as have semiautomated methods (Gentry and Liptrap, 1981;

Gentry et al., 1992; Kimura et al., 1994; Riipi and Carlson, 1990). Consistent results were reported for normal canine fibrinogen levels with the thrombin-time method irrespective of the instrumentation used to detect fibrin formation (Mischke and Menzel, 1994). Physicochemical methods are based on the selective precipitation of plasma fibrinogen following mild heat treatment (Blaisdell and Dodds, 1977; Miller et al., 1971). This type of methodology is widely used in veterinary clinical pathology, particularly with the current instrumentation that permits more precise quantification of fibrinogen compared to older methodologies (Evans and Duncan, 2003; Hart, 1997).

Immunological methods that are extensively used in human medicine generally detect circulating levels of fibrin or fibrinogen degradation products or the fibrinopeptides A and B generated during fibrin formation rather than the intact fibrinogen molecule (Marder et al., 1994). The antibodies generated against components of the human fibrinogen molecule generally show only partial cross-reactivity at best toward nonhuman fibrinogen and, hence, are not useful for nonhuman fibrinogen evaluation. In human medicine, immunological methods have proved useful in characterizing the many types of dysfibrinogenemia identified in the human population (McDonagh et al., 1994). Most of the over 200 human fibrinogen variants have been identified during routine laboratory hemostatic screening because the affected individuals appear clinically and hemostatically normal (McDonagh et al., 1994). This may explain, at least in part, why dysfibrinogenemias are infrequently identified in animals.

19.7.4 Pathophysiological Significance

Basal plasma fibrinogen values can be influenced by the physiological status of an animal, particularly by pregnancy. In many species, a characteristic increase in plasma fibrinogen is observed around the time of parturition (Gentry et al., 1990). In the dog, an earlier, transient increase in fibrinogen is also observed at midgestation, which can be used as a pregnancy marker in this species (Gentry and Liptrap, 1981; Hart, 1997).

The normal range for canine plasma fibrinogen has been determined as 0.9–2.9 mg/mL (Hart, 1997; Kaneko, 1997; Mischke and Menzel, 1994). In a study of healthy dogs, circulating fibrinogen values rose from 2.0 ± 0.1 mg/mL to 3.4 ± 0.4 mg/mL following heartworm implantation, which is typical of the extent of the fibrinogen response to inflammation in dogs (Boudreaux and Dillon, 1991). In dogs, rats, and rabbits, turpentine injection induced a two- to fivefold increase in plasma fibrinogen within 48 hours of treatment (French, 1989). In rabbits, administration of ACTH alone induced an increase in fibrinogen levels from 3.2 ± 0.3 mg/mL to 8.0 ± 1.9 mg/mL within 48 hours (Gentry et al., 1992). However, in this study, there appeared to be no correlation between the increase in circulating corticosterone and fibrinogen values induced by the ACTH treatment. This finding is consistent with observations in dogs that the extent of increase in plasma fibrinogen values does not necessarily correlate with the extent of inflammation (Eckersall and Conner, 1988). Similarly, in mice, the basal fibrinogen level of 1.8 ± 0.1 mg/mL rose to 4.5 ± 0.8 mg/mL following treatment of the animals with either 1 or 5 mg LPS per kg (Rofe et al., 1996). Under certain conditions, elevated plasma fibrinogen values can persist for extended periods of time. A chronic increase, lasting up to 2 months, was reported in both endotoxin-resistant mice (C3H/HeJ) and endotoxin-sensitive mice (C3H/HeN) following a single inoculation with *C. albicans* (Riipi and Carlson, 1990). In this study, there did not appear to be a corresponding decline in albumin, a negative APR (Baumann, 1990). This result is distinct from the acute response observed in turpentine-treated Wistar rats (Ballmer et al., 1992). In rats, the increased synthesis of fibrinogen inversely follows the time course of the decline in albumin synthesis (Ballmer et al., 1992). It is likely that the persistence of elevated fibrinogen values requires the continuous presence of inflammatory cytokines. For example, administration of daily doses of IL-6 to rhesus monkeys over a 4-week period was required to induce a twofold increase in plasma fibrinogen levels (Myers et al., 1995). In the monkeys, the fibrinogen values rose from an average of 2.5–5.4 mg/mL during the study period.

19.8 HAMSTER FEMALE PROTEIN

19.8.1 Properties

Hamster female protein (FP), so named because it was first identified in serum from female Syrian hamsters, is a member of the pentraxin family and shares many structural and immunological features with CRP and SAP (Coe, 1977; Coe et al., 1981). An intriguing observation is that the FPs isolated from Syrian (*Mesocricetus auratus*), Turkish (*Mesocricetus brandti*), and Armenian (*Cricetulus migratorius*) hamsters are structurally identical but exhibit different acute phase responses (Coe, 1977; Coe and Ross, 1990a; Coe et al., 1997).

The Syrian hamster female protein (FP-S), whether isolated from serum or amyloid deposits, is a pentameric molecule composed of covalently linked glycosylated 25.6 kDa subunits containing a single intrachain disulphide bridge (Tennet et al., 1993). Under physiological conditions, FP-S may circulate as a decamer, because like SAP, isolated five unit molecules aggregate to form 10 subunit molecules in the presence of calcium (Tennet et al., 1993). Female protein isolated from the Armenian hamster (FP-A) is also a pentameric oligomer of five identical nonconvalently assembled subunits (Coe and Ross, 1990a). The structural similarity between FP-S and FP-A has been demonstrated by the in vitro generation of a hybrid pentamer molecule consisting of both FP-S and FP-A monomer units (Coe and Ross, 1987) and by the observation that FP-S and FP-A share common antigens (Coe and Ross, 1990a). The Turkish female protein (FP-T) is also a 150 kDa pentameric molecule consisting of five identical 30 kDa subunits (Coe et al., 1997). Based on comparison of N-terminal amino acid sequences, FP-T and FP-A share 97.5% and 85.0% identity, respectively, with FP-S (Coe et al., 1997; Dowton and Waggoner, 1989). On the basis of amino acid composition, the FPs appear to be more closely related to SAP than CRP, with 77.5%, 72.5%, and 52.5% homology being found between FP-S and mouse SAP, human SAP, and human CRP, resepectively (Coe et al., 1981, 1997; Dowton et al., 1985; Ishikawa et al., 1987). However, on the basis of selective binding to phosphocholine and agarose, FP-S and FP-A exhibit characteristics of CRP (Coe et al., 1990a; Dowton et al., 1985; Etlinger and Coe, 1986). There are two calcium-binding sites on the FP-S molecule, and the changes in conformation following calcium or phosphocholine binding suggest that the physiological mechanism of ligand interaction is similar to other pentraxins (Dong et al., 1992).

19.8.2 Role/Function

In both Armenian and Turkish hamsters, FP responds as a positive acute phase protein in both males and females, with no gender differences being found in the hepatic FP-A-mRNA response during inflammation (Coe et al., 1997; Dowton and Waggoner, 1989). Although the regulation of expression of both Syrian and Armenian hamster FP genes occurs at the pretranslation level and the FP genes from both species are capable of responding to estrogen via an estrogen receptor mechanism, structural differences have been documented between the FP genes in these species (Coe and Ross, 1983, 1987; Dowton and Waggoner, 1989). The gene encoding for FP in Syrian hamsters is structurally similar to all reported pentraxin genes from many species, particularly in the intron/extron organization (Rudnick and Dowton, 1993).

The biological function of FP is not known. Like other pentraxins, it may have a role in clearing nuclear material from damaged cells because it shares the ability of CRP to bind to histones and chromatin in a PC-inhibitable manner, and like SAP, it can bind to DNA (Saunero-Nava et al., 1992). Also, like SAP, FP is a constituent of amyloid deposits. Amyloidosis is a common feature of aging Syrian hamsters, and the disease is more prevalent in females than males (Coe and Ross, 1985). The correlation between the appearance of amyloidosis and serum FP levels has been confirmed by hormonal manipulation of FP levels in Syrian hamsters with a corresponding increase or decrease in amyloid deposits (Coe and Ross, 1985, 1990b; Snel et al., 1989). Further, amyloidosis is a rare disease in Armenian and Turkish hamsters, which express low basals serum FP levels (Coe and Ross, 1985). In hamsters with amyloidosis, the metabolism of injected ^{125}I-FP is altered with FP rapidly entering and persisting in amyloid deposits (Coe and Ross, 1985).

19.8.3 Analytical Methods

Due to its binding characteristics, column chromatography techniques using substituted agarose, similar to the procedures used to isolate SAP, have been employed to isolate FP from both serum and amyloid deposits (Coe and Ross, 1987; Coe et al., 1997; Skinner and Cohen, 1988; Tennet et al., 1993). Quantitative determinations of serum FP levels in all strains of hamsters have utilized immunoelectrophoretic procedures and ELISA assays (Coe and Ross, 1990a, 1997; Rudnick and Dowton, 1993).

19.8.4 Pathophysiological Significance

Like CRP and SAP, FP is synthesized in the liver, but its regulation is unique in being under the dual control of sex hormones and cytokines (Coe and Ross, 1983, 1990a; Coe et al., 1997). In both Syrian and Turkish hamsters, FP synthesis is suppressed by testosterone (Coe and Ross, 1985; Coe et al., 1997; Rudnick and Dowton, 1993), while in Armenian hamsters, estrogen is the suppressor hormone (Coe and Ross, 1990a). As a consequence, in both Syrian and Turkish hamsters, basal serum FP levels are up to 1000-fold higher in females than in males (Coe and Ross, 1985; Coe et al., 1997). Species differences are also apparent in the FP response to inflammatory stimuli. In Syrian hamsters following turpentine administration, hepatic FP-mRNA levels rapidly decline in females, reaching a nadir within 12 hours, while FP-mRNA levels rise slowly in males only reaching maximal levels after 48 hours (Rudnick and Dowton, 1993). The difference in response is unrelated to circulating testosterone levels (Rudnick and Dowton, 1993). Following injection of ^{125}I-FP, a circulating half-life of 9–16 hours was found in both males and females (Coe and Ross, 1983). Nor do the gender differences appear to be related to an alteration in the rate of hepatic FP synthesis, because the transcription rates for the FP gene are similar in male and female hamsters (Dowton and Waggoner, 1989). Consequently, it has been suggested that like CRP, the gender differences in the steady state and acute phase mRNA concentrations may be related to altered FP-specific mRNA stability (Dowton and Waggoner, 1989). The in vivo administration of cytokines to Syrian Hamsters produces complex responses. While IL-6 or TNF administration to females induced a decrease in hepatic FP-mRNA levels within 8 hours of treatment, a decrease in FP-mRNA was not evident until 24 hours after IL-1 administration (Rudnick and Dowton, 1993). Moreover, the expected increase in hepatic FP-mRNA in male Syrian hamsters following cytokine administration did not occur (Rudnick and Dowton, 1993).

Adult Syrian female hamsters exhibit basal levels of FP in the 1.0–2.0 mg/mL range, while the range of values for Turkish female hamsters is 0.10–0.50 mg/mL (Coe and Ross, 1983; Coe et al., 1997; Etlinger and Coe, 1986). In both strains, the males exhibit similar values in the 0.01–0.02 mg/mL range. No gender differences have been observed in Armenian hamsters, with basal values of 0.05–0.30 mg/mL being reported for both sexes (Coe and Ross, 1990a). Seasonal sex-related variations in serum FP values have also been observed. In female Turkish hamsters, average FP values decreased to 0.15 ± 0.02 mg/mL in winter months, compared to 0.40 ± 0.05 mg/mL during summer months (Coe et al., 1997). In Armenian hamsters, a three- to fourfold increase over basal levels in serum FP values was observed in females but not in males during the winter period (Coe and Ross, 1990a). No age-related changes were observed for serum FP values in Armenian hamsters. In male Syrian hamsters, peak serum FP levels occurred at 21 days of age (0.4–0.5 mg/mL), which declined to adult values by 60–90 days of age, while in the females, adult values were reached by about 35 days of age (Coe and Ross, 1983; French, 1989).

In all types of hamsters (except the female Syrian hamster), FP acts as a positive APR. In both male and female Armenian hamsters, a 3–10-fold increase in serum FP values was observed following turpentine injection, which was independent of any seasonal variations (Coe and Ross, 1990a).

In Turkish hamsters, silver nitrate administration induced a transient fourfold increase in serum FP values in females and a 100-fold increase in males, which persisted for about 48 hours (Coe et al., 1997). A divergent response to inflammatory stimuli is observed in Syrian hamsters with serum FP values increasing 5–10-fold in males and decreasing by 50% in females (Coe and Ross, 1983). Prolonged administration of exogenous corticosteroids to female Syrian hamsters produced a similar response in serum FP levels as a single turpentine injection.

Castration of male Syrian hamsters induced an increase in hepatic FP-mRNA levels, which was translated into an increase in serum FP to average values of 1.43 ± 0.31 mg/mL (Coe and Ross, 1987). Estradiol administration to the castrated males further stimulated FP production to 2.54 ± 0.28 mg/mL, while both testosterone and dexamethasone administration reduced levels to 0.07 ± 0.02 mg/mL and 0.21 ± 0.03 mg/mL, respectively (Coe and Ross, 1987). These alterations in serum FP correlated with alterations in hepatic FP-mRNA levels induced by the hormones treatments.

19.9 MURINOGLOBULINS

19.9.1 Properties

Murinoglobulin is a member of the α_2M family that is unique to rodents, and in some species of rodents, it is the most prominent circulating α_2M-type protein (Geiger et al., 1987; Miyake et al., 1993; Saito and Sinohara, 1985a, 1985b; Van Leuven et al., 1992).

Murinoglobulins are monomeric glycoproteins with molecular weights ranging from 180 to 210 kDa (Saito and Sinohara, 1985a, 1985b) that are constitutively expressed in mice, rats, guinea pigs, and hamsters but are not present in rabbits or other nonrodent mammals (Ganrot, 1966; Miyake et al., 1993; Saito and Sinohara, 1985a, 1985b). Murinoglobulins and α_2M show only minor differences in inhibitory activity under in vitro conditions despite exhibiting markedly different primary structures in the reactive "bait" region (Overbergh et al., 1991, 1994).

19.9.2 Role/Function

Murinoglobulin interferes with the proteolytic activity of trypsin, papain, and thermolysin, but not with their esterolytic activity toward low-molecular-weight substrates (Saito and Sinohara, 1985b).

19.9.3 Analytical Methods

19.9.4 Pathophysiological Significance

In rats and mice, murinoglobulin is the major plasma constituent of the macroglobulin family with normal values ranging from 7 to 14 mg/mL in rats and around 2 mg/mL in mice (Cavus et al., 1996; Koj et al., 1995; Saito and Sinohara, 1985b; Yamamoto et al., 1985). In hamsters, the normal level of murinoglobulin is only approximately 1 µg/mL, and the trypsin inhibiting activity is weaker than that of the rat, mouse, and guinea pig homologs (Miyake et al., 1993). In addition to murinoglobulin and α_2M, rats constitutively express an α_1-macroglobulin, which shows a considerable degree of homology with mouse α_2M and remains unaltered during the acute phase response (Saito and Sinohara, 1985b; Van Leuven et al., 1992). Rat murinoglobulin partially cross-reacts with antibodies to mouse murinoglobulin and rat α_1-macroglobulin but not with human α_2M or rat α_2M (Saito and Sinohara, 1985b).

Following turpentine injection, a threefold decrease in circulating levels of murinoglobulin (also known as rat α_2-inhibitor 3) occurs in Sprague-Dawley rats, which corresponded to the decrease observed in murinoglobulin content in hepatocytes (Geiger et al., 1987). Murinoglobulin also responds as a negative APR in mice but not in guinea pigs (Miyake et al., 1993; Suzuki et al., 1990).

19.10 SERUM AMYLOID A

19.10.1 Properties

SAA proteins comprise a multigene regulated family of apolipoproteins that circulate in association with high-density lipoproteins (HDLs) (Benditt et al., 1989; French, 1989; Malle et al., 1993). In mice and people, SAA responds as a typical APR but not in rats or hamsters (Kushner and Mackiewicz, 1987). One form of circulating SAA is the precursor of secondary amyloid deposits in tissues.

In all species, the basic SAA protein is a single polypeptide chain with a molecular weight ranging from 11.4 to 16.0 kDa (Marhaug and Dowton, 1994). The prototype human and rabbit SAA proteins consist of 104 amino acid residues (Liepnieks et al., 1991; Parmelee et al., 1982), while murine and hamster SAA have 103 amino acid residues (De Beer et al., 1991, 1993; Webb et al., 1989). Dog and Abyssinian cat SAA molecules are larger due to an octapeptide insertion between the residues corresponding to 69–70 of the human sequence (Dwulet et al., 1988; Kluve-Beckerman et al., 1989; Sellar et al., 1991). The N-terminal part of the protein is hydrophobic, and confers lipid-binding properties to the molecule (Marhaug and Dowton, 1994).

Several isoforms of SAA have been identified in humans (Bausserman et al., 1980; Strachan et al., 1988), mice (Coetzee et al., 1986; Hoffman and Benditt, 1982; Lowell et al., 1986a), hamsters (Niewold and Tooten, 1990; Webb et al., 1989), rabbits (Brunn et al., 1995; Liepnieks et al., 1991; Rygg et al., 1991; Syversen et al., 1993; Tatum et al., 1990), and dogs (Sellar et al., 1991). In mice, the three distinct subfamilies of SAA proteins are produced in the liver and respond as APRs. They are classified as: (1) the isoforms, SAA_1 and SAA_2, which become major apolipoproteins in HDL in the circulation, (2) SAA_3, which is also produced in extrahepatic tissues, including macrophages, monocytes, Leydig cells of the testes and mononuclear cells of the spleen (Meek et al., 1992), and (3) SAA_5, the main isoform present in normal HDL (De Beer et al., 1996). The mouse SAA_5 isoform exhibits 48% amino acid sequence homology with the other mouse SAA proteins (De Beer et al., 1994). In Syrian hamsters, at least four distinct SAA isoforms have been identified (Niewold and Tooten, 1990; Webb et al., 1989). In rabbits, two SAA proteins characteristic of SAA_1 and SAA_2 have been identified (Brunn et al., 1995). Despite evidence that at least three SAA genes are present in the dog genome, canine SAA appears to circulate as a single homogenous 12.3 kDa protein (Sellar et al., 1991). In people, in addition to the SAA_1 and SAA_2 isoforms, there is a constitutively expressed isoform classified as SAA_4 (de Beer et al., 1995) that comprises 90% of the normal human serum SAA content and does not respond as an APR (Malle et al., 1993).

In humans, the SAA gene family is located on the short arm of chromosome 11 (Hoffman and Benditt, 1982). In mice, there are three genes and a pseudogene that are all located on the proximal arm of chromosome 7 (Butler et al., 1995; Lowell et al., 1986a; Sellar et al., 1991; Stearman et al., 1986; Stubbs et al., 1994; Taylor and Rowe, 1984). The mouse SAA_1 and SAA_2 genes show 96% nucleotide sequence homology over their entire length (Lowell et al., 1986a, 1986b; Yamamoto et al., 1987). The third gene, SAA_3, exhibits 70% homology in the translated exons but less that 25% homology in other nucleotide sequences (Huang et al., 1990; Yamamoto et al., 1987). The existence of multiple SAA gene families has also been found in the rabbit (Ray and Ray, 1991a, 1991b) and hamster genome (De Beer et al., 1993). Multiple factors are known to be involved in the induction of SAA genes. The mRNA expressed by each of the three SAA genes is elevated 200–500-fold in mice following either LPS or casein injections (Hoffman and Benditt, 1982; Lowell et al., 1986a; Meek and Benditt, 1986; Meek et al., 1989; Morrow et al., 1981). The increased SAA-mRNA expression in mice is accompanied by increased hepatocyte synthesis and secretion of both SAA_1 and SAA_2 (Benson and Kleiner, 1980; Hoffman and Benditt, 1982; Meek and Benditt, 1986; Meek et al., 1986; Selinger et al., 1980). In mice, despite evidence that SAA_1/SAA_2 is relatively uniformly distributed in all hepatocytes, it has been estimated that only 20% of hepatocytes participate in SAA synthesis (Hoffman and Benditt, 1982; Shirahama et al., 1984). In murine extrahepatic tissues, SAA_3-mRNA accumulates following LPS administration, but no increases in SAA-related mRNA occur in response to casein administration to mice (Hoffman and Benditt, 1982; Meek and Benditt, 1986; Meek et al., 1989). In Sprague-Dawley rats, both LPS and turpentine injections induce hepatocyte expression of SAA_1- and SAA_2-mRNAs (Meek and Benditt, 1989). Similarly, it has been shown that in dogs, rabbits, and Syrian hamsters, an acute phase response induces an increase in hepatocyte SAA-mRNA levels (De Beer et al., 1993; Ray and Ray, 1991a; Sellar et al., 1991). Additionally, several isoforms have been identified in dog serum, and the demonstration of highly alkaline SAA isoforms in synovial fluid, which suggest SAA is also produced locally in inflamed joints (Kjelgaard-Hansen et al., 2007).

19.10.2 Role/Function

The increase in hepatic SAA-mRNA expression is regulated at the transcriptional level (Lowell et al., 1986a) and is mediated by several cytokines, including IL-1 (Boraschi et al., 1990; Huang et al., 1990; Ramadori et al., 1985a, 1985b; Weinstein and Taylor, 1987). In vitro studies with cultured mouse hepatocytes or human primary liver cell cultures indicate that the presence of a combination of IL-1, IL-6, and glucocorticoids is required to fully stimulate SAA synthesis (Ganapathl et al., 1991; Prowse and Baumann, 1989). In primary hepatocyte cultures from *M. caroli*, IL-1 and IL-6 selectively induce an increase in the acidic, but not the basic, form of the SAA protein (Prowse and Baumann, 1989). The injection of either CNTF, IL-6, IL-11, LIF, oncostatin M, or cardotrophin-1 into CD-I mice each produced a 25-fold increase in serum SAA levels within 18 hours (Benigni et al., 1996). The similarity in the SAA response to the various cytokines is likely related to the fact that although these cytokines differ in structure and function, they share a common receptor subunit, referred to as gp 130. Similar to the alteration in transcription rates, the action of these cytokines may also be directed toward increasing SAA-mRNA stabilization because, several studies have shown that, following cytokine stimulation, there is a greater increase in SAA-mRNA accumulation than can be accounted for solely on the basis of the increased rate of SAA-mRNA transcription (Lowell et al., 1986a; Reinhoff and Groudine, 1988). The decreased stability of SAA-mRNA in normal mouse liver has been proposed as one of the mechanisms that acts to downregulate SAA production in vivo (Brisette et al., 1989; Lowell et al., 1986a; Sellar et al., 1991; Steel et al., 1993). Clearly, the factors contributing to the regulation of SAA expression are complex because transgenic IL-$1^{-/-}$ mice, which are incapable of expressing IL-1, exhibit a normal SAA response to LPS (Fantuzzi et al., 1996).

In extrahepatic tissues, such as macrophages and monocytes, that synthesize the SAA_3 isoform, IL-6 appears to activate a nuclear factor that binds to the promoter region of the SAA gene, resulting in increased accumulation of SAA_3-mRNA (Ray and Ray, 1993, 1996). In these cell types, glucocorticoids can further enhance the rate of SAA_3-mRNA transcription (Ishida et al., 1994; Urieli-Shoval et al., 1994). However, these effects may not be directly related to the acute phase response because there is no evidence of increased synthesis of the SAA_3 protein or its release into the circulation that accompanies the increase in tissue SAA-mRNA levels (Meek and Benditt, 1986).

In contrast to the relatively long circulating half-lives of other HDL apolipoproteins, radiolabeled SAA is rapidly cleared from the circulation in cynomologus monkeys, vervets, rats, and mice (Bausserman et al., 1984, 1987; Gollaher and Bausserman, 1990; Hoffman and Benditt, 1983; Parks and Rudel, 1983). The circulating half-life for SAA in mice is about 3.5 hours, compared to 11 hours for apoA-1 (Hoffman and Benditt, 1983; Tape and Kisilevsky, 1990). The degradation of SAA is mediated by cell-associated enzymes and is retarded by the association of SAA with lipoproteins. The catabolism of SAA is independent of other HDL lipoproteins (Bausserman et al., 1987). Hepatic catabolism of SAA occurs primarily in Kuppfer cells (Bausserman et al., 1987; Fuks and Zucker-Franklin, 1985; Meek et al., 1989), and the rate of degradation is depressed in both acute and chronic stages of inflammation (Gollaher and Bausserman, 1990).

The biological function(s) of SAA as an acute phase protein has still not been fully elucidated. It is likely, however, that SAA has a role in regulating lipid metabolism, particularly during the process of inflammation. The increased incorporation of SAA into HDL appears to accelerate the removal of these particles from the circulation (Watterson, 2009). During inflammation, there is an increased number of binding sites for SAA-HDL on macrophages and a reduction in binding sites on hepatocytes (Kisilevsky, 1991; Kisilevsky and Subrahamanyan, 1992). These changes are associated with a three- to fourfold higher macrophage affinity for SAA-rich HDL and a twofold reduction in hepatocyte affinity for the SAA-enriched HDL, compared to SAA-poor HDL (Kisilevsky and Subrahamanyan, 1992). The increased macrophage uptake of SAA coupled with the increased expression of SAA-mRNA in these cells during inflammation suggests that these SAA-mediated events may be one mechanism by which lipid debris is cleared from the circulation (Butler et al., 1995; Malle et al., 1993; Meek et al., 1989). In people, the marked decrease in both plasma HDL and esterified cholesterol during an acute phase reaction has been related to the changes in HDL apolipoprotein content, including the SAA content (Steinmetz et al., 1989). The reduction in plasma cholesterol levels may also be associated with a reduction in the activity of lecithin cholesterol acyltransferase as a result of SAA incorporation into phospholipid vesicles (Fielding et al., 1972; Steinmetz et al., 1989).

Another biological role for SAA proteins is to enhance the recruitment of white cells into inflammatory lesions. For example, SAA can function as a chemoattractant for human monocytes, neutrophils, and T lymphocytes and can also induce the adhesion of these cells to cultured umbilical cord vein endothelial cell monolayers (Badolato et al., 1994; Xu et al., 1995). However, unlike CRP, which activates neutrophils, SAA inhibits the oxidative burst in stimulated neutrophils (Foldes-Filep et al., 1992; Nunomura et al., 1990b). There is evidence that, at least in lymphocytes, the actions of SAA may be mediated through a G-protein-coupled receptor (Xu et al., 1995). This suggestion is supported by in vitro studies demonstrating that SAA inhibits platelet activation initiated by thrombin but not by other agonists (Zimlichman et al., 1990). Platelet aggregation is induced by thrombin through a specific membrane thrombin receptor, a G-type protein receptor, while other platelet agonists interact with different types of platelet receptors (Coughlin, 1995). It is, however, unlikely that the SAA platelet inhibitory effect has physiological significance, because it is only observed in isolated, protein-free platelet suspensions (Zimlichman et al., 1990).

Animal model studies have established the role of one of the SAA isoforms in the pathogenesis of amyloidosis. It appears that only the SAA_2 isoform of SAA is involved in the formation of amyloid deposits. In mice, as in people, the C-terminal portion of the SAA_2 molecule is cleaved to produce a 75 amino acid, the 8.5-kDa amyloid A (AA) protein (Cohen et al., 1983; Glenner, 1980; Miura et al., 1990). A serine protease derived from monocytes and neutrophils is thought to be responsible for this degradation of apo-SAA_2 (Lavie et al., 1978; Silverman et al., 1982). Precipitation of the released AA molecules to form the amorphous amyloid fibril is facilitated by their ability to bind to basement membrane constituents, such as heparan sulphate proteoglycans and laminin (Ancsin and Kisilevesky, 1997; Inoue et al., 1996). Partial degradation of apo-SAA_2 with the subsequent formation of AA molecules is observed in amyloid-susceptible CBA/J mice, while in amyloid-resistant CE/J mice, apo-SAA_2 is completely degraded with no release of AA molecules (Elliot-Bryant et al., 1996). It has been proposed that the variation in SAA_2 degradation is a function of the different isoforms of the SAA protein expressed among different mouse strains and is related to the different degrees of SAA-gene expression (De Beer et al., 1992; Gonnerman et al., 1995; Rokita et al., 1989; Taylor and Rowe, 1984). This suggestion is supported by the observation that the SAA-like protein expressed in both normal and acute phase rats lacks the N-terminal, or AA-related region of the SAA_2 molecule (Baltz et al., 1987). Rats, like Armenian hamsters, do not develop amyloidosis, and in these species, SAA is also not an apolipoprotein of HDL (Baltz et al., 1987; De Beer et al., 1993; Meek and Benditt, 1989).

Various other effects have been reported, which include detoxification of bacterial endotoxin, inhibition of lymphocyte and endothelial cell proliferation, inhibition of platelet aggregation, and inhibition of T lymphocyte adhesion to ECM proteins. It may also play a role in downregulation of the inflammatory process by inhibiting myeloperoxidase release and directed migration of phagocytes. Intestinal epithelial cells can release SAA upon stimulation by TNF-α, IL-1, and IL-6. The protein may also be involved in the local defence mechanism of the gut to endotoxin challenge. SAA has also been reported to bind to neutrophils and inhibit oxidative burst response suggesting it may help prevent oxidative tissue damage during inflammation. However, this effect may be concentration dependent as inhibition was restricted to lower concentrations. These results suggest that SAA may have different effects according to the local concentration, and that the anti-inflammatory effects may be selective and specific rather than systemic (Murata et al., 2004; Uhlar and Whitehead, 1999).

SAA can induce ECM-degrading enzymes such as collagenase, stromelysin, and matrix metallopreinases 2 and 3, which are important for repair processes after tissue damage. However, prolonged expression of SAA and the long-term production of these enzymes may play a role in degenerative diseases such as rheumatoid arthritis (Uhlar and Whitehead, 1999).

19.10.3 Analytical Methods

The majority of studies quantifying total plasma or serum SAA levels have used immunological procedures, including radioimmunoassays, ELISA, quantitative radial immunodiffusion, or solid-phase immunoradiometry (French, 1989; Hachem et al., 1991; Malle et al., 1993; Marhaug, 1983;McDonald et al., 1991; Sipe et al., 1989; Zuckerman and Surprenant, 1986). Several sandwich ELISA assays for quantifying serum SAA have been developed employing rabbit or rat antisera to human SAA (Dubois and Malmendier, 1988; McDonald et al., 1991), to AA protein (Sipe et al., 1976; Yamada et al., 1989), or to discrete SAA peptides (Saile et al., 1989). Both ELISA and micro-ELISA assays have been used to quantitate SAA in mouse serum using rat or rabbit polyclonal antibodies to mouse SAA (Vogels et al., 1993; Zuckerman and Suprenant, 1986). Despite the apparent lack of strong interspecies cross-reactivity for SAA (French, 1989), feline SAA has been detected in an ELISA assay using a rabbit anticanine SAA antibody, though the sensitivity of the antibody to the cat antigen was found to be lower than the sensitivity of the antibody to the homologous canine SAA (Kajikawa et al., 1996). A sandwich ELISA, along with Western blotting techniques, has also been used to quantitate canine serum SAA (Yamamoto et al., 1994c). Several investigators have noted that the precise quantitation of serum SAA levels is complicated due to its association in serum with HDL and that the procedures used to dissociate SAA from HDL tend to introduce increased variability to the reproducibility of the assays (Godenir et al., 1985; Malle et al., 1993; Saile et al., 1989). Isoelectrofocusing and two-dimensional electrophoresis are two techniques that have been used to visualize the isoforms of SAA in serum from various laboratory animals (Brunn et al., 1995; de Beer et al., 1991).

19.10.4 Pathophysiological Significance

Marked strain-dependent variation in serum SAA levels and in the serum SAA response to inflammatory stimuli have been reported in mice (French, 1989). In amyloid-resistant mouse strains, as in people, SAA responds as a prominent acute phase protein, with serum levels increasing 500–1000-fold following an inflammatory stimulus (Benson et al., 1977; Brandwein et al., 1985; Hoffman and Benditt, 1982; Malle et al., 1993; McAdam and Sipe, 1976; Nonogaki et al., 1996; Rokita et al., 1989). For example, in C57BL/6 mice, serum SAA levels change from being undetectable prior to treatment to 9.4 ± 1.0 μg/mL within 16 hours of administration of nerve growth factor (Nonogaki et al., 1996). Similarly, in Golden hamsters, which also exhibit amyloid resistance, serum SAA values increased from being nondetectable to 150 ± 1 mg/mL 24 hours after LPS treatment (Hol et al., 1987). In domestic cats, which rarely develop amyloidosis, SAA appears to be a weak APR protein. The mean serum SAA values in healthy cats were estimated as 1.2 ± 0.3 μg/mL, compared to 3.7 ± 0.3 μg/mL in animals with various inflammatory conditions (DiBartola et al., 1989). A biphasic change in serum SAA levels is frequently observed in animals with amyloidosis, with elevated values being observed in the early stages of the disease followed by a decline as amyloid deposits form (DiBartola et al., 1989; Rokita et al., 1989). Consequently, serum SAA values are not a useful indicator of amyloidosis.

A 9–20 increase in serum SAA values has been reported in beagle dogs following inoculation with *Bordetella bronchispetica* (Yamamoto et al., 1994b). Higher levels of SAA-mRNA than CRP-mRNA were detected in the liver of fetal, neonatal, and adult rabbits following LPS stimulation, suggesting that in this species (at least during the development phase), SAA rather than CRP may be the more important APR (Rygg et al., 1996).

Plasma levels of SAA can be used to predict the severity of acute pancreatitis significantly earlier than plasma CRP levels (Tape and Ksilevesky, 1990). Furthermore, SAA concentrations may be raised when CRP is not detectable in rheumatic disorders. Similarly, SAA is an early and sensitive marker for allograft organ rejection, being increased where as CRP levels are frequently within normal range or only slightly raised. The potential sensitivity of SAA has been demonstrated by its ability to predict myocardial infarction in the general population (Mayer et al., 2002). Changes of similar pattern and magnitude were observed in man and dog during an acute phase response, support this protein as a valuable diagnostic preclinical to clinical translational biomarker for toxicological studies (Watterson et al., 2008).

19.11 SERUM AMYLOID P

19.11.1 Properties

Serum amyloid P (SAP) was originally named on the basis of its identity with tissue amyloid-P component (Cathcart et al., 1965). The SAPs from different species share structural and functional similarities with both CRP and hamster FP, but among laboratory animals, only mouse SAP exhibits the characteristics of an APR.

Unlike CRP, which circulates as a single pentraxin molecule, SAP circulates as a glycoprotein composed of 10 identical, noncovalently linked subunits arranged as two stacked pentraxins bound "face-to-face" (Emsley et al., 1994; Pepys and Baltz, 1983; Siripont et al., 1988). The molecular weights of mouse, rat, and guinea pig SAP are similar, being in the range of 230–305 kDa (Baltz et al., 1982; Le et al., 1982; Nakada et al., 1986; Sarlo and Mortensen, 1987). Guinea pig SAP is composed of two types of subunits, only one of which is glycosylated (Maudsley et al., 1986). The SAP molecules from all species possess a high-affinity binding site for the 4,6-cyclic pyruvate acetal of the galactose residues present in agarose, which accounts for their preferential calcium-dependent binding to unsubstituted agarose rather than PC-substituted agarose (Baltz et al., 1982; Hind et al., 1984, 1985). Like CRP, both human and mouse SAP can bind to either phosphorylethanolamine or immobilized PC, though SAP has only one binding site per pentraxin, compared to the five per CRP molecule (Christner and Mortensen, 1994; Hawkins et al., 1991; Le et al., 1982).

Both human and mouse SAPs are coded by a single gene that is closely related to the CRP gene, located on chromosome 1 (Floyd-Smith et al., 1986; Mantzouranis et al., 1985; Whitehead et al., 1988; Yunis and Whitehead, 1990). The nucleotide sequences in the respective SAP genes from human, rabbit, mouse, hamster, guinea pig, and rat exhibit considerable homology, as do the amino acid sequences for the respective SAP proteins (Nakada et al., 1986; Rubio et al., 1993; Whitehead and Rits, 1990). The liver is the primary site of SAP synthesis, though not all hepatocytes constitutively express the SAP protein (Le and Mortensen, 1986). Like CRP, the rate of SAP synthesis is regulated at the transcription level. In mice, a single transcription initiation site on the SAP gene controls SAP-mRNA levels, regardless of the mouse strain or whether or not the animals are undergoing an inflammatory response (Itoh et al., 1992).

19.11.2 Role/Function

The administration of recombinant human IL-1 to C57BL/6 mice induced a dose-dependent increase in serum SAP levels (Mortensen et al., 1988). In this study, the serum SAP response to IL-1 was greater than that observed for either fibrinogen or the C3 complement component (Mortensen et al., 1988). In the C57BL/6 mice, recombinant TNFα alone induced a modest fourfold increase in serum SAP values, but when it was administered in combination with IL-1, an additive effect was observed (Mortensen et al., 1988). Results from hepatocyte culture studies suggest that the kinetics of SAP synthesis and secretion are similar in vivo and in vitro (Zahedi and Whitehead, 1993). In hepatocyte cultures, IL-1 is one of the primary cytokines that stimulates SAP synthesis by amplifying protein production in those hepatocytes that constitutively express SAP (Le and Mortensen, 1984a, 1984b, 1986). Secretions from activated macrophages that contain multiple cytokines can both enhance protein synthesis and induce a sevenfold increase in the number of SAP producing hepatocytes (Zahedi and Whitehead, 1993). The exposure of murine hepatocyte cultures to IL-1, IL-6, or a combination of the two induced an approximately threefold increase in cellular SAP-mRNA levels within 12 hours, and the increased expression was sustained for a further 24 hours (Lin et al., 1990; Zahedi and Whitehead, 1993).

Serum SAP levels appear to be governed by the rate of protein synthesis and hepatic secretion of SAP and not by the rate of catabolism or clearance of the molecule (Baltz et al., 1985b; Shirahama et al., 1984). The circulating half-life of SAP in mice is short, having been determined as 7.0–8.25 hours, and it is similar in normal mice expressing different genetically determined basal SAP levels, in mice undergoing an acute phase response, and in mice with casein-induced amyloidosis (Baltz et al., 1985b). In mice, the liver is the main site of SAP clearance and catabolism (Hutchinson et al., 1994).

Because IL-1 can induce an increase in SAP synthesis and secretion and, in turn, SAP can enhance IL-1 secretion by mononuclear phagocytes, it has been suggested that SAP has the potential to influence inflammatory and immunological events initiated by and dependent on IL-1 (Sarlo and Mortensen, 1985). Further, inflammatory responses may be mediated, at least in part, by the selective SAP enhancement of bactericidal activity of murine macrophages through calcium-dependent binding of SAP to mannose-6-phosphate type macrophage receptors (Le and Mortensen, 1986; Siripont et al., 1988). Although the role of SAP as a modulator of the immune response is still controversial, it has been shown that in C57BL/6 mice, SAP can suppress the antibody response to a T-dependent antigen by activating a nonspecific suppressor T-cell subpopulation (Sarlo and Mortensen, 1987). This action of SAP may contribute to the lowered antibody response reported in mice undergoing an inflammatory reaction or exhibiting elevated serum SAP values and also in mice genetically manipulated to endogenously express high levels of SAP (Sarlo and Mortensen, 1987). Alternatively, the primary role of SAP in modulating the immune mechanism may be related to its ability to form a complex with C4b-binding protein (C4BP), an inhibitor of complement (Evans and Nelsestuen, 1995; Schwalbe et al., 1990). When C4BP is complexed with SAP, its inhibitory activity is reduced (de Frutos and Dahlback, 1994).

Among the recognized physiological functions of SAP are its ability to bind to both chromatin and DNA (Butler et al., 1990; Pepys and Butler, 1987; Shephard et al., 1991) and to enhance the clearance of nuclear material from dying cells (Du Clos et al., 1988; Robey et al., 1984). The rate of chromatin clearance is higher in BALB/cJ mice, which constitutively express high amounts of SAP, compared to C57BL/10J mice, which exhibit low baseline serum SAP levels (Burlingame et al., 1996). When an inflammatory response was induced in the C57BL/10J mice, not only was an increase in serum SAP observed, but the rate of chromatin clearance increased to almost equivalent levels to those occurring in the BALB/cJ mice (Burlingame et al., 1996). It was noted that higher serum SAP levels were associated with a reduction of chromatin deposits in renal tissue and a concomitant increase in hepatic chromatin deposits. This SAP-induced redistribution of chromatin may serve to reduce chromatin exposure to the immune system and to protect the kidneys from the chromatin-containing immune complexes that have been implicated in the development of immune complex glomerulonephritis (Burlingame et al., 1996; Connolly et al., 1988).

In immunodeficient mice, elevations of SAP appear to be associated with degeneration of renal function (Connolly et al., 1988). In MRL lpr/lpr, B/W, and NZB mouse strains (which all spontaneously develop autoimmune disease, though at different rates), the relative increases in serum SAP and fibronectin values observed over time correspond to the rate of onset of the disease (Connolly et al., 1988). A similar correlation between serum SAP levels and the SAP inflammatory response has been found in A/J amyloid-resistant mice and CBA/J amyloid-susceptible mice (Zahedi et al., 1991). In both mouse strains, azocasein administration induced an increase in both SAP-mRNA and serum SAP levels during the early stages of inflammation, but during the later stages, the serum SAP levels in the A/J mice dropped to half those of the CBA/J mice (Zahedi et al., 1991). It has been estimated that SAP comprises 10%–15% of the protein in the amyloid deposits that develop as a consequence of chronic inflammation (Coe and Ross, 1985; Pepys and Baltz, 1983). The incorporation of SAP into amyloid deposits may be a function of its ability to interact with basement membrane components, such as collagen, sulfated polysaccharides, and fibronectin (Hamazaki, 1987, 1989; Schwalbe et al., 1991; Zahedi, 1996). The SAP molecule is inherently proteinase resistant, and the SAP in human amyloid deposits is neither degraded nor modified, thus rendering the amyloid deposit less sensitive to proteolysis.

19.11.3 Analytical Methods

Techniques used to quantitate serum SAP have included rocket immunoelectrophoresis (Connolly et al., 1988; Le et al., 1982), competitive binding radioimmunoassay (Sipe et al., 1982), rate nephelometry (Gertz et al., 1984), ELISA (Serban and Rordorf-Adam, 1986), and quantitative (Western) immunoblotting (Griswold et al., 1986). The rate nephelometery and Western blotting techniques are more sensitive than immunoelectrophoresis and superior to radioimmunoassay because the antigenic stability of radiolabeled SAP is lower than that of other APRs, for example, SAA (Gertz et al., 1984). The determination of serum SAP has been facilitated by the commercial availability of murine SAP protein standard and antibody preparations to murine SAP. Methods routinely used for isolating SAP from serum and tissues have been recently reviewed as have quantitative evaluation methods (Skinner and Cohen, 1988).

19.11.4 Pathophysiological Significance

There are considerable strain differences in the constitutively expressed serum SAP levels in mice (Table 19.3). Due to the structural similarities in the SAP genes from mice that are either high or low expressors of SAP, it has been speculated that trans-acting regulatory factor(s) may be involved in a suppressive manner in the transcriptional control of SAP-mRNA (Itoh et al., 1992). Peak hepatic SAP-mRNA levels were observed in female CBA/J mice 8 and 12 hours after thioglycollate and

TABLE 19.3
Serum Amyloid P-Component (SAP) in Different Mouse Strains Before and After Induction of an Inflammatory Response

Mouse Strain	SAP µg/mL	
	Normal Sera	Acute Phase Sera
C57BL/6, C57BL/10	15–37	275–403
MRL lpr/lpr, DBA1/LacJ	74–75	—
C3H/HeJ	82–126	158–170
BALB/cJ	84–138	—
DBA/2	150–180	210–230

azocasein administration, respectively (Zahedi and Whitehead, 1989), which is comparable to the time interval in which a 60-fold increase in SAP-mRNA was induced in C57BL/6 mice after LPS administration (Murakami et al., 1988). The SAP-mRNA response to LPS is approximately 10-fold greater than the CRP-mRNA response in the C57BL/6 mice, though it takes almost four times as long for the SAP-mRNA to reach maximum levels (Murakami et al., 1988). These results are compatible with the observation that the rate of SAP synthesis is generally fivefold higher in mice undergoing an acute phase response than in healthy mice (Le and Mortensen, 1984a). An increase in hepatic SAP-mRNA expression in rats has also been reported following LPS stimulation (Dowton and McGrew, 1990).

As shown in Table 19.3, baseline serum SAP values in mice show marked strain differences (Burlingame et al., 1996; French, 1989; Griswold et al., 1986; Le et al., 1982; Mortensen et al., 1983). The absolute serum SAP values determined for the same mouse strain can vary, depending on the methodology used for the determination. With Western blotting, the relative serum SAP values for BALB/c, DBA1/LacJ, MRL lpr/lpr, and C3H/HeJ strains were 33.7 ± 7.7 μg/mL, 35.4 ± 7.6 μg/mL, 45.6 ± 3.7 μg/mL, and 56.2 ± 4.2 μg/mL, respectively (Griswold et al., 1986). The higher values obtained with other laboratory methods are illustrated in Table 19.3. There appears to be only a modest correlation between basal hepatic SAP-mRNA levels and serum SAP levels in different mouse strains (Itoh et al., 1992). For example, in several strains of mice, LPS treatment induces a ninefold increase in SAP-mRNA that does not always correspond to the extent of the observed elevations in serum SAP values. In DBA/2J mice, only a 1.4-fold elevation in serum SAP occurred following LPS administration, while a ninefold increase was observed in C57BL/6 mice (Mortensen et al., 1983).

A similar lack of correlation between SAP-mRNA and serum SAP levels has been observed in rats. In Sprague-Dawley rats, turpentine treatment induced a 46-fold increase in hepatic SAP-mRNA levels while producing only a twofold increase in serum SAP (Nakada et al., 1986). In CBA/J mice, peak SAP-mRNA levels were recorded 8 and 12 hours after thioglycollate or azocasein injections, respectively, and the alterations in SAP-mRNA correlated with changes in other inflammatory parameters (Zahedi and Whitehead, 1989). In the CBA/J mice, SAP-mRNA levels had returned to near normal by 36 hours, at which time a 20-fold increase in serum SAP levels was detected (Zahedi and Whitehead, 1989). A lag phase between SAP-mRNA induction and increased serum SAP levels has also been noted in TO mice following endotoxin injection (Myers and Fleck, 1988). In both C57BL/6 and C57BL/10 mice, a single intraperitoneal injection of thioglycollate resulted in an 8- to 10-fold increase in serum SAP values within 24 hours (Burlingame et al., 1996; Sarlo and Mortensen, 1987). Similarly, casein administration to C57BL/10 mice caused serum SAP levels to rise to 340 ± 64 μg/mL from a baseline of 26 ± 11 μg/mL (Burlingame et al., 1996). Elevations in mouse serum SAP values also occur in response to parasitic and bacterial infections (French, 1989). Strain differences are also apparent in this type of response. Endotoxin administration to Parkes strain mice elevated serum SAP values from 89 ± 1 μg/mL to 248 ± 19 μg/mL, while the same treatment to C3H/HeJ mice had essentially no effect on serum SAP levels (Poole et al., 1984). In the C3H/HeJ mice, average serum SAP values only change from 109 ± 17 μg/mL to 164 ± 6 μg/mL following endotoxin treatment (Poole et al., 1984).

The baseline values of serum SAP in Dunkin–Hartley guinea pigs have been reported as 16 ± 4 μg/mL, which is similar to the basal values found for SAP in rat and human serum (Maudsley et al., 1986; Pepys et al., 1978). Subcutaneous administration of a 4% solution of silver nitrate to guinea pigs caused serum SAP to rise to only 25 ± 4 μg/mL within 24 hours, but lower doses were ineffective in raising serum SAP values (Maudsley et al., 1986). Hence, SAP is not considered to be a major APR protein in guinea pigs.

Human neonates have low serum SAP that rises to the adult range within a few weeks after birth (Pepys et al., 1982), while neonatal and adult mice exhibit similar serum SAP values (Waites et al., 1983). In female Wistar rats, age differences have been noted, with serum SAP levels rising from 29 μg/mL at 11 weeks of age to 107 μg/mL at 58 weeks (Hashimoto et al., 1995). Human males have been reported to have higher basal serum SAP levels than females (Pepys et al., 1978). In mice, no sex-related alterations in serum SAP levels have been found (Rordorf-Adam et al., 1985). In rats, variable results have been found with no gender-related differences being reported in one study (Nakada et al., 1986), while in another study, higher serum SAP values of 63 ± 18 μg/mL were reported for old females Wistar rats compared to values of 39 ± 10 μg/mL for age-matched males (Hashimoto and Migita, 1990). The gender- and age-related differences in serum SAP levels in Wistar rats have been attributed to the influence of estrogen, because estradiol administration to young males increased serum SAP levels from 26 ± 2 μg/mL to 49 ± 7 μg/mL while testosterone administration had no effect (Hashimoto and Migita, 1990; Hashimoto et al., 1995).

Syngenic pregnancy in C57BL/10 mice produces a transient increase in serum SAP levels in the 3 days before parturition (Waites et al., 1983). In contrast, allogeneic pregnancy (CBA/Ca males) produced triphasic serum SAP response in the C57BL/10 females with a transient twofold increase being observed at day 4 of pregnancy, a sustained threefold increase between days 8 and 12, and a maximum increase of five- to sixfold on day 18 of gestation (Waites et al., 1983). In both types of pregnancy, serum SAP returned to basal levels by day 8 postpartum.

ACKNOWLEDGMENT

I wish to thank Patricia A. Gentry, author of this chapter in the 2nd edition, for her vision and contributions to this chapter.

REFERENCES

Adib-Conquy, M., and Cavaillon, J. 2007. Stress molecules in sepsis and systemic inflammatory response syndrome. *FEBS Lett.* 581:3723–3733.

Aldred, A.R., Grimes, A., Schreiber, G., and Mercer, J.F.B. 1987. Rat ceruloplasmin. Molecular cloning and gene expression in liver, choroid plexus, yolk sac, placenta, and testis. *J Biol Chem.* 262:2875–2878.

Alving, B.M., Chung, S.I., Murano, G., Tang, D.B., and Finlayson, J.S. 1982. Rabbit fibrinogen: Time course of constituent chain production in vivo. *Arch Biochem Biophys.* 217:1–9.

Ancsin, J.B., and Kisilevesky, R. 1997. Characterization of high affinity binding between laminin and the acute phase protein, serum amyloid A. *J Biol Chem.* 272:406–413.

Andersen, P., and Eika, C. 1980. Inhibition of thrombin-induced platelet aggregation by crude and highly purified alpha 1-acid glycoprotein. *Scand J Haematol.* 25:202–204.

Andersen, V., Hansen, G.H., Olsen, J., Poulsen, M.D., Norén, O., and Sjöström, H. 1994. On the transfer of serum proteins to the rat intestinal juice. *Scand J Gastroeneterol.* 29:430–436.

Anderson, G.M., Shaw, A.R., and Shafer, J.A. 1993. Functional characterization of promoter elements involved in regulation of human Bb-fibrinogen expression. *J Biol Chem.* 268:22650–22655.

Andres, J.L., Stanley, K., Cheifetz, S., and Massague, J. 1989. Membrane-anchored and soluble forms of betaglycan, a polymorphic proteoglycan that binds transforming growth factor-β. *J Cell Biol.* 109:3137–3145.

Andrew, M., Paes, B., Milner, R., et al. 1987. Development of the coagulation system in the full-term infant. *Blood.* 70:167–172.

Andus, T., Geiger, T., Hirano, T., Kishimoto, T., and Heinrich, P.C. 1988. Action of recombinant human interleukin 6, interleukin 1β, and tumor necrosis factor α on the mRNA induction of acute-phase proteins. *Eur J Immunol.* 18:739–746.

Andus, T., Gross, V., Tran-Thi, T.-A., Schreiber, G., Nagashima, M., and Heinrich, P.C. 1983. The biosynthesis of acute-phase proteins in primary cultures of rat hepatocytes. *J Biochem.* 133:561–571.

Araujo-Jorge, T.C., de-Meirelles Mde, N., and Isaac, L. 1990. Trypanosoma cruzi: Killing and enhanced uptake by resident peritoneal macrophages treated with alpha-2-macroglobulin. *Parasitol Res.* 76:545–552.

Araujo-Jorge, T.C., Lage, M.-J.F., Rivera, M.T., Carlier, Y., and van Leuven, F. 1992. Trypanosoma cruzi: Enhanced alpha-macroglobulin levels correlate with the resistance of BALB/cj mice to acute infection. *Parasitol Res.* 78:215–221.

Arnaud, P., Gianazza, E., and Miribel, L. 1988. Ceruloplasmin. *Methods Enzymol.* 163:441–452.

Ashcom, J.D., Tiller, S.E., Dickerson, K., Cravens, J.L., Argraves, W.S., and Strickland, D.K. 1990. The human α_2 macroglobulin receptor: Identification of a 420-kD cell surface glycoprotein specific for the activated conformation of α_2 macroglobulin. *J Cell Biol.* 110:1041–1048.

Axelsson, L., Bergenfeldt, M., Björk, P., Olsson, R., and Ohlsson, K. 1991. Release of immunoreactive canine leukocytes elastase normally and in endotoxin and pancratitic shock. *Scand J Clin Lab Invest.* 50:35–42.

Badolato, R., Wang, J.M., Murphy, W.J., et al. 1994. Serum amyloid A is a chemoattractant: Induction of migration, adhesion, and tissue infiltration of monocytes and polymorphonuclear leukocytes. *J Exp Med.* 180:203–209.

Baker, R.J., and Valli, V.E.O. 1988. Electrophoretic and immunoelectrophoretic analysis of feline serum proteins. *Can J Vet Res.* 52:308–314.

Bala, S., and Failla, M.L. 1992. Copper deficiency reversibly impairs DNA synthesis in activated T lymphocytes by limiting interleukin 2 activity. *Proc Natl Acad Sci USA.* 89:6794–6797.

Ballmer, P.E., Ballmer-Hofer, K., Repond, F., Kohler, H., and Studer, H. 1992. Acute suppression of albumin synthesis in systemic inflammatory disease: An individually graded response of rat hepatocytes. *J Histochem Cytochem.* 40:201–206.

Ballou, S.P., Buniel, J., and MacIntyre, S.S. 1989. Specific binding of human C-reactive protein to human monocytes in vitro. *J Immunol.* 142:2708–2713.

Baltz, M.L., deBeer, F.C., Geinstein, A., et al. 1982. Phylogenetic aspects of C-reactive protein and related proteins. *Ann N Y Acad Sci.* 389:49–73.

Baltz, M.L., Dyck, R.F., and Pepys, M.B. 1985b. Studies of the in vivo synthesis and catabolism of serum amyloid P component SAP in the mouse. *Clin Exp Immunol.* 59:235–242.

Baltz, M.L., Rowe, I.F., Caspi, D., Turnell, W.G., and Pepys, M.B. 1987. Acute-phase high-density lipoprotein in the rat does not contain serum amyloid A protein. *Biochem J.* 242:301–303.

Baltz, M.L., Rowe, I.R., and Pepys, M.B. 1985a. In vivo turnover studies of C-reactive protein. *Clin Exp Immunol.* 59:243–250.

Banda, M.J., Rice, A.G., Griffin, G.L., and Senior, R.M. 1988. α_1-proteinase inhibitor is a neutrophil chemoattractant after proteolytic inactivation by macrophage elastase. *J Biol Chem.* 263:4481–4484.

Barbey-Morel, C., Pierce, J.A., Campbell, E.J., and Perlmutter, D.H. 1987. Lipopolysaccharide modulates the expression of alpha 1 proteinase inhibitor and other serine proteinase inhibitors in human monocytes and macrophages. *J Exp Med.* 166:1041–1054.

Barna, B.P., Deodhar, S.D., Gautam, S., Yen-Lieberman, B., and Roberts, D. 1984. Macrophage activation and generation of turmoridical activity by liposome-associated human C-reactive protein. *Cancer Res.* 44:305–310.

Barnes, G., and Frieden, E. 1984. Ceruloplasmin receptors of erythrocytes. *Biochem Biophys Res Commun.* 125:157–162.

Barrett, A.J., Brown, M.A., and Sayers, C.A. 1979. The electrophoretically "slow" and "fast" forms of the α_2-macroglobulin molecule. *Biochem J.* 181:401–418.

Barrett, A.J., and Starkey, P.M. 1973. The interaction of α_2 macroglobulin with proteinases. Characteristics and specificity of the reaction, and a hypothesis concerning its molecular mechanism. *Biochem J.* 133:709–724.

Bashir, M.S., Morrison, K., Wright, D.H., and Jones, D.B. 1992. Alpha-1 antitrypsin gene exon use in stimulated lymphoctyes. *J Clin Pathol.* 45:1776–1780.

Baumann, H. 1990. Transcriptional control of the rat alpha-1-acid glycoprotein gene. *J Biol Chem.* 265:19420–19423.

Baumann, H., and Berger, F.G. 1985. Genetics and evolution of the acute phase proteins in mice. *Mol Gen Genet.* 201:505–512.

Baumann, H., and Gauldie, J. 1990. Regulation of acute phase plasma protein genes by hepatocyte-stimulating factors and other mediators of inflammation. *Mol Biol Med.* 7:147–159.

Baumann, H., and Gauldie, J. 1994. The acute phase response. *Immunol Today.* 15:74–80.

Baumann, H., Held, W.A., and Berger, F.G. 1984. The acute phase response of mouse liver. *J Biol Chem.* 259:566–573.

Baumann, H., Jahreis, G.P., and Gaines, K.C. 1983. Synthesis and regulation of acute phase plasma proteins in primary cultures of mouse hepatocytes. *J Cell Biol.* 97:866–876.

Baumann, H., Jahreis, G.P., and Morella, K.K. 1990. Interaction of cytokine- and glucocorticoid-response elements of acute-phase plasma protein genes. *J Biol Chem.* 265:22275–22281.

Baumann, H., Jahreis, G.P., Morella, K.K., et al. 1991. Transcriptional regulation through cytokine and glucocorticoid response elements of rat acute phase plasma protein genes by C/EBP and Jun B. *J Biol Chem.* 266:20390–20399.

Baumann, H., Latimer, J.J., and Glibetic, M.D. 1986. Mouse α_1-protease inhibitor is not an acute phase reactant. *Arch Biochem Biophys.* 246:488–493.

Baumann, H., Morella, K.K., Campos, S.P., Cao, Z., and Jahreis, G.P. 1992. Role of CAAT-enhancer binding protein isoforms in the cytokine regulation of acute-phase plasma protein genes. *J Biochem.* 267:19744–19751.

Baumann, H., Morella, K.K., and Wong, G.H.W. 1993. TNF-α, IL-β, and hepatocyte growth factor cooperate in stimulating specific acute phase plasma protein genes in rat hepatoma cells. *J Immunol.* 151:4248–4257.

Baumann, H., Onorato, V., Gauldie, J., and Jahreis, G.P. 1987a. Distinct sets of acute phase plasma proteins are stimulated by separate human hepatocyte-stimulating factors and monokines in rat hepatoma cells. *J Biol Chem.* 262:9756–9768.

Baumann, H., Prowse, K.R., Marinkovic, S., Won, K.-A., and Jahreis, G.P. 1989. Stimulation of hepatic acute phase response by cytokines and glucocorticoids. *Ann N Y Acad Sci.* 557:280–295.

Baumann, H., Richards, C., and Gauldie, J. 1987b. Interaction among hepatocyte-stimulating factors, interleukin 1, and glucocorticoids for regulation acute phase plasma proteins in human hepatoma hepG-2 cells. *J Immunol.* 139:4122–4128.

Baumann, H., and Schendel, P. 1991. Interleukin-11 regulates the hepatic expression of the same plasma protein genes as interleukin-6. *J Biol Chem.* 266:20424–20427.

Baumann, H., and Wong, G.G. 1989. Hepatocyte-stimulating factor III shares structural and functional identity with leukemia-inhibitory factor. *J Immunol.* 143:1163–1167.

Bausserman, L.L., Herbert, P.N., and McAdam, K.P.W.J. 1980. Heterogeneity of human serum amyloid A proteins. *J Exp Med.* 152:641–656.

Bausserman, L.L., Herbert, P.N., Rodger, R., and Nicolosi, R.J. 1984. Rapid clearance of serum amyloid A from high-density lipoproteins. *Biochim Biophys Acta.* 792:186–191.

Bausserman, L.L., Saritelli, A.L., Zuiden, P.V., Gollaher, C.J., and Herbert, P.N. 1987. Degradation of serum amyloid A by isolated perfused rat liver. *J Biol Chem.* 262:1583–1589.

Beitel, G.J., Luft, A.J., Panrucker, D.E., and Lorscheider, F.L. 1986. Structural analysis of acute-phase α_2-macroglobulin. *Biochem J.* 238:359–364.

Belpaire, F., Braeckman, R.A., and Bogaert, M.G. 1984. Binding of oxpranolol and propranolol to serum, albumin, and α_1-acid glycoprotein in man and other species. *Biochem Pharmacol.* 33:2065–2069.

Belpaire, F.M., DeRick, A., Dello, C., Fraeyman, N., and Bogaert, M.G. 1987. α_1 acid glycoprotein and serum binding of drugs in healthy and diseased dogs. *J Vet Pharmacol Ther.* 10:43–48.

Benditt, E.P., Meek, R.L., and Eriksen, N. 1989. ApoSSA: Structure, tissue expression and possible function. In *Acute Phase Proteins in the Acute Phase Response.* Ed. M.B. Pepys, pp. 59–68. London: Springer-Verlag.

Benigni, F., Fantuzzi, G., Sacco, S., et al. 1996. Six different cytokines that share GP130 as a receptor subunit, induce serum amyloid A and potentiate the induction of interleukin-6 and the activation of the hypothalamus-pituitary-adrenal axis by interleukin-1. *Blood.* 87:1851–1854.

Bennett, M., and Schmidt, K. 1980. Immunosuppression by human plasma α_1-acid glycoprotein: Importance of the carbohydrate moiety. *Proc Natl Acad Sci USA.* 77:6109–6113.

Benson, M.D., and Kleiner, L. 1980. Synthesis and secretion of serum amyloid protein A SAA by hepatocytes in mice treated with casein. *J Immunol.* 124:495–499.

Benson, M.D., Scheinberg, M.A., Shirahama, T., Cathcart, E.S., and Skinner, M. 1977. Kinetics of serum amyloid protein A in casein-induced murine amyloidosis. *J Clin Invest.* 59:412–417.

Bhattacharya, A., Shepard, A.R., Moser, D.R., Roberts, L.R., and Holland, L.J. 1991. Molecular cloning of cDNA for the Bβ subunit of xenopus fibrinogen, the product of a coordinately-regulated gene family. *Mol Cell Endocrinol.* 75:111–121.

Bingle, C.D., Epstein, O., Srai, S.K.S., and Gitlin, J.D. 1991. Hepatic caeruloplasmin-gene expression during development in the guinea pig. *Biochem J.* 276:771–775.

Bingle, C.D., Kelly, F., Epstein, O., and Srai, S.K.S. 1992. Induction of hepatic and pulmonary caeruloplasmin gene expression in developing guinea pigs following premature delivery. *Biochem Biophys Acta.* 1139:217–221.

Bingle, C.D., Srai, S.K.S., and Epstein, O. 1990. Development changes in hepatic copper proteins in the guinea pig. *J Hepatol.* 10:138–143.

Bingley, J.B., and Dick, A.T. 1969. The pH optimum for ceruloplasmin oxidase activity in the plasma of several species of animals. *Clin Chim Acta.* 25:480–482.

Birch, H.E., and Schreiber, G. 1986. Transcriptional regulation of plasma protein synthesis during inflammation. *J Biol Chem.* 261:8077–8080.

Blaisdell, F.S., and Dodds, W.J. 1977. Evaluation of two microhematocrit methods for quantitating plasma fibrinogen. *J Am Vet Med Assoc.* 171:340–342.

Boraschi, D., Villa, L., Volpini, G., et al. 1990. Differential activity of interleukin la and interleukin 1b in the stimulation of the immune response in vivo. *Eur J Immunol.* 20:317–321.

Borth, W., and Luger, T.A. 1989. Identification of α_2-macroglobulin as a cytokine binding plasma protein. *J Biol Chem.* 264:5818–5825.

Boudreaux, M.K., and Dillon, A.R. 1991. Platelet function, antithrombin-III activity, and fibrinogen concentration in heartworm-infected and heartworm-negative dogs treated with thiacetarsamide. *Am J Vet Res.* 52:1986–1991.

Bouma, H., Kwan, S.-W., and Fuller, G.M. 1975. Radioimmunological identification of polysomes synthesizing fibrinogen polypeptide chains. *Biochemistry.* 14:4787–4792.

Bout, D., Joseph, M., Pontet, M., Vorng, H., Deslée, D., and Capron, A. 1986. Rat resistance to schistosomiasis: Platelet-mediated cytotoxicity induced by C-reactive protein. *Science.* 231:153–156.

Brandwein, S.R., Sipe, J.K., Skinner, M., and Cohen, A.S. 1985. Effect of colchicine on experimental amyloidosis in two CBA/J mouse models. Chronic inflammatory stimulation and administration of amyloid-enhancing factor during acute inflammation. *Lab Invest.* 52:319–325.

Brisette, L., Young, I., Narindrasorasak, S., Kisilevsky, R., and Deeley, R. 1989. Differential induction of the serum amyloid A gene family in response to an inflammatory agent and to amyloid-enhancing. *J Biol Chem.* 264:19327–19332.

Broadley, C., and Hoover, R.L. 1989. Ceruloplasmin reduces the adhesion and scavenger superoxide during the interaction of activated PMN leukocytes with endothelial cells. *Am J Pathol.* 135:647–655.

Brown, L.F., Lanir, N., McDonagh, J., Tognazzi, K., Dvorak, A.M., and Dvorak, H.F. 1993. Fibroblast migration in fibrin gel matrices. *Am J Pathol.* 142:273–283.

Brunn, C.F., Nordstoga, K., Sletten, K., Husby, G., and Marhaug, G. 1995. Serum amyloid A protein in humans and four animal species: A comparison by two dimensional electrophoresis. *Comp Biochem Physiol B.* 112:227–234.

Buchta, R., Gennaro, R., Pontet, M., Fridkin, M., and Romeo, D. 1988. C-reactive protein decreases protein phosphorylation in neutrophils. *FEBS Lett.* 237:173–177.

Burger, W., Schade, R., and Hirschelmann, R. 1987. The rat C-reactive protein—Isolation and response to experimental inflammation and tissue damage. *Agents Actions.* 21:93–97.

Burlingame, R.W., Volzer, M.A., Harris, J., and Du Clos, T.W. 1996. The effect of acute phase proteins on clearance of chromatin from the circulation of normal mice. *J Immunol.* 156:4783–4788.

Burton, S.A., Honor, D.J., Mackenzie, A.L., Eckersall, P.D., Markham, R.J.F., and Homey, B. S. 1994. C-reactive protein concentration in dogs with inflammatory leukograms. *Am J Vet Res.* 55:613–618.

Butler, A., Rochelle, J.M., Seldin, M.F., and Whitehead, A.S. 1995. The gene encoding the mouse serum amyloid A protein, Apo-SAA5, maps to proximal chromosome 7. *Immunogenetics.* 42:153–155.

Butler, P.J.G., Tennent, G.A., Pepys, M.B., Cook, R.B., and Caspi, D. 1990. Pentraxin-chromatin interactions: Serum amyloid P component specifically displaces H1 type histones and solubilizes native long chromatin. *J Exp Med.* 172:13–18.

Cabana, V.G., Gewurz, H., and Siegel, J.N. 1983. Inflammation-induced changes in rabbit CRP and plasma lipoproteins. *J Immunol.* 130:1736–1742.

Campbell, C.H., Brown, R., and Linder, M.C. 1981. Circulating ceruloplasmin is an important source of copper for normal and malignant animal cells. *Biochim Biophys Acta.* 678:27–38.

Campos, S.P., and Baumann, H. 1992. Insulin is a prominent modulator of the cytokine-stimulated expression of acute-phase plasma protein genes. *Mol Cell Biol.* 12:1789–1797.

Carlson, J., Eriksson, S., Alm, R., and Kjellstrom, T. 1984. Biosynthesis of abnormally glycosylated alpha 1-antitrypsin by a human hepatoma cell line. *Hepatology.* 4:235–241.

Carlson, J.A., Rogers, B.B., Sifera, R.N., Hawkins, H.K., Finegold, M.J., and Woo, S.L.C. 1988. Multiple tissues express alpha$_1$-antitrypsin in transgenic mice and man. *J Clin Invest.* 82:26–36.

Carrell, R.W., Jeppsson, J.-O., Laurell, C.-B., et al. 1982. Structure and variation of human α_1-antitrypsin. *Nature.* 298:329–334.

Caspi, D., Baltz, M.L., Snel, F., et al. 1984. Isolation and characterization of C-reactive protein from the dog. *Immunology.* 53:307–313.

Caspi, D., Snel, F.W.J.J., Batt, R.M., et al. 1987. C-reactive protein in dogs. *Am J Vet Res.* 48:919–921.

Castell, J.V., Gomez-Lechon, M.J., David, M., Hirano, T., Kishimoto, T., and Heinrich, P.C. 1988. Recombinant human interleukin-6 IL-6/BSF-2/HSF regulates the synthesis of acute phase proteins in human hepatocytes. *FEBS Lett.* 232:347–350.

Cathcart, E.S., Comerford, F.R., and Cohen, A.S. 1965. Immunologic studies on a protein extracted from human secondary amyloid. *N Engl J Med.* 273:143–146.

Cavarra, E., Martorana, P.A., Gambelli, F., de Santi, M., van Even, P., and Lungarella, G. 1996. Neutrophil recruitment in the lungs is associated with increased lung elastase burden, decreased lung elastin, and emphysema in α_1 proteinase inhibitor-deficient mice. *Lab Invest.* 75:273–280.

Cavus, I., Koo, P.H., and Teyler, T.J. 1996. Inhibition of long-term potentiation development in rat hippocampal slice by α_2-macroglobulin, an acute-phase protein in the brain. *J Neurolo Res.* 43:282–288.

Chao, S., Chai, K.X., Chao, L., and Chao, J. 1990. Molecular cloning and primary structure of rat α_1-antitrypsin. *Biochemistry.* 29:323–329.

Charlwood, P.A., Hatton, M.W.C., and Regoeczi, E. 1976. On the physiochemical and chemical properties of α_1-acid glycoproteins from mammalian and avian plasmas. *Biochem Biophys Acta.* 453:81–92.

Charo, I.F., Kieffer, N., and Phillips, D.R. 1994. Platelet membrane glycoproteins. In *Hemostasis and Thrombosis: Basic Principles and Clinical Practice*, 3rd edition. Eds. R.W. Colman, J. Hirsh, M.V. Marder, and E.W. Salzman, pp. 489–507. Philadelphia, PA: J. B. Lippincott.

Chauvelot-Moachon, L., Delers, F., Poüs, C., Engler, R., Tallet, F., and Giroud, J.P. 1988. Alpha-1-acid glycoprotein concentrations and protein binding of propranolol in Sprague-Dawley and Dark Agouti rat strains treated by pheobarbital. *J Pharmacol Exp Ther.* 244:1103–1108.

Chelladurai, M., MacIntyre, S.S., and Kushner, I. 1983. In vivo studies of serum C-reactive protein turnover in rabbits. *J Clin Invest.* 71:604–610.

Chen, Y., Saari, J.T., and Kang, Y.J. 1995. Expression of g-glutamylcysteine synthetase in the liver of copper-deficient rats. *Proc Soc Exp Biol Med.* 210:102–106.

Cheryk, L.A., Hayes, M.A., and Gentry, P.A. 1996. Modulation of bovine platelet function by C-reactive protein. *Vet Immunol Immunopathol.* 52:27–36.

Christner, R.B., and Mortensen, R.F. 1994. Binding of human serum amyloid P-component to phosphocholine. *Arch Biochem Biophys.* 314:337–343.

Ciliberto, G., Arcone, R., Wagner, E.F., and Ruther, U. 1987. Inducible and tissue-specific expression of human C-reactive protein in transgenic mice. *EMBO J.* 6:4017–4022.

Coe, J.E. 1977. A sex-limited serum protein of Syrian hamsters: Definition of female protein and regulation by testosterone. *Proc Natl Acad Sci USA.* 74:730–733.

Coe, J.E., Cieplak, W., Hadlow, W.J., and Ross, M.J. 1997. Female protein, amyloidosis, and hormonal carcinogenesis in Turkish hamster: Differences from Syrian hamster. *Am J Physiol.* 273:R934–941.

Coe, J.E., and Ross, M.J. 1983. Hamster female protein. A divergent acute phase protein in male and female Syrian hamsters. *J Exp Med.* 157:1421–1433.

Coe, J.E., and Ross, M.J. 1985. Hamster female protein, a sex-limited pentraxin, is a constituent of Syrian hamster amyloid. *J Clin Invest.* 76:66–74.

Coe, J.E., and Ross, M.J. 1987. Hamster female protein, a pentameric oligomer capable of reassociation and hybrid formation. *Biochemistry.* 26:704–710.

Coe, J.E., and Ross, M.J. 1990a. Armenian hamster protein: A pentraxin under complex regulation. *Am J Physiol.* 259:R341–349.

Coe, J.E., and Ross, M.J. 1990b. Amyloidosis and female protein in Syrian hamster. Concurrent regulation by sex hormones. *J Exp Med.* 171:1257–1267.

Coe, J.E., Morgossian, S.S., Slayter, H.S., and Sogn, J.A. 1981. Hamster female protein. A new Pentraxin structurally and functionally similar to C-reactive protein and amyloid A component. *J Exp Med.* 153:977–991.

Coetzee, G.A., Strachan, A.F., van der Westhuyzen, D.R., Hoppe, H.C., Jeenah, M.S., and de Beer, F.C. 1986. Serum amyloid A-containing human high density lipoprotein. 3. Density, size and apolipoprotein composition. *J Biol Chem.* 261:9644–9651.

Cohen, A.S., Shirahama, T., Sipe, J.D., and Skinner, M. 1983. Amyloid proteins, precursors, mediator, and enhancer. *Lab Invest.* 48:1–4.

Conner, J.G., and Eckersall, P.D. 1988. Acute phase response in the dog following surgical trauma. *Res Vet Sci.* 45:107–110.

Conner, J.G., Eckersall, P.D., and Douglas, T.A. 1988. Inhibition of elastase by canine serum: Demonstration of an acute phase response. *Res Vet Sci.* 44:391–393.

Conner, J.G., Eckersall, P.D., and Wiseman, A. 1986. The acute phase response in the cow and dog. *Protides Biol Fluids.* 34:509–512.

Connolly, K.M., Stecher, V.J., Rudofsky, U.H., and Pruden, D.J. 1988. Elevation of plasma fibronectin and serum amyloid P in autoimmune NZB, B/W, and MRL/lpr mice. *Exp Mol Pathol.* 49:388–394.

Cooper, R., and Papaconstantinou, J. 1986. Evidence for the existence of multiple α_1-acid glycoprotein genes in the mouse. *J Biol Chem.* 261:1849–1853.

Cornelissen, C.N., and Sparling, P.F. 1994. Iron piracy: Acquisition of transferrin-bound iron by bacterial pathogens. *Mol Microbiol.* 14:843–850.

Costello, M., Fiedel, B.A., and Gewurz, H. 1979. Inhibition of platelet aggregation by native and desialised alpha-1 acid glycoprotein. *Nature.* 281:677–678.

Costello, M.J., Gewurz, H., and Siegel, J.N. 1984. Inhibition of neutrophil activation by α_1-acid glycoprotein. *Clin Exp Immunol.* 55:465–472.

Coughlin, S.R. 1995. Platelet thrombin receptor. In *Molecular Basis of Thrombosis and Hemostasis.* Eds. K.A. High, and H.R. Roberts, pp. 639–649. New York, NY: Marcel Dekker.

Courtoy, P.J., Lombart, C., Feldmann, G., Moguilevsky, N., and Rogier, E. 1981. Synchronous increase of four acute phase proteins synthesized by the same hepatocytes during the inflammatory reaction: A combined biochemical and morphologic kinetics study in the rat. *Lab Invest.* 44:105–115.

Cox, D.W. 1966. Factors influencing serum ceruloplasmin levels in normal individuals. *J Lab Clin Med.* 68:893–904.

Crabtree, G.R., Comeau, C.M., Fowlkes, D.M., Fornace, A.J., Malley, J.D., and Kant, J.A. 1985. Evolution and structure of the fibrinogen genes. Random insertion of introns or selective loss? *J Mol Biol.* 185:1–19.

Crabtree, G.R., and Kant, J.A. 1982. Coordinate accumulation of the mRNAs for the alpha, beta, and gamma chains of rat fibrinogen following defibrination. *J Biol Chem.* 257:7277–7279.

Crowe, A., and Morgan, E.H. 1996. The effects of iron loading and iron deficiency on the tissue uptake of Cu during development in the rat. *Biochim Biophys Acta.* 1291:53–59.

Crowell, R.E., Du Clos, T.W., Montoya, G., Heaphy, E., and Mold, C. 1991. C-reactive protein receptors on the human monocytic cell line U-937. *J Immunol.* 147:3445–3451.

Danielpour, D., and Sporn, M.B. 1990. Differential inhibition of transforming growth factor $\beta 1$ and $\beta 2$ activity by α_2-macroglobulin. *J Biol Chem.* 265:6973–6977.

Davidsen, O., Christensen, E.I., and Gliemann, J. 1985. The plasma clearance of human α_1-macroglobulin-trypsin complex in the rat is mainly accounted for by uptake into hepatocytes. *Biochim Biophys Acta.* 846:85–92.

de Beer, F.C., Baltz, M.L., Munn, E.A., et al. 1982. Isolation and characterization of C-reactive protein and serum amyloid P component in the rat. *Immunology.* 45:55–70.

de Beer, M.C., Beach, C.M., Shedlofsky, S.I., and De Beer, F.C. 1991. Identification of a novel serum amyloid A protein in BALB/c mice. *Biochem J.* 280:45–49.

de Beer, M.C., de Beer, F.C., Beach, C.M., Carreras, I., and Sipe, J.D. 1992. Mouse serum amyloid A protein. *Biochem J.* 283:673–678.

de Beer, M.C., de Beer, F.C., Beach, C.M., Gonnerman, W.A., Carreras, I., and Sipe, J.D. 1993. Syrian and Armenian hamsters differ in serum amyloid A gene expression: Identification of novel Syrian hamster serum amyloid A subtypes. *J Immunol.* 150:5361–5370.

de Beer, M.C., de Beer, F.C., Gerardot, C.J., et al. 1996. Structure of the mouse SAA4 gene and its linkage to the serum amyloid A gene family. *Genomics.* 34:139–142.

de Boer, J.P., Creasey, A.A., Chang, A., et al. 1993. Alpha-2-macroglobulin functions as an inhibitor of fibrinolytic, clotting, and neutrophilic proteinases in sepsis: Studies using a baboon model. *Infect Immun.* 61:5035–5043.

de Beer, M.C., Kindy, M.S., Lane, W.S., and de Beer, F.C. 1994. Mouse serum amyloid A protein Sas structure and expression. *J Biol Chem.* 269:4661–4667.

de Beer, M.C., Yuan, T., Kindy, M.S., Asztalos, B.R., Roheim, P.S., and de Beer, F.C. 1995. Characterization of constitutive human serum amyloid A protein SAA4 as an apolipoprotein. *J Lipid Res.* 36:526–534.

de Frutos, P.G., and Dahlback, B. 1994. Interaction between serum amyloid P component and C4b-binding protein associated with inhibition of factor I-mediated C4b degradation. *J Immunol.* 152:2430–2437.

De Jong, F.A., Birch, H.E., and Schreiber, G. 1988. Effect of recombinant interleukin-1 on mRNA levels in rat liver. *Inflammation.* 12:613–617.

De Lorenzo, D., Williams, P., and Ringold, G. 1991. Identification of two distinct muclear factors with DNA binding activity within the glucocorticoid regulatory region of the rat alpha-1-acid glycoprotein promoter. *Biochem Biophys Res Commun.* 176:1326–1332.

de Santi, M.M., Martorana, P.A., Cavarra, E., and Lungarella, G. 1995. Pallid mice with genetic emphysema. *Lab Invest.* 73:40–47.

Debanne, M.T., Bell, R., and Dolovich, J. 1975. Uptake of proteinase-α-macroglobulin complexes by macrophages. *Biochim Biophys Acta.* 411:295–304.

Dello, C.P., Belpaire, F.M., De Rick, A., and Fraeyman, N.H. 1988. Influence of inflammation on serum concentration, molecular heterogeneity, and drug binding properties of canine alpha-1-acid glycoprotein. *J Vet Pharmacol Ther.* 11:71–76.

Dewey, M.J., Rheaume, C., Berger, F.G., and Baumann, H. 1990. Inducible and tissue-specific expression of rat a-1-acid glycoprotein in transgenic mice. *J Immunol.* 144:4392–4398.

Diarra-Mehrpour, M., Bourguignon, J., Leroux-Nicollet, I., et al. 1985. The effects of 17 α-ethynyloestradiol and of acute inflammation on the plasma concentration of rat α_1-acid glycoprotein and on the induction of its hepatic mRNA. *Biochem J.* 225:681–687.

DiBartola, S.P., Reiter, J.A., Cornacoff, J.B., Kociba, G.J., and Benson, M.D. 1989. Serum amyloid A protein concentration measured by radial immunodiffusion in Abyssinian and non-Abyssinian cats. *Am J Vet Res.* 50:1414–1417.

Dini, L., Carbonaro, M., Musci, G., and Calabrese, L. 1990. The interaction of ceruloplasmin with Kupffer cells. *Eur J Cell Biol.* 52:207–212.

DiSilvestro, R.A., Barber, E.F., David, E.A., and Cousins, R.J. 1988. An enzyme-linked immunoadsorbent assay for rat ceruloplasmin. *Biol Trace Elem Res.* 17:1–9.

Dong, A., Caughey, B., Caughey, W.S., Bhat, K.S., and Coe, J.E. 1992. Secondary structure of the pentraxin female protein in water determined by infrared spectroscopy: Effects of calcium and phosphorylcholine. *Biochemistry.* 31:9364–9370.

Doolittle, R.F. 1973. Structural aspects of the fibrinogen to fibrin conversion. *Adv Protein Chem.* 27:1–100.

Dougherty, T.J., Gewurz, H., and Siegel, J.N. 1991. Preferential binding and aggregation of rabbit C-reactive protein with arginine-rich proteins. *Mol Immunol.* 28:1113–1120.

Dowton, S.B., and Colten, H.R. 1988. Acute phase reactants in inflammation and infection. *Semin Hematol.* 25:84–89.

Dowton, S.B., and Holden, S.N. 1991. C-reactive protein CRP of the Syrian hamster. *Biochemistry.* 30:9531–9538.

Dowton, S.B., and McGrew, S.D. 1990. Rat serum amyloid P component. Analysis of cDNA sequence and gene expression. *Biochem J.* 270:553–556.

Dowton, S.B., and Waggoner, D.J. 1989. Armenian hamster female protein serum amyloid P component. Comparison with the sex-regulated homolog in Syrian hamster. *J Immunol.* 143:3776–3780.

Dowton, S.B., Waggoner, D.J., and Mandl, K.D. 1991. Developmental regulation of expression of rabbit C-reactive protein and serum amyloid A in Syrian hamsters. *Pediatr Res.* 30:444–449.

Dowton, S.B., Woods, D.E., Mantzouranis, E.C., and Coltern, H.R. 1985. Syrian hamster female protein: Analysis of female protein primary structure and gene expression. *Science.* 228:1206–1208.

Drechou, A., Perez-Gonzalez, N., Biou, D., Rouzeau, J.D., Feger, J., and Durand, G. 1989. One-step purification of rat plasma α1-acid glycoprotein by antibody affinity chromatography: Application to normal and inflamed rat sera. *J Chromatogr.* 489:271–281.

Du Bois, R.M., Bernaudin, J.-F., Paakko, P., et al. 1991. Human neutrophils express the alpha 1-antitrypsin gene and produce alpha 1-antitrypsin. *Blood.* 77:2724–2730.

Du Clos, T.W. 1989. C-reactive protein reacts with the U1 small nuclear ribonucleoprotein. *J Immunol.* 143:2553–2559.

Du Clos, T.W., Zlock, L.T., Hicks, P.S., and Mold, C. 1994. Decreased autoantibody levels and enhanced survival of NZB X NZW. F1 mice treated with C-reactive protein. *Clin Immunol Immunopathol.* 70:22–27.

Du Clos, T.W., Zlock, L.T., and Rubin, R.L. 1988. Analysis of the binding of C-reactive protein to histones and chromatin. *J Immunol.* 141:4266–4270.

Dubois, D.Y., and Malmendier, C.L. 1988. Non-competitive enzyme linked immunosorbent assay for human apolipoprotein SAA or S. *J Immunol Methods.* 112:71–75.

Dwulet, F.E., Wallace, D.K., and Benson, M.D. 1988. Amino acid structures of multiple forms of amyloid-related serum protein SAA from a single individual. *Biochemistry.* 27:1677–1682.

Dziegielewska, K.M., Saunders, N.R., Schejter, E.J., et al. 1986. Synthesis of plasma proteins in fetal, adult and neoplastic human brain tissue. *Dev Biol.* 115:93–104.

Eastman, E.M., and Gilula, N.B. 1989. Cloning and characterization of a cDNA for the B-beta chain of rat fibrinogen. *Gene.* 79:151–158.

Eckersall, P.D. 1995. Acute phase proteins as markers of inflammatory lesions. *Comp Haematol Int.* 5:93–97.

Eckersall, P.D., and Conner, J.G. 1988. Bovine and canine acute phase proteins. *Vet Res Commun.* 12:169–178.

Eckersall, P.D., Conner, J.G., and Harvie, J. 1991. An immunoturbidimetric assay for canine C-reactive protein. *Vet Res Commun.* 15:17–24.

Eckersall, P.D., Conner, J.G., and Parton, H. 1989. An enzyme-linked immunosorbent assay for canine C-reactive protein. *Vet Rec.* 124:490–491.

Eckersall, P.D., Sullivan, M., Kirkham, D., and Mohammed, N.A. 1985. The acute phase reaction detected in dogs by concanavalin a binding. *Vet Res Commun.* 9:233–238.

Elliot-Bryant, R., Liang, J.S., Sipe, J.D., and Cathcart, E.S. 1996. Degradation of serum amyloid A in amyloid-susceptible and amyloid-resistant mouse strains. *Scand J Immunol.* 44:223–228.

Emsley, J., White, H., O'Hara, B., et al. 1994. Structure of serumanyloid P component. *Nature.* 367:338–345.

Etlinger, H.M., and Coe, J.E. 1986. Complement activation by female protein, the hamster homologue of human C-reactive protein. *Int Arch Allergy Appl Immunol.* 81:189–191.

Evans, E.W., and Duncan, J.R. 2003. Proteins, lipids, and carbohydrates. In *Veterinary Laboratory Medicine Clinical Pathology,* 4th edition, Latimer, K.S., Mahaffey, E.A., and Prasse, K.W. (eds.) p. 166, Ames, IA: Iowa State Press.

Evans, G.W., Myron, D.R., Cornatzer, N.F., and Cornatzer, W.E. 1970. Age-dependent alterations in hepatic subcellular copper distribution and plasma ceruloplasmin. *Am J Physiol.* 218:298–300.

Evans T.C., Jr., and Nelsestuen, G.L. 1995. Dissociation of serum amyloid P from C4b-binding region and other sites by lactic acid: Potential role of lactic acid in the regulation of pentraxin function. *Biochemistry.* 34:10440–10447.

Evans, G.H., Nies, A.S., and Shand, D.G. 1973. The disposition of propranolol. III. Decreased half-life and volume of distribution as a result of plasma binding in man, monkey, dog, and rat. *J Pharmacol Exp Ther.* 186:114–122.

Fantuzzi, G., Zheng, H., Faggioni, R., et al. 1996. Effect of endotoxin in IL-1-β-deficient mice. *J Immunol.* 157:291–296.

Feldman, S.R., Rosenberg, M.R., Ney, K.A., Michalopoulos, G., and Pizzo, S.V. 1985. Binding of α_2-macroglobulin to hepatocytes: Mechanism of in vivo clearance. *Biochem Biophys Res Commun.* 128:795–802.

Feldmann, G., Bernuau, D., Scoazec, J.Y., and Maurice, M. 1989. Biosynthesis of acute phase proteins by the liver cells. In *Acute Phase Proteins in the Acute Phase Response.* Ed. M.B. Pepys, pp. 97–105. London: Springer-Verlag.

Fernandez-Moran, H., Marchalonjs, J., and Edelman, G.M. 1986. Electron microscopy of a hemaglutinin from *Limulus polyphemus. J Mol Biol.* 32:467–469.

Fiedel, B.A., and Gewurz, H. 1976. Effects of C-reactive protein on platelet function. I. Inhibition of platelet aggregation and release reactions. *J Immunol.* 116:1289–1294.

Fielding, C.J., Shore, V.G., and Fielding, P.E. 1972. A protein cofactor of lecithin cholesterol acyltransferase. *Biochem Biophys Res Commun.* 46:1493–1498.

Filep, J.G., Herman, F., Kelemen, E., and Foldes-Filep, E. 1991. C-reactive protein inhibits binding of platelet-activating factor to human platelets. *Thromb Res.* 61:411–421.

Fleming, R.E., and Gitlin, J.D. 1990. Primary structure of rat ceruloplasmin and analysis of tissue-specific gene expression during development. *J Biol Chem.* 265:7701–7707.

Fleming, R.E., and Gitlin, J.D. 1992. Structural and functional analysis of the 5'-flanking region of the rat ceruloplasmin gene. *J Biol Chem.* 267:479–486.

Fleming, R.E., Whitman, I.P., and Gitlin, J.D. 1991. Induction of ceruloplasmin in gene expresion in rat lung during inflammation and hyperoxia. *Am J Physiol.* 260:L68–L74.

Floyd-Smith, G., Whitehead, A.S., Colten, H.R., and Francke, U. 1986. The human C-reactive protein gene CRP and serum amyloid P component gene APCS are located on the proximal long arm of chromosome 1. *Immunogenetics.* 24:171–176.

Foldes-Filep, E., Filep, J.G., and Sirois, P. 1992. C-reactive protein inhibits intracellular calcium mobilization and superoxide production by guinea pig alveolar macrophages. *J Leukoc Biol.* 51:13–18.

Forti, G., Barni, T., Vannelli, B.G., Balboni, G.C., Orlando, D., and Serio, M. 1989. Sertoli cell proteins in the human seminiferous tubule. *J Steroid Biochem.* 32:135–144.

Fournier, T., Medjoubi-N.N., and Porquet, D. 2000. Alpha-1-acid glycoprotein. *Biochim Biophys Acta.* 1482(1–2):157–171.

Fournier, T., Vranckx, R., Mejdoubi, N., Durand, G., and Porquet, D. 1994. Induction of rat alpha-1-acid glycoprotein by pheobarbital is independent of a general acute-phase response. *Biochem Pharmacol.* 48:1531–1535.

Frazer, J.M., Nathoo, S.A., Katz, J., Genetta, T.L., and Finlay, T.H. 1985. Plasma protein and liver mRNA levels of two closely related murine a1-protease inhibitors during the acute phase reaction. *Arch Biochem Biophy.* 239:112–119.

French, T. 1989. Specific proteins D. Acute phase proteins. In *The Clinical Chemistry of Laboratory Animals.* Eds. W.F. Loeb, and F.W. Quimby, pp. 201–235. New York, NY: Pergamon Press.

Frost, S.J., and Weigel, P.H. 1990. Binding of hyaluronic acid to mammalian fibrinogens. *Biochim Biophys Acta.* 1034:39–45.

Fujise, H., Takanami, H., Yamamoto, M., et al. 1992. Simple isolation of canine C-reactive protein CRP by phosphorylcholine PC affinity chromatography. *J Vet Med Sci.* 54:165–167.

Fuks, A., and Zucker-Franklin, D. 1985. Impaired Kupffer cell function precedes development of secondary amyloidosis. *J Exp Med.* 161:1013–1028.

Fuller, G.M., Otto, J.M., Woloski, B.M., McGary, C.T., and Adams, M.A. 1985. The effects of hepatocyte stimulating factor on fibrinogen biosynthesis in hepatocyte monolayers. *J Cell Biol.* 101:1481–1486.

Ganapathl, M.K., Rzewnicki, D., Samols, D., Jiang, S.-L., and Kushner, I. 1991. Effect of combinations of cytokines and hormones on synthesis of serum amyloid A and C-reactive protein in HEP 3B cells. *J Immunol.* 147:1261–1265.

Ganrot, K. 1966. Determination of α_2-macroglotmlrn as trypsin-protein esterase. *Clin Chim Acta.* 14:493–501.

Ganrot, P.O. 1972. Variation of the concentrations of some plasma proteins in normal adults, in pregnant women, and in newborns. *Scand J Clin Lab Invest.* 29(Suppl. 124):83–88.

Ganrot, K. 1973a. Plasma protein response in experimental inflammation in the dog. *Res Exp Med.* 161:251–261.

Ganrot, K. 1973b. Rat α_2-acute phase globulin, a human α_2-macroglobulin homologue: Interaction with plasmin and trypsin. *Biochim Biophys Acta.* 322:62–67.

Ganrot, P.O. 1973c. Plasma protein response in experimental inflammation in the dog. *Res Exp Med.* 161:251–261.

Gauthier, F., and Mouray, F. 1976. Rat α_2 acute phase macroglobulin. Isolation and physicochemical properties. *Biochem J.* 159:661–665.

Gauldie, J., Northemann, W., and Fey, G.H. 1990. IL-6 functions as an exocrine hormone in inflammation. *J Immunol.* 144:3804–3808.

Ge, M., Tang, G., Ryan, T.J., and Malik, A.B. 1992. Fibrinogen degradation product fragment D induces endothelial cell detachment by activation of cell-mediated fibrinolysis. *J Clin Invest.* 90:2508–2516.

Gehring, M.R., Shiels, B.R., Northemann, W., et al. 1987. Sequence of rat liver α_2 macroglobulin and acute phase control of its messenger RNA. *J Biol Chem.* 262:446–454.

Geiger, T., Andus, T., Klapproth, J., Hirano, T., Kishimoto, T., and Heinrich, P.C. 1988b. Induction of rat acute-phase proteins by interleukin 6 in vivo. *Eur J Immunol.* 18:717–721.

Geiger, T., Andus, T., Klapproth, J., Northoff, H., and Heinrich, P.C. 1988a. Induction of alpha 1-acid glycoprotein by recombinant human interleukin-1 in rat hepatoma cells. *J Biol Chem.* 263:7141–7146.

Geiger, T., Lamri, Y., Tran-Thi, T.-A., et al. 1987. Biosynthesis and regulation of rat α1-inhibitor3, a negative acute-phase reactant of the macroglobulin family. *Biochem J.* 245:493–500.

Gentry, P.A. 1992. The mammalian platelet: Its role in haemostasis, inflammation, and tissue repair. *J Comp Pathol.* 107:243–270.

Gentry, P.A., and Downie, H.G. 1993. Blood coagulation and hemostasis. In *Dukes' Physiology of Domestic Animals.* Eds. M.J. Swenson, and W.O. Reece, 11th edition, pp. 49–63. New York, NY: Cornell University Press.

Gentry, P.A., Feldman, B.F., and Liptrap, R.M. 1990. Hemostasis and parturition revisited: Comparative profiles in mammals. *Comp Haematol Int.* 1:150–154.

Gentry, P.A., and Liptrap, R.M. 1981. Influence of progesterone and pregnancy on canine fibrinogen values. *J Small Anim Pract.* 22:185–194.

Gentry, P.A., Liptrap, R.M., Tremblay, R.R.M., Lichen, L., and Ross, M.L. 1992. Adrenocoricotrophic hormone fails to alter plasma fibrinogen and fibronectin values in calves but does so in rabbits. *Vet Res Commun.* 16:253–264.

Gertz, M.A., Sipe, J.D., Skinner, M., Cohen, A.S., and Kyle, R.A. 1984. Measurement of murine serum amyloid P component by rat nephelometry. *J Immunol Methods.* 69:173–180.

Giclas, P.C., Manthei, U., and Strunk, R.C. 1985. The acute phase response of C3, C5, ceruloplasmin, and C-reactive protein induced by turpentine pleurisy in the rabbit. *Am J Pathol.* 120:146–156.

Gilpin, D.A., Hsieh, C.-C., Kuninger, D.T., Herndon, D.N., and Papaconstantinou, J. 1996. Regulation of the acute phase response genes alpha$_1$-acid glycoprotein and alpha$_1$-antitrypsin correlates with sensitivity to thermal injury. *Surgery.* 119:664–673.

Gitlin, J.D. 1988. Transcriptional regulation of ceruloplasmin gene expression during inflammation. *J Biol Chem.* 263:6281–6287.

Gitlin, J.D., Schroeder, J.J., Lee-Ambrose, L.M., and Cousins, R.J. 1992. Mechanisms of caeruloplasmin biosynthesis in normal and copper-deficient rats. *Biochem J.* 282:835–839.

Glenner, G.G. 1980. Amyloid deposits and amyloidosis. The B fibrillosis. *N Engl J Med.* 302:1283–1333.

Glibetic, M.D., and Baumann, H. 1986. Influence of chronic inflammation on the level of mRNA for acute-phase reactants in the mouse liver. *J Immunol.* 137:1616–1622.

Glibetic, M., Bogojevic, D., Matic, S., and Sevaljevic, L. 1992. The expression of liver acute-phase protein genes during rat development and in response to inflammation of the dam. *Differentiation.* 50:35–40.

Godenir, N.L., Jeenah, M.S., Goetzee, G.A., Van der Esthuyzen, D., Strachan, A.F., and De Beer, F.C. 1985. Standardization of the quantitation of serum amyloid A protein SAA in human serum. *J Immunol Methods.* 83:217–225.

Godfrey, H.P., Atlas, A., Randazzo, B., and Angadi, C.V. 1984. Regulation of macrophage agglutination factor production by α_2-macroglobulin. *Immunology.* 51:503–510.

Goldberger, G., Bing, D.H., Sipe, J.D., Rits, M., and Colten, H.R. 1987. Transcriptional regulation of genes encoding the acute-phase proteins CRP, SAA, and C3. *J Immunol.* 138:3967–3971.

Goldstein, I.M., Kaplan, H.B., Edelson, H.S., and Weissmann, G. 1979. Ceruloplasmin. A scavenger of superoxide anion radicals. *J Biol Chem.* 254:4040–4045.

Gollaher, C.J., and Bausserman, L.L. 1990. Hepatic catabolism of serum amyloid A during an acute phase response and chronic inflammation. *Proc Soc Exp Biol Med.* 194:245–250.

Gonias, S.L., Balber, A.E., Hubbard, W.J., and Pizzo, S.V. 1983. Ligand binding conformational change and plasma elimination of human, mouse, and rat alpha-2-macroglobulin proteinase inhibitors. *Biochem J.* 209:99–105.

Gonias, S.L., and Pizzo, S. 1983. Conformation and protease binding activity of binary and ternary human α_2-macroglobulin-protease complexes. *J Biochem.* 258:14682–14685.

Gonnerman, W.A., Elliott-Bryant, R., Carreras, I., Sipe, J.D., and Cathcart, E.S. 1995. Linkage of protection against amyloid fibril formation in the mouse to a single, autosomal dominant gene. *J Exp Med.* 181:2249–2252.

Goode, C.A., Dinh, C.T., and Linder, M.C. 1990. Mechanism of copper transport and delivery in mammals. Review and recent findings. *Adv Exp Med Biol.* 258:131–144.

Goodwin, R.L., Baumann, H., and Berger, F.G. 1996. Patterns of divergence during evolution of α1-proteinase inhibitors in mammals. *Mol Biol Evol.* 13:346–358.

Goto, K., Suzuki, Y., Yoshida, K., Yamamoto, K., and Sinohara, H. 1994. Plasma α-1-antiproteinase from the Mongolian gerbil, *Meriones unguiculatus:* Isolation, partial characterization, sequencing of cDNA, and implications for molecular evolution. *J Biochem.* 116:582–588.

Gregoriadis, G., Morell, A.G., Sternlieb, I., and Scheinberg, I.H. 1970. Catabolism of desialylated ceruloplasmin in the liver. *J Biol Chem.* 245:5833–5837.

Gressner, A.M., and Peltzer, B. 1984. Amidolytic and immuno-nephelometric determination of α_1-proteinase inhibitor and α_2 macroglobulin in serum with calculation of specific inhibitor activities in health and disease. *J Clin Chem Clin Biochem.* 22:633–640.

Griswold, D.E., Hillegass, L., Antell, L., Shatzman, A., and Hanna, N. 1986. Quantitative Western blot assay for measurement of the murine acute phase reactant, serum amyloid P component. *J Immunol Methods.* 91:163–168.

Gross, N.J., Bublys, V., D'Anza, J., and Brown, C.L. 1995. The role of α_1-antitrypsin in the control of extracellular surfactant metabolism. *Am J Physiol.* 268:L438–445.

Gruys, E., Obwolo, M.J., and Toussaint, M.J.M. 1994. Diagnostic significance of the major acute phase proteins in veterinary clinical chemistry: A review. *Vet Bull.* 64:1009–1018.

Gubler, C.J., Lahey, M., Cartwright, C., and Wintrobe, M.M. 1953. Studies on copper metabolism. IX. The transport of copper in blood. *J Clin Invest.* 32:405–414.

Gutteridge, J.M.C. 1991. Plasma ascorbate levels and inhibition of the antioxidant activity of caeruloplasmin. *Clin Sci.* 81:413–417.

Gutteridge, J.M.C., and Stocks, J. 1981. Caeruloplasmin: Physiological and pathological perspectives. *Crit Rev Clin Lab Sci.* 14:257–329.

Gutteridge, J.M.C., Winyard, P.G., Blake, D.R., Lunee, J., Brailsford, S., and Halliwell, B. 1985. The behavior of caeruloplasmin in stored human extracellular fluids in relation to ferroxidase II activity, lipid peroxidation, and phenanthroline-detectable copper. *Biochem J.* 260:517–523.

Hachem, H., Saile, R., Favre, G., Bosco, R., Raynal, G., Fruchart, J.C., and Soula, G. 1991. A sensitive immunochemiluminescence assay for human serum amyloid A protein. *Clin Biochem.* 24:143–147.

Hamazaki, H. 1987. Ca2+-mediated association of serum amyloid P component with heparan sulfate and dermatan sulfate. *J Biol Chem.* 262:1456–1460.

Hamazaki, H. 1989. Calcim-dependent polymerization of human serum amyloid P component is inhibited by heparin and dextran sulfate. *Biochim Biophys Acta.* 998:231–235.

Handagama, P., Rappolee, D.A., Werb, Z., Levin, J., and Bainton, D.F. 1990. Platelet A—Granule fibrinogen, albumin, and immunoglobulin G are not synthesized by rat and mouse megakaryocytes. *J Clin Invest.* 86:1364–1368.

Hanover, J.A., Chjeng, S.-Y., Willingham, M.C., and Pastan, I.H. 1983. α_2 macroglobulin binding to cultured fibroblasts. *J Biol Chem.* 258:370–377.

Hantgan, R.R., Francis, C.W., and Marder, V.J. 1994. Fibrinogen structure and physiology. In *Hemostasis and Thrombosis: Basic Principles and Clinical Practice.* Eds. R.W. Colman, J. Hirsh, V.J. Marder, and E.W. Salzman, 3rd edition. Philadelphia, PA: J. B. Lippincott.

Harris, E.D. 1991. Copper transport: An overview. *Proc Soc Exp Biol Med.* 196:130–140.

Hart, A.H. 1997. A rapid, accurate in-house pregnancy test for dogs. *Vet Forum.* 14:40–43.

Hart, D.A., and Stein-Streilein, J. 1981. Hamster lymphoid cells responses in vitro. In *Advances in Experimental Medicine and Biology*, Vol. 134, pp. 7–22.

Hashimoto, S., Kato, M., Dong, Y., Terada, S., and Inoue, M. 1995. Effect of sex steroids on serum amyloid P-components female protein in rats. *Nippon Sanka Fujinka Gakkai Zasshi.* 47:1041–1047.

Hashimoto, S., and Migita, S. 1990. Serum amyloid P component regulation by sex steroids in rats. *Nippon Ketsueki Gakkai Zasshi.* 53:89–97.

Haston, L., FitzGerald, O., Kane, D., and Smith, K. 2002. Preliminary observations on the influence of rheumatoid alpha-1-acid glycoprotein on collagen fibril formation. *Biomed Chromatogr.* 16:332–342.

Hawkey, C.M., and Hart, M.G. 1987. Fibrinogen levels in mammals suffering from bacterial infections. *Vet Rec.* 121:519–521.

Hawkins, P., Tennent, G., Woo, P., and Pepys, M. 1991. Studies in vivo and in vitro of serum amyloid P component in normals and in a patient with AA amyloidosis. *Clin Exp Immunol.* 84:308–316.

Heegaard, P.M. 1992. Changes in serum glycoprotein glycosylation during experimental inflammation in mice are general, unrelated to protein type, and opposite changes in man and rat. *Inflammation.* 16:631–644.

Heinrich, P.C., Castell, J.C., and Andus, T. 1990. Interleukin-6 and the acute phase response. *Biochem J.* 265:621–636.

Henschen, A., Lottspeich, F., Kehl, M., and Southern, C. 1983. Covalent structure of fibrinogen. *Ann N Y Acad Sci.* 408:28–43.

Heuertz, R.M., Ahmed, N., and Webster, R.O. 1996. Peptides derived from C-reactive protein inhibit neutrophil alveolitis. *J Immunol.* 156:3412–3417.

Heuertz, R.M., Piquette, C.A., and Webster, R.O. 1993. Rabbits with elevated serum C-reactive protein exhibit diminished neutrophil infiltration and vascular permeability in C5a-induced alveolitis. *Am J Pathol.* 142:319–328.

Heuertz, R.M., Xia, D., Samols, D., and Webster, R.O. 1994. Inhibition of C5a des Arg-induced neutrophil alveolitis in transgenic mice expressing C-reactive protein. *Am J Physiol.* 266:L649–L654.

Hill, M.D., Briscoe, P.R., and Abramson, F.P. 1989. Comparison of propranolol-binding plasma proteins in sheep with those in humans, dogs, and rats. *Biochem Pharmacol.* 38:4199–4205.

Hill, R.E., Shaw, P.H., Barth, R.K., and Hastie, N.D. 1985. A genetic locus closely linked to a protease inhibitor gene complex controls the level of multiple RNA transcripts. *Mol Cell Biol.* 5:2114–2122.

Hilliker, C., Overbergh, L., Petit, P., Van Leuven, F., and Van den Berghe, H. 1992a. Assignment of mouse alpha-2-macroglobulin gene to chromosome 6 band F1–G3. *Mamm Genome.* 3:469–471.

Hilliker, C., Van Leuven, F., and Van den Berghe, H. 1992b. Assignment of the gene coding for the alpha-2-macroglobulin receptor to mouse chromosome 15 and to human chromosome 12q13-q14 by isotopic and nonisotopic in situ hybridization. *Genomics.* 13:472–474.

Hind, C.R.K., Collins, P.M., Baltz, M.L., and Pepys, M.B. 1985. Human serum amyloid P, a circulating lectin with specificity for the cyclic 4,6-pyruvate acetal galactose: Interactions with various bacteria. *Biochem J.* 225:107–111.

Hind, C.R.K., Collins, P.M., Renn, D., et al. 1984. Binding specificity of serum amyloid P component from the pyruvate acetal of galatose. *J Exp Med.* 159:1058–1069.

Hirose, S., Oda, K., and Ikehara, Y. 1988. Biosynthesis, assembly, and secretion of fibrinogen in cultured rat hepatocytes. *Biochem J.* 251:373–377.

Hirschelmann, R., Schade, R., and Bekemeier, H. 1990. Acute phase reaction in rats: Independent change of acute phase protein plasma concentration and macroscopic inflammation in primary rat adjuvant inflammation. *Agents Actions.* 30:412–417.

Hiyamuta, S., and Takeichi, N. 1993. Lack of copper binding sites in ceruloplasmin of LEC rats with abnormal copper metabolism. *Biochem Biophys Res Commun.* 197:1140–1145.

Hochepied, T., Berger, F., Baumann, H., and Libert, C. 2003. Alpha-1-acid glycoprotein: An acute phase protein with inflammatory and immunodulating properties. *Cytokine Growth Factor Rev.* 14(1):25–34.

Hoffman, J.S., and Benditt, E.P. 1982. Changes in high density lipoprotein content following endotoxin administration in the mouse. *J Biol Chem.* 257:10510–10517.

Hoffman, J.S., and Benditt, E.P. 1983. Plasma clearance kinetics of the amyloid-related high density lipoprotein apoprotein, aerum amyloid protein apoSAA in the mouse. *J Clin Invest.* 71:926–934.

Hol, P.R., Snel, F.W.J.J., Draaijer, M., and Grays, E. 1987. The serum amyloid A stimulating factor SAASF in the hamster. *J Comp Pathol.* 97:677–685.

Hood, J.M., Koep, L., Peters, R.F., et al. 1980. Liver transplantation for advanced liver disease with alpha-1-antitrypsin deficiency. *N Engl J Med.* 302:272–275.

Hovi, T., Mosher, D., and Vaheri, A. 1977. Cultured human monocytes synthesize and secrete α_2-macroglobulin. *J Exp Med.* 145:1581–1589.

Hu, S.I., MacIntyre, S.S., Schultz, D., Kushner, I., and Samols, D. 1988. Secretion of rabbit C-reactive protein by transfected human cell lines is more rapid than by cultured rabbit hepatocytes. *J Biol Chem.* 263:1500–1504.

Hu, S.I., Miller, S.M., and Samols, D. 1986. Cloning and characterization of the gene for rabbit C-reactive protein. *Biochemistry.* 25:7834–7839.

Huang, J.H., Rienhoff, H.Y., and Liao, W.S.L. 1990. Regulation of mouse serum amyloid A gene expression in transfected hepatoma cells. *Mole Cell Biol.* 10:3619–3625.

Huber, P., Laurent, M., and Dalmon, J. 1990. Human β-fibrinogen gene expression. *J Biol Chem.* 265:5695–5701.

Hughes, D., Elliot, D.A., Washabau, R.J., and Kueppers, F. 1995. Effects of age, sex, reproductive status, and hospitalization on serum a1-antitrypsin concentration in dogs. *Am J Vet Res.* 56:568–572.

Hunneyball, I.M., Spowage, M., Crossley, M.J., Rowe, I.F., and Baltz, M.L. 1986. Acute phase protein changes in antigen-induced mono-articular arthritis in rabbits and mice. *Clin Exp Immunol.* 65:311–318.

Hutchinson, W.L., Noble, G.E., Hawkins, P.N., and Pepys, M.B. 1994. The pentraxins, C-reactive protein and serum amyloid P component are cleared and catabolized by hepatocytes in vivo. *J Clin Invest.* 94:1390–1396.

Ichinose, A., and Davie, E.W. 1994. The blood coagulation factors: Their cDNAs, genes and expression. In *Hemostasis and Thrombosis: Basic Principles and Clinical Practice*., 3rd edition. Eds. R.W. Colman, J. Hirsh, V.J. Marder, and E.W. Salzman, pp. 19–54. Philadelphia, PA: J. B. Lippincott.

Ikawa, M., and Shozen, Y. 1990. Quantification of acute-phase proteins in rat serum and in the supernatants of a cultured rat hepatoma cell line and cultured primary hepatocytes by an enzyme-linked immunosorbent assay. *J Immunol Methods.* 134:101–106.

Imber, M.J., and Pizzo, S.V. 1981. Clearance and binding of two electrophoretic "fast" forms of human α_2 macroglobulin. *J Biol Chem.* 256:8134–8139.

Ingrassia, R., Savoldi, G.F., Caraffini, A., et al. 1994. Characterization of a novel transcription complex required for glucocorticoid regulation of the rat alpha-1-acid glycoprotein gene. *DNA Cell Biol.* 13:615–627.

Inoue, S., Hultin, P.G., Szarek, W.A., and Kisilevsky, R. 1996. Effect of polyvinylsulfonate on murine AA amyloid: A high-resolution ultrastructural study. *Lab Invest.* 74:1081–1090.

Ishida, T., Matsuura, K., Setoguchi, M., Higuchi, Y., and Yamamoto, S. 1994. Enhancement of murine serum amyloid A3 mRNA expression by glucocorticoids and its regulation by cytokines. *J Leukoc Biol.* 56:797–806.

Ishikawa, N., Shigemoto, K., and Maruyama, N. 1987. The complete nucleotide and deduced amino acid sequence of mouse serum amyloid P component. *Nucleic Acid Res.* 15:7186.

Itoh, Y., Takeuchi, S., Shigemoto, K., et al. 1992. The strain-dependent constitutive expression of murine serum amyloid-P component is regulated at the transcriptional level. *Biochim Biophys Acta.* 1131:261–269.

Jaeger, J.L., Shimizu, N., and Gitlin, J.D. 1991. Tissue specific ceruloplasmin gene expression in the mammary gland. *Biochem J.* 280:671–677.

James, K. 1980. Alpha-2-macroglobulin and its possible importance in immune systems. *Trends Biochem Sci.* 5:43–46.

James, K. 1990. Interactions between cytokines and α_2 macroglobulin. *Immunol Today.* 11:163–166.

James, H., and Cohen, A. 1978. Mechanism of inhibition of porcine elastase by human alpha-1-antitrypsin. *J Clin Invest.* 62:1344–1353.

Jamieson, J.C., and Ashton, F.E. 1973. Studies on acute phase proteins in rat serum. III. Site of synthesis of albumin and α_1-acid glycoprotein and the contents of these proteins in liver microsome fractions from rats suffering from induced inflammation. *Can J Biochem.* 51:1281–1291.

Jensen, P., Jorgensen, S., Datta, P., and Sorensen, P. 2004. Significantly increased fractions of transformed to total alpha-2- macroglobin concentrations in plasma from patients with multiple sclerosis. *Biochim Biophys Acta.* 1690:203–207.

Kajikawa, T., Furuta, A., Onishi, T., and Sugii, S. 1996. Enzyme-linked immunosorbent assay for detection of feline serum amyloid A potein by use of immunological cross-reactivity of polyclonal anti-canine serum amyloid A protein antibody. *J Vet Med Sci.* 58:1141–1143.

Kalmovarin, N., Friedrichs, E., O'Brien, H., Linehan, L.A., Bowman, B.H., and Yang, F. 1991. Extrahepatic expression of plasma protein genes during inflammation. *Inflammation.* 15:369–379.

Kaneko, J.J. 1997. Serum proteins and the dysproteinemias. In *Clinical Chemistry of Domestic Animals*, 5th edition. Eds. J.J. Kaneko, J.W. Harvey, and M.L. Bruss, pp. 117–138. New York, NY: Academic Press.

Kant, J.A., Fornace, A.J., Saxe, D., Simon, M.I., McBride, O.W., and Crabtree, G.R. 1985. Evolution and organization of the fibrinogen locus on chromosome 4. Gene duplication accompanied by transposition and inversion. *Proc Natl Acad Sci USA.* 82:2344–2348.

Kataoka, M., and Tavassoli, M. 1984. Ceruloplasmin receptors in liver cell suspensions are limited to the endothelium. *Exp Cell Res.* 155:232–240.

Kataoka, M., and Tavassoli, M. 1985. The role of liver endothelium in the binding and uptake of ceruloplasmin: Studies with colloidal gold probes. *J Ultrastruct Res.* 90:194–202.

Kempka, G., Roos, P.H., and Kolb-Bachofen, V. 1990. A membrane-associated form of C-reactive protein is the galactose-specific particle receptor on rat liver macrophages. *J Immunol.* 144:1004–1009.

Kent, J. 1992. Acute phase proteins: Their use in veterinary diagnosis. *Br Vet J.* 148:279–281.

Kerkay, J., and Westphal, U. 1968. Steroid-protein interactions. XIX. Complex formation between alpha-1 acid glycoprotein and steroid hormones. *Biochim Biophys Acta.* 170:324–333.

Kew, R.R., Hyers, T.M., and Webster, R.O. 1990. Human C-reactive protein inhibits neutrophil chemotaxis in vitro: Possible implications for the adult respiratory distress syndrome. *J Lab Clin Med.* 115:339–345.

Khan, M.M.H., Shibuya, Y., Kambara, T., and Yamamoto, T. 1995. Role of α-2-macroglobulin in bacterial elastase in guinea-pig pseudomonal septic shock. *Int J Exp Pathol.* 76:21–28.

Khan, M.M.H., Shibuya, Y., Nakagaki, T., Kambara, T., and Yamamoto, T. 1994. Alpha-2-macroglobulin as the major defence in acute pseudomonal septic shock in the guinea-pig model. *Int J Exp Pathol.* 75:285–293.

Kilpatrick, J.M., and Virella, G. 1985. Inhibition of platelet-activating factor by rabbit C-reactive protein. *Clin Immunol Immunopathol.* 37:276–281.

Kilpatrick, J.M., and Volanakis, J.E. 1985. Opsonic properties of C-reactive protein. Stimulation by phorbol myristate acetate enables human neutrophils to phagocytize C-reactive protein-coated cells. *J Immunol.* 134:3364–3370.

Kimura, M., Toth, L.A., Agostini, H., Cady, A.B., Majde, J.A., and Krueger, J.M. 1994. Comparison of acute phase responses induced in rabbits by lipopolysaccharide and double-stranded RNA. *Am J Physiol.* 267:R1596–1605.

Kimura-Takeuchi, M., Majde, J.A., Toth, L.A., and Krueger, J.M. 1992. Influenza virus-induced changes in rabbit sleep and acute phase responses. *Am J Physiol.* 263:R1115–1121.

Kingston, I.B., Kingston, B.L., and Putman, F.W. 1977. Chemical evidence that proteolytic cleavage causes the heterogeneity present in human ceruloplasmin preparations. *Proc Natl Acad Sci USA.* 74:5377–5381.

Kischinsky, M.L., Funk, W.D., VanOost, B.A., and MacGillivray, R.T.A. 1986. Complete cDNA sequence of human preceruloplasmin. *Proc Natl Acad Sci USA.* 83:5086–5090.

Kisilevsky, R. 1991. Serum amyloid A SAA, a protein without a function: Some suggestions with reference to cholesterol metabolism. *Med Hypotheses.* 35:337–341.

Kisilevsky, R., and Subrahmanyan, L. 1992. Serum amyloid A changes high density lipoprotein's cellular affinity. A clue to serum amyloid A's principle function. *Lab Invest.* 66:778–785.

Kjelgaard-Hansen, M., Christensen, M., Lee, M., Jensen, A., and Jacobsen, S. 2007. Serum amyloid A isoforms in serum and synovial fluid from spontaneously diseased dogs with joint diseases or other conditions. *Vet Immunol Immunopathol.* 117:296–301.

Klein, T.C., Doffinger, R., Pepys, M.B., Ruther, U., and Kyewski, B. 1995. Tolerance and immunity to the inducible self antigen C-reactive protein in transgenic mice. *Eur J Immunol.* 25:3489–3495.

Klomp, L.W.J., Farhangrazi, Z.S., Dugan, L.L., and Gitlin, J.D. 1996. Ceruloplasmin gene expression in the murine central nervous system. *J Clin Invest.* 98:207–215.

Kluve-Beckerman, B., Dwulet, F.E., DiBartola, S.P., and Benson, M.D. 1989. Primary structures of dog and cat amyloid proteins: Comparison to human AA. *Comp Biochem Physiol B.* 95:175–183.

Kodelja, V., Heisig, M., Northemann, W., Heinrich, P.C., and Zimmermann, W. 1986. Alpha-2-macroglobulin gene expression during rat development studied by in situ hybridization. *EMBO J.* 5:3151–3156.

Koj, A., Dubin, A., Kasperczyk, H., Bereta, J., and Gordon, A.H. 1982. Changes in the blood level and affinity to concanavalin A or rat plasma glycoprotein during acute inflammation and hepatoma growth. *Biochem J.* 206:543–553.

Koj, A., Gauldie, J., Regoeczi, E., Sauder, D.N., and Sweeney, G.D. 1984. The acute-phase response of cultured rat hepatocytes. *Biochem J.* 224:505–514.

Koj, A., Guzdel, A., Nakamura, R., and Kordula, T. 1995. Hepatocyte growth factor and retinoic acid exert opposite effects on synthesis of type 1 and type 2 acute phase proteins in rat hepatoma cells. *Int J Biochem Cell Biol.* 27:39–46.

Koj, A., Hatton, M.W.C., Wong, K.L., and Regoeczi, E. 1978. Isolation and partial characterization of rabbit plasma alphal-antitrypsin. *Biochem J.* 169:589–596.

Koj, A., Magielska-Zero, D., Kurdowska, A., and Bereta, J. 1988. Proteinase inhibitors as acute phase reactants: Regulation of synthesis and turnover. *Adv Exp Med Biol.* 240:171–181.

Koj, A., and Regoeczi, E. 1978. Effect of experimental inflammation on the synthesis and distribution of antithrombin III and α_1-antitrypsin in rabbits. *Br J Exp Pathol.* 59:473–481.

Koj, A., Rokita, H., Kordula, R., Kurdowska, A., and Travis, J. 1991. Role of cytokines and growth factors in the induced synthesis of proteinase inhibitors belonging to acute phase proteins. *Biomed Biochim Acta.* 50:421–425.

Kojima, E., Mitsuno, T., and Osawa, T. 1986. Immunological effects of mouse ceruloplasmin. *J Pharmacobiodyn.* 9:101–109.

Kolb-Bachofen, V. 1991. A membrane-bound form of the acute-phase protein C-reactive protein is the galactose-specific particle receptor on rat liver. *Pathobiolology.* 59:272–275.

Kolb-Bachofen, V. 1992. Uptake of toxic silica particles by isolated rat liver macrophages Kupffer cells is receptor-mediated and can be blocked by competition. *J Clin Invest.* 90:1819–1824.

Kolb-Bachofen, V., and Abel, F. 1991. Participation of D-galactose-specific receptors of liver macrophages in recognition of fibronectin-opsonized particles. *Carbohydr Res.* 213:202–213.

Kounnas, M.Z., Church, F.C., Argraves, W.S., and Strickland, D.K. 1996. Cellular internalization and degradation of antithrombin III-thrombin, heparin cofactor II-thrombin, and $\alpha 1$-antitrypsin-trypsin complexes is mediated by the low densitiy lipoprotein receptor-related protein. *J Biol Chem.* 271:6523–6529.

Kremer, J.M.H., Wilting, J., and Janssen, L.H.M. 1988. Drug binding to human alpha-1-acid glycoprotein in health and disease. *Pharmacol Rev.* 40:1–47.

Ku, N.O., and Mortensen, R.F. 1993. Cloning and tissue-specific expression of the gene for mouse C-reactive protein. *Biochem J.* 295:379–386.

Kudryk, B., Okada, M., Redman, C., and Blomback, B. 1982. Biosynthesis of dog fibrinogen. Characterization of nascent fibrinogen in the rough endoplasmic reticulum. *Eur J Biochem.* 125:673–682.

Kueppers, F., and Mills, J. 1983. Trypsin inhibition by mouse serum: Sexual dimorphism controlled by testosterone. *Science.* 219:182–184.

Kuranda, M.J., and Aronson, N.N., Jr. 1983. Tissue locations for the turnover of radioactively labelled rat orosomucoid in vivo. *Arch Biochem Biophys.* 224:526–533.

Kurokawa, S., Ishibashi, H., Hayashida, K., et al. 1987. Kupffer cell stimulation of alpha$_2$-macroglobulin synthesis in rat hepatocytes and the role of glucocorticoid. *Cell Struct Funct.* 12:35–42.

Kushner, I. 1988. The acute-phase response: An overview. *Methods Enzymol.* 163:373–383.

Kushner, I., and Mackiewicz, A. 1987. Acute phase proteins as disease markers. *Dis Markers.* 5:1–11.

Lacki, J.K., Klama, K., Mackiewicz, S.H., Mackiewicz, U., and Muller, W. 1994. Relation between IL-6 and acute phase proteins concentration in serum and synovial fluid. *Int J Immunopathol Pharmacol.* 7:87–93.

Lamarre, J., Wollenberg, G.K., Gauldie, J., and Hayes, M.A. 1990. α_2-Macroglobulin and serum preferentially counteract the mitoinhibitory effect of transforming growth factor-β2 in rat hepatocytes. *Lab Invest.* 62:545–551.

Lamarre, J., Wollenberg, G.K., Gonias, S.L., and Hayes, M.A. 1991. Cytokine binding and clearance properties of proteinase-activated α_2-macroglobulins. *Lab Invest.* 65:3–14.

Languino, L.R.A., Duperray, A., Joganic, K.J., Fornaro, M., Thornton, G.B., and Altieri, D. C. 1995. Regulation of leukocyte-endothelium interaction and leukocyte transendothelial migration by intercellular adhesion molecule 1-fibrinogen recognition. *Proc Natl Acad Sci USA.* 92:1505–1509.

Lanser, M.E., and Brown, G.E. 1989. Stimulation of rat hepatocyte fibronectin production by monocyte-conditioned medium is due to interleukin 6. *J Exp Med.* 170:1781–1786.

Laskowski, M. 1986. Protein inhibitors of serine proteinases: Mechanism and classification. *Adv Exp Med Biol.* 199:1–17.

Latimer, J.J., Berger, F.G., and Baumann, H. 1987. Developmental expression, cellular localization, and testosterone regulation of alpha 1-antitrypsin in *Mus caroli* kidney. *J Biol Chem.* 262:12641–12646.

Latimer, J.J., Berger, F.G., and Baumann, H. 1990. Highly conserved upstream regions of the α_1-antitrypsin gene in two mouse species govern liver-specific expression by different mechanisms. *Mol Cell Biol.* 10:760–769.

Laurell, C.B., and Rannevik, G. 1979. A comparison of plasma protein changes induced by danazol, pregnancy, and estrogens. *J Clin Endocrinol Metab.* 49:719–725.

Laurent, P.E. 1989. Clinical measurement of acute phase proteins to detect and monitor infectious disease. In *Acute Phase Proteins in the Acute Phase Response.* Ed. M.B. Pepys, pp. 151–159. New York, NY: Springer-Verlag.

Lavie, G., Zucker-Franklin, D., and Franklin, E.C. 1978. Degradation of serum amyloid A protein by surface-associated enzymes of human blood monocytes. *J Exp Med.* 148:1020–1031.

Le, P.T., and Mortensen, R.F. 1984a. In vitro induction of hepatocyte synthesis of the acute phase reactant mouse serum amyloid P-component by macrophages and IL 1. *J Leukoc Biol.* 35:587–603.

Le, P.T., and Mortensen, R.F. 1984b. Mouse hepatocyte synthesis and induction of the acute phase reactant: Serum amyloid P-component. *In Vitro.* 20:505–511.

Le, P.T., and Mortensen, R.F. 1986. Induction and regulation by monokines of hepatic synthesis of the mouse serum amyloid P-component SAP. *J Immunol.* 136:2526–2533.

Le, P.T., Muller, M.T., and Mortensen, R.F. 1982. Acute phase reactants of mice I. Isolation of serum amyloid P component SAP and its induction by a monokine. *J Immunol.* 129:665–672.

Lee, Y.-M., Miau, L.-H., Chang, C.-J., and Lee, S.-C. 1996. Transcriptional induction of the alpha-1 acid glycoprotein AGP gene by synergistic interaction of two alternative activator forms of AGP/enhancer-binding protein C/EBPb and NF-kB of noppl40. *Mol Cell Biol.* 16:4257–4263.

Lei, K-J., Liu, T., Zon, G., Soravia, E., Liu, T-Y., and Goldman, N.D. 1985. Genomic DNA sequence for human C-reactive protein. *J Biol Chem.* 160:13377–13383.

Levin, M.J., Tuil, D., Uzan, G., Dreyfus, J.C., and Kahn, A. 1984. Expression of the transferrin gene during development of nonhepatic tissues; high levels of transferrin mRNA in fetal muscle and rabbit brain. *Biochem Biophys Res Commun.* 122:212–217.

Li, S.P., and Goldman, N.D. 1996. Regulation of human C-reactive protein gene expression by two synergistic IL-6 responsive elements. *Biochemistry.* 35:9060–9068.

Li, S.P., Liu, T-Y., and Goldman, N.D. 1990. Cis-acting elements responsible for interleukin-6 inducible C-reactive protein gene expression. *J Biol Chem.* 265:4136–4142.

Li, Y., Togashi, Y., Sato, S., et al. 1991. Spontaneous hepatic copper accumulation in Long-Evans Cinnamon rats with hereditary hepatitis. A model of Wilson's disease. *J Clin Invest.* 87:1858–1861.

Liao, Y.C., Taylor, J.M., Vannice, J.L., Clawson, G.A., and Smuckler, E.A. 1985. Structure of the rat α_1-acid glycoprotein gene. *Mol Cell Biol.* 5:3634–3639.

Liepnieks, J.J., Dwulet, F.E., Benson, M.D., Kluve-Beckerman, B., and Kushner, I. 1991. The primary structure of serum amyloid A protein in the rabbit: Comparison with serum amyloid A proteins in other species. *J Lab Clin Med.* 118:570–575.

Lin, B.F., Ku, N.O., Zahedi, K., Whitehead, A.S., and Mortensen, R.F. 1990. IL-1 and IL-6 mediate increased production and synthesis by hepatocytes of acute-phase reactant mouse ser Interleukin-1-component SAP. *Inflammation.* 14:297–313.

Lin, L., and Liu, T-Y. 1993. Isolation and characterization of C-reactive protein CRP, cDNA, and genomic DNA from *Xenopus laevis*. *J Biol Chem.* 268:6809–6815.

Lin, C.S., Xia, D., Yun, J.S., et al. 1995. Expression of rabbit C-reactive protein in transgenic mice. *Immunol Cell Biol.* 73:521–531.

Liu, T-Y., Syin, C., Nguyen, N.Y., et al. 1987. Comparison of protein structure and genomic structure of human, rabbit and *Limulus* C-reactive proteins: Possible implications for function and evolution. *J Protein Chem.* 6:263–271.

Lobetti, R., Mohr, A., Dippenaar, T., and Myburgh, E. 2000. A preliminary study on the serum protein response in canine babesiosis. *S Afr Vet Assoc.* 71(1):38–42.

Logan, J.I., Harveyson, K.B., Wisdom, G.B., Hughes, A.E., and Archbold, G.P. 1994. Hereditary caeruloplasmin deficiency, dementia, and diabetes mellitus. *QJM.* 87:663–670.

Long, G.L., Chandra, T., Woo, S.L.C., Davie, E.W., and Kurachi, K. 1984. Complete sequence of the cDNA for human α1-antitrypsin and the gene for the S variant. *Biochemistry.* 23:4828–4837.

Lonky, S.A., Marsh, J., Steele, R., Jacobs, K., Konopka, R., and Moser, K.M. 1980. Protease and antiprotease responses in lung and peripheral blood in experimental canine pneumococcal pneumonia. *Am Rev Respir Dis.* 121:685–693.

Lord, S.T. 1995. Fibrinogen. In *Molecular Basis of Thrombosis and Hemostasis.* Eds. K.A. High, and H.R. Roberts, pp. 51–74. New York, NY: Marcel Dekker.

Lorent, K., Overbergh, L., Moechars, D., DeStrooper, B., Van-Leuven, F., and Van den Berghe, H. 1995. Expression in mouse embryos and in adult mouse brain of three members of the amyloid precursor protein family, of the alpha-2-macroglobulin receptor/low density lipoprotein lipase, alpha-2-macroglobulin, and the 40,000 molecular weight receptor-associated protein. *Neuroscience.* 65:1009–1025.

Lowell, C.A., Potter, D.A., Stearman, R.S., and Morrow, J.F. 1986b. Structure of the murine serum amyloid A gene family. *J Biol Chem.* 261:8442–8452.

Lowell, C.A., Stearman, R.S., and Morrow, J.F. 1986a. Transcriptional regulation of serum amyloid A gene expression. *J Biol Chem.* 261:8453–8461.

Macintyre, S.S. 1988. C-reactive protein. *Methods Enzymol.* 163:383–399.

Macintyre, S.S., Kushner, I., and Samols, D. 1985. Secretion of C-reactive protein becomes more efficient during the course of the acute phase response. *J Biol Chem.* 260:4169–4173.

Macintyre, S., Samols, D., and Dailey, P. 1994. Two carboxylesterases bind C-reactive protein within the endoplasmic reticulum and regulate its secretion during the acute phase response. *J Biol Chem.* 269:24496–24503.

Macintyre, S.S., Schultz, D., and Kushner, I. 1983. Synthesis and secretion of C-reactive protein by rabbit primary hepatocyte cultures. *Biochem J.* 210:707–715.

Mackiewicz, A., Ganapathi, M.K., Schultz, D., Samols, D., Reese, J., and Kushner, I. 1988. Regulation of rabbit acute phase protein biosynthesis by monokines. *Biochem J.* 253:851–857.

Mackiewicz, A., and Kushner, I. 1989. Interferon beta 2/B-cell stimulating factor 2/interleukin 6 affects glycosylation of acute phase proteins in human hepatoma cell lines. *Scand J Immunol.* 29:1–7.

Malle, E., Steinmetz, A., and Raynes, J.G. 1993. Serum amyloid A (SAA): An acute phase protein and apolipoprotein. *Atherosclerosis.* 102:131–146.

Mannhalter, J.W., Borth, W., and Eibl, M.M. 1986. Modulation of antigen-induced T-cell proliferation by α_2M-trypsin complexes. *J Immunol.* 136:2792–2799.

Mantzouranis, E.C., Dowton, S.B., Whitehead, A.S., Edge, M.D., Brans, G.A., and Colten, H. R. 1985. Human serum amyloid P component cDNA isolation, complete sequence of pre-serum amyloid P component, and localization of the gene to chromosome 1. *J Biol Chem.* 260:7752–7756.

Marder, V.J., Feinstein, D.I., Francis, C.W., and Colman, R.W. 1994. Consumptive thrombohemorrhagic disorders. In *Hemostasis and Thrombosis: Basic Principles and Clinical Practice*, 3rd edition. Eds. R.W. Colman, J. Hirsh, V.J. Marder, and E.W. Salzman, pp. 1023–1063. Philadelphia, PA: J. B. Lippincott.

Marhaug, G. 1983. Three assaays for the characterization and quantitation of human serum amyloid A. Scand J Immunol. 18:329–338.

Marhaug, G., and Dowton, S.B. 1994. Serum amyloid A: An acute phase apolipoprotein and precursor of AA amyloid. *Baillieres Clin Rheumatol.* 8:553–573.

Marinkovic, S., and Baumann, H. 1990. Structure, hormonal regulation, and identification of the interleukin-6- and dexamethasone-responsive element of the rat haptoglobin gene. *Mol Cell Biol.* 10:1573–1583.

Marinkovic, S., Jahreis, G.P., Wong, G.G., and Baumann, H. 1989. IL-6 modulates the synthesis of a specific set of acute phase plasma proteins in vivo. *J Immunol.* 142:808–812.

Marino, M.W., Fuller, G.M., and Elder, F.F. 1986. Chromosomal localization of human and rat Aα, Bβ, and γ fibrinogen genes by in situ hybridation. *Cytogenet Cell Genet.* 42:36–41.

Marnell, L., Mold, C., and Du Clos, T. 2005. C reactive protein: Ligands, receptors and role in inflammation. *Clin Immunol.* 117:104–111.

Martorana, P.A., Brand, T., Gardi, C., et al. 1993. The pallid mouse: A model of genetic α_1-antitrypsin deficiency. *Lab Invest.* 68:233–241.

Mast, A.E., Enghild, J.J., Pizzo, S.V., and Salvesen, G. 1991. Analysis of the plasma elimination kinetics and conformational stabilities of native, proteinase-complexed, and reactive site cleaved serpins: Comparison of alpha 1-proteinase inhibitor, alpha 1-antichymotrypsin, antithrombin III, alpha 2-antiplasmin, angiotensinogen, and ovalubmin. *Biochemistry.* 30:1723–1730.

Matsuda, T., Hirano, T., Nagasawa, S., and Kishimoto, T. 1989. Identification of α_2-macroglobulin as a carrier protein for IL-6. *J Immunol.* 142:148–152.

Maudsley, S., Hind, C.R.K., Munn, E.A., Buttress, N., and Pepys, M.B. 1986. Isolation and characterization of guinea-pig serum amyloid P component. *Immunology.* 59:317–322.

Mayer J., Raraty, M., Slavin, J., et al. 2002. Serum amyloid A is a better early predicator of severity than C reactive protein in acute pancreatitis. *Br J Surg.* 89:163–171.

McAdam, K.P.W.J., and Sipe, J.D. 1976. Murine model for human secondary amyloidosis: Genetic variability of the acute-phase serum protein SAA response to endotoxins and casein. *J Exp Med.* 144:1121–1127.

McDonald, T.L., Weber, A., and Smith, J.W. 1991. A monoclonal antibody sandwich immunoassay for serum amyloid A SAA protein. *J Immunol Methods.* 144:149–155.

McDonagh, J., Carrell, N., and Lee, M.H. 1994. Dysfibinogenemia and other disorders of fibrinogen structure and function. In *Hemostasis and Thrombosis: Basic Principles and Clinical Practice*, 3rd edition. Eds. R.W. Colman, J. Hirsh, V.J. Marder, and E.W. Salzman, pp. 314–334. Philadelphia, PA: J. B. Lippincott.

McGilligan, K., and Thomas, D.W. 1991. Evaluation of assays for detecting α-1-protease inhibitor during purification from rat serum. *Anal Biochem.* 193:260–265.

Medved, L.V., Gorkun, O.V., Manykov, V.F., and Belitser, V.A. 1985. The role of fibrinogen α-C domains in the fibrin assembly process. *FEBS Lett.* 181:109–112.

Meek, R.L., and Benditt, E.P. 1986. Amyloid A gene family expression in different mouse tissues. *J Exp Med.* 164:2006–2017.

Meek, R.L., and Benditt, E.P. 1989. Rat tissues express serum amyloid A protein-related mRNAs. *Proc Natl Acad Sci USA.* 86:1890–1894.

Meek, R.L., Eriksen, N., and Benditt, E.P. 1989. Serum amyloid A in the mouse. Sites of uptake and mRNA expression. *Am J Pathol.* 135:411–419.

Meek, R.L., Eriksen, N., and Benditt, E.P. 1992. Murine serum amyloid A3 is a high density apolipoprotein and is secreted by macrophages. *Proc Natl Acad Sci USA.* 89:4949–4952.

Meek, R.L., Hoffman, J.S., and Benditt, E.P. 1986. Amyloidogenesis: One serum amyloid A isotype is selectively removed from the circulation. *J Exp Med.* 163:499–510.

Meier, H., and MacPike, A.D. 1968. Levels and heritability of serum ceruloplasmin activity in inbred strains of mice. *Proc Soc Exp Biol Med.* 128:1185–1190.

Melgarejo, I., Williams, D.A., and Griffith, G. 1996. Isolation and characterization of α_1-protease inhibitor from canine plasma. *Am J Vet Res.* 57:258–263.

Milland, J., Tsykin, A., Thomas, T., Aldred, A.R., Cole, T., and Schreiber, G. 1990. Gene expression in regenerating and acute-phase rat liver. *Am J Physiol.* 259:G340–G347.

Miller, H.R., Simpson, J.G., and Stalker, A.L. 1971. An evaluation of the heat precipitation method for plasma fibrinogen estimation. *J Clin Pathol.* 24:827–830.

Min, K.S., Terano, Y., Onosaka, S., and Tanaka, K. 1991. Induction of hepatic metallothionein by nonmetallic compounds associated with acute-phase response in inflammation. *Toxicol Appl Pharmacol.* 111:152–162.

Mischke, R., and Menzel, D. 1994. Measuring fibrinogen concentrations in healthy dogs: Standardization, comparison of methods, and reference values. *J Vet Med.* 41:587–598.

Miura, K., Ju, S.T., Cohen, A.S., and Shirahama, T. 1990. Generation and use of site-specific antibodies to serum amyloid A for probing amyloid A development. *J Immunol.* 144:610–613.

Miyajima, H., Nishimura, Y., Mizoguchi, K., Sakamoto, M., Shimizu, T., and Honda, N. 1987. Familial apoceruloplasmin deficiency associated with blepharospasm and retinal degeneration. *Neurology.* 37:761–767.

Miyake, Y., Sinomura, M., Ito, T., et al. 1993. Hamster α-macroglobulin and murinoglobulin: Comparison of chemical and biological properties with homologs from other mammals. *J Biochem.* 114:513–521.

Miyanaga, O., Okubo, H., Kudo, J., Ikuta, T., and Hirata, Y. 1982. Effect of α_2 macroglobulin on the lymphocyte response. *Immunology.* 47:351–356.

Moak, S.A., and Greenwald, R.A. 1984. Enhancement of rat serum ceruloplasmin levels by exposure to hyperoxia. *Proc Soc Exp Biol Med.* 177:97–103.

Moestrup, S.K., Gliemann, J., and Pallesen, G. 1992. Distribution of the alpha 2-macroglobulin receptor/low density lipoprotein-related protein in human tissues. *Cell Tissue Res.* 269:375–382.

Mold, C., Du Clos, T.W., Nakayama, S., Edwards, K.M., and Gewurz, H. 1982. C-reactive protein reactivity with complement and effects on phagocytosis. *Ann N Y Acad Sci.* 389:251–259.

Mold, C., Nakayama, S., Holzer, T.J., Gewurz, H., and Du Clos, T.W. 1981. C-reactive protein is protective against *Streptococcus pneumoniae* infection in mice. *J Exp Med.* 154:1703–1708.

Monnet, D., Feger, J., Biou, D., et al. 1986. Effect of phenobarbital on the oligosaccharide structure of rat α_1-acid glycoprotein. *Biochim Biophys Acta.* 881:10–14.

Montaser, A., Tetreault, C., and Linder, M. 1992. Comparison of copper binding components in dog serum with those in other species. *Proc Soc Exp Biol Med.* 200:321–329.

Montgomery, K.T., Tardiff, J., Reid, L.M., and Krauter, K.S. 1990. Negative and positive cis-acting elements control the expression of murine α_1-protease inhibitor genes. *Mol Cell Biol.* 10:2625–2637.

Mookerjea, S., Francis, J., Hunt, D., Yang, C.Y., and Nagpurkar, A. 1994. Rat C-reactive protein causes a charge modification of LDL and stimulates its degradation by macrophages. *Arterioscler Thromb.* 14:282–287.

Mookerjea, S., and Hunt, D. 1995. A novel phosphatidylcholine hydrolysing action of C-reactive protein. *Biochem Biophys Res Commun.* 208:1046–1052.

Morgan, J.G., Holbrook, N.J., and Crabtree, G.R. 1987. Nucleotide sequence of the gamma chain of rat fibrinogen: Conserved intronic sequences. *Nucleic Acid Res.* 15:2774–2776.

Morrow, J.F., Stearman, R.S., Pelzman, C.G., and Potter, D.A. 1981. Induction of hepatic synthesis of serum amyloid A and actin. *Proc Natl Acad Sci USA.* 78:4718–4722.

Mortensen, R.F., Beisel, K., Zeleznik, N.J., and Le, P.T. 1983. Acute-phase reactants of mice. II. Strain dependence of serum amyloid-P component SAP levels and response to inflammation. *J Immunol.* 130:885–889.

Mortensen, R.F., Osmand, A.P., and Gewurz, H. 1975. Effects of C-reactive protein on the lymphoid system. *J Exp Med.* 141:821–839.

Mortensen, R.F., Shapiro, J., Lin, B., Douches, S., and Neta, R. 1988. Interaction of recombinant IL-1 and recombinant tumor necrosis factor in the induction of mouse acute phase proteins. *J Immunol.* 140:2260–2266.

Moshage, H.J., Kleter, B.E.M., vanPelt, J.F., Roelofs, H.M.J., Kleuskens, J.A.G.M., and Yap, S.H. 1988. Fibrinogen and albumin synthesis are regulated at the transcriptional level during the acute phase response. *Biochim Biophys Acta.* 950:450–454.

Mosher, D.F., and Wing, D.A. 1976. Synthesis and secretion of α_2-macroglobulin by cultured human fibroblasts. *J Exp Med.* 143:462–467.

Motie, M., Brockmeier, S., and Potempa, L.A. 1996. Binding of model soluble immune complexes to modified C-reactive protein. *J Immunol.* 156:4435–4441.

Mullins, R.E., Miller, R.L., Hunter, R.L., and Bennett, B. 1984. Standardized automated assay for functional α_1-antitrypsin. *Clin Chem.* 30:1857–1860.

Munck, A., Guyre, P.M., and Holbrook, N.J. 1984. Physiological functions of glucocorticoids in stress and their relation to pharmacological actions. *Endocr Rev.* 5:25–44.

Murakami, T., Ohnishi, S., Nishiguchi, S., Maeda, S., Araki, S., and Shimada, K. 1988. Acute-phase response of mRNAs for serum amyloid P component, C-reactive protein, and prealbumin transthyretin in mouse liver. *Biochem Biophys Res Commun.* 155:554–560.

Murakawa, M., Okamura, T., Kamura, T., Shibuya, T., Harada, M., and Niho, Y. 1993. Diversity of primary structures of the carboxy-terminal regions of mammalian fibrinogen Aα-chains. *Thromb Haemost.* 69:351–360.

Murata, H., Shimada, N., and Yoshioka, M. 2004. Current research on acute phase proteins in veterinary diagnosis: An overview. *Vet J.* 168(1):28–40.

Murtaugh, R.J., and Jacobs, R.M. 1985. Serum antiprotease concentration in dogs with sponatenous and experimentally induced pancreatitis. *Am J Vet Res.* 46:80–83.

Myers, L.A., Boyce, J.T., and Robison, R.L. 1995. The tolerability and pharmacology of interleukin-6 administered in combination with GM-CSF or G-CSF in the rhesus monkey. *Toxicology.* 101:157–166.

Myers, M.A., and Fleck, A. 1988. Observations on the delay in onset of the acute phase protein response. *Br J Exp Pathol.* 69:169–176.

Nagpurkar, A., Hunt, D., Yang, C.Y., and Mookerjea, S. 1993. Degradation of rat C-reactive protein by macrophages. *Biochem J.* 295:247–253.

Nagpurkar, A., and Mookerjea, S. 1981. A novel phosphorylcholine-binding protein from rat serum and its effect on heparin-lipoprotein complex formation in the presence of calcium. *J Biol Chem.* 256:7440–7448.

Nagpurkar, A., Randell, E., Choudhury, S., and Mookerjea, S. 1988. Effect of rat phosphorylcholine-binding protein on platelet aggregation. *Biochim Biophys Acta.* 967:76–81.

Nakada, H., Matsumoto, S., and Tashiro, Y. 1986. Biosynthesis and secretion of amyloid P component in the rat liver. *J Biochem.* 99:877–884.

Nakagawa, S., Fukata, Y., Nishida, K., Miyake, M., and Hama, T. 1993. Evidence for serum factors modulating antibody production in normal and macular mice. *Biol Pharm Bull.* 16:534–537.

Nakatani, T., Suzuki, Y., Yoshida, K., and Sinohara, H. 1995. Molecular cloning and sequence analysis of cDNA encoding plasma a-1-antiproteinase from Syrian hamster: Implications for the evolution of Rodentia. *Biochim Biophys Acta.* 1263:245–248.

Nathoo, S.A., and Finlay, T.H. 1986. Immunological and chemical properties of mouse a1-protease inhibitors. *Arch Biochem Biophys.* 246:162–174.

Nesbitt, J.E., Fuentes, N.L., and Fuller, G.M. 1993. Ciliary neurotrophic factor regulates fibrinogen gene expression in hepatocytes by binding to the interleukin-6 receptor. *Biochem Biophys Res Commun.* 190:544–550.

Nesbitt, J.E., and Fuller, G.M. 1991. Transcription and translation are required for fibrinogen mRNA degradation in hepatocytes. *Biochim Biophys Acta.* 1089:88–94.

Neubauer, K., Knittel, T., Armbrust, T., and Ramadori, G. 1995. Accumulation and cellular localization of fibrinogen/fibrin during short-term and long-term rat liver injury. *Gastroenterology.* 108:1124–1135.

Nicollet, I., Lebreton, J.-P., Fontaine, M., and Hiron, M. 1981. Evidence for alpha-1-glycoprotein populations of different pI values after concanavalin A affinity chromatography. Study of their evolution during inflammation in man. *Biochim Biophys Acta.* 668:235–245.

Nieuwenhuizen, W., Emeis, J., and Hemmink, J. 1979. Purification and properties of rat alpha 2 acute phase macroglobulin. *Biochim Biophys Acta.* 580:129–139.

Niewold, T.A., and Tooten, P.C.J. 1990. Purification and characterization of hamster serum amyloid A protein SAA by cholesteryl hemisuccinate affinity chromatography. *Scand J Immunol.* 31:389–396.

Noe, D.A., Murphy, P.A., Bell, W.R., and Siegel, J.N. 1989. Acute-phase behavior of factor Vm procoagulant and other acute-phase reactants in rabbits. *Am J Physiol.* 257:R49–R56.

Nonogaki, K., Moser, A.H., Shigenaga, J., Feingold, K.R., and Grunfeld, C. 1996. B-nerve growth factor as a mediator of the acute phase response in vivo. *Biochem Biophys Res Commun.* 219:956–961.

Northemann, W., Heisig, M., Kunz, D., and Heinrich, P.C. 1985. Molecular cloning of cDNA sequences for rat α_2 macroglobulin and measurement of its transcription during experimental inflammation. *J Biol Chem.* 260:6200–6205.

Nunomura, W. 1990. C-reactive protein in rat: In development, pregnancy and effect of sex hormones. *Comp Biochem Physiol A.* 96:489–493.

Nunomura, W. 1992. C-reactive protein CRP in animals: Its chemical properties and biological functions. *Zool Sci.* 9:499–513.

Nunomura, W., Hatakeyama, M., and Hirai, H. 1990a. Purification of human C-reactive protein by immunoaffinity chromatography using mouse monoclonal antibody. *J Biochem Biophys Methods.* 21:75–80.

Nunomura, W., Takakuwa, Y., and Higashi, T. 1994. Changes in serum concentration and mRNA level of rat C-reactive protein. *Biochim Biophys Acta.* 1227:74–78.

Nunomura, W., Watanabe, H.K., and Hirai, H. 1990b. Interaction of C-reactive protein with macrophages in rats. *Zool Sci.* 7:767–773.

Ohlsson, K. 1971. Isolation and partial characterization of two related trypsin binding α_2 macroglobulins of dog plasma. *Biochim Biophys Acta.* 236:84–91.

Ohnishi, S., Maeda, S., Shimada, K., and Arao, T. 1986. Isolation and characterization of the complete complementary and genomic DNA sequences of human serum amyloid P component. *J Biochem.* 100:849–858.

Okubo, H., Ishibashi, H., Shibata, K., Tsuda-Kawamura, K., and Yanase, T. 1984. Distribution of α_2 macroglobulin in normal, inflammatory, and tumor tissues in rats. *Inflammation.* 8:171–179.

Okubo, H., Miyanaga, O., Nagano, M., et al. 1981. Purification and immunological determination of α_2-macroglobulin in serum from injured rats. *Biochim Biophys Acta.* 668:257–267.

Oliveira, E.B., Gotschlich, E.C., and Liu, T.Y. 1980. Comparative studies on the binding properties of human and rabbit C-reactive proteins. *J Immunol.* 124:1396–1402.

Olman, M.A., Simmons, W.L., Pollman, D.J., et al. 1996. Polymerization of fibrinogen in murine bleomycin-induced lung injury. *Am J Physiol.* 271:L519–L526.

Omoto, E., and Tavassoli, M. 1990. Purification and partial characterization of ceruloplasmin receptors from rat liver endothelium. *Arch Biochem Biophys.* 282:34–38.

Onishi, T., Shimizu, T., and Kajikawa, T. 1994. Simple and efficient purification of C-reactive protein from canine serum. *J Vet Med Sci.* 56:417–419.

Osaki, S., Johnson, D.A., and Freiden, E. 1971. The mobilization of iron from the perfused mammalian liver by a serum copper enzyme, ferroxidase I. *J Biol Chem.* 246:3018–3023.

Osmand, A.P., Friedenson, B., Gewurz, H., Painter, R.H., Hofmann, T., and Shelton, E. 1977. Characterization of C-reactive protein and the complement subcomponent C1 as homologous proteins displaying cyclic pentameric symmetry pentraxins. *Immunology.* 74:739–743.

Otto, J.M., Grenet, H.E., and Fuller, G.M. 1987. The coordinated regulation of fibrinogen gene transcription by hepatocyte-stimulating factor and dexamethasone. *J Cell Biol.* 105:1067–1072.

Overbergh, L., Hilliker, C., Lorent, K., Van Leuven, F., and Van den Berghe, H. 1994. Characterization of four genes coding for isoforms of murinoglobulin, the monomeric mouse α_2 macroglobulin: Characterization of the exons coding for the bait region. *Genomics.* 22:530–539.

Overbergh, L., Lorent, K., Torrekens, S., Van Leuven, F., and Van den Berghe, H. 1995. Expression of mouse alpha-macroglobulins, lipoprotein receptor-related protein, LDL receptor, apolilpoprotein E, and lipoprotein lipase in pregnancy. *J Lipid Res.* 36:1774–1786.

Overbergh, L., Torrekens, S., Van Leuven, F., and Van den Berghe, H. 1991. Molecular characterization of the murinoglobulins. *J Biol Chem.* 266:16903–16910.

Pan, Y., Katula, K., and Failla, M.L. 1996. Expression of ceruloplasmin gene in human and rat lymphocytes. *Biochim Biophys Acta.* 1307:233–238.

Parks, J.S., and Rudel, L.L. 1983. Metabolism of the serum amyloid A proteins SAA in high-density lipoproteins and chylomicrons of nonhuman primates vervet monkey. *Am J Pathol.* 112:243–249.

Parmelee, D.C., Titani, K., Ericsson, L.H., Eriksen, N., Benditt, E.P., and Walsh, K.A. 1982. Amino acid sequence of amyloid related protein SAA complexed with serum lipoproteins apoSAA. *Biochemistry.* 21:3298–3303.

Paterson, T., and Moore, S. 1996. The expression and characterization of five recombinant murine α_1-protease inhibitor proteins. *Biochem Biophys Res Commun.* 219:64–69.

Pellegrini, A. 1994. Proteinase inhibitors in animal blood with special regard to equine pulmonary disease: α_1-proteinase inhibitor and α_2-macroglobulin. *Comp Haematol Int.* 4:121–129.

Penny, D., and Hendy, M. 1986. Estimating the reliability of evolutionary trees. *Mol Biol Evol.* 3:403–417.

Pepys, M., and Baltz, M.L. 1983. Acute phase proteins with special reference to C-reactive protein, related proteins pentraxins, and serum amyloid A protein. *Adv Immunol.* 34:141–212.

Pepys, M.B., Baltz, M.L., deBeer, F.C., et al. 1982. Biology of serum amyloid P component. *Ann N Y Acad Sci.* 389:286–297.

Pepys, M.B., and Butler, P.J.G. 1987. Serum amyloid P component is the major calcium-dependent specific DNA binding protein of the serum. *Biochem Biophys Res Commun.* 148:308–313.

Pepys, M.B., Dash, A.C., Markham, R.E., Thomas, H.C., Williams, B.C., and Petrie, A. 1978. Comparative clinical study of protein SAP amyloid P component and C-reactive protein in serum. *Clin Exp Immunol.* 32:119–124.

Percival, S.S., and Harris, E.D. 1988. Copper transport from ceruloplasmin. Charaterization of the cellular uptake mechanism. *Am J Physiol.* 258:C140–C146.

Perlmutter, D.H., May, L.T., and Sehgal, P.B. 1989. Interferon beta 2/interleukin 6 modulates synthesis of alpha 1-antitrypsin in human mononuclear phagocytes and in human hepatoma cells. *J Clin Invest.* 84:138–144.

Peters, M., Roeb, E., Pennica, D., zum Buschenfelde, K.H.M., and Rose-John, S. 1995. A new hepatocyte stimulating factor: Cardiotrophin-1 CT-1. *FEBS Lett.* 372:177–180.

Pierzchalski, P., Nakamura, T., Takehara, T., and Koj, A. 1992. Modulation of acute phase protein synthesis in cultured rat hepatocytes by human recombinant hepatocyte growth factor. *Growth Factors.* 7:161–165.

Poller, W., Willnow, T.E., Hilpert, J., and Herz, J. 1995. Differential recognition of α_1-antitrypsin-elastase and α_1-antichymotrypsin-cathepsin G complexes by the low density lipoprotein receptor-related protein. *J Biol Chem.* 270:2841–2845.

Poole, S., Gordon, A.H., Baltz, M., and Stenning, B.E. 1984. Effect of bacterial endotoxin on body temperature, plasma zinc, and plasma concentrations of the acute-phase protein serum amyloid P component in mice. *Br J Exp Pathol.* 65:431–439.

Potema, J., Korzus, E., and Travis, J. 1994. The serpin superfamily of proteinase inhibitors: Structure, function, and regulation. *J Biol Chem.* 269:15957–15960.

Potempa, L.A., Zeller, J.M., Fiedel, B.A., Kinoshita, C.M., and Gewurz, H. 1988. Stimulation of human neutrophils, monocytes, and platelets by modified C-reactive protein CRP expressing a neoantigenic specificity. *Inflammation.* 12:391–405.

Poüs, C., Giroud, J.-R., Damais, C., Raichvarg, D., and Chauvelot-Moachon, L. 1990. Effect of recombinant human interleukin-1 β and tumour necrosis factor α on liver cytochrome P-450 and serum α-1-acid glycoprotein concentrations in the rat. *Drug Metab Dispos.* 18:467–470.

Prowse, K.R., and Baumann, H. 1989. Interleukin-1 and interleukin-6 stimulates acute-phase protein production in primary mouse hepatocytes. *J Leukoc Biol.* 45:55–61.

Pruden, D.J., Connolly, K.M., and Stecher, V.J. 1988. Single-step purification of rat C-reactive protein and generation of monospecific C-reactive protein antibody. *J Chromatogr.* 437:399–410.

Ramadori, G., Sipe, J.D., and Colten, H.R. 1985a. Expression and regulation of the murine serum amyloid A SAA gene in extrahepatic sites. *J Immunol.* 135:3645–3647.

Ramadori, G., Sipe, J.D., Dinarello, C.A., Mizel, S.B., and Colten, H.R. 1985b. Pretranslational modulation of acute phase hepatic protein synthesis by murine recombinant interleukin 1 IL-1 and purified human IL-1. *J Exp Med.* 162:930–942.

Ramadori, G., Van Damme, J., Rieder, H., and zum Buschenfelde, K.H.M. 1988. Interleukin 6, the third mediator of acute-phase reaction, modulates hepatic protein synthesis in human and mouse. Comparison with interleukin 1 β and tumor necrosis factor-α. *Eur J Immunol.* 18:1259–1264.

Ramji, D.P., Vitelli, A., Tranche, F., Cortese, R., and Ciliberto, G. 1993. The two C/EBP isoforms, IL-6 DBP/NF-IL6 and C/EBP delta/NF-IL6 beta, are induced by IL-6 to promote acute phase gene transcription via different mechanisms. *Nucleic Acid Res.* 21:289–294.

Randell, E., Mookerjea, S., and Nagpurkar, A. 1990. Binding or rat serum phosphorylcholine binding protein to platelets. *Biochim Biophys Acta.* 1034:281–284.

Rassouli, M., Sambasivam, H., Azadi, P., et al. 1992. Derivation of the amino acid sequence of rat C-reactive protein from cDNA cloning with additional studies on the nature of its dimeric component. *J Biol Chem.* 267:2947–2954.

Rastogi, S.C., and Clausen, J. 1985. Kinetics of inhibition of mitogen-induced proliferation of human lymphocytes by α_2 macroglobulin in serum-free medium. *Immunobiology.* 169:37–44.

Ratajczak, T., Williams, P.M., DiLorenzo, D., and Ringold, G.M. 1992. Multiple elements within the glucocorticoid regulatory unit of the rat alpha-1-acid glycoprotein gene are recognition site for C/EPB. *J Biol Chem.* 267:1111–1119.

Ravin, H.A. 1961. An improved colorimetric enzymatic assay of ceruloplasmin. *J Lab Clin Med.* 58:161–168.

Ray, B.K., Gao, X., and Ray, A. 1994. Expression and structural analysis of a novel highly inducible gene encoding α_1-antitrypsin in rabbit. *J Biol Chem.* 269:22080–22086.

Ray, A., Gao, X., and Ray, B.K. 1996. Role of a distal enhancer containing a functional NF-kB-binding site in lipopolysaccharide-induced expression of a novel αl-antitrypsin gene. *J Biol Chem.* 270:29201–29208.

Ray, B.K., and Ray, A. 1991a. Complementary DNA cloning and nucleotide sequence of rabbit serum amyloid A protein. *Biochem Biophys Res Commun.* 178:68–72.

Ray, B.K., and Ray, A. 1991b. Rabbit serum amyloid A gene: Cloning, characterization, and sequence analysis. *Biochem Biophys Res Commun.* 180:1258–1264.

Ray, B.K., and Ray, A. 1993. Functional NF-κB element in rabbit serum amyloid A gene and its role in acute phase induction. *Biochem Biophys Res Commun.* 193:1159–1167.

Ray, A., and Ray, B.K. 1996. A novel CIS-acting element is essential for cytokine-mediated transcriptional induction of the serum amyloid A gene in nonhepatic cells. *Mol Cell Biol.* 16:1584–1594.

Reinhoff, H.R., and Groudine, M. 1988. Regulation of amyloid A gene expression in cultured cells. *Mol Cell Biol.* 8:3710–3716.

Reinke, R., and Feigelson, P. 1985. Rat α_1-acid glycoprotein. Gene sequence and regulation by glucocorticoids in transfected L-cells. *J Biol Chem.* 260:4397–4403.

Rheaume, D., Goodwin, R.L., Latimer, J.J., Baumann, H., and Berger, F.G. 1994. Evolution of murine α_1-proteinase inhibitors: Gene amplification and reactive center divergence. *J Mol Evol.* 38:121–131.

Rheaume, C., Latimer, J.J., Baumann, H., and Berger, F.G. 1988. Tissue- and species-specific regulation of murine α_1-antitrypsin gene transcription. *J Biol Chem.* 269:15118–15121.

Ricca, G.A., Hamilton, R.W., McLean, J.W., Conn, A., Kalinyak, J.E., and Taylor, J.M. 1981. Rat α_1-acid glycoprotein mRNA. Cloning of double-stranded cDNA and kinetics of induction of mRNA levels following acute inflammation. *J Biol Chem.* 256:10362–10368.

Richards, C.D., Brown, T.J., Shoyab, M., Baumann, H., and Gauldie, J. 1992. Recombinant oncostatin m stimulates the production of acute phase proteins in hepG2 cells and rat primary hepatocytes in vitro. *J Immunol.* 148:1731–1736.

Riipi, L., and Carlson, E. 1990. Tumor necrosis factor (TNF) is induced in mice by *Candida albicans:* Role of TNF in fibrinogen increase. *Infect Immun.* 58:2750–2754.

Rikihisa, Y., Yamamoto, S., Kwak, I., et al. 1994. C-reactive protein and α1-acid glycoprotein levels in dogs infected with Ehrlichia canis. *J Clin Microbiol.* 32:912–917.

Robey, F.A., Jones, K.D., Tanaka, T., and Liu, T-Y. 1984. Binding of C-reactive protein to chromatin and nucleosome core particles: A possible physiological role of C-reactive protein. *J Biol Chem.* 259:7311–7316.

Rofe, A.M., Philcox, J.C., and Coyle, P. 1996. Trace metal, acute phase and metabolic response to endotoxin in metallothionein-null mice. *Biochem J.* 314:793–797.

Rokita, H., Shirahama, T., Cohen, A.S., and Sipe, J.D. 1989. Serum amyloid A gene expression and AA amyloid formation in A/J and SJL/J mice. *Br J Exp Pathol.* 70:327–335.

Ronne, H., Anundi, H., Rask, L., and Peterson, P.A. 1979. Nerve growth factor binds to serum alpha-2-macroglobulin. *Biochem Biophys Res Commun.* 87:330–336.

Rordorf-Adam, C., Serban, D., Pataki, A., and Gruninger, M. 1985. Serum amyloid P component and autoimmune parameters in the assessment of arthritis activity in MRL/lpr/lpr mice. *Clin Exp Immunol.* 61:509–516.

Roux, K.H., Kilpatrick, J.M., Volanakis, J.E., and Kearney, J.F. 1983. Localization of the phosphocholine-binding sites on C-reactive protein by immunoelectron microscopy. *J Immunol.* 131:2411–2415.

Rowe, I.F., Baltz, M.L., Soutar, A.K., and Pepys, M.B. 1984c. In vivo turnover studies of C-reactive protein and lipoproteins in the rabbit. *Clin Exp Immunol.* 58:245–252.

Rowe, I.F., Soutar, A.K., Trayner, I.M., et al. 1984a. Rabbit and rat C-reactive proteins bind apolipoprotein B-containing lipoproteins. *J Exp Med.* 159:604–616.

Rowe, I.F., Soutar, A.K., Trayner, I.M., Thompson, G.R., and Pepys, M.B. 1984b. Circulating human C-reactive protein binds very low density lipoproteins. *Clin Exp Immunol.* 58:237–244.

Roy, S.N., Mukhopadhyay, G., and Redman, C.M. 1990. Regulation of fibrinogen assembly. Transfection of hep G2 cells with B beta cDNA specifically enhances synthesis of the three component chains of fibrinogen. *J Biol Chem.* 265:6389–6393.

Rubio, N., Sharp, P.M., Rits, M., Zahedi, K., and Whitehead, A.S. 1993. Structure, expression, and evolution of guinea pig serum amyloid P component and C-reactive protein. *J Biochem.* 113:277–284.

Rudnick, C.M., and Dowton, S.B. 1993. Serum amyloid P female protein. Of the Syrian hamster. Gene structure and expression. *J Biol Chem.* 268:21760–21769.

Ryan, T.P., Grover, T.A., and Aust, S.D. 1992. Rat ceruloplasmin: Resistance to proteolysis and kinetic comparison with human ceruloplasmin. *Arch Biochem Biophys.* 293:1–8.

Ryden, L. 1972. Comparison of polypeptide-chain structure of four mammalian ceruloplasmins by gel filtration in guanidine hydrochloride solution. *Eur J Biochem.* 28:46–50.

Ryffel, B., Car, B.D., Woerly, G., et al. 1994. Long-term interleukin-6 administration stimulates sustained thrombopoiesis and acute-phase protein synthesis in a small primate—The marmoset. *Blood.* 83:2093–2102.

Rygg, M., Alstad, H.K., and Marhaug, G. 1996. Developmental regulation of expression of rabbit C-reactive protein and serum amyloid A genes. *Biochim Biophys Acta.* 1307:89–96.

Rygg, M., Marhaug, G., Husby, G., and Dowton, S.B. 1991. Rabbit serum amyloid A: Expression and primary structure deduced from cDNA sequences. *Scand J Immunol.* 34:727–734.

Saenko, E.L., Skorobogat'ko, O.V., Tarasenko, P., et al. 1994. Modulatory effects of ceruloplasmin on lymphocytes, neutrophils, and monocytes of patients with altered immune states. *Immunol Invest.* 23:99–114.

Saile, R., Hocke, G., Tartar, A., Fruchart, J.-C., and Steinmetz, A. 1989. Antipeptide antibodies discriminate between different SAA protein in human plasma. *Biochim Biophys Acta.* 992:407–408.

Saito, A., and Sinohara, H. 1985a. Rat plasma murinoglobulin: Isolation, characterization, and comparison with rat alpha-1 and α_2 macroglobulins. *J Biochem.* 98:501–516.

Saito, A., and Sinohara, H. 1985b. Murinoglobulin, a novel protease inhibitor from murine plasma. Isolation, characterization, and comparison with murine alpha-macroglobulin and human α_2 macroglobulin. *J Biol Chem.* 260:775–781.

Saito, A., and Sinohara, H. 1988. Differential interactions of rabbit plasma alpha-1-antiproteinases S and F with porcine trypsin. *J Biochem.* 103:247–253.

Saito, A., and Sinohara, H. 1991. Cloning and sequencing of cDNA coding for rabbit α-1-antiproteinase F: Amino acid sequence comparison of α-1-antiproteinases of six mammals. *J Biochem.* 109:158–162.

Saito, A., and Sinohara, H. 1993. Rabbit plasma α_1-antiproteinase S-1: Cloning, sequiencing, expression, and proteinase inhibitory properties of recombinant protein. *J Biochem.* 113:456–461.

Saito, A., and Sinohara, H. 1995. Rabbit α-1-antiproteinase E: A novel recombinant serpin which does not inhibit proteinases. *Biochem J.* 307:369–375.

Salonen, E.M., Vartio, T., Hedman, K., and Vaheri, A. 1984. Binding of fibronectin by the acute phase reactant C-reactive protein. *J Biol Chem.* 259:1496–1501.

Samokyszyn, V.M., Miller, D.M., Reif, D.W., and Aust, S.D. 1989. Inhibition of superoxide and ferritin-dependent lipid peroxidation by ceruloplasmin. *J Biol Chem.* 264:21–26.

Sand, O., Folkersen, J., Westergaard, J.G., and Sottrup-Jensen, L. 1985. Characterization of human pregnancy zone protein. Comparison with human α_2 macroglobulin. *J Biol Chem.* 260:15723–15735.

Sarcione, E.J., and Bohne, M. 1969. Synthesis of alpha$_2$ acute phase globulin by fetal and neonatal rat liver in vitro. *Proc Soc Exp Biol Med.* 131:1454–1456.

Sarlo, K.T., and Mortensen, R.F. 1985. Enhanced interleukin IL-1 production mediated by mouse serum amyloid P component. *Cell Immunol.* 93:398–405.

Sarlo, K.T., and Mortensen, R.F. 1987. Regulation of the antibody response by the acute phase reactant: Mouse serum amyloid P-component SAP. *Cell Immunol.* 106:273–286.

Sato, M., Sasaki, M., and Hojo, H. 1994. Differential induction of metallothionein synthesis by interleukin-6 and tumor necrosis factor-α in rat tissues. *Int J Immunopharmacol.* 16:187–195.

Saunero-Nava, L., Coe, J.E., Mold, C., and Du Clos, T.W. 1992. Hamster female protein binding to chromatin histones and DNA. *Mol Immunol.* 29:837–845.

Schaeufele, J.T., and Koo, P.H. 1982. Structural comparison of rat α_1 and α_2 macroglobulin. *Biochem Biophys Res Commun.* 108:1–7.

Schmid, K. 1975. Alpha-1-acid glycoprotein. In *The Plasma Proteins.* Ed. F.W. Putnam, Vol. 1, pp. 183–228. New York, NY: Academic Press.

Schmid, K., Burgi, W., Collins, J.H., and Nanno, S. 1974. The disulfide bonds of alpha-1-acid glycoprotein. *Biochemistry.* 13:2694–2697.

Schmid, K., Kaufmann, H., Isemura, S., et al. 1973. Structure of α_1-acid glycoprotein. The complete amino acid sequence multiple amino acid subsitutions and homology with immunoglobulins. *Biochemistry.* 12:2711–2724.

Schooltink, H., Stoyan, T., Roeb, E., Heinrich, P.C., and Rose-John, S. 1992. Ciliary neurotrophic factor induces acute-phase protein expression in hepatocytes. *FEBS Lett.* 314:280–284.

Schreiber, G., Aldred, A.R., Thomas, T., et al. 1986. Levels of messenger ribonucleic acids for plasma protiens in rat liver during acute experimental inflammation. *Inflammation.* 10:59–66.

Schwalbe, R.A., Coe, J.E., and Nelsestuen, G.L. 1995. Association of rat C-reactive protein and other pentraxins with rat lipoproteins containing apolipoproteins E and A1. *Biochemistry.* 34:10432–10439.

Schwalbe, R.A., Dahlback, B., Coe, J.E., and Nelsestuen, G.L. 1992. Pentraxin family of proteins interact specifically with phosphorylcholine and/or phosphorylethanolamine. *Biochemistry.* 31:4907–4915.

Schwalbe, R.A., Dahlback, B., and Nelsestuen, G.L. 1990. Independent association of serum amyloid P component, protein S, and complement C4b with complement C4b binding protein and subsequent association of the complex with membranes. *J Biochem.* 265:21749–21757.

Schwalbe, R.A., Dahlback, B., and Nelsestuen, G.L. 1991. Heparin influence on the complex of amyloid P component and complement C4b binding protein. *J Biochem.* 266:12896–12901.

Schwarzenberg, S.J., Sharp, H.L., Berry, S.A., Manthei, R.D., and Seelig, S. 1987. Hormonal regulation of serum alpha$_1$-antitrypsin and hepatic alpha$_1$-antitrypsin mRNA in rats. *Biochem Biophys Res Commun.* 147:936–941.

Selinger, M.J., McAdam, K.P.W.J., Kaplan, M.M., Sipe, J.D., Vogel, S.N., and Rosenstreich, D.L. 1980. Monokine-induced synthesis of serum amyloid A protein by hepatocytes. *Nature.* 285:498–500.

Sellar, G.C., DeBeer, M.C., Lelias, J.M., et al. 1991. Dog serum amyloid A protein. *J Biol Chem.* 266:3505–3510.

Senior, R.M., Skogen, W.F., Griffin, G.L., and Wilner, G.D. 1986. Effects of fibrinogen derivatives upon the inflammatory response: Studies with human fibrinopeptide B. *J Clin Invest.* 77:1014–1019.

Serban, D., and Rordorf-Adam, C. 1986. Quantitation of serum amyloid P component by an enzyme-linked immunoassay. *J Immunol Methods.* 90:159–164.

Serbource-Goguel Seta, N., Durand, G., Corbie, M., Agneray, J., and Feger, J. 1986. Alterations in relative α_1-acid glycoprotein in liver disease. *J Hepatol.* 2:245–252.

Sevelius, E., Andersson, M., and Jönsson, L. 1994. Hepatic accumulation of alpha-1-antitrypsin in chronic liver disease in the dog. *J Comp Pathol.* 111:401–412.

Shephard, E.G., Kelly, S.L., Anderson, R., and Fridkin, M. 1992. Characterization of neutrophil-mediated degradation of human C-reactive protein and identification of the protease. *Clin Exp Immunol.* 87:509–513.

Shephard, E.G., Smith, P.J., Coetzee, S., Strachan, A.F., and de Beer, F.C. 1991. Pentraxin binding to isolated rat liver nuclei. *Biochem J.* 279:257–262.

Shephard, E.G., Van Helden, P.D., Strauss, M., Bohm, L., and De Beer, F.C. 1986. Functional effects of CRP binding to nuclei. *Immunology.* 58:489–494.

Shirahama, T., Skinner, M., and Cohen, A.S. 1984. Heterogenous participation of the hepatocyte population in amyloid protein AA synthesis. *Cell Biol Int.* 8:849–856.

Silverman, S.L., Cathcart, E.S., Skinner, M., and Cohen, A.S. 1982. The degradation of serum amyloid A protein by activated polymorphonuclear leukocytes: Participation of granulocytic elastase. *Immunology.* 46:737–744.

Silvestrini, B., Guglielmotti, A., Saso, L., et al. 1990. Development of an enzyme-linked immunosorbent assay with a monoclonal antibody prepared against α_1-antitrypsin for diagnostic screening of inflammatory disorders. *Clin Chem.* 36:277–282.

Sipe, J.D., Gonnerman, W.A., Loose, L.D., Knapschaefer, G., Xie, W.J., and Franzblau, C. 1989. Direct binding enzyme-linked immunosorbent assay ELISA for serum amyloid A SAA. *J Immunol Methods.* 125:125–135.

Sipe, J.D., Ignaczak, J.F., Pollock, S.P., and Glenner, G.G. 1976. Amyloid fibril protein AA: Purification and properties of the antigenically related serum component as determined by solid-phase radioimmunoassay. *J Immunol.* 116:1151–1156.

Sipe, J.D., Vogel, S.N., Sztein, M.B., Skinner, M., and Cohen, A.S. 1982. The role of interleukin 1 in acute phase serum amyloid A SAA and serum amyloid P SAP biosynthesis. *Ann N Y Acad Sci.* 389:137–149.

Siripont, J., Tebo, J.M., and Mortensen, R.F. 1988. Receptor-mediated binding of the acute-phase reactant mouse serum amyloid P-component SAP to macrophages. *Cell Immunol.* 117:239–252.

Skinner, M., and Cohen, A.S. 1988. Amyloid P component. *Methods Enzymol.* 163:523–537.

Skinner, M.K., and Griswold, M.D. 1983. Sertoli cells synthesize and secrete a ceruloplasmin-like protein. *Biol Reprod.* 28:1225–1229.

Smith, K., Pollacchi, A., Field, M., and Watson, J. 2002. The heterogeneity of the glycosylation of alpha-1-acid glycoprotein between the sera and synovial fluid in rheumatoid arthritis. *Biomed Chromatogr.* 16:261–266.

Snel, F.W., Niewold, T.A., Baltz, M.L., et al. 1989. Experimental amyloidosis in the hamster: Correlation between hamster female protein levels and amyloid deposition. *Clin Exp Immunol.* 76:296–300.

Snider, G.L., Cicolella, D.E., Morris, S.M., Stone, P.J., and Lucey, E. 1991. Putative role of neutrophil elastase in the pathogenesis of emphysema. *Ann N Y Acad Sci.* 624:45–59.

Solter, P.F., Hoffman, W.E., Hungerford, L.L., Siegel, J.P., St. Denis, S.H., and Dorner, J.L. 1991. Haptoglobin and ceruloplasmin as determinants of inflammation in dogs. *Am J Vet Res.* 52:1738–1742.

Song, C.S., Merkatz, I.R., Rifkind, A.B., Gillette, P.N., and Kappas, A. 1970. The influence of pregnancy and oral contraceptive steroids on the concentration of plasma proteins. *Am J Obstet Gynecol.* 108:227–231.

Sottrup-Jensen, L. 1989. Alpha macroglobulins: Structure, shape, and mechanism of proteinase complex formation. *J Biol Chem.* 264:11539–11542.

Sottrup-Jensen, L., and Birkedal-Hansen, H. 1989. Human fibroblast collagenase-α-macroglobulin interactions. *J Biol Chem.* 264:393–401.

Sottrup-Jensen, L., Sand, O., Kristensen, L., and Fey, G.H. 1989. The alpha-macroglobulin bait region: Sequence diversity and localization of cleavage sites for proteinases in five mammalian alpha-macroglobulins. *J Biol Chem.* 264:15781–15789.

Sottrup-Jensen, L., Stepanik, T.M., Kristensen, T., et al. 1984. Primary structure of human α_2-macroglobulin. *J Biol Chem.* 259:8318–8327.

Sottrup-Jensen, L., Stepanik, T.M., Kristensen, T., et al. 1985. Common evolutionary origin of α_2 macroglobulin and complement proteins C3 and C4. *Proc Natl Acad Sci USA.* 82:9–13.

Srai, S.K.S., Burroughs, A.K., Wood, B., and Epstein, O. 1986. The ontogeny of liver copper metabolism in the guinea pig. Clues to the etiology of Wilson disease. *Hepatology.* 6:427–432.

Starkey, P.M., and Barrett, A.J. 1982. Evolution of α_2 macroglobulin. The demonstarion in a variety of vertebrate species of a protein resembling human α_2 macroglobulin. *Biochem J.* 205:91–95.

Stearman, R.S., Lowell, C.A., Peltzman, G., and Morrow, J.F. 1986. The sequence and structure of a new amyloid gene. *Nucleic Acid Res.* 14:797–809.

Steel, D.M., Roger, J., De Beer, M.C., De Beer, F.C., and Whitehead, A.S. 1993. Biosynthesis of acute-phase serum amyloid A protein (A-SAA) in vitro: The roles of mRNA accumulation, poly(A), tail shortening, and translational efficiency. *Biochem J.* 291:701–707.

Steinmetz, A., Hocke, G., Saile, R., Puchois, P., and Fruchart, J.C. 1989. Influence of serum amyloid A on cholesterol esterification in human plasma. *Biochem Biophys Acta.* 1006:173–178.

Stern, R.V., and Frieden, E. 1990. Detection of rat ceruloplasmin receptors using fluorescence microscopy and microdensitometry. *Anal Biochem.* 190:48–56.

Stern, R.V., and Frieden, E. 1993. Partial purification of the rat erythrocyte ceruloplasmin receptor monitored by an electrophoresis mobility shift assay. *Anal Biochem.* 212:221–228.

Sternlieb, I., Morell, A.G., Tucker, W.E., Greene, M.W., and Scheinberg, I.H. 1961. The incorporation of copper into ceruloplasmin in vivo: Studies with copper^{64} and copper^{67}. *J Clin Invest.* 40:1960–1964.

Stevens, M.D., DiSilvestro, R.A., and Harris, E.D. 1984. Specific receptors for ceruloplasmin in membrane fragments of aortic and heart tissues. *Biochemistry.* 23:261–266.

Strachan, A.F., De Beer, F.C., van der Westhuyzen, D.R., and Coetzee, G.A. 1988. Identification of three isoform patterns of human serum amyloid A protein. *Biochem J.* 250:203–207.

Strickland, D.K., Ashcom, J.D., Williams, S., Burgess, W.H., Migliorini, M., and Argraves, W.S. 1990. Sequence identity between the α_2-macroglobulin receptor and low density lipoprotein receptor-related protein suggest that this molecule is a multifunctional receptor. *J Biol Chem.* 265:17401–17404.

Stubbs, L., Rinchik, F.M., Goldberg, R., Rudy, B., Handel, M.A., and Johnson, D. 1994. Clustering of six human Hp15 homologs within a 500 kb interval of proximal mouse chromosome 7. *Genomics.* 24:324–332.

Sui, S.F., Liu, Z., Li, W., et al. 1996. Two-dimensional crystallization of rabbit C-reactive protein on lipid monolayers. *FEBS Lett.* 388:103–111.

Suzuki, Y., and Sinohara, H. 1986. Isolation and characterization of α-macroglobulin from guinea pig plasma. *J Biochem.* 99:1655–1665.

Suzuki, Y., Yoshida, K., Ichimiya, T., Yamamoto, T., and Sinohara, H. 1990. Trypsin inhibitors in guinea pig plasma: Isolation and characterization of contrapsin and two isoforms of α-1 antiproteinase and acute phase response of four major trypsin inhibitors. *J Biochem.* 107:173–179.

Swanson, S.J., Lin, B-F., Mullenix, M.C., and Mortensen, R.F. 1991a. A synthetic peptide corresponding to the phosphorylcholine PC-binding region of human C-reactive protein possesses the TEPC-15 myeloma PC-idiotype. *J Immunol.* 146:1596–1601.

Swanson, S.M., McPeek, M.M., and Mortensen, R.F. 1989. Characteristics of the binding of human C-reactive protein CRP to laminin. *J Cell Biochem.* 40:121–132.

Swanson, S.J., and Mortensen, R.F. 1990. Binding and immunological properties of a synthetic peptide corresponding to the phosphorylcholine-binding region of C-reactive protein. *Mol Immunol.* 27:679–687.

Swanson, S.J., Mullenix, M.C., and Mortensen, R.F. 1991b. Monoclonal antibodies to the calcium-binding region peptide of human C-reactive protein alter its conformation. *J Immunol.* 147:2248–2252.

Syversen, P.V., Juul, J., Rygg, M., Sletten, K., Husby, G., and Marhaug, G. 1993. The primary structure of rabbit serum amyloid A protein isolated from acute phase serum. *Scand J Immunol.* 37:447–451.

Szalai, A.J., Briles, D.E., and Volanakis, J.E. 1995. Human C-reactive protein is protective against fatal *Streptococcus pneumoniae* infection in transgenic mice. *J Immunol.* 155:2557–2563.

Tagata, K., Yokoyama, S., Ginbo, T., et al. 1996. Quantitative capillary reversed passive latex agglutination test for C-reactive protein CRP in the dog. *Vet Res Commun.* 20:21–30.

Takahashi, N., Ortel, T.L., and Putman, F.W. 1984. Single-chain structure of human ceruloplasmin: The complete amino acid sequence of the whole molecule. *Proc Natl Acad Sci USA.* 81:390–394.

Takemura, S., Rossing, T.H., and Perlmutter, D.H.A. 1986. A lymphokine regulates expression of alpha-1-proteinase inhibitor in human monocytes and macrophages. *J Clin Invest.* 77:1207–1213.

Tamamizu, S., Miyake, Y., Ito, T., and Sinohara, H. 1989. Changes in trypsin binding properties and conformation of rabbit α_2-macroglobulin on reaction with methylamine. *J Biochem.* 105:898–904.

Tanaka, T., and Robey, F.A. 1983. A new sensitive assay for the calcium-dependent binding of C-reactive protein to phosphorylcholine. *J Immunol Methods.* 65:333–341.

Tang, L., Ugarova, T.P., Plow, E.P., and Eaton, J.W. 1996. Molecular determinants of acute inflammatory responses to biomaterials. *J Clin Invest.* 97:1329–1334.

Tape, C., and Kisilevsky, R. 1990. Apolipoprotein A-1 and apolipoprotein SAA half-lives during acute inflammation and amyloidogenesis. *Biochem Biophys Acta.* 1043:295–300.

Tatum, F., Alam, J., Smith, A., and Morgan, W.T. 1990. Molecular cloning, nucleotide sequence heterozygosity, and regulation of rabbit serum amyloid A cDNA. *Nucleic Acid Res.* 18:7447.

Tavassoli, M. 1985. Liver endothelium binds, transports, and desialates ceruloplasmin, which is then recognized by galactosyl receptors of hepatocytes. *Trans Assoc Am Physicians.* 98:370–377.

Tavassoli, M., Kishimoto, T., and Kataoka, M. 1986. Liver endothelium mediates the hepatocyte's uptake of ceruloplasmin. *J Cell Biol.* 102:1298–1303.

Taylor, J.A., Bruton, C.J., Anderson, J.K., et al. 1984. Amino acid sequence homology between rat and human C-reactive protein. *Biochem J.* 221:903–906.

Taylor, B.A., and Rowe, L. 1984. Genes for serum amyloid A proteins map to chromosome 7 in the mouse. *Mol Gen Genet.* 195:491–499.

Tebo, J.M., and Mortensen, R.F. 1991. Internalization and degradation of receptor bound C-reactive protein by U-937 cells: Induction of H_2O_2 production and tumoricidal activity. *Biochim Biophys Acta.* 1095:210–216.

Tennet, G.A., Baltz, M.L., Osborn, G.D., et al. 1993. Studies of the structure and binding properties of hamster female protein. *Immunology.* 80:645–651.

Terada, K., Kawarada, Y., Miura, N., Yasui, O., Koyama, K., and Sugiyama, T. 1995. Copper incorporation into ceruloplasmin in rat livers. *Biochim Biophys Acta.* 1270:58–62.

Thomas, J. 2000. Overview of plasma proteins. In *Schalms, Veterinary Haematology*. Eds. B. Feldman, J. Zinkl, and N. Jain, 5th edition, pp. 891–898. Philadelphia, PA: Lippincott Williams and Wilkins.

Thomas, T., Macpherson, A., and Rogers, P. 1995. Ceruloplasmin gene expression in the rat uterus. *Biochem Biophys Acta.* 1261:77–82.

Thomas, T., and Schreiber, G. 1988. The expression of genes coding for positive acute-phase proteins in the reproductive tract of the female rat. *FEBS Lett.* 243:381–384.

Thomas, T., and Schreiber, G. 1989. The expression of genes coding for positive acute-phase proteins in the reproductive tract of the female rat: High levels of ceruloplasmin mRNA in the uterus. *FEBS Lett.* 243:381–384.

Thomas, T., Schreiber, G., and Jaworowski, A. 1989. Developmental patterns of gene expression of secreted proteins in brain and choroid plexus. *Dev Biol.* 134:38–47.

Tillett, W.S., and Francis, T. 1930. Serological reactions in pneumonia with a non-protein somatic fraction of pneu-mococcus. *J Exp Med.* 52:561–571.

Titus, R.G., Sherry, B., and Cerami, A. 1991. The involvement of TNF, IL-1, and IL-6 in the immune response to protozoan parasites. *Immunol Today.* 12:A13–16.

Travis, J., and Salveson, G.S. 1983. Human plasma proteinase inhibitors. *Ann Rev Biochem.* 52:655–709.

Tseng, J., and Mortensen, R.F. 1988. Binding of human C-reactive protein CRP to plasma fibronectin occurs via the phosphorylcholine-binding site. *Mol Immunol.* 25:679–686.

Tseng, J., and Mortensen, R.F. 1989. The effect of human C-reactive protein on the cell-attachment activity of fibronectin and laminin. *Exp Cell Res.* 180:303–313.

Uhlar, C., and Whitehead, A. 1999. Serum amyloid A, the major vertebrates acute phase reactant. *Eur J Biochem.* 265(2):501–542.

Umans, L., Serneels, L., Stas, L., et al. 1994. Cloning of the mouse gene coding for alpha-2-macroglobulin and targeting of the gene in embryonic stem cells. *Genomics.* 22:519–529.

Umeda, M., Ishimori, Y., Yoshikawa, K., Takada, M., and Yasuda, T. 1986. Liposome immune lysis assay LILA. *J Immunol Methods.* 95:15–21.

Umeda, M., and Yasuda, T. 1994. A novel liposome immune lysis assay LILA for determination of CRP antigen using two monoclonal antibodies recognizing different antigenic determinants. *Acta Med Okayama.* 48:299–304.

Ungar-Waron, H., Gluckman, A., Spira, E., Waron, M., and Trainin, Z. 1978. Ceruloplasmin as a marker of neoplastic activity in rabbits bearing the VX-2 carcinoma. *Cancer Res.* 38:1296–1299.

Urieli-Shoval, S., Meek, R.L., Hanson, R.H., Eriksen, N., and Benditt, E.P. 1994. Human serum amyloid A genes are expressed in monocyte/macrophage cell lines. *Am J Pathol.* 145:650–660.

Van den Hamer, C.J.A., Morell, A.G., Scheinberg, I.H., Hickman, J., and Ashwell, G. 1970. Physical and chemical studies on ceruloplasmin. IX. The role of galactosyl residues in the clearance of ceruloplasmin from the circulation. *J Biol Chem.* 245:4397–4402.

Van Leuven, F., Stas, L., Raymakers, L., et al. 1993. Molecular cloning and sequencing of the murine alpha-2-macroglobulin receptor cDNA. *Biochim Biophys Acta.* 1173:71–74.

Van Leuven, F., Torrekens, S., Overbergh, L., Lorent, K., De Strooper, B., and Van den Berghe, H. 1992. The primary sequence and the subunit structure of mouse α-2-macroglobulin, deduced from protein sequencing of the isolated subunits and from molecular cloning of the cDNA. *Eur J Biochem.* 210:319–327.

Vannice, J.L., Taylor, J.M., and Ringold, G.M. 1984. Glucocorticoid-mediated induction of α_1-acid glycoprotein: Evidence for hormone-regulated RNA processing. *Proc Natl Acad Sci USA.* 81:4241–4245.

VanRuijven, I.A.M., and Nieuwenhuizen, W. 1978. Purification of rat fibrinogen and its constitutent chains. *Biochem J.* 169:653–658.

Venembre, P., Boutten, A., Seta, N., et al. 1994. Secretion of α_1-antitrypsin by alveolar epithelial cells. *FEBS Lett.* 346:171–174.

Venembre, P.C., Cong, H.N., Biou, D.R., and Durand, G.M. 1993. Changes in the glycoforms of rat alpha-1-acid glycoprotein during experimental polyarthritis. *Clin Chim Acta.* 221:59–71.

Verbanac, K.M., and Heath, E.C. 1983. Biosynthesis and processing of rat α1-antitrypsin. *Arch Biochem Biophys.* 223:149–457.

Versavel, C., Feve, A., Esnard, F., Lebreton de Vonne, T., and Mouray, H. 1983. The evolution of α-1 and α-2 macroglobulin in levels in the serum of rabbit fetus and newborn. *Comp Biochem Physiol B.* 75:701–702.

Vigo, C. 1985. Effect of C-reactive protein on platelet-activating factor-induced platelet aggregation and membrane stabilization. *J Biol Chem.* 260:3418–3422.

Vigushin, D.M., Pepys, M.B., and Hawkins, P.N. 1993. Metabolic and scintigraphic studies of radioiodinated human C-reactive protein in health and disease. *J Clin Invest.* 91:1351–1357.

Vogels, M.T.E., Cantoni, L., Carelli, M., Sironi, M., Ghezzi, P., and Van Der Meer, J.W.M. 1993. Role of acute-phase proteins in interleukin-1-induced nonspecific resistance to bacterial infections in mice. *Antimicrob Agents Chemother.* 37:2527–2533.

Wadsworth, C., Fasth, A., and Wadsworth, E. 1985. A critical analysis of commercially available latex particle reagents for C-reactive protein CRP slide agglutination tests. *J Immunol Methods.* 83:29–36.

Waites, G.T., Bell, A.M., and Bell, S.C. 1983. Acute phase serum proteins in syngeneic and allogeneic mouse pregnancy. *Clin Exp Immunol.* 53:225–232.

Warwas, M., and Osada, J. 1985. Changes of the level of proteinase inhibitors in rat plasma during turpentine-induced inflammation. *Experientia.* 41:633–634.

Watanabe, T. 1995. Analysis of a polyacrylamide gel electrophoretogram of beagle serum protein by laser densitometer. *Lab Anim Sci.* 45:295–298.

Watterson C. 2009. Proteins. In *Animal Clinical Chemistry: A Practical Handbook for Toxicologists and Biomedical Researchers—A Toxicology Primer for Veterinary Clinical Chemists*, 2nd edition. Ed. G. Evans, pp. 159–182. Boca Raton, FL: Taylor & Francis.

Watterson, C., Lanevschi, A., Horner, J., and Louden, C. 2008. A comparative analysis of acute phase proteins as inflammatory biomarkers in preclinical toxicology studies: Implications for preclinical to clinical translation. *J Soc Toxicol Pathol.* 37:28–33.

Webb, C.F., Tucker, P.W., and Dowton, S.B. 1989. Expression and sequence of serum amyloid A in the Syrian hamster. *Biochemistry.* 28:4785–4790.

Webster, R.O., Robinson-Hill, R., and Williams, D.A. 1994. Inhibition of neutrophil adherence by C-reactive protein: Association with decreased β_2-integrin expression. *Am J Respir Crit Care Med.* 149:A232–235.

Wegenka, U.M., Buschmann, J., Lutticken, C., Heinrich, P.C., and Horn, F. 1993. Acute-phase response factor, a nuclear factor binding to acute-phase response elements, is rapidly activated by interleukin-6 at the posttranslational level. *Mol Cell Biol.* 13:276–288.

Weimer, H.E., and Benjamin, D.C. 1965. Immunochemical detection of an acute-phase protein in rat serum. *Am J Physiol.* 209:736–744.

Weinstein, J.A., and Taylor, J.M. 1987. Interleukin-1 and the acute-phase response: Induction of mouse liver serum amyloid A mRNA by murine recombinant interleukin-1. *J Trauma.* 27:1227–1232.

Weisman, S., Goldsmith, B., Winzler, R., and Lepper, M.H. 1961. Turnover of plasma orosomucoid in man. *J Lab Clin Med.* 57:7.

Wenger, R.H., Rolfs, A., Marti, H.H., Bauer, C., and Gassmann, M. 1995. Hypoxia, a novel inducer of acute phase gene expression in a human hepatoma cell line. *J Biol Chem.* 27:27865–27870.

Whitehead, A.S. 1989. Organization, structure and expression of pentraxin genes. In *Acute Phase Proteins in the Acute Phase Response.* Ed. M.B. Pepys, pp. 47–57. London: Springer-Verlag.

Whitehead, A.S., and Rits, M. 1990. Characterization of the gene encoding mouse serum amyloid P component. *Biochem J.* 263:25–31.

Whitehead, A.S., Rits, M., and Michaelson, J. 1988. Molecular genetics of mouse serum amyloid P component SAP: Cloning and gene mapping. *Immunogenetics.* 28:388–390.

Whitehead, A.S., Zahedi, K., Rits, M., Mortensen, R.F., and Lelias, J.M. 1990. Mouse C-reactive protein. *Biochem J.* 266:283–290.

Wollenberg, G.K., Lamarre, J., Rosendal, S., Gonias, S.L., and Hayes, M.A. 1991a. Binding of tumor necrosis factor alpha to activated forms of human plasma $alpha_2$ macroglobulin. *Am J Pathol.* 138:265–272.

Wollenberg, G.K., Lamarre, J., Semple, E., Farber, E., Gauldie, J., and Hayes, M.A. 1991b. Counteracting effects of dexamethansone and α_2-macroglobulin on inhibition of proliferation of normal and neoplastic rat hepatocytes by transforming growth factors-β type 1 and type 2. *Int J Cancer.* 47:311–316.

Won, K., and Baumann, H. 1990. The cytokine response element of the rat α_1 acid glycoprotein gene is a complex of several interacting regulatory sequences. *Mol Cell Biol.* 10:3965–3978.

Xia, Z-F., Coolbaugh, M.I., He, F., Herndon, D.N., and Papaconstantinou, J. 1992. The effects of bum injury on the acute phase response. *J Trauma.* 32:245–251.

Xu, L., Badolato, R., Murphy, W.J., et al. 1995. A novel biologic function of serum amyloid A. Induction of T lymphocyte migration and adhesion. *J Immunol.* 155:1184–1190.

Yamada, T., Agui, E., Suzuki, Y., Sato, M., and Matsumoto, K. 1993. Inhibition of the copper incorporation into ceruloplasmin leads to the deficiency in serum ceruloplasmin activity in long-evans cinnamon mutant rat. *J Biol Chem.* 268:8965–8971.

Yamada, T., Uchiyama, K., Yakata, M., and Gejyo, F. 1989. Sandwich enzyme immunoassaay for serum amyloid A protein SAA. *Clin Chim Acta.* 179:169–175.

Yamamoto, S., Abe, N., Santsuka, H., et al. 1993a. Efficient preparation of monospecific anti-canine C-reactive protein serum and purification of canine C-reactive protein by affinity chromatography. *Vet Immunol Immunopathol.* 36:293–301.

Yamamoto, K.I., Goto, N., Kosaka, J., Shiroo, M., Yeul, Y.D., and Migita, S. 1987. Structural diversity of murine serum amyloid A genes. *J Immunol.* 139:1683–1688.

Yamamoto, S., Miyaji, S., Ashida, Y., Otabe, K., Momotani, E., and Rikihisa, Y. 1994c. Preparation of anti-canine serum amyloid A SAA serum and purification of SAA from canine high-density lipoprotein. *Vet Immunol Immunopathol.* 41:41–53.

Yamamoto, S., Tagata, K., Nagahata, H., Ishikawa, Y., Morimatsu, M., and Naiki, M. 1992. Isolation of canine C-reactive protein and characterization of its properties. *Vet Immunol Immunopathol.* 30:329–339.

Yamamoto, S., Shida, T., Honda, M., et al. 1994b. Serum C-reactive protein and immune responses in dogs inoculated with *Bordetella bronchiseptica* phase I cells. *Vet Res Commun.* 18:347–357.

Yamamoto, S., Shida, T., Miyaji, S., et al. 1993b. Changes in serum C-reactive protein levels in dogs with various disorders and surgical traumas. *Vet Res Commun.* 17:85–93.

Yamamoto, S., Shida, T., Okimura, T., et al. 1994a. Determination of C-reactive protein in serum and plasma from healthy dots and dogs with pneumonia by ELISA and slide reversed passive agglutination test. *Vet Quarterly.* 16:74–77.

Yamamoto, K.I., Tsujino, Y., Saito, A., and Sinohara, H. 1985. Concentrations of murinoglobulin and α_2 macroglobulin in the mouse serum: Variations with age, sex, strain, and experimental inflammation. *Biochem Int.* 10:463–469.

Yamashita, K., Fujinaga, T., Miyamoto, T., Hagio, M., Izumisawa, Y., and Kotani, T. 1994. Canine acute phase response: Relationship between serum cytokine activity and acute phase protein in dogs. *J Vet Med Sci.* 56:487–492.

Yang, C., Mookerjea, S., and Nagpurkar, A. 1992. Clearance of rat C-reactive protein in vivo and by perfused liver. *Glycobiology.* 2:41–48.

Yang, F., Naylor, S.L., Lum, J.B., et al. 1986. Characterization, mapping, and expression of human ceruloplasmin gene. *Proc Natl Acad Sci USA.* 83:3257–3261.

Yap, S.H., Moshage, H.J., Hazenberg, P.B.C., et al. 1991. Tumor necrosis factor TNF inhibits interleukin IL-1 and/or IL-6 stimulated synthesis of C-reactive protein CRP and serum amyloid A SAA in primary cultures of human hepatocytes. *Biochim Biophys Acta.* 1091:405–408.

Yiangou, M., Ge, X., Carter, K.C., and Papaconstantinou, J. 1991. Induction of several acute-phase protein genes by heavy metals: A new class of metal-responsive genes. *Biochem.* 30:3798–3806.

Yiangou, M., and Papaconstantinou, J. 1993. The differential induction of α1-acid glycoprotein and serum amyloid A genes by heavy metals. *Biochim Biophys Acta.* 1174:123–132.

Ying, S.C., Shephard, E., De Beer, F.C., et al. 1992. Localization of sequence-determined neoepitopes and neutrophil digestion fragments of C-reactive protein utilizing monoclonal antibodies and synthetic peptides. *Mol Immunol.* 29:677–687.

Yu, S., Sher, B., Kudryk, B., and Redman, C.M. 1983. Intracellular assembly of human fibrinogen. *J Biol Chem.* 258:13407–13410.

Yunis, I., and Whitehead, A.S. 1990. The mouse C-reactive protein gene maps to distal chromosome 1 and, like its human counterpart, is closely linked to the serum amyloid P component gene. *Immunogenetics.* 32:361–363.

Zahedi, K. 1996. Characterization of the binding of serum amyloid P to type IV collagen. *J Biol Chem.* 271:14897–14902.

Zahedi, K., Gonnerman, W.A., Debeer, F.C., et al. 1991. Major acute-phase reactant synthesis during chronic inflammation in amyloid-susceptible and -resistant mouse strains. *Inflammation.* 15:1–14.

Zahedi, K., and Mortensen, R.F. 1986. Macrophage tumoricidal activity induced by human C-reactive protein. *Cancer Res.* 46:5077–5083.

Zahedi, K., Tebo, J.M., Siripont, J., Klimo, G.F., and Mortensen, R.F. 1989. Binding of human C-reactive protein to mouse macrophages is mediated by distinct receptors. *J Immunol.* 142:2384–2392.

Zahedi, K., and Whitehead, A.S. 1989. Acute phase induction of mouse serum amyloid P component. correlation with other parameters of inflammation. *J Immunol.* 143:2880–2886.

Zahedi, K., and Whitehead, A.S. 1993. Regulation of mouse serum amyloid P gene expression by cytokines in vitro. *Biochim Biophys Acta.* 1176:162–168.

Zeineh, R.A., Barrett, B., Niemirowski, L., and Fiorella, B.J. 1972. Turnover rate of orosomucoid in the dog with sterile abscess. *Am J Physiol.* 222:1326–1332.

Zeller, J.M., Landay, A.L., Lint, T.F., and Gewurz, H., 1986. Enhancement of human peripheral blood monocyte respiratory burst activity by aggregated C-reactive protein. *J Leukoc Biol.* 40:769–783.

Zhang, D., Sun, M., Samols, D., and Kushner, I. 1996. STAT3 participates in transcriptional activation of the C-reactive protein gene by interleukin-6. *J Biol Chem.* 271:9503–9509.

Zhong, Z., Wen, Z., and Darnell, J.E. 1994. STAT3: A STAT family member activated by tyrosine phosphorylation in response to epidermal growth factor and interleukin-6. *Science.* 264:95–98.

Zimlichman, S., Danon, A., Nathan, I., Mozes, G., and Shainkin-Kestenbaum, R. 1990. Serum amyloid A, an acute phase protein, inhibits platelet activation. *J Lab Clin Med.* 116:180–186.

Zuckerman, S.H., and Surprenant, Y.M. 1986. Simplified microELISA for the quantitation of murine serum amyloid A protein. *J Immunol Methods.* 92:37–43.Claire L. ParryClaire L.

20 Carbohydrate Metabolism

Owen P. McGuinness and Masakasu Shiota

CONTENTS

20.1 INTRODUCTION

Defects in carbohydrate metabolism are the major focus of research because of the extremely high incidence of diabetes mellitus (DM) and obesity in the United States population. Based on the National Centers for Disease Diabetes Fact Sheet (www.cdc.gov/diabetes/library) ~11.3% of the adult (>20 years old) population in the United States has diabetes (25.6 million people). The two most common forms of diabetes mellitus (DM) are referred to as type 1 and type 2, ~90% have type 2 DM. In type 1 (previously called insulin-dependent diabetes mellitus [IDDM]), there is an absolute deficiency of insulin, generally due to an autoimmune destruction of the pancreatic β cells.

Type 2 (previously called non-insulin-dependent diabetes mellitus, NIDDM) is characterized by insulin resistance and inadequate compensatory increase in the secretion of insulin. Almost 90% of individuals with type 2 DM are overweight or obese. The rise in obesity and diabetes risk is also mirrored in companion animals (dogs and cats) although the relative contribution of type 1 versus type 2 DM varies depending on the species (German et al., 2010; German, 2006; Catchpole et al., 2008; Prahl et al., 2007). In cats, the most common form of DM is type 2 and is associated with islet amyloidosis (O'Brien, 2002). In canines, the primary cause is type 1 DM (Catchpole et al., 2008).

Other less common causes of defects in glucose homeostasis either target endocrine systems that modulate carbohydrate metabolism or directly affect organs that metabolize carbohydrates (primarily liver and muscle). Congenital defects in β-cell function can cause hypo- or hyperglycemia secondary to inappropriate insulin secretion (Hussain, 2010). An excess in thyroid hormone, growth hormone, or glucocorticoids can cause hyperglycemia and a deficiency on one or another can cause hypoglycemia. Glycogen storage diseases (GSD) can either limit the ability of the liver to release carbohydrate or store carbohydrate. This can have profound effects on glucose homeostasis. GSD can affect skeletal muscle function, which commonly manifests as exercise intolerance. Defects in the metabolism of fructose or galactose can dramatically affect liver function (Mayatepek et al., 2010).

Animal models are very powerful tools with which to understand the physiology and pathophysiology of metabolic disease. Rodents, canines, and nonhuman primates have been used extensively to understand how carbohydrate is metabolized and glucose homeostasis is maintained. Each species of laboratory animal has one or more particular area of strength most amenable for the study of carbohydrate metabolism. Research using canines was critical in the discovery of insulin in 1922, and dogs have been used extensively to study the regulation of hepatic and muscle glucose metabolism. Nonhuman primates, because of their evolutionary proximity to humans, and canines have been used extensively to test new therapeutics and to determine if observations made in other mammalian systems translate to other species (Cruzen and Colman, 2009; Saisho et al., 2010). For rodents and mice, in particular, the ability to genetically manipulate (spontaneous or genetically induced gene deletion or overexpression) has afforded development of many models of human disease that are not as easily generated in other animal models. In addition, rodent models have served as tools to evaluate potential therapeutic agents.

20.2 REGULATION OF GLUCOSE HOMEOSTASIS

Plasma glucose concentration is a tightly controlled physiologic variable. The mechanisms in place to prevent hypoglycemia are particularly critical, as hypoglycemia can cause metabolic dysfunction, neuroglycopenia, seizures, and even death. In our present Western society, carbohydrate and nutrient availability is high and predispose us to develop obesity and DM. The control systems to prevent hyperglycemia are less robust; therefore, hyperglycemia is more common. Chronic hyperglycemia can lead to end-organ damage (e.g., retinopathy, nephropathy, and neuropathy).

The three major sources of plasma glucose are dietary carbohydrate (glucose, galactose, and fructose), glycogenolysis (breakdown of glycogen, which is a polymerized storage from of glucose), and gluconeogenesis (formation of glucose from gluconeogenic precursors including lactate, gluconeogenic amino acids, and glycerol). Dietary carbohydrates, after being digested into monosaccharides in the lumen of the intestine, are readily absorbed and enter the portal circulation. Common carbohydrates in the diet are starch (amylose or amylopectin), sucrose, and lactose. The three monosaccharides that make up these carbohydrates are glucose, fructose, and galactose. Starch is a polymer of glucose. Sucrose (table sugar) is a disaccharide (glucose and fructose). Lactose is a disaccharide (glucose and galactose). All monosaccharides are not treated equally when metabolized. Fructose and to a lesser extent, galactose are preferentially metabolized by the liver (McGuinness and Cherrington, 2003; Tappy and Le, 2010; Leslie, 2003). Approximately one-third of dietary glucose is taken up by the liver. The remainder is metabolized by peripheral tissues (e.g., brain, muscle, and fat).

To maintain glucose homeostasis, physiologic mechanisms allow tight coupling between the rates of glucose entry into the circulation and the rates of glucose disposal. In the fasted state, the liver is the main source of glucose. The liver releases glucose from one of two pathways (glycogenolysis and gluconeogenesis) into the plasma at rates equal to the uptake of plasma glucose by peripheral (e.g., brain, muscle, and fat) tissues. Although the kidney produces glucose, it is a minor source compared with the liver. The brain and formed elements of the blood (e.g., erythrocytes) consume ~60% of the plasma glucose used in the sedentary, fasted person and their absolute rate of utilization is relatively constant. In contrast, glucose utilization in muscle, fat, and liver can change markedly depending on the physiologic setting.

The absolute rates of glucose production and the contribution of the brain to basal glucose uptake vary between species. The basal rate of glucose production is ~2 $mg{\cdot}kg^{-1}\ min^{-1}$ in humans, dogs, and nonhuman primates, ~7 $mg{\cdot}kg^{-1}\ min^{-1}$ in rats, and 15–20 $mg{\cdot}kg^{-1}\ min^{-1}$ in mice (Wasserman, 2009; Reivich et al., 1979; Nagle et al., 2007). The contribution of the brain to basal glucose uptake is substantially lower in rodents than in humans and nonhuman primates (Moore et al., 1999; Reivich et al., 1979). In the mouse and rat, the brain consumes only about 15% and 10%, respectively, of the basal rate of glucose utilization (Grunstein et al., 1985).

The endocrine pancreas plays an essential role in the minute regulation of glucose homeostasis. Insulin release by the β cell is very sensitive to changes in plasma glucose concentration. Insulin has effects on multiple tissues including the liver, muscle, and adipose tissue. It also has effects on specific brain regions that regulate feeding behavior and energy expenditure. Its release can be further amplified by incretins (e.g., glucagon-like peptides) released by endocrine cells in the intestine when nutrients are ingested. Insulin's primary effect is to lower plasma glucose concentration by promoting cellular uptake of insulin. The hormone opposing insulin is glucagon, which is released by the α-cells of the endocrine pancreas. Glucagon's primary site of action is the liver where it is a potent stimulator of liver glucose production; it is also a modest regulator of lipolysis.

The robustness of this glucose control system is readily demonstrated with the glucose response to ingestion of a meal or to exercise (Wasserman, 2009; Moore et al., 2003). Ingestion of a meal high in carbohydrates increases β-cell insulin secretion. Insulin suppresses the rate of liver glucose production and augments glucose uptake by muscle, liver, and fat. The result is that excursions in plasma glucose concentration are dampened. Exercise augments glucose uptake in the working muscle despite a fall in plasma insulin. The fall in insulin and rise in glucagon allow the liver to exactly match the increase in muscle glucose requirements, thus minimizing deviations in plasma glucose.

As animals do not eat continuously, a substantial portion of dietary carbohydrate must be stored and subsequently released during the postabsorptive state. While multiple tissues contribute to the disposal of dietary carbohydrate, the metabolic fate varies. In the liver, the primary metabolic fate is storage as glycogen. In response to the accompanying increase in insulin, arterial glucose, and delivery of glucose into the portal vein, the liver switches from a glucose producer to a glucose consumer and removes approximately one-third of the dietary glucose (Pagliassotti and Cherrington, 1992). The liver expresses hexokinase IV (i.e., glucokinase). In contrast to the other hexokinases found in muscle and fat, glucokinase has a low affinity for glucose (Km = 7 mM vs. <1 mM) and is associated with glucokinase-associated regulatory protein (GKRP). When bound to GKRP, glucokinase is inactive and is located in the nucleus. Metabolic intermediates (glucose-6-phosphate and fructose-1-phosphate) can compete with the binding of glucokinase to GKRP and thus activate glucokinase. This allows glucokinase and thus the liver to be very responsive to changes in glucose concentration (McGuinness and Cherrington, 2003; Van Schaftingen et al., 1994). The rapid entry of glucose facilitated by activation of glucokinase combined with the rise in insulin act to suppress hepatic glycogenolysis and augment glycogen synthesis. About 50% of the glycogen synthesized in the liver is from dietary glucose that is directly taken up by the liver in a process referred to as direct glycogen synthesis. The remaining 50% is from gluconeogenic precursors (e.g., lactate, alanine, and glycerol) taken up by the liver, which instead of being released as glucose, are diverted to glycogen storage (Pagliassotti and Cherrington, 1992; Moore et al., 1991; Giaccari and Rossetti,

1992; Chueh et al., 2006). Thus, the gluconeogenic pathway is continuously active during both the fed and fasted setting. What differs is the fate of the glucose that is synthesized. Less than 25% of the glucose taken up by the liver is completely oxidized. While the liver has the capacity to convert glucose carbon to lipid (i.e., de novo lipogenesis), which will then subsequently assembled into very low-density lipoprotein (VLDL) particles and released; this is a relatively minor metabolic pathway, except with carbohydrate over feeding (Lewis, 1997; Chong et al., 2007). The addition of fructose to the diet may amplify de novo lipogenesis, as the majority of dietary fructose is removed by the liver. The majority of the VLDL released by the liver is derived from free fatty acids taken up and reesterified by the liver. The glycerol used in the synthesis of the glycerol backbone of triglycerides can be derived from carbohydrates (glucose, galactose, and fructose) or gluconeogenic precursors taken up by the liver.

Muscle glucose uptake is very low in the fasted state and increases markedly following a carbohydrate-rich meal (Moore et al., 2003). The increase in muscle glucose uptake is driven by the increase in the prevailing glucose and insulin concentration and the decrease in circulating nonesterified fatty acids secondary to the suppression of adipose tissue lipolysis and enhancement of reesterification. The majority of the glucose taken up by the muscle is deposited as glycogen (Mandarino et al., 2001). The remaining is oxidized or released as lactate or alanine. The augmentation of muscle glucose uptake is facilitated by the increase in glucose delivery to the muscle and the direct effects of insulin on the muscle to augment fractional extraction of glucose from the plasma by the muscle. The increase in glucose delivery is due to the combined increase in glucose concentration and the insulin-mediated increase in muscle blood flow. The increase in fractional glucose extraction is due to the direct effect of insulin to stimulate muscle glucose transport (glucose transporter type 4 [GLUT4] translocation) and augment glucose phosphorylation and glycogen synthetic capacity (Wasserman, 2009).

In adipose tissue, glucose uptake in response to a meal increases markedly due to the ability of insulin to facilitate glucose entry by translocation of GLUT4 (a facilitated glucose transporter) to the plasma membrane. While adipose tissue is very sensitive to insulin, relative to skeletal muscle, adipose tissue plays less of a role on whole body glucose disposal. The majority of the glucose carbon taken up by the adipose tissue is used either to provide glycerol to esterify circulating lipid or for de novo lipogenesis (Bederman et al., 2009). As the carbohydrate content of the diet increases, the contribution of the de novo pathway for lipid synthesis in both the liver and, to a lesser extent adipose tissue, increases (Chong et al., 2007; Brown et al., 2005; Postic and Girard, 2008).

As individuals transition from the fed state into a fast, plasma glucose and insulin gradually diminish and the liver switches from a glucose consumer to a glucose producer. The hepatic glycogen stores are mobilized, and gluconeogenic carbon that was being diverted to glycogen during the absorptive period is released by the liver. Hepatic glycogen stores are limiting (~100 g in the human in the postabsorptive state) and would be depleted in 10 hours, if gluconeogenesis did not provide a significant portion of the glucose carbon. As the fast progresses beyond 12 hours, the absolute rate of glucose production gradually decreases and the contribution of gluconeogenesis to plasma glucose increases. The carbon used to support gluconeogenesis comes from lactate-derived hydrolysis of muscle glycogen (~400 g), glycerol from adipose tissue lipolysis, and amino acids derived from muscle protein breakdown. The rates of glucose uptake by fat and muscle diminish, while brain glucose uptake remains relatively constant after a brief fast in humans (24–48 hours). The equivalent fast to an overnight fast in humans is much shorter in rodents. Thus, because glucose uptake by peripheral tissues decreases as one progresses into a fast, the absolute rate of gluconeogenesis does not increase even after hepatic glycogen stores are depleted (Bjorkman and Eriksson, 1985). Adipose tissue breakdown gradually increases, allowing nonesterified fatty acids to become the major oxidative fuel of both the muscle and the liver. As the net rate of lipolysis exceeds, the immediate oxidative needs of the liver and muscle, the liver reesterifies the lipid and releases VLDL and ketones. Ketones are rapidly oxidized by metabolically oxidative tissues such as heart and muscle, and after a long-term fast, by brain. If the metabolic demands of peripheral tissues increase in the postabsorptive state, as is seen during exercise, glucose uptake, and oxidation increase in the working muscle. This is matched with an increase in hepatic glucose production derived from a combined increase in glycogenolysis and gluconeogenesis (Wasserman, 2009).

Problems in these homeostatic mechanisms can result in metabolic dysfunction. If glucose production does not increase during exercise or is not maintained during a fast, as sometimes happens in diabetics treated with too much insulin or drugs that augment insulin secretion or action, hypoglycemia ensues. As individuals gain adipose tissue mass, they generally become insulin resistant. Interestingly, the preferential accumulation of adipose in the visceral, as opposed to the subcutaneous, compartment confers a greater risk in developing insulin resistance, diabetes, and cardiovascular disease (Lam et al., 2011). In most individuals, insulin secretion increases to compensate for the insulin resistance and near-normal glucose homeostasis is maintained. Those individuals who cannot sustain this increase in β-cell insulin secretion develop DM. The medical management of the accompanying hyperglycemia either with pharmaceuticals or insulin will commonly result in iatrogenic hypoglycemia (Cryer, 2010; Banarer and Cryer, 2004).

The mechanism to protect against hypoglycemia (whether iatrogenic or pathophysiologic) requires responses to work in concert to augment hepatic glucose production, augment lipolysis, and impair glucose removal by peripheral tissues. These responses are suppression of endogenous insulin secretion, stimulation of glucagon secretion, and activation of the autonomic nervous system (epinephrine and neural drive) (Cryer, 2010; Banarer and Cryer, 2004). Other factors such as increases in growth hormone and cortisol (or corticosterone in rodents) play a relatively minor role in the acute (minutes to a few hours) protection against hypoglycemia, but play a more important role in prolonged periods of hypoglycemia, and when deficient, can predispose one to develop hypoglycemia. Humans and animals exposed to repeated bouts of hypoglycemia can develop autonomic failure that will predispose them to very severe and life threatening hypoglycemia. This is a major hurdle in the medical management of DM. Activation of these same stress-activated pathways explains the robust increase in glucose that occurs when an animal is under stress (e.g., physical restraint, novel environment, an infection, or toxin). Thus, understanding how to monitor and manage glucose homeostasis requires an understanding of the normal regulation of carbohydrate metabolism and how defects in carbohydrate metabolism, insulin action and β cell, and neuroendocrine function can impact glucose homeostasis.

20.3 LABORATORY ANIMAL MODELS OF CARBOHYDRATE METABOLIC DYSFUNCTION

Diabetes and obesity are the most common causes of defects in carbohydrate metabolism in humans; therefore, several animal models have been developed to mimic these conditions. Multiple animal models have been used to study endocrine disorders (cortisol and growth hormone excess or deficiency) or genetic disorders (GSD, defects in fatty acid oxidation) that can also cause either hypoglycemia or hyperglycemia. We focus on animal models of diabetes and obesity, but we have included a discussion of models that affect glycogen storage and fructose and galactose metabolism.

20.3.1 Type 1 Diabetes Mellitus

Type 1 DM is characterized by a specific destruction of pancreatic β cells and is, in many cases, associated with immune-mediated damage.

20.3.1.1 Spontaneous or Genetically Derived Type 1 DM Models

Spontaneous type 1 DM models have been developed by either identifying one or several genetic mutations or by selective outbreeding of nondiabetic animals for hyperglycemia (Rees and Alcolado, 2005). Typically, the animals present with basal insulin deficiency and a defect in the insulin response to glucose load (see Table 20.1).

TABLE 20.1
Animal Models of Type I Diabetes

- Nonobese diabetic (NOD) mouse (Thayer et al., 2010)
- Bio breeding (BB) rat (Parfrey et al., 1989)
- Long Evans Tokushima lean (LETL) rat (Shima et al., 1999)
- New Zealand white rabbit (Wang et al., 2010a)
- Keeshond dog (Kramer et al., 1980)
- Chinese hamster (Chang, 1981)
- Celebes black ape (*Macacca nigra*) (Stanhope and Havel, 2008)

The nonobese diabetic (NOD) mouse and bio breeding (BB) rat are the two most commonly used animals that spontaneously develop type 1 diabetes. These animals have been inbred in laboratories for many generations by selecting for hyperglycemia. In NOD mice, overt diabetes typically presents between 12 and 30 weeks of age. Ketoacidosis is relatively mild; affected animals can survive for weeks without the administration of insulin. In BB rats, weight loss, polyuria, polydipsia, hyperglycemia, and insulinopenia develop at around 12 weeks of age, often at the time of puberty. Ketoacidosis is severe and fatal unless exogenous insulin is administered. In both the NOD mouse and BB rat, the pancreatic islets are subjected to an immune attack, as T cells, B cells, macrophages, and natural killer cells are recruited to the islets. Diabetes in the Chinese hamster is inherited as a homozygous recessive trait. It exhibits no lymphocytic infiltration into the pancreatic islets and no evidence of autoimmunity.

20.3.1.2 Chemical-Induced Type 1 DM Models

Alloxan (ALX) and streptozotocin (STZ) are most commonly used to induce type 1 DM in experimental animals. Both cause selective loss of pancreatic β cells, while leaving pancreatic α and δ cells intact. The cytotoxic action of both these diabetogenic agents is mediated by reactive oxygen species; however, the source of their generation is different (Szkudelski, 2001). ALX is a uric acid derivative. ALX and the product of its reduction, dialuric acid, establish a redox cycle with the formation of superoxide radicals, which undergo dismutation to hydrogen peroxide. Highly reactive hydroxyl radicals are formed by Fenton reaction. The action of reactive oxygen species with a simultaneous massive increase in cytosolic calcium concentration causes rapid destruction of β cells. STZ is a nitrosourea derivative and a powerful alkylating agent that has been shown to interfere with the glucose transporter (GLUT2) and glucokinase. STZ may cause alkylation or breakage of DNA strands and a consequent increase in the activity of poly-ADP-ribose synthase, an enzyme that depletes NAD, leading to energy deprivation and death of β cells. The intravenous route of administration is preferred for ALX, because of its low stability and very short half-life (less than 1 minute). ALX is disadvantageous because the extent of β cell death and the severity of hyperglycemia and ketosis are quite variable and are not proportional to the dose of ALX that is used. In part, this is because the β cell damage can be reversible. Therefore, STZ has now replaced ALX for the induction of diabetes in most laboratory animal models. There is one exception. ALX is used in rabbits because STZ is ineffective for induction of diabetes in this species and has a well-characterized multiorgan (liver and kidney) toxicity (Rerup, 1970). Dogs exhibit a high mortality following the administration of diabetogenic doses of either ALX or STZ likely secondary to severe liver and kidney damage including necrosis and fatty infiltration (Rerup, 1970). Mortality can be avoided if diabetes is induced by a combination of the two compounds (Issekutz et al., 1974). The dosages when both drugs are used together are considerably below the diabetogenic doses required to induce diabetes and off target organ toxicity, if either drug is to be used individually. The combined drug approach has shown no evidence of any significant organ toxicity other than the intended toxicity to β cells in the pancreas (see Table 20.2).

TABLE 20.2
The Doses of Alloxan (ALX) and Streptozotocin (STZ) in Different Species Used to Induce Type 1 Diabetes

Species	Dose	Route	Reference
Dog	35 mg STZ/kg + 40 mg ALX/kg	IV	Issekutz et al. (1974), Black et al. (1980), and Anderson et al. (1993)
Rat	60 ~ 70 mg STZ/kg	IV	Beech et al. (1989), Gibson et al. (1993), Koopmans et al. (1996), Burcelin et al. (1995), Hough et al. (1982), and Dardevet et al. (1991)
	65 ~ 85 mg STZ/kg	IP	Napoli et al. (1995), Youn et al. (1994), and Webster et al. (1986)
Mouse	200 mg STZ/kg	IP	Kim et al. (2009), Kim et al. (2008), and Gronbaek et al. (2002)
	50 mg STZ/kg	IP 4–5 × daily injections	Amirshahrokhi et al. (2008), Kim et al. (2009), Yuan et al. (2008), and Karabatas et al. (2005)
Rabbit	65–100 mg STZ/kg	IV	Jablecka et al. (2009), Marrachelli et al. (2010), Shukla et al. (2008), and Kohli et al. (2004)
Pig (Gottingen minipig)	100 ~ 125 mg STZ/kg	IV	Larsen et al. (2002)

20.3.2 Type 2 Diabetes Mellitus

Type 2 DM models exhibit hyperglycemia with near normal or increased concentration of plasma insulin. The development of hyperglycemia is generally associated with insulin resistance in various tissues/organs, which can lead to impaired glucose disposal and inappropriate endogenous glucose production. In general, males have a more severe diabetic phenotype in most animal models of type 2 DM than do females.

20.3.2.1 Spontaneous or Genetically Derived Type 2 DM Models

Many spontaneous type 2 diabetic models exhibit hyperphagia and obesity. The most widely used mouse (an inbred C57BL/6J or a C57BLKS/J background) models carry a single mutation in either the leptin (*Lep*) or the leptin receptor (*Lepr*) genes. In a C57BL/6J background, hyperglycemia is transient, but plasma insulin concentration increase steadily with age. The time course and symptoms on a C57BLKS/J background are more severe; this is not related to the presence of a mutation in the NAD nucleotide transhydrogenase (*Nnt*) gene on the C57BL/6J background (Nicholson et al., 2010). Mice become diabetic by 6 weeks of age. They develop pancreatic islet degeneration and renal complications. This results in lethality as early as 16–20 weeks of age. KK mice (KK/HlJ) are an inbred mouse strain that become diabetic when they are maintained on a high-calorie diet. Obesity and hyperinsulinemia are not as prominent as in Lep^{ob}/Lep^{ob} (often referred to as ob/ob) mice, but hyperglycemia is generally higher. Insulin resistance and body weight increase considerably at 2–3 months of age, peak at about 5 months, and return to normal at 9–12 months. T-KK hybrid or KKBL mice were developed by crossing the KK mice with C57BL/6J. Yellow KK or KKA^{y} mice were developed by inserting the yellow agouti (A^{y}) gene from the yellow obese mice into the Japanese KK. T-KK and Yellow KK become diabetic when they are obese. In NZO (NZO/HlLtJ) mice, an inbred mouse strain, body weight rises considerably during the first 10 weeks of life and peaks at 12–14 months, together with the parallel manifestation of hyperglycemia and hyperinsulinemia.

The most widely used diabetic rat models include the Zucker Fatty rat (outbred ZUC-$Lepr^{fa}$) or the inbred Zucker diabetic fatty (ZDF-$Lepr^{fa}$) rat. In the Zucker Fatty rat, obesity is accompanied by mild hyperglycemia and significant hyperinsulinemia detectable as early as 2–3 weeks of age.

Profound insulin resistance persists throughout their life span. Ketosis is absent. The Zucker diabetic fatty rat is an inbred substrain of markedly hyperglycemic Zucker fatty rats (Friedman et al., 1991). Compared with Zucker fatty rats, this model is more hyperglycemic and less hyperinsulinemic. Fasting hyperglycemia increases gradually with a progressive decrease in plasma insulin concentration beginning approximately at 8 weeks of age. The Otsuka Long-Evans Tokushima fatty (OLETF) rat originates from an outbred colony of Long-Evans rats selectively bred for glucose intolerance and possesses a spontaneous mutation in the gene encoding the receptor for the brain–gut peptide cholecystokinin (gene symbol *Cckar*; Takiguchi et al., 1997). The rats are mildly obese and develop diabetes in adult life (Shafrir, 1992; Rees and Alcolado, 2005; Srinivasan and Ramarao, 2007).

Some rodent models are available with nonobese type 2 DM. The Akita mouse (C57BL/6-*Ins2*^{Akita}) is the nonobese mutant mouse derived from the colony of C57BL/6 (Shafrir, 1992; Rees and Alcolado, 2005; Srinivasan and Ramarao, 2007). The Akita (*Ins2*^{Akita}) spontaneous mutation is an autosomal dominant mutation in the insulin II gene (*Ins2*), which is the mouse homologue of human preproinsulin gene. This mutation disrupts normal insulin processing and causes a failure in secretion of mature insulin, which results in early development of hyperglycemia. The Goto-Kakisaki (GK/KyoSwe) rat was developed by the selective breeding of Wistar rats with abnormal glucose tolerance repeated up to 35 generations. The rats are nonobese and develop stable hyperglycemia in adult life. The fasting hyperglycemia is mild but rises further on challenge with glucose. Their impaired glucose tolerance neither improves with age nor deteriorates with further breeding, and it does not proceed to a ketotic stage. The Cohen diabetic rat expresses genetic susceptibility to a carbohydrate-rich diet. The Torii rat was derived from a Sprague-Dawley rat strain.

Three distinctive quantitative trait loci (QTLs) were identified for glucose intolerance and were highly associated with the development of diabetes. The Nagoya-Shibata-Yasuda (NSY) inbred mouse was developed by selective inbreeding using a laboratory strain of mouse termed Jcl:ICR. NSY mice develop diabetes in an age-dependent manner (see Table 20.3).

20.3.2.2 Chemical-Induced Type 2 DM Models

Gold thioglucose (150–350 or 200 mg/kg, intraperitoneal [IP]) injection into mice can induce type 2 DM associated with obesity. The gold thioglucose is transported to the cells of ventromedial Hypothalamus and causes necrotic lesions, which subsequently is responsible for the development of hyperphagia and obesity. Mice gradually develop obesity, hyperinsulinemia, hyperglycemia, and insulin resistance over a period of 16–20 weeks after gold thioglucose injection (Le Marchand et al., 1978).

Chemically induced type 2 DM can be induced in the absence of obesity by the neonatal injection of STZ into rats. A single injection of STZ (80–100 mg/kg; intravenously (IV) or IP or

TABLE 20.3
Animal Models of Type 2 Diabetes

Obese Models	Nonobese Models
ob/ob mouse	NSY mouse (Ueda et al., 1995)
db/db mouse	Akita mouse (Yoshioka et al., 1997)
KK mouse (Ikeda, 1994)	Goto Kakizaki (GK) rat
New Zealand obese (NZO) mouse (Subrahmanyam, 1960)	Torri rat (Miao et al., 2005)
NONcNZO10 mouse (Cho et al., 2007)	Cohen sucrose-induced diabetic rat (Rosenmann et al., 1975)
TSOD mouse (Hirayama et al., 1999)	
M16 mouse (Allan et al., 2004)	
Zucker fatty rat	
Zucker diabetic fatty rat	
The Otsuka Long-Evans Tokushima fatty (OLETF) rat	

subcutaneously [SC]) into 1- or 2- or 5-day old pups induces type 2 diabetes in outbred Wistar (WI) or Sprague-Dawley (SD) rats (Takada et al., 2007; Portha et al., 1989). The neonatal type 2 diabetic models can also be developed by injecting ALX (200 mg/kg, IP) to male neonatal rats at 2, 4, or 6 days after birth (Kodama et al., 1993). These models develop hyperglycemia, abnormal glucose tolerance, and mild hypoinsulinemia that does not manifest until the animals are adults. Adult male rats are more severely affected than female rats, while β cell susceptibility to STZ in vivo or in vitro during the neonatal period is not influenced by gender (Ostenson et al., 1989). Type 2 diabetic models have also been developed by injecting STZ (35 mg/kg) into animals that are genetically insulin resistant (e.g., Spontaneously Hypertensive Rat [SHR] and ZUC) (Reaven and Ho, 1991). These models develop mild hyperglycemia without altered plasma insulin concentration.

20.3.2.3 Diet/Nutrition-Induced Type 2 DM Models

Several nondiabetic animal species may acquire type 2 DM associated with obesity when they are exposed to energy-abundant diets (Shafrir, 1992; Rees and Alcolado, 2005; Srinivasan and Ramarao, 2007; Islam and Loots du, 2009). Although they do not appear to carry an overt genetic defect, they may be considered as carriers of a genetic trait, which limits the capacity of their metabolic system to adjust to the high nutrient intake. C57BL/6J mice, in contrast to other strains, develop hyperglycemia and hyperinsulinemia when they are exposed to high-fat diet (45%–60% of calories from fat). Since this mouse strain is shown to be mildly insulin resistant with a weak first phase of insulin release, latent genetic factors may become expressed in this mouse strain on high-fat diet. Sand rats remain normal in their natural habitat (e.g., fed their usual low-energy density vegetable diet). When placed on standard (e.g., higher energy density) laboratory chow, however, sand rats develop hyperphagia, obesity, hyperinsulinemia, and glucose intolerance. Over time, they exhibit β-cell degeneration and necrosis, resulting in profound insulin deficiency, overt diabetes and ketosis. Spiny mice (*Acomys* spp.) also develop obesity and marked pancreatic β-cell hyperplasia, hypertrophy, and increased pancreatic insulin content followed by an impaired insulin release mechanism when they are fed with rodent lab chow. Over time they develop overt hyperglycemia and fatal ketosis.

Type 2 DM can be induced by combining diet (high-fat or high-fructose diet) and STZ treatment in outbred rats (see Table 20.4). The diets induce hyperinsulinemia and insulin resistance. When treated with STZ to cause β-cell damage, hyperglycemia develops in the presence of almost normal insulin concentrations. The combination method has been used to induce obese-type 2 diabetes in canines (Bevilacqua et al., 1985; Ionut et al., 2009).

Golden hamsters fed a high-fat diet do not overeat, but they become obese because of decreases in energy expenditure (Wade, 1982, 1983). This decrease in energy expenditure is accompanied

TABLE 20.4
Diet-Induced Type 2 Diabetic Obese Models

High Energy Diet-Induced Type 2 Diabetic Obese Models (Srinivasan and Ramarao, 2007; Shafrir, 1992)

- Male C57BL/6J mouse by high-fat diet (40%–65% calorie as fat)
- Spiny mouse (*Acomys calirinus*): by standard laboratory chow
- Sand rat (*Psammomys obesus*): by standard laboratory chow

Type 2 Diabetic Models Induced by a Combination of Diet and Chemicals

- Injected with STZ (50 mg/kg IV) after high-fat diet (40% calories as fat) for 2 weeks (Reed et al., 2000)
- Injected with STZ (35 mg/kg, IV) after high-fat diet (33% calories as fat) for 2 weeks (Wang et al., 2011)
- Injected with STZ (45 mg/kg, IV) after high-fat diet (22% calories as fat) for 4 weeks (Zhang et al., 2003)
- Injected with STZ (15 mg/kg, IV) after high-fat diet (30% calories as fat) for two months (Zhang et al., 2003)
- Injected with STZ (25 mg/kg, IV) after high-fat (25.7 wt%) plus high fructose (46.5 wt%) for 6 weeks (Menard et al., 2010)

by increases in thermogenic capacity and brown adipose tissue mass, protein, and DNA content. They are hyperinsulinemic, hyperleptinemic, hypercholesterolemic, and hypertriglyceridemic (van Heek et al., 2001). The lipid and lipoprotein aspects of this model have been found to closely parallel lipid metabolism in humans (Spady et al., 1993; Dietschy, 1997; Kris-Etherton and Dietschy, 1997).

20.3.3 Surgically Induced DM Models

The entire pancreas or a portion of the pancreas can be removed to induce diabetes. The advantage of a total pancreatectomy is that it avoids the cytotoxic effects of chemical diabetogens on other body organs. The disadvantage of this technique is that it causes severe digestive problems, because the exocrine portion of the pancreas is also removed. To avoid malabsorption, the animals must receive pancreatic enzymes (Pancrease MT; Viokase®) with their diet. In addition, this technique removes α cells (glucagon-secreting cells) as well as β cells, leading to problems in the counter-regulatory response to hypoglycemia. Partial pancreatectomy (remove 70% or 90%) has been performed in dogs, pigs, rabbit, rats, and mice (Islam and Loots du, 2009; Srinivasan and Ramarao, 2007; Leahy et al., 1993). It is characterized by moderate hyperglycemia with neither a reduction in body weight nor in basal levels of plasma insulin.

A combined partial pancreatectomy with chemical treatment (e.g., ALX and STZ) is another model. The advantage of this technique is that it minimizes the adverse effect of chemicals on the body. In addition, it leads to a more stable form of chronic DM in the dog, pig, monkey, and other species. Another stable form of type 2 DM has been produced by combination of 50% partial pancreatectomy, NAD (350 mg/kg), and STZ (200 mg/kg) treatment in BALB/c mice (Kurup and Bhonde, 2000).

20.3.4 Other Disorders Affecting Carbohydrate Metabolism

Glycogen storage diseases (GSD) include a clinically heterogeneous group of disorders that are associated with inherited abnormalities of the carbohydrate metabolism. These abnormalities are caused by enzyme deficiencies, which give rise to the intracellular accumulation of structurally normal or abnormal glycogen or the decrease in normal glycogen in one or multiple tissues. As shown in Table 20.5, the GSD have been classified into 10 groups based on deficient genes. GSD have been verified in animals and mouse models of some types of GSD have been generated.

In most organisms, the utilization of galactose requires the Leloir pathway (Lai et al., 2009). The pathway converts galactose to UDP-glucose by a series of enzymatic reactions. In humans, deficiencies or mutations in one or more of these enzymes in the Leloir pathway will result in significant toxicity (e.g., cataracts, liver complications, hypotonia, and sepsis). In humans, newborn screening programs test for defects in this pathway. Defects in this pathway in other species have not been reported. In the rodent, targeted defects in this pathway have been generated (Leslie et al., 1996); however, the toxicity is not as severe as in humans, suggesting that alternative pathways may be active in rodents.

Fructose is a very popular addition to the Western diet (Mayes, 1993) and likely contributes to the prevalence of obesity, insulin resistance, and dyslipidemia. High-fructose diets are used to induce insulin resistance in a number of animal models (Coate et al., 2010; Wei et al., 2007; Zhang et al., 2009). In many cases, the insulin resistance is in the absence of accompanying obesity. In humans, hereditary fructose intolerance can occur; it is caused by the deficiency of either aldolase B or fructokinase (Mayatepek et al., 2010). While the absence of fructokinase has relatively silent phenotype, the absence of aldose B causes hypoglycemia because of the enzymes central role on the metabolism and synthesis of glucose. Animal models of these defects have not been reported.

TABLE 20.5
Glycogen Storage Disease

Type	Subtype	Gene	Protein	Human Metabolic Symptoms	Animal Models	Reference
GSD-0		*GYS2*	Hepatic isoform of glycogen synthase (glycogen synthase2)	Reduced glycogen storage in the liver, ketotic hypoglycemia, low lactatemia after prolong fasting. Hyperglycemia, hyperlactatemia and hyperlipidemia in the postprandial period		Orho et al. (1998), Wolfsdorf and Weinstein (2003), Weinstein et al. (2006), and Bachrach et al. (2002)
GSD-I	GSD-Ia	*G6PC*	Glucose-6-phosphatase-α	Hypoglycemia, hepatomegaly, nephromegaly, hyperlipidemia, hyperuricemia, lactic acidemia, growth retardation	Mouse (autosomal recessive) *G6pc*−/- mice (Kim et al., 2008; Lei et al., 1996) A naturally occurring dog model	Walvoort (1983), Wolfsdorf and Weinstein (2003), and Walvoort (1983)
	GSD-1b	SLC37A4	Glucose-6-phosphate transporter	Hypoglycemia, hepatomegaly, nephromegaly, hyperlipidemia, hyperuricemia, lactic acidemia, growth retardation, neutropenia, neutrophil dysfunction	*G6pt*−/- mice	Chen et al. (2003)
	G6Pase-β deficiency	G6PC3	Glucose-6-phosphatase-β	Neutropenia, neutrophil dysfunction	G6pc3$^{-/-}$ mice	Cheung et al. (2007)
GSD-II (Pompe disease)		*GAA*	Acid α-glucosidase	Impaired glycogen degradation and glycogen accumulation within the lysosomal, muscle weakness, and respiratory insufficiency	GAA$^{-/-}$ mice Animals with autosomal recessive (Cattle [shortthorn and Brahman], Sheep [Corriedale], cat, dog [Lapland], and Japanese Quail)	Ding et al. (2001), Raben et al. (2003), Wolfsdorf and Weinstein (2003), Zampieri et al. (2011), Walvoort (1983), and Walvoort et al. (1985)
GSD-III	GSD-IIIa	AGL	Loss of both debranching and glucosidase activities of glycogen debranching enzyme in liver, muscle, and heart	Hepatomegaly, fasting hypoglycemia with ketosis, hyperlipidemia, progressive muscle weakness	Dog (toy breed puppies, German shepherd, and Akita)	Wolfsdorf and Weinstein (2003) and Walvoort (1983)
	GSD-IIIb	AGL	Loss of both debranching and glucosidase activities of glycogen debranching enzyme in liver	Hepatomegaly, fasting hypoglycemia with ketosis, hyperlipidemia		
	GSD-IIIc	AGL	Loss of glucosidase activity of glycogen debranching enzyme			
	GSD-IIId	AGL	Loss of transferase activity of glycogen debranching enzyme			

(Continued)

TABLE 20.5 (*Continued*)
Glycogen Storage Disease

Type	Subtype	Gene	Protein	Human Metabolic Symptoms	Animal Models	Reference
GSD-IV		GBE1	Glycogen branching enzyme	Abnormal deposition of amylopectin-like glycogen in multiple organ Hepatosplenomegaly and failure to thrive	An inbred family of Norwegian forest cats	Bao et al. (1996), Greene et al. (1988), and Fyfe et al. (1992)
GSD-VI		PYGL	Hepatic glycogen phosphorylase	Hepatomegaly, growth retardation, ketotic hypoglycemia after an overnight fasting and mild hypoglycemia after prolong fasting, postprandial lactic acidosis		Wolfsdorf and Weinstein (2003)
GSD-V (McArdle disease)		PYGM	Glycogen phosphorylase, muscle form	Exercise intolerance		Martin et al. (1993)
GSD-VII (Tarui's disease)		PFKM	Human muscle phosphofructokinase		Iodoacetate-injected rats	Di Mauro (2007) and Brumback (1980)
GSD-VIII		PHKA1	Muscle isoform of phosphorylase b kinase	Exercise intolerance, mild myopathy, cognitive impairment	Autosomal recessive: Rat (NZR/Mh strain) X-linked: Mouse (I strain) Dog (toy breed puppies)	Orngreen et al. (2008), Echaniz-Laguna et al. (2010), and Walvoort (1983)
GSD-IX		PHKA2	Liver isoform of phosphorylase b kinase	Hypoglycemia, hepatomegaly, chronic liver disease, growth retardation, delayed motor development, hypercholesteroleamia, hypertriglyceridemia and hyperketosis following fasting		Wolfsdorf and Weinstein (2003)

20.4 MEASURING METABOLIC AND ENDOCRINE STATUS

20.4.1 Animal Husbandry and Experimental Design

Evaluation of the metabolic and endocrine status of an animal requires the collection of blood samples that are reflective of the physiology of the animal in its normal environment. The most important presampling procedure is to develop a standard protocol specific for the particular species of interest. The investigator should pay careful attention to a number of parameters when designing the protocol. These include the presampling status of the animal (i.e., fasting status, the environment, acclimation of the animal to the environment), the sampling procedure, the skill of the investigator/phlebotomist, blood sample handling, and reliability of the assays employed. To obtain reproducible baseline data, the animal should be fasted. For large species (e.g., nonhuman primates, dog), an overnight fast is appropriate (i.e., fasting glucose concentration), as these animals tend to eat during the day and are fed at predictable times. For example, canines are generally fed once a day and are slow absorbers, taking ~14–16 hours to absorb a chow meat meal (Davis et al., 1984). They should be trained to eat all of their meal in a defined period of time, so as to better control the duration of the fast prior to sample collection. Thus, feeding canines the afternoon prior to a study and assessing glucose metabolism after 18 hours is appropriate. Assessing glucose kinetics in the canine after fasting of much shorter duration (<16 hours) may not reflect basal metabolism as they will likely be still absorbing nutrients. For rodents (especially mice), an overnight fast is a major metabolic stress (Ayala et al., 2006). Mice have a very high metabolic rate, are typically housed in facilities well below their thermoneutral zone and are primarily nocturnal feeders. After an overnight fast, mice can lose a significant amount of lean body mass and, if individually housed during the fast, can go into a torpor state (McGuinness et al., 2009; Swoap et al., 2006; Geiser, 2004). A shorter 5–6-hour fast is often more appropriate for mice. For the rat, the current practice is to fast the animals overnight. While rats are not at risk of developing torpor, they, like mice, are nocturnal feeders. Thus, an overnight fast in rodents is metabolically similar to a 24–48 hours fast in primates or canines; the liver will be essentially glycogen depleted. In contrast, a 5–6 hours fasted mouse has a similar glycogen content as an overnight-fasted human and an 18 hours fasted dog (~30–40 mg/g liver). Once these variables are controlled, the plasma glucose sample is most likely to reflect the basal metabolic status of the animal. As will be discussed later, if the animal is metabolically stable, whole body insulin sensitivity (S_I) can be estimated from concurrent insulin and glucose concentrations.

Some investigators wish to assess endocrine status by collecting random and/or individual measures of glucose and/or insulin. The difficulty with this approach is that endocrine and metabolic parameters exhibit a high degree of diurnal variability. To assess endocrine status in the nonfasted state, the investigator should control for the time of day and the feeding patterns of the animal model, so as to minimize day-to-day variations in metabolic and endocrine status (Hut et al., 2011; Clifton, 2000). For rodents fed ad libitum, changes in diet composition can alter feeding patterns (e.g., rodents on a high-fat diet [40%–50% fat] tend to eat throughout the day and night, while rodents on a standard diet [e.g., 5%–7% fat] eat predominantly during the night). Unless accounted for when randomly assessing metabolic and endocrine parameters, data interpretation can be complicated. Alternatively, a 24-hour glucose profile can ameliorate the impact of diurnal variability on data interpretation.

The animal needs to be acclimated to the laboratory environment and sampling procedure (Ellacott et al., 2010). Frequently handled and trained animals will have fewer variations caused by the excitement and apprehension induced by unaccustomed handling and sampling. The phlebotomist must be experienced and able to obtain a sample with minimal disturbance. Individual housing, novel environments, restraint, and bright lights are all stressors for rodents that require acclimation to obtain reliable data.

Ideally, all samples should be taken from an artery as it reflects the blood that perfuses the major organs. Moreover, depending on the substrate (e.g., glucose, lactate, amino acids) venous plasma concentration may not be reflective of what is in arterial plasma (Sonnenberg and Keller, 1982; Jensen and Heiling, 1991). However, arterial access is difficult without surgical intervention, and common practice in a laboratory setting is to use venous blood. In general, the location from which blood is obtained (vein or artery) will not alter most metabolic or endocrine parameters, if animals are metabolically stable and the sample can be taken with minimal stress. Ideally, if blood is taken from a vein, the vein should drain tissues that are not very metabolically active (i.e., saphenous or cephalic, submandibular or tail vein in rodents) and are well perfused (Aasland et al., 2010; Christensen et al., 2009). As red blood cells are metabolically active, it is best that blood samples are immediately centrifuged and the plasma or serum should be quickly separated from the cells (see Section 20.4.2.1 for additional information on sampling handling for specific analytes).

20.4.2 Laboratory Analytes/Tests of Carbohydrate Metabolism

20.4.2.1 Glucose

While plasma glucose concentration is a tightly controlled parameter, it still changes throughout the day and is rapidly increased by stressful conditions. Once a sample is obtained, it is also important that glucose utilization by red blood cells be minimized. Therefore, the plasma or serum must be separated from the red cells as soon as possible, and if immediate separation is not feasible, the glucose in the blood sample must be protected from glycolysis by the red blood cells. This is best done by placing the blood sample in an ice bath followed by refrigeration and the addition of sodium fluoride (10 mg/mL of blood). Standard sodium fluoride-containing evacuated tubes are ideal for this purpose. Samples can be collected in serum separator tubes. In one study, human glucose concentration was stable for up to 24 hours after centrifugation (Landt et al., 1986). While it was unchanged, the authors recommend separating the plasma from the cells as soon as possible. Do not rely on fluoride or cold to completely inhibit glycolysis.

Of the many methods for glucose determination in plasma or serum, the enzymatic methods used in clinical analyzers are the most accurate (Johnson et al., 2009). However, despite the level of accuracy of enzymatic methods, many investigators rely upon handheld blood glucose meters to assess plasma glucose concentrations. Their ease of use, portability, and the very low blood volume requirements allows serial sampling for rodents, which have a very limited blood volume. While handheld glucometers are convenient to use, these instruments have significant drawbacks (D'Orazio et al., 2006). The majority of handheld glucose meters are standardized for human blood. The handheld glucose meters measure blood, not plasma, glucose concentration. This is important as the difference between blood and plasma glucose is substantial in some species because of the differences in erythrocyte glucose permeability (Rendell et al., 1985; Higgins et al., 1982). The order of erythrocyte glucose permeability across species occurs in the following descending order: primate>rodent>canine>pig. In primates, blood and plasma glucose are very similar, because their erythrocytes are relatively permeable to glucose. In canines, the red blood cell is relatively impermeable to glucose, such that blood glucose is ~70% of plasma glucose. This is important as the physiologically regulated variable is plasma glucose. In addition, blood glucose meters from different manufacturers can give different readings for the same blood sample (Cohn et al., 2000; Johnson et al., 2009). An additional confounding issue is that these meters as stated on the package insert are sensitive to the hematocrit and some pharmaceuticals (Mann et al., 2009; Boren and Clarke, 2010; Heinemann, 2010). For the dog, nonhuman primates and rat, blood volume is not a limitation, and plasma glucose concentration should be measured with a chemistry analyzer. For mice, if multiple samples need to be taken, such as during a glucose tolerance test (GTT), a blood glucose meter may be more practical. However, if blood glucose is monitored, the same meter should be used for a given experiment, and hematocrit should be checked to verify that it is not a variable in the study. In addition, the meter should be calibrated against a chemistry analyzer over the range of glucose concentration obtained in the study.

A plasma glucose concentration of 90 ± 12 mg/dL (SD) or 5 ± 1 mmol/L (SD) is a general reference value for the dog, cat, or nonhuman primate and is comparable to that of the adult human (Kaneko, 1997). For mice, glucose concentrations tend to be higher than in larger species and are strain and gender dependent. A database of typical glucose values in commonly used mice strains is available in the Jax phenome database (http://phenome.jax.org) (note the data use human and not rodent standardized meters). Mice with mixed backgrounds may have a higher variability in glucose concentration depending upon the relative contribution of the two strains in any given animal. Given the number of parameters that can influence glucose concentration it is best when making comparisons between groups that control and experimental groups be assayed together. Animals should be matched for genetic background, gender, and age. It is best to use littermates as controls; if it is possible.

20.4.2.2 Glycated Hemoglobins

Glycated hemoglobin or HbA1c is now widely used as an index of long-term average plasma glucose. The hemoglobins in the erythrocyte, when first formed, are not linked to glucose. If the red cell is permeable to glucose (note: permeability varies between species), a fraction of the hemoglobin, the HBA1, is glycosylated by a slow, nonenzymatic, and relatively irreversible mechanism. Multiple HbA1 fractions (HbA1a, HbA1b, and HbA1c) are slowly and irreversibly glycosylated. Of the fractions, HbA1c is the one that binds glucose in direct proportion to the plasma glucose concentration. Because the binding is irreversible, glucose remains bound to Hb over the life span of the red cell. Thus, HbA1c can be used as an index of the average plasma glucose concentration over a previous time period approximating half the life span of the red blood cell (Kaneko, 1997). The average red blood cell life span can range from 100 days in the dog and macaque, 70 days in the cat, and 40 days in the mouse (Bennett, 2002; Wang et al., 2010b). Therefore, HbA1c is used as an index of the average plasma glucose over the previous 30–60 days in most laboratory animals. The species-dependent differences in the permeability of the erythrocyte to glucose will markedly alter the rate of glycosylation (Higgins et al., 1982). For species whose erythrocytes are relatively impermeable to glucose, the basal rate of glycosylation is very low.

In veterinary clinical practice, HbA1c is used to monitor a patient's average plasma glucose control by sampling as infrequently as once every month or two, rather than having to measure blood glucose daily, which was common practice for animals with DM prior to the use of HbA1c. HbA1c is, however, insensitive to brief bouts of hypoglycemia and should not replace periodic plasma glucose monitoring.

In humans, an immunochemistry-based approach that detects HbA1c using a monoclonal antibody against human HbA1c has been widely used (e.g., DCA 2000 analyzer). The reference range for HbA1c in humans is ~3%–6% of the total Hb, and it is very closely correlated with reference plasma glucose concentration (Elliott et al., 1997; Wood and Smith, 1980). Significantly higher levels of HbA1c are associated with persistent hyperglycemia during the preceding months. This indirect method of monitoring plasma glucose is a valuable means to monitor glucose control (Nathan et al., 2008), and has been used in humans, nonhuman primates, rats, mice (Han et al., 2008), cats, and dogs (Marca and Loste, 2000; Bennett, 2002; Kaneko, 1997). However, the period that a given HbA1c reflects is dependent on the half-life of the red blood cell, which varies between species. Measurement of HbA1c is now the glycated protein of choice in humans and is used in animal models of DM to test the efficacy of new therapeutics. Controlling plasma glucose within narrow limits is highly beneficial to the well-being and survival of the patient, and measuring HbA1c is a valuable adjunct to maintaining this tight control therapeutically (Cohen and Smith, 2008). The applicability of this to mice has been examined (Han et al., 2008). HBA1c most closely correlates with 5–6 hours fasting glucose concentration in this species; however, the absolute value for HBA1c for any glucose level is mouse strain dependent. The mechanism for this difference is unclear.

20.4.2.3 Fructosamine

Fructosamine is a glycated serum protein that reflects glycemic control over the previous 1–3 weeks (Koga and Kasayama, 2010) in primates, dogs, and cats reflecting the higher rate of albumin turnover relative to red blood cells (Armbruster, 1987; Reusch et al., 1993). Glucose molecules are joined to protein molecules to form stable fructosamines, through glycation by a nonenzymatic mechanism (Armbruster, 1987). The assay assesses the formation of ketoamines in plasma proteins (Young et al., 1975; Schnedl et al., 2005). If a plasma sample is contaminated with hemoglobin or very lipemic, the data will not be accurate. Since albumin is the major plasma protein, alterations in albumin concentration or turnover will alter data interpretation.

20.4.2.4 Insulin

Insulin is secreted by the β cells of the endocrine pancreas and is released in a 1:1 molar ratio with C-peptide into the portal vein. Approximately 50% of the insulin is cleared on the first pass by the liver. Insulin half-life in primates is 3–5 minutes (Duckworth et al., 1998). Insulin is stable in plasma collected with EDTA or in serum if it is stored frozen (–70°C) until analyzed (Öberg et al., 2011). Because insulin's structure varies between species, investigators must use species-specific assays for analysis (Smith, 1966). Although the structure of insulin does differ across species, these structural differences do not affect insulin's biological activity. Occasionally, C-peptide is assayed, and, as with insulin, species-specific antibodies must be used. Basal insulin concentrations vary between species but are typically between 5 and 40 μU/mL in nonobese animals on a normal low-fat diet. Canines tend to have lower insulin concentrations than nonhuman primates and rodents. As insulin concentration is very sensitive to plasma (or serum) glucose concentration, both parameters should be measured and interpreted at the same time, and same procedures to control for fasting status and animal handling also apply.

20.4.2.5 C-peptide

C-peptide is secreted from the pancreatic β cell in equimolar concentration with insulin, but is not extracted by the liver. In contrast to insulin, C-peptide is primarily metabolized by the kidney and has a longer half-life (Castillo et al., 1994; Valera Mora et al., 2003). Thus, the absence of C-peptide is a more sensitive marker of residual insulin secretion in animal models of type 1 diabetes (Polonsky and Rubenstein, 1984). Moreover, peripheral C-peptide concentrations can be used as a marker of β cell secretory activity in a variety of clinical situations (Bonser et al., 1984; Polonsky and Rubenstein, 1984). The mouse and rat have two insulin genes (Shiao et al., 2008). The C-peptide released by the genes is not identical. C-peptide can be measured in the urine to obtain an index of daily C-peptide excretion, if renal function is normal and daily urine is accurately and quantitatively collected. This can be done by housing the animal in a metabolic cage that collects all of the urine, a second option is to measure urine creatinine and calculate the ratio of C-peptide to creatinine. As with insulin, the plasma should be stored (–70°C) frozen prior to being analyzed.

20.4.2.6 Glucagon

Glucagon is secreted primarily by the α cells of the endocrine pancreas. However, cells within the gastrointestinal tract can secrete glucagon in animals that are insulin deficient. This is most apparent in dogs (Vranic et al., 1974; Vranic et al., 1976). Normal plasma glucagon concentrations are ~50–100 pg/mL in mammalian species. The liver is exquisitely sensitive to both increases and decreases in glucagon. Like insulin, glucagon is secreted into the portal vein, resulting in an elevated glucagon concentration in the hepatic portal circulation. As such, changes in arterial or systemic plasma glucagon concentration will underestimate the accompanying changes in the portal vein (Wasserman and Cherrington, 1991; Cherrington, 1999). Stress can rapidly increase glucagon secretion into the blood; appropriate animal handling techniques are required to obtain accurate basal glucagon concentrations. In DM, plasma glucagon concentration can be normal or elevated in the basal state but are inappropriately elevated following a meal and inappropriately low during hypoglycemia (Cryer, 2012). Thus, inappropriate glucagon secretion contributes to the glucose dys-homeostasis in DM. The fact that basal plasma glucagon concentration is very low and glucagon is readily degraded requires that special care be taken following plasma collection. After separation of plasma from blood (preferably collected in EDTA-containing tubes), the plasma should be treated with aprotinin (500 Kallikrein Inhibitory Units/mL) to prevent proteolytic degradation and kept frozen (–70°C) until it is analyzed.

20.4.2.7 Catecholamines

The primary catecholamines in plasma are epinephrine and norepinephrine. Epinephrine is released by the adrenal medulla. Norepinephrine is released from both the adrenal medulla (although much less than the quantity of epinephrine released) and from spillover from noradrenergic nerve terminals. Epinephrine is a potent stimulator of hepatic glucose production and a potent stimulator of muscle glycogen breakdown with subsequent release of lactate. In individuals with longstanding diabetes, the adrenergic response to hypoglycemia is blunted (Cryer et al., 1989). In unstressed animals, plasma epinephrine concentration is less than 100 pg/mL, but it can increase to over 2000 pg/mL in stressful settings. Plasma norepinephrine concentration is higher than epinephrine (~300 pg/mL) and can increase to over 2000 pg/mL during stress (Wasserman and Cherrington, 1991; Stevenson et al., 1991; Cherrington, 1999). Baseline catecholamines are very sensitive to stress from handling. As such, it is very difficult to obtain reliable values when catecholamine concentrations are low, especially in mice. When handling stress is minimized, rodents, dogs, and nonhuman primates have very similar basal catecholamine concentrations (Ayala et al., 2006; Grouzmann et al., 2003). In general, measuring basal catecholamines are not very informative in ascribing changes in glucose metabolism to changes in adrenergic tone. Generally, they are measured in studies where a controlled stress (e.g., hypoglycemia) is induced to determine if the adrenergic response is altered (Jacobson et al., 2006; Davis et al., 1994, 1992). Because catecholamines are light sensitive, blood must be immediately treated with an antioxidant such as glutathione (1.0 mg/mL blood) with ethylene glycol tetraacetic acid (EGTA—1.8 mg/mL blood). The plasma should be separated from the blood cells and stored at –70°C until analyzed either via HPLC or enzymatic analysis (Macdonald and Lake, 1985).

20.4.2.8 Insulin-Like Growth Factor

Insulin-like growth factor (IGF) has two isoforms (IGF I and IGF II) (Annunziata et al., 2011). In plasma, the IGFs are associated with binding proteins (IGFBP I-VI), which dramatically increase their half-life (Clemmons, 1997). The affinity of IGF for their binding protein exceeds that of their affinity for their receptor. Thus, both IGF and the major binding partners should be measured (Quarmby et al., 1998). IGF-I (70 amino acids) is identical in human and porcine with three residues different in rodents (Humbel, 1990). IGFII (67 amino acids) is less homologous between species. Because of the binding proteins, standardization of IGF assays and assessing "Free" IGF has been challenging (Frystyk, 2007).

20.4.2.9 Glucagon-Like Peptide

Glucagon-like peptides are synthesized and secreted in response to nutrient ingestion (Drucker, 2007). GLP-1 is secreted from intestinal endocrine L-cells, which are located mainly in the distal ileum and colon (Baggio and Drucker, 2007). GLP-1 exists in multiple forms in vivo. GLP-1(1–37) and GLP-1(1–36)NH_2 are thought to be inactive. GLP-1(7–37) and GLP-1(7–36)NH_2 are biologically active. The active GLP-1 is rapidly cleared from circulation ($T_{1/2}$ < 2 minutes). It is rapidly inactivated by dipeptidyl peptidase-4 (DPP-4). Since DPP-4 is present in blood, when collecting blood, a DDP-4 or protease (aprotinin) inhibitor has to be directly added to the blood prior to centrifugation (Di Marino et al., 2011). Plasma should be frozen immediately and thawed on ice when the assay is performed.

20.4.3 Functional Evaluation of Insulin Action and Secretion

Insulin resistance is a characteristic of obesity, metabolic syndrome, and cardiovascular disease. When combined with defects in pancreatic insulin secretion, animals will progress from normal glucose tolerance to glucose intolerance and overt diabetes. Glucose tolerance is not a measure of insulin resistance. Obese individuals can have a normal GTT, but are typically insulin resistant.

Normal glucose tolerance is maintained because they hypersecrete insulin. If they are unable to do this, they become glucose intolerant. To quantify S_I/resistance and whole body glucose handling in animal models is of great importance. In humans, a number of approaches have been developed to assess insulin action from the most difficult (hyperinsulinemic-euglycemic clamp) to the simplest (calculation of basal insulin action) (Muniyappa et al., 2008). The hyperinsulinemic-euglycemic clamp is considered the "gold" standard to assess insulin action. However, it is not very practical for screening large populations for insulin resistance. Other tests were developed that were easier to perform and compared to the gold standard in humans. These approaches have been adapted to evaluate insulin action in other species with little or no critical analysis. No attempt was made to systematically compare the modified protocols to the "gold standard" (see Table 20.6).

20.4.3.1 Basal Insulin Action

In the fasting state, insulin serves to inhibit hepatic glucose production, limit mobilization of fat from adipose tissue and maintain basal glucose uptake in insulin-responsive tissues. In so doing, the liver can meet the glucose demands of tissues such as the brain. In insulin-resistant states, glucose requirements do not change, but pancreatic insulin secretion must increase to maintain the same rate of hepatic glucose production as basal glucose requirements by the brain and other tissues including muscle are not markedly altered. If it does not increase, the glucose concentration will rise. Thus, in insulin-resistant states, fasting hyperinsulinemia is commonly seen.

A commonly used approach to quantify insulin action is to measure fasting insulin and glucose concentration, and calculate an index of insulin action from those data (Table 20.6). In the human, a homeostasis model assessment (HOMA) is calculated from fasting plasma insulin (FPI) and fasting plasma glucose (FPG) data obtained from an overnight fasted individual. It can be used to predict β-cell function (HOMA—%B = [20 × FPI]/[FPG − 3.5]) and insulin action (HOMA-IR = [FPI × FPG]/22.5) (Wallace et al., 2004). A more improved HOMA (HOMA2) can be calculated using a computer model. This has been used in nonhuman primates with good success (Zhang et al., 2011). Other calculations can be made, such as quantitative S_I check index (QUICKI). This has been less commonly used in canines. The extent of the fasting hyperinsulinemia after a high-caloric diet is less consistent despite the presence of overt insulin resistance when a more sensitive and provocative test (intravenous or oral GTT or hyperinsulinemic-euglycemic clamp; see Section 20.4.3.4 for more details in these tests) can detect insulin resistance (Coate et al., 2010; Stefanovski et al., 2011). Recently, investigators have begun calculating HOMA-IR for mouse and rat studies (Muniyappa et al., 2009). However, this calculation assumes that the model parameters for mice are the same as for humans. One study found that the correlation between HOMA-IR and clamp estimates of insulin action was rather poor in mice and rats (Lee et al., 2008). The correlation could be improved,

TABLE 20.6
Measures of Insulin Sensitivity in Animal[a] Models

Direct Measure of Insulin Action	
Hyperinsulinemic-euglycemic clamp	M = steady state glucose infusion rate SI_{clamp} = M/(G × DI) where, G is the glucose concentration and DI is the difference in the insulin concentration between the clamp and basal insulin
Frequently sampled IVGTT	S_I calculated from MINMOD model
Basal Insulin Action	
G/I ratio	ratio of fasting plasma glucose (mg/dL) and insulin (μU/mL)
HOMA	HOMA-IR = fasting plasma insulin (μU/mL) × fasting plasma glucose (mM)/22.5
QUICKI	1/[Log (fasting plasma insulin, μU/mL) + Log (fasting plasma glucose, mg/dL)]

[a] The use of these calculations for mammals other than humans has not been critically evaluated.

if the data were normalized to body weight and log transformed. This approach is similar to the approach used in humans (Wallace et al., 2004). As mentioned in Section 20.4.1, in larger species, overnight fasting is appropriate. However, insulin and glucose concentration are markedly decreased in overnight-fasted mice resulting in an apparent marked improvement (decrease in HOMA-IR) in insulin action (Andrikopoulos et al., 2008). This improvement may or may not correlate with clamp assessment of insulin action (Lee et al., 2008; Ayala et al., 2006). A 6-hour fast allows for good discrimination of insulin action between chow and high-fat–fed mice, especially when HOMA-IR is calculated. Others have calculated the ratio of glucose to insulin (Dokmanovic-Chouinard et al., 2008) as a marker of insulin action. These surrogate indices of insulin action (many of which have not been validated for rodents) reflect basal insulin action. Since in large species (human, nonhuman primate, dog) the major fraction of the glucose is taken up by insulin-independent tissues (i.e., brain), basal estimates of insulin action are likely weighted to reflect hepatic as opposed to peripheral insulin action. In smaller species, such as the mouse, the brain is a relatively minor contributor to basal glucose utilization. A change in HOMA-IR in mice likely reflects the combined effects of insulin action in hepatic and peripheral tissues.

20.4.3.2 Glucose Tolerance Test

The term *glucose tolerance* describes the shape of the plasma glucose curve in the oral (OGTT) or intraperitoneal (IPGTT) glucose tolerance test or the shape and rate of disappearance of glucose in the intravenous glucose tolerance test (IVGTT). In comparison to a normal tolerance curve, the curve expressing glucose intolerance describes one with a very high peak and a slow return to fasting concentrations. The test was originally developed to identify individuals who have diabetes or have increased risk of developing diabetes (impaired glucose tolerance). Many investigators tried to quantify glucose tolerance so as to compare groups. However, it is important that investigators realize glucose tolerance and S_I are not synonymous. Glucose tolerance is influenced by the combined effects of three parameters:

- β-cell function
- Insulin action
- Glucose-mediated glucose disposal

As such, glucose tolerance is not a measure of insulin action. In the case of oral glucose delivery, the glucose excursion tends to be more variable, as it is also influenced by the rate of gastric emptying, glucose absorption, and any effects of incretins.

The GTT is commonly used to evaluate whether the animal can efficiently dispose of a defined glucose load. Many variations exist in GTTs conducted for diagnostic purposes in clinical medicine. They are generally not used to quantify glucose tolerance, but rather to detect glucose intolerance and diabetes. For the purpose of evaluating the laboratory animal, the need exists for establishing and defining a more narrowly reproducible result than is normally required so investigators can quantify glucose tolerance to assess whether their experimental manipulation improves or exacerbates glucose tolerance. Generally, one of two forms of the GTT is used: the oral (OGTT) or intravenous (IVGTT) test (in rodents; IPGTT).

Glucose tolerance can be assessed by administering glucose (IV, IP, or oral) and taking a limited number of blood samples in appropriately fasted animals. The IVGTT is widely used in the larger of the laboratory animals, particularly the dog, cat, and nonhuman primate, and it is also useful in the rabbit (Vicini and Cobelli, 2001; O'Brien et al., 1985; Leow, 1997; Beard et al., 1986; Finegood et al., 1984). For the IVGTT, a standard load of glucose is infused intravenously after a conditioning regimen similar to that for the OGTT. The standard glucose load of 0.5 g/kg body weight is sufficient to provoke a maximal insulin response and to permit reliable evaluations of glucose clearance in dogs, nonhuman primates and humans (Rottiers et al., 1981). Glucose loads greater than 0.5 g/kg are rapidly excreted in the urine and do not directly reflect the glucometabolic status of the dog (Kaneko, 1997). In the standard IVGTT, a preinfusion blood sample is taken, and the glucose load of 0.5 g/kg bw is infused as a sterile 50% solution in 30 seconds. Timing for the test is begun at the midpoint of the infusion period. Subsequent blood samples are taken at 5, 15, 25, 35, 45, and 60 minutes for glucose and insulin. The glucose concentrations are plotted on semilogarithmic coordinates versus time. The half-life ($T_{1/2}$) is calculated or can be graphically estimated from a linear segment of the disappearance curve (Rottiers et al., 1981). The time interval must be established for each species because the rate of glucose disappearance is truly a curve and is only quasilinear at certain time intervals. The half time is calculated or read from the linear portion of the curve, and the fractional turnover rate or *K* value can be calculated from the relationship:

$$\text{Fractional turnover rate}(K) = 0.693 / T_{1/2} \times 100 = \%/\text{m}$$

The fractional turnover rate has been described as the glucose turnover rate, glucose disappearance rate, glucose clearance rate, glucose disappearance coefficient, or simply the *K* value. In fact glucose clearance rate, turnover rate, and glucose disappearance rate are not the same as *K* or fractional turnover rate. Glucose clearance rate (mL/min or $mL \cdot kg^{-1}\ min^{-1}$) is equal to the product of *K* and the volume of distribution of glucose divided by 100. Glucose turnover rate and disappearance rate (= glucose clearance rate × plasma glucose concentration; mg/min or $mg \cdot kg^{-1}\ min^{-1}$) represent absolute fluxes of glucose and should not be used as a steady state is not present. In fact, their rate changes as the glucose concentration changes during the GTT. Using this standardized method, the reference range for $T_{1/2}$ in the dog is 15–45 minutes (25 ± 8 minutes) and a *K* value greater than 1.5%/min. The diabetic curve with its slower rate of glucose disappearance results in a half-time longer than 45 minutes, which calculates into a *K* value of less than 1.5%/min (Kaneko, 1997). In rats glucose (0.5–1 g/kg) can be injected via the tail vein and samples can be taken (5, 10, 15, 30, 60, 90, and 120 minutes) from the tail vein artery (Holemans et al., 2004; Lim et al., 2011). In mice, the dose of glucose is higher (1–2 g/kg; IP or per os [po]) and for practical reasons, it is only given by intraperitoneal injection or oral gavage. The glucose concentrations are monitored every 30 minutes between 0 and 120 minutes (Ayala et al., 2010). The glucose excursions are much higher in mice, but the renal glucose threshold is also higher (~400 mg/dL) (Noonan and Banks, 2000). As it is difficult to accurately calculate *K* from the limited time points using the rodent protocol, the area under the curve after subtracting the baseline glucose concentration can be used as an index of glucose tolerance. However, the kinetics of glucose disposal are rather fast after intravenous glucose delivery, and detecting impairments in glucose tolerance in insulin-resistant rat models is less reliable without accompanying insulin data (Varcoe et al., 2011). This helps to reinforce the fact that the GTT is not a measure of insulin action as compensatory increases in β-cell function can minimize any overt glucose intolerance. Generally, the glucose excursion is attenuated when glucose is given orally due to the combined effect of delayed gastric emptying, greater first pass hepatic glucose extraction and the effects of incretins (Andrikopoulos et al., 2008). In mice, higher doses of glucose may be better at allowing detection of impaired GTT in a high-fat–fed model (Morino et al., 2008). Interestingly, in cats, glucose tolerance is prolonged compared with other species. This is likely due in part to the fact the cat is an exclusive carnivore. Moreover, the feline liver has very little glucokinase or its binding partner glucokinase regulatory protein, which are essential for the liver to dispose of significant amounts of glucose (Ballard, 1965; Kienzle, 1994; Hiskett et al., 2009).

A number of factors should be considered when using the GTT. Glucose tolerance will be affected by the route of glucose delivery. Ideally, samples should be taken to define the rate of rise and fall in glucose until it returns to baseline values. Depending on the species and its metabolic state, the dose of glucose will have to be adjusted. It is important that the glucose concentration during the GTT not exceed the renal threshold, which is ~180 mg/dL in large species (canine and primate), ~270 mg/dL in rats and ~400 mg/dL in mice (López-Novoa et al., 1996; Noonan and Banks, 2000). Two groups could have differing baseline glucose values; baseline glucose values should be subtracted before calculating area under the curve. While area under the curve is informative in a manuscript, it is best to report the actual glucose values as well. The actual glucose values can give additional information as to the rate of rise and fall of glucose. This could give hints as to possible defects in pancreatic function or in the case of oral glucose delivery, changes in rate of glucose absorption.

The majority of exogenous glucose is disposed of by lean body tissues. If the dose of glucose is given on a per body weight basis, obese animals will be biased to have impaired glucose tolerance. If one is comparing animals with differing body composition, a fixed dose of glucose as is used in humans (e.g., 75 g) in mice could be used. In mice, a dose of 40 mg may suffice. Or ideally if lean body mass could be assessed, the dose could be normalized per lean body weight. In humans and primates, the dose can be normalized to body surface area.

To obtain more information from a GTT, the frequently sampled intravenous GTT (FSIGTT) can be used to assess β-cell function and insulin action. It requires rapid sampling of blood for both glucose and insulin following an intravenous glucose challenge. The data are then analyzed using the minimal model of Bergman and Cobelli, which was originally developed for the dog. It has since been adapted for humans and nonhuman primates (Bergman et al., 1985; Casu et al., 2008). After an overnight fast, an intravenous bolus of glucose (0.3–0.5 g/kg body wt) is infused over 2 minutes starting at time zero. Blood samples are taken for plasma glucose and insulin measurements at –10, –1, 1, 2, 3, 4, 5, 6, 7, 8, 10, 12, 14, 16, 20, 22, 23, 24, 25, 27, 30, 40, 50, 60, 70, 80, 90, 100, 120, 160, and 180 minutes. The approach requires a lot of blood samples and vascular access for injection and sampling. In addition, these data have to be analyzed using the computer program MINMOD to generate an index of S_I. The model, while robust, does oversimplify glucose homeostasis and lumps together hepatic and peripheral insulin action. Moreover, the accuracy of estimating S_I decreases in models where β-cell function or insulin action is low. The protocol was modified in humans with impaired β-cell function; exogenous insulin (4 $mU{\cdot}kg^{-1}$ min^{-1}) is infused over 5 minutes beginning 20 minutes after the intravenous glucose bolus (Quon et al., 1994; Ionut et al., 2009). In some studies, a bolus of insulin or a sulfonylurea is given to augment insulin availability, so a better estimate of S_I can be obtained. The FSIGTT was adapted for mice, pigs, and rats (Di Nardo et al., 2009; Christoffersen et al., 2009). However, the amount of blood required is substantial and will deplete total blood volume, if applied to mice (Ahren and Pacini, 2006).

20.4.3.3 Insulin Tolerance Test

In human studies, a quick test was developed to assess insulin action. This was termed the short insulin tolerance test (ITT). The basis of the test is to give overnight fasted humans an intravenous bolus of insulin (0.1–0.5 U/kg) and assess the rate of fall of plasma glucose. Glucose concentration is assessed every 2 minutes over a 15-minute period (Wallace and Matthews, 2002). Insulin action is calculated as the rate of fall of the log transformed glucose concentration. An important aspect of the design is to focus on the early rate of fall in glucose so as not to have the complicating effects of glucose counter-regulation and hypoglycemia. The ITT that is used in humans is relatively reliable and can be, but is rarely, used in nonrodent (e.g., canine) species.

The ITT has been adapted to the mouse, but the protocol has been substantially modified with no consistent approach (Cederroth et al., 2008; Dallaire et al., 2008; Duncan et al., 2008; Feral et al., 2008; Gomez-Valades et al., 2008; Jiang et al., 2008; Kebede et al., 2008; Li et al., 2008; Nieto-Vazquez et al., 2008; Oriente et al., 2008). Generally, mice are either not fasted or are fasted for a very brief period (0–3 hours). The dose of insulin is given intraperitoneally (0.5–2 U/kg), and the glucose is monitored over a longer duration (glucose assessed at 0, 20, 40, 60, and 120 minutes). Unfortunately, the modified design has major problems (McGuinness et al., 2009). Investigators did not consider that by 60 minutes most of the insulin injected has been metabolized and the higher doses of insulin increases the risk of hypoglycemia. Moreover, the abbreviated fast increases the risk of an unstable glucose baseline as food absorption abates, and the animal progresses into the fast. Thus, based on our experience, we do not recommend the modified ITT for mice. For larger species (rat, pig, dog, and primate) where limitations in blood volume is less of a concern and vascular access can be easily achieved, a short (<30 minutes) ITT can be used (Christoffersen et al.,

2009; Ropelle et al., 2009). A technical note is that insulin will stick to plastic further increasing the variability of the data. If insulin has to be diluted prior to injection, either obtain the insulin diluent from the company that provides the insulin (usually the pharmacy can obtain it) or dilute it with saline containing 0.3% serum from the species you are testing.

20.4.3.4 Hyperinsulinemic-Euglycemic Clamp

The hyperinsulinemic-euglycemic clamp is referred to as the gold standard upon which all other indices of insulin action are evaluated (Defronzo et al., 1979). Investigators recognized that the reliability and accuracy of the method depended upon standardization of procedures and the ability of the investigator to clamp glucose concentrations to obtain a metabolic steady state. The principle of the clamp is that a defined insulin infusion is given at a constant rate into a peripheral vein that will increase arterial insulin concentration. To prevent glucose concentration from decreasing, glucose is infused at a variable rate to maintain euglycemia. Typically, the clamp is ~120 minutes in duration and glucose is measured at least every 10 minutes. Usually, after 90 minutes into the clamp method, a steady state for the glucose infusion rate is reached, and the glucose infusion rate (GIR; mg·kg^{-1}/min^{-1}) is reflective of insulin action, if the insulin concentration during the clamp is measured and is comparable between groups. While there are algorithms available for clamping, an experienced investigator can empirically obtain a good clamp (Furler et al., 1986).

There are a number of important assumptions and considerations when designing and interpreting clamp data. At a given insulin concentration, GIR is a measure of insulin action, if endogenous (i.e., hepatic glucose production) is completely suppressed. Since a steady state is assumed to have been reached at the end of the clamp, whole body glucose utilization (= GIR + endogenous glucose production) will be underestimated by the amount of glucose still being released by the liver. Thus, enough insulin needs to be infused to be confident that endogenous glucose production is completely suppressed. However, if a very large insulin dose is used, it is difficult to see differences between models that are only moderately insulin resistant and the maximal rates of insulin-stimulated glucose disposal are very similar (i.e., shift in K_m but no change in V_{max}). If two groups are being compared, the glucose and insulin concentrations during the clamp should be matched. The insulin dose is typically given on a per body surface area in humans. In many rodent studies, the insulin dose is based on body weight. Increased adiposity can increase the insulin concentrations obtained during the clamp, if the dose is administered on a per body weight basis. Thus, it is critical that insulin concentration is measured in both in the basal and clamp periods. For animal models with severe insulin resistance, a much higher insulin concentration will have to be attained during the clamp to augment whole body glucose disposal so as to detect a change in insulin action. For individuals who wish to assess hepatic insulin action, lower doses of insulin and a glucose tracer will have to be infused. The tracer will allow the investigator to assess the extent of suppression of endogenous glucose production and the total rate of whole body glucose disposal.

In clamp studies, the ideal sites for glucose and insulin infusion are into a peripheral vein, and blood samples should be taken from an artery. If a vein is used for sampling, it should drain tissues that are not metabolically active. If the vein drains metabolically active tissues, the difference between arterial and venous glucose concentration during the clamp will be greatest in the most insulin-responsive animals. This will bias one to overestimate how insulin-responsive the most sensitive animals are, as they will be clamped at higher arterial glucose concentrations, even though the venous glucose concentrations will be equivalent. In humans, a heated hand vein is commonly used, as the glucose concentration in the vein reflects the arterial glucose concentration. In large animals, an artery is commonly used. In rodents, a tail vein can be used, if surgical implantation of an artery is not practical for the laboratory. Collecting blood from the tail is stressful in mice, if a significant volume of blood (>10 μL) has to be obtained at each time point.

Some specific comments should be made about clamp studies in mice. Performing clamp studies is not easy in mice, especially in conscious, unstressed mice. Their small size and limited blood volume severely limits the number of investigators who can successfully perform a clamp in mice

(McGuinness et al., 2009; Wasserman et al., 2009). Moreover, the genetic background can have a marked effect on insulin action and pancreatic function (Berglund et al., 2008). This can confound interpretation of studies using mice on mixed backgrounds. Ideally, litter mates of the same gender are the best controls.

20.4.3.5 Assessing β-Cell Function

As mentioned in Section 20.4.3.2, abnormal glucose tolerance could be due to defects in β cell function. There are three basic approaches to assess β-cell function. The first is to measure basal glucose and insulin concentrations and calculate HOMA%B using the HOMA model an estimate of β-cell function (Wallace et al., 2004). The appropriateness of this approach for species other than humans is unclear. Essentially, what the model allows one to do is determine if the insulin concentration is appropriate for the prevailing glucose concentration. If the insulin concentration is less than one might predict, a defect in β-cell function would be suspected. This calculation is very model dependent. In addition, in the basal state, β cells are not being challenged, thus this approach is very insensitive to small alterations in β-cell function. The two other approaches use provocative tests to evaluate the ability of the β cell to respond to a hyperglycemic stimulus. These are the hyperglycemic clamp and the FSIGTT; the latter was discussed in Section 20.4.3.2. In the FSIGTT, the time course of both insulin and glucose are assessed after an intravenous bolus of glucose. The data are put into a model (note using human parameters) and an estimate of β-cell function can be obtained. It has been used in mice to assess β-cell function (Alonso et al., 2012). Because of the large number of samples and the large amount of blood that will have to be taken, we do not recommend it for mice; unless blood is reinfused at each time point to minimize changes in blood volume and the hematocrit. The hyperglycemic clamp can be used to assess β-cell function. The study must be done in animals with direct vascular access. In large animals, a saphenous or cephalic vein can be cannulated. In rodents, a jugular cannula inserted 3–5 days in advance using sterile techniques will be required. This site will be used for the continuous infusion of glucose. A separate site for blood samples will be needed as well (e.g., artery). Typically, glucose is infused to approximately double the plasma glucose concentration. The glucose concentration is held at the target glucose concentration for ~90 minutes, and the insulin concentration is assessed at baseline and during the clamp. This approach allows one to assess both the first phase and second phase insulin secretion (Mager et al., 2004; Postic et al., 1999). In humans, it is the first-phase insulin secretion that is lost early in the progression of the type 2 DM (DeFronzo and Abdul-Ghani, 2011). Depending on whether one wants to assess first and/or second phase insulin secretion will determine the frequency of measurement of glucose and insulin concentrations.

20.5 SUMMARY

The basic control systems used by mammals to regulate carbohydrate metabolism are shared among species, and there are many different animal models available to study carbohydrate metabolism in normal and disease states. Each species and model has its advantages and disadvantages. If an investigator's goal is to translate observations made in a particular species to humans, appreciating the differences between species will be very helpful in optimizing experimental design. Thus, knowledge of the differences in species and appropriate research tools actually aids in understanding how these control systems regulate metabolism in all mammals.

REFERENCES

Aasland, K.E., Skjerve, E., and Smith, A.J. 2010. Quality of blood samples from the saphenous vein compared with the tail vein during multiple blood sampling of mice. *Lab Anim.* 44:25–29.

Ahren, B. and Pacini, G. 2006. A novel approach to assess insulin sensitivity reveals no increased insulin sensitivity in mice with a dominant-negative mutant hepatocyte nuclear factor-1{alpha}. *Am J Physiol Regul Integr Comp Physiol.* 291:R131–137.

Allan, M.F., Eisen, E.J., and Pomp, D. 2004. The M16 mouse: An outbred animal model of early onset polygenic obesity and diabesity. *Obes Res.* 12:1397–1407.

Alonso, L.C., Watanabe, Y., Stefanovski, D., et al. 2012. Simultaneous measurement of insulin sensitivity, insulin secretion, and the disposition index in conscious unhandled mice. *Obesity.* 20:1403–1412.

Amirshahrokhi, K., Dehpour, A.R., Hadjati, J., Sotoudeh, M., and Ghazi-Khansari, M. 2008. Methadone ameliorates multiple-low-dose streptozotocin-induced type 1 diabetes in mice. *Toxicol Appl Pharmacol.* 232:119–124.

Anderson, H.R., Stitt, A.W., Gardiner, T.A., Lloyd, S.J., and Archer, D.B. 1993. Induction of alloxan/streptozotocin diabetes in dogs: A revised experimental technique. *Lab Anim.* 27:281–285.

Andrikopoulos, S., Blair, A.R., Deluca, N., Fam, B.C., and Proietto, J. 2008. Evaluating the glucose tolerance test in mice. *Am J Physiol Endocrinol Metab.* 295:E1323–1332.

Annunziata, M., Granata, R., and Ghigo, E. 2011. The IGF system. *Acta Diabetologica.* 48:1–9.

Armbruster, D.A. 1987. Fructosamine: Structure, analysis, and clinical usefulness. *Clin Chem.* 33:2153–2163.

Ayala, J.E., Bracy, D., McGuinness, O.P., and Wasserman, D.H. 2006. Considerations in the design of hyperinsulinemic-euglycemic clamps in the conscious mouse. Diabetes. 55:390–397.

Ayala, J.E., Samuel, V.T., Morton, G.J., et al. 2010. Standard operating procedures for describing and performing metabolic tests of glucose homeostasis in mice. *Dis Model Mech.* 3:525–534.

Bachrach, B.E., Weinstein, D.A., Orho-Melander, M., Burgess, A., and Wolfsdorf, J.I. 2002. Glycogen synthase deficiency (glycogen storage disease type 0) presenting with hyperglycemia and glucosuria: Report of three new mutations. *J Pediatr.* 140:781–783.

Baggio, L.L. and Drucker, D.J. 2007. Biology of incretins: GLP-1 and GIP. *Gastroenterology.* 132:2131–2157.

Ballard, F.J. 1965. Glucose utilization in mammalian liver. *Comp Biochem Physiol.* 14:437–443.

Banarer, S. and Cryer, P.E. 2004. Hypoglycemia in type 2 diabetes. *Med Clin North Am.* 88:1107–1116.

Bao, Y., Kishnani, P., Wu, J.Y., and Chen, Y.T. 1996. Hepatic and neuromuscular forms of glycogen storage disease type IV caused by mutations in the same glycogen-branching enzyme gene. *J Clin Invest.* 97:941–948.

Beard, J.C., Bergman, R.N., Ward, W.K., and Porte, D. Jr. 1986. The insulin sensitivity index in nondiabetic man. Correlation between clamp-derived and IVGTT-derived values. *Diabetes.* 35:362–369.

Bederman, I.R., Foy, S., Chandramouli, V., Alexander, J.C., and Previs, S.F. 2009. Triglyceride synthesis in epididymal adipose tissue. *J Biol Chem.* 284:6101–6108.

Beech, J.S., Williams, S.R., Cohen, R.D., and Iles, R.A. 1989. Gluconeogenesis and the protection of hepatic intracellular pH during diabetic ketoacidosis in rats. *Biochem J.* 263:737–744.

Bennett, N. 2002. Monitoring techniques for diabetes mellitus in the dog and the cat. *Clin Tech Small Anim Pract.* 17:65–69.

Berglund, E.D., Li, C.Y., Poffenberger, G., et al. 2008. Glucose metabolism in vivo in four commonly used inbred mouse strains. *Diabetes.* 57:1790–1799.

Bergman, R.N., Finegood, D.T., and Ader, M. 1985. Assessment of insulin sensitivity in vivo. *Endocr Rev.* 6:45–86.

Bevilacqua, S., Barrett, E.J., Smith, D., et al. 1985. Hepatic and peripheral insulin resistance following streptozotocin-induced insulin deficiency in the dog. *Metabolism.* 34:817–825.

Bjorkman, O. and Eriksson, L.S. 1985. Influence of a 60-hour fast on insulin-mediated splanchnic and peripheral glucose metabolism in humans. *J Clin Invest.* 76:87–92.

Black, H.E., Rosenblum, I.Y., and Capen, C.C. 1980. Chemically induced (streptozotocin–alloxan) diabetes mellitus in the dog. Biochemical and ultrastructural studies. *Am J Pathol.* 98:295–310.

Bonser, A.M., Peter Garcia-Webb., and Harrison, L.C. 1984. C-Peptide measurement: Methods and clinical utility. *Crit Rev Clin Lab Sci.* 19:297–352.

Boren, S.A. and Clarke, W.L. 2010. Analytical and clinical performance of blood glucose monitors. *J Diabetes Sci Technol.* 4:84–97.

Brumback, R.A. 1980. Iodoacetate inhibition of glyceraldehyde-3-phosphate dehydrogenase as a model of human myophosphorylase deficiency (McArdle's disease) and phosphofructokinase deficiency (Tarui's disease). *J Neurol Sci.* 48:383–398.

Burcelin, R., Eddouks, M., Maury, J., Kande, J., Assan, R., and Girard, J. 1995. Excessive glucose production, rather than insulin resistance, accounts for hyperglycaemia in recent-onset streptozotocin-diabetic rats. *Diabetologia.* 38:283–290.

Castillo, M.J., Scheen, A.J., Letiexhe, M.R., and Lefebvre, P.J. 1994. How to measure insulin clearance. *Diabetes Metab Rev.* 10:119–150.

Casu, A., Bottino, R., Balamurugan, A., et al. 2008. Metabolic aspects of pig-to-monkey (*Macaca fascicularis*) islet transplantation: Implications for translation into clinical practice. *Diabetologia.* 51:120–129.

Catchpole, B., Kennedy, L.J., Davison, L.J., and Ollier, W.E.R. 2008. Canine diabetes mellitus: From phenotype to genotype. *J Small Anim Pract.* 49:4–10.

Cederroth, C.R., Vinciguerra, M., Gjinovci, A., et al. 2008. Dietary phytoestrogens activate AMP-activated protein kinase with improvement in lipid and glucose metabolism. *Diabetes.* 57:1176–1185.

Chang, A.Y. 1981. Biochemical abnormalities in the Chinese hamster (*Cricetulus griseus*) with spontaneous diabetes. *Int J Biochem.* 13:41–43.

Chen, L.Y., Shieh, J.J., Lin, B., et al. 2003. Impaired glucose homeostasis, neutrophil trafficking and function in mice lacking the glucose-6-phosphate transporter. *Hum Mol Genet.* 12:2547–2558.

Cherrington, A.D. 1999. Control of glucose uptake and release by the liver in vivo. *Diabetes.* 48:1198–1214.

Cheung, Y.Y., Kim, S.Y., Yiu, W.H., et al. 2007. Impaired neutrophil activity and increased susceptibility to bacterial infection in mice lacking glucose-6-phosphatase-beta. *J Clin Invest.* 117:784–793.

Cho, Y.R., Kim, H.J., Park, S.Y., et al. 2007. Hyperglycemia, maturity-onset obesity, and insulin resistance in NONcNZO10/LtJ males, a new mouse model of type 2 diabetes. *Am J Physiol Endocrinol Metab.* 293:E327–336.

Chong, M.F.F., Fielding, B.A., and Frayn, K.N. 2007. Metabolic interaction of dietary sugars and plasma lipids with a focus on mechanisms and de novo lipogenesis. *Proc Nutr Soc.* 66:52–59.

Christensen, S.D., Mikkelsen, L.F., Fels, J.J., Bodvarsdottir, T.B., and Hansen, A.K. 2009. Quality of plasma sampled by different methods for multiple blood sampling in mice. *Lab Anim.* 43:65–71.

Christoffersen, B., Ulla Ribel, K.R., Golozoubova, V., and Pacini, G. 2009. Evaluation of different methods for assessment of insulin sensitivity in Göttingen minipigs: Introduction of a new, simpler method. *Am J Physiol Regul Integr Comp Physiol.* 297:R1195–R1201.

Chueh, F.Y., Malabanan, C., and McGuinness, O.P. 2006. Impact of portal glucose delivery on glucose metabolism in conscious, unrestrained mice. *Am J Physiol Endocrinol Metab.* 291:E1206–1211.

Clemmons, D.R. 1997. Insulin-like growth factor binding proteins and their role in controlling IGF actions. *Cytokine Growth Factor Rev.* 8:45–62.

Clifton, P.G. 2000. Meal patterning in rodents: Psychopharmacological and neuroanatomical studies. *Neurosci Biobehav Rev.* 24:213–222.

Coate, K.C., Scott, M., Farmer, B., et al. 2010. Chronic consumption of a high-fat/high-fructose diet renders the liver incapable of net hepatic glucose uptake. *Am J Physiol.* 299:E887–E898.

Cohen, R.M. and Smith, E.P. 2008. Frequency of HbA1c discordance in estimating blood glucose control. *Curr Opin Clin Nutr Metab Care.* 11:512–517.

Cohn, L.A., McCaw, D.L., Tate, D.J., and Johnson, J.C. 2000. Assessment of five portable blood glucose meters, a point-of-care analyzer, and color test strips for measuring blood glucose concentration in dogs. *J Am Vet Med Assoc.* 216:198–202.

Cruzen, C. and Colman, R.J. 2009. Effects of caloric restriction on cardiovascular aging in non-human primates and humans. *Clin Geriatr Med.* 25:733–743, ix–x.

Cryer, P.E. 2010. Hypoglycemia in type 1 diabetes mellitus. *Endocrinol Metab Clin North Am.* 39:641–654.

Cryer, P.E. 2012. Minireview: Glucagon in the pathogenesis of hypoglycemia and hyperglycemia in diabetes. *Endocrinology.* 153:1039–1048.

Cryer, P.E., Binder, C., Bolli, G.B., et al. 1989. Hypoglycemia in IDDM. *Diabetes.* 38:1193–1199.

Dallaire, P., Bellmann, K., Laplante, M., et al. 2008. Obese mice lacking inducible nitric oxide synthase are sensitized to the metabolic actions of peroxisome proliferator-activated receptor-{gamma} agonism. *Diabetes.* 57:1999–2011.

Dardevet, D., Komori, K., Grunfeld, C., Rosenzweig, S.A., and Buse, M.G. 1991. Increased hepatic insulin proreceptor-to-receptor ratio in diabetes: A possible processing defect. *Am J Physiol.* 261:E562–571.

Davis, M.A., Williams, P.E., and Cherrington, A.D. 1984. Effect of a mixed meal on hepatic lactate and gluconeogenic precursor metabolism in dogs. *Am J Physiol.* 247:E362–369.

Davis, S.N., Dobbins, R., Tarumi, C., Colburn, C., Neal, D., and Cherrington, A.D. 1992. Effects of differing insulin levels on response to equivalent hypoglycemia in conscious dogs. *Am J Physiol.* 263 (Pt 1):E688–695.

Davis, S.N., Goldstein, R.E., Cherrington, A.D., and Price, L. 1994. Exaggerated epinephrine response to hypoglycemia in a physically fit, well-controlled IDDM subject. *Diabetes Res Clin Pract.* 22:139–146.

DeFronzo, R.A. and Abdul-Ghani, M.A. 2011. Preservation of β-cell function: The key to diabetes prevention. *J Clin Endocrinol Metab.* 96:2354–2366.

Defronzo, R.A., Tobin, J., and Andres, R. 1979. Glucose clamp technique a method for quantifying insulin secretion and resistance. *Am J Physiol.* 237:E214–E218.

Di Marino, L., Griffo, E., Maione, S., and Mirabella, M. 2011. Active glucagon-like peptide-1 (GLP-1): Storage of human plasma and stability over time. *Clin Chim Acta.* 412:1693–1694.

Di Mauro, S. 2007. Muscle glycogenoses: An overview. *Acta Myol.* 26:35–41.

Di Nardo, F., Burattini, R., Cogo, C.E., Faelli, E., and Ruggeri, P. 2009. Age-related analysis of insulin resistance, body weight and arterial pressure in the Zucker fatty rat. *Exp Physiol.* 94:162–168.

Dietschy, J.M. 1997. Theoretical considerations of what regulates low-density-lipoprotein and high-density-lipoprotein cholesterol. *Am J Clin Nutr.* 65:1581S–1589S.

Ding, E.Y., Hodges, B.L., Hu, H., et al. 2001. Long-term efficacy after [E1-, polymerase-] adenovirus-mediated transfer of human acid-alpha-glucosidase gene into glycogen storage disease type II knockout mice. *Hum Gene Ther.* 12:955–965.

Dokmanovic-Chouinard, M., Chung, W.K., Chevre, J.C., et al. 2008. Positional cloning of "Lisch-like," a candidate modifier of susceptibility to type 2 diabetes in mice. *PLOS Genet.* 4:e1000137.

D'Orazio, P., Burnett, R.W., Fogh-Andersen, N., et al. 2006. Approved IFCC recommendation on reporting results for blood glucose: International Federation of Clinical Chemistry and Laboratory Medicine Scientific Division, Working Group on Selective Electrodes and Point-of-Care Testing (IFCC-SD-WG-SEPOCT). *Clin Chem Lab Med.* 44:1486–1490.

Drucker, D.J. 2007. The role of gut hormones in glucose homeostasis. *J Clin Invest.* 117:24–32.

Duckworth, W.C., Bennett, R.G., and Hamel, F.G. 1998. Insulin degradation: Progress and potential. *Endocr Rev.* 19:608–624.

Duncan, E.R., Crossey, P.A., Walker, S., et al. 2008. Effect of endothelium-specific insulin resistance on endothelial function in vivo. *Diabetes.* 57:3307–3314.

Echaniz-Laguna, A., Akman, H.O., Mohr, M., et al. 2010. Muscle phosphorylase b kinase deficiency revisited. *Neuromuscul Disord.* 20:125–127.

Ellacott, K.L., Morton, G.J., Woods, S.C., Tso, P., and Schwartz, M.W. 2010. Assessment of feeding behavior in laboratory mice. *Cell Metab.* 12:10–17.

Elliott, D.A., Nelson, R.W., Feldman, E.C., and Neal, L.A. 1997. Glycosylated hemoglobin concentrations in the blood of healthy dogs and dogs with naturally developing diabetes mellitus, pancreatic beta-cell neoplasia, hyperadrenocorticism, and anemia. *J Am Vet Med Assoc.* 211:723–727.

Feral, C.C., Neels, J.G., Kummer, C., Slepak, M., Olefsky, J.M., and Ginsberg, M.H. 2008. Blockade of {alpha}4 integrin signaling ameliorates the metabolic consequences of high-fat diet-induced obesity. *Diabetes.* 57:1842–1851.

Finegood, D.T., Pacini, G., and Bergman, R.N. 1984. The insulin sensitivity index. Correlation in dogs between values determined from the intravenous glucose tolerance test and the euglycemic glucose clamp. *Diabetes.* 33:362–368.

Friedman, J.E., de Vente, J.E., Peterson, R.G., and Dohm, G.L. 1991. Altered expression of muscle glucose transporter GLUT-4 in diabetic fatty Zucker rats (ZDF/Drt-fa). *Am J Physiol Endocrinol Metab.* 261:E782–788.

Frystyk, J. 2007. Utility of free IGF-I measurements. *Pituitary.* 10:181–187.

Furler, S.M., Zelenka, G.S., and Kraegen, E.W. 1986. Development and testing of a simple algorithm for a glucose clamp. *Med Biol Eng Comput.* 24:365–370.

Fyfe, J.C., Giger, U., Van Winkle, T.J., et al. 1992. Glycogen storage disease type IV: Inherited deficiency of branching enzyme activity in cats. *Pediatr Res.* 32:719–725.

Geiser, F. 2004. Metabolic rate and body temperature reduction during hibernation and daily torpor. *Annu Rev Physiol.* 66:239–274.

German, A.J. 2006. The growing problem of obesity in dogs and cats. *J Nutr.* 136:1940S–1946S.

German, A.J., Ryan, V.H., German, A.C., Wood, I.S., and Trayhurn, P. 2010. Obesity, its associated disorders and the role of inflammatory adipokines in companion animals. *Vet J.* 185:4–9.

Giaccari, A. and Rossetti, L. 1992. Predominant role of gluconeogenesis in the hepatic glycogen repletion of diabetic rats. *J Clin Invest.* 89:36–45.

Gibson, R., Zhao, Y., Jaskiewicz, J., Fineberg, S.E., and Harris, R.A. 1993. Effects of diabetes on the activity and content of the branched-chain alpha-ketoacid dehydrogenase complex in liver. *Arch Biochem Biophys.* 306:22–28.

Gomez-Valades, A.G., Mendez-Lucas, A., Vidal-Alabro, A., et al. 2008. Pck1 gene silencing in the liver improves glycemia control, insulin sensitivity, and dyslipidemia in db/db mice. *Diabetes.* 57:2199–2210.

Greene, H.L., Brown, B.I., McClenathan, D.T., Agostini, R.M. Jr., and Taylor, S.R. 1988. A new variant of type IV glycogenosis: Deficiency of branching enzyme activity without apparent progressive liver disease. *Hepatology.* 8:302–306.

Gronbaek, H., Nielsen, B., Schrijvers, B., Vogel, I., Rasch, R., and Flyvbjerg, A. 2002. Inhibitory effects of octreotide on renal and glomerular growth in early experimental diabetes in mice. *J Endocrinol.* 172:637–643.

Grouzmann, E., Cavadas, C., Grand, D., et al. 2003. Blood sampling methodology is crucial for precise measurement of plasma catecholamines concentrations in mice. *Pflugers Arch.* 447:254–258.

Grunstein, H.S., James, D.E., Storlien, L.H., Smythe, G.A., and Kraegen, E.W. 1985. Hyperinsulinemia suppresses glucose utilization in specific brain regions: In vivo studies using the euglycemic clamp in the rat. *Endocrinology.* 116:604–610.

Han, B.G., Hao, C.M., Tchekneva, E.E., et al. 2008. Markers of glycemic control in the mouse: Comparisons of 6-h- and overnight-fasted blood glucoses to Hb A1c. *Am J Physiol Endocrinol Metab.* 295:E981–986.

Heinemann, L. 2010. Insulin assay standardization: Leading to measures of insulin sensitivity and secretion for practical clinical care: Response to Staten et al. *Diabetes Care.* 33:e83; author reply e84.

Higgins, P.J., Garlick R.L., and Bunn, H.F. 1982. Glycosylated hemoglobin in human and animal red cells. Role of glucose permeability. *Diabetes.* 31:743–748.

Hirayama, I., Yi, Z., Izumi, S., et al. 1999. Genetic analysis of obese diabetes in the TSOD mouse. *Diabetes.* 48:1183–1191.

Hiskett, E., Suwitheechon, O.U., Lindbloom-Hawley, S., Boyle, D., and Schermerhorn, T. 2009. Lack of glucokinase regulatory protein expression may contribute to low glucokinase activity in feline liver. *Vet Res Commun.* 33:227–240.

Holemans, K., Caluwaerts, S., Poston, L., and André van Assche, F. 2004. Diet-induced obesity in the rat: A model for gestational diabetes mellitus. *Am J Obstet Gynecol.* 190:858–865.

Hough, S., Russell, J.E., Teitelbaum, S.L., and Avioli, L.V. 1982. Calcium homeostasis in chronic streptozotocin-induced diabetes mellitus in the rat. *Am J Physiol.* 242:E451–E456.

Humbel, R.E. 1990. Insulin-like growth factors I and II. *Eur J Biochem.* 190:445–462.

Hussain, K. 2010. Mutations in pancreatic β -cell Glucokinase as a cause of hyperinsulinaemic hypoglycaemia and neonatal diabetes mellitus. *Rev Endocr Metab Disord.* 11:179–183.

Hut, R.A., Pilorz, V., Boerema, A.S., Strijkstra, A.M., and Daan, S. 2011. Working for food shifts nocturnal mouse activity into the day. *PLOS ONE* 6:e17527.

Ikeda, H. 1994. KK mouse. *Diabetes Res Clin Pract.* 24 (Suppl.):S313–S316.

Ionut, V., Liu, H., Mooradian, V., et al. 2009. Novel canine models of obese pre-diabetes and of mild type 2 diabetes. *Am J Physiol Endocrinol Metab.* 298:E38–48.

Islam, M.S. and Loots du, T. 2009. Experimental rodent models of type 2 diabetes: A review. *Methods Find Exp Clin Pharmacol.* 31:249–261.

Issekutz, B. Jr., Issekutz, T.B., Elahi, D., and Borkow, I. 1974. Effect of insulin infusions on the glucose kinetics in alloxan-streptozotocin diabetic dogs. *Diabetologia.* 10:323–328.

Jablecka, A., Czaplicka, E., Olszewski, J., Bogdanski, P., Krauss, H., and Smolarek, I. 2009. Influence of selected angiotensin-converting enzyme inhibitors on alloxan-induced diabetic cataract in rabbits. *Med Sci Monit.* 15:BR334–338.

Jacobson, L., Ansari, T., Potts, J., and McGuinness, O.P. 2006. Glucocorticoid-deficient corticotropin-releasing hormone knockout mice maintain glucose requirements but not autonomic responses during repeated hypoglycemia. *Am J Physiol.* 291:E15–E22.

Jensen, M.D. and Heiling, V.J. 1991. Heated hand vein blood is satisfactory for measurements during free fatty acid kinetic studies. *Metabolism.* 40:406–409.

Jiang, L., You, J., Yu, X., et al. 2008. Tyrosine-dependent and -independent actions of leptin receptor in control of energy balance and glucose homeostasis. *Proc Natl Acad Sci.* 105:18619–18624.

Johnson, B.M., Fry, M.M., Flatland, B., and Kirk, C.A. 2009. Comparison of a human portable blood glucose meter, veterinary portable blood glucose meter, and automated chemistry analyzer for measurement of blood glucose concentrations in dogs. *J Am Vet Med Assoc.* 235:1309–1313.

Kaneko, J.J. 1997. Carbohydrate metabolism and its diseases. In *Clinical Biochemistry of Domestic Animals.* Eds. J.W. Harvey, J.J. Kaneko, and M.L. Bruss, pp. 45–81. San Diego, CA: Academic Press.

Karabatas, L.M., Pastorale C., de Bruno, L.F., et al. 2005. Early manifestations in multiple-low-dose streptozotocin-induced diabetes in mice. *Pancreas.* 30:318–324.

Kebede, M., Alquier, T., Latour, M.G., Semache, M., Tremblay, C., and Poitout, V. 2008. The fatty acid receptor GPR40 plays a role in insulin secretion in vivo after high-fat feeding. *Diabetes.* 57:2432–2437.

Kienzle, E. 1994. Blood sugar levels and renal sugar excretion after the intake of high carbohydrate diets in cats. *J Nutr.* 124:2563S–2567S.

Kim, B., Backus, C., Oh, S., Hayes, J.M., and Feldman, E.L. 2009. Increased tau phosphorylation and cleavage in mouse models of type 1 and type 2 diabetes. *Endocrinology.* 150:5294–5301.

Kim, S.J., Nian, C., Doudet, D.J., and McIntosh, C.H. 2008. Inhibition of dipeptidyl peptidase IV with sitagliptin (MK0431) prolongs islet graft survival in streptozotocin-induced diabetic mice. *Diabetes.* 57:1331–1339.

Kim, S.Y., Weinstein, D.A., Starost, M.F., Mansfield, B.C., and Chou, J.Y. 2008. Necrotic foci, elevated chemokines and infiltrating neutrophils in the liver of glycogen storage disease type Ia. *J Hepatol.* 48:479–485.

Kodama, T., Iwase, M., Nunoi, K., Maki, Y., Yoshinari, M., and Fujishima, M. 1993. A new diabetes model induced by neonatal alloxan treatment in rats. *Diabetes Res Clin Pract.* 20:183–189.

Koga, M. and Kasayama, S. 2010. Clinical impact of glycated albumin as another glycemic control marker. *Endocr J.* 57:751–762.

Kohli, R., Meininger, C.J., Haynes, T.E., Yan, W., Self, J.T., and Wu, G. 2004. Dietary L-arginine supplementation enhances endothelial nitric oxide synthesis in streptozotocin-induced diabetic rats. *J Nutr.* 134:600–608.

Koopmans, S.J., Sips, H.C., Krans, H.M., and Radder, J.K. 1996. Pulsatile intravenous insulin replacement in streptozotocin diabetic rats is more efficient than continuous delivery: Effects on glycaemic control, insulin-mediated glucose metabolism and lipolysis. *Diabetologia.* 39:391–400.

Kramer, J.W., Nottingham, S., Robinette, J., Lenz, G., Sylvester, S., and Dessouky, M.I. 1980. Inherited, early onset, insulin-requiring diabetes mellitus of Keeshond dogs. *Diabetes.* 29:558–565.

Kris-Etherton, P.M. and Dietschy, J. 1997. Design criteria for studies examining individual fatty acid effects on cardiovascular disease risk factors: Human and animal studies. *Am J Clin Nutr.* 65:1590S–1596S.

Kurup, S. and Bhonde, R.R. 2000. Combined effect of nicotinamide and streptozotocin on diabetic status in partially pancreatectomized adult BALB/c mice. *Horm Metab Res.* 32:330–334.

Lai, K., Elsas, L.J., and Wierenga, K.J. 2009. Galactose toxicity in animals. *IUBMB Life.* 61:1063–1074.

Lam, Y.Y., Mitchell, A.J., Holmes, A J., et al. 2011. Role of the gut in visceral fat inflammation and metabolic disorders. *Obesity.* 19:2113–2120.

Landt, M., Norling, L.L., Steelman, M., and Smith, C.H. 1986. Monoject Samplette capillary blood container with serum separator evaluated for collection of specimens for therapeutic drug assays and common clinical-chemical tests. *Clin Chem.* 32:523–526.

Larsen, M.O., Wilken, M., Gotfredsen, C.F., Carr, R.D., Svendsen, O., and Rolin, B. 2002. Mild streptozotocin diabetes in the Gottingen minipig. A novel model of moderate insulin deficiency and diabetes. *Am J Physiol Endocrinol Metab.* 282:E1342–E1351.

Leahy, J.L., Bumbalo, L.M., and Chen, C. 1993. Beta-cell hypersensitivity for glucose precedes loss of glucose-induced insulin secretion in 90% pancreatectomized rats. *Diabetologia.* 36:1238–1244.

Le Marchand, Y., Freychet, P., and Jeanrenaud, B. 1978. Longitudinal study on the establishment of insulin resistance in hypothalamic obese mice. *Endocrinology.* 102:74–85.

Lee, S., Muniyappa, R., Yan, X., et al. 2008. Comparison between surrogate indexes of insulin sensitivity and resistance and hyperinsulinemic euglycemic clamp estimates in mice. *Am J Physiol Endocrinol Metab.* 294:E261–E270.

Lei, K.J., Chen, H., Pan, C.J., et al. 1996. Glucose-6-phosphatase dependent substrate transport in the glycogen storage disease type-1a mouse. *Nat Genet.* 13:203–209.

Leow, C.K. 1997. The effect of anesthesia on intravenous glucose tolerance test in the rat. *Hepatology.* 25:782–783.

Leslie, N.D. 2003. Insights into the pathogenesis of galactosemia. *Annu Rev Nutr.* 23:59–80.

Leslie, N.D., Yager, K.L., McNamara, P.D., and Segal, S. 1996. A mouse model of galactose-1-phosphate uridyltransferase deficiency. *Biochem Mol Med.* 59:7–12.

Lewis, G.F. 1997. Fatty acid regulation of very low density lipoprotein production. *Curr Opin Lipidol.* 8:146–153.

Li, M., Kim, D.H., Tsenovoy, P.L., et al. 2008. Treatment of obese diabetic mice with a heme oxygenase inducer reduces visceral and subcutaneous adiposity, increases adiponectin levels, and improves insulin sensitivity and glucose tolerance. *Diabetes.* 57:1526–1535.

Lim, J.S., Lee, J.A., Hwang, J.S., Shin, C.H., and Yang, S.W. 2011. Non-catch-up growth in intrauterine growth-retarded rats showed glucose intolerance and increased expression of PDX-1 mRNA. *Pediatr Int.* 53:181–186.

López-Novoa, J.M., Eleno, N., and Martínez-Maldonado, M. 1996. Dynamics of renal glucose reabsorption in rat. *Nephrology.* 2:155–160.

Macdonald, I.A. and Lake, D.M. 1985. An improved technique for extracting catecholamines from body fluids. *J Neurosci Meth.* 13:239–248.

Mager, D.E., Abernethy, D.R., Egan, J.M., and Elahi, D. 2004. Exendin-4 pharmacodynamics: Insights from the hyperglycemic clamp technique. *J Pharmacol Exp Ther.* 311:830–835.

Mandarino, L.J., Bonadonna, R.C., McGuinness, O.P., Halseth, A.E., and Wasserman, D.H. 2001. Regulation of muscle glucose uptake in vivo. In *The American Physiological Society Handbook of Physiology-Endocrine Pancreas*. Eds. L.S. Jefferson and A.D. Cherrington. Rockville, MD: Waverly Press.

Mann, E.A., Pidcoke, H.F., Salinas, J., Wolf, S.E., Wade, C.E., and Holcomb, J.B. 2009. Hematocrit causes the most significant error in point of care glucometers. *Crit Care Med.* 37:1530; author reply 1530–1531.

Marca, M.C. and Loste, A. 2000. Glycosylated haemoglobin assay of canine blood samples. *J Small Anim Pract.* 41:189–192.

Marrachelli, V.G., Miranda, F.J., Centeno, J.M., et al. 2010. Mechanisms involved in the relaxant action of testosterone in the renal artery from male normoglycemic and diabetic rabbits. *Pharmacol Res.* 61:149–156.

Martin, M.A., Lucia, A., Arenas, J., Andreu, A.L. 1993. Glycogen storage disease type V. In *GeneReviews(R)*, Pagon, R.A., Adam, M.P., Ardinger, H.H., Wallace, S.E., Amemiya, A., Bean, L.J.H. et al. (eds.). Seattle (WA): University of Washington, Seattle University of Washington, Seattle.

Mayatepek, E., Hoffmann, B., and Meissner, T. 2010. Inborn errors of carbohydrate metabolism. *Best Pract Res Clin Gastroenterol.* 24:607–618.

Mayes, P.A. 1993. Intermediary metabolism of fructose. *Am J Clin Nutr.* 58:754S–765S.

McGuinness, O.P., Ayala, J.E., Laughlin, M.R., and Wasserman, D.H. 2009. NIH experiment in centralized mouse phenotyping: The Vanderbilt experience and recommendations for evaluating glucose homeostasis in the mouse. *Am J Physiol Endocrinol Metab.* 297:E849–E855.

McGuinness, O.P. and Cherrington, A.D. 2003. Effects of fructose on hepatic glucose metabolism. *Curr Opin Clin Nutr Metab Care.* 6:441–448.

Menard, S.L., Croteau, E., Sarrhini, O., et al. 2010. Abnormal in vivo myocardial energy substrate uptake in diet-induced type 2 diabetic cardiomyopathy in rats. *Am J Physiol Endocrinol Metab.* 298:E1049–E1057.

Miao, G., Ito, T., Uchikoshi, F., et al. 2005. Development of islet-like cell clusters after pancreas transplantation in the spontaneously diabetic Torri rat. *Am J Transplant.* 5:2360–2367.

Moore, A.H., Cherry, S.R., Pollack, D.B., Hovda, D.A., and Phelps, M.E. 1999. Application of positron emission tomography to determine cerebral glucose utilization in conscious infant monkeys. *J Neurosci Methods.* 88:123–133.

Moore, M.C., Cherrington, A.D., and Wasserman, D.H. 2003. Regulation of hepatic and peripheral glucose disposal. *Best Pract Res Clin Endocrinol Metab.* 17:343–364.

Moore, M.C., Cherrington, A.D., Cline, G., et al. 1991. Sources of carbon for hepatic glycogen synthesis in the conscious dog. *J Clin Invest.* 88:578–587.

Morino, K., Neschen, S., Bilz, S., et al. 2008. Muscle-specific IRS-1 Ser->Ala transgenic mice are protected from fat-induced insulin resistance in skeletal muscle. *Diabetes.* 57:2644–2651.

Muniyappa, R., Chen, H., Muzumdar, R.H., et al. 2009. Comparison between surrogate indexes of insulin sensitivity/resistance and hyperinsulinemic euglycemic clamp estimates in rats. *Am J Physiol Endocrinol Metab.* 297:E1023–E1029.

Muniyappa, R., Lee, S., Chen, H., and Quon, M.J. 2008. Current approaches for assessing insulin sensitivity and resistance in vivo: Advantages, limitations, and appropriate usage. *Am J Physiol Endocrinol Metab.* 294:E15–E26.

Nagle, C.A., An, J., Shiota, M., et al. 2007. Hepatic overexpression of glycerol-sn-3-phosphate acyltransferase 1 in rats causes insulin resistance. *J Biol Chem.* 282:14807–14815.

Napoli, R., Hirshman, M.F., and Horton, E.S. 1995. Mechanisms and time course of impaired skeletal muscle glucose transport activity in streptozocin diabetic rats. *J Clin Invest.* 96:427–437.

Nathan, D.M., Kuenen, J., Borg, R., Zheng, H., Schoenfeld, D., and Heine, R.J. 2008. Translating the A1C assay into estimated average glucose values. *Diabetes Care.* 31:1473–1478.

Nicholson, A., Reifsnyder, P.C., Malcolm, R.D., et al. 2010. Diet-induced obesity in two C57BL/6 substrains with intact or mutant nicotinamide nucleotide transhydrogenase (Nnt) gene. *Obesity.* 18:1902–1905.

Nieto-Vazquez, I., Fernandez-Veledo, S., Le Alvaro, C., and Lorenzo, M. 2008. Dual role of interleukin-6 in regulating insulin sensitivity in murine skeletal muscle. *Diabetes.* 57:3211–3221.

Noonan, W.T. and Banks, R.O. 2000. Renal function and glucose transport in male and female mice with diet-induced type II diabetes mellitus. *Proc Soc Exp Biol Med.* 225:221–230.

Öberg, J., Fall, T., and Lilliehöök, I. 2011. Validation of a species-optimized enzyme-linked immunosorbent assay for determination of serum concentrations of insulin in dogs. *Vet Clin Pathol.* 40:66–73.

O'Brien, T.D. 2002. Pathogenesis of feline diabetes mellitus. *Mol Cell Endocrinol.* 197:213–219.

O'Brien, T.D., Hayden, D.W., Johnson, K.H., and Stevens, J.B. 1985. High dose intravenous glucose tolerance test and serum insulin and glucagon levels in diabetic and non-diabetic cats: Relationships to insular amyloidosis. *Vet Pathol.* 22:250–261.

Orho, M., Bosshard, N.U., Buist, N.R., et al. 1998. Mutations in the liver glycogen synthase gene in children with hypoglycemia due to glycogen storage disease type 0. *J Clin Invest.* 102:507–515.

Oriente, F., Fernandez Diaz, L.C., Miele, C., et al. 2008. Prep1 deficiency induces protection from diabetes and increased insulin sensitivity through a p160-mediated mechanism. *Mol Cell Biol.* 28:5634–5645.

Orngreen, M.C., Schelhaas, H.J., Jeppesen, T.D., et al. 2008. Is muscle glycogenolysis impaired in X-linked phosphorylase b kinase deficiency? *Neurology.* 70:1876–1882.

Ostenson, C.G., Grill, V., and Roos, M. 1989. Studies on sex dependency of B-cell susceptibility to streptozotocin in a rat model of type II diabetes mellitus. *Exp Clin Endocrinol.* 93:241–247.

Pagliassotti, M.J. and Cherrington, A.D. 1992. Regulation of net hepatic glucose uptake in vivo. *Ann Rev Physiol.* 54:847–860.

Parfrey, N.A., Prud'homme, G.J., Colle, E., et al. 1989. Immunologic and genetic studies of diabetes in the BB rat. *Crit Rev Immunol.* 9:45–65.

Polonsky, K.S. and Rubenstein, A.H. 1984. C-peptide as a measure of the secretion and hepatic extraction of insulin. Pitfalls and limitations. *Diabetes.* 33:486–494.

Portha, B., Blondel, O., Serradas, P., et al . 1989. The rat models of non-insulin dependent diabetes induced by neonatal streptozotocin. *Diabete Metab.* 15:61–75.

Postic, C. and Girard, J. 2008. Contribution of de novo fatty acid synthesis to hepatic steatosis and insulin resistance: Lessons from genetically engineered mice. *J Clin Invest.* 118:829–838.

Postic, C., Shiota, M., Niswender, K.D., et al. 1999. Dual roles for glucokinase in glucose homeostasis as determined by liver and pancreatic β cell-specific gene knock-outs using Cre recombinase. *J Biol Chem.* 274:305–315.

Prahl, A., Guptill, L., Glickman, N.W., Tetrick, M., and Glickman, L.T. 2007. Time trends and risk factors for diabetes mellitus in cats presented to veterinary teaching hospitals. *J Feline Med Surg.* 9:351–358.

Quarmby, V., Quan, C., Ling, V., Compton, P., and Canova-Davis, E. 1998. How much insulin-like growth factor I (IGF-I) circulates? Impact of standardization on IGF-I assay accuracy. *J Clin Endocrinol Metab.* 83:1211–1216.

Quon, M.J., Cochran, C., Taylor, S.I., and Eastman, R.C. 1994. Direct comparison of standard and insulin modified protocols for minimal model estimation of insulin sensitivity in normal subjects. *Diabetes Res.* 25:139–149.

Raben, N., Danon, M., Gilbert, A.L., et al. 2003. Enzyme replacement therapy in the mouse model of Pompe disease. *Mol Genet Metab.* 80:159–169.

Reaven, G.M. and Ho, H. 1991. Low-dose streptozotocin-induced diabetes in the spontaneously hypertensive rat. *Metabolism.* 40:335–337.

Reed, M.J., Meszaros, K., Entes, L.J., et al. 2000. A new rat model of type 2 diabetes: The fat-fed, streptozotocin-treated rat. *Metabolism.* 49:1390–1394.

Rees, D.A. and Alcolado, J.C. 2005. Animal models of diabetes mellitus. *Diabet Med.* 22:359–370.

Reivich, M., Kuhl, D., Wolf, A., et al. 1979. The [18F]fluorodeoxyglucose method for the measurement of local cerebral glucose utilization in man. *Circ Res.* 44:127–137.

Rendell, M., Stephen, P.M., Paulsen, R., et al. 1985. An interspecies comparison of normal levels of glycosylated hemoglobin and glycosylated albumin. *Comp Biochem Physiol B.* 81:819–822.

Rerup, C.C. 1970. Drugs producing diabetes through damage of the insulin secreting cells. *Pharmacol Rev.* 22:485–518.

Reusch, C.E., Liehs, M.R., Hoyer, M., and Vochezer, R. 1993. Fructosamine. A new parameter for diagnosis and metabolic control in diabetic dogs and cats. *J Vet Intern Med.* 7:177–182.

Ropelle, E.R., Pauli, J.R., Cintra, D.E., et al. 2009. Acute exercise modulates the Foxo1/PGC-1α pathway in the liver of diet-induced obesity rats. *J Physiol.* 587:2069–2076.

Rosenmann, E., Yanko, L., and Cohen, A.M. 1975. Comparative study of the pathology of sucrose-induced diabetes in the rat and adult-onset diabetes in man. *Isr J Med Sci.* 11:753–761.

Rottiers, R., Mattheeuws, D., Kaneko, J.J., and Vermeulen, A. 1981. Glucose uptake and insulin secretory responses to intravenous glucose loads in the dog. *Am J Vet Res.* 42:155–158.

Saisho, Y., Butler, A.E., Manesso, E., et al. 2010. Relationship between fractional pancreatic beta cell area and fasting plasma glucose concentration in monkeys. *Diabetologia.* 53:111–114.

Schnedl, W.J., Wallner, S.J., Piswanger, C., Krause, R., and Lipp, R.W. 2005. Glycated hemoglobin and liver disease in diabetes mellitus. *Wien Med Wochenschr.* 155:411–415.

Shafrir, E. 1992. Animal models of non-insulin-dependent diabetes. *Diabetes Metab Rev.* 8:179–208.

Shiao, M.S., Liao, B.Y., Long, M., and Yu, H.T. 2008. Adaptive evolution of the insulin two-gene system in mouse. *Genetics.* 178:1683–1691.

Shima, K., Zhu, M., and Mizuno, A. 1999. Pathoetiology and prevention of NIDDM lessons from the OLETF rat. *J Med Invest.* 46:121–129.

Shukla, N., Angelini, G.D., and Jeremy, J.Y. 2008. The administration of folic acid reduces intravascular oxidative stress in diabetic rabbits. *Metabolism.* 57:774–781.

Smith, L.F. 1966. Species variation in the amino acid sequence of insulin. *Am J Med.* 40:662–666.

Sonnenberg, G.E. and Keller, U. 1982. Sampling of arterialized heated-hand venous blood as a noninvasive technique for the study of ketone body kinetics in man. *Metabolism.* 31:1–5.

Spady, D.K., Woollett, L.A., and Dietschy, J.M. 1993. Regulation of plasma LDL-cholesterol levels by dietary cholesterol and fatty acids. *Annu Rev Nutr.* 13:355–381.

Srinivasan, K. and Ramarao, P. 2007. Animal models in type 2 diabetes research: An overview. *Indian J Med Res.* 125:451–472.

Stanhope, K.L. and Havel, P.J. 2008. Endocrine and metabolic effects of consuming beverages sweetened with fructose, glucose, sucrose, or high-fructose corn syrup. *Am J Clin Nutr.* 88:1733S–1737S.

Stefanovski, D., Richey, J.M., Woolcott, O., et al. 2011. Consistency of the disposition index in the face of diet induced insulin resistance: Potential role of FFA. *PLOS ONE* 6:e18134.

Stevenson, R.W., Steiner, K.E., Connolly, C.C., et al. 1991. Dose-related effects of epinephrine on glucose production in conscious dogs. *Am J Physiol.* 260:E363–E370.

Subrahmanyam, K. 1960. Metabolism in the New Zealand strain of obese mice. *Biochem J.* 76:548–556.

Swoap, S.J., Gutilla, M.J., Liles, L.C., Smith, R.O., and Weinshenker, D. 2006. The full expression of fasting-induced torpor requires {beta}3-adrenergic receptor signaling. *J Neurosci.* 26:241–245.

Szkudelski, T. 2001. The mechanism of alloxan and streptozotocin action in B cells of the rat pancreas. *Physiol Res.* 50:537–546.

Takada, J., Machado, M.A., Peres, S.B., et al. 2007. Neonatal streptozotocin-induced diabetes mellitus: A model of insulin resistance associated with loss of adipose mass. *Metabolism.* 56:977–984.

Takiguchi, S., Takata, Y., Funakoshi, A., et al. 1997. Disrupted cholecystokinin type-A receptor (CCKAR) gene in OLETF rats. *Gene.* 197:169–175.

Tappy, L. and Le, K.A. 2010. Metabolic effects of fructose and the worldwide increase in obesity. *Physiol Rev.* 90:23–46.

Thayer, T.C., Wilson, S.B., and Mathews, C.E. 2010. Use of nonobese diabetic mice to understand human type 1 diabetes. *Endocrinol Metab Clin North Am.* 39:541–561.

Ueda, H., Ikegami, H., Yamato, E., et al. 1995. The NSY mouse: A new animal model of spontaneous NIDDM with moderate obesity. *Diabetologia.* 38:503–508.

Valera Mora, M.E., Scarfone, A., Calvani, M., Greco, A.V., and Mingrone, G. 2003. Insulin clearance in obesity. *J Am Coll Nutrition.* 22:487–493.

Van Heek, M., Austin, T.M., Farley, C., Cook, J.A., Tetzloff, G.G., and Davis, H.R. 2001. Ezetimibe, a potent cholesterol absorption inhibitor, normalizes combined dyslipidemia in obese hyperinsulinemic hamsters. *Diabetes.* 50:1330–1335.

Van Schaftingen, E., Detheux, M., and Da Cunha, M.V. 1994. Short-term control of glucokinase activity: A role of a regulatory protein. *FASEB J.* 8:414–419.

Varcoe, T.J., Wight, N., Voultsios, A., Salkeld, M.D., and Kennaway, D.J. 2011. Chronic phase shifts of the photoperiod throughout pregnancy programs glucose intolerance and insulin resistance in the rat. *PLOS ONE* 6:e18504.

Vicini, P. and Cobelli, C. 2001. The iterative two-stage population approach to IVGTT minimal modeling: Improved precision with reduced sampling. Intravenous glucose tolerance test. *Am J Physiol Endocrinol Metab.* 280:E179–E186.

Vranic, M., Engerman, R., Doi, K., Morita, S., and Yip, C.C. 1976. Extrapancreatic glucagon in the dog. *Metabolism* 25:1469–1473.

Vranic, M., Pek, S., and Kawamori, R. 1974. Increased "glucagon immunoreactivity" in plasma of totally pancreatized dogs. *Diabetes.* 23:905–912.

Wade, G.N. 1982. Obesity without overeating in golden hamsters. *Physiol Behav.* 29:701–707.

Wade, G.N. 1983. Dietary obesity in golden hamsters: Reversibility and effects of sex and photoperiod. *Physiol Behav.* 30:131–137.

Wallace, T.M., Levy, J.C., and Matthews, D.R. 2004. Use and abuse of HOMA modeling. *Diabetes Care.* 27:1487–1495.

Wallace, T.M. and Matthews, D.R. 2002. The assessment of insulin resistance in man. *Diabet Med.* 19:527–534.

Walvoort, H.C. 1983. Glycogen storage diseases in animals and their potential value as models of human disease. *J Inherit Metab Dis.* 6:3–16.

Walvoort, H.C., Dormans, J.A., and van den Ingh, T.S. 1985. Comparative pathology of the canine model of glycogen storage disease type II (Pompe's disease). *J Inherit Metab Dis.* 8:38–46.

Wang, J., Wan, R., Mo, Y., Zhang, Q., Sherwood, L.C., and Chien, S. 2010a. Creating a long-term diabetic rabbit model. *Exp Diabetes Res.* 2010:>289614.

Wang, S., Dale, G.L., Song, P., Viollet, B., and Zou, M.H. 2010b. AMPKα1 deletion shortens erythrocyte life span in mice. *J Biol Chem.* 285:19976–19985.

Wang, Y., Campbell, T., Perry, B., Beaurepaire, C., and Qin, L. 2011. Hypoglycemic and insulin-sensitizing effects of berberine in high-fat diet- and streptozotocin-induced diabetic rats. *Metabolism.* 60:298–305.
Wasserman, D.H. 2009. Four grams of glucose. *Am J Physiol Endocrinol Metab.* 296:E11–E21.
Wasserman, D.H., Ayala, J.E., and McGuinness, O.P. 2009. Lost in translation. *Diabetes.* 59:1947–1950.
Wasserman, D.H. and Cherrington, A.D. 1991. Hepatic fuel metabolism during muscular work: Role and regulation [editorial]. [Review]. *Am J Physiol.* 260:E811–E824.
Webster, B.A., Vigna, S.R., and Paquette, T. 1986. Acute exercise, epinephrine, and diabetes enhance insulin binding to skeletal muscle. *Am J Physiol.* 250:E186–E197.
Wei, Y., Wang, D., Topczewski, F., and Pagliassotti, M.J. 2007. Fructose-mediated stress signaling in the liver: Implications for hepatic insulin resistance. *J Nutr Biochem.* 18:1–9.
Weinstein, D.A., Correia, C.E., Saunders, A.C., and Wolfsdorf, J.I. 2006. Hepatic glycogen synthase deficiency: An infrequently recognized cause of ketotic hypoglycemia. *Mol Genet Metab.* 87:284–288.
Wolfsdorf, J.I. and Weinstein, D.A. 2003. Glycogen storage diseases. *Rev Endocr Metab Disord.* 4:95–102.
Wood, P.A. and Smith, J.E. 1980. Glycosylated hemoglobin and canine diabetes mellitus. *J Am Vet Med Assoc.* 176:1267–1268.
Yoshioka, M., Kayo, T., Ikeda, T., and Koizumi, A. 1997. A novel locus, Mody4, distal to D7Mit189 on chromosome 7 determines early-onset NIDDM in nonobese C57BL/6 (Akita) mutant mice. *Diabetes.* 46:887–894.
Youn, J.H., Kim, J.K., and Buchanan, T.A. 1994. Time courses of changes in hepatic and skeletal muscle insulin action and GLUT4 protein in skeletal muscle after STZ injection. *Diabetes.* 43:564–571.
Young, D.S., Pestaner, L.C., and Gibberman, V. 1975. Effects of drugs on clinical laboratory tests. *Clin Chem.* 21:1D–432D.
Yuan, H., Lanting, L., Xu, Z.G., et al. 2008. Effects of cholesterol-tagged small interfering RNAs targeting 12/15-lipoxygenase on parameters of diabetic nephropathy in a mouse model of type 1 diabetes. *Am J Physiol Renal Physiol.* 295:F605–F617.
Zampieri, S., Buratti, E., Dominissini, S., et al. 2011. Splicing mutations in glycogen-storage disease type II: Evaluation of the full spectrum of mutations and their relation to patients' phenotypes. *Eur J Hum Genet.* 19:422–431.
Zhang, F., Ye, C., Li, G., et al. 2003. The rat model of type 2 diabetic mellitus and its glycometabolism characters. *Exp Anim.* 52:401–407.
Zhang, H.J., Zhou, F., Ji, B.P., et al. 2009. Effects of fructose and/or fat in the diet on developing the type 2 diabetic-like syndrome in CD-1 mice. *Horm Metab Res.* 41:40,45.
Zhang, X., Zhang, R., Raab, S., et al. 2011. Rhesus macaques develop metabolic syndrome with reversible vascular dysfunction responsive to pioglitazone. *Circulation.* 124:77–86.

21 Lipids

Dana Walker and Lindsay Tomlinson

CONTENTS

21.1 OVERVIEW OF LIPID FUNCTION

The physiologic importance of tissue lipids and lipid transport in the body is undeniably critical to life for all multicellular organisms. Lipids serve structural, functional, and metabolic roles within cells. Moreover, they provide insulation, protection (e.g., as waxes), and surfactant properties for various tissues. Structurally, the most generalized role of lipids is as the primary component of cell membranes. Notably, within membranes of different cell and organelle types, the specific lipid composition is highly diverse and dynamic. Some membrane lipids have further functional roles in organizing the cytoskeleton (Kwik et al., 2003) or as signaling or signal transduction molecules. Membrane lipids organized into heterogenous rafts can regulate major cellular events, including intracellular enzyme activity, electrolyte trafficking, exocytotic and endocytotic pathways, receptor presentation, ligand recruitment, cellular mobility, cell proliferation, membrane fusion, and even apoptosis (Gajate et al., 2009; Rosa and Fratangeli, 2010; Abbal et al., 2006; Knorr et al., 2009; Eum et al., 2009; Li et al., 2010). Extra-membrane lipids serve a tremendous range of other functional roles such as vitamins, hormones, local regulatory molecules (e.g., eicosanoids, sphingolipids [SLs]), specific ligands for the immune and nervous systems, and transcriptional factors. With inflammation, blood lipids act as acute phase reactants with purported direct bacteriostatic activity and as transporters for inflammatory mediators (e.g., C-reactive protein, serum amyloid A; Jahangiri, 2010; Taskinen et al., 2002). Lipids are the most concentrated source of energy for organisms, with β-oxidation of free fatty acids (FAs) to acetyl-CoA that then may enter the Krebs cycle for generating high-energy phosphates. Alternatively, acetyl-CoA can be recycled back for the synthesis of structurally new lipids.

Considering these broad functional roles, and variability in constitutive and inducible forms of lipids with physiologic needs, it is not surprising that tissue and blood lipid homeostasis is commonly altered in response to disease or toxicity. Accordingly, changes in serum/plasma lipid concentrations are most often attributable to a combination of influences, rather than a single cause. Importantly, circulating lipid values are also dependent upon metabolic rate, hormonal state, and relative age of the animal. Diet and nutritional state can have significant but often aleatoric and not fully predictable effects on circulating lipids. Species differences in baseline blood lipid concentrations and effects of pathologic states relative to such can be particularly prominent often due to phylogenetic differences in the predominant lipoprotein (LP) types and composition, and their associated channeling, regulation, and turnover. Hence, major species, sex, and age differences in blood lipid concentrations should be expected in both health and in response to pathologic states.

Useful interpretation of lipid data in laboratory animal species requires understanding of the differences in baseline states and factors influencing lipid transport and metabolism for the animals of interest and—as models of human disease—in comparison with human. A major reason for differences in circulating lipids between laboratory species and humans is due to dissimilar LP metabolism. In many laboratory species, blood cholesterol is predominantly carried by high-density lipoprotein (HDL) instead of low-density lipoprotein (LDL)—the major carrier of cholesterol in humans (Table 21.1). This is partly attributable to species differences in enzymes presence or activity (e.g., cholesterol ester transferase protein [CETP]) and LP synthesis and catabolism. The structure of most apolipoproteins (apos) also differs between nonhuman species and humans. In addition, the regulation of genes encoding proteins involved in lipid and LP metabolism is not identical between humans and studied laboratory species (e.g., peroxisome proliferator-activated receptors [PPARs]). Thus, the data obtained in nonhuman animals are often not directly relevant to humans.

TABLE 21.1
General Lipid Profiles across Species

Species	Detectable CETP	Inducible CYP7A1[b]	TG:TC Ratio[c]	Relative Absolute Serum Values for These Major Lipoproteins[d]: VLDL[e]	LDL-c	HDL-c	Predominant Cholesterol LP Carrier in Blood	Potential to Develop Atherosclerosis Spontaneously
Mouse (C57BL/6, CD1, BALB/c)	No	Yes (*though inhibition with very chronic cholesterol feeding in other strain[s]*)	1:1 to 1:3	Very low	Low	High	HDL	No (*except in a few strains [e.g., C57BL/6J] on chronic very high cholesterol, high-fat diet+ cholic acid*)
Rat (Sprague-Dawley, F344, Wistar)	No	Yes	1:1 to 1.5	Low	Low	Low–moderate	HDL	No
Hamster (Syrian Golden)	Yes	No	1:2 to 2:1	Very low	Low	High	HDL to 1:1, LDL:HDL	Yes (inconsistently in males on high cholesterol diet)
Rabbit(New Zealand White - NZW)	Yes (high)	No	1:1 to 2:1	Very low	Very low	Low	HDL to 1:1, LDL:HDL (LDL for some rabbit strains)	No
Guinea Pig	Yes	No	1:1 to 1:2	Very low	Low	Low	LDL	Yes (*especially with high cholesterol diet in susceptible lines*)
Dog (Beagle)	No	Yes	1:2 to 1:6	Very low	Low	Very high	HDL	No
Yucatan Miniature Pig	No	No	1:3 to 1:7	Very low	Low–moderate	Low–moderate	LDL	Yes (*some vessels [e.g., abdominal aorta], especially with chronic high cholesterol diet*)
Marmoset	Yes	No	1:1 to 1:2 (Crook et al., 1990)	Low	Moderate	Low–moderate	HDL (Crook et al., 1990)	Yes (*on high cholesterol diet*)
Cynomolgus monkey	Yes	No	1:2 to 1:6	Very low	Moderate	Moderate	1:1, LDL:HDL	Yes
African Green monkey	Yes	No (*inhibition with chronic high cholesterol feeding*)	1:2 to 1:2.5	Very low	Moderate	Low–moderate	LDL to 1:1, LDL:HDL	Yes
Rhesus monkey	Yes	No	1:3 to 1:7	Very low	Low–moderate	Low–moderate	1:1, LDL:HDL to LDL	Yes

(Continued)

TABLE 21.1 (*Continued*)
General Lipid Profiles across Species

Species	Detectable CETP	Inducible CYP7A1[b]	TG:TC Ratio[c]	Relative Absolute Serum Values for These Major Lipoproteins[d]			Predominant Cholesterol LP Carrier in Blood	Potential to Develop Atherosclerosis Spontaneously
				VLDL[e]	LDL-c	HDL-c		
Normal human[a]	Yes	No	1:1.1 to 1:3	Very low to low	Moderate to very high	Low–moderate	LDL	Yes
db/db mouse	No	Yes	2:1[d]	Very low	Very low	Very high	HDL	Yes
ApoE$^{-/-}$ mouse	No	Yes	1:4	Very high	Very high	Very low	LDL	Yes
LDLr$^{-/-}$ mouse	No	Yes	1:2	Very low	Very high	Moderate	LDL	Yes (*aged animals, or with high fat feeding*)
ZDF/+ rat	No	Yes	1:1 to 1:1.5	Very low	Low	Low–moderate	HDL	No
Hamster (high fat diet)	Yes	No	2 to 3:1	Low	Low–moderate	High	HDL	Yes (*lesion occurrence may be inconsistent and unrepeatable*)
Rabbit (cholesterol fed NZW)	Yes	No (*inhibition with high cholesterol feeding*)	1:>10	Very high	Very high	Low–moderate	HDL to LDL	Yes
Rhesus (diabetic)	Yes	No	1:1	Low	High	Low–moderate	LDL	Yes

Table values adapted from reference ranges and other data of a variety of private corporation animal clinical laboratories and from published resources (Loeb and Quimby, 2012).

CETP, cholesterol ester transfer protein; TG, triglyceride; CE, cholesterol ester; VLDL, very low-density lipoprotein; LDL, low-density lipoprotein; HDL, high-density lipoprotein; LP, lipoprotein.

[b] CYP7A1 inducibility with high cholesterol diet toward enhanced cholesterol catabolism to bile. (CYP7A1 inhibition/downregulation with high cholesterol feeding is also noted in Table 1 when known [Henkel et al., 2011; Rudel et al., 1994; Shang et al., 2006].)

[c] Ratio data based on SI units and primarily encompases that from fed states in young adult laboratory animals on normal commercial chow/pellet diet.

[d] "very low" = <+; "low" = +; "low–moderate" = ++; "moderate" = +++; "high" = ++++; "very high" = > to >>++++.

[e] Based on total lipid associated with apoB100-lipoprotein migration in fasted state.

[a] Human estimates including ranges for ratio of triglycerides: total cholesterol are based on fasted adults at least 20 years of age, multiple published commercial laboratory ranges and limited to general recommended ranges for health of fasting serum triglycerides 1.1–1.7 mmol/L and total cholesterol 3.2–5.2 mmol/L.

The lack of directly relevant animal models is one reason that the understanding of blood lipids and factors influencing their concentrations has been historically slower paced compared with that of other routinely measured circulating metabolites. This slower pace is also due to the many secondary variables influencing blood lipids and lipid changes, the cloudy definition of what constitutes a lipid, and the inconsistent and noncomparable methods to measure (and accordingly, classify) lipids. Indeed, there are still many aspects of lipid metabolism that are incompletely understood. The goal of this chapter is to aid the reader in understanding and interpreting measurable lipid concentrations in common laboratory species to the extent possible based on accumulated scientific knowledge. The focus is particularly on commonly evaluated lipids in serum/plasma, and factors that influence their concentrations. Circulating lipids that are not routinely evaluated and have primary functions in signaling, hormonal, enzyme/coenzyme or antioxidant activity (e.g., adrenocortical and sex steroids, and terpenes or isoprenols such as vitamin A, E, and K), or other complex roles (e.g., bile acids, oxidized lipids) or are absorbed plant-source lipids (phytosterols) will not be addressed in detail. Tissue lipids distinct from those in circulation greatly expand the complexity of physiologic and species differences in total lipid profile, and will not be addressed in detail in this chapter.

21.2 LIPID STRUCTURES

There are multiple ways for classifying mammalian blood lipids including blood transport form, function, or analytical properties. However, the most fundamental method is to consider physiologic lipids as subtypes of "simple" or "complex" lipids based on their structural components. This section provides a brief overview of lipid structure; more extensive and detailed information regarding lipid structures and anatomic and functional associations is readily available on several convenient websites including that on exogenous, and plant lipids at The LIPID Metabolites And Pathways Strategy (LIPID MAPS, http://www.lipidmaps.org), and on structures, sources, and analytical methods at Lipid Library (http://lipidlibrary.co.uk). Additional and complementary information on lipid structures, including steroids, waxes, vitamins, and those in bile are readily found at Lipid Bank (http://lipidbank.jp/). Moreover, particularly didactic websites of lipid structures and analysis are found at Cyberlipids (http://www.cyberlipid.org) and http://lipidlibrary.aocs.org. A literature search site for lipid physical and analytical information is available at LIPIDAT (http://www.lipidat.tcd.ie/SearchStart.htm).

21.2.1 Simple Lipids

Simple lipids (also called "neutral lipids") are composed exclusively of carbon chains, covalently bonded hydrogen, and a few oxygen atoms. These include lipids, which are predominantly linear carbon chains, including nonesterified fatty acid (NEFAs) and acylglycerols. Simple lipids also include those based upon a four-fused carbon ring structure, cholesterol, cholesterol esters (CEs, also known as cholesteryl esters), and other sterols, and variably straight-to-ringed five-carbon terpene (isoprene) polymers. (Representative simple lipid structures are presented in Figure 21.1a through f.)

21.2.2 Complex Lipids

Complex lipids (also called "polar" lipids) yield three or more products with hydrolysis: FA(s), an alcohol, and an additional polar/hydrophilic component that incorporates an inorganic phosphate or sphingosine group. Complex lipids in mammals are limited to phospholipids (PLs) or SLs, which are particularly concentrated (with PLs predominating overall) in cell membranes. PLs and SLs also show prominent differential tissue and organelle distribution. (Representative complex lipid structures are presented in Figure 21.2a through e.)

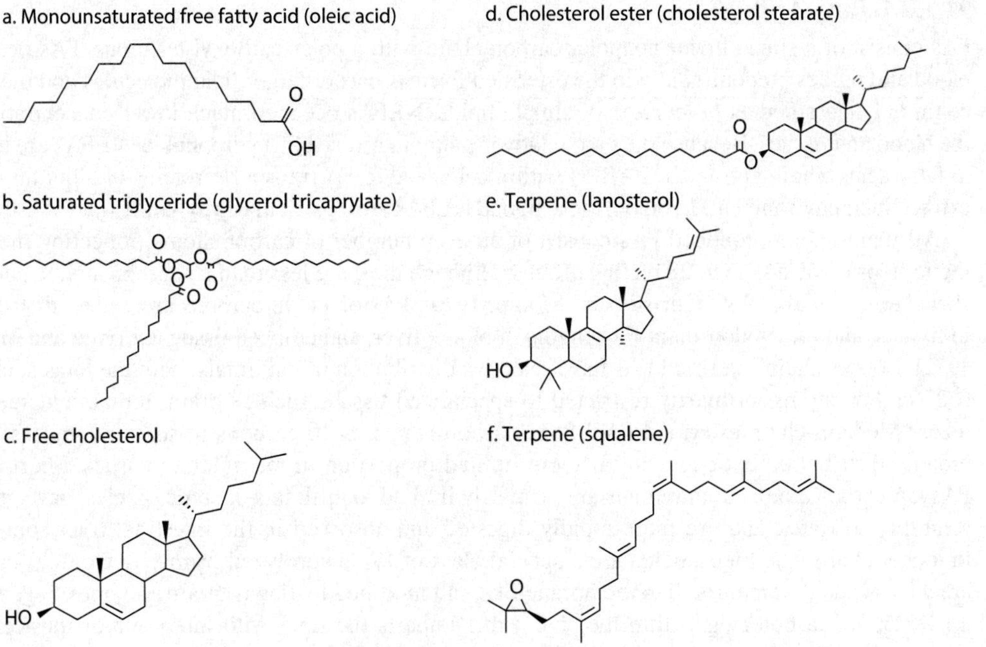

a. Monounsaturated free fatty acid (oleic acid)

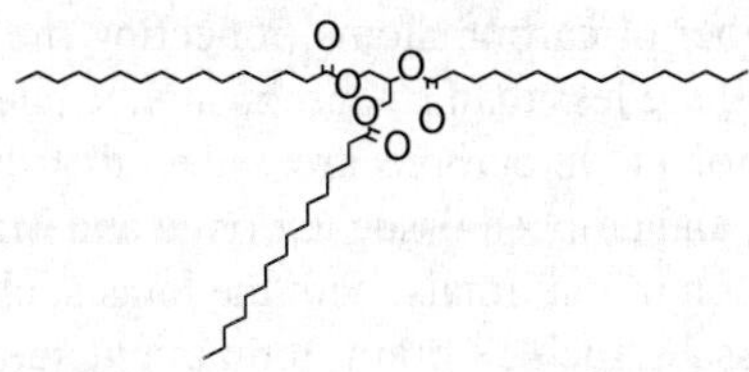

b. Saturated triglyceride (glycerol tricaprylate)

c. Free cholesterol

d. Cholesterol ester (cholesterol stearate)

e. Terpene (lanosterol)

f. Terpene (squalene)

FIGURE 21.1 Representative structure of simple lipids.

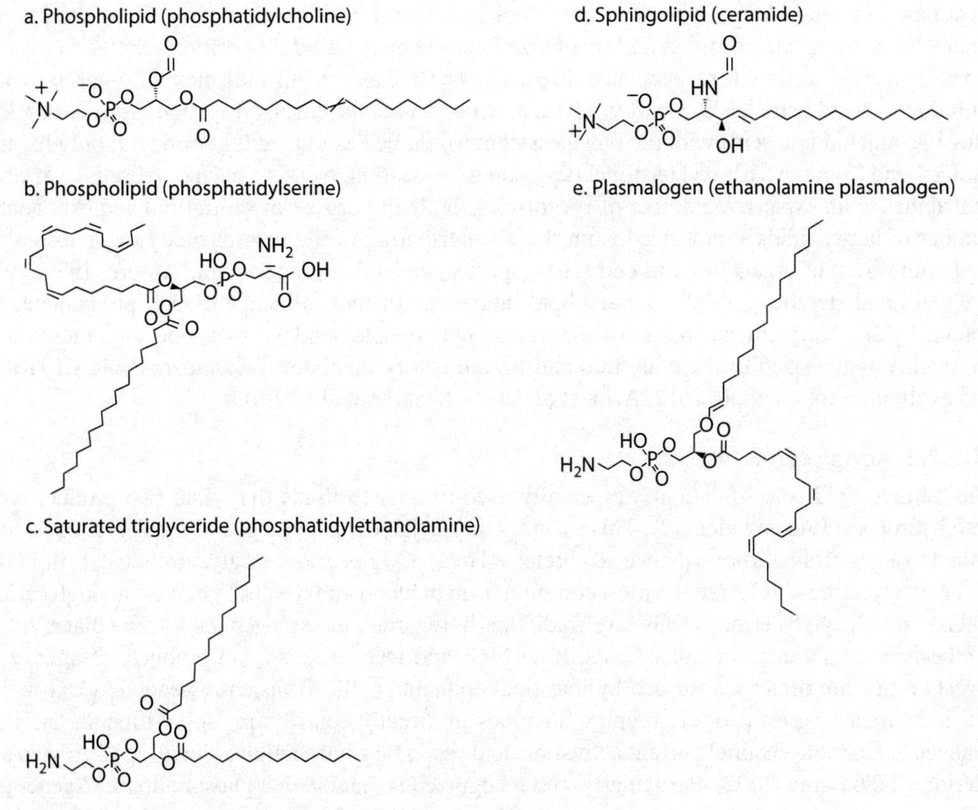

a. Phospholipid (phosphatidylcholine)

b. Phospholipid (phosphatidylserine)

c. Saturated triglyceride (phosphatidylethanolamine)

d. Sphingolipid (ceramide)

e. Plasmalogen (ethanolamine plasmalogen)

FIGURE 21.2 Representative structures of complex lipids.

21.2.2.1 Fatty Acids

FAs consist of a single linear nonpolar carbon chain with a polar carboxyl terminus. FAs occur in blood and tissues predominantly in the esterified form as part of larger lipid molecules and thus, are commonly classified as *precursor*s of simple lipids. NEFAs occur in much lower concentration in the blood and tissues. Because they are relatively, although variably, hydrophobic, NEFAs are bound to fatty acid–binding proteins (FABPs) within cells, and to FA transport proteins or albumin in the extracellular environment. In blood, these bound NEFAs are a particularly dynamic lipid constituent.

All mammalian-produced FAs consist of an even number of carbon atoms (reflecting the synthetic steps involved) up to 28 methyl groups, although most are less than 22 carbon atoms in length (Brockerhoff et al., 1966; Christie and Moore, 1970). FAs of 14–18 carbons are widely distributed in tissues, and the predominant FA lengths in blood, liver, and adipose tissue (Christie and Moore, 1972). Longer-chain esterified FAs have selective distribution in mammals, with the longest chains (≥22 carbon atoms) primarily restricted to specialized tissues such as brain, retina, and spermatozoa. Medium-chain esterified FAs (8–12 carbon atoms; 6–10 carbons in some references) have broader distribution but occur in far more limited proportion in mammalian tissues. Short-chain FAs (≤6 carbon atoms) in mammals are primarily limited to milk fats of some species, have greater solubility in water, and are more rapidly digested and absorbed in the intestinal tract compared to longer-chain fats. Eicosanoids are a special class of FAs hydrolyzed primarily from 20-carbon arachidonic acid in mammalian membrane PLs and modified by downstream enzymes to generate a five- or six-carbon ring within the chain; this imparts the lipid with inter- and/or intracellular signaling activity (e.g., as prostaglandins, prostacyclins, thromboxanes, leukotrienes, or lipoxins).

FAs are subclassified based on their length and degree of unsaturated carbon bonds. Unsaturated, naturally occurring FA bonds are generally *cis* configuration and separated by at least one unsaturated methyl group resulting in a 120° bend in the chain. There are multiple FA naming systems, most based on chain length and number, and/or location of unsaturated bonds. The delta (Δ) and omega (ω) systems are common and recognize double bonds based on position relative to the carboxyl or methyl terminal, respectively. Thus, C_{20}:4 in the Δ system indicates a 20-carbon chain with double bond between C-5-6, 8-9, 11-12, and 14-15 with the carboxyl carbon representing C-1. This FA (arachidonic acid) with the omega system would be designated C_{20}:4n-6 with only the first double bond from the carboxyl terminal designated by location. Notably, each of these FA variables contributes to an expansive number of FA forms (length and degree of saturation) and exponential number of larger lipids synthesized from them, contributing to the heterogeneity of lipids associated with different organelles and cell types, species, and so on (Christie and Moore, 1970, 1972; Sheppard and Herzberg, 1992). Dietary lipid intake can further influence tissue lipid content; the popularity of dietary omega 3n FAs (with three or more double bonds) is partly because these forms are readily synthesized in the body into anti-inflammatory mediators, such as resolvin E1 (RvE1) and oxylipins (Abbott et al., 2012; Arita et al., 2005; Shearer et al., 2010).

21.2.2.2 Acylglycerols

The "simple lipid" classification is especially used to refer to lipids that yield two product types with hydrolysis: FAs and alcohols. This includes the acylglycerols with one to three FAs covalently linked to a glycerol backbone (hence, also referred to as acylglycerides or glycerolipids). Within this group, triglycerides (TGs) are the most common form in blood and tissues, whereas monoglycerides (MGs) and diacylglycerides (DGs) are traditionally regarded as endogenous intermediates in the synthesis or degradation of other lipids. Both MGs and DGs are also end products of dietary fat digestion that are directly absorbed by intestinal epithelial cells. Transiently generated DG within cell membranes serves further complex functions in directly contributing to cell membrane fluid changes, membrane channel current activation, and secondary intracellular signaling (Carrasco and Mérida, 2007; Large, 2002). Particularly well recognized is the role that phospholipase C-generated DG serves as an activator of protein kinase C (Cai et al., 1997).

TGs serve as the primary intracellular lipid and are stored in specialized intracellular lipid droplet organelles. TG-containing lipid droplets are most abundant in adipose tissue, with much lower proportions in liver and striated muscle in most mammalian species. The constituent FAs of TGs in droplets vary, and the TG turnover within these intracellular stores is highly regulated. Intracellular TGs serve primarily as a source of components for other lipids and metabolizable energy. In contrast with most other major lipid types, TGs are not found in, and cannot cross through, cell membranes. In serum/plasma, TGs are second in concentration only to PLs of the major circulating lipids by class.

Structurally, the three different glycerol carbons of acylglycerols available for covalent linking with an FA are stereochemically identified by the (-*sn*-) numbering system (*sn*-1, -2, or -3), or α, β, or α‘. The *sn*-1, and *sn*-1 and *sn*-2 positions are typically acylated in MGs and DGs, respectively. These different carbons are also differentially recognized by endogenous enzymes of lipolysis and lipogenesis.

21.2.2.3 Sterols

A distinct category of simple lipids that also yield FAs and alcohols with hydrolysis are those composed of a four-fused carbon ring structure. This includes free cholesterol, CEs, and other sterols and sterol esters (e.g., steroid hormones: estrogens, androgens, glucocorticoids, and mineralocorticoids; bile acids and absorbed plant sterols) and five-carbon terpene (isoprene) polymers. Of all of these members, free cholesterol and CEs strongly predominate in mass in mammalian tissues, including blood.

Free cholesterol is abundant in cell membranes and has an important structural role in adding rigidity, and lateral organization by intercalating between other membrane lipids and proteins. The rings of cholesterol, as with most sterols are joined by *trans* junctions and give the molecule a planar conformation, with outside groups lying at the same angle away from the plane. The greatest relative proportion of cholesterol is in plasma membranes, while the less rigid membranes of mitochondria, endoplasmic reticulum (ER), and Golgi have much lower content. Free cholesterol content of membranes also varies between tissues, with the brain containing the greatest proportion by weight compared to all other organs. The distribution of the sterol in membranes also has functional, as well as structural purposes. The rigidity and planar nature enables free cholesterol to partition into membrane microdomains or "lipid rafts" variably organized with other lipids and proteins. Lipid rafts are essential for numerous membrane activities, including endocytosis, exocytosis, protein trafficking, signaling, and apoptosis. Conversely, free cholesterol in blood is the minor component; CEs are the major transport form of cholesterol in the circulation (Quehenberger et al., 2010).

CEs are covalently linked with long-chain FAs and are less polar than free cholesterol and thus, have a more limited role in cell membranes (Forrest and Cushley, 1977). Rather, intracellular CEs predominate within cytoplasmic lipid droplet organelles, and they are hydrolyzed in lysosomes and endosomes for component transfer to membranes, or metabolism/degradation (Wang et al., 2005). As with TGs, lipid droplet regulation of CE turnover is highly regulated. In adipocytes, CEs in lipid droplets are relatively low in concentration, likely due to their very active turnover in these cells (Radeau et al., 1995). Conversely, CE-containing droplets are particularly abundant in cells of the adrenal cortex (serving as precursor source for adrenal steroids) with some differences between species and sexes (Kraemer et al., 2002). With certain pathologic conditions (e.g., atherosclerotic plaques, xanthoma), CEs build up within (e.g., macrophage) lysosomes (Jerome, 2010).

21.2.2.4 Terpenes

Terpenes comprise a relatively miniscule proportion of blood lipids (Quehenberger et al., 2010). Polymers of five-carbon isoprene synthesized in mammals are generally limited to triterpenes and include lanosterol and squalene waxes and polyprenols (which mostly exist in cell membranes). Most, but not all of terpene structures contain carbon rings; in particular, squalene is a linear chain.

Notably, exogenous terpenes with other than three unit numbers are common in plants and bacterium, and include important essential nutrients such as vitamins A, E, and K. The carotenoids (α-carotene, lycopene, lutein, and zeaxanthin) taxol, limonene, and menthol are also among the plant terpenes with medicinal use.

21.2.2.5 Phospholipids

PLs are the major lipid components in blood, by concentration, comprising around 40% of total circulating lipids (Quehenberger et al., 2010; Quehenberger and Dennis, 2011). These complex lipids have a glycerol backbone linked to long-chain FAs on carbon (C)1 and C2, plus a phosphate group on C3, and may also be referred to as glycerophospholipids or phosphoglycerides (Goldfine, 2010). The most fundamental PL, phosphatidic acid has a simple, small, highly charged phosphate head and is relatively short-lived. Phosphatidic acid is a common precursor to other lipids within cells, including eicosanoids, DGs, and more extended PLs. Some PLs have their phosphate group further acetylated to an amino alcohol, such as choline, inositol, cephalin, or serine (i.e., phosphatidylcholine, phosphatidyl-inositol, phosphatidylethanolamine, or phosphatidylserine, respectively). Phosphotidylcholine (PL-C) is the most abundant PL in blood, cell membranes, and alveolar surfactant, and is termed "lecithin." Lysolecithin and other "lyso" PLs are phosphoglycerols esterified to only a single FA, and mostly serve as intermediates in interconversion of charged PLs with other structures. In lipid membranes, the combination and conversion of PLs with polar heads of different charge contribute to vesicle formation, fusion, and other aspects of membrane shape (Kooijman et al., 2003; Roelofsen et al., 1987; Weigert et al., 1999). In addition, PLs with cationic amino acids such as phosphatidic acid and PL-C tend to be in the outer bilayer leaflet, whereas anionic amino acid-containing PLs, such as phosphatidylethanolamine and phosphatidylserine tend to reside in the inner leaflet of resting membranes. Flip-flop of these charged PLs between leaflets has been linked to signaling events such as initiation of coagulation, apoptosis and specific binding, and phagocytosis by mononuclear phagocytes (Sapay et al., 2010).

Plasmalogens are a particularly unique PL found in high concentration in membranes of cardiac myocytes, adult nervous tissue, testes (especially spermatozoal acrosomes), and eye lenses (Goldfine, 2010; Lessig and Fuchs, 2009). Plasmalogens resemble phosphatidylethanolamine except that the *sn*-1 FA is linked by an ether bond with *cis* double bond on the adjacent alkyl chain. This difference allows plasmalogens to pack more closely in membranes making them less permeable and cleaved only by specific enzymes, which may account for their concentration in these specific tissues. Plasmalogens also facilitate membrane fusion and are a major reservoir of arachidonic acid for synthesis of lipid second messengers; functions that may also help explain their distinct tissue distribution (Lessig and Fuchs, 2009; Nagan and Zoeller, 2001).

21.2.2.6 Sphingolipids

SLs are also a major lipid component in blood. SLs consist of a sphingosine backbone linked by amide bond to a FA. The sphingosine molecule has a long (mainly 18 carbons in length) unsaturated hydrocarbon chain with C17 polar amino; thus, like the PLs, SLs consist of a polar group bound to two nonpolar tails (and are sometimes considered a form of PL, although lacking glycerol). Ceramide is the simplest SL, and a precursor to more complex SLs that are also referred to as glucosylceramides and galactosylceramides. For example, ceramide can react with phophatidylcholine to form sphingomyelin (ceramide phosphorylcholine), which is the most abundant SL in blood, and cell membranes overall (primarily in the outer bilayer leaflet) (Quehenberger et al., 2010; Merrill, 2011). Sphingomyelin is particularly concentrated in membranes of the central nervous system (CNS), and uniquely in erythrocytes of ruminants (Wood and Quiroz-Rocha, 2010). Other complex SLs are more selectively found in mammalian tissue-type membranes, and include cerebrosides, sulfatides, globosides, and gangliosides. Membrane SL content also varies within cells; plasma membranes generally have greater SL content compared with major organelles.

SLs in cell membranes have been shown to have bioactive roles in signal transduction, cell adhesion, intracellular and transcellular protein trafficking (e.g., transferrin endocytosis), modulating hormone responses, and/or antigen recognition (Merrill, 2011; Taniguchi and Okazaki, 2014). Some of these functions are mediated by SLs in combination with cholesterol as lipid membrane microdomains or rafts. A particularly well-studied signaling SL and downstream product of ceramide is sphingosine 1-phosphate (S1P). S1P is an example of a signaling lipid that retains this role within, and outside of cell membranes, including in circulating blood (Argraves and Argraves, 2007). This SL has a growing list of signaling roles including modulation of cellular immunity and cell growth, survival, differentiation, and migration (Rosen and Goetzl, 2005; Taha et al., 2006). SLs and their signaling role or metabolism have additionally been functionally associated in different contexts with a wide variety of human diseases including diabetes, and select neurodegenerative, cardiovascular, respiratory, neoplastic, and infectious diseases (Deevska and Nikolava-Karakasian, 2011; Haughey, 2010; Goldkorn and Filosto, 2010; Berenson et al., 2010; Xu et al., 2010).

21.3 LIPID SOURCES

21.3.1 Dietary Lipids

In the normal fed state, the primary source of tissue lipids of humans and most laboratory animals are derived from the diet. Dietary lipids require digestion to NEFAs, MGs, DGs, and free cholesterol for intestinal absorption. Ingested fats are first exposed to lipases in the oral cavity and stomach, and then to pancreatic acylglycerol lipases, phosholipases, carboxyl (cholesterol) ester lipases, and conjugated bile acids in the proximal small intestine (Hamosh et al., 1998; Hui and Howles, 2002; Kirby et al., 2002; Vaganay et al., 1998). Oral (lingual) lipase is a significant contributor to lipid digestion in adult mice and rats but appears to be less important in other tested species (rabbit, guinea pig, baboon, and humans) (DeNigris et al., 1988; Hamosh, 1978; Voigt et al., 2014); therefore, ingestion and gavage of lipid meals in most animals show limited difference in the products absorbed. Oral and gastric lipases vary in their efficiency with dietary long medium-chain versus medium-chain TGs and collectively enable some fat absorption even in the absence of pancreatic lipase. Pancreatic/small intestinal emulsification of the lipids with micelle formation is enabled by mixing with bile acids and is an essential process, as critical enzymes are generally active only at the oil–water interface. In addition, the quantity of each individual lipid type that can be absorbed depends upon the amount emulsified into, and size and content of the mixed micelles. In this way, although each lipid type is absorbed separately from the micelle, the amount of digestible TGs has an important positive influence on the amount of absorbed cholesterol. Conversely, the amount of select PLs in micelles may have a negative impact on cholesterol absorption (Rampone and Long, 1977). Importantly, absorbed lipid is also derived from enterocyte cell turnover and bile acids; these perpetual cholesterol-rich sources help explain why blood cholesterol concentration is far less affected than circulating TGs with fasting/anorexia, or loss of pancreatic enzyme activity (Tso et al., 2004).

Dietary FAs less than 12 carbons in length can be at least partly absorbed in the small and large intestine without micelle incorporation (Jørgensen et al., 2001; Ruppin and Middleton, 1980; You et al., 2008). These short- and medium-chain FAs are transported in portal circulation as albumin-bound NEFAs and are largely fated for hepatic β-oxidation in mitochondria (Section 21.7). Correspondingly, a diet rich in medium-chain FAs has been used to treat various human and animal malabsorption syndromes, and has reported benefit in upregulating metabolic oxidative processes (Beermann et al., 2003; Kuwahata et al., 2011; Pan et al., 2010; Wein et al., 2009).

Additional components of intestinal micelles are plant sterols, which are usually poorly absorbed and not utilized by mammalian cells; however, they displace cholesterol in micelles, inhibiting nonesterified cholesterol enterocyte uptake (Batta et al., 2006; Lu et al., 2001). Animals and patients with mutations in adenosine triphosphate (ATP)-binding cassette (ABC) transporter protein genes

(*ABCG5* and *ABCG8*) that encode for sterolin-1 and sterolin-2 enterocyte brush border transporter proteins lack the ability to restrict the amount or type of sterols absorbed, or to excrete sterols into bile, and have hypercholesterolemia as well as increased circulating plant sterols (Izar et al., 2011). Findings in these individuals provided early confirmation of the presence of enterocyte transporter proteins for specific lipid species.

Other specific enterocyte membrane transporter proteins for NEFAs, 2-MGs, and cholesterol have also now been reported (Murota and Storch, 2005; Nassir et al., 2007). These include the jejunal enterocyte brush border cholesterol transporter known as Nieman-Pick C1-like 1 (NPC1L1) protein (inhibited by the serum cholesterol-lowering drug ezetimbe), and cluster of differentiation 36 (CD36) and fatty acid transport protein 4 (FATP4), which have both shown measurable activity only under conditions of fasting and thus, may represent a redundant mechanism to ensure uptake of essential FAs when supply is limited (Garcia-Calvo et al., 2005; Tso et al., 2004). Enterocyte absorption of micellar lipids additionally occurs by passive diffusion facilitated by a low-pH microclimate lining the small intestinal villus surface that protonates NEFAs, reducing their solubility within micelles (Shia et al., 1985). Collectively, these findings indicate multiple mechanisms for intestinal lipid uptake with redundancy and supply-dependent mechanisms ensuring maintenance of essential nutrient absorption.

21.3.2 De Novo Lipid Synthesis

Both FAs and cholesterol (and a spectrum of simple and complex lipids derived from these products) are synthesized in mammalian tissues. Synthesis is particularly promoted in states of high insulin activity or excess dietary carbohydrates (with corresponding high mitochondrial Krebs cycle citrate and ATP production). Synthesis begins with the transport of citrate out of mitochondrion into the cytosol, where it is cleaved to form acetyl-CoA. These synthetic processes for both FAs and cholesterol are particularly active in hepatocytes. FA synthesis is also generally active in adipocytes (white and brown fat), lactating mammary gland and, to much a lesser extent, in striated muscle and skin (Harvey et al., 2005). However, cholesterol synthesis occurs in essentially all tissue cells, with prominent activity in intestine, adrenal gland, and reproductive tissues (e.g., ovaries, testes, placenta) in addition to liver (Tso et al., 2004; Turley et al., 1995).

21.3.2.1 Fatty Acid Synthesis

FA synthesis from acetyl-CoA occurs in two carbons at a time from the carboxyl end toward the carboxylic acid end via condensation with malonyl-CoA, and release of CO_2. This reaction is initiated by the rate-limiting enzyme, acetyl-CoA carboxylase (ACC), which is highly regulated by nutritional status and hormones (e.g., insulin, epinephrine, and glucagon) (Brownsey et al., 2006; Tso et al., 2004). Nearly all subsequent cytosolic FA-synthesizing enzyme reactions in mammals are catalyzed by a single, long peptide with multiple functional domains ("fatty acid synthase"). The product of these reactions is a saturated FA up to 16 carbons long (i.e., palmitic acid).

Further FA chain elongation and/or desaturation can occur through transport, and additional enzymes in mitochondria or ER. Regulation of these elongases and desaturases, and the role of specific FA chain length and saturation in physiological processes of cells are still poorly defined. However, a general role for nuclear hormone receptors in FA synthetic process has been reported for peroxisome proliferator-activated receptor α (PPARα), liver X receptor (LXR), sterol-regulatory element-binding protein-1 (SREBP-1), and others (Wang et al., 2006, 2008). These factors are, in turn, regulated by local levels of glucose, insulin, thyroid hormones, and leptin. Products of the FA synthesis pathway also bridge with FA catabolic pathways in regulating key enzymes (Section 21.7).

21.3.2.2 Cholesterol Synthesis

Cholesterol synthesis is initiated by condensation of acetyl-CoA with four-carbon-chain acetoacetyl-CoA to form the branched 3-hydroxy-3-methylglutaryl-CoA (HMG-CoA), catalyzed by cytosolic HMG-CoA synthase (an enzyme distinct from mitochondrial HMG-CoA synthase; Section 21.7). This six-carbon product is then reduced to mevalonate with release of coenzyme A (CoA) in a two-step reaction by the critical, rate-limiting enzyme, HMG-CoA reductase. HMG-CoA reductase is localized to the ER membrane, but with the catalytic domain exposed to the cytosol. HMG-CoA reductase is also highly regulated by certain hormones and end-product negative feedback. Stimulation of this enzyme's activity and ultimately, cholesterol synthesis is mediated by insulin, and inhibited by glucagon and epinephrine. Regulation by these hormones is rapid as it involves reversible protein phosphorylation of HMG-CoA reductase through a chain of upstream protein kinases. However, more long-term effects on the enzyme's activity by intracellular cholesterol levels involves the transcription factor SREBP and is mediated by complex multivalent regulation of HMG-CoA reductase gene transcription and translation, and mRNA degradation (Clarke and Hardie, 1990). Because of its pivotal role in cholesterol synthesis, HMG-CoA reductase is a major pharmaceutical target for blood cholesterol reduction (e.g., statins).

21.4 BLOOD LIPID TRANSPORT

Considering blood lipids based on their transport in circulation has particular relevance for understanding and interpreting serum/plasma lipid changes. The majority of blood lipids are transported in LPs. Structurally, LPs are disk shaped to spherical with a single outer layer of amphipathic lipids (PLs, SLs, and free cholesterol) surrounding a core of more hydrophobic TG, CEs, and sometimes terpenes (e.g., carotenes, vitamin D, E, K). Lipoproteins are classified based on their relative concentrations of each of these lipid structural types and surface-expressed apos. Laboratory classification of LPs is also by measurable particle size and density; however, the methods and cut-off values for these endpoints varies between methods, studies, and species. Importantly, the concentration of these LPs generally determines concentrations of plasma/serum simple and complex lipids, with the exception of NEFAs, which are transported, bound to other circulating components.

21.4.1 Apolipoproteins

Apos largely consist of amphipathic peptide helixes that have one face of hydrophobic amino acids associated with the particle surface lipids, and the other face of polar/hydrophilic amino acids variably exposed to interact with the environment. Apos in these particles serve as enzyme cofactors, activators, or inhibitors, and/or as ligands to facilitate membrane interactions, tissue secretion, or uptake. In this way, the proteins are the primary determinant of the fate of the circulating LP lipids. Notably, except for the larger apoB proteins, apos are only weakly associated with the outer layer lipids via hydrogen bonding and van der Waals forces enabling variable exchange of apos between particles. Similar weak bonding also enables considerable exchange of outer layer lipids between circulating LP types.

Among common laboratory species and humans, major apo classes and functions are generally comparable (Table 21.2). However, they have (often phylogenetically based) differences in amino acid sequence, thus requiring species-specific assays for accurate and optimal quantitation in collected samples (Luo et al., 1989). Also important for interpreting nonclinical lipid data and translating findings to humans is recognition of major species differences in (1) organ/tissue sources of some apos (e.g., apoB48), (2) lipid-metabolizing enzymes that interact with these proteins (e.g., CETP), and (3) common regulatory mechanisms of lipid metabolism (e.g., catecholamines).

21.5 LIPOPROTEIN SYNTHESIS AND METABOLISM

Lipoproteins are typically distinguished in the laboratory based on analytical properties (density, diameter, electrophoretic migration, and proportional lipid content). However, they are interdependent with each other and with regulators of lipid metabolism overall so that physiologic or pathologic

TABLE 21.2
Apoproteins of Animals and Humans

Apoprotein	Lipoproteins Associated	Tissue Source of Plasma Levels	Major/General Function	Associated Enzyme and Transporter Interactions	Disease Relationship(s)
A-I	HDL > chylomicron *(readily transferred to HDL in circulation)*	Enterocytes; hepatocytes	Promotes cholesterol efflux from tissue cells to HDL, and HDL uptake of free cholesterol from VLDL and LD in exchange for TG via LCAT	LCAT cofactor; additionally, interacts with cell transporters (*ABCA1* and *ABCG1*) and SR-B1 enabling selective cholesterol uptake from tissues	Human mutations have been associated with low blood HDL, Tangier-like disease, or variant of systemic amyloidosis. ApoA-I blood levels have also been negatively correlated with hepatic fibrosis (Bedossa et al., 1989; Vigushin et al., 1994)
	HDL >> chylomicron > VLDL	Hepatocyte; enterocytes	Role in HDL particle size and composition	Conflicting findings that ApoA-II inhibits or enhances hepatic lipase activity. (Bedossa et al., 1989; Vigushin et al., 1994)	Broad species differences in ApoA-II structure. ApoA-II is absent or only in very low concentrations in plasma of dogs, rabbits, pigs, and chickens. (Zhong et al., 1994) ApoA-II deficiency or over-expression in mice is associated with altered HDL size distribution, with no overt abnormalities. (Tso et al., 1999)
A-IV	Chylomicron *(nascent)*, HDL *(especially larger particles)*	Enterocytes, and in mice, rats, and rabbits, also hepatocytes	Modulates enterocyte and hepatocyte transcellular lipid transport and has role in appetite and satiety via CNS (inhibits food intake in rodent models). Synthesis upregulated by intestinal fat absorption and PYY hormone (Mowri et al., 1996)	Activates LCAT; inhibits LPL activation (Blanco-Vaca et al., 2001)	Humans with select ApoA-IV polymorphisms show delayed chylomicron clearance.
A-V	VLDL, chylomicron, HDL	Hepatocytes	Regulation of plasma TG levels	LPL activation	Mice lacking apoA-V have 4X increased blood TG; some human variants are associated with higher plasma TG (Tso et al., 1999)

(Continued)

TABLE 21.2 (*Continued*)
Apoproteins of Animals and Humans

Apoprotein	Lipoproteins Associated	Tissue Source of Plasma Levels	Major/General Function	Associated Enzyme and Transporter Interactions	Disease Relationship(s)
B-48	Chylomicrons, chylomicron remnants > and (in mice, rats, and dogs) VLDL	Enterocyte; and (in mice rats, dogs) hepatocytes	Enables synthesis and secretion of TG-rich LPs; truncated version of apoB-100 (and lacks the LDL receptor-binding domain)	Interacts intracellularly with the ER lipid transfer protein (MTP)	Genetic deficiency of both ApoB-48 and B-100 (abetalipoproteinemia) may be attributed to mutations in MTP gene. Clinical signs are due to impaired intestinal absorption of fat and fat-soluble vitamins. Blood levels of ApoB-48 have been purported to be a marker of metabolic syndrome risk
B-100	VLDL, IDL, LDL	Hepatocyte >> enterocyte	Aids synthesis and secretion of TG-rich LPs, and their uptake in tissues by the LDL receptor	Interacts intracellularly with the ER lipid transfer protein "MTP"; binds tissue LDL receptor	In addition to abetalipoproteinemia (above), mutations of the LDL receptor interfere with ApoB-100 function, generally impairing VLDL, IDL and especially LDL uptake (e.g., "familial hypercholesterolemia"). Selective deficiency of ApoB-100 has also been reported (Hockey et al., 2001)
C-I	HDL, chylomicrons, chylomicron remnants, VLDL, and IDL *(readily transferred between particles)*	Hepatocytes >>skin, testes, spleen, lung	Regulatory role in tissue lipid uptake from, and clearance of lipoproteins	Role in activating LCAT; and to a lesser degree, inhibiting LPL, HL, phospholipase A 2, CETP and ApoE-mediated binding to LRP, LDR, and VLDLR (may be due to ApoC-I ability to displace, mask or alter conformation of ApoE).	Familial chylomicronemia with deficiency in man (Kluger et al., 2008); Mice with deficiency show mildly impaired VLDL clearance. Knockout mice develop hypercholesterolemia with high cholesterol diet. ApoC-I overexpression in mice results in hypertriglyceridemia and hypercholesterolemia (Herbert et al., 1985)
C-II	Chylomicron remnants, VLDL, IDL, HDL		Regulatory role in tissue lipid uptake from, and clearance of lipoproteins	Activator of LPL > Role in inhibiting ApoE- and ApoB-mediated receptor binding, HL, and LCAT activity	Human deficiency: hyperlipoproteinemia type IB

(*Continued*)

TABLE 21.2 (*Continued*)
Apoproteins of Animals and Humans

Apoprotein	Lipoproteins Associated	Tissue Source of Plasma Levels	Major/General Function	Associated Enzyme and Transporter Interactions	Disease Relationship(s)
C-III	Chylomicron remnants, VLDL, IDL, HDL		Regulatory role in tissue lipid uptake from, and clearance of lipoproteins, and hepatic formation of VLDL	Inhibits activation of LPL, and ApoE- & ApoB-mediated receptor binding (with displacement of ApoE from small VLDL), inhibits HL, and LCAT activity; may enhance CETP and hepatic VLDL formation (Jong et al., 1999)	Human mutation associated with low blood triglycerides (King, 2007); knockout mice are hypotriglyceridemic; increased circulating ApoC-III levels have been linked with prolonged postprandial lipemia and metabolic syndrome in man (Qin et al., 2011)
D	HDL *(larger particle)* >> *VLDL* (Hofker, 2010)	A wide variety of tissues, including liver, adipose, heart, skeletal muscle, CNS, PNS, testes and ovaries	Function(s) unknown		ApoD in tissues have been associated with some pathologic, including psychiatric, conditions in man; Deficiency in mice associated with nonfasting hypertriglyceridemia and hyperinsulinemia (Clemente-Postigo et al., 2010)
E	Chylomicron remnants, VLDL, IDL > HDL	liver >>, macrophages; multiple other tissues	Receptor mediated clearance of apoE and apoB containing lipoproteins	High affinity ligand for the LDL receptor, the LDL receptor related protein 1 (LRP1), VLDL receptor, and the apoE receptor 2	Familial dysbetalipoproteinemia or type III hyperlipoproteinemia in humans with mutations; human deficiency also associated with atherosclerosis, Alzheimer's, shortened life span
H *(aka: β2-Glycoprotein I)*	Chylomicrons, HDL, VLDL very small quantities	Liver, human placenta (Perdomo et al., 2010)	Preferentially binds to negatively charged PLs: contributes to role in blood coagulation, platelet agglutination, and innate immunity; role in lipid metabolism is unclear		Major antigen for the circulating antibodies in the antiphospholipid syndrome (Jiménez-Palomares et al., 2011); deficiency may contribute to prothrombotic states or impaired innate immunity

(*Continued*)

TABLE 21.2 (*Continued*)
Apoproteins of Animals and Humans

Apoprotein	Lipoproteins Associated	Tissue Source of Plasma Levels	Major/General Function	Associated Enzyme and Transporter Interactions	Disease Relationship(s)
J *(aka: clusterin)*	HDL *(primarily smaller, more dense particles)*	Many tissues, including (human) smooth muscle cells associated with atherosclerotic lesions (Chamley et al., 1997)	May have a beneficial role in reverse cholesterol transport, and inactivation of complement C5b-9 complexes; however, has also been linked with amyloid β plaque formation (De Groot and Meijers, 2011; Schwarz et al., 2008)		Blood levels have been proposed as a negative risk factor for vascular disease
(a)	Covalently attached to ApoB100 in man and some nonhuman primate species	Hepatocytes	May have adverse role in inhibiting fibrinolysis, and promoting oxidation of PL and LDL within atherosclerotic lesions		Biomarker for cerebro-and cardio-vascular atherothrombosis risk (Gelissen et al., 1998)

Anglés-Cano et al. (2001).

changes are generally not isolated to a single LP. Lipid content within LPs is also generally comparable between common laboratory species and humans for the dominant lipid types (Table 21.3). However, the specific lipid and protein composition and proportions vary between species. These differences, as well as those in regulating enzymes, neurohormonal, nutritional, and other physiologic signals that affect LP metabolism account for many of the species differences in routine blood lipid data.

TABLE 21.3
Composition of Lipoproteins of Animals

Lipoprotein	Major Organ/Cell Synthesizing	Core Lipids (Approximate %)		Surface Components (Approximate %)			MW[a]/ Diameter[b]	Major Associated Apolipoproteins (apo)
		TG	CE	PL	FC	Protein		
Chylomicron	Small intestine enterocyte	≥85	<10	6–12	1–3	1–2	1000/ 100–1000	Major: B-48; E; Minor: A-I; A-II; A-IV; A-V; C-I; C-II; C-III
VLDL	Hepatocyte; enterocyte; cardiac myocyte	60	8	15	7	10	7500/ 30–80	B-100; E; C-I; C-II; C-III; A-II; A-V (B-48 in mice, rats and dogs)
IDL	VLDL degradation product	20	30	20	10	20	4000/ 25–35	B-100: E, C-I, C-II, C-III
LDL	VLDL degradation product	30	20	15	15	20	2000/ 15–25	B-100
HDL1	In circulation	12	20	30	8	30	200–400/ 10–14	A-I; A-II; A-IV; C-I; C-II; C-III; E, D
HDL2	In circulation	<5	20	30	5	40	200–400/ 8–11	A-I; A-II; A-IV; C-I; C-II; C-III; E, D
HDL3	In circulation (Hepatocyte/ enterocyte precursor origin)	<1	15	25	10	50	200–400/ 6–9	A-I; A-II; C-I; C-II; C-III; Major: E
Lp(a)	Liver	d	d	d	d	D	d	B-100; apo(a)
NEFAs	Adipose; skeletal muscle	–	–	–	–	–	–	Primarily bound to albumin

Lipid composition values adapted (rounded) from unpublished studies of rats and dogs, and published data for rat (Cartwright et al., 1982).

TG, triglyceride; CE, cholesterol ester; PL, phospholipid; FC, free cholesterol; MW, molecular weight; VLDL, very low-density lipoprotein; IDL, intermediate-density lipoprotein; LDL, low-density lipoprotein; Lp(a), lipoprotein A; NEFA, nonesterified fatty acid.

[a] MW; molecular weight (kilodaltons).

[b] Diameter in nanometers (nm); d: Lp(a) composition in nonhuman primates was not available, but expected to be similar to that of LDL in the respective species.

21.5.1 Chylomicron Assembly and Secretion

Chylomicron synthesis begins with enterocyte absorption of long-chain FAs that are bound to intestinal FABPs (Mansbach and Siddiqi, 2010). These are transported into the ER for reassembly into TGs. De novo TG synthesis through uptake of blood FAs and the α-glycerophosphate pathway is also utilized for chylomicron synthesis by enterocytes, especially when intracellular FA supply is inadequate (Gangl and Ockner, 1975; Guo et al., 2005; Shiau et al., 1985). The generated TGs are packaged via microsomal triglyceride transfer protein (MTP) with much smaller proportions of cholesterol, PLs, and LPs of apoB48, A-I, and A-IV within the ER to produce chylomicrons (Table 21.3) (Berriot-Varoqueaux et al., 2000). Mutations in MTP constitute the genetic basis for abetalipoproteinemia in humans and animal models (partly characterized by severe steatorrhea and reduced circulating lipids). Inhibitors of MTP have also been investigated as therapeutics to lower circulating blood lipid, especially TG concentrations (Aggarwal et al., 2005).

The nascent intracellular chylomicrons are transported by ER carrier proteins into the Golgi. Rare defects in these ER chylomicron transporter proteins have been demonstrated in human (e.g., Sar1b) resulting in chylomicron retention diseases characterized by severe fat malabsorption (Shoulders et al., 2004). Notably, these proteins are also being evaluated as drug targets for metabolic diseases. Chylomicrons reaching the Golgi complex are transferred to exocytotic vesicles, which are transported to the basolateral membrane, and their contents are secreted extracellularly. Secreted chylomicrons, aided by interstitial hydration, enter into mucosal lymphatics and ultimately into the bloodstream (Tso and Balint, 1986).

21.5.2 Chylomicron Catabolism

Of all the circulating LPs, nascent chylomicrons are the largest and least dense due to their predominance (≥85%) of unsaturated FA containing TGs (Table 21.3) (Kalogeris and Story, 1992). The wide range in size and density for chylomicrons is similarly linked to a wide range in TG content. The primary protein associated with chylomicrons, apoB48, is so called as it represents the N-terminal ~48% of apoB100 in humans. ApoB48 in laboratory species is similarly derived from the homologous apoB100 gene mRNA as a co- or posttranslationally modified protein (although variable amino acid sequences for these apos between species generally require distinct assays for detection/measurement) (Corsini et al., 1992; Greeve et al., 1993; Kendrick et al., 2001). The expression of apoB48 enables efficient synthesis and secretion of chylomicrons by small intestinal enterocytes. Importantly, mice lacking the capacity to produce apoB48 from apoB100 (due to knockout of the splicing gene, apobec-1) show little difference in lipid absorption and export in the fed state, but reduced capacity for particle production in the fasted state (Kalogeris and Story, 1992). Thus, the evolutionary change toward apoB48 in chylomicrons may have resulted from greater efficiency of TG utilization with this smaller apo in starvation conditions.

ApoB48 is exclusively produced by enterocytes in humans, rabbits, and hamsters in health (Liu et al., 1991; Greeve et al., 1993). However, apoB48-containing TG-rich particles are produced by the liver in dogs, rats, and mice (i.e., apoB48 very low density LPs or VLDLs). This difference has been purported to explain the prominent species differences in concentrations of circulating LDL cholesterol. ApoB48 particles (chylomicrons and some VLDLs in species with liver apoB48 production) are not metabolized to LDL (unlike apoB100-containing VLDLs). Therefore, apoB48 particles yield lower total downstream cholesterol-rich LDLs in the blood than comparable levels of apoB100 VLDLs (Greeve et al., 1993; Van't Hooft et al., 1982).

Nascent chylomicrons travel from intestinal lacteals to blood via the thoracic duct, bypassing the liver. In the process, they acquire apoCs (I, II, and III) and apoE transferred from HDL particles, while apoA-IV is displaced from the chylomicron surface. This exchange, which yields a "mature chylomicron," is critical for activation of enzymes essential for chylomicron metabolism and clearance. In tissue capillaries, particularly those of skeletal muscle and adipose, chylomicrons interact with the serine esterase lipoprotein lipase (LPL), which is secreted by endothelial cells and attached to their surfaces by heparan sulfate. Activity of LPL is enabled by cofactor apoC-II, and chylomicrons are the preferred enzyme substrate among all blood lipid transport vehicles (Bickerton et al., 2007). Interaction with LPL liberates NEFAs from the glycerol backbones of chylomicron core TGs. These NEFAs are partly absorbed by the endothelial cell and partly released into the surrounding blood (contributing to postprandial surge or "spillover" of NEFAs in blood). Deficiency of apoC-II, as the critical LPL cofactor, occurs as a rare autosomal hereditary disorder, and accordingly, is associated with hypertriglyceridemia and elevated chylomicron serum levels. Insulin is also important in enabling endothelial cell uptake of NEFAs from chylomicrons (Section 21.9). Water-soluble glycerol released with TG hydrolysis diffuses into blood and is readily absorbed by blood and tissue cells.

Among the other apos carried by chylomicrons, apoA-I is a cofactor, and apoA-IV and apoC-I are activators of lecithin:cholesterol acyltransferase (LCAT, also called phosphatidylcholine-sterol O-acyltransferase). This enzyme converts free cholesterol into more hydrophobic CE via transfer of FA to it from phosphatidylcholine (converting the latter into lysolecithin). Cholesterol can be retained in the core of a LP particle in the esterified form in greater proportion than as free cholesterol in the outer ring of amphipathic lipids encasing the particle. Thus, this enzyme enables enhanced cholesterol containment by chylomicrons, which acquire some CEs from other particles in transit. However, LCAT has an even greater role in formation and metabolism of cholesterol-containing HDL particles, which acquire the enzyme cofactors and activator apos from chylomicrons during chylomicrons lipolysis (see below) (Vigne and Havel, 1981). In humans, these transferred apos from chylomicrons include apoA-I and C-I; however, in contrast to rats and other laboratory species, the majority of human apoA-IV is released free into blood. This disinction for apoA-IV, as well as the highly variable LCAT activity in plasma among species have been proposed as additional factors accounting for some of the species differences in LP profiles and cholesterol metabolism (Lefevre et al., 1986; Ouguerram et al., 2004).

Another apoC carried by chylomicrons that undergoes exchange with HDL is apoC-III. This protein inhibits apoC-II activation of tissue LPL, as well as hepatic lipase, thereby slowing chylomicron degradation and premature hepatic uptake. Accordingly, increased circulating apoC-III concentrations have been linked with prolonged postprandial lipemia, metabolic syndrome, and other dyslipidemic conditions in human (Clemente-Postigo et al., 2010). Notably, the transfer of apoC and apoA proteins between chylomicrons and HDL particles is continuous and recycling; however, retention of these proteins by chylomicrons dwindles as the particles progressively shrink in size with lipid loss. The decreasing proportion of LPL-activating apoC-II in chylomicrons with degradation is likely particularly critical in initiating termination of chylomicron TG hydrolysis.

Additional functional roles for apoC-III, apoC-I, apoA-I, and apoA-IV that are important in other LP types are discussed below and listed in Table 21.2.

21.5.3 Chylomicron Remnants—Formation and Clearance

As chylomicrons lose TGs as FAs to peripheral tissues, and apoA and C to HDL, they also transfer a substantial portion of PLs to HDL. The proportional loss of apoA and apoC proteins renders the particles less capable of binding and activating LPL in capillaries, while the loss of PLs and the relative enrichment in apoB48 and apoE and CEs enhances hepatocyte uptake (Cooper, 1997). These chylomicron remnants are thus, distinct from their parent particle in both protein phenotype and lipid content. In particular, compared with parent chylomicrons, remnants are TG depleted and cholesterol- and lipid-soluble vitamin (terpene) enriched.

Hepatic uptake of these remnants is the final step in chylomicron clearance. This uptake occurs by multiple mechanisms. Most remnants reach a sufficiently small size to enter into the space of Dissé through the endothelial fenestre (Havel, 1998).These PL-depleted particles then interact with the microvillous hepatocyte surface LDL receptor via apoE and can undergo receptor-mediated endocytosis. A secondary slower apoE-dependent pathway (which takes precedence in conditions of defective LDL receptor-mediated uptake; e.g., familial hypercholesterolemia) is via the LDL receptor-related protein (LRP), a multifunctional receptor also known as α2 macroglobulin and found in many tissues in addition to liver (Hussain et al., 1991; Martins et al., 2000). Notably, the remnant particles may also be enriched with apoE secreted free into the space of Dissé or bound by heparan sulfate to the hepatocyte microvillar surface, both of which increase remnant affinity for LRP (Mahley and Ji, 1999; Willnow, 1997). Some chylomicron remnants in the space of Dissé may instead interact via their outer polar lipids with proteoglycan-bound sinusoidal endothelial-surface hepatic lipase and undergo nonreceptor-mediated (TG and PL) hydrolysis and hepatocyte absorption of their lipid content. A distinct chylomicron remnant clearance mechanism by hepatic Kupffer cells has been purported to take precedence with larger, oxidized, or overload remnant particles that do not enter the space of Dissé (Havel, 1998; Umeda et al., 1995). Notably, while apoB48 on chylomicrons is critical for particle assembly and secretion, it lacks the LDL-receptor binding domain that is present in the larger apoB100 protein, and thus lacks a functional role in remnant clearance (Hui et al., 1984).

Chylomicron clearance is generally rapid in health, occurring within ~30 minutes in a rodent, and a few hours in humans following a meal. Other relative species and strain differences in the capacity to generate and clear chylomicrons have been reported (Jeffery and Redgrave, 1982). Chylomicrons rich in polyunsaturated FAs are more rapidly cleared than those high in saturated FAs. A wide variety of pathologic conditions have also been associated with prolonged postprandial triglyceridemia due to delayed chylomicron clearance.

21.5.4 Other Lipoprotein Products of Enterocytes

In addition to chylomicrons, small intestinal enterocytes have been shown to produce small amounts of particles that correlate in size and lipid constituents with VLDLs. These are derived from scavenged products of intestinal cell turnover and bile acids during fasting/starvation, and under some hormonal influences (e.g., with late pregnancy in rats) (Lioi et al., 2010). This overlap in secretion of two distinct TG-rich particles from enterocytes likely ameliorates flux in circulating TG and cholesterol concentrations during fasting/starvation. However, the hallmark of VLDL particles and their metabolic successors (intermediate-density lipoprotein [IDL] and LDL) is the presence of apoB100. In human and most laboratory species, the reported capacity of apoB100 secretion by enterocytes is relatively low (Risser et al., 1978; Van't Hooft et al., 1982). Thus, the liver, with significantly greater capacity to generate apoB100, is still considered the primary organ capable of generating VLDL. Variable amounts of HDL particles have also been reported to be produced by enterocytes (Brunham et al., 2006). These functional overlaps in LP particle output between intestine and other tissues is primarily of consideration in analyzing samples and interpreting results from animals in the starved or physiologically stressed states.

21.5.5 VLDL—Assembly and Secretion

The other major TG-transporting LPs in blood are VLDLs, which are smaller and contain a lower proportion of TG, and greater total cholesterol by particle weight compared with chylomicrons. Accordingly, except for the postprandial state, a change in serum/plasma TGs can generally be attributed, in large part, to an alteration in VLDL metabolism (i.e., production, degradation, and/or clearance).

VLDLs are synthesized and secreted almost exclusively by the liver. Synthesis is highly dependent upon the available pool of metabolically active lipid constituents (especially FAs) with only a portion of hepatocellular lipid content contributing to this active pool (Gross et al., 1967). The assembly of lipids into VLDLs also depends upon the availability of apoB100; however, in mice, rats, dogs, and some other species, apoB48 (typically associated with chylomicrons) may be alternatively associated with VLDL-like particles produced by the liver (Greeve et al., 1993). A single nonexchangeable apoB100 (or apoB48) occurs with each VLDL particle. As with TG-rich chylomicrons, particle assembly is facilitated by the lipid transfer protein, MTP within the ER (Salter et al., 1998; Swift et al., 2003). Deficiency of MTP as a familial condition (abetalipoproteinemia) results in symptoms described above (associated with impaired chylomicron assembly), and also persistently and profoundly low blood TGs, and to a lesser magnitude, low circulating cholesterol attributed to impaired generation of VLDLs. Inability to transport lipid-soluble vitamins via these particles to peripheral tissues also contributes to clinical symptoms of the condition. The role of MTP further contributes to stepwise lipid loading of VLDL particles, with $VLDL_1$ and $VLDL_2$ representing TG-rich and TG-poor particles, respectively, secreted from the liver (Olofsson and Borèn, 2005).

Circulating VLDL concentrations also depend upon translational and posttranslational control of apoB100 synthesis and posttranslational degradation within hepatocytes. Altered degradation of apoB100 is a particularly common regulatory mechanism linked with hormonal, metabolic, and inflammation-related signaling. Increased ApoB intracellular degradation has been associated with insulin and choline deficiency, whereas reduced degradation has been linked with insulin resistance, endogenous glucocorticoids, dexamethasone administration, and activation of the inflammatory IκB kinase (IKK)–nuclear factor (NF)–κB signaling cascade (Wang et al., 1995; Tsai et al., 2009). These mechanisms are consistent with observed decreased or increased VLDL secretion associated with these conditions or treatments, accordingly.

Other apos that associate with VLDL particles include apoC-I, C-II, C-III, and E. These proteins are rapidly transferred from plasma and/or HDL to the nascent VLDL in the space of Dissé (Berbée et al., 2005; Cohn et al., 2002; Dolphin et al., 1986). This immediate transfer to VLDL within the peri-hepatocellular space is critical for blocking hepatic premature recapture or hydrolysis of VLDL via apoB100 (or apoE) binding to the LDL (or LRP) receptors (Jong et al., 1999). These apos further serve similar functions in VLDL as in chylomicrons. ApoC-I, as with apoC-III, has also been shown to delay VLDL catabolism via inhibiting LPL activity (Jong et al., 1999).

Notably, while VLDL is the predominant TG-carrying particle in blood in the postprandial state, the proportion of TG and cholesterol in VLDL is also species-, and diet-variable (Havel and Kane, 1995; Madani et al., 2003; Ramaswamy et al., 1999).

21.5.6 VLDL Catabolism

Catabolism of VLDL lipid content is similar to that of chylomicrons. As with chylomicrons, apoC-II serves as required cofactor for LPL on capillary endothelial surfaces (especially within adipose and skeletal muscle tissue). ApoE also has a critical role in VLDL lipid catabolism in peripheral tissue in aiding LP interaction with LPL though associating with endothelial cell-surface proteoglycans and slowing particle movement (Kowal et al., 1990). Loss of this function or deficiency of apoE in humans is associated with accumulation of an abnormal form of VLDL particles (Schaefer et al., 1986). Most apoC-I proteins are exchangeable with HDL, and readily transfer as VLDL particles circulate and shrink in diameter.

Notably, another peripheral tissue lipase, endothelial lipase (EL), which is putatively associated with endothelial surfaces via heparan sulfate binding similar to LPL, is a relatively newly identified lipase that facilitates catabolism of VLDL (as well as IDL, LDL, and HDL). Unlike LPL, this enzyme also has activity against PLs; its phospholipase activity is considered at least as potent as that against TGs (McCoy et al., 2002). PLs and free cholesterol in the outer shell of VLDLs are also lost during the process of lipolysis to other LPs, particularly HDLs through the activity of plasma phospholipid transfer protein (PLTP) (van Tol, 2002). Plasma PLTP activity has been reported to be significantly greater in mice, dogs, and pigs compared with humans (among tested species), a factor that has been proposed to contribute to differences in serum lipid concentrations, and atherogenesis between these species (Guyard-Dangremont et al., 1998; van Haperen et al., 2009).

As VLDLs lose lipids, apoE proteins gain exposure enabling them to undergo some TG hydrolysis by hepatic lipase and engage with apoE receptors, LRP or LDL receptors for hepatic uptake, or continue to be remodeled into IDLs. Notably, although apoB100 is also able to engage with the hepatic LDL receptor for particle uptake, the efficiency of this interaction is many times less than that of the apoE-LDL receptor, or -LRP, interactions; in addition, each LP carries only a single apoB100 protein, in contrast with multiple apoE proteins/particle.

21.5.7 Intermediate Density Lipoproteins

In general, IDLs are about half the diameter and contain about half as much TG, and twice as much cholesterol relative to particle weight as VLDLs. More simply, IDLs consist of roughly similar TG and cholesterol content by weight. These transient catabolic remnants are either ultimately taken up by the liver via similar hepatic receptor interactions as for VLDL, or undergo further hydrolysis with loss of apoE, and conversion to LDLs. In human, much of the IDL particles are converted to LDL. However, in rats and dogs, the majority of IDLs are cleared by the liver, a difference putatively attributable to lower apoB100 to apoB48 ratio in these species (Dupras et al., 1991; Gross et al., 1967).

21.5.8 Low-Density Lipoproteins

Unlike IDL, VLDL, or chylomicron particles described above, LDLs consist largely of cholesterol, and lack associated apoE. Hepatic uptake of LDL is therefore dependent upon interactions of a single apoB100 per particle with the LDL receptor. Accordingly, LDLs show relatively slow clearance from circulation among the Apo-B containing LPs.

In circulation, and once formed from IDL, LDL are remodeled via exchange of lipids with other LPs. As with VLDL particles, PLs and free cholesterol in the outer shell of LDLs undergo transfer to HDL via PLTP activity (an effect thought to ultimately stimulate hepatic uptake of HDL cholesterol) (van Haperen et al., 2009). In some species, LDLs also lose residual TGs via shuttling these to HDL in exchange for CEs via the actions of CETP. Plasma CETP among tested species has been found to be inversely correlated with HDL cholesterol concentration, and with the ratio of HDL, relative to total serum cholesterol (Tsutsumi et al., 2001). Accordingly, this difference in plasma CETP activity significantly contributes to species differences in serum cholesterol profile, and associated susceptibility to atherogenic conditions. It is noteworthy that mice and rats appear to lack a functional CETP gene altogether (Hogarth et al., 2003).

Final clearance of LDL particles requires interaction between apoB100 and hepatocellular LDL receptors. Dependency on the LDL receptor for clearance is exemplified in human and animal models that have deficiency or dysfunction of the LDL receptor. Both conditions are characterized by very high serum LDL cholesterol and excess cholesterol deposition in tissues. In humans, the condition (familial hypercholesterolemia) has been found to be caused by a mutation in the genes encoding the low-density lipoprotein receptor (LDLR), apolipoprotein B (APOB), a protein required for clathrin-mediated hepatic LDL receptor internalization, or recently, a member of the proprotein convertase family, (i.e., PCSK9 [proprotein convertase subtilisin/kexin type 9]) that has a role in mediating LDL-receptor protein degradation (Maxwell and Breslow, 2005), and is currently considered a novel target of cholesterol-lowering therapeutics.

21.5.9 High-Density Lipoproteins

HDLs are the smallest, most protein dense of the major LPs. These particles are 10–200-fold smaller than the diameter of chylomicrons, and particularly heterogenous among the LP types. Further classification of HDL is somewhat complex, with categories based on specific particle density, electrophoretic migration (single- or two-dimensional), size and/or apo content. There are animal species differences in HDL lipid and protein profiles, so that the relevance of more narrowly defined HDL properties/subclasses across species is not explicit or direct. However, the two major human HDL classes, HDL_3 and $HDL_{2,}$ show good correlation with HDL particles in laboratory species based on density and protein: lipid content (Edelstein et al., 1976; Haug and Høstmark, 1987). HDL_3 are nascent smaller, and more dense (and may be discoidal) particles that convert to larger, less dense, more spherical HDL_2 with LCAT-driven accumulation of CEs. Accordingly, HDL_3 consists of higher protein and less esterified cholesterol than the more spherical HDL_2. Both HDL_3 and HDL_2 contain predominantly apoA-1 as the apo component and lack detectable apoE.

A much more minor subtype, HDL_1, occurs in laboratory species with relative CETP deficiency in health (especially dog and pig), and humans with mutations resulting in CETP deficiency (Mori et al., 2011; Zak et al., 2002). A high cholesterol diet in these subjects can result increased circulating HDL_1 levels. HDL_1 are particularly rich in CE (as an outcome of reduced CETP-promoted CE exchange with other LPs), and also endowed with apoE, which can facilitate hepatic LP clearance. Another minor subtype, HDLc (cholesterol-enriched HDL-like particles), contains even greater concentrations of CEs than HDL_1, and almost exclusively apoE as the apo. HDLc LPs most often are found in human and animals with relative CETP deficiency and very high circulating cholesterol (e.g., >700 mg/dL or 18 mmol/L), such as dogs with hypothyroid conditions or high cholesterol feeding (Sloop et al., 1983; Wilson et al., 1986). Being highly enriched in CEs, these high apoE HDL_1 and HDLc particles are larger and lower in density than HDL_2 or HDL_3. Consistent with the reverse cholesterol transport function of apoE in facilitation of cholesterol efflux from macrophage foam cells and LP hepatic uptake (Table 21.2), formation of high apoE HDL_1 or HDLc may aid in limiting the relative risk of atherogenesis in these animals/subjects (Tietjen et al., 2012).

The majority of HDL particles originate with secretion by the liver or intestine of the major structural protein, apoA-I, as a proprotein (pro-apoA-I) in a lipid-poor particle (Gordon et al., 1982). These gradually acquire free cholesterol from cell membranes and apoB particles, and convert it to CEs via LCAT. With acquisition of CEs, pro-apoA-I is converted to the mature apoA-I, and lipid-poor pre-β HDL (based on surface charge with nondenaturing gel electrophoresis) becomes αHDL (HDL_3). These maturing HDL particles further acquire apoA-II and/or apoE in circulation. A minority of HDL particles also can form via intravascular metabolism of chylomicrons and hepatic VLDL; these begin as lipid-poor particles containing apoA-I or apoE, before acquiring sufficient CEs to be classified as αHDL (Zannis et al., 2008). All of these HDL particles lack apoB and generally contain a mixture of core CEs with outer shell of PLs, sphingomyelin, and free cholesterol.

ApoA-I is the major LP of HDL and serves as a cofactor for LCAT, enabling increased particle cholesterol-carrying capacity (as for chylomicrons discussed above). In lipid-poor HDL, apoA-I has the additional role of binding to the ABC subfamily A, member 1 (encoded by *ABCA1* gene) transporter of cells, including macrophages, to enable uptake of excess tissue cell cholesterol (Wróblewska, 2011). With this uptake, the lipid-poor HDL is converted to Pre-β-HDL, and with the action of LCAT, from thin discoid to spherical α-HDL. Pre-β-HDL and more mature α-HDL particles are capable of additional cholesterol uptake from cholesterol-laden peripheral tissue cells through facilitated diffusion mediated by the ABC subfamily G, member 1 (*ABCG1*) transporter, and the scavenger receptor class B type 1 (SR-B1) (Wang et al., 2004; Wróblewska, 2011). Discovery of these cellular HDL receptors/cholesterol transporters was an outcome of research in understanding the genetic basis for Tangier disease (TD). Patients with TD have a mutation of the *ABCA1* transporter gene and consequently, very low levels of circulating HDL and prominent cholesterol accumulation in cells (especially macrophages) with enlargement or discoloration of various organs (e.g., liver, spleen, lymph nodes) (Dechelotte et al., 1985; Kolovou et al., 2006).

The tissue distribution of these HDL receptors is broad, with redundant regulation of expression driven principally by intracellular cholesterol content. For *ABCA1* and *ABCG1* encoded transporters and possibly SR-B1, increased expression with increased cellular cholesterol is mediated by the LXR transcription pathway (Hu et al., 2010; Venkateswaran et al., 2000). For SR-B1, the receptor is distinct in being distributed especially in steroid hormone-producing tissues (e.g., adrenal gland, ovaries, testes, endometrium) with expression further regulated by systemic and tropic hormones, and being functionally unique in directing cholesterol transport both out of and into cells, and binding with LDL and VLDL proteins (Landschulz et al., 1996; Li et al., 1998; Rigotti et al., 1996, 1997). Collectively, these findings suggest that apoA-I binding to SR-B1 is part of a mechanism ensuring appropriate cholesterol supply to steroidogenic cells for hormone synthesis, as well as regulating cholesterol metabolism overall.

The role of apoA-II, the second most common apo of HDL, has been less clearly defined. This is partly due to prominent species differences (without apparent phylogenetic basis) in occurrence, and the activity of the protein and the enzymes and regulators with which it interacts (Blanco-Vaca et al., 2001; Fournier et al., 2002; Hime et al., 2006; Wróblewska et al., 2010). For example, apoA-II is readily detected in the plasma of humans, nonhuman primates, rats, mice, and fish, whereas it is expressed at either very low levels or absent in dogs, pigs, rabbits, and chickens. In humans, rats, and mice, the protein is produced by the liver and to a minor extent by the intestine; however, the amino acid sequence and protein structure is profoundly different, and the expression in response to the same regulatory transcription factors (e.g., PPARα) is contradictory between humans and these rodent species. Upregulating the murine apoA-II in mice is also associated with blood lipid findings distinct from those in transgenic mice expressing the human protein. Some of these functional species differences may also be due to dissimilar downstream enzymes that are regulated by apoA-II. Currently, the most scientifically supported proposals for the role of apoA-II is that it modifies interaction between apoA-I and LCAT, HDL and PLs (e.g., in cell membranes), and/or lipase-mediated degradation of HDLs. Collectively, the results of numerous studies suggest apoA-II does not facilitate, and may inhibit HDL-mediated cholesterol clearance from peripheral tissues. The multifaceted species differences in this apoA protein highlight the importance of considering such in interpreting blood lipid changes in general.

Several other apos that occur in human HDL, including apoE, apoC-I, C-II, and C-III, and apoA-IV and A-V are variably found in HDL of other species (Hollanders et al., 1986). The first five of these proteins are also associated, as described above, with chylomicrons and/or VLDLs; although, their expression and function(s) may have more or less of a prominent role with HDLs. The last of these, apoA-V is a recently discovered apo also found in chylomicrons and VLDLs, and purported to serve as regulator of LPL (affecting TG turnover in these LPs) (Ebara et al., 2010; Vaessen et al., 2009).

21.5.10 HDLs and Reverse Cholesterol Transport

HDL particles have a pivotal role in cholesterol metabolism by facilitating efflux of the lipid from peripheral tissue cells and ultimate delivery to the liver and biliary excretion. This process is credited with preventing accumulation of intracellular cholesterol from tissue cells, which can be cytotoxic and atherogenic. The process is termed reverse cholesterol transport (RCT) as it is considered a reversal of the effects cholesterol delivery to peripheral tissues via apoB LPs, especially LDL and VLDL. Much of the current research in RCT is focused on (1) the interaction of HDL apoA-I with peripheral tissue *ABCA1*and *ABCG1* encoded transporters, and the SR-B1 receptor enabling selective CE uptake; (2) HDL (and LDL) interactions with liver receptors important in whole particle clearance; (3) LCAT activity on HDL that enables increased quantity of cholesterol to be retrieved and transported per particle; and (4) HDL transfer of CEs to LDL and other particles through CETP.

Selective hepatocyte uptake of cholesterol from mature (cholesterol- and PL-rich) αHDL is considered the predominant means of RCT. This selective uptake is achieved primarily via interaction of apoA-I with specific receptors (e.g., SR-B1) (Trigatti et al., 2003). Notably, dogs have shown particularly prominent selective hepatic uptake of cholesterol from HDL (about twofold greater than even rats and mice) attributed to high activities of SR-B1 and LCAT and leading to very efficient RCT (Ouguerram et al., 2004). The remodeling of the HDL particle by this selective cholesterol uptake, as well as by hepatic and endothelial lipase and PLTP, results in a regeneration of lipid-poor HDL particles being returned to circulation.

Removal of cholesterol-rich whole HDL particles by the liver is another mechanism of RCT that can occur with HDL subtypes rich in apoE (HDL1 and especially HDLc). Clearance of these particles is mediated through interaction of apoE, as ligand for the LDL receptor or LRP on hepatocytes.

Transfer of cholesterol from HDL to LDL and other apoB particles, with subsequent clearance or degradation of the recipient particle by the liver is a third mechanism of RCT. As noted above, transfer of cholesterol (as CEs) to apoB particles is primarily catalyzed by CETP in exchange for TGs. The cholesterol in these recipient particles may then be delivered to the liver. However, the more common fate of the transferred cholesterol is delivery back to tissue cells, consistent with the dominant role of apoB particles in delivering lipids to peripheral tissue cells, and the converse of RCT. This reinforces the important difference in CETP activity between humans and common laboratory species (e.g., mice, rats, or dogs) (Groot et al., 2005). In the latter, the absence of significant plasma CETP activity results in HDL cholesterol captured from peripheral tissue to be delivered to the liver more consistently by the same particle, whereas in humans, CETP enables ready transfer of HDL CEs to other LPs. The influence of CETP on RCT has made it a target for antiatherogenic pharmaceutical development (De Grooth et al., 2004).

21.5.11 Lipoprotein(a)

Lipoprotein(a) [Lp(a)] is a particle that resembles LDL with an added apo(a) protein, synthesized by the liver and covalently attached to apoB100 via a single disulfide bond. The particle occurs in human and Old World monkeys (including macaques) and has also been detected in marmosets (Guo et al., 1991; Makino et al., 1989; Lawn, 1996), and has been associated a wide variety of human atherosclerotic conditions through epidemiological studies. Studies with evaluation of Lp(a) in transgenic mice and rabbits have also been reported; however, interpretation of results is confounded by the fact that the particle is not found in the wild-type animals. The hedgehog has an apo(a)-like protein that has evolved independently and is genetically distinct, with a distinct "Kringle" domain structure, characterized by large folded loops stabilized by three disulfide linkages (Lawn et al., 1995).

Numerous isoforms of Lp(a) are found in the plasma of human and Old world monkeys and their presence and concentration appear to be largely genetically determined (Boerwinkle et al., 1990; Taddei-Peters et al., 1993; Koschinsky, 2004). Isoforms differ in the number of repeated molecular "Kringle" units, which have also been shown to variably bind to biological substrates, including plasminogen and fibrinogen/fibrin and fibronectin. These binding properties contribute to proposals that Lp(a) is linked with vascular disease via inhibition of fibrinolysis, aortic smooth muscle cell proliferation, and oxidation of PL and LDL within atherosclerotic lesions. The absolute and relative concentration of different isoforms in plasma have shown better correlation with common human vascular diseases than nonspecific total Lp(a). Notably, commercial assays are nonstandardized and may vary in cross-reactivity to the nonhuman primate antigen.

21.5.12 Non-esterified Fatty Acids (NEFAs) in Blood—Transport and Clearance

In contrast with LPs, NEFAs are transported in blood as single hydrophobic carbon chains bound to a carrier molecule, primarily albumin. The plasma/serum concentration of NEFA is often a reflection of the extent of peripheral hydrolysis of TG-rich LPs (chylomicrons or VLDL). During hydrolysis, a portion of the resulting NEFAs are refluxed into surrounding capillary blood. This accounts for the rise in circulating NEFAs in the early postprandial state, and pathologic and physiologic states of hypertriglyceridemia. The other source of circulating NEFAs is attributable to intracellular TG lipolysis of regional depots of white adipose (and to a much lesser extent, intracellular lipids of muscle and glandular tissue). Prominent increases in circulating NEFAs from tissue lipolysis can occur with food restriction/anorexia, insulin deficiency or resistance, or excess β-adrenergic or thyroid hormone activity (Section 21.9) (Haude and Völcker, 1991; Horowitz, 2003).

Blood transport of NEFAs by albumin is efficient; a single albumin molecule can bind multiple NEFAs, with affinity and clearance correlated with chain length and saturation (Choi et al., 2002). However, NEFAs comprise only a minor fraction of total circulating lipids even in states of amplified lipolysis. There is little evidence that physiologic ranges of circulating NEFAs can significantly displace other albumin-bound (endogenous or exogenously administered) components, or that albumin-binding sites can reach saturation (Monks and Richens, 1979). The circulating half-life of individual NEFAs is generally very brief due to rapid tissue uptake, and accordingly, total blood NEFA concentration tends to be highly dynamic (Dole and Rizack, 1961).

21.6 PERIPHERAL TISSUE LIPID UPTAKE

Peripheral tissue uptake of circulating long-chain NEFAs from albumin, and TG-rich LPs (generated via endothelial LPL lipolysis) is considered to occur primarily through facilitated transport by specific membrane-associated, and cytoplasmic fatty acid transport proteins (FATPs), FABPs and fatty acid translocases (e.g., CD36/FATs) (Berk et al., 1994; Pownall and Hamilton, 2003). These proteins vary in type and distribution among tissues, depending partly on energy and hormonal state and circulating NEFA supply (Berk and Stump, 1999; Nickerson et al., 2009). Some FATPs and FATs may be regulated by physiologic factors to channel FAs toward esterification or oxidation (Consitt et al., 2009; Pohl et al., 2004). Despite such regulation, NEFA transport into tissue cells does not appear to be particularly rate limiting for clearance from blood; downstream metabolism is more likely limiting in tissue turnover of NEFA. Some NEFA uptake is also believed to occur by diffusive pathways.

Peripheral tissue cell uptake of cholesterol from circulating LPs has been most completely studied with steroid producing cells and adipocytes. Notably, pathways of such by these cells are likely more robust, with some differential aspects compared to other tissue cells. Cells of the adrenal, ovary, and other steroid-producing tissues have been shown to acquire cholesterol via the LDL receptor with endocytosis of ligand (apoB or apoE)-presenting LPs; albeit preferential uptake of LDL, over the other apoB LPs has been shown (Hu et al., 2010; Tsibulsky and Yakushkin, 1997). LDL receptor expression, and its regulation by fasting, has also been demonstrated on adipocytes (Kraemer et al., 1994). Conversely, uptake of HDL cholesterol by peripheral tissues occurs via the scavenger receptor class B type 1 (SR-B1) receptor (as noted above for hepatocytes) with selective removal of cholesterol and recycling of lipid-poor apoA-I HDL back into circulation (Reaven et al., 2004). The extent of reliance of steroid-producing cells on either LDL or HDL cholesterol for steroidogenesis appears to be species-dependent; that is, in rodents, steroid-producing cells preferentially utilize the SR-B1 pathway, while in humans, pigs, and cattle, these cells primarily utilize the LDL-receptor endocytic pathway for exogenous cholesterol supply. In adipocytes, there is also evidence of an SR-B1-independent mechanism that involves interaction of HDL apoE and the LRP receptor (Fazio and Linton, 2004).

Peripheral tissue uptake of PLs occurs by phospholipase hydrolysis to NEFAs and limited direct uptake of intact anionic (e.g., inner cell membrane) PLs via the SR-B1 and CD36 receptors (Rigotti et al., 1995; Ryeom et al., 1996).

21.7 INTRACELLULAR LIPID METABOLISM

Within tissue cells, FAs and cholesterol are generally esterified and may be (1) utilized for synthesis of more complex lipids, (2) released back into the blood, or (3) catabolized. Catabolism of FAs for energy occurs via oxidation in most cells of the body with metabolites entering into the Krebs cycle. Alternatively, FAs may be catabolized via ketogenesis to ketone bodies; a process essentially limited to hepatocytes. Catabolism of cholesterol is usually considered to involve the steps toward excretion into bile. These metabolic pathways are briefly described below.

21.7.1 Fatty Acid Oxidation

Fatty-acid degradation in the cell can occur by α-, β-, and ω-oxidation pathways, which take place in mitochondria, peroxisomes, and the ER. The major catabolic pathway is via β-oxidation in mitochondria, with α-, and ω-oxidation being far more minor routes. These processes rely on a multitude of enzymes and specific transport proteins. Deficiencies and impairment of these proteins can occur with familial disorders, chemical/drug toxicity, infectious diseases, and the cytokines of inflammation. Clinical deficiencies or impairment of some of the proteins shows a wide variety of symptoms that tend to be individualistic in their pattern (Moczulski et al., 2009). Because striated muscle and liver have especially high capacity for FA oxidation, these tissues tend to be particularly affected with such conditions. Some classic symptoms of impaired FA oxidation include skeletal muscle hypotonia, rhabdomyolysis, cardiomyopathy, cardiac arrhythmia, hypoketotic or ketotic hypoglycemia, metabolic acidosis, hyperammonemia, hepatic steatosis, and/or liver failure. Some marketed drugs (including aspirin, valproate, amiodarone, perhexiline, and tetracyclines) have been directly linked with impaired FA oxidation and associated clinical symptoms (Fréneaux et al., 1988; Fromenty and Pessayre, 1995; Silva et al., 2008; Spaniol et al., 2001; Vázquez et al., 2014; Ashrafian et al., 2007). Accordingly, understanding of lipid oxidative processes is important in interpretation of the collective laboratory data associated with such conditions.

21.7.1.1 β-Oxidation in Mitochondria

FAs undergo β-oxidation in mitochondria of most of the cells of the body (with known exceptions being erythrocytes and cells of the brain and adrenal medulla). The process enables straight chain FAs to be incorporated into the citric acid cycle for energy.

To enter the β-oxidation pathway, the carboxyl terminus of FAs must first be esterified to CoA in an ATP-dependent process. The acyl-CoA synthetases that catalyze this reaction are found in the cytosol, and within mitochondria, ER, and peroxisomes or their membranes, with most of these enzymes having specificity as to FA chain length (Watkins et al., 2007). Short- and medium-chain FA-CoAs may then diffuse into the mitochondria, while long-chain FAs (>16 carbons) require the acyl-CoA terminus to be esterified with carnitine for translocation (as acylcarnitine) across outer and inner mitochondrial membranes. This esterification occurs via a critical rate-limiting outer mitochondrial membrane enzyme, carnitine palmitoyltransferase (CPT) 1, and is followed by regeneration of the fatty acyl-CoA and free carnitine via the inner mitochondrial membrane enzyme, CPT 2 (also known as carnitine acyltransferase II) (Bonnefont et al., 2004). At the mitochondrial inner membrane or within the matrix (depending on chain length), the first step in β-oxidation of transferring electrons from the α- and β-carbon to the flavin cofactor occurs with generation of a C–C double bond. The electrons are, in turn, transferred to the electron transport chain with the production of ATP, and the double bond is hydrated with subsequent cleavage of a two-carbon molecule from the fatty acyl-CoA. The electron transfer is catalyzed by various dehydrogenases that are, again, specific for the FA chain length. Sequential cleavage of the FA chain then occurs with each two-carbon moiety combining with oxaloacetate in the Krebs cycle to form citrate. For those uncommon (diet-derived) odd-numbered FAs, the final three-carbon propional-CoA is reduced to succinyl-CoA, for entrance into a different step in the Krebs cycle. Unsaturated FAs require an additional step or two for isomerization at the double bond.

Lipid disorders attributed to deficiency of CPT 1, CPT 2, and mitochondrial medium-chain, long-chain, and very-long-chain acyl-CoA dehydrogenases are recognized in human. Several mouse models have been produced to study various defects in the FA oxidation pathway (Spiekerkoetter and Wood, 2010). Affected proteins (e.g., CPT 1) may have tissue-specific isoforms with differential regulation that help explain some of the varied clinical conditions associated with deficiency or inhibition (Eaton et al., 1996). Specific chemical/drug toxicity that results in impairment of β-oxidation are usually attributed to uncoupling of the electron transport system, mimicry of FA substrates, or inhibition of pathway enzymes or transporters, or their mitochondrial DNA transcription.

21.7.1.2 β-Oxidation in Peroxisomes

While mitochondria are the organelle responsible for the majority of FA oxidation within cells, peroxisomes are also capable of β-oxidation of long-chain and very-long-chain FAs. Fatty-acyl CoAs can diffuse across the peroxisomal membrane without involvement of carnitine, and where acyl-CoA oxidase transfers the electrons to oxygen, yielding hydrogen peroxide rather than ATP. Cleavage of the carbon chain in two-carbon sections is otherwise largely analogous to that described earlier, with production of a shortened fatty acyl (typically C9–C11) that is then exported to mitochondria for further β-oxidation. Peroxisomal β-oxidization also occurs for some unsaturated, branched, and ether FAs, eicosanoids, and bile acid intermediates.

Of note, these β-oxidation pathways, particularly those for long-chain FA oxidation in peroxisomes can be transcriptionally regulated and inducible by PPARα, and in rodents by the liver X receptor α (LXRα) (Van Veldhoven and Mannaerts, 1999; Braissant et al., 1996; Winegar et al., 2001; Hu et al., 2005) (see Section 21.12).

21.7.1.3 α-Oxidation

Alpha-oxidation is a minor process of FA catabolism by which certain dietary FAs branched at a β-carbon (e.g., phytanic acid in dairy products) cannot initially undergo β-oxidation in mitochondria, and are first catabolized in peroxisomes. Alpha-oxidation involves removal of the branched terminus of formyl-CoA, converting the new terminal carbon to an aldehyde, and then a carboxyl group for esterification with CoA and subsequent β-oxidation (Wierzbicki, 2007). The regulation of this process in peroxisomes is tissue and species variable (Singh et al., 1993).

21.7.1.4 ω-Oxidation

Omega oxidation is another minor pathway of FA oxidization. This pathway occurs almost exclusively in smooth ER, and involves (ω-1)-hydroxylation of medium- and long-chain FAs catalyzed by selected members of the cytochrome P450 (CYP) 4A enzyme family (Norlin and Wikvall, 2007). Hydroxylation is uniquely initiated at the carbon end opposite to the carboxyl group (Reddy and Hashimoto, 2001). The ω-hydroxy FA produced is ultimately converted into a substrate for β-oxidation. This becomes an alternative pathway of clinical significance in inherited mitochondrial FA β-oxidation deficiencies because of the generation of potentially toxic dicarboxylic acids.

21.7.1.5 Ketogenesis

FA ketogenesis occurs in hepatocyte mitochondria as a consequence of impaired cellular glucose utilization (e.g., hypoglycemia, insulin resistance), excessive energy demand (e.g., with illness, pregnancy), or excessive peripheral FA mobilization with delivery to the liver. Ketogenesis also occurs at a low rate under normal physiological conditions, and increases as an appropriate adaptive physiological response to glucose shortages (e.g., starvation, prolonged fasting).

In conditions of excessive FA delivery to the liver, the acetyl-CoA produced by mitochondrial β-oxidation may not readily enter the Krebs cycle due to substrate competition (for oxaloacetate). Instead, acetyl-CoA undergoes condensation to ketone bodies, which can serve as oxidizable fuels for extrahepatic tissues. In conditions of poor cellular glucose utilization, the decreased Krebs cycle flux limits the supply of oxaloacetate as substrate. With all of these conditions, ketone production provides an alternate energy source to carbohydrates primarily for the brain, heart, renal cortex, and skeletal muscle as an adaptive response for the survival of the organism (Laffel, 1999).

Three major ketone bodies are produced in liver mitochondria: acetoacetate, acetone, and 3-β-hydroxybutyrate (β-OHB). Their formation is initiated essentially as a reversal of the chain cleavage of β-oxidation, with condensation of two acetyl-CoAs to generate acetoacetyl-CoA. Addition of a third acetyl-CoA generates 3-hydroxy-3-methylglutaryl-CoA (HMG-CoA) via action of mitochondrial HMG-CoA synthase (an isozyme encoded by a distinct gene from that of cytosolic HMG-CoA synthase, Section 21.3). This product is then enzymatically degraded to acetoacetate and acetyl-CoA. Acetoacetate, if not oxidized to usable energy, is converted to β-OHB in another catalyzed reaction, or it degrades spontaneously to acetone. Acetoacetate and especially β-OHB released by the liver can be converted in peripheral tissues back to acetoacetyl-CoA for incorporation into the β-oxidation pathway. (The liver lacks the enzyme necessary to generate acetoacetyl-CoA, thus facilitating ketone body export to other tissues.) Hence, the ratio of circulating β-OHB to acetoacetate increases with progression of ketosis and shifts back with resolving severity of the condition. Accordingly, β-OHB is the predominant blood ketone with significant ketosis in mammals (Dedkova and Blatter, 2014). Ketoacidosis occurs if these ketone acids (H+) exceed the buffering capacity of bicarbonate.

The shift toward utilization of ketones as energy is somewhat tissue-dependent, and there are also age and species differences in tendency toward upregulation of ketogenic pathways (Hegardt, 1999; Spiekerkoetter and Wood, 2010; Thumelin et al., 1993). Ketogenesis is further subjected to hormonal influences (e.g., insulin, glucagon) and more long-term to nuclear-receptor-responsive elements of ketogenic enzymes. For example, expression of the rate-limiting enzyme, mitochondrial HMG-CoA synthase has been found to be regulated by PPARα, and the enzyme protein has been shown to translocate to the nucleus and potentiate PPARα-dependent activation of its own synthase gene promoter (Meertens et al., 1998). Ketone body production has additionally been reported to occur at low level in the neonatal kidney, intestine, and brain, and a few adult nonhepatic tissues (Hegardt, 1999; Thumelin et al., 1993).

21.8 CHOLESTEROL EXCRETION

Unlike FAs, mammals are not capable of catabolizing cholesterol intracellularly; rather, hepatic excretion into bile is the primary route of cholesterol elimination. Biliary excretion of cholesterol is in the form of bile acids and to a minor extent as free cholesterol. Bile acids are formed through modifying cholesterol to a more planar amphipathic molecule with distinct hydrophobic and hydrophilic surfaces that enable mixed-lipid micelle formation when secreted in the intestinal tract. Hence, bile acid formation serves to both protect against excess systemic cholesterol accumulation, as well as enable dietary lipid absorption, and other established functions (e.g., aid intestinal motility and limit bacterial growth in the small intestine and biliary tract). Bile acids further serve as ligands that signal through nuclear receptors and other transcription factors to regulate bile acid synthesis and transport, and other aspects of hepatic lipid metabolism.

Synthesis de novo of bile acids from cholesterol occurs predominantly in pericentral hepatocytes in health (Twisk et al., 1995) and involves multiple intracellular compartments, namely cytosol, ER, mitochondria, and peroxisomes, and numerous enzymatic steps with several alternative pathways. A review of these steps, and major species differences can be found in Chiang (2013), Lundell and Wikvall (2008), Norlin and Wikvall (2007), and Russell (2003). In all pathways, cholesterol requires three main modifications: (1) hydroxylation, (2) ring modification to eliminate the double bond, and (3) oxidation and shortening of the side chain. These steps vary in order among the different pathways. The two main pathways are the classical or "neutral," and "acidic," with the major primary bile acids synthesized via these pathways being cholic acid and chenodeoxycholic acid, respectively (Russell, 2003). Cholic acid is trihydroxylated and the more hydrophilic (and pH neutral), whereas chenodeoxycholic is dihydroxylated (i.e., "deoxy" terminology is relative to cholic acid) and the more hydrophobic (and acidic, with greater detergent properties). These primary bile acids can undergo further reactions to alter their properties; however, the ultimate ratio of hydrophilic to hydrophobic bile acids secreted in bile is critical to regulation of their synthesis and transport, as well as other aspects of systemic cholesterol metabolism.

Bile acid synthesis from cholesterol through the classical pathway initiates in the ER by the rate-limiting P450 cytochrome, cholesterol 7α-hydroxylase (CYP7A1), which drives the first required cholesterol modification, hydroxylation of cholesterol. Subsequent ring modification occurs via the microsomal enzyme required for synthesis of all bile acids: 3β-hydroxy-27-steroid dehydrogenase/isomerase (HSD3B7 or 3β-HSD). The intermediate formed by this latter enzyme in the classical pathway is "C4" (7α-hydroxy-4-cholestern-3-one), which also serves as a blood biomarker of CYP7A1 activity in human and animals (Chiang, 2013; Gälman et al., 2003). Another important downstream enzyme is sterol 12-α-hydroxylase (CYP8B1), the activity of which directs synthesis to cholic acid and essentially determines the ratio between cholic and chenodeoxycholic acid via the classical pathway. The alternative "acidic" pathway for bile acid synthesis is minor in humans, but significant in rats and mice (and human neonates) (Norlin and Wikvall, 2007; Repa et al., 2000; Vlahcevic et al., 1997). This pathway initiates with side-chain hydroxylation by the mitochondrial enzyme, sterol 27-hydroxylase or CYP27A1 resulting in an oxysterol that can then be hydroxylated by oxysterol 7α-hydroxylase (CYP7B1) with subsequent steps forming chenodeoxycholic acid. Chenodeoxycholic acid synthesized through either pathway can be further converted to more hydrophilic trihydroxylated muricholic acids and to additional dihydroxylated acids (e.g., hyocholic acid in pig). This further conversion of chenodeoxycholic acid is rapid and efficient in the mouse and rat (to muricholic acids) and occurs in some types of hepatobiliary disease but is otherwise negligible in humans and most other laboratory species (García-Cañaveras et al., 2012; Ellis et al., 1998; Hagey et al., 1998; Lundell and Wikvall, 2008; Russell, 2003). Additional alternative synthesis pathways that result in the conversion of cholesterol to an oxysterol intermediate can initiate extrahepatically (including in macrophages and cholangiocytes, brain, and lung). However, only the liver possesses the full enzyme complement to complete all molecular modifications of cholesterol for bile acid synthesis (Chiang, 2009, 2013; Xia et al., 2012; Russell, 2003).

Prior to secretion into hepatic canaliculi, the majority of bile acids are conjugated to taurine or glycine in peroxisomes. Conjugation converts bile acids to bile salts, decreasing cytotoxicity, and increasing their amphipathicity and solubility. As with bile acid constituents, there are species differences in conjugation. For example, conjugation is to taurine only in the dog and cat, predominantly taurine in rat, mouse, macaque, and squirrel monkey, predominantly glycine in rabbit and pig, and a variable mixture of glycine and taurine (diet-influenced) in human (García-Cañaveras et al., 2012; Lehman-McKeeman, 2013; Li and Chiang, 2013; Schwenk et al., 1978). Particularly, hydrophobic bile acids may also be conjugated to sulfate or glucuronidated by uridine diphosphate (UDP)-glucuronosyl N-transferases (with some species differences). Differences in whether taurine or glycine is the conjugated amino acid can affect the rate of active transport of a bile salt into canaliculi and enterocyte and hepatocyte uptake, as well as micelle structure (Hofmann and Mysels, 1992). However, these distinctions have less regulatory consequences on lipid metabolism than the overall ratio of conjugated to unconjugated bile acids (Ballatori et al., 2005; Carey et al., 1981; Parks et al., 1999; Russell, 2003; Van Der Meer and De Vries, 1985; Chiang, 2009; Solaas et al., 2004).

Conjugated bile salts are exported across the canalicular membrane by active transport (e.g., particularly by the bile salt export pump [BSEP]). Free cholesterol and other neutral sterols are transported out of hepatocytes into the canaliculi via liver ABC transporters, subfamily G, members 5 and 8 (encoded by *ABCG5* and *ABCG8* genes, the same sterolin-1 and sterolin-2 transporters that limit intestinal sterol absorption [Section 21.3, 21.4]). Free cholesterol transport into bile also depends upon an ABC transporter, multidrug resistance protein 3 (MDR3) in human (Mdr2 in mice, or PL flipase) for the transport of PLs into bile. As with bile acid constituents, there are some significant species differences in the role and/or regulation of bile acid and free cholesterol transporters in bile secretion. For example, human BSEP shows bile acid substrate differences compared with the rat homolog (Bsep), and functional differences between human and mouse are indicated by the finding that human BSEP deficiency results in severe liver disease with intrahepatic cholestasis, whereas *Bsep*-knockout mice develop only a mild form of cholestasis (reviewed in Stieger, 2009). Function and regulation of these transporters is still under concerted investigation.

Cholesterol excretion in bile is dependent not only on formation and ratio of bile salts and bile acids with PLs but also on the rate of bile flow. Bile flow is dependent upon the constituency and concentration of bile salts and acids (and their individual choleretic properties), as well as proportion of chloangiocyte secreted water and bicarbonate and osmotically active substances such as glutathione and glutathione conjugates (Kubegov and Karpen, 2008). Cholangiocyte stimulation and choloresis is also influenced by gastrointestine-associated hormones, such as cholecystokinin, secretin, bombesin, vasoactive intestinal polypeptide, and gastrin. In addition, bile concentration with water resorption occurs in the gall bladder in species that possess such. These collective factors contribute to the broad species differences in bile flow, including the significantly greater water content and relative bile flow in rat compared with other common laboratory species and human (Boyer, 2013). Bile that reaches the duodenum facilitates dietary lipid absorption throughout the small intestine. Unresorbed bile salts that reach anaerobic and facultative bacteria (mainly in the large intestine) can be deconjugated and oxidized converting them to secondary bile acids such as deoxycholic, lithocholic, and ursodeoxycholic acid (and murideoxycholic, hyodeoxycholic, and/or 7-oxolithocholic acid with some laboratory species) (Kasbo et al., 2002; Penno et al., 2013). Review of the factors involved in bile flow and enterohepatic circulation can be found in a number of current references (e.g., Chiang, 2013; Kubegov and Karpen, 2008; Steiger, 2011).

Excretion of cholesterol in bile is tightly regulated to support systemic cholesterol homeostasis and adequate intestinal lipid emulsification, as well as preclude bile acid-linked toxicity. This regulation is largely mediated by bile acid signaling through receptors that control the enzymes and transporters in the synthesis pathways. Distinctions in bile acid composition reaching enterocytes and returning to hepatocytes provide important feedback for regulation. Among the most well-established aspects of this signaling is that bile acids (particularly, the unconjugated hydrophobic bile acids, chenodeoxycholic, and lithocholic acids) are natural activating ligands for the nuclear receptor farnesoid X receptor α (FXRα). Expression of FXRα isoforms are found particularly in high concentration in the small intestine and liver (Zhang et al., 2003; Zhu et al., 2011). Accordingly, activation of small intestinal FXRα induces enterocyte release of fibroblast growth factor (FGF)19 (or FGF15 ortholog in mouse and rat) into portal blood, and upon reaching hepatocyte sinusoidal membrane receptors, signals downregulation of gene expression for key enzymes in bile acid synthesis, particularly CYP7A1 (reviewed in Chiang, 2013; Jones et al., 2012). Concomitantly, activation of liver FXRα independently induces the transcription factor, SHP ("small heterodimer partner"), which interacts with other proteins to repress transcription of CYP8B1, the key enzyme in regulating bile acid hydrophobicity (and to a lesser extent—at least in murine models, of CYP7A1) (Kong et al., 2012; Gardès et al., 2013). Intestinal and liver FXRα activation also induces transcription of genes that promotes bile acid conjugation and efflux from hepatocytes and enterocytes through transporter proteins, including upregulation of BSEP and MDR3 (for cholesterol) and terminal ileal organic solute transporter alpha and beta (OSTα and OSTβ, active in transporting bile acids from enterocytes into portal blood) (Ballatori et al., 2005; reviewed in Chiang, 2013; Zhu et al., 2011). Hepatic FXRα activation further downregulates hepatocellular uptake of recirculated conjugated bile acids. Collectively, these effects mediated through intestinal FXRα enable negative feedback for regulation of bile acid synthesis and resorption, and those mediated by hepatocellular FXRα activation are critical for protection of the liver from excessive exposure to cytotoxic hydrophobic bile acids such as with intrahepatic cholestasis. In support of these differential intestinal- and liver-specific FXRα functions, administration bile acids (taurocholate) into the duodenum of rats is more effective in suppressing hepatic CYP7A1 than with intravenous bile acid administration (Nagano et al., 2004). In contrast, intrahepatic cholestasis is associated with greater susceptibility to hepatotoxicity in FXR-null compared with wild-type mice (Cui et al., 2009; Shi et al., 2010). (Conversely, animals with extrahepatic cholestasis may be more susceptible to hepatoxicity, in association with the increased FXRα activity due to the induced increased bile acid efflux (Stedman et al., 2006). Of added consideration pertaining to FXRα regulation, the hydrophilic muricholic acids that form a major portion of bile in mice (and a significant component in rat) inhibit FXRα activation in opposition of the effects of hydrophobic bile acids on the nuclear receptor (Botham and Boyd, 1983; Hu et al., 2014); a finding that may explain some of the prominent *in vivo* species differences in lipid profile response to bile acid feeding and cholestasis.

Bile acids have additional important regulatory roles on systemic lipid metabolism and blood lipid profiles that are both dependent and independent of FXRα activation. Well established is that hydrophobic bile acid feeding decreases blood TG and liver VLDL, whereas reduction in recirculating bile acids through oral administration of bile acid-binding resins conversely increases circulating TG. These effects are considered at least partly FXRα-mediated, as $FXR^{-/-}$ mice have increased concentration of blood and liver TG, and FXR agonists decrease blood TG in mice. Studies have supported the mechanism for these findings to be linked with FXR/SHP inhibited transcription of the SREBP-1c, which promotes hepatic lipogenesis, and MTP, which enables hepatic VLDL efflux from the liver (Watanabe et al., 2004, Hirokane et al., 2004). In addition, FXR activation induces apoCII and inhibits apoCIII expression, which collectively promotes LPL activity and hence, tissue catabolism of circulating TG-rich LPs such as VLDL (Kast et al., 2001; Pineda Torra et al., 2003). FXR-mediated inhibition of apolipoprotein A-I (apoAI) and induction CETP expression are further associated with decreased blood HDL cholesterol levels (Gautier et al., 2013). Other reported effects of FXR that impact blood cholesterol include positive regulation of gene expression for PLTP, which facilitates transfer of PLs and cholesterol from other LPs to HDL, and negative regulation of hepatic lipase (HL), thereby decreasing hepatocyte TG and PL uptake from LDL and HDL (Urizar et al., 2000; Sirvent et al., 2004). These enzyme alterations collectively support increased LDL and HDL lipid accumulation and particle size. Conversely, studies have also shown that an increased bile acid pool promotes HDL lipid loss through upregulation of the scavenger lipid receptors SR-B1 and CD36, which enhance hepatic and adrenal uptake of cholesterol and PL from the LP (Gardès et al., 2013 and associated references; Li et al., 2012; Malerød et al., 2005; reviewed in Stanimirov et al., 2012). Overall, the effects of FXR activation and/or an increased bile acid pool on blood cholesterol have tended to result in decreased HDL and increased LDL cholesterol, although these changes seem dissociated from atherogenic effects (reviewed in Mazuy et al., 2015; Mudaliar et al., 2013; Hartman et al., 2009). Highly hydrophobic bile acids (e.g., lithocholic acid) can additionally affect blood lipid metabolism through activation of other important nuclear hormone transcription factors: pregnane X receptor (PXR) and vitamin D receptor (VDR) (Adachi et al., 2005; Wistuba et al., 2007; Khan et al., 2011).

One of the most remarkable differences between species in biliary cholesterol excretion associated with nuclear hormone receptor activation is that between both rats and mice and other common laboratory species (and humans) in response to a cholesterol-rich diet. In human and most other laboratory species, a high cholesterol diet expands the total pool of hydrophobic bile acids, which are natural ligands for activating FXR, triggering downregulation of CYP7A1 (and bile acid synthesis through the classical pathway). FXR activation in these species can also lead to increased liver and blood cholesterol concentration (Horton et al., 1995; Nguyen et al., 1999; Rudel et al., 1994; Xu et al., 2004) through some of the mechanisms mentioned previously. In contrast, mice and especially rats are resistant to increased hepatic synthesis of cholesterol-rich LPs and blood cholesterol due in part to high baseline and responsive induction of CYP7A1 through LXR activation (see Section 21.12.4) and lack of induction of FXR with cholesterol feeding (Xu et al., 2004). The activation of LXR is linked with increased formation of natural ligands, oxysterols that are formed through the alternative cholesterol metabolism pathways, while the lack of FXR activation in rats and mice is attributed to the significant formation of hydrophilic muricholic bile acids from cholesterol through the alternative pathways and which do not serve as FXR ligands. Hence, this important species difference is largely due to the distinctions in dominant bile acid synthesis pathways.

Other well-established factors that can affect cholesterol excretion through effects on key regulatory enzymes in bile acid synthesis include fasting/fed state, circadian cycles, hormones (e.g., estrogen, androgens, glucocorticoids, thyroid hormones, insulin, and glucagon) as well as inflammatory cytokines and disease pathology. These effects are generally described in other sections of this chapter.

21.9 PHYSIOLOGICAL ALTERATIONS IN BLOOD LIPIDS

21.9.1 Circadian Rhythm

Circadian rhythms of serum lipids and apos have been long-studied in humans and some animal species, both with and without fasting. Diurnal rhythms in rats have been reported for total serum TGs and cholesterol, as well as VLDL, IDL/LDL, and HDL lipid concentrations (Ahlers et al., 1980; Cayen et al., 1972; de Gasquet et al., 1977; Kalopissis et al., 1979; Marrino et al., 1987; Mondola et al., 1995). The lipid changes in these studies follow circadian rhythms of endogenous neurohormonal factors, especially insulin (Benavides et al., 1998; reviewed in Gnocchi et al., 2015). The pattern in fed rats typically shows a nadir in circulating NEFA, TG, and TG-rich LPs in the very early dark phase (corresponding with the early post prandial period) followed by increasing blood concentrations of these lipids during the later dark and early light phase (de Gasquet et al., 1977; Marrino et al., 1987). These early postprandial lipid decreases (which may be missed with less frequent evaluations) are linked with a rise in glucose and insulin with feeding and consequential inhibition of adipose secretion on NEFA and hepatic release of VLDL. Late in the postprandial phase, insulin-stimulated adipose LPL activity and increasing chylomicron catabolism lead to the increasing blood NEFA and TG (largely associated with increasing VLDL) levels. Total cholesterol changes tend to be less pronounced and more variable in this timecourse, with the upswing in HDL cholesterol from a nadir occurring at similar or slightly earlier intervals than for LDL cholesterol in the postprandial period, and with ApoB LPs also being a significant source of total cholesterol (Deshaies et al., 1990; Mondola et al., 1995; Miettinen, 1982; Rivera-Coll et al., 1994). This sequential pattern of changes in blood NEFA, TG, cholesterol, and associated LPs linked with postprandial periods are generally similar across species with adjustment of the diurnal periods and meal timing, that is, TG and NEFA nadir in the early light period, and peak values in the very late light to early dark phase in human and other diurnal species (Bertolucci et al., 2008; Miettinen, 1982; Karpe et al., 1998; Ishioka et al., 2005; van Oostrom et al., 2000).

However, the diurnal rhythms of blood lipids are not only substrate-driven but also more broadly regulated by complex molecular organization surrounding an organism's central circadian clock. Indeed, alterations in these normal lipid cycles are generally in magnitude and only incremental in time with short-term fasting or dietary changes (Kalopissis et al., 1979; Cayen et al., 1972; Mirani-Oostdijk et al., 1981; Mondola et al., 1995; Schlierf and Dorow, 1973). The central circadian clock controlling lipid metabolism is often described as beginning with the anterior hypothalamus (the suprachiasmatic nuclei or SCN) and its connection to the eye as part of a "retinohypothalamic tract" leading to both behavior and neuroendocrine patterned responses (reviewed in Gnocchi et al., 2015). Hence, master mediators of lipid metabolism throughout the body, including tissue-specific transcription factors (e.g., PPARs), bile acid and LP synthesis and uptake, and neurohormones are regulated by the SCN, in combination with environmental and physiologic cues (reviewed in Adamovich et al., 2014; Gooley and Chua, 2014; Hussain and Pan, 2012). The central circadian clock is also the source of some otherwise-unexplained diurnal differences in response to environmental (e.g., food, temperature) and physiologic factors (e.g., stress hormones). For example, the decline in insulin sensitivity in the evening relative to the light period in human has been proposed to be due to core clock genes regulating oscillating patterns of FA metabolism in adipose relative to skeletal muscle tissue (Yoshino et al., 2014). Similarly, differences in intestinal lipid absorption between the dark and light period may be partly due to SCN-mediated downstream variation in enterocyte capacity to absorb FAs and synthesize LPs (Hussain and Pan, 2012).

Hence, circadian rhythms in combination with diurnal patterns of nutrient intake and skeletal muscle activity explain both the relatively stable patterning of blood lipids over the course of a 24-hour day, as well as the differences between species and between daylight and nocturnal periods in these patterns. It is important to consider that these blood lipid cycles reflect cyclic fluctuations in the mediators of lipid metabolism, including expressed genes, enzyme activity, and circulating hormone levels—related endpoints that may be the specific focus of a study or target of a therapeutic. Evaluation of these specific mediators may also require consideration their circadian rhythm within the species evaluated.

21.9.2 Development and Aging

Aging has been positively associated with increasing levels of serum cholesterol and TGs in rats. In a study by Reaven and Reaven (1981), substantial increases in both cholesterol and TGs occurred in rats as early as 3–4 months of age compared with young adult rats at 1.5 months of age. In this same study, additional increases in theses serum lipids were evident at 6–8 months, while concentrations leveled off by 10–12 months. Boudet et al. (1988) similarly reported significant age-related higher concentrations of serum cholesterol, TGs and PLs when comparing adult (15–17 weeks of age) to aged (59 and 122 weeks of age) Wistar rats. Yet, Van Liew et al. (1993) reported an age-related increase in F344 rats in cholesterol in both sexes but with an increase in TG only in females. Overall, the majority of pertinent published data have indicated that age-related increases occur in both cholesterol and TGs in rats (Carlson et al., 1968; Ghezzi et al., 2012; Hubert et al., 2000; Matsuzawa et al., 1993; Nesic et al., 2013). Studies that do not show this pattern have usually involved animals on a restricted diet or of a distinct strain (Aguila et al., 2002; Hubert et al., 2000; Moriyama et al., 2006; Story et al., 1976).

While the mechanism(s) of increasing serum cholesterol and TGs with age in rats have not been clearly identified, some age-related lipid metabolism enzyme and hormone alterations may offer insight. Both Choi et al. (1988a) and Ståhlberg et al. (1991) observed a decline in HMG-CoA reductase (the rate-limiting enzyme for hepatic cholesterol biosynthesis) and more progressive and persistent decrease in CYP7A1 (the rate-limiting enzyme for bile acid synthesis via the classical pathway) in rats from early postweaning to middle-aged or geriatric stages. Nesic et al. (2013) further reported an increase in responsiveness of aged rats to selective effects of exogenous ghrelin, including an increase in white adipose mass, and circulating TGs, LDL cholesterol, and corticosterone levels compared with similarly treated younger rats. Age-related decreased insulin sensitivity and decrease in the hepatic expression of LDL receptor and LRP (resulting in relative delayed clearance of chylomicron remnants) has also been demonstrated in some rat studies (Field and Gibbons, 2000; Kazumi et al., 1989). Collectively, these enzyme, receptor, and hormonal findings suggest that multifactorial alterations in lipid metabolism homeostasis contribute to the age-related blood lipid changes in rats. Notably, cholesterol and/or TG increases in the aging rat have been prevented through dietary restriction or exercise training (Van Liew et al., 1993; Takeuchi et al., 2009; Reaven and Reaven, 1981; Hubert et al., 2000).

In Rhesus and African Green monkeys, mild increases in serum cholesterol have been associated with increasing age relatively consistently, whereas serum TGs have been found to increase (Mattison et al., 2012; Szymanski and Kritchevsky, 1980; Wolfe et al., 1991) or decrease (Kessler and Rawlins,1983) in association with age. In cynomolgus monkeys on standard chow diets, no consistent age-related pattern of change in blood lipids across studies or reference databases have been reported. However, a slight positive correlation between age and calculated plasma LDL cholesterol concentration in adult male cynomolgus monkeys fed a low cholesterol (0.04 mg/kcal) relatively high saturated fat diet for more than 2 years has been described (Colvin et al., 1994); the increase in LDL cholesterol was high in animals with the greatest body weight, which was also age-related. Hence, the authors suggested the interaction of age and bodyweight were most correlated with plasma LDL cholesterol.

In adult dogs, no consistent age-related pattern in total serum TGs and cholesterol concentrations was evident in a number of comparative studies with either beagles, or dogs of variable, including mixed breeds (Levine, 2009; Piccione et al., 2004; Uchiyama et al., 1985; Wolford et al., 1986). While in miniature swine (including Sinclair, Göttingen, and Hormel-Hanford variants), serum TGs and cholesterol were unchanged or decreased with age in one or both sexes (Berlin et al., 1985; Pond et al., 1968; Tumbleson et al., 1976; Zöllner and Tacconi, 1968).

The transition from immature to adult animal can show converse changes in serum lipids compared with aging. Indeed, serum lipids (TGs ± cholesterol and associated LPs) in very immature (suckling) animals of some species tend to be greater than those in the adult animals. In studies of juvenile Wistar or Sprague-Dawley (SD) rats (approximately 1–3 weeks postnatal), total serum cholesterol and TG, as well as circulating VLDL and LDL cholesterol (determined in one or both studies chemically or by ultracentrifugation) showed values notably greater than those in the adult animals (McMullin et al., 2008). Circulating levels of these lipids were reported to subsequently decline by around the end of the third or fourth week of age, presumably associated with weaning. Similarly, in mixed breed canine puppies, total plasma TGs, cholesterol, and β-lipoprotein cholesterol were considerably greater than the levels in the postpartum dams, especially up to about 3 weeks of age (Wright-Rodgers et al., 2005). Increases in TGs and cholesterol in preweaning piglets relative to adults has also been reported (Chen et al., 1982; Hollanders et al., 1985). Total TGs are generally more consistently or prominently affected than the other parameters evaluated in these juvenile animals. These greater lipid values in very young, rapidly growing animals partly reflect their overall high dietary lipid intake and downstream metabolism.

Serum TGs and correspondingly, β-lipoproteins are also higher in pregnant rat dams, dogs, and humans in the last half to third of pregnancy (Hachey, 1994; Konttinen et al., 1964; Liberati et al., 2004; McMullin et al., 2008; Wright-Rodgers et al., 2005; Sitadevi et al., 1981; Teichmann et al., 1988; Williams et al., 2009; Knopp et al., 1986). Higher β-lipoproteins in pregnancy are particularly attributed to hormonally mediated increased hepatic VLDL synthesis and decreased adipose LPL (Knopp et al., 1986; Wasfi et al., 1980; Herrera and Ortega, 2008; Martín-Hidalgo et al., 1994). Significantly increased cholesterol during late or the majority of gestation has also been reported for dogs (Wright-Rodgers et al., 2005), Sinclair miniature swine (Tumbleson et al., 1970), human (Sitadevi et al., 1981; Teichmann et al., 1988), and Wistar (but not CD) rats (McMullin et al., 2008). Conversely, lower cholesterol and TGs in cynomolgus monkeys, and lower cholesterol without significant difference in TGs in Rhesus macaques during pregnancy (stage inconsistently defined) compared with nonpregnant females have been reported (Gilbert and Rice, 1991; Kessler and Rawlins, 1983; Yoshida et al., 1988). Notably, maternal lipid profiles during late gestation do not correlate with fetal lipid values, as LPs do not freely cross the placenta (Herrera et al., 1988; Knopp et al., 1986). Rather, maternal circulating TGs are metabolized via LPL of the placental endothelium with release of NEFAs into the fetal circulation. The placenta also presents select receptors for regulated transfer of maternal cholesterol to the fetus, including the LDL receptor and scavenger receptor, SR-B1 (particularly important for HDL cholesterol uptake) (Wyne and Woollett, 1998; Ethier-Chiasson et al., 2007).

21.9.3 Gender

Gender differences in common laboratory species in mean fasting baseline total circulating TGs and/or cholesterol and corresponding LPs are common, but generally small in magnitude and not particularly consistent between reported studies. The limited differences in serum lipid profiles, despite overt differences in body mass, adipose distribution, energy metabolism, and hormonal influences between the sexes, partly reflects the inherently wide biological variability of blood LP concentrations and lipid content within and across individuals (including across age groups), along with the low "n" and timepoints commonly evaluated. Gender-related differences in blood lipids may also be more or less apparent with certain epidemiologic populations, strains, variants, and age categories within species but of limited relevance to other groups.

While gender differences in lipid profiles lack a universal pattern among species, a common reported finding among healthy fasted adult rats and mice is greater serum TGs in reproductively intact males compared with age-matched intact females (Matsuzawa et al., 1993; Moriyama et al., 2006; Wolford et al., 1986). Conversely, in other routinely studied species including human, nonhuman primates, and dogs, differences in serum TG values between the genders have not been consistent in either occurrence or pattern among published studies reference databases.

Sex-related differences in blood cholesterol concentrations in several laboratory species are suggested based on consistency of patterns across reported relevant studies. In particular, these studies suggest lower total and/or HDL cholesterol concentrations in adult males relative to females in Rhesus monkeys (Eggen et al., 1982; Mattison et al., 2012; Fless and Scanu, 1986), African Green monkeys (Wolfe et al., 1991), dogs (Pasquini et al., 2008; Barrie et al., 1993) rabbits (Hromadová and Hácik, 1984) guinea pigs (Roy et al., 2000), and miniature pigs (Tumbleson et al., 1976; Zamami et al., 1981). In a study of Hormel-Hanford miniature pigs (Berlin et al., 1985), serum TG, total cholesterol, and all cholesterol fractions (HDL, LDL, and VLDL) from puberty until old age were significantly lower in males than females. Consistent with these findings between sexes for HDL cholesterol, lower range for HDL cholesterol in men compared with women has been attributed to higher androgenic hormones. Concordantly in cynomolgus monkeys, increased HDL cholesterol in castrated males, and decreased HDL cholesterol in males administered exogenous testosterone or ovariectomized females administered 5α-dihydrotestosterone (DHT) have been observed (Greger et al., 1990; Leblanc et al., 2004; Nantermet et al., 2008; Weyrich et al., 1992). Two of these studies also showed a reduction in HDL particle size as reported in humans with increased androgen exposure (Weyrich et al., 1992; Nantermet et al., 2008). However, the induction of HL with increased androgen exposure seen in men (and associated with the HDL cholesterol change) was not detected in cynomolgus monkeys (Nantermet et al., 2008). Collectively, these studies suggest broadly similar sex-related hormonal influences on HDL cholesterol in cynomolgus monkeys as in human.

In association with estrogen flux and the menstrual cycle in females, several studies in women have shown aligned alterations in blood lipid profiles. However, no consistent cyclical changes in total cholesterol, or in HDL, LDL, or Lp(a) (analyzed by density-gradient ultracentrifugation, electrophoresis, and/or fast protein liquid chromatography) were seen in a large study of female Rhesus monkeys (Fless and Scanu, 1986) or in cynomolgus monkeys (Lehmann et al., 1993). Whether hormonal changes with the female reproductive cycle in other laboratory species impacts blood lipids is unclear, although published and other available information suggests that the effects are minor or not apparent.

Sex-related differences in lipid profile have additionally been reported in response to modified diets, aging, and disease states (Choi et al., 1988b; Galan et al., 1994; Rudel and Pitts, 1978; Priego et al., 2008; Thomàs-Moyà et al., 2006; Valle et al., 2007) and may be hormone-mediated, or secondary to gender-related differences in body composition and/or energy metabolism. These differences between males and females in responsive blood lipid profiles are commonly incremental in magnitude, timecourse, and/or balance of serum lipids/LP changes but still demonstrate the general utility of evaluating both sexes when investigating blood lipid effects. However, even in laboratory species susceptible to atherogenic diets (e.g., cynomolgus monkeys, baboons, pigs, New Zealand white rabbits, hamsters, guinea pigs), the gender-related changes in serum lipids with dietary manipulations or disease can, but often do not, clearly mimic the lipid profile differences observed between women and men with corresponding condition. Yet, understanding the gender differences in lipid profile within a species can enable translation of the findings from nonhuman species to human.

The outcome of functional gonadectomy or exogenously altered hormonal state in female or male animals can also result in hormone-related shifts in blood lipid. These are further addressed below in Section 21.9.12.

21.9.4 Fasting and Calorie/Nutrient Deficient Diets

Fasting for more than a few hours can measurably affect serum lipids and lipid metabolic pathways in small mammals with relatively high metabolic rates. Similar, albeit usually less prominent changes can be seen in larger laboratory species with short-term (e.g., overnight) fasting. In contrast, more prolonged calorie restriction results in progressive and adaptive changes in lipid turnover that orchestrate with the organism's metabolic needs. Accordingly, serum lipid patterns with prolonged calorie deficiency are distinct from both fed and acute fasting states, with, the extent of differences understandably variable with the level of macro- and micronutrient deficiencies as well as starting nutritional state, gender, hormonal state, age, species, and strain.

With acute fasting of monogastric species, the most consistent and prominent serum lipid change is a decrease serum TGs in association with decreased intestinally derived apoB chylomicrons and inhibition of hepatic VLDL secretion (Bertolucci et al., 2008; Ockner et al., 1969; Boudet et al., 1988). This decrease in TG is only partly ameliorated by a decrease in tissue uptake of TG-rich particles with the drop in adipose LPL activity (Bergö et al., 2002). Increase in NEFAs with peripheral tissue lipolysis and circulating ketones may also be seen, with the magnitude depending on the extent of fasting relative to metabolic rate and the animal's baseline nutritional level. However, changes in serum total cholesterol and cholesterol-rich particles are more minor or nondetectable mainly due to the continued efflux of cholesterol-rich LPs from the liver as well as intestinal cells (Section 21.5), and little to no change in the clearance of circulating LDL (Kraemer et al., 1994; Lane et al., 2000; Matsuzawa et al., 1993; Sokolović et al., 2010).

In contrast, more prolonged fasting/acute starvation may lead to increases in circulating TGs and/or cholesterol in association with more profound peripheral tissue lipolysis to meet energy needs, with resultant upregulation of hepatic VLDL synthesis (Iacono and Ammerman, 1966; Kalderon et al., 2000; Cahill et al., 1966; Parilla, 1978). The lipolysis-induced increased flux of NEFAs from peripheral (adipose, skeletal muscle) tissues is mediated primarily by a decrease in insulin activity and increase in circulating catecholamines, especially epinephrine (Jensen et al., 1987). Tissue NEFAs that are released into circulation in an animal that has undergone prolonged fasting/acute starvation are mostly consumed via oxidation for energy by a broad spectrum of peripheral tissues. However, those NEFAs that escape this process are absorbed by the liver and channeled (in individuals with adequate liver lipid stores) into VLDL correlating with the increased serum TG and cholesterol (Gibbons and Burnham, 1991; Kalderon et al., 2000; Lata et al., 2002). Prolonged fasting is also associated with insulin resistance, which further contributes to increased circulating TG through reduced inhibition of hepatic VLDL synthesis, reduced VLDL and LDL (receptor-mediated) uptake, and impaired peripheral tissue mitochondrial lipid oxidation (Chen et al., 2010; Hoeks et al., 2010; Markel et al., 1985; van der Crabben et al., 2008). These changes result in a relative increase in production and decrease in the clearance of VLDL and LDL. In some species (e.g., those with relatively high CETP; Sections 21.5 and 21.6, and Table 21.4), HDLs may be conversely decreased; a finding purported to reflect their increased clearance in association with insulin-resistance-triggered upregulated CETP activity (leading to loss of cholesterol from HDL) and increased TG transfer to HDL (due to increased circulating TG-rich VLDL) leading to increased hepatic HDL uptake (Borggreve et al., 2003; Lacombe et al., 1983; Markel et al., 1985; Rashid et al., 2002). Decreased peripheral lipid loading of HDL may also contribute to their decreases (Magun et al., 1988). Collectively, these insulin-resistant effects significantly contribute to the increases in TGs and cholesterol (and more variable LDL/HDL ratio) that can occur with prolonged fasting/acute starvation. However, some differences in extent and timecourse of these serum lipid and LP effects with differences in species, gender, nutritional state, NEFA re-esterification and oxidation, and hepatic LP synthesis rates should be expected (Lafontan, 1981; Lafontan et al., 1985; Levine, 2009; Piccione et al., 2004). As a general example of species differences, the overall NEFA flux in adipose tissue with comparable fasting is 5- to 15-fold higher in rats than in humans, while the extent of re-esterification of these NEFAs and the role of insulin resistance in hepatic VLDL synthesis appear to be greater in human.

More chronic calorie deficit leads to further adaptive changes in lipid metabolism, with a general shift toward enhanced peripheral tissue efficiency in lipid utilization. This shift is marked by enhanced LPL activity, NEFA uptake, and FA oxidation in nonadipose (i.e., energy consuming) peripheral tissues (e.g., skeletal muscle) (Bruss et al., 2010; Taskinen and

TABLE 21.4
Selective Enzymes and Proteins Important in Blood Lipid Transport

Enzyme	Abbreviation	Tissue Source/Site	Major/General Function	Species/Comments
Lipoprotein lipase	LPL	Capillary endothelial cells (particularly of adipose, skeletal, and cardiac muscle); Heparin bound to luminal surface	Hydrolyzes TGs in circulating large lipoproteins; chylomicrons are a preferred substrate	Activity is enabled by apoC-II and enhanced by A-V
Lecithin:cholesterol acyltransferase	LCAT	Hepatocytes	Catalyzes the transfer of long-chain FAs from PLs (mostly lecithin) to free cholesterol to form cholesterol esters (CEs); The FAs are mostly transferred from TG-rich LPs (chylomicrons, VLDL) and cells to HDLs. The CEs can then be stored and transported in the HDL core	ApoA-I is a cofactor, and apoA-IV and apoC-I are activators
Phospholipid transfer protein	PLTP	Synthesized by many tissues including lung, adipose, testis, brain, skeletal and heart muscle, liver, macrophages	Promotes transfer of PLs and free cholesterol between LPs Activity is particularly important during peripheral VLDL lipolysis to capture lipids released from the VLDL outer shell and transfer to HDLs (Schwarz et al., 2008)	Plasma PLTP activity is significantly greater in mice, dogs, and pigs compared with humans (among tested species), a factor that likely contributes to differences in serum lipid concentrations, and risk of atherogenesis between these species
Hepatic lipase	HL	Hepatocytes; heparin bound to sinusoidal endothelial surfaces in space of Dissé; also synthesized by macrophages; other tissues in some species (e.g., adrenal in rat)	Hydrolyzes both TGs and PLs from LPs, particularly LDL and HDL, generating small LDL and small HDL via nonreceptor-mediated catabolism with hepatocyte (macrophage) absorption of their lipid content	Species variability in HL expression level and tissue distribution; HL (mRNA) is particularly low in liver of rabbits
Endothelial lipase	EL	Synthesized by capillary endothelial and smooth muscle cells; heparin bound to luminal surfaces similar to LPL	Peripheral tissue lipase that hydrolyzes TGs and PLs of VLDL (as well as IDL, LDL, and HDL); has distincte sn-1 phospholipase activity	Increased expression in endothelial cells induced by inflammatory stimuli (e.g., TNFα, IL1β, LPS); and in macrophages and vascular smooth muscle cells with hypertension, angiotensin II

(Continued)

TABLE 21.4(*Continued*)
Selective Enzymes and Proteins Important in Blood Lipid Transport

Enzyme	Abbreviation	Tissue Source/Site	Major/General Function	Species/Comments
Cholesterol ester transfer protein	**CETP**	Expressed in various tissues: adipose, skeletal and heart muscle, hepatocyes, stomach, testis spleen (some species variability in distribution)	Mediates transfer of CEs from HDL to TG-rich lipoproteins, and shuttling of their TGs to HDL in exchange	Laboratory species widely vary in CETP activity (Section 21.5, Table 3). Plasma CETP among tested species has been found to be inversely correlated with HDL cholesterol concentration, and the ratio of HDL, relative to total serum cholesterol
Cholesterol 7α hydroxylase	**CYP7A1**	Hepatocytes (located in ER and mitochondria)	Rate-limiting enzyme in the conversion of cholesterol to bile acids via the classic pathway. Highly regulated by various circulating hormones and nuclear hormone receptors	Large species differences in baseline rate, and regulation of this classic enzyme pathway, and in occurrence of additional, alternative bile acid synthetic pathways
Hormone-sensitive lipase	**HSL**	Steroidogenic tissues (e.g., gonads, adrenal) where CEs are hydrolyzed for hormone synthesis. A truncated form is expressed in other tissues for intracellular hydrolysis of acylglycerides (e.g., adipose, skeletal and heart muscle, lung, pancreatic β cells, macrophages)	Hydrolyzes esters of TGs, DGs, MGs, and cholesterol. With TGs, only the initial esterase step is rate-limiting and regulated by the enzyme (and hormone signaling). The most important hormones in regulating this step are catecholamines, ACTH, and insulin	Some differences in tissue isoforms are associated with variable regulation between species and individuals

Nikkilä, 1979, 1987). These adaptations, together with decreases in hepatic lipid stores with prolonged calorie deficit eventually lead to decreased NEFA, TG, and VLDL serum levels. In contrast, decreases in peripheral tissue LDL receptor expression helps to maintain serum cholesterol levels for longer calorie-restricted periods, especially in species in which LDL is a prominent serum cholesterol-carrying LP. Greater efficiency of lipolysis within adipocytes has also been reported with chronic calorie restriction in rats, with increased white adipose capacity for basal and catecholamine-stimulated lipolysis (Lafontan et al., 1985). This adaptive effect in rats is attributed to increased response to β-adrenergic and hormonal lipase signaling, decreased inhibition of intracellular lipid droplet modulators, and decreased local LPL activity (and thus decreased adipose circulating lipid uptake) (Bertile et al., 2003; Taskinen and Nikkilä, 1987; Zechner, 1997). Incremental increases in lipolytic hormones such as circulating norepinephrine, growth hormone (GH), glucagon, and selective catecholamines also contribute to more efficient adipose lipolysis with chronic calorie restriction.

Effects of chronic calorie restriction can show additional sex-related differences in lipid metabolism and adaptive responses. For example, female rats and pigs have been reported to metabolize adipose stores and preserve lean body mass better than age-matched males during chronic undernutrition (Hill et al., 1986; Serrano et al., 2009; Smyers et al., 2015). Female Rhesus monkeys have also been shown to have lower energy expenditure than age-matched males with adaptation to long-term calorie restriction (Raman et al., 2007). These gender differences may explain some serum lipid distinctions between the sexes in caloric restriction studies, particularly the often more prominent TG changes in females of these species with food restriction (Cortright and Koves, 2000; Thomàs-Moyà et al., 2006; Hoyenga and Hoyenga, 1982; Hill et al., 1986). Dietary alterations (e.g., in carbohydrate and protein content) with chronic calorie restriction can further alter these common adaptive patterns of lipid metabolism. Effects of sustainable chronic food restriction have additionally been shown to interrupt typical age-related increases in serum TG and cholesterol levels in rodents and primates (Hubert et al., 2000; Roth et al., 2001).

Notably, short-term fasting (e.g., 12–24 hours in humans and large animal species; 6–12 hours in rodents) is commonly employed in evaluation of study animals. However, even short-term fasting can affect the magnitudes of normal diurnal changes in blood lipids and LP content (Ahlers et al., 1980; Mondola et al., 1995; Benavides et al.,1998). Hence, as in humans, fasting serum samples alone may not fully reflect, or can even mask effects of a treatment on blood lipids (Mora et al., 2008). Fasting also alters neurohormonal signaling in association with the changes in lipid metabolism; in particular, even short-term calorie deficiency is associated with increases in circulating GH, and catabolic hormones (e.g., glucagon, epinephrine, and cortisol) and decreases in insulin and insulin-like growth factor-1 (IGF-I) levels. More prolonged calorie restriction (or anorexia) can also impair functional activity of metabolic enzymes important for lipid, as well as xenobiotic metabolism (Zhang et al., 1999). Some specific nutrient deficiencies can lead to alterations in blood lipid profiles even with adequate caloric intake. One of the more classic changes is an increase in blood TG, and cholesterol in guinea pigs fed a diet deficient in ascorbic acid (Roomi, 1997). Deficiencies of zinc, copper, vitamin A, magnesium, or protein have also been associated with consistent alterations in blood lipid profiles in various laboratory species (Bouziane et al., 1994; Gatica et al., 2006; Hing and Lei, 1991; Lefevre et al., 1985; Rayssiguier et al., 1981; Schoenemann et al., 1990).

Refeeding after fasting or starvation also transiently alters serum lipid profile relative to that in health. As with the effects of fasting and starvation, these refeeding effects are mediated by neurohormonal and other variables, and can be especially species-variable in extent and timecourse. For example, the increase in serum TGs after refeeding is distinct in rats and mice (and to a lesser extent in dogs) compared with humans and nonhuman primates, in part, due to the capacity for hepatic apoB48 synthesis in the former (Baum et al., 1990; Greeve et al., 1993; Leighton et al., 1990).

21.9.5 Neurohormonal Signaling

Several neurohormones have a major regulatory role in lipid metabolism. The most potent and direct acting are catecholamines and insulin. Catecholamines primarily enhance TG hydrolysis and NEFA release into circulation by adipocytes, and can overcome the inhibitory effect on adipocyte lipolysis by insulin. Conversely, insulin is a potent antilipolytic hormone, inhibiting the activation of enzymes responsible for adipose lipolysis and promoting adipocyte uptake of glucose and NEFAs and de novo lipogenesis in hepatocytes. Other commonly measured circulating hormones have lesser but still significant impact on lipid metabolism and serum lipid levels. Most notably these include GH, glucocortocoids, thyroid hormone, estrogen, and testosterone—all of which partly to largely act through effects on catecholamine or insulin signaling. For example, thyroid hormone and testosterone (in rats) enhance adipocyte lipolysis largely by regulating cell sensitivity to β-adrenergic catecholamines (Fain and García-Sáinz, 1983; Arner, 2005). Estrogens also affect the signaling pathway of stimulatory catecholamine receptors (Lafontan and Berlan, 1993). Both corticosteroids and GH can promote NEFA generation partly through inhibition of insulin-mediated responses (Yang et al., 2004; Yip and Goodman, 1999; Burén et al., 2008).

A common mechanism of many of these neurohormones for stimulating lipid hydrolysis in adipocytes is upregulation of adenyl cyclase through G-protein-coupled receptors, with generation of cyclic adenosine monophosphate (cAMP) and protein kinase A (PKA) (reviewed in Carmen and Víctor, 2006; Fain and García-Sáinz, 1983; Strålfors and Honnor, 1989; Wang et al., 2008; Zechner et al., 2009). PKA-mediated phosphorylation of hormone-sensitive lipase (HSL) and coactivation of regulatory proteins surrounding intracellular TG-storing lipid droplets (e.g., perilipin-1) is associated with translocation (or enhanced docking) of HSL to the lipid droplet. HSL is found predominantly in (white and brown) adipocytes, with lower expression of HSL isoforms in other cell types, particularly muscle, steroidogenic cells, pancreatic β-cells, and macrophages (Yeaman, 2004). Hormones that directly stimulate HSL activity through intracellular cAMP/PKA generation include catecholamines (via β-adrenergic receptors), corticosteroids (e.g., dexamethasone) and (especially or exclusively in rodents) glucagon, adrenocorticotropic hormone (ACTH), parathyroid hormone, thyrotropin and α-melanocyte-stimulating hormone, and (in primates) atrial naturietic protein (Carmen and Víctor, 2006; Marcus et al., 1988; Sengenès et al., 2002; Xu et al., 2009; reviewed in Zechner et al., 2009, and in Wang et al., 2008). On the other hand, insulin suppresses lipolysis by activating an intracellular phosphodiesterase that degrades cAMP (reviewed in Kolditz and Langin, 2010).

While HSL serves a critical role in hormone-activated lipolysis, two other intracellular lipases coordinate to complete the process of adipocyte TG hydrolysis. Adipose triglyceride lipase (ATGL; also known as desnutrin) initiates the first step through cleavage of *sn*-2 FA from the glycerol backbone generating *sn*-1,3 diacylglycerol (preferred substrate for HSL) and a free FA (Eichmann et al., 2012; Rydén et al., 2007; Villena et al., 2004; Zechner et al., 2009). A less specific MG lipase completes the final hydrolytic step to cleave the remaining FA from glycerol (Kolditz and Langin, 2010; Nielsen et al., 2014). As with HSL, ATGL shows the highest expression and activity in adipose tissue and can be activated or repressed by similar neurohormonal signals. However, regulation and some responses of ATGL are distinct from that for HSL, including being increased with long-term calorie deficiency, upregulated by PPARγ agonists, and purportedly altered by obesity (Zechner et al., 2009; reviewed in Nielsen et al., 2014). Conversely, MG lipase has not been found to be directly under hormonal control. Notably, while these lipases are active in multiple cell types, only adipocytes are capable of releasing the generated NEFAs extracellularly (Kolditz and Langin, 2010).

Species differences in the extent of neurohormone responses of these intracellular lipases and lipid droplet docking sites (perilipins) have been reported and can be prominent (Arner, 2005; Castan et al., 1994; Lafontan et al., 1985; Bousquet-Mélou et al., 1995). An animal's age, fed/fasted state, energy expenditure, and activity of other lipomodulating hormones are also important variables affecting these molecular responses (Arner et al., 1990; Bertile and Raclot, 2011; Lafontan,

1981; Villena et al., 2004). The impact of some of these variables is noted below for specific neurohormones; however, all of these potential variables should be considered when designing studies and evaluating specific blood lipid data.

21.9.6 Catecholamines

Catecholamines are the primary activators of both fasting- and exercise-induced peripheral lipolysis, which is promoted through stimulation of adipocyte β-adrenergic receptors. Norepinephrine and epinephrine, as well as chemically synthesized catecholamimetics (e.g., isoproterenol, phenylephrine, theophylline), induce this adipose lipolytic effect, with norepinephrine and isproterenol having a greater overall potency than epinephrine (Fain and Garcĩa-Sáinz, 1983; Frisk-Holmberg and Ostman, 1977; Lafontan and Berlan, 1993). Stimulation of adipocyte β-adrenoceptors results in HSL activation (i.e., phosphorylation), intracellular lipolysis, and facilitated long-chain NEFA transport across the plasma membrane of white fat cells (Lafontan and Berlan, 1993). There are at least three functionally distinct β-adrenoceptor subtypes; all promote white and brown fat cell lipolysis with stimulation, but the distribution, participation, and functional importance of each receptor subtype in lipolysis varies with fat type, body region, gender, age, nutritional level (e.g., leanness vs. obesity), and species (Bousquet-Mélou et al., 1994; Carpéné et al., 1994a, 1994b, 1998; D'Allaire et al., 1995; Langin et al., 1991; Meyers et al., 1997).

Adrenoceptors β1 and β2 are the predominant β-adrenoceptor types in white adipose and induce lipolysis co-regulated by proteins surrounding intracellular lipid droplets. However, the β3-adrenoceptors predominate in brown fat where they promote thermogenesis, and have distinct regulation (Carpéné et al., 1998; D'Allaire et al., 1995). Accordingly, β3-adrenoceptors have prominent expression and functional importance in brown fat, as well demonstrated in certain rodents (rats, mice) and hibernating species (e.g., hamsters) (Carpéné et al., 1994a; Lafontan and Berlan, 1993; Carmen and Victor, 2006). In white fat, functional β3-adrenoceptors are lipolytic but, in some species, have lesser catecholamine responsiveness than the other β-adrenoceptors. The lipolytic responsiveness of white fat β3-receptors is relatively high in rats and hamsters; moderate in rabbits, dogs, and marmosets; and essentially absent in human, guinea pig, macaques, and baboons (Bousquet-Mélou et al., 1994; Sengenès et al., 2002; Langin et al., 1991; Meyers et al., 1997). These species distinctions in functional β-adrenoceptors, as well as those in α-receptors (described below), explain species differences in lipolytic response for a plethora of conditions that alter catecholamine activity.

White and brown fat cells also express α1- and α2-adrenoceptors that have distinct characteristics. Alphal-receptors are predominantly found in brown fat and, as with β3-adrenoceptors, have a role in thermogenesis (thus, less direct effect on blood lipid content), but a different signaling pathway involving protein kinase C (rather than PKA). In even greater contrast, α2-adrenoceptors have an inhibitory role on lipolysis through attenuation of adenylate cyclase generation. Thus, the lipolytic outcome of catecholamine stimulation of fat cells is a result of the interplay between the stimulatory and inhibitory effects of β- and α-adrenoceptors, respectively. The functional importance of α2-adrenoceptors in adipocytes is particularly dissimilar between species. In rats, there is a minor adrenoceptor with minimal to no functional activity in adipose. Moreover, in guinea pigs, hamsters, dormouse, and rabbits, the adrenoceptors do not appear to be involved in physiological control of lipolysis by catecholamines (Carpéné et al., 1994b; Pecquery et al., 1983; Castan et al., 1994). However, in humans and nonhuman primates, α2-adrenoceptors occur in relatively high density in fat cells—exceeding that of β-adrenoceptors in major adipose depots—and are functionally efficient and important in moderating lipolysis (Castan et al., 1994; Berlan and Lafontan, 1985; reviewed in Kolditz and Langin, 2010.). Not only do catecholamines (especially epinephrine), but also 3-β-OHB, the final product of ketogenesis stimulates this receptor in human (Wang et al., 2008). Thus, catecholamine stimulation and other mediators associated with fasting exert essentially an exclusively lipolytic effect in the rat, and a partly inhibitory effect on lipolysis in humans and nonhuman primates (Bousquet-Mélou et al., 1994). This moderating role of α2-adrenoceptors on lipolysis in humans has also been shown to be most prominent at rest (Arner et al., 1990).

Importantly, enhanced NEFA mobilization via catecholamine-mediated activation of adipocyte HSL is generally rapid in onset. However, increased adipose lipolysis via ATGL (which also occurs in rodents with fasting) appears to be triggered by a distinct signaling mechanism and follows a time-course uncorrelated with blood NEFAs (Bertile and Raclot, 2011; Zechner et al., 2009). Thus, ATGL activation has been proposed to be driven by glucocorticoids rather than to be stimulated by catecholamine and, accordingly, plays a particularly prominent role in severe starvation in rodents (Bertile and Raclot, 2011; Villena et al., 2004). In humans, ATGL has been reported to function in basal lipolysis but may have a less significant role in stimulated lipolysis than in rodents (Rydén et al., 2007).

21.9.7 Insulin

Insulin is the most potent inhibitory hormone on lipolysis. Acting primarily via the insulin receptor on adipocytes, insulin not only prevents HSL activation but also causes dephosphorylation of activated HSL (Strålfors and Honnor, 1982). Physiologic increases in insulin also upregulate peripheral lipid uptake through increased adipose LPL activity and intracellular NEFA re-esterification (Sadur and Eckel, 1982). Accordingly, blood NEFAs rapidly decrease postprandially due to the suppression of adipocyte NEFA secretion with increased plasma insulin (Karpe et al., 1998) (Figure 21.3a). However, in the late postprandial/postabsorptive phase (e.g., a few to several hours after a meal in primates [Figure 21.3b], and usually 1–2 hours postprandial in rats), NEFAs increase from this nadir

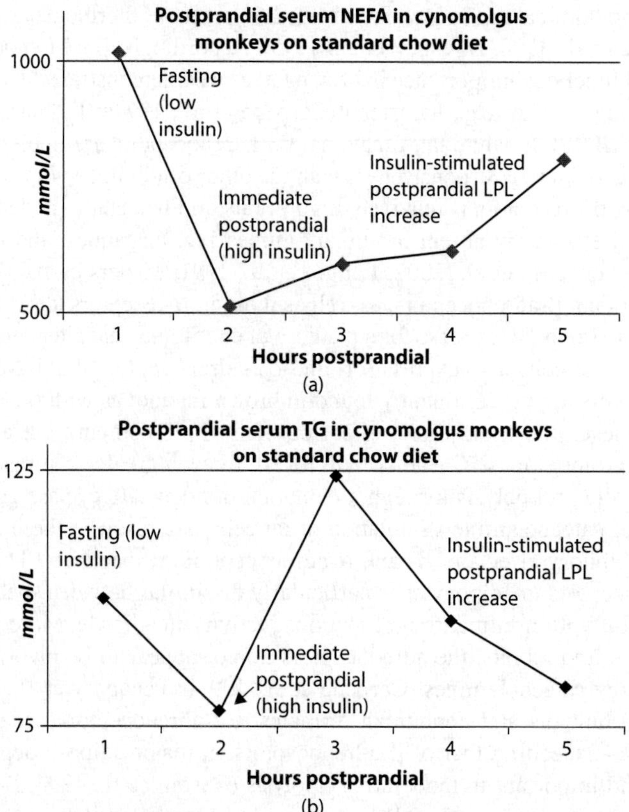

FIGURE 21.3 Pattern of serum NEFA (a) and TG (b) in cynomologous monkeys (pre- and postprandial on standard chow). *Note:* Associated relationship with expected normal insulin response across the same timecourse.

mainly due to insulin-mediated late increases in adipose LPL activity (through both transcriptional and posttranscriptional mechanisms) with resultant increased TG-rich LP catabolism and spillover of NEFAs into plasma (Chen et al., 2010; Fielding, 2011, Jelic et al., 2009; Karpe et al., 1998; Picard et al., 1999; Sadur and Eckel, 1982). This insulin-stimulated increase in adipose LPL is in contrast with skeletal muscle LPL activity, which is high during the fasting states. Blood NEFAs also peak during the fasting state predominantly due to low fasting insulin levels, which lift the inhibition on adipose NEFA secretion.

Physiologic increases in insulin are also associated with decrease in both tissue FA oxidation, and circulating VLDL (purportedly through inhibition of hepatic VLDL apoB secretion and increase in hepatic lipogenesis-related genes) (Chirieac et al., 2002; Malmström et al., 1997; reviewed in Kersten, 2001). Collectively, these changes contribute to the anabolic effect of insulin in promoting lipid uptake/retention and suppressing lipid degradation in adipose tissue and liver. In insulin-resistant states, the converse effects on apoB secretion and hepatic lipogenesis contribute to the hypertriglyceridemia commonly seen with this condition. Insulin resistance is also associated with a hampered upregulation of adipose tissue LPL activity; hence, peripheral tissue uptake of lipid from TG-rich VLDL and chylomicrons is slowed, augmenting the tendency toward hypertriglyceridemia.

The impact of insulin on serum lipids and lipid metabolism can be confounded by the concomitant influence of other hormones especially those that are responsive to, and/or directly influence insulin actions (e.g., glucagon, GH, IGF-1). Thus, the relative ratio of circulating insulin and these other hormones (and/or their receptors at the tissue level), rather than that of the individual hormones independently, is most relevant to the serum lipid profile (Frick et al., 2002; reviewed in Møller and Jørgensen, 2009).

21.9.8 Growth Hormone

GH is well established to have significant effects on lipid metabolism, with the expression of the GH receptor demonstrated on rodent and human adipocytes as well as hepatocytes (Vikman et al., 1991; Wei et al., 2006). However, the effects of the hormone on blood lipids and LPs are particularly complex in that they differ over time, as well as with gender, species, and age (Edén, 1979; Gabriel et al., 1992; Lado-Abeal et al., 2005). Lipid changes in response to endogenous GH alterations can also be challenging to directly link, because anterior pituitary release of the hormone occurs in oscillatory pulses of variable amplitude through the day so that frequent, serial time-point evaluations are required to measure functional circulating levels (Edén, 1979; Gabriel et al., 1992; Gobello et al., 2002; Lado-Abeal et al., 2005). The frequency and overall amplitude of these GH pulses, and some blood lipid responses are also strongly sexually dimorphic in many species (Edén, 1979; Edén et al., 2000; Oscarsson et al., 1991; Gabriel et al., 1992; Engström et al., 1998; Lado-Abeal et al., 2005). An added complexity in assessing GH effects on lipid metabolism is that the effects are often present in combination with other hormone abnormalities, which contribute especially to the chronic alterations in blood lipids.

Acute or short-term GH effects on lipid metabolism can be insulin-like in promoting adipose lipogenesis and have been shown to increase DNA synthesis and proliferation of islet β-cells and insulin secretion *in vitro*, and decrease glucose oxidation *in vivo* (Davidson, 1987; Frick et al., 2002; Møller et al., 1990; Nielsen, 1982). However, the long-term effects of GH are insulin-antagonistic, attributed to GH-upregulated adipose lipolysis, increased hepatic VLDL secretion, and increased nonadipose (skeletal muscle and heart) lipid uptake and oxidation (Frick et al., 2002; Oscarsson et al., 1999; reviewed in Nam and Marcus, 2000; Møller et al., 1993; Rathgeb et al., 1970). Adipose tissue lipolysis is partly mediated through enhanced HSL and β-adrenergic activity, which leads to increased circulating NEFA with downstream increased hepatic VLDL secretion and serum TG. Accordingly, increased blood NEFA and TG changes are common with acromegaly and reported as an effect of GH-treatment of growth hormone deficiency (GHD) in humans (reviewed in Frick et al., 2002). Increased blood NEFAs have also been reported in dogs and pigs with non-acute GH administration

(Rathgeb et al., 1970; Schneider et al., 2002) and hypophysectomized GH-administered rats after a two-day delay (McKee and Russell, 1968). Increased blood TGs have been further considered to be promoted through direct GH-enhanced hepatic secretion of ApoB (Apo48 in rats and ApoB100 in human) (Christ et al., 1999; Lindén et al., 2000). Increased circulating NEFAs and TGs may contribute to GH-associated insulin resistance through the same mechanisms as seen with obesity, particularly in inhibiting tissue glucose uptake and reducing hepatic insulin clearance.

Both chronic GH excess (acromegaly) and GHD in humans are additionally linked with increased risk for atherosclerosis, but only inconsistently with alterations in blood cholesterol typically associated with this condition. Untreated or active acromegaly has been most associated across studies with increased plasma concentration of LP(a), small dense LDL, and decreased HDL/LDL cholesterol ratio (Boero et al., 2012; Beentjes et al., 2000; Kostoglou-Athanassiou et al., 2013; Maldonado Castro et al., 2000; Oscarsson et al., 1999). Acromegalic patients have also been shown in some studies to have reduced plasma LCAT and PLTP, and decreased or increased CETP activity levels relative to a control population, which may collectively contribute to LDL cholesterol increases (Boero et al., 2012; Beentjes et al., 2000). While these findings are linked with GH excess, patients with untreated GHD have also been found to have an atherosclerotic lipid profile; most commonly, increased total and LDL and/or VLDL cholesterol levels (de Boer et al., 1994; Christ et al., 1999). One mechanism proposed for these findings in GHD patients is that, in addition to the role in ApoB secretion, the hormone has been found to upregulate LDL receptor expression in hypophysectomized rats and human liver tissue *in vitro* (Rudling et al., 1992). Hence, recovery of the expression of the hepatic LDL receptor following long-term GH replacement therapy may explain normalization of blood LDL cholesterol and HDL/LDL cholesterol ratio in treated GHD patients (Christ et al., 2006; de Boer et al., 1994).

These effects of GH on blood lipids are consistent with the hormone's role during prolonged fasting, significant physiologic (e.g., inflammatory) stress, or prolonged exercise. In such catabolic states, GH is anabolic for skeletal muscle tissue supporting protein preservation through increased availability and oxidation of FAs, and shifting energy generation away from glucose oxidation. In this role, GH directly and indirectly antagonizes the effects of insulin as a defense especially against hypoglycemia during these system challenges. While this role is similar across individuals and species, some differences in the effects of GH on blood lipids relative to age, gender, and diet and in animal models compared with acromegaly and GHD in humans deserve comment. The absolute secretion of GH in health is maximal (as with circulating IGF-1) at midpuberty. Circulating levels and the combined effects between GH and IGF-I gradually decline in adulthood and further with senescence. Hence, studies in very young animals may not duplicate effects seen in fully mature adult or aged animals (including human patient populations). Differences between genders in the baseline pulsatile pattern and the absolute amount of GH secreted, as well as sex-hormone influences on GH, and blood lipids are substantial in both humans and common laboratory animals (Edén, 1979; Edén et al., 2000; Ciresi et al., 2013); hence, GH-mediated blood lipid responses are generally not directly comparable between genders. Moreover, in rodent models, the differences in the GH effect on tissue LPL are considered as the potential cause of the differences in blood lipid responses with alterations of the hormone. In particular, GH robustly promotes increased LPL activity in skeletal muscle (including heart) in mice and rats, whereas GH-mediated decrease in adipose LPL activity with less distinct effect on muscles LPL has been reported in humans (Oscarsson et al., 1999; Frick et al., 2002; Richelsen et al., 2000; Khalfallah et al., 2001). These difference between species may explain the lack of increased blood NEFA, TG, and VLDL in a nonfasted GH transgenic mouse model and GH-mediated decreased LDL (with increased VLDL turnover) in a hypophysectomized female rat model in contrast with general GH-mediated blood lipid effects in humans (Frick et al., 2002). Moreover, short-term fasting alone has been associated with decreased GH in mice, in converse of the well-established findings in human (Steyn et al., 2012). These findings, as well as specific blood lipid responses to GH with altered diet in rodents, are complex in translation to human and in need of continued study. Some GH effects on blood lipids are also partly indirect in being secondary to insulin resistance or GH-stimulated IGF-1 synthesis and release.

21.9.9 Insulin-Like Growth Factor-1

Hepatic synthesis and secretion of IGF-1 are stimulated by GH. Indeed, the actions of IGF-1 are necessary for promoting the protein anabolic effects of GH, including for adipose tissue (promoting preadipocyte proliferation and differentiation). IGF-1 release is also dependent upon sufficient nutrient intake and availability, and portal insulin levels, with blood concentrations rapidly decreasing during fasting. In turn, IGF-1 negatively regulates the secretion of GH and insulin. Hence, there is a complex balance between the effects of GH, IGF-1, and insulin in the regulation of blood lipid and LP metabolism. Yet, the effects of IGF-1 on serum lipids in health are generally only indirect, and primarily mediated through stimulation of the insulin receptor. Administration of recombinant IGF-1, or chemical mimetics, to healthy or diabetic animals increases insulin sensitivity and can result in decreases in circulating TGs and VLDL as well as LDL cholesterol through mechanisms that are primarily the same as for insulin (Yuen and Dunger, 2006; Turkalj et al., 1992; Binoux, 1995). Exogenous IGF-1 can also result in (rapid, but temporary) hypoglycemia, and inhibition of insulin and GH secretion (with corresponding downstream impact on lipid metabolism). These, and relatively high incidence of other side effects of IGF-1 (e.g., arthralgia, edema), have limited the benefits of pharmaceutically enhanced IGF-1 activity in diabetic or dyslipoproteinemic conditions (Froesch and Hussain, 1994).

21.9.10 Glucocorticoids

Glucocorticoids (GCs), whether released endogenously in response to physiologic stress (e.g., starvation) or exogenously administered, have complex effects on lipid metabolism that are attributed to alterations primarily at the level of the adipocyte and hepatocyte.

In adipocytes, GCs have both lipolytic and anabolic effects. Lipolytic actions are principally indirect through a permissive effect on catecholamine-induced lipolysis and antagonism of insulin lipogenic response. Glucocorticoid response elements occur in regions of β-adrenergic receptor genes, and response to GCs have been shown to include increased adipocyte β receptor expression. Additionally, GCs appear to increase transcription of other elements of the β-adrenergic signaling cascade in the cells. The requisite protein synthesis explains the delayed onset and prolongation following withdrawal of exogenous steroids in adipocyte lipolytic effects (Vance and Vance, 2008; Campbell et al., 2011). This permissive effect of GCs on adrenergic activity, and the distinctions between species in adrenergic receptor expression, and brown and white fat content (see above on *Catecholamines*) may also explain the greater sensitivity of some species (e.g., rats and mice) to GC-mediated lipolysis compared with human.

Antagonism of insulin-induced adipocyte lipogenesis also contributes to lipolysis with long-term GC administration. A glucocorticoid receptor-dependent (transcription-independent) mechanism that attenuates insulin receptor (IRS-1) signaling for cell glucose uptake has been identified as one mechanism for this effect (Sakoda et al., 2000). GC-mediated upregulation of HSL and variable downregulation of LPL in adipose tissue also are considered to contribute to the insulin resistance (Slavin et al., 1994; Bagdade et al., 1976). Collectively, these lipolytic effects of GCs result in persistent increases in blood NEFA as well as impaired chylomicron and VLDL clearance.

Within hepatocytes, GCs promote uptake of the mobilized NEFA, and stimulation of VLDL synthesis and secretion (in animals with positive caloric balance) (Reaven et al., 1974; Mangiapane and Brindley, 1986). Thus, increases in blood VLDL and hypertriglyceridemia with GC excess is mediated by both decreased clearance and increased secretion of the LPs. Increase in LDL cholesterol is also common with GC excess, and likely represents an outcome of the impaired VLDL clearance

(Bagdade et al., 1976; Campbell et al., 2011). Consistent with these multiple contributing factors, the magnitude of circulating TG increase can be prominent. In a study of rats maintained for 5 days on a low dose of triamcinolone, serum TG concentration was doubled with a parallel rise in VLDL (Krausz et al., 1981). Of note, a much higher dose of triamcinolone for similar time period in this study produced a fall in serum TG and VLDL with increase in serum HDL cholesterol; a finding likely reflective of profound lipolytic effect and hyperinsulinism with concomitant negative caloric state as induced by high dose GCs in rats (You et al., 2009).

Glucocorticoids can also have an anabolic effect on adipose tissue in certain body regions, and in general, occurs through differentiation of preadipocytes in visceral fat. Thus, this effect likely has only muted impact on analyzed blood lipid content.

21.9.11 Thyroid Hormone (Triiodothyronine)

Triiodothyronine (T3) regulates, and predominantly promotes, adipose tissue lipolysis by both direct and indirect mechanisms. The effects of T3 on lipid metabolism have become particularly important to consider when evaluating blood chemistry data from animal studies where the administered drug or chemical toxicant inadvertently affects the hormone's function in the tested species (e.g., through upregulated T4 metabolism or impaired conversion to the active hormone). T3 directly influences the activity of critical enzymes in lipolytic pathways by acting on thyroid hormone-specific nuclear receptor isoforms. These receptor isoforms, and their corepressors/activators, are tissue specific and show age/development stage-dependent patterns in expression (reviewed in Zhu and Cheng, 2010). The hormone also promotes lipolysis indirectly through augmentation of local adrenergic, and (to a lesser extent) other hormone (e.g., GH) signaling in adipose tissue. Collectively, these T3-promoted processes enhance intracellular HSL-catalyzed lipolysis and β-oxidation. In animals with hyperthyroid conditions, increased FA uptake and β-oxidation in peripheral tissues are largely the reasons for the lack of prominent increase in circulating VLDL-TG despite the increased blood NEFA (Heimberg et al., 1985; Vance and Vance, 2008). Hyperthyroidism is also associated with the reduced hepatocyte esterification of FAs into TG, and the increased rate of clearance of circulating VLDL and chylomicron by peripheral tissues (Abrams et al., 1981; Erem et al., 1999; Jokinen et al., 1994; Wilcox and Heimberg, 1991). Thus, blood TG concentrations tend to be decreased to minimally increased with hyperthyroid conditions (Abrams et al., 1981; De Bruin et al., 1993; Erem et al., 1999; Heimberg et al., 1985). The slightly increased blood TG common in some species (typical with rats and mice) with hyperthyroidism may be partly due to an associated increased synthesis and release of intestinal apoB48 LPs (Davidson et al., 1988).

With conditions of low T3 (hypothyroidism), the change in blood TG shows a more species-distinct pattern. Hypothyroidism in humans and dogs is generally accompanied by increases in circulating TG with corresponding increases in VLDL (Dixon et al., 1999; Nikkilä and Kekki, 1972; Rogers et al., 1975; Schenck et al., 2004). However, in rats and mice (and most studied in the former), hypothyroidism results in rapid-onset, prominently and persistently decreased blood TG and VLDL (Dory et al., 1981; Patel et al., 2013; Meyer, et al., 1989; Davidson et al., 1988; Raheja et al., 1982). The reason for this species divergence, and the effect in other common laboratory species of hypothyroidism on TG have not been fully explored, although differences in α-adrenoceptor types in adipose tissue between these species is likely an important factor (see above on *Catecholamines*). In miniature pigs with experimental hypothyroidism, a response similar to rats (decreased serum TG), and in horses with spontaneous hypothyroidism, a pattern similar to human and dogs have been reported (Müller et al., 1983; Frank et al., 1999). In all evaluated species, hypothyroidism has generally been associated with slightly decreased to unchanged liver VLDL-TG secretion, and significantly decreased peripheral clearance of circulating VLDL (Dolphin and Forsyth, 1983; Fabbrini et al., 2012). In one study of hypothyroid rats, the rate of VLDL clearance from the plasma was about a third of that of pair-fed euthyroid controls (Dory et al., 1981). These factors are considered primary contributing factors to the increased serum TG in humans and dogs. However, in rats (and species with similar blood TG response), concomitant decreased intestinal synthesis of TG-rich apoB48 particles may be the most significant cause of the distinctly decreased VLDL-TG with low thyroid activity (Davidson et al., 1988).

One of the hallmark laboratory findings of thyroid hormone dysregulation in human and common laboratory species is altered serum cholesterol. Total blood cholesterol is typically decreased or increased inversely with change in thyroid hormone activity. These changes in total cholesterol predominantly reflect those in LDL cholesterol and are partly attributed to T3 augmentation of hepatocyte LDL receptor expression and function, and biliary excretion of cholesterol (Angelin and Rudling, 2010; Ness and Zhao, 1994; Staels et al., 1990; Salter et al., 1991; Thompson et al., 1981). A reduction in enterohepatic bile acid circulation is also reported with high T3 conditions. Thus, LDL cholesterol clearance is either enhanced or impaired with hyper- or hypo-thyroidism, respectively. These changes in blood LDL cholesterol occur despite counteracting thyroid hormone effects on cholesterol synthesis; that is, hyperthyroid conditions result in enhanced, and hypothyroidism exhibits reduced de novo cholesterol synthesis. These changes in blood LDL also occur in rats, despite the decrease in blood VLDL concentrations in this species with hypothyroidism (Dory et al., 1981).

Alterations in circulating HDL cholesterol concentration with thyroid dysfunction are less consistent or prominent than those in VLDL-TG or LDL cholesterol. Most commonly reported in human, dogs, and rats is a small increase in circulating HDL with hypothyroidism (Gross et al., 1987; Friis and Pedersen, 1987; Kung et al., 1995; Tan et al., 1998). The increase has been proposed to be due, in part, to greater apoA-I expression and decreased activity of HL and/or CETP (in species that express this enzyme; e.g., humans, rabbits, and guinea pigs) (Dory et al., 1981; Tan et al., 1998; Boone et al., 2011). Decreased HL can impair hepatic clearance of the LPs. While low CETP activity impairs net transfer of neutral lipids including CEs from HDL particles to the less dense apolipoprotein B (apoB)-containing LPs; hence decreased activity will prolong circulation time of some HDL forms (and may thus impair RCT in species that express the enzyme). Notably, these changes in HDL with thyroid dysfunction are generally small and not entirely consistent across published studies, especially in human in which HDL has also been reported to be decreased with hypothyroid conditions, and atypically increased with hyperthyroid conditions or unchanged in either endocrinopathy (Abrams et al., 1981; reviewed in Heimberg et al., 1985).

Although still under some debate, hypothyroidism has also been associated with increased blood Lp(a) in humans (De Bruin et al., 1993; Erem et al., 1999); whether this change is also seen in nonhuman (Old World) primates is unclear.

21.9.12 Testosterone and Estrogens

One of the most prominent effects of testosterone and estradiol in laboratory rodents is the effect of these hormones on adipose lipolysis. Castration or ovariectomy in adult rats is associated with a blunted lipolytic and corresponding blood lipid response to catecholamines (see section above on *Catecholamines*) (De Pergola et al., 1990; Xu et al., 1991). Conversely, testosterone and, to a lesser extent, estradiol administration to rats or mice of either sex enhances the lipolytic action on catecholamines with corresponding increase in blood NEFA and VLDL-TG (Uryszek et al., 1989; Tvorogova and Titov, 1986; Hansson et al., 1991). The predominance of these effects is species-specific in that, unlike primates and most other studied laboratory species, adipocytes of rats and mice express adrenoceptors that strongly promote lipolysis with catecholamine stimulation (see section on *Catecholamines*). In primates (and variably between adipose depots in all studied species), the lipolytic potential of testosterone varies with the regional balance of α- or β-adrenoceptors (Arner, 2005; Dicker et al., 2004; Hansson et al., 1991). Testosterone has also been shown in some species (e.g., hamsters) to alter tissue adrenoceptor balance over time (Arner, 2005). Administration of estradiol or testosterone to healthy rats has less pronounced impact and more select effects on lipolytic pathways in comparison with surgical castration and does not fully reverse effects of the latter on blood and tissue lipids.

In other species, both estrogens and testosterone at physiologic and supraphysiologic levels have mixed lipogenic and lipolytic effects with gender, age, and/or hormonal state and fat depot site as important variables. Accordingly, administration of exogenous estrogen or testosterone and/or gonadectomy in common non-rodent laboratory species (e.g., rabbit, dog, pig, and nonhuman primates (NHP), as in human, has not been associated with consistent pattern(s) in circulating NEFA, TG, or VLDL (Aydilek and Aksakal, 2005; Tvarijonaviciute et al., 2013; Hussein et al., 1999; Hromadová and Hácik, 1988a, 1988b; Pynadath and Chanapai, 1981).

In humans, the most well-established effect of testosterone and estrogens on blood lipids has been altered cholesterol levels, with correspondingly altered HDL and/or LDL cholesterol or LPs. More specifically, higher functional estrogen levels are linked with decreased (and testosterone levels with increased) total cholesterol, and/or LDL/HDL and/or HDL/total cholesterol ratio in humans. This hormonal influence has been long-studied, and variably supported by widely diverse animal models (some of which are discussed in Section 21.9.3). A very important consideration in the interpretation of the data from these animal models is that the effects of exogenous testosterone or estrogen on lipid metabolism (and blood lipids) partly depend upon whether the circulating hormone is in the physiologic or pharmacologic range. For example, Parini et al. (2000) described this as "biphasic" when presenting results in intact female rats, given 17β-estradiol (E2) for 1 week. At physiological doses in these animals, blood HDL cholesterol and apoA-I, and key liver enzymes activities for bile acid and cholesterol synthesis (HMG-CoA reductase and CYP7A1) were increased, whereas at higher (pharmacological) E2 doses, these hepatic enzyme activities were not increased, but hepatic LDL receptor protein and mRNA were increased and plasma total, HDL, and LDL cholesterol were decreased. Thus, the effects and mechanisms for estradiol-induced blood lipid changes in animal models can vary and even show contrasts depending upon the dose, although findings at all doses in this model (as commonly with animal models of estrogen effects on lipid metabolism) showed some consistencies with at least some effects of E2 in humans.

In animals, pharmacologic doses of estrogens and testosterone can also affect food consumption; and, as mentioned previously, in rodents, the doses can also be associated with adipose lipolysis and weight loss. These clinical effects affect the blood lipid profile and can confound assessment of the studied hormonal influence. In addition, and especially in rats, high-dose estrogens can also induce reduction of bile flow that can lead to intrahepatic cholestasis. The mechanisms for this are multifold and may overlap with those inducing cholestasis of pregnancy in women (Krell et al., 1987; Stieger et al., 2000). Blood lipid changes with the induced cholestasis in rats are also a consideration.

In summary, sex hormones can significantly affect blood lipid profiles in humans and animals, but the overall outcome is influenced by many factors, with species differences being one of the most important. Thus, while blood lipid changes with sex hormone administration can occur, the changes have not shown a consistent pattern.

21.9.13 Acute Phase Response

The acute phase response (APR) can have a profound effect on circulation lipids in all species. The APR is induced by a variety of pathologic stimuli, including infection, inflammation, necrosis, and some malignancies. The blood lipid changes with the response are rapid, occurring within 2 hours after administration of lipopolysaccharide (LPS) and are associated with the same cytokines that produce fever and anorexia (Feingold et al., 1992).

The most prominent, sensitive, and consistent APR blood lipid change is an increase in circulating TG (Nonogaki et al., 1995; Khovidhunkit et al., 2004). Hypertriglyceridemia has been shown to be induced by *in vivo* injection of bacterial cell wall components (e.g., LPS and lipoteichoic acid) and a broad range of proinflammatory cytokines (e.g., tumor necrosis factor (TNF) α, interleukin-1 [IL-1], IL-6) (reviewed in Khovidhunkit et al., 2004; Feingold et al., 1992; Nonogaki et al., 1995). The increase in TG is predominantly due to acute stimulated lipolysis with increased delivery of NEFA to the liver, and concomitant increased hepatic FA synthesis and VLDL secretion. However, with prominent APR, the increase in blood TG reflects TG enrichment of all circulating LP classes that is also associated with altered (generally reduced) FA oxidation and ketogenesis, and decreased clearance of TG-rich LPs attributed to reduced LPL and ApoE levels (Cabana et al., 1989, 1996; Khovidhunkit et al., 2004). Decreased clearance of TG-rich LPs is additionally a presumed cause of the significant APR-linked increase in blood IDL-TG and LDL-TG.

The effect of APR on increasing blood TG is similar in all species, with onset that is not only rapid but can be profound in magnitude. In rabbits injected intramuscularly with croton oil, serum TG increased 8- to 15-fold within 2–3 days (Cabana et al., 1983, 1989). African green monkeys given a subcutaneous injection of LPS showed increases in serum TG that reached sevenfold by 48 hours, and showed full resolution after 6 days (Auerbach and Parks, 1989). In rabbits given common water-in-oil adjuvants, one of the authors (DW) has observed that serum TG increased consistently between 5- and 12-fold within 24 hours and that fully resolved within 48–72 hours.

Importantly, the increases in TG-rich LPs are considered physiologically appropriate as part of the innate immune response offering some immediate protection against infection. As reviewed in Khovidhunkit et al. (2004), TG-rich VLDL, LDL, and chylomicrons have been shown to bind and neutralize LPS, lipoteichoic acid (LTA), certain bacterial toxicants, and a variety of DNA and RNA viruses. Lipoprotein bound to these bacterial components can also beneficially modify the inflammatory response by decreasing monocyte/macrophage activation, and accelerating the hepatocyte uptake and biliary excretion of these bacterial constituents (Feingold et al., 1998). Some apos and C-reactive protein (CRP) that are carried by TG-rich apoB-containing particles appear to have added beneficial roles for the host against infections.

In contrast to the overt change in blood TG, changes in serum cholesterol with inflammation are more subtle. In both primates and rodents, circulating HDL and HDL cholesterol have been shown to decrease, and the particles show APR-induced composition changes (Auerbach and Parks, 1989; Cabana et al., 1989, 1996; Fon Tacer et al., 2007; Khovidhunkit et al., 2004; Jahangiri et al., 2009). These composition changes include not only HDL enrichment with TG (noted above) but also with serum amyloid A (SAA; which binds to some bacterial toxins) and apoE (in contrast with decreased tissue and total circulating apoE). The increase in apoE and SAA likely contributes to lower HDL levels by enhancing uptake by hepatocytes (e.g., via apoE-LDL receptor binding) and scavenging by macrophages (via apoE-LDL-receptor and SAA-mediated mechanisms) (Artl et al., 2000; Auerbach and Parks, 1989; Cabana et al., 1996). With an APR, HDL is also typically depleted of cholesterol and apoA-I, II, and apoCs (negative APR proteins) (Auerbach and Parks, 1989). The decrease in HDL apoA-I content contributes to decreased cholesterol efflux from peripheral tissue to HDL, and, as enzyme cofactor, to decreased LCAT activity. Hence, there is decreased CE formation and capacity to absorb cholesterol from cells/other LPs. Directly decreased LCAT synthesis and activity with an APR have also been reported (Kitagawa et al., 1992). Collectively, these changes contribute to impaired RCT, a well-established APR effect.

Although these HDL alterations are generally consistent across species, APR effects on total serum cholesterol differ between several common laboratory species and primates, including humans (Artl et al., 2000; Cabana et al., 1996; Feingold et al., 1993; Kitagawa et al., 1992). In rodents and rabbits (nonstarved), serum total cholesterol concentration modestly increases, whereas in primates, total serum cholesterol shows no change to slight decreases with the APR. This converse effect appears to predominantly reflect species differences in baseline serum cholesterol concentration and metabolism. That is, the increase in total cholesterol in rodents and rabbits appears to largely represent the increase in VLDL particle number and VLDL cholesterol (that occurs with the APR in general) relative to the normally low baseline total cholesterol of the animals.

Additional reasons for the subtle, opposite change in total serum cholesterol between laboratory animal species (especially rodents) and primates can be attributed to species differences in the direction of change in LDL cholesterol content with the APR. Major proinflammatory cytokines (IL-1 and/or TNFα) have been shown to increase cholesterol content of LDL in rodents, and decrease cholesterol in LDL of primates (although decreases in blood LDL protein concentration are reported in both species with administration of the cytokines) (Cabana et al., 1996; Ettinger et al., 1992; Fon Tacer et al., 2007; Feingold et al., 1993). Changes in LDL cholesterol in all studied species are at least partly attributed to inflammation-induced increases in HMG-CoA reductase (the rate-limiting enzyme in hepatic cholesterol synthesis, Section 21.3), and decreases in CYP7A1 and CYP27A1 (the rate-limiting enzymes in the classic and alternative pathways for bile acid synthesis from cholesterol; Section 21.7) activity (reviewed in Khovidhunkit et al., 2004). The effects on these enzymes—in light of the known differences of the species in their enzyme regulation and cholesterol metabolism and catabolism—significantly explains the differences between rats and primates in blood LDL cholesterol content with the APR. Notably, the inhibition of these key enzymes, as well as transporters, for excretion of bile is believed to contribute to the intrahepatic cholestasis sometimes associated with inflammation (reviewed in Khovidhunkit et al., 2004).

An additional noteworthy mechanism for the differences of the species in the direction of the change in LDL cholesterol is the effect of inflammation on CETP. The concentration of CETP in plasma has been shown to significantly decrease with inflammation in humans (or following LPS injection in human CETP-transgenic mice) (Jahangiri et al., 2009; Masucci-Magoulas et al., 1995). Because CETP catalyzes the transfer of cholesterol from HDL to LDL (Section 21.5), the decreased enzyme protein is considered to contribute to decreased LDL cholesterol uptake. However, because CETP activity is virtually absent in the rat and several other laboratory animal species, this is not an important component of their altered blood lipids with the APR.

Additional mechanisms for changes in blood lipids and LPs with the APR have been described in the literature, although most are less well studied and/or consistent. These proposed mechanisms, collectively with known effects, indicate highly complex species-adaptive effects on lipid metabolism. It is therefore important to recognize the impact of inflammation/infection or proinflammatory cytokine administration when evaluating blood lipids in animals.

21.9.14 Hepatic Microsomal Enzyme Induction

There are relatively few published studies specifically addressing the potential for a link between general hepatic enzyme induction and blood lipid changes. Among them, small changes in blood TG and/or cholesterol have been reported with classic enzyme inducers, but the occurrence and direction of the changes has been inconsistent between studies and species (Elcombe et al., 2012; Ennulat et al., 2010; Goldberg et al., 1981; Heller et al., 1988; LaPorte et al., 1981; Luoma et al., 1982; Nousiainen and Ryhänen, 1984; Romaschin and Goldberg, 1987). Results of some studies on hepatic enzyme induction are also confounded by other factors affecting blood lipids independent of the induction (e.g., hepatic cirrhosis, inflammation, and/or altered food consumption or diet). Conversely, increased lipid content and/or synthesis in the liver has been fairly consistently reported in studies with various laboratory animals (mostly nonprimate) given phenobarbital or other inducers (de Haan et al., 2009; Ennulat et al., 2010; Je et al., 2015; Moreau et al., 2008). The increase in hepatic lipid content and blood lipid changes—when seen and directly associated—has been largely attributed to the inducing agents that activate certain hepatic nuclear receptors (e.g., PXR, FXR, and/or constitutive androstane receptor [CAR]), which have broad effects on metabolic pathways, including those of lipid metabolism. As an example, PXR induction with CYP3A-inducing agents (e.g., phenobarbital or rifampin) in rats has been closely associated with increased hepatic lipid content and also serum apoA-I and correspondingly, serum HDL cholesterol (Bachmann et al., 2004). This model has been considered representative of the increase in blood HDL cholesterol and apoA-I reported in humans administered antiepileptic CYP3A inducers (Luoma et al., 1988). However, the specific nuclear receptors targeted by hepatic enzyme inducers (or inhibitors) vary considerably between specific agents and animal species, and the associated downstream effects can be different even between individuals with the same signalment (see also Section 21.11). These differences, along with the role of other hepatic and nonhepatic factors in metabolism on blood lipid levels offers explanation for the lack of consistent or prominent changes in serum TG and cholesterol with hepatic microsomal enzyme induction.

Induction or inhibition of hepatic metabolizing enzymes can also affect enzymes critical to endogenous mediators, especially hormones. If this effect is adequate in severity and selectivity, blood lipid changes secondary to the altered mediator can result. A common example is induction of hepatic enzymes that catabolize circulating thyroxine (T4), or inhibit enzymes that convert T4 to T3 in rodents. Prominent effects on these enzymes in rats or mice are associated with a hypothyroid state and corresponding blood lipid alterations (Bookstaff et al., 1996; Gieger et al., 2000). Induction of a hypothyroid state in rats secondary to phenobarbital hepatic enzyme induction is well established. Alterations in testosterone or estrogen with enzyme induction have also been reported and could plausibly have some influence on blood lipid profile (Peakall, 1976).

21.10 PATHOPHYSIOLOGICAL ALTERATIONS IN BLOOD LIPIDS

21.10.1 Secondary Hyperlipidemia

Conditions that cause secondary hyperlipidemia are numerous. Some of the most common and/or well-established conditions, with particularly consistent lipid changes, are attributed to pathology that exacerbates physiologic influences on lipid metabolism (Section 21.8), for example, hypothyroidism, hyperadrenocorticism, diabetes mellitus, and inflammation. Other well-established causes include protein-losing nephropathy, acute pancreatitis, and cholestasis; these conditions are described in other chapters of this text pertaining to the major injured organ. However, due to the overlap in the pattern of altered blood lipids between pathologic conditions and confounding physiologic or pathologic factors (e.g., pregnancy, anorexia), only occasionally are the lipid changes specifically useful for a diagnosis. More often, the known condition can be helpful in explaining the pattern of blood lipid profile seen.

21.10.2 Primary Hyperlipidemia

Primary hyperlipidemia refers to a congenital, inherited, or idiopathic increase in fasting blood lipids that cannot be explained by other, including downstream or indirect, causes. The mechanism for primary conditions is usually due to deficiency or abnormality of an apo or its receptor, an LP transporter or a rate-limiting enzyme in lipid metabolism. Several of these conditions, especially those that are more common or scientifically significant in humans or animal models are described above (Section 21.5). Classically, these conditions are associated with persistent serum/plasma lactescence due to high serum concentration of TG (generally over 200 mg/dL to contribute to plasma turbidity) (Bauer, 1995). However, some primary hyperlipidemias are associated with more significant increases in blood cholesterol (e.g., some defects involving the LDL receptor or *CYP7A1* gene), or hypercholesterolemia without an abnormal TG concentration (e.g., HDL-associated primary hypercholesterolemia in Briard Dogs) (Watson et al., 1993). Not surprisingly, due to the many species differences in lipid metabolism and LP size and content, defects in a correlative apo, receptor, transporter, or enzyme is generally not associated with entirely identical lipid profile changes between species.

Compared with the number of established, spontaneously occurring, primary hyperlipidemias in human, those investigated in animals are relatively few. For most of these primary hyperlipidemias in nonhumans, the specific defect is still unclear; yet, they exhibit some consistent characteristics: occurrence at even a young age, persistence over time while consuming a normal diet, and absence of underlying hormonal or other contributing condition(s). Essentially, all recognized spontaneous primary hyperlipidemias in animals have also been reported only in purebred lines, with similar changes in litter mate(s) or others of the same breed or strain. It should be noted, due to species and analytical differences in measured baseline blood lipid levels, there are no universal cut-off values as to what classifies a significant increase in TGs or cholesterol in these animals. Depending on the lipid moieties affected, the condition can also be asymptomatic, or associated with a wide variety of clinical signs such as cutaneous and other tissue xanthomas (primarily seen in cats with hyperchylomicronemia), eye disorders (e.g., corneal lipid deposition, lipemia retinalis, lipid accumulation in aqueous humor), vomiting, diarrhea, pancreatitis, diabetes mellitus, peripheral neuropathies, seizures, vacuolar hepatopathy, and/or atherosclerosis (Johnstone et al., 1990; Crispin, 1993; Kluger et al., 2010; Watanabe, 1980; Whitney, 1992; Center, 1996; Williams, 2005). Recommended laboratory analysis for the investigation of potential primary lipidemic disorders has been reported (Whitney, 1992).

21.11 IMPORTANT NUCLEAR HORMONE RECEPTORS

21.11.1 Peroxisome Proliferator-Activated Receptor

Peroxisome proliferator-activated receptors are a group of nuclear hormone receptors that regulate lipid metabolism, and other cellular metabolic processes. Of the three PPAR subtypes, alpha (α), gamma (γ), and beta/delta (β/δ), the α subtype is the most relevant to lipid metabolism. PPARα is predominantly expressed in tissues that have a high level of FA catabolism, such as liver, heart, and skeletal muscle (Fruchart, 2009; Reddy and Hashimoto, 2001; Yoon, 2009). During a state of fasting, there is an increased release of NEFAs (the endogenous ligand of PPARα) from adipose tissue; consequently, PPARα induces expression of FA transport/translocase proteins, and increases mitochondrial and peroxisomal β-oxidation of the NEFAs delivered to these tissues (Fruchart, 2009; Reddy and Hashimoto, 2001). Influx of NEFA to the liver is accompanied by their complete catabolism and hepatic gluconeogenesis in response to the lower caloric intake (Reddy and Hashimoto, 2001). Thus, agonism of PPARα promotes lipolysis, lipid catabolism, and decreased hepatic synthesis of lipids and proteins for release to circulation. Accordingly, the agonism of PPARα is generally considered a therapy for dyslipidemia and atherosclerosis, and has been shown to lower blood TG, VLDL, and LDL, and increase circulating HDL.

Lower serum TGs with PPARα agonism is partly through upregulated expression of LPL (hydrolyzing circulating TGs at the tissue level), decreased apoC-III (which delays hepatic TG uptake; Section 21.5), and inhibition of hepatic VLDL synthesis (Yoon, 2009). Decreased serum TGs have been demonstrated in rodents and obese dogs, but only inconsistently in nonhuman primates administered PPARα agonists (Konig et al., 2009; Chen et al., 2008; Pugh et al., 2000).

PPARα agonism also can decrease circulating levels of small, dense LDL (which have lower affinity to the LDL receptor), and increased large, buoyant LDL (which display higher LDL receptor affinity; Sections 21.5 and 21.6) resulting in increased LDL clearance rate overall. PPARα agonists have also been shown to modestly increase HDL cholesterol through stimulating hepatic apoA-I and apoA-II expression (the two most abundant proteins in HDL particles; Section 21.5; Table 21.2) and promoting HDL-mediated cholesterol efflux from macrophages partly via enhanced expression of SR-B1 (Sections 21.5 and 21.6). Notably, PPARα agonism has also been associated with inhibition of CYP7A1 (Section 21.8; Table 21.4), and hence, decreased catabolism of cholesterol in bile and increased risk of gallstone formation in humans (Li and Chiang, 2009).

Species differences in tissue distribution and response to PPARα are significant (Braissant et al., 1996; Mukherjee et al., 1994; Van Veldhoven and Mannaerts, 1999). A number of responses to PPARs in regulated lipid metabolism moieties have been shown to be distinct or even converse between rodents and primates. Most notably, the receptor in rats is especially rich in hepatocytes, where agonism readily induces peroxisome proliferation. However, the primate PPARα expression is the greatest in the skeletal muscle followed by liver, kidney, and adrenal, and pharmacologic agonism shows far less potential for peroxisome proliferation (reviewed in Winegar et al., 2001; Mukherjee et al., 1994). Accordingly, several studies have shown that PPARα inducing agents elicit hepatic peroxisome proliferation, hepatocyte proliferation, hepatomegaly, and liver cancer in rats, while primates are considered resistant to these effects (Chopra et al., 2008; Holden and Tugwood, 1999; Mukherjee et al., 1994).

21.11.2 Liver X Receptor

LXR is a nuclear hormone receptor that is closely related to (and induced by some isoforms of) PPARs and similarly regulates multiple genes involved in lipid metabolism. In particular, LXR plays a pivotal role in controlling excess free cholesterol in the cells by enhancing cholesterol efflux and bile acid synthesis. As such, pharmacologic LXR agonists have been developed as a strategy in the treatment of atherosclerosis, to promote RCT and increase blood HDL cholesterol.

The nuclear hormone receptor has two isoforms, alpha (α) and beta (β), both of which regulate the expression of genes of cholesterol absorption, excretion, catabolism, and cellular efflux. The tissue distribution of these two isoforms differs: LXRα is expressed especially in liver, and predominantly in adipose tissue, intestine, macrophages, spleen, lung, and kidney, whereas LXRβ is an expression, which is essentially ubiquitous among tissues (reviewed in Wójcicka et al., 2007). Endogenous agonists for both isoforms consist of intracellular oxidized cholesterol (oxysterols; e.g., intermediates in cholesterol metabolism and steroid hormone synthesis); oxysterols can accumulate with increasing concentrations of cellular cholesterol (reviewed in Baranowski, 2008; Zhao and Dahlman-Wright, 2010). LXRα has a more significant regulatory role in cholesterol metabolism and RCT than LXRβ (reviewed in Steffensen and Gustafsson, 2004). Some of the genes regulated with LXRα activation include those involved in cholesterol absorption from the intestine, cholesterol biosynthesis, and incorporation of cholesterol in HDL (e.g., apoE) (Zhao and Dahlman-Wright, 2010; Steffensen and Gustafsson, 2004).

In addition to the beneficial role in maintaining cholesterol homeostasis, the agonism of LXR also activates hepatic FA synthesis and a liver-specific secretory protein that inactivates LPL. Thus, LXR activation tends to lead to increased liver and blood (VLDL) TG and PL (Groot et al., 2005). These deleterious effects of LXRα-mediated FA synthesis lead to hepatic steatosis and increased circulating LDL cholesterol. The effect on LDL cholesterol is especially seen in species that express CETP (including primates; Section 21.5) (Groot et al., 2005). An additional important species difference is in LXRα-mediated stimulation of CYP7A1. In rats and mice, LXRα stimulates transcription of CYP7A1, the rate-limiting enzyme in the classic bile acid biosynthetic pathway (Goodwin et al., 2003); thus, LXRα activation enhances the efficiency of cholesterol excretion via conversion to bile acids in these rodents. Conversely, the expression of the human hepatocyte CYP7A1 gene has been shown to be inhibited by LXRα (Goodwin et al., 2003). Further, LXR agonism has also been shown to regulate inflammatory processes through suppressing proinflammatory chemokine gene, and enhancing anti-inflammatory mediator gene induction. This LXR function may be a contributing factor in the link between inflammation and lipid metabolism pathways (Section 21.9).

21.12 NOVEL HORMONES OF LIPID METABOLISM

21.12.1 Leptin

Leptin is a cytokine-like hormone that is linked with lipid metabolism, as well as general energy homeostasis, neuroendocrine function, and immunity. The hormone is released into circulation in proportion to the amount of stored tissue lipid, and acts on the leptin receptors in the brain (principally, the hypothalamus) to regulate food intake and energy expenditure. In animals with normal body weight, leptin is readily transported into the CNS where it inhibits feeding and enhances thermogenesis. However, in obese animals, altered blood/brain concentration of leptin has been associated with the disruption of the feedback loop between hyperleptinemia and appetite, and with hyperglycemia, arterial hypertension, and diabetes mellitus type 1 and type 2. Thus, the replenishment of leptin specifically in the hypothalamus has been proposed as the target therapy for the metabolic syndrome (Kalra, 2011).

Leptin is produced predominantly in white adipose tissue, and to a lesser extent in other organs including the pituitary gland (reviewed in Sone and Osamura, 2001). Leptin activation of receptors in white adipose tissue mediates increased HSL activity resulting in lipolysis in lean (but not obese) animals, and induces adipocyte apoptosis. Leptin appears to have a role in regulating thermogenesis in brown fat as well, although the pathways are still not well defined (Baile et al., 2000; Richard et al., 2010). In the brain, leptin impacts central nervous system regulators that control food intake and energy balance such as neuropeptide Y (NPY), corticotropin-releasing hormone (CRH), proopiomelanocortin (POMC), melanin-concentrating hormone (MCH), and somatostatin (Baile et al., 2000). Overall, leptin appears to play a key role in the maintenance of serum TG. Several prominent animal models of hypertriglyceridemia are due to the defects in leptin signaling including the leptin deficient (ob) and leptin-receptor mutant (db) mouse, and the leptin receptor mutant Zucker rat.

Leptin concentrations in blood have diurnal variability that is impacted by body weight and gender (Baile et al., 2000). Circulating leptin levels are also affected by food intake with increases in postprandial levels of leptin that gradually decline hours after a meal. Fasting causes a proportionately greater decline in leptin levels in lean, compared with obese animals (Baile et al., 2000; Radin et al., 2009). Importantly, blood leptin concentrations do not directly reflect (and can be inversely) correlated with the hypothalamic concentrations, with the latter being the more significant regulator of food intake and energy homeostasis.

21.12.2 Ghrelin

Ghrelin is a signaling peptide that has a role in feeding behavior, energy expenditure, and obesity. Ghrelin blood levels have been shown to increase before meals and decrease after meals and is accordingly, believed to stimulate hunger. Ghrelin actions are also similar to (and may have evolved from the same peptide precursor as) motilin in inducing gastric acid secretion and gastric motility (reviewed in Asakawa et al., 2001; reviewed in Yin et al., 2009). Ghrelin effects in decreasing energy expenditure may be linked with an influence on GH and insulin secretion, adipocyte response to insulin and thermogenesis (Kojima et al., 1999; St-Pierre et al., 2004).

Ghrelin is primarily secreted by specialized cells in the gastric fundic mucosa and pancreas in response to a reduction in gastrointestinal contents, and its receptor is GH secretagogue receptor found in a variety of tissues including hypothalamus, pancreas, intestine, and adipose tissue (Kojima et al., 1999; reviewed in Yin et al., 2009). The transcriptional, translational, and post-translational modifications of the ghrelin gene are complex, with dissociated gene and protein expression, and with related hormones (including acyl ghrelin, des-acyl ghrelin, and obestatin) of differing activity also being released into the circulation (Ghelardoni et al., 2006; Yin et al., 2009). The amino acid sequence of ghrelin is well conserved across species, but the sequence and the number of these related hormones and secreting cell morphology is more variable among animals (Kojima et al., 1999; reviewed in Yin et al., 2009). In general, ghrelin and/or acyl ghrelin levels increase in blood with long-term fasting and insulin-induced hypoglycemia, and at night versus daylight hours. In humans and mice, levels of ghrelin (and/or acyl ghrelin) are higher in females compared with males, and decrease with age in both sexes (reviewed in Yin et al., 2009). In mice, the decrease with age is specific to acyl ghrelin and occurs after weaning is initiated. In humans, there is an inverse correlation between circulating ghrelin and body mass index (reviewed in Yin et al., 2009).

Ghrelin decreases have been proposed to be linked with increases in glycogen synthesis and tissue carbohydrate stores, and may result in decreased appetite stimulation. Blood glucose levels can impact ghrelin, with glucose infusions acutely decreasing circulating forms of ghrelin concentration in humans and rats (McCowen et al., 2002; Hotta et al., 2004). Less pronounced ghrelin decreases are also seen with increases in circulating long-chain NEFA (reviewed in Yin et al., 2009). Ghrelin also decreases with exercise training that may be linked with increased muscle glycogen stores; after 6 weeks of treadmill training in rats, there were decreases in ghrelin levels in plasma (Ghanbari-Niaki et al., 2009). In obesity, leptin and ghrelin have a negative correlation, with leptin generally accepted as an inhibitor of ghrelin synthesis, possibly through the ghrelin receptor in the stomach (reviewed in Yin et al., 2009). Notably, the physiology of ghrelin is not fully understood within, and across animal species at this time, complicating interpretation of blood levels.

21.12.3 Adiponectin

Adiponectin is a hormone produced by mature adipocytes, and its gene has been reported to be one of the most highly expressed in white adipose tissue (reviewed in Radin et al., 2009). It was discovered in mice and human adipose tissue in the same year by several laboratories and hence initially given various monikers (apM1, Acrp30, GBP28 and AdipoQ) (Scherer et al., 1995). Adiponectin is now considered an important mediator of lipid metabolism, involved in regulating both glucose levels and lipolysis and linking insulin resistance with obesity.

Adiponectin is induced by insulin and promotes insulin sensitivity and adipocyte differentiation. In humans, with insulin resistance, adiponectin plasma concentration shows a negative relationship with serum TGs and obesity and inverse relationship with fasting (Merl et al., 2005; Scherer et al., 1995; Vendrell et al., 2004; Weyer et al., 2001). In horses, dogs, cats, and rats, there is a similar inverse correlation between adiponectin levels and obesity, adiposity, and/or fat mass (Radin et al., 2009). However, the level of circulating adiponectin appears to be most closely related to the extent of insulin resistance rather than of adiposity or glucose intolerance (Weyer et al., 2001). Unlike ghrelin and leptin, adiponectin appears to have a random secretion pattern, unaltered by time of day or feeding (Yildiz et al., 2004).

Exercise may also have an effect on adiponectin levels; intermittent, repeated moderate aerobic exercise resulted in a rapid two- to threefold increase in circulating adiponectin in rats and men (Kriketos et al., 2004; Zeng et al., 2007). In one study of overweight men, multiple sessions of moderately intense aerobic exercise resulted in a 260% increase in circulating adiponectin levels within a week of baseline that remained elevated after 10 weeks of exercise (Kriketos et al., 2004). Authors of this study proposed that it may take repeated exercise to induce exercise-related changes in plasma adiponectin. However, while repeated intense exercise increased tissue mRNA adiponectin, no change in serum adiponectin was detected in rats (Zeng et al., 2007). Similarly, no change in the blood levels of adiponectin were detected in horses following repeated intense exercise (Gordon et al., 2007). Thus, the interpretation of blood adiponectin levels should be approached with understanding of these complexities and potential species distinctions.

21.12.4 Neuropeptide Y

Neuropeptide Y (NPY) is a neuromodulator produced in the hypothalamic arcuate nucleus (Malva et al., 2012). This neurotransmitter is considered to be one of the most orexigenic (appetite stimulating) peptides to play a role in the control of food intake and regulation of energy balance (Higuchi, 2012; Edelsbrunner et al., 2009). It signals through several NPY receptors, such as Y1 and Y5 in the paraventricular nucleus. A role in energy balance has been demonstrated in $NPY^{-/-}$ mice with decreased locomotion and exploratory behavior compared to wild-type mice. An associated decrease in food and water intake was evident in NPY and peptide YY (PYY short peptide with postprandial release by mucosal cells in the gastrointestinal tract that acts as an appetite suppressant in species including rats, nonhuman primates, and humans) double knockout mice (most consistently in females) compared to wild-type mice, but generally not in NPY or PYY knockouts alone. Consistent with the asynchronous effects in activity and feeding behavior, the knockouts (NPY and double NPY/PYY) were generally heavier than the wild-type mice (Edelsbrunner et al., 2009). Leptin deficient Lep^{ob}/Lep^{ob} mice exhibit a definitive role for NPY in stimulating food intake. NPY is normally overproduced in Lep^{ob}/Lep^{ob} mice, but Lep^{ob}/Lep^{ob} mice that are also deficient in NPY are less obese than Lep^{ob}/Lep^{ob} mice due to increased activity and decreased feed intake (Erickson et al., 1996). Systemic administration of leptin inhibits *NPY* gene expression and synthesis resulting in suppressed feed intake and decreased body weight in normal and *Lep^ob/Lep^ob* mice, but not *Lepr^db/Lepr^db* mice that lack a functional leptin receptor (Stephens et al., 1995).

21.12.5 Sterol Regulatory Element-Binding Protein

SREBPs (isoforms 1a, 1c, and 2) are transcription factors, which globally regulate intracellular levels of cholesterol, FAs, TGs, and PLs. The SREBP isoforms 1a and 1c are produced from a single gene (*SREBF1*) via alternate promoters, and isoform 2 is produced from a distinct gene (*SREBF2*) (Yokoyama et al., 1993). Essentially all cells produce one or more of these isoforms. The SREBP-1c isoform is expressed in especially high levels in liver, white adipose tissue, adrenal gland, and brain and skeletal muscles in adult animals (Shimomura et al., 1997).

These SREBP isoforms are inactive and bound to ER when cholesterol and FAs are available to the cell. However, when the cell is faced with low levels of cholesterol and/or FAs, the active NH_2-terminal fragments are released (via a number of steps: disassociation of Insig-1 (insulin-induced gene-1) protein from SCAP (SREBP cleavage activating protein), transport to the Golgi apparatus, and cleavage by proteases), allowing them to translocate to the nucleus (Ye and Debose-Boy, 2011). Translocation to the nucleus induces genes involved in synthesis and cellular uptake of lipids.

The three SREBP isoforms have differing efficiencies in FA and cholesterol lipid synthesis. Based on knockout mouse studies, SREBP 1c appears to primarily regulate FA- (and hepatic glucose-) synthesis-related genes, whereas the 1a isoform is involved in both FA and cholesterol synthesis, and SREBP-2 is more specific to cholesterol synthesis (Shimomura et al., 1997). Regulation of these transcription factors is controlled at the level of transcription, proteolytic cleavage of SREBP precursors, and posttranslational modification of nSREBPs, and varies between isoforms. Transcriptional regulation of liver SREBP-1c is a key for its role in lipid synthesis and can be induced by (1) feeding a high carbohydrate diet after a period of fasting (likely involving insulin signaling), (2) activation of LXR alpha, or (3) possibly through self-activation of the promoter of its own sterol response element (SRE) (Eberle et al., 2004). Activation of the promoter of its own SRE may also be involved in regulation of SREBP-2 (Schiavoni et al., 2010). Sterol-dependent regulation controls transport from the ER to the Golgi, where proteolytic cleavage occurs (Shao and Espenshade, 2012). The unique activity and regulation of each SREBP isoform is consistent with differences in isoform-related target gene specificity, and exemplifies the broad role of SREBP in lipid metabolism and homeostasis.

21.13 ANIMAL MODELS OF ALTERED LIPID METABOLISM

The number of animal models of altered lipid metabolism is vast and growing, perhaps because of the increasing recognition of lipid disorders in the most common of human diseases. The ideal animal model, with a lipid profile and response to challenge similar to that of humans does not exist. The relevance to humans of each animal model is often limited to specific lipid components or pathways. Thus, interpretation of data from these models for extrapolation to humans should always be couched with consideration of species/model differences in lipid metabolism. In addition, for a majority of these models, the age and sex reference ranges, and/or intra-study blood lipid values are not available, limiting constructive statements on general clinical pathology data interpretation. Thus, this section will discuss only some of the commonly used general models of dyslipidemia but will not focus on specific models of atherosclerosis or selective transgenic or knockout rodent strains that model specific lipid disorders.

Important factors to consider in selecting an acceptable model for study are the animal's predominant types of circulating LPs, hepatic predominance in cholesterol synthesis, and capacity for biliary excretion (Section 21.8), and the presence or absence of CETP and hepatic apoB48 production (Sections 21.4 and 21.5). Humans have a predominance of LDL cholesterol, as do a few common laboratory species including guinea pig, domestic pig, and some nonhuman primates (e.g., African green monkeys and macaques). Hamsters and rabbits have a predominance of HDL cholesterol in blood with a standard diet but convert to a predominance of circulating LDL cholesterol when exposed to a high fat diet. Hamsters and rabbits also tend to have a level of cholesterol synthesis in the liver relative to whole body cholesterol synthesis that is more similar to humans compared to that of rats or mice. Several other species, including dog, cat, horse, ruminants, rat, and mouse have predominantly HDL cholesterol and resist dietary cholesterol challenge (in contrast to humans). Laboratory species also significantly vary CETP activity (Table 21.1, Section 21.5, and Table 21.4) with rabbits, opossums, and trout having high levels, while rats, mice, dogs, cats, pigs, and sheep show little to no detectable CETP activity. Humans have an intermediate level of CETP activity (similar to guinea pigs, chickens, toads, and some reptile species). With low CETP activity, CEs are not readily transferred from HDL to other LPs, resulting in HDL being cholesterol-rich and less dense. In general, species with low CETP activity have high blood HDL cholesterol levels, and HDL/LDL ratio.

21.13.1 Leptin Receptor Mutant Mouse

The *db* mutation, one of the 14 known spontaneous mutations in the mouse leptin receptor (*Lepr*), is characterized by high plasma TGs and cholesterol, making it a good model of diabetic dyslipidemia (Kobayashi et al., 2000). The mouse becomes obese by 6 weeks of age with correlative increases in glucose, insulin, TGs, and cholesterol. The cholesterol levels are not only mainly due to relatively higher HDL cholesterol but also non-HDL cholesterol in the IDL/LDL cholesterol range. The non-HDL cholesterol proportion increased significantly with feeding of a high-fat or "Western" diet with 0.15% (wt/wt) cholesterol and 21% (wt/wt) fat. LPL in plasma and LPL mRNA expression in heart, muscle, and adipose tissue were substantially decreased in the db/db mice.

21.13.2 Fat-Fed Syrian Hamster

The fat-fed Syrian hamster [e.g., Crl:LVG(SYR)] has been compared to the fat-fed gerbils and guinea pigs and considered a good model to study hypertriglyceridemia since the serum concentrations of TGs will remain elevated with a high-fat, high-cholesterol diet (Sullivan et al., 1993). Several studies have used hamsters as an animal model for humans because they are touted as having similar levels of plasma LDL cholesterol, rates of sterol synthesis in the liver, and LP metabolism (Wang et al., 2001; Ohtani et al., 1990). This is partly due to the presence of CE-transfer protein (CETP) in hamsters but not in mice and rats (Groot et al., 2005).

21.13.3 Zucker Rat

The genetically obese Zucker rat, named after its founders, has a homozygous recessive mutation (*fa* for fatty) of the leptin receptor gene (*Lepr*) (Zucker and Zucker, 1963). This model is characterized by hyperphagia, hyperinsulinemia, insulin resistance, and juvenile onset obesity with hyperlipidemia due to elevated serum TGs (as early as 2 weeks of age) and cholesterol (Godbole et al., 1978; Boulange et al., 1981).

The plasma of these animals is milky in appearance, with TG that can be several-fold greater than that in the blood of non-homozygous lean Zucker rats (Aleixandre de Artiñano and Miguel Castro, 2009). The increased circulating TG is principally due to the accumulation of VLDL attributed to exaggerated hepatic synthesis and secretion of TG-rich LPs. Increases in the blood cholesterol also reflect the increases in VLDL and also HDL but not LDL. The clearance of TG-rich particles in these homozygous (fa/fa) animals is not consistently different from that of the lean counterparts; however, differential clearance between tissues may help predict distribution of adiposity in that LPL levels have been reported to be increased in white adipose, and normal to decreased in brown adipose and heart tissue in the rat (Horwitz et al., 1984; Wang et al., 1984).

21.13.4 Rabbits

Rabbits have been widely used as models of hypercholesterolemia and atherosclerosis. The well-characterized models are the homozygous and cholesterol-fed heterozygous Watanabe heritable hyperlipidemic rabbit (WHHL rabbit) (Aliev and Burnstock, 1998; Atkinson et al., 1989; Buja et al., 1990; Havel et al., 1989; Shiomi et al., 2000; Tanaka et al., 1995; Zhang et al., 2009). The WHHL rabbits have an in-frame deletion in the ligand-binding domain of the LDL receptors, which prevents LDL uptake and results in high serum cholesterol levels and spontaneous development of aortic atherosclerosis (Yamamoto et al., 1986; Li et al., 1995). Chow-fed WHHL rabbits had plasma cholesterol levels at 4 months of age of 260 ± 100 mg/dL, and at 15 months of 545 ± 178 mg/dL (Nolte et al., 1990). However, due to low availability of WHHL rabbits, many researchers have moved to more accessible rabbit strains such as New Zealand white rabbits and cholesterol-feeding regimens. Dutch belted rabbits provide an alternative strain for use in hypercholesterolemic modeling (Kritchevsky et al., 1971).

21.13.5 Minipigs

Minipigs have been promoted for lipid metabolism research due to ready availability and similarity with humans in having LDL as the dominant blood cholesterol carrier. Pigs, including minipigs, can also develop atherosclerosis even on a typical swine diet (Skold et al., 1966). The progression of these vascular lesions, from fatty streaks to fibrous plaques to more advanced atherosclerotic lesions is similar to humans and the severity and extent increase with age, and hypercholesterolemic diet as in human. Minipigs fed a low-cholesterol diet have plasma LPs that resemble humans in the relative levels of VLDL, LDL, and HDL (Mahley et al., 1975).

Several strains of minipig have been developed but the most well-characterized strains for lipid research are the Gottingen and Yucatan strains. The Göttingen minipig has been used as a model of postprandial hyperlidemia and metabolic syndrome (Olsen et al., 2002; Johansen et al., 2001). The Yucatan minipig has been utilized as a model of hypercholesterolemia and diabetic dyslipidemia (Sodha et al., 2008; Boullion et al., 2003). Other strains of minipig (Chinese Guizhou minipigs) have been utilized to evaluate diet-induced diabetes and atherosclerosis (Liu et al., 2007).

21.13.6 Cynomolgus Monkeys

The cynomolgus monkey (*Macaca fascicularis*) is a relatively good model for evaluation of hyperlipidemia because of similarities to humans in response to dietary lipid excess, and a susceptibility to type 2 diabetes mellitus, and naturally occurring (as well as experimentally induced) atherosclerosis. The atherosclerotic changes associated with high cholesterol also show gender-related differences as in humans (Weingand, 1989) (also see Section 21.9). The relatively low basal cholesterol synthesis in the liver of the cynomolgus monkey, which also limits capacity for hepatic bile synthesis, is similar to human and in contrast with rats and mice (Turley et al., 1995).

With cholesterol feeding of cynomolgus monkeys, hypercholesterolemia (and associated LDL cholesterol increases) occurs generally in proportion to the degree of dietary challenge (Marzetta and Rudel 1986; Rudel et al., 1986; Turley et al., 1995). However, the blood cholesterol increase is partly associated with an increase in LDL particle size in direct contrast with the pro-atherosclerotic small dense LDL profile of human (Bullock et al., 1975; Rudel et al., 1986). Cynomolgus monkeys also have a blood lipid composition that is generally similar to humans in health; however, relative concentrations of individual molecular lipid components differs (Shui et al., 2011).

21.13.7 African Green Monkeys

African Green Monkeys (*Cercopithecus aethiops*) have been proposed to be a relevant model of atherosclerosis, in part because they develop atherosclerotic lesions that follow a similar pathogenic course as in humans (Rudel et al., 1985). They also show lesser tendency than cynomolgus monkeys for LDL particle size increase with cholesterol feeding (i.e., LDL composition more comparable to higher risk of atherosclerosis in humans) (Rudel et al., 1985). However, African green monkeys are resistant to developing an atherosclerotic lipid profile with cholesterol feeding, and have an HDL-dominant blood lipid profile in health (Thomas and Rudel, 1996; Rudel et al., 1990).

Several other nonhuman primate species have also shown selective utility as animal models of lipid research and/or diet induced-atherosclerosis. This includes other species of macaques, such as pigtail macaques and obese Rhesus macaques (*Macaca nemestrina* and *Macaca mulatta*, respectively), patas monkeys (*Erythrocebus patas*), baboons (*Papio species*), Bornean orangutan (*Pongo pygmaeus*), and gorillas species (Kritchevsky et al., 1974; Rudel et al., 1985; Schmidt et al., 2006; Thomas and Rudel, 1996). Importantly, the composition of circulating LPs, LDL particle size, and HDL cholesterol concentration, as well as the extent of hyperlipoproteinemia in response to dietary cholesterol feeding is unique to each of these species.

21.14 LABORATORY ANALYSES OF BLOOD LIPIDS AND LIPOPROTEINS

21.14.1 Lipid Analysis

Samples for the analysis of blood lipids (TGs, cholesterol, NEFAs, or PLs) can be serum or plasma. For plasma, the preferred anticoagulant is disodium ethylenediaminetetraacetic acid (EDTA) or heparin. Lipid concentrations can be minimally (about 2%–5%) lower in EDTA plasma than corresponding serum (due to osmotic shift of water from cells to EDTA plasma) (Folsom et al., 1983). Samples are generally stable for up to 72 hours at 4°C, or frozen at ≤–20°C. Fasting, if indicated, should be for an appropriate time period for the animal to avoid blood lipid changes associated with physiologic lipolysis (Section 21.9).

Routine laboratory analysis of TGs and total cholesterol is conducted with enzymatic assays on an automated analyzer and requiring few microliters of sample. Most of the current commercial assays are useful for the analysis of the samples of any species. Chemical assays that differentiate between HDL and LDL cholesterol generally involve added reaction steps to precipitate or mask by inhibiting reactivity, or initial disruption of the nontarget LPs. Analysis of NEFA or PL concentrations is less routine but readily achieved with automated chemical assays. More specialized methods for some of these analyses are also briefly mentioned below.

21.14.1.1 Total Serum/Plasma TGs by Automated Chemical Analysis

TGs are measured with a two-step procedure initiated by lipase release of FAs from glycerol, which is subsequently quantified by oxidase-mediated production of hydrogen peroxide and peroxidase-linked colorimetric reaction:

1. Triglycerides + $3H_2O \xrightarrow[\text{Lipase}]{}$ glycerol and fatty acids
2. Glycerol + ATP $\xrightarrow[\text{glycerol kinase}]{}$ glycerol-3-phosphate + adenosine diphosphate (ADP)
3. Glycerol-3-phosphate + $O_2 \xrightarrow[\text{glycerol-3-phosphate oxidase}]{} 2H_2O_2$ + dihydroxyacetone phosphate
4. 2 H_2O_2 + 4-aminophenazone + 4-chlorophenol $\xrightarrow[\text{peroxidase}]{}$ quinoemine dye + $4H_2O$ + HCl

This method also measures other (mono- and di-)acylglycerides and free glycerol in serum samples; analytes that generally comprise ≤10% of the detected total TGs in healthy laboratory animals. Glycerol blanking to correct for free glycerol is a consideration, however, in animals with pathologic conditions associated with high peripheral lipolysis such as starvation, diabetes mellitus, high carbohydrate diet or catecholamine excess, or administration of mixed lipid preparations (Chatzipanteli et al., 1996; Ciraolo et al., 1995; Jessen et al., 1990).

Because the mg/dL unit is based on weight, and TGs are highly heterogenous in molecular weight due to variability in FA content, reporting in millimoles per liter (mmol/L; SI units) is the more precise unit measure (e.g., for investigative comparative assay/study purposes). If conversion is necessary for estimated value comparisons, mg/dL can be multiplied by 0.01129 (http://www.soc-bdr.org/rds/authors/unit_tables_conversions_and_genetic_dictionaries/e5196/index_en.html).

21.14.1.2 Total Serum/Plasma Cholesterol

For total cholesterol quantitation, cholesterol esterases are used to break the ester bond and release free cholesterol from LPs; this is followed by an oxidase step that generates hydrogen peroxide that together with a chromagen substrate and peroxidase generates a colorimetric reaction:

1. Cholesterol ester + $H_2O \xrightarrow[\text{cholesterol esterase}]{}$ cholesterol + FAs
2. Cholesterol + $O_2 \xrightarrow[\text{cholesterol oxidase}]{}$ cholestenone + H_2O_2
3. H_2O_2 + 4-aminophenazone + phenol + 4-aminoantipyrine $\xrightarrow[\text{peroxidase cholesterol oxidase}]{}$ quinoneimine dye + $2H_2O$

21.14.1.3 HDL and LDL Cholesterol

Commercial assays to measure HDL or LDL cholesterol on automated platforms utilize the same cholesterol esterase–cholesterol oxidase steps for analysis of total cholesterol, after first removing (by precipitation or disruption) or masking the nontargeted cholesterol containing LPs. The accuracy of the specific assay type, however, varies considerably between species and in cases of extremes in TG, cholesterol, or apo abnormalities. Thus, due to the numerous kits available and manufacturer changes made in components, validation with appropriate species samples to determine specific assay suitability is recommended. Notably, all HDL and LDL cholesterol commercial assays are calibrated with human standards, so that species differences from humans in LP content are an inevitable source of inaccuracy. Methods utilizing antibodies to immunoinhibit reactivity, or immunoprecipitate select LPs, are also not recommended for nonhuman samples if extent of cross-reactivity is unknown.

21.14.1.3.1 HDL Cholesterol

The precipitation-based method has long been utilized for HDL cholesterol analysis (Arranz-Pena et al., 1998; Tailleux and Staels, 2011). The method uses polyanions combined with divalent cations to aggregate particles with lower density than HDL cholesterol, while HDL cholesterol remains in solution (Warnick et al., 2001). The polyanions are complex carbohydrates (such as heparin, dextran sulfate or polyvinyl sulfate, and phosphotungstate Mg^{2+}) that complex with apoB-100 and apoB-48 under pH conditions that ensure these apos are positively charged. The interactions between the anionic sulfated glycans and cationic (arginine and lysine) amino acids of apoBs are believed to be primarily electrostatic. Notably, due to broad LP heterogeneity and despite assay improvements over time, precipitation methods remain somewhat imprecise.

Assay improvements have also led to homogeneous methods, for HDL cholesterol analysis without need for the added separation step of precipitation. One method (Kyowa assay) masks other LPs by the use of sulfated α-cyclodextrin and polyanion (dextran sulfate) with polyethylene glycol (PEG)-modified cholesterol esterase and cholesterol oxidase (Sugiuchi et al., 1995). The sulfated α-cyclodextrin reduces the reactivity of cholesterol in chylomicrons and VLDLs, without the need for precipitation. The modified enzymes show selective catalytic activities with increasing reactivity toward HDL over LDL and VLDL. This method may be especially appropriate for rat and rabbit samples (based on comparison of results with density ultracentrifugation (unpublished data). Another method uses a LP-selective reagent to release non-HDL cholesterol from apoB-particles, then catalyzes the esterase-oxidase reaction, and inhibits the resulting peroxidase prior to release cholesterol from HDL-particles by detergent. This method may be more accurate for mouse, hamster, cynomolgus monkey, and dog than the blocking method mentioned previously (unpublished data).

21.14.1.3.2 LDL Cholesterol

Evaluation of LDL cholesterol in nonhuman species can be even more challenging than that for HDL cholesterol, in that the specific lipid content of heterogenous LDL particles tends to overlap with a greater variety of LPs than HDL; that is LDL lipid content variably overlaps with HDL, VLDL, and IDL in all species. The extent of this overlap varies between species and lipid-altering conditions. In particular, LDL cholesterol assays do not distinguish between LDL, and IDL (and in primates, also Lp(a)) cholesterol. Thus, values obtained with all LDL cholesterol assays with laboratory animal samples are only estimations of true LDL cholesterol.

As with HDL cholesterol assays, the LDL cholesterol precipitation methods are being replaced by homogenous assays. The homogeneous assays use a variety of detergents and other chemicals to specifically block or solubilize LPs other than LDL, enabling LDL cholesterol to then be measured enzymatically. One homogeneous direct enzymatic methodology involves reducing the enzymatic reaction of the cholesterol measurement in VLDL and chylomicrons in the presence of magnesium. This, in combination with detergent, enables the determination of LDL cholesterol via selective micelle solubilization.

21.14.1.3.3 LDL Cholesterol by the Friedwald Formula

The Friedwald calculation is based on human blood lipid components, and the assumption that VLDLs carry the majority of serum TGs (in samples from a fasted animal). Therefore, the total TG concentration can be used to estimate VLDL cholesterol. This requires values for serum TG, total, and HDL cholesterol to estimate LDL cholesterol (Friedewald et al., 1972):

$$\text{LDL cholesterol} = \text{total serum cholesterol} - (\text{measured HDL cholesterol} + \text{estimated VLDL cholesterol})$$

With this calculation, human VLDL cholesterol is estimated as total serum TG divided by 5, a value that does not apply to nonhuman samples. However, because total serum VLDL cholesterol is proportionately minor compared to HDL and LDL cholesterol in many domestic species, the Friedwald formula without the VLDL cholesterol estimation has been commonly applied to samples from laboratory animals. Regardless, it should be emphasized that there are significant discrepancies in the calculated value compared with specific LDL cholesterol assay results with nonhuman serum samples. Further, the Friedwald formula is also not suitable for samples containing chylomicrons (which are present in health for some species and certain disease conditions even with fasting). For these reasons, in combination with the availability and ease of more direct chemical LDL cholesterol assays, the calculated value is not recommended for nonhuman samples.

21.14.1.4 Nonesterified Fatty Acids

In contrast to TG and cholesterol, NEFAs are transported in the blood bound to albumin rather than as a component of LPs. Low concentrations are found in the blood of healthy animals; increased concentrations most commonly indicate enhanced lipolysis. Serum or EDTA plasma NEFAs can be readily measured by automated chemical methods (as well as high-performance liquid chromatography [HPLC] and gas chromatography). Sample collection in heparin should be avoided to prevent increasing NEFA (and decreasing TG) values over time with endogenous LPL activation. Serum-separator tubes (SSTs) are also not ideal, because values have been reported to be artificially increased. With all collection methods, care must be taken to prevent release of FAs as the result of TG hydrolysis after specimen collections; preferably, samples are rapidly separated from cells and transferred to ice or refrigerated at 4°C. Specimens may also be mixed with paraoxon, a cholinesterase inhibitor, immediately after collection. NEFA concentrations in serum or plasma samples are generally stable at 4°C for up to 48 hours or frozen for up to 1 month but tend to increase over time, and especially when stored for even a few hours at room temperature (author experience; Menéndez et al., 2001).

Chemical (enzymatic) methods are simple (though somewhat less sensitive and do not provide information about the FA forms compared with research techniques mentioned). These assays are based on NEFAs forming acyl-CoA in the presence of acyl-CoA synthetase (and co-substrates);

generated Acyl CoA is enzymatically oxidized to produce hydrogen peroxide to form the final chromagen for spectrophotometric detection. With all of these methods, it is better to avoid samples with hemolysis or those collected immediately postprandial.

21.14.1.5 Phospholipids

PLs occur in blood in greater concentration than any other major lipid structural type; yet, their analysis is nonroutine. This may be largely due to the limited value of a single serum PL measurement because of broad and dynamic distribution of PLs in blood and among LPs even within an individual in health. This variability can confound interpretation of differences between intervals or groups. Broad species differences in circulating PLs are also well established (Diagne et al., 1984). Quantitation of total circulating (or LP fractions of) PLs, however, is sometimes conducted as an index of hepatobiliary disorders, nutritional status, dyslipoproteinemias, or in mediums other than blood (e.g., bile).

Quantification of total PLs can be achieved with automated direct, one-step chemical assays, in which PLs (and sphingomyelin) are hydrolyzed by phospholipase to phosphatidic acid and free choline. In the presence of choline oxidase and peroxidase, the free choline is then estimated colorimetrically. Analysis of specific PL forms (e.g., any of the major PLs in circulation: phosphotidylcholine [PL-C or lecithin], lysolysolecithin, or phosphatidyl ethanolamine) may be conducted by commercial chemical enzymatic assays or several research methods, including thin layer or gel chromatography, HPLC, and HPLC–mass spectrometry (MS) (Phillips, 1959; Subbaiah, 2000).

21.14.1.6 Sphingolipids

SLs, and specifically sphingomyelin, occur as a significant proportion of blood lipids. Analysis of serum/plasma sphingomyelin has been utilized to assess genetic dyslipoproteinemias and recently, to assess risk of atherosclerosis in humans and animal models with hyperlipidemia (Hidaka et al., 2008). Enzymatic assays for sphingomyelin are commercially available. These utilize sphingomyelinase to hydrolyze sphingomyelin to PL-C and ceramide. Subsequent steps are similar to those described earlier for PL quantitation. Additional (research) methods for broad SL analysis in blood and other fluids have been described in the published literature (Abnet et al., 2001).

21.14.2 Lipoprotein Analysis

21.14.2.1 Density-Gradient Ultracentrifugation

The gold standard for evaluation of LP levels, including the different major classes of serum LPs, is ultracentrifugation. The principal of ultracentrifugation is to separate LPs based on their hydrated density. Ultracentrifugation can also determine the predominant particle size distribution but does not provide concentrations of the LP particles themselves. Samples should be fresh or short-term refrigerated, thoroughly mixed plasma from EDTA-anticoagulated blood. Some assay methods also require smaller sample volumes that may enable in-life testing of small laboratory species. Common assay methodology has been described (Subbaiah, 2000).

However, ultracentrifugation is technically complex, and labor- and time-intensive and, except for utility as a research method and to validate new methods (e.g., HDL and LDL automated assays), is not practical for routine laboratory application. Due to broad differences in equipment, methodology, and conditions (such as salt concentrations and centrifugal forces) between laboratories, complete reproducibility between experiments is also difficult to achieve (Warnick et al., 2001; Wilcox and Heimberg, 1970). Thus, despite use as a gold standard, there are no standardized ultracentrifugation protocols, reference materials, or thresholds for subparticle distributions. Due to species differences in the specific composition of the different LP types, the density fractions collected are also highly variable between species, and can be difficult to interpret (especially if there are abnormal patterns) (Camus et al., 1983; Cole et al., 1984; Goulinet and Chapman, 1993; Hollanders et al., 1986; Lasser et al., 1973). In summary, although ultracentrifugation is useful as a research method, it is particularly technique-dependent and fairly subjective in results interpretation.

21.14.2.2 Gradient Gel Electrophoresis and Chromatography

Polyacrylamide or agarose gel electrophoresis, high-performance liquid chromatography (HPLC), fast-performance liquid chromatography (FPLC), and size exclusion or ion exchange chromatography are other methods used for analysis of plasma LPs. These methods base distinction between LP types on charge and/or particle size. The simplest and longest standing of these, electrophoresis, has given rise to the alternative common names of the LPs in association with their electrophoretic mobility: *a* (HDL), pre-β-VLDLs and β-LDLs. Compared with ultracentrifugation, they are more equipment-intensive but less laborious, and offer the advantage of being able to "observe" the extent of heterogeneity within LP types and significant atypical LPs. Electrophoresis may also be used to test suitability of other LP analytical methods, and to analyze fractions separated initially by ultracentrifugation. However, as with ultracentrifugation, particle separation with these methods is partly subjective and technique-variable. Methods have also had issues with equipment reliability and lot-to-lot reagent (e.g., gel) differences (author experience; Subbaiah, 2000). Not surprisingly, because the composition of LP types varies between species, the location and width of the corresponding LP bands also widely varies between species. Description of select electrophoresis methodology for lipid analysis with nonhuman samples has been published (Lehmann et al., 1993).

21.14.2.3 Nuclear Magnetic Resonance Spectroscopy and Ion-Mobility Analysis

Additional methods for LP analysis include nuclear magnetic resonance spectroscopy (NMR) and ion-mobility analysis. NMR enables quantification of VLDL, IDL, LDL, and HDL and their subfractions by both average particle concentration and size. Lipoprotein concentrations are derived from the amplitudes of their lipid methyl group signal, and particle sizes are derived from the summed diameter of each subclass multiplied by its relative mass percentage (also based on the amplitude of its methyl NMR signal).

Ion-mobility analysis measures both the size and concentrations of LP particle subclasses based on gas-phase differential electric mobility. These methods have valuable utility with LP analysis but require specialized equipment and expertise, and reported experience with nonhuman species have not been well investigated to date.

21.15 LABORATORY ANALYSIS OF KETONES AND SELECT MEDIATORS OF LIPID METABOLISM

21.15.1 Ketones

Increased blood ketone levels indicate a metabolism shift (Section 21.7) that could be a result of physiologically altered energy demands (e.g., fasting, and prolonged exercise), a high fat diet, disease (insulin deficiency or resistance, juvenile hypoglycemia), or toxicity (e.g., resulting hypoglycemia with salicylate administration). Of the three major ketone bodies produced (acetoacetate, β-OHB, and acetone), blood levels of β-OHB (the conversion product of acetoacetate) are considered the best indicator of significant ketosis or ketoacidosis (Laffel, 1999). Indeed, as ketosis progresses, the ratio between β-OHB and acetoacetate increases, with β-OHB being the predominant ketone body contributing to ketoacidosis (Bell et al., 2005). As the acidosis (i.e., ketosis or ketoacidosis) resolves with treatment, the β-OHB is oxidized to acetoacetate and the β-OHB:acetoacetate ratio returns toward 1:1. The other major ketone, acetone, is not metabolized for energy, does not contribute to acidosis and has little diagnostic utility (Laffel, 1999).

Ketone bodies can be analyzed by chemical (automated and manual) methods in serum, plasma (with EDTA, heparin, or citrate anticoagulant), whole blood, or urine. Assays for β-OHB first convert the ketone body to acetoacetate via 3-β-OHB dehydrogenase, which concomitantly reduces cofactor nicotinamide adenine dinucleotide (NAD). With spectrophotometric methods, the reduced NAD (NADH) and diaphorase enzyme convert a colorimetric detector to a colored product. Whole blood (point-of-care instrument) assays for β-OHB are based on the change in the electrochemical state mediated by NAD+/NADH and a redox mediator (Henderson and Schlesinger, 2010). Assays for acetoacetate (spectrophotometric) rely on the reverse reaction, oxidizing NADH; therefore, the chromogen is inversely related to the analyte concentration. Assays for determination of both of these ketone bodies ("total ketones") are also available. High concentrations of vitamin C or B (more common with urine) can interfere with the accuracy of the assays (Vianey-Liaud et al., 1987).

While blood β-OHB is the most specific test to assess ketonemia, the semiquantitative urine test strip (aka dipstick) or tablets for acetoacetate are also sometimes used, especially in clinical veterinary medicine. The urine tests are based on the use of a nitroprusside reaction and give a measure of trace, moderate or strong positivity to acetoacetate, react weakly with acetone, and do not detect β-OHB. The semiquantitative methods are quick and inexpensive but less sensitive than multistep enzymatic assays, and only semiquantitative at best. The urine test strips are inferior when compared with the tablets for ketone detection, and have a considerable variability. Strongly pigmented urine and some drugs (such as valproic acid) can cause false positive readings with either of these simple urine tests. In addition, with resolving acidosis, acetoacetate levels increase relative to β-OHB. Hence, the urine acetoacetate test may give the misleading impression that ketosis is not improving.

21.15.2 Carnitine and Aylcarnitine

Carnitines and acylcarnitines are crucial to the catabolism of FAs in mitochondria (Section 21.7). Due to the insolubility of FAs, carnitine and acylcarnitines move FAs into the mitochondria for catabolism with the assistance of carnitine palmitoyltransferase I (CPT 1), carnitine-acylcarnitine translocase (CACT), and carnitine palmitoyltransferase II (CPT 2). Once FAs are in the mitochondria, FA catabolism results in the formation of acetyl-CoA, which generates ATP from the Krebs cycle and oxidative phosphorylation (Longo et al., 2006).

In general, there are low levels of acylcarnitines in circulation, with carnitine levels being predominantly due to free carnitine (Reuter and Evans, 2012). However, alterations in the catabolism pathway of FAs can result in dramatically different carnitine and acylcarnitine profiles in the plasma and urine. For example, if there is deficiency or inhibition of one of the enzymes that is involved in removing pairs of carbon atoms from the acylcarnitine (e.g., short-, medium-, or long-chain acyl-coenzyme A dehydrogenases; SCAD, MCAD, or LCAD, respectively), then a characteristic pattern of plasma and urine metabolites is produced. SCAD results in the alternate metabolism of butyryl-CoA and large amounts of organic acids such as ethymalonic acid and methylsuccinic acid are excreted, resulting in an abnormal urine profile (Prieto et al., 2006).

Methods for laboratory evaluation of carnitine and acylcarnitines in plasma and/or urine include spectrophotometry, HPLC, and electrospray ionization tandem mass spectrometry (McEntyre et al., 2004; Mueller et al., 2003; Longo et al., 2006). Tandem mass spectrometry allows the evaluation of an extensive panel of acylcarnitine fractions (Mueller et al., 2003).

21.15.3 Leptin

Leptin homology is variable across species, and does not follow a direct evolutionary path (Doyon et al., 2001). Hence, serum (or plasma) leptin analysis requires species-specific assays. Enzyme-linked immunoassay (ELISA) and/or radioimmunoassay (RIA) kits are currently available for mice, rats, dogs, and humans. As expected, these assays vary in antibody sets and detection methods, and require validation for precision, linearity, dynamic range, and accuracy with expected highest and lowest leptin concentrations. Utility (apparent cross-reactivity) of some of these assays with other species has also been reported (Kitao et al., 2011; Tsubota et al., 2008).

21.15.4 Ghrelin

Ghrelin is highly homologous across species (Tvarijonaviciute et al., 2012), and cross-reactivity of human assays has been validated for other species (rat, mouse) by some manufacturers. However, species-specific ELISAs and/or RIAs for ghrelin are also available for mice, rats, and dogs.

21.15.5 Adiponectin

Adiponectin homology across species is relatively low (Jacobi et al., 2004; Li et al., 2008). Nonetheless, the published evaluations in animals have commonly relied on a commercially available human RIA, and only more recently on species-specific ELISAs for mouse/rat or for dogs. Assays for high molecular weight human adiponectin using a chemiluminescent enzyme immunoassay are also available; however, the significance of determining various molecular weight forms in dogs, cats, and horses has not been evaluated to date.

SUMMARY

Lipidology, including blood and tissue lipids and lipid transport, is a critical science in the study of human health. The differences between humans and other species, and across species overall in lipid metabolism in homeostasis, and response and adaption to physiologic whole body perturbations are often striking. These differences largely reflect, and are in themselves, a study of species differences in natural diet, environment, and physiology. Yet, understanding of these species differences and associated physiologic mechanisms can also significantly inform, and enable their translation, the human condition. Hence, this chapter provides a unique comprehensive synopsis of the basic measurable blood lipid components, lipid metabolism, and physiologic responses in blood lipids with system perturbation in nonclinical species, as well as major animal models of lipid disorders, and the assays used to measure and interpret circulating lipids in nonclinical species. This collective information provides a reference for readers toward understanding the complexity of lipid metabolism across species, the utility of associated endpoints, and comprehension of physiologic mechanisms behind, and interpretation of, blood lipid data.

REFERENCES

Abbal, C., Lambelet, M., Bertaggia, D., et al. 2006. Lipid raft adhesion receptors and Syk regulate selectin-dependent rolling under flow conditions. *Blood.* 108(10):3352–3359.

Abbott, S.K., Else, P.L., Atkins, T.A., and Hulbert, A.J. 2012. Fatty acid composition of membrane bilayers: Importance of diet polyunsaturated fat balance. *Biochim Biophys Acta.* 1818(5):1309–1317.

Abnet, C.C., Borkowf, C.B., Qiao, Y.L., et al. 2001. Sphingolipids as biomarkers of fumonisin exposure and risk of esophageal squamous cell carcinoma in china. *Cancer Causes Control.* 12(9):821–828.

Abrams, J.J., Grundy, S.M., and Ginsberg, H. 1981. Metabolism of plasma triglycerides in hypothyroidism and hyperthyroidism in man. *J Lipid Res.* 22(2):307–322.

Adachi, R., Honma, Y., Masuno, H., et al. 2005. Selective activation of vitamin D receptor by lithocholic acid acetate, a bile acid derivative. *J Lipid Res.* 46(1):46–57.

Adamovich, Y., Rousso-Noori, L., Zwighaft, Z., et al. 2014. Circadian clocks and feeding time regulate the oscillations and levels of hepatic triglycerides. *Cell Metab.* 19(2):319–330.

Aggarwal, D., West, K.L., Zern, T.L., Shrestha, S., Vergara-Jimenez, M., and Fernandez, M.L. 2005. JTT-130, a microsomal triglyceride transfer protein (MTP) inhibitor lowers plasma triglycerides and LDL cholesterol concentrations without increasing hepatic triglycerides in guinea pigs. *BMC Cardiovasc Disord.* 5:30–37.

Aguila, M.B., Loureiro, C.C., Pinheiro Ada, R., and Mandarim-De-Lacerda, C.A. 2002. Lipid metabolism in rats fed diets containing different types of lipids. *Arq Bras Cardiol.* 78(1):25–38.

Ahlers, I., Ahlersová, E., Smajda, B., and Sedláková, A. 1980. Circadian rhythm of serum and tissue lipids in fed and fasted rats. *Physiol Bohemoslov.* 29(6):525–533.

Aleixandre de Artiñano, A., and Miguel Castro, M. 2009. Experimental rat models to study the metabolic syndrome. *Br J Nutr*. 102(9):1246–1253.

Aliev, G., and Burnstock, G. 1998. Watanabe rabbits with heritable hypercholesterolaemia: A model of atherosclerosis. *Histol Histopathol*. 13(3):797–817.

Angelin, B., and Rudling, M. 2010. Lipid lowering with thyroid hormone and thyromimetics. *Curr Opin Lipidol*. 21(6):499–506.

Anglés-Cano, E., de la Peña Díaz, A., and Loyau, S. 2001. Inhibition of fibrinolysis by lipoprotein(a). *Ann N Y Acad Sci*. 936:261–275.

Argraves, K.M., and Argraves, W.S. 2007. HDL serves as a S1P signaling platform mediating a multitude of cardiovascular effects. *J Lipid Res*. 48(11):2325–2333.

Arita, M., Yoshida, M., Hong, S., et al. 2005. Resolvin E1, an endogenous lipid mediator derived from omega-3 eicosapentaenoic acid, protects against 2,4,6-trinitrobenzene sulfonic acid-induced colitis. *Proc Natl Acad Sci USA*. 102(21):7671–7676.

Arner, P. 2005. Effects of testosterone on fat cell lipolysis. Species differences and possible role in polycystic ovarian syndrome. *Biochimie*. 87(1):39–43.

Arner, P., Kriegholm, E., Engfeldt, P., and Bolinder, J. 1990. Adrenergic regulation of lipolysis in situ at rest and during exercise. *J Clin Invest*. 85(3):893–898.

Arranz-Pena, M.L., Tasende-Mata, J., and Martin-Gil, F.J. 1998. Comparison of two homogeneous assays with a precipitation method and an ultracentrifugation method for the measurement of HDL-cholesterol. *Clin Chem*. 44(12):2499–2505.

Artl, A., Marsche, G., Lestavel, S., Sattler, W., and Malle, E. 2000. Role of serum amyloid A during metabolism of acute-phase HDL by macrophages. *Arterioscler Thromb Vasc Biol*. 20(3):763–772.

Asakawa, A., Inui, A., Kaga, T., et al. 2001. Ghrelin is an appetite-stimulatory signal from stomach with structural resemblance to motilin. *Gastroenterology*. 120(2):337–345.

Ashrafian, H., Horowitz, J.D., and Frenneaux, M.P. 2007. Perhexiline. *Cardiovasc Drug Rev*. 25(1):76–97.

Atkinson, J.B., Hoover, R.L., Berry, K.K., and Swift, L.L. 1989. Cholesterol-fed heterozygous Watanabe heritable hyperlipidemic rabbits: A new model for atherosclerosis. *Atherosclerosis*. 78(2–3):123–136.

Auerbach, B.J., and Parks, J.S. 1989. Lipoprotein abnormalities associated with lipopolysaccharide-induced lecithin: Cholesterol acyltransferase and lipase deficiency. *J Biol Chem*. 264(17):10264–10270.

Aydilek, N., and Aksakal, M. 2005. Effects of testosterone on lipid peroxidation, lipid profiles and some coagulation parameters in rabbits. *J Vet Med A Physiol Pathol Clin Med*. 52(9):436–439.

Bachmann, K., Patel, H., Batayneh, Z., et al. 2004. PXR and the regulation of apoA1 and HDL-cholesterol in rodents. *Pharmacol Res*. 50(3):237–246.

Bagdade, J.D., Yee, E., Albers, J., and Pykalisto, O.J. 1976. Glucocorticoids and triglyceride transport: Effects on triglyceride secretion rates, lipoprotein lipase, and plasma lipoproteins in the rat. *Metabolism*. 25(5):533–542.

Baile, C.A., Della-Fera, M.A., and Martin, R.J. 2000. Regulation of metabolism and body fat mass by leptin. *Annu Rev Nutr*. 20:105–127.

Ballatori, N., Christian, W.V., Lee, J.Y., et al. 2005. OSTalpha–OSTbeta: A major basolateral bile acid and steroid transporter in human intestinal, renal, and biliary epithelia. *Hepatology*. 42:1270–1279.

Baranowski, M. 2008. Biological role of liver X receptors. *J Physiol Pharmacol*. 59(Suppl 7):31–55.

Barrie, J., Watson, T.D.G., Stear, M.J., and Nash, A.S. 1993. Plasma cholesterol and lipoprotein concentrations in the dog: The effects of age, breed, gender and endocrine disease. *J Sm Ani Prac*. 34:507–512.

Batta, A.K., Xu, G., Honda, A., Miyazaki, T., and Salen, G. 2006. Stigmasterol reduces plasma cholesterol levels and inhibits hepatic synthesis and intestinal absorption in the rat. *Metabolism*. 55(3):292–299.

Bauer, J.E. 1995. Evaluation and dietary considerations in idiopathic hyperlipidemia in dogs. *J AmerVet Med Assoc*. 206:1684–1688.

Baum, C.L., Teng, B.B., and Davidson, N.O. 1990. Apolipoprotein B messenger RNA editing in the rat liver. Modulation by fasting and refeeding a high carbohydrate diet. *J Biol Chem*. 265(31):19263–19270.

Bedossa, P., Poynard, T., Abella, A., et al. 1989. Apolipoprotein AI is a serum and tissue marker of liver fibrosis in alcoholic patients. *Alcohol Clin Exp Res*. 13(6):829–833.

Beentjes, J.A., van Tol, A., Sluiter, W.J., and Dullaart, R.P. 2000. Low plasma lecithin:Cholesterol acyltransferase and lipid transfer protein activities in growth hormone deficient and acromegalic men: Role in altered high density lipoproteins. *Atherosclerosis*. 153(2):491–498.

Beermann, C., Jelinek, J., Reinecker, T., Hauenschild, A., Boehm, G., and Klör, H.U. 2003. Short term effects of dietary medium-chain fatty acids and n-3 long-chain polyunsaturated fatty acids on the fat metabolism of healthy volunteers. *Lipids Health Dis*. 2:10.

Bell, P.M., Wiggam, M.I., and Hadden, D.R. 2005. Recent advances in the monitoring and management of diabetic ketoacidosis. *QJM*. 98(4):318.

Benavides, A., Siches, M., and Llobera, M. 1998. Circadian rhythms of lipoprotein lipase and hepatic lipase activities in intermediate metabolism of adult rat. *Am J Physiol*. 275(3 Pt 2):R811–817.

Berbée, J.F., van der Hoogt, C.C., Sundararaman, D., Havekes, L.M., and Rensen, P.C. 2005. Severe hypertriglyceridemia in human APOC1 transgenic mice is caused by apoC-I-induced inhibition of LPL. *J Lipid Res*. 46(2):297–306.

Berenson, C.S., Nawar, H.F., Yohe, H.C., et al. 2010. Mammalian cell ganglioside-binding specificities of E. coli enterotoxins LT-IIb and variant LT-IIb(T1+3I). *Glycobiology*. 20(1):41–54.

Bergö, M., Wu, G., Ruge, T., and Olivecrona, T. 2002. Down-regulation of adipose tissue lipoprotein lipase during fasting requires that a gene, separate from the lipase gene, is switched on. *J Biol Chem*. 277(14):11927–11932.

Berk, P.D., and Stump, D.D. 1999. Mechanisms of cellular uptake of long chain free fatty acids. *Mol Cell Biochem*. 192(1–2):17–31.

Berk, P.D., Zhou, S.L., Stump, D., Kiang, C.L., and Isola, L.M. 1994. Recent studies of the cellular uptake of long chain free fatty acids. *Trans Am Clin Climatol Assoc*. 105:179–189.

Berlan, M., and Lafontan, M. 1985. Evidence that epinephrine acts preferentially as an antilipolytic agent in abdominal human subcutaneous fat cells: assessment by analysis of beta and alpha 2 adrenoceptor properties. *Eur J Clin Invest*. 15(6):341--348.

Berlin, E., Khan, M.A., Henderson, G.R., and Kliman, P.G. 1985. Influence of age and sex on composition and lipid fluidity in miniature swine plasma lipoproteins. *Atherosclerosis*. 54(2):187–203.

Berriot-Varoqueaux, N., Aggerbeck, L.P., Samson-Bouma, M., and Wetterau, J.R. 2000. The role of the microsomal triglygeride transfer protein in abetalipoproteinemia. *Annu Rev Nutr*. 20:663–697.

Bertile, F., Criscuolo, F., Oudart, H., Le Maho, Y., and Raclot, T. 2003. Differences in the expression of lipolytic-related genes in rat white adipose tissues. *Biochem Biophys Res Commun*. 307(3):540–546.

Bertile, F., and Raclot, T. 2011. ATGL and HSL are not coordinately regulated in response to fuel partitioning in fasted rats. *J Nutr Biochem*. 22(4):372–379.

Bertolucci, C., Fazio, F., and Piccione, G. 2008. Daily rhythms of serum lipids in dogs: Influences of lighting and fasting cycles. *Comp Med*. 58(5):485–489.

Bickerton, A.S., Roberts, R., Fielding, B.A., et al. 2007. Preferential uptake of dietary fatty acids in adipose tissue and muscle in the postprandial period. *Diabetes*. 56(1):168–176.

Binoux, M. 1995. The IGF system in metabolism regulation. *Diabete Metab*. 21(5):330–337.

Blanco-Vaca, F., Escolà-Gil, J.C., Martín-Campos, J.M., and Julve, J. 2001. Role of apoA-II in lipid metabolism and atherosclerosis: Advances in the study of an enigmatic protein. *J Lipid Res*. 42(11):1727–1739.

Boero, L., Manavela, M., Meroño, T., Maidana, P., Gómez Rosso, L., and Brites, F. 2012. GH levels and insulin sensitivity are differently associated with biomarkers of cardiovascular disease in active acromegaly. *Clin Endocrinol (Oxf)*. 77(4):579--585.

Boerwinkle, E., Lee, S.S., Butler, R., Schumaker, V.N., and Chan, L. 1990. Rapid typing of apolipoprotein B DNA polymorphisms by DNA amplification. Association between Ag epitopes of human apolipoprotein B-100, a signal peptide insertion/deletion polymorphism, and a 3⊠flanking DNA variable number of tandem repeats polymorphism of the apolipoprotein B gene. *Atherosclerosis*. 81(3):225–232.

Bonnefont, J.P., Djouadi, F., Prip-Buus, C., Gobin, S., Munnich, A., and Bastin, J. 2004. Carnitine palmitoyltransferases 1 and 2: Biochemical, molecular and medical aspects. *Mol Aspects Med*. 25(5–6):495–520.

Bookstaff, R.C., Murphy, V.A., Skare, J.A., Minnema, D., Sanzgiri, U., and Parkinson, A. 1996. Effects of doxylamine succinate on thyroid hormone balance and enzyme induction in mice. *Toxicol Appl Pharmacol*. 141(2):584–594.

Boone, L.R., Lagor, W.R., de la Llera Moya, M., Niesen, M.I., Rothblat, G.H., and Ness, G.C. 2011. Thyroid hormone enhances the ability of serum to accept cellular cholesterol via the ABCA1 transporter. *Atherosclerosis*. 218(1):77–82.

Borggreve, S.E., De Vries, R., and Dullaart, R.P. 2003. Alterations in high-density lipoprotein metabolism and reverse cholesterol transport in insulin resistance and type 2 diabetes mellitus: Role of lipolytic enzymes, lecithin: Cholesterol acyltransferase and lipid transfer proteins. *Eur J Clin Invest*. 33(12):1051–1069.

Botham, K.M., and Boyd, G.S. 1983. The metabolism of chenodeoxycholic acid to beta-muricholic acid in rat liver. *Eur J Biochem*. 134(1):191–196.

Boudet, J., Roullet, J.B., and Lacour, B. 1988. Influence of fast, body weight and diet on serum cholesterol, triglycerides, and phospholipids concentrations in the aging rat. *Horm Metab Res*. 20(12):734–737.

Boulange, A., Planche, E., and de Gasquet, P. 1981. Onset and development of hypertriglyceridemia in the Zucker rat (fa/fa). *Metabolism*. 30(11):1045–1052.

Boullion, R.D., Mokelke, E.A., Wamhoff, B.R., et al. 2003. Porcine model of diabetic dyslipidemia: Insulin and feed algorithms for mimicking diabetes mellitus in humans. *Comp Med.* 53(1):42–52.

Bousquet-Mélou, A., Galitzky, J., Carpéné, C., Lafontan, M., and Berlan, M. 1994. Beta-adrenergic control of lipolysis in primate white fat cells: A comparative study with nonprimate mammals. *Am J Physiol.* 267(1 Pt 2):R115–123.

Bousquet-Mélou, A., Galitzky, J., Lafontan, M., and Berlan, M. 1995. Control of lipolysis in intra-abdominal fat cells of nonhuman primates: Comparison with humans. *J Lipid Res.* 36(3):451–461.

Bouziane, M., Prost, J., and Belleville, J. 1994. Changes in fatty acid compositions of total serum and lipoprotein particles, in growing rats given protein-deficient diets with either hydrogenated coconut or salmon oils as fat sources. *Br J Nutr.* 71(3):375–387.

Boyer, J.L. 2013. Bile formation and secretion. *Compr Physiol.* 3(3):1035–1078.

Braissant, O., Foufelle, F., Scotto, C., Dauça, M., and Wahli, W. 1996. Differential expression of peroxisome proliferator-activated receptors (PPARs): Tissue distribution of PPAR-alpha, -beta, and -gamma in the adult rat. *Endocrinology.* 137(1):354–366.

Brockerhoff, H., Hoyle, R.J., and Wolmark, N. 1966. Positional distribution of fatty acids in triglycerides of animal depot fats. *Biochim Biophys Acta.* 116(1):67–72.

Brownsey, R.W., Boone, A.N., Elliott, J.E., Kulpa, J.E., and Lee, W.M. 2006. Regulation of acetyl-CoA carboxylase. *Biochem Soc Trans.* 34(Pt 2):223–227.

Brunham, L.R., Kruit, J.K., Iqbal, J., et al. 2006. Intestinal ABCA1 directly contributes to HDL biogenesis in vivo. *J Clin Invest.* 116(4):1052–1062.

Bruss, M.D., Khambatta, C.F., Ruby, M.A., Aggarwal, I., and Hellerstein, M.K. 2010. Calorie restriction increases fatty acid synthesis and whole body fat oxidation rates. *Am J Physiol Endocrinol Metab.* 298(1):E108–116.

Buja, L.M., Clubb, F.J., Bilheimer, D.W., and Willerson, J.T. 1990. Pathobiology of human familial hypercholesterolaemia and a related animal model, the Watanabe heritable hyperlipidaemic rabbit. *Eur Heart J.* 11(Suppl E):41–52.

Bullock, B.C., Lehner, N.D., Clarkson, T.B., Feldner, M.A., Wagner, W.D., and Lofland, H.B. 1975. Comparative primate atherosclerosis. I. Tissue cholesterol concentration and pathologic anatomy. *Exp Mol Pathol.* 22(2):151–175.

Burén, J., Lai, Y.C., Lundgren, M., Eriksson, J.W., and Jensen, J. 2008. Insulin action and signalling in fat and muscle from dexamethasone-treated rats. *Arch Biochem Biophys.* 474(1):91–101.

Cabana, V.G., Gewurz, H., and Siegel, J.N. 1983. Inflammation-induced changes in rabbit CRP and plasma lipoproteins. *J Immunol.* 130(4):1736–1742.

Cabana, V.G., Lukens, J.R., Rice, K.S., Hawkins, T.J., and Getz, G.S. 1996. HDL content and composition in acute phase response in three species: Triglyceride enrichment of HDL a factor in its decrease. *J Lipid Res.* 37(12):2662–2674.

Cabana, V.G., Siegel, J.N., and Sabesin, S.M. 1989. Effects of the acute phase response on the concentration and density distribution of plasma lipids and apolipoproteins. *J Lipid Res.* 30(1):39–49.

Cahill, G.F., Herrera, M.G., Morgan, A.P., et al. 1966. Hormone–fuel interrelationships during fasting. *J Clin Invest.* 45(11):1751–1769.

Cai, H., Smola, U., Wixler, V., et al. 1997. Role of diacylglycerol-regulated protein kinase C isotypes in growth factor activation of the Raf-1 protein kinase. *Mol Cell Biol.* 17(2):732–741.

Campbell, J.E., Peckett, A.J., D'souza, A.M., Hawke, T.J., and Riddell, M.C. 2011. Adipogenic and lipolytic effects of chronic glucocorticoid exposure. *Am J Physiol Cell Physiol.* 300(1):C198–209.

Camus, M.C., Chapman, M.J., Forgez, P., and Laplaud, P.M. 1983. Distribution and characterization of the serum lipoproteins and apoproteins in the mouse, Mus musculus. *J Lipid Res.* 24(9):1210–1228.

Carey, M.C., Montet, J.C., Phillips, M.C., Armstrong, M.J., and Mazer, N.A. 1981. Thermodynamic and molecular basis for dissimilar cholesterol-solubilizing capacities by micellar solutions of bile salts: Cases of sodium chenodeoxycholate and sodium ursodeoxycholate and their glycine and taurine conjugates. *Biochemistry.* 20(12):3637–3648.

Carlson, L.A., Fröberg, S.O., and Nye, E.R. 1968. Effect of age on blood and tissue lipid levels in the male rat. *Gerontologia.* 14(1):65–79.

Carmen, G.Y., and Víctor, S.M. 2006. Signalling mechanisms regulating lipolysis. *Cell Signal.* 18(4):401–408.

Carpéné, C., Ambid, L., and Lafontan, M. 1994a. Predominance of beta 3-adrenergic component in catecholamine activation of lipolysis in garden dormouse adipocytes. *Am J Physiol.* 266(3 Pt 2):R896–904.

Carpéné, C., Bousquet-Mélou, A., Galitzky, J., Berlan, M., and Lafontan, M. 1998. Lipolytic effects of beta 1-, beta 2-, and beta 3-adrenergic agonists in white adipose tissue of mammals. *Ann N Y Acad Sci.* 839:186–189.

Carpéné, C., Castan, I., Collon, P., Galitzky, J., Moratinos, J., and Lafontan, M. 1994b. Adrenergic lipolysis in guinea pig is not a beta 3-adrenergic response: Comparison with human adipocytes. *Am J Physiol.* 266(3 Pt 2):R905–913.

Carrasco, S., and Mérida, I. 2007. Diacylglycerol, when simplicity becomes complex. *Trends Biochem Sci.* 32(1):27–36.

Cartwright, C.K., Ragland, J.B., Weidman, S.W., and Sabesin, S.M. 1982. Alterations in lipoprotein composition associated with galactosamine-induced rat liver injury. *J Lipid Res.* 23(5):667–679.

Castan, I., Valet, P., Quideau, N., et al. 1994. Antilipolytic effects of alpha 2-adrenergic agonists, neuropeptide Y, adenosine, and PGE1 in mammal adipocytes. *Am J Physiol.* 266(4 Pt 2):R1141–1147.

Cayen, M.N., Givner, M.L., and Kraml, M. 1972. Effect of diurnal rhythm and food withdrawal on serum lipid levels in the rat. *Experientia.* 28(5):502–503.

Center, S.A. 1996. Hepatic lipidosis, glucocorticoid hepatopathy, vacuolar hepatopathy, storage disorders, amyloidosis, and iron toxicity. In *Strombeck's Small Animal Gastroenterology*. Eds. D.R. Strombeck, W.G. Guilford, S.A. Center, D.A. Williams, and D.J. Meyer, 3rd edition, pp. 766–801. Philadelphia, PA: WB Saunders.

Chamley, L.W., Allen, J.L., and Johnson, P.M. 1997. Synthesis of beta2 glycoprotein 1 by the human placenta. *Placenta.* 18(5–6):403–410.

Chatzipanteli, K., Head, C., Megerman, J., and Axelrod, L. 1996. The relationship between plasma insulin level, prostaglandin production by adipose tissue, and blood pressure in normal rats and rats with diabetes mellitus and diabetic ketoacidosis. *Metabolism.* 45(6):691–698.

Chen, C.-Y., Huang, J-Y., and Huang, Y-T. 1982. Influences of age and breed on lipid and lipoprotein profiles in swine. In: *Pig Model for Biomedical Research,* Roberts, H.R. and Dodds, W.J. (Eds.), Taiwan: Pig. Research Institute, p. 65.

Chen, X., Matthews, J., Zhou, L., et al. 2008. Improvement of dyslipidemia, insulin sensitivity, and energy balance by a peroxisome proliferator-activated receptor alpha agonist. *Metabol.* 57(11):1516–1525.

Chen, Y.R., Fang, S.R., Fu, Y.C., Zhou, X.H., Xu, M.Y., and Xu, W.C. 2010. Calorie restriction on insulin resistance and expression of SIRT1 and SIRT4 in rats. *Biochem Cell Biol.* 88(4):715–722.

Chiang, J.Y. 2009. Bile acids: Regulation of synthesis. *J Lipid Res.* 50(10):1955–1966.

Chiang, J.Y. 2013. Bile acid metabolism and signaling. *Compr Physiol.* 3(3):1191–1212.

Chirieac, D.V., Cianci, J., Collins, H.L., Sparks, J.D., and Sparks, C.E. 2002. Insulin suppression of VLDL apoB secretion is not mediated by the LDL receptor. *Biochem Biophys Res Commun.* 297(1):134–137.

Choi, J.K., Ho, J., Curry, S., Qin, D., Bittman, R., and Hamilton, J.A. 2002. Interactions of very long-chain saturated fatty acids with serum albumin. *J Lipid Res.* 43(7):1000–1010.

Choi, Y.S., Goto, S., Ikeda, I., and Sugano, M. 1988a. Age-related changes in lipid metabolism in rats: The consequence of moderate food restriction. *Biochim Biophys Acta.* 963(2):237–242.

Choi, Y.S., Sugano, M., and Ide, T. 1988b. Sex-difference in the age related change of cholesterol metabolism in rats. *Mech Ageing Dev.* 44(1):91–99.

Chopra, B., Hinley, J., Oleksiewicz, M.B., and Southgate, J. 2008. Trans-species comparison of PPAR and RXR expression by rat and human urothelial tissues. *Toxicol Pathol.* 36(3):485–495.

Christ, E.R., Cummings, M.H., Stolinski, M., et al. 2006. Low-density lipoprotein apolipoprotein B100 turnover in hypopituitary patients with GH deficiency: A stable isotope study. *Eur J Endocrinol.* 154(3):459–466.

Christ, E.R., Wierzbicki, A.S., Cummings, M.H., Umpleby, A.M., and Russell-Jones, D.L. 1999. Dynamics of lipoprotein metabolism in adult growth hormone deficiency. *J Endocrinol Invest.* 22(Suppl 5):16–21.

Christie, W.W., and Moore, J.H. 1970. A comparison of the structures of triglycerides from various pig tissues. *Biochim Biophys Acta.* 210(1):46–56.

Christie, W.W., and Moore, J.H. 1972. The structures of adipose tissue and heart muscle triglycerides in the domestic chicken (*Gallus gallus*). *J Sci Food Agric.* 23(1):73–77.

Ciraolo, S.T., Previs, S.F., Fernandez, C.A., et al. 1995. Model of extreme hypoglycemia in dogs made ketotic with (R,S)-1,3-butanediol acetoacetate esters. *Am J Physiol.* 269(1 Pt 1):E67–75.

Ciresi, A., Amato, M.C., Pivonello, R., et al. 2013. The metabolic profile in active acromegaly is gender-specific. *J Clin Endocrinol Metab.* 98(1):E51–59.

Clarke, P.R., and Hardie, D.G. 1990. Regulation of HMG-CoA reductase: Identification of the site phosphorylated by the AMP-activated protein kinase in vitro and in intact rat liver. *EMBO J.* 9(8):2439–2446.

Clemente-Postigo, M., Queipo-Ortuño, M., Valdivielso, P., Tinahones, F.J., and Cardona, F. 2010. Effect of apolipoprotein C3 and apolipoprotein A1 polymorphisms on postprandial response to a fat overload in metabolic syndrome patients. *Clin Biochem.* 43(16–17):1300–1304.

Cohn, J.S., Tremblay, M., Batal, R., et al. 2002. Plasma kinetics of VLDL and HDL apoC-I in normolipidemic and hypertriglyceridemic subjects. *J Lipid Res.* 43(10):1680–1687.

Cole, T.G., Kuisk, I., Patsch, W., and Schonfeld, G. 1984. Effects of high cholesterol diets on rat plasma lipoproteins and lipoprotein–cell interactions. *J Lipid Res.* 25(6):593–603.

Colvin, P.L., Jr., Spray, B.J., and Miller, N.E. 1994. Plasma low density lipoprotein cholesterol concentration in cynomolgus monkeys; differing effects of age and body weight in animals consuming low and high cholesterol diets. *Atherosclerosis.* 111(2):191–197.

Consitt, L.A., Bell, J.A., and Houmard, J.A. 2009. Intramuscular lipid metabolism, insulin action, and obesity. *IUBMB Life.* 61(1):47–55.

Cooper, A.D. 1997. Hepatic uptake of chylomicron remnants. *J Lipid Res.* 38(11):2173–2192.

Corsini A., Mazzotti, M., Villa, A., et al. 1992. Ability of the LDL receptor from several animal species to recognize the human apoB binding domain: Studies with LDL from familial defective apoB-100. *Atherosclerosis.* 93(1–2):95–103.

Cortright, R.N., and Koves, T.R. 2000. Sex differences in substrate metabolism and energy homeostasis. *Can J Appl Physiol.* 25(4):288–311.

Crispin, S.M. 1993. Ocular manifestations of hyperlipoproteinemia. *J Small Anim Pract.* 34:500–506.

Crook, D., Weisgraber, K.H., Boyles, J.K., and Mahley, R.W. 1990. Isolation and characterization of plasma lipoproteins of common marmoset monkey. Comparison of effects of control and atherogenic diets. *Arteriosclerosis.* 10(4):633–647.

Cui, Y.J., Aleksunes, L.M., Tanaka, Y., Goedken, M.J., and Klaassen, C.D. 2009. Compensatory induction of liver efflux transporters in response to ANIT-induced liver injury is impaired in FXR-null mice. *Toxicol Sci.* 110(1):47–60.

D'Allaire, F., Atgié, C., Mauriège, P., Simard, P.M., and Bukowiecki, L.J. 1995. Characterization of beta 1- and beta 3-adrenoceptors in intact brown adipocytes of the rat. *Br J Pharmacol.* 114(2):275–282.

Davidson, M.B. 1987. Effect of growth hormone on carbohydrate and lipid metabolism. *Endocr Rev.* 8:115–131.

Davidson, N.O., Carlos, R.C., Drewek, M.J., and Parmer, T.G. 1988. Apolipoprotein gene expression in the rat is regulated in a tissue-specific manner by thyroid hormone. *J Lipid Res.* 29(11):1511–1522.

de Boer, H., Blok, G.J., Voerman, H.J., Phillips, M., and Schouten, J.A. 1994. Serum lipid levels in growth hormone-deficient men. *Metabolism.* 43(2):199--203.

de Bruin, T.W., van Barlingen, H., van Linde-Sibenius Trip, M., van Vuurst de Vries, A.R., Akveld, M.J., Erkelens, D.W. 1993. Lipoprotein(a) and apolipoprotein B plasma concentrations in hypothyroid, euthyroid, and hyperthyroid subjects. *J Clin Endocrinol Metab.* 76(1):121–126.

de Gasquet, P., Griglio, S., Pequignot-Planche, E., and Malewiak, M.I. 1977. Diurnal changes in plasma and liver lipids and lipoprotein lipase activity in heart and adipose tissue in rats fed a high and low fat diet. *J Nutr.* 107(2):199–212.

de Groot, P.G., and Meijers, J.C. 2011. β(2)-Glycoprotein I: Evolution, structure and function. *J Thromb Haemost.* 9(7):1275–1284.

de Grooth, G.J., Klerkx, A.H., Stroes, E.S., Stalenhoef, A.F., Kastelein, J.J., and Kuivenhoven, J.A. 2004. A review of CETP and its relation to atherosclerosis. *J Lipid Res.* 45(11):1967–1974.

de Haan, W., de Vries-van der Weij, J., Mol, I.M., et al. 2009. PXR agonism decreases plasma HDL levels in ApoE3-Leiden.CETP mice. *Biochim Biophys Acta.* 1791(3):191–197.

de Pergola, G., Holmäng, A., Svedberg, J., Giorgino, R., and Björntorp, P. 1990. Testosterone treatment of ovariectomized rats: Effects on lipolysis regulation in adipocytes. *Acta Endocrinol (Copenh).* 123(1):61–66.

Dechelotte, P., Kantelip, B., de Laguillaumie, B.V., Labbe, A., and Meyer, M. 1985. Tangier disease. A histological and ultrastructural study. *Pathol Res Pract.* 180(4):424–430.

Dedkova, E.N., and Blatter, L.A. 2014. Role of β-hydroxybutyrate, its polymer poly-β-hydroxybutyrate and inorganic polyphosphate in mammalian health and disease. *Front Physiol.* 5:260.

Deevska, G.M., and Nikolova-Karakashian, M.N. 2011. The twists and turns of sphingolipid pathway in glucose regulation. *Biochimie.* 93(1):

DeNigris, S.J., Hamosh, M., Kasbekar, D.K., Lee, T.C., and Hamosh, P. 1988. Lingual and gastric lipases: Species differences in the origin of prepancreatic digestive lipases and in the localization of gastric lipase. *Biochim Biophys Acta.* 959:38–45.

Deshaies, Y., Begin, F., Savoie, L., and Vachon, C. 1990. Attenuation of the meal-induced increase in plasma lipids and adipose tissue lipoprotein lipase by guar gum in rats. *J Nutr.* 120(1):64–70.

Diagne, A., Fauvel, J., Record, M., Chap, H., and Douste-Blazy, L. 1984. Studies on ether phospholipids. II. Comparative composition of various tissues from human, rat and guinea pig. *Biochim Biophys Acta.* 793(2):221–231.

Dicker, A., Ryden, M., Naslund, E., et al. 2004. Effect of testosterone on lipolysis in human pre-adipocytes from different fat depots. *Diabetologia.* 47:420–428.

Dixon, R.M., Reid, S.W., and Mooney, C.T. 1999. Epidemiological, clinical, haematological and biochemical characteristics of canine hypothyroidism. *Vet Rec.* 145:481–487.

Dole, V.P., and Rizack, M.A. 1961. On the turnover of long-chain fatty acids in plasma. *J Lipid Res.* 2:90–91.

Dolphin, P.J., and Forsyth, S.J. 1983. Nascent hepatic lipoproteins in hypothyroid rats. *J Lipid Res.* 24(5):541–551.

Dolphin, P.J., Forsyth, S.J., and Krul, E.S. 1986. Post-secretory acquisition of apolipoprotein E by nascent rat hepatic very-low-density lipoproteins in the absence of cholesteryl ester transfer. *Biochim Biophys Acta.* 875(1):21–30.

Dory, L., Krause, B.R., and Roheim, P.S. 1981. Plasma lipids, lipoproteins, and triglyceride turnover in eu- and hypo-thyroid rats and rats on a hypocaloric diet. *Can J Biochem.* 59(8):715–721.

Doyon, C., Drouin, G., Trudeau, V.L., and Moon, T.W. 2001. Molecular evolution of leptin. *Gen Comp Endocrinol.* 124(2):188–198.

Dupras, R., Brissette, L., Roach, P.D., Bégin, S., Tremblay, A., and Noël, S.P. 1991. The disappearance rate of human versus rat intermediate density lipoproteins from rat liver perfusion. *Biochem Cell Biol.* 69(8):537–543.

Eaton, S., Bartlett, K., and Pourfarzam, M. 1996. Mammalian mitochondrial beta-oxidation. *Biochem J.* 320(Pt 2):345–357.

Ebara, T., Hattori, H., Murase, T., and Okubo, M. 2010. Reduced plasma apolipoprotein A-V concentrations in two lecithin:Cholesterol acyltransferase deficient patients. *Clin Chem Lab Med.* 48(9):1359–1360.

Eberle, D., Hegarty, B., Bossard, P., Ferre, P., and Foufelle, F. 2004. SREBP transcription factors: Master regulators of lipid homeostasis. *Biochimie.* 86(11):839–848.

Edelsbrunner, M.E., Herzog, H., and Holzer, P. 2009. Evidence from knockout mice that peptide YY and neuropeptide Y enforce murine locomotion, exploration and ingestive behaviour in a circadian cycle- and gender-dependent manner. *Behav Brain Res.* 203(1):97–107.

Edelstein, C., Lewis, L.L., Shainoff, J.R., Naito, H., and Scanu, A.M. 1976. Isolation and characterization of a dog serum lipoprotein having apolipoprotein A-I as its predominant protein constituent. *Biochemistry.* 15(9):1934–1941.

Edén, S. 1979. Age- and sex-related differences in episodic growth hormone secretion in the rat. *Endocrinology.* 105:555–560.

Edén, S., Engström, B., Burman, P., Johansson, A.G., Wide, L., and Karlsson, F.A. 2000. Effects of short-term administration of growth hormone in healthy young men, women, and women taking oral contraceptives. *J Intern Med.* 247(5):570–578.

Eggen, D.A., Abee, C.R., Malcom, G.T., and Strong, J.P. 1982. Survey of serum cholesterol and triglyceride concentration and lipoprotein electrophoretic pattern in rhesus monkeys (*Macaca mulatta*). *J Med Primatol.* 11(1):1–9.

Eichmann, T.O., Kumari, M., Haas, J.T., et al. 2012. Studies on the substrate and stereo/regioselectivity of adipose triglyceride lipase, hormone-sensitive lipase, and diacylglycerol-O-acyltransferases. *J Biol Chem.* 287(49):41446–41457.

Elcombe, C.R., Elcombe, B.M., Foster, J.R., Chang, S.C., Ehresman, D.J., and Butenhoff, J.L. 2012. Hepatocellular hypertrophy and cell proliferation in Sprague-Dawley rats from dietary exposure to potassium perfluorooctanesulfonate results from increased expression of xenosensor nuclear receptors PPARα and CAR/PXR. *Toxicology.* 293(1–3):16–29.

Ellis, E., Goodwin, B., Abrahamsson, A., et al. 1998. Bile acid synthesis in primary cultures of rat and human hepatocytes. *Hepatology.* 27(2):615–620.

Engström, B.E., Karlsson, F.A., and Wide, L. 1998. Marked gender differences in ambulatory morning growth hormone values in young adults. *Clin Chem.* 44(6 Pt 1):1289–1295.

Ennulat, D., Walker, D., Clemo, F., et al. 2010. Effects of hepatic drug-metabolizing enzyme induction on clinical pathology parameters in animals and man. *Toxicol Pathol.* 38(5):810–828.

Erem, C., De⊠er, O., Bostan, M., et al. 1999. Plasma lipoprotein(a) in hypothyroid, euthyroid and hyperthyroid subjects. *Acta Cardiol.* 54(2):77–81.

Erickson, J.C., Hollopeter, G., and Palmiter, R.D. 1996. Attenuation of the obesity syndrome of ob/ob mice by the loss of neuropeptide Y. *Science.* 274(5293):1704–1707.

Ethier-Chiasson, M., Duchesne, A., Forest, J.C., et al. 2007. Influence of maternal lipid profile on placental protein expression of LDLr and SR-BI. *Biochem Biophys Res Commun.* 359(1):8–14.

Ettinger, W.H., Miller, L.A., Smith, T.K., and Parks, J.S. 1992. Effect of interleukin-1 alpha on lipoprotein lipids in cynomolgus monkeys: Comparison to tumor necrosis factor. *Biochim Biophys Acta.* 1128(2–3):186–192.

Eum, S.Y., Andras, I., Hennig, B., and Toborek, M. 2009. NADPH oxidase and lipid raft-associated redox signaling are required for PCB153-induced upregulation of cell adhesion molecules in human brain endothelial cells. *Toxicol Appl Pharmacol.* 240(2):299–305.

Fabbrini, E., Magkos, F., Patterson, B.W., Mittendorfer, B., and Klein, S. 2012. Subclinical hypothyroidism and hyperthyroidism have opposite effects on hepatic very-low-density lipoprotein-triglyceride kinetics. *J Clin Endocrinol Metab.* 97(3):E414–418.

Fain, J.N., and Garcĩa-Sáinz, J.A. 1983. Adrenergic regulation of adipocyte metabolism. *J Lipid Res.* 24:945–966.

Fazio, S., and Linton, M.F. 2004. Unique pathway for cholesterol uptake in fat cells. *Arterioscler Thromb Vasc Biol.* 24(9):1538–1539.

Feingold, K.R., Hardardottir, I., Memon, R., Krul, E.J.T., Moser, A.H., Taylor, J.M., and Grunfeld, C. 1993. Effect of endotoxin on cholesterol biosynthesis and distribution in serum lipoproteins in Syrian hamsters. *J. Lipid Res.* 34: 2147--2158.

Feingold, K.R., Hardardóttir, I., and Grunfeld, C. 1998. Beneficial effects of cytokine induced hyperlipidemia. *Z Ernahrungswiss.* 37(Suppl 1):66–74.

Feingold, K.R., Staprans, I., Memon, R.A., et al. 1992. Endotoxin rapidly induces changes in lipid metabolism that produce hypertriglyceridemia: Low doses stimulate hepatic triglyceride production while high doses inhibit clearance. *J Lipid Res.* 33(12):1765–1776.

Field, P.A., and Gibbons, G.F. 2000. Decreased hepatic expression of the low-density lipoprotein (LDL) receptor and LDL receptor-related protein in aging rats is associated with delayed clearance of chylomicrons from the circulation. *Metabolism.* 49(4):492–498.

Fielding, B. 2011. Tracing the fate of dietary fatty acids: Metabolic studies of postprandial lipaemia in human subjects. *Proc Nutr Soc.* 70(3):342–350.

Fless, G.M., and Scanu, A.M. 1986. Comparative study of density distribution of plasma lipoproteins of normo- and hypercholesterolemic rhesus monkeys and humans. *Arteriosclerosis.* 6(1):88–97.

Folsom, A.R., Kuba, K., Leupker, R.V., Jacobs, D.R., and Frantz, ID., Jr. 1983. Lipid concentrations in serum and EDTA-treated plasma from fasting and nonfasting normal persons, with particular regard to high-density lipoprotein cholesterol. *Clin Chem.* 29(3):505–508.

Fon Tacer, K., Kuzman, D., Seliskar, M., Pompon, D., and Rozman, D. 2007. TNF-alpha interferes with lipid homeostasis and activates acute and proatherogenic processes. *Physiol Genomics.* 31(2):216–227.

Forrest, B.J., and Cushley, R.J. 1977. Cholesterol esters and membrane permeability. A nuclear magnetic resonance (NMR) study. *Atherosclerosis.* 28(3):309–318.

Fournier, N., Cogny, A., Atger, V., et al. 2002. Opposite effects of plasma from human apolipoprotein A-II transgenic mice on cholesterol efflux from J774 macrophages and Fu5AH hepatoma cells. *Arterioscler Thromb Vasc Biol.* 22:638–643.

Frank, N., Sojka, J.E., Latour, M.A., McClure, S.R., and Polazzi, L. 1999. Effect of hypothyroidism on blood lipid concentrations in horses. *Am J Vet Res.* 60(6):730–733.

Fréneaux, E., Labbe, G., Letteron, P., et al. 1988. Inhibition of the mitochondrial oxidation of fatty acids by tetracycline in mice and in man: Possible role in microvesicular steatosis induced by this antibiotic. *Hepatology.* 8(5):1056–1062.

Frick, F., Lindén, D., Améen, C., Edén, S., Mode, A., and Oscarsson, J. 2002. Interaction between growth hormone and insulin in the regulation of lipoprotein metabolism in the rat. *Am J Physiol Endocrinol Metab.* 283(5):E1023–1031.

Friedewald, W.T., Levy, R.I., and Fredrickson, D.S. 1972. Estimation of the concentration of low-density lipoprotein cholesterol in plasma, without use of the preparative ultracentrifuge. *Clin Chem.* 18(6):499–502.

Friis, T., and Pedersen, L.R. 1987. Serum lipids in hyper- and hypothyroidism before and after treatment. *Clin Chim Acta.* 162(2):155–163.

Frisk-Holmberg, M., and Ostman, J. 1977. Differential inhibition of lipolysis in human adipose tissue by adrenergic beta receptor blocking drugs. *J Pharmacol Exp Ther.* 200(3):598–605.

Froesch, E.R., and Hussain, M. 1994. Recombinant human insulin-like growth factor-I: A therapeutic challenge for diabetes mellitus. *Diabetologia.* 37(Suppl 2):S179–185.

Fromenty, B., and Pessayre, D. 1995. Inhibition of mitochondrial beta-oxidation as a mechanism of hepatotoxicity. *Pharmacol Ther.* 67(1):101–154.

Fruchart, J.C. 2009. Peroxisome proliferator-activated receptor-alpha (PPARalpha): At the crossroads of obesity, diabetes and cardiovascular disease. *Atherosclerosis.* 205(1):1–8.

Gabriel, S.M., Roncancio, J.R., and Ruiz, N.S. 1992. Growth hormone pulsatility and the endocrine milieu during sexual maturation in male and female rats. *Neuroendocrinology.* 56(5):619–625.

Gajate, C., Gonzalez-Camacho, F., and Mollinedo, F. 2009. Lipid raft connection between extrinsic and intrinsic apoptotic pathways. *Biochem Biophys Res Commun.* 380(4):780–784.

Galan, X., Llobera, M., and Ramírez, I. 1994. Lipoprotein lipase and hepatic lipase in Wistar and Sprague-Dawley rat tissues. Differences in the effects of gender and fasting. *Lipids.* 29(5):333–336.

Gälman, C., Arvidsson, I., Angelin, B., and Rudling, M. 2003. Monitoring hepatic cholesterol 7-hydroxylase activity by assay of the stable bile acid intermediate 7-hydroxy-4-cholesten-3-one in peripheral blood. *J. Lipid Res.* 44:859–865.

Gangl, A., and Ockner, R.K. 1975. Intestinal metabolism of plasma free fatty acids. Intracellular compartmentation and mechanisms of control. *J. Clin. Invest.* 55:803–813.

Garcia-Calvo, M., Lisnock, J., Bull, H.G., et al. 2005. The target of ezetimibe is Niemann-Pick C1-Like 1 (NPC1L1). *Proc Natl Acad Sci USA.* 102(23):8132–8137.

García-Cañaveras, J.C., Donato, M.T., Castell, J.V., and Lahoz, A. 2012. Targeted profiling of circulating and hepatic bile acids in human, mouse, and rat using a UPLC-MRM-MS-validated method. *J Lipid Res.* 53(10):2231–2241.

Gardès, C., Chaput, E., Staempfli, A., Blum, D., Richter, H., and Benson, G.M. 2013. Differential regulation of bile acid and cholesterol metabolism by the farnesoid X receptor in Ldlr$^{-/-}$ mice versus hamsters. *J Lipid Res.* 54(5):1283–1299.

Gatica, L.V., Vega, V.A., Zirulnik, F., Oliveros, L.B., and Gimenez, M.S. 2006. Alterations in the lipid metabolism of rat aorta: Effects of vitamin A deficiency. *J Vasc Res.* 43(6):602–610.

Gautier, T., de Haan, W., Grober, J., et al. 2013. Farnesoid X receptor activation increases cholesteryl ester transfer protein expression in humans and transgenic mice. *J Lipid Res.* 54(8):2195–2205.

Gelissen, I.C., Hochgrebe, T., Wilson, M.R., et al. 1998. Apolipoprotein J (clusterin) induces cholesterol export from macrophage-foam cells: A potential anti-atherogenic function? *Biochem J.* 331(Pt 1):231–237.

Ghanbari-Niaki, A., Abednazari, H., Tayebi, S.M., Hossaini-Kakhak, A., and Kraemer, R.R. 2009. Treadmill training enhances rat agouti-related protein in plasma and reduces ghrelin levels in plasma and soleus muscle. *Metabolism.* 58(12):1747–1752.

Ghelardoni, S., Carnicelli, V., Frascarelli, S., Ronca-Testoni, S., and Zucchi, R. 2006. Ghrelin tissue distribution: Comparison between gene and protein expression. *J Endocrinol Invest.* 29(2):115–121.

Ghezzi, A.C., Cambri, L.T., Botezelli, J.D., Ribeiro, C., Dalia, R.A., and de Mello, M.A. 2012. Metabolic syndrome markers in wistar rats of different ages. *Diabetol Metab Syndr.* 4(1):16.

Gibbons, G.F., and Burnham, F.J. 1991. Effect of nutritional state on the utilization of fatty acids for hepatitic triacylglycerol synthesis and secretion as very-low-density lipoprotein. *Biochem J.* 275(Pt 1):87–92.

Gieger, T.L., Hosgood, G., Taboada, J., Wolfsheimer, K.J., and Mueller, P.B. 2000. Thyroid function and serum hepatic enzyme activity in dogs after phenobarbital administration. *J Vet Intern Med.* 14(3):277–281.

Gilbert, S.G., and Rice, D.C. 1991. Effects of chronic caffeine consumption in pregnant monkeys (*Macaca fascicularis*) on blood and urine clinical chemistry parameters. *Fundam Appl Toxicol.* 16(2):299–308.

Gnocchi, D., Pedrelli, M., Hurt-Camejo, E., and Parini, P. 2015. Lipids around the Clock: Focus on Circadian Rhythms and Lipid Metabolism. *Biology (Basel).* 4(1):104–132.

Gobellos, C., Corrada, Y.A., Castex, G.L., de la Sota, R.L., and Goya, R.G. 2002. Secretory patterns of growth hormone in dogs: Circannual, circadian, and ultradian rhythms. *Can J Vet Res.* 66(2):108–111.

Godbole, V., and York, D.A. 1978. Lipoprotein in situ in the genetically obese Zucker fatty rat (fa/fa): Role of hyperphagia and hyperinsulinaemia. *Diabetologia.* 14:191–197.

Goldberg, D.M., Roomi, M.W., Yu, A., and Roncari, D.A. 1981. Triacylglycerol metabolism in the phenobarbital-treated rat. *Biochem J.* 196(1):337–346.

Goldfine, H. 2010. The appearance, disappearance and reappearance of plasmalogens in evolution. *Prog Lipid Res.* 49(4):493–498.

Goldkorn, T., and Filosto, S. 2010. Lung injury and cancer: Mechanistic insights into ceramide and EGFR signaling under cigarette smoke. *Am J Respir Cell Mol Biol.* 43(3):259–268.

Goodwin, B., Watson, M.A., Kim, H., Miao, J., Kemper, J.K., and Kliewer, S.A. 2003. Differential regulation of rat and human CYP7A1 by the nuclear oxysterol receptor liver X receptor-alpha. *Mol Endocrinol.* 17:386–394.

Gooley, J.J., and Chua, E.C. 2014. Diurnal regulation of lipid metabolism and applications of circadian lipidomics. *J Genet Genomics.* 41(5):231–250.

Gordon, J.I., Smith, D.P., Andy, R., Alpers, D.H., Schonfeld, G., and Strauss, A.W. 1982. The primary translation product of rat intestinal apolipoprotein A-I mRNA is an unusual preproprotein. *J Biol Chem.* 257(2):971–978.

Gordon, M.E., McKeever, K.H., Betros, C.L., and Manso Filho, H.C. 2007. Exercise-induced alterations in plasma concentrations of ghrelin, adiponectin, leptin, glucose, insulin, and cortisol in horses. *Vet J.* 173(3):532–540.

Goulinet, S., and Chapman, M.J. 1993. Plasma lipoproteins in the golden Syrian hamster (*Mesocricetus auratus*): Heterogeneity of apoB- and apoA-I-containing particles. *J Lipid Res.* 34(6):943–959.

Greeve, J., Altkemper, I., Dieterich, J.H., Greten, H., and Windler, E. 1993. Apolipoprotein B mRNA editing in 12 different mammalian species: Hepatic expression is reflected in low concentrations of apoB-containing plasma lipoproteins. *J Lipid Res.* 34(8):1367–1383.

Greger, N.G., Insull, W., Jr., Probstfield, J.L., and Keenan. B.S. 1990. High-density lipoprotein response to 5-alpha-dihydrotestosterone and testosterone in Macaca fascicularis: A hormone-responsive primate model for the study of atherosclerosis. *Metabolism.* 39(9):919–924.

Groot, P.H., Pearce, N.J., Yates, J.W., et al. 2005. Synthetic LXR agonists increase LDL in CETP species. *J Lipid Res.* 46(10):2182–2191.

Gross, G., Sykes, M., Arellano, R., Fong, B., and Angel, A. 1987. HDL clearance and receptor-mediated catabolism of LDL are reduced in hypothyroid rats. *Atherosclerosis.* 66(3):269–275.

Gross, R.C., Eigenbrodt, E.H., and Farquhar, J.W. 1967. Endogenous triglyceride turnover in liver and plasma of the dog. *J Lipid Res.* 8(2):114–125.

Guo, H.C., Michel, J.B., Blouquit, Y., and Chapman, M.J. 1991. Lipoprotein(a) and apolipoprotein(a) in a New World monkey, the common marmoset (*Callithrix jacchus*). Association of variable plasma lipoprotein(a) levels with a single apolipoprotein(a) isoform. *Arterioscler Thromb.* 11(4):1030–1041.

Guo, Q., Avramoglu, R.K., and Adeli, K. 2005. Intestinal assembly and secretion of highly dense/lipid-poor apolipoprotein B48-containing lipoprotein particles in the fasting state: Evidence for induction by insulin resistance and exogenous fatty acids. *Metabolism.* 54(5):689–697.

Guyard-Dangremont, V., Desrumaux, C., Gambert, P., Lallemant, C., and Lagrost, L. 1998. Phospholipid and cholesteryl ester transfer activities in plasma from 14 vertebrate species; relation to atherogenesis susceptibility. *Comp Biochem Physiol B Biochem Mol Biol.* 120(3):517–525.

Hachey, D.L. 1994. Benefits and risks of modifying maternal fat intake in pregnancy and lactation. *Am J Clin Nutr.* 59(Suppl 2):454S–464S.

Hagey, L.R., Schteingart, C.D., Rossi, S.S., Ton-Nu, H.T., and Hofmann, A.F. 1998. An N-acyl glycyltaurine conjugate of deoxycholic acid in the biliary bile acids of the rabbit. *J Lipid Res.* 39(11):2119–2124.

Hamosh, M. 1978. Rat lingual lipase: Factors affecting enzyme activity and secretion. *Am J Physiol.* 235(4):E416–421.

Hamosh, M., Henderson, T.R., and Hamosh, P. 1998. Gastric lipase and pepsin activities in the developing ferret: Nonparallel development of the two gastric digestive enzymes. *J Pediatr Gastroenterol Nutr.* 26(2):162–166.

Hansson, P., Saggerson, D., and Nilsson-Ehle, P. 1991. Sex difference in triglyceride/fatty acid substrate cycling of rat adipose tissue: Indirect regulation by androgens. *Horm Metab Res.* 23(10):465–468.

Hartman, H.B., Gardell, S.J., Petucci, C.J., Wang, S., Krueger, J.A., and Evans, M.J. 2009. Activation of farnesoid X receptor prevents atherosclerotic lesion formation in $LDLR^{-/-}$ and $apoE^{-/-}$ mice. *J Lipid Res.* 50(6):1090–1100.

Harvey, R.A., Champe, P.C., and Ferrier, D.R. 2005. Integration of metabolism. In *Biochemistry.* Eds. R.A. Harvey, P.C. Champe, and D. Ferrier, 3rd edition, pp. 305–392. Baltimore, MD: Lippincott, Williams and Wilkins.

Haude, W., and Völcker, C.E. 1991. Hormonal effects on triacylglycerol secretion of rat liver. *Nahrung.* 35(10):1061–1066.

Haug, A., and Høstmark, A.T. 1987. Lipoprotein lipases, lipoproteins and tissue lipids in rats fed fish oil or coconut oil. *J Nutr.* 117(6):1011–1017.

Haughey, N.J. 2010. Sphingolipids in Neurodegeneration. *Neuromolecular Med.* 12(4):301–305.

Havel, R.J. 1998. Receptor and non-receptor mediated uptake of chylomicron remnants by the liver. *Atherosclerosis.* 141(Suppl 1):S1–7.

Havel, R., and Kane, J.P. 1995. Introduction: Structure and metabolism of plasma lipoproteins. In *The Metabolic and Molecular Basis of Inherited Diseases*. Eds. C.R. Scriver, A.L. Beaudet, W.S. Sly, and D. Valle, 7th edition, Vol. 11, pp. 1841–1850. New York, NY: McGraw-Hill.

Havel, R.J., Yamada, N., and Shames, D.M. 1989. Watanabe heritable hyperlipidemic rabbit. Animal model for familial hypercholesterolemia. *Arteriosclerosis.* 9(Suppl 1):I33–38.

Hegardt, F.G. 1999. Mitochondrial 3-hydroxy-3-methylglutaryl-CoA synthase: A control enzyme in ketogenesis. *Biochem J.* 338(Pt 3):569–582.

Heimberg, M., Olubadewo, J.O., and Wilcox, H.G. 1985. Plasma lipoproteins and regulation of hepatic metabolism of fatty acids in altered thyroid states. *Endocr Rev.* 6(4):590–607.

Heller, F.R., Desager, J.P., and Harvengt, C. 1988. Changes in plasma activities of lipolytic enzymes and lipids of normolipidemic subjects given phenobarbital, a strong microsomal inducer, alone or in combination with fenofibrate. *Int J Clin Pharmacol Ther Toxicol.* 26(3):138–142.

Henderson, D.W., and Schlesinger, D.P. 2010. Use of a point-of-care beta-hydroxybutyrate sensor for detection of ketonemia in dogs. *Can Vet J.* 51(9):1000–1002.

Henkel, A.S., Anderson, K.A., Dewey, A.M., Kavesh, M.H., and Green, R.M. 2011. A chronic high-cholesterol diet paradoxically suppresses hepatic CYP7A1 expression in FVB/NJ mice. *J Lipid Res.* 52(2):289–298.

Herbert, P.N., Hyams, J.S., Bernier, D.N., et al. 1985. Apolipoprotein B-100 deficiency. Intestinal steatosis despite apolipoprotein B-48 synthesis. *J Clin Invest.* 76(2):403–412.

Herrera, E., Lasunción, M.A., Gomez-Coronado, D., Aranda, P., López-Luna, P., and Maier, I. 1988. Role of lipoprotein lipase activity on lipoprotein metabolism and the fate of circulating triglycerides in pregnancy. *Am J Obstet Gynecol.* 158(6 Pt 2):1575–1583.

Herrera, E., and Ortega, H. 2008. Metabolism in normal pregnancy. In *Textbook of Diabetes and Pregnancy*. Eds. M. Hod, L. Jovanovich, G.C. Di Renzo, A. De Leiva, and O. Lange, 2nd edition, pp. 25–34. London: Informa Healthcare.

Hidaka, H., Yamauchi, K., Ohta, H., Akamatsu, T., Honda, T., and Katsuyama, T. 2008. Specific, rapid, and sensitive enzymatic measurement of sphingomyelin, phosphatidylcholine and lysophosphatidylcholine in serum and lipid extracts. *Clin Biochem.* 41(14–15):1211–1217.

Higuchi, H. 2012. Molecular analysis of central feeding regulation by neuropeptide Y (NPY) neurons with NPY receptor small interfering RNAs (siRNAs). *Neurochem Int.* 61(6):936–941.

Hill, J.O., Talano, C.M., Nickel, M., and DiGirolamo, M. 1986. Energy utilization in food-restricted female rats. *J Nutr.* 116:2000–2012.

Hime, N.J., Drew, K.J., Wee, K., Barter, P.J., and Rye, K.A. 2006. Formation of high density lipoproteins containing both apolipoprotein A-I and A-II in the rabbit. *J Lipid Res.* 47(1):115–122.

Hing, S.A., and Lei, K.Y. 1991. Copper deficiency and hyperlipoproteinemia induced by a tetramine cupruretic agent in rabbits. *Biol Trace Elem Res.* 28(3):195–211.

Hirokane, H., Nakahara, M., Tachibana, S., Shimizu, M., and Sato, R. 2004. Bile acid reduces the secretion of very low density lipoprotein by repressing microsomal triglyceride transfer protein geneexpression mediated by hepatocyte nuclear factor-4. *J Biol Chem.* 279:45685–45692.

Hockey, K.J., Anderson, R.A., Cook, V.R., Hantgan, R.R., and Weinberg, R.B. 2001. Effect of the apolipoprotein A-IV Q360H polymorphism on postprandial plasma triglyceride clearance. *J Lipid Res.* 42(2):211–217.

Hoeks, J., van Herpen, N.A., Mensink, M., et al. 2010. Prolonged fasting identifies skeletal muscle mitochondrial dysfunction as consequence rather than cause of human insulin resistance. *Diabetes.* 59(9):2117–2125.

Hofker, M.H. 2010. APOC3 null mutation affects lipoprotein profile APOC3 deficiency: From mice to man. *Eur J Hum Genet.* 18(1):1–2.

Hofmann, A.F., and Mysels, K.J. 1992. Bile acid solubility and precipitation in vitro and in vivo: The role of conjugation, pH, and Ca2+ ions. *J Lipid Res.* 33(5):617--626.

Hogarth, C.A., Roy, A., and Ebert, D.L. 2003. Genomic evidence for the absence of a functional cholesteryl ester transfer protein gene in mice and rats. *Comp Biochem Physiol B Biochem Mol Biol.* 135(2):219–229.

Holden, P.R., and Tugwood, J.D. 1999. Peroxisome proliferator-activated receptor alpha: Role in rodent liver cancer and species differences. *J Mol Endocrinol.* 22(1):1–8.

Hollanders, B., Audé, X., and Girard-Globa, A. 1985. Lipoproteins and apoproteins of fetal and newborn piglets. *Biol Neonate.* 47(5):270–279.

Hollanders, B., Mougin, A., N'Diaye, F., Hentz, E., Aude, X., and Girard, A. 1986. Comparison of the lipoprotein profiles obtained from rat, bovine, horse, dog, rabbit and pig serum by a new two-step ultracentrifugal gradient procedure. *Comp Biochem Physiol B.* 84(1):83–89.

Horowitz, J.F. 2003. Fatty acid mobilization from adipose tissue during exercise. *Trends Endocrinol Metab.* 14(8):386–392.

Horton, J.D., Cuthbert, J.A., and Spady, D.K. 1995. Regulation of hepatic 7 alpha-hydroxylase expression and response to dietary cholesterol in the rat and hamster. *J Biol Chem.* 270(10):5381–5387.

Horwitz, B.A., Inokuchi, T., Wickler, S.J., and Stern, J.S. 1984. Lipoprotein lipase activity and cellularity in brown and white adipose tissue in Zucker obese rats. *Metabolism.* 33(4):354–357.

Hotta, M., Ohwada, R., Katakami, H., Shibasaki, T., Hizuka, N., and Takano, K. 2004. Plasma levels of intact and degraded ghrelin and their responses to glucose infusion in anorexia nervosa. *J Clin Endocrinol Metab.* 89(11):5707–5712.

Hoyenga, K.B., and Hoyenga, K.T. 1982. Gender and energy balance: Sex differences in adaptations for feast and famine. *Physiol Behav.* 28(3):545–563.

Hromadová, M, and Hácik, T. 1984. Intersex differences in plasma lipid content and in various lipoprotein fractions in New Zealand albino rabbits. *Endocrinol Exp.* 18(4):255–261.

Hromadová, M., and Hácik, T. 1988a. Effect of short-term estrogen administration on some parameters of lipoprotein metabolism in male rabbits. *Exp Clin Endocrinol.* 91(1):91–96.

Hromadová, M., and Hácik, T. 1988b. Effect of short-term androgen administration to rabbit females on their lipoprotein metabolism. *Endocrinol Exp.* 22(3):181–186.

Hu, J., Zhang, Z., Shen, W.J., and Azhar, S. 2010. Cellular cholesterol delivery, intracellular processing and utilization for biosynthesis of steroid hormones. *Nutr Metab.* 7:47–71.

Hu, T., Foxworthy, P., Siesky, A., et al. 2005. Hepatic peroxisomal fatty acid beta-oxidation is regulated by liver X receptor alpha. *Endocrinology.* 146(12):5380–5387.

Hu, X., Bonde, Y., Eggertsen, G., and Rudling, M. 2014. Muricholic bile acids are potent regulators of bile acid synthesis via a positive feedback mechanism. *J Intern Med.* 275(1):27–38.

Hubert, M.F., Laroque, P., Gillet, J.P., and Keenan, K.P. 2000. The effects of diet, ad libitum feeding, and moderate and severe dietary restriction on body weight, survival, clinical pathology parameters, and cause of death in control Sprague-Dawley rats. *Toxicol Sci.* 58(1):195–207.

Hui, D.Y., and Howles, P.N. 2002. Carboxyl ester lipase: Structure-function relationship and physiological role in lipoprotein metabolism and atherosclerosis. *J Lipid Res.* 43(12):2017–2030.

Hui, D.Y., Innerarity, T.L., Milne, R.W., Marcel, Y.L., and Mahley, R.W. 1984. Binding of chylomicron remnants and beta-very low density lipoproteins to hepatic and extrahepatic lipoprotein receptors. A process independent of apolipoprotein B48. *J Biol Chem.* 259(24):15060–15068.

Hussain, M.M., Maxfield, F.R., Más-Oliva, J., et al. 1991. Clearance of chylomicron remnants by the low density lipoprotein receptor-related protein/alpha 2-macroglobulin receptor. *J. Biol Chem.* 266(21):13936–13940.

Hussain, M.M., and Pan , X. 2012. Clock regulation of dietary lipid absorption. *Curr Opin Clin Nutr Metab Care.* 15(4):336–341.

Hussein, S.A., Azab, M.E., and Abdel-Maksoud, H. 1999. Metabolic changes concerning the effect of castration on some blood constituents in male rabbits. *Dtsch Tierarztl Wochenschr.* 106(3):113–118.

Iacono, J.M., and Ammerman, C.B. 1966. The effect of calcium in maintaining normal levels of serum cholesterol and phospholipids in rabbits during acute starvation. *Am J Clin Nutr.* 18(3):197–202.

Ishioka, K., Hatai, H., Komabayashi, K., et al. 2005. Diurnal variations of serum leptin in dogs: Effects of fasting and re-feeding. *Vet J.* 169(1):85–90.

Izar, M.C., Tegani, D.M., Kasmas, S.H., and Fonseca, F.A. 2011. Phytosterols and phytosterolemia: Gene-diet interactions. *Genes Nutr.* 6(1):17–26.

Jacobi, S.K., Ajuwon, K.M., Weber, T.E., Kuske, J.L., Dyer, C.J., and Spurlock, M.E. 2004. Cloning and expression of porcine adiponectin, and its relationship to adiposity, lipogenesis and the acute phase response. *J Endocrinol.* 182(1):133–144.

Jahangiri, A. 2010. High-density lipoprotein and the acute phase response. *Curr Opin Endocrinol Diabetes Obes.* 17(2):156–160.

Jahangiri, A., de Beer, M.C., Noffsinger, V., et al. 2009. HDL remodeling during the acute phase response. *Arterioscler Thromb Vasc Biol.* 29(2):261–267.

Je, Y.T., Sim, W.C., Kim, D.G., Jung, B.H., Shin, H.S., and Lee, B.H. 2015. Expression of CYP3A in chronic ethanol-fed mice is mediated by endogenous pregnane X receptor ligands formed by enhanced cholesterol metabolism. *Arch Toxicol.* 89(4):579–589.

Jeffery, F., and Redgrave, T.G. 1982. Chylomicron catabolism differs between Hooded and albino laboratory rats. *J Lipid Res.* 23(1):154–160.

Jelic, K., Hallgreen, C.E., and Colding-Jørgensen, M. 2009. A model of NEFA dynamics with focus on the postprandial state. *Ann Biomed Eng.* 37(9):1897–1909.

Jensen, M.D., Haymond, M.W., Gerich, J.E., Cryer, P.E., and Miles, J.M. 1987. Lipolysis during fasting. Decreased suppression by insulin and increased stimulation by epinephrine. *J Clin Invest.* 79(1):207–213.

Jerome, W.G. 2010. Lysosomes, cholesterol and atherosclerosis. *Clin Lipidol.* 5(6):853–865.

Jessen, R.H., Dass, C.J., and Eckfeldt. J.H. 1990. Do enzymatic analyses of serum triglycerides really need blanking for free glycerol? *Clin Chem.* 36(7):1372–1375.

Jiménez-Palomares, M., Cózar-Castellano, I., Ganfornina, M.D., Sánchez, D., and Perdomo, G. 2011. Genetic deficiency of apolipoprotein D in the mouse is associated with nonfasting hypertriglyceridemia and hyperinsulinemia. *Metabolism.* 60:1767–1774.

Johansen, T., Hansen, H.S., Richelsen, B., and Malmlof, R. 2001. The obese Gottingen minipig as a model of the metabolic syndrome: Dietary effects on obesity, insulin sensitivity, and growth hormone profile. *Comp Med.* 51(2):150–155.

Johnstone, A.C., Jones, B.R., Thompson, J.C., and Hancock, W.S. 1990. The pathology of an inherited hyperlipoproteinaemia of cats. *J Comp Pathol.* 102(2):125–137.

Jokinen, E.V., Landschulz, K.T., Wyne, K.L., Ho, Y.K., Frykman, P.K., and Hobbs, H.H. 1994. Regulation of the very low density lipoprotein receptor by thyroid hormone in rat skeletal muscle. *J Biol Chem.* 269(42):26411–26418.

Jones, R.D., Repa, J.J., Russell, D.W., Dietschy, J.M., and Turley, S.D. 2012. Delineation of biochemical, molecular, and physiological changes accompanying bile acid pool size restoration in Cyp7a1–/– mice fed low levels of cholic acid. *Am J Physiol Gastrointest Liver Physiol.* 303(2):G263–274.

Jong, M.C., Hofker, M.H., and Havekes, L.M. 1999. Role of ApoCs in lipoprotein metabolism: Functional differences between ApoC1, ApoC2, and ApoC3. *Arterioscler Thromb Vasc Biol.* 19(3):472–484.

Jørgensen, J.R., Fitch, M.D., Mortensen, P.B., and Fleming, S.E. 2001. In vivo absorption of medium-chain fatty acids by the rat colon exceeds that of short-chain fatty acids. *Gastroenterology.* 120(5):1152–1161.

Kalderon, B., Mayorek, N., Berry, E., Zevit, N., and Bar-Tana, J. 2000. Fatty acid cycling in the fasting rat. *Am J Physiol Endocrinol Metab.* 279(1):E221–227.

Kalogeris, T.J., and Story, J.A. 1992. Lymph chylomicron size is modified by fat saturation in rats. *J Nutr.* 122(8):1634–1642.

Kalopissis, A.D., Girard, A., and Griglio, S. 1979. Diurnal variations of plasma lipoproteins and liver lipids in rats fed starch sucrose or fat. *Horm Metab Res.* 11(2):118–122.

Kalra, S.P. 2011. Pivotal role of leptin–hypothalamus signaling in the etiology of diabetes uncovered by gene therapy: A new therapeutic intervention? *Gene Ther.* 18(4):319–325.

Karpe, F., Olivecrona, T., Olivecrona, G., et al. 1998. Lipoprotein lipase transport in plasma: Role of muscle and adipose tissues in regulation of plasma lipoprotein lipase concentrations. *J Lipid Res.* 39(12):2387–2393.

Kasbo, J., Saleem, M., Perwaiz, S., et al. 2002. Biliary, fecal and plasma deoxycholic acid in rabbit, hamster, guinea pig, and rat: Comparative study and implication in colon cancer. *Biol Pharm Bull.* 25(10):1381–1384

Kast, H.R., Nguyen, C.M., Sinal, C.J., et al. 2001. Farnesoid x activated receptor induces apolipoprotein c-II transcription: A molecular mechanism linking plasma triglyceride levels to bile acids. *Mol Endocrinol.* 15:1720–1728.

Kazumi, T., Yoshino, G., Kasama, T., Iwatani, I., Iwai, M., and Baba, S. 1989. Effects of dietary sucrose on age-related changes in VLDL-triglyceride kinetics in the rat. *Diabetes Res Clin Pract.* 6(3):185–190.

Kendrick, J.S., Chan, L., and Higgins, J.A. 2001. Superior role of apolipoprotein B48 over apolipoprotein B100 in chylomicron assembly and fat absorption: An investigation of apobec-1 knock-out and wild-type mice. *Biochem J.* 356(Pt 3):821–827.

Kersten, S. 2001. Mechanisms of nutritional and hormonal regulation of lipogenesis. *EMBO Rep.* 2(4):282–286.

Kessler, M.J., and Rawlins, R.G. 1983. Age- and pregnancy-related changes in serum total cholesterol and triglyceride levels in the Cayo Santiago rhesus macaques. *Exp Gerontol.* 18 (1):1–4.

Khalfallah, Y., Sassolas, G., Borson-Chazot, F., Vega, N., and Vidal, H. 2001. Expression of insulin target genes in skeletal muscle and adipose tissue in adult patients with growth hormone deficiency: Effect of one year recombinant human growth hormone therapy. *J Endocrinol.* 171(2):285–292.

Khan, A.A., Chow, E.C., Porte, R.J., Pang, K.S., and Groothuis, G.M. 2011. The role of lithocholic acid in the regulation of bile acid detoxication, synthesis, and transport proteins in rat and human intestine and liver slices. *Toxicol In Vitro.* 25(1):80–90.

Khovidhunkit, W., Kim, M.S., Memon, R.A., et al. 2004. Effects of infection and inflammation on lipid and lipoprotein metabolism: Mechanisms and consequences to the host. *J Lipid Res.* 45(7):1169–1196.

King, K.C. 2007. Apolipoprotein (Apo) C1 mice as a model of nonalcoholic fatty liver disease. Dissertation. Available at: https://e-scholar.uncc.edu/dspace/bitstream/2029/93/1/umi-uncc-1058

Kirby, R.J., Zheng, S., Tso, P., Howles, P.N., and Hui, D.Y. 2002. Bile salt-stimulated carboxyl ester lipase influences lipoprotein assembly and secretion in intestine: A process mediated via ceramide hydrolysis. *J Biol Chem.* 277(6):4104–4109.

Kitagawa, S., Yamaguchi, Y., Imaizumi, N., Kunitomo, M., and Fujiwara, M. 1992. A uniform alteration in serum lipid metabolism occurring during inflammation in mice. *Jpn J Pharmacol.* 58(1):37–46.

Kitao, N., Fukui, D., Shibata, H., Saito, M., Osborne, P.G., and Hashimoto, M. 2011. Seasonality and fasting effect in raccoon dog Nyctereutes procyonoides serum leptin levels determined by canine leptin-specific enzyme-linked immunosorbent assay. *J Exp Zool A Ecol Genet Physiol A.* 315(2):84–89.

Kluger, E.K., Caslake, M., Baral, R.M., Malik, R., and Govendir, M. 2010. Preliminary post-prandial studies of Burmese cats with elevated triglyceride concentrations and/or presumed lipid aqueous. *JFMS.* 12:621–630.

Kluger, M., Heeren, J., and Merkel, M. 2008. Apoprotein A-V: An important regulator of triglyceride metabolism. *Inherit Metab Dis.* 31(2):281–288.

Knopp, R.H., Warth, M.R., Charles, D., et al. 1986. Lipoprotein metabolism in pregnancy, fat transport to the fetus, and the effects of diabetes. *Biol Neonate.* 50(6):297–317.

Knorr, R., Karacsonyi, C., and Lindner, R. 2009. Endocytosis of MHC molecules by distinct membrane rafts. *J Cell Sci.* 122(Pt 10):1584–1594.

Kobayashi, K., Forte, T.M., Taniguchi, S., Ishida, B.Y., Oka, K., and Chan, L. 2000. The db/db mouse, a model for diabetic dyslipidemia: Molecular characterization and effects of Western diet feeding. *Metabolism.* 49(1):22–31.

Kojima, M., Hosoda, H., Date, Y., Nakazato, M., Matsuo, H., and Kangawa, K. 1999. Ghrelin is a growth-hormone releasing acylated peptide from stomach. *Nature.* 402(6762):656–660.

Kolditz, C.I., and Langin, D. 2010. Adipose tissue lipolysis. *Curr Opin Clin Nutr Metab Care.* 13(4):377–381.

Kolovou, G.D., Mikhailidis, D.P., Anagnostopoulou, K.K., Daskalopoulou, S.S., and Cokkinos, D.V. 2006. Tangier disease four decades of research: A reflection of the importance of HDL. *Curr Med Chem.* 13(7):771–782.

Kong, B., Wang, L., Chiang, J.Y.L., Zhang, Y., Klaassen, C.D., and Guo, G.L. 2012. Mechanism of tissue-specific farnesoid X receptor in suppressing the expression of genes in bile-acid synthesis in mice. *Hepatology.* 56(3):1034–1043.

Konig, B., Koch, A., Spielmann, J., et al. 2009. Activation of PPARalpha and PPARgamma reduces triacylglycerol synthesis in rat hepatoma cells by reduction of nuclear SREBP-1. *Eur J Pharmacol.* 605(1–3):23–30.

Konttinen, A., Pyoeraelae, T., and Carpen, E. 1964. Serum lipid pattern in normal pregnancy and pre-eclampsia. *J Obstet Gynaecol Br Commonw.* 71:453–458.

Kooijman, E.E., Chupin, V., de Kruijff, B., and Burger, K.N. 2003. Modulation of membrane curvature by phosphatidic acid and lysophosphatidic acid. *Traffic.* 4(3):162–174.

Koschinsky, M.L. 2004. Lipoprotein(a) and the link between atherosclerosis and thrombosis. *Can J Cardiol.* 20(Suppl B):37B–43B.

Kostoglou-Athanassiou, I., Gkountouvas, A., Keramidas, I., Xanthakou, E., Chatjimarkou, F., and Kaldrymidis, P. 2013. Lipid levels in acromegaly. In Endocrine Abstracts from *15th European Congress of Endocrinology*, 32, p. 172.

Kowal, R.C., Herz, J., Weisgraber, K.H., Mahley, R.W., Brown, M.S., and Goldstein, J.L. 1990. Opposing effects of apolipoproteins E and C on lipoprotein binding to low density lipoprotein receptor-related protein. *J Biol Chem.* 265:10771–10779.

Kraemer, F.B., Laane, C., Park, B., and Sztalryd, C. 1994. Low-density lipoprotein receptors in rat adipocytes: Regulation with fasting. *Am J Physiol.* 266(1 Pt 1):E26–32.

Kraemer, F.B., Shen, W.J., Natu, V., et al. 2002. Adrenal neutral cholesteryl ester hydrolase: Identification, subcellular distribution, and sex differences. *Endocrinology.* 143(3):801–806.

Krausz, Y., Bar-On, H., and Shafrir, E. 1981. Origin and pattern of glucocorticoid-induced hyperlipidemia in rats. Dose-dependent bimodal changes in serum lipids and lipoproteins in relation to hepatic lipogenesis and tissue lipoprotein lipase activity. *Biochim Biophys Acta.* 663(1):69–82.

Krell, H., Metz, J., Jaeschke, H., Höke, H., and Pfaff, E. 1987. Drug-induced intrahepatic cholestasis: Characterization of different pathomechanisms. *Arch Toxicol.* 60(1–3):124–130.

Kriketos, A.D., Gan, S.K., Poynten, A.M., Furler, S.M., Chisholm, D.J., and Campbell, L.V. 2004. Exercise increases adiponectin levels and insulin sensitivity in humans. *Diabetes Care.* 27(2):629–630.

Kritchevsky, D., Davidson, L.M., Shapiro, I.L., et al. 1974. Lipid metabolism and experimental atherosclerosis in baboons: Influence of cholesterol-free, semi-synthetic diets. *Am J Clin Nutr.* 27(1):29–50.

Kritchevsky, D., Tepper, S.A., Vesselinovitch, D., and Wissler, R.W. 1971. Cholesterol vehicle in experimental atherosclerosis. Part II. Peanut oil. *Atherosclerosis.* 14(1):53–64.

Kubegov, A.C., and Karpen, S.J. 2008. Bile formation and cholestasis. In *Walker's Pediatric Gastrointestinal Disease*. Eds. R. Kleinman, O. Goulet, G. Mieli-Vergani, I. Sanderson, and P. Sherman, 5th edition, Chap. 28.1, pp. 757–766. Lewiston, NY: BC Decker, Inc.

Kung, A.W., Pang, R.W., Lauder, I., Lam, K.S., and Janus, E.D. 1995. Changes in serum lipoprotein(a) and lipids during treatment of hyperthyroidism. *Clin Chem.* 41:226–231.

Kuwahata, M., Kubota, H., Amano, S., et al. 2011. Dietary medium-chain triglycerides attenuate hepatic lipid deposition in growing rats with protein malnutrition. *J Nutr Sci Vitaminol (Tokyo).* 57(2):138–143.

Kwik, J., Boyle, S., Fooksman, D., Margolis, L., Sheetz, M.P., and Edidin, M. 2003. Membrane cholesterol, lateral mobility, and the phosphatidylinositol 4,5-bisphosphate-dependent organization of cell actin. *Proc Natl Acad Sci U S A.* 100(24):13964–13969.

Lacombe, C., Corraze, G., and Nibbelink, M. 1983. Increases in hyperlipoproteinemia, disturbances in cholesterol metabolism and atherosclerosis induced by dietary restriction in rabbits fed a cholesterol-rich diet. *Lipids.* 18(4):306–312.

Lado-Abeal, J., Robert-McComb, J.J., Qian, X.P., Leproult, R., Van Cauter, E., and Norman, R.L. 2005. Sex differences in the neuroendocrine response to short-term fasting in rhesus macaques. *J Neuroendocrinol.* 17(7):435–444.

Laffel, L. 1999. Ketone bodies: A review of physiology, pathophysiology and application of monitoring to diabetes. *Diabetes Metab Res Rev.* 15(6):412–426.

Lafontan, M. 1981. Alpha-adrenergic responses in rabbit white fat cells: The influence of obesity and food restriction. *J Lipid Res.* 22(7):1084–1093.

Lafontan, M., and Berlan, M. 1993. Fat cell adrenergic receptors and the control of white and brown fat cell function. *J Lipid Res.* 34(7):1057–1091.

Lafontan, M., Berlan, M., and Carpene, C. 1985. Fat cell adrenoceptors: Inter- and intraspecific differences and hormone regulation. *Int J Obes.* 9(Suppl 1):117–127.

Landschulz, K.T., Pathak, R.K., Rigotti, A., Krieger, M., and Hobbs, H.H. 1996. Regulation of scavenger receptor, class B1, type I, a high density lipoprotein receptor, in liver and steroidogenic tissues of the rat. *J Clin Invest.* 98:984–995.

Lane, M.A., Tilmont, E.M., De Angelis, H., et al. 2000. Short-term calorie restriction improves disease-related markers in older male rhesus monkeys (*Macaca mulatta*). *Mech Ageing Dev.* 112(3):185–196.

Langin, D., Portillo, M.P., Saulnier-Blache, J.S., and Lafontan, M. 1991. Coexistence of three beta-adrenoceptor subtypes in white fat cells of various mammalian species. *Eur J Pharmacol.* 199(3):291–301.

LaPorte, R., Valvo-Gerard, L., Kuller, L., et al. 1981. The relationship between alcohol consumption, liver enzymes and high-density lipoprotein cholesterol. *Circulation.* 64(3 Pt 2):III 67–72.

Large, W.A. 2002. Receptor-operated Ca2(+)-permeable nonselective cation channels in vascular smooth muscle: A physiologic perspective. *J Cardiovasc Electrophysiol.* 13(5):493–501.

Lasser, N.L., Roheim, P.S., Edelstein, D., and Eder, H.A. 1973. Serum lipoproteins of normal and cholesterol-fed rats. *J Lipid Res.* 14(1):1–8.

Lata, H., Ahuja, G.K., and Narang, A.P. 2002. Effect of starvation stress on lipid peroxidation and lipid profile in rabbits. *Indian J physiol pharmacol.* 46(3):371–374.

Lawn, R.M. 1996. How often has Lp(a) evolved? *Clin Genet.* 49(4):167–174.

Lawn, R.M., Boonmark, N.W., Schwartz, K., et al. 1995. The recurring evolution of lipoprotein(a). Insights from cloning hedgehog apolipoprotein(a). *J Biol Chem.* 270:24004–24009.

Leblanc, M., Bélanger, M.C., Julien, P., et al. 2004. Plasma lipoprotein profile in the male cynomolgus monkey under normal, hypogonadal, and combined androgen blockade conditions. *J Clin Endocrinol Metab.* 89(4):1849–1857.

Lefevre, M., Chuang, M.Y., and Roheim, P.S. 1986. ApoA-IV metabolism in the rat: Role of lipoprotein lipase and apolipoprotein transfer. *J Lipid Res.* 27(11):1163–1173.

Lefevre, M., Keen, C.L., Lönnerdal, B., Hurley, L.S., and Schneeman, B.O. 1985. Different effects of zinc and copper deficiency on composition of plasma high density lipoproteins in rats. *J Nutr.* 115(3):359–368.

Lehman-McKeeman, L. 2013. Biochemical and molecular basis of toxicity. In *Haschek and Rousseaux's Handbook of Toxicologic Pathology*. Eds. W.M. Haschek, C.G. Rousseaux, and M.A. Wallig, 3rd edition, pp. 15–38. Waltham, MA: Elsevier.

Lehmann, R., Bhargava, A.S., and Günzel, P. 1993. Serum lipoprotein pattern in rats, dogs and monkeys, including method comparison and influence of menstrual cycle in monkeys. *Eur J Clin Chem Clin Biochem.* 31(10):633–637.

Leighton, J.K., Joyner, J., Zamarripa, J., Deines, M., and Davis, R.A. 1990. Fasting decreases apolipoprotein B mRNA editing and the secretion of small molecular weight apoB by rat hepatocytes: evidence that the total amount of apoB secreted is regulated post-transcriptionally. *J Lipid Res.* 31(9):1663–1668.

Lessig, J., and Fuchs, B. 2009. Plasmalogens in biological systems: Their role in oxidative processes in biological membranes, their contribution to pathological processes and aging and plasmalogen analysis. *Curr Med Chem.* 16:2021–2041.

Levine, B.S. 2009. Animal clinical pathology. In *CRC Handbook of Toxicology*. Eds M.J. Derelanko, and M.A. Hollinger, pp. 517–537. Boca Raton, FL: CRC Press.

Li, C.J., Zhu, F.L., Sun, H.W., et al. 2008. Cloning of rabbit adiponectin and its relationship to age and high-cholesterol diet. *J Endocrinol Invest.* 31(9):755–759.

Li, G., Thomas, A.M., Williams, J.A., et al. 2012. Farnesoid X receptor induces murine scavenger receptor class B type I via intron binding. *PLoS One.* 7(4):e35895.

Li, J., Fang, B., Eisensmith, R.C., et al. 1995. In vivo gene therapy for hyperlipidemia: Phenotypic correction in Watanabe rabbits by hepatic delivery of the rabbit LDL receptor gene. *J Clin Invest.* 95 (2):768–773.

Li, T., and Chiang, J.Y. 2009. Regulation of bile acid and cholesterol metabolism by PPARs. *PPAR Res.* 2009:501739.

Li, T., and Chiang, J.Y. 2013. Nuclear receptors in bile acid metabolism. *Drug Metab Rev.* 45(1):145–155.

Li, X., Becker, K.A., and Zhang, Y. 2010. Ceramide in redox signaling and cardiovascular diseases. *Cell Physiol Biochem.* 26(1):41–48.

Li, X., Peegel, H., and Menon, K.M. 1998. In situ hybridization of high density lipoprotein (scavenger type 1) receptor messenger ribonucleic acid (mRNA) during folliculogenesis and luteinization: Evidence for mRNA expression and induction by human chorionic gonadotropin specifically in cell types that use cholesterol for steroidogenesis. *Endocrinology.* 139:3043–3049.

Liberati, T.A., Sansone, S.R., and Feuston, M.H. 2004. Hematology and clinical chemistry values in pregnant Wistar Hannover rats compared with nonmated controls. *Vet Clin Pathol.* 33(2):68–73.

Lindén, D., Sjöberg, A., Asp, L., Carlsson, L., and Oscarsson, J. 2000. Direct effects of growth hormone on production and secretion of apolipoprotein B from rat hepatocytes. *Am J Physiol Endocrinol Metab.* 279(6):E1335–1346.

Lioi, S.A., Rigalli, A., and Puche, R.C. 2010. Effect of rhGH on the synthesis and secretion of VLDL to lymph and plasma from the intestine of the female rat. *Growth Horm IGF Res.* 20(2):141–148.

Liu, G.L., Fan, L.M., and Redinger, R.N. 1991. The association of hepatic apoprotein and lipid metabolism in hamsters and rats. *Comp Biochem Physiol A Comp Physiol.* 99(1–2):223–228.

Liu, Y., Wang, Z., Yin, W., et al. 2007. Severe insulin resistance and moderate glomerulosclerosis in a minipig model induced by high-fat/ high-sucrose/ high-cholesterol diet. *Exp Anim.* 56(1):11–20.

Loeb, W.F., and Quimby, F.W(Eds.). 1999. *The Clinical Chemistry of Laboratory Animals*, 2nd edition. Philadelphia, PA: Taylor and Francis.

Longo, N., Amat di San Filippo, C., and Pasquali, M. 2006. Disorders of carnitine transport and the carnitine cycle. *Am J Med Genet C Semin Med Genet.* 142C(2):77–85.

Lu, K., Lee, M.H., and Patel, S.B. 2001. Dietary cholesterol absorption; more than just bile. *Trends Endocrinol Metab.* 12(7):314–320.

Lundell, K., and Wikvall, K. 2008. Species-specific and age-dependent bile acid composition: Aspects on CYP8B and CYP4A subfamilies in bile acid biosynthesis. *Curr Drug Metab.* 9(4):323–331.

Luo, C.C., Li, W.H., and Chan, L. 1989. Structure and expression of dog apolipoprotein A-I, E, and C-I mRNAs: Implications for the evolution and functional constraints of apolipoprotein structure. *J Lipid Res.* 30(11):1735–1746.

Luoma, P.V. 1988. Microsomal enzyme induction, lipoproteins and atherosclerosis. *Pharmacol Toxicol.* 62(5):243–249.

Luoma, P.V., Sotaniemi, E.A., Pelkonen, R.O., Arranto, A., and Ehnholm, C. 1982. Plasma high-density lipoproteins and hepatic microsomal enzyme induction. Relation to histological changes in the liver. *Eur J Clin Pharmacol.* 23(3):275–282.

Madani, S., Prost, J., Narce, M., and Belleville, J. 2003. VLDL metabolism in rats is affected by the concentration and source of dietary protein. *J Nutr.* 133(12):4102–4106.

Magun, A.M., Mish, B., and Glickman, R.M. 1988. Intracellular apoA-I and apoB distribution in rat intestine is altered by lipid feeding. *J Lipid Res.* 29(9):1107–1116.

Mahley, R.W., and Ji, Z.S. 1999. Remnant lipoprotein metabolism: Key pathways involving cell-surface heparan sulfate proteoglycans and apolipoprotein E. *J Lipid Res.* 40(1):1–16.

Mahley, R.W., Weisgraber, K.H., Innerarity, T., Brewer, H.B., Jr., and Assmann, G. 1975. Swine lipoproteins and atherosclerosis. Changes in the plasma lipoproteins and apoproteins induced by cholesterol feeding. *Biochemistry.* 14(13):2817–2823.

Makino, K., Abe, A., Maeda, S., Noma, A., Kawade, M., and Takenaka, O. 1989. Lipoprotein(a) in nonhuman primates. Presence and characteristics of Lp(a) immunoreactive materials using anti-human Lp(a) serum. *Atherosclerosis.* 78(1):81–85.

Maldonado Castro, G.F., Escobar-Morreale, H.F., Ortega, H., et al. 2000. Effects of normalization of GH hypersecretion on lipoprotein(a) and other lipoprotein serum levels in acromegaly. *Clin Endocrinol (Oxf).* 53(3):313–319.

Malerød, L., Sporstøl, M., Juvet, L.K., et al. 2005. Bile acids reduce SR-BI expression in hepatocytes by a pathway involving FXR/RXR, SHP, and LRH-1. *Biochem Biophys Res Commun.* 336(4):1096–1105.

Malmström, R., Packard, C.J., Watson, T.D., et al. 1997. Metabolic basis of hypotriglyceridemic effects of insulin in normal men. *Arterioscler Thromb Vasc Biol.* 17(7):1454–1464.

Malva, J.O., Xapelli, S., Baptista, S., et al. 2012. Multifaces of neuropeptide Y in the brain – neuroprotection, neurogenesis, and neuroinflammation. *Neuropeptides.* 46:299–308.

Mangiapane, E.H., and Brindley, D.N. 1986. Effects of dexamethasone and insulin on the synthesis of triacylglycerols and phosphatidylcholine and the secretion of very-low-density lipoproteins and lysophosphatidylcholine by monolayer cultures of rat hepatocytes. *Biochem J.* 233(1):151–160.

Mansbach, C.M., and Siddiqi, S.A. 2010. The biogenesis of chylomicrons. *Annu Rev Physiol.* 72:315–333.

Marcus, C., Ehrén, H., Bolme, P., and Arner, P. 1988. Regulation of lipolysis during the neonatal period. Importance of thyrotropin. *J Clin Invest.* 82(5):1793–1797.

Markel, A., Brook, J.G., and Aviram, M. 1985. Increased plasma triglycerides, cholesterol and apolipoprotein E during prolonged fasting in normal subjects. *Postgrad Med J.* 61(715):395–400.

Marrino, P., Gavish, D., Shafrir, E., and Eisenberg, S. 1987. Diurnal variations of plasma lipids, tissue and plasma lipoprotein lipase, and VLDL secretion rates in the rat. A model for studies of VLDL metabolism. *Biochim Biophys Acta.* 920(3):277–284.

Martín-Hidalgo, A., Holm, C., Belfrage, P., Scott, J., and Herrera, E. 1994. Lipoprotein lipase and hormone sensitive lipase activity and mRNA in rat adipose tissue during pregnancy. *Am. J. Physiol.* 266:E930–935.

Martins, I.J., Hone, E., Chi, C., Seydel, U., Martins, R.N., and Redgrave, T.G. 2000. Relative roles of LDLr and LRP in the metabolism of chylomicron remnants in genetically manipulated mice. *J Lipid Res.* 41(2):205–213.

Marzetta, C.A., and Rudel, L.L. 1986. A species comparison of low density lipoprotein heterogeneity in nonhuman primates fed atherogenic diets. *J Lipid Res.* 27(7):753–762.

Masucci-Magoulas, L., Moulin, P., Jiang, X.C., et al. 1995. Decreased cholesteryl ester transfer protein (CETP) mRNA and protein and increased high density lipoprotein following lipopolysaccharide administration in human CETP transgenic mice. *J Clin Invest.* 95(4):1587–1594.

Matsuzawa, T., Nomura, M., and Unno, T. 1993. Clinical pathology reference ranges of laboratory animals. Working Group II, Nonclinical Safety Evaluation Subcommittee of the Japan Pharmaceutical Manufacturers Association. *J Vet Med Sci.* 55(3):351–362.

Mattison, J.A., Roth, G.S., Beasley, T.M., et al. 2012. Impact of caloric restriction on health and survival in rhesus monkeys from the NIA study. *Nature.* 489(7415):318–321.

Maxwell, K.N., and Breslow, J.L. 2005. Proprotein convertase subtilisin kexin 9: The third locus implicated in autosomal dominant hypercholesterolemia. *Curr Opin Lipidol.* 16(2):167–172.

Mazuy, C., Helleboid, A., Staels, B., and Lefebvre, P. 2015. Nuclear bile acid signaling through the farnesoid X receptor. *Cell Mol Life Sci.* 72(9):1631–1650.

McCowen, K.C., Maykel, J.A., Bistrian, B.R., and Ling, P.R. 2002. Circulating ghrelin concentrations are lowered by intravenous glucose or hyperinsulinemic euglycemic conditions in rodents. *J Endocrinol.* 175(2):R7–11.

McCoy, M.G., Sun, G.S., Marchadier, D., Maugeais, C., Glick, J.M., and Rader, D.J. 2002. Characterization of the lipolytic activity of endothelial lipase. *J Lipid Res.* 43(6):921–929.

McEntyre, C.J., Lever, M., and Storer, M.K. 2004. A high performance liquid chromatographic method for the measurement of total carnitine in human plasma and urine. *Clin Chim Acta.* 344(1–2):123–130.

McKee, A., and Russell, J.A. 1968. Effect of acute hypophysectomy and growth hormone on FFA mobilization, nitrogen excretion and cardiac glycogen in fasting rats. *Endocrinology.* 83(6):1162–1165.

McMullin, T.S., Lowe, E.R., Bartels, M.J., and Marty MS. 2008. Dynamic changes in lipids and proteins of maternal, fetal, and pup blood and milk during perinatal development in CD and Wistar rats. *Toxicol Sci.* 105(2):260–274.

Meertens, L.M., Miyata, K.S., Cechetto, J.D., Rachubinski, R.A., and Capone, J.P. 1998. A mitochondrial ketogenic enzyme regulates its gene expression by association with the nuclear hormone receptor PPARalpha. *EMBO J.* 17(23):6972–6978.

Menéndez, L.G., Fernández, A.L., Enguix, A., Ciriza, C., and Amador, J. 2001. Effect of storage of plasma and serum on enzymatic determination of non-esterified fatty acids. *Ann Clin Biochem.* 38(Pt 3):252–255.

Merl, V., Peters, A., Oltmanns, K.M., et al. 2005. Serum adiponectin concentrations during a 72-hour fast in over- and normal-weight humans. *Int J Obes (Lond).* 29(8):998–1001.

Merrill, A.H., Jr. 2011. Sphingolipid and glycosphingolipid metabolic pathways in the era of sphingolipidomics. *Chem Rev.* 111(10):6387–6422.

Meyer, B.J., Ha, Y.C., and Barter, P.J. 1989. Effects of experimental hypothyroidism on the distribution of lipids and lipoproteins in the plasma of rats. *Biochim Biophys Acta.* 1004(1):73–79.

Meyers, D.S., Skwish, S., Dickinson, K.E., Kienzle, B., and Arbeeny, C.M. 1997. Beta 3-adrenergic receptor-mediated lipolysis and oxygen consumption in brown adipocytes from cynomolgus monkeys. *J Clin Endocrinol Metab.* 82(2):395–401.

Miettinen, T.A. 1982. Diurnal variation of cholesterol precursors squalene and methyl sterols in human plasma lipoproteins. *J Lipid Res.* 23(3):466–473.

Mirani-Oostdijk, C.P., van Gent, C.M., Terpstra, J., Hessel, L.W., and Frölich, M. 1981. Diurnal levels of lipids, glucose and insulin in type IV hyperlipidemic patients on high carbohydrate and high fat diet: comparison with normals. *Acta Med Scand.* 210(4):277–282.

Moczulski, D., Majak, I., and Mamczur, D. 2009. An overview of beta-oxidation disorders. *Postepy Hig Med Dosw.* 63:266–277.

Møller, N., and Jørgensen, J.O. 2009. Effects of growth hormone on glucose, lipid, and protein metabolism in human subjects. *Endocr Rev.* 30(2):152–177.

Møller, N., Jørgensen, J.O., Alberti, K.G., Flyvbjerg, A., and Schmitz, O. 1990. Short-term effects of growth hormone on fuel oxidation and regional substrate metabolism in normal man. *J Clin Endocrinol Metab.* 70(4):1179–1186.

Møller, N., Møller, J., Jørgensen, J.O., et al. 1993. Impact of 2 weeks high dose growth hormone treatment on basal and insulin stimulated substrate metabolism in humans. *Clin Endocrinol (Oxf).* 39(5):577–581.

Mondola, P., Gambardella, P., Santangelo, F., Santillo, M., and Greco, A.M. 1995. Circadian rhythms of lipid and apolipoprotein pattern in adult fasted rats. *Physiol Behav.* 58(1):175–180.

Monks, A., and Richens, A. 1979. Serum protein binding of valproic acid and its displacement by palmitic acid in vitro. *Br J Clin Pharmacol.* 8(2):187–189.

Mora, S., Rifai, N., Buring, J.E., and Ridker, P.M. 2008. Fasting compared with nonfasting lipids and apolipoproteins for predicting incident cardiovascular events. *Circulation.* 118(10):993–1001.

Moreau, A., Vilarem, M.J., Maurel, P., and Pascussi, J.M. 2008. Xenoreceptors CAR and PXR activation and consequences on lipid metabolism, glucose homeostasis, and inflammatory response. *Mol Pharmaceutics.* 5:35–41.

Mori, N., Lee, P., Kondo, K., Kido, T., Saito, T., and Arai, T. 2011. Potential use of cholesterol lipoprotein profile to confirm obesity status in dogs. *Vet Res Commun.* 35(4):223–235.

Moriyama, T., Miyazawa, H., Tomohiro, M., Fujikake, N., Samura, K., and Nishikibe, M. 2006. Beneficial effect of moderate food restriction in toxicity studies in rats. *J Toxicol Sci.* 31(3):197–206.

Mowri, O-H., Patsch, J.R., Gotto, A.M., and Wolfgang, W. 1996. Apolipoprotein A-II influences the substrate properties of human HDL2 and HDL3 for hepatic lipase. *Arterioscler Thromb Vasc Biol.* 16:755–762.

Mudaliar, S., Henry, R.R., Sanyal, A.J., et al. 2013. Efficacy and safety of the farnesoid X receptor agonist obeticholic acid in patients with type 2 diabetes and nonalcoholic fatty liver disease. *Gastroenterology.* 145(3):574–582.

Mueller, P., Schulze, A., Schindler, I., Ethofer, T., Buehrdel, P., and Ceglarek, U. 2003. Validation of an ESI-MS/MS screening method for acylcarnitine profiling in urine specimens of neonates, children, adolescents and adults. *Clin Chim Acta.* 327(1–2):47–57.

Mukherjee, R., Jow, L., Noonan, D., and McDonnell, D.P. 1994. Human and rat peroxisome proliferator activated receptors (PPARs) demonstrate similar tissue distribution but different responsiveness to PPAR activators. *J Steroid Biochem Mol Biol.* 51(3–4):157–166.

Müller, M.J., Paschen, U., and Seitz, H.J. 1983. Thyroid hormone regulation of glucose homeostasis in the miniature pig. *Endocrinology.* 112(6):2025–2031.

Murota, K., and Storch, J. 2005. Uptake of micellar long-chain fatty acid and sn-2-monoacylglycerol into human intestinal Caco-2 cells exhibits characteristics of protein-mediated transport. *J Nutr.* 135(7):1626–1630.

Nagan, N., and Zoeller, R.A. 2001. Plasmalogens: Biosynthesis and functions. *Prog Lipid Res.* 40(3):199–229.

Nagano, M., Kuroki, S., Mizuta, A., et al. 2004. Regulation of bile acid synthesis under reconstructed enterohepatic circulation in rats. *Steroids.* 69(10):701–709.

Nam, S.Y., and Marcus, C. 2000. Growth hormone and adipocyte function in obesity. *Horm Res.* 53(Suppl 1):87–97.

Nantermet, P., Harada, S., Liu, Y., et al. 2008. Gene expression analyses in cynomolgus monkeys provides mechanistic insight into high-density lipoprotein-cholesterol reduction by androgens in primates. *Endocrinology.* 149(4):1551–1561.

Nassir, F., Wilson, B., Han, X., Gross, R.W., and Abumrad, N.A. 2007. CD36 is important for fatty acid and cholesterol uptake by the proximal but not distal intestine. *J Biol Chem.* 282(27):19493–19501.

Nesic, D.M., Stevanovic, D.M., Stankovic, S.D., et al. 2013. Age-dependent modulation of central ghrelin effects on food intake and lipid metabolism in rats. *Eur J Pharmacol.* 710(1–3):85–91.

Ness, G.C., and Zhao, Z. 1994. Thyroid hormone rapidly induces hepatic LDL receptor mRNA levels in hypophysectomized rats. *Arch Biochem Biophys.* 315:199–202.

Nguyen, L.B., Xu, G., Shefer, S., Tint, G.S., Batta, A., and Salen, G. 1999. Comparative regulation of hepatic sterol 27-hydroxylase and cholesterol 7alpha-hydroxylase activities in the rat, guinea pig, and rabbit: Effects of cholesterol and bile acids. *Metabolism.* 48(12):1542–1548.

Nickerson, J.G., Alkhateeb, H., Benton, C.R., et al. 2009. Greater transport efficiencies of the membrane fatty acid transporters FAT/CD36 and FATP4 compared with FABPpm and FATP1 and differential effects on fatty acid esterification and oxidation in rat skeletal muscle. *J Biol Chem.* 284(24):16522–16530.

Nielsen, J.H. 1982. Effects of growth hormone, prolactin, and placental lactogen on insulin content and release, and deoxyribonucleic acid synthesis in cultured pancreatic islets. *Endocrinology.* 110:600–606.

Nielsen, T.S., Jessen, N., Jørgensen, J.O., Møller, N., and Lund, S. 2014. Dissecting adipose tissue lipolysis: Molecular regulation and implications for metabolic disease. *J Mol Endocrinol.* 52(3):R199–222.

Nikkilä, E.A., and Kekki, M. 1972. Plasma triglyceride metabolism in thyroid disease. *J Clin Invest.* 51(8):2103–2114.

Nolte, C.J., Tercyak, A.M., Wu, H.M., and Small, D.M. 1990. Chemical and physiochemical comparison of advanced atherosclerotic lesions of similar size and cholesterol content in cholesterol-fed New Zealand White and Watanabe Heritable Hyperlipidemic rabbits. *Lab Invest.* 62(2):213–222.

Nonogaki, K., Fuller, G.M., Fuentes, N.L., et al. 1995. Interleukin-6 stimulates hepatic triglyceride secretion in rats. *Endocrinology.* 136(5):2143–2149.

Norlin, M., and Wikvall, K. 2007. Enzymes in the conversion of cholesterol into bile acids. *Curr Mol Med.* 7(2):199–218.

Nousiainen, U., and Ryhänen, R. 1984. Serum lipids and hepatic microsomal enzymes with special reference to serum cholinesterase in Wistar rats. *Gen Pharmacol.* 15(2):123–127.

Ockner, R.K., Hughes, F.B., and Isselbacher, K.J. 1969. Very low density lipoproteins in intestinal lymph: Origin, composition, and role in lipid transport in the fasting state. *J Clin Invest.* 48(11):2079–2088.

Ohtani, H., Hayashi, K., Hirata, Y., et al. 1990. Effects of dietary cholesterol and fatty acids on plasma cholesterol level and hepatic lipoprotein metabolism. *J Lipid Res.* 31(8):1413–1422.

Olofsson, S.O., and Borèn, J. 2005. Apolipoprotein B: A clinically important apolipoprotein which assembles atherogenic lipoproteins and promotes the development of atherosclerosis. *J Intern Med.* 258(5):395–410.

Olsen, A.K., Bladbjerg, E.M., Marckmann, P., Larsen, L.F., and Hansen, A.K. 2002. The Gottingen minipig as a model for postprandial hyperlipidaemia in man: Experimental observations. *Lab Anim.* 36(4):438–444.

Oscarsson, J., Ottosson, M., and Edén S. 1999. Effects of growth hormone on lipoprotein lipase and hepatic lipase. *J Endocrinol Invest.* 22(Suppl 5):2–9.

Oscarsson, J., Olofsson, S.O., Vikman, K., and Edén, S. 1991. Growth hormone regulation of serum lipoproteins in the rat: Different growth hormone regulatory principles for apolipoprotein (apo) B and the sexually dimorphic apoE concentrations. *Metabolism.* 40(11):1191–1198.

Ouguerram, K., Nguyen, P., Krempf, M., et al. 2004. Selective uptake of high density lipoproteins cholesteryl ester in the dog, a species lacking in cholesteryl ester transfer protein activity; An in vivo approach using stable isotopes. *Comp Biochem Physiol B Biochem Mol Biol.* 138(4):339–345.

Pan, Y., Larson, B., Araujo, J.A., et al. 2010. Dietary supplementation with medium-chain TAG has long-lasting cognition-enhancing effects in aged dogs. *Br J Nutr.* 103(12):1746–1754.

Parilla, R. 1978. Flux of metabolic fuels during starvation in the rat. *Pfluegers Arch.* 374:3–7.

Parini, P., Angelin, B., Stavréus-Evers, A., Freyschuss, B., Eriksson, H., and Rudling, M. 2000. Biphasic effects of the natural estrogen 17beta-estradiol on hepatic cholesterol metabolism in intact female rats. *Arterioscler Thromb Vasc Biol.* 20(7):1817–1823.

Parks, D.J., Blanchard, S.G., Bledsoe, R.K., et al. 1999. Bile acids: Natural ligands for an orphan nuclear receptor. *Science.* 284(5418):1365–1368.

Pasquini, A., Luchetti, E., and Cardini, G. 2008. Plasma lipoprotein concentrations in the dog: The effects of gender, age, breed and diet. *J Anim Physiol Anim Nutr.* 92(6):718–722.

Patel, M., Mishra, V., Pawar, V., Ranvir, R., Sundar, R., and Dabhi, R. 2013. Evaluation of acute physiological and molecular alterations in surgically developed hypothyroid Wistar rats. *J Pharmacol Pharmacother.* 4(2):110–115.

Peakall, D.B. 1976. Effects of toxaphene on hepatic enzyme induction and circulating steroid levels in the rat. *Environ Health Perspect.* 13:117–120.

Pecquery, R., Leneveu, M.C., and Giudicelli, Y. 1983. Characterization of the β-adrenergic receptors of hamster white fat cells. Evidence against an important role for the α,-receptor subtype in the adrenergic control of lipolysis. *Biochim Biophys Acta.* 731:397–405.

Penno, C.A., Morgan, S.A., Vuorinen, A., Schuster, D., Lavery, G.G., and Odermatt, A. 2013. Impaired oxidoreduction by 11β-hydroxysteroid dehydrogenase 1 results in the accumulation of 7-oxolithocholic acid. *J Lipid Res.* 54(10):2874–2883.

Perdomo, G., Kim, D.H., Zhang, T., et al. 2010. A role of apolipoprotein D in triglyceride metabolism. *J Lipid Res.* 51(6):1298–1311.

Phillips, G.B. 1959. The phospholipid composition of human serum lipoprotein fractions separated by ultracentrifugation. *J Clin Invest.* 38(3):489.

Picard, F., Naïmi, N., Richard, D., and Deshaies, Y. 1999. Response of adipose tissue lipoprotein lipase to the cephalic phase of insulin secretion. *Diabetes.* 48(3):452–459.

Piccione, G., Fazio, F., Giudice, E., Grasso, F., and Caola, G. 2004. Blood lipids, fecal fat and chymotrypsin excretion in the dog: Influence of age, body weight and sex. *J Vet Med Sci.* 66(1):59–62.

Pineda Torra, I., Claudel, T., Duval, C., Kosykh, V., Fruchart, J-C., and Staels, B. 2003. Bile acids induce the expression of the human peroxisome proliferator-activated receptor alpha gene via activation of the farnesoid × receptor. *Mol Endocrinol.* 17:259–272.

Pohl, J., Ring, A., Hermann, T., and Stremmel, W. 2004. Role of FATP in parenchymal cell fatty acid uptake. *Biochim Biophys Acta.* 1686(1–2):1–6.

Pond, W.G., Banis, R.J., Van Vleck, L.D., Walker, E.F., Jr., and Chapman, P. 1968. Age changes in body weight and in several blood components of conventional versus miniature pigs. *Proc Soc Exp Biol Med.* 127(3):895–900.

Pownall, H.J. and Hamilton, J.A. 2003. Energy translocation across cell membranes and membrane models. *Acta Physiol Scand.* 178(4):357–365.

Priego, T., Sánchez, J., Picó, C., and Palou, A. 2008. Sex-differential expression of metabolism-related genes in response to a high-fat diet. *Obesity.* 16(4):819–826.

Prieto, J.A., Andrade, F., Aldamiz-Echevarria, L., and Sanjurjo, P. 2006. Determination of free and total carnitine in plasma by an enzymatic reaction and spectrophotometric quantitation spectrophotometric determination of carnitine. *Clin Biochem.* 39(10):1022–1027.

Pugh, G., Isenberg, J.S., Kamendulis, L.M., et al. 2000. Effects of di-isononyl phthalate, di-2-ethylhexyl phthalate, and clofibrate in cynomolgus monkeys. *Toxicol Sci.* 56(1):181–188.

Pynadath, T.I., and Chanapai S. 1981. Elevation of serum HDL and HDL cholesterol in cholesterol-fed male rabbits treated with estrogen. *Atherosclerosis.* 38(3–4):255–265.

Quehenberger, O., Armando, A.M., Brown, A.H., et al. 2010. Lipidomics reveals a remarkable diversity of lipids in human plasma. *J. Lipid Res.* 51(11):3299–3305.

Quehenberger, O., and Dennis, E.A. 2011. The human plasma lipidome. *N Engl J Med.* 365(19):1812–1823.

Radeau, T., Lau, P., Robb, M., McDonnell, M., Ailhaud, G., and McPherson, R. 1995. Cholesteryl ester transfer protein (CETP) mRNA abundance in human adipose tissue: Relationship to cell size and membrane cholesterol content. *J Lipid R*es. 36(12):2552–2561.

Radin, M.J., Sharkey, L.C., and Holycross, B.J. 2009. Adipokines: A review of biological and analytical principles and an update in dogs, cats, and horses. *Vet Clin Pathol.* 38(2):36–56.

Raheja, K.L., Linscheer, W.G., and Patel, D.G. 1982. Hypolipidemic and glycogenolytic effect of clofibrate (CPIB) in hypothyroid mice: Role of insulin and glucagon. *Gen Pharmacol.* 13(1):49–52.

Raman, A., Ramsey, J.J., Kemnitz, J.W., et al. 2007. Influences of calorie restriction and age on energy expenditure in the rhesus monkey. *Am J Physiol Endocrinol Metab.* 292(1):E101–106.

Ramaswamy, M., Wallace, T.L., Cossum, P.A., and Wasan, K.M. 1999. Species differences in the proportion of plasma lipoprotein lipid carried by high-density lipoproteins influence the distribution of free and liposomal nystatin in human, dog, and rat plasma. *Antimicrob Agents Chemother.* 43(6):1424–1428.

Rampone, A.J. and Long, L.W. 1977. The effect of phosphatidylcholine and lysophosphatidylcholine on the absorption and mucosal metabolism of oleic acid and cholesterol in vitro. *Biochim Biophys Acta.* 486(3):500–510.

Rashid, S., Uffelman, K.D., and Lewis, G.F. 2002. The mechanism of HDL lowering in hypertriglyceridemic, insulin-resistant states. *J Diabetes Complications.* 16(1):24–28.

Rathgeb, I., Winkler, B., Steele, R., and Altszuler, N. 1970. Effects of canine growth hormone on the metabolism of plasma glucose and free fatty acids in the dog. *Endocrinology.* 87(3):628–632.

Rayssiguier, Y., Gueux, E., and Weiser, D. 1981. Effect of magnesium deficiency on lipid metabolism in rats fed a high carbohydrate diet. *J Nutr.* 111(11):1876–1883.

Reaven, E., Cortez, Y., Leers-Schuta, S., Nomoto, A., and Azhar, S. 2004. Dimerization of the scavenger receptor class B type I: Formation, function, and localization in diverse cells and tissues. *J Lipid Res.* 45:513–528.

Reaven, E.P., Kolterman, O.G., and Reaven, G.M. 1974. Ultrastructural and physiological evidence for corticosteroid-induced alterations in hepatic production of very low density lipoprotein particles. *J Lipid Res.* 15(1):74–83.

Reaven, G.M., and Reaven, E.P. 1981. Prevention of age-related hypertriglyceridemia by caloric restriction and exercise training in the rat. *Metabolism.* 30(10):982–986.

Reddy, J.K., and Hashimoto, T. 2001. Peroxisomal beta-oxidation and peroxisome proliferator-activated receptor alpha: An adaptive metabolic system. *Annu Rev Nutr.* 21:193–230.

Repa, J.J., Lund, E.G., Horton, J.D., et al. 2000. Disruption of the sterol 27-hydroxylase gene in mice results in hepatomegaly and hypertriglyceridemia. Reversal by cholic acid feeding. *J Biol Chem.* 275:39685–39692.

Reuter, S.E., and Evans, A.M. 2012. Carnitine and acylcarnitines: Pharmacokinetic, pharmacological and clinical aspects. *Clin Pharmacokinet.* 51(9):553–72.

Richard, D., Carpentier, A.C., Doré, G., Ouellet, V., and Picard, F. 2010. Determinants of brown adipocyte development and thermogenesis. *Int J Obes.* 34(Suppl 2):S59–66.

Richelsen, B., Pedersen, S.B., Kristensen, K., et al. 2000. Regulation of lipoprotein lipase and hormone-sensitive lipase activity and gene expression in adipose and muscle tissue by growth hormone treatment during weight loss in obese patients. *Metabolism.* 49:906–11.

Rigotti, A., Acton, S.L., and Krieger, M. 1995. The class B scavenger receptors SR-BI and CD36 are receptors for anionic phospholipids. *J Biol Chem.* 270(27):16221–16224.

Rigotti, A., Edelman, E.R., Seifert, P., et al. 1996. Regulation by adrenocorticotropic hormone of the in vivo expression of scavenger receptor class B type 1 (SR- B1), a high density lipoprotein, in steroidogenic cells of the murine adrenal glands. *J Biol Chem.* 271:33545–33549.

Rigotti, A., Trigatti, B.L., Penman, M., Rayburn, H., Herz, J., and Krieger, M. 1997. A targeted mutation in the murine gene encoding the high density lipoprotein (HDL) receptor scavenger receptor class B type 1 reveals its key role in HDL metabolism. *Proc Natl Acad Sci USA.* 94:12610–12615.

Risser, T.R., Reaven, G.M., and Reaven, E.P. 1978. Intestinal contribution to secretion of very low density lipoproteins into plasma. *Am J Physiol.* 234(3):E277–281.

Rivera-Coll, A., Fuentes-Arderiu, X., and Díez-Noguera, A. 1994. Circadian rhythmic variations in serum concentrations of clinically important lipids. *Clin Chem.* 40(8):1549–1553.

Roelofsen, B., Op Den Kamp, J.A., and Van Deenen, L.L. 1987. Structural and dynamic aspects of red cell phospholipids; featuring phosphatidylcholine. *Biomed Biochim Acta.* 46(2–3):S10–15.

Rogers, W.A., Donovan, E.F., and Kociba, G.J. 1975. Lipids and lipoproteins in normal dogs and in dogs with secondary hyperlipoproteinemia. *J Am Vet Med Assoc.* 166(11):1092–1100.

Romaschin, A.D., and Goldberg, D.M. 1987. Effect of phenobarbital upon serum cholesterol lipoprotein fractions of three rodent species. *Clin Physiol Biochem.* 5(2):77–84.

Roomi, M.W. 1997. Association between hyperlipidemia and hepatic cytochrome P-450 in guinea pigs. *Res Commun Mol Pathol Pharmacol.* 97(2):139–150.

Rosa, P., and Fratangeli, A. 2010. Cholesterol and synaptic vesicle exocytosis. *Commun Integr Biol.* 3(4):352–353.

Rosen, H., and Goetzl, E.J. 2005. Sphingosine 1-phosphate and its receptors: An autocrine and paracrine network. *Nat Rev Immunol.* 5:560–570.

Roth, G.S., Ingram, D.K., and Lane, M.A. 2001. Caloric restriction in primates and relevance to humans. *Ann NY Acad Sci.* 928:305–315.

Roy, S., Vega-Lopez, S., and Fernandez, M.L. 2000. Gender and hormonal status affect the hypolipidemic mechanisms of dietary soluble fiber in guinea pigs. *J. Nutr.* 130:600–607.

Rudel, L.L., Bond, M.G., and Bullock, B.C. 1985. LDL heterogeneity and atherosclerosis in nonhuman primates. *Ann N Y Acad Sci.* 454:248–253.

Rudel, L., Deckelman, C., Wilson, M., Scobey, M., and Anderson, R. 1994. Dietary cholesterol and downregulation of cholesterol 7 alpha-hydroxylase and cholesterol absorption in African green monkeys. *J Clin Invest.* 93(6):2463–2472.

Rudel, L.L., Haines, J.L., and Sawyer, J.K. 1990. Effects on plasma lipoproteins of monounsaturated, saturated, and polyunsaturated fatty acids in the diet of African green monkeys. *J Lipid Res.* 31(10):1873–1882.

Rudel, L.L., Parks, J.S., Johnson, F.L., and Babiak, J. 1986. Low density lipoproteins in atherosclerosis. *J Lipid Res.* 27(5):465–474.

Rudel, L.L., and Pitts, L.L. 1978. Male-female variability in the dietary cholesterol-induced hyperlipoproteinemia of cynomolgus monkeys (*Macaca fascicularis*). *J Lipid Res.* 19:992–1003.

Rudling, M., Norstedt, G., Olivecrona, H.E., Reihner, E., Gustafsson, J.A., and Angelin, B. 1992. Importance of growth hormone for the induction of hepatic low density lipoprotein receptors. *Proc Natl Acad Sci USA.* 89:6983–6987.

Ruppin, D.C., and Middleton, W.R. 1980. Clinical use of medium chain triglycerides. *Drugs.* 20(3):216–224.

Russell, D.W. 2003. The enzymes, regulation and genetics of bile acid synthesis. *Annu Rev Biochem.* 72:137–174.

Rydén, M., Jocken, J., van Harmelen, V., et al. 2007. Comparative studies of the role of hormone-sensitive lipase and adipose triglyceride lipase in human fat cell lipolysis. *Am J Physiol Endocrinol Metab.* 292(6):E1847–1855.

Ryeom, S.W., Silverstein, R.L., Scotto, A., and Sparrow, J.R. 1996. Binding of anionic phospholipids to retinal pigment epithelium may be mediated by the scavenger receptor CD36. *J Biol Chem.* 271(34):20536–20539.

Sadur, C.N., and Eckel, R.H. 1982. Insulin stimulation of adipose tissue lipoprotein lipase. Use of the euglycemic clamp technique. *J Clin Invest.* 69:1119–1125.

Sakoda, H., Ogihara, T., Anai, M., et al. 2000. Dexamethasone-induced insulin resistance in 3T3–L1 adipocytes is due to inhibition of glucose transport rather than insulin signal transduction. *Diabetes.* 49:1700–1708.

Salter, A.M., Hayashi, R., Al-Seeni, M., et al. 1991. Effects of hypothyroidism and high-fat feeding on mRNA concentrations for the low density-lipoprotein receptor and on acyl-CoA: Cholesterol acyltransferase activities in rat liver. *Biochem J.* 276:825–832.

Salter, A.M., Wiggins, D., Sessions, V.A., and Gibbons, G.F. 1998. The intracellular triacylglycerol/fatty acid cycle: A comparison of its activity in hepatocytes which secrete exclusively apolipoprotein (apo) B100 very-low-density lipoprotein (VLDL) and in those which secrete predominantly apoB48 VLDL. *Biochem J.* 332(Pt 3):667–672.

Sapay, N., Bennett, W.F.D., and Tieleman, D.P. 2010. Molecular simulations of lipid flip-flop in the presence of model transmembrane helices. *Biochemistry.* 49(35):7665–7673.

Schaefer, E.J., Gregg, R.E., Ghiselli, G., et al. 1986. Familial apolipoprotein E deficiency. *J Clin Invest.* 78:1206–1219.

Schenck, P.A., Donovan, D., Refsal, K.N.R., and Rick, M. 2004. Incidence of hypothyroidism in dogs with chronic hyperlipidemia. *J Vet Intern Med.* 18:442.

Scherer, P.E., Williams, S., Fogliano, M., Baldini, G., and Lodish, H.F. 1995. A novel serum protein similar to C1q, produced exclusively in adipocytes. *J Biol Chem.* 270(45):26746–26749.

Schiavoni, G., Bennati, A.M., Castelli, M., et al. 2010. Activation of TM7SF2 promoter by SREBP-2 depends on a new sterol regulatory element, a GC-box, and an inverted CCAAT-box. *Biochim Biophys Acta.* 1801(5):587–592.

Schlierf, G., and Dorow, E. 1973. Diurnal patterns of triglycerides, free fatty acids, blood sugar, and insulin during carbohydrate-induction in man and their modification by nocturnal suppression of lipolysis. *J Clin Invest.* 52:732–740.

Schmidt, D.A., Ellersieck, M.R., Cranfield, M.R., and Karesh, W.B. 2006. Cholesterol values in free-ranging gorillas (*Gorilla gorilla gorilla* and *Gorilla beringei*) and Bornean orangutans (*Pongo pygmaeus*). *J Zoo Wildl Med.* 37(3):292–300.

Schneider, F., Kanitz, E., Gerrard, D.E., et al. 2002. Administration of recombinant porcine somatotropin (rpST) changes hormone and metabolic status during early pregnancy. *Domest Anim Endocrinol.* 23(4):455–474.

Schoenemann, H.M., Failla, M.L., and Steele, N.C. 1990. Consequences of severe copper deficiency are independent of dietary carbohydrate in young pigs. *Am J Clin Nutr.* 52(1):147–154.

Schwarz, M., Spath, L., Lux, C.A., et al. 2008. Potential protective role of apoprotein J (clusterin) in atherogenesis: Binding to enzymatically modified low-density lipoprotein reduces fatty acid-mediated cytotoxicity. *Thromb Haemost.* 100(1):110–118.

Schwenk, M., Hofmann, A.F., Carlson, G.L., Carter, J.A., Coulston, F., and Greim, H. 1978. Bile acid conjugation in the chimpanzee: Effective sulfation of lithocholic acid. *Arch Toxicol.* 40(2):109–118.

Sengenès, C., Zakaroff-Girard, A., Moulin, A., et al. 2002. Natriuretic peptide-dependent lipolysis in fat cells is a primate specificity. *Am J Physiol Regul Integr Comp Physiol.* 283(1):R257–265.

Serrano, M.P., Valencia, D.G., Fuentetaja, A., Lázaro, R., and Mateos, G.G. 2009. Influence of feed restriction and sex on growth performance and carcass and meat quality of Iberian pigs reared indoors. *J Anim Sci.* 87(5):1676–1685.

Shang, Q., Pan, L., Saumoy, M., et al. 2006. The stimulatory effect of LXRalpha is blocked by SHP despite the presence of a LXRalpha binding site in the rabbit CYP7A1 promoter. *Lipid Res.* 47(5):997–1004.

Shao, W., and Espenshade, P.J. 2012. Expanding roles for SREPB in metabolism. *Cell Metabolism.* 16: 414–419.

Shearer, G.C., Harris, W.S., Pedersen, T.L., and Newman, J.W. 2010. Detection of omega-3 oxylipins in human plasma and response to treatment with omega-3 acid ethyl esters. *J Lipid Res.* 51(8):2074–2081.

Sheppard, K., and Herzberg, G.R. 1992. Triacylglycerol composition of adipose tissue, muscle and liver of rats fed diets containing fish oil or corn oil. *Nutr Res.* 12(11):1405–1418.

Shi, Q.Y., Lin, Y.G., Zhou, X., Lin, Y.Q., and Yan, S. 2010. Expression of FXR mRNA, PPAR alpha mRNA and bile acid metabolism related genes in intrahepatic cholestasis of pregnant rats. *Zhonghua Gan Zang Bing Za Zhi.* 18(12):927--930.

Shiau, Y.F., Popper, D.A., Reed, M., Umstetter, C., Capuzzi, D., and Levine, G.M. 1985. Intestinal triglycerides are derived from both endogenous and exogenous sources. *Am J Physiol.* 248:G164–169.

Shimomura, I., Shimano, H., Horton, J.D., Goldstein, J.L., and Brown, M.S. 1997. Differential expression of exons 1a and 1c in mRNAs for sterol regulatory element binding protein-1 in human and mouse organs and cultured cells. *J Clin Invest.* 99(5):838–845.

Shiomi, M., Ito, T., Fujioka, T., and Tsujita, Y. 2000. Age-associated decrease in plasma cholesterol and changes in cholesterol metabolism in homozygous Watanabe heritable hyperlipidemic rabbits. *Metabolism.* 49(4):552–556.

Shoulders, C.C., Stephens, D.J., and Jones, B. 2004. The intracellular transport of chylomicrons requires the small GTPase, Sar1b. *Curr Opin Lipidol.* 15(2):191–197.

Shui, G., Stebbins, J.W., Lam, B.D., et al. 2011. Comparative plasma lipidome between human and cynomolgus monkey: Are plasma polar lipids good biomarkers for diabetic monkeys? *PLoS One.* 6(5):e19731.

Silva, MF1., Aires, C.C., Luis, P.B., et al. 2008. Valproic acid metabolism and its effects on mitochondrial fatty acid oxidation: A review. *J Inherit Metab Dis.* 31(2):205–216.

Singh, I., Pahan, K., Dhaunsi, G.S., Lazo, O., and Ozand, P. 1993. Phytanic acid alpha-oxidation. Differential subcellular localization in rat and human tissues and its inhibition by nycodenz. *J Biol Chem.* 268(14):9972–9979.

Sirvent, A., Verhoeven, A.J.M., Jansen, H., et al. 2004. Farnesoid X receptor represses hepatic lipase gene expression. *J Lipid Res.* 45:2110–2115.

Sitadevi, C., Patrudu, M.B., Kumar, Y.M., Raju, G.R., and Suryaprabha, K. 1981. Longitudinal study of serum lipids and lipoproteins in normal pregnancy and puerperium. *Trop Geogr Med.* 33(3):219–223.

Skold, B.H., Getty, R., and Ramsey, F.K. 1966. Spontaneous atherosclerosis in the arterial system of aging swine. *Am J Vet Res.* 27(116):257–273.

Slavin, B.G., Ong, J.M., and Kern, P.A. 1994. Hormonal regulation of hormone-sensitive lipase activity and mRNA levels in isolated rat adipocytes. *J Lipid Res.* 35:1535–1541.

Sloop, C.H., Dory, L., Krause, B.R., Castle, C., and Roheim, P.S. 1983. Lipoproteins and apolipoproteins in peripheral lymph of normal and cholesterol-fed dogs. *Atherosclerosis.* 49(1):9–21.

Smyers, M.E., Bachir, K.Z., Britton, S.L., Koch, L.G., and Novak, C.M. 2015. Physically active rats lose more weight during calorie restriction. *Physiol Behav.* 139:303–313.

Sodha, N.R., Boodhwani, M., Ramlawi, B., et al. 2008. Atorvastatin increases myocardial indices of oxidative stress in a porcine model of hypercholesterolemia and chronic ischemia. *J Card Surg.* 23(4):312–320.

Sokolović, M., Sokolović, A., van Roomen, C.P., et al. 2010. Unexpected effects of fasting on murine lipid homeostasis--transcriptomic and lipid profiling. *J Hepatol.* 52(5):737–744.

Solaas, K., Kase, B.F., Pham, V., Bamberg, K., Hunt, M.C., and Alexson, S.E. 2004. Differential regulation of cytosolic and peroxisomal bile acid amidation by PPAR alpha activation favors the formation of unconjugated bile acids. *J Lipid Res.* 45(6):1051–1060.

Sone, M., and Osamura, R.Y. 2001. Leptin and the pituitary. *Pituitary.* 4(1–2):15–23.

Spaniol, M., Bracher, R., Ha, H.R., Follath, F., and Krähenbühl, S. 2001. Toxicity of amiodarone and amiodarone analogues on isolated rat liver mitochondria. *J Hepatol.* 35(5):628–636.

Spiekerkoetter, U., and Wood, P.A. 2010. Mitochondrial fatty acid oxidation disorders: Pathophysiological studies in mouse models. *J Inherit Metab Dis.* 33(5):539–546.

Staels, B., Van Tol, A., Chan, L., et al. 1990. Alterations in thyroid status modulate apolipoprotein, hepatic triglyceride lipase, and low density lipoprotein receptor in rats. *Endocrinology.* 127:1144–1152.

Ståhlberg, D., Angelin, B., and Einarsson, K. 1991. Age-related changes in the metabolism of cholesterol in rat liver microsomes. *Lipids.* 26(5):349–352.

Stanimirov, B., Stankov, K., and Mikov, M. 2012. Pleiotropic functions of bile acids mediated by the farnesoid X receptor. *Acta Gastroenterol Belg.* 75(4):389–398.

Stedman, C., Liddle, C., Coulter, S., et al. 2006. Benefit of farnesoid X receptor inhibition in obstructive cholestasis. *Proc Natl Acad Sci USA.* 103:11323–11328.

Steffensen, K.R., and Gustafsson, J.A. 2004. Putative metabolic effects of the liver X receptor (LXR). *Diabetes.* 53(Suppl 1):S36–42.

Stieger B. 2009. Recent insights into the function and regulation of the bile salt export pump (ABCB11). *Curr Opin Lipidol.* 20(3):176--181.

Stieger, B. 2011. The role of the sodium-taurocholate cotransporting polypeptide (NTCP) and of the bile salt export pump (BSEP) in physiology and pathophysiology of bile formation. In *Drug Transporters, Handbook of Experimental Pharmacology 201*. Eds. M.F. Fromm, and R.B. Kim, pp. 205–259. Berlin Heidelberg: Springer-Verlag.

Stephens, T.W., Basinski, M., Bristow, P.K., et al. 1995. The role of neuropeptide Y in the antiobesity action of the obese gene product. *Nature.* 377(6549):530–532.

Steyn, F.J., Leong, J.W., Huang, L., et al. 2012. GH does not modulate the early fasting-induced release of free fatty acids in mice. *Endocrinology.* 153(1):273–282.

Stieger, B., Fattinger, K., Madon, J., Kullak-Ublick, G.A., and Meier, P.J. 2000. Drug- and estrogen-induced cholestasis through inhibition of the hepatocellular bile salt export pump (Bsep) of rat liver. *Gastroenterology.* 118(2):422–430.

Story, J.A., Tepper, S.A., and Kritchevsky, D. 1976. Age-related changes in the lipid metabolism of Fisher 344 rats. *Lipids.* 11(8):623–627.

Strålfors, P., and Honnor, R.C. 1989. Insulin-induced dephosphorylation of hormone-sensitive lipase. correlation with lipolysis and cAMP-dependent protein kinase activity. *Eur J Biochem.* 182(2):

St-Pierre, D.H., Karelis, A.D., Cianflone, K., et al. 2004. Relationship between ghrelin and energy expenditure in healthy young women. *J Clin Endocrinol Metab.* 89(12):5993–5997.

Strålfors, P., and Honnor, R.C. 1989. Insulin-induced dephosphorylation of hormone-sensitive lipase. Correlation with lipolysis and cAMP-dependent protein kinase activity. *Eur J Biochem.* 182(2):379–385.

Subbaiah, P.V. Determination and clinical significance of phospholipids. In *Handbook of Lipoprotein Testing*, Rifai, N., Warnick, G.R,. and Dominiczak, M.H. (Eds.), pp. 521--535. Washington, DC: AACC Press.

Sugiuchi, H., Uji, Y., Okabe, H., et al. 1995. Direct measurement of high-density lipoprotein cholesterol in serum with polyethylene glycol-modified enzymes and sulfated alpha-cyclodextrin. *Clin Chem.* 41(5):717–723.

Sullivan, M.P., Cerda, J.J., Robbins, F.L., Burgin, C.W., and Beatty, R.J. 1993. The gerbil, hamster, and guinea pig as rodent models for hyperlipidemia. *Lab Anim Sci.* 43(6):575–578.

Swift, L.L., Zhu, M.Y., Kakkad, B., et al. 2003. Subcellular localization of microsomal triglyceride transfer protein. *J Lipid Res.* 44(10):1841–1849.

Szymanski, E.S., and Kritchevsky, D. 1980. Serum lipid levels of young and old Rhesus monkeys. *Exp Gerontol.* 15(5):365–367.

Taddei-Peters, W.C., Butman, B.T., Jones, G.R., et al. 1993. Quantification of lipoprotein(a) particles containing various apolipoprotein(a) isoforms by a monoclonal anti-apo(a) capture antibody and a polyclonal anti-apolipoproteinB detection antibody sandwich enzyme immunoassay. *Cun Chem.* 39(7):1382–1389.

Taha, T.A., Hannun, Y.A., and Obeid, L.M. 2006. Sphingosine kinase: Biochemical and cellular regulation and role in disease. *J Biochem Mol Biol.* 39:113–131.

Tailleux, A., and Staels, B. 2011. Overview of the measurement of lipids and lipoproteins. *Curr Protoc Mouse Biol.* 1:265–277.

Takeuchi, H., Sekine, S., Noguchi, O., Murano, Y., Aoyama, T., and Matsuo, T. 2009. Effect of life-long dietary n-6/n-3 fatty acid ratio on life span, serum lipids and serum glucose in Wistar rats. *J Nutr Sci Vitaminol (Tokyo).* 55(5):394–399.

Tan, K.C., Shiu, S.W., and Kung, A.W. 1998. Plasma cholesteryl ester transfer protein activity in hyper- and hypothyroidism. *J Clin Endocrinol Metab.* 83(1):140–143.

Tanaka, M., Otani, H., Yokode, M., and Kita, T. 1995. Regulation of apolipoprotein B secretion in hepatocytes from Watanabe heritable hyperlipidemic rabbit, an animal model for familial hypercholesterolemia. *Atherosclerosis.* 114(1):73–82.

Taniguchi, M., and Okazaki, T. 2014. The role of sphingomyelin and sphingomyelin synthases in cell death, proliferation and migration-from cell and animal models to human disorders. *Biochim Biophys Acta.* 1841(5):692–703.

Taskinen, M.R., and Nikkilä, E.A. 1979. Effects of caloric restriction on lipid metabolism in man: Changes of tissue lipoprotein lipase activities and of serum lipoproteins. *Atherosclerosis.* 32(3):289–299.

Taskinen, M.R., and Nikkilä, E.A. 1987. Basal and postprandial lipoprotein lipase activity in adipose tissue during caloric restriction and refeeding. *Metabolism.* 36(7):625–630.

Taskinen, S., Kovanen, P.T., Jarva, H., Meri, S., and Pentikäinen, M.O. 2002. Binding of C-reactive protein to modified low-density-lipoprotein particles: Identification of cholesterol as a novel ligand for C-reactive protein. *Biochem J.* 367(Pt 2):403–412.

Teichmann, A.T., Wieland, H., Cremer, P., Kulow, G., and Mehle, U. 1988. Serum lipid and lipoprotein concentrations in pregnancy and at onset of labor in normal and complicated pregnancies caused by hypertensive gestosis and fetal growth retardation. *Geburtshilfe Frauenheilkd.* 48(3):134–139.

Thomas, M.J., and Rudel, L.L. 1996. Dietary fatty acids, low density lipoprotein composition and oxidation and primate atherosclerosis. *J Nutr.* 126(Suppl 4):1058S–1062S.

Thomàs-Moyà, E., Gianotti, M., Lladó, I., and Proenza, A.M. 2006. Effects of caloric restriction and gender on rat serum paraoxonase 1 activity. *J Nutr Biochem.* 17(3):197–203.

Thompson, G.R., Soutar, A.K., Spengel, F.A., et al. 1981. Defects of receptor-mediated low density lipoprotein catabolism in homozygous familial hypercholesterolemia and hypothyroidism in vivo. *Proc Natl Acad Sci USA.* 78:2591–2595.

Thumelin, S., Forestier, M., Girard, J., and Pegorier, J.P. 1993. Developmental changes in mitochondrial 3-hydroxy-3-methylglutaryl-CoA synthase gene expression in rat liver, intestine and kidney. *Biochem J.* 292(Pt 2):493–496.

Tietjen, I., Hovingh, G.K., Singaraja, R.R., et al. 2012. Segregation of LIPG, CETP, and GALNT2 mutations in Caucasian families with extremely high HDL cholesterol. *PLoS One.* 7(8): e37437.

Trigatti, B.L., Krieger, M., and Rigotti, A. 2003. Influence of the HDL receptor SR-BI on lipoprotein metabolism and atherosclerosis. *Arterioscler Thromb Vasc Biol.* 23(10):1732–1738.

Tsai, J., Zhang, R., Qiu, W., Su, Q., Naples, M., and Adeli, K. 2009. Inflammatory NF-kappaB activation promotes hepatic apolipoprotein B100 secretion: Evidence for a link between hepatic inflammation and lipoprotein production. *Am J Physiol Gastrointest Liver Physiol.* 296(6):G1287–1298.

Tsibulsky, V.P., Yakushkin, V.V., and Preobrazhensky, S.N. 1997. Immunoenzyme assessment of human apoB-lipoprotein binding to immobilized receptor of low density lipoproteins. 2. Binding of isolated lipoproteins. *Biochemistry.* 62(6):603–608.

Tso, P., and Balint, J.A. 1986. Formation and transport of chylomicrons by enterocytes to the lymphatics. *Am J Physiol.* 250(6 Pt 1):G715–726.

Tso, P., Liu, M., and Kalogeris, T.J. 1999. The role of apolipoprotein A-IV in food intake regulation. *J. Nutr.* 129(8):1503–1506.

Tso, P., Nauli, A., and Lo, C.M. 2004. Enterocyte fatty acid uptake and intestinal fatty acid-binding protein. *Biochem Soc Trans.* 32(Pt 1):75–78.

Tsubota, T., Sato, M., Okano, T., et al. 2008. Annual changes in serum leptin concentration in the adult female Japanese black bear (*Ursus thibetanus japonicus*). *J Vet Med Sci.* 70:1399–1403.

Tsutsumi, K., Hagi, A., and Inoue, Y. 2001. The relationship between plasma high density lipoprotein cholesterol levels and cholesteryl ester transfer protein activity in six species of healthy experimental animals. *Biol Pharm Bull.* 24(5):579–581.

Tumbleson, M.E., Burks M.F., Spate M.P., Hutcheson D.P., and Middleton C.C. 1970. Serum biochemical and hematological parameters of Sinclair(S-1) miniature sows during gestation and lactation. *Can J Comp Med.* 34:312–319.

Tumbleson, M.E., Hicklin, K.W., and Burks, M.F. 1976. Serum cholesterol, triglyceride, glucose and total bilirubin concentrations, as functions of age and sex, in Sinclair(S-1) miniature swine. *Growth.* 40(3):293–300.

Turkalj, I., Keller, U., Ninnis, R., Vosmeer, S., and Stauffacher, W. 1992. Effect of increasing doses of recombinant human insulin-like growth factor-I on glucose, lipid, and leucine metabolism in man. *J Clin Endocrinol Metab.* 75(5):1186–1191.

Turley, S.D., Spady, D.K., and Dietschy, J.M. 1995. Role of liver in the synthesis of cholesterol and the clearance of low density lipoproteins in the cynomolgus monkey. *J Lipid Res.* 36(1):67–79.

Tvarijonaviciute, A., Carrillo-Sanchez, J.D., and Ceron, J.J. 2013. Effect of estradiol and progesterone on metabolic biomarkers in healthy bitches. *Reprod Domest Anim.* 48(3):520–524.

Tvarijonaviciute, A., Martínez-Subiela, S., and Ceron, J.J. 2012. Validation of two ELISA assays for total ghrelin measurement in dogs. *J Anim Physiol Anim Nutr.* 96(1):1–8.

Tvorogova, M.G., and Titov, V.N. 1986. Metabolism of lipoproteins in rats treated with ethinyl estradiol. *Vopr Med Khim.* 32(1):42–49.

Twisk, J., Hoekman, M.F., Mager, W.H., et al. 1995. Heterogeneous expression of cholesterol 7 alpha-hydroxylase and sterol 27-hydroxylase genes in the rat liver lobulus. *J Clin Invest.* 95(3):1235–1243.

Uchiyama, T., Tokoi, K., and Deki, T. 1985. Successive changes in the blood composition of experimental normal beagle dogs associated with age. *Jikken Dobutsu.* 34(4):367–377.

Umeda, Y., Redgrave, T.G., Mortimer, B.C., and Mamo, J.C. 1995. Kinetics and uptake in vivo of oxidatively modified lymph chylomicrons. *Am J Physiol.* 268(4 Pt 1):G709–716.

Urizar, N.L., Dowhan, D.H., and Moore, D.D. 2000. The farnesoid X-activated receptor mediates bile acid activation of phospholipid transfer protein gene expression. *J Biol Chem.* 275:39313–39317.

Uryszek, W., Paluszak, J., Uryszek, E., and Soszy⊠ska, Z. 1989. Effect of estradiol on lipolytic processes in the blood and adipose tissue of female rats. *Endokrynol Pol.* 40(6):315–324.

Vaessen, S.F., Dallinga-Thie, G.M., Ross, C.J., et al. 2009. Plasma apolipoprotein AV levels in mice are positively associated with plasma triglyceride levels. *J Lipid Res.* 50(5):880–884.

Vaganay, S., Joliff, G., Bertaux, O., Toselli, E., Devignes, M.D., and Bénicourt C. 1998. The complete cDNA sequence encoding dog gastric lipase. *DNA Seq.* 8(4):257–262.

Valle, A., Guevara, R., García-Palmer, F.J., Roca, P., and Oliver, J. 2007. Sexual dimorphism in liver mitochondrial oxidative capacity is conserved under caloric restriction conditions. *Am J Physiol Cell Physiol.* 293(4):C1302–1308.

van der Crabben, SN., Allick, G., Ackermans, M.T., Endert, E., Romijn, J.A., and Sauerwein, H.P. 2008. Prolonged fasting induces peripheral insulin resistance, which is not ameliorated by high-dose salicylate. *J Clin Endocrinol Metab.* 93(2):638–641.

Van der Meer, R., and De Vries, H.T. 1985. Differential binding of glycine- and taurine-conjugated bile acids to insoluble calcium phosphate. *Biochem J.* 229(1):265–268.

Van Haperen, R., Samyn, H., van Gent, T., et al. 2009. Novel roles of hepatic lipase and phospholipid transfer protein in VLDL as well as HDL metabolism. *Biochim Biophys Acta.* 1791(10):1031–1036.

Van Liew, J.B., Davis, P.J., Davis, F.B., et al. 1993. Effects of aging, diet, and sex on plasma glucose, fructosamine, and lipid concentrations in barrier-raised Fischer 344 rats. *Gerontol.* 48(5):B184–190.

Van Oostrom, A.J., Castro Cabezas, M., Ribalta, J., Masana, L., Twickler, T.B., Remijnse, T.A., and Erkelens, D.W. 2000. Diurnal triglyceride profiles in healthy normolipidemic male subjects are associated to insulin sensitivity, body composition and diet. *Eur J Clin Invest.* 30(11): 964--971.

Van Tol, A. 2002. Phospholipid transfer protein. *Curr Opin Lipidol.* 13:135–139.

Van Veldhoven, P.P., and Mannaerts, G.P. 1999. Role and organization of peroxisomal beta-oxidation. *Adv Exp Med Biol.* 466:261–272.

Vance, J.E., and Vance, D.E (Eds.). 2008. *Biochemistry of Lipids, Lipoproteins, and Membranes*, 5th edition. Amsterdam, Netherlands: Elsevier.

Van't Hooft, F.M., Hardman, D.A., Kane, J.P., and Havel, R.J. 1982. Apolipoprotein B (B-48) of rat chylomicrons is not a precursor of the apolipoprotein of low density lipoproteins. *Proc Natl Acad Sci USA.* 79(1):179–182.

Vázquez, M., Fagiolino, P., Maldonado, C., et al. 2014. Hyperammonemia associated with valproic acid concentrations. *Biomed Res Int.* 2014:217269.

Vendrell, J., Broch, M., Vilarrasa, N., et al. 2004. Resistin, adiponectin, ghrelin, leptin, and proinflammatory cytokines: Relationships in obesity. *Obes Res.* 12(6):962–971.

Venkateswaran, A., Laffitte, B.A., Joseph, S.B., et al. 2000. Control of cellular cholesterol efflux by the nuclear oxysterol receptor LXR alpha. *Proc Natl Acad Sci USA.* 97(22):12097–12102.

Vianey-Liaud, C., Divry, P., Gregersen, N., and Mathieu, M. 1987. The inborn errors of mitochondrial fatty acid oxidation. *J Inherit Metab Dis.* 10(Suppl 1):159–200.

Vigne, J.L., and Havel, R.J. 1981. Metabolism of apolipoprotein A-I of chylomicrons in rats and humans. *Can J Biochem.* 59(8):613–618.

Vigushin, D.M., Gough, J., Allan, D., et al. 1994. Familial nephropathic systemic amyloidosis caused by apolipoprotein AI variant Arg26. *Q J Med.* 87(3):149–154.

Vikman, K., Carlsson, B., Billig, H., and Eden, S. 1991. Expression and regulation of growth hormone (GH) receptor messenger ribonucleic acid (mRNA) in rat adipose tissue, adipocytes, and adipocyte precursor cells: GH regulation of GH receptor mRNA. *Endocrinology.* 129:1155–1161.

Villena, J.A., Roy, S., Sarkadi-Nagy, E., Kim, K.H., and Sul, H.S. 2004. Desnutrin, an adipocyte gene encoding a novel patatin domain-containing protein, is induced by fasting and glucocorticoids: Ectopic expression of desnutrin increases triglyceride hydrolysis. *J. Biol. Chem.* 279:47066–47075.

Vlahcevic, Z.R., Stravitz, R.T., Heuman, D.M., Hylemon, P.B., and Pandak, W.M. 1997. Quantitative estimations of the contribution of different bile acid pathways to total bile acid synthesis in the rat. *Gastroenterology.* 113:1949–1957.

Voigt, N., Stein, J., Galindo, M.M., et al. 2014. The role of lipolysis in human orosensory fat perception. *J Lipid Res.* 55(5):870–882.

Wang, C.N., McLeod, R.S., Yao, Z., and Brindley, D.N. 1995. Effects of dexamethasone on the synthesis, degradation, and secretion of apolipoprotein B in cultured rat hepatocytes. *Arterioscler Thromb Vasc Biol.* 15:1481–1491.

Wang, C.S., Fukuda, N., and Ontko, J.A. 1984. Studies on the mechanism of hypertriglyceridemia in the genetically obese Zucker rat. *J Lipid Res.* 25(6):571–579.

Wang, N., Lan, D., Chen, W., Matsuura, F., and Tall, A.R. 2004. ATP-binding cassette transporters G1 and G4 mediate cellular cholesterol efflux to high-density lipoproteins. *Proc Natl Acad Sci USA*. 101(26):9774–9779.

Wang, P.R., Guo, Q., Ippolito, M., et al. 2001. High fat fed hamster, a unique animal model for treatment of diabetic dyslipidemia with peroxisome proliferator activated receptor alpha selective agonists. *Eur J Pharmacol*. 427(3):285–293.

Wang, S., Soni, K.G., Semache, M., et al. 2008. Lipolysis and the integrated physiology of lipid energy metabolism. *Mol Genet Metab*. 95(3):117–126.

Wang, Y., Botolin, D., Xu, J., et al. 2006. Regulation of hepatic fatty acid elongase and desaturase expression in diabetes and obesity. *J Lipid Res*. 47(9):2028–2041.

Wang, Y., Castoreno, A.B., Stockinger, W., and Nohturfft, A. 2005. Modulation of endosomal cholesteryl ester metabolism by membrane cholesterol. *J Biol Chem*. 280(12):11876–11886.

Warnick, G.R., Nauck, M., and Rifai, N. 2001. Evolution of methods for measurement of HDL-cholesterol: From ultracentrifugation to homogeneous assays. *Clin Chem*. 47(9):1579–1596.

Wasfi, I., Weinstein, I., and Heimberg, M. 1980. Increased formation of triglyceride from oleate in perfused livers from pregnant rats. *Endocrinology*. 107:584–596.

Watanabe, M., Houten, S.M., Wang, L., et al. 2004. Bile acids lower triglyceride levels via a pathway involving FXR, SHP, and SREBP-1c. *J Clin Invest*. 113:1408–1418.

Watanabe, Y. 1980. Serial inbreeding of rabbits with hereditary hyperlipidemia (WHHL-rabbit). *Atherosclerosis*. 36(2):261–268.

Watkins, P.A., Maiguel, D., Jia, Z., and Pevsner, J. 2007. Evidence for 26 distinct acyl-coenzyme A synthetase genes in the human genome. *J Lipid Res*. 48(12):2736–2750.

Watson, P., Simpson, K.W., and Bedford, P.G.C. 1993. Hypercholesterolaemia in Briards in the United Kingdom. *Res Vet Sci*. 54:80–85.

Wei, Y., Rhani, Z., and Goodyer, C.G. 2006. Characterization of growth hormone receptor messenger ribonucleic acid variants in human adipocytes. *J Clin Endocrinol Metab*. 91(5):1901–1908.

Weigert, R., Silletta, M.G., Spanò, S., et al. 1999. CtBP/BARS induces fission of Golgi membranes by acylating lysophosphatidic acid. *Nature*. 402(6760):429–433.

Wein, S., Wolffram, S., Schrezenmeir, J., Gasperiková, D., Klimes, I., and Seböková, E. 2009. Medium-chain fatty acids ameliorate insulin resistance caused by high-fat diets in rats. *Diabetes Metab Res Rev*. 25(2):185–194.

Weingand, K.W. 1989. Atherosclerosis research in cynomolgus monkeys (*Macaca fascicularis*). *Exp Mol Pathol*. 50(1):1–15.

Weyer, C., Funahashi, T., Tanaka, S., et al. 2001. Hypoadiponectinemia in obesity and type 2 diabetes: Close association with insulin resistance and hyperinsulinemia. *J Clin Endocrinol Metab*. 86(5):1930–1935.

Weyrich, A.S., Rejeski, W.J., Brubaker, P.H., and Parks, J.S. 1992. The effects of testosterone on lipids and eicosanoids in cynomolgus monkeys. *Med Sci Sports Exerc*. 24(3):333–338.

Whitney, M.S. 1992. Evaluation of hyperlipidemias in dogs and cats. *Semin Vet Med Surg (Small Anim)*. 7:292–300.

Wierzbicki, A.S. 2007. Peroxisomal disorders affecting phytanic acid alpha-oxidation: A review. *Biochem Soc Trans*. 35(Pt 5):881–886.

Wilcox, H.G., and Heimberg, M. 1970. Isolation of plasma lipoproteins by zonal ultracentrifugation in the B14 and B15 titanium rotors. *J Lipid Res*. 11(1):7–22.

Wilcox, H.G., and Heimberg, M. 1991. Effects of hyperthyroidism on synthesis, secretion and metabolism of the VLDL apoproteins by the perfused rat liver. *Biochim Biophys Acta*. 1081(3):246–252.

Williams, D.A., and Steiner, J.M. 2005. Canine pancreatic disease. In *Textbook of Veterinary Internal Medicine*. Eds. S.J. Ettinger, and E.C. Feldman, pp. 1482–1488. St. Louis, Missouri: Saunders Elsevier.

Williams, K., Slaughter, H., McAlister, J., Tomlinson, L., and Bounous, D. 2009. Clinical pathology reference ranges for pregnant rats: A comparison to non-pregnant rats. *Clin Chem*. 55(6) Suppl. A2 (Poster A-1).

Willnow, T.E. 1997. Mechanisms of hepatic chylomicron remnant clearance. *Diabet Med*. 14(Suppl 3):S75–80.

Wilson, D.E., Chan, I.F., Elstad, N.L., et al. 1986. Apolipoprotein E-containing lipoproteins and lipoprotein remnants in experimental canine diabetes. *Diabetes*. 35(8):933–942.

Winegar, D.A., Brown, P.J., Wilkison, W.O., et al. 2001. Effects of fenofibrate on lipid parameters in obese rhesus monkeys. *J Lipid Res*. 42:1543–1551.

Wistuba, W., Gnewuch, C., Liebisch, G., Schmitz, G., and Langmann, T. 2007. Lithocholic acid induction of the FGF19 promoter in intestinal cells is mediated by PXR. *World J Gastroenterol*. 13(31):4230–4235.

Wójcicka, G., Jamroz-Wi⊠niewska, A., Horoszewicz, K., and Bełtowski, J. 2007. Liver X receptors (LXRs). Part I: Structure, function, regulation of activity, and role in lipid metabolism. *Postepy Hig Med Dosw.* 61:736–759.

Wolfe, M.S., Parks, J.S., Morgan, T.M., and Rudel, L.L. 1991. Age and dietary polyunsaturated fat alter high density lipoprotein subfraction cholesterol concentrations in a pediatric population of African green monkeys. *Arterioscler Thromb.* 11(3):617–628.

Wolford, S.T., Schroer, R.A., Gohs, F.X., et al. 1986. Reference range data base for serum chemistry and hematology values in laboratory animals. *J Toxicol Environ Health.* 18(2):161–188.

Wood, D., and Quiroz-Rocha, G.F. 2010. Normal hematology of cattle. In *Schalms Hematology*. Eds. D.J. Weiss, and K.J. Wardrop, 6th edition, pp. 829. Ames, IA: Blackwell Publishing.

Wright-Rodgers, A.S., Waldron, M.K., Bigley, K.E., Lees, G.E., and Bauer, J.E. 2005. Dietary fatty acids alter plasma lipids and lipoprotein distributions in dogs during gestation, lactation, and the perinatal period. *J Nutr.* 135(9):2230–2235.

Wróblewska, M. 2011. The origin and metabolism of a nascent pre-β high density lipoprotein involved in cellular cholesterol efflux. *Acta Biochim Pol.* 58(3):275–285.

Wróblewska, M., Czy⊠ewska, M., Wolska, A., Kortas-Stempak, B., and Szutowicz A. 2010. ApoA-II participates in HDL-liposome interaction by the formation of new pre-beta mobility particles and the modification of liposomes. *Biochim Biophys Acta.* 1801(12):1323–1329.

Wyne, K.L., and Woollett, L.A. 1998. Transport of maternal LDL and HDL to the fetal membranes and placenta of the Golden Syrian hamster is mediated by receptor-dependent and receptor-independent processes. *J. Lipid Res.* 39:518–530.

Xia, X., Jung, D., Webb, P., et al. 2012. Liver X receptor β and peroxisome proliferator-activated receptor δ regulate cholesterol transport in murine cholangiocytes. *Hepatology.* 56(6):2288–2296.

Xu, C., He, J., Jiang, H., et al. 2009. Direct effect of glucocorticoids on lipolysis in adipocytes. *Ml Endocrinol.* 23(8):1161–1170.

Xu, G., Pan, L.X., Li, H., et al. 2004. Dietary cholesterol stimulates CYP7A1 in rats because farnesoid X receptor is not activated. *Am J Physiol Gastrointest Liver Physiol.* 286(5):G730–735.

Xu, X.F., De Pergola, G., and Björntorp, P. 1991. Testosterone increases lipolysis and the number of beta-adrenoceptors in male rat adipocytes. *Endocrinology.* 128(1):379–382.

Xu, Y.H., Barnes, S., Sun, Y., and Grabowski, G.A. 2010. Multi-system disorders of glycosphingolipid and ganglioside metabolism. *J Lipid Res.* 51(7):1643–1675.

Yamamoto, T.R., Bishop, W., Brown, M.S., Goldstein, J.L., and Russell, D.W. 1986. Deletion in cysteine-rich region of LDL receptor impedes transport to cell surface in WHHL rabbit. *Science.* 232(4755):1230–1237.

Yang, S., Mulder, H., Holm, C., and Edén, S. 2004. Effects of growth hormone on the function of beta-adrenoceptor subtypes in rat adipocytes. *Obes Res.* 12(2):330–339.

Ye, J., and Debose-Boyd, R.A. 2011. Regulation of cholesterol and fatty acid synthesis. *Cold Spring Harb Perspect Biol.* 3(7):pii: a004754.

Yeaman, S.J. 2004. Hormone-sensitive lipase--new roles for an old enzyme. *Biochem J.* 379(Pt 1):11–22.

Yildiz, B.O., Suchard, M.A., Wong, M.L., McCann, S.M., and Licinio, J. 2004. Alterations in the dynamics of circulating ghrelin, adiponectin, and leptin in human obesity. *Proc Natl Acad Sci USA.* 101(28):10434–10439.

Yin, W., Carballo-Jane, E., McLaren, D.G., et al. 2012. Plasma lipid profiling across species for the identification of optimal animal models of human dyslipidemia. *J Lipid Res.* 53(1):51–65.

Yin, X., Li, Y., Xu, G., An, W., and Zhang W. 2009. Ghrelin fluctuation, what determines its production? *Acta Biochim Biophys Sin.* 41(3):188–197.

Yip, R.G., and Goodman, H.M. 1999. Growth hormone and dexamethasone stimulate lipolysis and activate adenylyl cyclase in rat adipocytes by selectively shifting Gi alpha2 to lower density membrane fractions. *Endocrinology.* 140(3):1219–1227.

Yokoyama, C., Wang, X., Briggs, M.R., et al. 1993. SREBP-1, a basic-helix-loop-helix-leucine zipper protein that controls transcription of the low density lipoprotein receptor gene. *Cell.* 75(1):187–197.

Yoon, M. 2009. The role of PPARalpha in lipid metabolism and obesity: Focusing on the effects of estrogen on PPARalpha actions. *Pharmacol Res.* 60(3):151–159.

Yoshida, T., Ohtoh, K., Cho, F., Honjo, S., and Goto, N. 1988. Discriminant analyses for pregnancy-related changes in hematological and serum biochemical values in cynomolgus monkeys (*Macaca fascicularis*). *Jikken Dobutsu.* 37(3):257–262.

Yoshino, J., Almeda-Valdes, P., Patterson, B.W., et al. 2014. Diurnal variation in insulin sensitivity of glucose metabolism is associated with diurnal variations in whole-body and cellular fatty acid metabolism in metabolically normal women. *J Clin Endocrinol Metab.* 99(9):E1666–1670.

You, Y.N., Short, K.R., Jourdan, M., Klaus, K.A., Walrand, S., and Nair, K.S. 2009. The effect of high glucocorticoid administration and food restriction on rodent skeletal muscle mitochondrial function and protein metabolism. *PLoS One.* 4(4):e5283.

You, Y.Q., Ling, P.R., Qu, J.Z., and Bistrian, B.R. 2008. Effects of medium-chain triglycerides, long-chain triglycerides, or 2-monododecanoin on fatty acid composition in the portal vein, intestinal lymph, and systemic circulation in rats. *JPEN J Parenter Enteral Nutr.* 32(2):169–175.

Yuen, K.C., and Dunger, D.B. 2006. Impact of treatment with recombinant human GH and IGF-I on visceral adipose tissue and glucose homeostasis in adults. *Growth Horm IGF Res.* 16(Suppl A):S55–61.

Zak, Z., Lagrost, L., Gautier, T., et al. 2002. Expression of simian CETP in normolipidemic Fisher rats has a profound effect on large sized apoE-containing HDL. *J Lipid Res.* 43(12):2164–2171.

Zamami, T., Hirama, T., Unakami, S., Hattori, Y., Hirata, M., Nomura, G., Tanimoto, Y., and Tanioka, Y. 1981. [Hematochemical characteristics of miniature pig Göttingen (miniature pig G) (author's transl)]. *Jikken Dobutsu.* 30(4):435--443.

Zannis, VI., Koukos, G., Drosatos, K., et al. 2008. Discrete roles of apoA-I and apoE in the biogenesis of HDL species: Lessons learned from gene transfer studies in different mouse models. *Ann Med.* 40(Suppl 1):14–28.

Zechner, R. 1997. The tissue-specific expression of lipoprotein lipase: Implications for energy and lipoprotein metabolism. *Curr Opin Lipidol.* 8(2):77–88.

Zechner, R., Kienesberger, P.C., Haemmerle, G., Zimmermann, R., and Lass, A. 2009. Adipose triglyceride lipase and the lipolytic catabolism of cellular fat stores. *J Lipid Res.* 50(1):3–21.

Zeng, Q., Isobe, K., Fu, L., et al. 2007. Effects of exercise on adiponectin and adiponectin receptor levels in rats. *Life Sci.* 80(5):454–459.

Zhang, C., Jin, Y., Liu, T., Liu, F., and Ito, T. 2009. Hypertriglyceridemia in Watanabe heritable hyperlipidemic rabbits was associated with increased production and reduced catabolism of very-low-density lipoproteins. *Pathobiology.* 76(6):315–321.

Zhang, W., Parentau, H., Greenly, R.L., et al. 1999. Effect of protein-calorie malnutrition on cytochromes P450 and glutathione S-transferase. *Eur J Drug Metab Pharmacokinet.* 24(2):141–147.

Zhang, Y., Kast-Woelbern, H.R., and Edwards, P.A. 2003. Natural structural variants of the nuclear receptor farnesoid x receptor affect transcriptional activation. *J Biol Chem.* 278:104–110.

Zhao, C., and Dahlman-Wright, K. 2010. Liver X receptor in cholesterol metabolism. *J Endocrinol.* 204(3):233–240.

Zhong, S., Goldberg, I.J., Bruce, C., Rubin, E., Breslow, J.L., and Tall, A. 1994. Human apoA-II inhibits the hydrolysis of HDL triglyceride and the decrease of HDL size induced by hypertriglyceridemia and cholesteryl ester transfer protein in transgenic mice. *J Clin Invest.* 94:2457–2467.

Zhu, X., and Cheng, S.Y. 2010. New insights into regulation of lipid metabolism by thyroid hormone. *Curr Opin Endocrinol Diabetes Obes.* 17(5):408–413.

Zhu, Y., Li, F., and Guo, G.L. 2011. Tissue-specific function of farnesoid X receptor in liver and intestine. *Pharmacol Res.* 63(4):259–265.

Zöllner, N., and Tacconi, M. 1968. On the concentration of various lipids in the serum and organs of miniature pigs and their dependency on the age of the animal. *Z Gesamte Exp Med.* 145(4):326–334.

Zucker, T.F., and Zucker, L.M. 1963. Fat accretion and growth in the rat. *J Nutr.* 80:6–19.

22 Electrolytes, Blood Gases, and Acid–Base Balance

Isabel A. Lea, Susan J. Borghoff, and Gregory S. Travlos

CONTENTS

22.1 INTRODUCTION

Physiological maintenance of electrolytes, hydrogen ions, carbon dioxide, and oxygen is essential for providing a cellular environment conducive to optimal cell function. The absolute and relative amounts of these substances and their interrelationships determine the osmolality, state of hydration, and membrane potentials of the animal. They are integral to nerve conduction, muscle contraction, myocardial function, and bone formation, and they act as enzyme cofactors. Maintenance of pH within narrow limits is required for these functions and is achieved by manipulation of electrolyte and blood gas levels. Any deviation from a physiologically normal state produces a response in homeostatic mechanisms that attempt to return values to normal (Paulev and Zubieta-Calleja,

2005). Homeostatic responses are most often brought about by changes in ion channel activity. With this knowledge, manipulation of homeostatic mechanisms (such as ion channels, etc.) is sometimes utilized during drug development processes to produce pharmaceutical products. Moreover, it is important to be aware of the possibility of adverse effects drugs may have on electrolytes, blood gases, and acid–base parameters. For example, albuterol, a β agonist, can stimulate sodium–potassium adenosine triphosphatase (ATPase) pumps that result in an intracellular shift of potassium producing low blood potassium levels (Allon and Copkney, 1990). Moreover, the antiviral agent, fialuridine, has caused fatal acidosis in people by damaging mitochondrial DNA resulting in the inhibition of cellular respiration (Brahams, 1994; Honkoop et al., 1997; Guyader et al., 2002).

This chapter discusses the mechanisms resulting in changes in electrolyte and acid–base levels and the biochemical effects of these changes. Sample collection techniques and factors that influence the measurement of analytes are also addressed. Although laboratory animals are bred and housed in a uniform fashion, there are unexpected variations that can influence the electrolyte or blood gas balance. Knowledge of such conditions is essential for correct interpretation of data. Altitude, seasonal and diurnal changes, and breeding cycles need to be carefully assessed during the process of data interpretation; interspecies variation in effects should also be considered. The time at which samples are taken is an important consideration when interpreting data; intake of food, diurnal variation, and animal activity level can also produce significant changes in plasma electrolyte concentrations or acid–base parameters (Bar-Ilan and Marder, 1980; Janssen et al., 1992; Lee et al., 2003). To accurately interpret the results, data should always be considered within the framework of these factors. It should be recognized that there is little point in collecting samples for analyses of blood gases or electrolytes (or any analytes) using improper collection methodology or incomplete analysis of circumstance (e.g., inappropriate anticoagulant use, contamination with air, improper sample mixing, improper sample storage, or delayed analysis) as this will ultimately result in erroneous diagnoses and serious or fatal consequences.

22.2 ELECTROLYTES

22.2.1 Basic Concepts

The most abundant fluid in the body is water. Total body water (TBW) makes up approximately 60% of body weight in healthy adult animals and occupies three main locations: the intracellular compartment and the two extracellular compartments (interstitial fluid [ISF] and plasma). TBW volume is determined largely by water intake and renal output although metabolic synthesis of water (from cellular respiration) and dehydration synthesis contribute to water gains, and evaporation from the skin, exhalation from the lungs, and feces contribute to water losses. Typically, TBW volume remains constant with control mechanisms responding to changes in osmolarity or intravascular volume. When water losses are greater than gains, decreased blood volume leads to the activation of the renin–angiotensin–aldosterone system (RAAS) and a decrease in atrial natriuretic peptide (ANP). Osmoreceptors in the hypothalamus are activated by the increase in blood osmolality and increased angiotensin II. Baroreceptors respond to decreased arterial pressure for stimulating the thirst center in the hypothalamus and the restoration of fluid loss.

Intracellular fluid (ICF) comprises the largest percentage of the body's water (approximately 65%) and is composed primarily of a solution of potassium and magnesium ions (K^+, Mg^{2+}), anions (organic phosphates and negatively charged protein), and protein. Control of ICF constituents is brought about by cell membranes and cell metabolism. Extracellular fluid (ECF) is mainly a solution of sodium (Na^+), chloride (Cl^-), bicarbonate (HCO_3^-) ions, and proteins. ISF, the fluid surrounding cells, is the largest component of ECF and is separated from ICF and plasma by cell membranes and capillary endothelial cells, respectively. Movement of water between ICF and the extracellular compartments is primarily accomplished by osmosis with the direction of water movement determined by the concentration of electrolytes in these fluids. Movement of anions and cations across cell membranes not only allows cells to control levels of electrolytes but also to maintain cellular electroneutrality (a net charge of zero). There are three main mechanisms that are used to maintain fluid balance in the extracellular compartments: (1) concentration of electrolytes in ECF, (2) capillary blood pressure, and (3) concentration of protein in plasma.

The concentration of electrolytes, particularly Na^+, determines not only the balance of fluids in the body but also osmolarity. The physiological control of Na^+ excretion is therefore vital to homeostasis and is achieved by both neurohormonal mechanisms based on extracellular volume (volume natriuresis) and changes in arterial pressure (pressure natriuresis) (Bie et al., 2004). The concentration of protein in plasma should be included in a discussion of fluid balance because of the Gibbs–Donnan effect. Although water moves freely across cell membranes and the membrane permeability to Na^+ and Cl^- ions is high, the presence of high molecular weight plasma proteins causes the ionic composition of ISF and plasma to be different. Plasma proteins are not readily able to cross cell membranes and being negatively charged they attract positively charged cations into the plasma resulting in the movement of negatively charged anions to the ISF to preserve electroneutrality (Nguyen and Kurtz, 2005).

Reference ranges for serum levels of common electrolytes are provided in Table 22.1 for laboratory animals. These levels should be considered as a guide only; absolute values can be influenced by animal handling techniques, sample collection methodology, and technique used to determine electrolyte level and should be determined empirically by individual laboratories.

22.2.2 Ion Channels

Cells acquire all the ions they need from the ECF through the plasma membrane. There are two mechanisms of ion movement: passive/facilitated diffusion occurring down an electrochemical gradient and active transport occurring against a concentration gradient. Both types of movement occur through transmembrane, ion channel proteins that are both gated, to regulate the permeability of the membrane, and selective in which ions can be transported. Ion channels can be distinguished based on this selectivity, their gating mechanism, and sequence similarity (Jentsch et al., 2002; Camerino et al., 2007). Passive transport gating can be facilitated by intracellular or extracellular ligands (e.g., the neurotransmitter, acetylcholine, cyclic adenine monophosphate [cAMP], cyclic guanosine monophosphate [cGMP], or ATP) and voltage (operating in response to membrane potential) or

TABLE 22.1
Reference Ranges for Electrolyte Measurements

Species	Sodium (mmol/L)[a]	Potassium (mmol/L)[a]	Calcium (mmol/L)	Chloride (mmol/L)[a]	Phosphorous (mmol/L)[a]	REFS
Rhesus Macaque (*Mucaca mulatta*)	[151.72]	[4.78]	[2.67]	[107.14]	[0.07]	Chen et al. (2009)
Cynomologous Macaque (*Mucaca fascicularis*)	[158.5]	[5.48]	[2.63]	[113.4]	[1.74]	Schuurman and Smith (2005)
Cat	146–156	4.0–4.5	1.55–2.55	117–123	1.45–2.62	Kaneko et al. (1997)
Dog	141–152	4.37–5.35	2.25–2.83	105–115	0.84–2.00	Kaneko et al. (1997)
Rabbit: New Zealand White	138–148	3.4–5.1	3.22–3.75	96–109	0.88–2.35	Hewitt et al. (1989)
Guinea Pig: Hartley	130.9–160.7	8.02–23.11	2.35–3.65	102.4–130.7	2.62–4.85	Charles River (2008a)
Rat: Crl:CD(SD)	140.0–157.0	4.00–12.20	2.35–3.35	90.0–132.0	1.07–4.33	Charles River (2006)
Rat: Crl:WI(Han)	135–151	3.31–6.11	2.28–3.03	97–107	1.18–3.46	Charles River (2008b)
Mouse: Crl:CD1(ICR)	137.7–169.3	7.84–14.18	2.47–3.10	106.1–130.7	2.55–4.55	Charles River (2008-2011)

[a]Values are given either as a range or as [mean] for all ages and both sexes combined.

mechanical mechanisms (such as in response to stretch or pressure). In each case, when the channels are open, ions bind to the membrane protein and are transported down a concentration gradient.

For active transport of ions, ATP hydrolysis is coupled with the movement of ions against the concentration gradient (Glynn, 1993; Kaplan, 2002). In this way, the level of cytosolic ions can be maintained at a different level to the ECF. One example of this is the Na^+/K^+ ATPase pump that couples the hydrolysis of ATP with the movement of three Na^+ ions out of the cell followed by the import of two K^+ ions into the cell. These types of pumps are important to maintain cell membrane resting potentials and cell volume, and to drive secondary active transport mechanisms that bring glucose or amino acids into the cell using the Na^+ gradient (Lingrel et al., 1994; Jorgensen and Pedersen, 2001). Endogenous control over the activity of these pumps is exerted through hormones (thyroid hormone, aldosterone, catecholamines, and insulin); their activity may also be affected by drugs such as the cardiac glycosides (Clausen, 2002). Inherited mutations in the ion channel proteins cause diseases such as cystic fibrosis (involving chloride channel cystic fibrosis transmembrane conductance regulator (CTFR); Gadsby and Nairn, 1999), Liddle's syndrome (involving mutations in epithelial sodium channel [ENaC]; Oh and Warnock, 2000), deafness (involving mutations in potassium channel, potassium voltage-gated channel subfamily Q member 4 (KCNQ4); Nie, 2008), seizures (involving voltage gated sodium channels, sodium voltage-gated channel beta subunit 1 (SCN1B), sodium voltage-gated channel alpha subunit 1 (SCN1A) or potassium channels, potassium voltage-gated channel subfamily A member 1 (KCNA1), potassium voltage-gated channel subfamily Q member 2 (KCNQ2), potassium voltage-gated channel subfamily Q member 3 (KCNQ3); Lerche et al., 2001), or heart arrhythmias (reviewed by Delisle et al., 2004). Other types of active ion pumps include H^+/K^+ ATPase and Ca^{2+} ATPase. Not all active ion pumps use ATP hydrolysis to drive the movement of ions; in some cases, the passive movement of an ion (usually Na^+) down the concentration gradient into the cell is coincident with the movement of another molecule up a concentration gradient into the cell. These proteins are called symporters, one example being the Na^+/glucose transporter that moves glucose out of the gut and kidney and back into the blood (Abramson and Wright, 2009; Bakris et al., 2009). An antiporter is a protein that uses the downhill movement of Na^+ into the cell to provide the energy to move another molecule out of the cell; calcium ions are moved out of the cell in this way.

22.2.3 Physiological Functions

Steady intracellular water and osmolarity are essential for cell membrane integrity and optimal performance of cellular processes. The kidneys, specifically the proximal tubule and Loop of Henle, accomplish this by reabsorbing large quantities of sodium, water, potassium, organic solutes, urea, and phosphate. Following this large-scale reabsorption, small adjustments to the concentrations of these solutes occur in the distal tubule; it is here that homeostatic control mechanisms are focused. The first step in the filtration of blood to form urine occurs at the Bowman's capsule (glomerular capsule). Fluid from the blood is collected in the Bowman's capsule as a glomerular filtrate; this then passes through the nephrons to form urine. The glomerular filtrate contains all substances in plasma and at the same concentrations as in plasma except for high molecular weight proteins and anything bound to them. During passage through the tubules, substances move either from tubule to peritubular capillaries (reabsorption) or from peritubular capillaries to tubules (secretion). This movement occurs through channels that are regulated by hormones and neurotransmitters. For example, antidiuretic hormone (ADH, vasopressin) controls the process of water reabsorption in the collecting ducts. ADH stimulates the insertion of aquaporin-2 channels increasing water permeability and its reabsorption; low ADH levels leads to decreased water reabsorption (water diuresis). An additional form of diuresis, osmotic diuresis, occurs when urination is increased due to a rise in osmotically active substances (e.g., glucose, mannitol) in the renal tubules. This can be stimulated when hypothalamic osmoreceptors respond to increased serum osmolarity by increasing the circulating levels of ADH. ADH increases free water reabsorption from the urine yielding a low volume and relatively high osmolarity. Serum osmolarity, therefore, returns to normal. ADH is not the only hormone that regulates kidney function; aldosterone and parathyroid hormones (PTHs) can also regulate electrolyte balance. Aldosterone is secreted from the adrenal gland largely, as a response to hypovolemia through the renin–angiotensin–aldosterone axis; secretion is also directly stimulated by increased serum K^+ levels. Aldosterone increases the reabsorption of Na^+ in the distal renal tubule and the secretion of K^+. When this occurs, more water is retained and the hypovolemic state is corrected. Normal kidneys can maintain balanced sodium levels independently of ADH or aldosterone by varying the degree of Na^+ reabsorption in the distal tubule. PTH is responsible for the endocrine regulation of calcium and phosphorus by increasing calcium reabsorption in renal tubules and promoting phosphate excretion (Figure 22.1).

Osmolarity is a measure of solute concentration in a solution; it is related to the number of particles in the solution rather than to the solute weight or charge. Osmolarity is defined as the number of osmoles of solute per liter of solution. For nonionic compounds that do not dissociate in solution, 1 osmole is equal to the molecular weight (in grams). For ionic compounds such as salts that can dissociate in solution to their constituent ions, 1 osmole is equal to the molecular weight (in grams) divided by the number of ions formed. Multiple combinations of compounds contribute to the osmolarity of a single solution. For example, a 4 Osm solution might consist of 2 Osm NaCl, 2 Osm glucose and 1 Osm NaCl, or 3 Osm glucose and 0.5 Osm NaCl. Osmolality is a measure of the osmoles of solute per kilogram of solvent and represents the value most often measured in a clinical laboratory setting. It is defined more by the presence of electrolytes and small molecules (e.g., glucose) rather than the presence of larger proteins. The osmolality of serum and urine are indicators of an animal's ability to maintain a fluid balance. In conditions where urine cannot be concentrated appropriately, the osmolality of urine will be near that of plasma (approximately 290 mOsm/Kg for humans) and, in severe dehydration, serum osmolality will be increased. Changes in ECF osmolality cause water to move passively between the ECF and ICF to the compartment with lower osmolality.

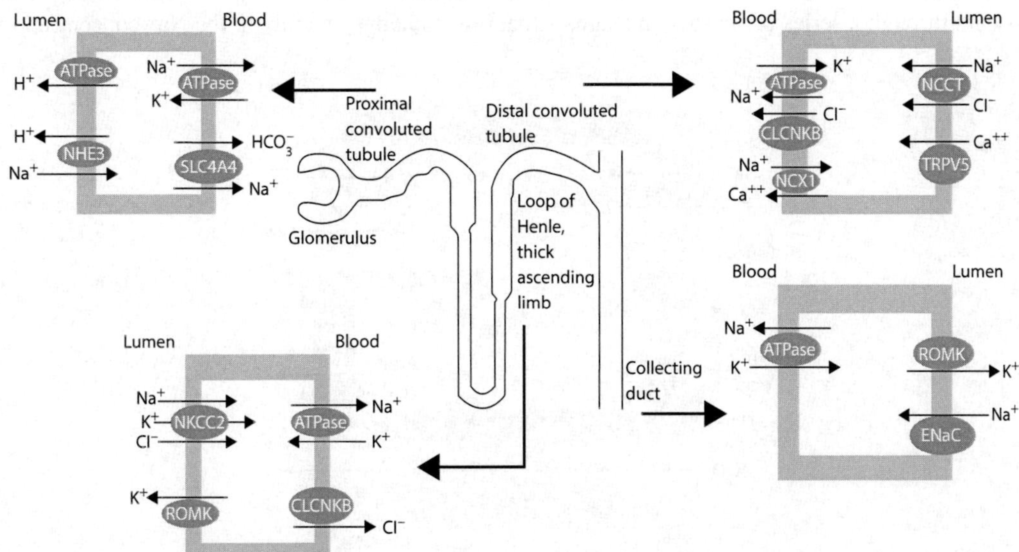

FIGURE 22.1 Selected ion transport proteins in tubules and collecting duct of the kidney. Apical reabsorption of Na^+ is effected by cotransporter proteins (NHE3, NKCC2, and NCCT) or the epithelial sodium channel, ENaC, and driven by Na^+/K^+ ATPase activity on the basolateral membrane. In the proximal convoluted tubule, HCO_3^- enters the blood via the Na^+-HCO_3^- cotransporter SLC4A4. Potassium is recycled over the apical membrane of the thick ascending limb and the cortical collecting duct through the ROMK channel. Chloride is reabsorbed in the thick ascending limb and distal tubule through the symporter proteins NKCC2 and NCCT and diffuses passively basolaterally through CLCNKB channels.

pH is a measure of the acidity or basicity of a solution; it is equal to the negative logarithm of the molar concentration of dissolved hydrogen ions:

$$pH = -\log\left[H^+\right]$$

Changes in hydrogen ion concentration, therefore, bring about changes in pH: when the concentration of the hydrogen rises, the drop in pH causes acidosis to develop; when the hydrogen concentration falls, the increase in pH brings about alkalosis. As different cellular components, enzymes, and other proteins have an optimal pH at which they function, the variation in pH levels is tightly regulated by acid–base homeostasis.

22.2.4 Cations

22.2.4.1 Sodium

Sodium is a naturally occurring mineral found in many foods and table salt. Its major role is to maintain the body's osmotic balance along with brain and neuron function. Sodium is absorbed in the small intestine in tandem with large quantities of water/fluid where it forms the major cation of the plasma. Absorption is made possible by the establishment of an electrochemical gradient for sodium across the enterocytes of the intestine. Na^+ enters through the luminal surface of epithelial cells via sodium channels and symporters (with glucose and amino acids) (Figure 22.2). Low intracellular Na^+ levels are then maintained by the presence of Na^+/K^+ ATPases on the basolateral membrane pumping Na^+ into the ICF from where it diffuses to the ECF (plasma of the villus capillaries). With the export of high concentrations of Na^+, an osmotic gradient is established that enables water to diffuse along the same pathway (Kiela et al., 2006). This Na^+/water balance is a major determinant of ECF osmolarity and volume.

Homeostatic control of ECF volume is vital to sustaining a constant cellular environment and occurs through a series of sensors and signals that effect changes mainly in the Na^+ concentration

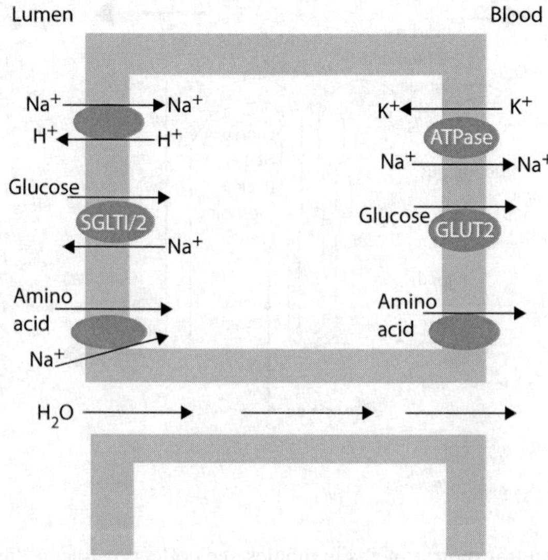

FIGURE 22.2 Intestinal absorption of sodium in the epithelial cells of the small intestine and colon. Sodium–glucose ligand transport proteins (SGLT1 and SGLT2) and sodium-coupled amino acid transport proteins move sodium across the apical membrane from the lumen into the cell. The sodium–potassium adenosine triphosphatase present on the basolateral membrane of the cell maintains a low intracellular sodium concentration and electronegative cell.

via neural, hormonal, and physical responses. Normal serum sodium concentrations in humans range from 136 to 145 mmol/L and normally are maintained at a constant level. Serum sodium levels in mice are slightly higher than other mammalian species with values in the range of 137.7–169.3 mmol/L (Finch and Foster, 1973); in comparison, rabbit sodium levels range from 138 to 148 mmol/L (Table 22.1). No age, sex, or strain differences have been observed for either species. The maintenance of serum sodium concentration can be illustrated in a study conducted in a group of five trained dogs where serum sodium was measured on alternate days over the course of a week. The maximum difference in serum sodium concentrations for an individual dog was 4 mmol/L with values ranging from 144 to 148 mmol/L (Riley and Cornelius, 1989). Homeostasis is achieved by a regulated excretion of water and salt, primarily via the kidneys but also at other epithelial sites such as the distal colon (Fuller and Young, 2005; Kiela et al., 2006). To preserve an electrochemical balance, this movement of sodium ions is coupled with that of hydrogen, potassium, and chloride ions; these will be discussed in later sections (de Wardener, 1978). There are multiple control systems involved in this regulated secretion including an ADH-mediated water-retaining mechanism and sodium-retaining systems dominated by the rennin–angiotensin–aldosterone cascade. Some of the most important hormones involved in the control of renal sodium excretion are aldosterone, urodilatin, ANP, and angiotensin II (Forssmann et al., 2001; Hall, 2003). These act to either stimulate (aldosterone and angiotensin II) or inhibit (ANP) Na^+ reabsorption principally in the proximal/distal tubules or collecting ducts of the kidney by activating Na^+/K^+ pumps, Na^+/H^+ antiporters, Na^+/glucose symporters, or Na^+ ion channels. An overview of the renal handling of sodium is shown in Figure 22.3 and Table 22.2.

Aldosterone and, to a minor degree, other mineralocorticoids and glucocorticoids bind to intra cellular receptors; the active hormone–receptor complex interacts with DNA through hormone-responsive elements to regulate transcription of genes encoding proteins such as RAS (proto-oncogene, GTPase), corticosteroid hormone-induced factor (CHIF), serum glucocorticoid-regulated kinase 1 (SGK1), and amiloride sensitive ENaC (Bhargava et al., 2004). The result of these changes

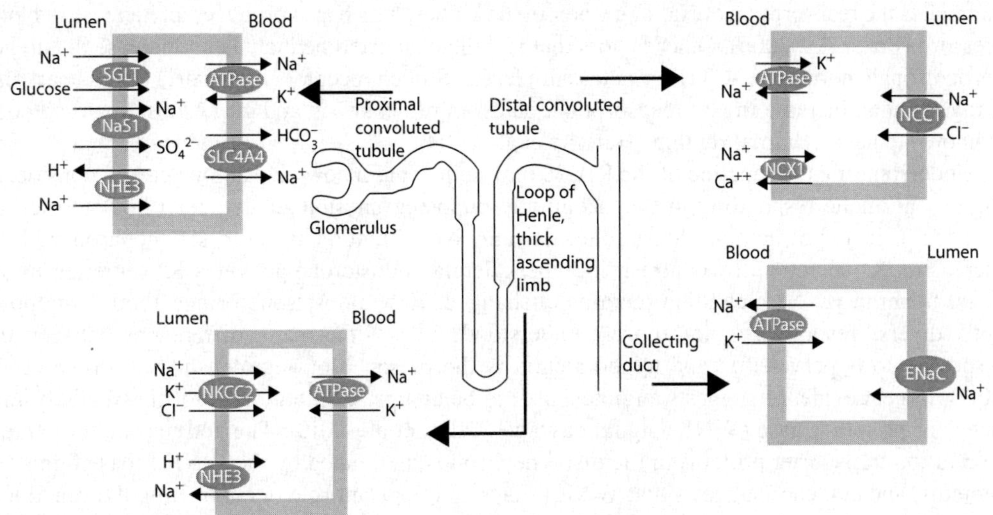

FIGURE 22.3 Renal sodium transport. Approximately 70% of filtered Na^+ is reabsorbed in the proximal tubule through apical transport proteins driven primarily by the Na^+/K^+ ATPase antiporter in the basolateral membrane. The thick ascending limb of the Loop of Henle reabsorbs approximately 15% of filtered Na^+ through the $Na^+/K^+/2Cl^-$ symporter, NKCC2 (SLC12A) on the apical surface of the cell; the distal convoluted tubule and collecting ducts collectively reabsorb approximately 15% of filtered Na^+ through the Na^+/Cl^- cotransporter, NCCT and the epithelial sodium channel, ENaC, respectively. In each tubule, segment Na^+ reabsorption is driven by Na^+/K^+ ATPase activity on the basolateral membrane.

TABLE 22.2
Control of Sodium Reabsorption in Different Segments of the Renal Tubule

Renal Tubule Segment	Stimulation of Sodium Reabsorption	Inhibition of Sodium Reabsorption
• Proximal Convoluted Tubule	• Angiotensin II • Epinephrine/norepinephrine	• Dopamine
• Thick Ascending Limb	• cAMP via the many hormones and mediators coupled to adenylyl cyclase, e.g., PTH, vasopressin, calcitonin, glucagon, and β-adrenergic agonists	• Negative modulation of cAMP/PKA signaling pathway via mediators such as angiotensin II, endothelin, cGMP and prostaglandin E_2
• Distal Convoluted Tubule	• Aldosterone	• ANP
• Collecting Duct	• Aldosterone • Vasopressin	• Dopamine • α2-Adrenergic agonists • Prostaglandins

Source: Feraille, E. and Doucet, A., *Physiol Rev*., 81, 345–418, 2001.

in gene expression is modulation of the activity or number of ion pumps and channels (Horisberger and Rossier, 1992; Fuller and Young, 2005). Aldosterone is part of the RAAS that regulates blood pressure and water balance. When blood volume is low, the kidneys secrete renin that stimulates the production of angiotensin that in turn stimulates the secretion of aldosterone from the adrenal cortex. Angiotensin constricts blood vessels causing an increase in blood pressure; aldosterone stimulates the reabsorption of Na^+ and water in the kidney, which also produces an increase in blood pressure (Rozansky, 2006). Other factors that stimulate aldosterone include an increase in adrenocorticotrophic hormone (ACTH) or potassium levels. Stretch receptors in the atria of the heart also bring about an increase in Na^+ reabsorption, but from urine, sweat, and gut. Aldosterone secretion is known to have a diurnal rhythm (Hurwitz et al., 2004).

Understanding the function of the RAAS may help explain how aldosterone can be considered the key hormone responding to two seemingly opposing physiological states (the "aldosterone paradox"). In hypovolemia, aldosterone activates Na^+ retention in the distal nephron without increasing K^+ secretion; by contrast, in hyperkalemia, aldosterone activates K^+ secretion in the distal nephron yet Na^+ retention remains unchanged. How aldosterone brings about two apparently diverse responses is not entirely understood. One of the major differences between the responses to hypervolemia and hyperkalemia is the presence of angiotensin II (Arroyo et al., 2011). Recent evidence suggests angiotensin II to be an upstream regulator for the WNK lysine-deficient protein kinase (WNK) signal cascade (Talati et al., 2010). The activity and/or expression of ion transporter proteins in the distal nephron is modulated by the WNK kinase family of proteins, and evidence suggests that WNK4 plays an important role in controlling the functional state of the Na^+ and K^+ transport proteins (NaCl co-transporter (NCCT) and renal outer-medullary K channel (ROMKt), thereby effecting the fine tuning of Na^+ and K^+ homeostasis (Verrey, 2007; McCormick et al., 2008).

ANP is produced and released from cardiac atrial myocytes and can counter the increase in blood volume stimulated by the RAAS (Inagami, 1994; Forssmann et al., 1998; Inoue et al., 2001). It is released in response to a variety of stimuli including distension of the atria, angiotensin II, endothelin, sympathetic stimulation of β-adrenoceptors, and raised sodium concentration (Harris et al., 1988). ANP binds to ANP transmembrane receptors and in the kidney increases the glomerular filtration rate (GFR) by dilating the afferent and constricting the efferent glomerular arterioles resulting in greater secretion of Na^+ and water. Sodium resorption in the distal convoluted tubule and collecting ducts is inhibited by the phosphorylation of ENaC; secretion of renin and aldosterone are also inhibited. Similar responses have been observed in dogs, rats, and humans (Haass et al., 1985; Dillingham and Anderson, 1986). Another member of this family of natriuretic peptides is urodilatin. This peptide is a differentially processed form of ANP (extended N-terminally by four amino acids compared to ANP) and is synthesized by the kidney tubular cells. It is secreted luminally where it binds to receptors ion the distal nephron, stimulates intracellular guanylyl cyclase, and activates cGMP-dependent protein kinases. In this way, urodilatin inhibits Na^+ reabsorption by closing amiloride sensitive Na^+ channels (ENaC) and enhancing dopamine-induced inhibition of Na^+/K^+ ATPase activity (Forssmann et al., 2001; Choi et al., 2011).

Pharmacologically sodium homeostasis can be influenced by the cardiac glycosides digitalis and ouabain. Both drugs bind to the alpha subunit of the Na^+/K^+ ATPase. Different isoforms of the alpha subunit can act as receptors of differing affinities but are typically used to treat congestive heart failure most likely acting by inhibiting the action of the sodium pump. More recently, endogenous ouabain has been isolated from the plasma of humans and several other mammals including rat, dog, and cow (Boulanger et al., 1993; Schneider et al., 1998). The mode of action and physiological significance of this finding is under investigation, but it has been suggested that ouabain acts to promote cell growth and stimulate the Na^+/K^+ pump (Gao et al., 2002).

22.2.4.1.1 Sodium Imbalance

22.2.4.1.1.1 Hypernatremia Hypernatremia is an electrolyte imbalance that is defined as an elevated plasma sodium level. In humans, hypernatremia occurs when the levels exceed 145 mmol/L; however, severe symptoms usually occur when the levels reach >158 mmol/L. In dogs, hypernatremia develops when sodium concentrations exceed 150 mmol/L, yet neurological symptoms are not usually evident until the levels reach 170 mmol/L. Hypernatremia is most often caused by a water deficiency relative to electrolyte content rather than a problem with sodium homeostasis (Chumlea et al., 1999; Adrogue and Madias, 2000). Usually, this occurs when there is inadequate access to water or the thirst mechanism is impaired; normally, thirst is stimulated by an increase in body fluid osmolarity. Less commonly, sodium excess can be a cause of hypernatremia usually through inappropriate ingestion or as a result of disease. Common causes of hypernatremia are presented in Table 22.3 (Agrawal et al., 2008). Higher mortality rates are associated with the acute form of the

TABLE 22.3
Causes of Hypernatremia

Water Deficit	Water and Sodium Loss	Sodium Gain
• Inadequate intake—either lack of access or improper thirst mechanism (adipsia)	• Cutaneous losses—sweating, burn injuries	• Consumption of seawater
• Panting, insensible losses (respiratory tract)	• Gastrointestinal disorders—diarrhea, gastroenteritis, or vomiting	• Iatrogenic (caused by treatment)
• Diabetes insipidus with restricted access to water	• Osmotic diuresis as a response to hyperglycemia, high protein diet, or mannitol	• Improperly formulated diet/salt poisoning/high salt diet with restricted access to water
• Vasopressin deficiency	• Renal disease—postobstructive diuresis, diuretic phase of acute tubular necrosis	• Hyperaldosteronism (Conn's syndrome)—either primary or secondary
–	• Diabetes mellitus	• Hyperadrenocorticism (Cushing's syndrome)

disease where cell dehydration leads to neuronal cell shrinkage, brain injury, and possible circulatory problems (Oh and Carroll, 1992; Darmon et al., 2010). Different forms of hypernatremia can be distinguished by the volume disturbance or tonicity (osmotic pressure) that they are associated with: hypovolemic, euvolemic, or hypervolemic, and hypertonic, isotonic, or hypotonic states.

22.2.4.1.1.1.1 Water Deficit A water deficit most commonly develops when impaired water intake is coupled with increased losses (e.g., respiratory or renal losses). The failure of the kidney to concentrate urine might also lead to a water deficit and can occur either through a failure in the hypothalamic–pituitary axis to synthesis or release sufficient levels of ADH hormone (neurogenic/central diabetes insipidus) or a failure of the kidney to respond appropriately to ADH (renal/nephrogenic diabetes insipidus). Most of the free water losses occur from intracellular and interstitial spaces, less from the ECF so blood volume usually remains within the normal range. Animals with diabetes insipidus generally do not develop hypernatremia if they are able to maintain adequate fluid intake to compensate for the losses (Agrawal et al., 2008). Rodent models of diabetes insipidus have been developed: hereditary neurogenic diabetes insipidus in the Brattleboro strain of Long-Evans rat (Moses and Miller, 1974), and nephrogenic diabetes in mice (Naik and Valtin, 1969). Experimental evidence from rats, dogs and cats in which lesions in the hypothalamus abolished the thirst centers demonstrate the development of severe hypernatremia (Gardiner et al., 1985; Morrison and Fales-Williams, 2006; Shimokawa Miyama et al., 2009). In general, any process that disrupts the hypothalamic–pituitary axis can lead to diabetes insipidus: pituitary injury, tumors, inflammatory states (encephalitis), aneurysms, drugs, or genetic defects.

22.2.4.1.1.1.2 Hypotonic Fluid Loss (Water and Sodium Loss) Loss of water in excess of electrolytes producing hypovolemia (decreased volume) results from anything that interferes with the ability of the kidney to concentrate urine. Postobstructive diuresis and the diuretic phase of acute tubular necrosis have both been shown to contribute to a hypernatremic state (de Morais and DiBartola, 2008). Other types of renal disease might also cause retention of sodium. The central feature of nephrotic syndrome is sodium retention and while the cause of this may not be completely understood, it has been attributed to an increase in aldosterone (Shapiro et al., 1990). More recently, the sodium retention in nephrotic syndrome has been associated with an increased activity of Na^+/K^+ ATPase and ENaC channels in conjunction with curtailment of the regulation of ANP-induced secretion of renal sodium in the collecting ducts (de Seigneux et al., 2006; Deschênes et al., 2003). In glomerulonephritis, the amount of sodium filtered is disproportionate to that reabsorbed; consequently, plasma sodium is increased. Osmotic diuresis, an increase in the osmotic pressure in kidney tubules due to the presence of substances such as glucose, causes retention of water in the tubule lumen and increased urination. This can also occur in animals fed a high protein diet where the increased production of urea acts as a diuretic and causes loss of water in excess of sodium (Godwin and Williams, 1984). Diabetes mellitus can also result in hypovolemic hypernatremia since glucose removed from the serum on administration of insulin is replaced by cellular sodium to maintain the osmotic equilibrium. Further to this, water leaves the plasma when the osmotic effects of glucose are removed. Ptyalism (profuse salivation) and diarrhea can both produce hypotonic fluid losses that result in dehydration and hypernatremia. In the dog and cat, salivary and digestive losses are more isotonic than they are in humans and other species, so they are less prone to develop hypernatremia by these means (Martin and Young, 1971).

22.2.4.1.1.1.3 Hypertonic Fluid Loss (Sodium Gain) Hypernatremia is caused less commonly by hypertonic fluid losses than by hypotonic fluid loss and water deficit (Tisdall et al., 2006). Hypertonic fluid loss can be the result of improperly formulated diets, iatrogenic induction (through administration or ingestion of salt or baking soda), or variations in aldosterone hormone level. Primary hyperaldosteronism (Conn's Syndrome) is a disease of the adrenal glands characterized by the secretion of excess aldosterone (Fardella and Mosso, 2002; Nadar et al., 2003). It can be caused by adrenal hyperplasia, adenoma, and rarely carcinoma. Increased aldosterone concentration causes an increase in Na^+ and water retention and K^+ secretion by the kidneys resulting in high blood pressure (arterial hypertension). The enhanced exchange of Na^+ for K^+ can also give rise to hypokalemia (see Section 22.2.4.2.1.2) and sometimes hypernatremia. Secondary hyperaldosteronism represent a diverse group of disorders that are characterized by the activation of the RAAS as a homeostatic mechanism to preserve serum electrolyte balance or fluid volume. As with primary hyperaldosteronism, hypokalemia is likely but hypernatremia may also occur. Possible causes include renin producing tumors, cardiac failure, and nephritic syndrome. Cushing's disease of the pituitary gland (hyperadrenocorticism) is caused by a tumor of the pituitary gland that produces large amounts of ACTH, which in turn stimulates the release of cortisol from the adrenal glands. When Cushing's disease is the result of adrenal gland hyperplasia or tumors, excess cortisol is secreted. This in turn inhibits Na^+ secretion by the kidney and leads to the development of hypernatremia.

22.2.4.1.1.2 Hyponatremia Hyponatremia is an electrolyte disturbance characterized by abnormally low sodium levels (<135 mmol/L) in the blood, most commonly because of an excess amount or effect of ADH (Pham et al., 2006; Kamel and Halperin, 2012). It is often a side effect of other conditions in which fluids rich in sodium are lost (vomiting or diarrhea) or water is accumulated at rate higher than it is excreted (syndrome of inappropriate ADH secretion). Serious hyponatremia occurs when the plasma sodium concentration is less than 120 mmol/L, and profound hyponatremia is seen at 100 mmol/L. In humans, clinical signs of slowly induced hyponatremia do not occur until serum sodium falls to less than 100 mmol/L. In dogs and cats, clinical central nervous system (CNS) signs are evident when serum sodium reaches ~115–120 mmol/L (Vexler et al., 1994; Brady et al., 1999). In male rats, chronic hyponatremia (induced by administration of vasopressin) with plasma Na^+ concentrations of 106–108 mmol/L results in 22%–23% mortality but no apparent changes in brain morphology. In hyponatremic male rabbits, brain edema was evident with plasma Na^+ concentrations of 118 mmol/L (Ayus et al., 2006; Vexler et al., 1994). The severities of the symptoms increase with the degree of the disease and the rapidity with which the condition develops. When sodium levels fall gradually, minimal symptoms may occur, as compensatory mechanisms have an opportunity to counterbalance the changes; for acute hyponatremia (developing in under 48 hours), a drop in the sodium level of a similar magnitude may have serious consequences (severe cerebral edema, coma, or brainstem herniation) (Soupart and Decaux, 1996; Fried and Palevsky, 1997; Tisdall et al., 2006). Different forms of hyponatremia can be distinguished by the volume disturbance or tonicity (osmotic pressure) that they are associated with: hypovolemic, euvolemic, or hypervolemic, and hypertonic, isotonic, or hypotonic states. Common causes of hyponatremia are given in Table 22.4.

TABLE 22.4
Causes of Hyponatremia

Water and Sodium Loss	Water Gain with Normal Sodium	Water and Sodium Gains
• Extrarenal Na^+ loss—diarrhea, vomiting, excessive sweating	• Disorders—"syndrome of inappropriate antidiuresis secretion," hypothyroidism, adrenal insufficiency	• Extrarenal disorders—heart failure, cirrhosis
• Na^+ loss—diuretics (thiazide and loop), osmotic diuresis, mineralocorticoid deficiency, cerebral salt wasting deficiency	• Other conditions—pulmonary infections, acute lung injury, CNS disorders such as demyelination, inflammatory disorders or lesions	• Renal disorders—nephrotic syndrome, chronic kidney disease, acute kidney dysfunction
–	• Drugs—diuretics, barbiturates, opioids, etc.	–
–	• Increased fluid intake—primary polydipsia	–

22.2.4.1.1.2.1 Water and Sodium Loss Water and sodium loss produces hypovolemic hyponatremia, when the Na+ loss proportionally exceeds that of water. Serum osmolarity is reduced (hypotonic) and a reduction in blood volume cautses an increase in ADH secretion. The resulting retention of water causes an increase in plasma dilution. Diuretics are an important cause of renal water loss. They act by inhibiting solute reabsorption in the diluting segment of the nephron and increasing Na^+ secretion. Once volume depletion occurs, the nonosmotic release of ADH causes water retention contributing to worsening hyponatremia. ADH release is enhanced by concurrent hypokalemia that causes the intracellular movement of Na^+ and worsens the state of hyponatremia (Agrawal et al., 2008).

22.2.4.1.1.2.2 Water Gain with Normal Sodium Hyponatremia where TBW is increased but Na^+ levels and ECF volume remain near normal (euvolemic/dilutional hyponatremia) can be caused by a variety of disorders. In the "syndrome of inappropriate antidiuresis" (SAID, also known as "syndrome of inappropriate antidiuretic hormone secretion" [SIADH]), ADH levels are elevated; this is associated with a variety of disorders such as cancer, CNS, pulmonary and endocrine disorders, or heartworm disease (Siragy, 2006; Agrawal et al., 2008). It is reported to occur in human and dog, but the importance of this condition in other species is unclear. Adrenal insufficiency arises when a mineralocorticoid deficiency causes increased secretion of Na^+ and decreased secretion of K^+. This results in an inability to concentrate urine and hyponatremia develops. Primary polydipsia occurs in humans and occasionally in animals when large quantities of water are consumed or there is an excretion deficiency in the kidneys. Hyponatremia can only develop when water intake exceeds the ability of the kidney to excrete water (Mallie et al., 1997). A variety of drugs can produce hyponatremia, and all operate through an ability to interfere in water excretion. Thiazide diuretics are the most common causes of drug-induced hyponatremia acting by inhibiting reabsorption of Na^+ and Cl^- through the Na^+/Cl^- symporter in the distal convoluted tubule (Hwang and Kim, 2010). In addition, a variety of drugs can precipitate increased vasopressin secretion; these include carbamazepine, chlorpropamide, clofibrate, opiates, tricyclic antidepressants, cyclophosphamide, and oxytocin (Kovacs and Robertson, 1992).

22.2.4.1.1.2.3 Water and Sodium Gains Hypervolemic hyponatremia is characterized by an increase in sodium (and therefore ECF volume) and TBW concentrations. Proportionally TBW increases are greater than Na^+. Hyponatremia occurs when a decrease in effective circulating volume caused by cardiac failure or decreased movement of water from the vasculature to the interstitial spaces results in the activation of compensatory mechanisms including the RAAS, ADH, and norepinephrine. Water and Na^+ are retained and hyponatremia develops. Disorders that cause this sequence of events include various edematous disorders (cirrhosis and heart failure) and nephrogenic diseases (Ali et al., 2007; de Morais and DiBartola, 2008; Farmakis et al., 2009).

22.2.4.1.1.2.4 Redistributive Hyponatremia Hyponatremia can also develop in cases where total body sodium and water concentrations are unchanged. In these situations, increased osmotic pressure in the extracellular compartment causes water to shift from the intracellular to the extracellular compartment. Extracellular Na^+ concentrations are diluted but total body sodium levels remain unchanged. This most often occurs with hyperglycemia and administration of osmotically active molecules with mannitol treatment for brain edema (Smith et al., 2000).

22.2.4.1.2 *Factors Influencing Measurement of Sodium Concentration*

Serum sodium is measured in all laboratory animal species by instruments requiring a relatively large sample volume: emission flame photometer, atomic absorption spectrophotometer, and ion specific electrode (Hansen et al., 1982). Measured as part of a profile with other electrolytes having similar volume requirements, it limits the profile choices particularly as fasted mice, young rats, and other very small laboratory animals do not yield a large volume of blood. Fractional clearance or excretion of sodium (FENa) can be determined in urine specimens at different time points daily and is often used as an estimation of sodium handling. FENa describes the proportion of sodium that is excreted in the urine compared with that filtered through the glomerulus. It may be quantified by comparison to the clearance of endogenous creatinine. This procedure simultaneously measures the electrolyte and creatinine concentration in single urine and serum samples and allows measurement of sodium clearance without knowledge of urine flow rate or volume. However, as with other methods, the small volume of blood that can be sampled daily from small laboratory animals can be a limit to experimental design using this method. FENa can be calculated using the following formula:

$$\text{FENa} = \frac{(\text{urine sodium/serum sodium})}{(\text{urine creatinine/serum creatinine})} \times 100$$

Instrument specific requirements must be taken into account. For example, lithium (lithium heparin is used an anticoagulant) interferes with Na^+ determination by the flame photometer, atomic absorption, and ion specific electrode; therefore, instruments should be adjusted to account for this potential error (van Suijlen et al., 1990). Moreover, measurements should always be performed within a linear, analytical range and within a fixed temperature range; outside of these ranges, the results may be erroneous. Metabolic disturbances that bring about hyperlipidemia, hyperproteinemia, hyperglycemia, or dehydration may produce spurious results (Roscoe et al., 1975; Dimeski et al., 2006). The practice of fasting rodents and removing drinking water during their active period should therefore be performed only when necessary and results interpreted with caution (Ramsay and Ganong, 1977; Kleeman, 1979). Ultimately, the decision to fast or not, prior to sample collection, must be based on individual study objectives and kept consistent within a particular study (Weingand et al., 1996). Rats require 72 hours of food deprivation to become nonabsorptive, comparable to the state achieved by dogs or humans in 10–14 hours (Loeb, 1999). Since rats are night feeders, removal of food overnight prior to specimen collection ostensibly results in a 24-hour fast. Shorter periods of food deprivation result in a progressive decrease in serum glucose, triglycerides, and alkaline phosphatase, but not of cholesterol (Waner and Nyska, 1994). To our knowledge, short-duration fasting does not affect serum electrolyte concentrations. However, fasting male adult Sprague Dawley rats for a longer duration (3–6 days) can result in a 20% decrease in serum potassium but no differences in sodium and chloride concentrations; carbon dioxide content was considered unaffected (Huth and Elkington, 1959). Severe diet restriction (feed intake 25% of controls) of Sprague Dawley rats for two weeks resulted in decreases in serum potassium (~18%) and calcium (~8%), and minimal increases in sodium and chloride concentration (<5%) (Levin et al., 1993).

22.2.4.2 Potassium

Potassium is a naturally occurring mineral found in many foods, particularly fruits and vegetables. It is absorbed from the intestine and excreted in both urine and feces (Klevay et al., 2007). Its primary role is in neuron, cardiac and skeletal muscle, and enzyme functions; it also plays a role in defining the osmotic balance between cells and the ISF. Potassium is the major cation of the ICF; approximately 2% of body K^+ is found in ECF, 98% is intracellular, located predominantly in muscle and bone (Greenlee et al., 2009). This intracellular store (150 mmol/L) can be used as a source through which the extracellular (3.5–5 mmol/L) potassium levels can be maintained at a constant level (Table 22.1). Movement of potassium between the different fluid compartments is mediated by Na^+/K^+ ATPase pumps and highly selective potassium ion channels in neurons and cardiac muscle (Doyle et al., 1998; Noskov and Roux, 2006).

Potassium homeostasis is principally maintained by feedback control of secretion from the kidney (90%) and gastrointestinal (GI) tract (10%) (Hayslett et al., 1982; Wang and Giebisch, 2009; Sorensen et al., 2010). The kidney is able to regulate K^+ levels by decreasing secretion when intake is low and increasing secretion when intake is high. Potassium continues to be lost even in the absence of any intake, in fact, K^+ homeostasis is able to be maintained until the GFR drops to 15–20 mL/min. When renal failure occurs, the colon becomes the major site of potassium secretion and is able to regulate K^+ levels. Renal secretion depends on free filtration at the glomerulus, extensive proximal tubule reabsorption, and highly regulated secretion at the distal tubule and collecting ducts (Palmer and Frindt, 2007). The collecting ducts contain two different cell types: principal cells and intercalated cells that mediate K^+ secretion and K^+ absorption, respectively. Principal cells mediate sodium reabsorption and potassium secretion, they are targets for angiotensin II, aldosterone, and potassium-sparing diuretics and use the basolateral N^+/K^+ ATPase to drive potassium secretion through apical potassium ion channels along a favorable electrochemical gradient. Several types of channels are involved in K^+ secretion including ROMK, the ATP-dependent renal out medullary potassium channel and potassium two pore domain channel subfamily K member 1 (KCNK1), the double-pore K^+ channel (Wang and Giebisch, 2009). Controlling the balance between renal potassium excretion and sodium reabsorption is achieved (at least in part) through WNK signaling, which modulates the activity of the Na^+Cl^- symporter, NCCT, and down regulates the expression of the ROMK channel at the cell surface (Welling and Ho, 2009; Cope et al., 2006; Kahle et al., 2003) (Figure 22.4).

Factors that can affect potassium secretion from these cells include K^+ intake, intracellular K^+ levels, urine flow rate, sodium levels, and hormones (aldosterone and β-catecholamines) (Field et al., 1984). Similar processes operate in the distal colon (Giebisch et al., 2007). When plasma potassium levels are high, aldosterone release stimulates the renal Na^+/K^+ ATPases to secrete excess K^+ into the collecting duct (Wang, 2004), and when plasma potassium concentrations are low, less aldosterone is released and renal potassium secretion is minimized.

In addition to renal control of homeostasis, transcellular redistribution can help maintain constant levels of potassium. Muscle contains the majority of the body's potassium, after ingestion, insulin stimulates increased activity of the sodium pump and increased potassium uptake (McDonough et al., 2002; McDonough and Youn, 2005). Other factors such as acid–base balance can also affect the balance between cellular and extracellular K^+ concentrations. Acidosis increases plasma K^+ concentration by inducing the movement of ions from the cellular to the extracellular compartment whereas alkalosis enhances cellular uptake of potassium (McDonough and Youn, 2005; Youn and McDonough, 2009).

22.2.4.2.1 Potassium Imbalance

22.2.4.2.1.1 Hyperkalemia Hyperkalemia is an electrolyte imbalance that is defined as an elevated plasma potassium level exceeding 5.5 mmol/L for most species; normal potassium levels range from 3.5 to 5.0 mmol/L in humans, 4.37 to 5.35 mmol/L in dogs, and 3.31 to 12.2 mmol/L in rats

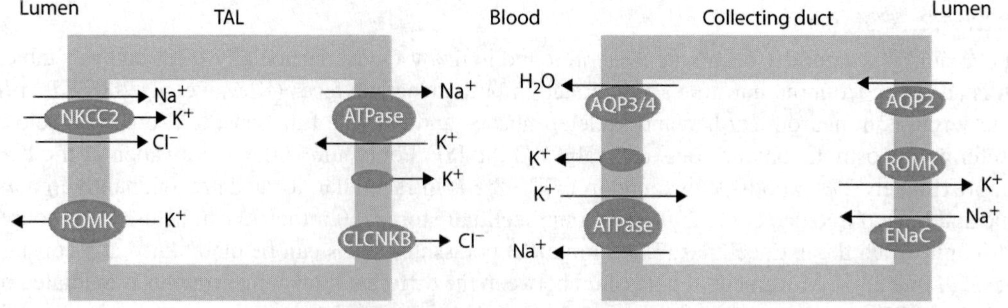

FIGURE 22.4 Renal handling of potassium. Potassium is recycled over the apical membrane of the thick ascending loop of Henle (TAL) through the ROMK channel and only a fraction on the potassium entering the cell apically exits the basolateral membrane (mechanism of transport unknown). In the collecting duct, sodium taken up by ENaC (apically) drives the secretion of potassium through the ROMK channel.

(Table 22.1) (Borok et al., 1987; Tran, 2005). It can arise by one of three mechanisms: decreased excretion of potassium (particularly when coupled with an excessive intake), potassium shift from intracellular to extracellular space, or excessive intake. The latter two mechanisms are rather less common than the first (Nyirenda et al., 2009). Common causes of hyperkalemia are given in Table 22.5.

22.2.4.2.1.1.1 Decreased Excretion Animals with chronic kidney disease are generally able to preserve near normal levels of K^+ as long as aldosterone secretion, aldosterone responsiveness, and the flow rate in the distal tubule of the kidney are maintained. This is in part due to the role the colon plays in the GI tract regulation of K^+ excretion. However, once the GFR drops to 15–20 mL/min or hypoaldosteronism (from with the lack or improper action of aldosterone) occurs, the ability to excrete K^+ is compromised and hyperkalemia develops (Karet, 2009). The conditions most often associated with this type of hyperkalemia are urethral obstruction, anuric, or oliguric renal failure; less commonly, it may also be caused by ruptured bladder, hyporeninemic hypoaldosteronism, and adrenal insufficiency (Kogika and de Morais, 2008). The use of drugs such as angiotensin-converting enzyme (ACE) inhibitors, NSAIDs (nonsteroidal anti-inflammatory drugs), and prostaglandin inhibitors can also play a role in the development of hyperkalemia. Failure of the RAAS alone rarely produces an increase in plasma potassium significant enough to cause hyperkalemia (Remuzzi et al., 2005).

22.2.4.2.1.1.2 Excessive Intake Excessive intake of potassium is an unlikely cause of hyperkalemia when coupled with normal renal or adrenal function. The kidney's ability to adapt to acute and chronic alterations in K^+ intake by renal secretion and shifts in the cellular balance of K^+ allow ingestion of almost unlimited quantities of potassium in healthy animals. Both animals and humans with impaired excretory mechanisms or transcellular K^+ mobility can develop hyperkalemia with excessive potassium intake, which also occurs with the administration of large doses of potassium penicillin or potassium salts of other drugs (Zietse et al., 2009).

22.2.4.2.1.1.3 Shift in Cellular Balance of Potassium Alone, the shift in cellular balance of K^+ (from ICF to ECF) is a relatively uncommon cause of hyperkalemia; however, when coupled with excessive intake or impaired excretion, elevated potassium levels can occur. These lead to the disruption of neuromuscular, cardiac, and GI systems due to the depolarization of membrane potentials in cells. One of the conditions in which the cellular balance of K^+ is often altered is diabetes mellitus where there is an insulin deficiency or resistance. Insulin enhances the entry of potassium into cells, and deficiency or resistance therefore limits the intracellular shift of K^+. As the major intracellular cation, K^+ is released into the extracellular space when any form of massive cell rupture occurs. Rhabdomyolysis (due to excessive exertion), tumor lysis, and hemolysis (due to blood transfusion,

TABLE 22.5
Causes of Hyperkalemia

Decreased Excretion	Excessive Intake	Shift in Cellular Balance
• Hypoaldosteronism/impaired responsiveness of distal tubule to aldosterone	• High dietary intake	• Massive tissue damage—tumor lysis, massive hemolysis, surgery, rhabdomyolysis, excessive burns
• Renal failure—anuric or oliguric	–	• Acute acidosis
• Hypoadrenocorticism (Addison's disease)	–	• Insulin deficiency or resistance
• GI disease—salmonellosis, perforated duodenal ulcer	–	• Drugs—digitalis toxicity, succinylcholine
• Drugs—potassium-sparing diuretics, prostaglandin inhibitors, NSAIDS, heparin	–	• Hyperosmolarity
	–	• Vigorous exercise

sickle cell disease) are all known causes of cell rupture. Mechanisms that inhibit the Na^+/K^+ ATPase pump can result in hyperkalemia; nonspecific beta blockers and digitalis inhibit Na^+/K^+ ATPase pumps, also succinylcholine, a membrane depolarizing drug, which leads to potassium efflux from the cells (Martyn and Richtsfeld, 2006). Hyperosmolarity can lead to hyperkalemia through loss of intracellular water. As water is lost from the cell, the increasing cellular potassium concentration creates a gradient down, which moves the potassium out of the cell. In dogs, this is known to occur in cases of diabetes mellitus.

Hyperkalemia can also develop in response to the administration of the synthetic amino acid, epsilon amino caproic acid (EACA). Studies performed in dogs suggest that the similarity of EACA structure to arginine and lysine allows the synthetic amino acid to enter cells in exchange for potassium leading to an increase in the concentration of extracellular potassium (Perazella and Biswas, 1999).

22.2.4.2.1.1.4 Pseudohyperkalemia Pseudohyperkalemia can occur when raised potassium levels are the result of a laboratory sampling error rather than a pathological condition. It can be defined as a serum potassium concentration exceeding that of plasma by more than 0.4 mmol/L, provided samples have been collected using appropriate sampling techniques, maintained at room temperature, and tested within 1 hour of collection. Under these conditions, pseudohyperkalemia appears to be the result of two independent mechanisms: (1) degranulation of aggregated platelets (providing a potassium load to the surrounding serum at the time of clot formation) and (2) transfer of a proportion of the potassium back to the red blood cells (to maintain homeostasis) leaving a significant amount of potassium in the serum (Sevastos et al., 2008). Typically, it occurs in species with a high red blood cell potassium concentration (cows, horses, and pigs), whereas erythrocytes with relatively low potassium levels (cats) rarely produce pseudohyperkalemia by hemolysis.

22.2.4.2.1.2 Hypokalemia Hypokalemia is defined as an electrolyte imbalance where the plasma potassium level is less than 3.5 mmol/L; severe hypokalemia is defined when plasma potassium is less than 2.5 mmol/L. It occurs relatively frequently in animals and may be brought about by three mechanisms: inadequate intake, excess excretion, or transcellular movement of K^+ from the extracellular to intracellular space. As potassium is largely an intracellular cation, the occurrence of hypokalemia does not always reflect a deficit in body potassium stores. Substantial losses in K^+ can be incurred without the development of hypokalemia; in humans (and most probably animals), the critical lower limit value is considered to be 2.8 mmol/L. Common causes of hypokalemia are given in Table 22.6.

TABLE 22.6
Causes of Hypokalemia

Inadequate Intake	Excess Excretion	Shift in Cellular Balance
• Prolonged poor nutrition—anorexia, bulimia, starvation, alcoholism	• Mineralocorticoid excess—hyperaldosteronism (Conn's syndrome) or hyperadrenocorticism (Cushing's syndrome)	• Insulin or glucose administration
• Potassium-free fluid therapy	• Osmotic diuresis and rapid rehydration therapy	• Metabolic alkalosis
–	• Drugs—diuretics, penicillins	• Beta-adrenergic stimulation
–	• Hypomagnesemia	–
–	• Gastrointestinal loss—vomiting, diarrhea	–
–	• Metabolic alkalosist	–

22.2.4.2.1.2.1 Inadequate Intake Inadequate potassium intake alone is a rare cause of hypokalemia. Even in the absence of potassium intake, potassium is excreted at between 10 and 15 mmol/day. In animals, particularly herbivores, if poor nutrition continues for extended periods of time such as with anorexia or starvation, a significant potassium deficit can occur.

22.2.4.2.1.2.2 Excess Excretion Excess K^+ excretion is the most common cause of hypokalemia, especially when accompanied with inadequate intake. The primary cause is from the use of diuretics, which produce elevated sodium levels in the collecting duct of the kidney with simultaneous K^+ secretion (Greenberg, 2000). In adrenal disorders that lead to mineralocorticoid excess (hyperaldosteronism), aldosterone causes the renal tubules to retain sodium and secrete high levels of potassium and chloride. Some potassium is conserved by exchange with hydrogen ions, but the level is insufficient to maintain homeostasis, and compensatory metabolic alkalosis and hypokalemia ensue. A similar enhanced mineralocorticoid effect is observed with excess ACTH occurring with hyperadrenocorticism. Increased loss of potassium in the urine (kaliuresis) is associated with polyuric states such as osmotic diuresis or rapid rehydration. Moreover, penicillin and its synthetic derivatives can also promote renal potassium secretion by increasing sodium delivery to the kidney. Both conditions can result in hypokalemia (Klastersky et al., 1973; Gill et al., 1977). Hypokalemia is both a cause and a frequent consequence of metabolic alkalosis; chronic metabolic alkalosis is seen when bicarbonate retention in the kidney is increased in response to plasma chloride deficits created by loss of gastric acid (HCl). This acute increase in HCO_3^- concentration can exceed the reabsorption capacity of the proximal tubule for this anion; bicarbonate and sodium pass to the distal tubule where sodium is reabsorbed in preference to K^+ leading to increased urinary excretion of potassium and decreased serum potassium (Walmsley and White, 1984). The increase in HCO_3^- reabsorption additionally causes ECF volume contraction that induces secondary hyperaldosteronism. Hypokalemia can therefore also be driven by aldosterone-mediated collecting tubule secretion of K^+ in response to enhanced Na^+ reabsorption. Alkalosis can also cause hypokalemia by changing the cellular balance of K^+. Potassium channels are inhibited by magnesium; therefore, low levels of magnesium (hypomagnesemia) result in a loss of intracellular K^+, which is excreted in the urine (Elisaf et al., 1997).

22.2.4.2.1.2.3 Shift in Cellular Balance The movement of K^+ from the extracellular to the intracellular space is associated with hypokalemia most often when it is accompanied by increased excretion of K^+. Intracellular shifts are often transient changes occurring with insulin or glucose therapy (glucose stimulates insulin release). Insulin increases the activity of the Na^+/K^+ pump in muscle stimulating the intracellular movement of potassium ions. Similarly, β-adrenergic stimulation enhances potassium entry into the cells. Metabolic alkalosis causes hypokalemia not only for increasing K^+ secretion but also for shifting the cellular K^+ balance to the intracellular space. This shift may be stimulated by Na^+/H^+ exchange and the subsequent activation of Na^+/K^+ ATPase; it is considered to be a minor cause of hypokalemia (Halperin and Kamel, 1998). Potassium entry into cells can be inhibited by glucagon, α-adrenergic stimulation, or acidosis.

22.2.4.2.2 Factors Influencing Measurement of Potassium Concentration

As potassium is predominantly an intracellular ion, serum potassium levels do not give a good indication of total body K^+ but rather, reflects both the movement of potassium between intracellular and ECFs and total body homeostasis. Fractional clearance or excretion of potassium (FEK) can be determined in urine specimens at different time points daily is often used as an estimation of potassium handling. FEK describes the proportion of potassium that is excreted in the urine compared with that filtered through the glomerulus. It may be quantified by comparison to the clearance of endogenous creatinine. This procedure simultaneously measures the electrolyte and creatinine concentration in single urine and serum samples and allows the measurement of potassium clearance without the knowledge of urine flow rate or volume. As with other methods of determining potassium concentration, the small volume of blood that can be sampled from small laboratory animals can be a limit to experimental design. FEK can be calculated using the following formula:

$$\text{FEK} = \left(\frac{\text{urine potassium}}{\text{serum potassium}}\right)\left(\frac{\text{urine creatinine}}{\text{serum creatinine}}\right) \times 100$$

When blood samples are collected, hemolysis during clot formation can increase serum potassium levels particularly in species with high intracellular potassium levels such as some dogs (Bergstrom, 1981; Nyirenda et al., 2009). This pseudohyperkalemia can be avoided by the measurement of plasma potassium (using lithium heparin) in normal cell samples, but it may not prevent it when the cells are neoplastic (O'Regan et al., 1977; Cohen, 1979). As muscle contains the bulk of body potassium, muscular activity before or at the time of blood collection can increase plasma/serum potassium levels. Animals should be taken quietly from their cages and handled gently to prevent overzealous muscular activity (Bergstrom, 1981). Erroneous values may also be obtained when animals have been treated with the penicillin family of antibiotics (especially in large doses) or when deproteinized serum or plasma samples are assayed using flame photometry (Cohen, 1979). As with the measurement of sodium levels, metabolic disturbances that bring about hyperlipidemia, hyperproteinemia, hyperglycemia, or dehydration may produce spurious results. The practice of fasting rodents and removing drinking water during their activity period should therefore be performed only when necessary, and the results should be interpreted with caution (Ramsay and Ganong, 1977; Kleeman, 1979).

22.2.4.3 Calcium

Calcium is an essential element, and it is the fifth most abundant element in the human body obtained solely from dietary sources (dairy foods and leafy green vegetables). The majority of body calcium (approximately 99%) is located in bones, and the remaining 1% is in the intracellular and extracellular compartments. Extracellular calcium occurs in three forms: free (active), protein bound complexes (binding principally to albumin, but also globulin and calmodulin), and anion bound complexes (citrate, phosphate, carbonate, lactate, or sulfate). Approximately 50% of serum calcium is in the ionized (free), active form, ~40% is protein bound, and ~10% exists as anion bound complexes. Nonbone, ionized calcium is responsible for a wide range of functions: cell signaling, nerve impulse transmission, blood coagulation, and muscle contraction; skeletal calcium is important in bone mineralization and it provides a reservoir from which intracellular and extracellular calcium levels can be maintained. Nonbone Ca^{2+} levels are homeostatically controlled within the range of 1.1–1.35 mmol/L in humans (serum Ca^{2+} levels: 2.2–2.5 mmol/L) (Peacock, 2010). In rabbits, nonbone (serum) Ca^{2+} levels are higher than other laboratory animals with normal values in the range of 3.22–3.75 mmol/L. In comparison, dogs have serum calcium levels ranging from 2.25 to 2.83 mmol/L and mice from 2.47 to 3.1 mmol/L (Table 22.1). Rabbits also differ from other laboratory animals by excreting a higher fraction of calcium in the urine; studies show New Zealand White rabbits excrete 47% calcium in the urine (and 53% in the feces), whereas urinary fractional excretion in rats is less than 2% (Buss and Bourdeau, 1984). Some variation of Ca^{2+} levels has been observed with age in BALB/c, C57BL/6, and outbred mice with higher levels occurring in younger animals. Likewise, some gender differences in nonbone Ca^{2+} levels have been observed in mice (Barrett et al., 1975; Frith et al., 1980).

Calcium is absorbed into the body through the small intestine and is excreted in the urine by the kidney. As bone is the major reservoir of calcium, maintaining metabolic balance in bone is an important aspect of Ca^{2+} homeostasis. The balance between the rate of bone formation and reabsorption changes throughout life; in young life, bone formation occurs in preference to reabsorption; in later life, this is reversed (Manolagas, 2000; Peacock, 2010). Homeostasis is regulated largely by hormones that maintain serum ionized (free) calcium levels while also allowing calcium to move in and out of the bone reservoir. Intracellular calcium does not appear to play an active role in homeostatic regulation except in the parathyroid gland where the intracellular concentration increases in response to changes in the extracellular concentration and alters the rate of PTH secretion. Hormones playing a role in homeostasis are as follows: PTH, calcitonin, and calcitriol (1,25-dihydroxyvitamin D; $1,25(OH)_2D$); they regulate Ca^{2+} transport in the gut, kidney, and bone (Jurutka et al., 2001; Potts and Gardella, 2007). A decrease in serum calcium concentration inactivates the calcium-sensing receptor (CaSR) in the parathyroid gland, increasing PTH secretion. PTH acts at three sites in the body by (1) increasing the production of calcitriol (the active form of vitamin D) from the proximal tubule of the kidney, which activates receptors in gut to increase intestinal absorption, (2) enhancing the reabsorption of calcium and magnesium in renal distal tubules of the kidney, and (3) releasing calcium from osseous tissue (Coetzee and Kruger, 2004; Poole and Reeve, 2005). The system is principally controlled by the negative feedback of calcium on PTH secretion; however, the calcium regulatory hormones also interact with each other providing a further level of regulation. Central to this process is the G-protein coupled CaSR located on the surface of the parathyroid cells and regulating the release of PTH (Taylor and Bushinsky, 2009) (Figure 22.5).

Calcium, phosphorous, and vitamin D metabolites play a role in regulating PTH release and synthesis (Kumar and Thompson, 2011). Phosphorous forms calcium phosphate complexes with serum calcium, thereby reducing the level of the free, ionized form and triggering CaSR to increase PTH secretion. Calcitonin, released from the thyroid gland, acts mostly by inhibiting osteoclastic activity. By preventing the resorption of bone, this hormone has the opposite effect to PTH of inhibiting Ca^{2+} release from bone. Vitamin D metabolites regulate expression of the calcitonin gene. Calcitonin effects a role in maintaining blood Ca^{2+} levels by inhibiting absorption in the gut and increasing reabsorption of both Ca^{2+} and Mg^{2+} in the kidney tubules (Carney, 1997). This hormone is important in counteracting the effects of PTH. Species differences in the importance of calcitonin as a factor affecting homeostasis occur. In rodents, calcitonin appears to play a significant role in calcium homeostasis; whereas, in humans, the role of calcitonin appears to be minor (Zaidi et al., 2002; Hoff et al., 2002).

22.2.4.3.1 Calcium Imbalance

22.2.4.3.1.1 Hypercalcemia Hypercalcemia is an electrolyte imbalance characterized by elevated serum calcium levels: greater than 2.5 mmol/L for serum calcium or 1.4 mmol/L for ionized (free) calcium in humans. It is a disorder commonly affecting dogs, most often as a result of neoplastic disease. The most severe symptoms are generally seen in animals with serum calcium levels greater than 4.0 mmol/L. Hypercalcemia not only develops as a direct result of an electrolyte imbalance but it can also occur secondary to disorders of serum proteins. It affects nearly every organ system, particularly the kidney and CNS; cardiac arrhythmias are also reported due the inotropic effect of calcium. The clinical signs of hypercalcemia depend on the rapidity of condition onset.

Hypercalcemia can be caused by three primary mechanisms: increased intestinal absorption of Ca^{2+}, decreased renal secretion, and excessive skeletal calcium release. These mechanisms can be either mediated by PTH (primary hyperparathyroidism) or non-PTH-mediated. Primary hyperparathyroidism is the excessive secretion of PTH and usually arises as a result of adenoma of the parathyroid gland. PTH regulates serum Ca^{2+} levels through effects on kidney, intestine, and bone. Nonhyperparathyroidism-mediated hypercalcemia is usually associated with malignancy (cancer in the absence of bone metastasis), most commonly squamous cell carcinoma, renal cell carcinoma, and mammary gland, prostate, or ovarian cancer. Tumors secrete PTH-related peptide (PTHrP), a protein in the same family as PTH. As both PTHrP and PTH stimulate the same receptor (PTHR1) in bone and kidney, they can both regulate calcium ion homeostasis. Malignancy can lead to changes in calcium homeostasis: excessive bone reabsorption and hypercalcemia (Strewler, 2000; Wysolmerski, 2012). Increase in Ca^{2+} concentration can also result from increased osteoclastic activity in bone or increased vitamin D levels (usually in granulomatous disorders). Common

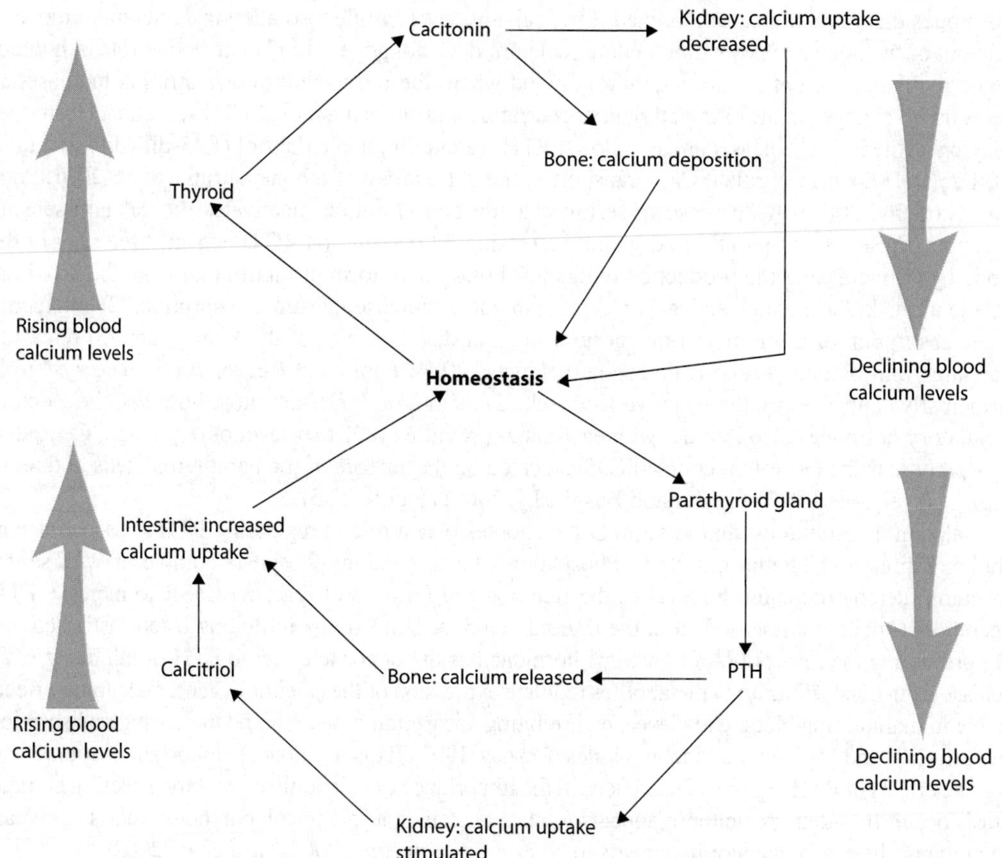

FIGURE 22.5 Calcium homeostasis is maintained through the action of three hormones: PTH, calcitonin, and calcitriol. Release of calcitonin from the thyroid gland in response to increased blood calcium levels inhibits renal absorption of calcium and promotes mineralization of bone, thereby effecting a reduction in blood calcium levels. Release of PTH in response to falling blood calcium levels stimulates bone demineralization, increases reabsorption of renal calcium, and stimulates the biosynthesis of calcitriol, thereby increasing intestinal uptake of calcium and raising blood calcium levels.

causes of hypercalcemia shown in Table 22.7 are grouped by the major organ effector sites although the development of hypercalcemia invariably involves multiple sites/mechanisms.

22.2.4.3.1.1.1 Increased Intestinal Absorption Primary hyperparathyroidism, the excessive secretion of PTH, occurs most often as a result of an adenoma of the parathyroid gland and as such it is not a common finding in young laboratory animals. Hyperplasia, carcinoma, or familial endocrine disorders are other known causes; all can lead to elevated Ca^{2+} levels. Neoplasia is the most common cause of hypercalcemia in dogs often associated with apocrine gland adenocarcinoma of the anal sac. Calcium absorption is not only regulated by PTH but also calcitriol, the biologically active form of vitamin D (Holick, 2004). Calcitriol mediates its effect by binding to the calcitriol (vitamin D) receptor (VDR). VDR is a member of the nuclear receptor family of transcription factors that regulate the transcription of hormone sensitive genes. In addition, VDR autoregulates its own expression by repressing the expression of the proximal activator of calcitriol, 1-α hydroxylase, and inducing the expression of the calcitriol inactivating enzyme 24-hydroxylase (CYP 24) (Fleet and Schoch, 2010; Xue and Fleet, 2009). Excess vitamin D can thereby lead to hypercalcemia. This can occur as a result of poisoning when calciferol-containing rodenticides or vitamin

TABLE 22.7
Causes of Hypercalcemia

Increased Intestinal Absorption	Bone Remodeling	Renal Excretion
• Primary hyperparathyroidism	• Primary hyperparathyroidism	• Primary hyperparathyroidism
• Chronic kidney disease	• Chronic kidney disease	• Chronic kidney disease
• Vitamin D poisoning/excess (hypervitaminosis D)	• Vitamin A excess	• Familial hypercalciuric hypercalcemia
• Granulomatous diseases—sarcoidosis, tuberculosis, Hodgkin's lymphoma, non-Hodgkin's lymphoma	• Malignancy	• Drugs—thiazide diuretics
–	• Immobilization	• Sodium depletion

D glycoside-containing plants are consumed. In granulomatous diseases, sarcoidosis, tuberculosis, Hodgkin's lymphoma, and non-Hodgkin's lymphoma increased intestinal Ca^{2+} absorption is induced by high serum calcitriol levels produced at extrarenal sites by macrophages within the granulomas (Barbour et al., 1981). Normally the activation of calcidiol to calcitriol in the kidney is under the control of PTH and serum phosphate concentration (Insogna et al., 1988). Physiological compensation for the extrarenal production of calcitriol by macrophages involves the suppression of PTH and prevents the development of hypercalcemia but may ultimately lead to hypoparathyroidism. This condition is exacerbated by high levels of estradiol and prolactin (Subramanian et al., 2004). Studies show the production of calcitriol is increased by prolactin in primary chick kidney cell cultures (Spanos et al., 1981) and estradiol has a stimulatory effect on the renal 1-α hydroxylase enzyme, which results in a positive correlation between serum calcitriol and estradiol levels (Verhaeghe and Bouillon, 1992; Cheema et al., 1989). Chronic kidney disease can lead to hypercalcemia by a combination of mechanisms that include vitamin D overdose and calcium ingestion; when the amount of Ca^{2+} absorbed in the gut exceeds the excretory ability of the kidneys, hypercalcemia develops (Pieper et al., 2006).

22.2.4.3.1.1.2 Bone Remodeling Primary hyperparathyroidism and malignancy are the two most common causes of bone remodeling sometimes associated with hypercalcemia. The excess secretion of PTH in hyperparathyroidism increases bone resorption by osteoclasts; however, this rarely induces elevated calcium levels or hypercalcemia because most of the PTH-induced breakdown of bone is balanced by hypercalcemic-induced bone deposition. Hypercalcemia is frequently associated with malignant tumors, in particular bone metastases that cause an imbalance between bone formation and bone resorption and result in the release of calcium to the blood; approximately 80% of malignancy-related hypercalcemias are caused by bone metastases. Cancers most likely to induce bone remodeling Ca^{2+} release are hematological cancers of the bone marrow (multiple myeloma, leukemia) and solid tumors that primarily metastasize to bone (breast, prostate, and lung cancers). The common mechanism of action for all malignancies is increased osteoclastic activity in the bone promoting calcium release; it may be brought about by either osteoclastic activating factors (produced by osteolytic metastasis of solid tumors) or a PTH-related protein that increases bone resorption. A third mechanism shown in animals (but not humans) is increased prostaglandin synthesis (Tashjian et al., 1972; Raisz et al., 1977). Chronic kidney disease can result in hypercalcemia when adynamic bone disease (low bone turnover) is present. In these cases, a reduced level of calcium uptake for bone formation produces excess serum calcium (Parfitt, 2003; Andress, 2008). Prolonged immobilization and hypervitaminosis A can also lead to the production of excess calcium due to bone loss (Gault et al., 1968).

22.2.4.3.1.1.3 Renal Excretion Dysregulation of renal calcium excretion can occur at two levels: either tubular reabsorption or calcium load. In chronic kidney disease with a reduced GFR, even calcium concentrations in the normal physiological range can give rise to hypercalcemia when the amount of calcium ingested exceeds the rate renal secretion (Goodman, 2005; Pieper et al., 2006). Other causes of increased tubular reabsorption of calcium include primary hyperparathyroidism and sodium depletion. Drugs such as thiazide diuretics increase Ca^{2+} reabsorption in the distal convoluted tubules by activation of transcellular Ca^{2+} transport systems and up regulation of the apical calcium channels transient receptor potential cation channel subfamily V member 5 (TRPV5), Calbindin 1 (CALB1), and S100 calcium binding protein G (CALB3) (Lee et al., 2004). In humans, familial hypercalciuric hypercalcemia is an autosomal defect that is most often associated with loss of function mutations in the CaSR gene expressed in parathyroid and kidney tissue. This is recognized as a lack of calcium by the parathyroid, which in turn produces constitutively high levels of PTH leading to hypercalcemia. Renal failure in dogs is a known cause of hypercalcemia; in other species, renal failure does not usually given rise to this condition (Ferguson and Hoenig, 2003).

22.2.4.3.1.1.4 Other Causes Hypercalcemia can occur secondary to disorders of serum proteins rather than as a consequence of changes in ionized (free) calcium levels. Any change in serum albumin level or binding capacity will be reflected as a change in total body calcium. However, as no changes occur in the ionized (free) fraction of calcium no clinical manifestations are apparent. Consequently, hypoalbuminemia occurring with normal serum calcium is interpreted as hypercalcemia. In acidosis, the amount of calcium bound to albumin is reduced; whereas, in alkalosis, the bound fraction of calcium is increased (Tietz, 1976; Girndt et al., 1979).

22.2.4.3.1.2 Hypocalcemia Hypocalcemia is an electrolyte disturbance characterized by low calcium levels: less than 2.1 mmol/L for serum calcium or 1.1 mmol/L for ionized (free) calcium in humans and 2 mmol/L for serum calcium or 0.31 mmol/L in dogs. Clinical signs are usually evident when serum levels fall below 1.62 mmol/L for both species. Hypocalcemia not only develops as a direct result of an electrolyte imbalance but also secondary to disorders of serum proteins. The main effect is seen in the contractility of muscles. The primary mechanisms that produce hypocalcemia include reduction in (1) plasma proteins, (2) absorption of calcium, (3) bone mobilization, (4) reabsorption of calcium in the kidney, (5) magnesium concentration, (6) concentration of calcitriol, and (7) increases in phosphate concentration. These are shown in Table 22.8 grouped by major organ effector sites although invariably, the development of hypocalcemia involves multiple mechanisms.

22.2.4.3.1.2.1 Reduced Intestinal Absorption Hypocalcemia is rarely caused by a low dietary intake of calcium; however, vitamin D deficiencies have been reported and these can lead to hypocalcemia through the reduction of calcium absorption in the gut (Linnebur et al., 2007). Dietary

TABLE 22.8
Causes of Hypocalcemia

Reduced Intestinal Absorption	Bone Remodeling	Renal Excretion
• Chronic kidney disease	• Postparathyroidectomy recalcification tetany	• Chronic kidney disease
• Hypoparathyroidism	• Hypoparathyroidism	• Hypoparathyroidism
• Hyperphosphatemia	• Hyperphosphatemia	• Hyperphosphatemia
• Acute pancreatitis	• Osteoblastic metastatic bone cancer	• Hypomagnesemia
• Low dietary intake		
• Vitamin D deficiency—small bowel diseases, liver disease		

vitamin D deficiency can be the result of reduced absorption in the intestine or a reduction in the conversion of calcidiol to active calcitriol. Numerous conditions can impair absorption or activation of vitamin D including celiac disease, gastric bypass, steatorrhea, liver, and pancreatic disease as well as inherited conditions such as pseudovitamin D deficiency rickets (type I) or hereditary vitamin D resistance rickets (Johnson et al., 2006). Chronic kidney disease leads to the development of hypocalcemia by two concurrent intestinal routes: first, a reduction in vitamin D activation; second, a decreased intestinal Ca^{2+} absorption. Hypoparathyroidism, common in dogs, is characterized by decreased secretion of PTH, and it causes a reduction in Ca^{2+} absorption. It may occur spontaneously or be induced by a variety of factors including neck irradiation therapy, surgical removal of parathyroid, and infiltrative diseases such as hemochromatosis or granulomatous diseases (Burch and Posillico, 1983). Acute pancreatitis in dogs is often associated with hypocalcemia. This inflammatory condition can reduce serum Ca^{2+} concentrations by causing calcium precipitation; decreased PTH secretion and calcitonin release may also play a role (Sánchez et al., 1996).

22.2.4.3.1.2.2 Bone Remodeling Hypocalcemia as a result of bone remodeling can occur when the rate of skeletal mineralization exceeds the rate of osteoclast-mediated bone resorption and occurs primarily when surgical correction of primary or secondary hyperparathyroidism produces a rapid drop in PTH levels and results in a rapid increase in bone remodeling (termed "hungry bone syndrome" in humans). Other conditions that cause mineralization of bone matrix include correction of thyrotoxicosis, vitamin D therapy for osteomalacia, and hematological or metastatic (to bone) tumors (Brasier and Nussbaum, 1988). Hypoparathyroidism causes hypocalcemia through bone remodeling because the reduction in PTH levels prevents the activation of osteoclasts and bone resorption, thereby preventing the release of calcium. Conditions that give rise to hypoparathyroidism are described in the previous section. Elevated levels of phosphorous (hyperphosphatemia) caused by phosphorous administration, tumor lysis, or rhabdomyolysis can also result in hypocalcemia as increased calcium deposition takes place in bone or extra-skeletal sites (Wilson and Berns, 2012; Peacock, 2010).

22.2.4.3.1.2.3 Renal Excretion Hypocalcemia arising from decreased tubular calcium reabsorption occurs primarily as a result of hypoparathyroidism. PTH has a calcium-retaining effect on the distal tubule of the kidney; when the levels of PTH are low, calcium reabsorption does not occur; ionized (free) calcium level in the serum is reduced and urinary calcium concentration increased. Hypomagnesemia is also associated with low PTH level, the loss of Mg^{2+} from the kidney or GI tract inhibits PTH secretion and decreases the function of the calcium pump. Hypocalcemia as a result of chronic kidney disease is produced by several mechanisms including decreased conversion of vitamin D to calcitriol and a reduction in the GFR (to below 30 mL/min); an increase in PTH level leads to increased calcium and phosphorous absorption and deposition at extraskeletal sites.

22.2.4.3.1.2.4 Other Causes Hypocalcemia can occur secondary to disorders of serum proteins rather than as a consequence of changes in ionized (free) calcium levels. Any change in serum albumin level or binding capacity will be reflected as a change in total body calcium. For example, in respiratory or metabolic alkalosis, the amount of calcium bound to albumin is increased resulting in decreased concentrations of ionized (free) calcium and pseudohypocalcemia.

22.2.4.3.2 Factors Influencing Measurement of Calcium Concentration

Although total calcium is a convenient measure of clinical conditions, it is ionized calcium that is physiologically active and under homeostatic control and therefore provides a better indicator of calcium imbalances. A variety of mathematical formulae have been proposed for calculating ionized calcium levels or total calcium corrected for serum albumin concentrations but these do not always provide accurate estimations (Clase et al., 2000). The equilibrium between total and ionized calcium fractions is dependent on a variety of factors including pH, temperature, and concentration of serum proteins particularly albumin. To accurately measure ionized calcium, samples must be procured anaerobically (to minimize loss of carbon dioxide) and processed quickly to reduce lactate generation. Total calcium concentration is not affected by changes in pH, yet a change in the pH of the assayed sample (e.g., a decrease caused by glycolysis) will affect the ionized calcium portion (Ng, 1987). Acidosis decreases binding of calcium to albumin and increases the ionized fraction; an acidotic animal may therefore have no clinical signs of hypocalcemia yet have a measured value that is sufficiently low to indicate the presence of hypocalcemia. Conversely, alkalosis decreases the ionized calcium fraction such that animals may show signs of hypocalcemia yet have a calcium value within the normal reference range. Moreover, as the degree of calcium dissociation increases with the rising temperature, samples should be measured at a constant temperature (Metzger and Kenny, 1987). Oxalate, EDTA, citrate, and heparin decrease calcium available for analysis by most methods of analysis because they bind calcium. The more common measurement of calcium level in serum is therefore total calcium (the sum of ionized and nonionized (primarily bound to albumin but also to other anions) components) and this should be used whenever serum albumin levels are not within normal ranges, or when a calcium disorder is suspected despite normal total calcium levels. The amount of total calcium varies with the level of plasma proteins (particularly albumin), such that a 250 mmol/L decrease in albumin raises the serum calcium by 0.2 mmol/L.

Measurement of total serum calcium can be performed using colorimetric methods but this method is not always reliable as it is affected by variables such as recent food ingestion (producing lipemia). Fasting animals prior to sample collection may be necessary (Ferguson and Hoenig, 2003). Ion selective electrodes can be used to measure ionized calcium based on changes in the thermodynamic activity of calcium ions. However, to ensure accurate electrolyte determination, samples must be maintained anaerobically at 37°C (Burnett et al., 2000). Urinary calcium excretion can be used to differentiate changes in calcium homeostasis. The amount of calcium excreted over a 24-hour period is measured in a 24-hour urine sample. Alternatively, the fractional clearance or excretion of calcium (FECa) on samples of serum and urine can be measured, although as discussed previously (for sodium and potassium) the amount of serum that can be collected daily from small laboratory animals (particularly mice) can be a limiting factor in experimental design. FECa can be calculated using the following formula:

$$\text{FECa} = \frac{(\text{urine calcium/serum calcium})}{(\text{urine creatinine/serum creatinine})} \times 100$$

22.2.4.4 Magnesium

Magnesium is an essential element and the fourth most abundant cation in the body obtained solely from dietary sources (green vegetables, nuts, whole grains, and seafood). It is the second most prevalent intracellular cation and plays a critical role in many cellular pathways including DNA and protein synthesis, enzyme activation (including most enzymes in phosphorylation reactions), and PTH synthesis (Soave et al., 2009). As Mg^{2+} is a cofactor for ATP, this element has wide-ranging effects on processes: muscle contraction, protein, fat and carbohydrate metabolism, cell growth and division, membrane permeability, and immune responses. Similar to calcium, the body's magnesium is distributed among bone, intracellular space, and extracellular space. Approximately 99% of total body magnesium is located in the bone and intracellular compartments. Only ~1% is found in the serum and ISF. The majority of intracellular Mg^{2+} is complexed with organic molecules (DNA, enzymes, etc.) or sequestered in organelles (mitochondria or endoplasmic reticulum); only ~1%–3% exists as the free, ionized (active) form, and this level is tightly regulated by the sequestration and organic molecule binding processes. Serum Mg^{2+} is also complexed, in this case, to either serum proteins or anions; however, the majority of serum magnesium exists in the free, ionized (active) form (Kulpmann and Gerlach, 1996; Thienpont et al., 1999).

Relatively little is known about the mechanisms involved in Mg^{2+} absorption by the GI tract. Vitamin D appears to play a role in increasing Mg^{2+} absorption, but significant absorption can occur independently of vitamin D (Hardwick et al., 1991). As with other cations, homeostatic control is brought about by the action of the kidneys. Ionized and complexed Mg^{2+} are approximately 70% of the total serum Mg^{2+} and are filtered freely by the glomerulus and then largely reabsorbed in the tubules such that only 3% of filtered Mg^{2+} is finally excreted in the urine, 97% is reabsorbed (Musso, 2009). Unlike sodium and potassium, reabsorption primarily occurs in the thick ascending Loop of Henle (TAL), and the fine control occurs in the distal convoluted tubules. High levels of natriuresis, osmotic load, and metabolic acidosis can all cause an elevation in the level of Mg^{2+} excreted from the kidney; whereas, a reduction in the level of Mg^{2+} excreted occurs in response to some hormones (PTH, calcitonin) and metabolic alkalosis.

22.2.4.4.1 Magnesium Imbalance

22.2.4.4.1.1 Hypermagnesemia Hypermagnesemia is an electrolyte imbalance characterized by the elevated levels of magnesium in the blood (greater than 0.95 mmol/L in humans). Plasma magnesium concentrations normally range from 0.75 to 0.95 mmol/L in human. Magnesium toxicity occurs in humans when levels exceed 1.74–2.61 mmol/L. This condition occurs rarely because the kidney is very effective at excreting excess magnesium (Musso, 2009). When it does occur, hypermagnesemia is almost exclusively associated with chronic kidney disease particularly when coupled with excessive Mg^{2+} intake (Moe, 2005). In this condition, Mg^{2+} levels can be maintained until the GFR falls to below 20 mL/min. At this point, hypermagnesemia can develop particularly when the fall in Mg^{2+} excretion is accompanied by increased intake (vitamins, antacids, laxatives). Other causes of decreased renal magnesium secretion leading to hypermagnesemia are lithium therapy, adrenal insufficiency (decreased levels of cortisol and aldosterone), and familial hypocalciuric hypercalcemia. In the latter condition, the loss of function mutations in the CaSR gene prevents the feedback inhibition of PTH, and it results in elevated blood calcium levels and increased Mg^{2+} reabsorption in the Loop of Henle (Pearce et al., 1995). As an intracellular cation, massive tissue damage can cause elevation of Mg^{2+} levels (also phosphorous and potassium), but this is an uncommon mechanism of hypermagnesemia unless accompanied by renal failure.

22.2.4.4.1.2 Hypomagnesemia Hypomagnesemia is an electrolyte imbalance characterized by abnormally low levels of magnesium in blood (less than 0.7 mmol/L in humans). It can be caused by three mechanisms: inadequate intake, redistribution from extracellular to intracellular space, or excessive gastrointestinal/renal loss. Common causes are given in Table 22.9.

22.2.4.4.1.2.1 Inadequate Intake Nutritional deficiency alone does not commonly cause hypomagnesemia; magnesium absorption in the gut can increase up to 40% compared to normal when low levels of magnesium are detected. Malnutrition, however, can lead to Mg^{2+} deficit and hypomagnesemia when coupled with alcohol dependency or enteric diseases (Molina-Perez et al., 2000).

22.2.4.4.1.2.2 Excess Excretion The most common causes of excessive loss of magnesium leading to hypomagnesemia are renal disease and diuretic use. Tubular dysfunction and increased tubular flow decrease magnesium reabsorption in the thick ascending limb of the Loop of Henle and cause hypomagnesemia in many renal conditions: the diuretic phase of acute tubular necrosis, postobstructive diuresis, and renal tubular acidosis. Experimental evidence in rats shows a similar mechanism of action whereby reabsorption of Mg^{2+} decreases with increased tubular flow (Levine et al., 1982). Increased tubular flow rates can be caused by volume expansion, which in turn may be brought about by saline infusion or hormonally by hyperaldosteronism (Topf and Murray, 2003). Drugs can also cause hypomagnesemia, the most common are loop diuretics. These block ion channels in the Loop of Henle, thereby preventing reabsorption of Mg^{2+} (Topf and Murray, 2003).

TABLE 22.9
Causes of Hypomagnesemia

Inadequate Intake	Excess Excretion	Shift in Cellular Balance
• Malnutrition • Enteric disease—chronic diarrhea, inflammatory bowel disease	• Gastrointestinal loss—vomiting, diarrhea • Inherited renal tubular defects • Drugs—diuretics, chemotherapeutics • Hypercalcemia • Chronic metabolic acidosis • Volume expansion • Osmotic diuresis • Primary hyperaldosteronism • Renal disease—diuretic phase of acute tubular necrosis, postobstructive diuresis, renal tubular acidosis	• Post parathyroid surgery recalcification tetany • Acute pancreatitis • Posttreatment of diabetic ketoacidosis • Excessive lactation

Similarly, when hypercalcemia is associated with hypomagnesemia, the activation of CaSRs in the ascending Loop of Henle closes the Na/K/2Cl pump and inhibits magnesium reabsorption. Osmotic diuresis produced by glycosuria in diabetes mellitus is also associated with hypomagnesemia (Schnack et al., 1992).

22.2.4.4.1.2.3 Shift in Cellular Balance Low serum Mg^{2+} as a consequence of a shift to the intracellular compartment is significant following parathyroidectomy to correct primary or secondary hyperparathyroidism. A rapid drop in the PTH level causes mineralization of osteoid and a rapid decrease in serum calcium, magnesium and potassium levels, hypocalcemia, and hypomagnesemia (Al-Ghamdi et al., 1994). Hypomagnesemia can also occur with acute pancreatitis (Liamis et al., 2001), excessive lactation or after insulin therapy for diabetic ketoacidosis where the insulin administered may drive magnesium, along with potassium and phosphorus, into the intracellular compartment.

22.2.4.4.2 Factors Influencing Measurement of Magnesium Concentration

Measurement of plasma magnesium levels does not always correlate with total body magnesium concentrations. Clinically, significant Mg^{2+} imbalance is more tightly correlated with intracellular magnesium levels than blood concentrations because of the roles this element plays. Accurate assessments can be obtained by measuring magnesium contained in erythrocytes or inferred from a 24-hour urine sample (Gullestad et al., 1992). For erythrocyte magnesium concentrations, the same site must always be used for collecting blood because of the erythrocyte volume differences between arterial and venous blood; magnesium may leak from erythrocytes under hypoxic conditions.

22.2.5 Anions

22.2.5.1 Chloride

Chloride is a naturally occurring mineral found in many foods and table salt. It is the principal anion in the body combining with sodium to form sodium chloride and potassium to form potassium chloride. Normal serum chloride levels in humans are in the range 98–108 mmol/L, tissue concentrations are almost negligible in normal circumstances; however, chloride enters damaged cells (Bergstrom, 1981). Little interspecies variation in the concentration of serum chloride is evident among common laboratory species (Table 22.1). In rat, chloride concentrations range from 90.0 to 132.0 mmol/L; whereas, in mice, chloride is present in the range 106.1–130.7 mmol/L (Table 22.1). With sodium, Cl^- shares the function of maintaining serum osmolarity and fluid balance; it also helps to maintain acid–base equilibrium and the electrical neutrality of extracellular bicarbonate and sodium. Chloride levels generally mirror sodium levels such that losses in sodium are usually followed by losses in chloride. Conversely, chloride has an inverse relationship with bicarbonate anions (Powers, 1999). The kidneys and gastrointestinal tract regulate chloride homeostasis. In the intestine, chloride is actively and passively absorbed. Passive absorption occurs when chloride follows sodium across the intestinal wall; active absorption occurs when bicarbonate moves from the blood to the intestine and is exchanged for chloride ions to maintain electrical neutrality. In the kidney, the majority of filtered chloride is passively reabsorbed with sodium in the proximal tubule. Active reabsorption of chloride occurs in the TAL, forcing the simultaneous passive movement of sodium to maintain electrical neutrality. In the distal tubule, passive and active reabsorption of smaller amounts of chloride refine chloride balance. Factors that regulate sodium reabsorption also control chloride levels. The WNK-SPAK (SPS1-related proline/alanine-rich kinase)/OSR1 (oxidative stress-responsive kinase 1) signaling pathway regulates cation-chloride coupled cotransporters Na+–K+–2Cl(–) cotransporter (NKCC) 1 (NKCC), solute carrier family 12 member 1 (NKCC2), and, under certain conditions, NCCT. Phosphorylation of these proteins by the WNK-regulated kinases OSR1 and SPAK is associated with their increased activation (Hoorn et al., 2011; Huang et al., 2008).

One of the most important functions of chloride is maintaining acid–base balance. One of the ways this can be achieved is through a process known as the chloride shift whereby chloride is exchanged for bicarbonate ions across the membranes of cells. Carbon dioxide dissolved in tissue fluid diffuses into capillaries where most reacts with water to produce carbonic acid (H_2CO_3). Immediately on entry into erythrocytes, this breaks down into H^+ and HCO_3^- increasing the intracellular bicarbonate concentration. The H^+ attaches to hemoglobin and the bicarbonate passes from the erythrocyte to the plasma. To maintain electrical neutrality, as bicarbonate ions enter the plasma, chloride ions move into the erythrocyte (Powers, 1999). The movement of these ions is effected through an anion antiporter, the chloride/bicarbonate exchangers. As a consequence of this exchange, a higher chloride value is found in arterial blood than in venous blood (Wagner et al., 2009).

Dysregulation of chloride movement can have profound effects as is seen with the genetic disease, cystic fibrosis. The cystic fibrosis transmembrane conductance regulator (CFTR) is a chloride channel located on the apical membranes of airway, intestine, sweat gland, and pancreas epithelial cells (Li and Naren, 2010). It plays a key role in determining ion concentration, fluid balance, and transepithelial salt transport by regulating the movement of Cl^- across the epithelium. Disruption of Cl^- movement has wide-ranging clinical effects in different organ systems (airway disease, pancreatic failure, infertility, and elevated levels of salt in sweat) (Sheppard and Welsh, 1999; Hwang and Sheppard, 2009).

22.2.5.1.1 *Chloride Imbalances*

22.2.5.1.1.1 Hyperchloremia Hyperchloremia is an electrolyte imbalance characterized by elevated serum chloride levels, greater than 108 mmol/L in humans. It is associated with a variety of clinical conditions, which can be grouped according to whether a proportional change in sodium concentration occurs with Cl^- excess or not. The primary cause of sodium associated hyperchloremia is a water loss in excess of sodium making the causes of hypernatremia also the primary causes of hyperchloremia. Elevated chloride concentrations that are not associated with a proportional increase in sodium are usually associated with acid–base imbalances such as hyperchloremic metabolic acidosis or respiratory alkalosis (Durward et al., 2001). The primary causes of hyperchloremia are shown in Table 22.10.

22.2.5.1.1.1.1 Increase in Chloride Proportional to Sodium Increase Conditions that cause an elevation of serum Cl^- concentration and a corresponding increase in serum Na^+ level generally result from fluid loss or Na^+ excess. Fluid losses may be pure water or hypotonic. Pure water losses

TABLE 22.10
Causes of Hyperchloremia

Increase in Cl^- Proportional to Na^+ Increase	Increase in Cl^- Disproportional to Na^+ Increase
• Pure water loss—dehydration, renal losses	• Recovery from diabetic acidoketosis
• Hypotonic fluid loss—diarrhea, burns, renal losses	• Respiratory alkalosis
• Sodium excess	• Hyperchloremic metabolic acidosis
	• Renal tubular acidosis
	• Urinary diversion
	• Early renal failure
	• Primary hyperparathyroidism

most often result from increased sweating, inadequate water intake, thyrotoxicosis, or conditions such as central or nephrogenic diabetes insipidus. Hypotonic fluid loss commonly occurs in diarrhea, burns, in renal conditions such as osmotic diuresis, postobstructive diuresis, or with diuretic use. As sodium concentration changes are mirrored by changes in the chloride level, the clinical conditions that give rise to these forms of hyperchloremia also produce hypernatremia and have been discussed in detail previously (Agrawal et al., 2008).

22.2.5.1.1.1.2 Increase in Chloride Disproportional to Sodium Increase Elevated serum chloride concentration without an increase in serum sodium is associated with hyperchloremic metabolic acidosis when the rise in Cl^- levels accompanies a fall in blood pH (to below pH 7.35). Disorders that give rise to hyperchloremia metabolic acidosis include renal tubule acidosis, ureteral diversion procedures, the early stages of chronic renal failure, the recovery phase of diabetic acidoketosis, and primary hyperparathyroidism (Batlle and Kurtzman, 1982; Basic et al., 2007; Liborio et al., 2008). These conditions all result in the inhibition of bicarbonate reabsorption, bicarbonate deficits, or the hyper absorption of Cl^-. Renal tubule acidosis can be caused by damage to renal tubules (e.g., interstitial nephritis) or drugs such as carbonic anhydrase inhibitors used as a diuretic or to treat a variety of other conditions. Bicarbonate reabsorption is blocked creating an acidemic blood pH in association with nonacidic urine. Hyperchloremic metabolic acidosis also occurs in the early stages of chronic renal failure especially in cases where renal damage is also present (Handy and Soni, 2008). The recovery phase of diabetic acidoketosis is responsible for elevated Cl^- because the loss of ketone bodies in the urine prevents their conversion to bicarbonate in the liver, thereby causing bicarbonate deficits. The reduction in plasma carbon dioxide in respiratory alkalosis (occurring with hyperventilation) lowers plasma bicarbonate concentration and results in increased serum Cl^- to replace lost bicarbonate (Unwin et al., 1997).

22.2.5.1.1.2 Hypochloremia Hypochloremia is an electrolyte imbalance characterized by serum chloride levels lower than their normal range. It is associated with a variety of clinical conditions that can be grouped according to whether a proportional change in sodium concentration occurs with Cl^- depletion or not. The main causes of hypochloremia associated with a decrease in sodium concentration are a total body depletion of Cl^- or retention of water causing dilutional hypochloremia (Madias et al., 1984). They are usually associated with acid–base imbalances such metabolic acidosis or compensated respiratory acidosis (Levitin et al., 1958). The primary causes of hypochloremia are shown in Table 22.11.

22.2.5.1.1.2.1 Decrease in Chloride Proportional to Sodium Loss Total body chloride depletion can be caused by extrarenal and renal conditions, Hypochloremia caused by extrarenal Cl^- loss results from inadequate intake, gastrointestinal loss and burns; these conditions produce low concentrations of Na^+ and Cl^- in the urine and ECF volume reduction (Madias et al., 1984). Renal

TABLE 22.11
Causes of Hypochloremia

Decrease in Cl^- Proportional to Na^+ Loss	Decrease in Cl^- Disproportional to Na^+ Loss
• Total body depletion Inadequate NaCl intake Fluid loss—vomiting, diarrhea, burns Drugs—diuretic use Interstitial nephritis Adrenal insufficiency	• Compensated respiratory acidosis
• Dilutional Increased effective circulatory blood volume—infusion, hyperglycemia Normal effective circulatory blood volume—excess water intake, hypothyroidism, renal disease, SIADH Decreased effective circulatory blood volume—edema	• Metabolic alkalosis

causes of hypochloremia include diuretic use (particularly loop diuretics), osmotic diuresis (from mannitol or diabetic acidoketosis), renal diseases, and deficiency in glucocorticoids or mineralocorticoids (adrenal insufficiency). In these conditions, the concentration of Na^+ and Cl^- in the urine is elevated yet the ECF volume is still reduced. Dilutional hypochloremia is associated with normal or increased total body content of sodium and chloride coupled with ECF volume expansion. As sodium concentrations changes are mirrored by changes in the chloride level, the clinical conditions that give rise to these forms of hypochloremia also produce hyponatremia and have been discussed in detail in the previous section (Agrawal et al., 2008).

22.2.5.1.1.2.2 Decrease in Chloride Disproportional to Sodium Loss Metabolic alkalosis occurs when metabolic increases in bicarbonate levels elevate the pH of the blood beyond the normal range (greater than pH 7.45). This occurs when chloride depletion results in ECF volume reduction and there are decreased levels of filtered chloride available for reabsorption by the kidney tubules. This leads to increased bicarbonate reabsorption and elevated blood pH. Metabolic alkalosis increases potassium secretion by the kidneys, which can also lead to hypokalemia (Galla, 2000). In respiratory acidosis, elevated carbon dioxide levels increase the secretion of H^+ in the kidney tubules. This leads to the retention of sodium as sodium bicarbonate rather than sodium chloride to resolve the acidemia. The increase in serum bicarbonate causes a reciprocal decrease in chloride concentration and hypochloremia can develop. Thiazide diuretics enhance sodium chloride excretion in the distal convoluted tubule causing metabolic alkalosis by chloride depletion (and enhancing potassium and hydrogen ion secretion).

22.2.5.1.2 Factors Influencing Measurement of Chloride Concentration

A wide variation in the normal range for chloride concentration makes it difficult to attach biological significance to changes in serum values except those at the extreme ends of the range. Determination of chloride in the serum or plasma can, however, be a useful indicator of the acid–base status of the animal. If chloride levels are high, bicarbonate is likely to be low, suggesting a metabolic acidemia. The reverse situation suggests metabolic alkalemia, but strict interpretation of these changes should be treated with caution owing to the wide, normal range for chloride. Ions such as Br^-, SH^-, CN^-, and CNS^- are not differentiated from chloride in most laboratory titrations; this interference can give spurious chloride levels and should be taken into account when assaying samples. A common use of bromide is potassium bromide given as an adjunct therapy for phenobarbital in dogs.

Postprandial hypochloremia can occur when measurement of chloride levels is performed after the administration of food. Two potential mechanisms operate to cause this effect: (1) chloride ions are secreted into the stomach lumen after a meal, along with hydrogen ions, (2) postprandial hyperlipidemia. The postprandial secretion of Cl^- into the stomach after a meal causing temporary depletion of chloride ions is not indicative of true hypochloremia. Pseudohypochloremia can be indicated in cases of hyperlipidemia or hyperproteinimia when chloride concentration is measured in a reference volume of fluid. The errors occur because both lipid and protein occupy part of the measured volume but do not contain chloride (Dimeski et al., 2006).

22.2.5.2 Bicarbonate/Total Carbon Dioxide

Biochemical processes that occur in all cells are dependent on a very narrow pH range. Carbon dioxide/bicarbonate plays a vital part in the pH buffering system that restricts changes in intracellular and extracellular pH. Carbonic acid maintains equilibrium with CO_2 and H_2O and, along with bicarbonate, constitutes the major buffer pair in body fluids. As CO_2 is acidic and can freely diffuse across membranes while bicarbonate is basic and moves through specific transport channels, cellular and extracellular pH can be maintained by the movement of these ions. Under normal physiological conditions, the majority of this buffer pair is found as bicarbonate (at approximately 25 mmol/L in humans) (Casey, 2006). Total carbon dioxide content is typically measured as an estimator of serum bicarbonate because of the labile nature of bicarbonate ions. Total CO_2 represents the amount of serum bicarbonate, carbonic acid, and dissolved carbon dioxide present.

Bicarbonate is one of the major anions of the ECF (the other being Cl^-) produced when CO_2 diffuses into erythrocytes and is converted by carbonic anhydrase to HCO_3^-. To prevent buildup of HCO_3^- in the cells, high levels of anion exchanger 1 (AE1, the HCO_3^- transport protein) are expressed, and these allow the movement of HCO_3^- out of the cell. To preserve electrical neutrality, Cl^- moves into the cells at the same rate (Alper et al., 2002). Movement of bicarbonate ions therefore affects three different processes: HCO_3^- metabolism, regulation of pH, and regulation of cell volume (effected by coordinated activation of Cl^-/HCO_3^- transporters with H^+/Na^+ transporters) (Mason et al., 1989; Cordat and Casey, 2009). Primary changes in plasma bicarbonate concentration lead to metabolic acid–base disorders. Moreover, decreased bicarbonate results in decreased carbon dioxide and hydrogen ions; whereas, increased bicarbonate results in increased CO_2 and hydrogen ions.

The process of bicarbonate reabsorption occurs predominantly in the proximal tubules of the kidney, the remainder in the thick ascending limb of the loop of Henle and the collecting duct (Boron, 2006). Under normal conditions, the kidney is able to reabsorb all filtered bicarbonate, which is important to maintain the acid–base balance. It is achieved by secreted H^+, combining with filtered HCO_3^- to form CO_2 and H_2O. These can be passively reabsorbed and the H_2O broke down intracellularly to OH^- and H^+. Reaction of OH^- and CO_2 then leads to the reformation of HCO_3^-. The net effect of this absorption is the loss of one H^+ in exchange for one HCO_3^-. Reabsorption of bicarbonate is affected by many factors: potassium balance, volume status, and renin/angiotensin levels (Boron, 2006) (Figure 22.6).

22.2.5.2.1 Hyperbicarbonatemia

Hyperbicarbonatemia is an electrolyte disturbance characterized by the elevated levels of bicarbonate in the blood, and it is almost always indicative of metabolic alkalosis; however, it can occur primary or secondary to respiratory acid–base disorders. Elevated bicarbonate levels are associated with hypercapnia, hypokalemia, or hyperchloremia. Metabolic alkalosis secondary to respiratory acidosis associated with an increase in the partial pressure of carbon dioxide (PCO_2) and decrease in pH due to the high levels of H^+ in the blood. This leads to the renal retention of bicarbonate, elevated serum bicarbonate, and metabolic alkalosis. The development of alkalosis occurs in an attempt to correct the primary respiratory acidosis. Metabolic alkalosis, respiratory acidosis, and hypercapnia are all indicative of hyperbicarbonatemia; they are not generally the cause. Elevated

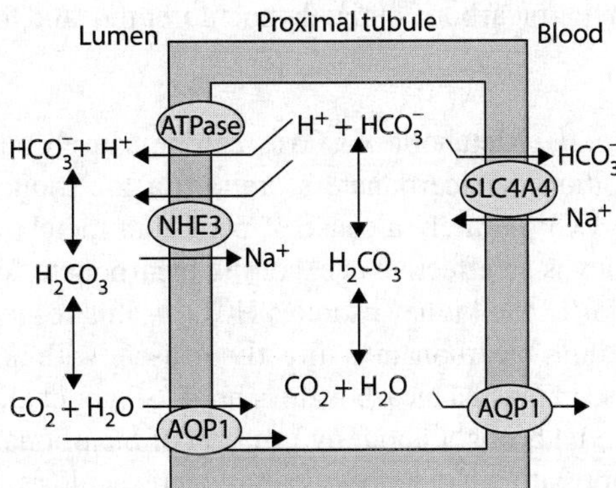

FIGURE 22.6 Bicarbonate reabsorption in the proximal tubule of the kidney. H^+ secreted into the tubule lumen is used to titrate the HCO_3^- to CO_2 and H_2O. These reenter the cell across the apical membrane and recombine to produce H^+ and HCO_3^- that moves out across the basolateral membrane.

TABLE 22.12
Causes of Hyperbicarbonatemia

Renal	Gastrointestinal
• Bicarbonate retention—compensation for respiratory acidosis	• Bicarbonate administration
• Diuretic use	• Gastrointestinal loss—vomiting, chloride diarrhea, gastric suction
• Mineralocorticoid excess—hyperaldosteronism, hyperadrenocorticism (Cushing's disease)	
• Potassium deficiency	

HCO_3^- concentrations are due to bicarbonate retention by the kidney, ingestion of bicarbonate, or loss of H^+ from the body (vomiting). Common causes of elevated HCO_3^- level are shown in Table 22.12.

22.2.5.2.1.1 Renal Respiratory acidosis is characterized by decreased respiration and causes a decrease in blood pH and an increase in PCO_2. Metabolic alkalosis developing secondary to this condition occurs when high levels of H^+ are present in blood promoting increased renal retention of HCO_3^-. This compensating response requires days to develop and results in a rise in the serum bicarbonate levels. The extent of the rise in plasma bicarbonate is determined by the increase in renal hydrogen secretion (Capasso et al., 2002). The factors that maintain elevation of bicarbonate levels are the same as those involved in the maintenance of metabolic alkalosis: chloride depletion, potassium depletion, ECF volume depletion, and reduction of GFR. Chloride depletion from the loss of bicarbonate-poor, chloride-rich ECF as occurs with thiazide or loop diuretics ultimately lead to a decrease in ECF volume (contraction alkalosis). As the original bicarbonate now exists in a smaller ECF volume, the elevation of bicarbonate concentration occurs. This mechanism of bicarbonate elevation however only causes small increases of at most, 2–4 mmol/L. In chloride depletion, there are also fewer chloride ions available to be exchanged with HCO_3^-, in the collecting duct of the kidney. This impairment of the kidney's ability to excrete bicarbonate leads to excess serum bicarbonate. Potassium depletion occurring in cases of mineralocorticoid excess/hyperaldosteronism (and hyperadrenocorticism) results in increased bicarbonate reabsorption in both the proximal and distal tubules of the kidney. Elevated aldosterone levels lead to increased distal tubular Na^+ reabsorption and increased K^+ and H^+ losses. The increased H^+ losses are matched by increased bicarbonate losses and can result in hyperbicarbonatemia, hypochloremia, and hypokalemia (Khanna and Kurtzman, 2001).

22.2.5.2.1.2 Gastrointestinal Metabolic alkalosis can be caused both by an increase in bicarbonate intake and an inhibition of bicarbonate secretion in the kidney. Increase in bicarbonate intake or alkali gain in the ECF is rarely a cause of persistent metabolic alkalosis or hyperbicarbonatemia because the kidney is so effective at excreting bicarbonate. Whenever plasma bicarbonate levels rise above 24 mmol/L, the kidney excretes HCO_3^-. This response effectively corrects the imbalance so even when sodium bicarbonate is directly infused, with normal renal function, bicarbonaturia follows and the rise in plasma bicarbonate is brief (Singer et al., 1955). Transient increases in bicarbonate level can also be brought about by infusion of bicarbonate base equivalents such as citrate in transfused blood or treatment of ketoacidosis or lactic acidosis. When these organic anions are metabolized to bicarbonate, a temporary increase in bicarbonate concentration ensues (Galla, 2000). Elevation of bicarbonate concentration can also be brought about by mechanisms that induce H^+ loss from the gut (through vomiting of acidic gastric contents). The loss of acidic gastric contents by vomiting can result in alkaline diuresis where the kidney reabsorbs sodium without chloride by an accelerated sodium–cation exchange. This process induces hyperbicarbonatemia and potassium depletion (Schwartz and Cohen, 1978). The sodium loss is small but volume is conserved, which is more important than the maintenance of normal acid–base or potassium balance (Kassirer and Schwartz, 1966).

22.2.5.2.2 Hypobicarbonatemia

Hypobicarbonatemia is an electrolyte disturbance characterized by abnormally depleted levels of bicarbonate in the blood. Bicarbonate concentrations of 8–10 mmol/L are incompatible with life in humans if they are maintained for more than a short period of time (Narins et al., 1980). Hypobicarbonatemia is almost always indicative of metabolic acidosis; it also occurs with progressive kidney disease (Shah et al., 2009). As with hyperbicarbonatemia, the metabolic changes associated with this condition may be primary or secondary to primary respiratory disorders. Causes of low plasma bicarbonate levels can be divided into renal and metabolic changes. The decrease in bicarbonate concentration can be due to loss from either the gastrointestinal tract or kidney. Additionally metabolic combination of bicarbonate with H^+ from acids such as lactic acid and keto acids can cause hypobicarbonatemia. These mechanisms are shown in Table 22.13.

22.2.5.2.2.1 Renal Excretion Renal loss of bicarbonate can be a compensatory mechanism for respiratory alkalosis or renal disease (renal failure or renal tubular acidosis). Respiratory alkalosis is associated with a decrease in PCO_2 and an increase in pH due to decreased circulating hydrogen ion concentration concurrent with a decrease in ionized calcium concentration causing symptoms of hypocalcemia. It is brought about by hyperventilation and may be seen in animals in pain, under psychological stress or in nonsweating animals, as they use respiratory evaporative processes for

TABLE 22.13
Causes of Hypobicarbonatemia

Renal Excretion	Metabolic
• Respiratory alkalosis—increased bicarbonate loss • Renal failure—decreased renal excretion • Renal tubular acidosis • Mineralocorticoid deficiency	• Increased acid production (acidosis)—diabetic ketoacidosis, lactic acidosis, ethanol consumption, salicylate, methanol, and ethylene glycol toxicity • Diarrhea, pancreatic fistula, urinary diversion—increased loss of bicarbonate

heat loss (Carlson, 1989). The initial response to respiratory alkalosis is a slight decline in ECF bicarbonate concentration; this occurs through cellular buffering. A slower renal response ensues to further decrease in HCO_3^- levels by decreasing renal bicarbonate reabsorption. The decline in bicarbonate is partially offset by chloride retention for preserving electrical neutrality. This mechanism can produce a 12–15 mmol/L (12–15 mmol/L) decrease in bicarbonate in humans (Carlson, 1989). In renal tubular acidosis, a defect in proximal tubule HCO_3^- reabsorption or distal tubule H^+ secretion (or both) cause low plasma bicarbonate levels and blood to remain considerably acidic (hyperchloremic metabolic acidosis). Mineralocorticoid deficiency also causes acidosis; low aldosterone levels result in a decline in sodium reabsorption by the distal tubule. Na^+ is lost in the urine and H^+ retained, so the normal acid load is not excreted. The buffering action of bicarbonate for this acid prevents normal regeneration reclamation from occurring and low plasma bicarbonate results.

22.2.5.2.2.2 Metabolic Metabolic acidosis is an acid–base disorder characterized by a decrease in pH that results from either a primary decrease in plasma bicarbonate concentration or an increase in hydrogen ion concentration (Kraut and Madias, 2010). ECF buffers, primarily bicarbonate–carbonic acid, bring about initial buffering of acid load. The most common causes of metabolic acidosis are shown in Table 22.14 and include ketoacidosis, lactic acidosis, diarrhea, and renal failure. In general, conditions that result in the excess production of acids cause a depletion of bicarbonate by the increased need for buffering. When coupled with a reduction in the GFR and a corresponding decrease in the kidney's capacity to reabsorb bicarbonate, the use of bicarbonate exceeds production and hypobicarbonatemia ensues. Ketoacidosis occurs when the body produces high levels of ketone bodies through the metabolism of fatty acids. It is often associated with diabetes mellitus as insulin production slows the process of ketosis. The body initially buffers the acidity of the ketone bodies with bicarbonate–carbonic acid; bicarbonate and ketones are lost in the urine. Common types of ketoacidosis are diabetic and alcoholic ketoacidosis; they occur with drug use (ethanol, ethylene glycol, methanol, aspirin, iron, and acetazolamide [a carbonic anhydrase inhibitor]), starvation, pregnancy, or myocardial infarction. Most animals (including dog, cat, rat, and guinea pig) develop only slight ketosis when starved; in humans and nonhuman primates, starvation ketosis is a regular phenomenon (Friedemann, 1926). Lactic acidosis is a state of acidosis characterized by the elevated levels of plasma lactate. The breakdown of lactate releases H^+, this is in turn buffered by bicarbonate and leads to bicarbonate depletion (Nadiminti et al., 1980). Fatal concentrations of lactate in humans are 7–8 mmol/L (Oliva, 1970). Normal concentrations in dogs range from 0.4 to 2.6 mmol/L, with a median value of 1.7 mmol/L (Thorneloe et al., 2007). Diarrhea (caused by infectious agents and osmotic effects), pancreatic fistula, or urine diversion can also lead to depleted bicarbonate levels.

TABLE 22.14
Causes of Metabolic Acidosis

High Anion Gap

- Ketoacidosis—diabetes, poor nutrition
- Lactic acidosis—shock, seizures, excessive exercise, carbon monoxide, or cyanide poisoning
- Renal failure
- Metabolism of toxins to acids—methanol, ethylene glycol, salicylates

Normal Anion Gap

- Gastrointestinal bicarbonate loss—diarrhea, uterosigmoidostomy
- Renal bicarbonate loss—renal tubule acidosis, hyperparathyroidism
- Ingestion or infusion—ammonium chloride, arginine, calcium chloride, magnesium sulfate
- Hypoaldosteronism
- Hyperkalemia

22.2.5.2.3 Factors Influencing Measurement of Bicarbonate/Total Carbon Dioxide Concentration

Measurement of total carbon dioxide represents the amount of serum bicarbonate, carbonic acid, and dissolved carbon dioxide present. It is typically measured as an estimator of serum bicarbonate because of the labile nature of bicarbonate ions. Bicarbonate concentration can then be calculated from PCO_2 and pH. A small error may occur when it is calculated rather than measured because the ionic strength of samples varies. An indirect titrimetric method determining total CO_2 can be used; however, it must be corrected for carbamate and carbonate. An altered bicarbonate value must be accompanied by other data for proper interpretation. Obtaining a satisfactory arterial sample from dogs, cats, rabbits, pigs, horses, cows, goats, sheep, and primates is not difficult. In rodents, it can probably be obtained by permanent surgical exteriorization of the carotid artery to permit arterial catheterization. The method of restraint used when obtaining cardiac blood from rats can have an effect on acid–base balance and plasma calcium and magnesium levels. Manual restraint can increase blood acidity and plasma calcium and magnesium levels whereas little difference in effect is observed when ether, pentobarbitone sodium, or fentanyl plus droperidol were used. In a study of Wistar rats treated with anesthesia, bicarbonate levels were between 19.44 and 22.25 mmol/L; however, when manually restrained the level was 14.44 mmol/L (Upton and Morgan, 1975). Changes in pH or temperature are important to accurately determine the values of bicarbonate; likewise the exposure of blood samples to air or plastic containers that absorb carbon dioxide produces a loss of this volatile acid; air bubbles erroneously lower PCO_2 by dilution (Beetham, 1982). When performing a complete clinical chemistry panel on samples, it is necessary to analyze a separate aliquot of blood for bicarbonate in order to minimize the amount of time the sample is exposed to air in the analyzer while other endpoints are determined. Acidic heparin should be avoided; heparin should be sterile, isotonic, and have a neutral pH (Beetham, 1982). Addition of heparin should be minimal and constant, as it is equilibrated with atmospheric gases. Normally, the proximal tubule reabsorbs almost all filtered bicarbonate so urinary bicarbonate is barely detectable and fractional excretion of bicarbonate ($FEHCO_3^-$) is <5% of the glomerular filtered load. However, $FEHCO_3^-$ is a useful measure of renal tubular acidosis. In proximal renal tubular acidosis, bicarbonate is increased, usually to approximately 15% and in distal renal tubular acidosis urine pH is high but plasma bicarbonate concentration remains low or normal (<5%–10%) (Bagga et al., 2005; Unwin, 2001). $FEHCO_3^-$ can be calculated using the following formula:

$$FEHCO_3^- = \frac{(\text{urine bicarbonate/serum bicarbonate})}{(\text{urine creatinine/serum creatinine})} \times 100$$

22.2.5.3 Inorganic Phosphorus (Phosphate)

Phosphorus is a naturally occurring element present in many foods. It is a major intracellular anion existing in two forms: dihydrogen phosphate ($H_2PO_4^-$) and mono-hydrogen phosphate ($H_2PO_4^-$) at normal blood pH levels. Approximately 85% of total body phosphorus is in the bone where it forms part of the mineralized extracellular matrix (crystalline hydroxyapatite) and creates a reservoir for maintaining homeostasis. The remaining phosphate is found in the soft tissues where the majority of the phosphorus is intracellular, complexed with carbohydrates, lipids, and proteins. It forms an essential part of cell structures including nucleic acids, cell membrane phospholipids, and mitochondria. Phosphate is necessary for many enzymatic reactions (in glycolysis, ammoniagenesis, and oxidative phosphorylation) and plays an important role in energy metabolism, storing energy in the chemical bonds between phosphate groups in ADP and ATP. In addition, it influences the oxygen carrying capacity of hemoglobin by its role in the regulation of 2,3-diphosphoglycerate (2,3-DPG) synthesis. Inorganic phosphate is present as a very minor component of serum, in the range 1.12–1.45 mmol/L in adult man. Inorganic phosphate levels are higher in rodent species than other laboratory animals, which are in the range of 2.55–4.55 mmol/L in mice (1.07–4.33 mmol/L in rats) compared to 0.88–2.35 mmol/L in rabbits. No diurnal variation or gender differences have been observed in phosphate levels; however, some differences have been observed between different breeds of rabbits. In mice, rats, and dogs, phosphate levels decrease with age (Loeb et al., 1996); younger animals have higher phosphate requirements due to active skeletal growth. Dietary intake and acid–base balance also play a role in determining the phosphate level of an animal.

Passive and active absorption of phosphate in the GI tract occurs by paracellular pathways (by passive diffusion between cells) and transport channels (antiporters). The uptake by luminal cells may be dependent on intraluminal sodium and is also vitamin D and calcium dependent. The kidney is the major route of phosphate secretion and controls homeostasis. Under normal conditions, approximately 85%–90% of filtered phosphorus is reabsorbed. The reabsorption is passive and linked to sodium transport, occurring largely in the proximal tubules. In some circumstances (in response to glucose and insulin administration), phosphate is reabsorbed independently of sodium. Reabsorption is inhibited by PTH, and may be influenced by vitamin D metabolites and calcium (Patel and Singh, 2009; Bergwitz and Juppner, 2010).

22.2.5.3.1 Phosphate Imbalances

22.2.5.3.1.1 Hyperphosphatemia Hyperphosphatemia is a rare electrolyte disturbance characterized by increased phosphate levels. Elevated serum phosphate levels occur by three general mechanisms: excess intake, reduced renal excretion, and shifts in cellular balance. One of the most common clinical conditions associated with hyperphosphatemia is chronic renal failure (Rosol and Capen, 1996; Moe, 2008). Common causes of hyperphosphatemia are shown in Table 22.15.

22.2.5.3.1.1.1 Excess Intake With properly functioning renal excretion mechanisms, an excess intake of dietary phosphorous is an uncommon cause of hyperphosphatemia. Mechanisms for renal excretion allow virtually unlimited intake of phosphate while still maintaining homeostatic control. In addition to the intake of phosphate, hypervitaminosis D can also cause increased gastrointestinal and renal absorption of phosphate (and calcium) and elevated phosphate levels. In conjunction with renal insufficiency, either mechanism can lead to hyperphosphatemia.

22.2.5.3.1.1.2 Reduced Renal Excretion Decreased excretion of phosphate, especially when accompanied by excess intake, is the most frequent cause of hyperphosphatemia; this is most commonly associated with reduced renal excretion in renal failure. When the GFR falls to below 25 mL/min, the excretion of ingested phosphate is insufficient to maintain homeostasis and hyperphosphatemia develops. In hypoparathyroidism, phosphate is retained through failure to inhibit proximal tubule reabsorption. Similar mechanisms are in action in severe hypomagnesemia and pseudohypoparathyroidism in which PTH secretion is impaired or there

TABLE 22.15
Causes of Hyperphosphatemia

Excess Intake	Reduced Renal Excretion	Shift in Cellular Balance
• High dietary phosphate	• Renal Failure	• Tumor lysis
• Hypervitaminosis D	• Hypoparathyroidism	• Rhabdomyolysis
• Phosphate enema	• Endocrine disorders—hyperthyroidism	• Respiratory acidosis
• Intravenous phosphate	• Pseudohypoparathyroidism	
	• Magnesium deficiency	
	• Tumoral calcinosis	

is a failure of PTH action in renal tubules; these all result in hyperphosphatemia. In other endocrine disorders such as acromegaly, excess growth hormone leads to increased tubular reabsorption of phosphate and high serum phosphate levels. Tumoral calcinosis is also characterized by decreased renal excretion of phosphate and hyperphosphatemia; this condition is caused by inactivating mutations in proteins that control urine phosphate levels (fibroblast growth factor 23 (FGF23), polypeptide *N*-acetylgalactosaminyltransferase 3 (GALNT3), or KL) (Prie et al., 2005).

22.2.5.3.1.1.3 Shift in Cellular Balance Alone, the movement of phosphate from the intracellular to the extracellular space is an uncommon cause of hyperphosphatemia. A shift in the cellular balance of phosphate causing hyperphosphatemia occurs with rhabdomyolysis or tumor lysis. Rarely, acidosis or insulin deficiency may cause cellular shifts in phosphate.

22.2.5.3.1.2 Hypophosphatemia Hypophosphatemia is a disturbed electrolyte balance characterized by a reduced serum phosphate level. Acute clinical manifestations are rare in laboratory animals; in human, clinical consequences are usually observed when hypophosphatemia is severe (<0.32 mmol/L). There are three primary mechanisms that lead to hypophosphatemia: low dietary intake, increased phosphate excretion (from the GI tract or kidney), and a shift in cellular balance from extracellular to intracellular compartments (Moe, 2008; Shaikh et al., 2008). Table 22.16 shows the common causes of hypophosphatemia.

22.2.5.3.1.2.1 Intake Deficiency Insufficient dietary intake of phosphate is an uncommon cause of hypophosphatemia because of the prevalence of phosphate in foods. However, in conditions of starvation (not uncommon in experimental animals used in drug development) or chronic alcoholism and in combination with renal insufficiency, hypophosphatemia may occur. Decreased intestinal absorption can also lead to a deficiency of phosphate; this can occur with diarrhea, severe vomiting, or malabsorption conditions. The use of large amounts of aluminum-containing antacids can cause depletion of phosphate by binding phosphate in the gut and preventing absorption of ingested and secreted phosphate (Bates, 2008). Vitamin D deficiency decreases gut absorption of calcium and phosphate. It also increases renal excretion of phosphate and decreases bone resorption resulting in hypophosphatemia and hypocalcemia.

22.2.5.3.1.2.2 Increased Renal Excretion The major cause of phosphate loss is increased renal excretion. Usually, this occurs as a result of excess PTH (primary or secondary hyperparathyroidism),

TABLE 22.16
Causes of Hypophosphatemia

Intake Deficiency	Increased Renal Excretion	Shift in Cellular Balance
• Poor dietary intake/starvation	• Hyperparathyroidism	• Respiratory alkalosis
• Malabsorption	• Sodium bicarbonate infusion/extracellular volume expansion	• Hyperalimentation
• Hypovitaminosis D	• Renal tubule defects—Fanconi syndrome	• High carbohydrate diet
• Phosphate binders—antacids	• Diuretic use—loop diuretics, thiazides, or carbonic anhydrases inhibitors	• Glucose ingestion/administration
• Diarrhea/vomiting	• Osmotic diuresis	• Insulin administration
	• Renal tubular acidosis	• Diabetic ketoacidosis
	• Hypokalemia/hypomagnesemia	

which stimulates the kidneys to excrete phosphate. Loss may also be the result of extracellular volume expansion with sodium or bicarbonate. The resulting dilution of serum calcium causes an increase in PTH release stimulating renal secretion of phosphate. Diuretic use can lead to phosphate depletion by interfering with the ability of the proximal tubule to reabsorb phosphate; hyperphosphaturia follows and hypophosphatemia can develop. Osmotic diuresis depletes phosphate by increasing its renal clearance, it can occur in conditions such as hyperosmolar hyperglycemic syndrome. Other conditions that can result in increased phosphate secretion by the kidney include Fanconi syndrome in dogs (characterized by failure to reabsorb amino acids, glucose, and phosphate), congenital defects, or estrogen down regulation of a renal sodium phosphate cotransporter (Faroqui et al., 2008; Rastegar, 2009).

22.2.5.3.1.2.3 Shift in Cellular Balance Hyperventilation leading to respiratory alkalosis can be caused by a variety of conditions including diabetic ketoacidosis or salicylate toxicity. It activates phosphofructokinase stimulating intracellular glycolysis, leading to phosphate consumption and the movement of phosphate from the extracellular to the intracellular compartment (Datta and Stone, 2009). A high carbohydrate diet or glucose administration lower serum phosphate levels by stimulating the release of insulin, which enhances the intracellular movement of phosphate and glucose into cells. It may also cause cells to switch to an anabolic state whereby serum phosphate is depleted through incorporation into the cells (Mehanna et al., 2009). Diabetic ketoacidosis is also an important cause of hypophosphatemia. In this condition, serum phosphate levels are initially higher due to metabolic acidosis and insulin deficiency shifting the intracellular phosphate stores to the extracellular compartment. This leads to urinary loss (Nowik et al., 2008). With insulin treatment, phosphate is translocated back into the cells resulting in a decrease in serum phosphate levels.

22.2.5.3.2 Factors Influencing Measurement of Phosphate Concentration

Since phosphate is predominantly an intracellular cation, hyperphosphatemia does not always reflect a true increase in total body phosphate stores. Moreover, cellular damage releases intracellular phosphate and can cause spurious hyperphosphatemia. Measurement of urine phosphate in samples obtained from the bottom of rodent cages has no credence; many detergents contain phosphate, and there is contamination by feces, hair, and microorganisms. As phosphate homeostasis is primarily regulated at the level of the proximal renal tubule, plasma phosphate levels are indicators of renal tubular handling. The fractional excretion of phosphate determined in urine specimens at different time points daily is often used as an estimation of phosphate handling. As tubular reabsorption of phosphate depends on plasma phosphate and GFR, it is not a good indicator of tubular phosphate handling. Increasingly, "tubular maximum for phosphate corrected for glomerular filtration rate" has been employed to assess renal phosphate handling. This provides an index of the renal threshold for phosphate that can be determined on timed urine samples and can be calculated as follows: plasma phosphate – (urine phosphate × plasma creatinine)/urine creatinine (Bagga et al., 2005). However, the small volume of blood that can be sampled daily from small laboratory animals can be a limit to experimental design when using this method.

22.2.5.4 Sulfate

Sulfate is the fourth most common anion in plasma, and it is known to play an essential role in a wide variety of physiological processes: particularly, the sulfation of exogenous and endogenous compounds (steroids, anti-inflammatory agents, and adrenergic blockers). Sulfation provides a mechanism of biotransformation of these compounds and in most cases leads to increased urinary excretion (Falany, 1997). One of the most important roles for sulfate is in the biosynthesis of 3′-phophoadenosine-5′-phosphosulfate (PAPS), which is the active sulfate used in the biosynthesis of many essential endogenous compounds (i.e., heparin and gastrin) that are necessary for the biosynthesis of cell membranes and tissues (proteoglycans) (Beck and Silve, 2001). Inorganic sulfate accounts for 90%–95% of naturally occurring sulfated compounds, the remaining 5%–10% of total body sulfate occurs as sulfoconjugates. Plasma sulfate concentration varies with age in mammals; in humans, it is 0.47 mmol/L at birth but decreases with age to 0.33 mmol/L in adults (Cole and Scriver, 1980; Bakhtian et al., 1993; Pena and Neiberger, 1997).

Although an essential anion, sulfate is infrequently assayed in clinical chemistry. Serum sulfate is strongly influenced by a variety of physiological factors such as age, diet, and drugs and is difficult to measure accurately. Quantitation of serum sulfate is achieved by ion conductimetry after anion-exchange chromatography (Cole and Evrovski, 1997, 2000). Little is known of the factors that regulate sulfate homeostasis in mammals; the role of changes in sulfate metabolism in the pathogenesis of disease is largely unknown. Sulfate homeostasis is achieved by three mechanisms: dietary intake, intestinal absorption, and renal secretion. In the intestine, approximately 90%–95% of sulfate ingested is absorbed. Uptake by the enterocytes occurs through Na^+-dependent transports and Na^+/Cl^- exchangers (Langridge-Smith and Field, 1981; Schron et al., 1987; Florin et al., 1991). The kidneys primarily control sulfate homeostasis; sulfate is freely filtered from the glomerulus and is reabsorbed in the proximal tubules. Approximately 80%–95% of filtered sulfate is reabsorbed; the remainder is excreted in the urine (Beck and Silve, 2001; Markovich, 2001). Regulation of proximal tubule reabsorption is largely unexplored. Factors known to regulate sulfate levels include vitamin D, which modulates Solute Carrier Family 13 Member 1 (NaS1) transport protein, thyroid hormone (hyperthyroidism in humans is associated with increased serum sulfate levels and hypothyroidism with decreased sulfate levels), and dietary sulfate intake (dietary sulfate levels regulate renal sulfate transport) (Markovich et al., 1998). More recently, knockout mouse models have highlighted factors that regulate sulfate homeostasis in mammals and the physiological consequence of homeostasis disruption. Functional characterization of the sulfate anion transporter, NaS1, knockout mouse model has shown the essential role played by this protein in mediating proximal tubule sulfate reabsorption. Targeted disruption of this gene leads to hyposulfatemia and hypersulfaturia in NaS1 knockout mice indicating that NaS1 is critical for maintaining sulfate homeostasis. Changes in blood sulfate levels affect a wide range of physiological functions including the metabolism, growth, fecundity, behavior, gut physiology, and liver detoxification (Markovich, 2011a, b).

22.2.5.4.1 Hypersulfatemia

Elevated levels of serum sulfate characterize hypersulfatemia; it occurs in chronic renal failure with reduced GFRs. The mechanisms involved in the development of hypersulfatemia are unknown but likely involve a decrease in the amount of sulfate transporter proteins, NaS1 and Sat1, leading to increased sulfate secretion (Beck and Silve, 2001).

22.2.5.4.2 Hyposulfatemia

Decreased levels of serum sulfate characterize hyposulfatemia; however, little is known about the clinical significance or factors that give rise to this condition. Studies in knockout mice show that the sodium-sulfate cotransporter NaS1 plays a pivotal role in maintaining serum sulfate levels within the normal physiological range. This gene is expressed predominantly in the kidney and intestine and is regulated by environmental factors (including diet and hormones); in NaS1 null mice, hyposulfatemia develops (Dawson et al., 2003; Markovich and Aronson, 2007).

22.3 Blood Gases

The process of respiration can be divided into four phases: ventilation, alveolar gas exchange, transport of gases in blood, and gas exchange in the tissues. Beginning with an exchange of air between the atmosphere and alveoli (ventilation), oxygen and carbon dioxide then move between alveolar air and capillary blood for transport to tissues. Ventilation is controlled by partial pressures of oxygen (PO_2) and carbon dioxide (PCO_2) and the concentration of hydrogen ions. Although gases are transported across the alveolar wall by passive diffusion, concentration gradient is not the primary determinant of rate of exchange. This is because when dissolved in body fluids, O_2 and CO_2 are mostly bound to hemoglobin (O_2) or exist as HCO_3^- (CO_2). As the bound molecules are not free to diffuse, partial pressure (measured in millimeters of mercury, mmHg or kilopascals, kPa) is considered a more accurate measure of the ability of the gas to move. Partial pressure (or tension) of a single gas (PO_2 or PCO_2) in a gaseous mixture is defined by the pressure exerted by that gas alone. Alveolar gases are comprised of oxygen, nitrogen, carbon dioxide, and water vapor. O_2 and CO_2 each rapidly diffuse down their own partial pressure gradient, which drives O_2 from the alveolus to the blood and CO_2 from the blood to the alveolus. The rate of O_2 diffusion is influenced by several factors: diffusion gradient, total surface area, respiratory membrane thickness, and respiratory rate. Diffusion rates can be reduced when the PO_2 gradient declines (reduced ventilation or perfusion), the surface area for gas exchange is reduced (emphysema), the respiratory membrane is abnormally thickened (pulmonary edema, pneumonia), or respiratory rates are depressed (barbiturates, anesthesia) (Misasi and Keyes, 1996).

Oxygen is transported in the blood primarily bound to hemoglobin (97%), ~3% of oxygen is dissolved in plasma, and it is this that accounts for the PO_2 of blood. A high PO_2 level in blood (occurring in the lungs) causes a rise in the amount of oxyhemoglobin formed; when PO_2 falls in the tissues, oxyhemoglobin breaks down and releases O_2. Oxyhemoglobin formation is also favored by lower PCO_2 and a rise in pH. Oxygen saturation is a measure of how much of the hemoglobin in red blood cells is carrying oxygen; it is typically >95%. Carbon dioxide is transported in three ways: the most important means is as bicarbonate ions (60%–80%); it is also attached to hemoglobin (23%) and dissolved in plasma (7%). The latter determines the PCO_2 value and obeys Henry's law stating that dissolved CO_2 increases linearly with PCO_2 (Wieth et al., 1982). Carbon dioxide in the form of bicarbonate ions represents one of the body's primary buffering systems for pH maintenance at a physiological optimum (pH 7.4) (Kellum, 2000; Dash and Bassingthwaighte, 2006); higher levels of CO_2 produce more H^+ and lower pH according to the equilibrium shown as follows:

$$CO_2 + H_2O \longleftrightarrow H_2CO_3 \longleftrightarrow H^+ + HCO_3^-$$

The Henderson–Hasselbalch equation applied to the HCO_3^-/H_2CO_3 buffer pair is expressed as follows:

$$pH = 6.1 + \log_{10}\left[\frac{HCO_3^-}{H_2CO_3}\right]$$

where 6.1 is the pK_a for the HCO_3^-/H_2CO_3 buffer pair at 37°C and pH 7.4 (Paulev and Zubieta-Calleja, 2005). [HCO_3^-] represents the bicarbonate concentration expressed in millimoles per liter. [H_2CO_3] consists of (1) physically dissolved carbon dioxide—99% (arterial PCO_2), and (2) hydrated carbon dioxide—1% (H_2CO_3). By controlling ventilation rates, the respiratory system therefore plays a primary role in regulating pH (Beetham, 1982). The role bicarbonate plays in acid–base balance will be discussed in more detail in a later section.

In tissues, O_2 and CO_2 diffuse down their partial pressure gradient defined by the fact that PO_2 in arterial blood > PO_2 of ISF > PO_2 ICF. The gradient is maintained because O_2 is continuously used in metabolism, and the release of O_2 from oxyhemoglobin maintains the PO_2 of blood. For carbon dioxide, the PCO_2 of arterial blood is less than that of ISF, which is less than that of ICF. CO_2 therefore moves out of the cell on a gradient maintained by the continual production of CO_2 by cellular processes.

Arterial blood gas is a collective term used to describe three measurements: pH, PCO_2, and PO_2. Although hydrogen is not present in blood as a gas and therefore does not exert a partial pressure, pH is a measure of hydrogen ion concentration and forms part of arterial blood gas measurements. Together, these measurements provide an assessment of acid–base status, ventilation, and arterial oxygenation. Each of these components is discussed individually below.

22.3.1 pH

Although hydrogen is not present in blood as a gas and therefore does not exert a partial pressure, pH is a measure of hydrogen ion concentration and forms part of arterial blood gas measurements. The normal range for blood pH varies little between species and is 7.32–7.5; a value less than 7.2 is considered life threatening in humans (Narins et al., 1980). Venous pH is lower than arterial pH. Moreover, in dog, the mean difference is 0.038 units (Zweens et al., 1977). Women have higher pH values than men, and pH decreases in old age (other species may be similar to humans in this respect). pH is defined as follows:

$$pH = -\log_{10}\left[H^+\right]$$

Normal H^+ concentration is 0.0004 mmol/L and is a measure of the acid–base status of blood. As enzymatic reactions operate within a tightly defined pH range, regulation of the acid–base balance is strictly controlled. Disturbances in pH result in abnormal respiratory and cardiac functions, abnormal blood clotting, and drug metabolism.

Small amounts of hydrogen ions are generated during the oxidation of amino acids and the anaerobic metabolism of glucose to lactic and pyruvic acid; however, the largest source of H^+ in the body is generated as a result of CO_2 production from metabolism according to the relationship below:

$$CO_2 + H_2O \longleftrightarrow H_2CO_3 \longleftrightarrow H^+ + HCO_3^-$$

This carbonic acid/bicarbonate equilibrium therefore forms one of the most important systems in the body for limiting changes in pH. H^+ homeostasis is maintained by three mechanisms: buffers that limit changes in H^+ concentration (especially carbonic acid/bicarbonate), the lungs (which control PCO_2), and the kidneys (which regulate plasma bicarbonate). As carbon dioxide is the primary source of H^+, the respiratory system is the primary regulator of H^+ concentration. Arterial PCO_2 is inversely proportional to alveolar ventilation, so profound changes in H^+ levels and pH are affected by changes in ventilation. The kidneys also play a role in H^+ homeostasis as tubule cells can excrete H^+ and regenerate bicarbonate ions (Gumz et al., 2010). Furthermore, the kidney is one of the primary sites for homeostatic control of electrolyte balance and therefore influences acid–base balance. Hydrogen ions are actively secreted into the kidney tubule lumen where they combine with bicarbonate to form carbonic acid. Carbonic acid dissociates to form CO_2 and H_2O catalyzed by luminal carbonic anhydrase. The CO_2 diffuses into the tubular epithelial cells where it combines with water again to form carbonic acid. Carbonic acid then dissociates into bicarbonate and H^+, which are excreted from the cell (McMurtrie et al., 2004; Purkerson and Schwartz, 2007). Hydrogen passes back into the blood in exchange for Na^+ and counter to Cl^- to maintain electrical neutrality. This elimination occurs by active secretion against a steep concentration gradient in the proximal and distal tubules. Urine is buffered from the constant influx of H^+ by phosphate and ammonia (Hamm and Simon, 1987).

22.3.2 Hydrogen Imbalance

22.3.2.1 Acidemia

Acidemia is defined as increased H^+ in blood plasma; it can be caused by metabolic or respiratory changes and can lead to acidosis. Moderate acidosis develops in most animals at pH 7.25–7.3, severe acidosis at pH 7.2–7.25 and grave acidosis at pH 7.0–7.1. In general, a rise in H^+ is associated with conditions such as lactic acidosis, ketosis, hyperventilation, urinary obstruction, or renal failure

(Charney and Feldman, 1984). Tubular dysfunction can cause hydrogen ion accumulation when electrolyte exchange or bicarbonate reclamation mechanisms fail or ammonia production is reduced and its buffering action lost (Bonilla-Felix, 1996).

22.3.2.2 Alkalemia

Alkalemia is defined as decreased H^+ in blood plasma; it can be caused by metabolic or respiratory changes and can lead to the development of alkalosis (blood pH >7.45). In general, a fall in H^+ is associated with a variety of factors including increased intake of bicarbonate, citrate or lactate, dehydration (contraction alkalosis), increased acid secretion, potassium depletion, gastrointestinal loss (vomiting), or decreased renal elimination (Tannen, 1987; Khanna and Kurtzman, 2001). Mechanistically, these conditions cause alkalemia in the following ways. Increased oral intake of weak bases (citrate, lactate) increases the total plasma base and causes secondary decrease in H^+ concentration. Loss of extracellular potassium can lead to hydrogen losses when the extracellular K^+ losses cause intracellular K^+ loss; as potassium is exchanged for H^+, the intracellular pH decreases and the extracellular pH rises. Vomiting causes the loss of H^+ and Cl^- from the gastric contents; this causes plasma bicarbonate to rise which in turn causes an alkali diuresis. Potassium and a small amount of sodium and chloride are lost in the urine promoting hydrogen secretion and bicarbonate reabsorption (Norris and Kurtzman, 1988). Loss of H^+ can also be a secondary or a compensatory response: increased arterial PCO_2 results in a decrease in H^+ concentration through increased urine excretion. Likewise, sodium and chloride depletion with the resultant secondary aldosteronism causes increased renal acid secretion, as sodium is retained under the influence of aldosterone while H^+ are lost.

22.3.2.3 Factors Influencing Measurement of Hydrogen Concentration

Accurate results for pH measurement depend on proper collection and handling techniques. The most common problems include nonarterial sampling, temperature, length of storage, improper sample mixing, and inappropriate use of anticoagulant. Precise pH levels require anaerobic collection of arterial blood samples from an undisturbed, unanesthetized animal. Consideration should be given to the use of heparin as an anticoagulant: in the acidic form it produces a small error in pH and, in large volumes it affects the PCO_2 and PO_2 levels as both are heparin soluble (Hamilton et al., 1978). On storage, glycolysis can increase the titratable hydrogen ion concentration by 0.5 mmol/L per hour at room temperature and 0.1 mmol/L per hour at 0–4°C. The increase is greater when leukocytosis is present (Siggaard Andersen, 1979). Performing blood gas analysis within 95 minutes of sample collection can minimize this effect (Brito et al., 2008). Additionally, hemolysis can cause an erroneously low pH (Siggaard Andersen, 1979); this can occur when samples are incorrectly mixed or place on ice. Blood pH decreases as the body temperature rises so sample analyzers should be adjusted to body temperature or a correction factor applied. Characterization of the physiological effects of isofluorane anesthesia on neonatal mice has shown significant changes in arterial pH in anesthetized animals (Loepke et al., 2006). Implanting arterial catheters has allowed blood gas analysis in conscious unrestrained animals (Lee et al., 2008; Brun-Pascaud et al., 1982). In one study of mice in which femoral arterial catheters were implanted, the measurement of pH was successfully performed by the rapid collection of blood samples (60 μL) and immediate analysis using an automated analyzer (Lee et al., 2008). The limitation of this technique is its cumbersome and invasive nature. Instrumentation used in measuring blood gases and pH is vital to obtain accurate results. In recent years, portable "point of care" systems (e.g., i-STAT 1 analyzer) have been validated for use in research laboratories. These typically require small volumes of blood and have been used successfully to assess pH in whole blood from dogs (Verwaerde et al., 2002) and blood gas CO_2 in mice (Sahbaie et al., 2006).

22.3.3 Carbon Dioxide

Carbon dioxide is present in blood in three different forms: bicarbonate ions (60%–80%), protein bound (23%), and dissolved in plasma (7%). The latter determines the PCO_2 value, which is typically in the range of 28–40 mmHg in arterial blood and 28–42 mmHg in venous blood in laboratory animals. It does not vary significantly with age but is lower at higher altitudes where ventilation is stimulated. Arterial PCO_2 values are fairly constant, venous values are higher and vary considerably, depending on the site, temperature, and muscular or metabolic activity. The most important CO_2 binding protein is hemoglobin; reversible binding of CO_2 to the amino groups of the polypeptide chain produce carbaminohemoglobin that transports CO_2 from the tissues after O_2 dissociation. Carbon dioxide can also bind to the amino groups of other plasma proteins.

Carbon dioxide homeostasis is achieved by three mechanisms: buffering of pH changes (largely achieved with the $H_2CO_3^-/HCO_3^-$ pair), control of arterial PCO_2 (effected by the lungs), and regulation of plasma bicarbonate level (by the kidneys). The fundamental relationship in this process is the equilibrium between dissolved CO_2, $H_2CO_3^-$, and HCO_3^- (shown above). The consequence of this is that dissolved CO_2 is directly proportional to arterial PCO_2. Processing of CO_2 occurs predominantly in erythrocytes (and renal tubular cells) catalyzed by the intracellular enzyme, carbonic anhydrase (Purkerson and Schwartz, 2007).

22.3.3.1 Carbon Dioxide Imbalances

22.3.3.1.1 Hypercapnia (Hypercarbia)

Hypercapnia is characterized by elevated CO_2 levels in blood (>50 mmHg results in moderate hypercapnia in most laboratory animal species), and it leads to a decrease in blood pH and acidosis. Respiratory acidosis is an associative effect to hypercapnia rather than a causative one, brought about by primary disturbances in arterial PCO_2. Changes in bicarbonate level can cause metabolic acid–base disorders. Both forms of acid–base disturbance bring about a compensatory response in an attempt to return blood pH to normal; this may cause hypercapnia. Elevated CO_2 levels develop when there is an imbalance between the CO_2 produced by the body and that excreted by the lungs. The source of this imbalance can occur anywhere from the initiation of ventilation to gas exchange at the alveolar membrane. Many clinical conditions contribute to inadequate removal of CO_2 from the blood including paralysis of the respiratory muscles, lung diseases, central respiratory drive depression, or exposure to unusually high levels of carbon dioxide. The ability of the body to adapt to these changes depends on whether the condition is acute or chronic; with chronic pulmonary diseases, the persistent elevation of PCO_2 leads to effective compensatory mechanisms and less of a clinical impact. Respiratory acidosis rarely develops because any increase in PCO_2 rapidly causes a large increase in ventilation.

Elevated PCO_2 can occur by three mechanisms: increased metabolic production of CO_2, decreased alveolar ventilation, and increased inspired carbon dioxide (Pahari et al., 2006). The most common cause is decreased alveolar ventilation; this can result from a defect in diaphragmatic and intercostal muscle contraction, paralysis, muscle degeneration, or pain. Increased resistance to air movement, as seen with obstruction, edema, bronchiolar constriction, and loss of surfactant, reduces minute volume and can also lead to hypercapnia. Increased inspired carbon dioxide produces a relatively small change in PCO_2 because of the strong opposing ventilatory response (Wasserman et al., 1975). A twofold increase in metabolism causes a 10% increase in PCO_2; however, this effect is offset by ventilation and rarely leads to hypercapnia. Deficiency or inhibition of carbonic anhydrase activity can produce hypercapnia, as the conversion of carbonic acid to CO_2 and water is slowed. Table 22.17 shows common causes of hypercapnia.

Biochemically, an increase in PCO_2 drives the CO_2/bicarbonate equilibrium to the right increasing the concentration of H^+ and HCO_3^- in erythrocytes. The rise in H^+ is buffered by hemoglobin preventing an increase in pH. HCO_3^- moves out of the cell to the plasma and to maintain electrical neutrality within the erythrocyte. Chloride ions move into the erythrocyte. This exchange

TABLE 22.17
Causes of Hypercapnia

- CNS related—central respiratory depression, trauma, infection, hypoxia, spinal trauma
- Nerve or muscle disorders—spinal muscular atrophy, muscle dystrophies
- Airway disorders—upper airway obstruction, asthma
- Lung or chest wall defects—pneumonia, pulmonary edema, trauma
- Hypercatabolic disorders—malignant hyperthermia
- Increased intake of CO_2—rebreathing of expired air, addition of CO_2 to inspired air

TABLE 22.18
Causes of Hypocapnia

- Hypoxemia—high altitudes, pulmonary disease
- Pulmonary disorders—pneumonia, pulmonary edema
- Cardiovascular disorders—congestive heart failure
- Metabolic disorders—acidosis, liver failure
- CNS related—pain, anxiety, fever, meningitis, encephalitis
- Endocrine related—pregnancy, hyperthyroidism
- Drugs—salicylates, progesterone

of bicarbonate and chloride ions across the erythrocyte membrane is known as the chloride shift (Hamburger shift). In acute hypercapnia, the movement of bicarbonate is small (3–4 mmol/L); in chronic hypercapnia, it is larger (~40 mmol/L) but in both cases the changes are physiological responses and not part of a buffering mechanism (Cogan, 1984; Hirakawa et al., 1993).

22.3.3.1.2 Hypocapnia (Hypocarbia)

Hypocapnia is a condition of unusually low arterial PCO_2 levels. If there is no compensation and no other acid–base disorder, this will lead to an increase in arterial pH and a corresponding decrease in bicarbonate concentration. As with hypercapnia, primary disturbances in arterial PCO_2 have an associative effect with respiratory acid–base imbalance (alkalosis), not a causative one. Hypocapnia develops when there is an imbalance between the CO_2 produced by the body and that excreted by the lungs (Laffey and Kavanagh, 2002). Under normal circumstances, the volume of inspired CO_2 is negligible and increased CO_2 production is unusual. Consequently, low PCO_2 is most often the result of an increased elimination of CO_2. The principal physiological causes of hypocapnia are related to hyperventilation. Hyperventilation is stimulated when chemoreceptors in the brain and carotid bodies sense an increase in hydrogen ions. The increased rate of alveolar ventilation is disproportional to the rate of metabolic carbon dioxide production. Common causes of hypocapnia are listed in Table 22.18 (Laffey and Kavanagh, 2002).

Biochemically, a decrease in PCO_2 drives the CO_2/bicarbonate equilibrium to the left. Indirectly, hypocapnia decreases renal bicarbonate resorption because low PCO_2 inhibits renal acid secretion (Schwartz and Cohen, 1978). The latter effect is a compensatory change brought about by alteration in the tubular chloride transport and is independent of plasma pH (Schwartz and Cohen, 1978). In dogs with chronic hypocapnia, the plasma bicarbonate is decreased 0.50 mmol/L for every millimeter of mercury decrease in PCO_2 (Schwartz and Cohen, 1978).

22.3.3.2 Factors Influencing Measurement of PCO_2 Concentration

Accurate results for PCO_2 measurement depend on proper collection and handling techniques. The most common problems include nonarterial sampling, air bubbles, temperature, length of storage, and inappropriate use of anticoagulant. Precise PCO_2 levels require anaerobic collection of arterial blood samples; contamination by a venous blood may produce a falsely increased PCO_2. The effect of sampling from different sites (arterial or venous) has been evaluated in dogs and horses and showed consistent differences between arterial and venous blood (Carlson, 1989). Removal of air bubbles from sampled blood is important in preventing the equilibration of CO_2 from the air with the collected sample as this would result in a reduction of the PCO_2 (air has essentially no CO_2). Likewise, the presence of liquid heparin in the collection syringe can sometimes cause erroneous PCO_2 measurements when carbon dioxide from the air equilibrates with heparin before sample collection (Higgins, 2007). When samples are stored at room temperature, glycolysis causes an increase in PCO_2 of approximately 5 mmHg/hour at 37°C. The rate is reduced by a factor of 10 if the sample is cooled to 2°C–4°C but the maximum storage time prior to analysis should be less than 1 hour at 2°C–4°C (Tietz, 1976). Since the measurement of PCO_2 is dependent on temperature, blood samples not measured at body temperature (preferable) will need a correction factor. The PCO_2 of blood decreases by approximately 5% per degree centigrade increase in temperature because the solubility of CO_2 in plasma is decreased (Beetham, 1982). Moreover, protein buffer dissociation affects the temperature response of PCO_2 (Beetham, 1982). Finally, significant errors arise when PCO_2 is calculated from the Henderson–Hasselbalch equation because samples with abnormal protein, lipid, and ionic composition alter the pK of carbonic acid and the solubility coefficient of CO_2. Optimally, arterial blood samples should be collected in a plastic syringe with a tight fitting cap (to prevent air equilibration) and processed immediately. Values collected from blood gas machines should be corrected for the body temperature of the animal (IFCC, 2001).

22.3.4 Oxygen

Oxygen is essential for aerobic metabolism, normal oxygen tension (normoxia) is usually approximately 80–100 mmHg for human arterial blood and 30–50 mmHg for venous blood. The arterial PO_2 is influenced by atmospheric pressure, composition of alveolar air, rate, and depth of breathing, cardiac function, and blood flow and distribution. Central and peripheral receptors control and modulate lung, heart, and vascular activity. The PO_2 is under both voluntary and involuntary control. Oxygen is carried in the blood in two forms: dissolved and bound to hemoglobin. Dissolved O_2 obeys Henry's law stating that the amount of dissolved O_2 is directly proportional to the PO_2 (Habler and Messmer, 1997). The solubility coefficient of oxygen at 37°C in plasma is 0.00126 mmol/L^{-1}/mmHg^{-1} and for whole blood, 0.00140 mmol/L^{-1}/mmHg^{-1} in humans (Thomas, 1997). It is reduced by increased ionic strength and protein concentration, and it is elevated by an increase in lipid content. The contribution of dissolved oxygen to arterial oxygen content is very small and does not provide sufficient amounts of O_2 to the tissues to sustain metabolism. Hemoglobin, the major oxygen transporting protein in the erythrocytes, carries oxygen bound reversibly to ferrous iron. It has four binding sites for oxygen and under normal conditions hemoglobin is approximately >95% saturated in arterial blood and 70% in venous blood. Oxygen saturation is the ratio of the amount of O_2 bound to hemoglobin to the oxygen carrying capacity of hemoglobin. The O_2 carrying capacity is determined by the amount of hemoglobin in the blood, and the amount of O_2 bound is determined by the partial pressure of O_2. In the lungs, PO_2 is high and therefore hemoglobin binds oxygen. In tissues, the PO_2 is lower and O_2 is released. This release and uptake of oxygen by hemoglobin is carefully controlled (Meldon, 1985; Jensen, 2004). The sigmoid shape of the oxyhemoglobin dissociation curve (Figure 22.7) reflects the changes in hemoglobin affinity for oxygen (Takano et al., 1979; Rees et al., 1996).

The position of the curve indicates the available oxygen supply to the tissues. Displacement to the right indicates decreased oxygen affinity and easier unloading of oxygen. The following conditions shift the curve to the right:

1. Increased hydrogen ion concentration (Bohr effect) (Δ log $PO_2/\Delta pH$ = 0.040 to 0.050 for most mammals) binds deoxyhemoglobin more actively than hemoglobin, which reduces the affinity of hemoglobin for O_2 and promotes O_2 dissociation (Kister et al., 1988).

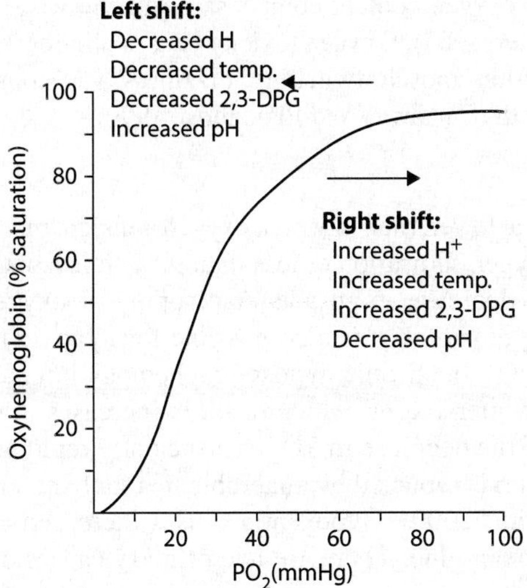

FIGURE 22.7 Oxyhemoglobin dissociation curve.

2. Increased CO_2 causes a decrease in blood pH as described previously (Jensen, 2004).
3. Increased temperature denatures the bond between O_2 and hemoglobin, which increases the amount of free O_2 and hemoglobin and decreases the concentration of oxyhemoglobin (Cambier et al., 2004).
4. Increased 2,3-DPG; as the primary organic phosphate in mammals, 2,3-DPG binds hemoglobin, modifies the conformation, and decreases its oxygen affinity (di Bella et al., 1996).
5. Hemoglobins with low oxygen affinity (human Hb Seattle and Kansas).
6. Increased ATP influences intracellular pH and may cause a conformation change in hemoglobin that reduces the binding to O_2 (Shappell and Lenfant, 1972).
7. Inorganic phosphate and other anions influence intracellular pH and may act in the same way as 2,3-DPG to modify hemoglobin conformation.
8. Anemia, the effects are mainly due to increased ATP.
9. Hyperthyroidism, the effect is mainly due to increased erythrocyte 2,3-DPG content.
10. Age of erythrocytes influences the affinity of hemoglobin for oxygen, and younger erythrocytes have lower affinity possibly as a result of 2,3-DPG level in the cells (Haidas et al., 1971).
11. Aldosterone and cortisol may decrease hemoglobin–oxygen affinity (rabbits) (Bauer and Rathschlag-Schaefer, 1968).

The curve is shifted to the left when the foregoing conditions are reversed and by the presence of fetal hemoglobin, abnormal hemoglobins (human Hb Yakima, Malmo, Rainier), or hexokinase deficiency (Jensen, 2004). Both carbon monoxide and methemoglobin increase oxygen affinity of the unused heme groups and shift the curve to the left (Sharan and Popel, 1989). For most species, PO_2 values increase from birth and reach adult values by several months of age. A slight aging-related decrease in PO_2 occurs in humans and may be present in other animals. There are no sex differences in oxygen pressures.

22.3.4.1 Oxygen Imbalances

22.3.4.1.1 Hyperoxemia

Hyperoxemia is defined as a higher than normal oxygen tension in the blood. It occurs when hyperbaric oxygen is administered. Administration of 100% oxygen under pressure saturates hemoglobin but also causes increased dissolved oxygen in the plasma (hyperoxygenation) due to Henry's law. The increased plasma oxygen content compensates for the vasoconstriction that occurs with hyperoxemia (Bird and Telfer, 1965). Oxygen toxicity causes blindness, chest pain, cough, tinnitus, decreased pulmonary function, muscle twitching, dizziness, vasoconstriction of cerebral vessels, convulsions, coma, and death (Carraway and Piantadosi, 1999).

22.3.4.1.2 Hypoxemia

Hypoxemia is defined as a lower than normal oxygen tension in arterial blood (<60 mmHg, 8 kPa) or a hemoglobin oxygen saturation of less than 90%. It is a pathological condition distinct from hypoxia, which is a decrease in an adequate supply of oxygen. Hypoxemia can be one of the characteristics of hypoxia but it is also possible for hypoxia to occur with a low oxygen content and high arterial PO_2. In chronic hypoxemia, hemoglobin has a reduced oxygen affinity and increased heme–heme interactions, which result in increases in the availability of O_2 to tissues (Waltemath, 1970). If the decrease in PO_2 is sufficiently rapid and falls below 35 mmHg in humans, aerobic metabolism is replaced by anaerobic metabolism, and lactic acid concentration rises (Forsythe and Schmidt, 2000). Hypoxemia causes increased concentrations of inorganic phosphate, urate, and hypoxanthine. There are five primary causes of hypoxemia, and these are shown in Table 22.19.

When alveolar ventilation is low, inadequate amounts of O_2 are delivered to the alveolar respiratory surfaces; this can cause hypoxemia and occurs as a result of a variety conditions (some shown in Table 22.19). A reduction in the partial pressure of inspired oxygen will also result in hypoxemia, and it can occur when breathing at high altitudes with reduced barometric pressure or with an accidental reduction in fractional oxygen content under anesthesia. The peripheral chemoreceptors, aortic, and carotid bodies respond immediately to a fall in PO_2 and stimulate respiration (Berger et al., 1973). Hyperventilation is not marked until the PO_2 falls to approximately 60 mmHg when it can cause hypocapnia. An anatomic shunt from the right side to the left side of the circulation can be intracardiac or intrapulmonary. It occurs when a portion of blood bypasses the lungs and can be caused by congenital abnormalities or disease states. In pneumonia or pulmonary edema, a portion of the cardiac blood enters the pulmonary vasculature without contacting the alveolar air because of fluid in the alveolar spaces. With both conditions blood is prevented from normal access to alveolar air and is improperly oxygenated. Ventilation–perfusion inequality is the most common cause of hypoxia. This is the result of a change in the relationship between alveolar PO_2 and PCO_2 caused by differences in the ratio of alveolar ventilation to perfusion. Rarely hypoxemia can occur because of impaired diffusion across alveolar membranes. Diseases such as interstitial lung disease can result in increased thickness of the gas exchange barrier; coupled with a shortened pulmonary transit time, reduced PO_2 can result.

Primary hemoglobin deficiency (anemia) is not generally considered a cause of hypoxemia because the reduced delivery of O_2 to the tissues is the result of a lack of O_2 binding protein rather than a decrease in the partial pressure of oxygen in blood (Habler and Messmer, 1997).

TABLE 22.19
Causes of Hypoxemia

- Hypoventilation (low alveolar ventilation)—diseases of respiratory muscles, depression of CNS, airway obstruction
- Low inspired oxygen (low PO_2)—decreased barometric pressure, decreased fractional oxygen content
- Right to left shunt—congenital abnormalities, pulmonary edema, pneumonia
- Ventilation–perfusion inequality—lung disease
- Diffusion impairment—interstitial lung disease

22.3.4.2 Factors Influencing Measurement of PO_2 Concentration

Accurate results for PO_2 measurement depend on proper collection and handling techniques. The most common problems include nonarterial sampling, exposure to air, temperature, length of storage, improper sample mixing, and inappropriate use of anticoagulant. Precise PO_2 levels require anaerobic collection of arterial blood samples; especially when the arteriolar PO_2 is high because of the inherent characteristics of hemoglobin–oxygen dissociation. Satisfactory blood gas samples may be obtained with relative ease from most laboratory species. Rats and mice present more of a problem because of their limited blood volume and small size but implantation of arterial catheters has been successfully utilized to intermittently sample and monitor blood gases in conscious and anesthetized animals (Pakulla et al., 2004; Lee et al., 2009). This technique, however, is limited by its cumbersome and invasive nature, requiring surgery, which unless performed sufficiently in advance of sampling, can affect the accuracy of blood gas measurement. Blood gas samples can also be obtained by cardiac puncture but the utility of this method is limited as continuous monitoring is not possible. An alternative, noninvasive technique that has been successfully utilized for blood gas analysis with dogs, mice, rats, rhesus monkeys, guinea pigs, and rabbits is transcutaneous monitoring in which a heated probe (comprised of a Clark-type polarographic electrode) is applied to the skin (Stout et al., 2001; Sahbaie et al., 2006). When sampling, exposure to air should be minimized to prevent equilibration of the sample with air; this can increase PO_2. Likewise, the presence of heparin can cause erroneous PO_2 measurements when oxygen from the air equilibrates with heparin before sample collection (Higgins, 2007). On storage, glycolysis causes an increase in PO_2, as it is liberated from oxyhemoglobin. The opposing effect of O_2 consumption in cellular respiration creates a net loss of PO_2 of approximately 0.4 kPa/hour at 37°C (Travis et al., 1971). As the PO_2 measurement is dependent on temperature, if the blood sample is not measured at body temperature (preferable), a correction factor needs to be applied. The O_2 solubility and equilibrium between oxyhemoglobin and dissolved oxygen are affected by temperature (Yamaguchi et al., 1987; Cambier et al., 2004).

22.4 ACID–BASE BALANCE

Acid–base balance is the balance of the body between acidity and alkalinity. Metabolic processes produce acid that must be excreted or metabolized to prevent a fall in pH. The acids produced by the body can be classified as either respiratory or metabolic (Kellum, 2000). One of the major respiratory acids produced is carbonic acid. Carbon dioxide, while strictly not an acid, is converted to carbonic acid and is often considered a respiratory acid. It is produced by cells in large quantities as an end product of metabolism and excreted from the lungs. All acids other than carbonic acid are metabolic and are not excreted by the lungs; they include lactate, phosphate, and sulfate. They are produced due to nutrient breakdown or as a normal intermediary to metabolism and are all excreted by the kidney. For acid–base balance to be maintained, the amount of acid produced must equal the amount excreted to sustain a physiologically normal pH. Free H^+ must be removed from the ECF and eliminated from the body, and mechanisms must be in place to compensate if the ECF becomes alkaline. Conditions that cause a rise in hydrogen ion concentration in the blood cause a pH decrease (acidosis) and a fall in H^+ causes a rise in pH (alkalemia). To prevent acid–base disturbances, the body responds in three ways: (1) intracellular and extracellular buffering, (2) respiratory control of alveolar ventilation to alter arterial PCO_2, and (3) renal regulation of HCO_3^-/H^+ secretion (Adrogue and Adrogue, 2001). By regulating blood chemistry, these systems are able to maintain electrical neutrality and a constant pH.

22.4.1 Buffer Systems

Buffering is an immediate physiochemical response to changes in body pH. A buffer consists of a weakly dissociated acid and the salt of that acid, and they are able to take up and release H^+ and thereby limit changes in pH. The buffering systems of the body include extracellular buffers, intracellular buffers, and bone. Extracellular buffers are bicarbonate (HCO_3^-/H_2CO_3), phosphate (HPO_4^{2-}/H_2PO^{4-}), and plasma proteins. The intracellular buffers include protein, organic and inorganic phosphates, and hemoglobin. In bone, carbonate forms a large buffer reservoir used particularly during chronic metabolic acidosis (Bushinsky, 2001; Arnett, 2008). Experimental evidence in the dog and cat shows that after 5 hours of acidosis, most of the tissue buffering is performed by bone (Bettice and Gamble, 1975). As bone contains no salts of acids weaker than carbonic acid, it buffers very little of the change in respiratory acidosis. Proteins (mainly intracellular) form the most important buffers in the body, and they possess both basic and acidic groups that can act either as H^+ acceptors or donors as needed. Hemoglobin buffers against changes associated with CO_2 transport. Buffers are most effective when the pH is equal to their p*K*; the phosphate buffer pair has a p*K* of 6.8. As this is near physiological normal, this is a moderately efficient buffer pair. It is mainly intracellular although its presence in the ECF makes it an important urinary buffer. Although H_2CO_3/HCO_3^- plays an integral role in regulating pH, their role is not as a buffer system. The p*K* of this pair is 6.1 and so far from normal physiological pH (7.4) that they are not effective buffers.

In the blood, hemoglobin acts as a primary intracellular buffer in erythrocytes. The exchange of oxygen with hemoglobin is associated with a simultaneous exchange of hemoglobin and hydrogen ion. Hemoglobin combines with oxygen and a hydrogen ion is released, whereas when oxygen is released, hydrogen ion is accepted. The result of this process is an arteriovenous pH difference of approximately 0.01–0.02 units (Siggaard Andersen, 1979). Hemoglobin–hydrogen ion exchange produces bicarbonate; carbonic acid (formed from erythrocytes by the continuous hydration of CO_2) donates a proton to hemoglobin, and the residual bicarbonate diffuses into the plasma. The departing bicarbonate is replaced by chloride from the plasma in a process known as the chloride shift (Hamburger shift) and as a result hemoglobin effectively buffers CO_2 (Crandall et al., 1981).

22.4.2 Respiratory Balance

Steady PCO_2 levels are important for reducing pH changes and are maintained by the excretion or retention of CO_2 by the lungs. Alterations in ventilation rate can rapidly bring about changes in PCO_2. Respiratory control can operate on two levels, preventing changes in PCO_2 and compensating for changes in PCO_2. By preventing changes in PCO_2 when alteration in other acids or bases occurs, a significant pH effect is prevented. Compensation by the respiratory system for changes in pH can be effected by corresponding changes in PCO_2. In this way, increased CO_2 excretion by hyperventilation results can correct respiratory acidosis, compensate for metabolic acidosis, and also produce respiratory alkalosis.

22.4.3 Renal Balance

The renal system controls ECF volume and composition through balance of electrolyte levels, and it assists in maintaining pH at 7.4. This process of control is considerably slower than respiratory control, taking days to effect change (Harrison, 1995). The kidneys excrete excess acids or bases (except carbonic acid) from the ECF to maintain homeostasis and maintain the pH in the normal range. If there is a deficiency of acid or base (other than carbonic acid), the kidneys are unable to restore normality. When high PCO_2 causes a low pH, the kidneys excrete acid, H^+ and Cl^-, NH_4 and Cl^-, or $2Na^+$ with Cl^- and H_2PO_4 to raise the pH to normal. The outcome is renal venous blood with a higher pH than normal and this raises the pH of systemic blood. As the H^+ concentration is lowered, the conversion of carbonic acid to bicarbonate and H^+ is increased.

22.4.4 Anion Gap

The anion gap (AG) represents the difference between the sum of the major anions and cations in the plasma. Under normal circumstances, in humans, routinely measured anions account for all

TABLE 22.20
Laboratory Animal Anion Gap Reference Values

Species	Anion Gap (mmol/L)
Cat[a]	13.0–27.0
Dog[a]	12.0–24.0
Sprague Dawley rat[b]	14.9–24.8
F344 rat[b]	15.2–23.7
ICR mouse[b]	23.3–27.3
Guinea pig[b]	13.7–23.2

[a] Kaae and deMarais (2008).
[b] Clinical chemistry values from Hilltop Lab. Animals, Inc. http://hilltoplabs.com/public/blood.html

except 8–16 mmol/L (mean 12) of the total anions (Emmett and Narins, 1977). Reference values for the AG in common laboratory species are shown in Table 22.20.

Negatively charged proteins make up the majority of the unmeasured anions with approximately 10% being plasma anions; acid anions such as lactate, sulfate, and pyruvate also contribute (Coude et al., 1982). Under most circumstances, the value of unmeasured cations (proteins, magnesium, calcium, and others) is small, and their contribution to a disturbance is usually not significant. AG can be calculated from the following formula:

$$AG = \left[Na^+\right] + \left[K^+\right] - \left[Cl^-\right] - \left[HCO_3^-\right]$$

The AG for most species of domestic animals appears to be similar to that defined for human subjects (10–20 mmol/L). In horses, age-related changes in AG have been reported with foals having a larger AG than horses (Gossett and French, 1983). The major use of AG measurements is in the interpretation of clinical data to enable categorization of acid–base disorders such as situations in which acidosis is not accompanied by decreased pH or an increase in free hydrogen (Kraut and Madias, 2007). This enables metabolic acidosis to be divided by the magnitude of the AG. For example, with inorganic metabolic acidosis (hyperchloremic acidosis) where Cl^- replaces HCO_3^-, the AG remains normal yet, and when lost bicarbonate ions are replaced by an unmeasured acid anion, the AG is increased. It is therefore apparent that while increased AG arises from conditions that cause acidosis, not all causes of acidosis increase the AG. Any decrease in routinely unmeasured cations and/or increase in unmeasured anions cause a raised AG; it can be associated with elevated organic acids (lactic acid, keto acids) in hypovolemia, shock, diabetes and ketosis, or raised nonmetabolizable acids (inorganic acid such as sulfate or phosphate) associated with excesses of compounds such as salicylates (Coude et al., 1982), methanol, or ethylene glycol. Acidoses that are the most common cause for increased AG include ketoacidosis, lactic acidosis, and uremic acidosis; additionally, salicylate, oxalate, or acetate toxicity can raise the AG (Fulop, 1993; Messa et al., 2001). Dehydration and alkalosis are minor causes of increased AG.

Decreased AG arises from increases in the unmeasured cations and/or decreases in the unmeasured anions. The most common cause of decreased AG is hypoalbuminemia. Albumin is the major unmeasured anion, making up almost the entire value of the AG. Hypoalbuminemia (reduced albumin concentration) therefore results in a low AG; a one gram decrease in albumin reduces the AG by 0.25 mmol/L (Figge et al., 1998; Carvounis and Feinfeld, 2000). Moreover, rarer causes include cationic protein (immunoglobulin) increases, which occur in polyclonal gammopathy or multiple myeloma (Qujeq and Mohiti, 2002).

22.4.5 Acid–Base Imbalance

Acid–base disturbances, characterized by changes in hydrogen ion concentration affect the ionization of molecules and reactive groups (Takeda et al., 1987). Proteins and other substances become more or less charged as pH is altered. Changes in acid–base balance can have wide-reaching effects on many organ systems in the body, as enzyme reactions are optimal at narrow pH ranges. Acid–base disturbances are diagnosed from arterial blood measurements because they reflect both respiratory and metabolic disturbances (Kellum, 2000).

22.4.5.1 Classification of Acid–Base Disturbances

Acid–base disturbances are classified in several ways according to the following:

1. The underlying cause. Acid–base disturbances are respiratory when the primary change is an alteration in the partial pressure of CO_2 and metabolic when the primary change is an alteration in bicarbonate concentration. Carbonic acid is produced endogenously, and its blood concentration is regulated by respiration. Metabolic conditions result from alterations in the nonvolatile or fixed acids. Respiratory and metabolic disturbances may be present concurrently as a mixed disturbance.
2. The course of the condition. Acid–base disturbances may be acute, or longer than a few hours in duration, in which case they are termed chronic.
3. The severity and response to the condition. Acid–base disturbances are uncompensated, partially compensated, and compensated. Metabolic disturbances are largely mitigated by respiratory compensation, whereas compensation for a respiratory disturbance is mainly by renal mechanisms.

Each condition should be identified by the primary cause, duration, and degree of compensation. A primary change in PCO_2 is a respiratory disturbance. Mechanisms that react to the altered PCO_2 by changing bicarbonate are secondary or compensatory mechanisms. A primary change in bicarbonate is a metabolic disturbance, and the mechanisms that operate to change the PCO_2 as a result of the bicarbonate change are secondary or compensatory mechanisms. Compensations for changes in blood pH are affected by respiratory and renal systems. Respiratory compensation is rapid, whereas renal compensation may take several days.

22.4.5.1.1 Metabolic Acidosis

Acidosis is an increased acidity in the blood where arterial pH is less than 7.35. Metabolic acidosis arises as a result of conditions that cause a primary decrease in bicarbonate concentration. Bicarbonate concentration can either be reduced by increased endogenous production of acids or reduced through gastrointestinal loss or failure of the kidney to excrete the normal acid load. Metabolic acidoses can be subdivided into high AG and normal AG forms. Common causes of metabolic acidosis are given in Table 22.14 (Kreisberg and Wood, 1983; Wagner, 2007).

Acidosis with a high AG can be caused by ketoacidosis and is associated, most commonly, with diabetes mellitus. Under these conditions, free fatty acids are converted to keto acids, acetoacetic acid, and β-hydroxybutyrate by the liver; as these are all unmeasured anions, they increase the AG. In lactic acidosis, lactate accumulates from both excess lactate formation and decreased usage. An increase in lactate formation occurs with anaerobic metabolism, and decrease in usage usually occurs with liver dysfunction. Renal failure can result in decreased acid excretion and decreased HCO_3^- reabsorption. In these cases, the high AG is caused by an accumulation of sulfates and phosphates.

Metabolic acidosis with a normal AG occurs when HCO_3^- is lost from the GI tract (diarrhea or uterosigmoidostomy) or kidney. In renal tubular acidosis, either tubular reabsorption of bicarbonate or tubular hydrogen ion secretion is defective or both. The inability to excrete H^+ load is also a cause for normal AG acidosis in cases of hypoaldosteronism. Likewise an increased H^+ load with the ingestion of ammonium chloride causes acidosis.

22.4.5.1.2 Compensation

The onset of metabolic acidosis causes a compensatory respiratory response; increased ventilation quickly reduces the PCO_2, which minimizes the fall in pH. This response is minimal in both humans and other animals because as PCO_2 falls, the cerebrospinal fluid pH rises and inhibits ventilatory drive. Maximal respiratory compensation occurs in humans in 24–36 hours. Other buffers, including bicarbonate, oxyhemoglobin, hemoglobin, phosphate, and protein buffers, act in defense of pH when a strong acid is added to the blood. Slower mechanisms of long-term correction for the acidosis require renal retention of bicarbonate and increased excretion of renal acid as the ammonium ion. The increase in ammonia formation takes several days to reach its maximum (Lane and Walker, 1987).

22.4.5.1.3 Respiratory Acidosis

Respiratory acidosis is defined as an increase in PCO_2 and subsequent to this, a proportionate increase in the carbonic acid concentration in blood (Epstein and Singh, 2001). The pH may remain unchanged, that is, acidemia may be absent. Elevated PCO_2 is caused by a greater tissue CO_2 output or (more commonly) as a consequence of inadequate alveolar ventilation; an immediate increase in bicarbonate concentration is produced. Moderate elevations in PCO_2 usually do not alter pH, however, when the PCO_2 is greater than 80 mmHg in humans, acidemia always develops (Adrogue and Madias, 1985). Elevated PCO_2 does not cause a corresponding increase in the metabolic acids in dogs or humans (Brackett et al., 1965). Intracellular acidosis is produced rapidly in this condition because dissolved CO_2 crosses cell membranes readily; in fact, the initial buffering of acid occurs by intracellular buffers. One third of the acute increase in hydrogen ions is buffered by hemoglobin and two thirds by tissue buffers (Bear and Gribik, 1974). The principal extracellular buffer system, carbonic acid/bicarbonate, is not able to respond to respiratory acidosis.

Respiratory acidosis can be caused by any disorder that interferes with effective ventilation and can result from CNS, pulmonary, or iatrogenic changes. Most commonly pulmonary diseases such as pneumonia, obstructive, or restrictive airway diseases are the basis of the condition. Diseases or drugs that impair the CNS respiratory drive and conditions that impair neuromuscular transmission or muscle weakness can also produce a profound respiratory acidosis.

22.4.5.1.4 Compensation

The compensating response for respiratory acidosis is the retention of bicarbonate by the kidney. As this response is slow to develop, it is only significant to conditions of chronic respiratory acidosis. Steady state chronic respiratory acidosis is reached in dogs in 3–5 days, in humans in 2–4 days, and even more rapidly in the rat (Carter et al., 1959). It induces less of a pH change than the acute condition owing to increased renal acid secretion and the generation of bicarbonate by the kidney. The tubular exchange of hydrogen is also stimulated by hypercapnia, and plasma bicarbonate is elevated (Schwartz and Cohen, 1978; Hansen et al., 1979). As the sodium exchanged for hydrogen ions is not reabsorbed with chloride, chloriuresis also occurs (Schwartz and Cohen, 1978). The amount of urinary ammonia excreted may increase 10-fold due to formation from glutamine in both acute and chronic acidoses in humans, rats, and dogs (Pollak et al., 1965; Fine, 1982; Garibotto et al., 2009).

22.4.5.2 Alkalosis

22.4.5.2.1 Metabolic Alkalosis

Metabolic alkalosis is characterized by an increase in bicarbonate ion concentration and pH and/or a decrease in hydrogen ion concentration (Khanna and Kurtzman, 2001; Foy and de Morais, 2008). It results from excessive loss of fixed acids, intracellular shift of H^+, HCO_3^- retention, or alkali administration. Regardless of the mechanism that causes alkalosis, maintenance of the state indicates that HCO_3^- reabsorption is increased in the kidneys. Metabolic alkalosis can be classified as follows:

1. Volume contracted, reduced ECF volume, loss of Na^+ and Cl^--containing fluid without loss of HCO_3^- (Kassirer, 1974).

2. Volume expanded, excreting large amounts of sodium chloride with bicarbonate production predominating over bicarbonate excretion (Adrogue and Madias, 1981).
3. Chloride wasting, caused by impaired chloride resorption and seen with hypercalcemia and severe hypokalemia (Narins et al., 1982).

Volume contraction and chloride wasting are the most important stimuli for increased HCO_3^- reabsorption, and the common causes of metabolic alkalosis are shown in Table 22.21.

The most common cause of metabolic alkalosis is gastrointestinal H^+ loss due to vomiting. Excessive renal acid loss associated with mineralocorticoid excess, diuretic use (particularly loop or thiazide diuretics), or low chloride intake can also contribute to the development of metabolic alkalosis. Most of these conditions are associated with Na^+ and Cl^- depletion and so also the result in volume contraction. Mineralocorticoid excess (Cushing's or Addison's disease) induced alkalosis is brought about by steroidal action on the distal tubule. Excess steroid enhances cation exchange, and hence both sodium and bicarbonate are retained, and hydrogen ions and potassium lost. Water retention and an expanded plasma volume result from the excess retained sodium. The expanded plasma volume, in turn, increases the GFR. This results in the filtration of more sodium chloride and so the loop continues at the expense of homeostasis. Potassium depletion (hypokalemia) can cause hydrogen loss through intracellular movement of ions from the ECF. Administration of excess bicarbonate is usually well tolerated by animals, however, coupled with volume contraction or potassium/chloride depletion, renal excretion of the excess base is impaired and alkalosis occurs.

Maintenance of metabolic alkalosis is characterized by the continued deficiency of renal bicarbonate excretion, which can be the result of decreased glomerular filtration or (more commonly) increased bicarbonate reabsorption. It is associated with potassium depletion and/or chloride depletion that are the renal response to volume contraction. Sodium reabsorption is increased to correct the low circulating volume, which leads to reabsorption of an anion (proximal tubule) and excretion of a cation (distal tubule) for preserving electrical neutrality. The anion is usually chloride; the cations are either H^+ or K^+. In the rat, uncomplicated potassium and chloride depletion produce metabolic alkalosis; however, in dogs and humans, these methods alone do not produce alkalosis (Aquino and Luke, 1973).

Urine pH is usually low with metabolic alkalosis. Once considered to be due to potassium depletion, this paradoxical aciduria is considered to be due to the pairing of bases such as sulfate with cations, Na^+, K^+, or H^+ before renal excretion. As neither sodium nor potassium is available, hydrogen ions perform this function and are excreted in the urine.

22.4.5.2.2 Compensation The respiratory center response to metabolic alkalosis is hypoventilation, increasing PCO_2. The degree of this compensatory response is proportional to the degree of arterial hydrogen ion depression (Aquino and Luke, 1973). Additionally, bicarbonate excretion by the kidney is enhanced within the first hour of the disturbance.

TABLE 22.21
Causes of Metabolic Alkalosis

Bicarbonate Excess	Cl^- Responsive	Cl^- Resistant
• Excess alkali administration—bicarbonate containing IV fluids	• Loss of gastric secretions—vomiting	• Hyperaldosteronism, excess mineralocorticoids
• Massive blood transfusion	• Loss of colon secretions—villous adenoma	• Diuretic use—thiazide and loop
• Intravenous penicillin	• Diuretic use—thiazide and loop	• Potassium depletion
–	• Posthypercapnia	• Hypomagnesemia
–	• Cystic fibrosis	–

TABLE 22.22
Causes of Respiratory Alkalosis

- Hypoxemia related—severe anemia, right to left shunts, high altitudes
- CNS related—pain, fear, anxiety, tumor, trauma
- Endocrine related—hyperthyroidism, pregnancy
- Pulmonary related—pneumonia, edema, asthma, emphysema
- Drug related—nicotine, salicylates, progesterone, catecholamines
- Congestive heart failure
- Hepatic failure
- Mechanical ventilation
- Heat exhaustion, panting

22.4.5.2.3 Respiratory Alkalosis Respiratory alkalosis is a reduction in PCO_2 in the blood and an increase in pH (Foster et al., 2001; Jensen, 2004); it develops when the lungs remove more carbon dioxide than is produced metabolically by the tissues. There is no renal loss of bicarbonate with this condition. The hyperventilation that produces respiratory alkalosis can be stimulated by a wide variety of conditions; these are described in Table 22.22.

22.4.5.2.4 Compensation The initial response to acute respiratory alkalosis is a decline in extracellular bicarbonate concentration as a result of cellular buffering (not renal loss). Bicarbonate is reduced by the release of hydrogen ions from hemoglobin and tissue buffers and by a small increase in lactic acid. Hemoglobin accounts for approximately one third of this effect; the remainder is tissue buffers. There is no loss of bicarbonate in acute respiratory alkalosis. Chronic respiratory alkalosis takes several days to develop and occurs when pH has been returned to normal while PCO_2 remains lowered. Renal reabsorption of bicarbonate is reduced, decreasing ECF bicarbonate concentrations in parallel with the fall in CO_2 (Bettice et al., 1984; Adrogue and Madias, 1985). To maintain electrical neutrality chloride retention partially compensates for HCO_3^- loss.

Paradoxical respiratory alkalosis accompanies rapid recovery from metabolic acidosis. It develops because the bicarbonate concentration is slow to equalize across the blood–brain barrier. The respiratory center remains stimulated by the acidic cerebrospinal fluid even though the plasma hydrogen ion concentration has normalized.

22.4.6 Mixed Acid–Base Disorders

Mixed acid–base disorders occur when several primary acid–base imbalances are present simultaneously (Adrogue, 2006). Some examples of this condition are high AG and normal AG acidosis, chronic respiratory acidosis and metabolic alkalosis, or normal AG acidosis and metabolic alkalosis. As a general rule, when a normal pH is seen with abnormal bicarbonate or CO_2, a mixed disorder is expected. When the pH moves in the opposite direction to that predicted for the primary disturbance, a mixed disturbance exists.

To interpret an acid–base disturbance correctly, the following information is required: (1) the environment, (2) state of hydration, (3) body temperature, (4) respiratory rate and character, (5) evidence of diarrhea, vomiting, and excoriation, (6) physical appearance, and (7) duration of the condition. The normal expected compensatory adjustments are calculated in order to categorize a set of acid–base values. Clinical input is needed to explain why compensation may not be as expected. For example, pain and decreased compliance hinder respiratory compensation, and urine retention limits renal compensation.

In summary, the complex interplay of electrolytes, hydrogen ions, carbon dioxide, and oxygen provides a framework in which optimal cell function is ensured. Homeostatic regulation of these parameters allows cells to function effectively in a broad range of conditions; however, when these are not maintained. there are serious clinical consequences. A change in the clinical chemistry profile of an animal therefore provides valuable information on the functional status of different organ systems. When multiple endpoints are assayed, disease- and treatment-related effects become evident; interpretation of results with respect to the normal reference range of values, however, should occur with the knowledge that variation in analytical technique can have profound effect on outcome.

Addendum: Gene Symbols and Descriptions

Gene Symbol Used in Chapter	HUGO Gene Nomenclature	Gene Name
AE1	SLC4A1	Solute carrier family 4, anion exchanger
AQP2	AQP2	Aquaporin 2
AQP3	AQP3	Aquaporin 3
AQP4	AQP4	Aquaporin 4
CALB1	CALB1	Calbindin 1, 28 kDa
CALB3	S100G	S100 calcium binding protein G
CaSR	CaSR	Calcium-sensing receptor
CHIF	FXYD4	FXYD domain containing ion transport regulator 4
CLCNKB	CLCNKB	Chloride channel, voltage-sensitive Kb
CFTR	CFTR	Cystic fibrosis transmembrane conductance regulator (ATP-binding cassette subfamily, C, member 7)
CYP24	CYP24A1	Cytochrome P450, family 24, subfamily A, polypeptide 1
ENaC	SCNN1	Sodium channel, nonvoltage gated 1
FGF23	FGF23	Fibroblast growth factor 23
GALNT3	GALNT3	UDP-N-acetyl-alpha-D-galactosamine: polypeptide N-acetylgalactosaminyltransferase 3
GLUT2	SLC2A2	Solute carrier family 2 (facilitated glucose transporter), member 2
KCNA1	KCNA1	Potassium voltage-gated channel, shaker-related subfamily, member 1
KCNK1	KCNK1	Potassium channel, subfamily K, member 1
KCNQ2	KCNQ2	Potassium voltage-gated channel, KQT-like subfamily, member 2
KCNQ3	KCNQ3	Potassium voltage-gated channel, KQT-like subfamily, member 3
KCNQ4	KCNQ4	Potassium voltage-gated channel, KQT-like subfamily, member 4
KLOTHO	KL	Klotho
NaS1	SLC13A1	Solute carrier family 13 (sodium/sulfate symporters), member 1
NCCT	SLC12A3	Solute carrier family 12 (sodium/chloride transporters), member 3
NCX1	SLC8A1	Solute carrier family 8 (sodium/calcium exchanger) member 1
NHE3	SLC9A3	Solute carrier family 9 (sodium/hydrogen exchanger), member 3
NKCC	SLC12A	Solute carrier family 12 (sodium/potassium/chloride transporters)
NKCC2	SLC12A2	Solute carrier family 12 (sodium/potassium/chloride transporters), member 1
OSR1	OSR1	Odd-skipped related 1
RAS	RAS	Rat sarcoma viral oncogene homolog
ROMK	KCNJ1	Potassium inwardly rectifying channel, subfamily J, member 1
SAT1	SAT1	Spermidine/spermine N1-acetyltransferase 1
SCN1A	SCN1A	Sodium channel, voltage-gated, type 1, alpha subunit
SCN1B	SCN1B	Sodium channel, voltage-gated, type 1, beta subunit
SGLT1	SLC5A1	Solute carrier family 5 (sodium/glucose cotransporter), member 1
SGLT2	SLC5A2	Solute carrier family 5 (sodium/glucose cotransporter), member 2
SGK1	SGK1	Serum/glucocorticoid-regulated kinase 1
SLC4A4	SLC4A4	Solute carrier family 4, sodium bicarbonate cotransporter, member 4
SPAK	STK39	Serine threonine kinase 39
TRPV5	TRPV5	Transient receptor potential cation channel, subfamily V, member 5
VDR	VDR	Vitamin D (1,25-dihydroxyvitamin D3) receptor
WNK	WNK	WNK lysine-deficient protein kinase

REFERENCES

Abramson, J. and Wright, E.M. 2009. Structure and function of Na(+)-symporters with inverted repeats. *Curr Opin Struct Biol.* 19:425–432.

Adrogue, H.J. 2006. Mixed acid–base disturbances. *J Nephrol.* 19:S97–S103.

Adrogue, H.E. and Adrogue, H.J. 2001. Acid–base physiology. *Respir Care.* 46:328–341.

Adrogue, H.J. and Madias, N.E. 1981. Changes in plasma potassium concentration during acute acid–base disturbances. *Am J Med.* 71:456–467.

Adrogue, H.J. and Madias, N.E. 1985. Influence of chronic respiratory acid–base disorders on acute CO_2 titration curve. *J Appl Physiol.* 58:1231–1238.

Adrogue, H.J. and Madias, N.E. 2000. Hypernatremia. *N Engl J Med.* 342:1493–1499.

Agrawal, V., Agarwal, M., Joshi, S.R., and Ghosh, A.K. 2008. Hyponatremia and hypernatremia: Disorders of water balance. *J Assoc Physicians India.* 56:956–964.

Al-Ghamdi, S.M., Cameron, E.C., and Sutton, R.A. 1994. Magnesium deficiency: Pathophysiologic and clinical overview. *Am J Kidney Dis.* 24:737–752.

Ali, F., Raufi, M.A., Washington, B., and Ghali, J.K. 2007. Conivaptan: A dual vasopressin receptor v1a/v2 antagonist [corrected]. *Cardiovasc Drug Rev.* 25:261–279.

Allon, M. and Copkney, C. 1990. Albuterol and insulin for treatment of hyperkalemia in hemodialysis patients. *Kidney Int.* 38:869–872.

Alper, S.L., Darman, R.B., Chernova, M.N., and Dahl, N.K. 2002. The AE gene family of Cl/HCO_3^- exchangers. *J Nephrol.* 15(Suppl 5):S41–S53.

Andress, D.L. 2008. Adynamic bone in patients with chronic kidney disease. *Kidney Int.* 73:1345–1354.

Aquino, H.C. and Luke, R.G. 1973. Respiratory compensation to potassium-depletion and chloride-depletion alkalosis. *Am J Physiol.* 225:1444–1448.

Arnett, T.R. 2008. Extracellular pH regulates bone cell function. *J Nutr.* 138:415S–418S.

Arroyo, J.P., Ronzaud, C., Lagnaz, D., Staub, O., and Gamba, G. 2011. Aldosterone paradox: Differential regulation of ion transport in distal nephron. *Physiology (Bethesda).* 26:115–123.

Ayus, J.C., Armstrong, D., and Arieff, A.I. 2006. Hyponatremia with hypoxia: Effects on brain adaptation, perfusion, and histology in rodents. *Kidney Int.* 69:1319–1325.

Bagga, A., Bajpai, A., and Menon, S. 2005. Approach to renal tubular disorders. *Indian J Pediatr.* 72:771–776.

Bakhtian, S., Kimura, R.E., and Galinsky, R.E. 1993. Age-related changes in homeostasis of inorganic sulfate in male F-344 rats. *Mech Ageing Dev.* 66:257–267.

Bakris, G.L., Fonseca, V.A., Sharma, K., and Wright, E.M. 2009. Renal sodium–glucose transport: Role in diabetes mellitus and potential clinical implications. *Kidney Int.* 75:1272–1277.

Barbour, G.L., Coburn, J.W., Slatopolsky, E., Norman, A.W., and Horst, R.L. 1981. Hypercalcemia in an anephric patient with sarcoidosis: Evidence for extrarenal generation of 1,25-dihydroxyvitamin D. *N Engl J Med.* 305:440–443.

Bar-Ilan, A. and Marder, J. 1980. Acid base status in unanesthetized, unrestrained guinea pigs. *Pflugers Arch.* 384:93–97.

Barrett, C.P., Donati, E.J., Volz, J.E., and Smith, E.B. 1975. Variations in serum calcium between strains of inbred mice. *Lab Anim Sci.* 25:638–640.

Basic, D.T., Hadzi-Djokic, J., and Ignjatovic, I. 2007. The history of urinary diversion. *Acta Chir Iugosl.* 54:9–17.

Bates, J.A. 2008. Phosphorus: A quick reference. *Vet Clin North Am Small Anim Pract.* 38:471–475, viii.

Batlle, D. and Kurtzman, N.A. 1982. Distal renal tubular acidosis: Pathogenesis and classification. *Am J Kidney Dis.* 1:328–344.

Bauer, C. and Rathschlag-Schaefer, A.M. 1968. The influence of aldosterone and cortisol on oxygen affinity and cation concentration of the blood. *Respir Physiol.* 5:360–370.

Bear, R.A. and Gribik, M. 1974. Assessing acid–base imbalances through laboratory parameters. *Hosp Pract.* 9:157.

Beck, L. and Silve, C. 2001. Molecular aspects of renal tubular handling and regulation of inorganic sulfate. *Kidney Int.* 59:835–845.

Beetham, R. 1982. A review of blood pH and blood–gas analysis. *Ann Clin Biochem.* 19(Pt 4):198–213.

Berger, A.J., Krasney, J.A., and Dutton, R.E. 1973. Respiratory recovery from CO_2 breathing in intact and chemodenervated awake dogs. *J Appl Physiol.* 35:35–41.

Bergstrom, J. 1981. Determination of electrolytes—Methodological problems. *Acta Med Scand Suppl.* 647:39–46.

Bergwitz, C. and Juppner, H. 2010. Regulation of phosphate homeostasis by PTH, vitamin D, and FGF23. *Annu Rev Med.* 61:91–104.

Bettice, J.A. and Gamble, J.L., Jr. 1975. Skeletal buffering of acute metabolic acidosis. *Am J Physiol.* 229:1618–1624.

Bettice, J.A., Owens, D., and Riley, S. 1984. The effects of hypocapnia on intracellular pH and bicarbonate. *Respir Physiol.* 55:121–130.

Bhargava, A., Wang, J., and Pearce, D. 2004. Regulation of epithelial ion transport by aldosterone through changes in gene expression. *Mol Cell Endocrinol.* 217:189–196.

Bie, P., Wamberg, S., and Kjolby, M. 2004. Volume natriuresis vs. pressure natriuresis. *Acta Physiol Scand.* 181:495–503.

Bird, A.D. and Telfer, A.B. 1965. Effect of hyperbaric oxygen on limb circulation. *Lancet.* 285:355–356.

Bonilla-Felix, M. 1996. Primary distal renal tubular acidosis as a result of a gradient defect. *Am J Kidney Dis.* 27:428–430.

Borok, Z., Schneider, S.M., Fraley, D.S., and Adler, S. 1987. A rat model for hyperkalemia. *Proc Soc Exp Biol Med.* 185:39–40.

Boron, W.F. 2006. Acid–base transport by the renal proximal tubule. *J Am Soc Nephrol.* 17:2368–2382.

Boulanger, B.R., Lilly, M.P., Hamlyn, J.M., Laredo, J., Shurtleff, D., and Gann, D.S. 1993. Ouabain is secreted by the adrenal gland in awake dogs. *Am J Physiol.* 264:E413–E419.

Brackett, N.C., Jr., Cohen, J.J., and Schwartz, W.B. 1965. Carbon dioxide titration curve of normal man. Effect of increasing degrees of acute hypercapnia on acid–base equilibrium. *N Engl J Med.* 272:6–12.

Brady, C.A., Vite, C.H., and Drobatz, K.J. 1999. Severe neurologic sequelae in a dog after treatment of hypoadrenal crisis. *J Am Vet Med Assoc.* 215:222–225, 210.

Brahams, D. 1994. Deaths in US fialuridine trial. *Lancet.* 343:1494–1495.

Brasier, A.R. and Nussbaum, S.R. 1988. Hungry bone syndrome: Clinical and biochemical predictors of its occurrence after parathyroid surgery. *Am J Med.* 84:654–660.

Brito, M.V., Cunha, I.C., Aragon, M.G., Braga, T.G., and Lima, F.D. 2008. Effects of blood storage on ice in biochemical and arterial blood gas analysis of rats. *Acta Cir Bras.* 23:462–468.

Brun-Pascaud, M., Gaudebout, C., Blayo, M.C., and Pocidalo, J.J. 1982. Arterial blood gases and acid base status in awake rats. *Resp Physiol.* 48:45–57.

Burch, W.M. and Posillico, J.T. 1983. Hypoparathyroidism after I-131 therapy with subsequent return of parathyroid function. *J Clin Endocrinol Metab.* 57:398–401.

Burnett, R.W., Christiansen, T.F., Covington, A.K., et al. 2000. IFCC recommended reference method for the determination of the substance concentration of ionized calcium in undiluted serum, plasma or whole blood. *Clin Chem Lab Med.* 38:1301–1314.

Bushinsky, D.A. 2001. Acid–base imbalance and the skeleton. *Eur J Nutr.* 40:238–244.

Buss, S.L. and Bourdeau, J.E. 1984. Calcium balance in laboratory rabbits. *Miner Electrolyte Metab.* 10:127–132.

Cambier, C., Wierinckx, M., Clerbaux, T., et al. 2004. Haemoglobin oxygen affinity and regulating factors of the blood oxygen transport in canine and feline blood. *Res Vet Sci.* 77:83–88.

Camerino, D.C., Tricarico, D., and Desaphy, J.F. 2007. Ion channel pharmacology. *Neurotherapeutics.* 4:184–198.

Capasso, G., Unwin, R., Rizzo, M., Pica, A., and Giebisch, G. 2002. Bicarbonate transport along the loop of Henle: Molecular mechanisms and regulation. *J Nephrol.* 15(Suppl 5):S88–S96.

Carlson, G.P. 1989. Fluid, electrolyte, and acid–base balance. In *Clinical Biochemistry of Domestic Animals.* Ed. J.J. Kaneko, 4th edition, pp. 543–575. New York, NY: Academic Press.

Carney, S.L. 1997. Calcitonin and human renal calcium and electrolyte transport. *Miner Electrolyte Metab.* 23:43–47.

Carraway, M.S. and Piantadosi, C.A. 1999. Oxygen toxicity. *Respir Care Clin N Am.* 5:265–295.

Carter, N.W., Seldin, D.W., and Teng, H.C. 1959. Tissue and renal response to chronic respiratory acidosis. *J Clin Invest.* 38:949–960.

Carvounis, C.P. and Feinfeld, D.A. 2000. A simple estimate of the effect of the serum albumin level on the anion gap. *Am J Nephrol.* 20:369–372.

Casey, J.R. 2006. Why bicarbonate? *Biochem Cell Biol.* 84:930–939.

Charney, A.N. and Feldman, G.M. 1984. Systemic acid–base disorders and intestinal electrolyte transport. *Am J Physiol.* 247:G1–G12.

Charles River. 2006. Clinical Chemistry Parameters for Crl:CD(SD) Rats. Available at: http://www.criver.com/EN-US/PRODSERV/BYTYPE/RESMODOVER/BASELINECOLONY/Pages/baselinecolonydatabystrain.aspx.

Charles River. 2008a. Baseline Colony Data for Charles River Hartley Guinea Pigs. Available at: http://www.criver.com/EN-US/PRODSERV/BYTYPE/RESMODOVER/BASELINECOLONY/Pages/baselinecolonydatabystrain.aspx.

Charles River. 2008b. Clinical Chemistry Parameters for Crl:WI(Han) Rats. Available at: http://www.criver.com/EN-US/PRODSERV/BYTYPE/RESMODOVER/BASELINECOLONY/Pages/baselinecolonydatabystrain.aspx.

Cheema, C., Grant, B.F., and Marcus, R. 1989. Effects of estrogen on circulating "free" and total 1,25-dihydroxyvitamin D and on the parathyroid-vitamin D axis in postmenopausal women. *J Clin Invest.* 83:537–542.

Chen, Y., Qin, S., Ding, Y., et al. 2009. Reference values of clinical chemistry and hematology parameters in rhesus monkeys (*Mucaca mulatta*). *Xenotransplantation.* 16:496–501.

Choi, M.R., Citarella, M.R., Lee, B.M., Lucano F., and Fernández, B.E. 2011. Urodilatin increases renal dopamine uptake: Intracellular network involved. *J Physiol Biochem.* 67:243–247.

Chumlea, W.C., Guo, S.S., Zeller, C.M., Reo, N.V., and Siervogel, R.M. 1999. Total body water data for white adults 18 to 64 years of age: The Fels Longitudinal Study. *Kidney Int.* 56:244–252.

Clase, C.M., Norman, G.L., Beecroft, M.L., and Churchill, D.N. 2000. Albumin-corrected calcium and ionized calcium in stable haemodialysis patients. *Nephrol Dial Transplant.* 15:1841–1846.

Clausen, T. 2002. Acute stimulation of Na/K pump by cardiac glycosides in the nanomolar range. *J Gen Physiol.* 119:295–296.

Coetzee, M. and Kruger, M.C. 2004. Osteoprotegerin-receptor activator of nuclear factor-kappaB ligand ratio: A new approach to osteoporosis treatment? *South Med J.* 97:506–511.

Cogan, M.G. 1984. Effects of acute alterations in PCO_2 on proximal HCO_3^-, Cl^-, and H_2O reabsorption. *Am J Physiol.* 246:F21–F26.

Cohen, J.J. 1979. Disorders of potassium balance. *Hosp Pract.* 14:119–128.

Cole, D.E. and Evrovski, J. 1997. Quantitation of sulfate and thiosulfate in clinical samples by ion chromatography. *J Chromatogr A.* 789:221–232.

Cole, D.E. and Evrovski, J. 2000. The clinical chemistry of inorganic sulfate. *Crit Rev Clin Lab Sci.* 37:299–344.

Cole, D.E. and Scriver, C.R. 1980. Age-dependent serum sulfate levels in children and adolescents. *Clin Chim Acta.* 107:135–139.

Cope, G., Murthy, M., Golbang, A.P., et al. 2006. WNK1 affects surface expression of the ROMK potassium channel independent of WNK4. *J Am Soc Nephrol.* 17:1867–1874.

Cordat, E. and Casey, J.R. 2009. Bicarbonate transport in cell physiology and disease. *Biochem J.* 417:423–439.

Coude, F.X., Ogier, H., Grimber, G., et al. 1982. Correlation between blood ammonia concentration and organic acid accumulation in isovaleric and propionic acidemia. *Pediatrics.* 69:115–117.

Crandall, E.D., Mathew, S.J., Fleischer, R.S., Winter, H.I., and Bidani, A. 1981. Effects of inhibition of RBC HCO_3^-/Cl^- exchange on CO_2 excretion and downstream pH disequilibrium in isolated rat lungs. *J Clin Invest.* 68:853–862.

Criver. 2008–2011. Baseline Colony Data for Charles River CD-1 Mice. Available at: http://www.criver.com/EN-US/PRODSERV/BYTYPE/RESMODOVER/BASELINECOLONY/Pages/baselinecolonydatabystrain.aspx.

Darmon, M., Timsit, J.F., Francais, A., et al. 2010. Association between hypernatraemia acquired in the ICU and mortality: A cohort study. *Nephrol Dial Transplant.* 25(8):2510–2515

Dash, R.K. and Bassingthwaighte, J.B. 2006. Simultaneous blood-tissue exchange of oxygen, carbon dioxide, bicarbonate, and hydrogen ion. *Ann Biomed Eng.* 34:1129–1148.

Datta, B.N. and Stone, M.D. 2009. Hyperventilation and hypophosphataemia. *Ann Clin Biochem.* 46:170–171.

Dawson, P.A., Beck, L., and Markovich, D. 2003. Hyposulfatemia, growth retardation, reduced fertility, and seizures in mice lacking a functional NaS_i-1 gene. *Proc Natl Acad Sci U S A.* 100:13704–13709.

de Morais, H.A. and DiBartola, S.P. 2008. Hypernatremia: A quick reference. *Vet Clin North Am Small Anim Pract.* 38:485–489, ix.

de Seigneux, S., Kim, S.W., Hemmingsen, S.C., Frøkiaer, J., and Nielsen, S. 2006. Increased expression but not targeting of ENaC in adrenalectomized rats with PAN-induced nephrotic syndrome. *Am J Physiol Renal Physiol.* 291:F208–F217.

de Wardener, H.E. 1978. The control of sodium excretion. *Am J Physiol.* 235:F163–F173.

Delisle, B.P., Anson, B.D., Rajamani, S., and January, C.T. 2004. Biology of cardiac arrhythmias: Ion channel protein trafficking. *Circ Res.* 94:1418–1428.

Deschênes, G., Feraille, E., and Doucet, A. 2003. Mechanisms of oedema in nephrotic syndrome: Old theories and new ideas. *Nephrol Dial Transplant.* 18:454–456.

di Bella, G., Scandariato, G., Suriano, O., and Rizzo, A. 1996. Oxygen affinity and Bohr effect responses to 2,3-diphosphoglycerate in equine and human blood. *Res Vet Sci.* 60:272–275.

Dillingham, M.A. and Anderson, R.J. 1986. Inhibition of vasopressin action by atrial natriuretic factor. *Science.* 231:1572–1573.

Dimeski, G., Mollee, P., and Carter, A. 2006. Effects of hyperlipidemia on plasma sodium, potassium, and chloride measurements by an indirect ion-selective electrode measuring system. *Clin Chem.* 52:155–156.

Doyle, D.A., Morais Cabral, J., Pfuetzner, R.A., et al. 1998. The structure of the potassium channel: Molecular basis of K^+ conduction and selectivity. *Science.* 280:69–77.

Durward, A., Skellett, S., Mayer, A., Taylor, D., Tibby, S.M., and Murdoch, I.A. 2001. The value of the chloride: Sodium ratio in differentiating the aetiology of metabolic acidosis. *Intensive Care Med.* 27:828–835.

Elisaf, M., Milionis, H., and Siamopoulos, K.C. 1997. Hypomagnesemic hypokalemia and hypocalcemia: Clinical and laboratory characteristics. *Miner Electrolyte Metab.* 23:105–112.

Emmett, M. and Narins, R.G. 1997. Clinical use of the anion gap. *Medicine (Baltimore)* 56:38–54.

Epstein, S.K. and Singh, N. 2001. Respiratory acidosis. *Respir Care.* 46:366–383.

Falany, C.N. 1997. Enzymology of human cytosolic sulfotransferases. *FASEB J.* 11:206–216.

Fardella, C.E. and Mosso, L. 2002. Primary aldosteronism. *Clin Lab.* 48:181–190.

Farmakis, D., Filippatos, G., Parissis, J., Kremastinos, D.T., and Gheorghiade, M. 2009. Hyponatremia in heart failure. *Heart Fail Rev.* 14:59–63.

Faroqui, S., Levi, M., Soleimani, M., and Amlal, H. 2008. Estrogen downregulates the proximal tubule type IIa sodium phosphate cotransporter causing phosphate wasting and hypophosphatemia. *Kidney Int.* 73:1141–1150.

Feraille, E. and Doucet, A. 2001. Sodium–potassium–adenosinetriphosphatase-dependent sodium transport in the kidney: Hormonal control. *Physiol Rev.* 81:345–418.

Ferguson, D.C. and Hoenig, M. 2003. Endocrine system. In *Duncan and Prasse's Veterinary Laboratory Medicine: Clinical Pathology*. Eds. K.S. Latimer, E.A. Mahaffey, and K.W. Prasse, 4th edition, pp. 231–259. Iowa, IA: Blackwell Publishing.

Field, M.J., Stanton, B.A., and Giebisch, G.H. 1984. Differential acute effects of aldosterone, dexamethasone, and hyperkalemia on distal tubular potassium secretion in the rat kidney. *J Clin Invest.* 74:1792–1802.

Figge, J., Jabor, A., Kazda, A., and Fencl, V. 1998. Anion gap and hypoalbuminemia. *Crit Care Med.* 26:1807–1810.

Finch, C.E. and Foster, J.R. 1973. Hematologic and serum electrolyte values of the C57BL-6J male mouse in maturity and senescence. *Lab Anim Sci.* 23:339–349.

Fine, A. 1982. Effects of acute metabolic acidosis on renal, gut, liver, and muscle metabolism of glutamine and ammonia in the dog. *Kidney Int.* 21:439–444.

Fleet, J.C. and Schoch, R.D. 2010. Molecular mechanisms for regulation of intestinal calcium absorption by vitamin D and other factors. *Crit Rev Clin Lab Sci.* 47:181–195.

Florin, T., Neale, G., Gibson, G.R., Christl, S.U., and Cummings, J.H. 1991. Metabolism of dietary sulphate: Absorption and excretion in humans. *Gut.* 32:766–773.

Forssmann, W.G., Meyer, M., and Forssmann, K. 2001. The renal urodilatin system: Clinical implications. *Cardiovasc Res.* 51:450–462.

Forssmann, W.G., Richter, R., and Meyer, M. 1998. The endocrine heart and natriuretic peptides: Histochemistry, cell biology, and functional aspects of the renal urodilatin system. *Histochem Cell Biol.* 110:335–357.

Forsythe, S.M. and Schmidt, G.A. 2000. Sodium bicarbonate for the treatment of lactic acidosis. *Chest.* 117:260–267.

Foster, G.T., Vaziri, N.D., and Sassoon, C.S. 2001. Respiratory alkalosis. *Respir Care.* 46:384–391.

Foy, D. and de Morais, H.A. 2008. Metabolic alkalosis: A quick reference. *Vet Clin North Am Small Anim Pract.* 38:435–438, vii.

Fried, L.F. and Palevsky, P.M. 1997. Hyponatremia and hypernatremia. *Med Clin North Am.* 81:585–609.

Friedemann, T.E. 1926. The starvation ketosis of a monkey. *Exp Biol Med.* 24:223–226.

Frith, C.H., Suber, R.L., and Umholtz, R. 1980. Hematologic and clinical chemistry findings in control BALB/c and C57BL/6 mice. *Lab Anim Sci.* 30:835–840.

Fuller, P.J. and Young, M.J. 2005. Mechanisms of mineralocorticoid action. *Hypertension.* 46:1227–1235.

Fulop, M. 1993. Alcoholic ketoacidosis. *Endocrinol Metab Clin North Am.* 22:209–219.

Gadsby, D.C. and Nairn, A.C. 1999. Control of CFTR channel gating by phosphorylation and nucleotide hydrolysis. *Physiol Rev.* 79:S77–S107.

Galla, J.H. 2000. Metabolic alkalosis. *J Am Soc Nephrol.* 11:369–375.

Gao, J., Wymore, R.S., Wang, Y., et al. 2002. Isoform-specific stimulation of cardiac Na/K pumps by nanomolar concentrations of glycosides. *J Gen Physiol.* 119:297–312.

Gardiner, T.W., Verbalis, J.G., and Stricker, E.M. 1985. Impaired secretion of vasopressin and oxytocin in rats after lesions of nucleus medianus. *Am J Physiol.* 249:R681–R688.

Garibotto, G., Verzola, D., Sofia, A., et al. 2009. Mechanisms of renal ammonia production and protein turnover. *Metab Brain Dis.* 24:159–167.

Gault, M.H., Dixon, M.E., Doyle, M., and Cohen, W.M. 1968. Hypernatremia, azotemia, and dehydration ue to high-protein tube feeding. *Ann Intern Med.* 68:778–791.

Giebisch, G., Krapf, R., and Wagner, C. 2007. Renal and extrarenal regulation of potassium. *Kidney Int.* 72:397–410.

Gill, M.A., DuBe, J.E., and Young, W.W. 1977. Hypokalemic, metabolic alkalosis induced by high-dose ampicillin sodium. *Am J Hosp Pharm.* 34:528–531.

Girndt, J., Henning, H.V., and Delling, G. 1979. Correlation of calcium and acid–base metabolism. *Horm Metab Res.* 11:587–588.

Glynn, I.M. 1993. Annual review prize lecture. All hands to the sodium pump. *J Physiol.* 462:1–30.

Godwin, I.R. and Williams, V.J. 1984. Renal control of plasma urea level in sheep: The diuretic effect of urea, potassium and sodium chloride. *Q J Exp Physiol.* 69:49–59.

Goodman, W.G. 2005. Calcium and phosphorus metabolism in patients who have chronic kidney disease. *Med Clin North Am.* 89:631–647.

Gossett, K.A. and French, D.D. 1983. Effect of age on anion gap in clinically normal Quarter Horses. *Am J Vet Res.* 44:1744–1745.

Greenberg, A. 2000. Diuretic complications. *Am J Med Sci.* 319:10–24.

Greenlee, M., Wingo, C.S., McDonough, A.A., Youn, J.H., and Kone, B.C. 2009. Narrative review: Evolving concepts in potassium homeostasis and hypokalemia. *Ann Intern Med.* 150:619–625.

Gullestad, L., Dolva, L.O., Waage, A., Falch, D., Fagerthun, H., and Kjekshus, J. 1992. Magnesium deficiency diagnosed by an intravenous loading test. *Scand J Clin Lab Invest.* 52:245–253.

Gumz, M.L., Lynch, I.J., Greenlee, M.M., Cain, B.D., and Wingo, C.S. 2010. The renal H^+-K^+-ATPases: Physiology, regulation, and structure. *Am J Physiol Renal Physiol.* 298:F12–F21.

Guyader, D., Poinsignon, Y., Cano, Y., and Saout, L. 2002. Fatal lactic acidosis in a HIV-positive patient treated with interferon and ribavirin for chronic hepatitis C. *J Hepatol.* 37:289–291.

Haass, M., Kopin, I.J., Goldstein, D.S., and Zukowska-Grojec, Z. 1985. Differential inhibition of alpha adrenoceptor-mediated pressor responses by rat atrial natriuretic peptide in the pithed rat. *J Pharmacol Exp Ther.* 235:122–127.

Habler, O.P. and Messmer, K.F. 1997. The physiology of oxygen transport. *Transfus Sci.* 18:425–435.

Haidas, S., Labie, D., and Kaplan, J.C. 1971. 2,3-diphosphoglycerate content and oxygen affinity as a function of red cell age in normal individuals. *Blood.* 38:463–467.

Hall, J.E. 2003. The kidney, hypertension, and obesity. *Hypertension.* 41:625–633.

Halperin, M.L. and Kamel, K.S. 1998. Potassium. *Lancet.* 352:135–140.

Hamilton, R.D., Crockett, R.J., and Alpers, J.H. 1978. Arterial blood gas analysis: Potential errors due to the addition of heparin. *Anaesth Intensive Care.* 6:251–255.

Hamm, L.L. and Simon, E.E. 1987. Roles and mechanisms of urinary buffer excretion. *Am J Physiol.* 253:F595–F605.

Handy, J.M. and Soni, N. 2008. Physiological effects of hyperchloraemia and acidosis. *Br J Anaesth.* 101:141–150.

Hansen, J.E., Stone, M.E., Ong, S.T., and Van Kessel, A.L. 1982. Evaluation of blood gas quality control and proficiency testing materials by tonometry. *Am Rev Respir Dis.* 125:480–483.

Hansen, A.C., Wamberg, S., Engel, K., and Kildeberg, P. 1979. Balance of net base in the rat: Adaptation to and recovery from sustained hypercapnia. *Scand J Clin Lab Invest.* 39:723–730.

Hardwick, L.L., Jones, M.R., Brautbar, N., and Lee, D.B. 1991. Magnesium absorption: Mechanisms and the influence of vitamin D, calcium and phosphate. *J Nutr.* 121:13–23.

Harris, P.J., Skinner, S.L., and Zhuo, J. 1988. The effects of atrial natriuretic peptide and glucagon on proximal glomerulo-tubular balance in anaesthetized rats. *J Physiol.* 402:29–42.

Harrison, R.A. 1995. Acid–base balance. *Respir Care Clin N Am.* 1:7–21.

Hayslett, J.P., Halevy, J., Pace, P.E., and Binder, H.J. 1982. Demonstration of net potassium absorption in mammalian colon. *Am J Physiol.* 242:G209–G214.

Hewitt, C.D., Innes, D.J., Savory, J., and Wills, M.R. 1989. Normal biochemical and hematological values in New Zealand White rabbits. *Clin Chem.* 35(8):1777–1779.

Higgins, C. 2007. The use of heparin in preparing samples for blood–gas analysis. *Med Lab Obs.* 39:16–18, 20; quiz 22–13.

Hirakawa, S., Shimabukuro, S., Asano, K., Minagawa, T., Iguchi, H., and Hiraoka, J. 1993. Transport of Na^+ and HCO_3^- out of red blood cells is simultaneous with a chloride shift in canine and human whole blood exposed to CO_2-rich gas. *Jpn J Physiol.* 43:35–49.

Hoff, A.O., Catala-Lehnen, P., Thomas, P.M., et al. 2002. Increased bone mass is an unexpected phenotype associated with deletion of the calcitonin gene. *J Clin Invest.* 110:1849–1857.

Holick, M.F. 2004. Sunlight and vitamin D for bone health and prevention of autoimmune diseases, cancers, and cardiovascular disease. *Am J Clin Nutr.* 80:1678S–1688S.

Honkoop, P., Scholte, H.R., de Man, R.A., and Schalm, S.W. 1997. Mitochondrial injury. Lessons from the fialuridine trial. *Drug Saf.* 17:1–7.

Hoorn, E.J., Walsh, S.B., McCormick, J.A., et al. 2011. The calcineurin inhibitor tacrolimus activates the renal sodium chloride cotransporter to cause hypertension. *Nat Med.* 17:1304–1309.

Horisberger, J.D. and Rossier, B.C. 1992. Aldosterone regulation of gene transcription leading to control of ion transport. *Hypertension.* 19:221–227.

Huang, C.L., Yang, S.S., and Lin, S.H. 2008. Mechanism of regulation of renal ion transport by WNK kinases. *Curr Opin Nephrol Hypertens.* 17:519–525.

Hurwitz, S., Cohen, R.J., and Williams, G.H. 2004. Diurnal variation of aldosterone and plasma renin activity: Timing relation to melatonin and cortisol and consistency after prolonged bed rest. *J Appl Physiol.* 96:1406–1414.

Huth, E.J. and Elkinton, J.R. 1959. Effect of acute fasting in the rat on water and electrolyte content of serum and muscle and on total body composition. *Am J Physiol.* 196:299–302.

Hwang, K.S. and Kim, G.H. 2010. Thiazide-induced hyponatremia. *Electrolyte Blood Press.* 8:51–57.

Hwang, T.C. and Sheppard, D.N. 2009. Gating of the CFTR Cl-channel by ATP-driven nucleotide-binding domain dimerisation. *J Physiol.* 587:2151–2161.

Inagami, T. 1994. Atrial natriuretic factor as a volume regulator. *J Clin Pharmacol.* 34:424–426.

Inoue, T., Nonoguchi, H., and Tomita, K. 2001. Physiological effects of vasopressin and atrial natriuretic peptide in the collecting duct. *Cardiovasc Res.* 51:470–480.

Insogna, K.L., Dreyer, B.E., Mitnick, M., Ellison, A.F., and Broadus, A.E. 1988. Enhanced production rate of 1,25-dihydroxyvitamin D in sarcoidosis. *J Clin Endocrinol Metab.* 66:72–75.

International Federation of Clinical Chemistry and Laboratory Medicine. IFCC Scientific Division, Working Group on Selective Electrodes. 2001. IFCC reference measurement procedure for substance concentration determination of total carbon dioxide in blood, plasma or serum. International Federation of Clinical Chemistry and Laboratory Medicine. *Clin Chem Lab Med.* 39:283–288.

Janssen, W.M., de Zeeuw, D., van der Hem, G.K., and de Jong, P.E. 1992. Atrial natriuretic factor influences renal diurnal rhythm in essential hypertension. *Hypertension.* 20:80–84.

Jensen, F.B. 2004. Red blood cell pH, the Bohr effect, and other oxygenation-linked phenomena in blood O_2 and CO_2 transport. *Acta Physiol Scand.* 182:215–227.

Jentsch, T.J., Stein, V., Weinreich, F., and Zdebik, A.A. 2002. Molecular structure and physiological function of chloride channels. *Physiol Rev.* 82:503–568.

Johnson, J.M., Maher, J.W., DeMaria, E.J., Downs, R.W., Wolfe, L.G., and Kellum, J.M. 2006. The long-term effects of gastric bypass on vitamin D metabolism. *Ann Surg.* 243:701–704; discussion 704–705.

Jorgensen, P.L. and Pedersen, P.A. 2001. Structure–function relationships of Na(+), K(+), ATP, or Mg(2+) binding and energy transduction in Na,K-ATPase. *Biochim Biophys Acta.* 1505:57–74.

Jurutka, P.W., Whitfield, G.K., Hsieh, J.C., Thompson, P.D., Haussler, C.A., and Haussler, M.R. 2001. Molecular nature of the vitamin D receptor and its role in regulation of gene expression. *Rev Endocr Metab Disord.* 2:203–216.

Kaae, J. and deMarais, H.A. 2008. Anion gap and strong ion gap: A quick reference. *Vet Clin North Am Small Anim Pract.* 38:43–47.

Kahle, K.T., Wilson, F.H., Leng, Q., et al. 2003. WNK4 regulates the balance between renal NaCl reabsorption and K^+ secretion. *Nat Genet.* 35:372–376.

Kamel, K.S. and Halperin, M.L. 2012. The importance of distal delivery of filtrate of residual water permeability in the pathophydiology of hyponatremia. *Nephrol Dial Transplant.* 27:872–875.

Kaneko, J.J., Harvey, J.W., and Bruss, M.L. Eds. 1997. *Clinical Biochemistry of Domestic Animals*, 5th edition. San Diego, CA: Academic Press.

Kaplan, J.H. 2002. Biochemistry of Na,K-ATPase. *Annu Rev Biochem.* 71:511–535.

Karet, F.E. 2009. Mechanisms in hyperkalemic renal tubular acidosis. *J Am Soc Nephrol.* 20:251–254.

Kassirer, J.P. 1974. Serious acid–base disorders. *N Engl J Med.* 291:773–776.

Kassirer, J.P. and Schwartz, W.B. 1966. The response of normal man to selective depletion of hydrochloric acid. Factors in the genesis of persistent gastric alkalosis. *Am J Med.* 40:10–18.

Kellum, J.A. 2000. Determinants of blood pH in health and disease. *Crit Care.* 4:6–14.

Khanna, A. and Kurtzman, N.A. 2001. Metabolic alkalosis. *Respir Care.* 46:354–365.

Kiela, P.R., Xu, H., and Ghishan, F.K. 2006. Apical NA^+/H^+ exchangers in the mammalian gastrointestinal tract. *J Physiol Pharmacol.* 57(Suppl 7):51–79.

Kister, J., Marden, M.C., Bohn, B., and Poyart, C. 1988. Functional properties of hemoglobin in human red cells: II. Determination of the Bohr effect. *Respir Physiol.* 73:363–378.

Klastersky, J., Vanderklen, B., Daneau, D., and Mathiew, M. 1973. Carbenicillin and hypokalemia. *Ann Intern Med.* 78:774–775.

Kleeman, C.R. 1979. The kidney in health and disease: X. CNS manifestations of disordered salt and water balance. *Hosp Pract.* 14:59–68, 73.

Klevay, L.M., Bogden, J.D., Aladjem, M., et al. 2007. Renal and gastrointestinal potassium excretion in humans: New insight based on new data and review and analysis of published studies. *J Am Coll Nutr.* 26:103–110.

Kogika, M.M. and de Morais, H.A. 2008. Hyperkalemia: A quick reference. *Vet Clin North Am Small Anim Pract.* 38:477–480, viii.

Kovacs, L. and Robertson, G.L. 1992. Syndrome of inappropriate antidiuresis. *Endocrinol Metab Clin North Am.* 21:.859–875.

Kraut, J.A. and Madias, N.E. 2007. Serum anion gap: Its uses and limitations in clinical medicine. *Clin J Am Soc Nephrol.* 2:162–174.

Kraut, J.A. and Madias, N.E. 2010. Metabolic acidosis: pathophysiology, diagnosis and management. *Nat Rev Nephrol.* 6:274–285.

Kreisberg, R.A. and Wood, B.C. 1983. Drug and chemical-induced metabolic acidosis. *Clin Endocrinol Metab.* 12:391–411.

Kulpmann, W.R. and Gerlach, M. 1996. Relationship between ionized and total magnesium in serum. *Scand J Clin Lab Invest Suppl.* 224:251–258.

Kumar, R. and Thompson, J.R. 2011. The regulation of parathyroid hormone secretion and synthesis. *J Am Soc Nephrol.* 22:216–224.

Laffey, J.G. and Kavanagh, B.P. 2002. Hypocapnia. *N Engl J Med.* 347:43–53.

Lane, E.E. and Walker, J. 1987. *Clinical Arterial Blood Gas Analysis.* St. Louis, MO: Mosby.

Langridge-Smith, J.E. and Field, M. 1981. Sulfate transport in rabbit ileum: Characterization of the serosal border anion exchange process. *J Membr Biol.* 63:207–214.

Lee, J.I., Hong, S.H., Lee, S.J., Kim, Y.S., and Kim, M.C. 2003. Immobilization with ketamine HCl and tiletamine-zolazepam in cynomolgus monkeys. *J Vet Sci.* 4:187–191.

Lee, C.T., Shang, S., Lai, L.W., Yong, K.C., and Lien, Y.H. 2004. Effect of thiazide on renal gene expression of apical calcium channels and calbindins. *Am J Physiol Renal Physiol.* 287:F1164–F1170.

Lee, E.J., Woodske, M.E., Zou, B., and O'Donnell, C.P. 2008. Dynamic arterial blood gas analysis in conscious, unrestrained C57BL/6J mice during exposure to intermittent hypoxia. *J Appl Physiol.* 107:290–294.

Lerche, H., Jurkat-Rott, K., and Lehmann-Horn, F. 2001. Ion channels and epilepsy. *Am J Med Genet.* 106:.146–159.

Levin, S., Semler, D., and Ruben, Z. 1993. Effects of two weeks of feed restriction on some common toxicologic parameters in Sprague-Dawley rats. *Toxicol Pathol.* 21:1–14.

Levine, D.Z., Roinel, N., and de Rouffignac, C. 1982. Flow-correlated influx of K, Ca, P, and Mg during continuous microperfusion of the loop of Henle in the rat. *Kidney Int.* 22:634–639.

Levitin, H., Branscome, W., and Epstein, F.H. 1958. The pathogenesis of hypochloremia in respiratory acidosis. *J Clin Invest.* 37:1667–1675.

Li, C. and Naren, A.P. 2010. CFTR chloride channel in the apical compartments: Spatiotemporal coupling to its interacting partners. *Integr Biol (Camb).* 2:161–177.

Liamis, G., Gianoutsos, C., and Elisaf, M. 2001. Acute pancreatitis-induced hypomagnesemia. *Pancreatology.* 1:74–76.

Liborio, A.B., Daher, E.F., and de Castro, M.C. 2008. Characterization of acid–base status in maintenance hemodialysis: Physicochemical approach. *J Artif Organs.* 11:156–159.

Lingrel, J.B., Van Huysse, J., O'Brien, W., Jewell-Motz, E., Askew, R., and Schultheis, P. 1994. Structure-function studies of the Na,K-ATPase. *Kidney Int Suppl.* 44:S32–S39.

Linnebur, S.A., Vondracek, S.F., Vande Griend, J.P., Ruscin, J.M., and McDermott, M.T. 2007. Prevalence of vitamin D insufficiency in elderly ambulatory outpatients in Denver, Colorado. *Am J Geriatr Pharmacother.* 5:1–8.

Loeb, W.F. 1999. The Rat. In *The Clinical Chemistry of Laboratory Animals.* Eds. W.F. Loeb and F.W. Quimby, 2nd edition, pp. 33–48. Philadelphia, PA: Taylor & Francis.

Loeb, W.F., Das, S.R., Harbour, L.S., Turturro, A., Bucci, T.J., and Clifford, C.B. 1996. Clinical biochemistry. In *Pathobiology of the Aging Mouse.* Eds. U. Mohr, D.L. Dungworth, C.C. Capen, W.W. Carlton, J.P. Sundberg, and J.M. Ward, pp. 3–19. Washington, DC: ILSI Press.

Loepke, A.W., McCann, J.C., Kurth, D., and McAuliffe, J.J. 2006. The physiologic effects of isofluorane anesthesia in neonatal mice. *Anesth Analg.* 102:.75–80.

Madias, N.E., Homer, S.M., Johns, C.A., and Cohen, J.J. 1984. Hypochloremia as a consequence of anion gap metabolic acidosis. *J Lab Clin Med.* 104:15–23.

Mallie, J.P., Bichet, D.G., and Halperin, M.L. 1997. Effective water clearance and tonicity balance: The excretion of water revisited. *Clin Invest Med.* 20:16–24.

Manolagas, S.C. 2000. Birth and death of bone cells: Basic regulatory mechanisms and implications for the pathogenesis and treatment of osteoporosis. *Endocr Rev.* 21:115–137.

Markovich, D. 2001. Physiological roles and regulation of mammalian sulfate transporters. *Physiol Rev.* 81:1499–1533.

Markovich, D. 2011a. Physiological roles of mammalian sulfate transporters NaS1 and Sat1. *Arch Immunol Ther Exp (Warsz).* 59:113–116.

Markovich, D. 2011b. Physiological roles of renal anion transporters NaS1 and Sat1. *Am J Physiol Renal Physiol.* 300:F1267–F1270.

Markovich, D., and Aronson, P.S. 2007. Specificity and regulation of renal sulfate transporters. *Annu Rev Physiol.* 69:361–375.

Markovich, D., Murer, H., Biber, J., Sakhaee, K., Pak, C., and Levi, M. 1998. Dietary sulfate regulates the expression of the renal brush border Na/Si cotransporter NaSi-1. *J Am Soc Nephrol.* 9:1568–1573.

Martin, C.J. and Young, J.A. 1971. Electrolyte concentrations in primary and final saliva of the rat sublingual gland studied by micropuncture and catheterization techniques. *Pflugers Arch.* 324:344–360.

Martyn, J.A. and Richtsfeld, M. 2006. Succinylcholine-induced hyperkalemia in acquired pathologic states: Etiologic factors and molecular mechanisms. *Anesthesiology.* 104:158–169.

Mason, M.J., Smith, J.D., Garcia-Soto, J.J., and Grinstein, S. 1989. Internal pH-sensitive site couples Cl^-(–) HCO_3^- exchange to Na^+–H^+ antiport in lymphocytes. *Am J Physiol.* 256:C428–C433.

McCormick, J.A., Yang, C.L., and Ellison, D.H. 2008. WNK kinases and renal sodium transport in health and disease: An integrated view. *Hypertension.* 51:588–596.

McDonough, A.A., Thompson, C.B., and Youn, J.H. 2002. Skeletal muscle regulates extracellular potassium. *Am J Physiol Renal Physiol.* 282:F967–F974.

McDonough, A.A. and Youn, J.H. 2005. Role of muscle in regulating extracellular [K^+]. *Semin Nephrol.* 25:335–342.

McMurtrie, H.L., Cleary, H.J., Alvarez, B.V., et al. 2004. The bicarbonate transport metabolon. *J Enzyme Inhib Med Chem.* 19:231–236.

Mehanna, H., Nankivell, P.C., Moledina, J., and Travis, J. 2009. Refeeding syndrome—awareness, prevention and management. *Head Neck Oncol.* 1:4.

Meldon, J.H. 1985. Blood gas transport and 2,3-DPG. *Adv Exp Med Biol.* 191:63–73.

Messa, P., Mioni, G., Maio, G.D., et al. 2001. Derangement of acid–base balance in uremia and under hemodialysis. *J Nephrol.* 14:S12–S21.

Metzger, G. and Kenny, M. 1987. Temperature-dependent results with the ChemPro-1000. *Clin Chem.* 33:443–444.

Misasi, R.S. and Keyes, J.L. 1996. Matching and mismatching ventilation and perfusion in the lung. *Crit Care Nurse.* 16:23–27, 31–28; quiz 39–40.

Moe, S.M. 2005. Disorders of calcium, phosphorus, and magnesium. *Am J Kidney Dis.* 45:213–218.

Moe, S.M. 2008. Disorders involving calcium, phosphorus, and magnesium. *Prim Care.* 35:215–237, v–vi.

Molina-Perez, M., Gonzalez-Reimers, E., Santolaria-Fernandez, F., et al. 2000. Relative and combined effects of ethanol and protein deficiency on bone histology and mineral metabolism. *Alcohol.* 20:1–8.

Morrison, J.A. and Fales-Williams, A. 2006. Hypernatremia associated with intracranial B-cell lymphoma in a cat. *Vet Clin Pathol.* 35:362–365.

Moses, A.M. and Miller, M. 1974. Drug-induced dilutional hyponatremia. *N Engl J Med.* 291:1234–1239.

Musso, C.G. 2009. Magnesium metabolism in health and disease. *Int Urol Nephrol.* 41:357–362.

Nadar, S., Lip, G.Y., and Beevers, D.G. 2003. Primary hyperaldosteronism. *Ann Clin Biochem.* 40: 439–452.

Nadiminti, Y., Wang, J.C., Chou, S.Y., Pineles, E., and Tobin, M.S. 1980. Lactic acidosis associated with Hodgkin's disease: Response to chemotherapy. *N Engl J Med.* 303:15–17.

Naik, D.V. and Valtin, H. 1969. Hereditary vasopressin-resistant urinary concentrating defects in mice. *Am J Physiol.* 217:1183–1190.

Narins, R.G. 1977. Clinical use of the anion gap. *Medicine (Baltimore).* 56:38–54.

Narins, R.G., Jones, E.R., Stom, M.C., Rudnick, M.R., and Bastl, C.P. 1982. Diagnostic strategies in disorders of fluid, electrolyte and acid–base homeostasis. *Am J Med.* 72:496–520.

Narins, R.G., Rudnick, M.R., and Bastl, C.P. 1980. Lactic acidosis and the elevated anion gap (I). *Hosp Pract.* 15:125–129, 133–126.

Ng, R.H. 1987. Quality performance in the physician's office. *Med Clin North Am.* 71:677–690.

Nguyen, M.K. and Kurtz, I. 2005. A new formula for predicting alterations in plasma sodium concentration in peritoneal dialysis. *Am J Physiol Renal Physiol.* 288:F1113–F1117.

Nie, L. 2008. KCNQ4 mutations associated with nonsyndromic progressive sensorineural hearing loss. *Curr Opin Otolaryngol Head Neck Surg.* 16:441–444.

Norris, S.H. and Kurtzman, N.A. 1988. Does chloride play an independent role in the pathogenesis of metabolic alkalosis? *Semin Nephrol.* 8:101–108.

Noskov, S.Y. and Roux, B. 2006. Ion selectivity in potassium channels. *Biophys Chem.* 124:279–291.

Nowik, M., Picard, N., Stange, G., et al. 2008. Renal phosphaturia during metabolic acidosis revisited: Molecular mechanisms for decreased renal phosphate reabsorption. *Pflugers Arch.* 457:539–549.

Nyirenda, M.J., Tang, J.I., Padfield, P.L., and Seckl, J.R. 2009. Hyperkalaemia. *BMJ.* 339:b4114.

Oh, M.S. and Carroll, H.J. 1992. Disorders of sodium metabolism: Hypernatremia and hyponatremia. *Crit Care Med.* 20:94–103.

Oh, Y.S. and Warnock, D.G. 2000. Disorders of the epithelial Na(+) channel in Liddle's syndrome and autosomal recessive pseudohypoaldosteronism type 1. *Exp Nephrol.* 8:320–325.

Oliva, P.B. 1970. Lactic acidosis. *Am J Med.* 48:209–225.

O'Regan, S., Carson, S., Chesney, R.W., and Drummond, K.N. 1977. Electrolyte and acid–base disturbances in the management of leukemia. *Blood.* 49:345–353.

Pahari, D.K., Kazmi, W., Raman, G., and Biswas, S. 2006. Diagnosis and management of metabolic alkalosis. *J Indian Med Assoc.* 104:630–634, 636.

Pakulla, M.A., Obal, D., and Loer, S.A. 2004. Continuous intra-arterial blood gas monitoring in rats. *Lab Anim.* 38:133–137.

Palmer, L.G. and Frindt, G. 2007. Na+ and K+ transport by the renal connecting tubule. *Curr Opin Nephrol Hypertens.* 16:477–483.

Parfitt, A.M. 2003. Renal bone disease: A new conceptual framework for the interpretation of bone histomorphometry. *Curr Opin Nephrol Hypertens.* 12:387–403.

Patel, T.V. and Singh, A.K. 2009. Role of vitamin D in chronic kidney disease. *Semin Nephrol.* 29:113–121.

Paulev, P.E. and Zubieta-Calleja, G.R. 2005. Essentials in the diagnosis of acid–base disorders and their high altitude application. *J Physiol Pharmacol.* 56(Suppl 4):155–170.

Peacock, M. 2010. Calcium metabolism in health and disease. *Clin J Am Soc Nephrol.* 5(Suppl 1):S23–S30.

Pearce, S.H., Trump, D., Wooding, C., et al. 1995. Calcium-sensing receptor mutations in familial benign hypercalcemia and neonatal hyperparathyroidism. *J Clin Invest.* 96:2683–2692.

Pena, D.R. and Neiberger, R.E. 1997. Renal brush border sodium-sulfate cotransport in guinea pig: Effect of age and diet. *Pediatr Nephrol.* 11:724–727.

Perazella, M.A. and Biswas, P. 1999. Acute hyperkalemia associated with intravenous epsilon-aminocaproic acid therapy. *Am J Kidney Dis.* 33:782–785.

Pham, P.C., Pham, P.M., and Pham, P.T. 2006. Vasopressin excess and hyponatremia. *Am J Kidney Dis.* 47:727–737.

Pieper, A.K., Haffner, D., Hoppe, B., et al. 2006. A randomized crossover trial comparing sevelamer with calcium acetate in children with CKD. *Am J Kidney Dis.* 47:625–635.

Pollak, V.E., Mattenheimer, H., Debruin, H., and Weinman, K.J. 1965. Experimental metabolic acidosis: The enzymatic basis of ammonia production by the dog kidney. *J Clin Invest.* 44:169–181.

Poole, K.E. and Reeve, J. 2005. Parathyroid hormone—A bone anabolic and catabolic agent. *Curr Opin Pharmacol.* 5:612–617.

Potts, J.T. and Gardella, T.J. 2007. Progress, paradox, and potential: Parathyroid hormone research over five decades. *Ann N Y Acad Sci.* 1117:196–208.

Powers, F. 1999. The role of chloride in acid–base balance. *J Intraven Nurs.* 22:286–291.

Prie, D., Beck, L., Urena, P., and Friedlander, G. 2005. Recent findings in phosphate homeostasis. *Curr Opin Nephrol Hypertens.* 14:318–324.

Purkerson, J.M. and Schwartz, G.J. 2007. The role of carbonic anhydrases in renal physiology. *Kidney Int.* 71:103–115.

Qujeq, D. and Mohiti, J. 2002. Decreased anion gap in polyclonal hypergammaglobulinemia. *Clin Biochem.* 35:73–75.

Raisz, L.G., Simmons, H.A., Gworek, S.C., and Eilon, G. 1977. Studies on congenital osteopetrosis in microphthalmic mice using organ cultures: Impairment of bone resorption in response to physiologic stimulators. *J Exp Med.* 145:857–865.

Ramsay, D.J. and Ganong, W.F. 1977. CNS regulation of salt and water intake. *Hosp Pract.* 12:63–69.

Rastegar, A. 2009. New concepts in pathogenesis of renal hypophosphatemic syndromes. *Iran J Kidney Dis.* 3:1–6.

Rees, S.E., Andreassen, S., Hovorka, R., Summers, R., and Carson, E.R. 1996. Acid–base chemistry of the blood—a general model. *Comput Methods Programs Biomed.* 51:107–119.

Remuzzi, G., Perico, N., Macia, M., and Ruggenenti, P. 2005. The role of renin–angiotensin–aldosterone system in the progression of chronic kidney disease. *Kidney Int Suppl.* 99:S57–S65.

Riley, J.H. and Cornelius, L.M. 1989. Electrolytes, blood gases and acid base balance. In *The Clinical Chemistry of Laboratory Animals*. Eds. W.F. Loeb and F.W. Quimby, pp. 345–413. New York, NY: Pergamon Press.

Roscoe, J.M., Halperin, M.L., Rolleston, F.S., and Goldstein, M.B. 1975. Hyperglycemia-induced hyponatremia: Metabolic considerations in calculation of serum sodium depression. *Can Med Assoc J.* 112:452–453.

Rosol, T.J. and Capen, C.C. 1996. Pathophysiology of calcium, phosphorus, and magnesium metabolism in animals. *Vet Clin North Am Small Anim Pract.* 26:1155–1184.

Rozansky, D.J. 2006. The role of aldosterone in renal sodium transport. *Semin Nephrol.* 26:173–181.

Sahbaie, P., Madanlou, S., Gharagozlou, P., Clark, J.D., Lameh, J., and Delorey, T.M. 2006. Transcutaneous blood gas CO_2 monitoring of induced ventilatory depression in mice. *Anesth Analg.* 103:620–625.

Sánchez, J., Aguilera-Tejero, E., Estepa, J.C., Almadén, Y., Rodríguez, M., and Felsenfeld, A.J. 1996. A reduced PTH response to hypocalcemia after a short period of hypercalcemia: A study in dogs. *Kidney Int Suppl.* 57:S18–S22.

Schnack, C., Bauer, I., Pregant, P., Hopmeier, P., and Schernthaner, G. 1992. Hypomagnesaemia in type 2 (non-insulin-dependent) diabetes mellitus is not corrected by improvement of long-term metabolic control. *Diabetologia.* 35:77–79.

Schneider, R., Wray, V., Nimtz, M., Lehmann, W.D., Kirch, U., Antolovic, R., and Schoner, W. 1998. Bovine adrenals contain, in addition to ouabain, a second inhibitor of the sodium pump. *J Biol Chem.* 273:784–792.

Schron, C.M., Knickelbein, R.G., Aronson, P.S., and Dobbins, J.W. 1987. Evidence for carrier-mediated Cl–SO_4 exchange in rabbit ileal basolateral membrane vesicles. *Am J Physiol.* 253:G404–G410.

Schuurman, H.-J. and Smith, H.T. 2005. Reference values for clinical chemistry and clinical hematology parameters in cynomologous monkeys. *Xenotransplantation.* 15:72–75.

Schwartz, W.B. and Cohen, J.J. 1978. The nature of the renal response to chronic disorders of acid–base equilibrium. *Am J Med.* 64:417–428.

Sevastos, N., Theodossiades, G., and Archimandritis, A.J. 2008. Pseudohyperkalemia in serum: A new insight into an old phenomenon. *Clin Med Res.* 6:.30–32.

Shah, S.N., Abramowitz, M., Hostetter, T.H., and Melamed, M.L. 2009. Serum bicarbonate levels and the progression of kidney disease: A cohort study. *Am J Kidney Dis.* 54:270–277.

Shaikh, A., Berndt, T., and Kumar, R. 2008. Regulation of phosphate homeostasis by the phosphatonins and other novel mediators. *Pediatr Nephrol.* 23:1203–1210.

Shapiro, M.D., Hasbargen, J., Hensen, J., and Schrier, R.W. 1990. Role of aldosterone in the sodium retention of patients with nephrotic syndrome. *Am J Nephrol.* 10:44–48.

Shappell, S.D., and Lenfant, C.J. 1972. Adaptive, genetic, and iatrogenic alterations of the oxyhemoglobin-dissociation curve. *Anesthesiology.* 37:127–139.

Sharan, M. and Popel, A.S. 1989. Algorithm for computing oxygen dissociation curve with pH, PCO_2, and CO in sheep blood. *J Biomed Eng.* 11:48–52.

Sheppard, D.N. and Welsh, M.J. 1999. Structure and function of the CFTR chloride channel. *Physiol Rev.* 79:S23–S45.

Shimokawa Miyama, T., Iwamoto, E., Umeki, S., Nakaichi, M., Okuda, M., and Mizuno, T. 2009. Magnetic resonance imaging and clinical findings in a miniature Schnauzer with hypodipsic hypernatremia. *J Vet Med Sci.* 71:1387–1391.

Siggaard Andersen, O. 1979. Hydrogen ions and blood gases. In *Chemical Diagnosis of Disease*. Eds. S.S. Brown, F.L. Mitchell, and D.S. Young. Amsterdam: Elsevier/North Holland Biomedical Press.

Singer, R.B., Clark, J.K., Barker, E.S., Crosley, A.P., Jr., and Elkinton, J.R. 1955. The acute effects in man of rapid intravenous infusion of hypertonic sodium bicarbonate solution. I. Changes in acid–base balance and distribution of the excess buffer base. *Medicine (Baltimore).* 34:51–95.

Siragy, H.M. 2006. Hyponatremia, fluid-electrolyte disorders, and the syndrome of inappropriate antidiuretic hormone secretion: Diagnosis and treatment options. *Endocr Pract.* 12:446–457.

Smith, D.M., McKenna, K., and Thompson, C.J. 2000. Hyponatraemia. *Clin Endocrinol (Oxf).* 52:667–678.

Soave, P.M., Conti, G., Costa, R., and Arcangeli, A. 2009. Magnesium and anaesthesia. *Curr Drug Targets.* 10:734–743.

Sorensen, M.V., Matos, J.E., Praetorius, H.A., and Leipziger, J. 2010. Colonic potassium handling. *Pflugers Arch.* 459:645–656.

Soupart, A. and Decaux, G. 1996. Therapeutic recommendations for management of severe hyponatremia: Current concepts on pathogenesis and prevention of neurologic complications. *Clin Nephrol.* 46:149–169.

Spanos, E., Brown, D.J., Stevenson, J.C., and MacIntyre, I. 1981. Stimulation of 1,25-dihydroxycholecalciferol production by prolactin and related peptides in intact renal cell preparations in vitro. *Biochim Biophys Acta.* 672:7–15.

Stout, R.W., Cho, D.Y., Gaunt, S.D., Taylor, W., and Baker, D.G. 2001. Transcutaneous blood gas monitoring in the rat. *Comp Med.* 51:524–533.

Strewler, G.J. 2000. The physiology of parathyroid hormone-related protein. *N Engl J Med.* 342:177–185.

Subramanian, P., Chinthalapalli, H., Krishnan, M., et al. 2004. Pregnancy and sarcoidosis: An insight into the pathogenesis of hypercalciuria. *Chest.* 126:995–998.

Takano, N., Lever, M.J., and Lambertsen, C.J. 1979. Acid–base curve nomogram for chimpanzee blood and comparison with human blood characteristics. *J Appl Physiol.* 46:381–386.

Takeda, N., Niwa, T., Tatematsu, A., and Suzuki, M. 1987. Identification and quantification of a protein-bound ligand in uremic serum. *Clin Chem.* 33:682–685.

Talati, G., Ohta, A., Rai, T., et al. 2010. Effect of angiotensin II on the WNK-OSR1/SPAK-NCC phosphorylation cascade in cultured mpkDCT cells and in vivo mouse kidney. *Biochem Biophys Res Commun.* 393:844–888.

Tannen, R.L. 1987. Effect of potassium on renal acidification and acid–base homeostasis. *Semin Nephrol.* 7:263–273.

Tashjian, A.H., Jr., Voelkel, E.F., Levine, L., and Goldhaber, P. 1972. Evidence that the bone resorption-stimulating factor produced by mouse fibrosarcoma cells is prostaglandin E 2. A new model for the hypercalcemia of cancer. *J Exp Med.* 136:1329–1343.

Taylor, J.G. and Bushinsky, D.A. 2009. Calcium and phosphorus homeostasis. *Blood Purif.* 27:387–394.

Thienpont, L.M., Dewitte, K., and Stockl, D. 1999. Serum complexed magnesium—A cautionary note on its estimation and its relevance for standardizing serum ionized magnesium. *Clin Chem.* 45:154–155.

Thomas, P.D. 1997. Fluid, electrolyte and metabolic management. In *Head Injury: Pathophysiology and Management of Severe Closed Head Injury*. Eds. P. Reilly and R. Bullock. London: Chapman and Hall.

Thorneloe, C., Bedard, C., and Boysen, S. 2007. Evaluation of a hand-held lactate analyzer in dogs. *Can Vet J.* 48:283–288.

Tietz, N.W. Ed. 1976. *Fundamentals of Clinical Chemistry*. Philadelphia, PA: W.B. Saunders Co.

Tisdall, M., Crocker, M., Watkiss, J., and Smith, M. 2006. Disturbances of sodium in critically ill adult neurologic patients: A clinical review. *J Neurosurg Anesthesiol.* 18:57–63.

Topf, J.M. and Murray, P.T. 2003. Hypomagnesemia and hypermagnesemia. *Rev Endocr Metab Disord.* 4:195–206.

Tran, H.A. 2005. Extreme hyperkalemia. *South Med J.* 98:729–732.

Travis, S.F., Morrison, A.D., Clements, R.S., Jr., Winegrad, A.I., and Oski, F.A. 1971. Metabolic alterations in the human erythrocyte produced by increases in glucose concentration. The role of the polyol pathway. *J Clin Invest.* 50:2104–2112.

Unwin, R.J. and Capasso, G. 2001. The renal tubular acidoses. *J R Soc Med.* 94:221–225.

Unwin, R.J., Stidwell, R., Taylor, S., and Capasso, G. 1997. The effects of respiratory alkalosis and acidosis on net bicarbonate flux along the rat loop of Henle in vivo. *Am J Physiol.* 273:F698–F705.

Upton, P.K. and Morgan, D.J. 1975. The effect of sampling technique on some blood parameters in the rat. *Lab Anim.* 9:85–91.

van Suijlen, J.D., Berrevoets, C.A., and Leijnse, B. 1990. A candidate reference method for coupled sodium-water determination in human serum. *J Clin Chem Clin Biochem.* 28:817–824.

Verhaeghe, J. and Bouillon, R. 1992. Calciotropic hormones during reproduction. *J Steroid Biochem Mol Biol.* 41:469–477.

Verrey, F. 2007. WNK4, as thiazides, shuts off NaCl reabsorption to stimulate Na/K exchange. *Nephrol Dial Transplant.* 22:.1305–1308.

Verwaerde, P., Malet, C., Lagente, M., de la Farge, F., and Braun, J.P. 2002. The accuracy of the I-STAT portable analyzer for measuring blood gases and pH in whole-blood samples from dogs. *Res Vet Sci.* 73:71–75.

Vexler, Z.S., Ayus, J.C., Roberts, T.P., Fraser, C.L., Kucharczyk, J., and Arieff, A.I. 1994a. Hypoxic and ischemic hypoxia exacerbate brain injury associated witth metabolic encephalopathy in laboratory animals. *J Clin Invest.* 93:.256–264.

Vexler, Z.S., Roberts, T.P., Kucharczyk, J., and Arieff, A.I. 1994b. Severe brain edema associated with cumulative effects of hyponatremic encephalopathy and ischemic hypoxia. *Acta Neurochir Suppl (Wien).* 60:246–249.

Wagner, C.A. 2007. Metabolic acidosis: new insights from mouse models. *Curr Opin Nephrol Hypertens.* 16:471–476.

Wagner, C.A., Devuyst, O., Bourgeois, S., and Mohebbi, N. 2009. Regulated acid–base transport in the collecting duct. *Pflugers Arch.* 458:137–156.

Walmsley, R.N. and White, G.H. 1984. Occult causes of hypokalemia. *Clin Chem.* 30:1406–1408.

Waltemath, C.L. 1970. Oxygen, uptake, transport, and tissue utilization. *Anesth Analg.* 49:184–203.

Waner, T. and Nyska, A. 1994. The influence of fasting on blood glucose, triglycerides, cholesterol and alkaline phosphatase in rats. *Vet Clin Pathol.* 23:78–80.

Wang, W. 2004. Regulation of renal K transport by dietary K intake. *Annu Rev Physiol.* 66:547–569.

Wang, W.H. and Giebisch, G. 2009. Regulation of potassium (K) handling in the renal collecting duct. *Pflugers Arch.* 458:157–168.

Wasserman, K., Whipp, B.J., Casaburi, R., Huntsman, D.J., Castagna, J., and Lugliani, R. 1975. Regulation of arterial PCO_2 during intravenous CO_2 loading. *J Appl Physiol.* 38:651–656.

Weingand, K., Brown, G., Hall, R., et al. 1996. The influence of fasting on blood glucose, triglycerides, cholesterol and alkaline phosphatase in rats. *Fundam Appl Toxicol.* 29:198–201.

Welling, P.A. and Ho, K. 2009. A comprehensive guide to the ROMK potassium channel: Form and function in health and disease. *Am J Physiol Renal Physiol.* 297:F849–F863.

Wieth, J.O., Andersen, O.S., Brahm, J., Bjerrum, P.J., and Borders, C.L., Jr. 1982. Chloride—bicarbonate exchange in red blood cells: physiology of transport and chemical modification of binding sites. *Philos Trans R Soc Lond B Biol Sci.* 299:383–399.

Wilson, F.P. and Berns, J.S. 2012. Onco-nephrology: Tumor lysis syndrome. *Clin J Am Soc Nephrol.* August 9;7(10):1730–1739.

Wysolmerski, J.J. 2012. Parathyroid hormone-related protein: An update. *J Clin Endocrinol Metab.* 97:2947–2956.

Xue, Y. and Fleet, J.C. 2009. Intestinal vitamin D receptor is required for normal calcium and bone metabolism in mice. *Gastroenterology.* 136:1317–1327.

Yamaguchi, K., Glahn, J., Scheid, P., and Piiper, J. 1987. Oxygen transfer conductance of human red blood cells at varied pH and temperature. *Respir Physiol.* 67:209–223.

Youn, J.H. and McDonough, A.A. 2009. Recent advances in understanding integrative control of potassium homeostasis. *Annu Rev Physiol.* 71:381–401.

Zaidi, M., Moonga, B.S., and Abe, E. 2002. Calcitonin and bone formation: A knockout full of surprises. *J Clin Invest.* 110:1769–1771.

Zietse, R., Zoutendijk, R., and Hoorn, E.J. 2009. Fluid, electrolyte and acid–base disorders associated with antibiotic therapy. *Nat Rev Nephrol.* 5:193–202.

Zweens, J., Frankena, H., van Kampen, E.J., Rispens, P., and Zijlstra, W.G. 1977. Ionic composition of arterial and mixed venous plasma in the unanesthetized dog. *Am J Physiol.* 233:F412–F415.

23 Hormones

Jerome M. Goldman, Lori K. Davis, and Ralph L. Cooper

CONTENTS

23.1 INTRODUCTION

The rudimentary concept of internal secretions can be traced back to the second century AD in writings of the Greek physician Galen. His idea of *bodily humors* and the relationships between imbalances in them and disease (termed *dyscrasia,* from the Greek, *a bad mixture*) continued, in one form or another, to be prevalent through the medieval period and into the eighteenth century. During that time, blood letting and other purges were employed medically to rid the body of a harmful surplus of *humor.* In fact, use of the adjective *humoral* has persisted in reference to elements in the blood or other body fluids. However, it was not until Claude Bernard described his work on the release of glucose from liver glycogen in the mid-nineteenth century (reviewed by Young, 1957) that the first convincing demonstration of systemic effects from the secretion of chemical substances into the blood was provided.

Fascination with this idea of chemical messengers quickly began to surface in both the scientific and lay communities at the conclusion of the nineteenth century with the (subsequently disproven) claim by physiologist Charles–Edouard Brown–Séquard that his self-administration of extracts of animal testes caused an increase in physical strength, improvements in intellectual capacity, and an augmentation in sexual prowess (Brown-Séquard, 1899a,b). At the same time, the English physician George Murray presented evidence (Murray, 1891) that thyroid extracts were able to improve myxoedema, a skin and tissue disorder that typically developed in response to severe, prolonged hypothyroidism. Many physiologists have come to believe that these two reports were seminal to the emergence of the new field of Endocrinology. However, it was not until a 1904 address to the Royal College of Physicians by Ernest Starling, professor of physiology at the University College, London, describing collaborative work on the pancreatic response to intestinal secretin that the term *hormone*, from the Greek word *to excite* or *arouse*, entered the medical lexicon (Starling, 1905). Endocrinology then began to acquire an identity with a foothold as a separate discipline.

23.2 DEFINITIONS AND CLASSIFICATION OF HORMONES

As originally characterized during those early, heady days of endocrine discovery, hormones were chemical substances secreted by glandular tissue and carried through the circulation to impose regulatory effects on other cell populations. This classic mechanism of hormone action has expanded to include forms of paracrine communication between adjacent or nearby cells and autocrine signaling involving individual cells. Various terms, such as *cybernins* and *intracrines*, have been proposed to capture the extent of these types of communication. Neurotransmitters secreted from neurons are also known to act as blood-borne endocrine factors. Dopamine, for example, functions as an inhibitory regulator of prolactin (Prl) secretion following its release from brain hypothalamic nerve terminals into the portal vasculature that extends to the anterior pituitary. Under the large umbrella of hormonal chemicals, three basic criteria are classically met: (1) the biological activity must be established, (2) a specific and saturable receptor needs to be identified, and (3) with the notable exception of hormones binding to nuclear receptors, a second messenger has to be determined. Although this broadened definition of signaling molecules encompasses a considerable range of endogenous chemicals, endocrine factors tend to populate one of the three classes: (1) Protein and polypeptide hormones comprised of chains of amino acids, (2) lipid or phospholipid hormones, including the steroid hormones, generated from cholesterol, and (3) the amine-related hormones, containing an NH_2 group at the end of the molecule that are derivatives of the amino acids tyrosine and tryptophan. The abovementioned neurotransmitter dopamine falls into this group, along with epinephrine, norepinephrine, and serotonin (discussed in Section 23.4.4.4).

23.2.1 Hormone Receptors

The binding of a hormone to a specific protein receptor initiates its appropriate cellular response. With the exception of the members of the nuclear receptor superfamily (encompassing steroid androgen, estrogen, progesterone, and thyroid hormone receptors), amino acid-derived receptors and peptide hormone receptors are present in the plasma membrane. Multiple receptor isoforms have been discovered for different hormones and amine-related neurotransmitters that serve functionally diverse roles. The structures of these receptors vary, with some being present as single membrane-spanning configurations, while others are polypeptide chains that stretch multiple times back and forth through the membrane. The binding of the hormone ligand to the receptor will then initiate a metabolic response via second messenger and phosphorylated protein transducers.

Steroid hormone receptors can be present as multiple isoforms. They are intracellular in location, although there is now good evidence for androgen, estrogen, and progesterone receptors that are also resident in the plasma membrane (e.g., Boonyaratanakornkit and Edwards, 2004; Michels and Hoppe, 2008; Prossnitz et al., 2008; Roepke et al., 2009) and exert rapid effects on intracellular signaling pathways independent of gene transcription. Intracellularly, steroid receptors are present in the cytosol and, upon binding to their particular steroid ligand, translocated together to the nucleus. These receptors may also reside in the nucleus until activated by an individual steroid hormone. In the nucleus, the hormone–receptor complex associates with cofactors, general transcription factors and RNA polymerase II, binding to particular sequences on DNA to stimulate or suppress the activity of individual genes that direct the synthesis of specific proteins (see Trapman and Dubbink, 2007 for review).

23.2.2 Bound versus Free Hormones

Hormones that are released into the blood circulate as either free hormone or bound to carrier or binding proteins. In general, the protein and peptide hormones (in addition to the amine-derived factors) circulate in their free form, while the tyrosine-derived hormones thyroxine (T4) and triiodothyronine (T3) are mostly carrier bound. This binding functions to impede hormonal degradation by plasma proteases, thereby increasing the half-lives of the hormones. In contrast, circulating steroid hormones exist primarily in a bound form, with only 1%–10% of individual hormones in plasma present in the free state, the fraction considered to be the biologically active form. Here, the bound fractions tend to regulate steroid activity by limiting the biological availability of the hormone. Furthermore, free steroid molecules are poorly soluble in aqueous media. By increasing the solubility of the normally hydrophobic steroids, the carrier molecules also serve to increase circulating plasma concentrations beyond what would otherwise be possible.

23.3 HORMONE ASSESSMENT

Although gas chromatographic/mass spectrometric (GC/MS) and liquid chromatographic techniques have been employed to assess hormonal concentrations, immunoassays have been the standard analytical approach in veterinary medicine and animal research. They have mostly replaced bioassays, which provided a quantifiable cellular response to hormonal stimulation, but were frequently difficult to properly validate (Kalia et al., 2004). Unlike immunoassays, such bioassays are able to provide an indication of the biological activity of a hormone, which may vary depending upon a number of factors, including the degree of glycosylation/sialylation (discussed further in Sections 23.4.3.1.2 and 23.4.3.3.2) or the presence of cofactors required for steroid receptor binding. On the other hand, immunoassays are typically rapid, sensitive, and cost effective, with a diverse assortment of commercial kits appearing regularly that require a relatively modest degree of expertise for proper use.

23.3.1 Polyclonal versus Monoclonal Antibodies

The distinguishing nature of the immunoassay is based on the ability of a specific immunoglobulin antibody to recognize and bind to a particular three-dimensional configuration on the surface of a molecule (the epitope). This configuration exists as an orientation of residues that can be shaped by a folding within the structure of the molecule. Both polyclonal and monoclonal antibodies are commonly used in various types of immunoassays. For protein and polypeptide hormones, they are typically species-specific, although some degree of cross-species reactivity can exist. Polyclonal antibodies raised in host animals are derived from different lymphocyte B-cell lines that are mixtures of immunoglobulins recognizing various epitopes on a hormonal antigen. In contrast, monoclonal antibodies are monospecific, recognizing a single epitope. This antibody is produced by a single B-lymphocyte clone, and all are therefore identical. Each has distinctive advantages for hormonal assessment. Polyclonal antibodies typically have a higher affinity and wider reactivity, but a lower specificity than monoclonals. They are able to detect multiple epitopes in different orientations. In general, polyclonal antibodies are easier to produce. However, there is considerable animal-to-animal variability in antibodies from noninbred animals, meaning that dissimilar epitopes can be recognized and the potencies can be quite different. Consequently, an individual animal host generating a particularly valued polyclonal is highly coveted. Moreover, such an antibody from a larger animal will provide a sizeable volume of antibody-rich serum. Nevertheless, a healthy animal is limited by its lifespan to serve as a source of that antibody, and recurring immunizations with a particular antigen may generate a new mixture of polyclonal antibodies against that antigen. Should that animal die and the antibody stock become depleted, alternative sources must be sought that will likely produce antibodies with different reactivities and titers. Monoclonals, on the other hand, are very specific and can be generated as a potentially inexhaustible supply from a continuous culture. Their production had been time consuming and often frustrating, but the market for the therapeutic application of monoclonal antibodies has rapidly grown and the early technical difficulties in their preparation in numerous cases have been overcome (reviewed by Tabrizi et al., 2009).

23.3.2 Competitive versus Sandwich Immunoassays

The great majority of immunoassays fall into one of two groups, competitive and sandwich-type assays. Competitive radioimmunoassays (RIAs) originated from the groundbreaking work of Berson and Yalow (1957, 1959) and are based on the competition of a hormone sample with a radiolabeled form of the same hormone (the tracer) for binding to an immunoglobulin antibody (Figure 23.1, upper panel). The greater the amount of hormone in the sample to be measured, the greater is the ability of this antigen to compete with a known level of tracer radioactivity. Unknown samples are run in parallel with a standard series with identified hormone concentrations. A second antibody generated by a different animal species against the first or primary antibody will then bind to the primary antibody–hormone or primary antibody–tracer combinations, forming a large complex. This complex can then be precipitated by centrifugation, and the supernatant, containing unbound standards or sample hormone, and unbound radioactivity is aspirated off. Alternatively, staphylococcal protein A (Gupta and Morton, 1979) and polyethylene glycol (PEG) have been employed as a precipitant instead of a second antibody. Staph protein A has the property of binding to immunoglobulin antibodies of a wide variety of mammalian species (Grov et al., 1970), and most immunoglobulins are insoluble in 20% PEG, unlike smaller, soluble albumins and other antigens (Creighton et al., 1973). PEG combined with a second antibody has also been used for increasing the rate of precipitation. Radioactivity remaining in the precipitated pellet can subsequently be counted. As mentioned above, increasing concentrations of the hormone to be measured will be better able to compete against the tracer for the primary antibody and show corresponding decreases in the pellet radioactivity. Units of radioactivity can then be compared against the standard series to quantify the unknown concentrations. Instead of adding hormones and antibodies separately, some commercial kits are supplied with the antibody previously coated to the walls of tubes provided in the kit, precluding the need to precipitate the antibody–antigen complexes. Such kits also typically include vials containing a radionuclide-labeled hormone and a defined standard series against which the unknown samples are compared. One reservation with this type of immunoassay, however, is that the antibody adsorption to the tube can potentially mask immunoreactive sites.

Competitive immunoassays are still commonly employed today for the measurement of steroids and peptide hormones of varying sizes, although there has been a trend away from the use of radioactive-labeled materials, toward the broad application of enzyme-linked sandwich assays and increasing numbers of chemiluminescent immunoassays that have undergone validation for use (e.g., Singh et al., 1997; Scott-Moncrieff et al., 2003; Russell et al., 2007). Sandwich immunoassays, in contrast, employ a *capture antibody* that binds one site on the sample and a *detection antibody* directed against a second site. In the kit form, they are typically supplied with a monoclonal antibody adsorbed on to a plastic microtiter plate (Figure 23.1, lower panel). This *capture antibody* will bind the target antigen from a sample. A *detection antibody* is then added, and it binds to a separate site on the target antigen, forming a sandwich of the antigen between the two antibodies. It is common to have an enzyme attached to the detection antibody (known as enzyme-linked

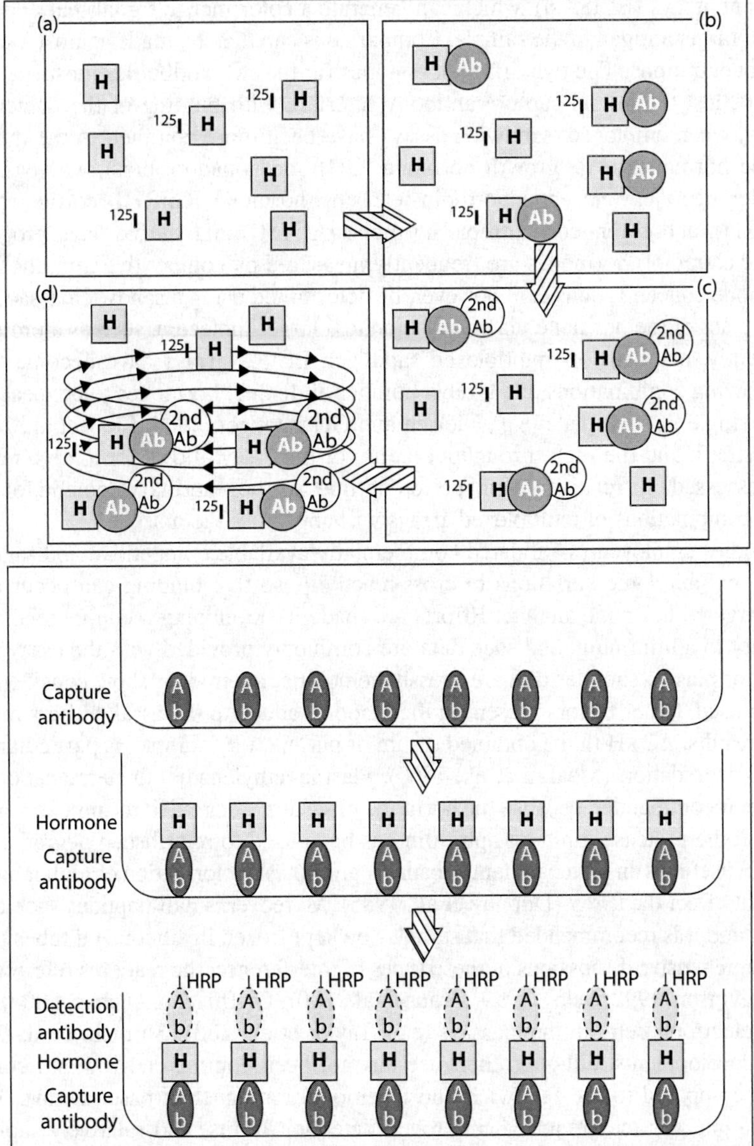

FIGURE 23.1 (Upper panel) Illustration depicting the basic steps in a classic competitive radioimmunoassay. A mixture (a) of both the hormone to be quantified and a defined radioactive (^{125}I) aliquot of that hormone are exposed to a specific antibody (first antibody), allowing both hormones to compete for the antibody (b). A second antibody targeted to the immunoglobulin configuration of the first antibody (c) creates a large structure that can be pelleted by centrifugation (d), thus separating hormone–antibody complex from non-antibody-bound hormones. Following aspiration of the supernatant containing the unbound hormone, radioactivity in the pellet is then counted and compared against the radioactivity present in a series of concurrently run standards containing defined concentrations of that hormone. (Lower panel) As opposed to the competitive immunoassay, sandwich assays in kit form are provided with a microtiter plate containing a capture antibody that recognizes an epitope on the hormone. A second or detection antibody conjugated to a detection enzyme (in this example, horseradish perioxidase [HRP]) then recognizes a separate epitope on the hormone, sandwiching the hormone between the two antibodies. After washing out unbound HRP, the substrate for the enzyme is added and allowed to incubate for a defined period of color development before the reaction is stopped. A readout of the detection signal is then performed. In this case, the amount of color generated by a reaction to the signaling molecule is compared against a standard series of known hormone concentrations.

immunosorbant assays [ELISAs]), which can generate a colorimetric signal that is proportional to the amount of target antigen in the sample. Comparisons can then be made against a standard series of known concentrations. The two different epitopes for the two antibodies must spatially be some distance apart, lest the bound capture antibody interfere with binding of the detection antibody. Consequently, when employed, sandwich assays have been more confined to the measurement of larger peptide hormones (e.g., growth hormone [GH] and gonadotropins), whereas, as indicated above, smaller peptides (e.g., gonadotropin-releasing hormone [GnRH], corticotropin-releasing hormone [CRH], and adrenocorticotropic hormone [ACTH]) and steroid (e.g., progesterone, testosterone, and estradiol) hormones are frequently measured by competitive immunoassay. Smaller peptide hormone concentrations can, however, be determined using a sandwich assay by increasing the apparent mass of the hormone via conjugation to a larger molecule, such as a protein.

More recently, platforms of multiplexed sandwich ELISA arrays have become commercially available, allowing combinations of a sizable number of distinct hormones to be measured simultaneously on a single 96-well plate (e.g., Nielsen and Geierstanger, 2004; Liew et al., 2007). Sample volumes are small, and the high throughput nature of the assay allows for a large number of hormones to be assessed in a relatively rapid period of time. As the veterinary demand for such ELISAs grows, more combinations of multiplexed arrays will appear on the market.

The antibodies employed in validated commercially available competitive and sandwich immunoassays will exhibit some variations in cross-reactivity, so that binding can occur to substances beyond the targeted hormone analyte. Efforts are made in developing a commercial assay to keep cross-reactivity to a minimum, and such data are commonly provided with the assay materials. As a rule, serum or plasma samples that are grossly hemolytic, lipemic, or show considerable turbidity should not be used. Other factors present in the blood or added to the assay buffers may also affect the obtained results. ACTH in the obtained serum or plasma, for example, is particularly vulnerable to proteolytic degradation (Meakin et al., 1960). Plasma–ethylenediaminetetraacetic acid (EDTA) collections are recommended because the hormone in serum is degraded to some extent while blood is clotting, and the protease inhibitor aprotinin has been used to retard such degradation. Heparin, however, is not useful as an anticoagulant because it promotes the formation of high molecular weight aggregates that affect the assay (Dupouy et al., 1986). Moreover, small peptides such as ACTH can stick to glass, and it is recommended that samples be kept frozen in siliconized tubes prior to assay. For more comprehensive discussions of these types of interference, the reader is referred to a number of reviews (Levinson, 1992; Selby, 1999; Evans et al., 2001; Griffin and Auchus, 2004).

Capillary electrophoretic immunoassays (e.g., Taylor et al., 2001; Shinichi et al., 2005) are the more recent developments, although their use has not been commercialized and consequently is more limited compared to the sandwich and traditional radionuclide-based assays. However, the very small sample volumes required, improved detection limits, and relatively rapid results are attractive possibilities for specific needs.

Kit materials obtained from different commercial sources using a diversity of polyclonal or monoclonal antibodies will commonly exhibit discrepant results with the same samples, something that is discussed further in Section 23.4.2. Nevertheless, in the conduct of all such immunoassays, an understanding of a particular assay's specificity and sensitivity is paramount. In this regard, it is essential to define the appropriate assay performance criteria. For an individual assay, the incorporation of defined quality control samples is necessary to ensure consistency of results both within and among multiple assay runs. When comparing the samples of interest against a known series of standards covering a range of hormonal concentrations, it is imperative that the unknown samples not fall at the extremes of the standard series, something that would meaningfully impair the accuracy of the data. Moreover, as mentioned previously, it is also important to know the extent to which any confounding factor(s) may impact the utility of the results. For a further discussion of issues and requirements concerning the quality of the different endocrine assay techniques, there are several publications (e.g., Rosner et al., 2007; Stenman, 2013) and websites (e.g., Center for Disease Control and Prevention [www.cdc.gov/labstandards/hs.html]) that detail the best laboratory practices needed for an accurate detection and interpretation of hormonal values.

23.4 ENDOCRINE PHYSIOLOGY

23.4.1 Endocrine Homeostasis

23.4.1.1 Insulin, Glucagon, and Glucose

The ability to maintain an internal physiological environment within a tolerable range is a fundamental characteristic of living systems. The interaction and integration of the extensive variety of hormonal signals in the mammalian body are the essential components of homeostatic regulation. The classic example of a physiological homeostatic relationship is the balance between insulin and glucagon to maintain blood glucose within a narrow range. Both hormones are secretory products of the pancreas, insulin by the pancreatic beta cells and glucagon by the alpha cells. As the blood glucose level increases, after a meal for example, insulin secretion increases, causing cellular glucose uptake. Glucagon secretion then is very low or absent. However, when circulating glucose is low, insulin production is suppressed and there is an increase in alpha cell glucagon secretion, stimulating the liver to release glucose stored as the glucose polymer glycogen. This classic interactive mechanism of homeostatic regulation is now known to involve in the participation of a family of gut hormones, which includes glucose-dependent insulinotropic polypeptide (GIP), glucagon-like peptide-1 (GLP-1), and peptide YY (PYY). They are secreted in response to nutrient absorption—GIP by K cells of the upper small intestine, GLP-1, and PYY cosecreted from L cells of the distal intestine (reviewed by Dumoulin et al., 1995; Gautier et al., 2008; Bauer et al., 2016). GIP and GLP-1 are able to stimulate the biosynthesis and secretion of insulin in a glucose-dependent manner, and GLP-1 has been found to suppress glucagon seretion, although the mechanism of effect, be it direct or indirect, is still being investigated. Moreover, GLP-1, but not GIP, acts to inhibit gastric emptying (Hansotia and Drucker, 2005). Both have a short half-life and are rapidly degraded by the enzyme dipeptidyl-peptidase IV. PYY, which has also been identified in the brain hypothalamic region (Ekblad and Sundler, 2002), is essentially an antisecretory peptide. It has been found to mediate satiety signaling and inhibit many gastrointestinal functions, including gastric acid secretion, gastric emptying, and small bowel and colonic chloride secretion (Ballantyne, 2006; Ueno et al., 2008).

One of the most frequently diagnosed endocrine disorders in cats and dogs is diabetes mellitus, characterized by an elevation in blood glucose. In dogs, the more common form is type 1 or insulin-dependent diabetes, in which activated lymphocytes target pancreatic islets destroying the β-cells and abolishing insulin production. Type 1 has been reported in approximately half of diabetic dogs (Elle and Hoenig, 1995). Type 2, or noninsulin-dependent diabetes, is more frequently seen in cats, accounting for 80%–95% of cases (Rand, 1999). It is referred to as adult-onset and involves an insulin resistance, wherein cells are unable to use insulin properly. The condition may be accompanied by a reduction in insulin secretion.

23.4.1.2 Rhythmic Secretions and Singular Events

The secretory activity of a diverse variety of endocrine factors that maintain physiological homeostasis commonly exhibits a characteristic pulsatility. This is true for a growing number of hormones, including hypothalamic, pituitary peptide (Figure 23.2), adrenal, and thyroid hormones (e.g., Moor and Younglai, 1975; Dluzen and Ramirez, 1987; Larsen and Odell, 1987; Martin and Thiéry, 1987; Irvine and Alexander, 1988; Günzel-Apel et al., 1994; Kemppainen and Peterson, 1996; Kooistra and Okkens, 2001; Gan and Quinton, 2010). For various peptide hormones, this pulsatile secretion, characterized by recurrent peaks and valleys, acts to prevent the emergence of a desensitization of second messenger mechanisms caused by a constant exposure of receptors to increased levels of a hormone (Li and Goldbeter, 1989; Goldbeter et al., 2000). However, such is not the case for all hormones that exhibit rhythmic secretion. For example, gonadal hormones, which are pulsatile in nature, exhibit comparable effects with rhythmic or continuous exposure. Their secretion is a consequence of the upstream pulses of pituitary gonadotropins, which themselves are a response to secretory variations in brain hypothalamic GnRH (a relationship detailed in Section 23.4.3.1).

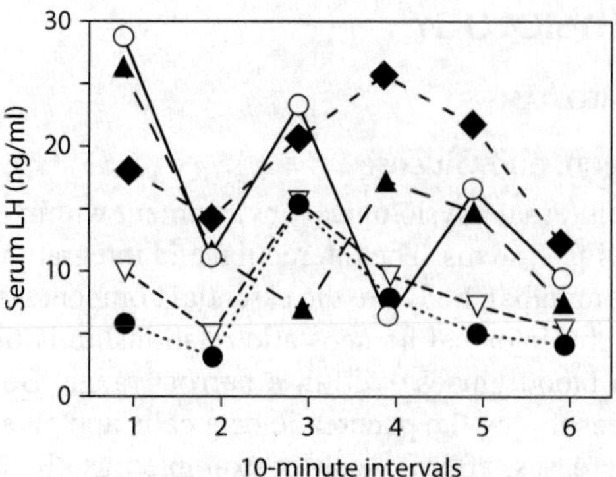

FIGURE 23.2 Pulsatile secretion of luteinizing hormone (LH) in the adult female Fischer 344 rat. In the five individual examples shown, animals were ovariectomized 4 weeks prior to sampling of blood from surgically implanted jugular catheters. Ovariectomy abolished the negative feedback by ovarian steroids, causing an enhancement in the concentrations of circulating LH. Small quantities of blood, with saline replacement, were withdrawn every 10 minutes over the course of 1 hour. Values were determined by radioimmunoassay using the following materials provided by the National Hormone and Pituitary Program: iodination preparation I-9, reference preparation RP-3, and rabbit anti-rat antiserum S-11.

The pulsatile secretion of a hormone can also be embedded within a diurnal rhythm. Corticosterone secretion in the female rat, for example, shows pulses that occur approximately every hour over the course of the day. Pulse amplitude increases during the latter half of the light portion of the photoperiod, resulting in an overall rise in circulating concentrations over the day (Lightman et al., 2000). Similar diurnal patterns have been reported for pulsatile luteinizing hormone (LH) and testosterone in young adult male rhesus monkeys (Winters et al., 1991; Schlatt et al., 2008). Some pulsatile secretion can also have marked valley-to-peak excursions. For example, beagle dogs can show three to nine pulses of GH over a 6-hour period that can rise as much as fivefold greater than nadir concentrations (Lee et al., 2003).

The pulsatile secretion of hormones may show differences between genders. For example, during the summer breeding season for horses, mares tend to exhibit about one large amplitude pulse of GH every 6 hours that can be in excess of ninefold over baseline, while stallions show 2–2.5 smaller amplitude pulses over the same time (Thompson et al., 1992). In rats, it is the male that shows a marked pulsatile elevation in GH with large bursts occurring at 3–4 hour intervals. In contrast, pulse amplitudes are lower in females, but the interpulse concentration of GH is higher than in the male (see Jansson et al., 1985 for a review of this sexual dimorphism).

However, the most salient differences in endocrine homeostasis between males and females are those changes that are tied to the ovarian cycle. In spontaneously cycling animals, circulating concentrations of the gonadotropins (LH and follicle-stimulating hormone [FSH]) exhibit sharp midcycle elevations or surges that serve as functional endocrine events, stimulating ovarian follicles to ovulate (LH) or undergo maturational changes (FSH). A further discussion of the importance of the gonadotropin surge in females and the consequences of various forms of insult will be presented in Sections 23.4.3.1.2 and 23.4.3.1.5.

23.4.2 Sampling of Analytes

Given that hormonal concentrations can show diurnal variations or alterations over an ovarian cycle, it is imperative that the sampling of biological material for analysis be performed with an understanding of the nature of these normative changes. Consequently, the most appropriate sampling parameters can vary, depending upon what is to be measured and, for various diagnostic tests, the purpose of a reaction to a challenge. The focus can be on a stimulation or suppression at various time points in response of one hormone to an administration of another. For the test to be useful, a selection of sampling times must allow for a definitive characterization of the response.

Species differences can exist in the periodicity of hormonal concentrations, which can dictate when samples are taken. For example, there is an apparent absence of rhythmic diurnal glucocorticoid changes in dogs and cats (e.g., Johnston and Mather, 1978, 1979), while rats will show basal corticosterone levels during the early morning period, which begin to rise at midday and exhibit elevated concentration late in the afternoon (e.g., Allen and Kendall, 1967; Allen-Rowlands et al., 1980). In animals that show a diurnal rhythm for a particular hormone, nadir concentrations of that hormone may fall at or near the level of sensitivity for that individual assay. For a condition in which the hormone is decreased, the lower circulating concentrations may not be detectable or be of questionable validity, providing no indication of the magnitude of the effect. In this situation, it may be more appropriate to sample during the period in which concentrations would normally be elevated. The opposite would then be true for a suspected condition that caused a marked increase. Sampling at a time when the synthesis of an individual hormone is typically activated and the secretory levels are highest may not show a comparable percentage rise in concentration as a sample taken during the diurnal nadir.

Hormones that respond to nutrient ingestion will show dramatic postprandial changes, so that sampling after meals will not provide any indication of basal values but may show alterations in the normative endocrine responsiveness to a defined quantity of nutrient. Adult male rhesus monkeys, for example, will show a diurnal rhythm of LH, with elevated nighttime circulating concentrations that begin to rise in response to an afternoon meal. Consequently, sampling for baseline values needs to take this into consideration. Elimination of that meal revealed an absence of the rhythm, and a delay in the meal time showed a corresponding shift in the diurnal rise (Mattern et al., 1993). Fasting in dogs has been reported to attenuate ACTH-stimulated serum cortisol concentrations, but not thyroid hormones increased by thyroid-stimulating hormone (TSH; Reimers et al., 1986). If a short-lived rise in the circulating concentrations of a hormone serves as the impetus for other critical changes, which occurs with the gonadotropin surges, any concerns about a suppression in this elevation would require that samples be obtained over a window of time that would normally encompass the event.

Animals diagnosed with various endocrinopathies may require hormonal treatments. Dogs suffering from hypothyroidism (discussed in Section 23.4.3.3.4) that are treated with thyroid hormone supplements must be monitored for circulating thyroid hormone and TSH concentrations. The time of sampling relative to the treatment has a major influence on the obtained hormone concentrations and dosing adjustments, with 4–6 hours postadministration optimal for testing (e.g., Dixon et al., 2002; Le Traon et al., 2009).

The responsiveness of a variety of hormones to novel and/or stressful situations is a factor of concern in endocrine assessments. Stress as a category, however, is not easily definable. It was originally conceptualized by Hans Selve in the 1930s as the state of the organism as it responded and adapted to the environment. Although definitions are imprecise, it is well-established that stressful conditions will cause increases in the circulating concentrations of glucocorticoids (see section 23.4.3.2). Other endocrine factors, moreover, have been found to be altered as a consequence of the glucocorticoid elevation (see Section 23.4.3.2.4). Stressors and stressful conditions come in many forms, and a diversity of mammalian species can exhibit distinctive patterns of endocrine responses to these stressors (e.g., Lenox et al., 1980). Introduction to a novel environment can be stressful in various species and cause elevations in glucocorticoid levels (Coe et al., 1982; Brett et al., 1983; Weinberg and Wong, 1986; Gust et al., 1994) that may obscure the cause of other effects on adrenal homeostasis. Disease states are undoubtedly stressful and cause independent disruptions in an endocrine profile. Such medical conditions may be the focus of a diagnostic evaluation or cause unwelcome disruptive effects on other assessments.

Administered anesthetics also constitute a form of insult to the system. Sampling under anesthesia can reveal significant alterations in circulating hormone concentrations, and the effects can vary with the type of inhaled or injected anesthetic employed. For example, pentobarbital, ketamine, halothane, and isoflurane have been found to stimulate adrenal activity and elevate glucocorticoid concentrations in various species, which include monkeys, dogs, cats, rabbits, and rats (e.g., Puri et al., 1981; Fox et al., 1994; Illera et al., 2000; Ambrisko et al., 2005; Gil et al., 2007). A number of anesthetics are also able to alter the levels of circulating Prl (e.g., Quadri et al., 1978; Puri et al., 1981; Furudate, 1991); in mated female rabbits, ketamine–xylazine was reported to attenuate the rise in blood concentrations of FSH (Mills and Copland, 1982). Pentobarbital will suppress the preovulatory surge of luteinizng hormone in female rats (Gosden et al., 1976; ter Haar and MacKinnon, 1976), something that has also been seen in the baboon (Hagino, 1979). These findings underscore the caution that must be exercised in evaluations of hormonal concentrations obtained by sampling under anesthesia.

For the subsequent discussion of individual hormones, values for those that are considered to be clinically important will not be provided, since the normal ranges can vary for diverse species at different sampling times and for assorted immunoassays of the same hormone using different polyclonal or monoclonal antibodies (e.g., Taylor et al., 1994; Barbé et al., 1995; Niccoli et al., 1996; Boots et al., 1998; Steinberger et al., 1998; Stanczyk et al., 2003). For example, reference materials provided by the US National Hormone and Pituitary Program that had previously been used (reference preparation-1) and are currently being employed (reference preparation-2 or -3) to set up standards for a rat LH RIA will generate concentrations for identical samples that differ by 61-fold. Rat and mouse serum estradiol concentrations showed wide variation when samples for each were split into aliquots and run using different commercial kits (Ström et al., 2008; Haisenleder et al., 2011). In women taking the oral estradiol Estrace®, assay values in serum using a commercial chemiluminescent kit were reported to be approximately 1/3 of those estradiol concentrations determined with an RIA kit (Hershlag et al., 2000). Whether the discrepancies in this study were attributable to differences in antibody specificity, the nature of the assay platform employed, or a contribution of both, were not clear. It is important, then, for referencing of immunoassay results to normative endocrine levels for individual hormones that the same assay materials and parameters be employed.

A number of hormones, as indicated above, will exhibit rhythmic changes over the day; in cycling females, the circulating concentrations of sex steroids and some peptide hormones will shift quite markedly over the cycle. Consequently, it is critical for any hormonal evaluations to reference concentrations to the appropriate controls, which for clinical purposes are frequently established historically. Again, it must be reemphasized that referencing clinical results against such historical values should be restricted to a common assay platform and its provider. For this chapter, most of the descriptive information about the various hormones and normal endocrine homeostatic interactions will rely on the rat as a representative mammalian species. Although various interspecies disparities do exist, rodents have been commonly employed as valued model systems for describing endocrine functions and interrelationships, which in the main hold true for other mammals. Nevertheless, information about other species has been included as well, particularly in those subsections that focus on pathological alterations in the various endocrine axes.

23.4.3 Endocrine Axes

As indicated above, maintenance of physiological homeostasis relies heavily on the systems of communication among organs and tissues. The overarching term *endocrine system* really embraces multiple, yet interrelated, systems, within which feedback loops of hormonal messengers serve to regulate activity among organs subserving particular physiological functions. These subsystems of hormones have been termed *axes* that are typically identified by the individual network of organs involved. The pituitary is an integral component of these axes and, unless otherwise indicated, refers to the anterior pituitary (adenohypophysis). During embryogenesis it arises from Rathke's pouch, a depression in the roof of the developing mouth and, unlike the posterior pituitary (neurohypophysis), receives no neuronal fibers from the brain hypothalamic region, only blood-borne contact.

23.4.3.1 Hypothalamic–Pituitary–Gonadal Axis

Communication among the hypothalamus, pituitary, and gonads is essential for the regulation of reproductive activity. The principal hormones involved are GnRH, LH, and FSH and, in the female, the gonadal steroids progesterone and estradiol (Figure 23.3). In the male, the primary circulating androgen is testosterone; whereas, in the prostate, the concentration of 5α-dihydrotestosterone (DHT) is the principal and most potent form (Bruchovsky, 1971). A range of factors also is able to influence activity within the axis. Noradrenergic input from neurons whose cell bodies reside in the brain stem locus coeruleus acts as a permissive factor, allowing other processes to proceed. Excess or insufficient input will adversely affect axis functions. γ-Aminobutyric acid (GABA) and opioid input have inhibitory roles, as dose increasing the activity of CRH neurons.

In the females of all mammalian species, an abrupt rise in the blood concentrations of LH serves as a trigger for the process of ovulation. Those species that give birth to live young have been traditionally dichotomized into spontaneous or induced ovulators. Spontaneous ovulators (e.g., rat, mouse, hamster, guinea pig, dog, horse, cow, sheep, human, and nonhuman primates) undergo hormonally regulated ovarian cycles at recurrent intervals. Some cycles, as those in dogs, exhibit periods of anestrus with minimal ovarian activity between cycles. Such anestrous intervals may be seasonal, as in sheep and horses. In contrast to spontaneous ovulators, induced ovulators (e.g., rabbits, cats, ferrets, mink, voles, llamas, and camels) show a surge of LH and ovulate in response to sensory stimuli associated with mating. However, there are various examples of different regularly cycling species (Jöchle, 1975) undergoing ovulatory induction. Female rats, for example, that exhibit a persistent anestrus under constant light exposure can be induced to ovulate by coitis (Brown-Grant et al., 1973).

23.4.3.1.1 Gonadotropin-Releasing Hormone

GnRH (also referred to as LH-releasing hormone [LHRH]) is a decapeptide that is cleaved post-translationally to its final form from a higher molecular weight prohormone.

In evolutionary terms, GnRH is an ancient peptide and forms have been identified in a wide range of invertebrates, including mollusks, nematodes, and even coral (reviewed by Kah et al., 2007). As the name indicates, mammalian GnRH acts to stimulate the pituitary secretion of the gonadotropins, LH, and FSH. In primitive species, it is believed to initiate gamete release either directly or indirectly by an effect on nerve cells. In mammals, GnRH neurons migrate during embryogenesis

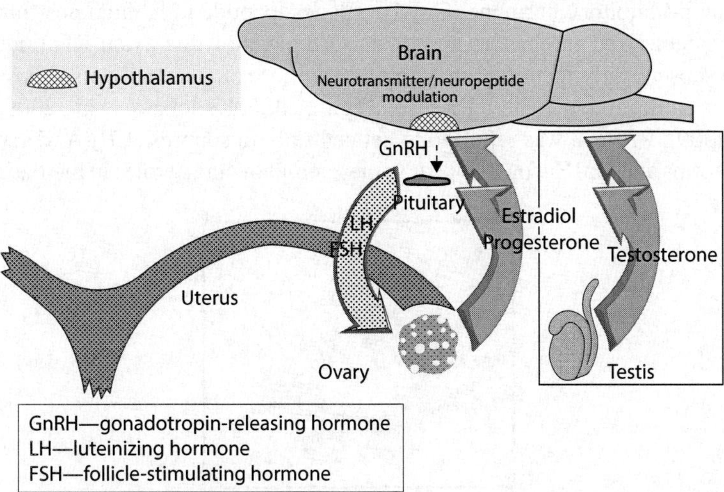

FIGURE 23.3 Using the rat as a representative example, the hypothalamic–pituitary–ovarian axis showing stimulatory and feedback relationships among gonadotropin-releasing hormone (GnRH), LH/follicle-stimulating hormone (FSH), and estradiol and progesterone. Feedback from the testis in the male to pituitary and hypothalamus is shown in the box at the right.

from the olfactory placode into the brain, ending their journey in the rostral portion of the hypothalamus (Schwanzel-Fukuda and Pfaff, 1989; Torbet et al., 1997). Nerve fibers from these cell bodies reach the median eminence at the base of the brain (Figure 23.4) where the hormone is released from terminals into a discrete grouping of portal vessels that descend to the anterior pituitary. Although GnRH has been found to bind to gonadal receptors (e.g., Bourne et al., 1980; Clayton et al., 1980; Uemura et al., 1994), systemic circulating concentrations are uniformly low, frequently difficult to quantify accurately and are typically of limited diagnostic value. In mammalian females that exhibit recurring ovarian cycles, a shift in the pulsatile secretion of GnRH in response to ovarian steroid feedback parallels a large surge in the release of both gonadotropins from the pituitary (e.g., Clarke et al., 1987; Gore, 2002). Castrated, testosterone-replaced males also show an increase in responsiveness (defined as an increase in the expression of LH subunit mRNA) that is dependent upon the frequency of exogenously applied pulses of GnRH (Haisenleder et al., 1987).

In mammals, two forms of GnRH, designated types I and II, have been found in distinct GnRH neurons and differ one from the other by three amino acid residues. The functional relationship between these two forms, GnRH-I and GnRH-II, still remains to be completely resolved (Pawson et al., 2003; Urbanski, 2012), although there is recent evidence in female rhesus macaques that these two types of neurons respond differently to estradiol (Urbanski, 2015). The data suggest that it is the GnRH-II neurons that play a predominant role in stimulating the female ovulatory surge of LH described in Section 4.3.1.2.

One type of input to GnRH neurons has now emerged as a major factor in GnRH secretion. Kisspeptin peptides released from neurons (termed KiSS1 neurons) concentrated in the hypothalamic periventricular region appear to be the most potent endogenous stimuli for GnRH release that serves to initiate the LH surge. They were originally identified as metastatic inhibitors in cultures of human melanoma cells and are members of the growing RFamide family of peptides that contain the Arg–Phe–NH_2 sequence at their amino-terminus. Fibers from these neurons have been demonstrated to terminate at GnRH neurons, and the secreted kisspeptins bind there to resident G-protein receptors (GPR54 receptors, currently designated as KiSS1 receptors), triggering pro-GnRH synthesis and GnRH secretion into the portal vasculature (e.g., Navarro et al., 2005; Seminara, 2007). Moreover, in mammals, it now appears that this relationship between kisspeptins and GnRH is a major factor in the transition through puberty (Kuohung and Kaiser, 2006). Another hypothalamic RFamide neuropeptide has recently been found to exert a suppressive effect on GnRH secretion. This gonadotropin-inhibitory hormone (GnIH), a dodecapeptide in its final posttranslational form, was initially characterized in chicken and quail. Orthologs of this avian RFamide (RFRP-1 and RFRP-3) were subsequently identified in a growing number of mammalian species, including rats, hamsters, sheep, cattle, and primates (Kriegsfeld et al., 2006; Kadokawa et al., 2009; Tsutsui, 2009; Ubuka et al., 2009); RFRP-3 was reported to act centrally to suppress LH (Anderson et al., 2009). Both the kisspeptins and GnIH would appear to play complementary roles in mediating the feedback

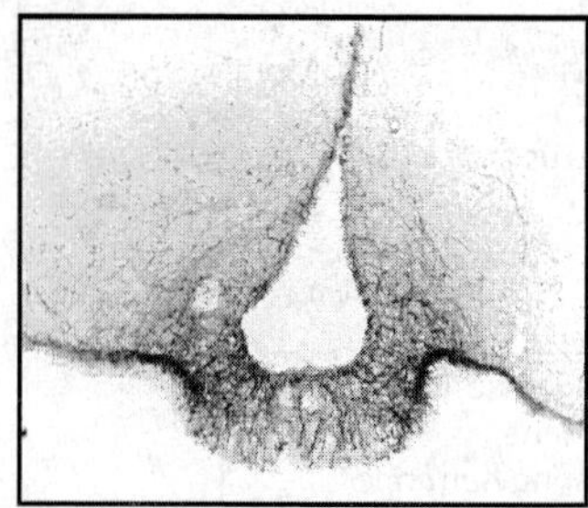

FIGURE 23.4 Photomicrograph of the rat median eminence, located at the base of the third ventricle. It is the site of release for hormones that in turn affect the secretion of the various pituitary peptide hormones. This particular image shows immunostaining of GnRH axons that project from neuronal cell bodies located primarily within a region termed the organum vasculosum of the lamina terminalis.

effects of sex steroids at the hypothalamus (Kriegsfeld, 2006; Wahab et al., 2015), although the complex of relationships in mammals among GnRH, kisspeptins, neurotransmitters/neuromodulators, and these GnIH orthologs under different physiological conditions still remains to be clarified.

23.4.3.1.2 Luteinizing Hormone and Follicle-Stimulating Hormone

LH is a glycoprotein that is composed of two α- and β-subunits connected by disulfide bridges. The α-subunits are common to both LH and FSH, along with TSH, whereas the β-subunits differ among the three hormones and confer specific biologic action in response to binding to their hormone-associated receptors. The α-subunit has been preserved throughout evolution, with some modifications in amino acid sequences. In an extension of the work cited above, demonstrating a relationship between GnRH pulse frequency and LH subunit transcription, Burger et al. (2008) have indicated that differential changes in pulse frequency regulate the transcription of either the β-subunit for LH (8–60-minute pulse intervals) or the β-subunit for FSH (>120-minute pulse intervals). Subunits of LH and the other glycoprotein hormones contain oligosaccharides that show different degrees of sulfation and sialylation, the basis for multiple isoforms of each hormone (Wilson et al., 1990a). This also results in a charge heterogeneity, with the more sialylated forms being more acidic and having longer circulatory half-lives (e.g., Burgon et al., 1996; Ulloa-Aguirre et al., 1999). On the other hand, the less sialylated variants exhibit higher receptor binding and greater biological activity (Ulloa-Aguirre et al., 2001a), although at least one oligosaccharide moiety is required for the full expression of bioactivity (Sairam, 1989). Families of LH isoforms have been described in humans (Ulloa-Aguirre et al., 2001b), nonhuman primates (Khan et al., 1985), horses (Irvine, 1979), pigs (Nomura et al., 1989), sheep (Keel et al., 1987), goats (Rojas-Maya et al., 2007), cattle (Zalesky and Grotjan, 1991), and rodents (Robertson et al., 1982). The relative proportions of these isoforms in males and females are not stable and are influenced by alterations in the endogenous steroid milieu.

LH principally functions in the male to promote the production of androgens in the testes. In the female, it stimulates ovarian follicular androgen synthesis. Aromatase activity then converts the androgens to estrogens. As indicated above, females who are spontaneous ovulators show a distinctive large midcycle surge of LH that serves to initiate the final stages of follicular and oocytic maturation that culminate in the release of one or more oocytes. Female rats have a cycle of 4–5 days and will typically ovulate 10–12 hours after the surge. In dogs, ovulation will take place about 48 hours from the surge peak (Bouchard et al., 1991). For rhesus monkeys, the time between the onset of the surge and follicle rupture is 36–40 hours (Stouffer, 2002), while the interval from the peak LH concentration to ovulation was reported to be approximately 22 hours (Pauerstein et al., 1978). Cats are considered to be induced ovulators, but have a cycle of 2–3 weeks, with a seasonal anestrus during the short days of autumn and winter. As in rabbits, they will only show a surge and ovulation in response to male cervical stimulation. The rise in LH in cats occurs within minutes of copulation, and ovulation will take place within 24–32 hours post coitum (Shille et al., 1983), whereas the postcopulatory interval in rabbits is about 11–12 hours (Milligan, 1982). For induced ovulators, genital stimulation activates brainstem noradrenergic neurons, which project to the hypothalamus to promote the secretion of GnRH from median eminence nerve terminals (Caba et al., 2000; Bakker and Baum, 2000). This pathway in primate, rodent, and canine spontaneous ovulators is also a component of the mechanisms involved in the secretion of GnRH (see Section 23.4.4.4).

The LH surge, then, is a functional endocrine event, and a suppression will block ovulation (discussed below in Section 23.4.3.1.5). Eliminating recognition of GnRH pulses by the pituitary with a constant exposure to elevated GnRH concentrations will cause a desensitization of the mechanisms of LH secretion. This would effectively suppress the gonadotropins and cause a chemical castration. In young girls exhibiting a precocious puberty caused by a premature activation of hypothalamic GnRH neurons, the administration of long-acting GnRH agonists has been used to postpone the emergence of menses, ovulation, and secondary sexual development (reviewed by Mansfield et al.,

1983; Boepple et al., 1986; Mul and Hughes, 2008). In precocious puberty, these agonists also serve to slow the increased maturational tempo of skeletal growth that would then be followed by an accelerated senescence at the bone growth plates.

As previously mentioned, the second gonadotropin, FSH, is also a glycoprotein, sharing a common α-subunit with LH. Both are secreted from gonadotrophs in the anterior pituitary and together in the mammalian female serve a coordinate function. LH functions to trigger the final maturational changes in ovarian follicles that conclude in ovulation. FSH, following a surge-like rise and fall, stimulates the growth of a cohort of immature follicles to a mature preovulatory stage to await action by a surge of LH during the next cycle. In the male, FSH supports the function of the testicular Sertoli cells, which sustain the maturing spermatozoa. FSH receptor knockout mice show underdeveloped testes, poor sperm quality, and a 50% reduction in Sertoli cells (Krishnamurthy et al., 2000; Sairam and Krishnamurthy, 2001).

As a glycoprotein, FSH also exists as different isoforms. When compared to LH, it tends to contain more sialic acid moieties on its oligosaccharide structures (Ulloa-Aguirre et al., 1995; Green and Baenziger, 1988), consequently increasing its circulating half-life. In adult male rats, multiple isoforms exhibited half-lives between 13 minutes and several hours, with the longer-lived forms that were more heavily sialylated predominating (Blum and Gupta, 1985).

23.4.3.1.3 Gonadal Hormones

The steroidogenic pathway synthesizing the sex steroids begins with the translocation of cholesterol from the outer to the inner mitochondrial membrane. This is a rate-determining process involving a signaling complex composed of steroidogenic acute regulatory protein (StAR) and a translocator protein (the peripheral benzodiazepine receptor) (Liu et al., 2006). After transport through the membrane, cholesterol is converted to pregnenolone by cytochrome P450scc (P450 side chain cleavage, or CYP11A) before entering the Δ4 or Δ5 pathway (Figure 23.5). In the Δ4 path, pregnenolone is converted first to progesterone by 3β-hydroxysteroid dehydrogenase (3β-HSD) and then to 17α-hydroxyprogesterone. In the Δ5 direction, 17α-hydroxylase/17,20 lyase (CYP17) converts pregnenolone to 17α-hydroxypregnenolone and dihydroepiandrosterone. Species differences exist in the substrate preferences of the 17,20 lyase. In humans (Weusten et al., 1987), rabbits, dogs, and cows (Fortune, 1986), the preferred substrate is 17α-hydroxypregnenolone; whereas, in the rodent (Brock and Waterman, 1999), ferret (Kintner and Mead, 1983), chicken, mare, and some macaques (Weusten et al., 1990), the preference is for 17α-hydroxyprogesterone. This preference can be influenced by shifts in concentrations of other hormones. For example, in hamster preovulatory ovarian follicles, Δ5 predominates before and up to 2 hours after exposure in vitro to LH. There then occurs a switch to the Δ4 direction as the major pathway (Makris et al., 1983), markedly increasing the formation of progesterone from exogenously provided pregnenolone. Both paths will generate androstenedione, which can then be converted to testosterone by the action of 17β-hydroxysteroid dehydrogenase (17β-HSD), or to estrone by P450arom (P450aromatase, CYP19). CYP19 will also catalyze testosterone to estradiol, whereas estrone and estradiol can be interconverted by 17β-HSD. In the prostate, 5α-reductase will catalyze the production of 5α-DHT from testosterone.

23.4.3.1.3.1 Estrogens As mentioned above, the two most common circulating estrogens are estradiol and estrone. A third, estriol, is short acting and in women likely has some role in parturition (e.g., Inoue et al., 1971; Lintner et al., 1988), being produced in large quantities by the feto-placental unit during the latter stages of pregnancy. The affinity of estriol to the estrogen receptor, however, is reduced relative to the other estrogens. 17β-Estradiol is the principal estrogen and is produced in ovarian granulosa cells from androgen precursors transported from the thecal layer (see Figure 23.6a). During particular segments of the estrous/menstrual cycle, it serves to increase the responsiveness of participating hypothalamic mechanisms, a shift possibly associated with a lessening of an inhibitory restraint on GnRH neuronal activity (Gibson et al., 2008). In addition, estradiol (a) has a role in pubertal development and

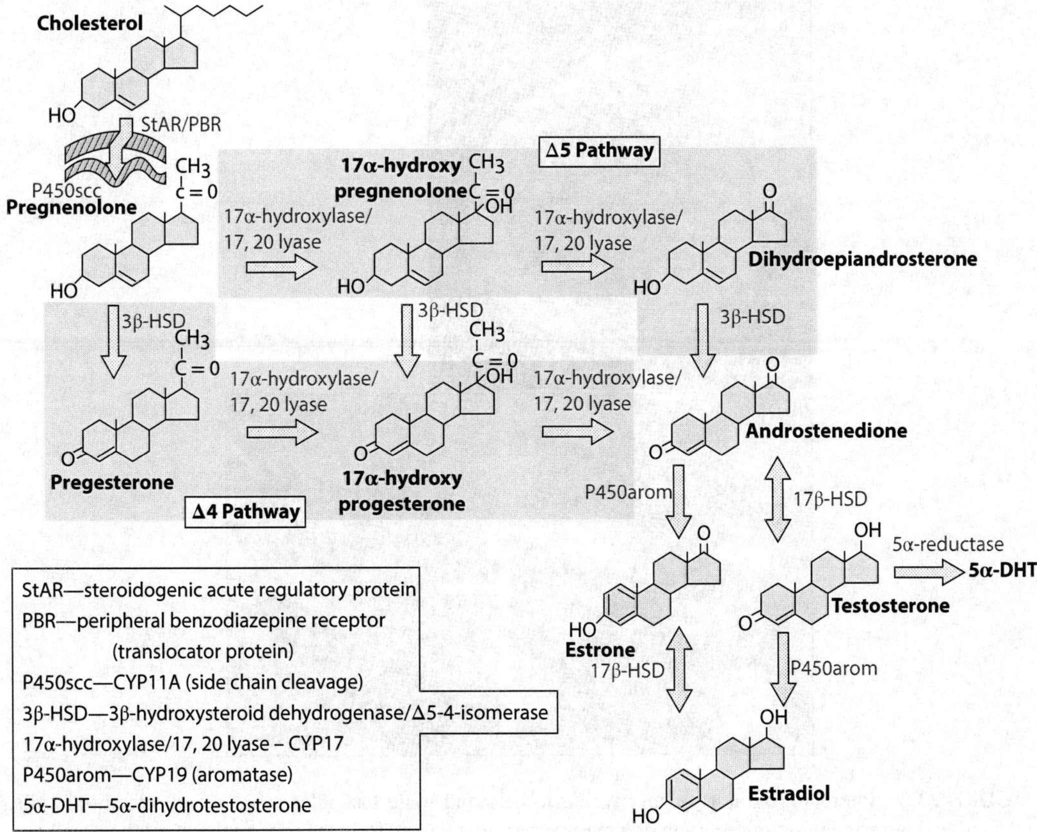

FIGURE 23.5 Steroidogenic pathway, depicting cholesterol transport from the outer to the inner mitochondrial membrane, with steps up through the synthesis of the testosterone, estrone, and estradiol. Both the Δ4 and Δ5 paths (see text) are shown against a shaded background. (Redrawn from Elsevier Press, Vol. 11, 2nd edition, Perreault, S.D. et al., Targeting female reproductive function during follicular maturation, ovulation, and fertilization: Critical windows for pharmaceutical or toxicant action, pp. 399–417, 2010, with permission from Elsevier.)

sexual behavior (e.g., Ojeda et al., 1983, 1986), (b) induces progesterone receptors to prepare the uterine endometrium for the action of progesterone (e.g., Okulicz et al., 1989; Kurita et al., 2001), (c) plays an important role in regulating the uterine immune system (Wira and Sullivan, 1981), (d) helps maintain the size and density of mammary tissue (e.g., Pompei et al., 2005; Fendrick et al., 1998), although excess amounts will increase the risk of some forms of breast cancer, (e) decreases the development and activity of bone-clearing osteoclast cells and increases the bone-building ability of osteoblast cells (e.g., Lafferty et al., 1964; Ernst et al., 1988; Saintier et al., 2006), and (f) acts as a neuroprotective factor within the brain (e.g., Green et al., 2001; Fujita et al., 2006). In laboratory animals, estradiol is also known to affect food intake, acting as a modulatory factor to decrease consumption. Daily food intake in female rats will differ over the estrous cycle, with the lowest consumption taking place during the periovulatory period, when circulating estradiol concentrations show proestrus peaks and then begin to fall over the evening transition to estrus (e.g., Asarian and Geary, 2006). Gonadectomized females will eat more, in contrast to gonadectomized males, who will decrease their consumption (Gentry and Wade, 1976; Chai et al., 1999). During meals, a peptide hormone, cholecystokinin, is released from the small intestine and binds to receptors in the brain, providing satiety signals. Results from studies using ovariectomized rats have demonstrated that estradiol will increase the potency of exogenously administered cholecystokinin (Butera et al., 1993).

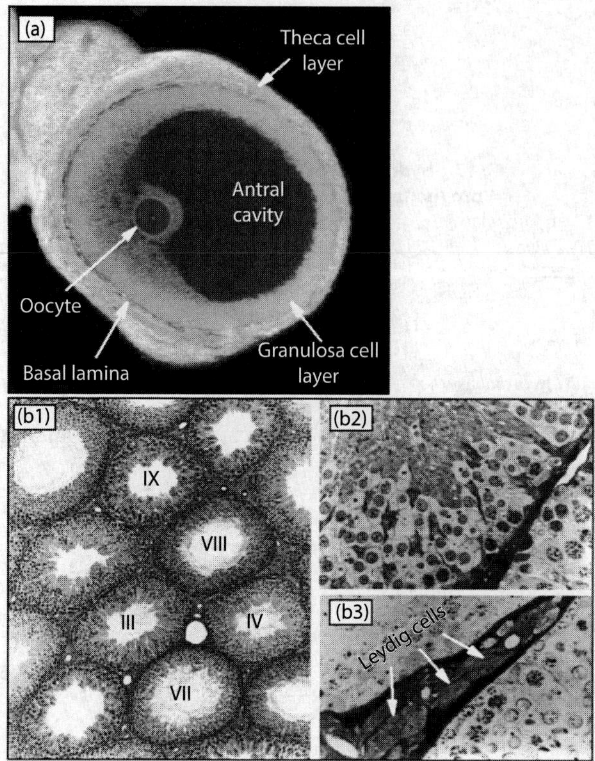

FIGURE 23.6 Photomicrographs of an ovarian follicle and male testicular tubules and interstitial cells. (a) Confocal laser scanning micrograph of a mature rat preovulatory follicle showing the outer theca cell layers and inner granulosa cells separated by the basal lamina. The oocyte, within the antral cavity, is surrounded by cumulous cells. (b1) Photomicrograph of tubules within the rat testis are shown at different maturational stages of spermiation designated with roman numerals; (b2) An enlarged portion of seminiferous epithelium of one tubule containing spermatocytes and Sertoli cells; (b3) A further enlargement of the interstitial space between tubules showing the testosterone-secreting Leydig cells. (Testicular images courtesy of Dr. Gary Klinefelter, US EPA, Follicular image in (a). Reprinted from Elsevier Press, Vol. 11, 2nd edition, Perreault, S.D. et al., Targeting female reproductive function during follicular maturation, ovulation, and fertilization: Critical windows for pharmaceutical or toxicant action, pp. 399–417, 2010, with permission from Elsevier.)

A single intravenous administration of ^{3}H-17β-estradiol in the female rat showed two component clearance curves. The first pool was cleared relatively rapidly (5.5 minutes, plasma half-life), while the second pool disappeared more slowly (half-life of 31 minutes in plasma) (Littleton and Anderson, 1972). Table 23.1 shows metabolic clearance rates (MCR, expressed as L/day/kg) for estradiol in female rat, rabbit, dog, and nonhuman primates.

In the cell nucleus, signaling by estrogens is mediated by two types of evolutionarily conserved receptors, estrogen receptor-α (ERα), and estrogen receptor-β (ERβ), which are produced from separate genes located on different chromosomes (Pavao and Traish, 2001). Both are members of the nuclear receptor family of transcription factors and serve to translocate estrogens into the cell nucleus to link with DNA. In a form unbound to its estrogen ligand, cytosolic estrogen receptors are associated with a complex of chaperones, including heat-shock protein 90, which maintains the receptor in an inactive condition, but prepared for binding to the hormone (Pratt and Toft, 1997). Estrogen receptors can also be present in the plasma membrane and induce a rapid nongenomic signal (e.g., Márquez and Pietras, 2001; Micevych and Mermelstein, 2008). ERα and ERβ can coexist in populations of neurons, although they also show distinctive distributions and selectivity to estrogenic compounds in addition to a differential transcriptional regulation (Laflamme et al., 1998; Shughrue et al., 1998; Haeger et al.,

TABLE 23.1
Metabolic Clearance Rates (L/day/kg) of Gonadal Steroid Hormones in Various Animals

	Rabbit	Rat	Dog	Nonhuman Primate
Testosterone—males	[a]42 ± 8 (Bourget et al., 1984 [intact, *inf*]) [a]39 ± 2.6 (Mahoudeau et al., 1973 [intact, *inf*])	[a]52.5 (Lee et al., 1975 [intact, *inf*]) [a]66 ± 17 (Heinrichs et al., 1979 [cast, *inf*])	[a]76 ± 37 (Tremblay et al., 1972 [intact, *inf*])	14 ± 2 (Franz and Longcope, 1979 [intact, inf]) (rhesus) 7.4 ± 0.6 (Bourget et al., 1988 [intact, inf]) (cynomolgus) 8.2 ± 0.4 (Heinrichs et al., 1979 [cast, *inf*]) (rhesus) 7.1 ± 1.8 (Heinrichs et al., 1979 [cast, *inf*]) (rhesus)
Estradiol—females	[a]88 (Fraser et al., 1976 [intact, *inf*])	[a]129 ± 46 (Petroff and Mizinga, 2003 [ovx, *inj*])	136 ± 8 (Longcope et al., 1980 [intact, p *inj*]) [a]51 ± 14 (Dupuy et al., 1982 [intact, *inf*])	30 ± 5.2 (Longcope et al., 1988 [ovx, *inf*]) (baboon)
Progesterone—females	[a]130 ± 10 (Corbo et al., 1988 [intact, *inj*])	[a]27 ± 7.8 (Petroff and Mizinga, 2003 [ovx, *inj*]) [a]66 ± 10 (Corbo et al., 1988 [intact, *inj*]) [a]76 (Mannino et al., 2005 [ovx., *silast*])	88 ± 6 (Runic et al., 1976 [pregnant, *inj*])	87 ± 6 (Albrecht and Townsley, 1976 [intact, *inf*]) (baboon) 53 ± 3.5 (Albrecht and Townsley, 1976 [intact, *inf*]) (baboon)

Note: Published metabolic clearance rates (L/day/kg ± SEM, if available) of testosterone in male; estradiol and progesterone in female rabbits, rats, dogs, and nonhuman primates determined by constant infusion (*inf*), single injection (*inj*), pulse injection (*p inj.*), or silastic implant (*silast*).

[a] Indicates values where L/day have been extrapolated to L/day/kg based on animal weights stated in the publication. cast, castrated; ovx, ovariectomized.

2006). ERα is now understood to mediate effects of estradiol on the hypothalamic periventricular kisspeptin neurons that coordinate with GnRH in initiating the LH surge (Roa et al., 2008).

In males, the presence of testicular aromatase activity (Dorrington et al., 1978; Valladares and Payne, 1979) and concentrations of male gonadal fluid estrogens in various species (e.g., Ganjam and Amann, 1976; Eiler and Graves, 1977; Claus et al., 1992) have been reported since the 1970s. Estrogen receptors are also present in testicular tissue. Of the two estrogen receptor subtypes, ERβ appears to be much more prevalent than ERα (Saunders et al., 1998; Nie et al., 2002). The function of male gonadal estrogens is still unclear, but they may play some role within the efferent ductules positioned between the rete testis and caput region of the epididymis, contributing to the reabsorption of rete testis fluid that concentrates sperm prior to their entry into the tubules of the epididymis (Hess, 2003), the structure in which sperm gain motility and fertilizing capacity.

23.4.3.1.3.2 Progesterone The name progesterone is a compilation of the term *progestational steroidal ketone* (Allen, 1970). Discovered in the 1930s, it is synthesized from pregnenolone by the action of 3β-HSD (see Figure 23.5) and is a product of both ovarian granulosa and adrenal cortical cells (e.g., Armstrong, 1968; De Geyter et al., 2002) and placenta (e.g., Schubert and Schade, 1977), in addition to some synthesis by brain astrocytes (Micevych and Sinchak, 2008) and cerebellar Purkinje cells (Tsutsui, 2008). It binds to a receptor that exists in three isoforms (Kastner et al., 1990; Wei et al., 1997), each with a high affinity for the hormone and each having a differential specificity for target genes in the nucleus.

Work performed in the rat has shown that the disappearance curve for progesterone consists of two components (Pepe and Rothchild, 1973). The first component is rapidly cleared, with a half-life in ovariectomized females of 2.7 minutes, whereas the second disappears more slowly, having a half-life of 18 minutes. In the cow, this can range up to 36 minutes (Pineda, 2003). MCRs for progesterone in L/day/kg body weight for female rabbit, rat, dog, and nonhuman primate are listed in Table 23.1.

As is true for estradiol, progesterone serves a number of functions. It (a) prepares the uterus to receive the embryo (e.g., Glasser and Clark, 1975; Yochim, 1986), (b) maintains the uterus during pregnancy (Csapo and Wiest, 1969; Takayama and Greenwald, 1972), (c) stimulates mammary gland growth (e.g., Humphreys et al., 1997; Ismail et al., 2003), (d) acts to increase the loss of sodium in the kidney (e.g.,Wambach and Higgins, 1978), (e) has a mild catabolic effect (Landau and Lugibihl, 1961a,b), and (f) is involved in mechanisms regulating gonadotropin secretion (e.g., Karsch, 1987; Evans et al., 2002). During pregnancy, an increased level of progesterone receptor transcriptional activity maintains a uterine quiescence (Mendelson and Condon, 2005). In pregnancies of subprimate placental mammals, a significant fall in circulating progesterone occurs near term (reviewed by Zakar and Hertelendy, 2007). As contractions increase at labor, all progesterone receptor isoforms show a sharp decrease (Goldman et al., 2005), which parallels a series of biochemical events that serve to lower progesterone receptor function (Mendelson and Condon, 2005).

Over the course of the normal ovarian cycle in regularly cycling mammals, the feedback of ovarian estradiol (augmented by progesterone) sensitizes or upregulates the hypothalamic mechanisms stimulating the increase in the pulsatile release of GnRH from the median eminence into the portal vessels, triggering the LH surge. It has been argued that the role of estradiol in the surge is secondary to that of progesterone (Zalányi, 2001), with estradiol feedback serving to increase the production of hypothalamic neuroprogesterone (Micevych et al., 2003; Micevych and Sinchak, 2008). Around the appearance of the surge, progesterone rises in concert with the fall in estradiol. In dogs, the elevation has been reported to be greater than 100-fold over the anestrous nadir (Olson et al., 1982). Circulating concentrations secreted from ovulated follicles (transformed to corpora lutea) will initiate a series of cellular changes in the uterine endothelia, both permitting embryonic blastocysts to adhere initially to the endometrial surface of the uterus and inducing a decidualization of endometrial stromal fibroblasts that converts them into secretory cells to provide the blastocyts with early nutrient support as they penetrate and settle within the endometrium. If the implantation of one or more fertilized ova takes place, the progesterone will remain elevated and serve to maintain the pregnancy and also suppressing the LH surges during this time. If implantation does not occur, the corpora lutea will undergo luteolysis, and progesterone levels will decline, removing the restraint on the ovulatory LH stimulus. In fact, a number of third generation progestin-only oral contraceptives for women have been demonstrated to target the hypothalamus and pituitary, mimicking this progesterone restraint on the surge and ovulation (Faundes et al., 1991; Couzinet et al., 1999).

An additional source of progesterone is the placenta, and there are marked species differences in the relative contributions of luteal and placental progesterone in pregnancy maintenance. For example, in the pig, goat, dog, and rat, the progesterone secreted from the corpora lutea is required throughout the pregnancy, whereas a shift to placental progesterone during the second half of pregnancy occurs in the ewe and mare (reviewed by Geisert and Conley, 1998).

23.4.3.1.3.3 Testosterone Testosterone, the principal male sex steroid, is synthesized from androstenedione by the action of 17β-hydroxysteroid dehydrogenase and has a reported half-life in the rat of about 30 minutes (Nett, 1989). In the male, it is secreted from the interstitial Leydig cells within the testis (Figures 23.6b1 through 23.6b3). In the female testosterone produced in the ovarian theca cells is transported into the granulosa cell layer (Figure 23.6a), where it is aromatized to estradiol. The growth and differentiated function of the Leydig cells are dependent upon the stimulatory effect of LH from the pituitary (Ewing and Zirkin, 1983). Within the prostate, testosterone is rapidly converted to a number of metabolites, the major one being DHT. MCRs for testosterone in male rabbit, rat, dog, and nonhuman primate are shown in Table 23.1.

The primary action of androgens is to regulate gene expression through the androgen receptor (AR), which, like the estrogen receptors, belongs to the superfamily of nuclear receptors. Two isoforms of the AR (A and B) exist. They appear to be structurally similar to the two progesterone receptor isoforms (Wilson and McPhaul, 1996). The B isoform is present in much lower levels than the A form, and its role is unclear. As is the case for the other sex steroids, when the AR is inactive, it is bound to heat-shock proteins in the cytoplasm. Binding of testosterone to the receptor dissociates the heat-shock proteins, and the hormone-bound receptor is translocated into the nucleus to activate genes involved in cell growth (e.g., Veldscholte et al., 1992; Zoubeidi et al., 2007).

In the male, testosterone is the androgenic hormone that is primarily responsible for the normal growth and development of male reproductive organs and spermatogenesis (e.g., Sharpe et al., 1990; Kerr et al., 1993; Walker, 2009), along with the development of secondary sexual characteristics. A suppression of testosterone in male rats caused a depletion of elongated spermatids that is apparently due to a detachment of the round spermatid precursors from their association with testicular Sertoli cells (O'Donnell et al., 1996), which normally provide nutritional and structural support (Figure 23.6b3) for germ cell spermatogenic maturation. The hormone promotes protein biosynthesis that underlies the hormone's anabolic characteristics. As such, it accelerates the building of muscle (Florini, 1970), increases erythropoiesis (Fisher et al., 1971), promotes the catabolism of body fat (Xu et al., 1990), and shortens the recovery time after injuries (Ehrlich and Hunt, 1969; Brown et al., 1999). In prostate, DHT is the principal androgen that stimulates normal prostatic development, growth, and function (e.g., Tenniswood et al., 1982). In men, the production of DHT is also involved in androgenic pattern baldness, although this condition appears to have no homolog in nonhuman primates, and an androgen-associated alopecia normally is absent in other species. Dog hair follicles only exhibit a minor conversion of DHT from testosterone (Bamberg et al., 2004). In mice, treatment with DHT has been reported to affect hair follicle growth, and AR knockout mice show fur that is longer and thicker than wildtype littermates (Naito et al., 2008).

23.4.3.1.4 Activins, Inhibins, and Follistatin

Although not typically presented as components of the hypothalamic–pituitary–gonadal (H–P–G) axes, the integrated actions of activin, inhibin, and follistatin hormones contribute to homeostatic regulation of the reproductive system in both males and females. Both activin and inhibin are dimeric glycoproteins that have a similar β-subunit, with activin being a homodimer (β/β-subunits) and inhibin a heterodimer (α/β-subunits). The β-subunits have been shown to exhibit a remarkable degree of homology across mammalian species and show a good deal of structural conservation throughout vertebrate evolution (Ge et al., 1993). The two glycoproteins are both members of the transforming growth factor-β (TGF-β) superfamily, which acts to modulate growth and developmental processes in most tissues, including the pituitary. They were originally discovered to stimulate (activins) or inhibit (inhibins) the secretion of FSH (for review, see Vale et al., 1990), although gene expression is present elsewhere, including mammary and adrenal tissues. In mammary tissue, activin is generally characterized as an inhibitor of cell proliferation, since activin treatment in vitro will arrest the growth of breast cancer cells (Reis et al., 2004). Beyond a role in FSH secretion, it appears to participate as an early component of the inflammatory cascade (Phillips et al., 2005).

Activin is present in two biologically active forms, A and B (Vale et al., 1990). Activin A has been shown to have marked stimulatory effects on the secretion of pituitary FSH that principally occur via gene transcription of the FSH β-subunit (Suszko et al., 2003). In male rat gonads, activin A is produced in the seminiferous epithelium, particularly in Sertoli cells. In the testes, activin A predominantly has a local paracrine action, regulating Sertoli cell number and germ cell maturation (e.g., de Kretser et al., 2001; Sofikitis et al., 2008). It may have a similar paracrine effect on FSH, since subunits are expressed locally in adult pituitary gland (Roberts et al., 1989). In the female rodent, activin A is produced in granulosa cells and has a stimulatory effect on granulosa cell proliferation and the growth of preantral follicles (Findlay et al., 2001). As in the male, it likely serves a similar local regulatory effect on pituitary FSH. The contributions of activin B to gonadal activity are still unclear, although some evidence suggests that it also plays a paracrine role in pituitary FSH production (Corrigan et al., 1991). Greater clarification requires the development of more specific activin B immunoassays, which have now only begun to appear (Ludlow et al., 2008).

Whereas activin stimulates the synthesis of FSH and its secretion from pituitary gonadotropes, the inhibins act as potent activin antagonists. There are two forms of inhibin, A and B, which have inhibitory effects on ovarian folliculogenesis (Findlay, 1993) and pituitary FSH secretion (Woodruff et al., 1993). In males, inhibin production by Sertoli cells provides endocrine feedback to the pituitary to antagonize activin signaling in gonadotropes. Increased inhibin-like immunoreactivity was reported in dogs with a Sertoli cell tumor that correlated with reductions in FSH, LH, and testosterone concentrations (Peters et al., 2000). Inhibin A and B antagonism of activin is mediated by membrane polysaccharides known as betaglycans that act as co-receptors (Lewis et al., 2000; Chapman et al., 2002), so that a stable complex is formed with activin receptors and interferes with the ability of activin to bind. The extent of inhibin glycosylation will decrease its bioactivity, something that is apparently due to a reduced affinity for betaglycan (Makanji et al., 2007).

The third of the glycoproteins in this category of FSH regulatory factors is follistatin. These molecules are ubiquitous throughout the body in nearly all higher animals and in the pituitary are produced by the folliculostellate cells (Gospodarowicz and Lau, 1989). Over the reproductive cycle, they act in conjunction with the activins to adjust a differential production of FSH from gonadotropes via their ability bind activins and bioneutralize them. Two molecules of follistatin have been reported to envelop the activin dimer, covering a large portion of its surface and preventing activin from associating with its receptor (Thompson et al., 2005).

23.4.3.1.5 *Pathological Alterations in the H–P–G Axis*

Adverse effects on the process of ovulation can be the result of insult to one or more sites within the H–P–G axis. A direct impairment in the hypothalamic mechanisms underlying the increase in the secretion of GnRH is not subject to in-life assessments, particularly since concentrations of GnRH entering the circulation are frequently too low to assess by common immunological methods. Alternatively, plasma or serum levels of the gonadotropins are measurable and can often provide valuable information, since they are conveyed to the gonads via the general circulation. In cycling females, alterations in the midcycle LH and FSH surges can be assessed by serially sampling blood (or possibly urinary [Jeffcoate and England, 1997]) gonadotropin concentrations over the over the normal window of appearance. A number of compounds, including opiates, dithiocarbamate, and formamidine pesticides, shown to target mechanisms of GnRH secretion will suppress the LH surge and block an ensuing ovulation (e.g., Gosden et al., 1976; Parvizi et al., 1976; Hagino, 1979; Goldman and Cooper, 1993, 2010; Goldman et al., 1994, 2008; Cooper et al., 2000; Stoker et al., 2005).

A distinction between a primary site of impairment within an endocrine axis and one that represents a secondary response to the primary insult can often be made by evaluating whether stimulation can elicit a normal endocrine response from components of the axis. For example, a single exposure in female rats to the fungicide metam sodium (sodium N-methyldithiocarbamate) during a sensitive window hours prior to the anticipated appearance of the LH surge was found to block the surge and ovulation (Goldman et al., 1994). Its effectiveness when administered during this time indicated that the primary target was either at the level of the hypothalamus or the pituitary. In this case, a concurrent treatment with GnRH was able to overcome the effect of metam sodium and induce a normal ovulatory response, indicating that the hypothalamus and not the pituitary was the target site for the insult.

In the normally functioning male H–P–G axis, normal gonadotropin and steroid concentrations, along with spermatogenesis, are under close regulation. Dysfunctional alterations in the hypothalamus or pituitary can lower the circulating gonadotropin and testosterone concentrations, decreasing testicular stimulation and affecting sperm production. Conversely, should damage occur to the testes, for example by chemical or physical trauma, a decline in gonadal Leydig or Sertoli cell activity would cause a persistent gonadotropin elevation by lowering negative feedback to the pituitary. Such an elevation in response to two-week treatments with LH in both intact and hypophysectomized male rats, in addition to increasing testosterone production, caused Leydig cells to undergo hyperplastic alterations (Kerr and Sharpe, 1986; Mendis-Handagama et al., 1998).

Testicular Leydig and Sertoli cell tumors are both frequently found in mature and old dogs and in the latter can be as high as 60% (Mosier, 1989). In those dogs with Leydig cell tumors, circulating concentrations of LH were decreased and negatively correlated with testosterone, estradiol, and inhibin. Dogs with Sertoli cell tumors, as previously mentioned in Section 23.4.3.1.4 showed reductions in FSH, LH, and testosterone, along with increases in inhibin immunoreactivity (Peters et al., 2000).

Measures of male serum testosterone have been an integral part of assessments of insults caused by endocrine-disrupting chemicals. The alkylating agent ethane dimethane sulfonate (EDS) has been found to be a Leydig cell toxicant, and the resultant decline in testosterone in response to EDS exposure will eliminate the negative feedback and cause a rise in LH and FSH (Bartlett et al., 1986). A number of environmental toxicants (e.g., phthalates and dicarboximide fungicides) have also been found to act as antiandrogens. In developmental studies of male rats, the antagonism of AR activity has been reported to reduce anogenital distance, cause nipple retention, and induce genital malformations such as cleft phallus and hypospadias (Gray et al., 1994; Hotchkiss et al., 2002; Foster, 2006). Sertoli cell toxicants, such as 2,5-hexanedione, will induce long-lasting testicular atrophy with the almost complete absence of spermatogonia from seminiferous tubules (Allard and Boekelheide, 1996).

Pubertal development in both sexes can be affected by environmental compounds that interfere with those endocrine mechanisms underlying this transition to sexual maturity. The nonsteroidal estrogen, diethylstilbestrol, will advance puberty in female mice (Honma et al., 2002) and rats and disrupt subsequent estrous cyclicity (Nass et al., 1984). For reviews of the processes of normal pubertal development and the effects of endocrine disrupting chemicals on sexual maturity that have been a focus of the US Environmental Protection Agency (US EPA) under its Endocrine Disruptors Screening Program, the reader is referred to two companion monographs (Goldman et al., 2000; Stoker et al., 2000).

In the prostate, the binding of the androgen–nuclear receptor complex to androgen-regulated genes is essential for normal prostatic development and can also be responsible for the pathogenesis of the prostate neoplasms in humans and prostatic hyperplasia, for example, in humans, dogs, and rodents (e.g., Berry and Isaacs, 1984; Bartsch et al., 2002; Nantermet et al., 2004). In contrast, pharmacological agents with antiandrogenic properties can produce atrophy of the prostate (e.g., Iswaran et al., 1997; Mylchreest et al., 1998), in addition to Leydig cell hyperplasia due to the suppression of inhibitory testosterone feedback to the pituitary.

23.4.3.2 Hypothalamic–Pituitary–Adrenal Axis

The hypothalamic–pituitary–adrenal (H–P–A) axis is an endocrine unit that functions to maintain basal and stress-related homeostasis by incorporating a wide variety of signals. The integrative core components of the axis are hypothalamic corticotrophin-releasing hormone (CRH), pituitary ACTH, and the adrenal glucocorticoids (the corticotropins cortisol and/or corticosterone; Figure 23.7). Input to the axis from peripheral sympathetic neuronal activity, circulating cytokines (e.g., interleukins and tumor necrosis factor alpha), posterior pituitary hormones (oxytocin and vasopressin), and central noradrenergic stimulation will collectively initiate a behavioral reaction, encompassing what is

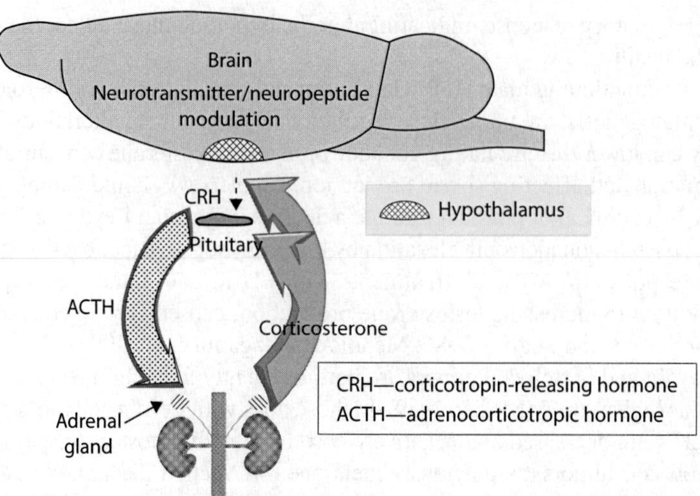

FIGURE 23.7 Representative rat hypothalamic–pituitary–adrenal axis depicting the relationships among corticotrophin-releasing hormone (CRH), adrenocorticotropic hormone (ACTH), and corticosterone, along with central modulatory effects from neurotransmitters and neuropeptides.

termed the stress response. In addition, activity within the H–P–A axis serves other roles beyond reactions to distress. For example, glucocorticoids have an important role both peripherally and centrally in the control of energy homeostasis by regulating carbohydrate and protein metabolism (e.g., Hopgood et al., 1981; McMahon et al., 1988; O'Callaghan et al., 1989; Wang, 2005).

23.4.3.2.1 Corticotropin-Releasing Hormone

CRH is a member of the corticoliberin family of related neuropeptides that includes the urocortins and urotensin. In evolutionary terms, its 41-amino acid sequence is fairly well conserved, with a primary structure that is identical in primates, carnivores, and rodents (Shibahara et al., 1983; Mol et al., 1994; Rivier et al., 1983). In the hypothalamus, it is first synthesized as a larger prohormone and then transported to nerve terminals in the median eminence for release into the portal vasculature, where it is conveyed to the pituitary, stimulating the secretion of ACTH. Measurements of CRH, using immunohistochemical methods, western blot peptide identification, or northern blot detection of the prohormone message are not performed "in-life," which make them much less useful than clinical assessments of other factors linked to correlative activity within the axis.

CRH and its related peptides are found in the gastrointestinal, cardiovascular, reproductive, and immune systems, being involved in a wide spectrum of stress-associated responses. Members of this family fall into one of three groupings based upon their receptor binding. The CRH subfamily will selectively bind to CRFR1 receptors, whereas urocortins II and III bind to CRFR2 receptors. Urocortin I and urotensin I are nonselective for the CRF receptors (Dautzenberg and Hauger, 2002). In mediating the stress response, the two CRF/urocortin receptors were found to have distinctive roles in both the regulation of behavioral reactions (Bale et al., 2002) and centrally and peripherally mediated energy homeostasis (Carlin et al., 2006; Kuperman and Chen, 2008). They show conspicuous differences in their distribution. The location of CRFR1 mRNA in mouse is basically comparable to that in rat and is widely expressed in the brain, predominating in the pituitary, cerebral cortex, arcuate nucleus, hippocampus, amygdala, olfactory bulb, and cerebellum. In the pituitary, rat and mouse displayed a CRFR1 mRNA signal throughout the intermediate lobe and in a subset of anterior lobe cells. The highest density of CRFR2 neuronal expression was found in the lateral septal nucleus, bed nucleus of the stria terminalis, ventromedial hypothalamic nucleus, olfactory bulb, amygdala, and mesencephalic raphe nuclei. In the pituitary, CRFR2 transcripts were expressed mainly in the posterior lobe (Van Pett et al., 2000).

23.4.3.2.2 *Adrenocorticotropic Hormone*

ACTH, also known as corticotropin, was the first pituitary hormone to be synthesized (Li et al., 1955). It is proteolytically cleaved from a larger glycosylated precursor protein, proopiomelanocortin (POMC), which is expressed in the pituitary by two cell types, corticotropic cells and melanotropic cells. In addition to ACTH, a variety of biologically active products are generated: β-lipotropin, α- and β-melanocyte stimulating hormones, and the endogenous opioids β-endorphin and met-enkephalin. POMC has likely emerged from an ancestral gene, and among mammalian species, there is a considerable degree of sequence homology in the active core of ACTH (e.g., Stewart and Channabasavaiah, 1979).

Classically, the role of ACTH is to stimulate the adrenal glands to release glucocorticoids in situations of stress. In this capacity, it stimulates the transcriptional activity of those genes involved throughout the steroidogenic pathway (e.g., Waterman and Bischof, 1996; Sewer and Waterman, 2003). In adrenal cortical cell cultures, cholesterol transport from the outer to the inner mitochondrial membrane was promptly enhanced following ACTH exposure, along within an increase in side chain cleavage activity (DiBartolomeis and Jefcoate, 1984). It also has indirect mitogenic effects on capillary epithelial cells. Adrenal cortical tissue is abundantly vascularized with a dense blood capillary network, and ACTH has been reported to be involved in the development of this vasculature via an induction of the angiogenic signaling protein, vascular endothelial growth factor (VEGF) (Thomas et al., 2003).

The presence of ACTH immunoreactivity in the brain was reported in the 1970s and 1980s (Larsson, 1978; Joseph, 1980), findings that have been observed, with some variation in ACTH fiber distribution, in a variety of mammalian species (e.g., Abrams et al., 1980; Coveñas et al., 1996; Pesini et al., 2004). The role of these fibers still remains to be elucidated, although there are apparent relationships to various neurotransmitter systems (Azmitia and de Kloet, 1987; Liang et al., 1992).

23.4.3.2.3 *Cortisol and Corticosterone*

The mammalian adrenal gland is composed of two developmentally dissimilar tissues, the adrenal cortex and a core region, the adrenal medulla. The cortex is comprised of three concentric zones, first labeled by Julius Arnold in 1866 as the zona glomerulosa, zona fasciculata, and zona reticularis. These zones have functionally distinct roles in steroid hormone production. The glucocorticoids cortisol and corticosterone are synthesized in the zona fasciculata, whereas the zona glomerulosa synthesizes mineralocorticoids and the zona reticularis produces adrenal androgens (although in rats this appears at best to be quite limited). The synthetic pathway for these two glucocorticoids is shown in Figure 23.8. The ratio of one to the other varies among mammals. Rats, mice, and rabbits, for example, secrete corticosterone, with little or no cortisol, unlike in dogs, sheep, humans, and nonhuman primates where cortisol predominates. Hamsters produce both glucocorticoids (Ottenweller et al., 1985); wheras, dairy cows show different ratios, depending upon the breed (Venkataseshu and Estergreen, 1970). The absence of cortisol in the adult rat has generally been considered to be due to a repressed adrenal expression of the CYP17 gene (Van Weerden et al., 1992; Brock and Waterman, 1999). Recent evidence has implicated DNA methylation in silencing of the gene (Missaghian et al., 2009). There is, however, cortisol production in prepubertal males and females (Pignatelli et al., 2006), along with some reports of adult rat adrenal tissue steroid production from 17-hydroxylation (e.g., Vinson et al., 1978; Bell et al., 1979).

As mentioned in Section 23.4.1, corticosterone secretion is pulsatile in nature, something that is also true for cortisol. In the female rat, a pulse of corticosterone occurs approximately once every hour. This secretion reflects an episodic activation and inhibition of the H–P–A axis and results in a refractory period, during which the axis becomes nonresponsive to the presence of a mild stressor (Windle et al., 1998). The activity of the H–P–A axis is also dampened during the latter portion of pregnancy, reflecting a reduced activation of CRH neurons (Brunton et al., 2008). This may function

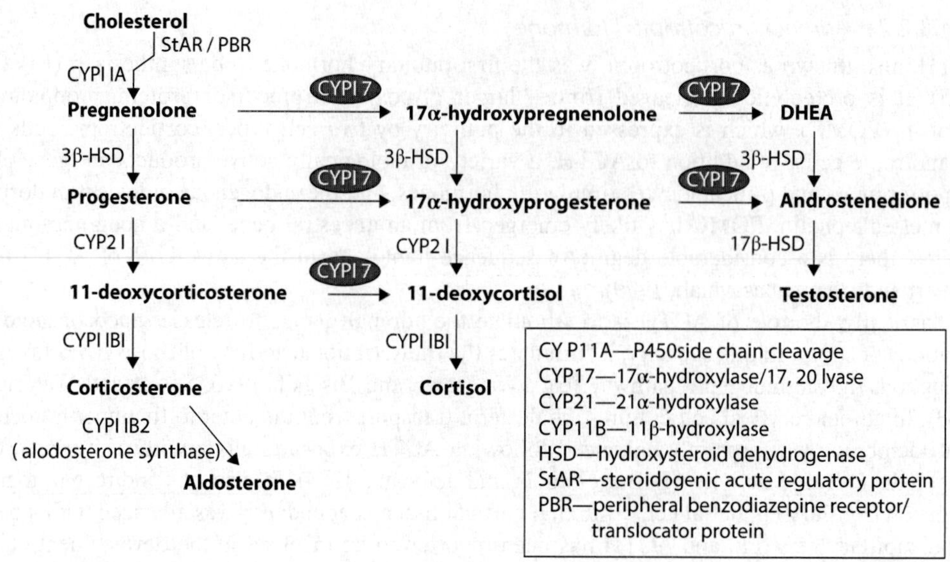

FIGURE 23.8 Steps in the adrenal synthesis of the glucocorticoids cortisol and corticosterone and the mineralocorticoid aldosterone. Unlike human adrenals, rat adrenals show a repressed (or negligible) expression of the gene for CYP17 (17α-hydroxylase/17,20 lyase), blocking 17-hydroxylation and preventing (or almost entirely impeding) the production of cortisol.

to avert the adverse influence of stress on the mother and offspring. The underlying mechanism still remains to be elucidated, but now appears to involve an upregulated endogenous opioid response to allopregnanolone, the neuroactive steroid metabolite of progesterone (Brunton et al., 2009).

The great majority of circulating cortisol is bound to a plasma protein, termed transcortin (or corticosteroid-binding protein [CBP]). In dogs, for example, only 5%–12% exists in the biologically active free form (Meyer and Rothuizen, 1993). A product of the liver, this protein is also able to bind aldosterone (Section 23.4.4.6) and shows varying degrees of glycosylation, affecting its half-life (Avvakumov, 1995). The physiological effects of glucocorticoids are mediated via binding to its intracellular receptor, which is predominantly present in the cytoplasm. When activated by glucocorticoid binding, this receptor undergoes a conformational change and is translocated to the cell nucleus (Picard and Yamamoto, 1987), where it initiates transcriptional activity by associating with specific DNA response elements. In the liver, glucorticoids serve an important regulatory role in energy metabolism/glucose utilization, and the translocated receptors appear to target directly more than 50 genes (Phuc Le et al., 2005). The hormones are also able to influence fat deposition, but show differential effects for peripheral and central lipids, increasing lipolysis in peripheral fats (Slavin et al., 1994), while promoting lipogenic pathway activity in central fat (Gaillard et al., 1991). Their anti-inflammatory role is well known, and pharmacological glucocorticoid doses are effective in immunosuppressing macrophage activation and T-cell receptor expression (reviewed by Sternberg, 2001).

23.4.3.2.4 Pathological Alterations in the H–P–A Axis

The significance of adverse effects on the functioning of the H–P–A axis has long been known. Human adrenal insufficiency was first described in 1849 by Thomas Addison (reviewed by Bishop, 1950) and is typically caused by an autoimmune attack on the adrenal glands (primary hypoadrenocorticism). Its symptoms include low blood pressure, constipation or diarrhea, nausea, vomiting, weight loss, increased desire for salty foods, lack of appetite, and hyperpigmentation. An Addison-like hypoadrenocorticism, with accompanying lethargy, anorexia and weight loss has been described in dogs and cats (reviewed by Greco, 2007). An experimental animal model of Addison's disease (experimental autoimmune adrenalitis) has also been produced in guinea pigs, rabbits, rats, monkeys, and mice by an injection of adrenal homogenates mixed with various adjuvants (e.g., Fujii et al., 1992).

In humans, a hyperadrenocorticism syndrome is characterized by a prompt gain in weight, excess sweating, polyuria, persistent hypertension, gastrointestinal problems, hyperglycemia, osteoporosis, and possible hirsutism. Harvey Cushing first described such a condition in the 1930s that was due to a benign pituitary ACTH-secreting adenoma (Cushing, 1932), and it has since come to bear his name. Pituitary adenomas have been found to be the cause of a majority of the cases of Cushing's syndrome. There also is an adrenal Cushing's syndrome, in which elevated concentrations of cortisol are attributable to adrenal gland tumors, hyperplastic adrenal glands, or adrenal glands with nodular adrenal hyperplasia. Hyperadrenocorticism with alterations in ACTH secretion, hyperglycemia, polyuria, polydipsia, and polyphagia is also observed in cats and dogs (more commonly in middle or old age). There are elevations in serum alkaline phosphatase and cholesterol, low urine specific gravity, and proteinuria. Diagnostically, the condition is identified by ACTH stimulation and cortisol analysis and a low dose dexamethasone suppression test (LDDS). In the latter test, the normal decline in cortisol seen after an injection of dexamethasone is not present in dogs with Cushing's disease, and these levels remain high. The tests can, however, generate some false-negative and false-positive results. Some dogs have shown classic signs of hyperadrenocorticism with a typical biochemical profile, but exhibit a normal response to ACTH administration or an LDDS test. This atypical Cushing's disease may be due to increased levels of intermediate steroids within the adrenal steroidogenic pathway. For a more comprehensive presentation of adrenocortical pathology, its diagnosis and treatment in dogs and cats, along with discussions of other endocrinopathies, the reader is referred to the text, "Endocrinology for the Small Animal Practitioner" by Panciera and Carr (2006).

As in humans, the hyperadrenocorticism can be due to hyperplastic changes in the pituitary or adrenals (reviewed by Feldman and Nelson, 1994; Meij et al., 1997; Chiaramonte and Greco, 2007). Rats have also been reported to exhibit an adrenocortical hyperplasia (Kaspareit-Rittinghausen et al., 1990). In horses, a Cushing's-like syndrome, characterized by excessive ACTH secretion, is due to a benign tumor of the pituitary pars intermedia (for review, see Love, 1993; Schott, 2002).

In the rat brain hippocampal dentate gyrus, granule cells are enriched with glucocorticoid receptors. It appears that these cells require corticosterone levels to be within a physiological range, since in the absence of corticosteroids, apoptotic cell death is enhanced (Joëls, 2007). However, a prolonged excess of corticosterone will suppresses neurogenesis in the region and could make the cells more vulnerable to delayed cell death (Sapolsky et al., 1988; McEwen and Magarinos, 1997) and impair learning (Luine et al., 1994).

The H–P–G axis will show suppression in activity in response to stress. Cycling rodents and nonhuman primates with normal menstrual cycles may stop ovulating (e.g., Roozendaal et al., 1995; Cameron, 1997). Central administration of CRH inhibits pulsatile LH (Rivier and Vale, 1984; Williams et al., 1990), and the effect can be reversed by antagonists to CRH (Tsukahara et al., 1999). This suppression appears to be mediated, at least in part, by CRFR2 receptors, since the central administration of urocortin II, which specifically binds to these receptors, resulted in a dose-related inhibition of the pulses (Li et al., 2005).

23.4.3.3 Hypothalamic–Pituitary–Thyroid Axis

The thyroid is one of the largest endocrine glands in the body. Interest in its functions as a focal point in human health and disease dates back to the middle ages, when surgical explorations in pigs were conducted at the southern Italian Medical School of Salerno (Scuola Medica Salernitana), modern civilization's oldest school of medicine (see de Divitiis et al., 2004; Bifulco and Cavallo, 2007). Similar to the gonads, thyroid activity is under hypothalamic–pituitary control, functioning within a classic physiological axis that comprises signaling among thyrotropin-releasing hormone, TSH and the two thyroid hormones, thyroxine and triiodothyronine (Figure 23.9).

23.4.3.3.1 Thyrotropin-Releasing Hormone

Hypophysiotropic thyrotropin-releasing hormone (TRH) neurons are located in the periventricular region of the hypothalamus. The hormone, whose primary structure pGlu-His-Pro-NH2 is conserved across vertebrates, undergoes processing in the cell bodies from a translated prohormone and is axonally transported to the median eminence region. There, it is released in the portal vessels and binds to receptors on pituitary thyrotrophs, triggering secretion of TSH. Using GH_3 rat anterior pituitary cells, two TRH receptor isoforms have been reported that appear to be functionally comparable (de la Peña et al., 1992). TRH neurons receive input from various neuronal populations, coordinating effects on feeding behavior and energy homeostasis, autonomic regulation, thermogenesis, and locomotor activation (reviewed by Lechan and Fekete, 2006; Chiamolera and Wondisford, 2009). In addition to its stimulatory effect on TSH, this hormone is also able to trigger Prl release from pituitary lactotrophs (e.g., Takahara et al., 1974; Chen and Meites, 1975; Smith and Convey, 1975).

23.4.3.3.2 Thyroid-Stimulating Hormone

TSH is a glycoprotein secretory product of pituitary thyrotrophs. As is the case for LH and FSH, TSH possesses a common α-subunit, with the β-subunit conferring receptor specificity. Free α- and β-subunits, however, have essentially no biological activity. Moreover, TSH is also produced and released into the circulation as multiple isoforms with different oligosaccharide configurations. The half-life in the rat of deglycosylated bovine TSH has been reported to be 3.8 minutes (Constant and Weintraub, 1986), although as for the other glycoprotein hormones, the number will be influenced by the extent of glycosylation. However, the prolongation in half-life with increased glycosylation is correlated with a diminished intrinsic bioactivity (Szkudlinski et al., 1993).

Circulating TSH is commonly used as a reliable index of thyroid status in humans and various other mammalian species. That said, it should be reemphasized that competitive immunoassays employing different antibodies can yield quite discrepant results, so it is important that the values for referenced normal ranges be generated using the same primary antibody. TSH functions primarily to stimulate the synthesis and release of thyroid hormones by binding to receptors on the surface of thyroid epithelial cells. One critical component of the TSH receptor is the presence of a disialoganglioside glycolipid, which forms a tight complex with the glycoprotein component of

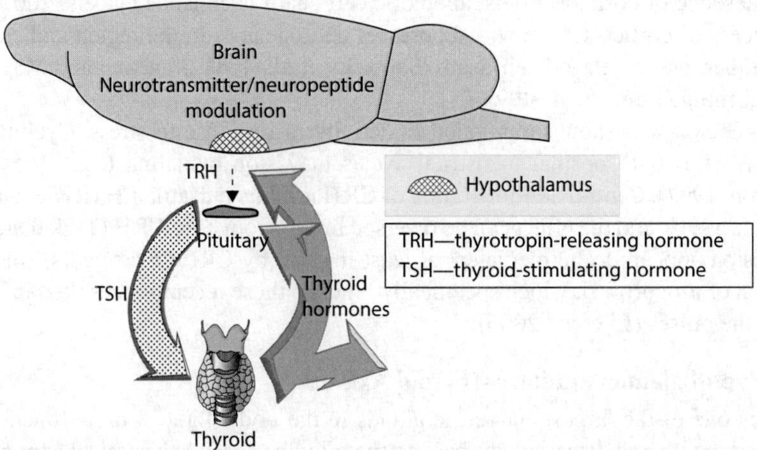

FIGURE 23.9 Representative rat hypothalamic–pituitary–thyroid endocrine axis showing relationships among thyrotropin-releasing hormone (TRH), thyroid stimulating hormone (TSH), and the thyroid hormones (THs) T3 and T4, with TH feedback to brain and pituitary, along with an additional arrow indicating TH impacts on other tissue and organ systems. As in Figures 23.3 and 23.7, central modulatory effects from neurotransmitters and neuropeptides are indicated.

the receptor and is involved in the coupling of the receptor to its second messenger complex (Kohn et al., 1989). The binding of TSH to the receptor initiates the first step in the thyroid hormone synthetic process—the uptake of iodide from the blood by the thyroid gland. In addition, TSH is also involved in the regulation of skeletal morphogenesis and remodeling (see Iqbal et al., 2009 for review of this role).

23.4.3.3.3 Thyroid Hormones: Thyroxine (T4) and Triiodothyronine (T3)

Thyroid epithelial cells have an iodide trap or sodium-iodide symporter on their outer plasma membrane that serves to convey iodine into the cell. The synthesis of the thyroid hormone thyroxine (T4) by the enzyme thyroperoxidase is based upon the iodination of tyrosines on a large epithelial cell glycoprotein, thyroglobulin. This glycoprotein prohormone is the most abundant protein in the thyroid and is the only protein in the mammalian body to contain significant amounts of iodine. Thyroperoxidase acts on thyroglobulin to generate T4 from two iodotyrosines. The more biologically active thyroid hormone, triiodothyronine or T3, is produced within the thyroid gland and in extrathyroidal tissues by a deiodination of T4 (reviewed by Köhrle et al., 1999). A large percentage of circulating T4 is bound to proteins in the serum. In dogs, for example, only about 0.1% in the blood is present in the free form (Ferguson, 1995). The major carrier of thyroid hormones in humans and nonhuman primates is thyroxine-binding globulin (TBG). Dogs have only about 15% of the TBG present in humans, while cats and rabbits have none and instead show binding to a thyroxine binding prealbumin (Larsson et al., 1985). In rats, TBG shows an initial postnatal surge, but then is virtually absent in the adult (Rouaze-Romet et al., 1992), with T4 principally bound to transthyretin and the prealbumin (Chanoine et al., 1992).

In the pituitary, the activity of T4-5′-deiodinase type II (T4-5′-DII) is primarily responsible for the conversion of T4 to T3, and the presence of T3 concentrations there is the main inhibitor of TSH secretion (e.g., Larsen et al., 1981). In addition, both T3 and T4 feed back directly on TRH neurons within the brain periventricular nucleus to inhibit the biosynthesis of pro-TRH (Dyess et al., 1988; Kakucska et al., 1992). Hypothyroidism, then, will cause both an increase in the content of pro-TRH mRNA in this area and an elevation in blood levels of TSH (Segerson et al., 1987). Overall, the deiodination of T4 also generates a number of iodothyronines. Both diiodothyronines (T2) and a monoiodothyronine (T1) are present in the circulation (DiStefano and Feng, 1988), but are physiologically of minor importance. An isomer of T3, termed reverse triiodothyronine (rT3) is also generated that has been found to be a potent inhibitor of T4-5′-DII (St Germain, 1986; Gavin et al., 1988).

In rat, the half-life of the thyroid hormones is significantly affected by their binding to the above-mentioned serum proteins. It ranges up to 24 hours for T4 and approximately 6 hours for T3, much shorter than the 5–9 days and 1 day reported, respectively, for T4 and T3 in humans (Tucker, 1997; Jahnke et al., 2004). The metabolism and action of thyroid hormone takes place within the cell, and the uptake of T4 and T3 into cells within different tissues is facilitated by the participation of several forms of transporters. A number of those transporters belong to the monocarboxylate family, so named because the first four members of the family are able to transport lactate and pyruvate (Halestrap and Meredith, 2004). One member, monocarboxylate transporter 8 (MCT8), has been found to be an active transporter of thyroid hormones in rats (Friesema et al., 2005). Within the cell, the thyroid hormones interact with their nuclear receptor and then bind to specific recognition sequences on DNA, resulting in a transcription/translation of DNA/RNA to increase protein synthesis specific for that cell. In the rat, thyroid hormone receptors are present in two primary isoforms, with splice variants of different amino acid lengths existing for each (Tomura et al., 1995).

Thyroid hormones are important for normal growth and development, regulating intermediary metabolism in order to maintain metabolic stability. They are involved in mitochondrial oxygen consumption and gene expression (Mutvei et al., 1989a,b; Wrutniak-Cabello et al., 2001), thermogenesis (e.g., Dauncey, 1990; Bianco et al., 2005), and serve as a major physiological regulator of mammalian brain, bone, and body development, coordinating diverse developmental events (e.g., Anderson et al., 2003; Bassett and Williams, 2008; Sanders and Harvey, 2008). For example, T3 appears to be important in the proliferation and further differentiation of precursor brain cerebellar GABAergic cells (Manzano et al., 2007). Thyroid hormones are critical to neuronal migration, myelination (Gravel et al., 1990; Schoonover et al., 2004), and synaptogenesis in the developing brain. The process of neuronal migration involves the presence of an actin cytoskeleton, and it now appears that T4 and rT3 function nongenomically to modulate this organization (Farwell et al., 2005; Leonard, 2008). In this context, T3, the transcriptional activator, is inert. On the other hand, T3 is acknowledged as a major regulator of mitochondrial activity, and mitochondrial T3 receptors have been identified (e.g., Scheller et al., 2003; Psarra et al., 2006). The hormone is also able to upregulate the number of β-adrenergic receptors in cells of the heart, increasing their sensitivity to catecholamines (Bahouth, 1991).

23.4.3.3.4 Pathological Alterations in the H–P–T Axis

Pathological alterations in thyroid activity can be genetically based, a consequence of chemical exposure, or assigned categorically to uncertain etiology. The most common hormonal dysfunctions seen by veterinary medical personnel in both dogs and cats are thyroid disorders. In dogs, autoimmune thyroiditis appears to be present in the great majority of cases and has a genetic basis (Bush, 1969). Autoantibodies can be present against thyroglobulin, thyroid hormones, and thyroid peroxidase. But because T4 and T3 are small molecules, they will not by themselves cause an immune response, and a thyroid hormone epitope must be linked to an immunogenic molecule like thyroglobulin.

In hypothyroidism, low thyroid hormone concentrations typically fall well before outward signs (e.g., weakness, lethargy, weigh gain, hair loss, cardiac arrhythmias, gastrointestinal disorders, diarrhea, and vomiting) appear. TSH concentrations are elevated, which is at least partly attributable to an increase in TSH subunit transcription (Shupnik and Ridgeway, 1985) and partly to an enhancement in TSH glycosylation (DeCherney et al., 1989) prolonging the metabolic clearance of the hormone. Testing for the condition can be performed after puberty and during the quiescent anestrous period of the cycle in female dogs, when the influence of sex steroids is minimal. A TSH test, given primarily to dogs and horses, involves an intravenous administration of bovine TSH, which can often provide a clear distinction between a euthyroid condition and hypothyroidism. Thyroid hormones are then sampled at particular times postdosing (Beale et al., 1990; Sojka et al., 1993), revealing that hypothyroid animals are relatively nonresponsive to TSH administration.

In cats, hypothyroidism is rarely present, while hyperthyroidism is the thyroid disorder more commonly seen in the clinic, occurring most often in older animals. It can be present in males and females, neutered or intact. This hyperthyroid condition is dissimilar from the autoimmune hyperthyroid Graves disease and appears to be linked to an excessive growth of some thyroid cells (Peterson, 2014). The condition causes weight loss, an increase in blood pressure, cardiac arrhythmia, hyperactivity, polyuria, kidney damage, and intestinal problems (Bustad and Fuller, 1970; Peterson et al., 1983). Often an enlargement of the heart, vomiting and diarrhea are present. T4 concentrations can be as high as threefold greater than normal, although a growing number of cats have clinical signs of hyperthyroidism, with enlarged thyroid glands, but have baseline serum total thyroid hormone values within the normal or borderline range (Peterson et al., 1987). While TSH is normally able to induce a marked increase in thyroid hormone secretion, hyperthyroid cats will typically show minimal elevations after administration of bovine TSH (Mooney et al., 1996). This lack of a robust response has been attributed to either a dysregulation in the relationship between TSH and T4, or to a near maximal rate of T4 production that has depleted its reserve capacity.

Goiter has been identified in all domestic mammals and is a non-neoplastic, noninflammatory enlargement of the thyroid gland. There is a hyperplasia of thyroid follicular cells that can be a response to diets deficient in iodine, an iodide excess, or inherited enzymatic defects in thyroid hormone synthesis, all of which will result in a decrease of circulating thyroid hormones and a responsive increase in TSH. In adults, goiter typically does not have the clinical impact that the condition does in the developing fetus or newborn, and an iodine deficiency can be treated with iodized salt. Large goiters in pregnant females can prolong gestation, and the fetal placenta is often retained. Newborns frequently show hair loss and have an increased incidence of mortality. For a more comprehensive review of the thyroid and thyroid disorders, the reader is referred to Capen and Martin (2003).

Some rat strains are genetically susceptible to autoimmune thyroiditis. This is true for inbred Biobreeding rats (e.g., Wilson et al., 1990b) and, when provided with excessive amounts of dietary iodine, the Buffalo rat (Cohen and Weetman, 1988). However, most of the published descriptions of rodent thyroid disorders have been from chemically induced alterations. It is their ability to decrease circulating concentrations of thyroid hormones, by affecting their biosynthesis, storage, transport or catabolism that has been the defining characteristic of thyroid toxicants (Brucker-Davis, 1998). Perchlorate has been found in the groundwater in the near industries of the United States that involved in the manufacture of rockets, explosives, and fireworks (Motzer, 2001). Its toxicity appears to be caused by an inhibition in thyroid iodide uptake (Van Sande et al., 2003); in the rat, increasing doses will disrupt homeostatsis in the hypothalamic–pituitary–thyroid (H–P–T) axis (Wolff, 1998). However, there are species differences in the susceptibility to perchlorate, with rats being much more susceptible to thyroid disruption than rabbits (Lewandowski et al., 2004).

Probably the best known of the thyrotoxicants is 6-propyl-2-thiouracil (PTU). It is used pharmaceutically in humans to treat hyperthyroidism (including Graves disease), decreasing the amount of thyroid hormone produced by the thyroid gland. It inhibits the activity of thyroperoxidase that catalyzes the addition of iodide to tyrosine residues on thyroglobulin thereby generating T4 (Shiroozu et al., 1983). In animal research, it has been employed as the prototypical thyroid toxicant, either as a positive control in toxicological studies or for investigations of thyroid hormone physiology. Its effect, however, is not likely restricted to thyroid function. There have been reported alterations in the steroidogenic pathway (Chiao et al., 2002; Chen et al., 2003, 2010), and PTU can cause disruptions in the rat estrous cycle (Hatsuta et al., 2004). Thyroidectomy will also cause similar cyclic alterations in both rat (Hatsuta et al., 2004) and Japanese macaque (Nozaki et al., 2002). In ewes, fertility was reduced, but not completely eliminated, suggesting to the authors that there was a reduction in gonadal hormones and possibly gonadotropins (Brooks et al., 1964). At least in rats, the impact on cyclicity was reversed after T4 administration, a treatment that also improved the fertility of hypothyroid males of the mutant *rdw* line (Jiang et al., 2000), implying a role for thyroid hormones in the regulation of reproductive activity.

A variety of other chemicals, both pharmaceutical and environmental, have been shown to affect circulating levels of thyroid hormones. As pharmaceuticals, the abovementioned perchlorates have been used to treat thyroid disorders for more than 50 years (e.g., Godley and Stanbury, 1954; Crooks and Wayne, 1960). Along with their use as oxidizers in rocket fuel and explosives, potassium perchlorate and ammonium perchlorate are employed extensively within the pyrotechnics industry. They have been found to be inhibitors of the sodium-iodide symporter, blocking the uptake of iodide into the cell. Polychlorinated biphenyls (PCBs) have been reported in rats to decrease thyroid hormone concentrations and induce ultrastructural lesions in thyroid follicular cells, effects that were time- and dose dependent (e.g., Collins et al., 1977; Kasza et al., 1978). There is some evidence that the decrease in circulating thyroid hormones is linked, at least partly, to an increase in hepatic metabolism (Bastomsky and Murthy, 1976; Yang et al., 2008) and/or a tissue accumulation (Kato et al., 2007). The herbicide, thiazopyr, has been found to cause rat thyroid follicular-cell tumors by a putative effect on thyroid homeostasis. The postulated pathway of effect (Dellarco et al., 2006) begins with an induction of hepatic T4-uridine diphosphate glucuronyl transferase (UGT) activity, leading to a subsequent increase in T4 metabolism. T4 levels then fall, triggering an increase in pituitary TSH synthesis and secretion. A prolonged elevation in concentrations of circulating TSH causes a similar increase in thyroid hormone production and receptor-mediated follicular cell hypertrophy and potential hyperplasia (e.g., Thomas and Williams, 1999).

23.4.3.4 Growth Hormone Axis

The classic characterization of the GH axis encompasses, at core, hypothalamic growth hormone releasing hormone (GHRH), pituitary GH, and a hypothalamic GH release-inhibiting hormone

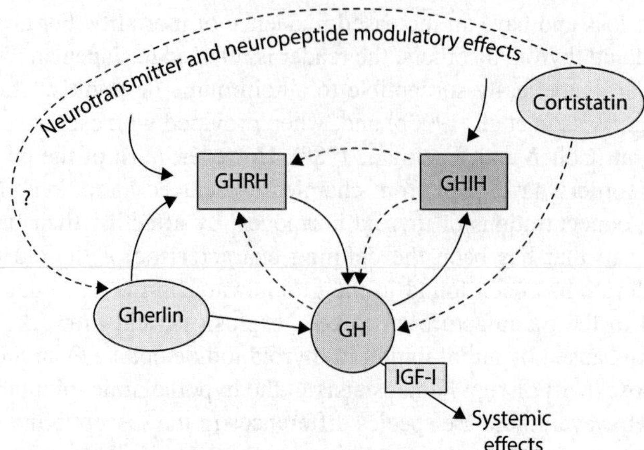

FIGURE 23.10 Generalized depiction of relationships among hypothalamic growth hormone releasing hormone (GHRH), somatostatin or growth hormone inhibitory hormone (GHIH), and pituitary GH, along with input from circulating gastric ghrelin, brain cortistatin, and other modulatory neurotransmitters and neuropeptides. GH influence on growth and metabolism are mediated via effects on insulin-like growth factor-1 (IGF-1). Unbroken lines with filled arrowheads indicate stimulatory effects, whereas dotted lines with open arrowheads show reported inhibition.

(GHIH) or somatostatin. The organization of these relationships is unlike the H–P–G, H–P–A, and H–P–T axes in that it is not based on a tripartite regulatory structure involving three distinct organs. Its signaling activity fundamentally involves endocrine interrelationships among the two hypothalamic releasing and inhibiting hormones and the pituitary, in addition to regulatory input from a number of brain-gut peptides. Figure 23.10 shows a simplified depiction of various interrelationships. For a more detailed discussion of the axis, the reader is referred to a review by Giustina and Veldhuis (1998).

23.4.3.4.1 Growth Hormone Releasing Hormone

GHRH is a peptide related to the "brain-gut" family of peptides. Members include glucagon, gastric inhibitory peptide, vasoactive intestinal polypeptide, and the intestinal peptide secretin. It is initially produced as a prohormone, primarily in neurons residing within the hypothalamic arcuate nucleus. GHRH neurons have also been found in other brain regions (i.e., ventromedial nucleus, periventricular nucleus, and amygdala (Muller et al., 1999), from which GHRH projections have no direct involvement in the control of pituitary secretion. It has also been detected in the pancreas (Bosman et al., 1984) and human gastrointestinal tract (Shibasaki et al., 1984).

GHRH plays a critical role in the cellular proliferation of pituitary somatotrophs during development and stimulates the synthesis and secretion of GH from secretory granules in these cells by binding to its transmembrane receptor, a member of cytokine receptor superfamily. GHRH receptor expression in the rat pituitary is sexually dimorphic (Ono et al., 1995; Mayo et al., 2000), suggesting that this may contribute to the sex difference observed in postpubertal GH secretion. In addition to its effect on GH synthesis and secretion, GHRH has been reported to augment the stimulation by FSH of ovarian granulosa cell steroidogenesis (Moretti et al., 1990) and amplify the effect of gonadotropins on male testicular Leydig cells (Ciampani et al., 1992). Although the role of GHRH is fundamental to the activity of the GH axis, other assessments of functioning within this axis are employed diagnostically.

23.4.3.4.2 Somatostatin (Growth Hormone Inhibiting Hormone)

In this axis, somatostatin and GHRH have been depicted as classic opposing forces in the regulation of GH. However, the regulatory mechanisms influencing GH release involve levels of various factors beyond a straightforward stimulation and suppression by these two peptides. A range of neurotransmitters (e.g., norepinephrine, GABA, and glutamate) and neuropeptides (e.g., TRH, CRH, galanin, and neuropeptide Y [NPY]) are now known to exert functional control over GH. In addition to coverage of TRH and CRH as part of the respective H–P–T and H–P–A axes, two of these neuropeptides, ghrelin and cortistatin will be briefly discussed in Section 23.4.3.4.4.

The peptide somatostatin is synthesized as two bioactive peptides (SRIF-14 and SRIF-28) in populations of neurons located within various hypothalamic areas, including the periventricular and paraventricular nuclei, along with scatterings in the suprachiasmatic, arcuate, dorsomedial, and ventromedial regions. Fibers from periventricular and paraventricular somatostatinergic neurons project to the median eminence, where the hormone is released into the portal vessels. Upon reaching the pituitary, somatostatins bind to the members of a family of five somatostatin receptor subtypes (SSTR1–5) (e.g., Guillermet-Guibert et al., 2005). The receptors are located on various types of pituitary cells, and there appears to some differential specificity for the somatostatin peptides. While SSTR1–4 have been reported to show similar affinities for both SRIF-14 and SRIF-28, SSTR5 has a greater affinity for SRIF-28 (Reisine and Bell, 1995).

The simplified depiction of the GH axis depicted in Figure 23.10 showing interrelationships among GHRH, somatostatin (GHIH), and GH, with inputs from ghrelin and cortistatin (see section 23.4.3.4.4), also includes the umbrella category of modulatory factors (mentioned above) found to colocalize with GHRH or GHIH perikarya/fibers (for review, see Muller et al., 1999; Cocchi et al., 1999; Fodor et al., 2006).

23.4.3.4.3 GH and Insulin-Like Growth Factor

With the exception of humans and old world monkeys, GHs in other mammalian species are closely conserved, differing among most only by up to four amino acids in the mature 190 amino acid peptides. However, discrepancies between humans/rhesus monkeys and nonprimate mammalian GHs can range up to 33% (Liu et al., 2001), with the majority of the amino acid substitutions occurring over a short period of primate evolution. This hormone is a secretory product of pituitary somatotropes and is structurally and evolutionarily also homologous to Prl. It functions in the regulation of a variety of complex physiological growth and metabolic processes. GH stimulates the liver and other tissues to secrete insulin-like growth factor (IGF-1), resulting in protein anabolic effects in many tissues (e.g., Isaksson et al., 1991; Florini et al., 1996). It counteracts the effects of insulin on glucose and lipid metabolism (Møller et al., 1991), increases the utilization of fat by augmenting triglyceride breakdown and adipocyte oxidation (e.g., Keller and Miles, 1991), and acts as an immunomodulatory factor (Savino et al., 2002). GH also strengthens and increases bone mineralization either directly or indirectly through IGF-1 (e.g., Giustina et al., 2008). IGF-1 is a potent mitogen that promotes proliferative activity by stimulating cell cycle progression. There is evidence in mammals that GH increases T3 concentrations, while decreasing levels of T4 (Brixen et al., 1992; Møller et al., 1992). However, whether the cause is a peripheral action on thyroid hormone metabolism or a direct thyrotropic effect on the thyroid gland is uncertain.

Mammalian GH is present in multiple isoforms generated during posttranslational processing. These isoforms may exist as monomers, or various oligomers composed of noncovalently associated or disulfide-connected isoforms (Baumann, 2009). Under basal conditions, approximately 50% of circulating GH is bound to growth hormone binding protein (GHBP). GHBP serves as a buffer/reservoir for the GH isoforms, prolonging their half-lives in plasma (Baumann, 2001). As previously mentioned, GH secretion shows bursts of release and in the rat exhibits a sex difference, with male peak-to-valley excursions much larger than those seen in females. The bursts in males are unchanged throughout the day and night, while female rats shift at night from more extended secretory valleys to rapid, short duration bursts of increased amplitude (Clark et al., 1987). This pulsatile secretion can also be seasonally dissimilar. For example, during the autumn and early winter (April–June in the southern hemisphere), red deer stags had frequent GH pulses of low amplitude. In contrast, the amplitude of pulses in spring (August and September) were higher and more frequent, resulting in a high mean plasma level of circulating GH, effects that were tied to an increase in antler growth (Suttie et al., 1989).

Dog breeds can differ markedly in circulating concentrations of both GH and IGF-1. In large breeds, the relatively extended persistence of elevated levels of GH and IGF-1 at a young age is a primary factor in their increased body size (e.g., Eigenmann et al., 1984; Rijnberk et al., 2003). In poodles, the short stature of the miniature breed is associated with low serum levels of IGF-I. Standard poodles are taller and have considerably higher serum levels of IGF-1 (Guler et al., 1989).

The receptor for GH belongs to the superfamily of transmembrane proteins that includes the Prl receptor and a number of cytokine receptors. GH causes a dimerization of this receptor at the cell surface and this appears to be a prerequisite for biological activity of the hormone (see Postel-Vinay and Finidori, 1995 for review). The extracellular domain of the full-length membrane receptor is also found soluble in the circulation and has been identified as the above-described GH-binding protein (Postel-Vinay, 1996).

23.4.3.4.4 Ghrelin and Cortistatin

Ghrelin (from *ghre*, the Indo-European root of the word grow) is a peptide that is produced mainly in the stomach, but has also been found to be expressed in the hypothalamus, pituitary, gonads, intestine, kidney, pancreas, and heart. It is a member of a group of brain-gut peptides that have GH-stimulating properties, although the effects are not limited to GH; ghrelin is also able to stimulate the secretion of pituitary Prl and CRH (Arvat et al., 2001; Wren et al., 2002). It acts as an appetite stimulant by what appears to be a complex response that involves an increase in NPY (see Section 23.4.4.7) and inhibition of POMC (Toshinai et al., 2003). Ghrelin and other growth hormone secretagogues (GHS) are endogenous ligands for a previously discovered orphan receptor, originally cloned in 1996 and now abbreviated as GHS-R. GHS-R is also expressed in the hypothalamus, pituitary, neuronal cells of the gut, stomach tissue, gonads, and heart, in addition to adrenals, thyroid, spleen, and pancreas (Shuto et al., 2001; Gnanapavan et al., 2002), suggesting that the GHS peptides have paracrinic effects.

Cortistatin was initially identified in rat as a cortical hormone structurally related to GHIH/somatostatin, and its mRNA was reported to be restricted to GABA neurons in the cerebral cortex and hippocampus (de Lecea et al., 1997), but also appears, with somatostatin, to be present in cells of the immune system (Dalm et al., 2003). Cortistatin binds with high affinity to all of the somatostatin receptor subtypes, and like somatostatin, it inhibits in vivo GH release in man and rats (Luque et al., 2006). It also has been found, at least in humans, to bind to GHS-R and inhibit ghrelin secretion (Broglio et al., 2002), an effect not seen for GHIH/somatostatin, adding an additional layer of regulatory complexity to the GH axis.

23.4.3.4.5 Pathological Alterations in the GH Axis

Acromegaly is characterized by a chronic excessive secretion of GH by the pituitary. Although infrequently seen in cats, the most common cause in these animals is a hypophyseal tumor, which when present can often occur with a GH-induced insulin-resistant diabetes mellitus (e.g., Hurty and Flatland, 2005; Niessen et al., 2007). The detection of elevated circulating concentrations of both GH and IGF-1 are both useful in the diagnosis of the condition.

GH undersecretion in dogs is relatively uncommon, but can occur in adults and puppies. In the puppy, it results in dwarfism, while hair loss is the major symptom in adults. In cats, progestins can stimulate the production of GH from mammary tissue and the induction of mammary fibroadenomas (Mol et al., 2000). This is also true for dogs. As opposed to pituitary GH secretion, progestin-induced mammary GH is not released in a pulsatile pattern, and is not stimulated by GHRH or inhibited by GHIH/somatostatin (Mol et al., 1996). Acromegaly is also seen in dogs, but the condition is more commonly attributable to progesterone-induced hypersecretion of GH from mammary tissue and not to a pituitary tumor, as seen in cats. In this case, a demonstration of an inability to suppress these high GH levels is important for the diagnosis (Eigenmann, 1984), and the condition can be treated with a progesterone receptor antagonist (Bhatti et al., 2006). In contrast, the induction of mammary GH production by progestin administration has been employed for the treatment of GH deficiency (Rijnberk et al., 2003).

As the main regulator of IGF-1 production, GH may also be an important factor in the incidence of at least some types of mammalian cancer (e.g., Waters and Conway-Campbell, 2004). Experiments in the rat have shown that advanced mammary cancers are dependent on GH and/or IGF-1 for their survival (Shen et al., 2007). Moreover, GH receptors are expressed, for example, in a number of canine mammary tumor cell types (Van Garderen et al., 1999). The administration of GHRH receptor antagonists has been reported to decrease serum and tumor IGF-1 and inhibit the growth of and enhance apoptosis in estrogen-independent methotrexate (MTX) mouse mammary cancers (Kahan et al., 2000; Szepeshazi et al., 2001). GH production can be induced by progestins in the dog mammary gland (Selman et al., 1994), and female dogs treated with progestins show in a dose-dependent development of mammary tumors, suggesting a potential role of GH in the tumor formation. Such interactions in various mammalian species among local mammary progesterone, GH, and the GH receptor have also contributed to the debate on the risk of breast cancer in postmenopausal women on hormone replacement therapy (reviewed by Rijnberk et al., 2003).

23.4.4 Other Hormones

The list of endogenous biochemicals acting as endocrine factors has been continuously expanding. However, rather than attempting to be all-encompassing, this section will focus on a shorter list of additional hormone/endocrine factors that have been shown to be important participants in various physiological activities.

23.4.4.1 Prolactin

Prl is a pituitary peptide hormone that is principally secreted by the lactotropes. It is closely related to GH and belongs to a large family that, in addition to these two hormones, also includes placental lactogens and Prl-like proteins. As had been found for GH, changes in Prl occurred more rapidly during a period of primate evolution, leading to marked differences in amino acid sequences between human and nonprimate mammalian Prl (Wallis et al., 2005). In addition to its presence in lactotropes, Prl has also been found to colocalize with GH in a small population of anterior pituitary cells termed mammosomatotrophs (Nikitovitch-Winer et al., 1987; Yeung et al., 2006). It appears likely that both were the result of duplication of an ancestral gene. As is the case for the other pituitary peptide hormones, Prl is synthesized as a prohormone and posttranslationally cleaved. In male rats, it has a reported half-life of about 7 minutes (Chi and Shin, 1978).

The conventional role of Prl, for which it was named, is the stimulation of lobuloalveolar growth in the mammary gland and milk production by the alveoli. However, its metabolic actions are much more widespread, and its functions can be subsumed under two general headings, reproduction and homeostasis. Prl has been demonstrated to have a role in the transition to sexual maturity in female rats. When introduced into the median eminence region of immature females, it was able to advance puberty (Clemens et al., 1969). In contrast, a chronic suppression of Prl from prepubertal day 22 onward caused a marked delay (Advis et al., 1981)

In addition to its lactational role in reproduction, Prl has a luteotrophic function in some species. For example, in rodents, dogs, and skunks, it is required for pregnancy maintenance. Rodents, for example, exhibit diurnal and nocturnal surges of Prl that are required during the early stages of the pregnancy to sustain necessary progesterone secretion from the corpora lutea. Prl may also be luteolytic and induce programmed cell death in the rat corpora lutea if copulatory cervical stimulation does not occur (Wuttke and Meites, 1971). The influence of Prl on parenting behavior has been extensively studied, most frequently in the rat, and its effect has been reported for mice, rabbit, hamsters, and sheep (Bridges, 1994; Numan, 1994). The hormone is also involved in a variety of other functions, including the suppression of lipid storage, growth support of pancreatic islets, stimulation of insulin secretion, and an increase in citrate production in the prostate (reviewed by Ben-Jonathan et al., 2006).

Prl has also been observed to have marked effects on immune function. Mouse lymph node lymphocytes have Prl receptors (Gala and Shevach, 1993), and antibodies to Prl were shown in vitro to inhibit lymphocyte proliferation (Hartmann et al., 1989). In humans, the hormone has been demonstrated to homeostatically enhance the restoration of immunity after chemotherapy and bone marrow transplantation (reviewed by Redelman et al., 2008). Prl has also been reported to have effects on the development of blood vessels and appears to have opposing actions, in that the parent Prl molecule can promote angiogenesis, whereas proteolytic processing results in a peptide fragment that has antiangiogenic properties (Corbacho et al., 2002). Overall, it appears that Prl has a modulatory role in several aspects of immune function, but data have indicated that it is not strictly required for immune activity.

The neurotransmitter dopamine, released into the portal blood from neurons within the arcuate nucleus that project to the median eminence (the tuberoinfundibular pathway) serves as a negative regulator of lactotrope Prl secretion, binding to the dopamine D2 receptor. TRH, in addition to its role in TSH secretion, will also trigger Prl release (e.g., Takahara et al., 1974; D'Angelo et al., 1975). Beginning in 1998, Hinuma and colleagues first reported the existence of another prolactin-releasing peptide (PrRP), an RFamide family member whose cell bodies were located in the dorsomedial hypothalamus, among other brain regions (Hinuma, 1998; Matsumoto et al., 1999). However, unlike the other classical hypophysiotropic hormones, no immunopositive PrRP fibers were detected in the external layer of the median eminence (Yamakawa et al., 1999), and the Prl-releasing potency of PrRP has been reported to be less than that of TRH (Samson et al., 1998), raising doubts about its physiological importance as a Prl-releasing factor.

The receptor for Prl belongs to the cytokine receptor superfamily, and isoforms have been described in different tissues (e.g., Davis and Linzer, 1989), but having extracellular domains that are identical (Kelly et al., 1991). In the rat ovary, short and long forms of Prl receptor mRNA are present and appear to be involved in different functions during ovulation. It is believed that mRNA for the long form of the receptor is involved in folliculogenesis, whereas mRNA for the short form may play a role in the formation and maintenance of the corpus luteum (Kinoshita et al., 2001).

Chronic hyperprolactinemia can be induced in rats by grafting pituitary fragments under the kidney capsule, removing inhibitory dopaminergic regulation. This protocol has been used to advance puberty in immature female rats (Gonzalez et al., 1984), an effect consistent with the aforementioned administration of Prl into the median eminence. The same protocol for producing elevated levels of Prl was employed in adult male rats and mice and was found to reduce levels of copulatory behavior (Svare et al., 1979). In cycling female rats, the administration of ovine Prl over the course of the estrous cycle completely blocked the LH surge and ovulation (Wise, 1986). Similar results were seen in females innoculated with a Prl/GH-secreting pituitary tumor (Nass et al., 1983). In these rats, ovarian estradiol decreased, while circulating progesterone was elevated.

Dogs have been reported to show an elevation in Prl in a pituitary-dependent hyperadrenocorticism that was considered to be due to a neoplastic transformation of pituitary corticotropic cells that then co-secreted ACTH and Prl (Meij et al., 1997). There also has been speculation that Prl is involved in the growth of mammary tumors in dogs and mice. Mice with grafted pituitary fragments were found to have areas of mammary hyperplasia within dilated ducts (Huseby et al., 1985), and those with transplanted mammary tumors have shown modest responsive growth to the hormone (Koseki et al., 1987). Furthermore, Prl receptors have been found in approximately 28% of dog mammary tumors (Rutteman et al., 1986), and it is possible that, in some dogs, tumor growth may be linked to a hyperresponsiveness of Prl secretion to stimulation (Rutteman et al., 1989). However, the relationship between Prl and tumorigenesis is still unclear.

23.4.4.2 Oxytocin and Vasopressin

In the supraoptic and paraventricular nuclei of the hypothalamus are several thousand magnocellular neurons that project to the neurohypophysis or posterior lobe of the pituitary. Roughly, half of these primarily make one of two hormones, oxytocin, or vasopressin. They are peptide hormones and, similar to others in this class, are initially synthesized as larger prohormones. Both of these hormones are, respectively, stored within large numbers of vesicles in the terminal axonal regions and released in response to electrical action potentials at the terminals. Vasopressin is also synthesized and secreted by the adrenal medulla in many species including humans and is often referred to as *antidiuretic hormone* because one of its principal physiologic effects is the retention of water by the kidney. It also increases the resistence to vascular blood flow, elevating arterial blood pressure. A deficiency in vasopressin or a failure of the kidney to respond to the hormone is the pathological basis for diabetes insipidus.

Oxytocin is one of the most potent agents able to overcome relaxation of the muscular wall of the uterus and in pharmaceutical form has been used clinically to induce labor in mammals. Uterine oxytocin receptors are regulated by the steroid environment (e.g., Soloff, 1975), and before the onset of labor there is an increase in the sensitivity of the uterus to oxytocin that is accompanied by an upregulation of myometrium oxytocin receptors (Gimpl and Fahrenholz, 2001). This is also the case in decidual tissue where the hormone stimulates prostaglandin F2α (PGF2α) secretion (see Section 23.4.4.5.3). Binding to its receptors in the brain, oxytocin plays an important role in milk ejection (e.g., Nishimori et al., 1996) and establishing maternal behavior around the time of parturition (see Poindron, 2005 for review). It also has been reported to be synthesized in the ovaries and may serve as a luteolytic factor, stimulating prostaglandin (PG) secretion (Luck, 1989). Oxytocin is produced within the mammalian male hypothalamus in similar quantities to the female. In several species, an increase in circulating oxytocin appears to be associated with ejaculation, stimulating smooth muscle cells (Ivell et al., 1997). Studies have also shown that oxytocin is synthesized locally within the testis, where it likely serves, via an autocrine/paracrine action, to modulate steroid metabolism (Nicholson et al., 1991) and affect seminiferous tubule contractibility (Harris and Nicholson, 1998). Recent studies on both vasopressin and oxytocin have focused on their potential roles in social bond formation (e.g., Young and Wang, 2004; Lim and Young, 2006) and speculation that human genetic variations in them may contribute to the dysregulation seen in autism spectrum disorders (Lim et al., 2005; Hammock and Young, 2006).

23.4.4.3 Natriuretic Peptides

Atrial natriuretic peptide (ANP), brain natriuretic peptide (BNP), and C-type natriuretic peptide (CNP) are hormonal factors that serve important functions in the regulation of cardiovascular homeostasis, causing both arterial and venous dilatation that serves to control blood pressure and extracellular fluid volume (reviewed by Woodard and Rosado, 2008). They are processed from larger pro-forms, and along with their receptor subtypes, NPR-A, NPR-B, and NPR-C, all are found in the hypothalamus, pituitary, and adrenals. ANP and BNP bind to NPR-A, whereas CNP will preferentially bind to NPR-B and the three peptides have similar affinities for NPR-C. Natriuretic peptides in the hypothalamus have been found to inhibit oxytocin and vasopressin, along with CRH and GnRH (Samson et al., 1993). BNP can increase the glomerular filtration rate and thus alter kidney hemodynamics. Also, ANP and CNP have been identified in the gastrointestinal tract and are able to stimulate basal as well as induced pancreatic secretion and alter the secretion of bicarbonate and chloride (Sabbatini, 2009). Moreover, CNP and NPR-B are present in uterus and ovaries, and marked CNP mRNA expression has been found in the placenta, suggestive of a role in gestation, antagonizing the vasoconstrictive function of angiotensin II (Walther and Stepan, 2004; see Section 23.4.4.6).

There are indications that elevations in one or more of these natriuretic peptides can serve as useful indicators of cardiac pathology. Dogs and cats with clinical signs of heart failure were found to have had signficantly elevated pro-forms of ANP and BNP (Boswood et al., 2003; Connolly et al., 2008; Tarnow et al., 2009). Whereas, these pro-natriuretic peptides may be informative as biomarkers, recent research has suggested that BNP infusion can have beneficial effects on cardiac functioning following the induction of acute myocardial infarction (He et al., 2009; George et al., 2010).

23.4.4.4 Neurotransmitters as Endocrine Agents

Neurotransmitters had traditionally been described as local tissue factors located and released in the brain that convey an impulse from one nerve cell to another by means of an association with specific receptors. However, the distinction between local tissue factors and blood-borne secretions acting at a distance has become less clear. Some neurotransmitters are now known to fill both roles. The classic neurotransmitter dopamine is concentrated within various brain regions and has been reported to participate in motor activity, attention and learning, sleep, and reward. In terms of a traditional role as a hormone, it was previously mentioned to be an inhibitory regulator of Prl secretion. It is released from nerve terminals in the median eminence for transport in the portal blood to the anterior pituitary, where it binds to one particular form of the five identified dopamine receptors, the D2 variant. Dopamine is generated within a synthetic pathway that is shared by epinephrine and norepinephrine. L-tyrosine is first converted to L-dihydroxyphenylalanine (L-DOPA) by the enzyme tyrosine hydroxylase (Figure 23.11a). DOPA decarboxylase then catalyzes L-DOPA to form dopamine, which in the presence of dopamine-β-hydroxylase, can be further converted to norepinephrine (noradrenaline [NE]). Epinephrine (adrenaline) can then be generated by the action of phenylethanolamine N-methyltransferase (PNMT). Dopamine and norepinephrine are two of the principal transmitters in the brain. Although it is primarily localized in the adrenal medulla, PNMT activity has also been demonstrated in kidney, spleen, lung, skeletal muscle, thymus, retina, and different parts of the brain (e.g., Ziegler et al., 2002).

In the brain, NE functions as a classical neurotransmitter, modulating the activity of the hypothalamic components of the aforementioned axes (see Figures 23.3, 23.7, and 23.8; e.g., Kalra and Kalra, 1983; Tapia-Arancibia et al., 1985; Alonso et al., 1986; Malozowski et al., 1990; Goldman et al., 2008). Its modulatory responses can be excitatory or inhibitory, and in some cases noradrenergic input provides a necessary permissive tone that allows other processes to proceed. Perturbations of NE in either direction can be disruptive. Acute stress can activate noradrenergic neuronal pathways extending to various brain regions from cell populations residing in the area of the brain stem locus coeruleus that, along with adrenal secretory activity, elicit a variety of neuroendocrine, autonomic, behavioral, and cognitive participants in the organism's response to stress (for review, see Morilak et al., 2005). Chromaffin cells in the adrenal medulla synthesize and secrete both NE and epinephrine, whereupon the two chemicals act as blood-borne hormonal factors that (1) increase heart rate, (2) stimulate lipolysis in fat cells, contributing fatty acids to the production of energy, (3) induce lung bronchiole and pupil dilation, (4) cause widespread vasoconstriction that elevates arterial blood pressure, and (4) increase the body's metabolic rate.

NE binds to two main groups of adrenergic receptors, α or β, each of which has several subtypes. α1 and α2 receptors are principally involved in smooth muscle contraction, causing vasoconstriction in many blood vessels. In addition to vasoconstriction, α1 receptors participate in GnRH secretion (Le et al., 1997), the inhibition of insulin release in pancreas (e.g., Drews et al., 1990; Debuyser et al., 1991) and induction of glucagon release from the pancreas (e.g., Vieira et al., 2004). The involvement of β-adrenergic activity in cardiac function has been known for some time, and a persistent elevation in β-adrenergic receptor stimulation is believed to contribute to congestive heart failure (Lefkowitz et al., 2000).

The monoamine serotonin (5-hydroxytryptamine [5-HT]) has traditionally been identified as a neurotransmitter that is synthesized in brain stem neurons from the amino acid L-tryptophan (Figure 23.11b). These neurons extend throughout the central nervous system and comprise an expansive neurochemical network. In addition to the central nervous system, serotonin is present in the intestinal wall (e.g., Hansen and Witte, 2008) and large blood vessels (e.g., Ramage and Villalón, 2008). Functionally, it is involved in the control of appetite, sleep, memory, and learning, temperature regulation, cardiovascular function, muscle contraction, and the regulation of other endocrine factors. In humans, a large number of publications have shown a link to mood and depression (see Lowry et al., 2008 for review). As an endocrine factor itself, serotonin acting through 5-HT2B receptors has a role in bone metabolism (Collet et al., 2008) and gastrointestinal cell proliferation (Wouters et al., 2007). Serotonin associations with this same receptor subtype have also been reported to contribute to pulmonary cell proliferative activity (Esteve et al., 2007). Both serotonin receptors and estrogen receptors are present in cells within various tissues, and it has been argued that many estrogenic effects in these tissues may be mediated by estradiol's stimulative effect on serotonin synthesis (Rybaczyk et al., 2005). Neuronal projections of serotonergic fibers from the brain stem raphe nuclei to the basal hypothalamus are known to cause elevations in pituitary Prl

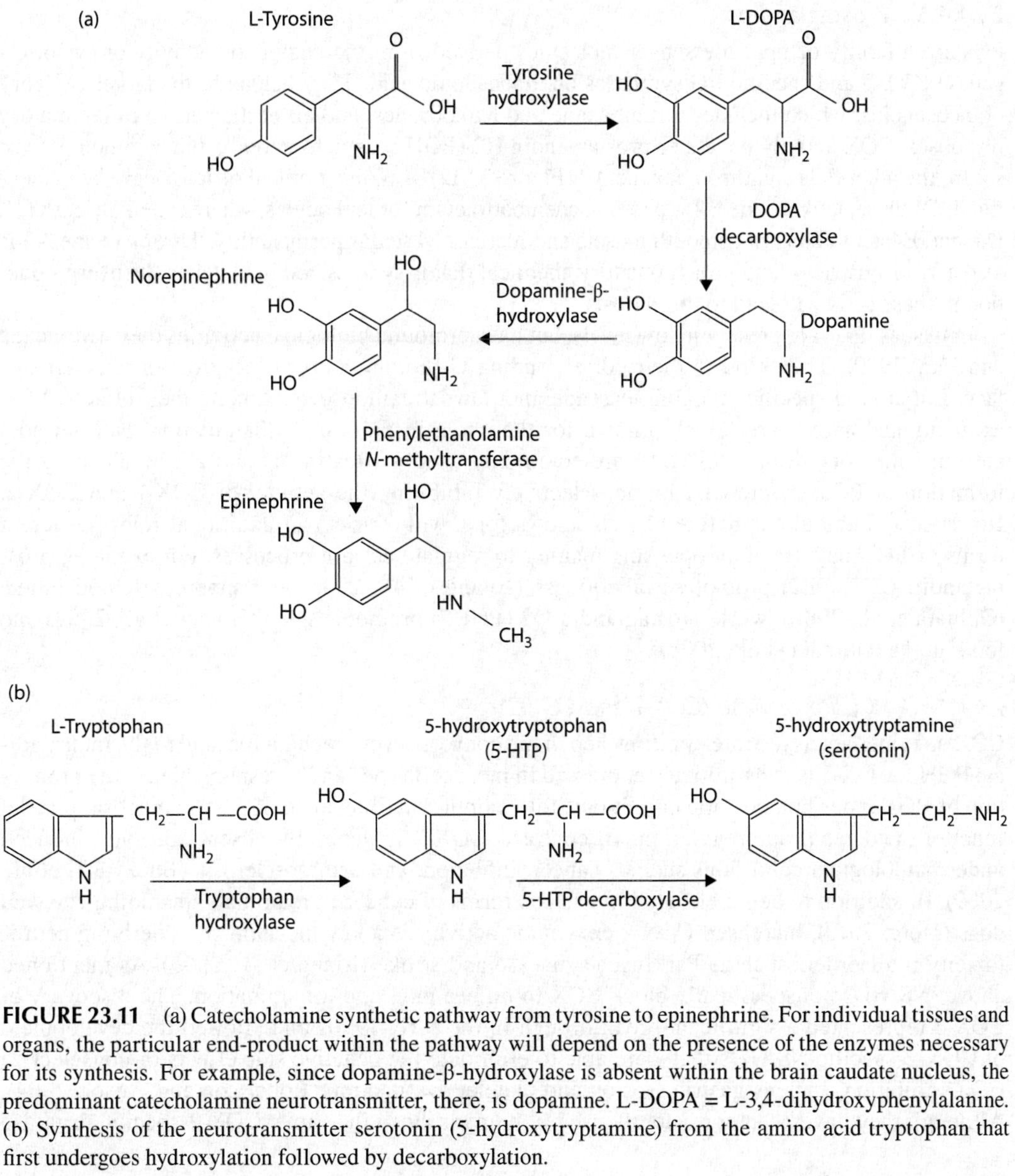

FIGURE 23.11 (a) Catecholamine synthetic pathway from tyrosine to epinephrine. For individual tissues and organs, the particular end-product within the pathway will depend on the presence of the enzymes necessary for its synthesis. For example, since dopamine-β-hydroxylase is absent within the brain caudate nucleus, the predominant catecholamine neurotransmitter, there, is dopamine. L-DOPA = L-3,4-dihydroxyphenylalanine. (b) Synthesis of the neurotransmitter serotonin (5-hydroxytryptamine) from the amino acid tryptophan that first undergoes hydroxylation followed by decarboxylation.

secretion (Fessler et al., 1984), an effect mediated through the 5-HT4 receptors that likely involves a disinhibition of dopamine regulation.

The acetylcholine is a neurotransmitter generated from the amino acid choline by the action of choline acetyltransferase. It is involved in autonomic nervous system stimulation of the heart and smooth muscles, in both complementary parasympathetic (muscle relaxation, slowing of heart rate) and sympathetic (heart rate acceleration, blood vessel constriction, and increase in blood pressure) activity. Cholinergic receptors are present in two forms, nicotinic and muscarinic, both of which exist in multiple subtypes. They were named according to their responsiveness to the acetylcholine agonist drugs, muscarine, and nicotine. Although their tissue distributions can overlap, these receptors subserve different functional roles. For a review of the relationships of these two receptors to acetylcholine activity, the reader is referred to chapters by Sastry and Robertson (2004) and Taylor (2004), both in the same volume.

23.4.4.5 Prostaglandins

PGs are a family of lipid messenger molecules derived from the enzymatic activity of cyclooxygenase (COX) and specific PG synthases on arachadonic acid. They belong to the larger category of eicosanoids, which includes thromboxane and leukotrienes, and all participate in inflammatory responses. COX activity generates prostaglandin H2 (PGH2), which serves as the common precursor for the other PGs and thromboxane A2 (Figure 23.12). A number of leukotrienes have been identified. Of those, leukotriene B4 is a strong chemoattractant for leukocytes, whereas leukotrienes C4, D4, and E4 act to constrict smooth muscle and increase vascular permeability. Thromboxane A2 is also a vasoconstrictor and proaggregatory chemical that is synthesized in platelets. Its overproduction in these cells will lead to thrombosis.

In tissues, PGs are present in low levels, but have profound biological activities there (Moncada and Van, 1979). They bind to their corresponding G-protein coupled receptors on the cell surface, initiating a specific signaling cascade and downstream effects. Among their effects, PGs, as mentioned above, are largely known for their role in pain and inflammation. Nonsteroidal anti-inflammatory drugs (NSAIDs) are commonly used as treatments and act by blocking the formation of PGs, specifically by nonselectively inhibiting the activity of COX-1 and COX-2. However, the ubiquitous nature of PGs allows for a wide variety of additional roles. Different forms of PGs may act in an opposing manner to regulate certain processes. For example, prostaglandin E2 (PGE2) promotes wakefulness (Huang et al., 2003) and suppresses food intake (Ohinata et al., 2006), while prostaglandin D2 (PGD2) promotes sleep (Huang et al., 2007) and food intake (Ohinata et al., 2008).

23.4.4.5.1 Cycloxygenase (COX-1 and COX-2)

COX enzymes act as the rate-limiting step in the conversion of arachadonic acid to the intermediate PGH2. COX-1 is constitutively expressed in most cell types and is responsible for the production of PGs under homeostatic conditions, for example, maintenance of gastric mucosa, platelet function, and renal autoregulation. In contrast, COX-2 is generally absent and only induced under pathological conditions such as cancer, infection, and artherosclerosis (Buczynski et al., 2009). In addition to being elevated in various forms of cancer in mammals, including cats and dogs (Dore, 2010), increased COX-2 enzymatic activity is a key mechanism underlying neurotoxicity in disorders such as Parkinson's disease and stroke (Liang et al., 2005). As mentioned above, NSAIDs nonspecifically block COX to relieve pain and inflammation. The discovery of COX-2 represented a significant breakthrough in the early 1990s and allowed the development of COX-2-specific NSAIDs that were able to eliminate the negative side effects of nonselective COX inhibition, such as gastric erosion and platelet dysfunction (Robertson and Taylor, 2004). Although they have been consistently used in humans since that time, COX-2-specific drug use

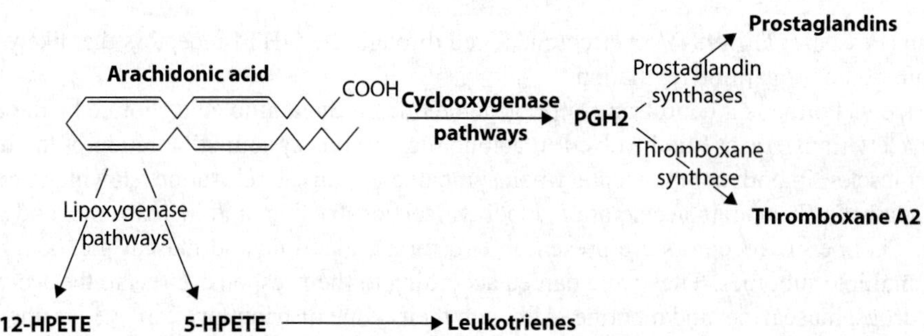

FIGURE 23.12 Prostaglandin, thromboxane, and leukotriene mediators of inflammation are generated via the cyclooxygenase and lipooxygenase pathways from the 20-carbon unsaturated fatty acid, arachidonic acid. Both 5- and 12-hydroperoxyeicosatetraenoic acids (HPETEs) are within the lipoxygenase pathway.

in veterinary medicine did not emerge until a decade later. However, marked interspecies differences have been found in clearance and elimination. A third form, COX-3, a splice variant of COX-1, was subsequently discovered to be involved in the regulation of fever. Recent studies have demonstrated that acetaminophen apparently exhibits both COX-3 (Botting et al., 2005) and COX-2 (Hinz et al., 2008) inhibition.

23.4.4.5.2 Prostaglandin E2

PGE2 is the most thoroughly characterized PG and is widely studied for its roles in parturition, bronchial dilation, pain, cancer, inflammation, atherosclerosis, and smooth muscle control (Buczynski et al., 2009). There are four G-protein coupled receptors (EP 1–4) that mediate PGE2 actions. In general, EP1 and EP3 induce smooth muscle contraction, while EP2 and EP4 induce smooth muscle relaxation. PGE2 is also important in renal homeostasis, with different receptor isoforms mediating opposing functions. EP1 and EP3 mediate PGE2-induced salt excretion and dieresis, while EP4 mediates salt and water absorption (Breyer et al., 1998). In dogs, PGE2 contracts the urinary bladder and relaxes the urethra and differences in gene and protein expression of the receptors there has been reported to differ between sexes, and among regions of the urinary tract (Ponglowhapan et al., 2010). As mentioned above, it has also been shown that PGE2 suppresses food intake via the EP4 receptor and promotes wakefulness (Ohinata et al., 2008). Moreover, PGE2 acts as an immunosuppressant by inhibiting production of inflammatory cytokines and helper T cell differentiation (Sakata et al., 2010). In the pig endometrium, PGE2 is thought to increase vascularization and support early pregnancy (Kaczmarek et al., 2008). Via binding to its EP1 receptor, PGE2 is also responsible for maintenance and cytoprotective actions in the gastrointestinal tract of rats, reducing the degree of damage done by harmful agents or conditions (Araki et al., 2000).

23.4.4.5.3 Prostaglandin F2α

PGF2α is largely recognized for its involvement in the mammalian female reproductive system. It is present in corpora lutea from a wide range of mammalian species, including horses, cows, rabbits, sheep, rats, pigs, and primates (Wiltbank and Ottobre, 2003). It has a prominent role in the regression of ovarian corpora lutea, increasing over the later luteal stages and serving as a luteolytic signal for the decrease in progesterone (Diaz et al., 2002). The secretion of PGF2α by luteal cells can also feed back on corpora lutea to further amplify PGF2α during the luteolytic process (Tsai and Wiltbank, 1997). PGF2α is also known to cause contraction of smooth muscle in the uterus (Crankshaw and Gaspar, 1995), gastrointestinal (Stein et al., 1994), and respiratory (Karlsson et al., 1993) tracts, effects that also involve the participation of oxytocin (Russ et al., 1992; Qin et al., 2009). A knockout of the gene encoding the receptor for PGF2α showed a failure of normal parturition in pregnant mice (Sugimoto et al., 1997), an effect that was attributable to the absence of the progressive decline in progesterone late in pregnancy (see Section 4.3.1.3.2). In the 1970s, PGs were also discovered to modulate intraocular pressure and blood flow. Since then, a variety of synthetic analogs of PGF2α have emerged for the treatment of glaucoma and other eye conditions in both human and veterinary medicine (Lee et al., 1984; Gum et al., 1991; Kurashima et al., 2010).

Uterine diseases in dogs are typically accompanied by elevations in PGF2α. Such is the case in canine pyometra, which is seen within weeks of a female's period of heat. In the condition, abnormal sex steroid levels will stimulate a thickening of the uterus, accompanied by an increase in uterine fluid that can lead to an infection and accumulation of pus. Plasma levels of endotoxin are increased and correlate with elevations in the PGF2α metabolite 15-keto-(13,14)-dihydro-PGF2α (Hagman et al., 2006). An increased presence of this metabolite has also been observed in cat inflammatory uterine diseases (Hagman et al., 2009).

23.4.4.5.4 Prostaglandin D2

PGD2 is the most abundant PG in the central nervous system, having roles in sleep (Hayaishi, 1991), pain, and as a key mediator of allergic inflammatory response. There are two receptor forms to which PGD2 binds. Initially, it was believed that most of the biological actions of PGD2 were mediated by what is now known as DP1. However, a second receptor, DP2, was found to be expressed on Th2 cells, a subset of T-lymphocytes. These lymphocytes secrete a number of interleukin signaling molecules that in the immune system serve as cytokine chemical messengers in the cross-talk among leukocytes. A major role of PGD2 is the promotion of an allergic reaction, with each receptor mediating unique responses (Pettipher, 2008). Peripherally, PGD2 promotes vasodilatation, constriction of the bronchioles, and inhibits platelet aggregation (Liang et al., 2005).

In addition to those discussed above, other eicosanoids exist, including prostacyclin (PGI2) and thromboxane A2. In general, research on PGs is largely conducted with human interests in mind, with less known about PGs in domesticated species. Some work that has been done, however, suggests that homology exists in PGs and COX enzymes across species (Lin and London, 2010; Bhattacherjee et al., 1997; Bennett and Moore, 1991; Setty et al., 1991). Nonetheless, species differences in PG activity or responses have also been shown (Chand and Altura, 1980; Taniguchi et al., 1982; Lee et al., 1984; Henderson et al., 1988), so cross-species generalizations about this highly functional family of lipids can be inappropriate.

23.4.4.6 Aldosterone and Cardiac Glycosides

Aldosterone is a mineralocorticoid hormone, a designation that is derived from an effect on mineral metabolism. It is generated within the adrenal cortex zona glomerulosa from progesterone through deoxycorticosterone and corticosterone, with aldosterone synthase catalyzing the final conversion from corticosterone (see Figure 23.8). Aldosterone acts on the nuclear mineralocorticoid receptors in the distal tubule and collecting ducts of the kidney, increasing sodium reabsorption, potassium secretion and water retention by the kidneys. An rise in the level of circulating potassium ions, a drop in the level of sodium ions, or a persistant fall in blood pressure stimulates the release of the peptide renin from the kidneys and the globulin angiotensinogen from the liver. Angiotensinogen is converted in sequence to angiotensins I and II, and the latter directly raises blood pressure by vasoconstriction and stimulates the adrenals to produce aldosterone and the posterior pituitary to secrete vasopressin. Aldosterone, in turn, promotes sodium and water retention by the kidneys, which then serves to increase blood pressure. The secretion of aldosterone, both basal and stimulated, is inhibited by natriuretic peptides (e.g., Richards et al., 1993), and is potentiated by serotonin (Rocco et al., 1990). Serotonin is directly able as well to stimulate aldosterone synthesis from adrenocortical cells (Al-Dujaili et al., 1982). Renin and angiotensin also have a role in the regulation of water balance by stimulating the release of vasopressin from the posterior pituitary to increase the permeability of the kidney collecting ducts to water.

Given their interrelationships, renin, angiotensin, and aldosterone are physiologically often grouped as a single system (i.e., the renin–angiotensin–aldosterone system), which is central to the pathogenesis of hypertension, cardiovascular disease, and kidney disease. Pathological changes in the levels of aldosterone are more often than not entwined with alterations in the other two participants. The development of chronic renal failure and proteinuria is frequently associated with an elevation in adrenal aldosterone production that can be attributable to an upregulation in the renin–angiotensin system (Endemann et al., 2004). Elevated circulating aldosterone levels and dysregulation in renin and angiotensin activity are also associated with impaired cardiovascular function (e.g., Rossi et al., 2005; Cachofeiro et al., 2008; Gaddam et al., 2009).

Cardiac glycosides are a class of adrenal steroid hormones that influence the active sodium pump and intracellular free calcium concentrations. They enhance the vagal tone in the heart, affecting the force of cardiac muscle contraction and slowing the heart rate. The existence of such substances in nature has long been known. Herbal concoctions that influenced the functioning of the heart were employed by the ancient Romans, Syrians, and Chinese. In 1775, the English physician William Withering reported using extracts from the foxglove plant to treat patients suffering from dropsy, an earlier term for congestive heart failure (see Norman, 1985 for review). The effectiveness of the treatments, although initially given by him in excessive dosages, was attributable to the fact that the plant contained the glycoside digitalis. The discovery that digitalis and other similar steroids inhibited the sodium pump, leading to an increase in intracellular calcium ions and hypertension, was an early impetus for a search for endogenous cardiotonic substances. One digitalis-like steroid, similar to the plant toxin ouabain, was reported to be synthesized in adrenals, although it has also been identified in the hypothalamus and pituitary (Hamlyn et al., 1998). It appears that progesterone and pregnenolone can serve as intermediate precursors (Perrin et al., 1997; Komiyama et al., 2001) for this ouabain-like compound (OLC). However, the synthetic pathway has been reported to diverge in different cultured cell types (Perrin et al., 1997; Lichtstein et al., 1998). The endogenous OLC is regulated by both catecholamines and angiotensin II (Laredo et al., 1997, 2000), indicating a functional interplay with the renin–angiotensin system.

In addition to foxglove, a variety of plants contain glycosides that are toxic upon ingestion, and this accounts for many cases of animal poisonings and death due to heart failure. The evergreen ornamental shrub oleander, for example, contains the glycoside oleandrin, and all parts of the plant are toxic. Pheasant's eye is a perennial plant, and its many stems and serrated leaves contain toxic cardiac glycosides similar to those of digitalis. Other plants include milkweed, Christmas rose, lilly of the valley, and white water lily. The animals that appear most affected by ingesting these plants are cattle, sheep, and goats, although poisonings have been detected in horses and deer. As a rule, herbivores in the wild will avoid the plants, making cases of such poisonings relatively rare (for review, see Joubert, 1989). The venom gland of cane toad (*Bufo marinus*) contains large quantities of cardiac glycosides, and toad venom poisoning is similar to digitalis toxicity. All toads produce venom, but the toxicity varies by species and is attributable to several chemicals, including catecholamines in addition to glycosides. These chemicals are expressed onto the surface of the skin when the toads are under threat. Toads are a common cause of dog poisonings, although toxic exposures have also been reported in cats, which typically occur in both when they mouth the toad. Symptoms begin promptly and usually consist of abundant drooling and vomiting, which can persist for hours. Affected animals can also exhibit seizures or convulsions.

23.4.4.7 Leptin and Neuropeptide Y (NPY)

Leptin is a hormone that was first identified in the laboratory of Jeffrey Friedman at Rockefeller University (Zhang et al., 1994) in mice from the Jackson Laboratory that showed a random mutation, causing them to become markedly obese (Ingalls et al., 1950), as much a four times heavier than littermates. It is principally described as a hormone of white fat, tissue which has also been found to secrete a variety of endocrine factors (i.e., adipokines and cytokines), including adiponectin, resistin and tumor necrosis factor-α (reviewed by Rondinone, 2006). In addition, leptin has been observed in placental syncytiotrophoblasts, ovaries, skeletal muscle, stomach, mammary epithelial cells, bone marrow, pituitary, and liver (Margetic et al., 2002). Its receptors exist in at least five different isoforms. One form of the receptor, OB-Rb, has a long intracellular domain, essential for intracellular signal transduction, and is highly expressed in brain hypothalamus and cerebellum (Burguera et al., 2000).

Leptin is now known to have various roles that encompass the regulation of energy balance, (1) conveying information to the hypothalamus about energy stores, (2) acting as a permissive factor for puberty, (3) being involved as a satiety hormone in the attenuation of food intake, and (4) interacting with other hormonal metabolic regulators as insulin, glucagon, cholecystokinin, POMC, GH, and IGF-1 (for review, see Moschos et al., 2002; Meier and Gressner, 2004). The metabolic signaling conveyed by leptin now appears to act as a gating factor for the maturational processes taking place during puberty. This hormone provides cues to the brain that sufficient energy stores are available to meet the metabolic demands needed for the transition to sexual maturity. As mentioned in Section 23.4.3.1.1, this transition is now believed to require kisspeptin activity, and recent evidence has implicated a serine/threonine kinase (also known as the mammalian target of rapamycin, or mTOR) as a critical intermediary in linking leptin signals to kisspeptin activation during this time (Roa et al., 2009).

One of the more intriguing lines of research in recent years has focused on the role of leptin in the assembly of tubulin into microtubules. Leptin has been found to regulate the phosphorylation of the microtubule-associated tau protein, whilch promotes this assembly. A hyperphosphorylation of tau results in the formation of tangles of microtubule filaments, something that is implicanted in the pathogenesis of Alzheimer's disease in humans. Treatment of human and rat neuronal cell lines with leptin (Greco et al., 2008, 2009) was found to inhibit tau phosphorylation and reduce the levels of amyloid β that is a component of the neuritic plaques present in the Alzheimer's brain, suggesting a potential therapeutic approach to the disease (reviewed by Signore et al., 2008; Tezapsidis et al., 2009). Amyloid β deposits are found in the brains of aged dogs and cats (e.g., Head et al., 2005; Bernedo et al., 2009), and the senile dementias do show neurodegenerative changes and cognitive impairments. In dogs, amyloid plaques are present, although they diffuse and are conformationally different than those seen in Alzheimer's disease. Tau protein hyperphosphorylation has been reported, and as in humans, the process of phosphorylation presumably involves the participation of leptin. However, the hyperphosphorylation was not related to any neurofibrillary and neurtic changes and was not observed to be localized in the area of these diffuse plaques (Pugliese et al., 2006).

NPY is the most abundant peptide in the brain and appears to be highly conserved throughout evolution. It functions there, in sympathetic neurons and in various other organ systems, as a neurotransmitter that is implicated in several physiological processes through binding to five different forms of the receptor: Y1, Y2, Y4, Y5, and Y6. Activation of the sympathetic nervous system in physical exercise, stressful situations, and hypoxia will stimulate NPY release from peripheral nerves or the adrenal medulla (reviewed by Pedrazzini et al., 2003). It has a role in the interaction between cardiac sympathetic and parasympathetic nerves (Ilebekk et al., 2005), and its cardiovascular effects could be related to modulation of the renin–angiotensin system (Pedrazzini et al., 2003). In the renal vasculature, NPY and NE have been found to be colocalized, and NPY contributes, with an activation of sympathetic neurons by the renin–angiotensin system, to the development of high blood pressure (Pedrazzini et al., 2003).

NPY is additionally present in the plexus of enteric nerves in the submucous coat of the intestine, where it functions, along with its related PYY (see Section 23.4.1.1), in the coordination of intestinal motility and in the regulation of ion and water transport (Cox, 2008). As an appetite stimulant, NPY is a principal factor in the regulation of food intake. The combination of NPY and leptin, with profusion of inputs from insulin, glucagon, cholecystokinin, GIP, GLP-1, PYY, GH, IGF-1, and POMC, in addition to TRH, CRH, and oxytocin, comprise a complex interactive system of central and peripheral signals that modulate the individual response to nutrient ingestion (for review, see Valassi et al., 2008).

Mammalian reproduction is a physiological process that consumes significant amounts of energy. It is well known that marked reductions in body weight that deplete energy reserves can both suppress female adult reproductive functions and inhibit sexual maturation in immature animals (see Wade and Schneider, 1992 for review). Information about metabolic status is communicated to the brain from both central (e.g., NPY) and peripheral (e.g., leptin, ghrelin, and insulin) signaling. In general, these signals are not inducers, but are seen more as factors that convey the availability of sufficient or insufficient metabolic stores to support reproductive activity.

23.5 SUMMARY

The broadened description of a hormone as any endogenous chemical that controls and regulates the activity of organs or specific cell groups means that the individual hormones presented here comprise only a portion of this category. A more inclusive coverage could easily be expanded beyond a chapter into an entire book, particularly as these chemicals more specifically relate to individual laboratory animal species. Those endocrine factors not discussed in this chapter include the following:

- Placental chorionic gonadotropins—equine, porcine, and human chorionic gonadotropins that help prevent degeneration of the corpora lutea and maintain progesterone production during pregnancy
- Pineal melatonin—important in the regulation of circadian rhythms
- Melanocyte-stimulating hormone—pituitary hormone that stimulates melanin production
- Parathyroid hormone—acts to increase Ca^{2+} concentrations in the blood
- Calcitonin—reduces blood Ca^{2+}, opposing the action of parathyroid hormone
- Gastrin—stimulates the secretion of acid by the stomach
- Secretin—intestinal hormone that stimulates bicarbonate secretion by the pancreas, inhibiting gastrin production
- Vitamin D3 (cholecalciferol)—a steroid-like prohormone that, through conversion to 1,25-dihydroxyvitamin D3, regulates calcium and phosphorus levels in the blood and promotes phagocytosis
- Neuromedin B—widely distributed and is involved in cell growth, body temperature, and glucose regulation
- Placental lactogens—related to Prl and acts in concert with it in various animal species to stimulate maternal behavior, maintain luteal progesterone secretion, and facilitate energy supply to the growing fetus
- Galanin—wide tissue distribution, released from hypothalamus into portal vessels and involved in regulating secretion of other hypothalamic hormones
- Vasoactive intestinal peptide—plays a role in muscle relaxation, coronary vasodilation, adrenal activity, LH, and Prl gene expression
- Nesfatin-1—a satiety peptide present in several brain areas, involved in energy balance and H–P–A activation
- Thymosins—peptides originally identified in thymus, although there is wide tissue distribution, involved in modulating immune activity, cellular growth/survival
- Erythropoietin—glycoprotein hormone promoting red blood cell production
- Endogenous opioid peptides—functional roles in pain and analgesia, drug tolerance, reproductive regulation, learning and memory, food intake, immunological responses, and gastrointestinal, renal, and hepatic functions

This list will continue to expand along with our progressive understanding of the intricacies of cellular communication and the normal roles for (and aberrant shifts in) the multiplicity of endocrine factors across species.

ACKNOWLEDGMENTS

The authors wish to express their appreciation to Ms. Ashley Murr (US EPA) for her excellent technical contributions and to Dr. Michael Narotsky (US EPA) for providing valuable comments on the manuscript. Material described in this chapter has been reviewed by the National Health and Environmental Effects Research Laboratory, US EPA and approved for publication. Approval does not signify that the contents necessarily reflect the views and policies of the Agency, nor does the mention of trade names or commercial products constitute endorsement or recommendation for use.

REFERENCES

Abrams, G.M., Nilaver, G., Hoffman, D. et al. 1980. Immunocytochemical distribution of corticotrophin (ACTH) in monkey brain. *Neurology.* 30:1106–1110.

Advis, J.P., White, S.S., and Ojeda, S.R. 1981. Delayed puberty induced by chronic suppression of prolactin release in the female rat. *Endocrinology.* 109:1321–1330.

Albrecht, E.D. and Townsley, J.D. 1976. Metabolic clearance and production rates of progesterone in non-pregnant and pregnant baboons (*Papio papio*). *Endocrinology.* 99:1291–1294.

Al-Dujaili, E.A., Boscaro, M., and Edwards, C.R. 1982. An in vitro stimulatory effect of indoleamines on aldosterone biosynthesis in the rat. *J. Steroid Biochem.* 17:351–355.

Allard, E.K. and Boekelheide, K. 1996. Fate of germ cells in 2,5-hexanedione-induced testicular injury. *Toxicol Appl Pharmacol.* 137:149–156.

Allen, C. and Kendall, J.W. 1967. Maturation of the circadian rhythm of plasma corticosterone in the rat. *Endocrinology*. 80:926–930.

Allen, W.M. 1970. Progesterone: How did the name originate? *South Med J.* 63:1151–1155.

Allen-Rowlands, C.F., Allen, J.P., and Greer, M.A. 1980. Circadian rhythmicity of ACTH and corticosterone in the rat. *J Endocrinol Invest.* 3:371–377.

Alonso, G., Szafarczyk, A., Balmefrézol, M. et al. 1986. Immunocytochemical evidence for stimulatory control by the ventral noradrenergic bundle of parvocellular neurons of the paraventricular nucleus secreting corticotropin releasing hormone and vasopressin in rats. *Brain Res.* 397:297–307.

Ambrisko, T.D., Hikasa, Y., and Sato, K. 2005. Influence of medetomidine on stress-related neurohormonal and metabolic effects caused by butorphanol, fentanyl, and ketamine administration in dogs. *Am J Vet Res.* 66:406–412.

Anderson, G.M., Relf, H.L., Rizwan, M.Z. et al. 2009. Central and peripheral effects of RFamide-related peptide-3 on luteinizing hormone and prolactin secretion in rats. *Endocrinology.* 150:1834–1840.

Anderson, G.W., Schoonover, C.M., and Jones, S.A. 2003. Control of thyroid hormone action in the developing rat brain. *Thyroid.* 13:1039–1056.

Araki, H., Ukawa, H., Sugawa, Y. et al. 2000. The roles of prostaglandin E receptor subtypes in the cytoprotective action of prostaglandin E2 in rat stomach. *Aliment Pharmacol Ther.* 14(Suppl 1):116–124.

Armstrong, D.T. 1968. In vitro synthesis of progesterone. *J Anim Sci.* 27:181–203.

Arnold, J. 1866. Ein Beitrag zu der feiner Struktur und dem Chemismus der Nebennieren. *Virchows Arch Pathol Anat Physiol Klin Med.* 35:64–107.

Arvat, E., Gianotti, L., Giordano, R. et al. 2001. Growth hormone-releasing hormone and growth hormone secretagogue-receptor ligands: Focus on reproductive system. *Endocrine.* 14:35–43.

Asarian, L. and Geary, N. 2006. Modulation of appetite by gonadal steroid hormones. *Phil Trans R Soc B.* 361:1251–1263.

Avvakumov, G.V. 1995. Structure and function of corticosteroid-binding globulin: Role of carbohydrates. *J Steroid Biochem Mol Biol.* 53:515–522.

Azmitia, E.C. and de Kloet, E.R. 1987. ACTH neuropeptide stimulation of serotonergic neuronal maturation in tissue culture: Modulation by hippocampal cells. *Prog Brain Res.* 72:311–318.

Bahouth, S.W. 1991. Thyroid hormones transcriptionally regulate the beta 1-adrenergic receptor gene in cultured ventricular myocytes. *J Biol Chem.* 266:15863–15869.

Bakker, J. and Baum, M.J. 2000. Neuroendocrine regulation of GnRH release in induced ovulators. *Front Neuroendocrinol.* 21:220–262.

Bale, T.L., Picetti, R., Contarino, A. et al. 2002. Mice deficient for both corticotropin-releasing factor receptor 1 (CRFR1) and CRFR2 have an impaired stress response and display sexually dichotomous anxiety-like behavior. *J Neurosci.* 22:193–199.

Ballantyne, G.H. 2006. Peptide YY(1-36) and peptide YY(3-36): Part I. Distribution, release and actions. *Obes Surg.* 16:651–658.

Bamberg, E., Aichinger, A., and Mitteregger, G. 2004. In vitro metabolism of dehydroepiandrosterone and testosterone by canine hair follicle cells. *Vet Dermatol.* 15:19–24.

Barbé, F., Legagneur, H., Watrin, V. et al. 1995. Undetectable luteinizing hormone levels using a monoclonal immunometric assay. *J Endocrinol Invest.* 18:806–808.

Bartlett, J.M.S., Kerr, J.B., and Sharpe, R.M. 1986. The effect of selective destruction and regeneration of rat Leydig cells on the intratesticular distribution of testosterone and morphology of the seminiferous epithelium. *J Androl.* 7:240–253.

Bartsch, G., Rittmaster, R.S., and Klocker, H. 2002. Dihydrotestosterone and the concept of 5α-reductase inhibition in human benign prostatic hyperplasia. *World J Urol.* 19:413–425.

Bassett, J.H. and Williams, G.R. 2008. Critical role of the hypothalamic–pituitary–thyroid axis in bone. *Bone.* 43:418–426.

Bastomsky, C.H. and Murthy, P.V. 1976. Enhanced in vitro hepatic glucuronidation of thyroxine in rats following cutaneous application or ingestion of polychlorinated biphenyls. *Can J Physiol Pharmacol.* 54:23–26.

Bauer, P.V., Hamr, S.C., and Duca, F.A. 2016. Regulation of energy balance by a gut–brain axis and involvement of the gut microbiota. *Cell Mol Life Sci.* 73:737–755.

Baumann, G. 2001. Growth hormone binding protein. 2001. *J Pediatr Endocrinol Metab.* 14:355–375.

Baumann, G.P. 2009. Growth hormone isoforms. *Growth Horm IGF Res.* 19:333–340.

Beale, K.M., Helm, L.J., and Keisling, K. 1990. Comparison of two doses of aqueous bovine thyrotropin for thyroid function testing in dogs. *J Am Vet Med Assoc.* 197:865–867.

Bell, J.B., Gould, R.P., Hyatt, P.J. et al. 1979. Properties of rat adrenal zona reticularis cells: Production and stimulation of certain steroids. *J Endocrinol.* 83:435–447.

Ben-Jonathan, N., Hugo, E.R., Brandebourg, T.D. et al. 2006. Focus on prolactin as a metabolic hormone. *Trends Endocrinol Metab.* 17:110–116.

Bennett, P.R. and Moore, G.E. 1991. Genetic conservation of cyclo-oxygenase. *Prostaglandins.* 41:135–142.

Bernedo, V., Insua, D., Suárez, M.L. et al. 2009. Beta-amyloid cortical deposits are accompanied by the loss of serotonergic neurons in the dog. *J Comp Neurol.* 513:417–429.

Berry, S.J. and Isaacs, J.T. 1984. Comparative aspects of prostatic growth and androgen metabolism with aging in the dog versus the rat. *Endocrinology.* 114:511–520.

Berson, S.A. and Yalow, R.S. 1957. Kinetics of reaction between insulin and insulin-binding antibody. *J Clin Invest.* 36:873.

Berson, S.A. and Yalow, R.S. 1959. Quantitative aspects of reaction between insulin and insulin-binding antibody. *J Clin Invest.* 38:1996–2016.

Bhattacherjee, P., Smithson, M., and Paterson, C.A. 1997. Generation second messengers by prostanoids in the iris-sphincter and ciliary muscles of cows, cats and humans. *Prostaglandins Leukot Essent Fatty Acids.* 56: 443–449.

Bhatti, S.F., Duchateau, L., Okkens, A.C. et al. 2006. Treatment of growth hormone excess in dogs with the progesterone receptor antagonist aglépristone. *Theriogenology.* 66:797–803.

Bianco, A.C., Maia, A.L., da Silva, W.S. et al. 2005. Adaptive activation of thyroid hormone and energy expenditure. *Biosci Rep.* 25:191–208.

Bifulco, M. and Cavallo, P. 2007. Thyroidology in the medieval medical school in Salerno. *Thyroid.* 17:39–40.

Bishop, P.M.F. 1950. The history of the discovery of Addison's disease. *Proc R Soc Med.* 43:35–42.

Blum, W.F. and Gupta, D. 1985. Heterogeneity of rat FSH by chromatofocusing: Studies on serum FSH, hormone released in vitro and metabolic clearance rates of its various forms. *J Endocrinol.* 105:29–37.

Boepple, P.A., Mansfield, M.J., Wierman, M.E. et al. 1986. Use of a potent, long acting agonist of gonadotropin-releasing hormone in the treatment of precocious puberty. *Endocr Rev.* 7:24–33.

Boonyaratanakornkit, V. and Edwards, D.P. 2004. Receptor mechanisms of rapid extranuclear signalling initiated by steroid hormones. *Essays Biochem.* 40:105–120.

Boots, L.R., Potter, S., Potter, D. et al. 1998. Measurement of total serum testosterone levels using commercially available kits: High degree of between-kit variability. *Fertil Steril.* 69:286–292.

Bosman, F.T., Van Assche, C., Nieuwenhuyzen Kruseman, A.C. et al. 1984. Growth hormone releasing factor (GRF) immunoreactivity in human and rat gastrointestinal tract and pancreas. *J Histochem Cytochem.* 32:1139–1144.

Boswood, A., Attree, S., and Page, K. 2003. Clinical validation of a proANP 31-67 fragment ELISA in the diagnosis of heart failure in the dog. *J Small Anim Pract.* 44:104–108.

Botting, R. and Ayoub, S.S. 2005. COX-3 and the mechanism of action of paracetamol/acetaminophen. Prostaglandins Leukot Essent Fatty Acids. 72:85–87.

Bouchard, G.F., Solorzano, N., Concannon, P.W. et al. 1991. Determination of ovulation time in bitches based on teasing, vaginal cytology, and elisa for progesterone. *Theriogenology.* 35:603–611.

Bourget, C., Femino, A., Franz, C. et al. 1988. Estrogen and androgen dynamics in the cynomolgus monkey. *Endocrinology.* 122:202–206.

Bourget, C., Flood, C., and Longcope, C. 1984. Steroid dynamics in the rabbit. *Steroids.* 43:225–233.

Bourne, G.A., Regiani, S., Payne, A.H. et al. 1980. Testicular GnRH receptors-characterization and localization on interstitial tissue. *J Clin Endocrinol Metab.* 51:407–409.

Brett, L.P., Chong, G.S., Coyle, S. et al. 1983. The pituitary–adrenal response to novel stimulation and ether stress in young adult and aged rats. *Neurobiol Aging.* 4:133–138.

Breyer, M.D., Zhang, Y., Guan, Y.F. et al. 1998. Regulation of renal function by prostaglandin E receptors. *Kidney Int.* 67:S88–94.

Bridges, R.S. 1994. The role of lactogenic hormones in maternal behavior in female rats. *Acta Paediatr.* 83(Suppl 397):33–39.

Brixen, K., Nielsen, H.K., Bouillon, R. et al. 1992. Effects of short-term growth hormone treatment on PTH, calcitriol, thyroid hormones, insulin and glucagon. *Acta Endocrinol (Copenh.).* 127:331–336.

Brock, B.J. and Waterman, M.R. 1999. Biochemical differences between rat and human cytochrome P450c17 support the different steroidogenic needs of these two species. *Biochemistry.* 38:1598–1606.

Broglio, F., Koetsveld, Pv.Pv., Benso, A. et al. 2002. Ghrelin secretion is inhibited by either somatostatin or cortistatin in humans. *J Clin Endocrinol Metab.* 87:4829–4832.

Brooks, J.R., Ross, C.V., and Turner, C.W. 1964. Effect of thyroidectomy on reproductive performance of ewes and semen quality of rams. *J Anim Sci.* 23:54–58.

Brown, T.J., Khan, T., and Jones, K.J. 1999. Androgen induced acceleration of functional recovery after rat sciatic nerve injury. *Restor Neurol Neurosci.* 15:289–295.

Brown-Grant, K., Davidson, J.M., and Greig, F. 1973. Induced ovulation in albino rats exposed to constant light. *J Endocrinol.* 57:7–22.

Brown-Séquard, C.E. 1899a. The effects produced in men by the injection of extracts of the testes of guinea pigs and dogs. *Compte Rendu Societe de Biologie.* 1(Series 9):415–419.

Brown-Séquard, C.E. 1899b. The effects produced on man by subcutaneous injection of a liquid obtained from the testicles of animals. *Lancet.* 2:105–107.

Bruchovsky, N. 1971. Comparison of the metabolites formed in rat prostate following the in vivo administration of seven natural androgens. *Endocrinology.* 89:1212–1222.

Brucker-Davis, F. 1998. Effects of environmental synthetic chemicals on thyroid function. *Thyroid.* 8:827–856.

Brunton, P.J., McKay, A.J., Ochedalski, T. et al. 2009. Central opioid inhibition of neuroendocrine stress responses in pregnancy in the rat is induced by the neurosteroid allopregnanolone. *J Neurosci.* 29:6449–6460.

Brunton, P.J., Russell, J.A., and Douglas, A.J. 2008. Adaptive responses of the maternal hypothalamic–pituitary–adrenal axis during pregnancy and lactation. *J Neuroendocrinol.* 20:764–776.

Buczynski, M.W., Dumlao, D.S., and Dennis, E.A. 2009. Thematic review series: Proteomics. An integrated omics analysis of eicosanoid biology. *J Lipid Res.* 50:1015–1038.

Burger, L.L., Haisenleder, D.J., Aylor, K.W. et al. 2008. Regulation of intracellular signaling cascades by GnRH pulse frequency in the rat pituitary: Roles for CaMK II, ERK, and JNK activation. *Biol Reprod.* 79:947–953.

Burgon, P.G., Stanton, P.G., and Robertson, D.M. 1996. In vivo bioactivities and clearance patterns of highly purified human luteinizing hormone isoforms. *Endocrinology.* 137:4827–4836.

Burguera, B., Couce, M.E., Long, J. et al. 2000. The long form of the leptin receptor (OB-Rb) is widely expressed in the human brain. *Neuroendocrinology.* 71:187–195.

Bush, B.M. 1969. Thyroid disease in the dog—a review. I. *J Small Anim Pract.* 10:95–109.

Bustad, L.K. and Fuller, J.M. 1970. Thyroid function in domestic animals. *Lab Anim Care.* 20:561–581.

Butera, P.C., Bradway, D.M., and Cataldo, N.J. 1993. Modulation of the satiety effect of cholecystokinin by estradiol. *Physiol Behav.* 53:1235–1238.

Caba, M., Pau, K.-Y F., Beyer, C. et al. 2000. Coitus-induced activation of c-fos and gonadotropin-releasing hormone in hypothalamic neurons in female rabbits. *Mol Brain Res.* 78:69–79.

Cachofeiro, V., Miana, M., de Las Heras, N. et al. 2008. Aldosterone and the vascular system. *J Steroid Biochem Mol Biol.* 109:331–335.

Cameron, J.L. 1997. Stress and behaviorally induced reproductive dysfunction in primates. *Semin Reprod Endocrinol.* 15:37–45.

Capen, C.C. and Martin, S.L. 2003. The thyroid gland. In *McDonald's Veterinary Endocrinology and Reproduction*. Ed. M.H. Pineda, and M.P. Dooley, 5th edition, pp. 35–70. Ames, IA: Blackwell Publishing.

Carlin, K.M., Vale, W.W., and Bale, T.L. 2006. Vital functions of corticotropin-releasing factor (CRF) pathways in maintenance and regulation of energy homeostasis. *Proc Natl Acad Sci.* 103:3462–3467.

Chai, J.K., Blaha, V., Meguid, M.M. et al. 1999. Use of orchiectomy and testosterone replacement to explore meal number-to-meal size relationship in male rats. *Am J Physiol.* 276:R1366–1373.

Chand, N. and Altura, B.M. 1980. Reactivity of isolated rat and canine pulmonary arteries to prostaglandins. *Prostaglandins Med.* 5:59–67.

Chanoine, J.P., Alex, S., Fang, S.L. et al. 1992. Role of transthyretin in the transport of thyroxine from the blood to the choroid plexus, the cerebrospinal fluid, and the brain. *Endocrinology.* 130:933–938.

Chapman, S.C., Bernard, D.J., Jelen, J. et al. 2002. Properties of inhibin binding to betaglycan, InhBP/p120 and the activin type II receptors. Mol Cell Endocrinol. 196:79–93.

Chen, H.J. and Meites, J. 1975. Effects of biogenic amines and TRH on release of prolactin and TSH in the rat. *Endocrinology.* 96:10–14.

Chen, J.J., Wang, S.W., Chien, E.J. et al. 2003. Direct effect of propylthiouracil on progesterone release in rat granulosa cells. *Br J Pharmacol.* 139:1564–1570.

Chen, M.-C., Wang, S.W., Kan, S.-F. et al. 2010. Stimulatory effects of propylthiouracil on pregnenolone production through upregulation of steroidogenic acute regulatory protein expression in rat granulosa cells. *Toxicol Sci.* 118:667–674.

Chi, H.J. and Shin, S.H. 1978. The effect of exposure to ether on prolactin secretion and the half-life of endogenous prolactin in normal and castrated male rats. *Neuroendocrinology.* 26:193–201.

Chiamolera, M.I. and Wondisford, F.E. 2009. Thyrotropin-releasing hormone and the thyroid hormone feedback mechanism. *Endocrinology.* 150:1091–1096.

Chiao, Y.C., Cho, W.L., and Wang, P.S. 2002. Inhibition of testosterone production by propylthiouracil in rat Leydig cells. *Biol Reprod.* 67:416–422.

Chiaramonte, D. and Greco, D.S. 2007. Feline adrenal disorders. *Clin Tech Small Anim Pract.* 22:26–31.

Ciampani, T., Fabbri, A., Isidori, A. et al. 1992. Growth hormone-releasing hormone is produced by rat Leydig cell in culture and acts as a positive regulator of Leydig cell function. *Endocrinology.* 131:2785–2792.

Clark, R.G., Carlsson, L.M., and Robinson, I.C. 1987. Growth hormone secretory profiles in conscious female rats. *J Endocrinol.* 114:399–407.

Clarke, I.J., Thomas, G.B., Yao, B. et al. 1987. GnRH secretion throughout the ovine estrous cycle. *Neuroendocrinology.* 46:82–88.

Claus, R., Dimmick, M.A., Gimenez, T. et al. 1992. Estrogens and prostaglandin F2α in the semen and blood plasma of stallions. *Theriogenology.* 38:687–693.

Clayton, R.N., Katikineni, M., Chan, V. et al. 1980. Direct inhibition of testicular function by gonadotropin-releasing hormone: Mediation by specific gonadotropin-releasing hormone receptors in interstitial cells. *Proc Natl Acad Sci.* 77:4459–4463.

Clemens, J.A., Minaguchi, H., Storey, R. et al. 1969. Induction of precocious puberty in female rats by Prolactin. *Neuroendocrinology.* 4:150–156.

Cocchi, D., De Gennaro Colonna, V., Bagnasco, M. et al. 1999. Leptin regulates GH secretion in the rat by acting on GHRH and somatostatinergic functions. *J Endocrinol.* 162:95–99.

Coe, C.L., Franklin, D., Smith, E.R. et al. 1982. Hormonal responses accompanying fear and agitation in the squirrel monkey. *Physiol Behav.* 29:1051–1057.

Cohen, S.B. and Weetman, A.P. 1988. The effect of iodide depletion and supplementation in the Buffalo strain rat. *J Endocrinol Invest.* 11:625–627.

Collet, C., Schiltz, C., Geoffroy, V. et al. 2008. The serotonin 5-HT2B receptor controls bone mass via osteoblast recruitment and proliferation. *FASEB J.* 22:418–427.

Collins, W.T., Jr., Capen, C.C., Kasza, L. et al. 1977. Effect of polychlorinated biphenyl (PCB) on the thyroid gland of rats. Ultrastructural and biochemical investigations. *Am J Pathol.* 89:119–136.

Connolly, D.J., Magalhaes, R.J., Syme, H.M. et al. 2008. Circulating natriuretic peptides in cats with heart disease. *J Vet Intern Med.* 22:96–105.

Constant, R.B. and Weintraub, B.D. 1986. Differences in the metabolic clearance of pituitary and serum thyrotropin (TSH) derived from euthyroid and hypothyroid rats: Effects of chemical deglycosylation of pituitary TSH. *Endocrinology.* 119:2720–2727.

Cooper, R.L., Stoker, T.E., Tyrey, L. et al. 2000. Atrazine disrupts the hypothalamic control of pituitary–ovarian function. *Toxicol Sci.* 53:297–307.

Corbacho, A.M., Martínez De La Escalera, G., and Clapp, C. 2002. Roles of prolactin and related members of the prolactin/growth hormone/placental lactogen family in angiogenesis. *J Endocrinol.* 173:219–238.

Corbo, D.C., Huang, Y.C., and Chien, Y.W. 1988. Nasal delivery of progestational steroids in ovariectomized rabbits. I. Progesterone—comparison of pharmacokinetics with intravenous and oral administration. *Int J Pharm.* 46:133–140.

Corrigan, A.Z., Bilezikjian, L.M., Carroll, R.S. et al. 1991. Evidence for an autocrine role of activin B within rat anterior pituitary cultures. *Endocrinology.* 128:1682–1684.

Couzinet, B., Young, J., Kujas, M. et al. 1999. The antigonadotropic activity of a 19-nor-progesterone derivative is exerted both at the hypothalamic and pituitary levels in women. *J Clin Endocrinol Metab.* 84:4191–4196.

Coveñas, R., de León, M., Narváez, J.A. et al. 1996. An immunocytochemical mapping of ACTH/CLIP in the cat diencephalon. *J Chem Neuroanat.* 11:191–197.

Cox, H.M. 2008. Endogenous PYY and NPY mediate tonic Y1- and Y2-mediated absorption in human and mouse colon. *Nutrition.* 24:900–906.

Crankshaw, D.J. and Gaspar, V. 1995. Pharmacological characterization in vitro of prostanoid receptors in the myometrium of nonpregnant ewes. *J Reprod Fertil.* 103:55–61.

Creighton, W.D., Lambert, P.H., and Mieschner, P.A. 1973. Detection of antibodies and soluble antigen–antibody complexes by precipitation with polyethylene glycol. *J Immunol.* 111:1219–1227.

Crooks, J. and Wayne, E.J. 1960. A comparison of potassium perchlorate, methylthiouracil, and carbimazole in the treatment of thyrotoxicosis. *Lancet.* 1(7121):401–404.

Csapo, A.I. and Wiest, W.G. 1969. An examination of the quantitative relationship between progesterone and the maintenance of pregnancy. *Endocrinology.* 85:735–746.

Cushing, H.W. 1932. The basophil adenomas of the pituitary body and their clinical manifestations (pituitary basophilism). *Bull Johns Hopkins Hosp.* 50:137–195.

D'Angelo, S.A., Wall, N.R., Bowers, C.Y. et al. 1975. Effects of acute and chronic administration of TRH on TSH and prolactin secretion in normal and hypothyroid rats. *Neuroendocrinology.* 18:161–175.

Dalm, V.A., van Hagen, P.M., van Koetsveld, P.M. et al. 2003. Expression of somatostatin, cortistatin, and somatostatin receptors in human monocytes, macrophages, and dendritic cells. *Am J Physiol Endocrinol Metab.* 285:E344–353.

Dauncey, M.J. 1990. Thyroid hormones and thermogenesis. *Proc Nutr Soc.* 49:203–215.

Dautzenberg, F.M. and Hauger, R.L. 2002. The CRF peptide family and their receptors: Yet more partners discovered. *Trends Pharmacol Sci.* 23:71–77.

Davis, J.A. and Linzer, D.I.H. 1989. Expression of multiple forms of the prolactin receptor in mouse liver. *Mol Endocrinol.* 3: 674–680.

de Divitiis, E., Cappabianca, P., and de Divitiis, O. 2004. The "schola medica salernitana": The forerunner of the modern university medical schools. *Neurosurgery.* 55:722–744.

De Geyter, C., De Geyter, M., Huber, P.R. et al. 2002. Progesterone serum levels during the follicular phase of the menstrual cycle originate from the crosstalk between the ovaries and the adrenal cortex. *Hum Reprod.* 17:933–939.

de Kretser, D.M., Loveland, K.L., Meehan, T. et al. 2001. Inhibins, activins and follistatin: Actions on the testis. Mol Cell Endocrinol. 180:87–92.

de la Peña, P., Delgado, L.M., del Camino, D. et al. 1992. Two isoforms of the thyrotropin-releasing hormone receptor generated by alternative splicing have indistinguishable functional properties. *J Biol Chem.* 267:25703–25708.

de Lecea, L., del Rio, J.A., Criado, J.R. et al. 1997. Cortistatin is expressed in a distinct subset of cortical interneurons. *J Neurosci.* 17:5868–5880.

Debuyser, A., Drews, G., and Henquin, J.C. 1991. Adrenaline inhibition of insulin release: Role of the repolarization of the B cell membrane. *Pflugers Arch.* 419:131–137.

DeCherney, G.S., Gesundheit, N., Gyves, P.W. et al. 1989. Alterations in the sialylation and sulfation of secreted mouse thyrotropin in primary hypothyroidism. *Biochem Biophys Res Commun.* 159:755–762.

Dellarco, V.L., McGregor, D., Berry, S.C. et al. 2006. Thiazopyr and thyroid disruption: Case study within the context of the 2006 IPCS Human Relevance Framework for analysis of a cancer mode of action. *Crit Rev Toxicol.* 36:793–801.

Diaz, F.J., Anderson, L.E., Wu, Y.L. et al. 2002. Regulation of progesterone and prostaglandin F2α production in the CL. *Mol Cell Endocrinol.* 191:65–80.

DiBartolomeis, M.J., and Jefcoate, C.R. 1984. Characterization of the acute stimulation of steroidogenesis in primary bovine adrenal cortical cell cultures. *J Biol Chem.* 259:10159–10167.

DiStefano, J.J., 3rd. and Feng, D. 1988. Comparative aspects of the distribution, metabolism, and excretion of six iodothyronines in the rat. *Endocrinology.* 123:2514–2525.

Dixon, R.M., Reid, S.W., and Mooney, C.T. 2002. Treatment and therapeutic monitoring of canine hypothyroidism. *J Small Anim Pract.* 43:334–340.

Dluzen, D.E. and Ramirez, V.D. 1987. In vivo activity of the LHRH pulse generator as determined with push–pull perfusion of the anterior pituitary gland of unrestrained intact and castrate male rats. *Neuroendocrinology.* 45:328–332.

Dore, M. 2010. Cyclooxygenase-2 expression in animal cancers. In press. *Vet Pathol.* Available at: http://vet.sagepub.com/content/early/2010/09/25/0300985810379434.

Dorrington, J.M., Fritz, B., and Armstrong, D.T. 1978. Control of testicular estrogen synthesis. *Biol Reprod.* 18:55–64.

Drews, G., Debuyser, A., Nenquin, M. et al. 1990. Galanin and epinephrine act on distinct receptors to inhibit insulin release by the same mechanisms including an increase in K+ permeability of the B-cell membrane. *Endocrinology.* 126:1646–1653.

Dumoulin, V., Dakka, T., Plaisancie, P. et al. 1995. Regulation of glucagon-like peptide-1-(7-36) amide, peptide YY, and neurotensin secretion by neurotransmitters and gut hormones in the isolated vascularly perfused rat ileum. *Endocrinology.* 136:5182–5188.

Dupouy, J.P., Godaut, M., and Chatelain, A. 1986. [Influence of heparin on the radioimmunological assay of ACTH]. *Ann Endocrinol (Paris).* 47:429–434.

Dupuy, G.M., Roberts, K.D., Bleau, G. et al. 1982. Sites of *in vivo* extraction and interconversion of estrone and estradiol in the dog. *Steroids.* 39:201–219.

Dyess, E.M., Segerson, T.P., Liposits, Z. et al. 1988. Triiodothyronine exerts direct cell-specific regulation of thyrotropin-releasing hormone gene expression in the hypothalamic paraventricular nucleus. *Endocrinology.* 123:2291–2297.

Ehrlich, H.P. and Hunt, T.K. 1969. The effects of cortisone and anabolic steroids on the tensile strength of healing wounds. *Ann Surg.* 170:203–206.

Eigenmann, J.E. 1984. Acromegaly in the dog. *Vet Clin North Am Small Anim Pract.* 14:827–836.

Eigenmann, J.E., Patterson, D.F., Zapf, J. et al. 1984. Insulin-like growth factor I in the dog: A study in different dog breeds and in dogs with growth hormone elevation. *Acta Endocrinol (Copenh.).* 105:294–301.

Eiler, H. and Graves, C.N. 1977. Oestrogen content of semen and the effect of exogenous oestradiol-17α on the oestrogen and androgen concentration in semen and blood plasma of bulls. *J Reprod Fertil.* 50:17–21.

Ekblad, E. and Sundler, F. 2002. Distribution of pancreatic polypeptide and peptide YY. *Peptides.* 23:251–261.

Elle, M. and Hoenig, M. 1995. Canine immune mediated diabetes mellitus: A case report. *J Am Anim Hosp Assoc.* 31:295–299.

Endemann, D.H., Wolf, K., Boeger, C.A. et al. 2004. Adrenal aldosterone biosynthesis is elevated in a model of chronic renal failure—role of local adrenal renin–angiotensin system. *Nephron Physiol.* 97:37–44.

Ernst, M., Schmid, C., and Froesch, E.R. 1988. Enhanced osteoblast proliferation and collagen gene expression by estradiol. *Proc Natl Acad Sci USA.* 85:2307–2310.

Esteve, J.M., Launay, J.M., Kellermann, O. et al. 2007. Functions of serotonin in hypoxic pulmonary vascular remodeling. *Cell Biochem Biophys.* 47:33–44.

Evans, M.J., Livesey, J.H., Ellis, M.J. et al. 2001. Effect of anticoagulants and storage temperatures on stability of plasma and serum hormones. *Clin Biochem.* 34:107–112.

Evans, N.P., Richter, T.A., Skinner, D.C. et al. 2002. Neuroendocrine mechanisms underlying the effects of progesterone on the oestradiol-induced GnRH/LH surge. *Reproduction.* 59:57–66.

Ewing, L.L. and Zirkin, B.R. 1983. Leydig cell structure and steroidogenic function. *Recent Prog Horm Res.* 39:599–635.

Farwell, A.P., Dubord-Tomasetti, S.A., Pietrzykowski, A.Z. et al. 2005. Regulation of cerebellar neuronal migration and neurite outgrowth by thyroxine and 3,3′,5′-triiodothyronine. *Dev Brain Res.* 154:121–135.

Faundes, A., Brache, V., Tejada, A.S. et al. 1991. Ovulatory dysfunction during continuous administration of low-dose levonorgestrel by subdermal implants. *Fertil Steril.* 56:27–31.

Feldman, E.C. and Nelson, R.W. 1994. Comparative aspects of Cushing's syndrome in dogs and cats. *Endocrinol Metab Clin North Am.* 23:671–691.

Fendrick, J.L., Raafat, A.M., and Haslam, S.Z. 1998. Mammary gland growth and development from the postnatal period to postmenopause: ovarian steroid receptor ontogeny and regulation in the mouse. *J Mammary Gland Biol Neoplasia.* 3:7–22.

Ferguson, D.C. 1995. Free thyroid hormone measurement in the diagnosis of thyroid disease. In *Current Veterinary Therapy XII.* Eds. J.D. Bonagura, and R.W. Kirk, pp. 360–364. Philadelphia, PA: W.B. Saunders.

Fessler, R.G., Deyo, S.N., Meltzer, H.Y. et al. 1984. Evidence that the medial and dorsal raphe nuclei mediate serotonergically-induced increases in prolactin release from the pituitary. *Brain Res.* 299:231–237.

Findlay, J.K. 1993. An update on the roles of inhibin, activin, and follistatin as local regulators of folliculogenesis. *Biol Reprod.* 48:15–23.

Findlay, J.K., Drummond, A.E., Dyson, M. et al. 2001. Production and actions of inhibin and activin during folliculogenesis in the rat. *Mol Cell Endocrinol.* 180:139–144.

Fisher, J.W., Samuels, A.I., and Malgor, L.A. 1971. Androgens and erythropoiesis. *Isr J Med Sci.* 7:892–900.

Florini, J.R. 1970. Effects of testosterone on qualitative pattern of protein synthesis in skeletal muscle. *Biochemistry.* 9:909–912.

Florini, J.R., Ewton, D.Z., and Coolican, S.A. 1996. Growth hormone and the insulin-like growth factor system in myogenesis. *Endocr Rev.* 17:481–517.

Fodor, M., Kordon, C., and Epelbaum, J. 2006. Anatomy of the hypophysiotropic somatostatinergic and growth hormone-releasing hormone system minireview. *Neurochem Res.* 31:137–143.

Fortune, J.E. 1986. Bovine theca and granulose cells interact to promote androgen production. *Biol Reprod.* 35:292–299.

Foster, P.M. 2006. Disruption of reproductive development in male rat offspring following in utero exposure to phthalate esters. *Int J Androl.* 29:140–147.

Fox, S.M., Mellor, D.J., Firth, E.C. et al. 1994. Changes in plasma cortisol concentrations before, during and after analgesia, anaesthesia and anaesthesia plus ovariohysterectomy in bitches. *Res Vet Sci.* 57:110–118.

Franz, C. and Longcope, C. 1979. Androgen and estrogen metabolism in male rhesus monkeys. *Endocrinology.* 105:869–874.

Fraser, I.S., Challis, J.R.G., and Thorburn, G.D. 1976. Metabolic clearance rate and production rate of oestradiol in conscious rabbit. *J Endocrinol.* 68:313–320.

Friesema, E.C., Jansen, J., Milici, C. et al. 2005. Thyroid hormone transporters. *Vitam Horm.* 70:137–167.

Fujii, Y., Kato, N., Kito, J. et al. 1992. Experimental autoimmune adrenalitis: A murine model for Addison's disease. *Autoimmunity.* 12:47–52.

Fujita, K., Kato, T., Shibayama, K. et al. 2006. Protective effect against 17β-estradiol on neuronal apoptosis in hippocampus tissue following transient ischemia/recirculation in mongolian gerbils via down-regulation of tissue transglutaminase activity. *Neurochem Res.* 31:1059–1068.

Furudate, S. 1991. Suppression of the prolactin surges in the pseudopregnant rat by urethane anesthesia. *Jikken Dobutsu.* 40:77–82.

Gaddam, K.K., Pimenta, E., Husain, S. et al. 2009. Aldosterone and cardiovascular disease. *Curr Probl Cardiol.* 34:51–84.

Gaillard, D., Wabitsch, M., Pipy, B. et al. 1991. Control of terminal differentiation of adipose precursor cells by glucocorticoids. *J Lipid Res.* 32:569–579.

Gala, R.R. and Shevach, E.M. 1993. Identification by analytical flow cytometry of prolactin receptors on immunocompetent cell populations in the mouse. *Endocrinology.* 133:1617–1623.

Gan, E.-H. and Quinton, R. 2010. Physiological significance of the rhythmic secretion of hypothalamic and pituitary hormones. *Progr Brain Res.* 181:111–126.

Gangrade, N.K., Boudinot, F.D., and Price, J.C. 1992. Pharmacokinetics of progesterone in ovariectomized rats after a single dose intravenous administration. *Biopharm Drug Dispos.* 13:703–709.

Ganjam, V.K. and Amann, R.P. 1976. Steroids in fluids and sperm entering and leaving the bovine epididymis, epididymal tissue, and accessory sex gland secretions. *Endocrinology.* 99:1618–1630.

Gautier, J.F., Choukem, S.P., and Girard, J. 2008. Physiology of incretins (GIP and GLP-1) and abnormalities in type 2 diabetes. *Diabetes Metab.* 34(Suppl 2):S65–72.

Gavin, L.A., Moeller, M., Shoback, D. et al. 1988. Reverse T3 and modulators of the calcium messenger system rapidly decrease T4-5′-deiodinase II activity in cultured mouse neuroblastoma cells. *Thyroidology.* 1:5–12.

Ge, W., Gallin, W.J., Strobeck, C. et al. 1993. Cloning and sequencing of goldfish activin subunit genes: Strong structural conservation during vertebrate evolution. *Biochem Biophys Res Commun.* 193:711–717.

Geisert, R.D. and Conley, A.J. 1998. Secretion and metabolism of steroids in subprimate mammals during pregnancy. In *Endocrinology of Pregnancy*. Ed. F.W. Bazer, pp. 291–318. Totowa, NJ: Humana Press.

Gentry, R.T. and Wade, G.N. 1976. Androgenic control of food intake and body weight in male rats. *J Comp Physiol Psychol.* 90:747–754.

George, I., Xydas, S., Klotz, S. et al. 2010. Long-term effects of B-type natriuretic peptide infusion after acute myocardial infarction in a rat model. *J Cardiovasc Pharmacol.* 55:14–20.

Gibson, E.M., Humber, S.A., Jain, S. et al. 2008. Alterations in RFamide-related peptide expression are coordinated with the preovulatory luteinizing hormone surge. *Endocrinology.* 149:4958–4969.

Gil, A.G., Silván, G., and Illera, J.C. 2007. Pituitary–adrenocortical axis, serum serotonin and biochemical response after halothane or isoflurane anaesthesia in rabbits. *Lab Anim.* 41:411–419.

Gimpl, G. and Fahrenholz, F. 2001. The oxytocin receptor system: Structure, function, and regulation. *Physiol Rev.* 81:629–683.

Giustina, A. and Veldhuis, J.D. 1998. Pathophysiology of the neuroregulation of growth hormone secretion in experimental animals and the human. *Endocr Rev.* 19:717–797.

Giustina, A., Mazziotti, G., and Canalis, E. 2008. Growth hormone, insulin-like growth factors, and the skeleton. *Endocr Rev.* 29:535–559.

Glasser, S.R. and Clark, J.H. 1975. A determinant role for progesterone in the development of uterine sensitivity to decidualization and ovo-implantation. *Symp Soc Dev Biol.* 33:311–345.

Gnanapavan, S., Kola, B., Bustin, S.A. et al. 2002. The tissue distribution of the mRNA of ghrelin and subtypes of its receptor, GHS-R, in humans. *J Clin Endocrinol Metab.* 87:2988–2991.

Godley, A.F. and Stanbury, J.B. 1954. Preliminary experience in the treatment of hyperthyroidism with potassium perchlorate. *J Clin Endocrinol Metab.* 14:70–78.

Goldbeter, A., Dupont, G., and Halloy, J. 2000. The frequency encoding of pulsatility. *Novartis Foundation Symp.* 227:19–36.

Goldman, J.M. and Cooper, R.L. 1993. Assessment of toxicant-induced alterations in the luteinizing hormone control of ovulation in the rat. In *Methods in Toxicology*, Vol. 1, Part B, *Female Reproductive Toxicology*. Eds. J.J. Heindel, and R.E. Chapin, pp. 79–91. San Diego, CA: Academic Press.

Goldman, J.M. and Cooper, R.L. 2010. The impact of centrally acting pesticidal/environmental toxicants on the neuroendocrine regulation of reproductive function in the female rat: Relevance to human reproductive risk assessment. In *Endocrine Toxicology*. Eds. J.C. Eldridge, and J.T. Stevens, 3rd edition, pp. 210–239. London: Informa Healthcare.

Goldman, J.M., Laws, S.C., Balchak, S.K. et al. 2000. Endocrine disrupting chemicals: Prepubertal exposures and effects on sexual maturation and thyroid activity in the female rat. A focus on the EDSTAC recommendations. *Crit Rev Toxicol.* 30:135–196.

Goldman, J.M., Murr, A.S., Buckalew, A.R. et al. 2008. Suppression of the steroid-primed luteinizing hormone surge in the female rat by sodium dimethyldithiocarbamate: Relationship to hypothalamic catecholamines and GnRH neuronal activation. *Toxicol Sci.* 104:107–112.

Goldman, J.M., Stoker, T.E., Cooper, R.L. et al. 1994. Blockade of ovulation in the rat by the fungicide sodium *N*-methyldithiocarbamate: Relationship between effects on the luteinizing hormone surge and alterations in hypothalamic catecholamines. *Neurotoxicol Teratol.* 16:257–268.

Goldman, S., Weiss, A., Almalah, I. et al. 2005. Progesterone receptor expression in human decidua and fetal membranes before and after contractions: Possible mechanism for functional progesterone withdrawal. *Mol Hum Reprod.* 11:269–277.

Gonzalez, M.D., López, F., and Aguilar, E. 1984. Involvement of prolactin in the onset of puberty in female rats. *J Endocrinol.* 101:63–68.

Gore, A.C. 2002. GnRH pulsatility. In *GnRH: The Master Molecule of Reproduction*, Chap. 2, pp. 29–52. Dordrecht, Netherlands: Kluwer Academic Publication.

Gosden, R.G., Everett, J.W., and Tyrey, L. 1976. Luteinizing hormone requirements for ovulation in the pentobarbital-treated proestrous rat. *Endocrinology.* 99:1046–1053.

Gospodarowicz, D. and Lau, K. 1989. Pituitary follicular cells secrete both vascular endothelial growth factor and follistatin. *Biochem Biophys Res Commun.* 165:292–298.

Gravel, C., Sasseville, R., and Hawkes, R. 1990. Maturation of the corpus callosum of the rat: II. Influence of thyroid hormones on the number and maturation of axons. *J Comp Neurol.* 291:147–161.

Gray, L.E., Jr., Ostby, J.S., and Kelce, W.R. 1994. Developmental effects of an environmental antiandrogen: The fungicide vinclozolin alters sex differentiation of the male rat. *Toxicol Appl Pharmacol.* 129:46–52.

Greco, D.S. 2007. Hypoadrenocorticism in small animals. *Clin Tech Small Anim Pract.* 22:32–35.

Greco, S.J., Sarkar, S., Johnston, J.M. et al. 2008. Leptin reduces Alzheimer's disease-related tau phosphorylation in neuronal cells. *Biochem Biophys Res Commun.* 376:536–541.

Greco, S.J., Sarkar, S., Johnston, J.M. et al. 2009. Leptin regulates tau phosphorylation and amyloid through AMPK in neuronal cells. *Biochem Biophys Res Commun.* 380:98–104.

Green, E.D. and Baenziger, J.U. 1988. Asparagine-linked oligosaccharides on lutropin, follitropin, and thyrotropin. *J Biol Chem.* 263:36–44.

Green, P.S., Yang, S.H., Nilsson, K.R. et al. 2001. The nonfeminizing enantiomer of 17beta-estradiol exerts protective effects in neuronal cultures and a rat model of cerebral ischemia. *Endocrinology.* 142:400–406.

Griffin, J.E. and Auchus, R.J. 2004. Assessment of endocrine function. In *Textbook of Endocrine Physiology*. Eds. J.E. Griffin, and S.R. Ojeda, pp. 101–119. New York, NY: Oxford University Press.

Grov, A., Oeding, P., Myklestad, B. et al. 1970. Reactions of staphylococcal antigens with normal sera, gamma G-globulins, and gamma G-globulin fragments of various species origin. *Acta Pathol Microbiol Scand B Microbiol Immunol.* 78:106–111.

Guillermet-Guibert, J., Lahlou, H., Cordelier, P. et al. 2005. Physiology of somatostatin receptors. *J Endocrinol Invest.* 28 (11 Suppl International):5–9.

Guler, H.P., Binz, K., Eigenmann, E. et al. 1989. Small stature and insulin-like growth factors: Prolonged treatment of mini-poodles with recombinant human insulin-like growth factor I. *Acta Endocrinol (Copenh.).* 121:456–464.

Gum, G.G., Kingsbury, S., Whitley, R.D. et al. 1991. Effect of topical prostaglandin PGA2, isopropyl ester, and PGF2α isopropyl ester on intraocular pressure in normotensive and glaucomatous canine eyes. *J Ocul Pharmacol.* 7:107–116.

Günzel-Apel, A.R., Hille, P., and Hoppen, H.O. 1994. Spontaneous and GnRH-induced pulsatile LH and testosterone release in pubertal, adult and aging male beagles. *Theriogenology.* 41:737–745.

Gupta, R.K. and Morton, D.L. 1979. Double-antibody method and the protein-A-bearing *Staphlylococcus aureus* cells method compared for separating bound and free antigen in radioimmunoassay. *Clin Chem.* 25:752–756.

Gust, D.A., Gordon, T.P., Brodie, A.R. et al. 1994. Effect of a preferred companion in modulating stress in adult female rhesus monkeys. *Physiol Behav.* 55:681–684.

Haeger, P., Andrés, M.E., Forray, M.I. et al. 2006. Estrogen receptors alpha and beta differentially regulate the transcriptional activity of the Urocortin gene. *J Neurosci.* 26:4908–4916.

Hagino, N. 1979. Effect of Nembutal on LH release in baboons. *Horm Metab Res.* 11:296–300.

Hagman, R., Karlstam, E., Persson, S. et al. 2009. Plasma PGF 2 alpha metabolite levels in cats with uterine disease. *Theriogenology.* 72:1180–1187.

Hagman, R., Kindahl, H., and Lagerstedt, A.S. 2006. Pyometra in bitches induces elevated plasma endotoxin and prostaglandin F2α metabolite levels. *Acta Vet Scand.* 47:55–67.

Haisenleder, D.J., Khoury, S., Zmielli, S.M. et al. 1987. The frequency of gonadotropin-releasing hormone secretion regulates expression of alpha and luteinizing hormone beta-subunit messenger ribonucleic acids in male rats. *Mol Endocrinol.* 1:834–838.

Haisenleder, D.J., Schoenfelder, A.H., Marcinko, E.S., Geddis, L.M., and Marshall, J.C. 2011. Estimation of estradiol in mouse serum samples: Evaluation of commercial estradiol immunoassays. *Endocrinology.* 152:4443–4447.

Halestrap, A.P. and Meredith, D. 2004. The SLC16 gene family- from monocarboxylate transporters (MCT) to aromatic amino acid transporters and beyond. *Pflugers Arch.* 447:619–628.

Hamlyn, J.M., Lu, Z., Manunta, P. et al. 1998. Observations onn the nature, biosynthesis, secretion and significance of endogenous ouabain. *Clin Exp Hypertens.* 20:523–533.

Hammock, E.A. and Young, L.J. 2006. Oxytocin, vasopressin and pair bonding: Implications for autism. *Philos Trans R Soc Lond B Biol Sci.* 361:2187–2198.

Hansen, M.B. and Witte, A.B. 2008. The role of serotonin in intestinal luminal sensing and secretion. *Acta Physiol (Oxf).* 193:311–323.

Hansotia, T. and Drucker, D.J. 2005. GIP and GLP-1 as incretin hormones: Lessons from single and double incretin receptor knockout mice. *Regul Peptides.* 128:125–134.

Harris, G.C. and Nicholson, H.D. 1998. Stage-related differences in rat seminiferous tubule contractility in vitro and their response to oxytocin. *J Endocrinol.* 157:251–257.

Hartmann, D.P., Holaday, J.W., and Bernton, E.W. 1989. Inhibition of lymphocyte proliferation by antibodies to prolactin. *FASEB J.* 3:2194–2202.

Hatsuta, M., Abe, K., Tamura, K. et al. 2004. Effects of hypothyroidism on the estrous cycle and reproductive hormones in mature female rat. *Eur J Pharmacol.* 486:343–348.

Hayaishi, O. 1991. Molecular mechanisms of sleep–wake regulation: Roles of prostaglandins D2 and E2. *FASEB J.* 5:2575–2581.

He, J., Chen, Y., Huang, Y. et al. 2009. Effect of long-term B-type natriuretic peptide treatment on left ventricular remodeling and function after myocardial infarction in rats. *Eur J Pharmacol.* 602:132–137.

Head, E., Moffat, K., Das, P. et al. 2005. Beta-amyloid deposition and tau phosphorylation in clinically characterized aged cats. *Neurobiol Aging.* 26:749–763.

Heinrichs, W.L., Tabei, T., Kuwabara, Y. et al. 1979. Differentiation and regulation of peripheral androgen metabolism in rats and rhesus monkeys. *Am J Obstet Gynecol.* 135:974–983.

Henderson, R.F., Leung, H.W., Harmsen, A.G. et al. 1988. Species differences in release of arachidonate metabolites in response to inhaled diluted diesel exhaust. *Toxicol Lett.* 42:325–332.

Hershlag, A., Zinger, M., Lesser, M. et al. 2000. Is chemiluminescent immunoassay an appropriate substitution for radioimmunoassay in monitoring estradiol levels? *Fertil Steril.* 73:1174–1178.

Hess, R.A. 2003. Estrogen in the adult male reproductive tract: A review. *Reprod Biol Endocrinol.* 1:1–14.

Hinuma, S., Habata, Y., Fujii, R. et al. 1998. A prolactin-releasing peptide in the brain. *Nature.* 393:272–276.

Hinz, B., Cheremina, O., and Brune, H. 2008. Acetaminophen (paracetamol) is a selective cyclooxygenase-2 inhibitor in man. *FASEB J.* 22:383–390.

Honma, S., Suzuki, A., Buchanan, D.L. et al. 2002. Low dose effect of in utero exposure to bisphenol A and diethylstilbestrol on female mouse reproduction. *Reprod Toxicol.* 16:117–122.

Hopgood, M.F., Clark, M.G., and Ballard, F.J. 1981. Stimulation by glucocorticoids of protein degradation in hepatocyte monolayers. *Biochem J.* 196:33–40.

Hotchkiss, A.K., Ostby, J.S., Vandenbergh, J.G. et al. 2002. Androgens and environmental antiandrogens effect reproductive development and play behavior in the sprague-dawley rat. *Environ Hlth Perspect.* 110(Suppl 3):435–439.

Huang, Z.L., Sato, Y., Mochizuki, T. et al. 2003. Prostaglandin E2 activates the histaminergic system via the EP4 receptor to induce wakefulness in rats. *J Neurosci.* 23:5975–5983.

Huang, Z.L., Urade, Y., and Hayaishi, O. 2007. Prostaglandins and adenosine in the regulation of sleep and wakefulness. *Curr Opin Pharmacol.* 7:33–38.

Humphreys, R.C., Lydon, J.P., O'Malley, B.W. et al. 1997. Use of PRKO mice to study the role of progesterone in mammary gland development. *J Mammary Gland Biol Neoplasia.* 2:343–354.

Hurty, C.A. and Flatland, B. 2005. Feline acromegaly: A review of the syndrome. *J Am Anim Hosp Assoc.* 41:292–297.

Huseby, R.A., Soares, M.J., and Talamantes, F. 1985. Ectopic pituitary grafts in mice: Hormone levels, effects on fertility, and the development of adenomyosis uteri, prolactinomas, and mammary carcinomas. *Endocrinology.* 116:1440–1448.

Ilebekk, A., Björkman, J.A., and Nordlander, M. 2005. Influence of endogenous neuropeptide Y (NPY) on the sympathetic-parasympathetic interaction in the canine heart. *J Cardiovasc Pharmacol.* 46:474–480.

Illera, J.C., González Gil, A., Silván, G. et al. 2000. The effects of different anesthetic treatments on the adreno-cortical functions and glucose levels in NZW rabbits. *J Physiol Biochem.* 56:329–336.

Ingalls, A.M., Dickie, M.M., and Snell, G.D. 1950. Obese, a new mutation in the house mouse. *J Hered.* 41:317–318.

Inoue, M., Oishi, T., Fujita, F. et al. 1971. Influence of estriol on the onset of labor. *Acta Obstet Gynaecol Jpn.* 18:150–154.

Iqbal, J., Davies, T.F., Sun, L. et al. 2009. Skeletal morphofunctional considerations and the pituitary–thyroid axis. *Front Biosci.* S1:92–107.

Irvine, C.H. 1979. Kinetics of gonadotrophins in the mare. *J Reprod Fertil Suppl.* 27: 131–141.

Irvine, C.H. and Alexander, S.L. 1988. Secretion rates and short-term patterns of gonadotrophin-releasing hormone, FSH and LH in the normal stallion in the breeding season. *J Endocrinol.* 117:197–206.

Isaksson, O.G., Ohlsson, C., Nilsson, A. et al. 1991. Regulation of cartilage growth by growth hormone and insulin-like growth factor I. *Pediatr Nephrol.* 5:451–453.

Ismail, P.M., Amato, P., Soyal, S.M. et al. 2003. Progesterone involvement in breast development and tumorigenesis–as revealed by progesterone receptor "knockout" and "knockin" mouse models. *Steroids.* 68:779–787.

Iswaran, T.J., Imai, M., Betton, G.R., and Siddall, R.A. 1997. An overview of animal toxicology studies with bicalutamide (ICI 176,334). *J Toxicol Sci.* 22:75–88.

Ivell, R., Balvers, M., Rust, W. et al. 1997. Oxytocin and male reproductive function. *Adv Exp Med Biol.* 424:253–264.

Jahnke, G.D., Choksi, N.Y., Moore, J.A. et al. 2004. Thyroid toxicants: Assessing reproductive health effects. *Environ Hlth Perspect.* 112:363–368.

Jansson, J.O., Edén, S., and Isaksson, O. 1985. Sexual dimorphism in the control of growth hormone secretion. *Endocr Rev.* 6:128–150.

Jeffcoate, I.A. and England, G.C. 1997. Urinary LH, plasma LH and progesterone and their clinical correlates in the periovulatory period of domestic bitches. *J Reprod Fertil Suppl.* 51:267–275.

Jiang, J.Y., Umezu, M., and Sato, E. 2000. Characteristics of infertility and the improvement of fertility by thyroxine treatment in adult male hypothyroid rdw rats. *Biol Reprod.* 63:1637–1641.

Jöchle, W. 1975. Current research in coitus-induced ovulation: A review. *J Reprod Fertil Suppl.* 22:165–207.

Joëls, M. 2007. Role of corticosteroid hormones in the dentate gyrus. *Prog Brain Res.* 163:355–370.

Johnston, S.D. and Mather, E.C. 1978. Canine plasma cortisol (hydrocortisone) measured by radioimmunoassay: Clinical absence of diurnal variation and results of ACTH stimulation and dexamethasone suppression tests. *Am J Vet Res.* 39:1766–1770.

Johnston, S.D. and Mather, E.C. 1979. Feline plasma cortisol (hydrocortisone) measured by radioimmunoassay. *Am J Vet Res.* 40:190–192.

Joseph, S.A. 1980. Immunoreactive adrenocorticotropin in rat brain: A neuroanatomical study using antiserum generated against synthetic ACTH. *Am J Anat.* 158:533–548.

Joubert, J.P.J. 1989. Cardiac glycosides. In *Toxicants of Plant Origin, Glycosides*. Ed. P.R. Cheeke, Vol. 2, pp. 61–96. Boca Raton, FL: CRC Press.

Kaczmarek, M.M., Blitek, A., Kaminska, K. et al. 2008. Assessment of VEGF-receptor system expression in the porcine endometrial stromal cells in response to insulin-like growth factor-I, relaxin, oxytocin and prostaglandin E2. *Mol Cell Endocrinol.* 291:33–41.

Kadokawa, H., Shibata, M., Tanaka, Y. et al. 2009. Bovine C-terminal octapeptide of RFamide-related peptide-3 suppresses luteinizing hormone (LH) secretion from the pituitary as well as pulsatile LH secretion in bovines. *Domest Anim Endocrinol.* 36:219–224.

Kah, O., Lethimonier, C., Somoza, G. et al. 2007. GnRH and GnRH receptors in metazoa: A historical, comparative, and evolutive perspective. *Gen Comp Endocrinol.* 153:346–364.

Kahan, Z., Varga, J.L., Schally, A.V. et al. 2000. Antagonists of growth hormone-releasing hormone arrest the growth of MDA-MB-468 estrogen-independent human breast cancers in nude mice. *Breast Cancer Res Treat.* 60:71–79.

Kakucska, I., Rand, W., and Lechan, R.M. 1992. Thyrotropin-releasing hormone gene expression in the hypothalamic paraventricular nucleus is dependent upon feedback regulation by both triiodothyronine and thyroxine. *Endocrinology.* 130:2845–2850.

Kalia, V., Jadhav, A.N., and Bhutani, K.K. 2004. Luteinizing hormone estimation. *Endocr Res.* 30:1–17.

Kalra, S.P. and Kalra, P.S. 1983. Neural regulation of luteinizing hormone secretion in the rat. *Endocr Rev.* 4:311–351.

Karlsson, J.A., Sant'Ambrogio, F.B., Forsberg, K. et al. 1993. Respiratory and cardiovascular effects of inhaled and intravenous bradykinin, PGE2, and PGF2 alpha in dogs. *J Appl Physiol.* 74:2380–2386.

Karsch, F.J. 1987. Central actions of ovarian steroids in the feedback regulation of pulsatile secretion of luteinizing hormone. *Ann Rev Physiol.* 49:365–382.

Kaspareit-Rittinghausen, J., Hense, S., and Deerberg, F. 1990. Cushing's syndrome- and disease-like lesions in rats. *Z Versuchstierkd.* 33:229–234.

Kastner, P., Krust, A., Turcotte, B. et al. 1990. Two distinct estrogen-regulated promoters generate transcripts encoding the two functionally different human progesterone receptor forms A and B. *EMBO J.* 9:1603–1614.

Kasza, L., Collins, W.T., Capen, C.C. et al. 1978. Comparative toxicity of polychlorinated biphenyl and polybrominated biphenylin the rat thyroid gland: Light and electron microscopic alterations after subacute dietary exposure. *J Environ Pathol Toxicol.* 1:587–599.

Kato, Y., Ikushiro, S., Takiguchi, R. et al. 2007. A novel mechanism for polychlorinated biphenyl-induced decrease in serum thyroxine level in rats. *Drug Metab Dispos.* 35:1949–1955.

Keel, B.A., Schanbacher, B.D., and Grotjan, H.E., Jr. 1987. Ovine luteinizing hormone. I. Effects of castration and steroid administration on the charge heterogeneity of pituitary luteinizing hormone. *Biol Reprod.* 36:1102–1113.

Keller, U. and Miles, J.M. 1991. Growth hormone and lipids. *Horm Res.* 36(Suppl 1):36–40.

Kelly, PA., Djiane, J., Postel-Vinay, M.-C. et al. 1991. The prolactin/growth hormone receptor family. *Endocr Rev.* 12:235–251.

Kemppainen, R.J. and Peterson, M.E. 1996. Domestic cats show episodic variation in plasma concentrations of adrenocorticotropin, alpha-melanocyte-stimulating hormone (alpha-MSH), cortisol and thyroxine with circadian variation in plasma alpha-MSH concentrations. *Eur J Endocrinol.* 134:602–609.

Kerr, J.B. and Sharpe, R.M. 1986. Effects and interactions of LH and LHRH agonist on testicular morphology and function in hypophysectomized rats. *J Reprod Fertil.* 76:175–192.

Kerr, J.B., Millar, M., Maddocks, S. et al. 1993. Stage-dependent changes in spermatogenesis and Sertoli cells in relation to the onset of spermatogenic failure following withdrawal of testosterone. *Anat Rec.* 235:547–559.

Khan, S.A., Syed, V., Fröysa, B. et al. 1985. Influence of gonadectomy on isoelectrofocusing profiles of pituitary gonadotropins in rhesus monkeys. *J Med Primatol.* 14:177–194.

Kinoshita, H., Yasui, T., Ushigoe, K. et al. 2001. Expression of ovarian prolactin receptor in relation to hormonal changes during induction of ovulation in the rat. *Gynecol Obstet Invest.* 52:132–138.

Kintner, P.J. and Mead, R.A. 1983. Steroid metabolism in the corpus luteum of the ferret. *Biol Reprod.* 29:1121–1127.

Kohn, L.D., Saji, M., Akamizu, T. et al. 1989. Receptors of the thyroid: The thyrotropin receptor is only the first violinist of a symphony orchestra. In *Control of the Thyroid Gland. Regulation of Its Normal Function and Growth (Adv. Exp. Med. Biol.).* Ed. R. Ekholm, L.D. Kohn, and S.H. Wollman, pp. 151–209. New York, NY: Plenum Press.

Köhrle, J. 1999. Local activation and inactivation of thyroid hormones: The deiodinase family. *Mol Cell Endocrinol.* 151:103–119.

Komiyama, Y., Nishimura, N., Munakata, M. et al. 2001. Identification of endogenous ouabain in culture supernatant of PC12 cells. *J Hypertens.* 19229–19236.

Kooistra, H.S. and Okkens, A.C. 2001. Role of changes in the pulsatile secretion pattern of FSH in initiation of ovarian folliculogenesis in bitches. *J Reprod Fertil Suppl.* 57:11–14.

Koseki, Y., Cole, D., Matsuzawa, A. et al. 1987. Prolactin regulation of estrogen and progesterone receptors in normal and neoplastic mouse mammary tissue. *Jpn J Cancer Res.* 78:1105–1111.

Kriegsfeld, L.J. 2006. Driving reproduction: RFamide peptides behind the wheel. *Horm Behav.* 50:655–666.

Kriegsfeld, L.J., Mei, D.F., Bentley, G.E. et al. 2006. Identification and characterization of a gonadotropin-inhibitory system in the brains of mammals. *Proc Natl Acad Sci U S A.* 103:2410–2415.

Krishnamurthy, H., Danilovich, N., Morales, C.R. et al. 2000. Qualitative and quantitative decline in spermatogenesis of the follicle-stimulating hormone receptor knockout (FORKO) mouse. *Biol Reprod.* 62:1146–1159.

Kuohung, W. and Kaiser, U.B. 2006. GPR54 and KiSS-1: Role in the regulation of puberty and reproduction. *Rev Endocr Metab Disord.* 7:257–263.

Kuperman, Y. and Chen, A. 2008. Urocortins: Emerging metabolic and energy homeostasis perspectives. *Trends Endocrinol Metab.* 19:122–129.

Kurashima, K., Watabe, H., Sato, N. et al. 2010. Effects of prostaglandin F2a analogues on endothelin-1-induced impairment of rabbit ocular blood flow: Comparison among tafluprost, travoprost, and latanoprost. *Exp Eye Res.* 91:853–859.

Kurita, T., Lee, K., Saunders, P.T. et al. 2001. Regulation of progesterone receptors and decidualization in uterine stroma of the estrogen receptor-alpha knockout mouse. *Biol Reprod.* 64:272–283.

Laflamme, N., Nappi, R.E., Drolet, G. et al. 1998. Expression and neuropeptidergic characterization of estrogen receptors (ERalpha and ERbeta) throughout the rat brain: Anatomical evidence of distinct roles of each subtype. *J Neurobiol.* 36:357–378.

Lafterty, F.N., Spencer, G.E., and Pearson, O.H. 1964. Effects of androgens, estrogens, and high calcium intakes on bone formation and resorption in osteoporosis. *Am J Med.* 36:514–528.

Landau, R.L. and Lugibihl, K. 1961a. The catabolic and natriuretic effects of progesterone in man. *Recent Prog Horm Res.* 17:249–292.

Landau, R.L. and Lugibihl, K. 1961b. The effect of dietary protein on the catabolic influence of progesterone. *J Clin Endocrinol Metab.* 21:1345–1354.

Laredo, J., Shah, J.R., Hamilton, B.P. et al. 2000. Alpha-1 adrenergic receptors stimulate secretion of endogenous ouabain from human and bovine adrenocortical cells. In *Na/K-ATPase and Related ATPases*. Ed. K. Taniguchi, and S. Kayas, pp. 671–679. Amsterdam: Elsevier Science.

Laredo, J., Shah, J.R., Lu, Z. et al. 1997. Angiotensin II stimulates secretion of endogenous ouabain from bovine adrenal cortical cells via angiotensin II receptors. *Hypertension.* 29:401–407.

Larsen, J.L. and Odell, W.D. 1987. Prolactin alters luteinizing hormone pulsation characteristics in the intact and castrate male rabbit. *Neuroendocrinology.* 45:446–450.

Larsen, P.R., Silva, J.E., and Kaplan, M.M. 1981. Relationships between circulating and intracellular thyroid hormones: Physiological and clinical implications. *Endocr Rev.* 2:87–102.

Larsson, L.-I. 1978. Distribution of ACTH-like immunoreactivity in rat brain and gastrointestinal tract. *Histochemistry.* 55:225–233.

Larsson, M., Pettersson, T., and Carlström, A. 1985. Thyroid hormone binding in serum of 15 vertebrate species: Isolation of thyroxine-binding globulin and prealbumin analogs. *Gen Comp Endocrinol.* 58:360–375.

Le Traon, G., Brennan, S.F., Burgaud, S. et al. 2009. Clinical evaluation of a novel liquid formulation of L-thyroxine for once daily treatment of dogs with hypothyroidism. *J Vet Intern Med.* 23:43–49.

Le, W.W., Berghorn, K.A., Smith, M.S. et al. 1997. Alpha1-adrenergic receptor blockade blocks LH secretion but not LHRH cFos activation. *Brain Res.* 747:236–245.

Lechan, R.M. and Fekete, C. 2006. The TRH neuron: A hypothalamic integrator of energy metabolism. *Progr Brain Res.* 153:209–235.

Lee, D.K.H., Bird, C.E., and Clark, A.F. 1975. *In vivo* metabolism 3H-testosterone in adult male rats: Effects of estrogen administration. *Steroids.* 26:137–147.

Lee, P., Podos, S.M., and Severin, C. 1984. Effect of prostaglandin F2a on aqueous humor dynamics of rabbit, cat, and monkey. *Invest Ophthalmol Vis Sci.* 25:1087–1093.

Lee, W.M., Meij, B.P., Bhatti, S.F.M. et al. 2003. Pulsatile secretion pattern of growth hormone in dogs with pituitary-dependent hyperadrenocorticism. *Domestic Anim Endocrinol.* 24:59–68.

Lefkowitz, R.J., Rockman, H.A., and Koch, W.J. 2000. Catecholamines, cardiac ß-adrenergic receptors, and heart failure. *Circulation.* 101:1634–1637.

Lenox, R.H., Kant, G.J., Sessions, G.R. et al. 1980. Specific hormonal and neurochemical responses to different stressors. *Neuroendocrinology.* 30:300–308.

Leonard, J.L. 2008. Non-genomic actions of thyroid hormone in brain development. *Steroids.* 73:1008–1012.

Levinson, S.S. 1992. Antibody multispecificity in immunoassay interference. *Clin Biochem.* 25:77–87.

Lewandowski, T.A., Seeley, M.R., and Beck, B.D. 2004. Interspecies differences in susceptibility to perturbation of thyroid homeostasis: A case study with perchlorate. *Regul Toxicol Pharmacol.* 39:348–362.

Lewis, K.A., Gray, P.C., Blount, A.L. et al. 2000. Betaglycan binds inhibin and can mediate functional antagonism of activin signalling. *Nature.* 404:411–414.

Li, C.H., Geschwind, I.I., Cole, R.D. et al. 1955. Amino-acid sequence of alpha-corticotropin. *Nature.* 176:687–689.

Li, X.F., Bowe, J.E., Lightman, S.L. et al. 2005. Role of corticotropin-releasing factor receptor-2 in stress-induced suppression of pulsatile luteinizing hormone secretion in the rat. *Endocrinology.* 146:318–322.

Li, Y. and Goldbeter, A. 1989. Frequency specificity in intercellular communication. Influence of patterns of periodic signaling on target cell responsiveness. *Biophys J.* 55:125–145.

Liang, C.L., Kozlowski, G.P., Joseph, S.A. et al. 1992. ACTH1-39 inputs to mesocorticolimbic dopaminergic neurons: Light and electron microscopic examination. *Neurosci Lett.* 146:79–83.

Liang, X., Wu, L., Hand, T. et al. 2005. Prostaglandin D2 mediates neuronal protection via the DP1 receptor. *J Neurochem.* 92: 477–486.

Lichtstein, D., Steinitz, M., Gati, I. et al. 1998. Biosynthesis of digitalis-like compounds in rat adrenal cells: Hydroxycholesterol as possible precursor. *Life Sci.* 62:2109–2126.

Liew, M., Groll, M.C., Thompson, J.E. et al. 2007. Validating a custom multiplex ELISA against individual commercial immunoassays using clinical samples. *BioTechniques.* 42:327–333.

Lightman, S.L., Windle, R.J., Julian, M.D. et al. 2000. Significance of pulsatility in the HPA axis. In *Mechanisms and Biological Significance of Pulsatile Hormone Secretion (Novartis Foundation Symposium 227).* Eds. D.J. Chadwick, and J.A. Goode, pp. 244–257. Hoboken, NJ: Wiley Interscience.

Lim, M.M. and Young, L.J. 2006. Neuropeptidergic regulation of affiliative behavior and social bonding in animals. *Horm Behav.* 50:506–517.

Lim, M.M., Bielsky, I.F., and Young, L.J. 2005. Neuropeptides and the social brain: Potential rodent models of autism. *Int J Dev Neurosci.* 23:235–243.

Lin, T.Y. and London, C.A. 2010. Characterization and modulation of canine mast cell derived eicosanoids. *Vet Imm Immunopath.* 135:118–127.

Lintner, F., Hertelendy, F., and Zsolnai, B. 1988. Endocrine regulation of the onset of parturition in rats. *Acta Physiol Hung.* 71:337–346.

Littleton, G.K. and Anderson, R.R. 1972. Characterization of 17β-estradiol- ^{3}H single-injection disappearance curves in rat plasma and red cells. *Proc Soc Exptl Biol Med.* 140:1015–1020.

Liu, J., Rone, M.B., and Papadopoulos, V. 2006. Protein–protein interactions mediate mitochondrial cholesterol transport and steroid biosynthesis. *J Biol Chem.* 281:38879–38893.

Liu, J.C., Makova, K.D., Adkins, R.M. et al. 2001. Episodic evolution of growth hormone in primates and emergence of the species specificity of human growth hormone receptor. *Mol Biol Evol.* 18:945–953.

Longcope, C., Femino, A., and Johnston, J.O. 1988. Androgen and estrogen dynamics in the female baboon (*Papio anubis*). *J Steroid Biochem.* 31:195–200.

Longcope, C., Yesair, D.W., Williams, K.I.H. et al. 1980. Comparison of the metabolism in dogs of estradiol-17β following its intravenous and oral administration. *J Steroid Biochem.* 13:1047–1055.

Love, S. 1993. Equine Cushing's disease. *Br Vet J.* 149:139–153.

Lowry, C.A., Hale, M.W., Evans, A.K. et al. 2008. Serotonergic systems, anxiety, and affective disorder: Focus on the dorsomedial part of the dorsal raphe nucleus. *Ann NY Acad Sci.* 1148:86–94.

Luck, M.R. 1989. A function for ovarian oxytocin. *J Endocrinol.* 121:203–204.

Ludlow, H., Muttukrishna, S., Hyvönen, M. et al. 2008. Development of a new antibody to the human inhibin/activin betaB subunit and its application to improved inhibin B ELISAs. *J Immunol Methods.* 329:102–111.

Luine, V., Villegas, M., Martinez, C., and McEwen, B.S. 1994. Repeated stress causes reversible impairments of spatial memory performance. *Brain Res.* 639:167–170.

Luque, R.M., Peinado, J.R., Gracia-Navarro, F. et al. 2006. Cortistatin mimics somatostatin by inducing a dual, dose-dependent stimulatory and inhibitory effect on growth hormone secretion in somatotropes. *J Mol Endocrinol.* 36:547–556.

Mahoudeau, J.A., Corvol, P., and Bricare, H. 1973. Rabbit testosterone-binding globulin. II Effect on androgen metabolism *in vivo*. *Endocrinology.* 92:1120–1125.

Makanji, Y., Harrison, C.A., Stanton, P.G. et al. 2007. Inhibin A and B in vitro bioactivities are modified by their degree of glycosylation and their affinities to betaglycan. *Endocrinology.* 148:2309–2316.

Makris, A., Olsen, D., and Ryan, K.J. 1983. Significance of the delta 5 and delta 4 steroidogenic pathways in the hamster. *Steroids.* 42:641–651.

Malozowski, S., Hao, E.H., Ren, S.G. et al. 1990. Effects of inhibition of norepinephrine synthesis on spontaneous and growth hormone-releasing hormone-induced GH secretion in cynomolgus macaques: Evidence for increased hypothalamic somatostatin tone. *Neuroendocrinology.* 51:455–458.

Mannino, C.A., South, S.M., Inturrisi, C.E. et al. 2005. Pharmacokinetics and effects of 17beta-estradiol and progesterone implants in ovariectomized rats. *J Pain.* 6:809–816.

Mansfield, M.J., Beardsworth, D.E., Loughlin, J.S. et al. 1983. Long-term treatment of central precocious puberty with a long-acting analogue of luteinizing hormone-releasing hormone. Effects on somatic growth and skeletal maturation. *N.E J Med.* 309:1286–1290.

Manzano, J., Cuadrado, M., Morte, B. et al. 2007. Influence of thyroid hormone and thyroid hormone receptors in the generation of cerebellar gamma-aminobutyric acid-ergic interneurons from precursor cells. *Endocrinology.* 148:5746–5751.

Margetic, S., Gazzola, C., Pegg, G.G. et al. 2002. Leptin: A review of its peripheral actions and interactions. *Int J Obes Relat Metab Disord.* 26:1407–1433.

Márquez, D.C. and Pietras, R.J. 2001. Membrane-associated binding sites for estrogen contribute to growth regulation of human breast cancer cells. *Oncogene.* 20:5420–5430.

Martin, G.B. and Thiéry, J.C. 1987. Hypothalamic multiunit activity and LH secretion in conscious sheep. *Exp Brain Res.* 67:469–478.

Matsumoto, H., Noguchi, J., Horikoshi, Y. et al. 1999. Stimulation of prolactin release by prolactin-releasing peptide in rats. *Biochem Biophys Res Commun.* 259:321–324.

Mattern, L.G., Helmreich, D.L., and Cameron, J.L. 1993. Diurnal pattern of pulsatile luteinizing hormone and testosterone secretion in adult male rhesus monkeys (Macaca mulatta): Influence of the timing of daily meal intake. *Endocrinology.* 132:1044–1054.

Mayo, K.E., Miller, T., DeAlmeida, V. et al. 2000. Regulation of the pituitary somatotroph cell by GHRH and its receptor. *Recent Prog Horm Res.* 55:237–266.

McEwen, B.S. and Magarinos, A.M. 1997. Stress effects on morphology and function of the hippocampus. *Ann NY Acad Sci.* 821:271–284.

McMahon, M., Gerich, J., and Rizza, R. 1988. Effects of glucocorticoids on carbohydrate metabolism. *Diabetes Metab Rev.* 4:17–30.

Meakin, J.W., Tingey, W.H., Jr., and Nelson, D.H. 1960. The catabolism of adrenocorticotropic hormone: The stability of adrenocorticotropic hormone: The stability of adrenocorticotropic hormone in blood, plasma, serum, and saline. *Endocrinology.* 66:59–72.

Meier, U. and Gressner, A.M. 2004. Endocrine regulation of energy metabolism: Review of pathobiochemical and clinical chemical aspects of leptin, ghrelin, adiponectin, and resistin. *Clin Chem.* 50:1511–1525.

Meij, B.P., Mol, J.A., Bevers, M.M. et al. 1997. Alterations in anterior pituitary function in dogs with pituitary-dependent hyperadrenocorticism. *J Endocrinol.* 154:505–512.

Mendelson, C.R. and Condon, J.C. 2005. New insights into the molecular endocrinology of parturition. *J Steroid Biochem Mol Biol.* 93:113–119.

Mendis-Handagama, S.M., Watkins, P.A., Gelber, S.J. et al. 1998. The effect of chronic luteinizing hormone treatment on adult rat Leydig cells. *Tissue Cell.* 30:64–73.

Meyer, H.P. and Rothuizen, J. 1993. Determination of the percentage of free cortisol in plasma in the the dog by ultrafiltration/dialysis. *Domest Anim Endocrinol.* 10:45–53.

Micevych, P. and Sinchak, K. 2008. Estradiol regulation of progesterone synthesis in the brain. *Mol Cell Endocrinol.* 290:44–50.

Micevych, P. and Sinchak, K. 2008. Synthesis and function of hypothalamic neuroprogesterone in reproduction. *Endocrinology.* 149:2739–2742.

Micevych, P., Sinchak, K., Mills, R.H. et al. 2003. The luteinizing hormone surge is preceded by an estrogen-induced increase of hypothalamic progesterone in ovariectomized and adrenalectomized rats. *Neuroendocrinology.* 78:29–35.

Micevych, P.E. and Mermelstein, P.G. 2008. Membrane estrogen receptors acting through metabotropic glutamate receptors: An emerging mechanism of estrogen action in brain. *Mol Neurobiol.* 38:66–77.

Michels, G. and Hoppe, U.C. 2008. Rapid actions of androgens. *Front Neuroendocrinol.* 29:182–198.

Milligan, S.R. 1982. Induced ovulation in mammals. *Oxford Rev Reprod Biol.* 4:1–46.
Mills, T.M. and Copland, J.A. 1982. Effects of ketamine–xylazine anesthesia on blood levels of luteinizing hormone and follicle stimulating hormone in rabbits. *Lab Anim Sci.* 32:619–621.
Missaghian, E., Kempná, P., Dick, B. et al. 2009. Role of DNA methylation in the tissue-specific expression of the CYP17A1 gene for steroidogenesis in rodents. *J Endocrinol.* 202:99–109.
Mol, J.A., Lantinga-van Leeuwen, I., van Garderen, E. et al. 2000. Progestin-induced mammary growth hormone (GH) production. *Adv Exp Med Biol.* 480:71–76.
Mol, J.A., van Garderen, E., Rutteman, G.R. et al. 1996. New insights in the molecular mechanism of progestin-induced proliferation of mammary epithelium: Induction of the local biosynthesis of growth hormone (GH) in the mammary glands of dogs, cats and humans. *J Steroid Biochem Mol Biol.* 57:67–71.
Mol, J.A., van Wolferen, M., Kwant, M. et al. 1994. Predicted primary and antigenic structure of canine corticotropin-releasing hormone. *Neuropeptides.* 27:7–13.
Møller, J., Jorgensen, J.O., Christiansen, J.S. et al. 1992. Effects of growth hormone administration on fuel oxidation and thyroid function in normal man. *Metabolism.* 41:728–731.
Møller, N., Jørgensen, J.O., Abildgård, N. et al. 1991. Effects of growth hormone on glucose metabolism. *Horm Res.* 36(Suppl 1):32–35.
Moncada, S. and Vane, J.R. 1979. Pharmacology and endogenous roles of prostaglandin endoperoxidases, thromboxane A2, and prostacyclin. *Pharmacol Rev.* 30:293–331.
Mooney, C.T., Thoday, K.L., and Doxey, D.L. 1996. Serum thyroxine and triiodothyronine responses of hyperthyroid cats to thyrotropin. *Am J Vet Res.* 57:987–991.
Moor, B.C. and Younglai, E.V. 1975. Variations in peripheral levels of LH and testosterone in adult male rabbits. *J Reprod Fertil.* 42:259–266.
Moretti, C., Bagnato, A., Solan, N. et al. 1990. Receptor-mediated actions of growth hormone releasing factor on granulosa cell differentiation. *Endocrinology.* 127:2117–2126.
Morilak, D.A., Barrera, G., Echevarria, D.J. et al. 2005. Role of brain norepinephrine in the behavioral response to stress. *Prog Neuropsychopharmacol Biol Psychiatry.* 29:1214–1224.
Moschos, S., Chan, J.L., and Mantzoros, C.S. 2002. Leptin and reproduction: A review. *Fertil Steril.* 77:433–444.
Mosier, J.E. 1989. Effect of aging on body systems of the dog. *Vet Clin North Am.* 19:1–12.
Motzer, W.E. 2001. Perchlorate: problems, detection and solutions. *Environ Forensics.* 2:301–311.
Mul, D. and Hughes, I.A. 2008. The use of GnRH agonists in precocious puberty. *Eur J Endocrinol.* 159:S3–S8.
Muller, E.E., Locatelli, V., and Cocchi, D. 1999. Neuroendocrine control of growth hormone secretion. *Physiol Rev.* 79:511–607.
Murray, G.R. 1891. Note on the treatment of myxoedema by hypodermic injections of an extract of the thyroid gland of a sheep. *Brit Med J.* 2:796.
Mutvei, A., Husman, B., Andersson, G. et al. 1989a. Thyroid hormone and not growth hormone is the principal regulator of mammalian mitochondrial biogenesis. *Acta Endocrinol.* 121:223–228.
Mutvei, A., Kuzela, S., and Nelson, B.D. 1989b. Control of mitochondrial transcription by thyroid hormone. *Eur J Biochem.* 180:235–240.
Mylchreest, E., Cattley, R.C., and Foster, P.M. 1998. Male reproductive tract malformations in rats following gestational and lactational exposure to di(n-butyl) phthalate: An antiandrogenic mechanism? *Toxicol Sci.* 43:47–60.
Naito, A., Sato, T., Matsumoto, T. et al. 2008. Dihydrotestosterone inhibits murine hair growth via the androgen receptor. *Br J Dermatol.* 159:300–305.
Nantermet, P.V., Xu, J., Yu, Y. et al. 2004. Identification of genetic pathways activated by the androgen receptor during the induction of proliferation in the ventral prostate gland. *J Biol Chem.* 279:1310–1322.
Nass, T.E., Lapolt, P.S., Judd, H.L. et al. 1983. Gonadotropin secretion during prolonged hyperprolactinemia: Basal secretion and the stimulatory feedback effect of estrogen. *Biol Reprod.* 28:1140–1147.
Nass, T.E., Matt, D.W., Judd, H.L. et al. 1984. Prepubertal treatment with estrogen or testosterone precipitates the loss of regular estrous cyclicity and normal gonadotropin secretion in adult female rats. *Biol Reprod.* 31:723–731.
Navarro, V.M., Castellano, J.M., Fernández-Fernández, R. et al. 2005. Characterization of the potent luteinizing hormone-releasing activity of KiSS-1 peptide, the natural ligand of GPR54. *Endocrinology.* 146:156–163.
Nett, T.M. 1989. Hormonal evaluation of testicular function: Species variation. *Int J Toxicol.* 8:539–549.
Niccoli, P., Ferrand, V., Lejeune, P.J. et al. 1996. Interest of epitopic dissection in immunoanalysis of proteins and peptides: Review of theoretical and practical aspects. *Eur J Clin Chem Clin Biochem.* 34:741–748.
Nicholson, H.D., Guldenaar, S.E., Boer, G.J., and Pickering, B.T. 1991. Testicular oxytocin: Effects of intratesticular oxytocin in the rat. *J Endocrinol.* 130:231–238.

Nie, R., Zhou, Q., Jassim, E. et al. 2002. Differential expression of estrogen receptors α and β in the reproductive tracts of adult male dogs and cats. *Biol Reprod.* 66:1161–1168.

Nielsen, U.B. and Geierstanger, B.H. 2004. Multiplexed sandwich assays in microarray format. *J Immunol Methods.* 290:107–120.

Niessen, S.J., Petrie, G., Gaudiano, F. et al. 2007. Feline acromegaly: An underdiagnosed endocrinopathy? *Vet Intern Med.* 21:899–905.

Nikitovitch-Winer, M.B., Atkin, J., and Maley, B.E. 1987. Colocalization of prolactin and growth hormone within specific adenohypophyseal cells in male, female, and lactating female rats. *Endocrinology.* 121:625–630.

Nishimori, K., Young, L.J., Guo, Q. et al. 1996. Oxytocin is required for nursing but is not essential for parturition or reproductive behavior. *Proc Natl Acad Sci U S A.* 93:11699–11704.

Nomura, K., Ohmura, K., Nakamura, Y. et al. 1989. Porcine luteinizing hormone isoform(s): Relationship between their molecular structures, and renotropic versus gonadotropic activities. *Endocrinology.* 124:712–719.

Norman, J.M. 1985. William Withering and the purple foxglove: A bicentennial tribute. *J Clin Pharmacol.* 25:479–483.

Nozaki, M., Shimizu, K., Mitsunaga, F. et al. 2002. Blockade of menstrual cycle by thyroidectomy in Japanese monkeys (Macaca fuscata fuscata). *Endocrine.* 19:131–137.

Numan, M. 1994. Maternal behavior. In *The Physiology of Reproduction.* Ed. E. Knobil, and J.D. Neill, pp. 221–302. New York, NY: Raven.

O'Callaghan, J.P., Brinton, R.E., and McEwen, B.S. 1989. Glucocorticoids regulate the concentration of glial fibrillary acidic protein throughout the brain. *Brain Res.* 494:159–161.

O'Donnell, L., McLachlan, R.I., Wreford, N.G. et al. 1996. Testosterone withdrawal promotes stage-specific detachment of round spermatids from the rat seminiferous epithelium. *Biol Reprod.* 55:895–901.

Ohinata, K., Suetsugu, K., Fujiwara, Y. et al. 2006. Activation of prostaglandin E receptor EP4 subtype suppresses food intake in mice. *Prostagland Other Lipid Mediat.* 81:31–36.

Ohinata, K., Takagi, K., and Biyajima, K. 2008. Central prostaglandin D2 stimulates food intake via the neuropeptide Y system in mice. *FEBS Lett.* 582:679–684.

Ojeda, S.R., Aguado, L.I., and Smith, S. 1983. Neuroendocrine mechanisms controlling the onset of female puberty: The rat as a model. *Neuroendocrinology.* 37:306–313.

Ojeda, S.R., Urbanski, H.F., Katz, K.H. et al. 1986. Activation of estradiol-positive feedback at puberty: Estradiol sensitizes the LHRH-releasing system at two different biochemical steps. *Neuroendocrinology.* 43:259–265.

Okulicz, W.C., Savasta, A.M., Hoberg, L.M. et al. 1989. Immunofluorescent analysis of estrogen induction of progesterone receptor in the rhesus uterus. *Endocrinology.* 125:930–934.

Olson, P.N., Bowen, R.A., Behrendt, M.D. et al. 1982. Concentrations of reproductive hormones in canine serum throughout late anestrus, proestrus and estrus. *Biol Reprod.* 27:1196–1206.

Ono, M., Miki, N., Murata, Y. et al. 1995. Sexually dimorphic expression of pituitary growth hormone-releasing factor receptor in the rat. *Biochem Biophys Res Commun.* 216:1060–1066.

Ottenweller, J.E., Tapp, W.N., Burke, J.M. et al. 1985. Plasma cortisol and corticosterone concentrations in the golden hamster (*Mesocricetus auratus*). *Life Sci.* 37:1551–1558.

Panciera, D.L. and Carr, A.P. 2006. *Endocrinology for the Small Animal Practitioner.* Jackson, WY: Teton NewMedia.

Parvizi, N., Elsaesser, F., Smidt, D. et al. 1976. Plasma luteinizing hormone and progesterone in the adult female pig during the oestrous cycles, late pregnancy and lactation, and after ovariectomy and pentobarbitone treatment. *J Endocrinol.* 69:193–203.

Pauerstein, C.J., Eddy, C.A., Croxatto, M.D. et al. 1978. Temporal relationships of estrogen, progesterone, and luteinizing hormone levels to ovulation in women and infrahuman primates. *Am J Obstet Gynecol.* 130:876–886.

Pavao, M. and Traish, A.M. 2001. Estrogen receptor antibodies: Specificity and utility in detection, localization and analyses of estrogen receptor α and β. *Steroids.* 66:1–16.

Pawson, A.J., Morgan, K., Maudsley, S.R. et al. 2003. Type II gonadotropin-releasing hormone (GnRH-II) in reproductive biology. *Reproduction.* 126:271–278.

Pedrazzini, T., Pralong, F., and Grouzmann, E. 2003. Neuropeptide Y: The universal soldier. *Cell Mol Life Sci.* 60:350–377.

Pepe, G.J. and Rothchild, I. 1973. Metabolic clearance rate of progesterone: Comparison between ovariectomized, pregnant, pseudopregnant and deciduoma-bearing pseudopregnant rats. *Endocrinology.* 93:1200–1205.

Perreault, S.D., Goldman, J.M., Luderer, U., and Hunt, P.A. 2010. Targeting female reproductive function during follicular maturation, ovulation, and fertilization: Critical windows for pharmaceutical or toxicant action. In *Comprehensive Toxicology—Reproductive and Endocrine Toxicology*. Eds. J. Richburg, and P. Hoyer, 2nd edition, Vol. 11, pp. 399–417. Oxford, England: Elsevier Press.

Perrin, A., Brasmes, B., Chambaz, E.M. et al. 1997. Bovine adrenocortical cells in culture synthesize an ouabain-like compound. *Mol Cell Endocrinol.* 126:7–15.

Pesini, P., Pego-Reigosa, R., Tramu, G. et al. 2004. Distribution of ACTH immunoreactivity in the diencephalon and the brainstem of the dog. *J Chem Neuroanat.* 27:275–282.

Peters, M.A., de Jong, F.H., Teerds, K.J. et al. 2000. Ageing, testicular tumours and the pituitary–testis axis in dogs. *J Endocrinol.* 166:153–161.

Peterson, M.E. 2014. Animal models of disease: Feline hyperthyroidism: an animal model for toxic nodular goiter. *J. Endocrinol.* 223:T97–114.

Peterson, M.E., Graves, T.K., and Cavanagh, I. 1987. Serum thyroid hormone concentrations fluctuate in cats with hyperthyroidism. *J Vet Intern Med.* 1:142–146.

Peterson, M.E., Kintzer, P.P., Cavanagh, P.G. et al. 1983. Feline hyperthyroidism: Pretreatment clinical and laboratory evaluation of 131 cases. *J Am Vet Med Assoc.* 183:103–110.

Petroff, B.K. and Mizinga, K.M. 2003. Pharmacokinetics of ovarian steroids in Sprague-Dawley rats after acute exposure to 2,3,7,8-tetrachlorodibenzo-p-dioxin (TCDD). *Reprod Biol.* 3:131–141.

Pettipher, R. 2008. The roles of the prostaglandin D2 receptors DP1 and CRTH2 in promoting allergic responses. *Br J Pharmacol.* 153:S190–199.

Phillips, D.J., Jones, K.L., Clarke, I.J. et al. 2005. Activin A: From sometime reproductive factor to genuine cytokine. *Vet Immunol Immunopathol.* 108:23–27.

Phuc Le, P., Friedman, J.R., Schug, J. et al. 2005. Glucocorticoid receptor-dependent gene regulatory networks. *PLoS Genet.* 1:e16. doi:10.1371/journal.pgen.0010016.

Picard, D. and Yamamoto, K.R. 1987. Two signals mediate hormone-dependent nuclear localization of the glucorticoid receptor. *EMBO J.* 6:3333–3340.

Pignatelli, D., Xiao, F., Gouveia, A.M. et al. 2006. Adrenarche in the rat. *J Endocrinol.* 191:301–308.

Pineda, M.H. 2003. Female reproductive system. In *McDonald's Veterinary Endocrinology and Reproduction*, Eds. M.H. Pineda, and M.P. Dooley, 5th edition, pp. 283–340. Ames, IA: Blackwell Publishing.

Poindron, P. 2005. Mechanisms of activation of maternal behaviour in mammals. *Reprod Nutr Dev.* 45:341–351.

Pompei, L., Carvalho, F., Ortiz, S. et al. 2005. Morphometric evaluation of effects of two sex steroids on mammary gland of female rats. *Maturitas.* 51:370–379.

Ponglowhapan, S., Church, D.B., and Khalid, M. 2010. Expression of prostaglandin E2 receptor subtypes in the canine lower urinary tract varies according to the gonadal status and gender. *Theriogenology.* 74:1450–1466.

Postel-Vinay, M.C. 1996. Growth hormone- and prolactin-binding proteins: Soluble forms of receptors. *Horm Res.* 45:178–181.

Postel-Vinay, M.C. and Finidori, J. 1995. Growth hormone receptor: Structure and signal transduction. *Eur J Endocrinol.* 133:654–659.

Pratt, W.B. and Toft, D.O. 1997. Steroid receptor interactions with heat shock protein and immunophilin chaperones. *Endocr Res.* 18:306–360.

Prossnitz, E.R., Arterburn, J.B., Smith, H.O. et al. 2008. Estrogen signaling through the transmembrane G protein-coupled receptor GPR30. *Ann Rev Physiol.* 70:165–190.

Psarra, A.M., Solakidi, S., and Sekeris, C.E. 2006. The mitochondrion as a primary site of action of steroid and thyroid hormones: Presence and action of steroid and thyroid hormone receptors in mitochondria of animal cells. *Mol Cell Endocrinol.* 246:21–33.

Pugliese, M., Mascort, J., Mahy, N. et al. 2006. Diffuse beta-amyloid plaques and hyperphosphorylated tau are unrelated processes in aged dogs with behavioral deficits. *Acta Neuropathol.* 112:175–183.

Puri, C.P., Puri, V., and Anand Kumar, T.C. 1981. Serum levels of testosterone, cortisol, prolactin and bioactive luteinizing hormone in adult male rhesus monkeys following cage-restraint or anaesthetizing with ketamine hydrochloride. *Acta Endocrinol (Copenh).* 97:118–124.

Qin, J., Feng, M., Wang, C. et al. 2009. Oxytocin receptor expressed on the smooth muscle mediates the excitatory effect of oxytocin on gastric motility in rats. *Neurogastroenterol Motil.* 21:430–438.

Quadri, S.K., Pierson, C., and Spies, H.G. 1978. Effects of centrally acting drugs on serum prolactin levels in rhesus monkeys. *Neuroendocrinology.* 27:136–147.

Ramage, A.G. and Villalón, C.M. 2008. 5-hydroxytryptamine and cardiovascular regulation. *Trends Pharmacol Sci.* 29:472–481.

Rand, J.S. 1999. Current understanding of feline diabetes mellitus: Part 1, pathogenesis. *J Feline Med Surg.* 1:143–153.

Redelman, D., Welniak, L.A., Taub, D. et al. 2008. Neuroendocrine hormones such as growth hormone and prolactin are integral members of the immunological cytokine network. *Cell Immunol.* 252:111–121.

Reimers, T.J., McGarrity, M.S., and Strickland, D. 1986. Effect of fasting on thyroxine, 3,5,3′-triiodothyronine, and cortisol concentrations in serum of dogs. *Am J Vet Res.* 47:2485–2490.

Reis, F.M., Luisi, S., Carneiro, M.M. et al. 2004. Activin, inhibin and the human breast. *Mol Cell Endocrinol.* 225:77–82.

Reisine, T. and Bell, G.I. 1995. Molecular biology of somatostatin receptors. *Endocr Rev.* 16:427–442.

Richards, A.M., Crozier, I.G., Holmes, S.J. et al. 1993. Brain natriuretic peptide: Natriuretic and endocrine effects in essential hypertension. *J Hypertens.* 11:163–170.

Rijnberk, A., Kooistra, H.S., and Mol, J.A. 2003. Endocrine diseases in dogs and cats: Similarities and differences with endocrine diseases in humans. *Growth Horm IGF Res.* 13(Suppl A):S158–164.

Rivier, C. and Vale, W. 1984. Influence of corticotropin-releasing factor on reproductive functions in the rat. *Endocrinology.* 114:914–921.

Rivier, J., Spiess, J., and Vale, W. 1983. Characterization of rat hypothalamic corticotropin-releasing factor. *Proc Natl Acad Sci.* 80:4851–4855.

Roa, J., Garcia-Galiano, D., Varela, L. et al. 2009. The mammalian target of Rapamycin as novel central regulatory of puberty onset via modulation of hypothalamic Kiss1 system. *Endocrinology.* 150:5016–5026.

Roa, J., Vigo, E., Castellano, J. et al. 2008. Opposite roles of estrogen receptor (ER)-alpha and ERbeta in the modulation of luteinizing hormone responses to kisspeptin in the female rat: Implications for the generation of the preovulatory surge. *Endocrinology.* 149:1627–1637.

Roberts, V., Meunier, H., Vaughan, J. et al. 1989. Production and regulation of inhibin subunits in pituitary gonadotropes. *Endocrinology.* 124:552–554.

Robertson, D.M., Foulds, L.M., and Ellis, S. 1982. Heterogeneity of rat pituitary gonadotropins on electrofocusing; differences between sexes and after castration. *Endocrinology.* 111:385–391.

Robertson, S.A. and Taylor, P.M. 2004. Pain management in cats-past, present and future. Part 2. Treatment of pain-clinical pharmacology. *J Feline Med Surg.* 6:321–333.

Rocco, S., Ambroz, C., and Aguilera, G. 1990. Interaction between serotonin and other regulators of aldosterone secretion in rat adrenal glomerulosa cells. *Endocrinology.* 127:3103–3110.

Roepke, T.A., Qiu, J., Bosch, M.A. et al. 2009. Cross-talk between membrane-initiated and nuclear-initiated oestrogen signalling in the hypothalamus. *J Neuroendocrinol.* 21:263–270.

Rojas-Maya, S., González-Padilla, E., Murcia-Mejía, C. et al. 2007. Caprine luteinizing hormone isoforms during the follicular phase and anestrus. *Anim Reprod Sci.* 100:280–290.

Rondinone, C.M. 2006. Adipocyte-derived hormones, cytokines, and mediators. *Endocrine.* 29:81–90.

Roozendaal, M.M., Swarts, H.J., Wiegant, V.M. et al. 1995. Effect of restraint stress on the preovulatory luteinizing hormone profile and ovulation in the rat. *Eur J Endocrinol.* 133:347–353.

Rosner, W., Auchus, R.J., Azziz, R. et al. 2007. Position Statement: Utility, limitations, and pitfalls in measuring testosterone: An Endocrine Society position statement. *J Clin Endocrinol Metab.* 92:405–413.

Rossi, G., Boscaro, M., Ronconi, V. et al. 2005. Aldosterone as a cardiovascular risk factor. *Trends Endocrinol Metab.* 16:104–107.

Rouaze-Romet, M., Vranckx, R., Savu, L. et al. 1992. Structural and functional microheterogeneity of rat thyroxine-binding globulin during ontogenesis. *Biochem J.* 286(Pt 1):125–130.

Runic, S., Miljkovic, M., Bogumil, R.J. et al. 1976. The *in vivo* metabolism of progestins. I. The metabolic clearance rates of progesterone and medroxyprogesterone acetate in the dog. *Endocrinology.* 99:108–113.

Russ, R.D., Resta, T.C., and Walker, B.R. 1992. Pulmonary vasodilatory response to neurohypophyseal peptides in the rat. *J Appl Physiol.* 73:473–478.

Russell, N.J., Foster, S., Clark, P. et al. 2007. Comparison of radioimmunoassay and chemiluminescent assay methods to estimate canine blood cortisol concentrations. *Aust Vet J.* 85:487–494.

Rutteman, G.R., Bevers, M.M., Misdorp, W. et al. 1989. Anterior pituitary function in female dogs with mammary tumors: II. Prolactin. *Anticancer Res.* 9:241–245.

Rutteman, G.R., Willekes-Koolschijn, N., Bevers, M.M. et al. 1986. Prolactin binding in benign and malignant mammary tissue of female dogs. *Anticancer Res.* 6:829–835.

Rybaczyk, L.A., Bashaw, M.J., Pathak, D.R. et al. 2005. An overlooked connection: Serotonergic mediation of estrogen-related physiology and pathology. *BMC Women's Hlth.* 5:12.

Sabbatini, M.E. 2009. Natriuretic peptides as regulatory mediators of secretory activity in the digestive system. *Regul Peptides.* 154:5–15.

Saintier, D., Khanine, V., Uzan, B. et al. 2006. Estradiol inhibits adhesion and promotes apoptosis in murine osteoclasts in vitro. *J Steroid Biochem Mol Biol.* 99:165–173.

Sairam, M.R. 1989. Role of carbohydrates in glycoprotein hormone signal transduction. *FASEB J.* 3:1915–1926.

Sairam, M.R. and Krishnamurthy, H. 2001. The role of follicle-stimulating hormone in spermatogenesis: Lessons from knockout animal models. *Arch Med Res.* 32:601–608.

Sakata, D., Yao, C., and Narumiya, S. 2010. Prostaglandin E2, an immunoactivator. *J Pharmacol Sci.* 112:1–5.

Samson, W.K., Huang, F.L., and Fulton, R.J. 1993. C-type natriuretic peptide mediates the hypothalamic actions of the natriuretic peptides to inhibit luteinizing hormone secretion. *Endocrinology.* 132:504–509.

Samson, W.K., Resch, Z.T., Murphy, T.C. et al. 1998. Gender-biased activity of the novel prolactin releasing peptides: Comparison with thyrotropin releasing hormone reveals only pharmacologic effects. *Endocrine.* 9:289–291.

Sanders, E.J. and Harvey, S. 2008. Peptide hormones as developmental growth and differentiation factors. *Dev Dyn.* 237:1537–1552.

Sapolsky, R.M., Packan, D.R., and Vale, W.W. 1988. Glucocorticoid toxicity in the hippocampus: in vitro demonstration. *Brain Res.* 453:367–371.

Sastry, B.V.R. and Robertson, D. 2004. Acetylcholine and muscarinic receptors. In *Primer on the Autonomic Nervous System*. Ed. D. Robertson, pp. 70–72. Elsevier Science: Amsterdam.

Saunders, P.T., Fisher, J.S., Sharpe, R.M. et al. 1998. Expression of oestrogen receptor beta (ER beta) occurs in multiple cell types, including some germ cells, in the rat testis. *J Endocrinol.* 156:R13–17.

Savino, W., Postel-Vinay, M.C., Smaniotto, S. et al. 2002. The thymus gland: A target organ for growth hormone. *Scand J Immunol.* 55:442–452.

Scheller, K., Seibel, P., and Sekeris, C.E. 2003. Glucocorticoid and thyroid hormone receptors in mitochondria of animal cells. *Int Rev Cytol.* 222:1–61.

Schlatt, S., Pohl, C.R., Ehmcke, J. et al. 2008. Age-related changes in diurnal rhythms and levels of gonadotropins, testosterone, and inhibin B in male rhesus monkeys (*Macaca mulatta*). *Biol Reprod.* 79:93–99.

Schoonover, C.M., Seibel, M.M., Jolson, D.M. et al. 2004. Thyroid hormone regulates oligodendrocyte accumulation in developing rat brain white matter tracts. *Endocrinology.* 145:5013–5020.

Schott, H.C. 2nd. 2002. Pituitary pars intermedia dysfunction: Equine Cushing's disease. *Vet Clin North Am Equine Pract.* 18:237–270.

Schubert, K. and Schade, K. 1977. Placental steroid hormones. *J Steroid Biochem.* 8:359–365.

Schwanzel-Fukuda, M. and Pfaff, D.W. 1989. Origin of luteinizing hormone-releasing hormone neurons. *Nature.* 338:161–164.

Scott-Moncrieff, J.C., Koshko, M.A., Brown, J.A. et al. 2003. Validation of a chemiluminescent enzyme immunometric assay for plasma adrenocorticotropic hormone in the dog. *Vet Clin Pathol.* 32:180–187.

Segerson, T.P., Kauer, J., Wolfe, H.C. et al. 1987. Thyroid hormone regulates TRH biosynthesis in the paraventricular nucleus of the rat hypothalamus. *Science.* 238:78–80.

Selby, C. 1999. Interference in immunoassay. *Ann Clin Biochem.* 36:704–721.

Selman, P.J., Mol, J.A., Rutteman, G.R. et al. 1994. Progestin-induced growth hormone excess in the dog originates in the mammary gland. *Endocrinology.* 134:287–292.

Seminara, S.B. 2007. Kisspeptin in reproduction. *Semin Reprod Med.* 25:337–343.

Setty, B.N.Y., Phelps, D.L., Walenga, R.W. et al. 1991. Identification of prostaglandins and hydroxyeicosatetraenoic acids in kitten retina: Comparison with other species. *Exp Eye Res.* 53:81–88.

Sewer, M.B. and Waterman, M.R. 2003. ACTH modulation of transcription factors responsible for steroid hydroxylase gene expression in the adrenal cortex. *Microsc Res Tech.* 61:300-307.

Sharpe, R.M., Maddocks, S., and Kerr, J.B. 1990. Cell–cell interactions in the control of spermatogenesis as studied using Leydig cell destruction and testosterone replacement. *Am J Anat.* 188:3–20.

Shen, Q., Lantvit, D.D., Lin, Q. et al. 2007. Advanced rat mammary cancers are growth hormone dependent. *Endocrinology.* 148:4536–4544.

Shibahara, S., Morimoto, Y., Furutani, Y. et al. 1983. Isolation and sequence analysis of the human corticotrophin-releasing factor precursor gene. *EMBO J.* 2:775–776.

Shibasaki, T., Kiyosawa, Y., Masuda, A. et al. 1984. Distribution of growth hormone-releasing hormone-like immunoreactivity in human tissue extracts. *J Clin Endocrinol Metab.* 59:263–268.

Shille, V.M., Munro, C., Farmer, S.W. et al. 1983. Ovarian and endocrine responses in the cat after coitus. *J Reprod Fertil.* 68:29–39.

Shinichi, M., Kaneta, T., and Imasaka, T. 2005. Capillary electrophoresis immunoassay based on an on-column immunological reaction. *J Chromatogr A.* 1066:197–203.

Shiroozu, A., Taurog, A., Engler, H. et al. 1983. Mechanism of action of thioureylene antithyroid drugs in the rat: Possible inactivation of thyroid peroxidase by propylthiouracil. *Endocrinology.* 113:362–370.

Shughrue, P.J., Lane, M.V., Scrimo, P.J. et al. 1998. Comparative distribution of estrogen receptor-alpha (ER-alpha) and beta (ER-beta) mRNA in the rat pituitary, gonad, and reproductive tract. *Steroids.* 63:498–504.

Shupnik, M.A. and Ridgway, E.C. 1985. Triiodothyronine rapidly decreases transcription of the thyrotropin subunit genes in thyrotropic tumor explants. *Endocrinology.* 117:1940–1946.

Shuto, Y., Shibasaki, T., Wada, K. et al. 2001. Generation of polyclonal antiserum against the growth hormone secretagogue receptor (GHS-R): Evidence that the GHS-R exists in the hypothalamus, pituitary and stomach of rats. *Life Sci.* 68:991–996.

Signore, A.P., Zhang, F., Weng, Z. et al. 2008. Leptin neuroprotection in the CNS: Mechanisms and therapeutic potentials. *J Neurochem.* 106:1977–1990.

Singh, A.K., Jiang, Y., White, T. et al. 1997. Validation of nonradioactive chemiluminescent immunoassay methods for the analysis of thyroxine and cortisol in blood samples obtained from dogs, cats, and horses. *J Vet Diagn Invest.* 9:261–268.

Slavin, B.G., Ong, J.M., and Kern, P.A. 1994. Hormonal regulation of hormone-sensitive lipase activity and mRNA levels in isolated rat adipocytes. *J Lipid Res.* 35:1535–1541.

Smith, V.G. and Convey, E.M. 1975. TRH-stimulation of prolactin release from bovine pituitary cells. *Proc Soc Exp Biol Med.* 149:70–74.

Sofikitis, N., Giotitsas, N., Tsounapi, P. et al. 2008. Hormonal regulation of spermatogenesis and spermiogenesis. *J Steroid Biochem Mol Biol.* 109:323–330.

Sojka, J.E., Johnson, M.A., and Bottoms, G.D. 1993. Serum triiodothyronine, total thyroxine, and free thyroxine concentrations in horses. *Am J Vet Res.* 54:52–55.

Soloff, M.S. 1975. Uterine receptor for oxytocin: Effects of estrogen. *Biochem Biophys Res Commun.* 65:205–212.

St Germain, D.L. 1986. Hormonal control of a low Km (type II) iodothyronine 5′-deiodinase in cultured NB41A3 mouse neuroblastoma cells. *Endocrinology.* 119:840–846.

Stanczyk, F.Z., Cho, M.M., Endres, D.B. et al. 2003. Limitations of direct estradiol and testosterone immunoassay kits. *Steroids.* 68:1173–1178.

Starling, E.H. 1905. Croonian lecture: On the chemical correlation of the functions of the body I. *Lancet.* 2:339–341.

Stein, J., Zeuzem, S., Uphoff, K. et al. 1994. Effects of prostaglandins and indomethacin on gastric emptying in the rat. *Prostaglandins.* 47:31–40.

Steinberger, E., Ayala, C., Hsi, B. et al. 1998. Utilization of commercial laboratory results in management of hyperandrogenism in women. *Endocr Pract.* 4:1–10.

Stenman, U.-H. 2013. Standardization of hormone determinations. *Best Pract Res Clin Endocrinol Metab.* 27:823–830.

Sternberg, E.M. 2001. Neuroendocrine regulation of autoimmune/inflammatory disease. *J Endocrinol.* 169:429–435.

Stewart, J.M. and Channabasavaiah, K. 1979. Evolutionary aspects of some neuropeptides. *Fed Proc.* 38:2302–2308.

Stoker, T.E., Parks, L.G., Gray, L.E. et al. 2000. Endocrine-disrupting chemicals: Prepubertal exposures and effects on sexual maturation and thyroid function in the male rat. A focus on the EDSTAC recommendations. *Crit Rev Toxicol.* 30:197–252.

Stoker, T.E., Perreault, S.D., Bremser, K. et al. 2005. Acute exposure to molinate alters neuroendocrine control of ovulation in the rat. *Toxicol Sci.* 84:38–48.

Stouffer, R.L. 2002. Pre-ovulatory events in the rhesus monkey follicle during ovulation induction. *Reprod Biomed Online.* 4(Suppl 3):1–4.

Ström, J.O., Theodorsson, A., and Theodorsson, E. 2008. Substantial discrepancies in 17β-oestradiol concentrations obtained with three different commercial direct radioimmunoassay kits in rat sera. *Scand J Clin Lab Invest.* 68:806–813.

Sugimoto, Y., Yamasaki, A., Segi, E. et al. 1997. Failure of parturition in mice lacking the prostaglandin F receptor. *Science.* 277:681–683.

Suszko, M.I., Lo, D.J., Suh, H. et al. 2003. Regulation of the rat follicle-stimulating hormone β-subunit promoter by activin. *Mol Endocrinol.* 17:318–332.

Suttie, J.M., Fennessy, P.F., Corson, I.D. et al. 1989. Pulsatile growth hormone, insulin-like growth factors and antler development in red deer (*Cervus elaphus scoticus*) stags. *J Endocrinol.* 121:351–360.

Svare, D., Bartke, A., Doherty, P. et al. 1979. Hyperprolactinemia suppresses copulatory behavior in male rats and mice. *Biol Reprod.* 21:529–535.

Szepeshazi, K., Schally, A.V., Armatis, P. et al. 2001. Antagonists of GHRH decrease production of GH and IGF-I in mxt mouse mammary cancers and inhibit tumor growth. *Endocrinology.* 142:4371–4378.

Szkudlinski, M.W., Thotakura, N.R., Bucci, I. et al. 1993. Purification and characterization of recombinant human thyrotropin (TSH) isoforms produced by Chinese hamster ovary cells: The role of sialylation and sulfation in TSH bioactivity. *Endocrinology.* 133:1490–1503.

Tabrizi, M.A., Bornstein, G.G., Klakamp, S.L. et al. 2009. Translational strategies for development of monoclonal antibodies from discovery to the clinic. *Drug Discov Today.* 14:298–305.

Takahara, J., Arimura, A., and Schally, A.V. 1974. Stimulation of prolactin and growth hormone release by TRH infused into a hypophysial portal vessel. *Proc Soc Exp Biol Med.* 146:831–835.

Takayama, M. and Greenwald, G.S. 1972. Hormonal requirements for the maintenance of deciduomata and pregnancy in the same rat. *J Endocrinol.* 53:507–508.

Taniguchi, M., Akiawa, M., and Sakagami, T. 1982. Comparative studies on hemolysis in the erythrocytes from various animals: Inhibitory effect of prostaglandins and phospholipid content. *Comp Biochem Physiol A.* 73:445–458.

Tapia-Arancibia, L., Arancibia, S., and Astier, H. 1985. Evidence for alpha 1-adrenergic stimulatory control of in vitro release of immunoreactive thyrotropin-releasing hormone from rat median eminence: In vivo corroboration. *Endocrinology.* 116:2314–2319.

Tarnow, I., Olsen, L.H., Kvart, C. et al. 2009. Predictive value of natriuretic peptides in dogs with mitral valve disease. *Vet J.* 180:195–201.

Taylor, A.E., Khoury, R.H., Crowley, W.F., Jr. 1994. A comparison of 13 different immunometric assay kits for gonadotropins: Implications for clinical investigation. *J Clin Endocrinol Metab.* 79:240–247.

Taylor, J., Picelli, G., and Harrison, D.J. 2001. An evaluation of the detection limits possible for competitive capillary electrophoretic immunoassays. *Electrophoresis.* 22:3699–3708.

Taylor, P. 2004. Nicotinic acetylcholine receptors: Structure and functional properties. In *Primer on the Autonomic Nervous System*. Ed. D. Robertson, pp. 70–76. Amsterdam: Elsevier Science.

Tenniswood, M., Bird, C.E., and Clark, A.F. 1982. The role of androgen metabolism in the control of androgen action in the rat prostate. *Mol Cell Endocrinol.* 27:89–96.

ter Haar, M.B. and MacKinnon, P.C. 1976. Effects of sodium pentobarbitone on serum gonadotrophin levels and on the incorporation of 35S from methionine into protein in the brain and anterior pituitary during the oestrous cycle of the rat. *J Endocrinol.* 68:289–296.

Tezapsidis, N., Johnston, J.M., Smith, M.A. et al. 2009. Leptin: A novel therapeutic strategy for Alzheimer's disease. *J Alzheimers Dis.* 16:731–740.

Thomas, G.A. and Williams, E.D. 1999. Thyroid stimulating hormone (TSH)-associated follicular hypertrophy and hyperplasia as a mechanism of thyroid carcinogenesis in mice and rats. *IARC Sci Publ.* 147:45–59.

Thomas, M., Keramidas, M., Monchaux, E. et al. 2003. Role of adrenocorticotropic hormone in the development and maintenance of the adrenal cortical vasculature. *Microsc Res Tech.* 61:247–251.

Thompson, D.L., Jr., Rahmanian, M.S., DePew, C.L. et al. 1992. Growth hormone in mares and stallions: Pulsatile secretion, response to growth hormone-releasing hormone, and effects of exercise, sexual stimulation, and pharmacological agents. *J Anim Sci.* 70:1201–1207.

Thompson, T.B., Lerch, T.F., Cook, R.W. et al. 2005. The structure of the follistatin:Activin complex reveals antagonism of both type I and type II receptor binding. *Dev Cell.* 9:535–543.

Tomura, H., Lazar, J., Phyillaier, M. et al. 1995. The N-terminal region (A/B) of rat thyroid hormone receptors alpha 1, beta 1, but not beta 2 contains a strong thyroid hormone-dependent transactivation function. *Proc Natl Acad Sci U S A.* 92:5600–5604.

Torbet, S.A., Lower, S.A., and Schwarting, G.A. 1997. Gonadotropin-releasing hormone containing neurons and olfactory fibers during development: From lamprey to mammals. *Brain Res Bull.* 44:479–486.

Toshinai, K., Date, Y., Murakami, N. et al. 2003. Ghrelin-induced food intake is mediated via the orexin pathway. *Endocrinology.* 144:1506–1512.

Trapman, J. and Dubbink, H.J. 2007. The role of cofactors in sex steroid action. *Best Pract Res Clin Endocrinol Metab.* 21:403–414.

Tremblay, R.R., Forest, M.G., Shalf, J. et al. 1972. Studies on the dynamics of plasma androgens and on the origin of dihydrotestosterone in dogs. *Endocrinology.* 91:556–561.

Tsai, S.-J. and Wiltbank, M.C. 1997. Prostaglandin F2α induces expression of prostaglandin G/H synthase-2 in the ovine corpus luteum: A potential positive feedback loop during luteolysis. *Biol Reprod.* 57:1016–1022.

Tsukahara, S., Tsukamura, H., Foster, D.L. et al. 1999. Effect of corticotropin-releasing hormone antagonist on oestrogen-dependent glucoprivic suppression of luteinizing hormone secretion in female rats. *J Neuroendocrinol.* 11:101–105.

Tsutsui K. 2008. Progesterone biosynthesis and action in the developing neuron. *Endocrinology.* 149:2757–2761.

Tsutsui, K. 2009. A new key neurohormone controlling reproduction, gonadotropin-inhibitory hormone (GnIH): Biosynthesis, mode of action and functional significance. *Prog Neurobiol.* 88:76–88.

Tucker, M.J. 1997. The endocrine system. In *Target Organ Pathology: A Basic Text.* Eds. J. Turton, and J. Hooson, pp. 311–334. London: Informa Healthcare.

Ubuka, T., Morgan, K., Pawson, A.J. et al. 2009. Identification of human GnIH homologs, RFPR-1 and RFRP-3, and the cognate receptor, GPR147 in the human hypothalamic pituitary axis. *PLOS ONE.* 4:e8400.

Uemura, T., Namiki, T., Kimura, A. et al. 1994. Direct effects of gonadotropin-releasing hormone on the ovary in rats and humans. *Horm Res.* 41(Suppl 1):7–13.

Ueno, H., Yamaguchi, H., Mizuta, M. et al. 2008. The role of PYY in feeding regulation. *Regul Peptides.* 145:12–16.

Ulloa-Aguirre, A., Maldonado, A., Damián-Matsumura, P. et al. 2001a. Endocrine regulation of gonadotropin glycosylation. *Arch Med Res.* 32:520–532.

Ulloa-Aguirre, A., Midgley, A.R., Jr., Beitins, I.Z. et al. 1995. Follicle-stimulating isohormones: Characterization and physiological relevance. *Endocr Rev.* 16:765–787.

Ulloa-Aguirre, A., Timossi, C., and Méndez, J.P. 2001b. Is there any physiological role for gonadotrophin oligosaccharide heterogeneity in humans? I. Gondatrophins are synthesized and released in multiple molecular forms. A matter of fact. *Hum Reprod.* 16:599–604.

Ulloa-Aguirre, A., Timossi, C., Damián-Matsumura, P. et al. 1999. Role of glycosylation in function of follicle-stimulating hormone. *Endocrine.* 11:205–215.

Urbanski, H.F. 2012. Differential roles of GnRH-I and GnRH-II neurons in the control of the primate reproductive axis. *Front Endocrinol.* 3:1–7.

Urbanski, H.F. 2015. Selective targeting of GnRH-II neurons to block ovulation. *Contraception.* 91:423–425.

Valassi, E., Scacchi, M., and Cavagnini, F. 2008. Neuroendocrine control of food intake. *Nutr Metab Cardiovasc Dis.* 18:158–168.

Vale, W., Hsueh, A., Rivier, C. et al. 1990. The inhibin/activin family of growth factors. In *Peptide Growth Factors and Their Receptors (Handbook of Experimental Pharmacology).* Eds. M.A. Sporn, and A.B. Roberts, pp. 211–248. Heidelberg: Springer-Verlag.

Valladares, L.E. and Payne, A.H. 1979. Induction of testicular aromatization by luteinizing hormone in mature rats. *Endocrinology.* 105:431–436.

Van Garderen, E., van der Poel, H.J., Swennenhuis, J.F. et al. 1999. Expression and molecular characterization of the growth hormone receptor in canine mammary tissue and mammary tumors. *Endocrinology.* 140:5907–5914.

Van Pett, K., Viau, V., Bittencourt, J.C. et al. 2000. Distribution of mRNAs encoding CRF receptors in brain and pituitary of rat and mouse. *J Comp Neurol.* 428:191–212.

Van Sande, J., Massart, C., Beauwens, R. et al. 2003. Anion selectivity by the sodium iodide symporter. *Endocrinology.* 144:247–252.

Van Weerden, W., Bierings, H., Steenbrugge, G. et al. 1992. Adrenal glands of mouse and rat do not synthesize androgens. *Life Sci.* 50:857–861.

Veldscholte, J., Berrevoets, C.A., Zegers, N.D. et al. 1992. Hormone-induced dissociation of the androgen receptor-heat-shock protein complex: Use of a new monoclonal antibody to distinguish transformed from nontransformed receptors. *Biochemistry.* 31:7422–7430.

Venkataseshu, G.K. and Estergreen, V.L., Jr. 1970. Cortisol and corticosterone in bovine plasma and the effect of adrenocorticotropin. *J Dairy Sci.* 53:480–483.

Vieira, E., Liu, Y.J., and Gylfe, E. 2004. Involvement of alpha1 and beta-adrenoceptors in adrenaline stimulation of the glucagon-secreting mouse alpha-cell. *Naunyn Schmiedebergs Arch Pharmacol.* 369:179–183.

Vinson, G.P., Whitehouse, B.J., and Goddard, C. 1978. Steroid 17-hydroxylation and androgen production by incubated rat adrenal tissue. *J Steroid Biochem Mol Biol.* 9:677–683.

Wade, G.N. and Schneider, J.E. 1992. Metabolic fuels and reproduction in female mammals. *Neurosci Biobehav Rev.* 16:235–272.

Wahab, F., Shahab, M., and Behr, R. 2015. The involvement of gonadotropin inhibitory hormone and kisspeptin in the metabolic regulation of reproduction. *J Endocrinol.* 225:R49–66.

Walker, W.H. 2009. Molecular mechanisms of testosterone action in spermatogenesis. *Steroids.* 74:602–607.

Wallis, O.C., Mac-Kwashie, A.O., Makri, G. et al. 2005. Molecular evolution of prolactin in primates. *J Mol Evol.* 60:606–614.

Walther, T. and Stepan H. 2004. C-type natriuretic peptide in reproduction, pregnancy and fetal development. *J Endocrinol.* 180:17–22.

Wambach, G. and Higgins, J.R. 1978. Antimineralocorticoid action of progesterone in the rat: Correlation of the effect on electrolyte excretion and interaction with renal mineralocorticoid receptors. *Endocrinology.* 102:1686–1693.

Wang, M. 2005. The role of glucocorticoid action in the pathophysiology of the Metabolic Syndrome. *Nutr Metab (Lond.).* 2:3. doi:10.1186/1743-7075-2-3.

Waterman, M.R. and Bischof, L.J. 1996. Mechanisms of ACTH(cAMP)-dependent transcription of adrenal steroid hydroxylases. *Endocr Res.* 22:615–620.

Waters, M.J. and Conway-Campbell, B.L. 2004. The oncogenic potential of autocrine human growth hormone in breast cancer. *Proc Natl Acad Sci USA.* 101:14992–14993.

Wei, L.L., Norris, B.M., and Baker, C.J. 1997. An N-terminally truncated third progesterone receptor protein, PR(C), forms heterodimers with PR(B) but interferes in PR(B)-DNA binding. *J Steroid Biochem Mol Biol.* 62:287–297.

Weinberg, J. and Wong, R. 1986. Adrenocortical responsiveness to novelty in the hamster. *Physiol Behav.* 37:669–672.

Weusten, J.J., Smals, A.G., Hofman, J.A. et al. 1987. Early time sequence in pregnenolone metabolism to testosterone in homogenates of human and rat testis. *Endocrinology.* 120:1909–1913.

Weusten, J.J., van der Wouw, M.P., Smals, A.G. et al. 1990. Differential metabolism of pregnenolone by testicular homogenates of human and two species of macaques. Lack of synthesis of the human sex pheromone precursor 5,16-androstadien-3beta-ol in nonhuman primates. *Horm Metab Res.* 22:619–621.

Williams, C.L., Nishihara, M., Thalabard, J.C. et al. 1990. Corticotropin-releasing factor gonadotropin-releasing hormone pulse generator activity in the rhesus monkey: Electrophysiological studies. *Neuroendocrinology.* 52:133–137.

Wilson, C.A., Jacobs, C., Baker, P. et al. 1990b. IL-1 beta modulation of spontaneous autoimmune diabetes and thyroiditis in the BB rat. *J Immunol.* 144:3784–3788.

Wilson, C.A., Leigh, A.J., and Chapman, A.J. 1990a. Gonadotrophin glycosylation and function. *J Endocrinol.* 125:3–14.

Wilson, C.M. and McPhaul, M.J. 1996. A and B forms of the androgen receptor are expressed in a variety of human tissues. *Mol Cell Endocrinol.* 120:51–57.

Wiltbank, M.C. and Ottobre, J.S. 2003. Regulation of intraluteal production of prostaglandins. *Repro Biol Endocrinol.* 1:91.

Windle, R.J., Wood, S.A., Shanks, N. et al. 1998. Ultradian rhythm of basal corticosterone release in the female rat: Dynamic interaction with the response to acute stress. *Endocrinology.* 139:443–450.

Winters, S.J., Medhamurthy, R., Gay, V.L. et al. 1991. A comparison of moment to moment and diurnal changes in circulating inhibin and testosterone concentrations in male rhesus monkeys (Macaca mulatta). *Endocrinology.* 129:1755–1761.

Wira, C.R. and Sullivan, D.A. 1981. Effect of estradiol and progesterone on the secretory immune system in the female genital tract. *Adv Exp Med Biol.* 138:99–111.

Wise, P.M. 1986. Effects of hyperprolactinemia on estrous cyclicity, serum luteinizing hormone, prolactin, estradiol, and progesterone concentrations, and catecholamine activity in microdissected brain areas. *Endocrinology.* 118:1237–1245.

Wolff, J. 1998. Perchlorate and the thyroid gland. *Pharmacol Rev.* 50:89–105.

Woodard, G.E. and Rosado, J.A. 2008. Natriuretic peptides in vascular physiology and pathology. *Int Rev Cell Mol Biol.* 268:59–93.

Woodruff, T.K., Krummen, L.A., Lyon, R.J. et al. 1993. Recombinant human inhibin A and recombinant human activin A regulate pituitary and ovarian function in the adult female rat. *Endocrinology.* 132:2332–2341.

Wouters, M.M., Gibbons, S.J., Roeder, J.L. et al. 2007. Exogenous serotonin regulates proliferation of interstitial cells of Cajal in mouse jejunum through 5-HT2B receptors. *Gastroenterology.* 133:897–906.

Wren, A.M., Small, C.J., Fribbens, C.V. et al. 2002. The hypothalamic mechanisms of the hypophysiotropic action of ghrelin. *Neuroendocrinology.* 76:316–324.

Wrutniak-Cabello, C., Casas, F., and Cabello, G. 2001. Thyroid hormone action in mitochondria. *J Mol Endocrinol.* 26:67–77.

Wuttke, W. and Meites, J. 1971. Luteolytic role of prolactin during the estrous cycle of the rat. *Proc Soc Exp Biol Med.* 137:988–991.

Xu, X., De Pergola, G., and Björntorp, P. 1990. The effects of androgens on the regulation of lipolysis in adipose precursor cells. *Endocrinology.* 126:1229–1234.

Yamakawa, K., Kudo, K., Kanba, S. et al. 1999. Distribution of prolactin-releasing peptide-immunoreactive neurons in the rat hypothalamus. *Neurosci Lett.* 267:113–116.

Yang, F., Xu, Y., Pan, H. et al. 2008. Induction of hepatic cytochrome P4501A1/2B activity and disruption of thyroglobulin synthesis/secretion by mono-ortho polychlorinated biphenyl and its hydroxylated metabolites in rat cell lines. *Environ Toxicol Chem.* 27:220–225.

Yeung, C.M., Chan, C.B., Leung, P.S. et al. 2006. Cells of the anterior pituitary. *Int J Biochem Cell Biol.* 38:1441–1449.

Yochim, J.M. 1986. Progesterone action in preparation for decidualization. *Ann N Y Acad Sci.* 476:122–135.

Young, F.G. 1957. Claude Bernard and the discovery of glycogen. *Br Med J.* 1(5033):1431–1437.

Young, L.J. and Wang, Z. 2004. The neurobiology of pair bonding. *Nat Neurosci.* 7:1048–1054.

Zakar, T. and Hertelendy, F. 2007. Progesterone withdrawal: Key to parturition. *Am J Obstet Gynecol.* 196:289–296.

Zalányi, S. 2001. Progesterone and ovulation. *Eur J Obstet Gynecol Reprod Biol.* 98:152–159.

Zalesky, D.D. and Grotjan, H.E. 1991. Comparison of intracellular and secreted isoforms of bovine and ovine luteinizing hormone. *Biol Reprod.* 44:1016–1024.

Zhang, Y., Proenca, R., Maffei, M. et al. 1994. Positional cloning of the mouse obese gene and its human homologue. *Nature.* 372:425–32.

Ziegler, M.G., Bao, X., Kennedy, B.P. et al. 2002. Location, development, control, and function of extraadrenal phenylethanolamine *N*-methyltransferase. *Ann N Y Acad Sci.* 971:76–82.

Zoubeidi, A., Zardan, A., Beraldi, E. et al. 2007. Cooperative interactions between androgen receptor (AR) and heat-shock protein 27 facilitate AR transcriptional activity. *Cancer Res.* 67:10455–10465.

24 Vitamins, Selected Diet-Derived Factors, and Minerals

Robert B. Rucker, Andrea J. Fascetti, and Jennifer A. Larsen

CONTENTS

24.1 INTRODUCTION AND BRIEF HISTORY

The initial indications that food components may be linked to health are described in the writings of ancient Greek philosophers in the fourth and fifth centuries BC. An Egyptian medical text, the *Papyrus Ebers* (written about 1550–1570 BC) contains references that described liver as a potential treatment to improve vision including night blindness. In China, descriptions related to the husbandry and nutritional care of horses also occurred at about this time (Lusk, 1922).

In the mid-1700s, a number of documents focusing on the treatment of specific diseases acknowledged the curative effects of given foods. As an example, James Lynn, a physician in England, developed his treatise that fresh fruits and vegetables seemed effective in treating scurvy (Carpenter, 1986). By the late 1800s, an association between corn and pellagra (niacin deficiency) was made. Another conceptually important observation was the connection between the consumption of polished rice and polyneuritis (associated with the nutrition disease beriberi). Although the concept of vitamins was not fully established at this time, studies in the late 1800s and early 1900s that focused on defining food components relevant to disease were the first to utilize experimental animals in controlled settings (Goldblith and Joslyn, 1964). Concerning essential minerals, French agricultural chemist Jean Boussingault first suggested that iodine compounds might be able to cure goiter only 50 years after its discovery as an element in 1811 (Hetzel, 1996). A key factor in this advance was analytical procedures were in place for iodine by the mid-1800s. Thus, relationships between low iodine levels and goiter could be made.

The next advance in identifying essential functions and requirements came in the early to mid-1900s. In the United States, the Bureau of Animal Industries accelerated both governmental and academic research to combat major animal diseases and improve animal food production. Much of this work represented the underpinnings and early financial success of many current vitamin and pharmaceutical manufacturers and feed companies.

Now, there is constant awareness and sensitivity to the possibility of dietary vitamin deficiencies (and excesses), particularly diets containing a limited (or restricted) number of dietary ingredients. Or, when subsidiary and contributory factors lead to vitamin-related diseases (compromised food intake), loss of appetite (anorexia), impaired absorption and/or utilization, and the presence of antagonists.

24.2 DEFINITIONS, NOMENCLATURE, AND GENERAL PROPERTIES

24.2.1 VITAMINS

Vitamins have been defined as organic substances present in minute amounts in natural foodstuffs that are essential to normal metabolism, the lack of which causes given deficiency signs and syndromes. For a compound to be considered a vitamin it must be shown to be a dietary essential; that is, its elimination from the diet must result in defined sets of deficiency-related signs and symptoms. Restoration or repletion must be able to reverse the disorder. Merely demonstrating that a compound has a pharmacological activity, however, does not classify a compound as a vitamin, even when found in common foodstuffs. Moreover, the broad range of vitamin functions has also made the development of a systematic nomenclature even more challenging. Likewise, classifications based on chemical properties have proved problematic, although noting the solubility in aqueous or lipid solvents has been useful as a starting point, even for the development of physiological concepts. For example, vitamins that are soluble in lipid solvents (vitamins A, D, E, and K) are absorbed and transported physiologically by conventional lipid transport processes. For water-soluble vitamins, their respective solubility coefficients are major factors that dictate bioavailability and ease of absorption.

When the vitamins were originally discovered they were isolated as chemically or physically defined fractions or factors from selected foods, but their exact chemical composition was seldom known. The designation of vitamins by letters was not systematically pursued in many cases (Goldblith and Joslyn, 1964), particularly when functions ascribed to given factors were discovered to be due to other substances (e.g., an essential amino acid). What are in place today are designations and nomenclature that have evolved somewhat independently for each of the compounds designated as a vitamin. The International Union of Pure and Applied Chemistry and the International Union of Biochemistry (IUPAC-IUB) Joint Commission on Biochemical Nomenclature (JCBN) are responsible for nomenclature designations. In some cases, trivial names were maintained and utilized along with a letter designation (e.g., pyridoxine for the vitamin B-6 family of vitamers). The commission, as needed, rectifies controversies and inconsistencies in nomenclature.

24.2.2 Minerals

Of the 103 elements in the periodic table, about 30 are presently considered essential or important for the normal health and growth of animals. Of these, 16 are often described as "essential trace elements," a classification initially based on the difficulty of measuring such elements with precision (Reilly, 2004). As the designation implies, trace minerals are found and needed in relatively low concentrations in cells and tissues. Herein, 6 of the 16 trace elements are highlighted, because nutritional or toxicological concerns involving them are encountered.

Regarding functions, essential elements are distinguished because of their association with the functions of specific organic molecules, mostly proteins with enzymatic properties. When metals function to facilitate enzymatic catalysis they usually fall into two categories, metals necessary to metalloenzymes or metal–enzyme complexes. The stability of the interaction (e.g., the magnitude of the association or disassociation constants) helps to define whether metalloenzyme or metal–enzyme complex is the best designation. Metalloenzymes have metal-binding constants of 108–109 or greater. Metal–protein complexes have constants of 105 or less (Harris, 2014). Trace elements that are nutritionally essential are localized to the fourth and fifth rows of the periodic table and have incompletely filled *d* orbitals, except for Cu and Zn. How a given metal facilitates catalytic functions is related in part to its ability to engage in redox, act as a Lewis acid, or modulate an energy excitable transition state during a catalytic event. Like the vitamins, the designation of given minerals as essential requires that their elimination from the diet result in a defined set of deficiency-related signs. It is also critical to identify a mechanism of action in association with a metalloprotein or metal complex with a known function.

24.2.3 Requirements

For both vitamins and minerals, when expressed on an energy basis, metabolic requirements are most often of the same order of magnitude from one species to the next. When differences in the dietary requirement for a given nutrient between species do occur, in contrast to a physiological or metabolic need, the differences are usually due to the presence of unique pathways for production, degradation, and/or disposal of the nutrient. In some cases (e.g., requirements for ferrets, rabbits, dogs), more data may be needed to define an actual dietary, physiological, or minimum need. A particular concern is the expression of requirements for various breeds of dogs. Differing species of dogs can vary in body weight by two orders of magnitude. Expression of requirements based directly on body weight (e.g., amount/kg) grossly overestimates the need in large species and underestimates the need in smaller species (Subcommittee on Dog and Cat Nutrition et al., 2006).

Some examples are given in Tables 24.1 through 24.3. Note that requirements of trace elements also scale allometrically in a manner that is similar in principle to scaling algorithms for basal metabolism (e.g., kWt3/4, Figure 24.1). Given that a common set of biological or evolutionary principles are involved in the selection of the elements essential to life, it follows that nutritional requirements might also be influenced by the same principles (Rucker and Storms, 2002; Rucker, 2007). Indeed, a strong case can be made that when expressed per unit of food-derived energy or relative to metabolic body size; requirements for essential elements and vitamins are similar to a diverse

TABLE 24.1
Fat-Soluble Vitamin Requirements[a,b]

	Vitamin							
	A		D		E		K	
Species[d]	Amount/kg Diet or Dry Matter (~3,200 kcal/kg DM)[c]	Amount/ 1,000 kcal (4.2 MJ)	Amount/kg Diet or Dry Matter (~3,200 kcal/kg DM)[c]	Amount/1,000 kcal (4.2 MJ)	Amount/kg Diet or Dry Matter (~3,200 kcal/kg DM)[c]	Amount/ 1,000 kcal (4.2 MJ)	Amount/kg Diet or Dry Matter (~3200 kcal/ kg DM)[c]	Amount/1,000 kcal (4.2 MJ)
Mouse[a] 15–25 g	2,000–4,000 Units (0.7–1.4 mg as retinol)	625–1,250 Units (0.22–0.44 mg as retinol)	1,000 Units (0.025 mg as D_3)	312 Units (0.008 mg as D_3)	20–50 mg	6.25–16 mg	1 mg as phylloquinone	0.33 mg as phylloquinone
Rat[a] 175–250 g	2,300 Units (0.8 mg as retinol)	720 Units (0.22 mg as retinol)	1,000 Units (0.025 mg as D_3)	312 Units (0.008 mg as D_3)	18–26 mg	5.6–8.1 mg	1 mg as phylloquinone	0.33 mg as phylloquinone
Hamster[a] 75–125 g	9,000 Units (18 mg as retinoyl palmitate)	2,812 (5.63 mg as retinoyl palmitate)	480 Units (0.012 mg as D_3)	150 Units (0.004 mg as D_3)	180.0 mg	56 mg	2.4 mg as menadione	0.75 mg as menadione
Guinea pig[a] 500–850 g	6.6 mg as retinol (28 mg as β-carotene)	2.06 mg as retinol (8.75 mg as β-carotene)	1,000 Units (0.025 mg as D_3)	312 Units (0.008 mg as D_3)	27 mg	8.3 mg	5 mg as menadione	1.6 mg as menadione
Dog[a] 1–50 kg	4,040 Units (1.2 mg as retinol)	1,263 Units (0.38 mg as retinol)	442 Units (0.01 mg as D_3)	136 Units (0.003 mg as D_3)	24 mg	7.5 mg	1.3 mg as menadione	0.41 mg as menadione
Cat[a] 4–8 kg	2,664 Units (0.8 mg as retinol)	833 Units (0.25 mg as retinol)	224 Units (0.006 mg as D_3)	70 Units (0.002 mg as D_3)	30.4 mg	10 mg	0.8 mg as menadione	0.25 mg as menadione
Ferret[a,b] 500–2,000 g	~30,000 Units (9 mg as retinol)	9,375 Units (2.8 mg as retinol)	~3,000 Units (0.075 mg as D_3)	~940 Units (0.024 mg as D_3)	167 mg	52 mg	3.3 mg as menadione	~1 mg as menadione

(Continued)

TABLE 24.1 (*Continued*)
Fat-Soluble Vitamin Requirements[a,b]

	Vitamin							
	A		D		E		K	
Species[d]	Amount/kg Diet or Dry Matter (~3,200 kcal/kg DM)[c]	Amount/ 1,000 kcal (4.2 MJ)	Amount/kg Diet or Dry Matter (~3,200 kcal/kg DM)[c]	Amount/1,000 kcal (4.2 MJ)	Amount/kg Diet or Dry Matter (~3,200 kcal/kg DM)[c]	Amount/ 1,000 kcal (4.2 MJ)	Amount/kg Diet or Dry Matter (~3200 kcal/ kg DM)[c]	Amount/1,000 kcal (4.2 MJ)
Pig[a] 10–20 kg	1,750–2,000 Units (0.5–0.7 mg as retinol)	550–625 Units (0.19–0.22 mg as retinol)	200 Units (0.005 mg as D_3)	62.5 Units (0.0016 mg as D_3)	7–24 mg	2.2–7.5 mg	0.5 mg as menadione	0.16 mg as menadione
Nonhuman primate[a] 1–15 kg	6,000–10,000 Units (1.8–3.0 mg as retinol)	1,875–3,125 Units (0.72–0.93 as retinol)	1,000 Units (0.025 mg as D_3)	312 Units (0.008 mg as D_3)	10–50 mg	3–16 mg	0.2–5.0 mg as phylloquinone	0.066–1.6 mg as phylloquinone
Rabbits[a] 3–5 kg	600–1,200 Units (0.18–0.36 mg as retinol)	188–375 Units (0.05–0.94 mg as retinol)	250–550 Units (0.007–0.014 mg as retinol)	63–134 Units (0.002–0.044 mg as retinol)	18–32 mg	5.6–10 mg	0.45–0.9 mg	0.14–0.28 mg as phylloquinone

[a] The sources for nutrient requirements were for the mouse, rat, hamster, and guinea pig, Reports from the Subcommittees for Nutrient the Requirements of Laboratory Animals (1995); the dog, cat, and ferret, Nutrient Requirements of Dogs and Cats (2006); the pig, Nutrient Requirements of Swine (1998); the nonhuman primate, Nutrient Requirements of Nonhuman Primates (2003); the rabbit, Nutrient Requirements of Rabbits (1977).

[b] Additional sources for the nutrient requirements for ferrets: Fekete et al. (2005); Bell (1999).

[c] Metabolic energy per kg dry matter (DM) in typical laboratory diets. MJ, megajoule.

[d] Typical weight at sexual maturity or adulthood for species used as laboratory animals.

TABLE 24.2
Water-Soluble Vitamin Requirements[a,b]

	Vitamin							
	Ascorbic Acid		Niacin		Riboflavin		Thiamin	
Species[d]	Amount/kg Diet or Dry Matter (~3,200 kcal/kg DM)[c]	Amount/ 1,000 kcal (4.2 MJ[e])	Amount/kg Diet or Dry Matter (~3,200 kcal/kg DM)[c]	Amount/ 1,000 kcal (4.2 MJ)	Amount/kg Diet or Dry Matter (~3,200 kcal/kg DM)[c]	Amount/ 1,000 kcal (4.2 MJ)	Amount/kg Diet or Dry Matter (~3,200 kcal/kg DM)[c]	Amount/ 1,000 kcal (4.2 MJ)
Mouse[a] 15–25 g	NR[e]	NR[e]	15	4.7	7	2.2	4	1.25
Rat[a] 175–250 g	NR[e]	NR[e]	15	4.7	3	0.9	5	1.6
Hamster[a] 75–125 g	NR[e]	NR[e]	15	4.7	8.2	2.6	7.2	2.25
Guinea Pig[a] 500–850 g	200	62.3	10	3.1	3	0.9	2	0.63
Dog[a] 1–50 kg	NR[e]	NR[e]	13.6	4.25	4.2	1.3	1.8	0.56
Cat[a] 4–8 Kg	NR[e]	NR[e]	32	10	3.2	1	4.48	1.4
Ferret[a,b] 500–2,000 g	NR[e]	NR[e]	130	41	23	7.2	56	17.5
Pig[a] 10–20 Kg	NR[e]	NR[e]	12	3.8	3	0.9	1–2	0.3–0.6
Nonhuman primate[a] 1–15 Kg	200	62.3	10	3.1	3	0.9	2	0.6

(*Continued*)

TABLE 24.2 (*Continued*)
Water-Soluble Vitamin Requirements[a,b]

	Vitamin							
	Ascorbic Acid		Niacin		Riboflavin		Thiamin	
Species[d]	Amount/kg Diet or Dry Matter (~3,200 kcal/kg DM)[c]	Amount/ 1,000 kcal (4.2 MJ)	Amount/kg Diet or Dry Matter (~3,200 kcal/kg DM)[c]	Amount/ 1,000 kcal (4.2 MJ)	Amount/kg Diet or Dry Matter (~3,200 kcal/kg DM)[c]	Amount/ 1,000 kcal (4.2 MJ)	Amount/kg Diet or Dry Matter (~3,200 kcal/kg DM)[c]	Amount/ 1,000 kcal (4.2 MJ)
Rabbits[a] 3–5 Kg	NR[e]	NR[e]	11	3.4	3–5*	0.9–1.6	3	0.9

	Vitamin									
	Vitamin B6		Pantothenic Acid		Biotin		Folic Acid (Folacin)		Vitamin B12	
Species[d]	Amount/kg Diet or Dry Matter (~3,200 kcal/kg DM)	Amount/ 1,000 kcal (4.2 MJ)	Amount/kg Diet or Dry Matter (~3,200 kcal/kg DM)	Amount/ 1,000 kcal (4.2 MJ)	Amount/kg Diet or Dry Matter (~3,200 kcal/kg DM)	Amount/ 1,000 kcal (4.2 MJ)	Amount/kg Diet or Dry Matter (~3,200 kcal/kg DM)	Amount/ 1,000 kcal (4.2 MJ)	Amount/kg Diet or Dry Matter (~3,200 kcal/ kg DM)	Amount/ 1,000 kcal (4.2 MJ)
Mouse[a] 15–25 g	8	2.5	16	5	0.2	0.063	1	0.3	0.01	0.003
Rat 175–250 g	6	1.9	10	3.1	0.2	0.063	1	0.3	0.05	0.016
Hamster[a] 75–125 g	8.4		19	2.6	0.24		2.4	0.75	0.012	0.004
Guinea pig[a] 500–850 g	3	0.94	20	6.2	0.2	0.063	3	0.94	NE[e]	NE[e]
Dog[a] 1–50 Kg	1.2	0.38	12	3.75	NE[e]	NE[e]	0.22	0.07	0.028	0.009

(Continued)

TABLE 24.2 (*Continued*)
Water-Soluble Vitamin Requirements[a,b]

	Vitamin									
	Vitamin B6		Pantothenic Acid		Biotin		Folic Acid (Folacin)		Vitamin B12	
Species[d]	Amount/kg Diet or Dry Matter (~3,200 kcal/kg DM)	Amount/ 1,000 kcal (4.2 MJ)	Amount/kg Diet or Dry Matter (~3,200 kcal/kg DM)	Amount/ 1,000 kcal (4.2 MJ)	Amount/kg Diet or Dry Matter (~3,200 kcal/kg DM)	Amount/ 1,000 kcal (4.2 MJ)	Amount/kg Diet or Dry Matter (~3,200 kcal/kg DM)	Amount/ 1,000 kcal (4.2 MJ)	Amount/kg Diet or Dry Matter (~3,200 kcal/ kg DM)	Amount/ 1,000 kcal (4.2 MJ)
Cat[a] 4–8 Kg	2	0.63	4.6	1.44	0.06	0.02	0.6	0.19	0.02	0.006
Ferret[a,b] 500–2,000 g	19		26	8,1	0.43	0.134	4.7	1.5	0.025	0.0078
Pig[a] 10–20 Kg	1.5	5.9	9	2.8	0.05	0.016	0.3	0.9	0.015	0.047
Nonhuman primate[a] 1–15 Kg	2–3	0.6–0.94	20	6.2	0.2	0.063	3	0.94	0.01	0.003
Rabbits[a] 3–5 Kg	40	12.5	NE[e]	NE[e]	NE[e]	NE[e]	NE[e]	NE[e]	NE[e]	NE[e]

[a] The sources for nutrient requirements were for the mouse, rat, hamster, and guinea pig, Nutrient Requirements of Laboratory Animals (1995); the dog, cat, and ferret, Nutrient Requirements of Dogs and Cats (2006); the pig, Nutrient Requirements of Swine (1998); the non-human primate, Nutrient Requirements of Nonhuman Primates (2003); the rabbit, Nutrient of Rabbits (1977). All numerical values listed in this table are in milligrams.

[b] Additional sources for the nutrient requirements for ferrets: Fekete et al. (2005) and Bell (1999).

[c] Metabolic energy per kg dry matter (DM) in typical laboratory diets. MJ = megajoule.

[d] Typical weight at sexual maturity or adulthood for species used as laboratory animals.

[e] NR = not required in the diet for normal growth. NE = requirement is not well documented or established.

TABLE 24.3
Mineral Requirements[a,b]

	Minerals											
	Co[e]		Cu		Mo[f]		Mn		Se		Zn	
Species[d]	Amount/kg Diet or Dry Matter (~3,200 kcal/kg DM)[c]	Amount/ 1,000 kcal (4.2 MJ)	Amount/Kg Diet or Dry Matter (~3,200 kcal/kg DM)[c]	Amount/ 1,000 kcal (4.2 MJ)	Amount/Kg Diet or Dry Matter (~3,200 kcal/kg DM)[c]	Amount/ 1,000 kcal (4.2 MJ)	Amount/Kg Diet or Dry Matter (~3,200 kcal/kg DM)[c]	Amount /1,000 kcal (4.2 MJ)	Amount/Kg Diet or Dry Matter (~3,200 kcal/kg DM)[c]	Amount/ 1,000 kcal (4.2 MJ)	Amount/Kg Diet or Dry Matter (~3,200 kcal/kg DM)[c]	Amount/ 1,000 kcal (4.2 MJ)
Mouse[a] 15–25 g	NE	NE	6	1.9	0.15	0.047	10	3.1	0.15	0.047	10	3.1
Rat[a] 175–250 g	NE	NE	5	1.6	0.15	0.047	10	3.1	0.15	0.047	12	3.75
Hamster[a] 75–125 g	NE	NE	6	1.9	NE	NE	10	3.1	0.15	0.047	10	3.1
Guinea Pig[a] 500–850 g	NE	NE	6	1.9	0.15	0.047	40	9.4	0.15	0.047	20	6.2
Dog[a] 1–50 Kg	NE	NE	4.8	1.5	NE	NE	3.84	1.2	0.28	0.09	48	15
Cat[a] 4–8 Kg	NE	NE	4	1.2	NE	NE	3.84	1.2	0.24	0.08	59.2	18.5
Ferret[a,b] 500–2,000 g	NE	NE	5	1.6	NE	NE	8	2.5	0.1	0.03	75	23.4

(Continued)

TABLE 24.3 (*Continued*)
Mineral Requirements[a,b]

	Minerals											
	Co[e]		Cu		Mo[f]		Mn		Se		Zn	
Species[d]	Amount/kg Diet or Dry Matter (~3,200 kcal/kg DM)[c]	Amount/ 1,000 kcal (4.2 MJ)	Amount/Kg Diet or Dry Matter (~3,200 kcal/kg DM)[c]	Amount/ 1,000 kcal (4.2 MJ)	Amount/Kg Diet or Dry Matter (~3,200 kcal/kg DM)[c]	Amount/ 1,000 kcal (4.2 MJ)	Amount/Kg Diet or Dry Matter (~3,200 kcal/kg DM)[c]	Amount /1,000 kcal (4.2 MJ)	Amount/Kg Diet or Dry Matter (~3,200 kcal/kg DM)[c]	Amount/ 1,000 kcal (4.2 MJ)	Amount/Kg Diet or Dry Matter (~3,200 kcal/ kg DM)[c]	Amount/ 1,000 kcal (4.2 MJ)
Pig[a] 10–20 Kg	NE	NE	5	1.6	NE	NE	4	1.25	0.25	0.08	80	25
Nonhuman primate[a] 1–15 Kg	NE	NE	~10	3.2	NE	NE	20	6.25	0.15	0.047	10–20	3.1–6.2
Rabbits[a] 3–5 Kg	1	0.3	4	1.25	NE	NE	30	9.4	0.1	0.03	40	12.5

[a] The sources for nutrient requirements were for the mouse, rat, hamster, and guinea pig, Nutrient Requirements of Laboratory Animals (1995); the dog, cat, and ferret, Nutrient Requirements of Dogs and Cats (2006); the pig, Nutrient Requirements of Swine (1998); the nonhuman primate, Nutrient Requirements of Nonhuman Primates (2003); the rabbit, Nutrient Requirements of Rabbits (1977). All numerical values listed in this table are in milligrams.

[b] Additional sources for the nutrient requirements for ferrets: Fekete et al. (2005) and Bell (1999).

[c] Metabolic energy per kg dry matter in typical laboratory diets.

[d] Typical weight at sexual maturity or adulthood for species used as laboratory animals.

[e] A need for cobalt beyond that found in vitamin B12 has not been defined for most animals. The value indicated for the rabbit reflects the ability of nonruminant herbivores to synthesis vitamin B12. Synthesis occurs in the cecum and the vitamin is acquired by direct absorption from the intestine or by reingestion and absorption following coprophagy. If a requirement exists in nonherbivores beyond the need for vitamin B12, it is most likely less than 200 μg/1,000 kcal dry matter (DM) consumed. MJ, megajoule; NE, requirement is not well documented or established.

[f] The need for the molybdenum is most likely less than 200 μg/1,000 kcal **dry matter** (DM) consumed; the amount required to produce the Molybdenum cofactor. NE = requirement is not well documented or established.

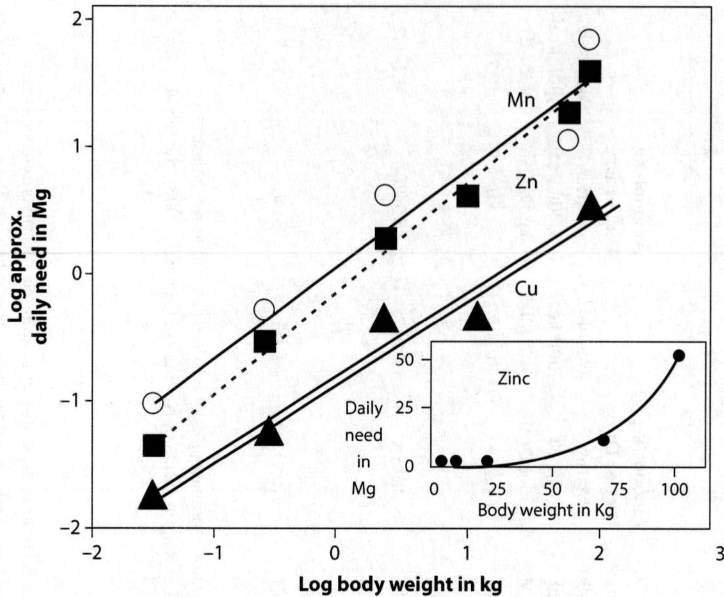

FIGURE 24.1 Daily intake of selected minerals for mice, rats, chickens, dogs, humans, and pigs versus their respective body weights in kilograms. The data for individual minerals plotted in this fashion result in reasonably linear plots with slopes that range from 0.6 to 0.8. A slope of ~0.75 represents the active tissue mass or metabolic mass. As noted in the small figure insert, for any given mineral, plots of daily intake versus body weight are not linear and require polynomial equations to describe the function. (From Rucker, R., and Storms, D., *J Nutr,* 132, 2999–3000, 2002.)

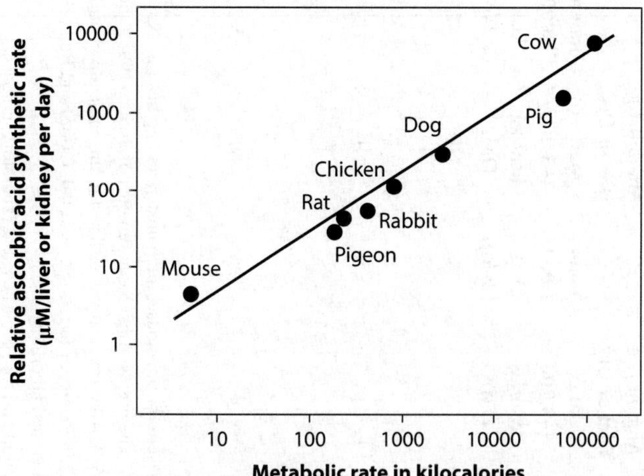

FIGURE 24.2 Ascorbic acid production and basal energy expenditure are functions of metabolic size. The principles that control ascorbic acid production appear to follow the same allometric relationships as energy expenditure among homeothermic animals (e.g., as a function of $(Wt_{kg})^{3/4}$). (From Rucker, R.B., *J Anim Physiol Anim Nutr (Berl)*, 91, 148–156, 2007.)

array of species. To illustrate this point, the relationship between the ascorbic acid (vitamin C) requirements is given in Figure 24.2. Most mammals that require ascorbic acid meet their needs at intakes of 20–80 mg per 1000 kcal (4.184 megajoule or MJ). This amount corresponds to what may be extrapolated from synthetic rates in animals that are known to produce ascorbic acid (Rucker, 2007). Examination of genetic animal models, such as the gulonolactone oxidase null mouse and the osteogenic disorder Shionogi (ODS) rat, both of which cannot synthesize ascorbic acid, is also illustrative of the concept. The L-ascorbic acid requirement for normal growth and metabolism in these two animal models is of the same order as the amount produced by normal rats and mice (Rucker, 2007), as well as that needed by guinea pigs for optimal growth (Table 24.2).

24.2.4 Nutritional Deficiencies and Toxicities

Why do deficiencies or excesses occur? Primary deficiencies often happen when monotonous diets or limited combinations of foods are consumed. For certain mineral elements (e.g., selenium), a deficiency may arise if the foodstuff comes from a single region deficient in the nutrient. Secondary mineral and vitamin deficiencies can also result through a variety of mechanisms that include poor bioavailability, interactions with other competing substances, and genetic influences (e.g., polymorphisms that dictate an increased need for given nutrients). Table 24.4 provides a list of mechanisms underlying the development of deficiencies and interactions that will be amplified in each of the sections that follow. Tables 24.5 and 24.6 highlight deficiencies and toxicities in dogs and cats. Note that in many cases, the signs for specific mineral and vitamin deficiencies are similar to those observed in other mammals and common laboratory animals.

24.3 FAT-SOLUBLE VITAMINS

Vitamins A, D, E, and K are unlike the water-soluble vitamins because of their lipid solvent solubility, diverse nonenzymatic functions, sequestration in lipid vacuoles and adipose, and greater risk for toxicity. Like dietary triglycerides, fat-soluble vitamins are solubilized in the duodenal lumen in the presence of bile and pancreatic enzymes. They are then maintained within the lipophilic core of mixed micelles. Next, pancreatic esterases, in the presence of bile salts, catalyze the release of fat-soluble vitamins from their esters. Together with fatty acids derived from triglycerides, fat-soluble vitamins are released from micelles at the enterocyte brush border membrane. At high doses, vitamins A and E can be absorbed directly from water-miscible emulsions. The next steps involve incorporation into chylomicrons for secretion into lymphatics and ultimate uptake by the liver. Intestinal, biliary, and pancreatic diseases that cause decreased dietary lipid absorption may cause a decrease in the absorption of fat-soluble vitamins.

TABLE 24.4
Potential Causes of Vitamin and Mineral Deficiencies

Cause	Mechanism
Food processing	Loss of a nutrient due to isolation and/or refinement of selected food components
Prolonged or inappropriate storage of feed stuffs or components	Exposure to UV light, heat, excessive moisture
Dietary interactions	Competitive interactions between nutrients for transport or chemical modification processes that are in common
Drug interactions	Alterations in metabolism that affect absorption (chelators and structural analogs) and/or excretion (e.g., laxatives, diuretics) redistribution among tissue pools; induction of phase 1 and 2 enzyme systems important to the metabolism of a given vitamin or mineral
Physiological state	Change in requirement due to reproduction, growth, lactation, or aging
Disease	Alterations in metabolism that affect absorption and/or excretion; rates of energy expenditure
Genetic	Polymorphism or alteration in genes important to specific steps in nutrient metabolism and/or transport

TABLE 24.5
Clinical Signs of Nutrient Deficiency and Toxicity, Diagnostic Tests, and Blood Concentrations in Dogs

Nutrient	Clinical Signs of Deficiency	Clinical Signs of Toxicity	Diagnostics for Status Assessment	Blood/Urine or Organ Concentrations[a,b]
		Fat-Soluble Vitamins		
Vitamin A	Anorexia, weight loss, ataxia, xerophthalmia, conjunctivitis, corneal opacity and ulceration, skin lesions, metaplasia of the bronchiolar epithelium, pneumonitis, and increased susceptibility to infections	Poor bone growth, reluctance to walk, depression, anorexia, gingivitis, fetal malformations	Serum or liver retinol concentrations	Retinol; 642 ± 36 ng/mol (P) (Schweigert et al., 1990) Retinyl palmitate; 609 ± 67 ng/mol (P) (Schweigert et al., 1990) Retinyl sterate; 916 ± 101 ng/mol (P) (Schweigert et al., 1990) Liver retinol; 794–1,129 IU/g retinol (wet tissue) (Goldy et al., 1996)
Vitamin D	Rickets: osteomalacia, orthopedic pain, impaired growth, malformation of long bones	Lethargy, anorexia, vomiting, polydipsia, hypercalcemia	Radiographic imaging of skeletal bones, serum 25-hydroxyvitamin D	Cholecalciferol; 153 ± 50 pmol/L (P)[#] (Gerber et al., 2003)
Vitamin E	Muscle weakness, reproductive failure, nodular adipose tissue (associated with steatitis)	Growth depression, degreased bone growth increased prothrombin time (associated with vitamins D and K antagonism)	Plasma α- tocopherol	α- tocopherol; 7.54 ± 0.4 μg/mL (P) (Schweigert et al., 1990)
Vitamin K	Excessive bleeding, prolonged clotting times	Anemia	Prothrombin times (PT), PIVKA (Proteins induced by vitamin K antagonism)	PT; 11–15 sec (P) (Rozanski et al., 1999) PIVKA; 18–24 sec (P) (Rozanski et al., 1999)
		Water-Soluble Vitamins		
Thiamin	Inappetance, weight loss, coprophagia, cardiac hypertrophy, bradycardia, muscle weakness, ataxia, paraparesis, torticollis, circling, tonic-clonic convulsions, death	None reported with oral ingestion in dogs. Intravenous injection can cause a decrease in blood pressure and bradycardia	Plasma concentration of thiamin phosphorylated esters, erythrocyte transketolase saturation	Thiamin; 46–112 ng/mL (WB) (Baker et al., 1986)
Riboflavin	Anorexia, weight loss, periauricular alopecia, epidermal trophy, cataracts	None reported in dogs	Erythrocyte glutathione reductase activity coefficient, urine riboflavin	Riboflavin; 185–420 ng/mL (WB) (Baker et al., 1986)

(Continued)

TABLE 24.5 (*Continued*)
Clinical Signs of Nutrient Deficiency and Toxicity, Diagnostic Tests, and Blood Concentrations in Dogs

Nutrient	Clinical Signs of Deficiency	Clinical Signs of Toxicity	Diagnostics for Status Assessment	Blood/Urine or Organ Concentrations[a,b]
Pyridoxine (vitamin B6)	Anorexia, microcytic hypochromic anemia, convulsions, cardiac dilation, and hypertrophy	Ataxia, muscle weakness, tonic convulsions	Pyridoxal blood concentration, aminotransferase activity, kynureninase activity	Pyridoxine; 40–270 ng/mL (P) (Baker et al., 1986)
Niacin	Black tongue, stomatitis, 4 D's = dermatitis, diarrhea, dementia, and death	High doses reported to cause bloody feces, convulsions, and death in dogs	Nicotinamide loading test: urine N′-methylnicotinamide concentration	Niacin; 2.7–12 μg/mL (WB) (Baker et al., 1986)
Folic acid	Macrocytic hypochromic anemia, poor appetite and weight gain, cleft palates in Boston Terriers	None reported in dogs	Serum folic acid concentration	Folic acid; 4–26 ng/mL (P) (Baker et al., 1986)
Vitamin B12	Macrocytic hypochromic anemia, inappetance, failure to thrive	None reported in dogs	Serum vitamin B12 concentration, serum or urine methylmalonic acid	Vitamin B12; 135–950 pg/mL (WB) (Baker et al., 1986)
Pantothenic acid	Anorexia, diarrhea, locomotive incoordination	None reported in dogs	Urinary output of pantothenate	Pantothenic acid; 104–270 ng/mL (WB) (Baker et al., 1986)
Biotin	Dermatitis	None reported in dogs	Serum biotin concentration, acetyl CoA carboxylase and propionyl CoA carboxylase activities, urine biotin	Biotin; 530–5,000 pg. mL (WB) (Baker et al., 1986)
		Vitamin-Like Compounds		
Choline	Weight loss, vomiting, fatty liver	Possible depression in erythropoiesis	Plasma choline and phosphatidylcholine	Choline; 235–800 μg/mL (P) (Baker et al., 1986)
		Macro Minerals		
Calcium	Reluctance to move, posterior lameness, uncoordinated gait and painful enlarged joints, osteopenia, rickets, osteoporosis, spontaneous fractures, facial pruritis, agitation, tetany, cardiac arrhythmias, seizures	Inappetance, poor growth	Radiographic imaging of skeleton, parathyroid hormone levels, serum ionized calcium concentration	Calcium; 9.0–11.3 mg/dL (S, P) (Kaneko et al., 2008) Ionized calcium 1.2–1.35 mmol/L (S) (Unterer et al., 2004)

(*Continued*)

TABLE 24.5 (*Continued*)
Clinical Signs of Nutrient Deficiency and Toxicity, Diagnostic Tests, and Blood Concentrations in Dogs

Nutrient	Clinical Signs of Deficiency	Clinical Signs of Toxicity	Diagnostics for Status Assessment	Blood/Urine or Organ Concentrations[a,b]
Phosphorus	Hemolytic anemia, locomotor disturbances, metabolic acidosis	None reported in dogs, effects appear to be more related to calcium excess rather than phosphorus deficiency	Plasma concentration (not a good assessment of body stores)	Phosphorus; 2.6–6.2 mg/dL (S, P) (Kaneko et al., 2008)
Potassium	Depression, weakness, neck ventroflexion, weight loss	None reported, hypothesized to cause cardiac abnormalities and arrest at very high doses	Plasma concentration (not a good assessment of body stores)	Potassium; 4.35–5.35 mg/dL (S, P) (Kaneko et al., 2008)
Sodium	Inappetance, polyuria/polydypsia, increased hematocrit and hemoglobin concentrations	Vomiting	Increased plasma and urine aldosterone concentration (serum levels not a reliable indicator of nutritional deficiency)	Sodium; 141–152 mmol/L (S, P) (Kaneko et al., 2008)
Chloride	Deficiency leads to excess potassium excretion in the kidneys; therefore, clinical signs of potassium deficiency may occur, metabolic acidosis	None reported in dogs	Plasma concentration (not a good assessment of body stores)	Chloride; 105–115 mmol/L (S, P) (Kaneko et al., 2008)
Magnesium	Tetany, tremors, hyperexcitability, tachycardia, and seizures	None reported in dogs	Ionized serum magnesium concentration	Total magnesium: 1.8–2.4 mg/dL (S) (Kaneko et al., 2008) Ionized magnesium; 0.42–0.58 mmol/L (S) (Unterer et al., 2004)
		Trace Minerals		
Iron	Hypochromic, microcytic anemia, lethargy, weakness, weight loss or lack of weight gain, hematuria, melena	Vomiting (acute toxicity)	Total serum iron-binding capacity, serum iron concentration	Iron-binding capacity, total (unbound); 170–222 µg/dL (S) (Kaneko et al., 2008) Total iron-binding capacity; 165–418 µg/dL (S) (Kaneko et al., 2008) Iron; 30–180 µg/dL (S) (Kaneko et al., 2008) Liver; 400–1,200 ppm (dry weight) (Schultheiss et al., 2002)

(*Continued*)

TABLE 24.5 (*Continued*)
Clinical Signs of Nutrient Deficiency and Toxicity, Diagnostic Tests, and Blood Concentrations in Dogs

Nutrient	Clinical Signs of Deficiency	Clinical Signs of Toxicity	Diagnostics for Status Assessment	Blood/Urine or Organ Concentrations[a,b]
Zinc	Decreased appetite, parakeratosis, reproductive failure, decreased wound healing	Acute gastroenteritis, hemolytic anemia, and lethargy	Plasma or WB zinc concentration (may not be a reliable indicator of zinc stores), liver concentration	Zinc; 1.2–0.4 mg/L (S)[#](Kazmierski et al., 2001) Liver; 120–300 ppm (dry weight) (Schultheiss et al., 2002)
Manganese	Suspected retarded bone growth, lameness, enlarged joints, poor locomotor function based on studies in other species	None reported in dogs	Manganese lymphocyte concentration	None available
Copper	Neurological signs, anemia, hypochromotricia	Hemolytic anemia, liver disease	Liver concentration, RBC Cu/Zn SOD activity	RBC SOD; 40 ± 6 U/mg Hb[#] (Desilvestro et al., 2005) Copper; 100–200 μg/dL (S) (Kaneko et al., 2008) Liver: 120–400 ppm (dry weight) (Schultheiss et al., 2002)
Iodine	Goiter, alopecia, dry sparse overall hair coat, weight gain	Excessive lacrimation, salivation, nasal discharge, flaky, dry skin, and hair coat	Urine iodine excretion, thyroid hormone	Iodine; 5–20 μg/dL (S) (Kaneko et al., 2008) Thyroxine (T_4—RIA); 0.6–3.6 μg/dL (S) (Kaneko et al., 2008) Triiodothyronine (T_3—RIA); 82–138 ng/dL (S) (Kaneko et al., 2008)
Selenium	Anorexia, depression, dyspnea, "white muscle disease"	Microcytic, hypochromic anemia, liver necrosis, and cirrhosis	Plasma concentration of Se and activity of glutathione peroxidase (GPx) in plasma	Selenium; 2.29–2.45 μmol/L (S) (Wedekind et al., 2004) GSHpx; 1.25–1.32 nmol/NAPDH (S) (Wedekind et al., 2004)

Note: Serum Se and plasma GSHpx from kittens consuming a diet containing 0.15 mg Se/kg diet.

[a] Reference ranges will vary with laboratory, please consult the ranges provided by the lab you are using. In some cases, samples from normal animals may need to be provided to serve as controls. Validation of a given assay for the species in question should be confirmed. In many cases, there are no reference ranges available for the diagnostic tests listed in column 4.

[b] GPx = glutathione peroxidase, WB = whole blood, P = plasma, S = serum. Values are expressed as ranges or mean ±SE with the exception that those noted (#) are expressed as mean ±SD.

TABLE 24.6
Clinical Signs of Nutrient Deficiency and Toxicity, Diagnostic Tests, and Blood Concentrations in Cats

Nutrient	Clinical Signs of Deficiency	Clinical Signs of Toxicity	Diagnostics for Status Assessment	Blood/Urine or Organ Concentrations[a,b]
		Fat-Soluble Vitamins		
Vitamin A	Anorexia, weight loss, ataxia, xerophthalmia, conjunctivitis, corneal opacity and ulceration, skin lesions, metaplasia of the bronchiolar epithelium, pneumonitis, and increased susceptibility to infections	Extensive osseocartilagenous hyperplasia of the first three cervical vertebrae, poor bone growth, gingivitis, tooth loss, fetal malformations	Serum or liver retinol concentrations	Retinol; 240 ± 65 ng/mL (P) (Raila et al., 2001) Retinyl palmitate; 275 ± 282 ng/mL (P) (Raila et al., 2001) Retinyl stereate; 433 ± 290 ng/mL (P) (Raila et al., 2001) Liver retinol; 11 ± 4 μg/g retinol (wet tissue) (Raila et al., 2001)
Vitamin D	Rickets: osteomalacia, orthopedic pain, impaired growth, malformation of long bones	Lethargy, anorexia, vomiting, polydipsia, hypercalcemia	Radiographic imaging of skeletal bones, serum 25-hydroxyvitamin D	Cholecalciferol; 36.5 ± 4.8 nmol/L (P) (Sih et al., 2001)
Vitamin E	Muscle weakness, reproductive failure, nodular adipose tissue (associated with steatitis)	Growth depression, degreased bone growth increased prothrombin time (associated with vitamins D and K antagonism)	Plasma α-tocopherol	α- tocopherol; 9.86 ± 1.66 μg/mL (P) (Schweigert et al., 1990)
Vitamin K	Excessive bleeding, prolonged clotting times	None reported in cats	Prothrombin times (PT), PIVKA (Proteins Induced by Vitamin K Antagonism)	PT; <11 sec (P) (Center et al., 2000) PIVKA; 16.6–25.2 sec (P) (Center et al., 2000)
		Water-Soluble Vitamins		
Thiamin	Inappetance, weight loss, coprophagia, muscle weakness, ataxia, paraparesis, torticollis, circling, tonic-clonic convulsions, neck ventroflexion, death	None reported in cats	Plasma concentration of thiamin phosphorylated esters, erythrocyte transketolase saturation	Thiamin; 20–90 ng/mL (WB) (Baker et al., 1986)
Riboflavin	Anorexia, weight loss, periauricular alopecia, epidermal trophy, cataracts, fatty liver	None reported in cats	Erythrocyte glutathione reductase activity coefficient, urine riboflavin	Riboflavin; 196–660 ng/mL (WB) (Baker et al., 1986)
Pyridoxine (vitamin B6)	Anorexia, microcytic hypochromic anemia, convulsions, enhanced oxalate excretion	None reported in cats	Pyridoxal blood concentration, aminotransferase activity, kynureninase activity	Pyridoxine; 86–350 ng/mL (P) (Baker et al., 1986)

(Continued)

TABLE 24.6 (*Continued*)
Clinical Signs of Nutrient Deficiency and Toxicity, Diagnostic Tests, and Blood Concentrations in Cats

Nutrient	Clinical Signs of Deficiency	Clinical Signs of Toxicity	Diagnostics for Status Assessment	Blood/Urine or Organ Concentrations[a,b]
Niacin	Black tongue, stomatitis, 4 D's = dermatitis, diarrhea, dementia, and death	None reported in cats	Nicotinamide loading test: urine N′-methylnicotinamide concentration	Niacin; 1.8–5.8 µg/mL (WB) (Baker et al., 1986)
Folic acid	Macrocytic hypochromic anemia	None reported in cats	Serum folic acid concentration	Folic Acid; 3.2–34 ng/mL (P) (Baker et al., 1986)
Vitamin B12	Macrocytic hypochromic anemia	None reported in cats	Serum vitamin B12 concentration, serum, or urine methylmalonic acid	Vitamin B12; 120–1,200 pg/mL (WB) (Baker et al., 1986)
Pantothenic acid	Dermal lesions (dermatitis and alopecia), anorexia, diarrhea, locomotive incoordination, ketoacidiosis	None reported in cats	Urinary output of pantothenate	Pantothenic acid; 104–270 ng/mL (WB) (Baker et al., 1986)
Biotin	Alopecia, dermatitis, metabolic acidosis	None reported in cats	Serum biotin concentration, Acetyl CoA carboxylase and propionyl CoA carboxylase activities, urine biotin	Biotin; 1,000–3,000 pg. mL (WB) (Baker et al., 1986)
		Vitamin-Like Compounds		
Choline	Fatty liver	None reported in cats	Serum alanine aminotransferase activity (rises approximately 1 week after the feeding a choline-deficient diet), plasma choline, and phosphatidylcholine	Choline; 180–490 µg/mL (P) (Baker et al., 1986)
		Macro Minerals		
Calcium	Reluctance to move, posterior lameness, uncoordinated gait and painful enlarge joints, osteopenia, rickets, osteoporosis, spontaneous fractures, agitation, tetany, cardiac arrhythmias, seizures	Inappetance, poor growth	Radiographic imaging of skeleton, parathyroid hormone levels, serum ionized calcium concentration	Calcium; 6.2–10.22 mg/dL (S, P) (Kaneko et al., 2008) Ionized calcium 1.18–1.38 mmol/L (S) (Schenck and Chew, 2010)
Phosphorus	Hemolytic anemia, locomotor disturbances, metabolic acidosis	Depression, dehydration, metabolic acidosis	Plasma concentration (not a good assessment of body stores)	Phosphorus; 4.5–8.1 mg/dL (S, P) (Kaneko et al., 2008)

(*Continued*)

TABLE 24.6 (*Continued*)
Clinical Signs of Nutrient Deficiency and Toxicity, Diagnostic Tests, and Blood Concentrations in Cats

Nutrient	Clinical Signs of Deficiency	Clinical Signs of Toxicity	Diagnostics for Status Assessment	Blood/Urine or Organ Concentrations[a,b]
Potassium	Depression, weakness, neck ventroflexion, weight loss	None reported in cats, hypothesized to cause cardiac abnormalities and arrest at very high doses	Plasma concentration (not a good assessment of body stores)	Potassium; 4.0–4.5 mg/dL (S, P) (Kaneko et al., 2008)
Sodium	Inappetance, polyuria/polydypsia in kittens	None reported in cats	Increased plasma and urine aldosterone concentration (serum levels not a reliable indicator of nutritional deficiency)	Sodium; 147–156 mmol/L (S, P) (Kaneko et al., 2008)
Chloride	Deficiency leads to excess potassium excretion in the kidneys; therefore, clinical signs of potassium deficiency may occur	None reported in cats	Plasma concentration (not a good assessment of body stores)	Chloride; 117–123 mmol/L (S, P) (Kaneko et al., 2008)
Magnesium	Tetany, tremors, hyperexcitability, tachycardia, and seizures	Struvite urolithiasis	Ionized serum magnesium concentration	Total magnesium; 2–2.59 mg/dL (S) (Shin et al., 2004) Ionized magnesium; 1.1–1.44 mg/dL (S) (Shin et al., 2004)
		Trace Minerals		
Iron	Hypochromic, microcytic anemia, lethargy, weakness, weight loss or lack of weight gain, hematuria, melena	Vomiting (acute toxicity)	Total serum iron-binding capacity, serum iron concentration	Iron-binding capacity, total (unbound); 105–205 μg/dL (S) (Kaneko et al., 2008) Total iron-binding capacity; 209 μg/dL (mean) (S) (Kaneko et al., 2008) Iron; 68–215 μg/dL (S) (Kaneko et al., 2008)
Zinc	Decreased appetite, parakeratosis, reproductive failure, decreased wound healing	None reported in cats	Plasma or WB zinc concentration (may not be a reliable indicator of zinc stores), liver concentration	Zinc; 8.2–14.7 μmol/L (P) (Van den Broek et al., 1992)
Manganese	Suspected retarded bone growth, lameness, enlarged joints, poor locomotor function based on studies in other species	None reported in cats	Manganese lymphocyte concentration	None available

(*Continued*)

TABLE 24.6 (*Continued*)
Clinical Signs of Nutrient Deficiency and Toxicity, Diagnostic Tests, and Blood Concentrations in Cats

Nutrient	Clinical Signs of Deficiency	Clinical Signs of Toxicity	Diagnostics for Status Assessment	Blood/Urine or Organ Concentrations[a,b]
Copper	Neurological signs, anemia (kittens), ypochromotricia	None reported in cats	Liver concentration, RBC Cu/Zn SOD activity	RBC SOD; 2.2–11.6 U/mg Hb (Fascetti et al., 2002) Plasma Cu; 8.6–18 μmol/L (P) (Fascetti et al., 2002) Liver: 0.82 ± 0.03 μmol/g (wet weight) (Fascetti et al., 2000)
Iodine	Goiter, alopecia, dry sparse overall hair coat, weight gain	Excessive lacrimation, salivation, nasal discharge, flaky, dry skin, and hair coat	Urine iodine excretion, thyroid hormone	Iodine; 3.23 μmol/L (U) (Wedekind et al., 2010) Thyroxine (T_4—RIA); 0.1–2.5 μg/dL (S) (Kaneko et al., 2008) Triiodothyronine (T_3-RIA); 15–104 ng/dL (S) (Kaneko et al., 2008)
Selenium	Anorexia, depression, dyspnea, "white muscle disease" based on studies in other species	None reported in cats	Plasma concentration of Se and activity of glutathione peroxidase (GPx) in plasma	Selenium; 3.95–8.70 mmol/L (P) (Wedekind et al., 2003) GSHpx; >2 mU/L (P) (Foster et al., 2001)

Notes: Cats were consuming 50 ug/kg diet (DM) cholecalciferol; urinary iodine reported in cats consuming a diet containing 0.47 mg/kg diet (DM) supplied as KI; plasma GSHpx from kittens consuming 0.15 mg Se/kg diet.

[a] Reference ranges will vary with laboratory, please consult the ranges provided by the lab you are using. In some cases, samples from normal animals may need to be provided to serve as controls. Validation of a given assay for the species in question should be confirmed. In many cases, there are no reference ranges available for the diagnostic tests listed in column 4.

[b] WB = whole blood, P = plasma, S = serum, U = urine. Values are expressed as ranges or mean ±SE.

24.3.1 Vitamin A

24.3.1.1 Overview

Vitamin A includes the provitamin dietary carotenoid precursors of retinol and dietary retinol in its esterified form (Figure 24.3). Retinol in the form of retinyl esters is found in liver, eggs, and milk products, while carotenoids are present in oils, fruits, and vegetables. When released, retinol is transported into enterocytes by a specific carrier protein. Carotenoids comprise a group of more than 600 compounds (most often red, yellow, and orange pigments in their isolated states). Carotenoids are split into two classes, xanthophylls (contain oxygen) and carotenes (purely hydrocarbon in nature). A carotenoid must contain a β-ionone structure to act as a provitamin. Of the carotenoids, six are known to be biologically important: α-carotene, lycopene, lutein, zeaxanthin, cryptoxanthin, and β-carotene (Krinsky and Johnson, 2005). Carotenoid pigments in combination with given proteins or fats can produce blue, green, purple, or brown pigments in addition to yellow, orange, and red. Typically, if an animal's skin or feather color comes from carotenoids, and it is not available in food, some or all of the color fades.

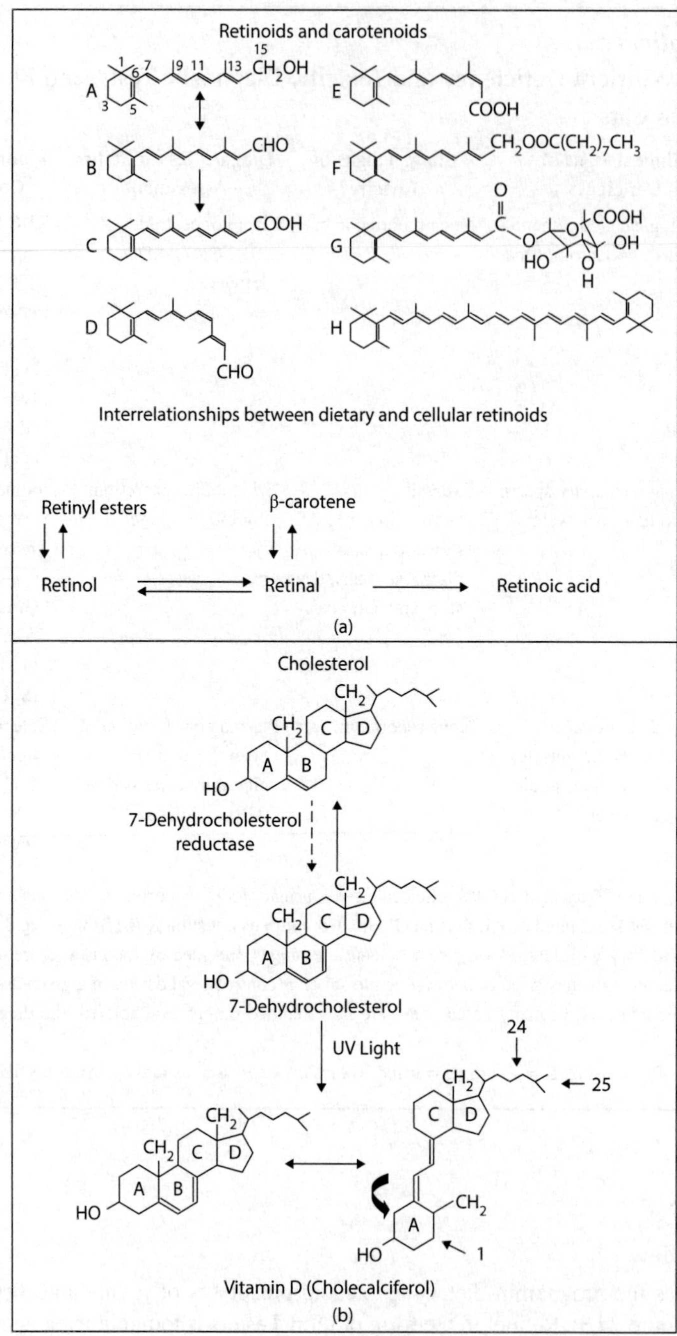

FIGURE 24.3 Absorption and cellular metabolism of carotenoids and retinoids. In the intestinal mucosal cell, some carotenoids are oxidized to both carotenals and retinals. Retinal is reduced by alcohol dehydrogenases (RolDH) to retinol and reesterified by lecithin retinol acyl transferase (LRAT). Retinol and associated esters are incorporated into chylomicrons or into intestinal very low-density lipoprotein particles (not shown), which are released into the lymph. Retinol released from retinyl esters by the action of retinyl ester hydrolase (REH) may also be oxidized to retinal by short-chain dehydrogenases/reductases (SDR). Retinoic acid is formed from retinal by the action of retinal dehydrogenase (RalDH). Retinoic acid-derived products are sufficiently polar that they may be transported directly into blood, whereas carotenoid pigments and retinyl esters are partitioned into chylomicrons for delivery into lymph.

24.3.1.2 Metabolism

The intestinal transport of retinoids is active and saturable at physiological concentrations (Ross and Zolfaghari, 2004; Harrison, 2005). For most monogastric animals, the overall availability of pure β-carotene in oil is about half that of retinol. However, because the average availability of dietary β-carotene is about 8% or less in mixed vegetable and fruit diets after absorption and bioconversion, 20 μg or more of mixed dietary carotenoids are often required to yield the equivalent of ~1 μg of retinol. In nonruminant animals, poor digestion of complex plant organelle structures, such as chloroplasts, where carotenoids are concentrated, can lead to poor digestibility of carotenoid components, even though their concentrations are sufficient to meet requirements. Concerning carnivores, such as cats and ferrets, their digestive systems are best suited for digesting and absorbing nutrients from animal-based proteins and fats, because they are descended from carnivores (Raila et al., 2002). Although early studies were unable to detect significant amounts of β-carotene in the blood of cats given oral doses, more recent studies have found β-carotene absorption to be relatively efficient in cats, which brings into question issues regarding the limits of detection and specificity of earlier methods used for retinoid and carotenoid detection. For example, Schweigert et al. (2002) have reported that cats are able to absorb β-carotene from the diet, but it is not efficiently converted to vitamin A. Unlike most mammals, cats have little capacity to convert carotenoids to vitamin A, because of low levels of β-carotene 15,15'-monooxygenase, an enzyme essential for the conversion of carotenoids to retinol (Figure 24.4). Cats and ferrets should be fed animal sources rich in retinyl ester or vitamin A as retinyl palmitate or acetate in supplements (Lederman et al., 1998; White et al., 1993). Further, it is also noteworthy that cats may potentially serve as a model for the study of β-carotene independent of its role as a vitamin A precursor (e.g., its putative role as an antioxidant or mediator of certain types of immune responses).

24.3.1.3 Absorption and Transport

Efficient entry of carotenoids and retinol in enterocytes is dependent on normal biliary and pancreatic secretion, the presence of dietary lipid, and the formation of intestinal micelles. Sufficient dietary lipid for most animals is achieved if the diet contains more than 10% lipid. The various

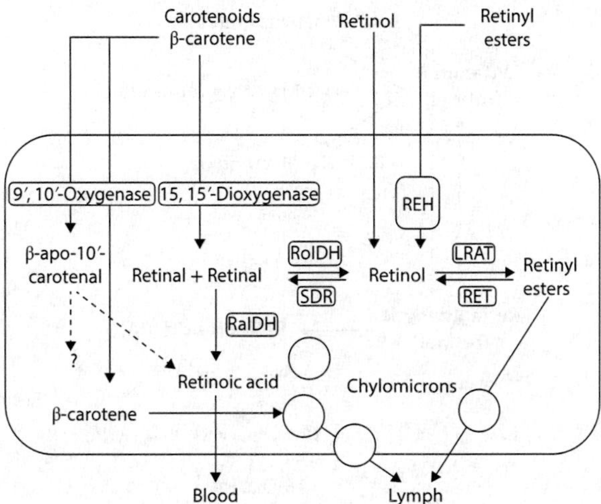

FIGURE 24.4 (a) Structures and relationships for selected retinoids, β-carotene and (b) cholecalciferol. The structures are A, retinol, which can be converted in reversible reactions to B, retinal; retinal can be irreversibly converted to C, all-trans retinoic acid; C can isomerize to D, 11-cis, or E, 13-cis retinoic acids, respectively; F, retinyl palmitate; G, retinoyl glucuronic acid; H, β-carotene. Important interrelationships for the interconversion of retinoids and carotene are also shown. The steps related to the conversion of cholesterol in skin to cholecalciferol are given in (b).

retinoids and carotenoids that enter intestinal cells are transported next by cytosolic retinol-binding proteins (CRBPs) to the smooth endoplasmic reticulum (Ross and Zolfaghari, 2004, Krinsky and Russell, 2001, Wang and Krinsky, 1998, Harrison, 2005). They are next reesterified and incorporated into chylomicrons and very-low-density lipoproteins (VLDLs). Some of the steps are shown in Figure 24.5. Intact carotenoids that reach the liver and other target tissues are converted to retinoids in most animals by tissue β-carotene 15,15′-monooxygenase (EC 1.14.99.36), which catalyzes the chemical reaction:

$$\beta\text{-carotene} + O_2 \rightarrow 2 \text{ retinal}$$

In liver, there is active exchange of retinyl and other retinoids between stellate (also known as Ito cells) and parenchymal cells. Retinol is converted to retinyl esters to aid in buffering cells from an excess of vitamin A, for which retinyl palmitate is usually the most predominant form of the ester. When vitamin A is needed, retinyl ester in the liver is hydrolyzed and released as retinol bound to retinol-binding protein (RBP), which exists complexed to transthyretin, a thyroxine-binding protein. The purpose of this complex is to protect vitamin A from oxidation, facilitate renal reabsorption, and provide selectivity and delivery to targeted epithelial cells.

Regarding turnover and disposal, liver microsomal CYP2E1 and various phase 2 enzymes enhance catabolism and biliary excretion of hepatic retinoids by converting them to glucuronides or various oxidized forms (Figure 24.5). Drugs that stimulate microsomal and xenobiotic metabolism (e.g., barbiturates) have as a secondary effect the acceleration of retinoid metabolism.

24.3.1.4 Functions

The biologic functions of vitamin A primarily include the maintenance of vision and the orchestration of genes important to immune function, development, and epithelial cell functions (Krinsky and Johnson, 2005). Retinol delivered to the eye helps to sustain rod vision. In rod cells, retinol is converted to retinal, which next binds reversibly via an imine bond to a lysyl moiety in the protein, opsin. Isomerization of 11-cis-retinal into all-trans-retinal by light induces a conformational change in opsin to form rhodopsin (Lamb, 2009). The conformational changes

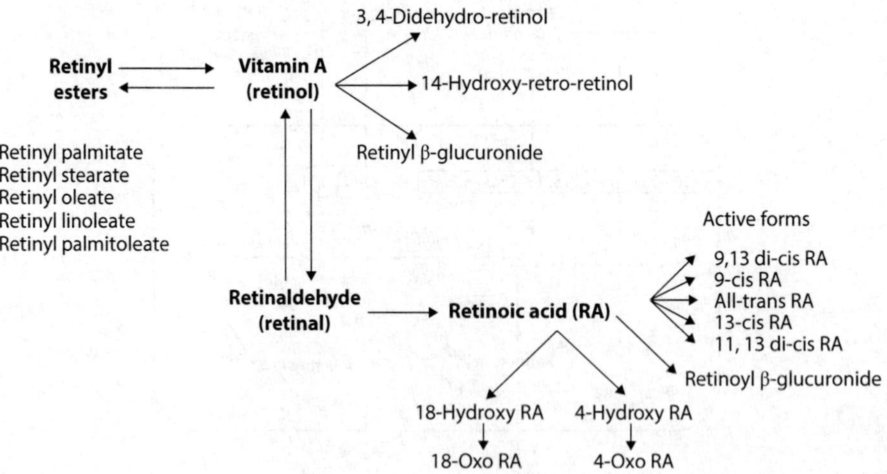

FIGURE 24.5 Retinoid metabolism. Microsomal enzymes (cytochrome P-450 hydroxylases and various transferases) catalyze the conversion of retinyl esters to active cellular forms of vitamin A (the isomers of retinoic acid, RA) or initiate catabolism for eventual excretion by converting them to glucuronides or various oxidized forms.

associated with the transition from opsin to rhodopsin initiate a secondary messenger cascade that alters rod cell membrane potential, which leads to activation of visual signaling via the optic nerve (Figure 24.6).

With regard to control of gene expression, retinoic acid via the retinoic acid receptor influences the process of cell differentiation. Changes in the concentration gradient of retinoic acid along the embryonic anterior–posterior (head-tail) axis, the layers of dermis, and structures containing secretory epithelial cells (e.g., lung, intestine) have been associated with regulation of over 600 genes. Accordingly, the signs of vitamin A deficiency include failure of dark adaptation

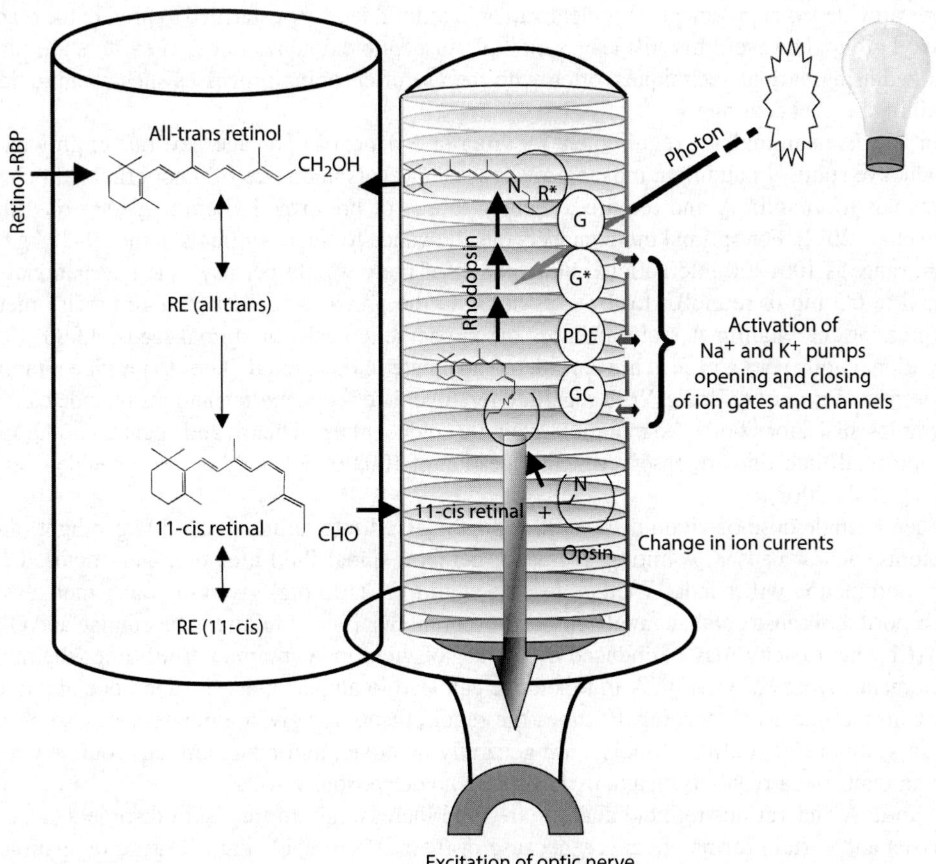

FIGURE 24.6 Vitamin A and vision. All-trans retinol is transported to the eye by retinol-binding protein (RBP) and is converted in epithelial cells to all-trans retinyl esters. Next, cleavage of the ester and isomerization to 11-cis retinal occurs. The 11-cis form is either reesterified or transported into rod cells; wherein it combines with opsin to form rhodopsin. The rod cell is designed for highly efficient transfer of energy from photons of light to rhodopsin. The series of events includes structural changes in rhodopsin (e.g., to metarhodopsin and other conformations) with subsequent deprotonation. The deprotonated metarhodopsin interacts with transducin, one of the proteins in the transmembrane G-protein family (depicted as G and G*) and all-trans-retinal is released for utilization. This interaction causes stimulation of cGMP phosphodiesterase activity (PDE) that results in a decrease in the cGMP formed by guanidylic cyclase (GC) and signal amplification. The local changes in cGMP concentration, in turn, result in cation flux across rod cell membranes to initiate excitation of the optic nerve.

(night blindness), a follicular hyperkeratotic rash of the extremities, and impaired resistance to infections, in addition to congenital ocular malformations in the case of poor maternal vitamin A status.

24.3.1.5 Requirements, Pharmacology, and Toxicity

Cereal grains, with some exceptions (e.g., corn) are minor sources of provitamin A. Among the legume, grains, chickpeas, green, and black beans are the best sources of provitamin A. Because carotenoids are rich in conjugated double bonds and susceptible to oxidation, they are easily destroyed by exposure to intense light, particularly ultraviolet (UV) light. For example, when hay, grasses, and grains are stored for long periods (e.g., months or more), the carotenoid content can be markedly reduced due to chemical or physical (UV light) oxidation. Likewise, retinoid compounds provided as supplements in tablet form or in animal feed are esterified to protect the reactive hydroxyl group; however, this still leaves multiple susceptible double bonds. The esters are further stabilized using various techniques, often with the use of enrobing processes such as antioxidant-containing beadlet coatings.

For any given animal, the requirement for vitamin A depends upon age, sex, rate of growth, and reproductive status. In addition, most carnivores such as cats and ferrets do not efficiently convert carotenoids to vitamin A and require a dietary source of preformed vitamin A (Morris, 2002a, Green et al., 2012). For optimal maintenance, the allowance for many animals in the 10–30 kg body weight range is 100–200 international units per kg of body weight per day (one international unit is equal to 0.3 mg of retinol). However, as noted in the previous section, a more precise method of expressing the vitamin A requirement is on an energetic basis. In animal feeds, 4,000–10,000 international units per kg of feed are considered adequate in the United States to provide vitamin A requirements for most animals. With regard to teratogenic effects, malformations include cleft palate, cranioschisis, foreshortened mandible, stenotic colon, enlarged heart, and agenesis of the spinal cord and small intestine are observed with ingestion of 100,000 RE/kg diet over extended periods (Freytag et al., 2003).

When a single dose of vitamin A (>100 mg) is injected into animals (20–50 kg weight range), symptoms such as nausea, vomiting, increased cerebral spinal fluid pressure, and impaired muscular coordination will result. A lethal dose of vitamin A (100 mg) given to young monkeys has been reported to cause coma, convulsions, and eventual respiratory failure (Macapinlac and Olson, 1981). Chronic toxicity may be induced by intakes of vitamin A in amounts 10 times the normal requirements. Doses of vitamin A in this range can lead to alopecia, ataxia, and bone and muscle pain. Chronic intakes (exceeding 10 times the requirements for given animals) can also be teratogenic. Carotenoids, unlike retinoids, are generally nontoxic, and many animals routinely ingest gram amounts of carotenoids on a daily basis with no deleterious effects.

Vitamin A and various retinoid analogs are used increasingly to treat skin disorders (acne and psoriasis) and certain forms of cancer, because of their role in epithelial cell gene regulation. As an example, vitamin A responsive dermatitis in cocker spaniels is well recognized and described. Retinoyl-β-glucuronide and hydroxyethyl retinamide are commercial preparations of retinoids are sometimes used in treating the dermatitis. In this regard, retinoyl-β-glucuronide and hydroxyethyl retinamide are less toxic than retinoic acid.

24.3.2 Vitamin D

24.3.2.1 Overview

Vitamin D is the generic term for a group of sterols that regulate calcium absorption and homeostasis (Norman and Henry, 2007). The forms of vitamin D include vitamin D_3 (cholecalciferol), which is the naturally active form of the vitamin, and vitamin D_2 (ergocalciferol), its synthetic form and a form also found in plants, fungi, and yeast. When UV light from the sun interacts with the leaf of a plant, ergosterol is converted into ergocalciferol or vitamin D_2. Vitamin D_3 is a provitamin that is synthesized in skin from endogenous 7-dehydrocholesterol upon exposure to sunlight and is found in the diet in oily fish, egg yolks, and fortified milk (Figure 24.4). The dietary requirements for the intake of vitamin D are not precise because they depend in part on the degree of exposure to the sun. The differences in the side chains of vitamin D_3 and vitamin D_2 also result in compounds with different potencies.

Most animals can synthesize sufficient quantities of cholecalciferol 7-dehydrocholesterol if they receive adequate exposure to UV light of wavelength 280–320 nm. The skin of dogs and cats and other carnivores (e.g., ferrets), however, contains only small quantities of 7-dehydrocholesterol, which does not permit adequate synthesis of vitamin D or cholecalciferol. As such, both species are solely dependent on the diet for this vitamin (How et al., 1994; Morris et al., 1999; Morris, 1999, 2002b; Hazewinkel and Tryfonidou, 2002). Cats can utilize ergocalciferol to meet these needs with an efficiency of about 70% that of cholecalciferol (Morris, 2002b); research is lacking in dogs but presumably the utilization is at least as high as that of the cat.

With the exception of animal products, most natural foods contain low vitamin D activity. Fish liver oils (mainly sardines, salmon, and herring) contain high amounts of vitamin D. Ergosterol derivatives are present in many plants, some of which have potent vitamin D activities.

24.3.2.2 Metabolism

Like other fat-soluble vitamins, dietary vitamin D is absorbed after micellar solubilization in the upper intestine. It is then incorporated into chylomicrons for entry into the circulation via lymphatics followed by uptake by the liver. Several hydroxylation steps are required for the activation of vitamin D. The product of the hydroxylations is 25-(OH)-D_3. 25-(OH)-D3 is synthesized in the liver and serves as the precursor for 1α,25-$(OH)_2$-D_3, the active form of the vitamin that is synthesized in response to hypocalcemic states, and 24,25-$(OH)_2$-D_3, which is synthesized in response to hypercalcemic states. Synthesis of both forms occurs in the proximal renal tubular cells of mammals. The main action of 1α,25-$(OH)_2$-D_3 is to maintain blood calcium levels by aiding in the regulation of calcium absorption from the intestine and by suppressing the release of parathyroid hormone (PTH). 1α,25-$(OH)_2$-D_3 also regulates gene transcription by interacting with vitamin D membrane receptors and nuclear receptors in many different tissues. Alternatively, when calcium regulation is normal, the metabolism of 1-(OH)-D_3 or 1-(OH)-D_2 is diverted to 24,25-$(OH)_2$-D_3 or 24,25-$(OH)_2$-D_2 formation, respectively, by the action of a renal 24-hydroxylase (Norman and Henry, 2007). The derivative 24,25-$(OH)_2$-D_3 metabolite has been shown to be crucial to bone fracture healing. The renal 24-hydroxylase becomes elevated after a fracture, thereby increasing the blood concentrations of 24,25(OH_2)-D_2 or D_3 (Norman and Henry, 2007). Also, more than 20 other hydroxylated intermediates and end products have been identified. Most of these derivatives are routed into elimination pathways, although some may be potentially functional (e.g., 1,24,25-trihydroxycholecalciferolthat has some vitamin D activity).

24.3.2.3 Functions

Dietary vitamin D deficiency reduces calcium absorption, secondarily increasing PTH, and the risk for osteopenic bone disorders. The two major sites of action of 1,25-$(OH)_2$-D_3 (1,25-$(OH)_2$-cholecalciferol, also called calcitriol) are in bone, where it acts rapidly in concert with PTH in response to hypocalcemia, and at the intestine, where the response time is longer (Xue et al., 2005). Calbindin, a calcium-binding protein, is a major product synthesized in intestinal cells in response to calcitriol. Calbindin influences the movement of calcium across the intestinal cell. Binding of calcium to this protein allows the intracellular concentration of calcium to be elevated. The hormone forms of cholecalciferol also stimulate the production of the calcium, sodium-dependent ATPases, which reside on the luminal surface of the intestinal cell, and facilitate the movement of calcium out into circulation.

Vitamin D receptors (VDRs) have also been found in a large number of cell types, ranging from skeletal muscle to cells important to immune and phagocytic functions, for example, macrophages (Norman and Henry, 2007). In pancreatic β-cells, 1,25-(OH)2-D3 has also been observed to be important to normal insulin secretion. Vitamin D increases insulin release from isolated perfused pancreatic cells. Moreover, vitamin D metabolites can suppress immunoglobulin production by activated B lymphocytes. T cells are also affected by vitamin D metabolites. 1,25-(OH)2-D3 exhibits permissive or enhancing effects on T-cell suppressor activity. Naturally occurring deficiencies of vitamin D occur in lambs born to ewes not supplemented prepartum with D3 in northern latitudes during the winter months (Figure 24.7). Vitamin D deficiency also occurs in animals reared in rooms with artificial light (Morris et al., 1999).

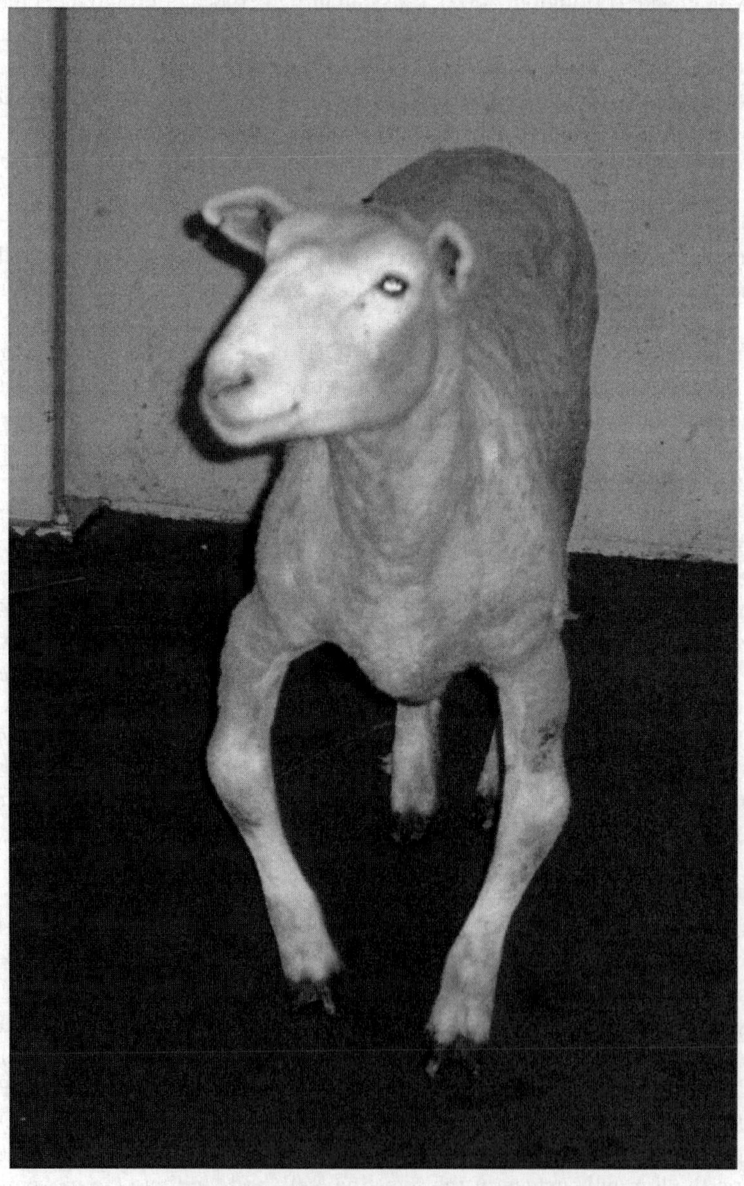

FIGURE 24.7 Vitamin D deficient rachitic sheep. (Courtesy of James Morris, School of Veterinary Medicine, UC Davis.)

More recently, Titmarsh et al. (2015a, 2017) demonstrated a negative relationship between serum 25-hydroxyvitamin D concentrations and neutrophil, monocyte, lymphocyte, and eosinophil counts, duodenal histopathology scores, and serum IL-2, IL-6, IL-8, and TNFα concentrations in dogs with histologically confirmed chronic enteropathies. In a related publication, this group also reported that low serum 25-hydroxyvitamin D concentrations at the time of diagnosis were associated with negative outcomes in dogs with chronic enteropathies (Titmarsh et al., 2015b). Also, a study by some of the same authors reported an inverse relationship between serum 25-hydroxyvitamin D and neutrophil counts in hospitalized cats (Titmarsh et al., 2017). They also reported low serum 25-hydroxyvitamin D concentrations in cats with feline immunodeficiency virus (FIV) compared to healthy controls (Titmarsh et al., 2015c). Further research is necessary to determine how vitamin D status influences the immune system and disease outcomes in dogs and cats.

24.3.2.4 Requirements, Pharmacology, and Toxicity

Most adult animals require approximately 7.5 μg cholecalciferol or more per 1000 kcal of diet. When intake exceeds 10–20 times that amount on a chronic basis, there is a risk of toxicity, characterized by hypercalcemia, hypercalciuria, and soft-tissue calcification, in particular, the blood vessels of the lung, kidney, and heart. Acute doses of vitamin D (>100 times the requirement) can eventually result in a negative calcium balance because bone resorption is accelerated. As noted, some plants (e.g., *Solanum malacoxylon*, *Cestrum diurnum*, and *Trisetum flavescens*) contain compounds with vitamin D activity (mostly glycosylated forms of ergocalciferols), and vitamin D intoxication can follow their ingestion (Norman et al., 2002). Naturally occurring toxicity has occurred in dog and cats given commercial diets containing large amounts of vitamin D or rodenticides (Morita et al., 1995, Studdert, 1990). The viscera of some fish, particularly liver, may contain high amounts of vitamin D. Administration of pamidronate, in the bisphosphonate family, has been used to treat vitamin D toxicosis in dogs (Rumbeiha et al., 1999).

24.3.3 Vitamin E

24.3.3.1 Overview

Vitamin E comprises eight tocopherols, of which two, α- and γ-tocopherol, appear to be the most significant (Figure 24.8). The predominant natural form of vitamin E is the RRR isomer of α-tocopherol. Compounds with vitamin E activity are found in polyunsaturated vegetable and seed oils. In addition to the tocopherols, tocotrienols are also a part of the family but differ because of the presence of an unsaturated side chain. Tocotrienols occur at lower levels in nature.

Tocopherols act primarily at a chemical level as antioxidants and because of their function in stabilizing cell membranes also have a facilitative role in cell signaling (Mustacich et al., 2009). Compounds with the properties of vitamin E protect unsaturated fatty acids in the phospholipids of cell membranes from oxidation. The quinone moiety of tocopherols is capable of quenching free radicals, such as free radicals of hydrogen (H•), superoxide radicals (O2•-), hydroxyl radicals (OH•), and other lipid-derived radical species (LOO•). Vitamin E, in the course of its action, is sacrificed in acting as a free radical scavenger, although there is evidence that the monomeric forms of the vitamin may be recovered following reduction.

Cell membranes contain vitamin E at a concentration of approximately 1 mg per 5–10 g of lipid membranes. Membrane lipids are constantly engaged in the process of turnover and repair. By prolonging the initiation time, before a free-radical chain reaction occurs (Figure 24.9), vitamin E gives cells time to replace damaged membrane lipids and lipid island domains through the process of normal cell turnover (Rucker, 2015).

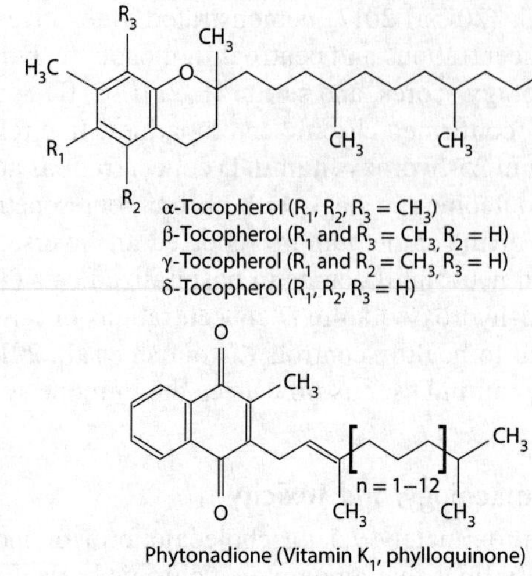

α-Tocopherol (R_1, R_2, R_3 = CH_3)
β-Tocopherol (R_1 and R_3 = CH_3, R_2 = H)
γ-Tocopherol (R_1 and R_2 = CH_3, R_3 = H)
δ-Tocopherol (R_1, R_2, R_3 = H)

n = 1–12
Phytonadione (Vitamin K_1, phylloquinone)

n = 3
Menaquinone (Vitamin K_2)

FIGURE 24.8 Tocopherol isomers, phylloquinone, and menaquinone.

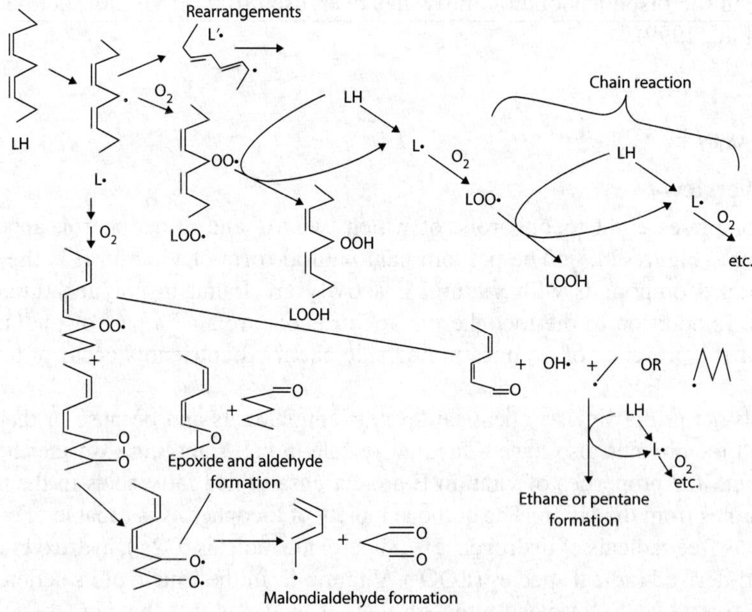

Rearrangements
Chain reaction
Epoxide and aldehyde formation
Ethane or pentane formation
Malondialdehyde formation

FIGURE 24.9 Steps in lipid oxidative cascade reactions. Hydrogen atoms associated with nonconjugated double bonds, allylic H atoms (–C=C–HCH–C=C–) in fatty acids (LH) are particularly susceptible to abstraction. A large amount of oxygen is taken up, leading to the formation of hydroperoxides (LO·), which can decompose into alkoxy and peroxy free radicals, followed by the formation of cross-links and various short-chain cleavage products (malondialdehyde, ethane, and pentane). The process leads to an amplified chain of reactions and cellular damage if the process is not diverted or quenched by an antioxidant.

24.3.3.2 Metabolism

The intestinal absorption of dietary vitamin E (natural and synthetic forms) includes de-esterification of vitamin E esters by pancreatic esterases, followed by bile-dependent incorporation into intraluminal micelles (Traber, 2014). Manufacturers of synthetic vitamin E convert the phenol form of the vitamin to esters (usually as the acetate or succinate), which makes them more stable and easier to use in vitamin supplements. Intralumenal micelle incorporation is followed by the uptake of vitamin E into enterocytes and incorporation into chylomicrons for the eventual transfer to the lymphatics for transport to targeted tissues.

Once the chylomicrons are broken down by lipoprotein lipase, the vitamin E equilibrates with both high-density (HDL) and low-density lipoproteins (LDL) and vitamin E remaining in the chylomicron returns to the liver for reuptake. In this regard, the reuptake and redistribution from the liver to peripheral tissues has some unusual dimensions. The vitamin E returned to circulation from the liver is mostly associated with hepatic VLDL. RRR-α-tocopherol now constitutes over 80% of the vitamin E in the VLDL fraction. The predominance of RRR-α-tocopherol is due to the preference of hepatic alpha-tocopherol transfer protein (ATTP) for RRR-α-tocopherol (Traber, 2007). ATTP is essential for the transfer of vitamin E to VLDL during hepatic VLDL assembly. Following release from the liver and the action of lipoprotein lipase, the VLDL fractions equilibrate to LDL containing RRR-α-tocopherol. Peripheral tissues then take up the LDL by LDL-receptor mediated endocytosis.

24.3.3.3 Functions

Because vitamin E is ubiquitous in most mixed diets, a deficiency occurs primarily with malabsorptive disorders involving the biliary circulation, pancreas, and intestinal mucosa (Traber, 2014). Young animals are more susceptible to a deficiency than older animals. In its most severe forms, vitamin E deficiency results in neurological damage involving the posterior columns, cranial nerves, brainstem, and peripheral nerves. Retinal damage may also occur. Vitamin E deficiency presents clinically with loss of balance, peripheral neuropathy, or possible visual field defects. Deficiency signs also include immune system compromise (including periportal mononuclear infiltration in the liver), dermatitis, cardiomyopathy, and focal interstitial and myositis of muscle.

In horses, neuronal axonal dystrophy, equine degenerative myeloencephalopathy, and equine motor neuron disease are associated with a temporal deficiency of α-tocopherol (Finno et al., 2016). The former two can occur in genetically susceptible horses if α-tocopherol deficiency occurs during the first year of life (Finno et al., 2015). Comparatively, equine motor neuron disease occurs in adult horses after a long period of α-tocopherol deficiency (Mohammed et al., 2007). It is still not clear what role α-tocopherol plays in the pathogenesis of equine degenerative diseases. The major dietary source of α-tocopherol for the horse is grass. It has been speculated that many horses could be deficient in α-tocopherol secondary to reductions in pasture due to drought and urban housing of horses (Finno et al., 2016).

Because vitamin E acts as a defense for lipid oxidation, other compounds capable of residing in lipid membrane may substitute for vitamin E (e.g., various flavonoids). Enzymes such as superoxide dismutase, catalase, glutathione peroxidase (GPx), and related systems for oxidant defense can moderate the absolute need for vitamin E (Figure 24.10; Rucker, 2015).

As noted, vitamin E can also influence cell signal transduction pathways. Changes in the activities of protein kinase C and phosphatidylinositol 3-kinase have been reported and associated with changes in cell proliferation, platelet aggregation, and nicotinamide adenine dinucleotide phosphate (NADPH)-oxidase activation. Vitamin E status also influences genes that are involved in the uptake and degradation of tocopherols and antioxidant defense (e.g., α-tocopherol transfer protein, cytochrome P450-3A, γ-glutamyl-cysteine synthetase heavy subunit, and glutathione-S-transferase), and genes that are involved in the modulation of extracellular matrix proteins, cell adhesion, and inflammation (Traber, 2007, 2014).

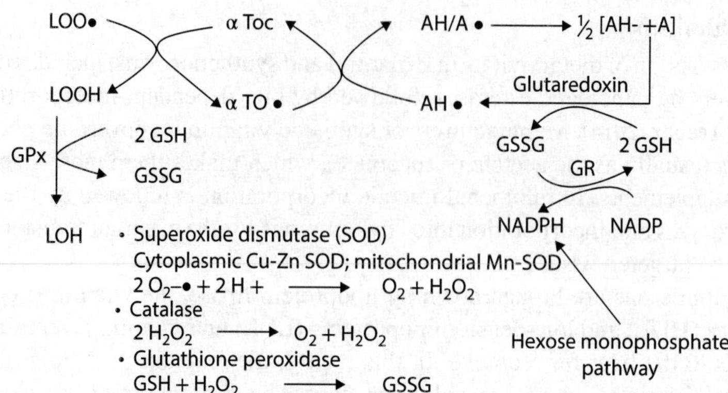

FIGURE 24.10 Vitamin E and antioxidant defense. A number of factors can influence the need for tocopherols in cells and its utilization at a cellular level. Vitamin E acts as the last line of defense for lipid oxidation, primarily residing in lipid membranes. Tocopherols quench lipid-derived free radicals (LOO·, see Figure 24.9). Ascorbic acid is capable of regenerating vitamin E as long as ample reduced glutathione (GSH) and glutatredoxin are available to regenerate ascorbic acid. Free radical scavenging enzymes, such as superoxide dismutase (catalyzes super oxide radicals to hydrogen peroxide), catalase (catalyzes hydrogen peroxide to water and oxygen), and glutathione peroxidase (GPx, catalyzes lipid and/or hydrogen peroxides to water or hydroxy fatty acids) assist in the process. Related systems for oxidant defense (generation of reductants, such as NADPH), via the indirect oxidation of glucose (e.g., the hexose monophosphate shunt pathway) and reduced GSH (maintained by glutathione reductase, GR) also play essential roles. Without intracellular control of reactive oxygen species, polyunsaturated lipids are targets for oxidation (see Figure 24.9).

In domestic and laboratory animals, naturally occurring deficiencies of vitamin E do occur. "Brown bowel syndrome" is the condition that has been used to describe inadequate vitamin E intake owing to ulcerative and degenerative changes in intestinal tissue. In addition, the cells of the eyes and testes can be affected. In cats, especially those fed fish diets that are not usually fortified with vitamin E, the condition is sometimes referred to as "yellow fat disease" or pansteatitis. Pansteatitis is often caused by the consumption of high levels of unsaturated fatty acids or the insufficient intake of vitamin E (Niza et al., 2003). Proper handling of fish is essential to prevent the polyunsaturated fatty acids (PUFAs) in fish oil from readily oxidizing following their harvest and processing. Consumption and deposition of oxidized lipids and PUFAs can accelerate tissue oxidation.

24.3.3.4 Requirements, Pharmacology, and Toxicity

The requirement of vitamin E varies with the intake of PUFA, and for most animals is on the order of 25–50 mg per kg dry diet or 4–8 mg per 1000 kcal or 4.184 MJ. A water-soluble form of vitamin E, RRR-α-tocopherol glycol (Aquasol E), is better absorbed than the dietary, fat-soluble natural vitamin, and hence is more useful in the treatment or prevention of vitamin E deficiency in malabsorption diseases. There are few data on vitamin E toxicities (Traber, 2014). In the human clinical literature, there is the concern that pharmacologic doses of vitamin E (gram quantities per day) may displace or interfere with vitamin K metabolism, but very high and sustained intakes are required.

24.3.4 Vitamin K

24.3.4.1 Overview

Vitamin K is derived from dietary phylloquinone (K_1, from plants) and menaquinones (K_2, synthesized by intestinal bacteria). The primary dietary sources of phylloquinone are green leafy vegetables; dairy products are minor sources. All members of the vitamin K group of vitamins share a methylated naphthoquinone ring structure (menadione, sometimes designated K_3), but vary in the aliphatic side chain attached at the 3-position of menadione (Figure 24.7). Phylloquinone (vitamin K_1) contains in its side chain four isoprenoid residues, one of which is unsaturated. Menaquinones have side chains composed of a variable number of unsaturated isoprenoid residues and are designated as MK-*n*, where *n* specifies the number of isoprenoids. As a class of compounds, vitamin K facilitates the posttranslational γ-carboxylation of proteins involved in blood clotting: prothrombin and factors VII, IX, and X. The presence of γ-carboxyglutamic acid (GLA) residues is essential for calcium binding, as required in blood clotting. Vitamin K also enhances γ-carboxylation of osteocalcin, and vitamin K deficiency contributes to osteoporosis, whereas vitamin K supplementation has been shown to prevent bone fractures (Suttie, 2014).

24.3.4.2 Metabolism

Menaquinone is absorbed from the distal ileum in the presence of bile salts and less efficiently from the colon of most animals. In contrast, phylloquinone undergoes micellar incorporation, after which it is transported into the enterocytes. Comparative studies of the forms of vitamin K in the liver suggest that menaquinone from bacterial synthesis provides substantially less vitamin K than dietary phylloquinone for most monogastric animals. Regarding turnover, unlike other fat-soluble vitamins, the total pool of vitamin K in the body is replaced rapidly within hours to days in contrast to weeks or months (Suttie, 2014).

24.3.4.3 Functions

Although a detailed history related to the discovery of vitamin K is beyond the scope of this section, it is important to note that much of the early progress toward discovery was accelerated when it was demonstrated that hemorrhagic disease in animals could be reversed by extracts of alfalfa. A connection between spoiled clover and grasses that seemed to cause hemorrhagic disorders in animals was also known. It is now appreciated that some compounds in the 1,4-napthoquinone series possess vitamin K activity, as well as relatively simple compounds, such as menadione. For example, an active "vitamin K" can be synthesized from menadione when combined with isoprenoids from the cholesterol synthesis pathway.

Vitamin K serves as a cofactor for microsomal carboxylases (Stafford, 2005), which are responsible for GLA formation (Figure 24.11). GLA residues serve as calcium binding sites in the proforms of proteinases associated with blood coagulation and bone formation. Calcium binding is a requisite for their eventual activation. The vitamin K-dependent (VKD) carboxylase utilizes oxygen and bicarbonate as cosubstrates, and the reaction only occurs if glutamic acid is a part

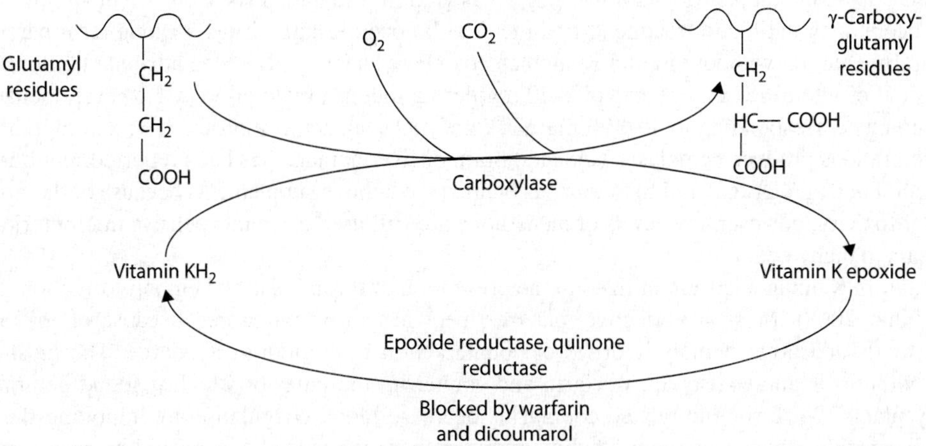

FIGURE 24.11 The role of vitamin K in γ-carboxyglutamyl residue formation.

of a polypeptide. The levels of reduced vitamin K available for the reactions control the rate of carboxylation. Carboxylation requires the abstraction of a proton from the 4-carbon of glutamate by reduced vitamin K and results in the conversion of reduced vitamin K to a vitamin K epoxide, which can be recycled to vitamin K (Stafford, 2005).

Vitamin K regulation is linked to control of blood coagulation owing to its role as a cofactor for the activities of factor X and prothrombin. The system comprises membrane-bound and circulating proteins that assemble into multimolecular complexes on cell surfaces. Vitamin K-dependent protein C also is a key component of the system. VKD protein circulates in blood as a zymogen with potential anticoagulant serine protease activity. It is activated on the surface of endothelial cells by thrombin bound to the membrane protein thrombomodulin; an endothelial protein C receptor further stimulates the protein C activation. Moreover, activated protein C together with another protein, cofactor protein S, can also slow coagulation by degrading FVIIIa and FVa on the surface of negatively charged phospholipid membranes, providing a level of reversible control (Suttie, 2014). Recent interest in vitamin K has also stimulated a search for physiological roles beyond that of coagulation and control of mineralization. Vitamin K and VKD proteins have been suggested to be involved in regulation of energy metabolism and inflammation. However, the evidence for many of these proposed roles in the maintenance of animal health remains equivocal or appears indirectly related to the well-established functions of this vitamin (Booth, 2009).

In bone, GLA-containing proteins (osteocalcins) are involved in the regulation of new bone growth and formation. The presence of GLA protein in bone helps to explain why administration of the vitamin K antagonist at levels that cause hemorrhagic diseases may result in bone defects, particularly in neonates. Vitamin K-related mineralization disorders are characterized by complete fusion of the proximal tibia growth plate and cessation of longitudinal bone growth (Suttie, 2014).

24.3.4.4 Requirements, Pharmacology, and Toxicity

The establishment of the dietary requirement for many animals has been difficult due to vitamin K's short half-life and possible synthesis of vitamin K by intestinal bacteria. The extent to which animal species practice coprophagy is another factor. Birds tend to have relatively high requirements for vitamin K; thus, chickens have been used extensively as experimental animal models in vitamin K-related studies. Recent work suggests that the vitamin K requirement is dependent upon the relative content of vitamin K epoxide reductase activity. A low level of epoxide reductase activity can result in an increased requirement for vitamin K. Ruminal microorganisms synthesize large amounts of vitamin K; thus, ruminants do not need an external source for this reason.

Recent assessments of nutritional requirements suggest that small animals should obtain approximately 500–1000 μg as phylloquinone per kg diet (Table 24.1 and references cited). Oxidized squalene and high intakes of vitamin E may act as vitamin K antagonists. Insufficient vitamin K can also occur with antibiotic treatment, treatment with coccidiostatic drugs, or long-term parenteral hyperalimentation without vitamin K supplements. Few hazards have been attributed to long-term ingestion of vitamin K in amounts of 1–10 mg per kg diet as phylloquinone. However, menadione in amounts corresponding to 10–100 mg per kg of diet may act as a prooxidant, and high dietary concentrations produce hemolysis. Neonatal brain or liver damage has been reported. For humans, the U.S. Food and Drug Administration has banned menadione supplements because of their potential for toxicity; however, low levels of menadione are still used as an inexpensive micronutrient for animals in many countries.

Vitamin K antagonists are utilized in the prevention of thrombosis and emboli formation (Merli and Fink, 2008). Most are effective, but treatment has to be monitored because of interaction with foods and other hemolytic drugs or counteraction by a vitamin K source. The most common vitamin K antagonists are warfarin and coumarin, the latter of which is found naturally in many plants. Warfarin and related coumarins decrease blood coagulation by inhibiting the vitamin K epoxide reductase system. Phylloquinone, rather than menadione, should be used parenterally to treat animals that have ingested warfarin or other anticoagulants. The clinical settings for vitamin K deficiency include a combination of dietary inadequacy and prolonged antibiotic use, lipid malabsorption syndromes such as cholestatic liver disease (including biliary obstruction), or exposure to vitamin K antagonists.

24.3.5 Fat-Soluble Vitamin Assessment

Vitamin A status can be measured by HPLC methods using plasma or serum samples. Blood levels of RBP can be measured by radial immunodiffusion (Eitenmiller and Landen, 1998, Weinmann et al., 1999). The relative dose–response assay is used in field studies and consists of measuring RBP before and after a standard oral dose of vitamin A. Apo-RBP accumulates in the liver during vitamin A deficiency. Thus, an increase of circulating holo-RBP following treatment is indicative of vitamin A deficiency. Assessment using plasma RBP, however, is complicated when there is accompanying protein–calorie malnutrition, severe infections, or trauma. In particular, malnutrition decreases the expression and release of RBP (Vesterberg, 1994). The content of vitamin A in a liver biopsy is the gold standard for assessment of vitamin A status (Eitenmiller and Landen, 1998).

Reliable assays for the measurement of vitamin D and its calcidiol and calcitriol metabolites in plasma are available (Higashi et al., 2008, 2010). The best index is 25-OH vitamin D, which has a half-life of about 3 weeks and provides a useful index of vitamin D status, making it the measurement of choice. Plasma concentrations of 25-OH vitamin D of 20–150 nmol/L or 8–60 ng/mL cover the normal range of most animals. Specific ranges to support distinctions for sufficiency, insufficiency, and deficiency have recently been advocated in both humans and animals (Holick, 2007; Selting et al., 2014). Calcitriol is present in picomolar concentrations (normal values range from 40 to 150 pmol/L or 16 to 60 pg/mL), and has a half-life of about 4–6 hours in a large (50–100 kg) animal. Concentrations of vitamin D in plasma after oral administration are often a 1000-fold higher in the nanomolar range. Vitamin D has a half-life of 24 hours, so the plasma concentration reflects immediate intake, rather than overall status.

Plasma levels of α-tocopherol are also routinely determined by high-performance liquid chromatography (HPLC) methods (Karppi et al., 2008, Bompadre et al., 2008) and vary according to the total plasma lipid concentration because α-tocopherol is transported mostly in association with LDL particles. While α-tocopherol can readily be separated from other tocopherols, the separation of δ and γ isomers is difficult. For nutritional assessment of vitamin E, the current indices are based on changes in total tocopherol concentrations in plasma and serum. Measurement of tocopherol concentration in erythrocytes or platelets is also a good indicator of vitamin E status. Although the measurement of adipose levels of tocopherols may seem to be a reliable index for assessing vitamin E status, vitamin E partitions primarily into the membrane lipid compartments. Thus, the concentration of vitamin E per adipose tissue mass may increase when there is a loss of nonmembrane-stored triglycerides. As the plasma tocopherol concentration is affected by lipid concentration, an α-tocopherol/total lipid ratio of 0.6–0.8 mg/g of total lipids has been suggested as indicating adequate nutritional status. Functional tests, such as the hemolysis of erythrocytes in the presence of 2% peroxide, are also used to indicate vitamin E status. Malondialdehyde, 8-hydroxy-2′-deoxyguanosine, 4-hydroxy-2-nonenal-modified proteins, and ethane or pentane exhalation (see Figure 24.9) have also been used as indirect measures of vitamin E. Of note, malondialdehyde can be measured as a thiobarbituric acid or 1-methyl-2-phenylindole adduct to yield colored fluorescent derivatives that can be assayed spectrophotometrically.

Vitamin K deficiency can be assessed by a prolonged prothrombin time that responds to parenteral vitamin K administration and by direct measurement of circulating phylloquinone by HPLC methods (Eitenmiller and Landen, 1998, Kamao et al., 2005).

24.4 WATER-SOLUBLE VITAMINS

Most water-soluble vitamins serve as enzymatic cofactors (Rucker and Chowanadisai, 2016). For example, ascorbic acid, niacin, and riboflavin serve primarily as redox cofactors. The roles of thiamin, pyridoxine (vitamin B-6), and pantothenic acid (as a component of coenzyme A [CoA]) are distinguished because of their importance to carbohydrate, amino acid, and acyl and acetyl transport, respectively. Biotin, folic acid, and vitamin B-12 (cobalamin) have roles in single-carbon metabolism. Regarding functions, the most limiting events that control or regulate function are specific step(s) in cofactor formation, for example, a phosphorylation reaction or adenosine triphosphate (ATP) addition. From a nutrition perspective, the availability of vitamins from foods often requires complex processes and specialized transport mechanisms (Figure 24.12).

24.4.1 Vitamins Involved in Reduction–Oxidation

Redox, or reduction–oxidation, reactions describe chemical reactions in which atoms or intermediates in a process have their oxidation number (oxidation state) changed, although the actual transfer of electrons may not always be apparent, such as reactions and processes involving covalent bonds. With the cofactors derived from ascorbic acid, niacin, and riboflavin (Figure 24.13), it is possible for cellular systems to carry out a range of redox reactions utilizing mechanisms that involve ion hydride transfers (via NAD or NADP), radical hydrogen ion transfers (via flavin mononucleotide [FMN] or flavin adenine dinucleotide [FAD] or ascorbic acid), and one electron plus one proton transfers (via FMN or FAD). Enzymes utilizing these vitamins catalyze reactions over a wide range of chemical potentials (Johnston et al., 2014; Kirkland, 2014; McDonell, 2001; Pinto and Rivlin, 2014; Rucker and Chowanadisai, 2016).

24.4.1.1 Ascorbic Acid

24.4.1.1.1 Overview

Ascorbic acid (vitamin C) is one of the most important redox cofactors in animal systems. Although most animals make sufficient ascorbic acid, for some, ascorbic acid is a true vitamin because of an inability to carry out adequate synthesis or production. This is true for higher primates, a small

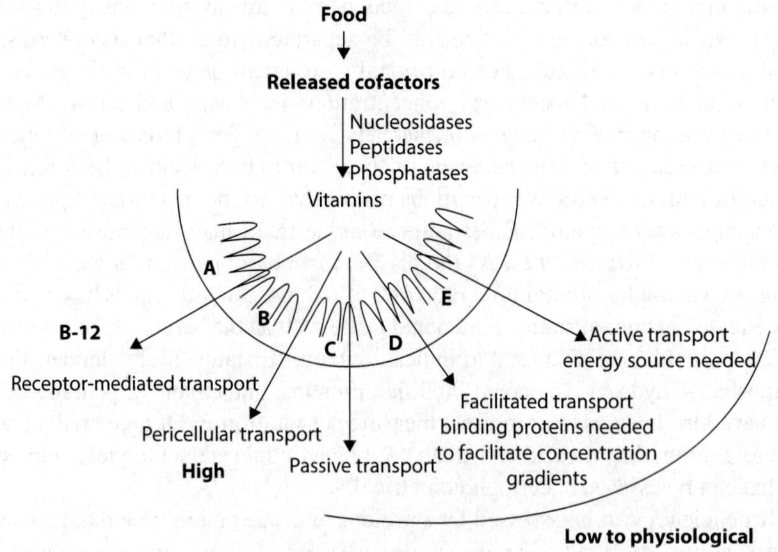

FIGURE 24.12 Vitamin absorption. Vitamins in foods are usually present as cofactors or attached to proteins. Pancreatic and intestinal enzymes, nucleosidases, phosphatases, and peptidases are key factors in processing cofactors to vitamins in the intestinal lumen. Transport of given vitamins next occurs by receptor receptor-mediated or pericellular-related processes, passive transport (usually at high luminal concentrations), active transport, or facilitated processes (requiring a transporter or chaperone). (From Rucker et al., In N. Van Alfen (ed.), *Encyclopedia of Agriculture and Food Systems*, San Diego, 2014.)

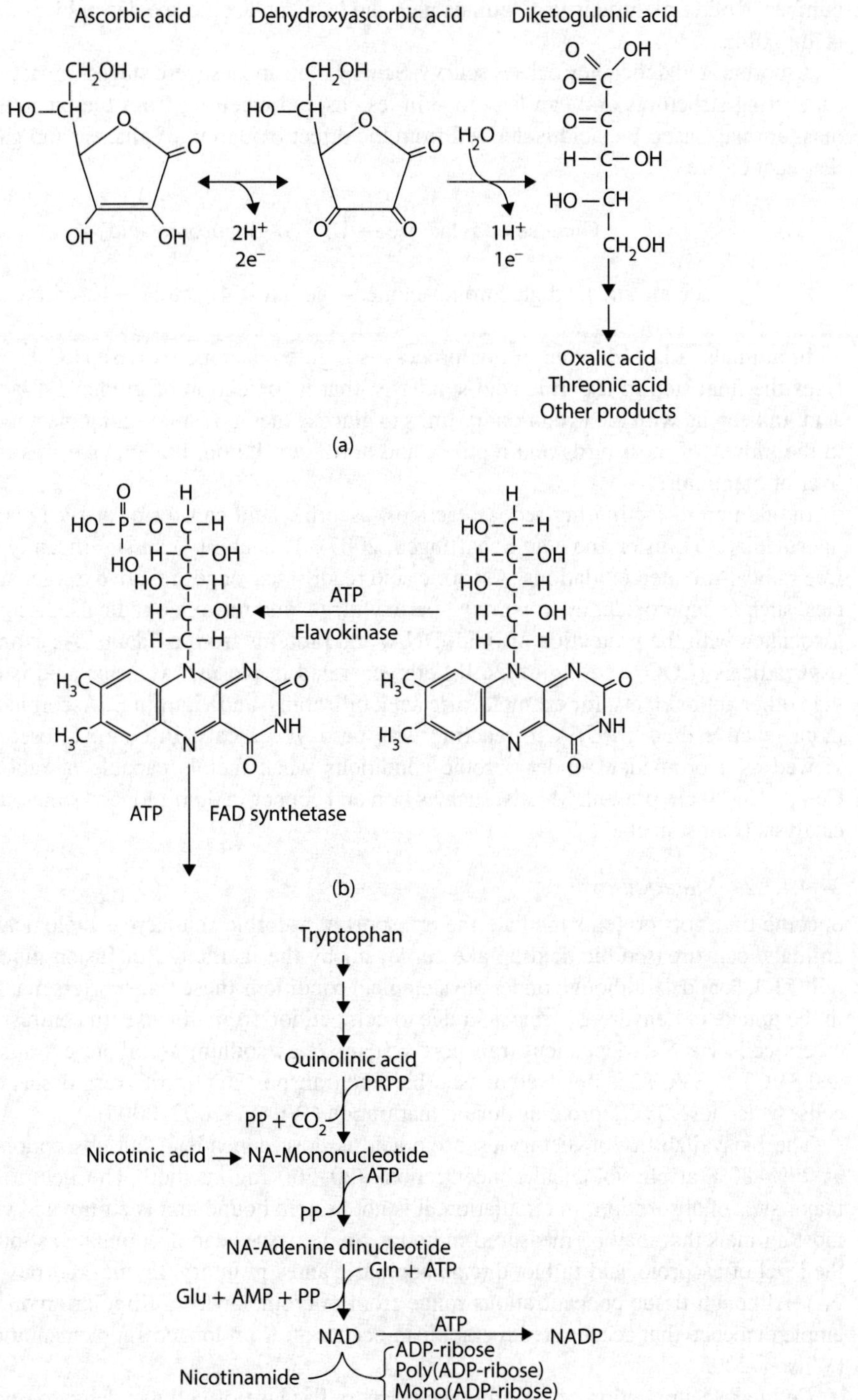

FIGURE 24.13 Vitamins necessary to redox. (a) The relationship between ascorbic acid, dehydroascorbic acid, and various products of ascorbic acid oxidation; (b) the relationship of riboflavin to flavin mononucleotide (FMN) and flavin adenine dinucleotide (FAD); (c) the relationship of tryptophan degradation to nicotinic acid, niacin, and NAD production and function.

number of other mammals (e.g., guinea pigs and bats), and some species of birds and fish (Johnston et al., 2014).

Ascorbic acid deficiency causes scurvy. Scurvy in its most severe stages impacts collagen-related supporting structures and can lead to skin lesions and bleeding from the mucous membranes. In most animals, ascorbic acid is derived from the direct oxidation of glucose and galactose. Steps in the reaction are

$$\text{Glucose or galactose} \rightarrow \text{UDP-D-glucuronic acid} \rightarrow$$

$$\text{Glucuronic acid/glucuronolactone} \rightarrow \text{gulono-1,4-lactone} \rightarrow \text{ascorbic acid}$$

In animals, a key enzyme in this process is L-gulonolactone oxidase (EC 1.1.3.8), which catalyzes the final step in ascorbic acid synthesis, that is, oxidation of gulono-1,4-lactone to ascorbic acid. In keeping with the evolutionary links to glucose metabolism, L-gulonolactone oxidase resides in the kidney of most birds and reptiles, and during evolution, the enzyme was transferred to the liver of mammals.

In addition to facilitating redox reactions, ascorbic acid can form relatively stable free radical intermediates (Linster and Van Schaftingen, 2007). This ability can significantly delay or prevent free radical-initiated oxidations. Ascorbic acid readily scavenges reactive oxygen and nitrogen species, such as superoxide, hydroperoxyl, peroxynitrite, and nitroxide radicals. Ascorbic acid is often associated with the protection of lipid, DNA, and proteins from oxidants. As examples, when peroxyl radicals (LOO·, see Figure 24.10) are generated in plasma, ascorbic acid is consumed faster than other antioxidants, for example, uric acid, bilirubins, and vitamin E. Ascorbic acid is 100 times more reactive than a PUFA in reacting with peroxyl radicals. In contrast, ascorbic acid can be viewed as a prooxidant under aerobic conditions when metals capable of redox (Fe+2↔Fe+3; Cu+1↔Cu+2) are present. Metals, such as iron and copper in their reduced states, are useful Fenton catalysts (Johnston et al., 2014).

24.4.1.1.2 Metabolism

Specific transport proteins mediate the transport of ascorbic acid across biological membranes. In animals, dehydroascorbic acid uptake can occur by the facilitated-diffusion glucose transporters (GLUT 1, 3, and 4), although under physiological conditions these transporters may play minor roles in the uptake of dehydroascorbic acid due to competition from glucose. In contrast, L-ascorbic acid enters cells via Na^+-dependent transport systems (e.g., sodium-ascorbate cotransporters (SVCT1 and SVCT2). SVCT2 is involved in ascorbic acid transport in almost every tissue, except red blood cells, which lose SVCT proteins during maturation (Wilson, 2002, 2005).

The bioavailability of dietary ascorbic acid is dose dependent, but absorption can be as high as 70%–80% at physiological concentrations (20–200 mg/kg diet). The ileum and jejunum are major sites of absorption. In circulation, it is not protein bound and is eliminated with a half-life in most animals that may be measured in hours. Some tissues can accumulate as much as 100 times the level of ascorbic acid in blood (e.g., adrenal glands, pituitary, thymus, corpus luteum, and retina). Although tissue concentrations range from micromolar to millimolar amounts, there is also ample evidence that accelerated metabolism occurs after prolonged supplementation at high doses (Wilson, 2005).

Cellular accumulation of ascorbic acid occurs because of cellular dehydroascorbate reduction systems that are capable of rapidly generating reduced ascorbic acid (Wilson, 2002). The ascorbate reduction systems are also important in reducing the ascorbic acid radical. This is important because excess ascorbate radicals may initiate free radical cascade reactions or nonspecific oxidations. The reduction system is dependent on maintaining NADPH and reduced glutathione levels. An aspect of this relationship is given in Figure 24.11 and involves mechanisms in which decreased glutathione levels may stimulate ascorbic acid synthesis in animals that can produce it. During the postnatal period, animals adapt from a relatively hypoxic to a relatively hyperoxic environment. In this regard, one of the glutathione's many functions is to keep ascorbic acid in a reduced form. In adult animals that make ascorbic acid, a reduction in glutathione levels can lead to a rapid increase in liver dehydroascorbic acid. An adequate ascorbic acid intake is particularly important in newborns and neonates, for which the potential to synthesize ascorbate is less than adults.

Vitamin C homeostasis is also facilitated by the induction of ascorbic acid decarboxylase activity, which initiates degradation of ascorbate to CO_2 and C-4 or C-5 fragments. Significant amounts of ascorbic acid, particularly in fish, may also exist as the 2-sulfate derivative. In rats, about 5% of a labeled dose of ascorbic acid is recovered in urine as 2-O-methyl ascorbic acid. Cellular modification of ascorbic acid is important for compartmentalization or modulation of functional ascorbic acid levels.

24.4.1.1.3 Functions

In addition to serving as a general antioxidant and reductant, ascorbic acid also functions as a cofactor in many mono- and dioxygenases to maintain metals (specifically iron and copper) in a reduced state (Rucker, 2015). Important reactions and processes that require ascorbic acid include: (1) norepinephrine synthesis by functioning in dopamine-β-hydroxylase, (2) hormone activation by functioning in peptidyl glycine—amidating monooxygenase, which carries out α-amidation and is found in secretory granules of neuroendocrine cells, (3) carnitine biosynthesis by serving as a cofactor for two of the hydroxylation steps in the pathway of carnitine biosynthesis, γ-butyrobetaine hydroxylase, and ε-N-trimethyllysine hydroxylase, and (4) collagen, elastin, C1q complement, and acetylcholine esterase hydroxylations by functioning as a cofactor for prolyl and lysyl hydroxylases. In scurvy, poor wound healing, bruising, and osteopenic abnormalities, impaired lipid metabolism, and behavioral changes occur because of perturbations largely due to the inability to carry out appropriate levels of prolyl and lysyl hydroxylations (Johnston et al., 2014; Linster and Van Schaftingen, 2007).

24.4.1.1.4 Requirements, Pharmacology, and Toxicity

To maintain normal functions, most animals generate 10–60 mg of ascorbic acid per 1000 kcal utilized in the course of normal metabolism. The requirement for animals that need dietary sources is in the same range of 30–60 mg per 1000 kcal or 4.2 MJ. Because of the mechanisms in place to homeostatically regulate ascorbic acid, evidence of toxicity, other than gastric upset, is seldom observed (Hathcock et al., 2005). Evidence of toxicity, however, may be manifest when ascorbic acid is consumed in near gram quantities per 1000 kcal. Of interest, ascorbic acid intake in this range can result in decreased histamine production and facilitate reduction of nitrosamines and other putative cancer-promoting agents with similar chemical characteristics. The interaction with nitrosamines occurs primarily in the stomach.

It is also important to reiterate the interaction between ascorbic acid and glutathione (Linster and Van Schaftingen, 2007). Although glutathione's primary function is to reduce disulfide bonds formed within cytoplasmic proteins to cysteinyl residues (by acting as an electron donor), along with ascorbic acid, glutathione is also essential in protecting cells from reactive oxygen species (ROS). Like ascorbic acid, glutathione is found almost exclusively in its reduced form. Indeed, the ratio of reduced glutathione to oxidized glutathione within cells is often used as a measure of cellular toxicity. Also, like ascorbic acid, glutathione is often maintained in the millimolar range in some cells. A deficiency of both ascorbic acid, whether dietary or metabolic, and glutathione (e.g., inhibition by buthionine sulfoximine or acetaminophen) can cause pathologic changes to liver and other organs.

Ascorbic acid is widely distributed in fruits and vegetables; however, it is relatively unstable and easily destroyed during food processing and storage. Ascorbic acid is labile in alkali, heat, intense light, and prolonged exposure to oxygen. The rate of decomposition is accelerated by the presence of metals, especially iron and copper, and by enzymes, such as peroxidases.

24.4.1.2 Niacin

24.4.1.2.1 Overview

Normally, niacin (Figure 24.13) is derived from nicotinamide adenosyl dinucleotide (NAD) and nicotinamide adenosyl phosphodinucleotide (NADP) in food by the action of pancreatic or intestinal nucleosides and phosphatases (Figure 24.12). With the exception of cats and other carnivores, niacin may also be derived from the degradation of tryptophan. Up until the 1930s, niacin deficiency (pellagra) was relatively common and endemic in some human populations. As most mixed diets now contain adequate tryptophan plus available NAD and NADP, niacin deficiency is seldom observed, although it remains a possibility in animals fed monotonous diets containing a limited number of foodstuffs (Kirkland, 2014).

24.4.1.2.2 Metabolism

Following NAD/NADP hydrolysis in the intestinal lumen, niacin is actively taken up by enterocytes. Transporters for subsequent cellular uptake have been identified, but are not as well characterized. About half the niacin present in cells as NAD or NADP is associated with enzymes and the remainder is available as a substrate for mono- and polyribosylation reactions that are important in the regulation of a broad range of enzymes. In the nuclei of cells, polyribosylation of specific histones precedes the normal process of DNA repair. It is this nonredox function of NAD that accounts for the rapid turnover of NAD in cells. Some estimates suggest that as much as 40%–60% of the NAD in cells (Kirkland, 2014; Koch-Nolte et al., 2009) is involved in mono- or polyribosylation reactions (Figure 24.13). When niacin is in excess, most mammals convert it to N-methylnicotinamide, which has a low renal threshold and is excreted (Kirkland, 2014).

24.4.1.2.3 Functions

In 1937, Elvehjem discovered that dogs with "black tongue" responded dramatically both to nicotinic acid and to nicotinamide, which was isolated from liver extracts that had previously been found to have relatively high antipellagra activity. The acid and the amide were tested in humans with pellagra and relief from the irritation of lesions associated with the mucous membrane of the mouth and digestive tract, and the disappearance of acute mental symptoms occurred within a few days.

Virtually, all cells are capable of converting niacin to NAD/NADP. Most enzymes that require NAD are oxidoreductases (dehydrogenases). NAD catalyzes a diverse array of reactions, such as the conversion of alcohols and polyols to aldehydes or ketones. Moreover, cells delegate NAD to enzymes in catabolic pathways, whereas NADP is utilized in synthetic pathways (Kirkland, 2014). An additional and equally important function of NAD is its role as a substrate in mono- and polyribosylation reactions. Mono- and polyribosylation posttranslational chemical modifications are important in many cellular regulatory functions. In the nuclei of cells, polyribosylation of histone precedes the normal process of DNA repair (Koch-Nolte et al., 2008). For example, pellagra-related skin lesions following exposure to sunlight, UV damage of epidermal cell DNA is an underlying mechanism for the dark pigmented lesions associated with pellagra. Lack of niacin and therefore NAD is thought to be a contributing factor to the skin lesions because of the inability of cells to carry out polyribosylation reactions (Koch-Nolte et al., 2008). NAD is also the substrate for cyclic ADP-ribose, which acts as a Ca^{2+} mobilizing second messenger in steps necessary to activating intracellular Ca^{2+} release (Koch-Nolte et al., 2009).

24.4.1.2.4 Requirements, Pharmacology, and Toxicity

Niacin is needed in amounts corresponding to 3–5 mg per 1000 kcal or 4.2 MJ for most monogastric omnivores. The requirement for carnivores is three- to fourfold higher. Carnivores have high protein requirements and appear to have evolved enzyme functions that are less adaptive than in other species (e.g., cats do not downregulate urea cycle enzymes when dietary protein is reduced below requirements). With regard to niacin, the cat also does not decrease α-amino-β-carboxymuconate-ε-semialdehyde decarboxylase (a lyase, which is commonly referred to as picolinic carboxylase) to force tryptophan toward the niacin-synthetic pathway, which in effect makes niacin a dietary essential in carnivores (McDonell, 2001; MacDonald et al., 1884).

Omnivores: Tryptophan→→L-Kynurenine→→3-Hydroxyanthranilic acid→Quinolinic acid→→→NAD

Carnivores: Tryptophan→→L-Kynurenine→→3-Hydroxyanthranilic acid→2-aminomuconic acid-6-semialdehyde→Picolinic acid or TCA cycle oxidation

Niacin requirements are often expressed as equivalents, where one equivalent corresponds to 1 mg of niacin. In many animals, the conversion of 50–60 mg of tryptophan to niacin produces about 1 mg. Accordingly, a diet containing high-quality protein may contribute as much as 10–15 mg of niacin for NAD/P production. Niacin is found in high levels in animal tissues (chicken, fish, beef—especially liver) and peanuts. Niacin is also present in moderate amounts in whole grains such as wheat and barley, enriched cereal products, mushrooms, and some vegetables such as corn and peas. With regard to pellagra and corn, however, niacin is not highly available unless the corn is finely ground or processed under alkaline conditions, for example, ground in the presence of limestone. Niacin is chemically stable. Thus, treatments such as moderate heat and alkali can result in greater niacin availability.

There are some therapeutic uses for pharmacologic doses of niacin-derived compounds when increased blood flow is desirable. Nicotinic acid can cause vasodilatation. In humans, nicotinic acid in gram quantities per day is an effective lipid-lowering agent (increases HDL).

24.4.1.3 Riboflavin

24.4.1.3.1 Overview

Riboflavin (Figure 24.13) exists in coenzyme forms as FMN and FAD. Riboflavin deficiency is manifested by glossitis, seborrheic dermatitis, and peripheral neuropathies. Riboflavin was one of the first of the B vitamins to be identified. FAD and FMN are cofactors in aerobic processes, usually functioning as cofactors for oxidases, although FAD also can operate in anaerobic environments as a dehydrogenase cofactor (Pinto and Rivlin, 2014).

24.4.1.3.2 Metabolism

FMN and FAD in foods are hydrolyzed in the upper gut to free riboflavin. Riboflavin is absorbed by active processes and is transported in blood to target tissues in association with albumin. The solubility of flavins per se is poor, but the presence of ribose and phosphorylation at the 5 position (riboflavin-5′-phosphate) improves solubility. Riboflavin is chemically stable, although it can be degraded in alkali and by prolonged exposure to UV light.

Enterocytes play a significant role in the rephosphorylation of riboflavin (e.g., the total FMN and FAD prevail over the free form as >50% of the total flavins). Both riboflavin and FMN may be released for utilization by other cells. Because flavin cofactors are tightly bound to the enzymes that they serve, and in some cases even covalently bound, turnover is slower than that for ascorbic acid and niacin (both easily dissociated). The recycling of riboflavin is more a function of the turnover of enzymes that it serves (Mewies et al., 1998) and it does not undergo rapid oxidative destruction (e.g., as is the case for ascorbic acid). Urine is the major route of excretion for riboflavin, although some FAD is excreted in bile. In this regard, riboflavin transport occurs via the bile/arsenite/riboflavin transporter (BART) and putative signaling family of proteins, which includes transporters for bile salts, organic anions, and riboflavin (Mansour et al., 2007).

24.4.1.3.3 Functions

Many flavin-containing proteins are found in the smooth endoplasmic reticulum of cells associated with microsomal phase 1 and 2 processes and xenobiotic metabolism (De Colibus and Mattevi, 2008). Flavoproteins have been discovered that are implicated in a variety of biological processes, including cell signaling, chromatin remodeling, and cell development. Enzymes containing flavin moieties are distinguished because they are capable of transferring hydrogen directly to molecular oxygen with often the formation of hydrogen peroxide as a product (pinto and Rivlin, 2014; De Colibus and Mattevi, 2008).

Riboflavin deficiency is classically associated with the so-called oral-ocular-genital syndrome. When signs of riboflavin deficiency are observed, they usually include lesions of the oral cavity (cheilitis), inflammation of the tongue (glossitis), and accompanying seborrhea and dermatitis in the genital area. In severe cases of riboflavin deficiency, the filiform papillae are lost, and the tongue changes color from its usual pink to magenta. The ocular lesions include corneal opacity and lenticular cataracts. Riboflavin deficiency also results in lack of growth and failure to thrive. During the deficiency state, dermatitis may develop together with hair loss. One of the more striking signs of riboflavin deficiency in birds is "curled toe syndrome." Curled toe paralysis has been of economic significance to the broiler industry (McDonell, 2001). Riboflavin deficiency is rarely found in isolation; it frequently occurs in combination with deficiencies of other water-soluble vitamins.

24.4.1.3.4 Requirements, Pharmacology, and Toxicity

Drugs with chemical structures that are similar to riboflavin (e.g., chlorpromazine, imipramine, amitriptyline, penicillin, and theophylline) can displace riboflavin from binding proteins that are important to riboflavin and FMN transport. Flavoproteins are also targets for polymorphic alterations, which can result in higher levels of systemic riboflavin for activation (Shane, 2008). Requirements for riboflavin are lower than those for niacin or ascorbic acid (e.g., 2–6 mg of riboflavin per kg of diet or 0.5–2.0 mg per 1000 kcal). Lean meats, eggs, legumes, nuts, green leafy vegetables, dairy products, and milk are good sources; grains are a poor source of riboflavin. Thus, deficiencies can occur in animals given diets based on primarily cereal grains.

24.4.2 Vitamins Important to Specific Features of Carbohydrate, Protein, and Lipid Metabolism

24.4.2.1 Thiamin

24.4.2.1.1 Overview

Thiamin, in its active form as thiamin pyrophosphate, is involved in carbohydrate metabolism as a coenzyme for pyruvate dehydrogenase, transketolase reactions, and for the decarboxylation of α-keto acids (Figure 24.14). The five-member (thiazole) ring of thiamin contains an arrangement of atoms (–N=CH–S–) called an ylid. The central carbon has carbanion character that acts as an electron-rich center for reactions that are commonly characterized as decarboxylations and transketolations, reactions key to TCA cycle and pentose phosphate pathway regulation.

24.4.2.1.2 Metabolism

Thiamin occurs in cells as free thiamin and mono- (TMP), di- (TDP), and triphosphorylated (TTP) derivatives. For example, a thiamine adenine nucleotide has been described (Bettendorff et al., 2007; Makarchikov et al., 2003). As is the case for the other vitamins in their cofactor forms, thiamin is released from foods by the action of phosphatases and pyrophosphatases in the upper small intestine. The active transport of thiamin is greatest in the jejunum and ileum. The majority of thiamin present in the intestine is TDP, but when thiamin is released into circulation, the majority is present as free thiamin. On the serosal side of intestinal cells, egress into plasma is dependent on Na^+-dependent ATPases.

The majority of thiamin in serum is bound to albumin (Itokawa et al., 1982). Usually, over 80% of total thiamin in blood is found in erythrocytes. A thiamine-binding protein in serum has also been identified and appears to be a hormonally regulated carrier protein. Uptake of thiamin by cells occurs by active transport; about 80% of intracellular thiamin is phosphorylated (Bettendorff and Wins, 2009).

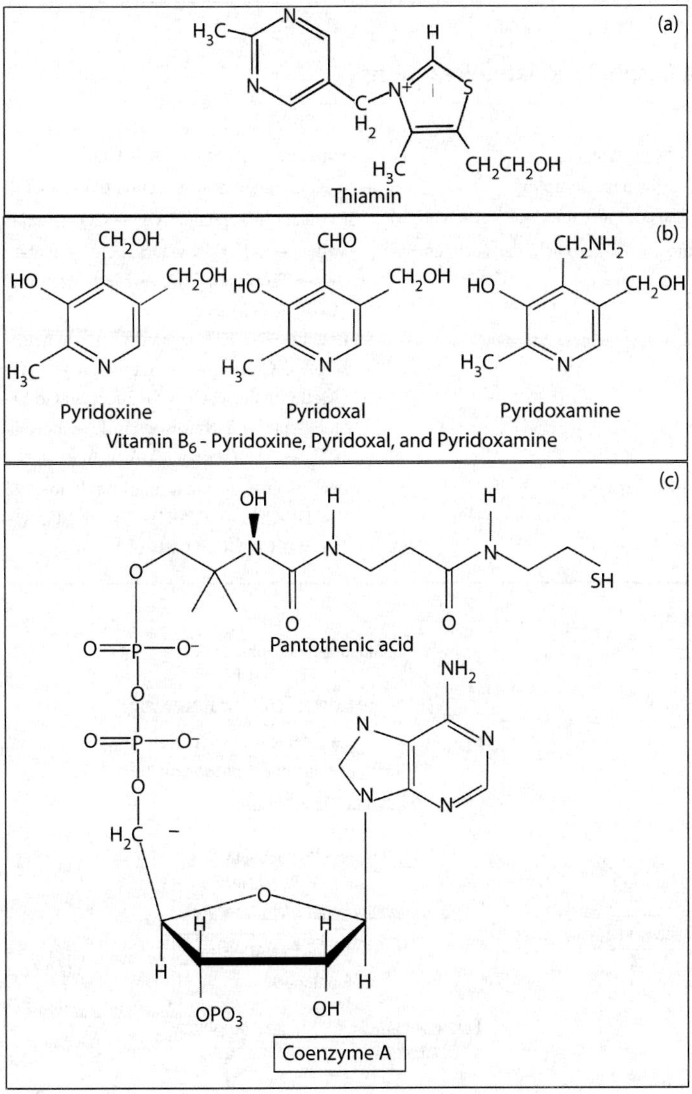

FIGURE 24.14 Chemical structures for (a) thiamin, (b) the vitamers of B-6, pyridoxal, pyridoxine, and pyridoxamine, and (c) the relationship of pantothenic acid to coenzyme A.

24.4.2.1.3 *Functions*

TDP works as a coenzyme in enzymatic reactions that are involved in oxidative decarboxylations of α-keto acids (Makarchikov et al., 2003). Some examples are given in Table 24.7. These reactions take place in mitochondria and peroxisomes (particularly those involved in the oxidation of branched-chained amino acid and fatty acid-derived products). Also, TDP is also an essential cofactor in transketolase reactions (Figure 24.15). Transketolase reactions (Zhao and Zhong, 2009), in the pentose phosphate pathway, result in the formation of ribose-5-phosphate, which is essential in the production of high-energy ribonucleotides (e.g., synthesis of ATP, GTP, and nucleic acids for DNA and RNA synthesis). An indirect product of such thiamin-related reactions is the production of the coenzyme NADPH, necessary for biosynthetic reactions. A deficiency of thiamin can lead to decreased production of NADPH. In neural tissue, TTP seems to play a role in ion transport (maintenance of Na^+ and K^+ gradients). It is evident from the neurological disorders caused by thiamin

TABLE 24.7
Thiamine Pyrophosphate-Related Reactions

Enzyme	Reaction
Pyruvate dehydrogenase complex	Pyruvate → Acetyl CoA + CO_2
α-Ketoglutarate dehydrogenase complex	α-Ketoglutarate → Succinyl CoA + CO_2
Pyruvate decarboxylase complex (ethanol fermentation)	Pyruvate → Acetaldehyde + CO_2 (Acetaldehyde → Ethanol)
Branched-chain amino acid/α-keto acid dehydrogenase complexes	Valine → 2-Ketoisovaleric acid → Isobutyryl CoA + CO_2 → → → Propionyl CoA → Methylmalonyl CoA → Succinyl CoA → TCA cycle
	Leucine → 2-Keto-3-methylvaleric acid → 2 Methylbutyryl CoA + CO_2 → → → Acetyl CoA or [Propionyl CoA → Methylmalonyl CoA → Succinyl CoA] → TCA cycle
	Isoleucine → 2-Ketoisocaproic acid → Isovaleryl CoA + CO_2 → → → Acetyl CoA or Acetoacetate → TCA cycle
2-Hydroxyphytanoyl-CoA lyase	Peroxisomal α-oxidation of phytanoic acid R–CH(–CH3)–CH(OH)–C(=O)–SCoA → R–CH(–CH3)–C(=O)H + HC=O–SCoA

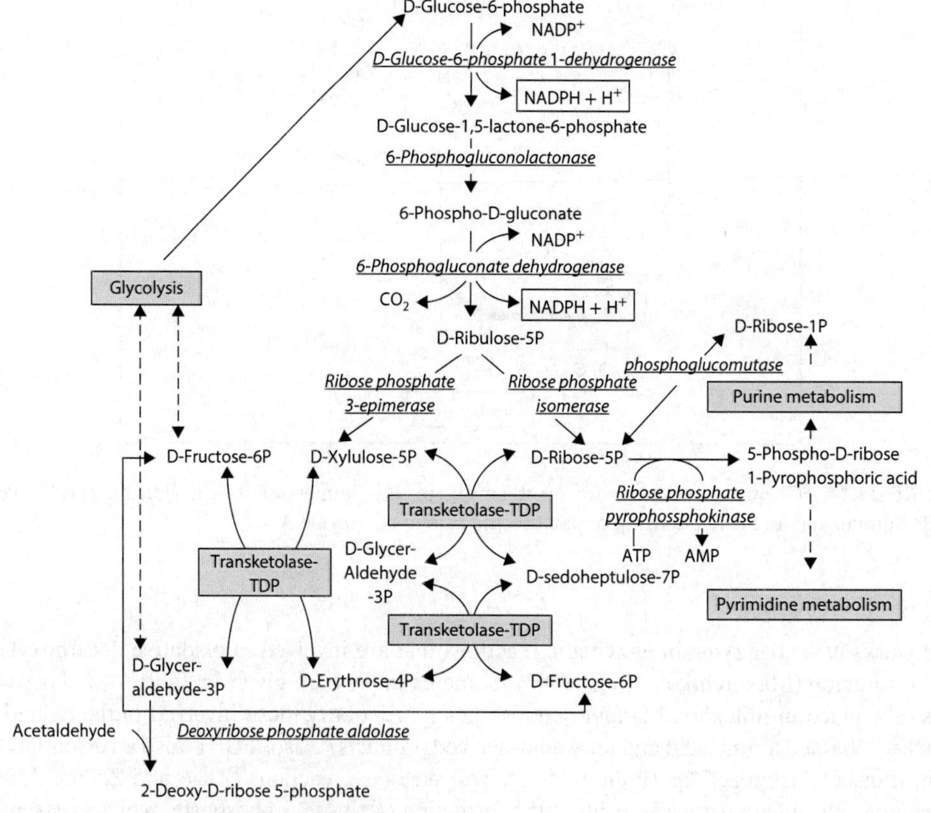

FIGURE 24.15 Transketolation reactions and products. The process is initiated by the direct oxidation of glucose-6-phosphate, which results in the production of NADPH. Next, transkelatoses are essential to the transformations that take place in the pentose phosphate shunt pathway, which in turn are important to the production of purines and pyrimidines. Transketolation allows for the transfer of aldol and ketol moieties that results in a mix of three, five, and seven carbon sugars.

deficiency that thiamin plays a vital role in nerve function (Makarchikov et al., 2003, Bettendorff, 1994; Bettendorff et al., 1993).

Thiamin deficiency causes the condition beriberi, which is characterized by peripheral neuropathy including abnormal (exaggerated) reflexes, diminished sensations, and cardiac failure (due to impaired oxidative metabolism). Thiamin deficiency is common in animals; poultry are particularly susceptible (McDonell, 2001; Lanska, 2009). Mature chickens show signs of thiamin deficiency in 3–4 weeks and young chicks after 2 weeks when fed diets deficient in thiamin. Signs include apparent paralysis of the flexor of the toes (similar to that what observed in riboflavin deficiency and avian encephalomyelitis) along with a characteristic head retraction. A therapeutic diagnosis is achieved if the afflicted birds respond in a few hours to thiamin supplementation.

Polioencephalomalacia is the most common thiamin deficiency disorder in young ruminant animals. Diarrhea, listlessness, head retraction, and muscle tremors are symptoms. The most common cause is overgrowth of thiaminase-producing bacteria, ingestion of thiaminases (e.g., in bracken fern), or inhibition of thiamin absorption from diets containing high sulfur. Other examples involving thiaminase exposure include thiamin deficiency in fish-eating birds, seals, and dolphins, and when spoiled or uncooked fish has been routinely fed (Geraci, 1974). Thiaminase activity is strikingly high in fish, particularly in tuna, saminoids, and sardines (Ceh et al., 1964). Idiopathic paralytic disease in wild birds is also associated with thiamin deficiency (Balk et al., 2009; De Roode et al., 2000). The birds have difficulty in keeping their wings folded and loss of their ability to fly. Other examples include foxes fed uncooked fish products and cats fed food in which thiamin has been lost due to excessive processing or preserved by sodium metabisulfite treatment (Okajima et al., 2007). All of the published case reports of thiamin deficiency in cats eating commercially available diets have involved canned foods, which are subjected to relatively high temperatures during processing. Anorexia and vomiting are often reported in these animals, which can exacerbate the thiamine deficiency. Clinical signs in the cat include impaired vision, mydriasis, ataxia, vestibular signs, ventroflexion of the neck, and seizures which progress to coma and death. In both humans and cats, characteristic findings on magnetic resonance imaging (MRI) support a diagnosis of thiamin deficiency; these changes resolve with repletion (White et al., 2005; Palus et al., 2010, Marks et al., 2011, Markovich et al., 2013).

24.4.2.1.4 Requirements, Pharmacology, and Toxicity

The requirement for thiamin is 0.5–1.0 mg per 1000 kcal or 4.2 MJ of diet. As noted above, factors that most often influence the need for thiamin are exposure to antagonists and thiaminases. Antagonists that are used in experimental settings are pyrithiamine and oxythiamine, which act to inhibit the phosphorylation of thiamin. Amprolium is a coccidiostat that can inhibit thiamin absorption. Thiamin is present in most animal and plant foods but is especially prominent in whole grains and organ meats. Similar to other water-soluble vitamins, alkaline conditions, heat, and oxidants can reduce or chemically modify active forms of thiamin. Milling of whole grains to remove the bran reduces the thiamin content. Feedstuffs rich in tannins can bind and facilitate oxidation of thiamin, which leads to reduced availability (Vimokesant et al., 1982).

24.4.2.2 Pyridoxine

24.4.2.2.1 Overview

The family of B-6 vitamers includes pyridoxine, pyridoxal, and pyridoxamine (Figure 24.14). Pyridoxine is most abundant in plants, and pyridoxal and pyridoxamine are most abundant in animal tissues. Each can be converted to the other. The active form of pyridoxal is phosphorylated (e.g., pyridoxal-5-phosphate). Vitamin B-6 is essential for amino acid and sphingolipid metabolism and glycogen hydrolysis (Mooney et al., 2009).

24.4.2.2.2 Metabolism

Vitamin B-6 is absorbed in the upper gut by energy-dependent pathways (Said, 2004). As the cofactor forms present in foods, B-6 vitamers are first dephosphorylated by alkaline phosphatases. From the intestine, the bulk of B-6 vitamers is transported to target cells by albumin. Following active cellular uptake, rephosphorylation of the various B-6 vitamers (to corresponding 5′-phosphates) occurs via cellular pyridoxal kinases. The pyridoxine and pyridoxamine forms may then be oxidized, if needed, to pyridoxal phosphate. Muscle, kidney, and liver (the primary sites for amino acid metabolism) are abundant in the B-6 vitamers.

The products of vitamin B-6 metabolism are excreted in the urine, the major product of which is 4-pyridoxic acid (Dakshinamurti and Dakshinamurti, 2014). Other products of vitamin B-6 metabolism that are excreted in the urine include pyridoxal, pyridoxamine, and pyridoxine and their phosphates when high doses (10–20× requirements) are administered.

24.4.2.2.3 Functions

The major types of reactions involving amino acids that are catalyzed by vitamin B-6 fall into three categories: (1) transaminase reactions (essential to the interconversion of amino acids to corresponding α-keto acids), (2) decarboxylations, and (3) aldol reactions (electron withdrawal from the α,β-carbons of amino acids). Vitamin B-6 (as pyridoxal 5′-phosphate, PLP) is also a cofactor for glycogen phosphorylase (Palm et al., 1990), which catalyzes the hydrolysis of ether bonds in glycogen to form 6-phosphoglucose (Dakshinamurti and Dakshinamurti, 2014; Mooney et al., 2009; Rucker and Chowanadisai, 2016).

PLP is also an essential component of two enzymes that convert methionine to cysteine, as well as enzymes involved in the metabolism of selenomethionine to selenohomocysteine and selenohomocysteine to hydrogen selenide. Regarding specific amino acid transformations, vitamin B-6 is required for the conversion of tryptophan to niacin. The decarboxylation reactions catalyzed by vitamin B-6 are important to the production of neural signaling compounds such as histidine to histamine, tryptophan to serotonin, glutamate to GABA (γ-aminobutyric acid), and dihydroxyphenylalanine to dopamine (Mooney et al., 2009).

The formation of heme is also vitamin B-6 dependent. The pathway is initiated by the synthesis of D-aminolevulinic acid (ALA) from glycine and succinyl-CoA. The rate-limiting enzyme responsible for this reaction, ALA synthase, requires vitamin B-6 (Dakshinamurti and Dakshinamurti, 2014). As a final example, vitamin B-6 is an essential component of enzymes that catalyze the formation of sphingolipids; particularly, the synthesis of ceramide via a reaction in which serine is decarboxylated and combined with palmitoyl-CoA (Mooney et al., 2009).

Neurological signs and symptoms occur with vitamin B-6 deficiency as a result of the inability to synthesize important biogenic amines from amino acid precursors (Plecko and Stockler, 2009), and anemia results from decreased heme synthesis. In experimental settings, some animals may show signs of oxaluria with a long-term deficiency.

24.4.2.2.4 Requirements, Pharmacology, and Toxicity

Vitamin B-6 deficiency is rarely observed as most diets provide adequate amounts. Typically, the vitamin B-6 requirement is met at about 0.3 mg per 1000 kcal (4.2 MJ) of diet. The richest sources of vitamin B-6 are meats and whole grains. Heat and light negatively affect the stability, and milling to remove bran can result in losses of B-6 from grains.

Drug-induced vitamin B-6 deficiency can also occur following administration of tuberculostatic drugs, such as isoniazid (isonicotinic acid hydrazide). This drug forms hydrazone derivatives with the pyridoxal forms of B-6. Penicillamine (β-dimethylcysteine), a copper chelator, may also interfere with normal B-6 metabolism due to the formation of thiazole derivatives. A naturally occurring antagonist to vitamin B-6, linatine (1-amino-D-proline), is present in flax seed, which forms a stable product with pyridoxal phosphate (Dakshinamurti and Dakshinamurti, 2014).

24.4.2.3 Pantothenic Acid

24.4.2.3.1 Overview

Although the widespread occurrence of pantothenic acid in food makes a dietary deficiency of pantothenic acid unlikely, the use of experimental animal models and antagonistic analogs has helped to define its functions. Pantothenic acid is composed of pantoic acid linked to β-alanine. Pantothenic acid is one of the components comprising CoA and acyl carrier protein (ACP), important in fatty acid synthesis and metabolism (Figure 24.14). Pure pantothenic acid is water soluble, viscous, and yellow. It is stable at neutral pH but is readily destroyed by acid, alkali, and heat. Calcium pantothenate is the form most often found in commercial vitamin supplements due to greater stability than the pure acid (Rucker and Bauerly, 2014).

24.4.2.3.2 Metabolism

To be absorbed, pantothenic acid in food is released from CoA and ACP by the actions of intestinal phosphatases and nucleosidases (Figure 24.12). In rats, pantothenic acid is absorbed in all sections of the small intestine at high concentrations by simple diffusion; however, at low or physiological levels absorption occurs by saturable, sodium-dependent transport mechanisms, which are used in common by both pantothenic acid and biotin (Said, 2004).

The most important control step in this process is the phosphorylation of pantothenic acid to 4′-phosphopantothenic acid by pantothenic acid kinase. Feedback inhibition of the kinase by CoA or CoA derivatives governs flux and defines the upper threshold for intracellular CoA cofactor levels. Moreover, L-carnitine, important for the transport of fatty acids into mitochondria, is a nonessential activator of pantothenic acid kinase.

24.4.2.3.3 Functions

Pantothenic acid deficiency results in generalized malaise, perturbations in CoA and lipid metabolism, and mitochondrial dysfunction. In animals, a mild pantothenate deficiency in which abnormal weight differences are not observed causes serum triglyceride and free fatty acid levels to be elevated, which is a reflection of reduced CoA levels. In deficient states, pantothenate is reasonably conserved, particularly when there is prior exposure to the vitamin. CoA acts as an acetyl and acyl group carrier and allows pyruvate to enter the tricarboxylic acid (TCA) cycle. CoA also allows α-ketoglutarate to be transformed to succinyl-CoA in the TCA cycle. In addition, ACP is also an important component to both fatty acid and polyketide biosynthetic complexes, where 4′-phosphopantethiene serves as the essential prosthetic group (Rucker and Bauerly, 2009).

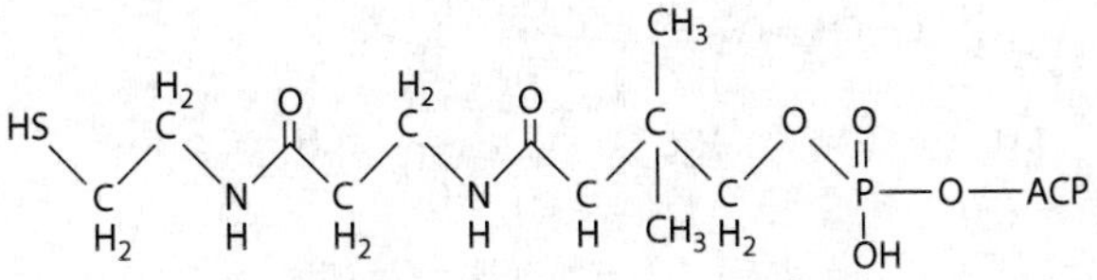

Neurological, immunological, hematological, reproductive and gastrointestinal pathologies, and hair loss and graying occur with pantothenic acid deficiency in part related to decreased levels of CoA. For example, acetylcholine synthesis is impaired, which may account for the numbness associated with a deficiency in pantothenic acid. Hypoglycemia and increased sensitivity to insulin may also occur along with adrenal insufficiency.

24.4.2.3.4 Requirements, Pharmacology, and Toxicity

Pantothenic acid deficiency has been induced in animals by administration of the pantothenic acid kinase inhibitor,γ-methyl pantothenate, in combination with a diet low in pantothenic acid. Another pantothenic acid antagonist, calcium hopantenate, has been shown to induce encephalopathy with hepatic steatosis and a Reye-like syndrome in both dogs and humans. The loss of pantothenic acid is 1%–2% of the body pool per day. The requirement is met at about 3–5 mg per 1000 kcal of dietary intake.

24.4.3 Vitamins Involved in Single-Carbon Transfer Reactions

24.4.3.1 Biotin

24.4.3.1.1 Overview

Biotin is a coenzyme in the metabolism of fatty acids and branched-chain amino acids (Figure 24.16). Biotin also plays a significant role in enzymes involved in gluconeogenesis by acting as a catalyst essential to certain types of carboxylation reactions. Biotin is composed of an ureido

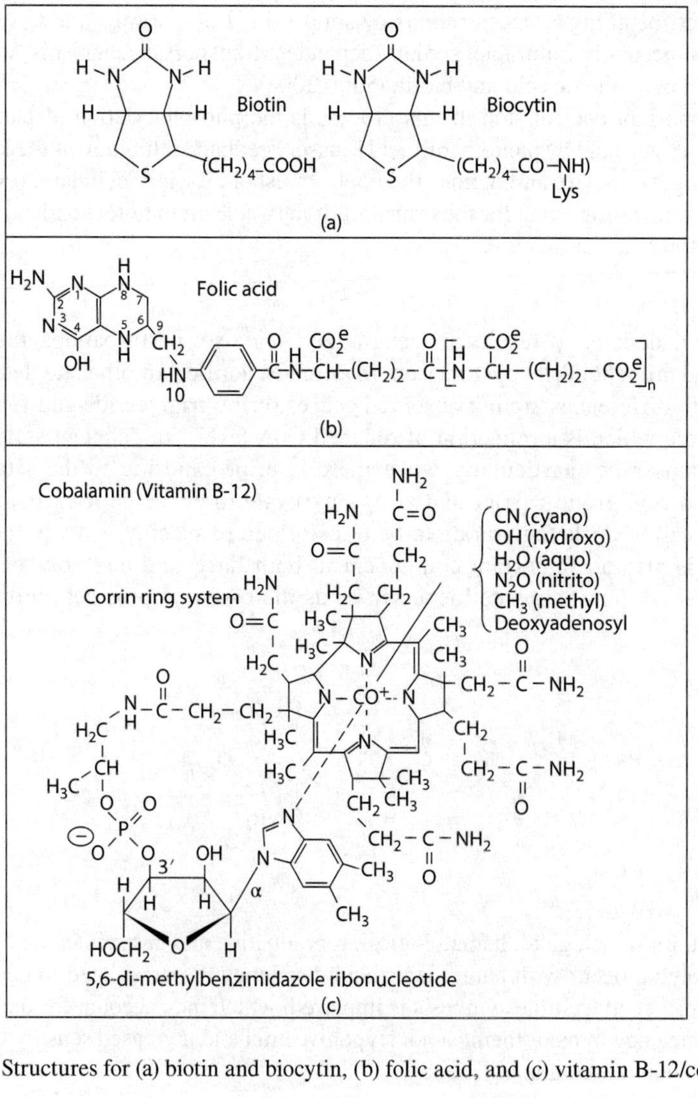

FIGURE 24.16 Structures for (a) biotin and biocytin, (b) folic acid, and (c) vitamin B-12/cobalamin.

(tetrahydroimidizalone) ring fused with a tetrahydrothiophene ring. A valeric acid substituent is attached to one of the carbon atoms of the tetrahydrothiophene ring (Zempleni et al., 2008b, 2009b).

24.4.3.1.2 Metabolism

Biotin is found in highest concentrations in the liver. In food, biotin is present in relatively high concentrations in cereals including soybeans, rice, barley, oats, corn, and wheat. Bioavailability of biotin from cereals varies widely.

The first steps in absorption involve proteolysis of biotin-containing enzymes to release biocytin (biotin linked to lysine via a peptide bond) and free biotin (Said, 2004). Nutritional problems often arise because biotin and biocytin have affinity for certain proteins, particularly avidin in egg white, which is not easily digested, and as a consequence, biotin is not released in regions of the small intestine where efficient absorption occurs. Inclusion of raw eggs in diets can cause biotin deficiency (Zempleni et al., 2008b). The response in fur-bearing animals to ingestion of significant quantities of raw egg white has been described as "egg white injury." Native (nondenatured) avidin in eggs causes egg white injury because it binds very tightly to biotin, preventing its absorption (Whitehead, 1981, 1985).

In cells, when biotin-containing carboxylases are degraded, biotin is released as biocytin. Biocytin is an important liver enzyme that catalyzes the cleavage of the peptide linkage between biotin and lysine to release free biotin for utilization. Biotin turnover and requirements can be estimated by concentrations of biotin and metabolites in body fluids, activities of biotin-dependent carboxylases, and the urinary excretion of organic acids that are formed at increased rates in amino acid catabolic pathways if biotin-related carboxylase activities are compromised.

24.4.3.1.3 Functions

Biotin serves as a cofactor for three CO_2-fixing enzymes: acetyl-CoA carboxylase, which is essential for fatty acid synthesis; propionyl-CoA carboxylase, which participates in odd chain fatty acid metabolism; and pyruvate carboxylase, which is involved in the formation of oxaloacetate, an important obligatory step in reverse glycolysis and gluconeogenesis (Rucker and Chowanadisai, 2016). Biotin deficiency is rare as intestinal bacteria produce biotin. Symptoms of overt biotin deficiency include hair loss and a red scaly rash around the eyes, nose, mouth, and genital area. Neurological symptoms include lethargy, numbness, and tingling of the extremities. Perosis is observed in the skeleton. Hepatic steatosis also can occur. The biochemical manifestation of biotin deficiency includes ketolactic acidosis, organic aciduria, and hyperammonemia. Mice fed with dried raw egg to induce biotin deficiency during gestation have a high (>80%) incidence of malformations. Biotinylation of histones also occurs and appears to play a role in cell proliferation, gene silencing, and the cellular response to DNA repair (Zempleni et al., 2008a, 2009a, 2009b).

24.4.3.1.4 Requirements, Pharmacology, and Toxicity

The relationship of biotin to avidin is important, particularly to industries that utilize fur-bearing animals for profit. It was found that egg white injury could be cured by a liver factor, which was first called protective factor X. Factor X was later determined to be biotin. Because biotin cured the skin disorder of egg white injury, biotin was called vitamin H (for Haut, the German word for skin). For most monogastric animals, 50–100 μg of biotin per 1000 kcal or ~0.2–0.4 mg per kg of diet is probably sufficient.

24.4.3.2 Folic Acid

24.4.3.2.1 Overview

Knowledge regarding folic acid evolved initially from efforts to understand macrocytic anemias and certain degenerative neurological disorders. By the late 1940s, folic acid was recognized as one of the factors associated with macrocytic anemias, and large-scale efforts by some pharmaceutical companies led to the isolation of folic acid (Goldblith and Joslyn, 1964).

Folic acid is one in a family of compounds with a pteridine moiety associated with aminobenzoic acid and a series of conjugated glutamyl residues. Folic acid along with vitamin B-12 is central to one-carbon transfer reactions (Figure 24.16). The reactions include the generation and utilization of formaldehyde and formimino groups in the synthesis of pyridine nucleotides, interconversion of some amino acids, and eventual reduction of the methylene form of tetrahydrofolic acid (THF) to methyl THF (MTHF) to facilitate the conversion of homocysteine to methionine (Figure 24.17). The formyl, methenyl, and methylene forms are utilized for purine synthesis and steps in thymidylate, that is, DNA-related synthesis (Baily, 2014). These reactions are therefore of obvious importance and are essential to cell division and proliferation. As a final step, 5-MTHF transfers its methyl moiety to vitamin B-12. The resulting product is oxidized folic acid, which must be again reduced to reinitiate the cycle.

24.4.3.2.2 Metabolism

The steps in the absorption, transport, and utilization of folic acid (i.e., folacin, the more inclusive term) are more complex than many of those for other water-soluble vitamins. Dietary sources include green leafy vegetables, fruit juices, some grains, and organ meats. Folylpolyglutamates present in the diet are cleaved to folylmonoglutamate by endopeptidases. The various folacins are absorbed in the duodenum and upper jejunum. During the process of intestinal absorption, dietary folylpolyglutamates are hydrolyzed, which is followed by active transport of the folylmonoglutamate derivative, folic acid, which refers to the oxidized monoglutamyl form of the vitamin. Absorption of folic acid is about 85%, compared to 50% or less for the more complex dietary forms of folylpolyglutamates (Baily, 2014).

Two proteins, glutamate γ-carboxypeptidase (formerly designated as folate conjugase) and reduced folate carrier (RFC) protein are essential to the absorption process (Halsted et al., 2002; Villanueva et al., 1998). Following deconjugation or hydrolysis of glutamyl residues, folic acid is taken up by enterocytes and reduced to its THF form. This step is followed by methylation to 5-methyl-THF (Figure 24.17). It is the 5-methyl-THF form that is transported across the intestinal basolateral membrane. RFC protein next carries 5-methyl-THF to target organs, such as the liver.

In the liver, the uptake of 5-methyl-THF by hepatocytes involves carrier-mediated transport. Within the hepatocyte, as well as other cells, 5-methyl-THF uptake is immediately followed by conversion to folylpolyglutamate, which serves to keep the coenzyme inside cells or bound to the appropriate enzymes. The pteridine portion of the coenzyme and the p-aminobenzoic acid portion participate directly in the metabolic reactions of folate. Further, to carry out the transfer of 1-carbon units, NADPH must reduce folic acid two times in the cell. The "rightmost" pyrazine ring of 6-methylpterin is reduced at each of the two N-C double bonds (Baily, 2014).

From 5% to 20% of liver folate undergoes biliary secretion (as 5-methyl-THF) and is subject to enterohepatic recirculation, while most of the remaining passes into the systemic circulation (Tamura and Halsted, 1983). Maintenance of body pools is also dependent on renal filtration and reuptake. About 1% of the total body folate pool is excreted daily in the urine and 0.1% in the feces (Halsted, 1975, 1979, 1980; Halsted et al., 1976, 1977, 1978).

24.4.3.2.3 Functions

Folacins serve as substrates or cofactors in the transfer of single-carbon moieties in amino acid metabolism and nucleic acid synthesis. In the methyltransferase pathway, 5-methyl-THF, which is derived from both dietary and endogenous sources, is also the substrate for methionine synthesis (Baily, 2014; Toohey, 2006). Some of the methionine is converted to S-adenosylmethionine (SAM) by methionine adenosyltransferase. A primary function of SAM is methyl transfer reactions. SAM is metabolized to S-adenosylhomocysteine (SAH), which is also generated from homocysteine through the reversible SAH hydrolase reaction (Figure 24.17).

Other functions of SAM include glutathione regulation by up-regulating cystathionine-β-synthase. Further, SAM can provide negative regulatory feedback to the methylene tetrahydrofolate reductase

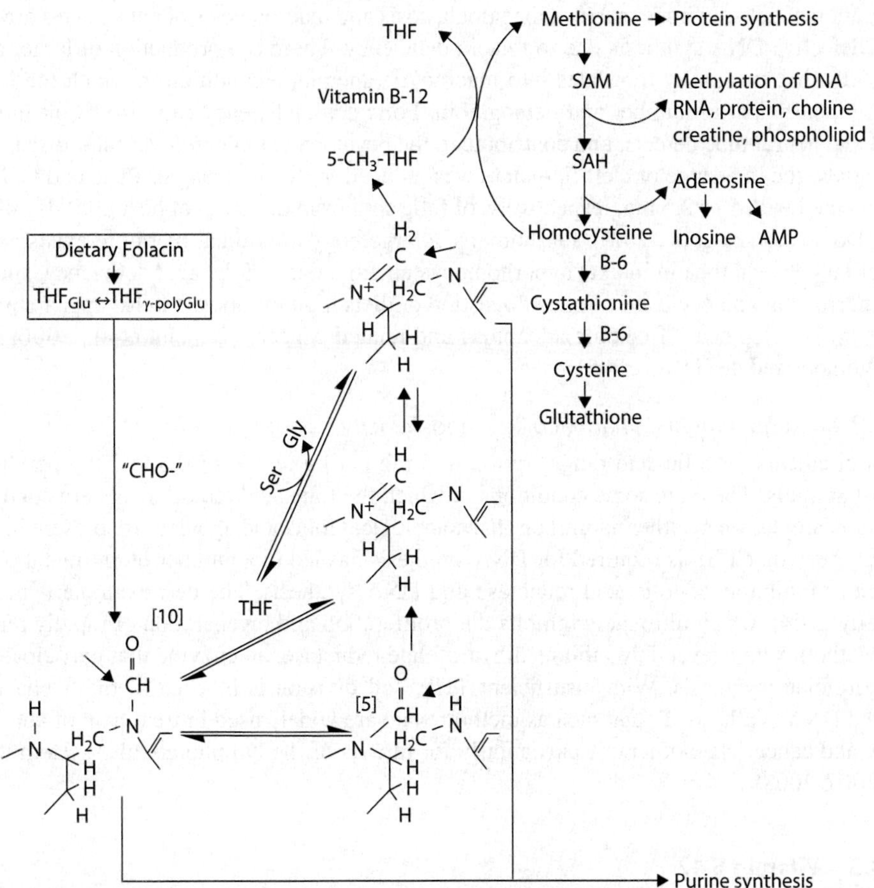

FIGURE 24.17 Folacin and key steps in single-carbon transfer reactions. Folylpolyglutamates are converted to the monoglutamate by intestinal endopeptidases. In the enterocyte, the oxidized forms of folacin are reduced, and single carbon units derived from formyl groups and formimino groups (from the degradation of L-histidine) are directed to the N10 position of THF. Next, the single carbon is transferred to the N5 position and oxidized to methenyl-THF. Following reduction to N5,N10-methylene-THF, depending on the biosynthetic pathway involved, any of these species can donate the one-carbon group to an acceptor. The methylene form donates its methyl group during the biosynthesis of thymidine nucleotides for DNA synthesis; the methenyl form donates its group as a formyl group during purine biosynthesis, and the methyl form is the donor of the methyl group to sulfur during methionine formation. Intermediates that serve as substrates for transmethylation reactions depend on the continuous synthesis of methionine. S-adenosylmethionine (SAM) is made from L-methionine and adenosine triphosphate (ATP) by methionine adenosyltransferase. Transmethylation, transsulfuration, and aminopropylation are the metabolic pathways that use SAM. These reactions are anabolic and occur throughout the body. More than 40 metabolic reactions involve the transfer of a methyl group from SAM to various substrates such as nucleic acids, proteins, and lipids. The resulting homocysteine is either reutilized for methionine regeneration or converted to cystathionine. It can also be inferred that these processes influence glutathione generation. (From Rucker et al., In N. Van Alfen (ed.), *Encyclopedia of Agriculture and Food Systems*, San Diego, 2014.)

reaction that converts 5,10-methyl-THF to 5-methyl-THF. Thus, adequate SAM ensures sufficient 5,10-methyl-THF as a substrate for thymidylate synthase, which provides the nucleotide balance of deoxyuridine monophosphate and deoxythymidine monophosphate for DNA synthesis (Toohey, 2006; Baily, 2014).

Because folacin is required for maintaining nucleotide balance during DNA synthesis, its deficiency is expressed by increased cell death and in some cases by compensatory increased proliferation of cells. In bone marrow, megaloblastosis and macrocytosis of enterocytes are a reflection of defective DNA synthesis due to folacin deficiency. There is a production of larger dysfunctional cells that eventually translates into macrocytic anemia, a condition in which the larger red cells are insufficient in number and hemoglobin. Folic acid deficiency can also result in developmental and neural tube defects, and contribute to the development of cardiovascular disease. In one recent study, the incidence of cleft lip/palate was reduced in the offspring of Pugs and Chihuahuas supplemented with 5 or 2.5 mg, respectively, of folic acid from the onset of heat until day 40 of gestation (Domoslawska et al., 2013). For humans, a large body of clinical literature exists noting the connection between folacin intake, hyperhomocysteinemia due to folic acid deficiency, and carotid artery narrowing and occlusive strokes. Ingestion of diets high in folic acid also appears protective against the development of colonic adenomas and related cancers (Depeint et al., 2006; Verhoef, 2007; Verhoef and de Groot, 2005).

24.4.3.2.4 Requirements, Pharmacology, and Toxicity

The requirements for folic acid range from 2 to 5 mg per kg of diet or 0.5 to 3 mg per 1000 kcal for most animals. There are some conditions in which the folic acid requirements are conditionally high, for example, when either natural or pharmacological folic acid agonists are present in the diet. The discovery that THF is required for DNA synthesis has led to a number of antimetabolites that function as inhibitors of folic acid reductase and DNA synthesis. The best example is methotrexate (Baily, 2014), which ultimately inhibits the proliferation and regeneration of rapidly replicating cells. Methotrexate irreversibly inhibits dihydrofolate reductase, an enzyme that participates in the tetrahydrofolate synthesis. With insufficient THF, cell division is blocked in the S phase due to impaired DNA synthesis. Drugs such as methotrexate are widely used in treatment of autoimmune disease and cancer chemotherapy, particularly for tumors of the lymphoreticular system (Gangjee et al., 2007, 2008).

24.4.3.3 Vitamin B-12

24.4.3.3.1 Overview

Vitamin B-12, also called cobalamin, is another water-soluble vitamin that plays a key role in the formation of blood and brain and nervous system (Figure 24.16). Vitamin B-12 helps to link many of the functions of folic acid to the THF-homocysteine transmethylase system (Green and Miller, 2014). Other reactions involving vitamin B-12 utilize the vitamin in the form of the deoxyadenosylcobalamine derivative. An example is methylmalonyl-CoA mutase, which catalyzes the conversion of methylmalonic acid to succinyl-CoA for ultimate use as a metabolic fuel. Vitamin B-12 is a class of chemically related compounds, which is structurally more complex than the other vitamins, and novel in that it contains cobalt. Biosynthesis of vitamin B-12 is only accomplished by bacteria, but conversion between different forms of the vitamin can occur in many types of cells.

24.4.3.3.2 Metabolism

Vitamin B-12 associated with food is released in the stomach by proteolysis and acid denaturation. In animals with simple stomachs, "R-proteins" (haptocorrins and cobalaphilins) are secreted, which bind to free vitamin B-12 (Festen, 1991, Green and Miller, 2014). Intrinsic factor (IF) is a protein synthesized by the gastric parietal cells of most animals. However, the pancreas can also be a site of synthesis (e.g., in dogs and cats; Vaillant et al. 1990; Fyfe et al., 1991). IF is secreted in response to food consumption and binds vitamin B-12 released in response to gastric digestion. In the small intestine, R-proteins are digested, and B-12 is released. The released vitamin B-12 then binds to IF, to form a B-12-IF complex. B-12 must be attached to IF to be recognized by receptors on the enterocytes in the terminal ileum, where uptake involves endocytotic mechanisms. IF protects B-12 from catabolism by intestinal bacteria. The B-12-IF complex that is recognized by ileal receptors is next transported into the portal circulation where it is transferred to transcobalamin.

Vitamin B-12 is transported in plasma by one of three known transport proteins: transcobalamins I, II, or III (Seetharam and Yammani, 2003). The transcobalamins carry vitamin B-12 to cells where it is again transferred into given cells by endocytotic mechanisms. Interference with R protein or IF production can influence the availability of vitamin B-12. With bacterial overproduction, there is competition between the host and bacteria for vitamin B-12. Many animals obtain vitamin B-12 through coprophagy. In ruminants, vitamin B-12 is synthesized in ample quantities by ruminal bacteria. Within cells, vitamin B-12 is transported by specific chaperons to specific organelles and the locations of vitamin B-12 requiring enzymes (Banerjee, 2006). Once associated with targeted enzymes, the vitamin B-12 in cells is relatively stable. Approximately 0.1% of the pool is lost per day, and bile is the principal route for B-12 excretion (Green and Miller, 2014).

As a final point, malabsorption of B-12 can be a problem in aging animals. Analogous to pernicious anemia in humans, in old animals, autoimmune diseases that affect the gastric parietal cells result in their destruction. Such events can curtail the production of IF and limits absorption. Accordingly, autoimmune diseases should be considered in aging animals with signs of macrocytic or megaloblastic anemia.

24.4.3.3.3 Functions

Because methylated folacins and cobalamin are required as substrates and cofactors for the methionine synthase reaction and DNA synthesis, the clinical expression of cobalamin deficiency as megaloblastic anemia or hyperhomocysteinemia is not distinguishable from severe folate deficiency (Figure 24.17). Cobalamin is also required in the methylmalonyl-CoA mutase reaction and methylation of branched-chain fatty acids necessary for neural membrane assembly. The substrate for methylmalonyl-CoA mutase, methylmalonyl-CoA, is primarily derived from propionyl-CoA, a substance formed from the catabolism and digestion of isoleucine, valine, threonine, methionine, thymine, cholesterol, or odd-chain fatty acids (Banerjee, 2006).

As a consequence, prolonged vitamin B-12 deficiency can result in neurologic disorders, for example, degeneration of the myelin sheath, because of the inability to produce complex lipids for membrane assembly. The clinical signs include loss of position and vibratory sensation in the extremities, ataxia, and paresthesis, even in the absence of anemia.

24.4.3.3.4 Requirements, Pharmacology, and Toxicity

Vitamin B-12 deficiency should be suspected in macrocytic anemia, particularly when the mean corpuscular red cell volume is elevated. The need for vitamin B-12 for most animals is in the 2–15 μμg per kg of diet range. Although deficiencies are uncommon in free-ranging animals, diseases of the proximal duodenum or stomach and ileum and pancreatic insufficiency can decrease vitamin B-12 absorption. Studies have shown low serum cobalamin concentrations are present in most dogs and all cats with exocrine pancreatic insufficiency (Batchelor et al., 2007; Hall et al., 1991; Steiner and Williams, 1995; Thompson et al., 2009). Moreover, cobalt deficiency can result in vitamin B-12 deficiency in ruminants, because of the need for cobalt by rumen microorganisms to synthesize vitamin B-12 (McDonell, 2001).

The daily requirement of cobalamin is very small compared to the body pool size (1–2 mg); therefore, it takes many weeks or months to become deficient from dietary inadequacy alone. Of conditions to note, total gastrectomy in animals places a strain on vitamin B-12 metabolism, because of the loss in IF and R factor production. Autoimmune disorders related to destruction of parietal cells and characterized by the absence of IF and achlorhydria can have a profound effect on vitamin B-12 absorption. Chronic use of antacid medications is also a risk factor for deficiency as release of vitamin B-12 is impaired (Howden, 2000; Andrès et al., 2003). In addition, chronic duodenal hyperacidity may inactivate pancreatic trypsin and prevent the transfer of cobalamin from gastric haptocorrin (R factor) to IF. Further, inflammation of the terminal ileum may impact the receptor-mediated uptake of the IF-B-12 complex. Two drugs, colchicine and p-aminosalicylic acid, may also cause cobalamin deficiency by inhibiting receptor interactions.

Dogs and cats with chronic enteropathies are frequently deficient in cobalamin. Historically, parenteral administration of cobalamin has been recommended in these cases. However, findings of a recent retrospective study suggest that oral cobalamin supplementation is effective in normalizing cobalamin concentrations in dogs with chronic enteropathies (Toresson et al., 2015). However, further studies are needed to compare cobalamin status in dogs receiving oral versus parenteral supplementation before this approach can be widely recommended.

24.4.4 Water-Soluble Vitamin Assessment

Approaches to vitamin assessment may be found in several sources. An excellent series, the *Methods in Enzymology* (particularly volumes: 18, 62, 66, 67, 81, 105, 122, 190, 123, 234, 279, 281, 282, 299) published by Elsevier (http://www.elsevier.com/) provide descriptions of numerous approaches for individual water-soluble vitamin determination. HPLC methods using differing detection approaches (e.g., tandem and quadrupole mass spectrometry) are also available. The use of accelerated mass spectrometry constitutes a seminal breakthrough in that physiological concentrations of vitamins (both fat and water soluble) can be detected in the attomolar range (Kim et al., 2009; Ebeler et al., 2005; Ross et al., 2004; Lemke et al., 2003). With approaches currently in use, it is often possible to be noninvasive or carry out multiple sampling on the same subject.

24.5 VITAMIN-LIKE COMPOUNDS

24.5.1 Lipotropic Factors

Nutritional requirements exist for a number of compounds at specific periods in development, particularly neonatal development, and periods of rapid growth. These compounds often perform specialized transport functions, particularly in relation to fatty acids. Examples include choline, inositol, carnitine, and taurine (Figure 24.18).

24.5.1.1 Choline

Choline is particularly noteworthy, because it plays a key role in methyl group metabolism, carcinogenesis, and lipid transport as a component of lecithin (Garrow, 2007). Choline is normally

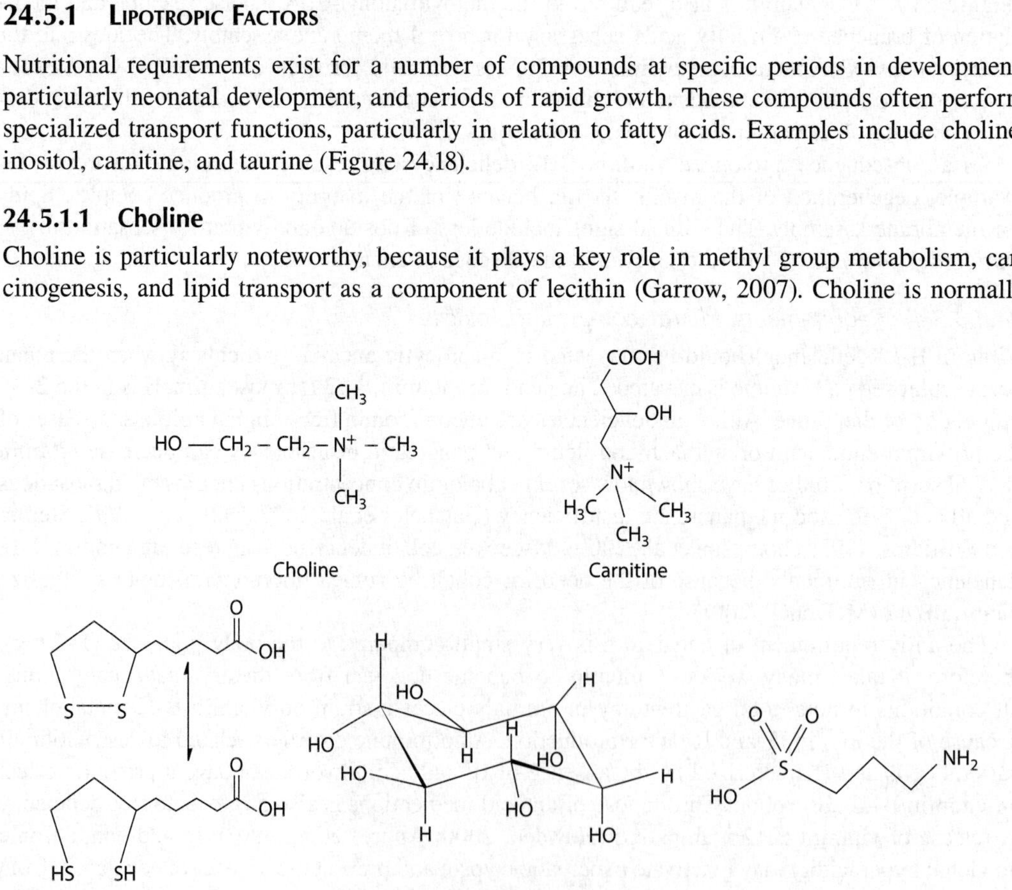

Choline

Carnitine

Lipoic acid

Inositol

Taurine

FIGURE 24.18 Chemical structures for choline, inositol, carnitine, and taurine.

produced in sufficient amounts from the transmethylation pathways involving S-adenosyl methionine (Figure 24.17); however, in young growing animals a positive growth response can occur upon addition of choline. Commercially available forms of choline are available as the trimethyl hydroxyethylammonium chloride or as the bitartrate. Choline is generally added to diets to reduce the need for activated methyl groups supplied by methionine. It is more economical to add choline for these methyl groups than to add methionine. The most abundant source of choline in the diet is lecithin.

The primary sign of choline deficiency is fatty liver and cirrhosis. Choline is a component of sphingomyelin and lecithin. Formation of betaine from choline provides another important source of labile methyl groups for transmethylation reactions. In mice and rats, a novel observation is that a prolonged deficiency of choline can result in hepatocellular cancer. This is a unique example of a nutritional deficiency leading to a neoplasm without having to expose the animal to known liver carcinogens or promoters (Zeisel, 1995, 1996). Five hundred to 1000 mg of choline is often added per kg of diet to promote growth and optimize phospholipids production.

24.5.1.2 Inositol

Inositol is synthesized using glucose-6-phosphate as a precursor. Inositol is particularly important in cellular signal transduction and phospholipid assembly. Like choline, a case may be made that it is required to some degree (e.g., to optimize growth in adolescent gerbils and hamsters), although most animals appear able to produce or derive sufficient inositol from dietary sources (Chu and Hegsted, 1980a, 1980b; Holub, 1992). The estimated daily intake of inositol for large animals can be as high as 1 or 2 g per day. It is also noteworthy that a relationship exists between inositol ingestion and its distribution as inositol-6-phosphate in various tissues, and that a depletion of extracellular inositol-6-phosphate occurs at higher rates when inositol-deficient diets are consumed.

24.5.1.3 Carnitine

Carnitine comes both from the diet and synthesis from lysine by a process that is ascorbic acid and iron dependent. Carnitine concentrations in mammalian milk (as carnitine plus acylcarnitine) are in the 100 μM range. The distribution and levels are affected by a number of factors ranging from changes in the metabolic state (e.g., ketosis) to the stage of lactation (e.g., transition from colostrum to whole milk). These points are important, because carnitine production is not sufficient in newborns, particularly animals that are weaned too early to ill-defined diets. Dogs with the genetic disorder cystinuria may have increased renal excretion of carnitine; monitoring or dietary supplementation is advisable (Sanderson et al., 2001). Carnitine is required for the transport of fatty acids from the cytosol into the mitochondria for the generation of metabolic energy (Kittleson et al., 1997). There is a growing literature in humans that suggests carnitine supplementation may be helpful to improve glucose utilization and fatty acid oxidation (Challem, 1999). Amounts of 100 mg/kg of diet are often suggested, which is similar to the concentration of dried milk or milk solids of most animals (Blanchard et al., 2002; Doberenz et al., 2006; Kidd et al., 2005; Peebles et al., 2007). Much higher doses (2–3 g daily) are advised as a therapy for American Cocker Spaniel dogs with dilated cardiomyopathy, as this has been reported to result in significant improvement in disease parameters, at least when used with taurine (Kittleson et al., 1997).

24.5.1.4 Taurine

Taurine (2-aminoethanesulfonic acid) is derived from cysteine and is one of the few known naturally occurring sulfonic acids. Taurine is present in all animal tissues. Most animals can synthesize taurine; however, some animals, particularly domesticated and wild felids, do not synthesize adequate amounts. In cats and some species of dogs (Kittleson et al., 1997), defective synthesis is a result of low activity of two enzymes in the synthetic pathway: cysteine dioxygenase and cysteine sulfinic acid decarboxylase. Losses occur because of an obligatory requirement for taurine to conjugate bile acids.

An array of clinical signs has been described in taurine-deficient cats including central retinal degeneration, reversible dilated cardiomyopathy, and reproductive failure in queens, teratogenic defects, and abnormal brain development in kittens (Backus et al., 1995; Edgar et al., 1998; Hickman et al., 1990b; Hickman et al., 1992; Kittleson et al., 1997; Pion et al., 1992). Low blood taurine concentrations and dilated cardiomyopathy have been identified in dogs that do not have a genetic predilection to this disease (Backus et al., 2003; Fascetti et al., 2003). Suggested mechanisms for taurine deficiency in these dogs were considered to be (1) insufficient synthesis of taurine, (2) extraordinary loss of taurine or its precursors in urine, (3) extraordinary gastrointestinal loss of taurine in bile acid conjugates (as found in cats), or (4) a reduction in protein digestibility (Morris et al. 1994). Meats, dairy products, and especially seafood in contrast to plant foods are good sources of taurine. Dietary concentrations of taurine that are required to maintain adequate levels in plasma and whole blood in cats are dependent on a function of type of diet, which affects the degree of microbial degradation that occurs during enterohepatic circulation. Plasma and whole blood concentrations of 40 and 300 mM of taurine, respectively, appear to be adequate in cats for reproduction. Intakes of taurine from 1 to 2.5 g taurine/kg of diet may be needed to sustain plasma and blood concentrations in this range.

24.5.2 Novel Cofactors, Electron Transporters, Bioflavonoids, and Polyphenolics

The following compounds are highlighted because of their known roles as coenzymes in prokaryotes and potential roles as probiotics and growth-promoting substances in higher animals. These compounds include quesuosine, coenzyme Q (CoQ), pteridines (other than folic acid), such as biopterin and the pteridine cofactor for the Mo-Fe flavoproteins (see Section 24.6.4), lipoic acid (LA), pyrroloquinoline quinone (PQQ), and bioflavonoids and related plant pigments (Figure 24.19). Increasing or decreasing dietary exposure to these compounds is known to produce a number of systemic effects, most of which are considered healthful.

24.5.2.1 Queuosine

Queuosine is included because it is a novel product arising from microbe–host interactions. Queuine is a nucleoside base made by bacteria, which is modified to queuosine (Boland et al., 2009; Kang et al., 2009). Germ-free animals seem to survive without a source of queuine or queuosine, yet

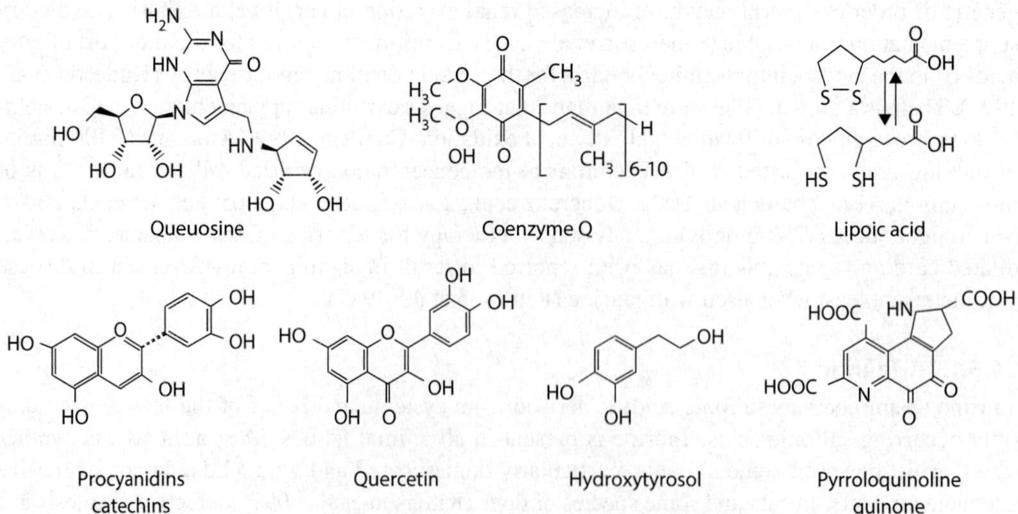

FIGURE 24.19 Chemical structures for queuosine, coenzyme Q, lipoic acid, procyanidins catechin, quercetin, hydroxytyrosol, and pyrroloquinoline quinone.

it is found in measurable amounts in animals with a normal intestinal microflora (Farkas, 1980; Reyniers et al., 1981). Queuosine resembles guanidine and is preferentially utilized in some t-RNAs. The importance of this interaction has yet to be fully understood, although it is known that tRNAs of the queuosine-family (Q-tRNA) are completely modified in terminally differentiated somatic cells and that modification of Q-tRNA is associated with cell proliferation, control of aerobic and anaerobic metabolism, and perhaps malignancy.

24.5.2.2 Coenzyme Q

Although claims have been made for a nutritional requirement for CoQ, more work is needed to fully clarify an exact nutritional role for this compound. CoQ, or ubiquinone, is found in mitochondria and is structurally similar to vitamins E and K. As a quinone, CoQ is ideally suited to interact with cytochromes to affect the flow of electrons in the mitochondrial respiratory chain. CoQ can be synthesized and is readily absorbed from the intestine by the same route as other fat-soluble vitamins. CoQ is found mainly in the mitochondrial intermembrane. Although there is no apparent dietary requirement, CoQ is present in food and promoted for various health benefits in which improving the efficiency of oxidative metabolism is a concern. If used therapeutically (based mostly on human and rodent studies), effective doses are one or more g/kg of the dry diet. In dogs, tachycardia-induced cardiac failure is not associated with reduced CoQ levels, but CoQ-treated dogs have less hypertrophy compared with untreated dogs. CoQ that is absorbed from the intestine is transported by the same transport system as vitamin E and vitamin K.

24.5.2.3 Pteridines (Biopterin and the Mo-Fe Pteridine Cofactor)

In animals, tetrahydrobioterin (commonly abbreviated BH_4) is a redox cofactor, best known for its role at the catalytic site for phenylalanine, tryptophan, and tyrosine hydroxylases, and more recently endothelial NO synthase (Ozkor and Quyyumi, 2008). Tetrahydrobiopterin (BH4) is synthesized from guanosine triphosphate by GTP cyclohydrolase I, 6-pyruvoyltetrahydropterin synthase (PTS), and sepiapterin reductase (SPD). GTP cyclohydrolase I is the rate-limiting enzyme (Nagatsu and Ichinose, 1999). A related cofactor is the molybdenum cofactor, also in the pterin family, which is a cofactor for xanthine oxidase and aldehyde oxidase (important in purine metabolism) and sulfite oxidase (important in sulfur amino acid metabolism). Dietary intervention with tetrahydrobioterin may be useful when there are signs of perturbed phenylalanine or tyrosine metabolism that are genetic in origin. The production of the molybdenum cofactor is directly dependent on adequate molybdenum intake (see Section 24.6.4).

24.5.2.4 Lipoic Acid

LA is made in the liver of most animals. This coenzyme is linked by amide linkage to lysyl residues within transacetylases and functions in the transfer of electrons and activated acyl groups as a part of the pyruvate dehydrogenase complex, that is, the initial step important to the regulation and function of the TCA cycle. Reduction of oxidative stress by LA supplementation has been demonstrated in animal models. Mice deficient in LA synthase have been generated. The heterozygotes have significantly reduced erythrocyte glutathione levels, indicating that their endogenous antioxidant capacity is lower than those of wild-type mice (Yi et al., 2009). Homozygous embryos die by day 8–12 of gestation. Of nutritional interest, supplementing the diet of heterozygous mothers with LA during pregnancy fails to prevent the prenatal deaths of homozygous embryos. Apparently, an endogenous LA synthesis is essential for developmental survival and cannot be replaced by LA in maternal tissues and blood via the diet (Yi et al., 2009; Yi and Maeda, 2005). Further, although LA is often supplemented as an antioxidant, toxicity with changes in liver function is more easily observed in felids than in humans and rodents (Hill et al., 2004, 2005). An oral dose of LA produces hepatocellular toxicity in cats when given at 30 mg or more per kg body weight. In dogs, hypoglycemia, acute renal failure, and hepatic injury have also been reported at doses of 1000 mg LA/kg body weight (Hill et al., 2004). The LD 50 for rodents is >2000 mg LA/kg body weight.

24.5.2.5 PQQ, Bioflavonoids, and Dietary Polyphenolic Pigments

Various phytochemicals and biofactors are worth mention, because they are capable of influencing mitochondrial function and oxidative metabolism. Examples include several plant-derived flavonoids (quercetin and the procyanidins, epicatechins, and catechins), and two tyrosine-derived quinones (hydroxytyrosol in olive oil and PQQ). These compounds serve in plants as pigments, phytoalexins, or growth factors. In animals, positive nutritional and physiological attributes have been established for each, especially in the respect to their ability to affect energy metabolism, cell signaling, and mitochondrial function. At least one, PQQ, has been shown to stimulate growth and development in rodents when added to highly purified diets (Akagawa et al., 2015; Chowanadisai et al., 2010; Rucker et al., 2009, 2014; Steinberg et al., 2003; Stites et al., 2006). Regarding possible mechanisms of action, PQQ, quercetin, and hydroxytyrosol have been shown to influence cell signaling and regulators of mitochondrial biogenesis, such as the peroxisome proliferator-activated receptor gamma family of transcriptional coactivators (abbreviated: PGC-1α, PGC-1β, and the PGC-related coactivator (Rasbach and Schnellmann, 2008; Davis et al., 2009; Chowanadisai et al., 2010). PGC-1α is thought to be the principal regulator in this family, although all are important. PGC-1α helps to regulate many of the genes involved in energy metabolism by interacting with other factors and nuclear receptors. PGC-1α is an important coactivator of the PPAR family of nuclear receptors, in addition to nuclear respiratory factor 1 and 2. These factors, in turn, are a part of transcriptional complexes that activate other mitochondrial-related transcription factors (Chowanadisai et al., 2010; Tchaparian et al., 2010; Harris et al., 2013; Zhang et al., 2015).

To add to this complex arrangement, another family of factors, silent information regulators or sirtuins (SIRTs), function in the nucleus by acting as histone deacetylase and monoribosyltransferases. Histone deacylation and monoribosylation affect DNA and histone organization, making exposure to transcription complexes and related synthesis machinery possible (Zhang et al., 2015). Hydroxytyrosol and quercetin also seem to influence aspects of sirtuin regulation (Shoba et al., 2009; Rasbach and Schnellmann, 2008; Hirschey et al., 2009; Davis et al., 2009; Rucker et al., 2009).

In addition, Akagawa et al. (2016) have demonstrated that some mammalian NAD-dependent dehydrogenases have PQQ-binding domains. For example, in purified rabbit muscle lactate dehydrogenase (LDH), PQQ inhibits the formation of lactate from pyruvate in the presence of NADH and enhances the conversion of lactate to pyruvate in the presence of NAD(+) (Akagawa et al., 2015, 2016). The oxidation of NADH to NAD(+) is attributed to PQQ's redox-cycling activity. PQQ also attenuated cellular lactate release and increased intracellular ATP levels in cells.

The polyphenolics in the catechin family, particularly specific isomers of epigallocatechin-3-gallate, impact on mitochondrial processes appears more related to apoptosis and the expression and regulation of Bcl-2-associated proteins (Keen et al., 2005). The family of Bcl-2 proteins acts as both anti- and proapoptotic regulators. One protein in this family, Bcl-2–associated X or BAX, functions by competing with Bcl-2-proper (another member of the Bcl-2 family of proteins that acts as an antiapoptotic regulator). BAX can also insert itself into organelle membranes, primarily the outer mitochondrial membrane, to induce the opening of voltage-dependent channels, which results in the release of cytochrome c and other proapoptotic factors from the mitochondria. This action eventually leads to activation of caspaces, enzymes that are essential to mitochondrial outer membrane permeabilization, as well as other steps important to the initiation of apoptosis and eventual cell death (Rasbach and Schnellmann, 2008).

In addition to the effects on mitochondria, many flavonoids influence endothelial function by activating endothelial nitric oxide synthase. Consumption has also been associated with inhibition of platelet activity, and decreasing blood pressure in animal models and humans because of endothelium-dependent flow-mediated dilation of arteries. Although antioxidant activity is often ascribed as the principal physiological effect of flavonoid and polyphenolic exposure, most studies indicate that antioxidant capacity of blood seen after the consumption of flavonoid-rich foods is not a direct effect of flavonoids, but rather due to other factors, such as improved mitochondrial function or amplification of other antioxidant processes or factors (e.g., increasing uric acid levels). For the most part, the biological effects of flavonoids appear related more to their ability to modulate cell-signaling pathways than their antioxidant activity (Rasbach and Schnellmann, 2008).

Regarding the intakes that need to be added to diets to obtain physiological effects, quercetin, hydroxytyrosol, and isomers of catechin and epicatechin (e.g., epigallocatechin-3-gallate) are functional in the 20–100 mg/kg diet range. PQQ is effective in promoting growth and reproduction in rodents when fed highly purified diets, if provided at ~0.3 mg or more per kg of diet (Steinberg et al., 2003). Taken together, bioflavonoids, carotenoids, anthocyanins, and other phytochromes are consumed on the order of 2–4 g per kg of conventional diets comprised of whole foods and components. In plants, these compounds provide protective camouflage, facilitate transformation of light into chemical energy, or act as protective chemicals and repellents to predators (e.g., phytoalexins). In animals, plant pigments are also utilized for some of the same purposes, although their importance as absolute nutritional essentials remains unclear.

24.6 TRACE MINERALS

Six elements: cobalt (Co), copper (Cu), manganese (Mn), molybdenum (Mo), selenium (Se), and zinc (Zn) will be used to illustrate concepts relevant to metabolism and function of trace minerals. The importance of iron, calcium, magnesium, sodium, potassium, and other essential minerals is discussed elsewhere in this volume. Discussions of vanadium, chromium, silicon, nickel, and tin are not included because nutritional essentiality remains to be established. If there is a nutritional need for these elements, it is likely to be in the μg per kg of diet range (Reilly, 2004), whereas the relative need for Co, Cu, Mn, Mo, Se, and Zn approach or exceed amounts in the mg per kg of diet range. The essential elements are distinguished because they are usually associated with the functions of specific proteins, peptides, and enzymes. As noted previously, they usually fall into two categories, metalloenzymes and metal–enzyme complexes, depending upon the stability constants that define metal binding. In simple metal complexes, the basicity of the electron donating group and the ability to approach the metal ion (steric effects) are the primary factors that influence stability (Reedijk and Bouwman, 1999, Harris, 2014).

24.6.1 Cobalt

24.6.1.1 Overview

Compounds containing Co are stabilized by complex ion formation. In tissues, Co is normally found associated with vitamin B-12 in animals that require preformed vitamin B-12. Co is novel because there is no evidence that any organism needs the Co ion, either in the free form or as a simple protein complex. Plants contain Co, but there is no indication that Co occurs as a cobalamide, that is, vitamin B-12. However, in plants, Co is important because of the symbiotic relationship with nitrogen-fixing Rhizobia in legume nodules (O'Dell and Sunde, 1997).

A somewhat parallel in animals is the role of cobalt in the propagation of microflora cofactors, specifically vitamin B-12, in those animals with reticulorumen pouches (Kennedy et al., 1995, 1997). In ruminants, Co is a primary gluconeogenic precursor for ruminants is propionic acid. Propionyl-CoA cannot enter β-oxidation-related pathways or the TCA cycle unless it is converted to succinyl-CoA via vitamin B-12-dependent steps (Kennedy et al., 1995). A way of thinking about Co from a mechanistic perspective is that as a component of vitamin B-12, it functions as a Grignard reaction catalyst acting as a nucleophile and in the addition of a single carbon moiety to another electrophilic carbon atom to form a new carbon–carbon bond.

24.6.1.2 Metabolism

As noted, Co is most important to ruminant animals, because of the rumen microflora. Ruminants can be fed ionic Co and rumen microbes will synthesize cobalamin for absorption. Nevertheless, the relative inefficiency of vitamin B-12 production in the rumen and poor absorption of B-12 can predispose ruminants to deficiency. Soils comprised of calcareous sands are commonly associated with Co deficiency in grazing animals, and applications of superphosphate have been related to reduced vitamin B-12 concentrations in ruminants. Seasonal variations in Co nutrition may also be significant.

Although roles for Co beyond vitamin B-12 production have not been defined, Co is absorbed and shares the same pathways as iron (Fe) for absorption. High amounts of Fe in the diet can depress Co absorption and vice versa. Co absorption is enhanced in Fe deficiency. Excretion of Co is primarily via the kidneys and bile and is linearly related to the ingested dose (Barceloux, 1999; Lauwerys and Lison, 1994). Other aspects important to the absorption of Co are similar to those described for vitamin B-12.

24.6.1.3 Functions

The signs and biochemical lesions that are manifested in Co deficiency correspond to those of vitamin B-12 deficiency. The pathways that are most severely impaired are those of purine biosynthesis and gluconeogenesis. A primary defect in Co deficiency underlying the above has been attributed to a reduction in the activity of methylmalonyl CoA mutase in ruminants. The hepatic lipidosis observed in Co-deficient animals has been attributed to a reduction in choline biosynthesis caused by a decrease in the activity of homocysteine methyltransferase. Accordingly, Co deficiency eventually leads to a loss of appetite, anemia, decreased fertility, and decreased milk production. Sheep are more susceptible to Co deficiency than cattle (McDonell, 2001). In this species, there is loss of wool production, and even the accumulation of fat in the liver of vitamin B-12 deficient sheep, but not cattle, may be related to a methyl-group deficiency affecting liver lipid metabolism. Another metabolic anomaly of Co-deficient lambs is the accumulation of homocysteine in the plasma, which leads to an accumulation of oxidation products, depletion of vitamin E, and damage to the mitochondria. Reduction in the ability to produce normal levels of choline (see Sections 24.4.3.2 and 24.4.3.3) can lead to the inability to export triglycerides as a component of VLDL.

24.6.1.4 Requirements, Pharmacology, and Toxicity

Co deficiency in ruminants occurs when pasture Co concentrations are less than 0.10 mg/kg dry edible matter (Ellison, 2002). Toxicity in animals under natural conditions has not been reported. Toxic levels appear to be at least 300–1000 times the requirement in most species.

24.6.2 Copper

24.6.2.1 Overview

Cu serves as a redox cofactor for a number of oxidases and monooxygenases that are essential for life. Perturbations in the activity of these enzymes are linked to a number of unusual biochemical steps and lesions. Cu deficiency results in reduced rates of growth, impaired reproduction, and defects in skeletal and vascular formation, as well as decreased production of nitric oxide (NO). Impaired immunity, neurological function, and depigmentation may also result from Cu deprivation. Table 24.8 lists processes related to these events.

24.6.2.2 Metabolism

Cu is found in meats, grains, and nuts. Milk and dairy products, however, are low in Cu. Environmental factors, such as soil, water source, fertilizer use, processing, and cooking, may affect the Cu content of food. Cu absorption from diets is relatively efficient, although some dietary constituents can affect bioavailability (Harris, 2014). Cu hydroxides, iodides, glutamates, and citrates are more easily

TABLE 24.8
Physiological Processes Directly Influenced by Dietary Copper Intake

Function	Mechanism
Hematopoiesis	Two copper-containing enzymes, ceruloplasmin (ferroxidase I) and ferroxidase II have the capacity to reduce and oxidize ferrous iron (Fe^{2+}) to ferric iron (Fe^{3+}). Fe^{2+} complexes are two to four orders of magnitude more soluble than Fe^{3+} complexes. Iron mobilization from storage sites is impaired in copper deficiency and microcytic anemia can occur.
Collagen and elastin stability	Copper is a cofactor for lysyl oxidase, an enzyme involved in the intra- and intermolecular cross-linking of collagen and elastin. Defective cross-linking can cause friable skin, bone fragility, and vascular lesions.
Antioxidant defense	Copper functions at the catalytic site of the antioxidant enzyme, superoxide dismutase.
Energy metabolism	The redox potential of ionic copper gives it a role in energy metabolism as a component of the cytochromes that participate in electron transport (e.g., cytochrome *c* oxidase).
Neurotransmitter production and metabolism	A number of reactions essential to normal function of the brain and nervous system are catalyzed by cuproenzymes. For example, dopamine-β-monooxygenase catalyzes the conversion of dopamine to the neurotransmitter norepinephrine inhibitors as antidepressants.
Pigmentation	The cuproenzyme, tyrosinase, is required for the formation of the pigment melanin important to the pigmentation of hair, skin, and eye.

absorbed than molybdates, sulfates, and phytates. High intakes (100 or more mg/kg of diet) of silver (Ag) and Zn can interfere with intestinal Cu transport. Moreover, the extended use of supplements that contain Fe can negatively affect Cu status. Cu absorption is greater in neonates than in adults. Another interaction involves the relationship between Cu, Mo, and sulfate. In ruminants, dietary sulfate intensifies the harmful effects of Mo on Cu absorption. $CuSO_4$ and Na_2MoO_4 react to form insoluble thiomolybdate complexes, which render Cu biologically less active and bioavailable (Nederbragt et al., 1984). Dietary reducing agents, such as ascorbic acid, may also lower Cu absorption because the intestinal transfer of divalent cupric ion is substantially greater the monovalent cuprous ion.

Cu absorption occurs by active transport (see Figure 24.20). For most species, absorption takes place in the upper small intestine, but in sheep, considerable absorption also occurs in the large intestine. In many animals, uptake of Cu is about 30%–60% with a net absorption of about 5%–10% owing to the rapid excretion of newly absorbed Cu into the bile (Ammerman et al., 1995). Cu uptake by cells occurs via high- and low-affinity transport systems (La Fontaine et al., 2010). Cupric ion (Cu^{+1}) is the primary substrate for the transport systems that take Cu across plasma membranes.

Recent studies in yeast have shed light on proteins involved in the process of Cu transport. In mammalian cells, the entry of Cu into cells is first orchestrated by the action of a reductase and then contact with a high-affinity Cu transporter, currently designated as Ctrl and Ctr3 (Ctr2 is a low-affinity transporter). Under Cu-limiting conditions, the transporters and proteins involved in Cu redox are up-regulated. In addition to the transporters, cellular chaperones specific for Cu deliver Cu to specific cellular proteins (La Fontaine et al., 2010). Other important features of Cu regulation include the role for metallothionein, which acts to buffer shifts in the cellular concentrations of Cu (and Zn). Alternatively, Cu egress or transport out of cells is controlled by membrane transporters in the family of P-type ATPases (P-ATPases). Precise control of the regulation of Cu is necessary, in that free cuprous (as well as ferric) ions react readily with hydrogen peroxide to yield harmful hydroxyl radicals. Accordingly, unbound Cu is extremely low in concentration (~one atom/cell). In addition to the transporters, cellular chaperones specific for Cu deliver Cu to specific cellular proteins (La Fontaine et al., 2010). Other important features of Cu regulation include the role of metallothionein, a metal-binding protein for Cu, Zn, and cadmium that acts to buffer abnormal shifts in the cellular concentrations of Cu, and the proteins and transporters involved in the egress of Cu from cells.

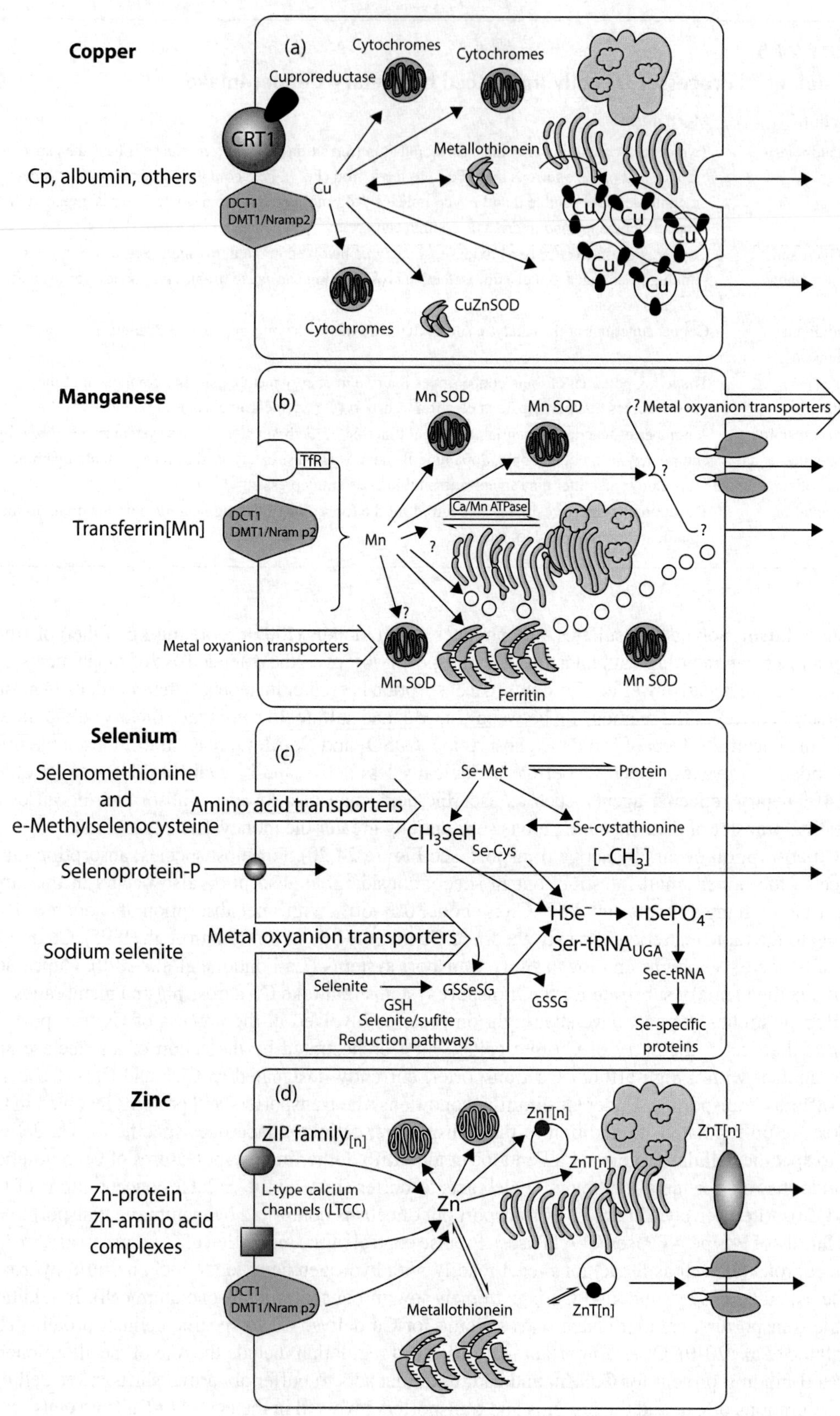
Copper
(a)
Cytochromes
Cytochromes
Cuproreductase
CRT1
Metallothionein
Cp, albumin, others
Cu
DCT1
DMT1/Nramp2
Cu
Cu
Cu
Cu
Cu
CuZnSOD
Cytochromes
Manganese
(b)
Mn SOD
Mn SOD
? Metal oxyanion transporters
TfR
Ca/Mn ATPase
Transferrin[Mn]
DCT1
DMT1/Nram p2
Mn
Metal oxyanion transporters
Mn SOD
Ferritin
Mn SOD
Selenium
(c)
Selenomethionine
and
e-Methylselenocysteine
Amino acid transporters
Se-Met
Protein
CH3SeH
Se-cystathionine
Se-Cys
[–CH3]
Selenoprotein-P
HSe⁻
HSePO4⁻
Ser-tRNAUGA
Metal oxyanion transporters
Sodium selenite
Selenite
GSSeSG
GSH
GSSG
Sec-tRNA
Selenite/sufite
Reduction pathways
Se-specific
proteins
Zinc
(d)
ZIP family[n]
ZnT[n]
ZnT[n]
ZnT[n]
L-type calcium
channels (LTCC)
Zn-protein
Zn-amino acid
complexes
Zn
DCT1
DMT1/Nram p2
Metallothionein
ZnT[n]

Regarding systemic regulation, from the intestine, a case can be made for the transport of Cu on albumin and in the form of low molecular weight complexes (e.g., histidine) to target tissues, particularly the liver. From the liver, ceruloplasmin transports Cu to other tissues. Ceruloplasmin is the predominant Cu containing protein in mammalian serum, a glycosylated multi-Cu ferroxidase that carries >95% of total serum Cu. Although ceruloplasmin may function in Cu transport, the absence of ceruloplasmin has not been shown to alter Cu levels in the peripheral tissues. Such observations come from what is known about individuals and animal models that are aceruloplasminemic, a genetic disorder of ceruloplasmin deficiency (Shim and Harris, 2003; Meyer et al., 2001). Moreover, analbuminemic rats do not have significantly impaired Cu metabolism (Vargas et al., 1994). The whole body regulation of Cu is also mediated in part by biliary Cu excretion; about 15% of the Cu excreted in bile is reabsorbed through the enterohepatic circulation. A large animal can contain 50–120 mg (780–1889 μmol) of Cu, about one-third of which is found in the liver and brain. Most nonruminant species have liver Cu concentrations that are between 2 and 10 μg/g liver. Skeletal muscle, although considered low in Cu, represents about one-third of the total body Cu because of its mass.

Ruminants have relatively high levels of liver Cu compared to nonruminants. Typical liver Cu concentrations in sheep and cattle range from 20–150 μg/g liver. Similarly, high liver Cu levels have been reported for ducks and some fish. For most species, liver Cu concentrations are highest in the newborn (Harris, 2014).

FIGURE 24.20 Cellular transport of copper, manganese, zinc, and selenium. (a) Dietary copper is presented to intestinal cells most probably in the form of amino acid complexes. In plasma, Cu is most often associated with albumin and ceruloplasmin. A high-affinity copper transporter (CTR1) is utilized for Cu's entry into cells. It is induced at low copper levels and degraded at high copper levels. Associated with this transporter is a copper reductase that maintains Cu in the +1 state (its most soluble form) while in the vicinity of the transporter. In cells, Cu is next transferred to chaperones whose functions are to carry copper to specific proteins with in the cell (e.g., cytochromes, vesicular P-ATPases, or SOD). A novel process accomplishes Cu efflux from cells. There is transport of Cu into secretory vesicles, which occurs coincidently with efflux of specific apocuproproteins (lysyl oxidase, ceruloplasmin) that are localized to the same vesicles. Two Cu-transporting ATPase enzymes, ATP7A and ATP7B, are responsible for the transfer of Cu to such intracellular vesicles. In response to high levels of cellular Cu, there is a higher rate of recycling of the vesicles to remove copper. Within the vesicles, apocuproproteins can also become activated. Consequently, the amounts of activity of cuproproteins secreted, such as lysyl oxidase (if from connective tissue cells) or ceruloplasmin (if from liver or neural cells), often reflect Cu status or dietary intake. Some evidence also suggests DMT or Nramp transporters essential to iron transport can play a minor role in copper uptake. (b) Intestinal and systemic cellular manganese transport is mediated mostly by divalent metal transporter 1 (DMT1) and is up-regulated in iron deficiency. Within the body, Mn bound to transferrin is taken up transferrin receptors. Unlike other transition metals, Mn is dissociable; thus less is known currently about specific chaperones for Mn. A Golgi-derived ATPase has been described to facilitate the movement of Mn from and to the nucleus and cis- and trans-Golgi compartments. Given that MnO_4 anion can be transported into and out of cells, a role for oxyanion transport is indicated. (c) Selenium is delivered to cells via amino acid and oxyanion transporters, and when present in plasma via processes that recognize selenoprotein P. The selenite and selenate forms must first be reduced (via a glutathione reduction system) to HSe- before Se can be utilized as a cofactor. Selenomethionine, if not incorporated into protein, can also be eventually converted to HSe-. Next, for incorporation into specific Se-proteins (e.g., GPx, 5′-ID, or Se-protein P), HSe- is phosphorylated (requires ATP). Next, following transfer to Ser-$tRNA_{UGA}$ to form Se-Cys-$tRNA_{UGA}$ the stage is set for translation of Se-containing proteins. Regarding cellular efflux, Se is lost from cells as secreted Se-proteins, such selenoprotein P, Se-cystathionine, or as volatile forms of methylated Se (e.g., CH_3–Se–CH_3). (d) Zinc uptake and cellular translocation are controlled by two large families of metal transporters for which there were over two-dozen variants. More specifically, the two solute-linked carrier (SLC) gene families encode the zinc transporters: ZnT (SLC30) and Zip (SLC39). The ZnT transporters reduce intracellular zinc availability by promoting zinc efflux from cells or into intracellular vesicles, while Zip transporters increase intracellular zinc promote extracellular zinc uptake. The ZnT and Zip transporter families exhibit unique tissue-specific expression and differential responsiveness to dietary Zn intake and physiologic stimuli. Temporary influxes of Zn are buffered by the induction of metallothionein. DMT1 and over ion channels can play minor roles in Zn transport.

24.6.2.3 Functions

Anemia (microcytic hypochromic or normocytic hypochromic) is probably the most frequent sign associated with chronic Cu deficiency. Cu deficiency results in impaired Fe absorption, mobilization, and utilization due to Cu's role as a redox cofactor in various membrane-associated ferrioxidases that oxidize Fe^{+2} and Fe^{+3}. ALA dehydrase, critical to the first step in heme synthesis, is also decreased in Cu deficiency. Heinz body anemia caused by ROS is also associated with a significant depression of Cu, Zn superoxide dismutase activity (Hickman et al., 1990a). Neutropenia and myelodysplasia are also associated with Cu deficiency, perhaps related to the importance of adequate Fe to Cu metabolism.

In ruminants, neonatal ataxia (also referred to as enzootic ataxia or swayback) is the most recognized of the naturally occurring Cu deficiency diseases. For example, it is frequently observed in areas of Australia where soil and plant sources of Cu are low. The disorder is characterized by spastic paralysis, especially of the hind limbs, severe incoordination of movement, blindness in some cases, and anemia (Ellison, 2002).

Cardiovascular defects are also associated with Cu deficiency. Cu deficiency can result in degeneration of the myocardium with fibrosis. Cardiac failure may also occur due to decreased cytochrome oxidase activity and abnormalities in elastin and collagen structures. The most severe manifestation of the latter is aortic aneurysms due to decreased elastin and collagen lysine-derived cross-linking, because of reductions in lysyl oxidase activity (Tchaparian et al., 2000; Rucker et al., 1999, 1998; Cui et al., 2004). Moreover, cardiac norepinephrine levels are sensitive to changes in Cu status. Changes in norepinephrine production result in decreased coronary resistance and reduced systolic pressure. Also, skeletal defects have been reported in Cu-deficient dogs, sheep, chicks, cattle, foals, and humans. The primary biochemical lesion is again a reduction in the activity of lysyl oxidase, leading to a reduction in cross-linking of bone collagen.

Increased rates of tissue lipid peroxidation, compromised NO metabolism, and impaired immune response are additional features of Cu deficiency. Lipid peroxidation can occur, because two major components of the cells' antioxidant defense system are affected: Cu, Zn superoxide dismutase, and Se-dependent GPx activities. Because of the increase in various reactive oxidant species resulting from Cu deficiency, NO levels may also be altered (Wu and Meininger, 2002). NO is converted to products, such as peroxynitrite, thus altering NO-dependent cell signaling. Impaired immunity (including defects in neutrophil and lymphocyte function) appears due to the inability to carry out effective oxidative burst reactions and secondary effects, such as the reduced leukocyte trafficking between the blood and tissues. It has been demonstrated that decreased levels of vascular adhesion protein 1 (VAP-1) are associated with deviations in the mucosal immune system (Smith and Vainio, 2007). VAP-1, or semicarbazide-sensitive amine oxidase, is a Cu-containing amine oxidase. VAP-1 alters the expression of molecules involved in the leukocyte extravasation cascade and can prime the vessels for an enhanced inflammatory response. VAP-1 is found in the smooth muscle of blood vessels. Although not all physiological functions of VAP-1 are understood, development of blood vessels, lipolysis regulation, and detoxication are all suggested features.

Moreover, altered insulin secretion and glucose regulation occur during Cu deficiency that can result from peroxidative damage to pancreatic cells. Total cholesterol and free cholesterol levels may also be elevated. A biochemical lesion underlying the hypercholesterolemia is a reduction in hepatic HDL binding. This results in a slower turnover of HDL and leads to an accumulation of apo E-rich HDL. The lipid peroxidation and abnormal lipid transport are important features that can lead to abnormal membrane function.

24.6.2.4 Requirements, Pharmacology, and Toxicity

Most animals meet their requirements if the levels of available Cu exceed 4 mg Cu per kg of diet or 1 mg per 1000 kcal (4.2 MJ) (Doong et al., 1983; Fascetti et al., 2002). Acute Cu toxicity is rare and usually is caused by the consumption of contaminated foods or beverages, or by the accidental or deliberate ingestion of large quantities of Cu salts (Subcommittee on Mineral Toxicity in Animals and Board on Agricultures and Renewable Resources, 1980). Sheep are more sensitive than cattle, with toxicosis being reported in herds of sheep fed cattle rations or provided water from copper-containing plumbing lines. Clinical signs include gastrointestinal distress followed by hemolytic crises.

Two genetic conditions, Menkes' and Wilson's diseases are worthy of mention because the understanding of each has contributed to the understanding of general Cu transport processes (Harris, 2000). In Menkes' disease, there is poor Cu absorption and Cu transport in mesenchymal cells. In Wilsons disease, there is an increased liver Cu content, leading to severe hepatic damage, followed by increased brain Cu levels and neurological lesions. Menkes' disease results in pathology resembling Cu deficiency, as opposed to the pathology of Wilson's disease, which resembles Cu toxicity. Both the Wilson and Menkes' genes code for one of the P-ATPases involved in Cu egress (Harris, 2000).

In Menkes' disease, the mutation prevents Cu transport across the basal lamina of the intestine. JH Menkes first described this Cu transport disorder in 1962 in a family of English–Irish descent. It was recognized immediately as an X-linked recessive disorder, characterized by retardation, impaired growth, peculiar hair, and focal cerebral and cerebellar degeneration. Oral treatment with Cu is ineffective because the genetic defect is due to altered expression of ATPase A7, the enzyme necessary to Cu egress in mesenchymal-derived cells. The condition is often lethal, with death occurring in the first or second year of life, usually from a vascular accident, that is, aneurysm or stroke. Menkes' patients also show signs of osteopenia (poor bone development) and vascular disease. In cell culture, mesenchymal, epithelial, and neural cells from Menkes' patients abnormally sequester Cu. Moreover, the ability to transfer Cu to some Cu-requiring enzymes, for example, lysyl oxidase, is lacking or abnormal (La Fontaine et al., 2010; Rucker et al., 1998). In humans, the frequency of Menkes' disease is estimated to be about one in 35,000–40,000 live births among those of English–Irish descent. The mottled mouse is an animal model analog for Menkes' disease (Shim and Harris, 2003).

In contrast, Wilson's disease is an inherited, autosomal recessive disorder of Cu accumulation and toxicity that occurs in about one of every 40,000 people (Schilsky, 2009a, 2009b). The responsible gene (P-ATP-7B, a homolog to P-ATP-7A) also codes for a vesicular membrane-bound Cu transport protein, but, unlike the Menkes' gene, it is expressed primarily in the liver. As in Menkes' disease, there are mutations in ATP7B that account for symptoms associated with Wilson's disease. Owing to its location in liver, when ATP7B is altered by mutations, biliary excretion of Cu is impaired. An important detail is that the vesicles to which P-ATPase-7B is localized also appear to transport ceruloplasmin from cells. In cells adjacent to biliary canaliculi, some of the vesicular movement is to the cellular membrane that is exposed to the biliary canaliculus; while in other cells, the movement is to the cell membrane exposed to sinusoids and distensible vascular channels. It has therefore been postulated that the liver "packages" Cu for excretion into the bile by binding Cu to ceruloplasmin for release into bile or plasma. This process accounts for the observations that defects in P-ATPase-7B activity often result in low levels of Cu bound to ceruloplasmin in blood and eventually failure of whole body Cu regulation, due to a hepatic accumulation of Cu.

The analog of this disorder in animals is Cu toxicosis in Bedlington Terriers, which affects 60% of the breed (Haywood, 2006). Dogs homozygous for the gene are characterized by extremely high liver Cu concentrations, often exceeding 500 μg/g (7.87 μmol/g) compared to normal values of less than 75 μg/g (1.180 μmol/g). The associated hepatic injury is thought to be due to free radical damage and lysosomal rupture. Several other breeds, including West Highland White Terriers, Skye Terriers, Dobermans, Dalmatians, Keeshonden, and Labrador Retrievers have also been identified as having Cu-associated liver disease.

The treatment strategies for both Wilson's disease and Cu-associated liver disease in dogs include chelation therapy with drugs such as penicillamine and trientine, or high oral doses of Zn (40–50 mg/d in humans, equivalent to 100–150 mg Zn/kg of typical animal rations). Excess Zn can inhibit Cu absorption (Schilsky, 2009a, 2009b). Recent work in a population of Labrador Retrievers with subclinical hepatic copper accumulation demonstrated that feeding a copper restricted (1.3 ± 0.3 mg Cu/Mcal), zinc enhanced (64.3 ± 5.9 mg Zn/Mcal) diet reduced hepatic copper concentrations (Fieten et al., 2015). The genetic background of this group of dogs may influence their response to dietary treatment.

In summary, several complex strategies are used to maintain Cu homeostasis at the cellular and organismal level. The complexities are in part related to maintaining Cu in an appropriate redox state and the need to accommodate a diverse array of enzymatic functions. Fortunately, Cu deficiency is a rare occurrence, but genetic polymorphisms involving Cu transporters can occur, which mimic the signs of Cu deficiency and toxicity observed in animal models.

As a final comment, transmissible spongiform encephalopathies (TSEs) are a family of neurodegenerative diseases characterized by their long incubation periods, progressive neurological changes, and spongiform appearance in the brain. There is now evidence that TSEs are caused by an isoform of the normal cellular surface prion protein PrPC. The function of PrPC is still unknown, but it exhibits properties of a cupro-protein, capable of binding Cu ions (Viles et al., 2008; Leach et al., 2006). In sheep, scrapie is one of several forms of TSE and related to bovine spongiform encephalopathy or "mad cow disease." There are two differing views on Cu's role in prion diseases. While one view looks at the PrPC Cu binding as the trigger for conversion to PrPSc (the scrapie-associated isoform), the opposing viewpoint suggests it is a lack of PrPC Cu-binding that results in the disease-causing isoform. Moreover, Mn and Zn have also been shown to interact with PrPC; thus, the mechanism remains unresolved.

24.6.3 Manganese

24.6.3.1 Overview

Mn is an essential trace element that is required for the activity of enzymes with transferase or hydrolase functions. The mitochondrial form of superoxide dismutase also requires Mn. Maintaining regular Mn status is also important to glucose metabolism, insulin function, and cholesterol regulation. Manifestations of Mn deficiency in domestic animals include impaired growth, skeletal abnormalities, disturbed or depressed reproductive function, ataxia of the newborn, and defects in lipid and carbohydrate metabolism (Aschner et al., 2007).

24.6.3.2 Metabolism

In intestinal cells, the uptake and transport of Mn appear controlled by active transporters (Figure 24.20). The transport characteristics under steady-state conditions at the intestine can exhibit two components that probably reflect transcellular (carrier-mediated) and paracellular (diffusional) pathways. Calcium, calcium antagonists, ATP synthesis inhibitors, and high levels of Fe decrease Mn absorption. Reducing agents, such as ascorbic acid, do not influence uptake. However, compounds that affect solubility (e.g., phytates) decrease Mn absorption (Ammerman et al., 1995). In general, the efficiency of Mn absorption is relatively low. Mn entering portal blood from the gastrointestinal tract can either remain free or rapidly become bound to α-2-macroglobulin and transferrin, particularly as Mn^{+3}. Mn uptake by cells is usually unidirectional and saturable.

The cellular transport of Mn involves transporters in the natural resistance-associated macrophage protein (Nramp) solute carrier family that are involved in proton-coupled divalent metal ion transport (Aschner et al., 2007). The divalent metal transporter-1 (DMT-1) that transports Fe also seems to play a significant role in Mn transport (Fitsanakis et al., 2010). Analogous to the regulation of Zn and Cu transporters, the differential regulation of DMT-1 occurs at the level of protein stability and trafficking through the various secretory pathways. For example, it undergoes regular turnover in cells with sufficient Mn but accumulates in Mn-deficient cells. Moreover, animal models with Fe transporter defects also have impaired Mn transport. For example, homozygous Belgrade rats have hypochromic anemia (due to reduced Fe transport) as well as abnormalities in Mn metabolism (Chua and Morgan, 1997).

Mitochondria have a large capacity for Mn^{+2} uptake and it has been suggested that mitochondrial Mn^{+2} and Ca^{+2} uptakes are linked. Nuclear, cytoskeletal (microsomal), and cytosolic pools of Mn^{+2} also exist. In contrast to Zn, Cu, and Fe for which only a few atoms per cell exist in free form, an easily measurable portion of Mn is dissociable (Reilly, 2004), more analogous to Ca^{+2} and Mg^{+2}.

The metabolic fate of newly absorbed Mn entering the hepatocyte has not been well defined, although several cellular pools of Mn can be identified. The first represents Mn taken up by the lysosomes. Lysosomal uptake of Mn is also considered to be an essential step to egress as it is thought that lysosomes concentrate Mn for delivery to the bile.

Expressed as a percentage of total, skeletal Mn can account for up to 25% of the total body pool. Bone Mn can be raised or lowered by substantially varying dietary Mn, but skeletal pools of Mn exchange slowly; thus they are not thought to constitute a major pool for rapid mobilization. The fetus does not typically accumulate liver Mn before birth, and the levels of Mn in fetal liver are lower than in adult liver, which mainly follows the expression of Mn enzymes such as arginase, pyruvate carboxylase, and Mn-superoxide dismutase.

24.6.3.3 Functions

Mn functions as an enzyme activator and as a constituent of metalloenzymes (Reilly, 2004). For Mn-activated reactions, Mn binds either to a substrate (such as ATP) or to the protein directly, to facilitate subsequent conformational changes. While there are relatively few Mn metalloenzymes, there are a large number of enzymes that can be activated upon Mn additions (e.g., various hydrolases, kinases, decarboxylases, and transferases). Although the extent to which such activation is specifically related to Mn can be questioned (e.g., Mg can replace Mn in many of the reactions), some appear Mn specific (e.g., several glycosyltransferases). For example, it has been suggested that xylosyl transferase is specifically activated by Mn (Liu et al., 1994). Cartilage isolated from Mn-deficient chicks is xylose poor, and fetuses born of Mn-deficient rats have limb deformities that can be related to reduced glycosylation (Liu et al., 1994).

The effects of Mn deficiency on skeletal development have been extensively described (Keen et al., 1999, 2000). Mn deficiency results in limbs that are shortened and thickened, and joints that are swollen and enlarged. The basic biochemical lesion is a reduction in proteoglycan biosynthesis, which is secondary to a decrease in the activities of glycosyltransferases. Ataxia in the offspring of Mn-deficient animals also appears to be related to defects in proteoglycan synthesis. Ataxia is the result of impaired vestibular function caused by abnormal cartilage formation in otoliths present in the utricular and secular maculae.

Further, defects in carbohydrate and lipid metabolism have been observed in Mn-deficient animals due to pancreatic pathology characterized by aplasia or marked hypoplasia of cellular components, including fewer and less intensely granulated pancreatic islet cells than in normal animals. When glucose is given either orally or intravenously to Mn-deficient animals, diabetic-like glucose tolerance curves are observed, which are reversed upon Mn repletion (Keen et al., 1999, 2000). In the pancreas, Mn in islet cells is associated with two pools: a readily exchangeable pool associated with the cell surface, and an intracellular pool. Mn fluxes between these pools can affect insulin release. Accumulation of Mn within the islet cell membrane inhibits insulin release while increases in the intracellular concentration of Mn are associated with a stimulation of insulin synthesis and release. In vivo, Mn deficiency depresses pancreatic insulin synthesis and secretion and enhances intracellular insulin degradation. Also, Mn can activate phosphoenolpyruvate carboxykinase and influence pyruvate carboxylase activity, important to gluconeogenesis (Keen et al., 1999, 2000).

Mn-deficient animals often have excess fat accumulation in the liver. This may be due to alterations in mitochondrial assembly. Mn-deficient animals develop abnormally elongated mitochondria with stacked cristae and decreased capacities to oxidize lipid. Mn is also critical for lipid metabolism as a cofactor in steroid biosynthesis. Mn is thought to be required in farnesyl pyrophosphate synthase, a key step in cholesterol and steroid hormone biosynthesis (Klimis-Tavantzis et al., 1983).

24.6.3.4 Requirements, Pharmacology, and Toxicity

Diets containing less than 1 mg Mn/kg are unable to support normal reproduction. The minimum dietary Mn requirement for poultry for growth and egg production and hatchability is about 40 mg/kg. The concentration of Mn in feedstuffs is dependent on soil conditions and fertilizer practice (Zheljazkov and Warman, 2004). Foods considered high in Mn include nuts, whole cereals, dried fruits, and leafy vegetables. Meats and dairy products are poor sources of Mn. In typical animal feeds, Mn can range from 10 mg/kg in corn and grain-based diets to 100 mg/kg in diets based on ryegrass and clover.

Although excessive Mn can produce toxic effects, it is considered to be among the less toxic of the essential trace elements. For example, chicks, calves, pigs, and sheep can tolerate diets up to 3000, 1000, 500, and 200 mg Mn/kg, respectively. In animals, the primary lesion associated with dietary Mn toxicosis is an induction of Fe deficiency, which is thought to result from Mn and Fe sharing similar transporters (Aschner et al., 2007). In humans working in environments contaminated with Mn, overt signs of toxicity (usually by inhalation) can occur after months of chronic exposure. These signs are characterized by psychiatric disorders that include memory impairment, disorientation, hallucination, speech disturbances, and compulsive behavior and signs of Parkinson-like tremors and gait (Keen et al., 1999). Disturbance in carbohydrate metabolism may also occur. With acute Mn toxicity, there is a rapid uptake of Mn by the pancreas, a sharp reduction in circulating insulin, and an increase in plasma glucose. Thus, similar to Mn deficiency, Mn toxicity can affect insulin production or release from the pancreas (Keen et al., 2000, Harris, 2014). Acute manganese toxicity has been recently reported in a dog that consumed 100 joint supplements containing manganese ascorbate (Borchers et al., 2014). It was determined that the dog consumed 86 mg Mn/kg of body weight. Progression to fulminant liver failure prompted euthanasia in this case.

24.6.4 Molybdenum

24.6.4.1 Overview

The most important function of Mo is as a cofactor for xanthine dehydrogenase/oxidase, aldehyde oxidase, and sulfite oxidase (Brondino et al., 2006). Mo is present in these enzymes as molybdopterin or Mo cofactor (Figure 24.21).

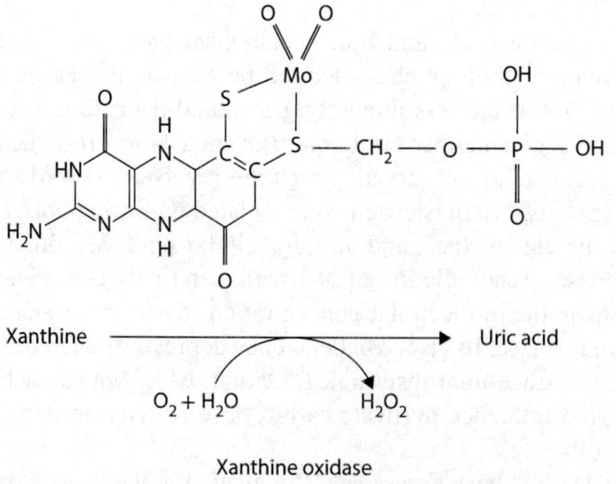

O O
Mo
OH
O
S
H
N C S — CH_2 — O — P — OH
HN C
O
H_2N N N
H
O
Xanthine → Uric acid
$O_2 + H_2O$ H_2O_2
Xanthine oxidase

FIGURE 24.21 Molybdenum cofactor. Mo as molybdate enters cells by way of oxyanion transporters. A series of complex condensation and reductive steps (e.g., formation of the pterin precursor from guanidine triphosphate and condensation with Mo) results in the formation of the molybdenum cofactor. The cofactor is essential for the activities of sulfite oxidase, xanthine dehydrogenase, and aldehyde oxidase.

24.6.4.2 Metabolism

Other than thiomolybdates (see Section 24.6.2), Mo is well absorbed by all species. It has been proposed that a carrier-mediated process transports Mo and that sulfate and Mo (as molybdate) compete for the same carrier. Excretion in nonruminants appears to be mostly via the kidney, in contrast to ruminants, wherein fecal and milk losses are more significant.

24.6.4.3 Functions

Mo-containing xanthine dehydrogenase exists in two interconvertible forms, xanthine dehydrogenase and xanthine oxidase. In its dehydrogenase form, xanthine dehydrogenase catalyzes the reaction:

$$XH + 1/2\,[H_2O] + NAD^{+} \rightarrow XO + NADH + H^{+}$$

The common substrate (XH) is a purine. Uric acid is a metabolic endpoint (XO). In its oxidase form, the enzyme transfers the reducing equivalent generated by oxidation of substrates to molecular oxygen, with the resultant production of superoxide anion and hydrogen peroxide. For example, during ischemia, reperfusion and/or reoxygenation of an injured tissue can occur, and xanthine dehydrogenase can be converted to xanthine oxidase. In the oxidase form, the reaction sequence is

$$XH + H_2O + O_2 \rightarrow HXO + H_2O_2$$

Given that in such conditions, ATP is usually depleted and there is an increase in the purine pool, increased quantities of superoxide radicals may be released and can be a major source of tissue peroxidation.

Aldehyde oxidase is a related Mo enzyme that catalyzes many of the same reactions as xanthine dehydrogenase. Both of these enzymes are needed in ruminants to catabolize exogenous pyrimidines. The third known Mo enzyme is sulfite oxidase, a mitochondrial enzyme that catalyzes the oxidation of sulfite to sulfate during the degradation of sulfur amino acids.

24.6.4.4 Requirements, Pharmacology, and Toxicity

Deficiencies of Mo are rare. The requirement is no more than 0.15–0.3 mg/kg of diet for most animals. Genetic disorders involving Mo cofactor production are also rare (e.g., 100 cases have been reported in humans). Low levels of the Mo cofactor cause toxic levels of sulfite with accompanying neurological damage (Schwarz and Mendel, 2006).

The clinical signs of Mo toxicity are characterized by achromotrichia, anemia, cartilaginous dysplasia, abnormal endochondrial ossification, subperiosteal ossification, and abnormal fibrogenesis. The clinical signs of molybdenosis also include lameness, weight loss, anorexia, loss of color, and quality of the wool or hair, and in cattle, diarrhea. These lesions are characteristic signs of an induced Cu deficiency.

24.6.5 Selenium

24.6.5.1 Overview

A nutritional need for selenium (Se) is now well established, although before 1950 Se was viewed as a potential carcinogen. Se plays an important role in thyroid hormone metabolism, antioxidant defense, and immune function (Foster and Sumar, 1997). Se as selenocysteine is at the active site of a wide range of selenoproteins. Many provocative clinical studies suggest putative roles for Se in cancer protection, ROS protection, and even relationships involving viral exposure.

24.6.5.2 Metabolism

Both organic and inorganic forms of Se can be utilized in the body. The order of uptake is SeO_3^{-2} < or = to selenocysteine < selenomethionine < SeO_4^{-2}. Both amino acid related and anion transporters are involved in Se transport (Figure 24.20). Many of the details, however, have yet to be resolved. The transport of SeO_4^{-2} is inhibited by thiosulfate, but not sulfate. A Na^+, K^+-ATPase is probably responsible for energizing the brush-border transport of selenate, where the ileum is the site of absorption. Some inflammatory intestinal diseases and short-bowel syndrome can lead to Se deficiency. In contrast to intestinal cells, selenate, selenite, selenomethionine, and selenocysteine, or selenite injected intravenously is each taken up rapidly and selectively through an anion-exchange carrier or transporter (Burk and Hill, 2009).

Absorption of Se occurs mainly in the duodenum with little evidence of uptake by the rumen, abomasums, stomach, jejunum, or ileum. In monogastric animals, absorption of soluble forms of Se is very high (>80%) and does not appear to be homeostatically controlled (Foster and Sumar, 1997). Absorption of Se in ruminants is lower than in nonruminants (about 40%), presumably because of the reduction of selenite to insoluble forms of Se in the rumen. Elemental Se and Se sulfide are not absorbed to any appreciable degree. After absorption, there appears to be a rapid distribution of water-soluble Se compounds to most organs. Transport in plasma to various organs seems to involve a specific selenoprotein, selenoprotein P. Se is found throughout the body with highest concentrations in the kidney and liver (0.5–1.5 and 0.2–0.8 µg/g, respectively). Skeletal muscle has a mean Se concentration of about 0.0.1–0.2 µg/g and accounts for about 50% of the total body pool (Sunde, 1990).

A novel aspect of Se regulation is that its insertion into protein occurs posttranscriptionally (Lu and Holmgren, 2009). Such occurrence of this element in protein is widespread. The knowledge that Se is incorporated as SeCys has modified our understanding of the genetic code (Lu and Holmgren, 2009). The formation of SeCys with its novel codon expanded to 21 the codon usage for the naturally occurring amino acids. Although it was recognized in the mid-1960s that the codon, AUG, had a dual role of initiating protein synthesis and inserting methionine at protein translation start sites, the possibility that a second codon also had two functions was not considered at the time. It is now known that UGA serves both as a termination and a SeCys codon. SeCys can be attached to tRNACys by cysteinyl-tRNA synthetase and can be incorporated nonspecifically into protein in

TABLE 24.9
Selenium-Containing Proteins

Protein	Function
Glutathione peroxidase (GPx) 1–8	An enzyme family with peroxidase activity lipid hydroperoxides and H_2O_2 is reduced to its corresponding alcohols and water, respectively. GPx1 is the most abundant with H_2O_2 as the preferred substrate. GPx4 has a preference for lipid hydroperoxides. GPx2 is an intestinal and extracellular enzyme. GPx3 is extracellular and abundant in plasma. Four other variants have also been identified.
Iodothyronine deiodinase (ID) 1–3	In the tissues, deiodinase either activates thyroid hormones by converting thyroxin (T4) to the active hormone triiodothyronine (T3) through the removal of an iodine on the outer ring or inactivates by removal of iodine on the inner ring, which converts T3 to the inactive diiodothyroxine (T2). ID 1 is found in liver and kidney, ID 2 in the thyroid and adipose, and ID 3 in fetal tissue and placenta.
Selenoproteins and variants	SEPN1, associated with respiratory distress and muscular dystrophy. SEPP1, a heparin-binding protein that appears to be associated with endothelial cells and has been suggested to function as an antioxidant in the extracellular space and in extracellular transport of selenium to targeted cells. SEPW1, found in skeletal muscle and acts as a methionine sulfoxide reductase. SMCP, sperm mitochondrial-associated cysteine-rich protein.
Thioredoxin reductases 1–3	Thioredoxin reductases catalyze the reduction of thioredoxin using NADPH as a reducing agent.

response to Cys codons, which is the reason why many proteins contain Se at sites other than the Se-containing active sites in selenoenzymes.

The translation of selenoprotein mRNAs requires both cis-acting and trans-acting factors (Lu and Holmgren, 2009; Burk and Hill, 2009). SeCys is inserted into nascent selenopeptides in mammals using a unique amino acid insertion system. Distinct 3′-UTR mRNA structures, designated SECIS elements, function in recruiting SBP2, a SeCys-specific elongation factor, and selenocysteine-tRNASer, SeCys, into the SeCys insertion complex, designated the selenosome. SeCys tRNASer, SeCys is used both as the site for SeCys biosynthesis and its incorporation into the active site of specific selenoproteins. Recent work also suggests considerable complexity in the regulation of specific selenoenzymes (Burk and Hill, 2009), for example, transcriptional as well as translational regulatory controls exist for GPx.

24.6.5.3 Functions

Examples of important selenoproteins are noted in Table 24.9. The best defined functionally is GPx. GPx catalyzes the reduction of hydrogen and organic peroxides (ROOH) to their respective alcohols and water (Margis et al., 2008). It is now recognized that there are two different GPx activities in tissues, one that is Se-dependent and a second, which is not. The non-Se-dependent GPx enzymes are referred to as GSH S-transferases, and their activities can increase under conditions of severe Se deficiency. There are several isozymes encoded by different genes that vary in cellular location and substrate specificity. GPx1 is the most abundant and is found in the cytoplasm. Although H_2O_2 is the preferred substrate ($2GSH + H_2O_2 \rightarrow GS–SG + 2H_2O$, where GSH represents reduced monomeric glutathione, and GS–SG represents glutathione disulfide), fatty acid and other lipid peroxides (ROOH) also function as substrates. The product is an acyl moiety wherein the [-OOH] group is converted to a [-OH] group. Mice genetically designed to lack GPx1 are in many respects phenotypically normal, indicating that the enzyme is not critical for life. However, GPx1 belongs to the family of GPxs, which consists of eight known mammalian isoenzymes. Mice lacking GPx4, which differs from the other GPx family members regarding its protein structure and less restricted dependence on glutathione, die during early embryonic development. GPx4 can reduce lipid-hydroperoxides, specifically phospholipids, inside biological membranes (Burk and Hill, 2009).

Another family of selenoproteins is the 1,5′-iodothyronine deiodinases (Beckett and Arthur, 2005). The 5′-monodeiodination of thyroxin, the major secretory product of the thyroid gland, to its active form 3, 3′, and 5-triiodothyronine is catalyzed by 1,5′-ID. In Se deficiency, the activity of 1,5′-ID is decreased along with the concentration of thyroxin. Also, a 5′-ID occurs in peripheral tissues (e.g., liver, kidney, and muscle), which can remove the remaining iodine group at the five position.

Moreover, there are also proteins that have been identified that are important to Se transport and delivery to organelles and tissues (Burk and Hill, 2009), for example, the plasma protein; selenoprotein P. Selenoprotein P is an abundant extracellular glycoprotein that is rich in selenocysteine. At least four isoforms of selenoprotein P have been identified. In rats, it has been estimated that 25% of whole-body Se passes through selenoprotein P each day. Selenoprotein P knockout mice have low Se concentrations in the brain, testis, and fetus. Measurement of selenoprotein P in human plasma has shown that it is depressed by Se deficiency and by cirrhosis. Of potential importance, Se supplementation optimizes GPx activity before Se in selenoprotein P is optimized, indicating that plasma selenoprotein P can be a useful index for assessing Se nutritional status (Burk and Hill, 2009).

The primary biochemical lesions that are associated with Se deficiency are low GPx and 5′-ID activities. Excess cellular free radical damage can be the initial lesion underlying the widespread pathologies. Consistent with this idea are the observations that simultaneous deficiencies of other antioxidants (i.e., hypovitaminosis E and A) amplify the signs of Se deficiency when they occur (Foster and Sumar, 1997). Nutritional muscular dystrophy (white muscle disease) is a Se-responsive disorder that can affect farm animals (sheep, cattle, pigs, horses, and poultry). This myopathy is associated with excessive peroxidation of lipids, particularly the mitochondrial lipids, resulting in degeneration, necrosis, and subsequent fibrosis of myofibers (Lenz and Lens, 2009). Often this is associated with cardiac involvement and, depending on the species, hepatic necrosis. Poultry and swine can be affected by exudative diathesis and edematous conditions that respond to supplemental Se. Testicular degeneration and impaired sperm production and infertility occur with Se deficiency. In humans, Keshan disease is an endemic congestive cardiomyopathy that affects primarily children and women of childbearing age with lesions that are very similar to the characteristic lesions of nutritional cardiomyopathy associated with white muscle disease in animals (Foster and Sumar, 1997).

The study of Keshan disease also led to an association between Se and increased susceptibility to infection with certain enteroviruses. The discovery that the cardiomyopathy of Keshan disease likely had a dual etiology (nutritional and infectious) provided impetus for additional studies of relationships between Se nutritional status and viral infection. It was observed that an amyocarditic strain of coxsackievirus B3, CVB3/0, was converted to a highly virulent strain when it was inoculated into Se-deficient mice. Similar alterations in virulence and genomic composition of CVB3/0 were next observed in GPx knockout mouse models (Beck et al., 2003).

24.6.5.4 Requirements, Pharmacology, and Toxicity

Plants are the primary dietary sources of Se. In general, requirements for Se range from 200 to 400 μg/kg of diet for most species. Although rare, there is also a health risk of too much Se (selenosis). Symptoms include gastrointestinal irritation, hair loss, changes in hoof and nail texture, and nerve damage (Schrauzer, 2003). Three types of Se toxicity have been identified in livestock: acute and chronic blind staggers and chronic alkali disease. Abnormal movement and posture, breathing difficulties, diarrhea, and rapid death characterize acute Se toxicity. Chronic Se toxicity of the blind staggers type occurs when animals consume Se-toxic accumulator plants (usually over a period of weeks or months).

24.6.6 Zinc

24.6.6.1 Overview

Zn functions at the active site of many enzymes by facilitating strong, but readily exchangeable, substrate or ligand binding (Harris, 2014). Zn is not capable of redox. Thus, it can be used biologically in novel ways at the functional sites of proteins without causing oxidative changes. Zn also plays important structural roles in proteins. One example is the Zn-finger motif, the most common recurring motif in proteins that serve as transcription factors.

24.6.6.2 Metabolism

The primary site of absorption of exogenous Zn is the proximal small bowel, either the distal duodenum or proximal jejunum. Absorption studies in animal models indicate an inverse relationship between the percentage of Zn absorbed and dietary Zn intake (Harris, 2014; O'Dell and Sunde, 1997). In cattle, about one-third of the Zn is absorbed from the abomasum. In most species, the initial absorption of Zn is about 10%–20%. Phytate (myoinositol hexaphosphate), which is found in all plant seeds and most roots and tubers, can significantly inhibit Zn absorption. Moreover, high dietary Fe decreases Zn absorption, although its significance concerning overall Zn balance can be questioned. Several amino acids form Zn complexes with high stability constants and it has been suggested that such complex formation facilities Zn uptake. Zn absorption is higher in neonates than in adults and is increased in Zn-deficient animals. The physiological state also affects absorption; pregnancy and lactation can enhance absorption.

Plasma Zn is associated with albumin (about 90%) and α-2 macroglobulin (about 10%). Less than 1% is complexed to other plasma components. Zn homeostasis is achieved largely by enterohepatic recirculation. A primary source of Zn in the intestinal lumen is also from pancreatic secretions, because of Zn's importance as a cofactor for pancreatic peptidases, various hydrolases, and proteinases.

As is the case for other essential metals, several transporter systems have been identified for Zn based on corresponding homologs in yeasts (Figure 24.20). Two distinct families of Zn transporters are known: the ZIP family that imports Zn and the ZnT family that functions in releasing Zn or sequestering Zn internally (Lichten and Cousins, 2009). The ZIP transporters are found in the duodenum in the crypts and lower villi and appear available for the uptake of several metal ions, including Zn. Uptake assays demonstrate that Cu^{+1} and Fe^{+2} can be potential substrates, as they inhibit Zn+2 uptake, whereas Co^{+2}, Mn^{+2}, Mg^{+2}, and Ni^{+2} have no effect on Zn^{+2} uptake. Given that about 10% of the total proteome has Zn binding domains, the importance of Zn^{+2} transporters and their regulation becomes very clear (Kambe et al., 2015). Such transporters help to regulate processes ranging from proteolytic to neurological functions (Kambe et al., 2015; Chowanadisai et al., 2013).

The ZIP transporters are under transcriptional control based on the observation that one of the family of ZIP transporters, ZRT1, is inversely expressed relative to cellular Zn+2 levels; Zn^{+2} depleted cells have 10-fold more ZRT1 mRNA than do Zn^{+2}-repleted cells. There is also evidence for posttranslational regulation. When cellular Zn is elevated, there is degradation of the transporters by vacuolar proteases (Lichten and Cousins, 2009; Kambe et al., 2015).

24.6.6.3 Functions

Specific biochemical changes associated with the clinical features of Zn deficiency are not easy to identify. As a general rule, epithelial cells and cells involved in immune function are most affected by Zn deprivation. The principal biochemical lesion centers on the non-coordination of events critical to the differentiation of cells; perhaps related to the important function that Zn plays in transcription factor integrity and structure (Harris, 2014; Failla, 2003; Keen and Gershwin, 1990). Of interest, there are greater changes in immune responsiveness than in changes in the activities of Zn-requiring enzymes. Zn deficiency can also have a significant impact on the hormonal regulation of cell division, specifically alterations in the pituitary growth hormone (GH) and insulin-like growth factor-I (IGF-I) axes. Changes in the concentrations of GH are observed in Zn deficiency and circulating IGF-I is decreased. Other evidence suggests that Zn deficiency can also alter cell membrane integrity and membrane-signaling systems as well as coordination of intracellular second messengers critical to cell proliferation (Keen and Gershwin, 1990; MacDonald, 2000). Moreover, circulating IGF-I concentrations are decreased.

Zn is essential for the function of more than 200 enzymes. Zn-containing enzymes are found in all of the major metabolic pathways involved in carbohydrate, lipid, protein, and nucleic acid metabolism. Zn functions as a structural component of proteins, as a proton donor at the active site of enzymes, and as a bridging atom between substrates and their enzymes (e.g., carboxypeptidases, alkaline phosphatase, alcohol dehydrogenase, carbonic anhydrase, and superoxide dismutase).

Zn is also involved in stabilizing the structures of RNA, DNA, and ribosomes, wherein Zn facilitates conformational transformations of DNA (e.g., from beta to the Z forms). Further, a large number of nuclear binding proteins (mostly transcription factors) have Zn-binding domains (so-called Zn-binding fingers) (Harris, 2014).

Because of the wide range of functions, Zn deficiency signs are nonspecific and include periorificial (oral, anal, genital) and acral dermatitis, diarrhea, and behavioral and mental changes. Indices of normal immune function are also depressed. An early effect of severe Zn deficiency in many species is anorexia and cyclic feeding. The cyclical food intake patterns of Zn-deficient animals may represent an adaptation of the animal to the Zn-deficient state. During the periods of low food intake, there is muscle catabolism and measurable release of Zn into the plasma pool.

To reiterate, the most striking effect of an acute or marginal prenatal Zn deficiency is on the ontogeny of the immune system. In mice and rhesus monkeys, marginal prenatal Zn deficiency results in impairment in immunoglobulin M production and a decreased sensitivity to specific mitogens. Of interest are the observations that these immune defects can persist well into adulthood despite the introduction of Zn-replete diets at birth. Immune defects associated with postnatal Zn deficiency include reduced thymic hormone production and activity, impaired lymphocyte, natural killer cell and neutrophil function, and impaired antibody-dependent cell mediated cytotoxicity. Postulated defects include impaired cell replication, gene expression and cell motility, and alterations in cell surface recognition sites.

Genetic disorders of Zn metabolism are rare. However, at least five genetic errors in Zn metabolism that mimic Zn deficiency have been identified in mammals. They are Adema disease (inherited parakeratosis) of cattle (Yuzbasiyan-Gurkan and Bartlett, 2006), chondrodysplasia, congenital Zn deficiency (lethal acrodermatitis) in bull terriers (McEwan et al., 2000), acrodermatitis enteropathica (AE) in humans (MacDonald, 2000), and lethal milk syndrome in mice (Lee et al., 1992). AE responds dramatically to oral Zn supplementation when it occurs in children. AE is autosomal recessive and results from a mutation of the SLC39A4 gene on chromosome 8 q24.3. SLC39A4 encodes for ZIP4 in the family of Zn transporters (Lichten and Cousins, 2009). Bovine hereditary Zn deficiency, Adema disease, is an autosomal recessive disorder that also results in inadequate amounts of Zn being absorbed from the gastrointestinal tract and leads to a number of clinical abnormalities. The first manifestation is diarrhea, followed by skin lesions, poliosis, and a decreased ability to sustain a suckle reflex. It is similar in many respects to AE in humans. The oral administration of Zn acetate causes a reversal of biochemical abnormalities in affected calves. Adema disease occurs predominately in black pied cattle of Friesan descent. An additional sign of the disease is delayed sexual maturation, which is common in many species that are Zn deprived. Mature dwarfs produce spermatozoa with 45% acrosomal defects compared to 5% in controls. Significantly, this defect in spermatozoa is reportedly reversed by dietary Zn supplementation. Lethal milk syndrome is an autosomal recessive disorder caused by a mutant gene in the C57BL/6J(B6) mouse strain (Lee et al., 1992). Offspring which suckle from affected dams exhibit stunted growth, alopecia, dermatitis, immune incompetence, and rarely survive past weaning.

Zn responsive dermatosis is a well-documented disease in dogs. When congenital, it is an autosomal recessive disorder in bull terriers (MacDonald, 2000; McEwan et al., 2000). The phenotypic expression of lethal acrodermatitis in Bull Terriers is very similar to experimental Zn deficiency in dogs. A similar disorder has also been reported in northern-breed dogs (Alaskan Malamute, Samoyed, and Siberian Husky). Although these dogs are consuming Zn-adequate diets, they frequently require Zn supplementation, either orally or parenterally, in some cases throughout their entire life span. Chondrodysplasia (short-limbed dwarfism) is a sign related to the phenomenon in Alaskan Malamute.

Fortunately, the risk for Zn toxicity and the likelihood of achieving excessive dietary intakes of Zn are both low. Zn has been characterized as a relatively nontoxic element with a wide margin of safety. One notable exception is consumption of zinc-containing foreign bodies, which has been documented in humans as well as a wide variety of wild and companion animals. Everyday items associated with zinc toxicity include batteries, zinc-containing creams, zippers, screws/nuts (usually from pet carriers), and pennies minted in the United States in 1983 and later. Investigating the potential presence of a gastrointestinal metallic foreign object is prudent in any case of unexplained hemolytic anemia. For more chronic intakes, toxicity is usually not diagnosed until Zn intake exceeds about 700 mg or more per kg of diet (O'Dell and Sunde, 1997; Harris, 2014). Gastrointestinal, renal, hepatic, pancreatic, and pulmonary systems are the most consistently and severely involved.

24.6.7 Trace Mineral Assessment

Good analytical methodology is essential to data interpretation regarding trace mineral nutritional or toxicological status. Similar to the accelerator mass spectrometry approaches used to assess vitamin status (see Section 24.4.4), inductively coupled plasma mass spectrometry, and newer methods employing atomic absorption or chemical X-ray fluorescence analyses allow determinations that extend to femtomole range (Tranter et al., 2000; Taylor, 2001; Todoli and Mermet, 2008). It is no longer tolerable to base judgments using methods that introduced error so that values vary substantially from experiment to experiment. As an example, this was the case for chromium measurements during the first two decades of work that was used to define its putative importance, during which errors of two orders of magnitude were tolerated (Mertz, 1993).

Regarding approaches to assessment, tissue concentrations of given minerals can be measured; however, of the six metals discussed only selenium plasma or serum levels reflect prior dietary history with any reliability (Burk and Hill, 2009). Tissue and cellular compartments may also be used. For given well-defined studies, the levels of metals in leukocyte, lymphocyte, and neutrophil compartments may have value for assessment, although as general biomarkers there is currently inadequate validation (Hambidge, 2003). For example, erythrocyte-membrane zinc has been found to be sensitive to dietary zinc restriction, although there are exceptions that have been reported. Moreover, the use of urine or fecal metal concentrations as a biomarker requires a good understanding of the homeostatic mechanisms related to absorption transport and elimination of the given mineral. In some cases, the activity of a metalloenzyme of serum level of a metalloprotein can be used, but again as markers, they may be only specific in the context of well-defined guidelines. The measurement of ceruloplasmin or lysyl oxidase activities for the assessment of copper is an example. Both proteins bind more copper than is needed for optimal activity (Harris, 2000; Rucker et al., 1998). In certain conditions, such as Wilson's disease in which copper is sequestered in cells, the activity of the enzyme in plasma or serum may be quite variable. Likewise, the insensitivity of plasma zinc to reductions in dietary zinc reflects the capacity of the organism to conserve tissue zinc by reductions in zinc excretion, reductions in the rate of growth, or utilization of zinc from sequestration sites (e.g., bone). Accordingly, metallothionein plasma concentrations have been used to reflect hepatic Zn concentrations analogous to the use of ferritin levels, the degree of transferrin iron saturation, or transferrin receptors levels as indirect measures of iron status. For metallothionein, however, the caveats are that its plasma levels change in response to stress, infection, and other metabolic conditions (Hambidge, 2003). Similarly, lymphocyte metallothionein or changes in metallothionein lymphocyte mRNA levels have been suggested as a marker for zinc status (Hambidge, 2003), however, there are examples wherein lymphocyte metallothionein mRNA concentrations do not reflect the differences in dietary zinc supplementation (Carlson et al., 2007).

24.7 CONCLUDING COMMENTS

As is the case for all substances that are relevant to given biological functions, a limitation or excess of an essential vitamin or mineral can result in specific pathological signs and symptoms. That applies particularly to any given vitamin, dietary growth factor, or mineral when there is a loss due to processing, storage, or as often is the case, the consumption of monotonous or nutritionally limiting diet. Concerning each of the nutrients described in this chapter, it may be inferred that fundamental evolutionary processes have led to a physiological need that for most animals are similar on a metabolic basis. Usually, dietary requirements differ depending on the animal's ability to produce the substance. Indeed, there is usually a good biological question to be asked when an organism deviates markedly from an allometric scale that defines metabolic or physiological need. New analytical tools have increased sensitivity in some cases to the attomole to femtomole range along with the ability to carry out high-throughput assays. There is no doubt that the next decades will allow expansion of our current understanding of vitamin and mineral function, particularly in areas such as epigenetics, cell signaling, nuclear organization and regulation, and species systematics.

REFERENCES

Akagawa, M., Minematsu, K., Shibata, T., Kondo, T., Ishii, T., and Uchida, K. 2016. Identification of lactate dehydrogenase as a mammalian pyrroloquinoline quinone (PQQ)-binding protein. *Sci Rep.* 6:26723.

Akagawa, M., Nakano, M., and Ikemoto, K. 2015. Recent progress in studies on the health benefits of pyrroloquinoline quinone. *Biosci Biotechnol Biochem.* 80:13–22.

Ammerman, C., Baker, D., and Lewis, A. 1995. *Bioavailability of Nutrient for Animals: Amino Acids, Minerals, and Vitamins*, pp. 1–443. New York, NY: Academic Press.

Andrès, E., Noel, E., and Ben Abdelghani, M. 2003. Vitamin B12 deficiency associated with chronic acid suppression therapy. *Ann Pharmacother.* 37:1730–1735.

Aschner, M., Guilarte, T.R., Schneider, J.S., and Zheng, W. 2007. Manganese: Recent advances in understanding its transport and neurotoxicity. *Toxicol Appl Pharmacol.* 221:131–147.

Backus, R.C., Cohen, G., Pion, P.D., Good, K.L., Rogers, Q.R., and Fascetti, A.J. 2003. Taurine deficiency in Newfoundlands fed commercially available complete and balanced diets. *J Am Vet Med Assoc.* 223:1130–1136.

Backus, R.C., Rogers, Q.R., Rosenquist, G.L., Calam, J., and Morris, J.G. 1995. Diets causing taurine depletion in cats substantially elevate postprandial plasma cholecystokinin concentration. *J Nutr.* 125:2650–2657.

Baily, L. 2014. Folic acid. In *Handbook of Vitamins*. Eds. J. Zempleni, J. Suttie, J. Gregory, and P.J. Stover, 5th edition, pp. 421–446. New York, NY: Taylor & Francis.

Baker, H., Schor, S.M., Murphy, B.D., De Angelis, B., Feigngold, S., and Frank, O. 1986. Blood vitamin and choline concentrations in healthy domestic cats, dogs and horses. *AJVR.* 47:1468–1471.

Balk, L., Hagerroth, P.A., Akerman, G., et al. 2009. Wild birds of declining European species are dying from a thiamine deficiency syndrome. *Proc Natl Acad Sci U S A.* 106:12001–12006.

Banerjee, R. 2006. B12 trafficking in mammals: A for coenzyme escort service. *ACS Chem Biol.* 1:149–159.

Barceloux, D. 1999. Cobalt. *J Toxicol Clin Toxicol.* 37:201–206.

Batchelor, D.J., Noble, P.J., Taylor, R.H., Cripps, P.J., and German, A.J. 2007. Prognostic factors in canine exocrine pancreatic insufficiency: Prolonged survival is likely if clinical remission is achieved. *J Vet Intern Med.* 21:54–60.

Beck, M.A., Levander, O.A., and Handy, J. 2003. Selenium deficiency and viral infection. *J Nutr.* 133: 1463S–1467S.

Beckett, G.J., and Arthur, J.R. 2005. Selenium and endocrine systems. *J Endocrinol.* 184:455–465.

Bell, J. 1999. Ferret nutrition. *Vet Clin North Am Exot Anim Pract.* 2:169–192.

Bettendorff, L. 1994. Thiamine in excitable tissues: Reflections on a non-cofactor role. *Metab Brain Dis.* 9:183–209.

Bettendorff, L., and Wins, P. 2009. Thiamin diphosphate in biological chemistry: New aspects of thiamin metabolism, especially triphosphate derivatives acting other than as cofactors. *FEBS J.* 276:2917–2925.

Bettendorff, L., Kolb, H.A., and Schoffeniels, E. 1993. Thiamine triphosphate activates an anion channel of large unit conductance in neuroblastoma cells. *J Membr Biol.* 136:281–288.

Bettendorff, L., Wirtzfeld, B., Makarchikov, A.F., et al. 2007. Discovery of a natural thiamine adenine nucleotide. *Nat Chem Biol.* 3:211–212.

Blanchard, G., Paragon, B.M., Milliat, F., and Lutton, C. 2002. Dietary L-carnitine supplementation in obese cats alters carnitine metabolism and decreases ketosis during fasting and induced hepatic lipidosis. *J Nutr.* 132:204–210.

Boland, C., Hayes, P., Santa-Maria, I., Nishimura, S., and Kelly, V.P. 2009. Queuosine formation in eukaryotic tRNA occurs via a mitochondria-localized heteromeric transglycosylase. *J Biol Chem.* 284:18218–18227.

Bompadre, S., Tulipani, S., Romandini, S., Giorgetti, R., and Battino, M. 2008. Improved HPLC column-switching determination of Coenzyme Q and vitamin E in plasma. *Biofactors.* 32:257–262.

Booth, S.L. 2009. Roles for vitamin K beyond coagulation. *Annu Rev Nutr.* 29:89–110.

Borchers, A., Epstein, S.E., Gindiciosi, B., Cartoceti, A., and Puschner, B. 2014. Acute enteral manganese intoxication with hepatic failure due to ingestion of a joint supplement overdose. *J Vet Diag Invest.* 25:658–663.

Brondino, C.D., Romao, M.J., Moura, I., and Moura, J.J. 2006. Molybdenum and tungsten enzymes: The xanthine oxidase family. *Curr Opin Chem Biol.* 10:109–114.

Burk, R., and Hill, K. 2009. Selenoprotein P-expression, functions, and roles in mammals. *Biochim Biophys Acta.* 1790:1441–1447.

Carlson, D., Beattie, J., and Poulsen, H. 2007. Assessment of zinc and copper status in weaned piglets in relation to dietary zinc and copper supply. *J Anim Physiol Anim Nutr (Berl).* 91:19–28.

Carpenter, K.J. 1986. *The History of Scurvy and Vitamin C*, Chap. 3, pp. 43–74. London: Cambridge University Press.

Ceh, L., Helgebostad, A., and Ender, F. 1964. Thiaminase in capelin (*Mallotus villosus*), an arctic fish of the salmonidae family. *Int Z Vitaminforsch.* 34:189–196.

Center, S.A., Warner, K., Corbett, J., Randolph, J.F., and Erb, H.N. 2000. Proteins invoked by vitamin K absence and clotting times in clinically ill cats. *JVIM.* 14:292–297.

Challem, J.J. 1999. Toward a new definition of essential nutrients: Is it now time for a third 'vitamin' paradigm? *Med Hypotheses.* 52:417–422.

Chowanadisai, W., Bauerly, K.A., Tchaparian, E., Wong, A.. Cortopassi, G.A., and Rucker, R.B. 2010. Pyrroloquinoline quinone stimulates mitochondrial biogenesis through cAMP response element-binding protein phosphorylation and increased PGC-1alpha expression. *J Biol Chem.* 285:142–152.

Chowanadisai, W., Graham, D.M., Keen, C.L., Rucker, R.B., and Messerli, M.A. 2013. Neurulation and neurite extension require the zinc transporter ZIP12 (slc39a12). *Proc Natl Acad Sci U S A.* 110:9903–9908.

Chu, S.H., and Hegsted, D.M. 1980a. Myo-inositol deficiency in gerbils: Changes in phospholipid composition of intestinal microsomes. *J Nutr.* 110:1217–1223.

Chu, S.H., and Hegsted, D.M. 1980b. Myo-inositol deficiency in gerbils: Comparative study of the intestinal lipodystrophy in *Meriones unguiculatus* and *Meriones libycus*. *J Nutr.* 110:1209–1216.

Chua, A.C., and Morgan, E.H. 1997. Manganese metabolism is impaired in the Belgrade laboratory rat. *J Comp Physiol B.* 167:361–369.

Cui, C.T., Uriu-Adams, J.Y., Tchaparian, E.H., Keen, C.L., and Rucker, R.B. 2004. Metavanadate causes cellular accumulation of copper and decreased lysyl oxidase activity. *Toxicol Appl Pharmacol.* 199:35–43.

Dakshinamurti, S., and Dakshinamurti, K. 2014. Vitamin B6. In *Handbook of Vitamins*. Eds. J. Zempleni, J. Suttie, J. Gregory, and P.J. Stover, 5th edition, pp. 351–396. New York, NY: Taylor & Francis.

Davis, J.M., Murphy, E.A., Carmichael, M.D., and Davis, B. 2009. Quercetin increases brain and muscle mitochondrial biogenesis and exercise tolerance. *Am J Physiol Regul Integr Comp Physiol.* 296:R1071–R1077.

De Colibus, L., and Mattevi, A. 2008. New frontiers in structural flavoenzymology. *Curr Opin Struct Biol.* 16:722–728.

De Roode, D.F., Balk, L., and Koeman, J.H. 2000. Development of a bioassay to test the possible role of thiamine disturbance as a mechanism behind pollution-induced reproductive failures in birds. *Arch Environ Contam Toxicol.* 39:386–391.

Depeint, F., Bruce, W.R., Shangari, N., Mehta, R., and O'Brien, P.J. 2006. Mitochondrial function and toxicity: Role of B vitamins on the one-carbon transfer pathways. *Chem Biol Interact.* 163:113–132.

Desilvestro, R.A., Hinchcliff, K.W., and Blostein-Fujii, A. 2005. Sustained strenuous exercise in sled dogs depresses three copper enzyme activities. *Bio Trace Element Res.* 105:87–96.

Doberenz, J., Birkenfeld, C., Kluge, H., and Eder, K. 2006. Effects of L-carnitine supplementation in pregnant sows on plasma concentrations of insulin-like growth factors, various hormones and metabolites and chorion characteristics. *J Anim Physiol Anim Nutr (Berl).* 90:487–499.

Domoslawska, A., Jurczak, A., and Janowski, T. 2013. Oral folic acid supplementation decreases palate and/or lip cleft occurrence in Pug or Chihuahua puppies and elevates folic acid blood levels in pregnant bitches. *Pol J Vet Sci.* 16:33–37.

Doong, G., Keen, C.L., Rogers, Q., Morris, J., and Rucker, R.B. 1983. Selected features of copper metabolism in the cat. *J Nutr.* 113:1963–1971.

Ebeler, S.E., Dingley, K.H., Ubick, E., et al. 2005. Animal models and analytical approaches for understanding the relationships between wine and cancer. *Drugs Exp Clin Res.* 31:19–27.

Edgar, S.E., Kirk, C.A., Rogers, Q.R., and Morris, J.G. 1998. Taurine status in cats is not maintained by dietary cysteinesulfinic acid. *J Nutr.* 128:751–757.

Eitenmiller, E., and Landen, W. 1998. *Vitamin Analysis for the Health and Food Sciences*, pp. 1–544. Cambridge: Woodhead Publishing Limited.

Ellison, R.S. 2002. Major trace elements limiting livestock performance in New Zealand. *N Z Vet J.* 50:35–40.

Failla, M.L. 2003. Trace elements and host defense: Recent advances and continuing challenges. *J Nutr.* 133:1443S–1447S.

Farkas, W.R. 1980. Effect of diet on the queuosine family of tRNAs of germ-free mice. *J Biol Chem.* 255: 6832–6835.

Fascetti, A.J., Reed, J.R., Rogers, Q.R., and Backus, R.C. 2003. Taurine deficiency in dogs with dilated cardiomyopathy: 12 cases (1997–2001). *J Am Vet Med Assoc.* 223:1137–1141.

Fascetti, A.J., Rogers, Q.R., and Morris, J.G. 2000. Dietary copper influences reproduction in cats. *J Nutr.* 130:1287–1290.

Fascetti, A.J., Rogers, Q.R., and Morris, J.G. 2002. Blood copper concentrations and cuproenzyme activities in a colony of cats. *Vet Clin Pathol.* 31:183–188.

Fekete, S.G., Fodor, K., Prohászik, A., and Andrásofszky, E. 2005. Comparison of feed preference and digestion of three different commercial diets for cats and ferrets. *J Anim Physiol Anim Nutr (Berl).* 89:199–202.

Festen, H.P. 1991. Intrinsic factor secretion and cobalamin absorption. Physiology and pathophysiology in the gastrointestinal tract. *Scand J Gastroenterol Suppl.* 188:1–7.

Fieten, H., Hooijer-Nouwens, B.D., Biourge, V.C., et al. 2015. Association of dietary copper and zinc levels with hepatic copper and zinc concentration in Labrador Retrievers. *J Vet Int Med.* 29:822–827.

Finno, C.J., Estell, K., Katzman, S., et al. 2015. Blood and cerebrospinal fluid alpha-tocopherol and selenium concentrations in neonatal foals with neuroaxonal dystrophy. *J Vet Intern Med.* 29(6):1667–1675.

Finno, C.J., Miller, A.D., Sisó, S., et al. 2016. Concurrent equine degenerative myeloencephalopathy and equine motor neuron disease in three young horses. *J Vet Int Med.* 30:1344–1350.

Fitsanakis, V.A., Zhang, N., Garcia, S., and Aschner, M. 2010. Manganese (Mn) and iron (Fe): Interdependency of transport and regulation. *Neurotox Res.* 18:124–131.

Foster, D.J., Thoday, K.L., Arthur, J.R., et al. 2001. Selenium status of cats in four regions of the world and comparison with reported incidence of hyperthyroidism in cats in those regions. *AJVR.* 62:934–937.

Foster, L.H., and Sumar, S. 1997. Selenium in health and disease: A review. *Crit Rev Food Sci Nutr.* 37:211–228.

Freytag, T.L., Liu, S.M., Rogers, Q.R., and Morris, J.G. 2003. Teratogenic effects of chronic ingestion of high levels of vitamin A in cats. *J Anim Physiol Anim Nutr (Berl).* 87:42–51.

Fyfe J.C., Ramanujam, K.S., Ramaswamy, K., Patterson, D.F., and Seetharam, B. 1991. Defective brush-border expression of intrinsic factor-cobalamin receptor in canine inherited intestinal cobalamin malabsorption. *J Biol Chem.* 266:4489–4494.

Gangjee, A., Jain, H.D., and Kurup, S. 2007. Recent advances in classical and non-classical antifolates as antitumor and antiopportunistic infection agents: Part I. *Anticancer Agents Med Chem.* 7:524–542.

Gangjee, A., Jain, H.D., and Kurup, S. 2008. Recent advances in classical and non-classical antifolates as antitumor and antiopportunistic infection agents: Part II. *Anticancer Agents Med Chem.* 8:205–231.

Garrow, T. 2007. Choline. In *Handbook of Vitamins*. Eds. J. Zempleni, R.B. Rucker, J.W. Suttie, and D.B. McCormick, 4th edition, pp. 459–488. New York, NY: Taylor & Francis.

Geraci, J.R. 1974. Thiamine deficiency in seals and recommendations for its prevention. *J Am Vet Med Assoc.* 165:801–803.

Gerber, B., Hassig, M., and Reusch, C.E. 2003. Serum concentrations of 1,25-dihydroxycholecalciferol and 25-hydroxycholecalciferol in clinically normal dogs and dogs with acute and chronic renal failure. *AJVR.* 64:1161–1166.

Goldblith, S., and Joslyn, M. 1964. *Milestones in Nutrition*, Chap. 11, pp. 479–538. Westport, CT: Avi Publishing.

Goldy, G.G., Burr, J.R., Longardner, C.N., Hirakawa, D.A.S., and Norton, S.A. 1996. Effects of measured doses of vitamin A fed to healthy beagle dogs for 26 weeks. *Vet Clin Nutr.* 3:29–42.

Green, A.S., Tang, G., Lango, J., Klasing, K.C., and Fascetti, A.J. 2012. Domestic cats convert [2H8]-B-carotene to [2H4]-retinol following a single oral dose. *J Anim Physio Anim Nutr (Berl).* 96:681–692.

Green, R., and Miller, J. 2014. Vitamin B-12. In *Handbook of Vitamins*. Eds. J. Zempleni, J. Suttie, J. Gregory, and P.J. Stover, 5th edition, pp. 447–491. New York, NY: Taylor & Francis.

Hall, E.J., Bond, P.M., Mclean, C., Batt, R.M., Mclean, L. 1991. A survey of the diagnosis and treatment of canine exocrine pancreatic insufficiency. *J Sm Anim Pract.* 32:613–618.

Halsted, C.H. 1975. The small intestine in vitamin B12 and folate deficiency. *Nutr Rev.* 33:33–37.

Halsted, C.H. 1979. The intestinal absorption of folates. *Am J Clin Nutr.* 32:846–855.

Halsted, C.H., Ling, E.H., Luthi-Carter, R., Villanueva, J.A., Gardner, J.M., and Coyle, J.T. 2000. Folylpoly-gamma-glutamate carboxypeptidase from pig jejunum. Molecular characterization and relation to glutamate carboxypeptidase II. *J Biol Chem.* 275:30746.

Halsted, C.H., Reisenauer, A., Back, C., and Gotterer, G.S. 1976. In vitro uptake and metabolism of pteroylpolyglutamate by rat small intestine. *J Nutr.* 106:485–492.

Halsted, C.H., Reisenauer, A.M., Romero, J.J., Cantor, D.S., and Ruebner, B. 1977. Jejunal perfusion of simple and conjugated folates in celiac sprue. *J Clin Invest.* 59:933–940.

Halsted, C.H., Reisenauer, A.M., Shane, B., and Tamura, T. 1978. Availability of monoglutamyl and polyglutamyl folates in normal subjects and in patients with celiac sprue. *Gut.* 19:886–891.

Halsted, C.H., Villanueva, J.A., Devlin, A.M., et al. 2002. Folate deficiency disturbs hepatic methionine metabolism and promotes liver injury in the ethanol-fed micropig. *Proc Natl Acad Sci U S A.* 99:10072–10077.

Hambidge, M. 2003. Biomarkers of trace mineral intake and status. *J Nutr.* 133:948S–955S.

Harris, C.B., Chowanadisai, W., Mishchuk, D.O., Satre, M.A., Slupsky, C.M., and Rucker, R.B. 2013. Dietary pyrroloquinoline quinone (PQQ) alters indicators of inflammation and mitochondrial-related metabolism in human subjects. *J Nutr Biochem.* 24:2076–2084.

Harris, E.D. 2000. Cellular copper transport and metabolism. *Annu Rev Nutr.* 20:291–310.

Harris, E.D. 2014. *Minerals in Foods: Nutrition, Metabolism, Bioactivity*, pp. 1–361. Lancaster, PA: DEStech Publications.

Harrison, E.H. 2005. Mechanisms of digestion and absorption of dietary vitamin A. *Annu Rev Nutr.* 25:87–103.

Hathcock, J., Azzi, A., Blumberg, J., et al. 2005. Vitamins E and C are safe across a broad range of intakes. *Am J Clin Nutr.* 81:736–745.

Haywood, S. 2006. Copper toxicosis in Bedlington Terriers. *Vet Rec.* 159:687–689.

Hazewinkel, H.A.W., and Tryfonidou, M.A. 2002. Vitamin D3 metabolism in dogs. *Mol Cell Endo.* 197:23–33.

Hetzel, B.S. 1996. Iodine deficiency: A global problem. *Med J Aust.* 165:28–29.

Hickman, M.A., Rogers, Q.R., and Morris, J.G. 1990a. Effect of diet on Heinz body formation in kittens. *Am J Vet Res.* 51:475–478.

Hickman, M.A., Rogers, Q.R., and Morris, J.G. 1990b. Effect of processing on fate of dietary [14C]taurine in cats. *J Nutr.* 120:995–1000.

Hickman, M.A., Rogers, Q.R., and Morris, J.G. 1992. Taurine balance is different in cats fed purified and commercial diets. *J Nutr.* 122:553–559.

Higashi, T., Shibayama, Y., Fuji, M., and Shimada, K. 2008. Liquid chromatography-tandem mass spectrometric method for the determination of salivary 25-hydroxyvitamin D3: A noninvasive tool for the assessment of vitamin D status. *Anal Bioanal Chem.* 391:229–238.

Higashi, T., Shimada, K., and Toyo' oka, T. 2010. Advances in determination of vitamin D related compounds in biological samples using liquid chromatography-mass spectrometry: A review. *J Chromatogr B Analyt Technol Biomed Life Sci.* 878:1654–1661.

Hill, A.S., Rogers, Q.R., O'Neill, S.L., and Christopher, M.M. 2005. Effects of dietary antioxidant supplementation before and after oral acetaminophen challenge in cats. *Am J Vet Res.* 66:196–204.

Hill, A.S., Werner, J.A., Rogers, Q.R., O'Neill, S.L., and Christopher, M.M. 2004. Lipoic acid is 10 times more toxic in cats than reported in humans, dogs or rats. *J Anim Physiol Anim Nutr (Berl).* 88:150–156.

Hirschey, M.D., Shimazu, T., Huang, J.Y., and Verdin, E. 2009. Acetylation of mitochondrial proteins. *Methods Enzymol.* 457:137–147.

Holick, M.F. 2007. Vitamin D deficiency. *N Engl J Med.* 357:266–281.

Holub, B.J. 1992. The nutritional importance of inositol and the phosphoinositides. *N Engl J Med.* 326: 1285–1287.

How, K.L., Hazewinkel, H.A.W., and Mol, J.A. 1994. Dietary vitamin D dependence of cat and dog due to inadequate cutaneous synthesis of vitamin D. *Gen Comp Endo.* 96:12–18.

Howden, C.W. 2000. Vitamin B12 levels during prolonged treatment with proton pump inhibitors. *J Clin Gastroenterol.* 30:29–33.

Itokawa, Y., Kimura, M., and Nishino, K. 1982. Thiamin-binding proteins. *Ann N Y Acad Sci.* 378:327–336.

Johnston, C., Steinberg, F., and Rucker, R. 2014. Ascorbic acid. In *Handbook of Vitamins*. Eds. J. Zempleni, J. Suttie, J. Gregory, and PJ. Stover, 5th edition, pp.515–550. New York, NY: Taylor & Francis.

Kamao, M., Suhara, Y., Tsugawa, N., and Okano, T. 2005. Determination of plasma Vitamin K by high-performance liquid chromatography with fluorescence detection using Vitamin K analogs as internal standards. *J Chromatogr B Analyt Technol Biomed Life Sci.* 816:41–48.

Kambe, T., Tsuji, T., Hashimoto, A., and Itsumura, N. 2015. The physiological, biochemical, and molecular roles of zinc transporters in zinc homeostasis and metabolism. *Physiol Rev.* 95:749–784.

Kaneko, J.J., Harvey, J.W., and Bruss, M.L. 2008. Appendix. In *Clinical Biochemistry of Domestic Animals*. Eds. J.J. Kaneko, J.W. Harvey, and M.L. Bruss, 6th edition, pp. 889–895. New York, NY: Elsevier.

Kang, M., Peterson, R., and Feigon, J. 2009. Structural insights into riboswitch control of the biosynthesis of queuosine, a modified nucleotide found in the anticodon of tRNA. *Mol Cell.* 33:784–790.

Karppi, J., Nurmi, T., Olmedilla-Alonso, B., Granado-Lorencio, F., and Nyyssonen, K. 2008. Simultaneous measurement of retinol, alpha-tocopherol and six carotenoids in human plasma by using an isocratic reversed-phase HPLC method. *J Chromatogr B Analyt Technol Biomed Life Sci.* 867:226–232.

Kazmierski, K.J., Ogilvie, G.K., Fettman, M.J., et al. 2001. Serum zinc, chromium and iron concentrations in dogs with lymphoma and osteosarcoma. *JVIM.* 15:585–588.

Keen, C.L., Ensunsa, J.L., Watson, M.H., et al. 1999. Nutritional aspects of manganese from experimental studies. *Neurotoxicology.* 20:213–223.

Keen, C.L., and Gershwin, M.E. 1990. Zinc deficiency and immune function. *Annu Rev Nutr.* 10:415–431.

Keen, C.L., Ensunsa, J.L., and Clegg, M.S. 2000. Manganese metabolism in animals and humans including the toxicity of manganese. *Met Ions Biol Syst.* 37:89–121.

Keen, C.L., Holt, R.R., Oteiza, P.I., Fraga, C.G., and Schmitz, H.H. 2005. Cocoa antioxidants and cardiovascular health. *Am J Clin Nutr.* 81:298S–303S.

Kennedy, D., Young, P., Kennedy, S., et al. 1995. Cobalt-vitamin B12 deficiency and the activity of methylmalonyl CoA mutase and methionine synthase in cattle. *Int J Vitam Nutr Res.* 65:241–247.

Kennedy, S., McConnell, S., Anderson, H., Kennedy, D., Young, P., and Blanchflower, W. 1997. Histopathologic and ultrastructural alterations of white liver disease in sheep experimentally depleted of cobalt. *Vet Pathol.* 34:575–584.

Kidd, M.T., McDaniel, C.D., Peebles, E.D., et al. 2005. Breeder hen dietary L-carnitine affects progeny carcass traits. *Br Poult Sci.* 46:97–103.

Kim, S.H., Kelly, P.B., and Clifford, A.J. 2009. Accelerator mass spectrometry targets of submilligram carbonaceous samples using the high-throughput Zn reduction method. *Anal Chem.* 81:5949–5954.

Kirkland, J. 2014. Niacin. In *Handbook of Vitamins*. Eds. J. Zempleni, J. Suttie, J. Gregory, P.J. Stover, 5th edition, pp. 149–190. New York, NY: Taylor & Francis.

Kittleson, M.D., Keene, B., Pion, P.D., and Loyer, C.G. 1997. Results of the multicenter spaniel trial (MUST): Taurine- and carnitine-responsive dilated cardiomyopathy in American cocker spaniels with decreased plasma taurine concentration. *J Vet Intern Med.* 11:204–211.

Klimis-Tavantzis, D.J., Leach, R.M., Jr., and Kris-Etherton, P.M. 1983. The effect of dietary manganese deficiency on cholesterol and lipid metabolism in the Wistar rat and in the genetically hypercholesterolemic RICO rat. *J Nutr.* 113:328–336.

Koch-Nolte, F., Haag, F., Guse, A.H., Lund, F., and Ziegler, M. 2009. Emerging roles of NAD+ and its metabolites in cell signaling. *Sci Signal.* 2:mr1.

Koch-Nolte, F., Kernstock, S., Mueller-Dieckmann, C., Weiss, M.S., and Haag, F. 2008. Mammalian ADP-ribosyltransferases and ADP-ribosylhydrolases. *Front Biosci.* 13:6716–6729.

Krinsky, N. and Russell, R.M. 2001. Regarding the conversion of beta-carotene to vitamin A. *Nutr Rev.* 59:309.

Krinsky, N.I., and Johnson, E.J. 2005. Carotenoid actions and their relation to health and disease. *Mol Aspects Med.* 26:459–516.

La Fontaine, S., Ackland, M., and Mercer, J. 2010. Mammalian copper-transporting P-type ATPases, ATP7A and ATP7B: Emerging roles. *Int J Biochem Cell Biol.* 42:206–209.

Lamb, T.D. 2009. Evolution of vertebrate retinal photoreception. *Philos Trans R Soc Lond B Biol Sci.* 364:2911–2924.

Lanska, D.J. 2009. Chapter 30 Historical aspects of the major neurological vitamin deficiency disorders: The water-soluble B vitamins. *Handb Clin Neurol.* 95:445–476.

Lauwerys, R., and Lison, D. 1994. Health risks associated with cobalt exposure—An overview. *Sci Total Environ.* 150:1–6.

Leach, S.P., Salman, M.D., and Hamar, D. 2006. Trace elements and prion diseases: A review of the interactions of copper, manganese and zinc with the prion protein. *Anim Health Res Rev.* 7:97–105.

Lederman, J.D., Overton, K.M., Hofmann, N.E., Moore, B.J., Thornton, J., and Erdman, J.W. 1998. Ferrets (*Mustela putoius furo*) inefficiently convert beta-carotene to vitamin A. *J Nutr.* 128:271–279.

Lee, D.Y., Shay, N.F., and Cousins, R.J. 1992. Altered zinc metabolism occurs in murine lethal milk syndrome. *J Nutr.* 122:2233–2238.

Lemke, S.L., Dueker, S.R., Follett, J.R., et al. 2003. Absorption and retinol equivalence of beta-carotene in humans is influenced by dietary vitamin A intake. *J Lipid Res.* 44:1591–1600.

Lenz, M., and Lens, P.N. 2009. The essential toxin: The changing perception of selenium in environmental sciences. *Sci Total Environ.* 407:3620–3633.

Lichten, L.A., and Cousins, R.J. 2009. Mammalian zinc transporters: Nutritional and physiologic regulation. *Annu Rev Nutr.* 29:153–176.

Linster, C.L., and Van Schaftingen, E. 2007. Vitamin C. Biosynthesis, recycling and degradation in mammals. *FEBS J.* 274:1–22.

Liu, A.C., Heinrichs, B.S., and Leach, R.M., Jr. 1994. Influence of manganese deficiency on the characteristics of proteoglycans of avian epiphyseal growth plate cartilage. *Poult Sci.* 73:663–669.

Lu, J., and Holmgren, A. 2009. Selenoproteins. *J Biol Chem.* 284:723–727.

Lusk, G. 1922. A history of metabolism. *Endocrinol Metab.* 3:3–78.

Macapinlac, M.P., and Olson, J.A. 1981. A lethal hypervitaminosis A syndrome in young monkeys (*Macacus fascicularis*) following a single intramuscular dose of a water-miscible preparation containing vitamins A, D2 and E. *Int J Vitam Nutr Res.* 51:331–341.

Macdonald, M., Rogers, Q., and Morris, J. 1984. Nutrition of the domestic cat, a mammalian carnivore. *Annu Rev Nutr.* 4:521–562.

Macdonald, R.S. 2000. The role of zinc in growth and cell proliferation. *J Nutr.* 130:1500S–1508S.

Makarchikov, A.F., Lakaye, B., Gulyai, I.E., et al. 2003. Thiamine triphosphate and thiamine triphosphatase activities: From bacteria to mammals. *Cell Mol Life Sci.* 60:1477–1488.

Mansour, N., Sawhney, M., Tamang, D., Vogl, C., and Saier, M. 2007. The bile/arsenite/riboflavin transporter (BART) superfamily. *FEBS J.* 274:612–629.

Margis, R., Dunand, C., Teixeira, F.K., and Margis-Pinheiro, M. 2008. Glutathione peroxidase family - an evolutionary overview. *FEBS J.* 275:3959–3970.

Markovich, J.E., Heinze, C.R., and Freeman, L.M. 2013. Thiamine deficiency in dogs and cats. *J Am Vet Med Assoc.* 243:649–656.

Marks, S.L., Lipsitz, D., Vernau, K.M., et al. 2011. Reversible encephalopathy secondary to thiamine deficiency in 3 cats ingesting commercial diets. *J Vet Int Med.* 25:949–953.

McDonell, L. 2001. *Vitamins in Animal and Human Nutrition*, 2nd edition, pp. 1–793. Ames, IA: Iowa State Press.

McEwan, N.A., Mcneil, P.E., Thompson, H., and Mccandlish, I.A. 2000. Diagnostic features, confirmation and disease progression in 28 cases of lethal acrodermatitis of bull terriers. *J Small Anim Pract.* 41:501–507.

Merli, G., and Fink, J. 2008. Vitamin K and thrombosis. *Vitam Horm.* 78:265–279.

Mertz, W. 1993. Chromium in human nutrition. A review. *J. Nutr.* 123:626–633.

Mewies, M., Mcintire, W.S., and Scrutton, N.S. 1998. Covalent attachment of flavin adenine dinucleotide (FAD) and flavin mononucleotide (FMN) to enzymes: The current state of affairs. *Protein Sci.* 7:7–20.

Meyer, L.A., Durley, A.P., Prohaska, J.R., and Harris, Z.L. 2001. Copper transport and metabolism are normal in aceruloplasminemic mice. *J Biol Chem.* 276:36857–36861.

Mohammed, H.O., Divers, T.J., Summers, B.A., Omar, A.H., White, M.E., de Lahunta, A. 2007. Vitamin E deficiency and risk of equine motor neuron disease. *Acta Vet Scand.* 49:17.

Mooney, S., Leuendorf, J.E., Hendrickson, C., and Hellmann, H. 2009. Vitamin B6: A long known compound of surprising complexity. *Molecules.* 14:329–351.

Morita, T., Awakura, T., Shimada, A., Umemura, T., Nagai, T., and Haruna, A. 1995. Vitamin D toxicosis in cats: Natural outbreak and experimental study. *J Vet Med Sci.* 57:831–837.

Morris, J.G. 1999. Ineffective vitamin D synthesis in cats is reversed by an inhibitor of 7-dehydrocholestrol-delta7-reductase. *J Nutr.* 129:903–908.

Morris, J.G. 2002a. Idiosyncratic nutrient requirements of cats appear to be diet-induced evolutionary adaptations. *Nutr Res Rev.* 15:153–168.

Morris, J.G. 2002b. Cats discriminate between cholecalciferol and ergocalciferol. *J Anim Physiol Anim Nutr (Berl).* 86:229–238.

Morris, J.G., Earle, K.E., and Anderson, P.A. 1999. Plasma 25-hydroxyvitamin D in growing kittens is related to dietary intake of cholecalciferol. *J Nutr.* 129:909–912.

Morris, J.G., Rogers, Q.R., Kim, S.W., and Backus, R.C. 1994. Dietary taurine requirement of cats is determined by microbial degradation of taurine in the gut. In *Taurine in Health and Disease*. Eds. R.J. Huxtable, D. Michalk, pp. 59–70. New York, NY: Plenum Press.

Mustacich, D.J., Gohil, K., Bruno, R.S., et al. 2009. Alpha-tocopherol modulates genes involved in hepatic xenobiotic pathways in mice. *J Nutr Biochem.* 20:469–476.

Nagatsu, T., and Ichinose, H. 1999. Regulation of pteridine-requiring enzymes by the cofactor tetrahydrobiopterin. *Mol Neurobiol.* 19:79–96.

Nederbragt, H., Van den Ingh, T., and Wensvoort, P. 1984. Pathobiology of copper toxicity. *Vet Q.* 6:179–185.

Niza, M.M., Vilela, C.L., and Ferreira, L.M. 2003. Feline pansteatitis revisited: Hazards of unbalanced home-made diets. *J Feline Med Surg.* 5:271–277.

Norman, A., and Henry, H. 2007. Vitamin D. In *Handbook of Vitamins*. Eds. J. Zempleni, R.B. Rucker, D.B. McCormick, and J.W. Suttie, 4th edition, Chap. 2, pp. 41–110. Boca Raton, FL: CRC Press.

Norman, A., Okamura, W., Bishop, J., and Henry, H. 2002. Update on biological actions of 1alpha,25(OH)2-vitamin D3 (rapid effects) and 24R,25(OH)2-vitamin D3. *Mol Cell Endocrinol.* 197:1–19.

O'Dell, B., and Sunde, R. 1997. *Handbook of Nutritionally Essential Mineral Elements*, pp. 1–680. New York, NY: Dekker Publishing.

Okajima, M., Shimada, A., Kimura, T., Morita, T., Hikasa, Y., and Yao, M. 2007. Chastek paralysis in two wild foxes (*Vulpes vulpes japonica*). *Vet Rec.* 161:206–207.

Ozkor, M.A., and Quyyumi, A.A. 2008. Tetrahydrobiopterin. *Curr Hypertens Rep.* 10:58–64.

Palm, D., Klein, H.W., Schinzel, R., Buehner, M., and Helmreich, E.J. 1990. The role of pyridoxal 5′-phosphate in glycogen phosphorylase catalysis. *Biochemistry.* 29:1099–1107.

Palus, V., Penderis, J., Jakovljevic, S., and Cherubini, G.B. 2010. Thiamine deficiency in a cat: Resolution of MRI abnormalities following thiamine supplementation. *J Fel Med Surg.* 12:807–810.

Peebles, E.D., Kidd, M.T., Mcdaniel, C.D., et al. 2007. Effects of breeder hen age and dietary L-carnitine on progeny embryogenesis. *Br Poult Sci.* 48:299–307.

Pinto, J.T., and Rivlin, R. 2014. Riboflavin. In *Handbook of Vitamins*. Eds. J. Zempleni, J. Suttie, J. Gregory, and P.J. Stover, 5th edition, pp. 191–267. New York, NY: Taylor & Francis, NYC.

Pion, P.D., Kittleson, M.D., Skiles, M.L., Rogers, Q.R., and Morris, J.G. 1992. Dilated cardiomyopathy associated with taurine deficiency in the domestic cat: Relationship to diet and myocardial taurine content. *Adv Exp Med Biol.* 315:63–73.

Plecko, B., and Stockler, S. 2009. Vitamin B6 dependent seizures. *Can J Neurol Sci.* 36(Suppl 2):S73–S77.

Raila, J., Gomez, C., and Schweigert, F.J. 2002. The ferret as a model for vitamin A metabolism in carnivores. *J Nutr.* 132:1787S–1789S.

Raila, J., Mathews, U., and Schweigert, F.J. 2001. Plasma transport and tissue distribution of β-carotene, vitamin A and retinol-binding protein in domestic cats. *Comp Biochem Physiol A Mol Integr Physiol.* 130:849–856.

Rasbach, K.A., and Schnellmann, R.G. 2008. Isoflavones promote mitochondrial biogenesis. *J Pharmacol Exp Ther.* 325:536–543.

Reedijk, J., and Bouwman, E. 1999. *Bioinorganic Catalysis*, 2nd edition, pp. 1–595. New York, NY: Marcel Dekker.

Reilly, C. 2004. *The Nutritional Trace Elements*, pp.1–233. Oxford: Blackwell Publishing.

Reyniers, J.P., Pleasants, J.R., Wostmann, B.S., Katze, J.R., and Farkas, W.R. 1981. Administration of exogenous queuine is essential for the biosynthesis of the queuosine-containing transfer RNAs in the mouse. *J Biol Chem.* 256:11591–11594.

Ross, A.C., and Zolfaghari, R. 2004. Regulation of hepatic retinol metabolism: Perspectives from studies on vitamin A status. *J Nutr.* 134:269S–275S.

Ross, S.A., Srinivas, P.R., Clifford, A.J., Lee, S.C., Philbert, M.A., and Hettich, R.L. 2004. New technologies for nutrition research. *J Nutr.* 134:681–685.

Rozanski, E.A., Drobatz, K.J., Hughes, D., Scotti, M., and Giger, U. 1999. Thrombotest (PIVKA) test results in 25 dogs with acquired and hereditary coagulopathies. *JVECC.* 9:73–78.

Rucker, R., and Bauerly, K. 2014. Pantothenic acid. In *Handbook of Vitamins*. Eds. J. Zempleni, J. Suttie, J. Gregory, and P.J. Stover, 5th edition, pp. 325–351. New York, NY: Taylor & Francis.

Rucker, R., and Storms, D. 2002. Interspecies comparisons of micronutrient requirements: Metabolic vs. absolute body size. *J Nutr.* 132:2999–3000.

Rucker, R., Chowanadisai, W., and Nakano, M. 2009. Potential physiological importance of pyrroloquinoline quinone. *Altern Med Rev.* 14:268–277.

Rucker, R.B. 2007. Allometric scaling, metabolic body size and interspecies comparisons of basal nutritional requirements. *J Anim Physiol Anim Nutr (Berl).* 91:148–156.

Rucker, R.B. 2015. Reactive oxygen species: Regulation and essential functions. In *Antioxidants in Health and Disease*. Eds. A. Zampelas and E. Micha, Chap. 1, pp. 3–22. New York, NY: Taylor & Francis (CRC Press).

Rucker, R.B., and Chowanadisai, W. 2016. Coenzymes and cofactors. In: *The Encyclopedia of Food and Health*. Eds. B. Caballero, P. Finglas, and F. Toldrá, Vol. 2, pp. 206–224. Oxford: Academic Press.

Rucker, R.B., Keen, C.L., and Steinberg, F.M. 2014. Vitamins and food-derived biofactors. In *Encyclopedia of Agriculture and Food Systems*. Ed. N. Van Alfen, Vol. 5, pp. 356–377. San Diego, CA: Elsevier.

Rucker, R.B., Kosonen, T., Clegg, M.S., et al. 1998. Copper, lysyl oxidase, and extracellular matrix protein cross-linking. *Am J Clin Nutr.* 67:996S–1002S.

Rucker, R.B., Rucker, B.R., Mitchell, A.E., et al. 1999. Activation of chick tendon lysyl oxidase in response to dietary copper. *J Nutr.* 129:2143–2146.

Rumbeiha, W.K., Kruger, J.M., Fitzgerald, S.F., et al. 1999. Use of pamidronate to reverse vitamin D3-induced toxicosis in dogs. *Am J Vet Res.* 60:1092–1097.

Said, H. 2004. Recent advances in carrier-mediated intestinal absorption of water-soluble vitamins. *Annu Rev Physiol.* 66:419–446.

Sanderson, S.L., Osborne, C.A., Lulich, J.P., et al. 2001. Evaluation of urinary carnitine and taurine excretion in 5 cystinuric dogs with carnitine and taurine deficiency. *J Vet Intern Med.* 15:94–100.

Schenck, P.A., and Chew, D.J. 2010. Prediction of serum ionized calcium concentration by serum total calcium measurement in cats. *Can Vet J.* 74:209–213.

Schilsky, M. 2009a. Zinc treatment for symptomatic Wilson disease: Moving forward by looking back. *Hepatology.* 50:1341–1343.

Schilsky, M.L. 2009b. Wilson disease: Current status and the future. *Biochimie.* 91:1278–1281.

Schrauzer, G.N. 2003. The nutritional significance, metabolism and toxicology of selenomethionine. *Adv Food Nutr Res.* 47:73–112.

Schultheiss, P.C., Bedwell, C.L., Hamar, D.W., and Fettman, M.J. 2002. Canine liver iron, copper and zinc concentrations and association with histologic lesions. *J Vet Diag Invest.* 14:396–402.

Schwarz, G., and Mendel, R.R. 2006. Molybdenum cofactor biosynthesis and molybdenum enzymes. *Annu Rev Plant Biol.* 57:623–647.

Schweigert, F.G., Raila, J., Wichert, B., and Kienzle, E. 2002. Cats absorb β-carotene, but it is not converted to vitamin A. *J. Nutr.* 132:1610S–1612S.

Schweigert, F.J., Ryder, O.A., Rambeck, W.A., and Zucker, H. 1990. The majority of vitamin A is transported as retinyl esters in the blood of most carnivores. *Comp Biochem Physiol A.* 95:573–578.

Seetharam, B., and Yammani, R. 2003. Cobalamin transport proteins and their cell-surface receptors. *Expert Rev Mol Med.* 5:1–18.

Selting, K.A., Sharp, C.R., Ringold, R., Thamm, D.H., and Backus, R. 2014. Serum 25-hydroxyvitamin D concentrations in dogs – correlation with health and cancer risk. *Vet Comp Oncol.* 14:295–305.

Shane, B. 2008. Folate and vitamin B12 metabolism: Overview and interaction with riboflavin, vitamin B6, and polymorphisms. *Food Nutr Bull.* 29:S5–16; discussion S17–S19.

Shim, H., and Harris, Z.L. 2003. Genetic defects in copper metabolism. *J Nutr.* 133:1527S–1531S.

Shin, E.D., Delaney, S.J., Kass, P.H., Christopher, M.M., and Fascetti, A.J. 2004. Serum ionized magnesium reference intervals and storage effects in cats. *The American Academy of Veterinary Nutrition Clinical Nutrition and Research Symposium.* Minneapolis, MN, June 9.

Shoba, B., Lwin, Z.M., Ling, L.S., Bay, B.H., Yip, G.W., and Kumar, S.D. 2009. Function of sirtuins in biological tissues. *Anat Rec (Hoboken).* 292:536–543.

Sih, T.R., Morris, J.G., and Hickman, M.A. 2001. Chronic ingestion of high concentrations of cholecalciferol in cats. *AJVR.* 62:1500–1506. (Note: Cats were consuming 50 ug/kg diet (DM) cholecalciferol.

Smith, D.J., and Vainio, P.J. 2007. Targeting vascular adhesion protein-1 to treat autoimmune and inflammatory diseases. *Ann N Y Acad Sci.* 1110:382–388.

Stafford, D.W. 2005. The vitamin K cycle. *J Thromb Haemost.* 3:1873–1878.

Steinberg, F., Stites, T.E., Anderson, P., et al. 2003. Pyrroloquinoline quinone improves growth and reproductive performance in mice fed chemically defined diets. *Exp Biol Med (Maywood).* 228:160–166.

Steiner, J.M., and Williams, D.A. 1995. Validation of a radioimmunoassay for feline trypsin-like imunoreactivity (fTLI) and serum cobalamin and folate concentrations in cats with exocrine pancreatic insufficiency. *J Vet Int Med.* 9:193.

Stites, T., Storms, D., Bauerly, K., et al. 2006. Pyrroloquinoline quinone modulates mitochondrial quantity and function in mice. *J Nutr.* 136:390–396.

Studdert, V.P. 1990. Toxicity of cholecalciferol--containing rodenticides for dogs and cats. *Aust Vet J.* 67:N218.

Subcommittee (Ad Hoc) on Nonhuman Primate Nutrition, Committee on Animal Nutrition, and National Research Council, Board on Agriculture. 2003. *Nutrient Requirements of Nonhuman Primates*, pp. 1–308. Washington, DC: National Research Council National Academy Press.

Subcommittee on Dog and Cat Nutrition, Committee on Animal Nutrition, and National Research Council. 2006. *Nutrient Requirements of Dogs and Cats*, pp. 1–424. Washington, DC: National Research Council National Academy Press.

Subcommittee on Laboratory Animal Nutrition, Committee on Animal Nutrition, National Research Council, and Board on Agriculture. 1995. *Nutrient Requirements of Laboratory Animals*, 4th edition, pp. 1–176. Washington, DC: National Research Council National Academy Press.

Subcommittee on Mineral Toxicity in Animals, C.O.A.N. and Board on Agricultures and Renewable Resources. 1980. *Mineral Tolerance of Domestic Animals.* pp. 1–577. Washington, DC: National Research Council, National Academy of Sciences.

Subcommittee on Rabbit Nutrition, Committee on Animal Nutrition, National Research Council, and Board on Agriculture. 1977. *Nutrient Requirements of Rabbits*, 2nd edition, pp. 1–30. Washington, DC: National Research Council National Academy Press.

Subcommittee on Swine Nutrition, Committee on Animal Nutrition, National Research Council, and Board on Agriculture. 1998. *Nutrient Requirements of Swine*, 10th edition, pp. 1–210. Washington, DC: National Research Council National Academy Press.

Sunde, R. 1990. Molecular biology of selenoproteins. *Annu Rev Nutr.* 10:451–474.

Suttie, J.W. 2014. Vitamin K. In *Handbook of Vitamins*. Eds. J. Zempleni, J. Suttie, J. Gregory, and P.J. Stover, 5th edition, pp. 89–125. New York, NY: Taylor & Francis.

Tamura, T., and Halsted, C.H. 1983. Folate turnover in chronically alcoholic monkeys. *J Lab Clin Med.* 101:623–628.

Taylor, H. 2001. *Inductively Coupled Plasma-Mass Spectrometry*, pp. 1–294. San Diago, CA: Academic Press.

Tchaparian, E., Marshal, L., Cutler, G., et al. 2010. Identification of transcriptional networks responding to pyrroloquinoline quinone dietary supplementation and their influence on thioredoxin expression, and the JAK/STAT and MAPK pathways. *Biochem J.* 429:515–526.

Tchaparian, E.H., Uriu-Adams, J.Y., Keen, C.L., Mitchell, A.E., and Rucker, R.B. 2000. Lysyl oxidase and P-ATPase-7A expression during embryonic development in the rat. *Arch Biochem Biophys.* 379:71–77.

Thompson, K.A., Parnell, N.K., Hohenhaus, A.E., Moore, G.E., and Rondeau, M.P. 2009. Feline exocrine pancreatic insufficiency: 16 cases (1992–2007). *J Feline Med Surg.* 11:935–940.

Titmarsh, H., Cartwright, J.A., Kilpatrick, S., et al. 2017. Relationship between vitamin D status and leukocytes in hospitalized cats. *J Feline Med Surg.* 19:364–369.

Titmarsh, H., Gow, A.G., Kilpatrick, S., et al. 2015a. Low vitamin D status is associated with systemic and gastrointestinal inflammation in dogs with a chronic enteropathy. *PLOS ONE.* 10(9):e0137377.

Titmarsh, H., Gow, A.G., Kilpatrick, S., et al. 2015b. Association of vitamin D status and clinical outcome in dogs with chronic enteropathy. *J Vet Int Med.* 29:1473–1478.

Titmarsh, H., Lalor, S., Tasker, S., et al. 2015c. Vitamin D status in cats with feline immunodeficiency virus. *Vet Med Sci.* 1:72–78.

Todoli, J-L., and Mermet, J-M. 2008. *Liquid Sample Introduction in ICP Spectrometry*, pp. 1–300. New York, NY: Academic Press.

Toohey, J.I. 2006. Vitamin B12 and methionine synthesis: A critical review. Is nature's most beautiful cofactor misunderstood? *Biofactors.* 26:45–57.

Toresson, L., Steiner, J.M., Suchodolsk, J.S., and Spillmann, T. 2015. Oral cobalamin supplementation in dogs with chronic enteropathies and hypocobalanemia. *J Vet Int Med.* 30:101–107.

Traber, M. 2007. Vitamin E regulatory mechanisms. *Annu Rev Nutr.* 27:347–362.

Traber, M. 2014. Vitamin E. In *Handbook of Vitamins*. Eds. J. Zempleni, J. Suttie, J. Gregory, and P.J. Stover, 5th edition, pp. 125–148. New York, NY: Taylor & Francis.

Tranter, E., Lindon, J., and Holmes, J.E. 2000. *Encyclopedia of Spectroscopy and Spectrometry, Three-Volume Set*, pp. 1–2581. New York, NY: Academic Press.

Unterer, S., Lutz, H., Gerber, B., Glaus, T.M., Hassig, M., and Reusch, C.E. 2004. Evaluation of an electrolyte analyzer for measurement of ionized calcium and magnesium concentrations in blood, plasma and serum of dogs. *AJVR.* 65:183–187.

Vaillant, C., Horadagoda, N.U., and Batt, R.M. 1990. Cellular localization of intrinsic factor in pancreas and stomach of the dog. *Cell Tissue Res.* 260:117–122.

Van den Broek, A.H.M., Stafford, W.L., and Keay, G. 1992. Zinc and copper concentrations in the plasma and hair of normal cats. *Vet Rec.* 131:512–513.

Vargas, E.J., Shoho, A.R., and Linder, M.C. 1994. Copper transport in the Nagase analbuminemic rat. *Am J Physiol.* 267:G259–269.

Verhoef, P. 2007. Homocysteine--an indicator of a healthy diet? *Am J Clin Nutr.* 85:1446–1447.

Verhoef, P., and De Groot, L.C. 2005. Dietary determinants of plasma homocysteine concentrations. *Semin Vasc Med.* 5:110–123.

Vesterberg, O. 1994. Specific, sensitive and accurate quantification of albumin, retinol binding protein and transferrin in human urine and serum by zone immunoelectrophoresis assay (ZIA). *Electrophoresis.* 15:589–593.

Viles, J.H., Klewpatinond, M., and Nadal, R.C. 2008. Copper and the structural biology of the prion protein. *Biochem Soc Trans.* 36:1288–1292.

Villanueva, J., Ling, E.H., Chandler, C.J., and Halsted, C.H. 1998. Membrane and tissue distribution of folate binding protein in pig. *Am J Physiol.* 275:R1503–1510.

Vimokesant, S., Kunjara, S., Rungruangsak, K., Nakornchai, S., and Panijpan, B. 1982. Beriberi caused by antithiamin factors in food and its prevention. *Ann N Y Acad Sci.* 378:123–136.

Wang, X.D., and Krinsky, N.I. 1998. The bioconversion of beta-carotene into retinoids. *Subcell Biochem.* 30:159–180.

Wedekind, K.J., Yu, S., and Combs, G.F. 2004. The selenium requirement of the puppy. *J Anim Physiol Anim Nutr (Berl).* 88:340–347. (Note: Serum Se and plasma GSHpx from kittens consuming a diet containing 0.15 mg Se/kg diet).

Wedekind, K.J., Howard, K.A., Backus, R.C., Yu, S., Morris, J.G., and Rogers, Q.R. 2003. Determination of the selenium requirement in kittens. *J Anim Physiol Anim Nutr (Berl).* 87:315–323. (Note: Plasma GSHpx from kittens consuming 0.15 mg Se/kg diet).

Wedekind, K.J., Blumer, M.E., Huntinton, C.E., Spate, V., and Morris, J.S. 2010. The feline iodine requirement is lower than the 2006 NRC recommended allowance. *J Anim Physiol Anim Nutr (Berl).* 94:527–539. (Note: Urinary iodine reported in cats consuming a diet containing 0.47 mg/kg diet (DM) supplied as KI).

Weinmann, A.R., Oliveira, M.S., Jorge, S.M., and Martins, A.R. 1999. Simultaneous high-performance liquid chromatographic determination of retinol by fluorometry and of tocopherol by ultraviolet absorbance in the serum of newborns. *J Chromatogr B Biomed Sci Appl.* 729:231–236.

White, M.L., Zhang, Y., Andrew, L.G., and Hadley, W.L. 2005. MR imaging with diffusion-weighted imaging in acute and chronic Wernicke encephalopathy. *AJNR Am J Neuroradiol.* 26:2306–2310.

White, W.S., Peck, K.M., Ulman, E.A., and Erdman, J.W., Jr. 1993. The ferret as a model for evaluation of the bioavailabilities of all-trans-beta-carotene and its isomers. *J Nutr.* 123:1129–1139.

Whitehead, C.C. 1981. The assessment of biotin status in man and animals. *Proc Nutr Soc.* 40:165–172.

Whitehead, C.C. 1985. Assessment of biotin deficiency in animals. *Ann N Y Acad Sci.* 447:86–96.

Wilson, J.X. 2002. The physiological role of dehydroascorbic acid. *FEBS Lett.* 527:5–9.

Wilson, J.X. 2005. Regulation of vitamin C transport. *Annu Rev Nutr.* 25:105–125.

Wu, G., and Meininger, C. 2002. Regulation of nitric oxide synthesis by dietary factors. *Annu Rev Nutr.* 22:61–86.

Xue, Y., Karaplis, A., Hendy, G., Goltzman, D., and Miao, D. 2005. Genetic models show that parathyroid hormone and 1,25-dihydroxyvitamin D3 play distinct and synergistic roles in postnatal mineral ion homeostasis and skeletal development. *Hum Mol Genet.* 14:1515–1528.

Yi, X., and Maeda, N. 2005. Endogenous production of lipoic acid is essential for mouse development. *Mol Cell Biol.* 25:8387–8392.

Yi, X., Kim, K., Yuan, W., et al. 2009. Mice with heterozygous deficiency of lipoic acid synthase have an increased sensitivity to lipopolysaccharide-induced tissue injury. *J Leukoc Biol.* 85:146–153.

Yuzbasiyan-Gurkan, V., and Bartlett, E. 2006. Identification of a unique splice site variant in SLC39A4 in bovine hereditary zinc deficiency, lethal trait A46: An animal model of acrodermatitis enteropathica. *Genomics.* 88:521–526.

Zeisel, S. 1995. Nutrients, signal transduction and carcinogenesis. *Adv Exp Med Biol.* 369:175–183.

Zeisel, S. 1996. Choline. A nutrient that is involved in the regulation of cell proliferation, cell death, and cell transformation. *Adv Exp Med Biol.* 399:131–141.

Zempleni, J., Chew, Y.C., Bao, B., Pestinger, V., and Wijeratne, S.S. 2009a. Repression of transposable elements by histone biotinylation. *J Nutr.* 139:2389–2392.

Zempleni, J., Chew, Y.C., Hassan, Y.I., and Wijeratne, S.S. 2008a. Epigenetic regulation of chromatin structure and gene function by biotin: Are biotin requirements being met? *Nutr Rev.* 66(Suppl 1):S46–48.

Zempleni, J., Hassan, Y.I., and Wijeratne, S.S. 2008b. Biotin and biotinidase deficiency. *Expert Rev Endocrinol Metab.* 3:715–724.

Zempleni, J., Wijeratne, S.S., and Hassan, Y.I. 2009b. Biotin. *Biofactors.* 35:36–46.

Zhang, J., Meruvu, S., Bedi, Y.S., et al. 2015. Pyrroloquinoline quinone increases the expression and activity of Sirt1 and -3 genes in HepG2 cells. *Nutr Res.* 35:844–849.

Zhao, J., and Zhong, C.J. 2009. A review on research progress of transketolase. *Neurosci Bull.* 25:94–99.

Zheljazkov, V.D., and Warman, P.R. 2004. Phytoavailability and fractionation of copper, manganese, and zinc in soil following application of two composts to four crops. *Environ Pollut.* 131:187–195.

25 Development of Biomarkers

Holly L. Jordan

CONTENTS

25.1 DEFINITION OF "BIOMARKER" AS IT APPLIES TO LABORATORY ANIMAL CLINICAL CHEMISTRY

In 2001, the Biomarkers Definitions Working Group convened by the National Institutes of Health defined a biomarker as "a characteristic that is objectively measured and evaluated as an indicator of normal biological processes, pathogenic processes, or pharmacologic responses to a therapeutic intervention" (Atkinson et al., 2001; see Table 25.1). Although this has become a very popular area of research in recent years, the modern notion of biomarkers essentially evolved from the field of clinical chemistry. Clinical chemistry parameters—biomarkers—that are very familiar to veterinary clinical pathologists and laboratory animal clinicians, such as serum alanine aminotransferase (ALT) activity, urine specific gravity, and plasma glucose, have been utilized for decades to diagnose and prognosticate disease, determine responses to experimental conditions, monitor health status, and define phenotypic characteristics. Clinical chemistry tests are now just one facet of the field of biomarkers that encompasses not only biochemical measurements (e.g., proteins, enzymatic activity, nucleic acids, metabolic products), but also structural (e.g., organ weights), anatomical, (e.g., ventricular wall thickness), physicochemical (e.g., bone densitometry), and functional endpoints (e.g., arterial blood pressure).

Innovation in laboratory technology is, and will continue to be, one of the strongest drivers in biomarker development. In the past half century, clinical chemistry methods have transformed from predominantly manual bench-top chemistry testing to high throughput, fully automated analyses. Technological tools derived from immunology, genomics, protein biochemistry, and metabolomics have significantly contributed to expanding the range of possible measurements. In some cases, these technologies have broadened our understanding of traditional biomarkers. For example, ALT is typically measured in terms of serum activity based on an enzymatic reaction. However, there are now experimental methods for measuring specific ALT isoenzyme proteins, ALT1 and ALT2 in serum by immunoassay and isoenzyme messenger RNA in tissues that are enhancing our understanding of the fundamental biology of this enzyme in animals and humans (Lindblom et al., 2007; Miyazaki et al., 2009; Rajamohan et al., 2006).

In the context of laboratory animal clinical chemistry, biomarkers usually represent endpoints measured in serum, plasma, urine, and other body fluids. Advances in assay and technology miniaturization and in sample collection have broadened the range of biomarker alternatives for laboratory animal species in which body fluids may be limited in volume or accessibility. For example, glucose monitoring has historically required repeated collection of serum by venipuncture, but now can be accomplished by continuous microsampling of interstitial tissue fluid with portable miniature analyzers (Woderer et al., 2007). Availability of assays for glycated proteins, such as hemoglobin A1c and fructosamine, supports that serial blood glucose testing no longer remains the only or necessarily the optimal measure of glucose status depending on species and application.

25.2 GENERAL PRINCIPLES OF AN "OPTIMAL" BIOMARKER

Characterizing an optimal biomarker requires clearly defining its intended purpose and use. For example, of the circulating cardiac biomarkers currently available, troponin I is a highly sensitive and specific marker of acute myocardial cell necrosis in multiple species, but it has more limited value in heart conditions that are not associated with myocardial cell disruption, such as non-ischemic ventricular dysfunction (Nishijima et al., 2005). Conversely, natriuretic peptides, which respond to changes in ventricular stretch, may have less value in assessing cardiac injury that is not accompanied by altered cardiac afterload (Oyama et al., 2007). In some cases, diagnostic utility may be optimized with a panel of biomarkers, a common approach in evaluating derangements of systems such as the hepatobiliary and renal systems. In any case, the more diverse and complex the process being evaluated, the more complicated and time consuming are the validation and qualification efforts required.

To this end, Lee et al. (2006) proposed that rational biomarker development should be "fit for purpose" (Table 25.1). Specifically, assay validation should be tailored to meet the intended purpose of the biomarker with a level of rigor commensurate with the intended use of the results. Thus, the most important step in biomarker evaluation is to clarify the purpose of the proposed data and to understand the impact on subsequent decision-making. This shapes the validation and qualification process and ultimately guides determination of the best candidate. As an example, the study design, test groups and outcome measures needed to evaluate a biomarker intended to diagnose osteoarthritis in an experimental mouse model may differ from those needed to evaluate a marker intended to predict efficacy of a novel osteoarthritis treatment, or of a prognostic biomarker intended to predict the course of injury in this model (Bauer et al., 2006; Soreide, 2009). In addition, an optimal "fit-for-purpose" biomarker must be technically feasible, technically sound, and meet the established biologic criteria appropriate to the use of the biomarker.

There are a number of scientific and practical considerations when determining whether an assay is appropriate for a given disease or toxicity and is technically feasible for a given laboratory (Table 25.2). It is important to understand as much as possible about the biology of the biomarker and the process of the disease or toxicity to be evaluated, although valuable biomarkers (such as kidney injury molecule-1 [KIM-1], renal papillary antigen-1, and even ALT) were identified in the

TABLE 25.1
Definitions

Term	Definition	Reference
Biomarker	A characteristic that is objectively measured and evaluated as an indicator of normal biological processes, pathogenic processes, or pharmacologic responses to a therapeutic intervention.	Atkinson et al. (2001)
Fit for purpose	Assay validation that is tailored to meet the intended purpose of the biomarker with a level of rigor commensurate with the intended use of the data.	Lee et al. (2006)
Validation	The process of assessing the assays and its measurement performance characteristics, and determining the range of conditions under which the assay will give reproducible and accurate data.	Wagner et al. (2008)
Qualification	The evidentiary process of linking a biomarker with biological processes and clinical end points.	Wagner (2002, 2008)

TABLE 25.2

Factors in Assessing the Technical Feasibility of a Proposed Biomarker for Laboratory Animals

Biological and Species Rationale

- What is the biological rationale for the biomarker?
- Is the analyte appropriate/measurable in the species of interest?

Assay Availability

- Is an assay available?
- Are reagents and instrumentation available?
- Is the assay validated for the species of interest?
- Is the vendor likely to discontinue the assay?

Technology Availability

- Does it require specialized training?
- Does it require special facilities or capabilities?

Cost Effectiveness

- What is the assay cost?
- How much is the labor cost to perform the analysis?

Sample Collection

- Can it be measured in a body fluid?
- How much volume is required?
- How invasive is sample collection?
- Is it sufficiently stable in the matrix of interest?

absence of detailed mechanistic information. In veterinary species, an obvious limitation may be whether the analyte is even measurable in the species of interest. For example, circulating cortisol can be assayed in humans, monkeys, dogs, and other species, but it is not appropriate in rats or mice in which the primary glucocorticoid is corticosterone.

Availability of species-appropriate assays can be challenging for laboratory animal species. Commercial tests are often designed for human samples and may or may not be applicable in veterinary species, and assays developed for one animal species may not be valid in another species. This is especially true for immunoassays in which cross-reactivity of antibody reagents must be demonstrated for the species of interest. A good example of the variability in assay performance that can be observed when analyzing animal specimens with human commercial reagents was provided by Apple et al. (2008) who found considerable differences across multiple cardiac troponin platforms tested with rat, dog, and monkey samples. Because the veterinary market is relatively small, assay availability may be hampered by vendor decisions to alter or discontinue assays, irrespective of veterinary customer needs.

An optimal biomarker assay must meet the resource capabilities of a given laboratory: the assay, reagents, instrumentation, and labor requirements should be affordable. Some methods require special facilities or training, such as those using radioactive materials (e.g., radioimmunoassays) or hazardous substances (e.g., paraoxon reagent for measuring serum paraxonase-1 activity). Proprietary intellectual property restrictions may also restrict availability of unique assay materials.

Sample requirements must be reasonable and attainable for laboratory animal species. For example, methods requiring serum volumes of 2 mL and greater are not practical in mice, but are reasonable for dogs, pigs, monkeys, and other larger species. Many diagnostic applications in laboratory animals are best suited to minimally invasive procedures. Thus, assays that can be performed with peripheral blood, urine, or saliva are advantageous. It is important to confirm that a new assay is appropriate with the matrix of interest. For example, ethylenediaminetetraacetic acid (EDTA) plasma may not be suitable for a test developed with heparinized plasma, and a serum assay may not work with urine samples. Species differences may also be present across the same sample type. For instance, unless a species-specific calibrator is used, serum albumin as measured by the bromcresol green method may be inaccurate in the rabbit and other species due to inherent differences in protein binding affinity of this dye (Stokol et al., 2001). Stability of the analyte in the matrix of interest must also be confirmed. For example, some urine analytes require overnight collection at low temperature and/or addition of preservatives. If potential interfering conditions, such as hemolysis and lipemia are likely in the test system, then effects of these preanalytical variables on assay results should also be evaluated (Jacobs et al., 1992).

Once there is sufficient technical support and justification to implement a biomarker assay, it must be shown to be technically sound. The term "biomarker validation" has been used interchangeably with terms such as biomarker development, correlation, and evaluation. However, in its guidance on bioanalytical method validation, the Food and Drug Administration (FDA) (2001) defined validation specifically as the procedures that demonstrate that a particular method used for quantitative measurement of analytes in a biological matrix is reliable and reproducible for the intended use. For drug development applications, Wagner (2008) expanded this slightly by describing validation as the process of assessing the assay and its measurement performance characteristics, and determining the range of conditions under which the assay will provide reproducible and accurate data to meet the individual study objectives (Table 25.1).

The assay performance characteristics most commonly evaluated are listed in Table 25.3 and are further discussed in Chapter 26 and by Lee et al. (2005, 2006). Assay performance characteristics should be tailored to the type of analytical method and endpoints. For example, analytical accuracy and dilutional linearity can be assessed in quantitative assays which have reference standards and continuous numeric units (e.g., serum glucose or plasma fibrinogen), but cannot be evaluated for semiquantitative or qualitative methods that lack reference standards and may be reported in discontinuous (discrete) units (e.g., urine protein as measured by reagent pad). Also, immunoassays are inherently nonlinear and may be less precise when compared with an analytical method, such as liquid chromatography/mass spectrometry (LC/MS), necessitating different approaches to validation and acceptance criteria (Findlay et al., 2000; FDA, 2001).

25.3 PROCESS OF IDENTIFYING POTENTIAL BIOMARKERS

Once the biologic, pathologic, or therapeutic process of interest has been defined and an objective criterion or "gold standard" benchmark has been agreed, there are many avenues for identifying potential clinical chemistry biomarkers. Some analytes like HbA1c have been identified as a result of elucidating specific pathobiological effects of the disease (Bunn et al., 1975). Other biomarkers like lipocalin-2, a general marker of inflammation (Devarajan, 2008; Hoo et al., 2008), have been identified by comparing constituents in biological samples from healthy and diseased individuals using technologies that can generate hundreds and even thousands of possible candidates. Such platforms may employ proteomic (analysis of global protein profiles, i.e., using MS or electrophoretic-based methods), genomic (analysis of gene expression profiles, i.e., using DNA or oligonucleotide microarrays), or metabolomic (analysis of endogenous metabolites, i.e., using LC/MS) methods (Marrer and Dieterle, 2007). Emerging techniques using peptidomics (identifying and quantifying peptide fragments, as opposed to proteins), histomics (raising antibodies against peripheral body fluids of diseased or treated subjects and using them to stain tissues of interest), and epigenetics (reversible, heritable changes in gene regulation which occur without a change in DNA sequence) are also under investigation (Marrer and Dieterle, 2007). With the evolution of these high-throughput technologies, multivariate data sets are becoming more widely available in the public arena, facilitating a growing number of *in silico* avenues for potential biomarker identification based on data mining and biostatistical computations (Klee, 2008).

TABLE 25.3
Performance Characteristics in the Technical Validation of a Biomarker

Performance Characteristic	Definition	Quantitative Method	Semiquantitative or Qualitative Method
Analytical accuracy	The closeness of mean test results to the true amount of the analyte.	√[a]	–
Precision (within run and between run)	The closeness of individual measures of an analyte when the procedure is applied repeatedly to multiple aliquots of a single homogenous volume of sample.	√	√/–
Analytical sensitivity	The lowest analyte concentration detectable with acceptable precision and accuracy.	√ (LLOQ[b])	√
Assay specificity	Ability of the assay to unequivocally distinguish the analyte from other substances in the sample.	√	√
Dilutional linearity	Ability to dilute samples originally above upper limit of quantification with acceptable precision and accuracy.	√	–
Working range (linearity)	The range of values over which the analyte is measurable with acceptable levels of precision and accuracy.	√ (LLOQ and ULOQ[c])	√
Analyte stability	Stability should be assessed for storage time and temperature conditions relevant to intended use. May also need to include freeze–thaw cycles.	√	√
Limit of detection	The minimum concentration that can be distinguished from background.	√	√
Cross-validation (inter-method or inter-laboratory)	Comparison of validation characteristics when two or more methods or two or more labs are used to generate the same endpoint.	√	√
Interference	Characterize negative or positive effects of common interfering substances, such as hemoglobin, lipid, or bilirubin.	√	√

[a] √ required.
[b] LLOQ, lower limit of quantification: the lowest measurable concentration with acceptable precision and accuracy.
[c] ULOQ, upper limit of quantification: the highest measurable concentration with acceptable precision and accuracy.
Source: Adapted from Lee, J.W. et al., *Pharm Res*, 22, 2495–2499, 2005.

A common approach with these types of broad-based molecular profiling tools is to generate a reference data set from animals with known positive conditions (i.e., exposed to known toxicants or expressing a well-characterized disease, etc.). The specificity and reproducibility of these results are further refined by comparing these responses to responses from animals with known negative conditions (i.e., healthy animals as well as animals with unrelated conditions) and to responses from an independent set of animals with the condition of interest (a validation set). Subsequently, results from animals with unknown conditions can be queried against the defined pattern or "signature" for that condition. Molecular profiling has been used to identify biomarker candidates especially in the areas of cancer staging, classification, and prognosis and in toxicology and drug development (Bailey and Ulrich 2004; Marrer and Dieterle, 2007).

Although "-omics" methods offer the advantages of speed, high throughput, and generation of large numbers of possible candidates, they require appropriate analytical and statistical expertise and can be expensive. The reproducibility and generalizability of molecular profiling methods can be hampered by poor study design. Common mistakes include experimental bias, use of validation sets that are too small, and validation sets that lack independence from the training set (Ransohoff, 2004, 2007). Discriminating changes due to factors unrelated to the biologic process of interest, such as interindividual variation (e.g., due to hormonal status), unique experimental factors (e.g., effects of fasting), posttranslational modifications, and artifacts continues to be challenging (Sinhaa et al., 2007). Due to this inherent biological and technical variability, "false positives" are common with these "shotgun" approaches and can complicate efforts to produce scientifically robust markers in a timely and efficient manner (Carr, 2008; Ransohoff, 2007). "False negatives" may occur with assays that lack sufficient dynamic range and fail to identify constituents that are present at very high or very low concentrations. The relevance of changes in a new marker must be fully evaluated in relation to changes in the specified gold standard (i.e., functional endpoint, histomorphologic change, disease condition, etc.), as well as normal biological variability of the marker in the population of interest.

One example of a successful biomarker is KIM-1 (Bonventre, 2008, 2009) (Table 25.4). This renal injury marker, also known as TIM-1 or T-cell immunoglobulin and mucin-containing molecule, was first identified through a polymerase chain reaction technique comparing gene expression in renal tissue from healthy and postischemic rats. This was followed by tissue localization with *in situ* hybridization and immunohistochemistry (Ichimura et al., 1998). The gene encoding this type 1 transmembrane protein was an optimal choice to pursue as a renal injury marker as it is present in very low levels in healthy kidney and is strongly upregulated in proximal tubular epithelial cells after ischemia or toxic injury. In addition, the KIM-1 ectodomain is cleaved and the protein can be detected in urine using immunoassay-based methods (Zhou et al., 2008). Subsequent work has shown that urinary KIM-1 is elevated in rodents and humans with a variety of renal pathologies, but not in healthy individuals nor in individuals with other types of injury (Sabbisetti et al., 2013; Bonventre, 2008; Vaidya et al., 2010).

TABLE 25.4
Example of Progression of Novel Biomarker Development

Step	KIM-1 Example
Define need	Biomarker needed for early diagnosis of acute kidney injury and for monitoring proximal tubular injury
Identify a novel biomarker	A PCR method using representational difference analysis identified highly upregulated renal mRNA for KIM-1 in rats with renal ischemia compared with normal rats
Develop and optimize detection method(s) for technical feasibility and soundness	Gene cloned and antibody generated for detection of KIM-1 protein in tissues by immunohistochemistry and in urine by ELISA. Technical attributes of ELISA assessed as noninvasive application
Define biological attributes in healthy and diseased subjects and in species of interest	Assess tissue, cellular localization by in situ methods Evaluate in human specimens as well as animal
Test against current gold standard, other markers in known positive and negative conditions and perform appropriate statistical testing [e.g., Received Operator Curves (ROC) analysis, likelihood ratios].	Test in animals given well-characterized nephrotoxicants and compare with renal histology, serum urea, and creatinine Test as a diagnostic and prognostic marker in cross-sectional and longitudinal studies in healthy volunteers and in human patients with ischemic and acute kidney injury documented by biopsy. Evaluate as a prognostic marker in patients with renal graft rejection

25.4 BIOLOGICAL QUALIFICATION

After a biomarker assay has been optimized analytically, it must be "qualified" for the purposes intended. In contrast to validation which is the evaluation of assay technical performance, assay qualification is "the evidentiary process linking a biomarker with the intended biological processes or clinical endpoint" (Wagner, 2008) (see Table 25.1). Like validation, assay qualification must be tailored to each biomarker application, but in general requires characterizing attributes of the analyte in healthy animals, in animals with the injury or disease of interest, and in animals with unrelated conditions.

Most clinical chemistry biomarker applications in laboratory animals require an understanding of the range of analyte values within normal, healthy individuals (see Table 25.5). The analyte should be measured in a sufficient number of individuals to provide a working reference interval that can be refined as experience with the marker grows. Reference intervals can be stratified as needed to best represent the population of interest, that is, by gender, strain, age, and so on. It is important to also include characterization of the variability of the analyte within the same individual over time (e.g., over 24 hours, over a week, or over the life span of the animal as needed), as this can be substantial for some constituents (e.g., reproductive and adrenocortical hormones). It may also be important to assess effects of external variables, such as environmental conditions, diet, housing, social influences, sample collection site, and sample handling, depending on the range of intended applications for the biomarker.

To fully understand their specificity, sensitivity, and predictive value, new biomarker assays must be evaluated in animals that have the condition (injury, disease, toxicity, etc.) of interest as well as in animals without the condition. To accomplish this, it is essential to evaluate the biomarker against an agreed objective "gold standard" as stated earlier (e.g., histopathology, a measurable functional change, or a physiological endpoint). To demonstrate that changes in a novel marker correlate with the magnitude of a response (i.e., severity of injury), validation studies should be designed to generate a wide range of responses (i.e., minimal to severe injury). For predictive markers that are expected to demonstrate changes that precede changes in the gold standard, longitudinal studies with serial sampling are required. As an example, Zhou et al. (2008) found very good correlation between the magnitude of increase in urinary KIM-1 levels and renal histopathology severity scores by studying rats exposed to several well-characterized rodent nephrotoxicants administered across multiple doses. To provide evidence that KIM-1 is specific for renal injury, rats were also exposed to a known hepatotoxicant with no renal effects (negative treatment control) and no change in urinary KIM-1 was detected. The reversibility of KIM-1 responses was evaluated in a longitudinal study in rats with adriamycin-induced chronic nephropathy. Renoprotective treatment lowered urine KIM-1 levels which was correlated with improved renal morphologic measures (Kramer et al., 2009). As a

TABLE 25.5
Biological Qualification: Characterization in Healthy Animals

Determine Reference Ranges for Population of Interest

- Assess intra-animal variability
- Assess inter-animal variability

Evaluate potential preanalytic effects of interest

- Gender, age, strain
- Physiologic effects: stress, handling, diurnal or seasonal variation
- Dietary effects: fasting, nonfasting
- Environmental effects: housing, light, social structure, etc.
- Sampling site: tail vein, cardiac puncture, abdominal vessel, etc.
- Sample handling: anticoagulant, temperature, preservatives, etc.
- Anesthesia: isoflurane, ketamine, etc.

potential predictive application, urinary KIM-1 has also been demonstrated to independently predict graft loss in a prospective study of renal transplant patients (van Timmeren et al., 2007).

Developing a biomarker for acceptance by the wider scientific or medical community requires a rigorous iterative evidentiary process of testing the biomarker in multiple studies across multiple laboratories. Because this is very time consuming and resource intensive, there is a growing number of collaborative initiatives in laboratory animal and human biomarker development (Wagner, 2008). For instance, KIM-1 is one of several nephrotoxicity markers that have been evaluated by the Nephrotoxicity Working Group of the Predictive Safety Testing Consortium established by the FDA and the Critical Path Institute in collaboration with the pharmaceutical industry (Goodsaid et al., 2008, Mendrick, 2008). Whether accomplished through the focused efforts of a consortium or via an unstructured process of repeated testing in diverse independent laboratories, biological qualification of an assay requires generating sufficient positive and negative data to fully evaluate its diagnostic attributes (Table 25.6). Sensitivity ("positivity in disease") is the proportion of animals with the condition that have positive results. Specificity ("negativity in health") is the proportion of animals without the condition that have negative results. Thus, a highly sensitive assay is an ideal "rule-out" test and a highly specific test is an ideal "rule-in" test (Florkowski, 2008). Predictive values can also be calculated, though they vary with the prevalence of the condition in the particular population being studied. Positive predictive value is the proportion of positive results that are true positives, while negative predictive value is the proportion of negative results that are true negatives.

Because this type of assay evaluation requires a dichotomous outcome (the animal does or does not have the condition), a cut-off value must be selected for assays that generate continuous data (as do most clinical chemistry assays). Sensitivity and specificity will necessarily vary with the specific threshold chosen. For example, when a 1350 fmol/mL cut-off value for a proANP ELISA is used to screen dogs for the presence of congestive heart failure (in which the theoretical prevalence is 10%), only 38% of positive results represent true cases, though 99% of negative results are correct. Raising the cut-off value to 1750 fmol/mL results in 79% correct positive results and 98% correct negative results (Boswood et al., 2003).

Receiver operator curves (ROCs) are an accepted method for describing and comparing the accuracy of diagnostic assays for each possible cut-off value (Metz, 1978; Zou et al., 2007; Soreide, 2009). Their use in veterinary clinical pathology is growing (Gardner and Greiner, 2006). A ROC curve is a graphical display of the sensitivity (true positive rate) of a diagnostic test over all possible false-positive rates (1 − specificity; false detection of the condition) (see hypothetical ROC curve in Zou et al., 2007). The area under the curve (AUC) is a summary statistic of test accuracy also known as the c-statistic or c-index wherein an AUC of 0.50 indicates that the test has no ability to discriminate animals with the condition from those without the condition, while an AUC of 1.00

TABLE 25.6
Diagnostic Test Attributes Table

	Gold Standard			
	Condition Present	**Condition Absent**	**Total**	
Assay Result Positive	True Positive (TP)	False Positive (FP)	TP + FP	Positive Predictive Value = TP/(TP + FP)
Assay Result Negative	False Negative (FN)	True Negative (TN)	TN + FN	Negative Predictive Value = TN/(TN + FN)
Total	TP + FN	TN + FP	–	–
–	Sensitivity = TP/(TP + FN)	Specificity = TN/(TN + FP)	–	Prevalence = TP + FN/TP + FP + TN + FN

Source: Modified from Florkowski, C.M., *Clin Biochem Rev*, 29, S83–S87, 2008.

perfectly discriminates. Tests considered to have moderate to high discrimination have an AUC in the range of 0.80–0.90 (Gardner and Greiner, 2006).

The ROC curve and the measures of accuracy derived from it have several advantages over other measures of diagnostic performance: (1) they are independent of the prevalence of the condition; (2) both components of accuracy, that is, sensitivity and specificity, are incorporated into an AUC as a single measure of accuracy, and (3) two or more diagnostic assays can be compared (Obuchowski et al., 2004). Results from ROC analysis that are typically reported in addition to the AUC include confidence intervals (CIs) for the AUC, and the sensitivity and specificity at selected cut-off points.

Study design that minimizes bias and ensures proper patient selection and classification is essential for optimal ROC analysis (Gardner and Greiner, 2006; Zweig and Campbell 1993). Sample size is a key factor affecting the precision of estimation of AUC for a single assay and the ability to identify differences between AUCs for multiple tests (Gardner and Greiner, 2006). For example, at least 33 control animals and 33 animals with the condition of interest are needed if a given diagnostic test is expected to have fair accuracy (e.g., AUC = 0.70) (Obuchowski 2004). Sample sizes that are too small may result in overly optimistic measures of accuracy (Leeflang et al., 2008). Specific recommendations for sample size calculation for ROC analysis have been published (Obuchowski and McClish, 1997; Obuchowski et al., 2004).

For clinical biomarkers that are specifically intended to be used to diagnose a condition in an individual animal, defining a likelihood ratio (LR) may be helpful (Gardner and Greiner, 2006; Kim and Pak, 2008). This ratio is an index of diagnostic utility that incorporates sensitivity and specificity and provides the diagnostician an estimate of how much a test result will change the odds that the individual has the condition. LRs can be calculated for a positive (LR+) and for a negative (LR–) test result. LR+ is sensitivity/(1 – specificity) and ranges from 1 to infinity. It conveys how much the odds of having the condition increase when the test is positive. LR– is (1 – sensitivity)/specificity and ranges from 0 to 1. It conveys how much the odds of having the condition decrease when a test is negative. The LR can then be used to inform clinical decision-making by providing an estimate of the "posttest" odds that the individual animal has the condition by multiplying the LR by the "pretest" odds. Pretest odds have some level of uncertainty, but can be estimated based on the prevalence of the condition, patient risk factors, and the clinician's assessment of that individual patient's status. Examples of applications of likelihood ratios can be found in Gardner and Greiner (2006), Glas et al. (2003), and Parikh et al. (2009).

When multiple biomarkers are compared or a novel biomarker is developed to address limitations of a traditional marker, verifying improved accuracy, sensitivity, and specificity is a key, but not the only consideration in qualification. Additional advantages of a potentially superior candidate might include a greater dynamic range of response, improved correlation with the course injury (e.g., more closely follows changes from baseline, peak, and recovery of the condition of interest), exhibits more consistent premonitory changes prior to manifestation of the condition of interest (e.g., for a predictive biomarker), improved correlation between the magnitude of change in the analyte and the severity of injury, and/or a distinct dose relationship (e.g., for pharmaceutical studies). When urinary KIM-1 was compared to serum urea nitrogen and creatinine in rats with renal toxicity, the traditional markers were less sensitive, exhibited smaller dynamic ranges, and demonstrated less consistent correlation with the course of injury providing support for the practical utility and biological superiority of the new marker (Zhou et al., 2008).

25.5 SUMMARY

Biomarker research is a dynamic interdisciplinary field driven by novel technologies and by advances in basic biological science and comparative medicine. Development of a successful biomarker in laboratory animals can lead to applications in humans and vice versa. Such "bridging" biomarkers must undergo rigorous technical validation and qualification efforts tailored to the intended use in the species of interest. Markers that progress from research to clinical settings are often described as translational markers. Examples of these types of biomarkers in recent years include KIM-1, troponin I, and natriuretic peptides. Whatever the specific application may be, the key attributes of an optimal biomarker assay are that it is fit for purpose, e.g., technically feasible, technically sound, and meet the established biologic criteria appropriate to the use of the assay.

REFERENCES

Apple, F.S., Murakami, M.M., Ler, R., et al. 2008. Analytical characteristics of commercial cardiac troponin I and T immunoassays in serum from rats, dogs, and monkeys with induced acute myocardial injury. *Clin Chem.* 54:1982–1989.

Atkinson Jr., A.J., Colburn, W.A., DeGruttola,V.G., et al. 2001. Biomarkers and surrogate endpoints: Preferred definitions and conceptual framework. *Clin Pharmacol Ther.* 69:89–95.

Bailey, W.J. and Ulrich, R. 2004. Molecular profiling approaches for identifying novel biomarkers. *Expert Opin Drug Saf.* 3:137–151.

Bauer, D.C., Hunter, D.J., Abramson, S.B., et al. 2006. Classification of osteoarthritis biomarkers: A proposed approach. *Osteoarthritis Cartilage.* 14:723–727.

Bonventre, J.V. 2008. Kidney injury molecule-1 (KIM-1): A specific and sensitive biomarker of kidney injury. *Scand J Clin Lab Invest.* 241:78–83.

Bonventre, J.V. 2009. Kidney injury molecule-1 (KIM-1): A urinary biomarker and much more. *Nephrol Dialysis Transpl.* 24:3265–3268.

Boswood, A., Attree, S., and Page, K. 2003. Clinical validation of a proANP 31-67 fragment ELISA in the diagnosis of heart failure in the dog. *J Small Anim Pract.* 44:104–108.

Bunn, H.F., Haney, D.N., Gabbay, K.H., et al. 1975. Further identification of the nature and linkage of the carbohydrate in hemoglobin A1c. *Biochem Biophys Res Commun.* 67:103–109.

Carr, S.A. and Anderson, L. 2008. Protein quantitation through targeted mass spectrometry: The way out of biomarker purgatory? *Clin Chem.* 54:1749–1752.

Devarajan, P. 2008. Neutrophil gelatinase-associated lipocalin (NGAL): A new marker of kidney disease. *Scand J Clin Invest Suppl.* 24:89–94.

Findlay, J.W.A., Smith, W.C., Lee, J.W., et al. 2000. Validation of immunoassays for bioanalysis: A pharmaceutical industry perspective. *J Pharm Biomed Anal.* 21:1249–1273.

Florkowski, C.M. 2008. Sensitivity, specificity, receiver-operating characteristic (ROC) curves and likelihood ratios: Communicating the performance of diagnostic tests. *Clin Biochem Rev.* 29(Suppl 1):S83–S87.

Food and Drug Administration. 2001. Guidance for industry on bioanalytical method validation. *Fed Regist.* 66:28526–28527.

Gardner, I.A. and Greiner, M. 2006. Receiver-operating characteristic curves and likelihood ratios: Improvements over traditional methods for the evaluation and application of veterinary clinical pathology tests. *Vet Clin Pathol.* 35:8–17.

Glas, A.S., Lijmer, J.G., Prins, M.H. et al. 2003.The diagnostic odds ratio: a single indicator of test performance. *J Clin Epidemiol.* 56:1129--1135.

Goodsaid, F.M., Frueh, F.W., and Mattes, W. 2008. Strategic paths for biomarker qualification. *Toxicology.* 245:219–223.

Hoo, R.L.C., Yeung, D.C.Y., Lam, K.S.L., et al. 2008. Inflammatory biomarkers associated with obesity and insulin resistance: A focus on lipocalin-2 and adipocyte fatty acid-binding protein. *Expert Rev Endocrinol Metab.* 3:29–41.

Ichimura, T., Bonventre, J.V., Bailly, V., et al. 1998. Kidney injury molecule-1 (KIM-1), a putative epithelial cell adhesion molecule containing a novel immunoglobulin domain, is up-regulated in renal cells after injury. *J Biol Chem.* 273:4135–4142.

Jacobs, R.M., Lumsden, J.H., and Grift, E. 1992. Effects of bilirubinemia, hemolysis, and lipemia on clinical chemistry analytes in bovine, canine, equine, and feline sera. *Can Vet J.* 33:605–608.

Kim, E. and Pak, S. 2008. Use of likelihood ratios in evidence-based clinical decision making. *J Vet Clin.* 25:146–151.

Klee, E.W. 2008. Data mining for biomarker development: A review of tissue specificity analyses. *Clin Lab Med.* 28:127–143.

Kramer, A.B., van Timmeren, M.M., Schuurs, T.A., et al. 2009. Reduction of proteinuria in adriamycin-induced nephropathy is associated with reduction of renal kidney injury molecule (Kim-1) over time. *Am J Physiol Renal Physiol.* 296:F1136–F1145.

Lee, J.W. Devanarayan, V., Barrett, Y.C., et al. 2006. Fit-for-purpose method development and validation for successful biomarker measurement. *Pharm Res.* 23:312–328.

Lee, J.W., Weiner, R.S., Sailstad, J.M, et al. 2005. Method validation and measurement of biomarkers in nonclinical and clinical samples in drug development: A conference report. *Pharm Res.* 22:2495–2499.

Leeflang, M.M.G., Moons, K.G.M., Reitsma, J.B., et al. 2008. Bias in sensitivity and specificity caused by data-driven selection of optimal cutoff values: Mechanisms, magnitude, and solutions. *Clin Chem.* 54:729–737.

Lindblom, P., Rafter, I., Copley, C., et al. 2007. Isoforms of alanine aminotransferases in human tissues and serum-differential tissue expression using novel antibodies. *Arch Biochem Biophys.* 466:66–77.

Marrer, E. and Dieterle, F. 2007. Promises of biomarkers in drug development—a reality check. *Chem Biol Drug Des.* 69:381–394.

Mendrick, D.L. 2008. Genomic and genetic biomarkers of toxicity. *Toxicology.* 245:175–181.

Metz, C.E. 1978. Basic principles of ROC analysis. *Semin Nucl Med.* 8:282–298.

Miyazaki, M, Rosenblum, J.S., Kasahara, Y., et al. 2009. Determination of enzymatic source of alanine aminotransferase activity in serum from dogs with liver injury. *J Pharmacol Toxicol Meth.* 60:307–315.

Nishijima, Y., Feldman, D.S., Bonagura, J.D., et al., 2005. Canine nonischemic left ventricular dysfunction: A model of chronic human cardiomyopathy. *J Cardiac Failure.* 11:638–644.

Obuchowski, N.A. and McClish, D.K. 1997. Sample size determination for diagnostic accuracy studies involving binormal ROC curve indices. *Stat Med.* 16:1529–1542.

Obuchowski, N.A., Leiber, M.L., and Wians, F.H., Jr. 2004. ROC curves in clinical chemistry: Uses, misuses, and possible dolutions. *Clin Chem.* 50:1118–1125.

Oyama, M.A., Sission, D.D., and Solter, P.E. 2007. Prospective screening for occult cardiomyopathy in dogs by measurement of plasma atrial natriuretic peptide, B-type natriuretic peptide, and cardiac troponin-I concentrations. *Am J Vet Res.* 68:42–47.

Parikh, R. Parikh, S., Arun, E., and Thomas, R. 2009. Likelihood ratios; Clinical application in day-to-day practice. *Indian J Ophthalmol* 57:217–221.

Rajamohan, F., Nelms, L., Joslin, D.L., et al, 2006. cDNA cloning, expression, purification, distribution, and characterization of biologically active canine alanine aminotransferase-1. *Prot Express Purif.* 48:81–89.

Ransohoff, D.F. 2004. Rules of evidence for cancer molecular-marker discovery and validation. *Nature Rev Cancer.* 4:309–314.

Ransohoff, D.F. 2007. How to improve reliability and efficiency of research about molecular markers: Roles of phases, guidelines and study design. *J Clin Epidemiol.* 60:1205–1219.

Sabbisetti, V.S., Ito, K., Wang, C. et al. 2013. Novel assays for detection of urinary KIM-1 in mouse models of kidney injury. *Toxicol Sci.* 131:13–25.

Sinhaa, A., Singha, C., Parmara, D., et al. 2007. Proteomics in clinical interventions: Achievements and limitations in biomarker development. *Life Sci.* 80:1345–1354.

Soreide, K. 2009. Receiver-operating characteristic curve analysis in diagnostic, prognostic and predictive biomarker research. *J Clin Path.* 62:1–5.

Stokol, T., Tarrant, J.M., and Scarlett, J.M. 2001. Overestimation of canine albumin concentration with the bromcresol green method in heparinized plasma samples. *Vet Clin Pathol.* 30:170–176.

Vaidya, V.S., Ozer, J.S., Dieterle, F., et al. 2010. Kidney injury molecule-1 outperforms traditional biomarkers of kidney injury in preclinical biomarker qualification studies. *Nat Biotechnol.* 28:478–485.

Van Timmeren, M.M., Vaidya, V.S., van Ree, R.M., et al. 2007. High urinary excretion of kidney injury molecule-1 is an independent predictor of graft loss in renal transplant recipients. *Transplantation.* 84:1625–1630.

Wagner, J.A. 2002. Overview of biomarkers and surrogate endpoints in drug development. *Dis Markers.* 18:41–46.

Wagner, J.A. 2008. Strategic approach to fit-for-purpose biomarkers in drug development. *Annu Rev Pharmacol Toxicol.* 48:631–651.

Woderer, S., Henninger, N., Garthe, C.-D., et al. 2007. Continuous glucose monitoring in interstitial fluid using glucose oxidase-based sensor compared to established blood glucose measurement in rats. *Anal Chim Acta.* 581:7–12.

Wu, Y., Boonloed, A., Sleszynski, N., et al. 2015. Clinical chemistry measurements with commercially available test slides on a smartphone platform: colorimetric determination of glucose and urea. *Clin Chem.* 448:133–138.

Zhou, Y., Vaidya, V.S., Brown, R.P., et al. 2008. Comparison of kidney injury molecule-1 and other nephrotoxicity biomakers in urine and kidney following acute exposure to gentamicin, mercury, and chromium. *Toxicol Sci*. 101:159–170.

Zou, K.H., O'Malley, A.J., and Mauri, L. 2007. Receiver-operating characteristic analysis for evaluating diagnostic tests and predictive models. *Circulation*. 115:654–657.

Zweig, M.H. and Campbell, G. 1993. Receiver-operating characteristic (ROC) plots: A fundamental evaluation tool in clinical medicine. *Clin Chem*. 39:561–577.

26 Statistical Methods

Grace E. Kissling

CONTENTS

Clinical chemistry assays produce either quantitative or qualitative results. Because most statistical issues involve quantitative results, this chapter primarily focuses on quantitative assays; however, where applicable, statistical treatment of qualitative assays will also be described.

26.1 STATISTICS FOR EVALUATION OF ANALYTICAL METHODS

26.1.1 QUANTITATIVE ASSAYS

To best understand quantitative assay results, it is helpful to review the numerical development of the assay. Typically, a range of known quantities of the analyte is processed and the assay instrumentation produces numeric results (analytic values or analytic signals). A plot of the analytic values versus the known quantities of the analyte is the calibration or standard curve (Figure 26.1a). While some standard curves are based on as few as six distinct known concentrations, more are recommended, especially if the standard curve departs from linearity (FDA, 2001). In addition to known concentrations, samples lacking the analyte, or blanks, are also included to determine the lower limit of detection (LOD). Once the standard curve is established, unknown concentrations can be determined from analytic values as shown in Figure 26.1b. Standard curves are highly dependent on the assay methodology and laboratory, so each laboratory develops its own standard curve for each assay.

The accuracy of an assay refers to its ability to produce correct values, while the precision refers to its ability to produce consistent, reproducible values. A good assay is both accurate and precise. While it may be reassuring to get similar numbers from different runs on the same sample, these numbers are not useful if they are incorrect. Likewise, if an assay produces correct results, on average, but any given measurement greatly varies around the average, the assay results are also not useful. The precision of an assay is commonly expressed as a coefficient of variation, CV, which is the standard deviation (SD) divided by the mean ($\overline{x}$), expressed as a percentage.

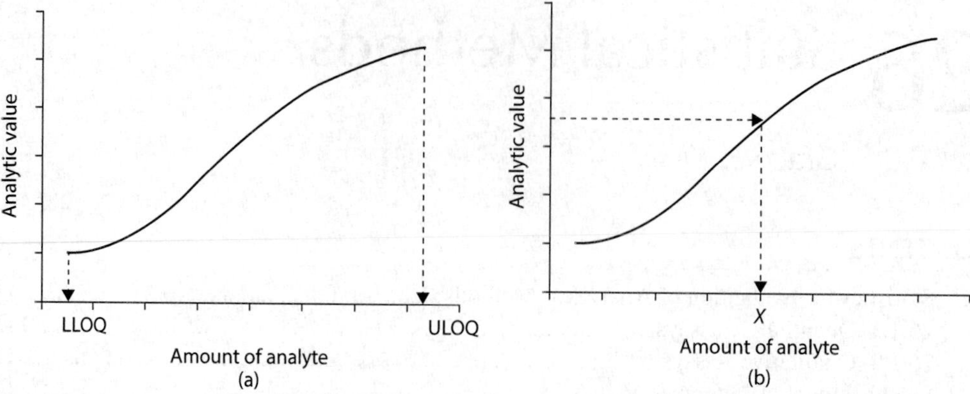

FIGURE 26.1 Standard curve or calibration curve. (a) Using a range of known concentrations of the analyte, the standard curve is a plot of the instrumentation's analytic value versus the amount of the analyte. The standard curve is valid for analyte amounts between the lower limit of quantitation (LLOQ) and the upper limit of quantitation (ULOQ). (b) Once the standard curve is generated, the amount of analyte in a new sample, *X*, can be determined from the analytic value by following the analytic value horizontally to the curve, then reading down to the analyte axis.

$$\mathrm{CV} = \frac{\mathrm{SD}}{\bar{x}} \times 100\%$$

Coefficients of variation for quantitative assays should be small, ideally, less than 10%–15%. *CVs* are useful for quantifying both intra- and interassay variability. Intra-assay variability is assessed from technical replicates (e.g., aliquots from the same sample) that are run simultaneously; interassay variability is assessed from technical replicates that are run sequentially over time. For establishing both intra- and interassay variability, the technical replicates are drawn from samples having known concentrations that span the range of the assay, and runs are repeated several times.

Over time, analytic values may drift due to instrumentation idiosyncrasies and/or local environmental conditions. Therefore, laboratories routinely include calibration runs periodically to check for drift. In these runs, known concentrations of the analyte are processed to verify that they still fall along the standard curve. If the readings are found to be out of calibration, adjustments are made either to the assay or to the standard curve. To minimize potential drift, it is common during assay development to identify factors that affect the readings so that these can be controlled to the extent possible (e.g., temperature, humidity, etc.).

The standard curve is monotonic increasing (or decreasing) for which a one-to-one correspondence exists between analytic values and analyte concentrations. A linear standard curve indicates that analyte concentrations are proportional to the assay's measured values; this contributes to greater assay accuracy. Furthermore, linear standard curves may be converted to formulas that are less prone to error than concentrations read from a plot. Because of the quantitation advantages of linear standard curves, authoritative guidelines describe methods of assuring linearity (EMEA, 1995; FDA, 1998).

All quantitative assays have a specific range within which they provide analytic values. The limits of this range are laboratory-specific and will be determined during the development of the standard curve. In most assays, a blank (absence of the analyte) will still produce a measurement, and if blanks are run repeatedly, these measurements will exhibit variability (e.g., standard deviation of blanks, $\mathrm{SD}_{\mathrm{blanks}}$) around a mean ($\bar{x}_{\mathrm{blanks}}$). The LOD is defined as the smallest concentration of the analyte that will produce measurements that are statistically significantly higher than the blank and it is determined from the distribution of blanks measurements. The LOD is calculated as t SDs above the mean of the blanks.

$$\text{LOD} = \bar{x}_{\text{blanks}} + t \times \text{SD}_{\text{blanks}}$$

There are various recommendations about how to determine t. Some authors recommend selecting t from the Student's t-distribution at the 0.01 level of significance, while others set t to a specific number such as 6 or 8 (e.g., see discussions in ACS, 1980; Long and Winefordner, 1983). The lower limit of quantitation (LLOQ) is the lowest concentration that can be reliably measured, while the upper limit of quantitation (ULOQ) is the highest concentration that can be reliably measured. These limits of quantitation are determined during the development of the standard curve and may be laboratory dependent. The interval between the LLOQ and the ULOQ is the dynamic range of the assay.

In research studies, analyte concentrations that are determined to be below the LLOQ or LOD or above the ULOQ present a challenge because numeric values are not immediately available for calculations. These measurements should not be discarded; they indicate that the amount of analyte is very low or very high even if it cannot be reliably quantified. For concentrations below the LLOQ, a usual practice is to substitute LLOQ/2 or LLOQ/$\sqrt{2}$ (EPA, 2000; Croghan and Egeghy, 2003; Clayton et al., 2003). Substitution is reasonable as long as not more than 10%–15% of the values are below LLOQ. If more than 15% are below the LLOQ, substitution will artificially reduce the variability of the sample, and other methods should be considered. An alternative to substitution is to use likelihood methods, such as profile likelihood estimation. These methods are also applicable when measurements exceed the ULOQ. Likelihood methods rely on specifying the shape of the distribution of measurements (such as log-normal) and using the observed values along with the numbers of values below the LLOQ and above the ULOQ to estimate the mean and standard deviation of the group (Helsel, 1990; EPA, 2000; Koo et al., 2002).

During the development and distribution of a new assay, a round-robin test is often conducted for which a common set of samples are sent to several laboratories to determine the extent to which measurements agree across different laboratories (Youden, 1963). These tests may require that the same assay is used at each laboratory, or they may allow each laboratory to select the assay to use. In either case, the goal is to determine the validity and reproducibility of determining analyte concentrations in a variety of settings.

26.1.2 Qualitative Assays

Qualitative assays, such as dipstick assays, usually indicate the presence or absence of an analyte. For these assays, sensitivity and specificity are of primary importance. Sensitivity of the assay is the proportion of tests that are positive when the analyte is present; specificity is the proportion of tests that are negative when the analyte is absent. An informative assay should be both sensitive and specific. Three additional measures of qualitative assay performance are positive predictive value, negative predictive value, and accuracy. The positive predictive value is the proportion of positive tests that correctly determined that the analyte is present; the negative predictive value is the proportion of negative tests that correctly determined that the analyte is absent. The accuracy is the proportion of all tests that correctly determined that the analyte is present or absent. These measures are summarized in Table 26.1.

26.2 ESTABLISHMENT OF REFERENCE VALUES

A clinician or researcher who obtains an assay value on an animal will usually want to interpret that value in the context of what is typical. There are several ways to determine this. Many diagnostic laboratories maintain reference values (or reference ranges) of "normal" or "control" animals. Research facilities may establish historical control databases in which data from control animals are recorded. These values are species-, sex-, and strain-specific, and they may also depend on a

TABLE 26.1
Sensitivity, Specificity, Positive Predictive Value, Negative Predictive Value, and Accuracy of Qualitative Assays Having Binary Outcomes

	In Reality		
Assay Result	**Analyte Is Present**	**Analyte Is Absent**	**Total**
Positive	n_{P+}	n_{A+}	n_+
Negative	n_{P-}	n_{A-}	n_-
Total	n_P	n_A	n

n_{P+} is the number of samples for which the analyte is present and the assay is positive.
n_{A+} is the number of samples for which the analyte is absent and the assay is positive.
n_{P-} is the number of samples for which the analyte is present and the assay is negative.
n_{A-} is the number of samples for which the analyte is absent and the assay is negative.
n_P is the number of samples for which the analyte is present; it is also called the number of "true positives."
n_A is the number of samples for which the analyte is absent; it is also called the number of "true negatives."
n_+ is the number of samples for which the assay is positive.
n_- is the number of samples for which the assay is negative.
n is the number of samples assayed.
Sensitivity = n_{P+}/n_P.
Specificity = n_{A-}/n_A.
Positive Predictive Value (PPV) = n_{P+}/n_+.
Negative Predictive Value (NPV) = n_{A-}/n_-.
Accuracy = $(n_{P+} + n_{A-})/n$.

multitude of factors including age, diet, route of exposure, housing arrangements, animal husbandry practices, season, and year. Therefore, these factors, and any other potential influences, should be examined and accounted for when compiling reference ranges.

In the past, the range of typical values has been referred to as "normal values" or the "normal range"; this terminology may be somewhat confusing in that it seems to imply that these are ranges for healthy individuals, or possibly that they follow the statistical normal distribution (e.g., see Sunderman, 1975 and its references). A better term is "reference values" or "reference range." The reference values are obtained from a well-defined set of individuals (the reference sample) in terms of age, sex, species/strain, condition of health, and so on. Furthermore, these values may be specific to a particular laboratory and the analytical instrumentation that they use. Reference ranges should be periodically verified with new data and updated to adjust for unanticipated drift.

The reference range spans the middle 95% of values obtained from the reference sample; this is sometimes referred to as a "tolerance interval" (Wald and Wolfowitz, 1946; Proschan, 1953). Determination of the endpoints of the reference range depends on the shape of the distribution of measurements in the reference sample. Many biological measurements have a normal or Gaussian distribution. Normal distributions are characterized by their mean, μ, and standard deviation, σ, and by their bell-curve shape (see Figure 26.2a). When $\mu = 0$ and $\sigma = 1$, the distribution is known as the standard normal distribution. The normal distribution has been well studied and its properties are also useful in parametric statistical testing, as described later in this chapter. A useful property of the family of normal distributions is that approximately 68% of the distribution lies within one standard deviation of the mean; approximately 95% lies within two standard deviations of the mean; and over 99% lies within three standard deviations of the mean. Thus, if reference sample measurements are normally distributed, as in Figure 26.2a, the upper and lower reference values are 1.96 (or 2) standard deviations above and below the mean

$$\bar{x} \pm 1.96 \times \text{SD}$$

This will encompass the middle 95% of values. One should keep in mind that 5% of the reference sample values will be outside of this range.

More typically for clinical chemistry, measurements from the reference sample are not normally distributed, so other methods for determining the reference range must be considered. Often, analyte concentrations are skewed to the right (skewed upward) and the logarithm of the concentrations are normally distributed. In this case, the concentrations are log-normally distributed (Figure 26.2b). Reference values of the log-transformed distribution (i.e., a normal distribution) can be found as described above, then antilog transformed to return to the original unit of measure. If the reference sample values do not reasonably fit a normal or log-normal distribution, the 2.5th and 97.5th percentiles can still be determined, provided that the sample is large enough (Figure 26.2c).

The number of individuals needed to establish the reference range will depend on the nature of the distribution of values. Reed et al. (1971) suggested that data from 120 individuals is usually adequate for establishing reference values. If the values are strongly skewed, however, 120 will not be sufficient to precisely capture the extreme percentiles (Reed et al., 1971; Miller et al., 1984).

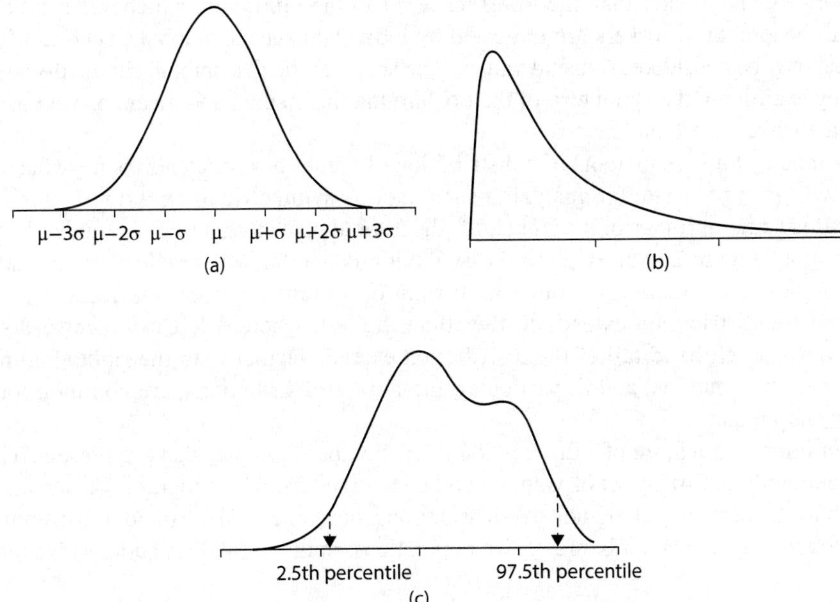

FIGURE 26.2 Examples of analyte distributions. (a) The normal distribution is symmetric and unimodal. It is centered around the mean, μ, and variability is described by the standard deviation, σ. Approximately 68% of the distribution is within 1σ of the mean; 95% is within 2σ of the mean; and over 99% is within 3σ of the mean. (b) The log-normal distribution is skewed to the right. It is a common distribution for clinical chemistry endpoints. (c) This non-normal distribution has two modes, which may suggest that two populations are present. The 95% tolerance interval extends from the 2.5th to the 97.5th percentile.

26.3 METHODS FOR EVALUATING STUDY DATA

Research studies on laboratory animals often involve clinical chemistry endpoints. The statistical methods selected for evaluation of study data will depend on a number of factors including the study design, the hypotheses, the data type (quantitative or qualitative), the sample size, and the shape of the distribution of values. For this discussion, the term, sample, refers to the collection of values obtained from an assay, rather than the biological material that is assayed.

26.3.1 Descriptive Statistics

The initial step in any statistical analysis is to summarize the data. Three characteristics of the data are of primary interest: central or typical value, variability relative to the center, and shape of the distribution of values. The most appropriate methods for summarizing center and variability depend on the shape of the distribution, so that will be the first topic.

26.3.1.1 Shape of the Distribution

Graphical statistical tools are useful for characterizing the shape of the distribution of an endpoint. These tools include histograms, bar charts, and boxplots. Boxplots convey several important features of a distribution. The box indicates the range of the middle 50% of the values, with endpoints ranging from the 25th to the 75th percentiles (Figure 26.3). The magnitude of this middle 50% is the interquartile range (IQR) and is sometimes used as a measure of variability. Within the box, the median is indicated by a horizontal line. The mean is indicated with a special symbol, usually a plus sign (+). The upper and lower fences are, respectively, 1.5 IQRs above and below the box. A line above the box (also known as a whisker) extends to the value closest to, and less than, the upper fence or to the maximum, whichever is reached first; the line below the box extends to the value closest to, and greater than the lower fence, or to the minimum, whichever is reached first. Any values beyond the whiskers are indicated by individual special symbols, such as asterisks or circles, and may be considered unusual values. The shape of the distribution can be discerned from boxplots by examining the symmetry of the box around the median and mean, as well as the symmetry of the whiskers around the box.

The symmetry (or lack thereof) of a distribution of values has implications for what statistical methods will be appropriate for analyzing such data. A symmetric distribution is one for which the left half is a mirror image of the right half; the normal distribution is an example of a symmetric distribution (Figure 26.2a). A skewed distribution is one for which values in one half extend farther along the scale than in the other half; right or upward skewness indicates that the right-hand tail of the distribution extends farther than the left, whereas left or downward skewness indicates that the left-hand tail of the distribution extends farther than the right (Figure 26.2b). Right-skewed distributions, and in particular, log-normal distributions, are common for clinical chemistry endpoints.

Another important feature of a distribution is the number of modes that are present. The mode, or most commonly occurring set of values, can be identified from a histogram. Unimodal distributions, such as the normal and log-normal distributions, have one mode. Bimodal distributions have two modes and may reflect a mixture of two populations; multimodal distributions also may reflect

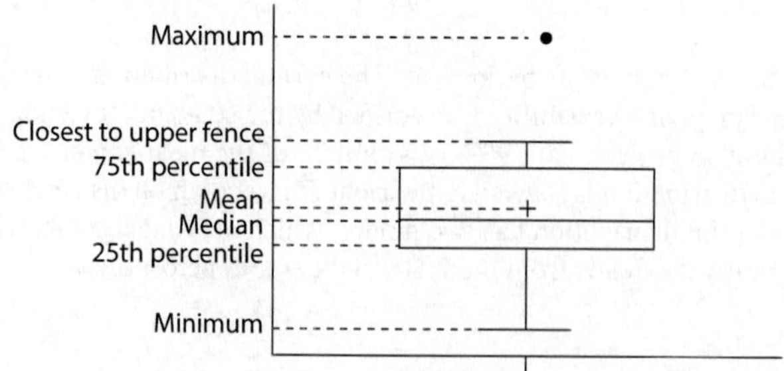

FIGURE 26.3 Example of a boxplot. Boxplots are useful graphical tools for illustrating several characteristics of a distribution. The box extends from the 25th to the 75th percentiles, capturing the middle 50% of the data; the length of the box is the interquartile range (IQR). The median and mean are indicated by a horizontal line and a plus sign (+), respectively. Whiskers extend from the box to indicate the range of values within 1.5 IQRs. Values beyond 1.5 IQRs of the box are indicated by special symbols, such as a dot, and may be considered outliers.

a mixture of populations. Samples having bimodal or multimodal distributions may be difficult to interpret in experimental investigations without intensive statistical treatment.

As previously mentioned, the normal distribution is commonly observed in biological systems. It is a unimodal, symmetric distribution that has sometimes been characterized as a bell curve. Because many parametric statistical methods rely on properties of the normal distribution, statistical researchers have developed a number of formal tests for normality. These include the chi-square goodness-of-fit test (Cochran, 1952), Kolmogorov–Smirnov test (Massey, 1951), Lilliefors test (Lilliefors, 1967), Shapiro–Wilk test (Shapiro and Wilk, 1965), among others. In addition, graphical methods such as Q–Q plots are helpful in establishing normality (Samuels and Witmer, 2002). In these plots, the sample percentiles are plotted against theoretical percentiles that would result if the data were normally distributed. If the points fall on or near a straight line at a 45° angle, the data are considered normally distributed.

Another concern about the distribution of an endpoint is the presence of outliers. There are a number of methods for detecting outliers (e.g., see Barnett and Lewis, 1994). As described above for boxplots, values that are more than 1.5 IQRs beyond the 25th and 75th percentiles are unusual and may be considered possible outliers. Formal statistical outlier tests are based on distances between the potential outlier and the rest of the data. For example, if the maximum is suspected to be an outlier, Dixon's Q test is based on the ratio of the gap between the highest and next highest values and the range.

$$\frac{\text{Maximum} - \text{Next Highest Value}}{\text{Maximum} - \text{Minimum}}$$

If this difference exceeds tabled values, the maximum is declared an outlier (Dean and Dixon, 1951; Dixon, 1953). Other outlier tests are based on properties of the normal distribution, such as Grubbs' test (Grubbs, 1969). If the maximum is the suspected outlier, the quantity

$$\frac{\text{Maximum} - \overline{x}}{s}$$

is calculated and compared to tabled critical values (Grubbs, 1969). If the minimum is the suspected outlier, it replaces the maximum in the above formula.

When an outlier is found, it is natural to consider whether to retain the value for further statistical analyses. Generally, an outlier should be removed only if there is evidence that it is a result of an error in the execution of the study. These errors may include instrumentation problems, record-keeping errors, insufficient sampling, implausible values, and serious deviations from protocol. Outliers that are likely due to biological variation may be informative to the study and should not be discarded.

26.3.1.2 Measures of the Center

For notational ease, suppose that there are n values, labeled $x_1, x_2, \ldots, x_n$. When the distribution of values is symmetric and unimodal, the mean (or arithmetic average) is the preferred measure of the center of the data:

$$\overline{x} = \frac{\sum_{i=1}^{n} x_i}{n}$$

If, however, the distribution is skewed to the right (left), the mean will be unduly influenced by the higher (lower) values and will not be a good representative of the center. In this case, the median is preferred. The median is the value for which half of the measurements are higher and half are lower. This middle value is said to be a "resistant" measure of center because it is not influenced by outliers or skewness. For bimodal and multimodal distributions, the mode(s) will be the most appropriate measure of center.

The geometric mean is used for data that have a log-normal distribution. By definition, the geometric mean is the *n*th root of the product of the values, and it is easily calculated as the exponential of the mean of the log-transformed values:

$$x_{geo} = \sqrt[n]{\prod_{i=1}^{n} x_i}$$

$$= \exp\left(\frac{\sum_{i=1}^{n} \log_e(x_i)}{n}\right)$$

26.3.1.3 Measures of Variability

Measures of variability are generally paired with a measure of center. The standard deviation and standard error of the mean are typically associated with the mean, while the range and IQR are associated with the median. The modal percentage, or percentage of the sample belonging to the modal set, describes the variability associated with the mode(s).

The standard deviation (SD) describes an average deviation of individual values around the mean:

$$SD = \sqrt{\frac{\sum_{i=1}^{n} (x_i - \bar{x})^2}{n-1}}$$

The denominator, $n - 1$, is referred to as the degrees of freedom or *df*. As previously described, normally distributed endpoints have very predicable properties; in that ~68% of the values will be between $\bar{x} - SD$ and $\bar{x} + SD$; ~95% will be between $\bar{x} - 2 \times SD$ and $\bar{x} + 2 \times SD$; and nearly all of the distribution will be between $\bar{x} - 3 \times SD$ and $\bar{x} + 3 \times SD$. Endpoints that are not normally distributed do not follow this 68%–95%–99% rule.

The standard error of the mean (SEM or SE) originates from the properties of the mean, $\bar{x}$. Hypothetically, if one were to repeat an experiment infinitely many times and calculate the mean each time, the set of means would vary around a true mean. The standard deviation of these infinitely many means is the standard error of the mean. Thus, the SEM quantifies the variation in the sample mean that we would expect to see if we were to repeat the experiment many times. For normally distributed endpoints

$$SEM = \frac{SD}{\sqrt{n}}$$

Whether to use the SD or the SEM in a given situation will depend on the purpose of the numerical summary. If the purpose is to describe how individuals vary, the SD should be selected. For example, for normally distributed endpoints, the SD is used to derive reference values used to interpret individual measurements. On the other hand, if a goal of the study is to describe the mean of a group and how it might differ from other groups, the SEM should be selected.

For log-normally distributed endpoints, use of the SEM is not entirely straightforward. The SEM of the log-transformed data can be calculated using the formula above, but taking the antilog to return to the original unit of measure will give a value that has no context with the log-normal distribution. Instead, calculations using the SEM of the log-transformed data, such as confidence interval construction described below, should be carried out before the result is antilog transformed (Bland and Altman, 1996).

Statistical calculations should always use the original, unrounded data to avoid round-off errors. The final result, however, should be rounded off to reflect the accuracy of the measurements. There is no standard rule for how much to round off. However, some considerations in deciding how much to round off include the precision of the measurements and the sample size.

26.4 CONFIDENCE INTERVALS

Confidence intervals are a useful inferential tool to describe a likely range within which a parameter is likely to belong. The idea behind confidence intervals is very similar to that of the SEM. If an experiment were to be repeated infinitely many times, and a parameter (e.g., mean, area under the curve, proportion) is estimated each time, the parameter estimates would vary and their distribution could be determined. In reality, the experiment is conducted only once and the parameter is estimated only once. By statistical theory, we can predict the distribution of values and construct a confidence interval that will have a prescribed probability of capturing the true parameter value. Generally, this probability is high, such as 95% or 99%. For example, the mean of n normally distributed values has a 95% confidence interval of the form

$$\bar{x} \pm t_{n-1} \times \text{SEM}$$

where t_{n-1} is a critical value from the student's t-distribution having n−1 df and probability 0.025 to the right. While this confidence interval is symmetric around $\bar{x}$, confidence intervals, such as those for the standard deviation or for the geometric mean, may be asymmetric. To construct a 95% confidence interval for the geometric mean, we first construct a confidence interval for the log-transformed mean, using the same critical t_{n-1} value as before. For notational ease, let $z_i = \log_e(x_i)$:

$$\bar{z} \pm t_{n-1}\sqrt{\frac{\sum_{i=1}^{n}(z_i - \bar{z})^2}{n-1}}$$

Labeling the lower limit of this interval as z_L and the upper limit as z_U, the 95% confidence interval for the geometric mean will be

$$(\exp(z_L), \exp(z_U))$$

Confidence intervals can also be useful for qualitative endpoints, such as for the proportion showing a positive response. Within a homogeneous group, statistical theory predicts that the number of positive responders has a binomial distribution, so the formula for the 95% confidence interval reflects this underlying distribution.

$$\hat{p} \pm z \times \sqrt{\frac{\hat{p}(1-\hat{p})}{n}}$$

Here, $\hat{p}$ is the proportion of responders in the sample, n is the total number of individuals in the sample, and z is a critical value from the standard normal distribution having probability 0.025 to the right. For 95% confidence, z = 1.96. The square-root quantity is the standard error of the proportion.

26.5 HYPOTHESIS TESTING

Many excellent introductory statistics texts describe hypothesis testing (Sokal and Rohlf, 1995; Moore and McCabe, 2002; Samuels and Witmer, 2002), so only a brief summary is given here. In statistical hypothesis testing, two hypotheses (statements) are under consideration: the null hypothesis, H_0, and the alternative hypothesis, H_1. H_0 states that there is no difference or no effect, while H_1 is usually the research hypothesis and states that there is a difference or effect and may even specify the nature of the difference (e.g., an increase). It is always the null hypothesis that is tested, in the spirit of assuming no effect unless there is adequate evidence to the contrary. The test statistic is a number calculated from the data, assuming that H_0 is true. In most situations, the distribution of this test statistic when H_0 is true is known, so that the probability of the observed value or a value more extreme when H_0 is true (i.e., the *p*-value) can be easily found. If the *p*-value is large, it indicates that the observed test statistic value or something more extreme was likely when H_0 is true; thus, the data are consistent with H_0, and H_0 is accepted. On the other hand, if the *p*-value is small, the observed test statistic value or something more extreme is unlikely when H_0 is true, the data are not very consistent with H_0 and, therefore, H_0 is rejected in favor of H_1.

The level of significance of the test, α, serves as the cutpoint between "small" and "large," and is usually set at 0.05, or sometimes, 0.01. Researchers should keep in mind, however, that this choice is arbitrary, especially when p only slightly exceeds α. In some instances, the researcher is fairly certain of being able to predict the direction of the effect. Thus, H_1 is directional, in the sense that it specifies an increase (or a decrease). When this is the case, the *p*-value should be one-sided in the direction that the test statistic would go in the event of an increase (decrease). Directional alternatives should be used with care, however, because if an increase is expected, but the data showed a dramatic decrease, a one-sided *p*-value (in the "wrong" direction) would lead to acceptance of the null hypothesis of no difference. If the researcher is not fairly certain of the direction of the outcome, a two-sided *p*-value should be used.

The statistical decision to accept or reject H_0 is based on probabilities of making the correct decision. In reality, the truth of H_0 is never completely known. If H_0 is rejected, there is still the possibility that H_0 is actually true. Rejection of a true H_0 is a Type I error or a false positive. On the other hand, if H_0 is accepted, it is possible that H_0 is actually false. Acceptance of a false H_0 is a Type II error or a false negative. Using statistical theory, it is possible to quantify the probabilities of Type I and Type II errors, and by careful study design, minimize them. As shown in Table 26.2, the probability of a Type I error is the significance level of the test, α, and is usually set by the researcher to be a small number such as 0.05 or 0.01. When H_0 is actually false, the probability of making a Type II error is β and the probability of making a correct decision to reject H_0 is the power of the test, $1 - \beta$.

TABLE 26.2
Hypothesis Testing Outcomes

	In Reality:	
Statistical Decision	**H_0 Is True**	**H_0 Is False**
Accept H_0	Correct decision	Type II error False negative, β
Reject H_0	Type I error False positive, α	Correct decision Power = $1 - \beta$

Note: The null hypothesis, H_0, may be true or it may be false. The statistical decision based on evidence from an experiment will be to Accept H_0 or to Reject H_0. While the truth of H_0 is not known with certainty, the probability of making an incorrect decision can be controlled to a low level. The significance level of the test, α, is the probability of rejecting H_0 when it is actually true, i.e., the probability of a false positive result. β is the probability of accepting H_0 when it is actually false, i.e., the probability of a false negative result. The power of the test is $1 - \beta$, the probability of correctly rejecting H_0 when it is false; the power is usually controlled by the sample size and study design, and should be high.

The goal of a good experimental design is to maintain both the Type I and Type II probabilities low, in other words, to maintain the probabilities of a false positive and of a false negative low. When the probability of a false negative is low, the power is high. Holding everything else constant, the Type I and Type II error probabilities are inversely related; that is, if α is decreased, β will increase and if β is decreased, α will increase. Because of interrelationships among α, β, σ (the variability of the endpoint), n (the sample size), and D (the difference to be detected), however, there are several approaches to reduce β and thus increase power, while keeping α small. The exact interrelationship will depend on the experimental design and the statistical test to be used, but generally, the power will increase with increasing n and with decreasing variation in the endpoint. Therefore, strategies to reduce false positives and increase statistical power will include having a relatively large sample size and removing as much extraneous variability from each endpoint as possible. Furthermore, the size of the effect to be detected, D, should be an amount that is biologically meaningful. With a sufficiently large sample size, it is possible to declare that even small differences are statistically significant. However, if these small differences are not biologically meaningful, time and resources will have been wasted in conducting such a large study. On the other hand, if the sample size is too small, it is possible to observe a meaningful biological effect that does not reach statistical significance. Again, time and resources will have been wasted in conducting an underpowered study. Therefore, when designing an experiment, it is critical to investigate the statistical power and required sample sizes, as well as control extraneous sources of variability so that effects of biological significance will also be statistically significant.

26.5.1 Quantitative Endpoints

The statistical test applied to data in any given situation will depend on the experimental design, the hypotheses, and the distribution of the endpoint. Suppose that administration of Compound X to an animal is suspected to change the mean level of analyte A. A study might be designed in which animals are randomly assigned to either receive Compound X or to receive a placebo/control (Figure 26.4a). If A is normally distributed, a two-sample t-test is the test of choice. Alternatively, suppose that the design calls for A to be measured on all animals, then Compound X is administered to all animals, then A is measured again on all animals (Figure 26.4b). In this design, the pretreatment and posttreatment measurements on each animal are statistically treated as a pair, and a paired t-test is the preferred test. More complicated designs, such as a cross-over design, would require more complicated statistical tests.

If A is not normally distributed, either the data may be transformed or a nonparametric method may be used. Mathematical transformations, such as taking the logarithm (natural or common) of each value, may result in a distribution that is approximately normal so that parametric tests, such as t-tests, can be applied. Log-transformations reduce upward skewness and pull high outliers closer to the center of the data. The log-transformation not only tends to improve normality of an endpoint, but it may also equalize variances across groups. The Box–Cox family of power transformations may be useful as they estimate the most effective transformation directly from the data (Box and Cox, 1964). However, there are certainly cases in which even the best transformation does not sufficiently improve normality and other approaches must be considered.

Nonparametric statistical methods, sometimes known as distribution-free methods, include a broad collection of methods and approaches (e.g., see Conover, 1998; Hollander and Wolfe, 1999). Some methods, such as the Mann–Whitney test (Mann and Whitney, 1947) and the Kruskal–Wallis analysis of variance (Kruskal and Wallis, 1952), are based on ranks of the data, while other methods are based on resampling techniques, such as randomization t-tests and permutation tests (Conover, 1998). Recent ease of computing has also led to computing-intensive resampling methods, such as bootstrapping, jackknifing, and Monte Carlo sampling (Efron, 1979, 1981; Efron and Tibshirani, 1993).

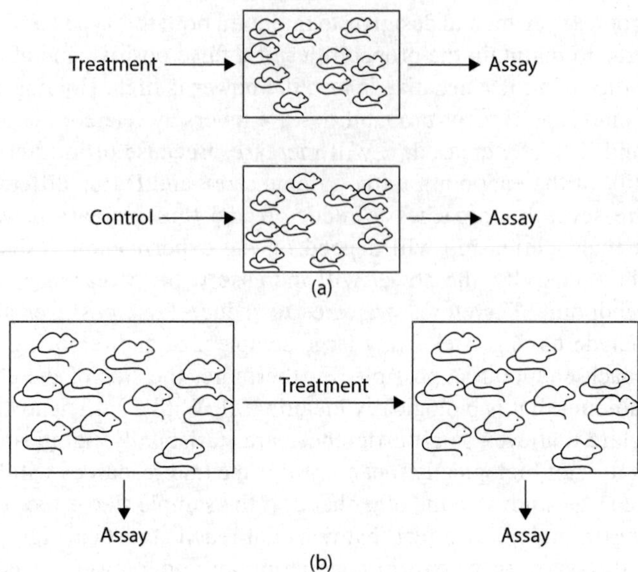

FIGURE 26.4 Illustration of two study designs. (a) Animals are randomly assigned to two independent groups. One group receives a treatment while the other group receives a placebo or control. At some time after treatment, all animals in both groups are assayed. (b) In this pretreatment, posttreatment design, a single group of animals are assayed before treatment. Then, the treatment is applied. After treatment, the animals are assayed again. Because the same animals were measured twice, their pretreatment and posttreatment values are paired and the statistical analysis should acknowledge this pairing.

For non-normally distributed data obtained from the design in Figure 26.4a, the Mann–Whitney test is a nonparametric analog of the two-sample *t*-test (Mann and Whitney, 1947). Because this test statistic is based on the ranks of the data values rather than on the data values, themselves, it is less influenced by skewness and outliers. For the paired design (Figure 26.4b), the Wilcoxon signed-ranks test, a nonparametric analog of the paired *t*-test, is a reasonable choice for a non-normally distributed endpoint. Alternatively, a resampling-based test could be applied to data from either experimental design.

Regardless of whether a parametric or nonparametric test is selected in the examples above, the *p*-value would be two-tailed because Compound X is expected to change A, but the change is not specified as an increase or a decrease. If, on the other hand, Compound X is expected to *increase* A, a one-tailed *p*-value should be used. Likewise, if Compound X is expected to *decrease* A, a one-tailed *p*-value should be used.

A common experimental design is the dose–response study. This design includes a placebo or control group along with two or more groups, each receiving a specified dose of Compound X. Animals are randomized to these groups. Moreover, a reasonable alternative hypothesis may be that analyte A increases with dose versus the null hypothesis that A does not change with dose. In this case, a trend statistic should be used to test H_0. If the data are normally distributed, linear regression or Pearson's correlation coefficient (Neter et al., 1996) are reasonable choices. If the data are not normally distributed, nonparametric tests of trend, such as Jonckheere's test (Jonckheere, 1954) or Spearman's rho (Spearman, 1904) would be more appropriate. If H_0 is rejected, a logical next step is to determine which dose group or groups differ from the control group. Dose groups are then statistically compared, pairwise with the control group. Because this involves testing multiple hypotheses, an adjustment for doing multiple comparisons is usually employed. Such adjustments ensure that the Type I error rate (false positive rate) is controlled; without control, the false positive rate grows with the number of comparisons, possibly approaching certainty. For normally distributed data, Williams' test (Williams, 1971, 1972) and Dunnett's test (Dunnett, 1955, 1964) are good approaches to multiple comparisons with the control group. If other pairs of dosed groups are to be compared, other multiple comparisons procedures are preferable, for example, Tukey's honestly significant difference (HSD) test (see Neter et al., 1996). For multiple pairwise comparisons with the control group with non-normally distributed data, Shirley's test (Shirley, 1977; Williams, 1986) and Dunn's test (Dunn, 1964) are commonly used.

Table 26.3 provides some guidance about selecting test statistics for specific experimental designs and hypotheses.

26.5.2 Qualitative Endpoints

The same hypothesis testing framework extends to qualitative assay data (e.g., present/absent, yes/no). The null and alternative hypotheses are specified, a test statistic is calculated from the data, a *p*-value is derived, and a decision about acceptance or rejection of H_0 is made. For qualitative data, the most common tests used are Fisher's exact test and chi-square tests (Fisher, 1922, 1954). As with quantitative measurements, the study design and hypotheses are integral to selecting which statistical test should be used.

In dose–response studies, dose-related trends in proportions of positives, for example, can be tested. The Cochran–Armitage trend test (Armitage, 1955) is usually a good choice in this setting. If a significant trend is detected, Fisher's exact test or chi-square statistics may be used to individually compare each dose group to the control group. To control the false positive rate for multiple comparisons, the Bonferroni correction of dividing α by the number of tests performed may be used to set the significance level for each individual pairwise comparison.

TABLE 26.3
Recommended Statistical Methods for Specific Experimental Designs

	Distribution of the Endpoint		
	Normally Distributed	**Not Normally Distributed**	**Categorical**
Two independent groups	Two-sample *t*-test	Mann–Whitney test, Resampling methods	Chi-square test, Fisher's exact test
Two related groups (e.g., pre–post treatment	Paired *t*-test	Wilcoxon signed ranks test, Resampling methods	McNemar's chi-square test
Three or more independent groups	Analysis of variance (ANOVA)	Kruskal–Wallis ANOVA, Resampling methods	Chi-square test
Dose–response with three or more groups	Linear regression, Correlation	Jonckheere–Terpstra test, Spearman's correlation, Resampling methods	Cochran–Armitage trend test
Cross-over design	Repeated measures ANOVA	a	a
Multiple pairwise comparisons with a control group	Dunnett's test if no trend, Williams' test if there is a trend	Dunn's test if no trend, Shirley's test if there is a trend	Categorical data analysis[a]

[a] Seek advice from a statistician.

Note: Most of these statistical tests are widely available in standard statistical software. For non-normally distributed data, resampling methods are also very useful and may take the form of permutation tests, randomization tests, bootstrapping, or Monte Carlo tests; these tests require specialized software.

26.6 SUMMARY

The statistical analysis of clinical chemistry endpoints benefits from an understanding of how analytic measurements are made and translated to analyte concentrations. A good assay determines these concentrations with accuracy and precision. When the assay is performed on a large, well-defined set of animals, reference ranges can be determined to describe typical values and how much variation might be expected for that population. Reference ranges are useful in interpreting the results from assays on individuals and must be updated as characteristics of the population of interest or the assay change. Assay results are also used in research studies. The appropriate statistical methods to be selected for a study will depend on the experimental design, the hypotheses, and the shape of the distribution of analyte concentrations. For complex studies, it is always advisable to involve a statistician, starting from the beginning of the planning stages.

REFERENCES

ACS. 1980. Guidelines for data acquisition and data quality evaluation in environmental chemistry. *Anal Chem.* 52:2242–2249.

Armitage, P. 1955. Tests for linear trends in proportions and frequencies. *Biometrics.* 11:375–386.

Barnett, V. and Lewis, T. 1994. *Outliers in Statistical Data.* New York, NY: John Wiley & Sons.

Bland, J.M. and Altman, D.G. 1996. Transformations, means, and confidence intervals. *BMJ.* 312:1079.

Box, G.E.P. and Cox, D.R. 1964. An analysis of transformations. *J R Stat Soc Series B.* 26:211–252.

Clayton, C., Mosquin, P., Pellizzari, E., and Quackenboss, J. 2004. Limitations on the uses of multimedia exposure measurements for multipathway exposure assessment—Part I: Handling observations below detection limits. *Qual Assur.* 10:123–159.

Cochran, W.G. 1952. The chi-square test of goodness of fit. *Ann Math Stat.* 23:315–345.

Conover, W.J. 1998. *Practical Nonparametric Statistics*. New York, NY: John Wiley & Sons.

Croghan, C.W. and Egeghy, P.P. 2003. *Methods of Dealing with Values Below the Limit of Detection Using SAS.* St. Petersburg, FL: Presentation at the Southeastern SAS User Group, September.

Dean, R.B. and Dixon, W.J. 1951. Simplified statistics for small numbers of observations. *Anal Chem.* 23:636–638.

Dixon, W.J. 1953. Processing data for outliers. *Biometrics.* 9:74–89.

Dunn, O.J. 1964. Multiple comparisons using rank sums. *Technometrics.* 6:241–252.

Dunnett, C.W. 1955. A multiple comparisons procedure for comparing several treatments with a control. *J Am Stat Assoc.* 50:1096–1121.

Dunnett, C.W. 1964. New table for multiple comparisons with a control. *Biometrics.* 20:482–491.

Efron, B. 1979. Bootstrap methods: Another look at the jackknife. *Ann Stat.* 7:1–26.

Efron, B. 1981. Nonparametric estimates of standard error: The jackknife, the bootstrap and other methods. *Biometrika.* 68:589–599.

Efron, B. and Tibshirani, R.J. 1993. *An Introduction to the Bootstrap*. New York, NY: Chapman & Hall.

Environmental Protection Agency (EPA). 2000. *Assigning Values to Non-Detected/Non-Quantified Pesticide Residues in Human Health Food Exposure Assessments*. Washington, DC: U.S. Environmental Protection Agency Office of Pesticide Programs.

European Medicines Agency (EMEA).1995. *ICH Topic Q2 (R1) Validation of Analytical Procedures: Text and Methodology*. London: EMEA.

Fisher, R.A. 1922. On the interpretation of χ^2 from contingency tables, and the calculation of P. *J R Stat Soc.* 85:87–94.

Fisher, R.A. 1954. *Statistical Methods for Research Workers*. Edinburgh: Oliver and Boyd.

Food and Drug Administration (FDA). 1998. *Guidance for Industry: Validation of Analytical Procedures: Methodology*. Rockville, MD: U.S. Food and Drug Administration Center for Drug Evaluation and Research.

Food and Drug Administration (FDA). 2001. *Guidance for Industry: Bioanalytical Method Validation*. Rockville, MD: U.S. Food and Drug Administration Center for Drug Evaluation and Research.

Grubbs, R.E. 1969. Procedures for detecting outlying observations in samples. *Technometrics.* 11:1–21.

Helsel, D.R. 1990. Less than obvious: Statistical treatment of data below the detection limit. *Environ Sci Technol.* 24:1766–1774.

Hollander, M. and Wolfe, D.A. 1999. *Nonparametric Statistical Methods*. New York, NY: Wiley-Interscience.

Jonckheere, A.R. 1954. A distribution-free k-sample test against ordered alternatives. *Biometrika.* 41:133–145.

Koo, J-W., Parham, F., Kohn, M.C., et al. 2002. The association between biomarker-based exposure estimates for phthalates and demographic factors in a human reference population. *Environ Health Perspect.* 110:405–410.

Kruskal, W.H. and Wallis, W.A. 1952. Use of ranks in one-criterion variance analysis. *J Am Stat Assoc.* 47:583–621.

Lilliefors, H.W. 1967. On the Kolmogorov–Smirnov test for normality with mean and variance unknown. *J Am Stat Assoc.* 62:399–402.

Long, G.L. and Winefordner, J.D. 1983. Limit of detection. A closer look at the IUPAC definition. *Anal Chem.* 55:712A–724A.

Mann, H.B. and Whitney, D.R. 1947. On a test of whether one of two random variables is stochastically larger than the other. *Ann Math Stat.* 18:50–60.

Massey, F.J. 1951. The Kolmogorov–Smirnov test for goodness of fit. *J Am Stat Assoc.* 46:68–78.

Miller, W.G., Chinchilli, V.M., Gruemer, H-D., Nance, W.E. 1984. Sampling from a skewed population distribution as exemplified by estimation of the creatine kinase upper reference limit. *Clin Chem.* 30:18–23.

Moore, D.S. and McCabe, G.P. 2002. *Introduction to the Practice of Statistics*, 4th edition. New York, NY: W.H. Freeman.

Neter, J., Kutner, M.H., Nachtsheim, C.J., Wasserman, W. 1996. *Applied Linear Statistical Models*, 4th edition. Boston, MA: WCB McGraw-Hill.

Proschan, F. 1953. Confidence and tolerance intervals for the normal distribution. *J Am Stat Assoc.* 48:550–564.

Reed, A.H., Henry, R.J., Mason, W.B. 1971. Influence of statistical method used on the resulting estimate of normal range. *Clin Chem.* 17:275–284.

Samuels, M.L. and Witmer, J.A. 2002. *Statistics for the Life Sciences*, 3rd edition. Upper Saddle River, NJ: Prentice Hall.

Shapiro, S.S. and Wilk, M.B. 1965. An analysis of variance test for normality (complete samples). *Biometrika.* 52:591–611.

Shirley, E. 1977. A non-parametric equivalent of Williams' test for contrasting increasing dose levels of a treatment. *Biometrics.* 33:386–389.

Spearman, C. 1904. The proof and measurement of association between two things. *Am J Psychol.* 15:72–101.

Sunderman, F.W. 1975. Current concepts of "normal values," "reference values," and "discrimination values" in clinical chemistry. *Clin Chem.* 21:1873–1877.

Wald, A. and Wolfowitz, J. 1946. Tolerance limits for a normal distribution. *Ann Math Stat.* 17:208.

Williams, D.A. 1971. A test for differences between treatment means when several dose levels are compared with a zero dose control. *Biometrics.* 27:103–117.

Williams, D.A. 1972. The comparison of several dose levels with a zero dose control. *Biometrics.* 28:519–531.

Williams, D.A. 1986. A note on Shirley's nonparametric test for comparing several dose levels with a zero-dose control. *Biometrics.* 42:183–186.

Youden, W.J. 1963. Ranking laboratories by round-robin tests. *Mater Res Stand.* 3:9–13.

Index

B

C

D

H

J

K

L

M

P

T

U

V

W

X

Y

Z